LIFESTYLE MEDICINE

LIFESTYLE MEDICINE

Edited by
James M. Rippe, MD

Founder and Director
The Center for Clinical and Lifestyle Research
Shrewsbury, Massachusetts
Associate Professor of Medicine (Cardiology)
Tufts University School of Medicine
Boston, Massachusetts
Founder and Director
Rippe Health Assessment at Celebration Health
Orlando, Florida
Medical Director
TBG Development
St. Louis, Missouri

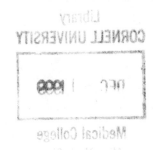
b
Blackwell
Science

©1999 by James M. Rippe

Blackwell Science
Editorial Offices:
Commerce Place, 350 Main Street, Malden, Massachusetts 02148, USA
Osney Mead, Oxford OX2 0EL, England
25 John Street, London WC1N 2BL, England
23 Ainslie Place, Edinburgh EH3 6AJ, Scotland
54 University Street, Carlton, Victoria 3053, Australia
Other Editorial Offices:
Blackwell Wissenschafts-Verlag GmbH, Kurfürstendamm 57, 10707 Berlin, Germany
Blackwell Science KK, MG Kodenmacho Building, 7–10 Kodenmacho Nihombashi, Chuo-ku, Tokyo 104, Japan

Distributors:
USA

 Blackwell Science, Inc.
 Commerce Place
 350 Main Street
 Malden, Massachusetts 02148
 (Telephone orders: 800-215-1000 or 781-388-8250; fax orders: 781-388-8270)

Canada

 Login Brothers Book Company
 324 Saulteaux Crescent
 Winnipeg, Manitoba, R3J 3T2
 (Telephone orders: 204-224-4068)

Australia

 Blackwell Science Pty, Ltd.
 54 University Street
 Carlton, Victoria 3053
 (Telephone orders: 03-9347-0300;
 fax orders: 03-9349-3016)

Outside North America and Australia

 Blackwell Science, Ltd.
 c/o Marston Book Services, Ltd.
 P.O. Box 269
 Abingdon
 Oxon OX14 4YN
 England
 (Telephone orders: 44-01235-465500;
 fax orders: 44-01235-465555)

Acquisitions: James Krosschell
Production: Andover Publishing Services
Manufacturing: Lisa Flanagan
Cover design by Crane Graphics
Typeset by Best-set Typesetter Ltd., Hong Kong
Printed and bound by Braun-Brumfield, Inc.

Printed in the United States of America
99 00 01 02 5 4 3 2 1
The Blackwell Science logo is a trade mark of Blackwell Science Ltd., registered at the United Kingdom Trade Marks Registry
Library of Congress Cataloging-in-Publication Data
Lifestyle medicine / edited by James M. Rippe.
     p. cm.
  Includes index.
  ISBN 0-86542-294-X
  1. Medicine, Preventive. 2. Health promotion. 3. Health behavior. I. Rippe, James M.
  [DNLM: 1. Primary Prevention. 2. Health Behavior. 3. Health
Promotion. 4. Life Style. WA 108 L722 1999]
  RA427.L54 1999
  610—dc21
  DNLM/DLC
  for Library of Congress   99-13000
                                                             CIP

To Stephanie, Hart, and Jaelin

Contents

Contents   ix

Contents

Contributors

Steven G. Aldana, PhD
Department of Physical Education
Brigham Young University
Provo, Utah

Sandra Anderson, BSc
Département d'éducation physique
Université de Montréal
Montréal, Quebec, Canada

James D. Anholm, MD
Pulmonary and Intensive Care Section
Department of Internal Medicine
Loma Linda University School of Medicine and the
   Jerry L. Pettis Veterans Medical Center
Loma Linda, California

Louis J. Aronne, MD
Clinical Associate Professor of Medicine
Cornell University Medical College
Director of the Comprehensive Weight Control Program
The New York Hospital-Cornell Medical Center
New York, New York

Judith M. Ashley, PhD, RD
Nutrition Education and Research Program
Department of Internal Medicine
University of Nevada School of Medicine
Reno, Nevada

E. Wayne Askew, PhD
Professor and Chair
Division of Foods and Nutrition
College of Health
University of Utah
Salt Lake City, Utah

Richard L. Atkinson, MD
Departments of Medicine and Nutritional Sciences
University of Wisconsin
Madison, Wisconsin

Donald A. Bailey
Professor
College of Kinesiology
University of Saskatchewan
Saskatoon, Canada
Department of Human Movement Studies
University of Queensland
Brisbane, Australia

Isabela Bensenor, MD, PhD
Division of Preventive Medicine
Brigham and Women's Hospital
Boston, Massachusetts

Joan E. Benson MS, RD
Division of Public Health Sciences
School of Medicine
University of Utah
Salt Lake City, Utah

Susan Bittenbender, MD
West Chester, Pennsylvania

James A. Blumenthal, PhD
Department of Psychiatry and Behavioral Sciences
Duke University Medical Center
Durham, North Carolina

Kimberly Bonzheim, MSA
Assistant Director
Cardiac Rehabilitation and Exercise Laboratories
William Beaumont Hospital
Royal Oak, Michigan

David R. Brown, PhD
Behavioral Scientist
Centers for Disease Control and Prevention
National Center for Chronic Disease Prevention and
    Health Promotion
Division of Nutrition and Physical Activity
Atlanta, Georgia

Catherine Buchanan
Medical Student
Wake Forest University School of Medicine
Winston-Salem, North Carolina

Janet Buckworth, PhD
Assistant Professor
Department of Sport and Exercise Sciences
The Ohio State University
Columbus, Ohio

Kevin Burroughs, MD
Resident Physician
Sports Medicine Fellowship Program
Moses Cone Family Practice Residency
University of North Carolina at Chapel Hill School of Medicine
Greensboro, North Carolina

Jill A. Bush, MS
Laboratory for Sports Medicine/Kinesiology Department
The Pennsylvania State University
University Park, Pennsylvania

Karen J. Calfas, PhD
Assistant Clinical Professor
Family and Preventive Medicine
University of California, San Diego
San Diego, California

Joseph J. Carlson, PhD
Postdoctoral Research Fellow
Stanford Center for Research in Disease Prevention
Stanford University School of Medicine
Stanford, California

Richard Casaburi, PhD, MD
Division of Respiratory and Critical Care Physiology and
    Medicine
Harbor-UCLA Medical Center
Torrance, California

Carl J. Caspersen, PhD, MPH
Associate Director for Science
Division of Diabetes Translation
National Center for Chronic Disease Prevention and
    Health Promotion
Centers for Disease Control and Prevention
Atlanta, Georgia

Frank J. Cerny, PhD
Chair, Department of Physical Therapy & Exercise Science
SUNY at Buffalo
Buffalo, New York

Linda Chapin, DDS
Executive Director
National Wellness Institute
Stevens Point, Wisconsin

Larry S. Chapman, MPH
Chairman of the Board
SUMMEX
Seattle, Washington

David E. Ciccolella, MD
Associate Professor of Medicine
Division of Pulmonary and Critical Care Medicine
Temple University School of Medicine
Philadelphia, Pennsylvania

Matthew M. Clark, PhD
Brown University Center for Behavioral and Preventive Medicine
The Miriam Hospital
Providence, Rhode Island

Priscilla M. Clarkson, PhD
Chair and Associate Dean
Department of Exercise Science
University of Massachusetts
Amherst, Massachusetts

Gilbert E. D'Alonzo, DO
Professor of Medicine
Division of Pulmonary and Critical Care Medicine
Temple University School of Medicine
Philadelphia, Pennsylvania

Adam deJong, BAA
Exercise Physiologist
Cardiac Rehabilitation and Exercise Laboratories
William Beaumont Hospital
Royal Oak, Michigan

Eric J. DeMaria, MD
Medical College of Virginia
Virginia Commonwealth University
Richmond, Virginia

Mary Jane De Souza, PhD
Department of Medicine
Bone Health and Osteoporosis Center
New Britain General Hospital
New Britain, Connecticut

Nikhil V. Dhurandhar, PhD
Department of Medicine
University of Wisconsin
Madison, Wisconsin

Rod K. Dishman, PhD
Professor
University of Georgia
Department of Exercise Science
Athens, Georgia

Elen Casso Donahue, MD
Fall River, Massachusetts

Barbara L. Drinkwater, PhD
Department of Medicine
Pacific Medical Center
Seattle, Washington

Patricia M. Dubbert, PhD
Veterans Affairs Medical Center
University of Mississippi School of Medicine
Jackson, Mississippi

Robert H. DuRant, PhD
Professor of Pediatrics and Public Health Service
Vice Chair for Health Services Research
Department of Pediatrics
Brenner Children's Hospital
Wake Forest University School of Medicine
Winston-Salem, North Carolina

Johanna T. Dwyer, DSc, RD
Professor of Medicine and Community Health
Schools of Nutrition and Medicine
Senior Scientist, Jean Mayer US Department of Agriculture
    Human Nutrition
Center on Aging
Tufts University
Director, Frances Stern Nutrition Center
New England Medical Center
Boston, Massachussets

Charles B. Eaton, MD, MS
Associate Professor of Family Medicine
Department of Family Medicine
Memorial Hospital of Rhode Island
Pawtucket, Rhode Island
Brown University School of Medicine
Providence, Rhode Island

Karen M. Emmons, PhD
Harvard School of Public Health
The Dana Farber Cancer Institute
Center for Community-Based Research
Boston, Massachusetts

Avery D. Faigenbaum, EdD
Department of Human Performance and Fitness
University of Massachusetts
Boston, Massachusetts

Jonathan E. Fielding, MD, MPH, MBA
Department of Health Services
School of Public Health
University of California, Los Angeles
Los Angeles, California

Karl Fields, MD
Professor, Associate Chairman
Department of Family Medicine
University of North Carolina at Chapel Hill School of
    Medicine
Greensboro, North Carolina

Aaron R. Folsom, MD
Professor
Division of Epidemiology
University of Minnesota
Minneapolis, Minnesota

John P. Foreyt, PhD
Professor
Department of Medicine
Baylor College of Medicine
Houston, Texas

Daniel E. Forman, MD
Assistant Professor
Division of Cardiology
The Miriam Hospital
Brown University School of Medicine
Providence, Rhode Island

Michael J. Fotheringham, PhD
Postdoctoral Research Fellow
School of Human Movement
Deakin University
Burwood, Victoria, Australia

Barry A. Franklin, PhD
Director, Cardiac Rehabilitation and Exercise Laboratories
William Beaumont Hospital
Royal Oak, Michigan
Professor of Physiology
Wayne State University School of Medicine
Detroit, Michigan

Patty S. Freedson, PhD
Department of Exercise Science
University of Massachusetts
Totman Gymnasium
Amherst, Massachusetts

Christine M. Friedenreich, PhD
Research Scientist/National Health Research Scholar
Division of Epidemiology, Prevention and Screening
Alberta Cancer Board
Calgary, Alberta
Canada

Victor Froelicher, MD
Cardiology Division
VA Palo Alto Health Care System
Palo Alto, California

Janet E. Fulton, PhD
Department of Health and Human Services
Public Health Service
Centers for Disease Control
Division of Nutrition and Physical Activity
Atlanta, Georgia

Carol Ewing Garber, PhD, FACSM
Division of Cardiology
Memorial Hospital of Rhode Island
Pawtucket, Rhode Island
Brown University School of Medicine
Providence, Rhode Island

Andrew W. Gardner, PhD
Department of Medicine, Division of Gerontology
University of Maryland
Baltimore, Maryland

Lise Gauvin, PhD
Associate Professor
Department of Social and Preventive Medicine
Université de Montréal
Montréal, Quebec, Canada

Veronica F. Gilligan
Regional Manager, Health Promotion
AT&T
Basking Ridge, New Jersey

Karen Glanz, PhD, MPH
Professor
Cancer Research Center of Hawaii
University of Hawaii
Honolulu, Hawaii

Scott Going, PhD
Department of Physiology
The University of Arizona
Tucson, Arizona

Robert J. Goldberg, PhD
Professor of Medicine and Epidemiology
University of Massachusetts Medical School
Worcester, Massachusetts

Michael G. Goldstein, MD
Professor
Department of Psychiatry
The Miriam Hospital
Brown University School of Medicine
Providence, Rhode Island

Henry Gong, Jr., MD
Chief, Department of Medicine and Environmental
    Health Service
Rancho Los Amigos Medical Center
Professor of Medicine
University of Southern California School of Medicine
Downey, California

Elizabeth C.D. Gullette, MA
Department of Psychiatry and Behavioral Sciences
Duke University Medical Center
Durham, North Carolina

Bernard Gutin, PhD
Georgia Prevention Institute
The Medical College of Georgia
Augusta, Georgia

C. Keith Haddock, PhD
Department of Psychology
University of Missouri-Kansas City
Kansas City, Missouri

William L. Haskell, PhD
Professor of Medicine
Stanford Center for Research in Disease Prevention
Stanford University School of Medicine
Palo Alto, Claifornia

Ashraf M. Hassanein, MD, PhD
Assistant Professor
Departments of Pathology and Dermatology
Director, Division of Dermatopathology
University of Florida College of Medicine
Gainesville, Florida

Susan Hellerstein, MD, MPH
Department of Obstetrics and Gynecology
Beth Israel Deaconess Medical Center
Boston, Massachusetts

Bill Hettler, MD
Director, UWSP Health Service
University of Wisconsin, Stevens Point
Stevens Point, Wisconsin

Joeli Hettler, MD
Chief Resident, Pediatrics
Rochester General Hospital
Rochester, New York

Robert J. Heyka, MD
Department of Nephrology and Hypertension
Cleveland Clinic Foundation
Cleveland, Ohio

Mike Hilts, MD
Sports Medicine Fellow
Moses Cone Family Practice Residency
University of North Carolina at Chapel Hill School of Medicine
Greensboro, North Carolina

Elizabeth Harper Howze, ScD, CHES
Associate Director for Health Promotion
Division of Nutrition and Physical Activity
Centers for Disease Control & Prevention
Atlanta, Georgia

Toni Huebscher, MD
Department of Obstetrics and Gynecology
Beth Israel Deaconess Medical Center
Boston, Massachusetts

Rebecca Jaffe, MD
Instructor
Thomas Jefferson University School of Medicine
Philadelphia, Pennsylvania

Leonard A. Kaminsky, PhD
Professor and Director
Adult Fitness/Cardiac Rehabilitation Program
Human Performance Laboratory
Ball State University
Muncie, Indiana

Gary R. Kantor, MD
Professor of Dermatology and Pathology and Laboratory
Medicine
Department of Dermatology
MCP Hahnemann University
Philadelphia, Pennsylvania

Betsy Keller, PhD
Department of Exercise and Sport Sciences
Ithaca College
Ithaca, New York

John M. Kellum, MD
Medical College of Virginia
Virginia Commonwealth University
Richmond, Virginia

Donald W. Kemper
Healthwise, Incorporated
Boise, Idaho

Abby C. King, Ph.D.
Division of Epidemiology
Department of Health Research & Policy
Stanford Center for Research in Disease Prevention
Department of Medicine
Stanford University
School of Medicine
Palo Alto, California

Teresa K. King, PhD
Brown University Center for Behavioral and Preventive Medicine
The Miriam Hospital
Providence, Rhode Island

Harold W. Kohl, III, PhD
Director of Research
Baylor Sports Medicine Institute
Baylor College of Medicine
Houston, Texas

William J. Kraemer, PhD
The Human Performance Laboratory
Ball State University
Muncie, Indiana

Jacqueline Kral, MPH
Senior Program Coordinator
Violence Prevention Programs
Division of Public Health Practice
Harvard School of Public Health
Boston, Massachusetts

J. Stuart Krause, PhD
Crawford Research Institute
Shepherd Center
Atlanta, Georgia

Jean L. Kristeller, PhD
Department of Psychology
Indiana State University
Department of Psychiatry
Indiana State University School of Medicine
Terre Haute, Indiana

David Kritchevsky, PhD
Wistar Institute
Philadelphia, Pennsylvania

Lisa S. Krivickas, MD
Instructor, Harvard Medical School
Department of Physical Medicine and Rehabilitation
Spaulding Rehabilitation Hospital
Boston, Massachusetts

Shiriki Kumanyika, PhD, RD, MPH
Professor and Head
Department of Human Nutrition and Dietetics
College of Associated Health Professions
University of Illinois at Chicago
Chicago, Illinois

Idamarie Laquatra, PhD, RD
Shape Up America!
Bethesda, Maryland

Meryl S. LeBoff, MD
Associate Professor
Harvard Medical School
Director, Skeletal Health and Osteoporosis Program
Endocrine-Hypertension Division, Department of Medicine
Brigham and Women's Hospital
Boston, Massachusetts

Alice H. Lichtenstein, DSc
Professor
School of Nutrition Science and Policy
Jean Mayer US Department of Agriculture Human Nutrition
Center on Aging
Tufts University
Boston, Massachusetts

Devora Lieberman, MD, MPH
Department of Obstetrics and Gynaecology
Royal North Shore Hospital
University of Sydney
Sydney, Australia

Gila Lindsley, PhD
Department of Psychiatry
Tufts School of Medicine
Boston, Massachusettes

William S. Linn, MA
Senior Project Scientist
Rancho Los Amigos Medical Center
Clinical Associate Professor of Preventive Medicine
University of Southern California School of Medicine
Downey, California

Elizabeth E. Lloyd, PhD
Brown University Center for Behavioral and Preventive Medicine
The Miriam Hospital
Providence, Rhode Island

David Neubauer Lombard, PhD
Tinker Air Force Base
United States Air Force

Tamara Neubauer Lombard, PhD
Tinker Air Force Base
United States Air Force

Carol London, RNC, MS
Department of Obstetrics and Gynecology
Beth Israel Deaconess Medical Center
Boston, Massachusetts

Laurel T. Mackinnon, PhD
Associate Professor
Department of Human Movement Studies
The University of Queensland
Queensland, Australia

Stefania Maggi, MA
The Dana Farber Cancer Institute
Center for Community-Based Research
Boston, Massachusetts

Donald A. Mahler, MD
Professor of Medicine
Dartmouth Medical School
Section of Pulmonary and Critical Care Medicine
Dartmouth-Hitchcock Medical Center
Lebanon, New Hampshire

JoAnn E. Manson, MD, DrPH
Division of Preventive Medicine
Brigham and Women's Hospital
Boston, Massachusetts

Bess H. Marcus, PhD
Brown University Center for Behavioral and Preventive Medicine
The Miriam Hospital
Providence, Rhode Island

Kathryn A. Martin, MD
Instructor of Medicine
Harvard Medical School
Director, Reproductive Endocrine Associates
Reproductive Endocrine Unit
Massachusetts General Hospital
Boston, Massachusetts

Ursula A. Matulonis, MD
Assistant Professor of Medicine
Harvard Medical School
Department of Adult Oncology
Dana Farber Cancer Institute
Boston, Massachusetts

Robert S. Mazzeo, PhD
Department of Kinesiology
University of Colorado
Boulder, Colorado

Mary P. McGowan, MD
Medical Director
Cholesterol Management Center
New England Heart Institute
Manchester, New Hampshire
Assistant Professor of Medicine
University of Massachusetts Medical School
Worcester, Massachusetts

Lisa Litchfield McSherry, RN, BSN, IB, CLC
Department of Obstetrics and Gynecology
Beth Israel Deaconess Medical Center
Boston, Massachusetts

Roberto Mejia, MD
Visiting Scientist in Medicine
Dartmouth Medical School
Lebanon, New Hampshire
Faculty, National Institute of Respiratory Diseases
Mexico City, Mexico

Lisa M. Menard
Third Year Medical Student
Brown University School of Medicine
Providence, Rhode Island

Molly Mettler
Healthwise, Incorporated
Boise, Idaho

Felise Milan, MD
Clinical Associate Professor
Rhode Island Hospital
Brown University School of Medicine
Providence, Rhode Island

Brian E. Miller, PhD
Center for Fertility and Reproductive Endocrinology
New Britain General Hospital
New Britain, Connecticut

Sanford A. Miller, PhD
Professor and Dean
Graduate School of Biomedical Sciences
The University of Texas Health Science Center at San Antonio
San Antonio, Texas

Karen D. Mittleman, PhD
Design Write, Inc
Princeton, New Jersey

Lori Moger, MS
Department of Kinesiology
Indiana University-Bloomington
Bloomington, Indiana

Scott J. Montain, PhD
US Army Research Institute of Environmental Medicine
Thermal & Mountain Medicine Division
Natick, Massachusetts

Barbara Moore, PhD
Shape Up America!
Bethesda, Maryland

Robert J. Nicolosi, PhD
Director, Center for Chronic Disease Control and Prevention
University of Massachusetts, Lowell
Lowell, Massachusetts

David C. Nieman, DrPH
Professor, Department of Health, Leisure, and
   Exercise Science
Appalachian State University
Boone, North Carolina

Bradley C. Nindl, MS
Laboratory for Sports Medicine/Kinesiology Department
The Pennsylvania State University
University Park, Pennsylvania

Diane O'Brien, RN, BSN
Laboratory Research Director
The Center for Clinical and Lifestyle Research
Shrewsbury, Massachusetts

Patrick J. O'Connor, PhD
Associate Professor
Department of Exercise Science
University of Georgia
Athens, Georgia

Michael P. O'Donnell, PhD, MBA, MPH
Editor in Chief and President
American Journal of Health Promotion
Keego Harbor, Michigan

David M. Orenstein, MD
Professor of Pediatrics
School of Medicine
Professor of Health, Physical, and Recreation Education
School of Education
University of Pittsburgh
Pittsburgh, Pennsylvania

Neville Owen, PhD
Professor of Human Movement Science
Head, School of Human Movement
Deakin University
Burwood, Victoria, Australia

Gary M. Owens, MD
Vice President for Patient Care Management
Independence Blue Cross/Keystone Health Plan East
Philadelphia, Pennsylvania

Scott Owens, PhD
Georgia Prevention Institute
The Medical College of Georgia
Augusta, Georgia

Russell R. Pate, PhD
Department of Exercise Science
University of South Carolina
Columbia, South Carolina

Bente Klarland Pedersen, PhD, MD
The Copenhagen Muscle Research Centre
Department of Infectious Diseases
Rigshospitalet
Copenhagen
Denmark

Mark A. Pereira, PhD
School of Public Health
Division of Epidemiology
University of Minnesota
Minneapolis, Minnesota

Steven J. Petruzzello, PhD
Associate Professor
Department of Kinesiology
University of Illinois at Urbana-Champaign
Urbana, Illinois

Bernadine M. Pinto, PhD
Assistant Professor
Department of Psychiatry
The Miriam Hospital
Brown University School of Medicine
Providence, Rhode Island

Walker S. Carlos Poston, PhD
Department of Medicine
Baylor College of Medicine
Houston, Texas

Deborah Prothrow-Stith, MD
Professor, Public Health Practice
Division of Public Health Practice
Harvard School of Public Health
Boston, Massachusetts

Charles T. Pu, MD
Instructor in Medicine
Harvard Medical School Senior Research Associate
Jean Mayer US Department of Agriculture Human Nutrition
Center on Aging
Tufts University
Boston, Massachusetts

Charles P. Quesenberry, Jr., PhD
Senior Biostatistician
Division of Research
The Permanente Medical Group, Inc.
Oakland, California

John S. Raglin, PhD
Associate Professor
Department of Kinesiology
Indiana University
Bloomington, Indiana

Kathryn M. Rexrode, MD, MPH
Division of Preventive Medicine
Brigham and Women's Hospital
Boston, Massachusetts

Hope A. Ricciotti, MD
Department of Obstetrics and Gynecology
Beth Israel Deaconess Medical Center
Boston, Massachusetts

Andrew L. Ries, MD, MPH
Professor of Medicine
University of California, San Diego
San Diego, California

James M. Rippe, MD
Founder and Director
The Center for Clinical and Lifestyle Research
Shrewsbury, Massachusetts
Associate Professor of Medicine (Cardiology)
Tufts University School of Medicine
Boston, Massachusetts
Founder and Director
Rippe Health Assessment at Celebration Health
Orlando, Florida
Medical Director
TBG Development
St. Louis, Missouri

Penny Harris Rosenzweig, MS
Department of Nutrition
University of Massachusetts
Amherst, Massachusetts

Contributors

Thomas W. Rowland, MD
Director of Pediatric Cardiology
Baystate Medical Center Children's Hospital
Springfield, Massachusetts

Joseph E. Scherger, MD, MPH
Associate Dean for Clinical Affairs
Professor and Chair
Department of Family Medicine
College of Medicine
University of California, Irvine
Orange, California

Laura Schmitt, MSPT, ATC
Department of Physical Therapy
University of Delaware
Newark, Delaware

Chris Scholes, MD
Twin Falls, Idaho

Jon P. Schrage, MD
Nutrition Education and Research Program
Department of Internal Medicine
University of Nevada School of Medicine
Reno, Nevada

Richard M. Schwartzstein, MD
Division of Pulmonary and Critical Care Medicine
Beth Israel Deaconess Medical Center
Boston, Massachusetts

Michael Schweitzer, MD
Medical College of Virginia
Virginia Commonwealth University
Richmond, Virginia

Daniel J. Sheehan, MD
Resident, Physical Medicine and Rehabilitation
Spaulding Rehabilitation Hospital and Harvard Medical School
Boston, Massachusetts

Roy J. Shephard
Professor
Faculty of Physical Education and Health
Department of Public Health Sciences
Faculty of Medicine, University of Toronto
Toronto Rehabilitation Centre
Toronto, Ontario, Canada

Madeleine Sigman-Grant, PhD, RD
Associate Professor of Maternal and Child Nutrition
Cooperative Extension
University of Nevada-Reno
Las Vegas, Nevada

James S. Skinner, PhD
Department of Kinesiology
Indiana University
Bloomington, Indiana

Angela Smith, MD
Adjunct Professor
University of Delaware
Newark, Delaware

J. Carson Smith, BS
Department of Exercise Science
University of Georgia
Athens, Georgia

L. Kent Smith, MD, MPH
Arizona Heart Institute and Foundation
Phoenix, Arizona

Lynn Snyder-Mackler, ScD, PT
Department of Physical Therapy
University of Delaware
Newark, Delaware

Marjorie Speers, PhD
Behavioral and Social Sciences Coordinator
Centers for Disease Control and Prevention
Atlanta, Georgia

John C. Spence, PhD
Senior Research Associate
Alberta Centre for Well-Being
University of Alberta
Edmonton, Alberta, Canada

Sachiko St. Jeor, PhD, RD
Nutrition Education and Research Program and
   Department of Internal Medicine
University of Nevada School of Medicine
Reno, Nevada

Risa J. Stein, PhD
Department of Psychology
Rockhurst College
Kansas City, Missouri

Lou A. Stephenson, PhD
US Army Research Institute of Environmental Medicine
Thermal & Mountain Medicine Division
Natick, Massachusetts

Barbara A. Stetson, PhD
Department of Psychiatry and Behavioral Sciences
University of Louisville
Louisville, Kentucky

Jodie M. Stocks, MSc
Department of Biomedical Science
University of Wollongong
Wollongong, Australia

Harvey J. Sugerman, MD
Medical College of Virginia
Virginia Commonwealth University
Richmond, Virginia

Kathleen Taylor, RN
Manager, Cardiovascular Health Management Operations
Long Term Care Marketing
Key Pharmaceuticals
Schering-Plough Corporation
Kenilworth, New Jersey

Nigel A.S. Taylor, PhD
Department of Biomedical Science
University of Wollongong
Wollongong, Australia

Beti Thompson, PhD
Member and Professor
Fred Hutchinson Cancer Research Center
School of Public Health and Community Medicine
University of Washington
Seattle, Washington

Malani R. Trine, MS
Department of Kinesiology
University of Wisconsin-Madison
Madison, Wisconsin

Stewart G. Trost, PhD
Department of Health and Human Performance
Auburn University
Auburn, Alabama

Brian N. Victoroff, MD
Assistant Professor
Department of Orthopedic Surgery
Case Western Reserve University
Cleveland, Ohio

Stella L. Volpe, PhD, RD
Department of Nutrition
University of Massachusetts
Amherst, Massachusetts

Ann Ward, PhD
Department of Kinesiology
University of Wisconsin-Madison
Madison, Wisconsin

Andrea Watson, RN, BSN
Nurse Clinician
Cardiac Rehabilitation and Exercise Laboratories
William Beaumont Hospital
Royal Oak, Michigan

C. Bruce Wenger, MD, PhD
Research Pharmacologist
US Army Research Institute of Environmental Medicine
Military Peformance Division
Natick, Massachusetts

Nanette K. Wenger, MD
Professor of Medicine
Department of Medicine
Division of Cardiology
Emory University School of Medicine
Consultant, Emory Heart Center
Director, Cardiac Clinics
Grady Memorial Hospital
Atlanta, Georgia

Mitchell H. Whaley, PhD
Associate Professor
Adult Fitness/Cardiac Rehabilitation Program
Human Performance Laboratory
Ball State University
Muncie, Indiana

Robbin Wickham, MSPT
Department of Physical Therapy
University of Delaware
Newark, Delaware

Thomas A. Wilson, PhD, MPH
Center for Chronic Disease Control
Department of Clinical Science
University of Massachusetts, Lowell
Lowell, Massachusetts

Mark G. Wilson, HSD
Department of Health Promotion & Behavior
University of Georgia
Athens, Georgia

Christine L. Williams, MD, MPH
Director, Children's Cardiovascular Health Center
Professor of Clinical Pediatrics
Columbia-Presbyterian Medical Center
New York, New York

Jeffrey A. Woods, PhD
Department of Kinesiology
University of Illinois at Urbana/Champaign
Urbana, Illinois

Jorge L. Yarzebski, MD, PhD
Research Assistant Professor of Medicine
Department of Medicine
University of Massachusetts Medical School
Worcester, Massachusetts

Mimi R. Yum, MD
Department of Obstetrics and Gynecology
Beth Israel Deaconess Medical Center
Boston, Massachusetts

Preface

There is no longer any serious doubt that daily lifestyle decisions and practices exert a profound impact on both short and long-term health and quality of life. Scientific and medical advances over the last 20 years, and particularly over the last 5 years, have solidified the evidence that positive lifestyle measures are vitally important to good health. While this body of literature has grown stronger and its breadth wider, keeping up with it, and assimilating it into clinical practice, has presented a unique and seemingly almost insurmountable challenge to the average health care practitioner. To further complicate matters, the literature supporting positive lifestyle behavior has emerged from a bewilderingly wide variety of areas related to health including medicine, public health, epidemiology, nutrition, psychology, exercise physiology, sports medicine, and pediatrics, to name only a few of the disciplines involved.

As this literature has grown more complex, and the implications more important to the daily practice of medicine, a need has arisen to bring the key findings and disciplines together in one major medical textbook. This is the fundamental goal and challenge of *Lifestyle Medicine*.

I am proud to serve as the editor of the first comprehensive medical textbook bringing diverse disciplines related to lifestyle and health together in a clinically relevant, comprehensive textbook. It is my hope, and the hope of the talented group of section editors assembled to complete the monumental effort to write and edit *Lifestyle Medicine*, that it will open an entire new branch of medicine emphasizing the important linkages between clinical practice and the recommendation of positive lifestyle behaviors for patients.

Medical professionals in general, and physicians in particular, occupy a uniquely powerful position from which to encourage patients to change their behaviors. In fact, in many surveys, physician recommendation has been shown to be the leading reason why individuals change actions and behaviors. Unfortunately, a distinct minority of physicians wield this power wisely, or at all. Clearly there is a challenge in front of us to bring the power of lifestyle decisions and practices together with modern medical practices, innovative pharmaceutical care, and advanced surgical techniques to improve not only outcomes but also efficiency of health care delivery.

So what is "lifestyle medicine?" As defined in this textbook, and by this editor, "lifestyle medicine" involves the integration of lifestyle practices into the modern practice of medicine both to lower the risk factors for chronic disease and/or, if disease is already present, serve as an adjunct in its therapy. Lifestyle medicine brings together sound, scientific evidence in diverse health-related fields to assist the clinician in the process of not only treating disease, but also promoting good health.

This definition of lifestyle medicine provided the organizational framework for our textbook. We divided the vast area into segments that we felt were relevant to the practicing clinician and in which sound science concerning lifestyle and health exists. *Lifestyle Medicine* is divided into 21 sections, each ably organized and edited by a talented section editor. The textbook opens with a section looking at how lifestyle practices impact on the *management and prevention of cardiovascular disease*. It seems appropriate to inaugurate this textbook with a section on cardiovascular disease, not only because the editor is a cardiologist, but also because the area of lifestyle and risk factor management in the clinical management of cardiovascular disease has taken a prominent position amongst lifestyle interventions in American medicine.

The second section, on *nutrition*, underscores the multiple links between nutrition and disease prevention and therapy. The section on *sports medicine and orthopedics* deals not only with injury prevention and rehabilitation, but also metabolic issues related to good health and prevention of bone and joint disease.

The section on *preventive medicine* emphasizes partnerships that can be developed between physician and patient to enhance good health and outlines exciting new information access available through the Internet, on CD-ROM, and from other electronic resources to improve patient access to information on preventive measures.

The section on *women's health* brings together an emphasis on both prevention and treatment of the most common diseases of women. Also emphasized are such critically important issues as physical activity and the prevention of violence against women. The related section on *obstetrics and gynecology* focuses on how daily lifestyle practices combined with good medical care are critically important throughout all phases of pregnancy and the postpartum period.

The *pulmonary medicine* section provides a state-of-the-art summary of key pulmonary conditions and their interface with lifestyle measures both for prevention and treatment. The section on *behavioral psychology* provides fundamental behavioral psychological theory as well as practical applications of this theory that provides the underpinnings common to all lifestyle practices.

If we are ever to have a serious impact on chronic disease, it is critically important that strong and consistent efforts be undertaken to influence habits and practices among children. The section on *pediatric medicine* not only provides an overview of how this might be accomplished, but also explores some of the specific lifestyle related areas in which prevention and treatment can be implemented in the practice of every clinician who sees children. The *pediatric fitness* section builds on these principles of prevention and provides an exhaustive view of what is known about various aspects of strength training, physical activity, and other fitness-related issues in children.

Family practitioners represent frontline health professionals dealing with virtually every aspect of lifestyle as it relates to disease prevention and treatment. The section on *family medicine* provides specific recommendations for how lifestyle practices can be incorporated into a busy family practice environment. The section on *cardiovascular rehabilitation and secondary prevention* provides a state-of-the-art summary of cardiac rehabilitation and secondary prevention of coronary artery disease. In addition, it provides a look forward to directions that this important field will take in the 21st century.

The section on *epidemiology* provides a wide-ranging survey of how epidemiologic studies have affected virtually every aspect of medicine and applies this information to several specific disease categories including cardiovascular disease, diabetes, and reduction in cancer risk.

In addition to the setting of the office practice, other important venues in which positive lifestyle should be emphasized include the workplace and managed care environments. The section on *health promotion* summarizes the important literature that has emerged in this wide-ranging field. The section on *exercise and sport psychology* points to the important interfaces

between mind and body. Certainly these linkages represent powerful tools for the clinician to utilize to change behavior.

The section on *obesity and weight management* provides an up-to-date summary of advances in this critically important health related field. A variety of lifestyle measures including proper exercise and dietary management as well as pharmaceutical therapy and surgery are skillfully discussed in this section. The section on *fitness and exercise* provides excellent, clinically oriented information for clinicians about the multiple contributions that exercise physiology has made to patient care over the last 25 years. Included in this area are specific recommendations for physical fitness evaluation, body composition, assessment, and exercise prescription.

The section on *immunology* provides cutting-edge information on the emerging field of how physical activity interacts with the immune system both in apparently healthy individuals and in individuals who are immunocompromised. Often clinicians do not pay proper credence to the effect of the environment on good health. The section on *environmental stress* elucidates some of the key environmental stressors, including heat, cold, high altitude, air pollution, and sleep, and provides clinically relevant discussions that will be of great use to all health care providers.

The section on *dermatology* addresses the important and often neglected interactions between lifestyle and skin conditions. Included in this section are excellent discussions on nutrition, aging, the sun and exercise, and their effects on the skin. The final section of the textbook deals with *public policy* issues and reminds us that clinicians do not practice in a vacuum. Rather, clinical medicine is practiced in an environment in which public policy decisions can dramatically affect the health of not only populations, but also individual patients. In this section policy issues related both to physical activity and obesity are discussed.

Textbook writing is a collaborative undertaking. I have been blessed with the privilege of working with 20 superb section editors who have devoted great energy and talent to the difficult task of organizing sections that are not only scientifically accurate, but also clinically relevant. I am deeply grateful to all of these individuals.

What has emerged from their efforts and those of the 148 distinguished contributors is a textbook that we hope will be clinically useful to the practicing health care professional as well as provide a state of the art summary of modern scientific and medical understandings related to the interface between lifestyle practices, modern medicine, and good health.

In any textbook of this size, certain editorial decisions had to be made. When faced with the task of determining overall direction for the book, I challenged the section editors to focus their attention largely on clinical issues and perhaps somewhat less so on theory, without sacrificing scientific precision. All of them have risen ably to this challenge.

Editing a major textbook also relies on the superb efforts and dedication of people working closely with me. I would like to particularly acknowledge a few people without whom this textbook would never have been possible. First, and foremost, the Editorial Director in my laboratory, Elizabeth Porcaro, has guided this book through every step of the editorial and prepublication process. Without Beth's good humor, intelligence, and superb organizational skills, this book could never have been accomplished. Carol Moreau, my Executive Assistant, manages to keep my complex life in some semblance of order, which allows me to carve out time for major editorial projects. Diane O'Brien, RN, BSN, Laboratory Director of the Center for Clinical and Lifestyle Research, and Deirdre Morrissey, the laboratory Research Development Director, managed multiple research projects while this editorial process was taking place.

My longtime friend and colleague at Blackwell Science, James Krosschell, Senior Vice President and Publisher, was an early champion of this book and never doubted that it would take its rightful place as a major entry into clinical medicine. Bill Gibson, the former President of Blackwell Science, was also a staunch supporter of this project and exhibited great patience over some early delays. Susan Catterall has played a key role in managing diverse aspects of the publication process.

Finally, I am grateful to my family, my loving wife Stephanie Hart Rippe, our "oldest daughter" Natasha Koeberg, and my two younger daughters, Hart Elizabeth Rippe and Jaelin Davis Rippe, for loving and supporting me through the arduous process of editing another major textbook.

If there are errors or limitations in *Lifestyle Medicine* the responsibility is mine. If there is credit due for this project, it belongs to the numerous people who have helped along the way.

James M. Rippe, MD
Boston, Massachusetts

Part I.

LIFESTYLE MANAGEMENT AND PREVENTION OF CARDIOVASCULAR DISEASE

Edited by
James M. Rippe

Introduction to Lifestyle Management and Prevention of Cardiovascular Disease

James M. Rippe

It seems fitting that a textbook devoted to how daily habits and practices impact on both short- and long-term health and quality of life would start with a section on the management and prevention of cardiovascular disease. It is in this critically important area that lifestyle medicine has, perhaps, advanced the furthest. There has been a significant and encouraging downward trend in death rates from coronary artery disease in the United States since the 1960s. Between 1960 and 1990, mortality from coronary artery disease fell over 50% and accounted for half of the decline in total mortality rate in the United States during this period of time. This sharp decline coincided with elucidation of risk factors for coronary artery disease and a national effort to reduce these risk factors, largely based on lifestyle issues, which has taken place over the last 40 years.

The section on lifestyle management and prevention of cardiovascular disease starts with a review of the epidemiology of risk factors and their temporal trends by Goldberg and Yarzebski. In the next chapter, Nicolosi provides the underpinnings for why elevated blood cholesterol plays such a key role in the pathobiology of atherosclerosis. The chapters by Rippe, O'Brien, and Taylor provide an overall rationale for why it is worthwhile to intervene in the area of coronary artery disease as well as specific lifestyle strategies for accomplishing this intervention.

The next five chapters deal with specific lifestyle issues related to the prevention and/or treatment of coronary heart disease. Kristeller provides an up-to-date summary on how managing cigarette smoking can reduce the risk of cardiovascular disease. Glanz surveys the literature on nutrition intervention, Ward provides a concise survey of exercise intervention, and McGowan provides a clinically oriented chapter on managing dyslipidemias. Heyka examines the various lifestyle modalities that have been proven effective in prevention and treatment of hypertension. The section closes with a comprehensive chapter on how community efforts can be focused to lower the risk of cardiovascular disease in population groups.

Although cardiovascular disease remains the leading killer in the United States and other industrialized countries, encouraging progress has been made. Now it is up to the medical community to apply proven strategies for lifestyle intervention to continue the downward trend of cardiovascular disease, morbidity, and mortality.

Chapter 1

Coronary Heart Disease: Epidemiology, Risk Factors, and Temporal Trends

Robert J. Goldberg
Jorge L. Yarzebski

Despite continuing declines in the mortality rates attributed to coronary heart disease in the United States over the past nearly 3 decades, coronary atherosclerosis and the clinical expressions of this disease process remain the leading cause of death in the United States and in many industrialized countries (1,2). Many of the adverse sequelae associated with coronary atherosclerosis could be prevented, or at least forestalled, in persons identified as being at high risk for coronary disease since an increasing array of tailored pharmacologic and lifestyle interventions are presently available.

A number of modifiable risk factors as well as nonmodifiable risk markers have been associated with the occurrence of coronary heart disease (CHD). Coronary disease, however, is best conceptualized as a multifactorial disease with no individual risk factor essential or sufficient for causation (3,4). Data collected from prospective epidemiological investigations and studies of migrant populations have established a clear and increased risk for CHD with increasing levels of blood pressure, serum cholesterol, and cigarette smoking. These risk factors have been shown to be singly important and interactively multiplicative in the development of CHD. Recent attention has focused on the important role of physical inactivity and obesity in the development of coronary disease, as well as other chronic diseases of major public health importance. Given the overall prevalence and increasing magnitude of these two conditions, and the increased risk of CHD associated with these predisposing factors, physical inactivity and obesity are presently considered as major modifiable risk factors by national scientific advisory committees (5–7).

Given the extensive wealth of information compiled about the risk factors for CHD, this chapter will provide an overview of the primary as well as secondary risk factors for CHD, with a particular focus on those factors that may be alterable through lifestyle changes and/or pharmacologic interventions. In general, the major coronary risk factors are related to each of the principal clinical manifestations of CHD including angina pectoris, acute myocardial infarction (AMI), and sudden cardiac death, although their predictive utility varies according to the clinical condition examined as well as according to sociodemographic characteristics and comorbid conditions.

MAGNITUDE OF CORONARY HEART DISEASE

Since the turn of the twentieth century, when the epidemic of CHD in the United States first appeared, the cardiovascular diseases have been the leading cause of death as well as a significant contributor to personal disability and an impaired quality of life. As a group, the cardiovascular diseases exact an enormous toll. In 1995, cardiovascular disease was the leading contributor to hospital discharges with 5.8 million persons hospitalized with a first listed diagnosis of cardiovascular disease during that year. It is estimated that more than one in five men and women in the United States have some form of cardiovascular disease. In 1995, the various forms of cardiovascular disease claimed more than 960,000 lives.

Of the several different diseases that comprise cardiovascular disease, CHD is the most prevalent. More than 480,000 persons died from CHD in 1995, leading to its unenviable position as the leading cause of death among all persons in the United States and claiming approximately one of every five deaths (1,2). Approximately one half of the deaths attributed to CHD occur as sudden deaths, usually within 1 hour of the onset of acute symptoms and before the patient can reach a hospital. Of the different manifestations of heart disease—rheumatic and hypertensive heart disease, diseases of the pulmonary circulation, heart failure, cardiomyopathies, and others—CHD, or atherosclerotic heart disease, is the principal disease entity discussed in this chapter.

Coronary heart disease is highly prevalent among adults in the United States and has a significant impact on use of health care resources and services. In 1995, approximately 2.1 million persons were hospitalized with CHD. These persons spent an average of 4.3 days in the hospital, and several million visits were made to physicians' offices due to coronary atherosclerosis in 1995 (2). Approximately 1.1 million Americans will experience a heart attack annually and about one third of them will die from AMI. Coronary disease is the leading cause of death in Caucasian men and women and is the second leading cause of death in African-American men and women. Nearly 13.9 million Americans alive today have a history of AMI or angina pectoris. These estimates emphasize the high prevalence of this disease process and the important public health and clinical implications associated with coronary artery disease.

Although CHD remains of epidemic proportion in the United States, despite the encouraging and ongoing declines in CHD mortality described later in this chapter, concern has been raised that a number of developing countries may soon be undergoing the epidemiologic transition to the more chronic degenerative diseases including CHD (Table 1-1) (8,9). Although the United States and a number of industrialized countries are firmly entrenched in the third or fourth stages of this epidemiologic transition, limited data from several developing countries suggest the emergence of cardiovascular diseases in these countries (10,11). These findings are of particular concern given the increased life expectancies at birth that are taking place in a number of developing countries and the preventability of coronary atherosclerosis through use of pharmacologic and lifestyle interventions. Although it remains of importance to carefully monitor trends in CHD incidence and/or mortality in countries experiencing significant financial and sociocultural changes, increased attention needs to be paid by the ministries of health and health practitioners in these countries to forestalling, or preventing, this impending epidemic of CHD and other chronic diseases.

EPIDEMIOLOGY OF CORONARY HEART DISEASE

Beginning in the late 1940s with the establishment and screening of the first cohort of a general population sample of men and women in Framingham, Mass (12,13), a number of workplace and community-based studies investigating factors associated with the occurrence of CHD were initiated. These investigations included the Chicago Peoples Gas Company Study (14) and Chicago Western Electric Company Study (15), the Tecumseh Health Study (16), the Albany Cardiovascular Health Center Study (17), the Los Angeles Heart Study (18), the Minnesota Business and Professional Men's Study (19), and the Western Collaborative Group Study (20). These studies ranged from relatively small select samples of middle-aged men to more extensive community-based samples designed to provide a representative overview of the risk factors for CHD and associated morbidity and mortality.

The seminal Framingham Heart Study has identified a host of nonmodifiable (e.g., family history, male gender, advancing age) risk markers and modifiable (e.g., elevated total serum cholesterol and low levels of high-density lipoprotein cholesterol, cigarette smoking, elevated blood pressure, physical inactivity) risk factors associated with the development of CHD. This National Heart, Lung, and Blood Institute–funded investigation recently celebrated its fiftieth anniversary, during which time highlights and accomplishments of the Framingham study were reviewed. This prospective epidemiologic study has also provided a systematic framework for assessing the magnitude of risk associated with identified coronary risk factors singly and in combination. Based on the absolute, relative, and attributable risks associated with the major coronary risk factors, what in the past may have been considered as usual or normal has now been revised downward to provide more optimal levels associated with a reduced risk of disease (21).

The landmark prospective epidemiologic investigations of CHD in the United States were complimented by additional cohort studies in other parts of the world, including Great Britain (22), Hawaii (23), Israel (24), Japan (25), and Scandinavia (26). A particularly ambitious undertaking of the determinants of CHD was the Seven Countries Study (27). This multicohort study, initiated in the mid 1950s, examined the morbidity and mortality rates of CHD, as well as host and

Table 1-1 The Epidemiologic Transition

PHASE OF EPIDEMIOLOGIC TRANSITION	DEATHS FROM CIRCULATORY DISEASE (%)	CIRCULATORY PROBLEMS	RISK FACTORS
Age of Pestilence and Famine	5–10	Rheumatic heart disease; infectious and deficiency-induced cardiomyopathies	Uncontrolled infection; deficiency conditions
Age of Receding Pandemics	10–35	As above, plus hypertensive heart disease and hemorrhagic stroke	High-salt diet leading to hypertension; increased smoking
Age of Degenerative and Man-Made Diseases	35–55	All forms of stroke; ischemic heart disease	Atherosclerosis from fatty diets; sedentary lifestyle; smoking
Age of Delayed Degenerative Diseases	<50 (probably)	Stroke and ischemic heart disease	Education and behavioral changes leading to lower levels of risk factors

environmental factors associated with its occurrence, in over 12,000 middle-aged (40 to 59 years) men from seven countries differing in their cultural and lifestyle habits.

These national and international observational epidemiologic investigations established a methodologic and logistical framework for the study of CHD and its natural history from a broad population-based perspective, providing clues to factors associated with its occurrence and ultimately its prevention. These methodologically rigorous studies firmly established the credibility and usefulness of the epidemiologic approach to the study of the cardiovascular diseases in general and CHD in particular and of the use of representative population samples to more systematically study the occurrence of chronic disease and its precursors.

Further support for the integral role of environmental factors associated with the occurrence of CHD was provided by migrant studies carried out in Israel, New Zealand, and Japan. Perhaps the most compelling of these studies was the Ni-Hon-San study (from *Nip*pon, *Hon*olulu, and *San* Francisco) of middle-aged Japanese men migrating to Honolulu, Hawaii, and to San Francisco, Calif. In comparison to those remaining behind in Japan, the CHD death rates of migrants came to resemble those of their country of adoption within several decades of migration (28). These varying death rates were attributed to likely changes in dietary habits and the adoption of adverse lifestyle and other habits, different from those of their country of birth, associated with an increased risk for the development of, and/or risk of dying from, CHD.

Each of the risk factors described subsequently has been shown to be associated with various clinical manifestations of coronary atherosclerosis. Although these predisposing factors may or may not be causally related to CHD, their presence increases the likelihood that a person has, or will develop, CHD within a defined period of time. It may very well be that there is a single "causal" risk factor, such as an underlying lipid abnormality, and that all other known or suspected risk factors are "accelerators," namely agents that cannot by themselves initiate the atherosclerotic process, but which promote its course with varying degrees of strength (29). The recent investigation of the role of potential triggers, or precipitating factors, such as extreme physical exertion or acute psychosocial distress, are discussed in later sections of this chapter in relation to the acute onset of CHD. Conversely, it should not be inferred that persons free from the established coronary risk factors, risk markers, or precipitating factors identified to date are immune from the risk of developing CHD. In the United States many men and women have none of the currently identified and established risk factors for CHD, yet the incidence of CHD in these groups is much higher than that observed in groups of similar individuals from other parts of the world where CHD is of lesser magnitude. It is widely accepted and generally acknowledged that CHD is a multifactorial disease and that a multiplicity of interacting factors are involved in its development.

Natural History of Atherosclerotic Heart Disease

Clinically apparent coronary disease is the end result of an underlying atherosclerosis whose focal lesions lead to myocardial ischemia. This disease process has a multiple decade–long latency period that starts in the relatively young and culminates in the onset of clinically detectable disease most typically in the fifth through the seventh decades of life.

The focal lesions of coronary atherosclerosis, which primarily affect the intima of normal arteries, are the fatty streaks, fibrous plaques, and complicated lesions (30,31). The fibrous plaques and complicated lesions are collectively referred to as *raised lesions*. As the raised lesions increase in size, they may impede or cut off blood flow in affected coronary arteries and are responsible for the clinical signs and symptoms of CHD. In contrast, the sessile fatty streak is not associated with significant obstruction of the coronary vessels. Although no definitive agreement has been reached concerning the precise progression of change from the earliest recognizable lesions of coronary atherosclerosis to the raised or calcified lesions and eventual onset of clinically detectable disease, the "response to injury" hypothesis (32), subsequently modified and updated based on more recent findings (33), places the probable sequence of events in an understandable and working context (Figure 1-1).

In recent years, considerable attention has focused on the concept of plaque vulnerability as a key determinant of acute coronary disease. Biochemical and pathologic studies suggest that a number of characteristics associated with the atherosclerotic plaque likely contribute to the development of acute coronary disease, even in the presence of minimally obstructive underlying disease (34,35). These characteristics include a thin fibrous cap, a soft lipid-rich core with predominantly more liquid rather than crystalloid cholesterol, and the presence of subintimal inflammation, superimposed on a substrate of mild to moderate coronary atherosclerosis. The presence of these and other factors presently under active study is speculated to lead to plaque vulnerability, eventual plaque disruption or fissuring under selected conditions, and subsequent development of CHD. On the other hand, coronary vessels complicated by plaques not prone to vulnerability are presently characterized by a thick calcified fibrous cap, large amounts of crystalline as opposed to liquid cholesterol, and lack of inflammatory cells in the subintimal region. These recent observations have provided valuable insights into the pathogenesis of CHD and have led to increased efforts to identify factors associated with plaque vulnerability and strategies by which their impact might be minimized.

The well-established risk factors for CHD may become involved in the pathway to atherosclerosis in a number of ways. They may be intimately involved (e.g., serum cholesterol) in leading to the earliest lesions of coronary atherosclerosis, they may facilitate changes in the earliest lesions to the more complicated or raised lesions (e.g., cholesterol, blood pressure), and they may be involved in transforming the underlying subclinical state to that of overt, clinically detectable disease through acute pathophysiologic changes in susceptible coronary vessels (e.g., cigarette smoking).

In a further effort to conceptualize the interplay of risk factors in the onset of clinical CHD, a working theory has been proposed by which physical and mental stressors may trigger coronary thrombosis in susceptible individuals with vulnerable atherosclerotic plaques (36) (Figure 1-2). It has been proposed that, in persons with underlying atherosclerosis and vulnerable atherosclerotic lesions that may be susceptible to plaque rupture, coronary thrombosis may be set into motion through a complex and incompletely understood

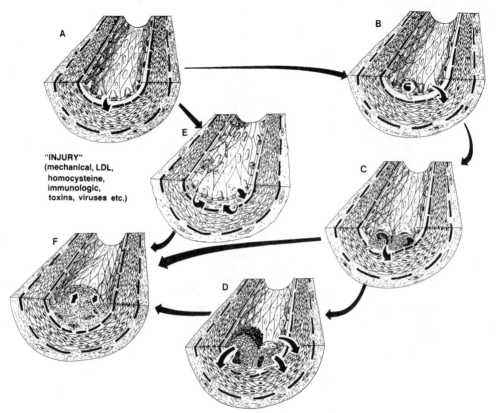

Figure 1-1 Response to injury hypothesis.

interaction of stressor agents and accompanying hemodynamic changes. Although there are few data to support or refute this hypothesis, it places into further perspective the role of potential acute triggers in the development of myocardial necrosis and provides a fertile base from which further investigative and interventional activities might arise. The existence of triggers for AMI is suggested by the occurrence of a prominent circadian rhythm of this disorder, with an increased onset of AMI in the morning hours; similar observations have been documented in patients with sudden cardiac death (37–41). Excess physical exertion and psychosocial factors have been shown in recent studies to act as possible triggers for AMI. These studies have used a novel methodologic approach, the case-crossover design, in which the patient is used as his or her own control to address these and other potential associations (42–44). Triggering agents may also be involved in the acute onset of unstable angina.

The following section provides an overview of the descriptive epidemiology of CHD with a primary focus on the relation of age, gender, race, and socioeconomic status to the attack and mortality rates of CHD.

Age

Each of the major prospective epidemiologic investigations carried out over the past several decades has shown a marked increase in the risk of CHD with advancing age. This finding is to be expected given the well-known association of age with the development of the chronic diseases of major public health importance and the decades-long latency period required for the clinical expression of CHD. During the first 14 years of follow-up in the Framingham study, among individuals initially free from CHD, every eighth man 40 to 44 years of age at the time of study entry had developed some form of coronary disease during this follow-up period; the percentage of men developing CHD increased with age to approximately every sixth man aged 45 to 49 years at entry, every fifth man 50 to 54, and every fourth man 55 years of age or older (45). Among women free from CHD at the time of their baseline examination, women under 50 years of age experienced about one sixth the CHD incidence rate among men; the incidence of CHD rose dramatically after menopause. By 60 years of age, approximately every fifth man and every seventeenth woman had developed CHD during the first 14 years of this study.

Death rates from CHD rise in an essentially linear fashion with increasing age. Heart disease is the leading cause of death in men by their fourth decade and in women by their sixth and seventh decades of life (1,2). In part because of declining CHD death rates, by 1991 there were more deaths attributed to cancer, however, than there were to CHD in white and African-American men and women. Although some of the well-accepted risk factors for CHD have smaller risk ratios with advancing age, these lower relative risks are counterbalanced by the high absolute risk of CHD in the elderly.

Gender

CHD is a major health concern for men and women. In the United States, men typically exhibit higher age-specific inci-

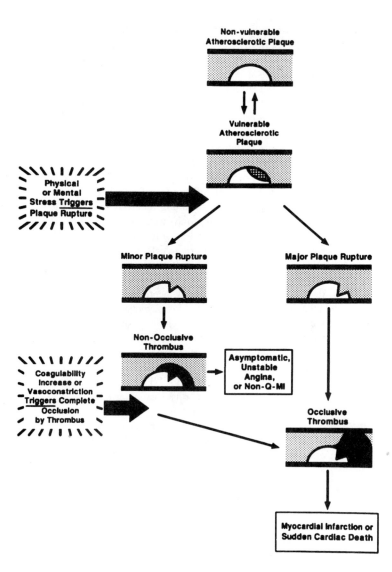

Figure 1-2 Triggering of acute coronary thrombosis.

dence rates of CHD than women throughout life although the difference in attack rates of CHD tends to narrow after menopause, with CHD becoming a major cause of morbidity and mortality among women beyond their mid to late fifties (46,47). Whether or not menopause in and of itself, however, is responsible for the increased attack rates of CHD in women remains controversial. In the Framingham study, the incidence rates of CHD increased in both men and women with advancing age, with the incidence rates of CHD being greater among men than women; these gender differences in the incidence of CHD, however, diminished with incremental increases in age (46,47). In general, the recognized risk factors for CHD tend to be operative in men and women, although obesity, low serum levels of high-density lipoprotein choles- terol, and diabetes mellitus appear to have a relatively greater adverse impact in women.

Race

Limited data exist examining differences in the predisposing factors for CHD as well as in the incidence rates of, and mor- tality from, CHD in African-Americans as compared to whites in the United States. In terms of mortality rates from CHD,

deaths from CHD were lower in African-American than white men in the United States in the 1940s, and then increased rapidly until the late 1960s, after which time marked declines have been observed in these two races (1,2,48). In 1995, the age-adjusted death rates from CHD were slightly higher in African-American men than in white men, whereas the death rates from CHD were appreciably higher in African-American women than in white women (2). The mortality rates from CHD were between 1.5- and 2-fold higher in men as in women irrespective of race. In examining age-specific death rates from CHD, mortality is slightly greater in African-American than white men until approximately 70 years of age, after which the death rates from CHD rise to a greater degree in whites than in African-Americans. The death rates from CHD tend to be consistently higher in African-American than in white women up until the eighth decade of life, after which the death rates tend to run an essentially parallel course.

Despite lingering questions as to the relevance of the usual risk factors for CHD in African-American, as well as Hispanic populations, given the dearth of investigative activity in this area, African-American adults tend to have higher prevalence rates of elevated blood pressure and cigarette smoking, although the prevalence rates of heavy smoking are less among African-Americans than whites (2,49–51). The incidence of hypercholesterolemia tends to be relatively similar between the races, whereas obesity is highly prevalent among African-American women. On the other hand, African-American men tend to have a more favorable lipoprotein profile than white men; these differences are less striking among women. In an attempt to explain some of the paradoxical observations with regard to the highly prevalent distribution of risk factors in African-Americans and occurrence rates of CHD, it has been suggested that African-Americans may have higher levels of risk factors that protect against CHD, including higher work-related patterns of physical activity, lower triglyceride levels, higher alcohol intake, and possibly familial and other factors that may protect them from coronary atherosclerosis. Differences in hemostatic factors between African-Americans and whites have not been systematically explored. The multisite Atherosclerosis Risk in Communities (ARIC) study is examining racial differences in risk factors for underlying atherosclerosis through noninvasive measurement of carotid intimal thickness. This large epidemiologic study should provide valuable insights to the differential impact, if any, of several coronary risk factors in African-Americans as compared to whites on extent of underlying atherosclerosis (52).

Limited incidence data exist that would allow for a systematic determination of differences in the annual incidence or hospitalization rates for AMI in African-Americans as compared to whites. In general, the incidence rates of AMI tend to be lower in African-American men as compared to white men, with inconsistent trends observed in African-American women relative to white women. African-Americans in the Coronary Artery Surgery Study were shown to have less coronary artery disease than their white counterparts, including multivessel and left main coronary artery disease (53). The lower rates of anatomic coronary artery disease in African-Americans were seen despite higher levels of modifiable risk factors than among whites.

Socioeconomic Status

Low social class, low educational attainment, and other indicators of socioeconomic status have been associated with CHD morbidity and mortality, as well as all-cause mortality (54). The consensus of the many published reports in this area suggests an inverse association between socioeconomic status and many of the important CHD risk factors, as well as an inverse relation with the attack and mortality rates of CHD.

RISK FACTORS FOR CORONARY HEART DISEASE

The following section will overview the primary and secondary risk factors associated with CHD, as well as the role of familial and genetic factors in the development of premature atherosclerosis.

Cigarette Smoking

Cigarette smoking has been consistently and in a dose-related manner shown to be related to the development of fatal and nonfatal CHD events (55–58). Despite the general strength

and consistency of these observations, data from the Framingham Heart Study has shown a lack of association between cigarette smoking and angina pectoris in both men and women. Consumption of cigarettes, however, was clearly related to the risk of myocardial infarction, sudden cardiac death, and CHD mortality in both men and women.

On the other hand, cigarette smoking has not been shown to be a potent risk factor for CHD in populations, such as the Japanese, that are characterized by low serum cholesterol levels. These observations, in conjunction with results from studies in men and women that have shown a markedly decreased risk of CHD after quitting smoking (59,60), with the excess risk of CHD declining relatively quickly after quitting, suggest that smoking may act as a triggering agent, rather than as a necessary and sufficient factor, for CHD. Even among patients suffering AMI, the risk of subsequent mortality and reinfarction is dramatically lower among ex-smokers as opposed to continuing smokers (61). Nicotine and the smoking of cigarettes have been shown to have a multiplicity of adverse affects on the cardiovascular system, including undesirable effects on platelet adhesiveness and clotting factors, increased heart rate, catecholamine levels, myocardial oxygen demand, and decreased oxygen carrying capacity of the blood. Pipe and cigar smokers appear to have only a slight, if any, increase in risk for CHD with the observed absolute and relative risks considerably lower than those observed for smoking cigarettes.

Passive exposure to secondary cigarette smoke has been associated with clinically manifest as well as subclinical CHD and carotid atherosclerosis through a number of pathophysiologic mechanisms (62,63). Although the relative risks of CHD associated with passive smoking are less than those attributed to direct inhalation, the large proportion of the population exposed to environmental tobacco smoke suggests that the adverse health consequences for a large number of persons may be affected by even small increases in the risk of coronary disease, as well as possibly selected cancers.

Blood Pressure

Elevation of either systolic or diastolic blood pressure has been shown to be predictive of the subsequent risk of CHD, with hypertension consistently and independently established as one of the major coronary risk factors in national and international studies (2–4). The risk of morbid and fatal CHD events is related to increasing levels of blood pressure in a direct and continuous manner with no clear cut-off point below which risk becomes negligible. From a clinical point of view, definite as well as borderline hypertension is highly correlated with the development of CHD even within the so-called "mild" range. Actuarial studies published by the insurance companies have shown higher all-cause mortality rates with increasing levels of either systolic or diastolic blood pressure.

Despite favorable trends in the management and control of hypertension, the benefits of reductions in blood pressure through pharmacologic means in mildly hypertensive individuals in terms of reduced CHD morbidity and mortality, nonetheless, remain controversial. A pooled analysis of the data from nine controlled clinical trials suggested a decrease in the incidence rates of fatal and nonfatal coronary events among treated hypertensives although a clear-cut benefit of antihypertensive treatment on these events was lacking (64,65). The lack of compelling benefit on CHD outcomes may be, in part, attributed to the undesirable effects on serum lipids and other important metabolic parameters associated with the antihypertensive agents used in these trials.

Serum Lipids

Evidence accumulated from observational epidemiologic studies over the past several decades has provided strong support for total serum cholesterol as a major predictive factor in the development of CHD (2–4). Data collected from observations between countries, population-based investigations within the United States, and additional prospective epidemiologic investigations summarized in the Pooling Project, have established in a clear, dose-responsive, and temporal manner the important role for total serum cholesterol in the development of CHD (66,67). Evidence has also been collected from prospective population-based studies suggesting an increased risk of dying from CHD among persons with preexisting coronary disease who have elevated cholesterol levels and need for dietary and/or pharmacologic interventions (68,69).

Epidemiologic observations of the atherogenicity of elevated serum cholesterol levels are consistent with information obtained from randomized clinical trials that suggest a beneficial effect of lowering blood cholesterol levels on the risk of developing clinical CHD even among persons with what are presently considered average cholesterol levels (70–74). Data obtained from treatment studies in humans also suggest that, through the use of dietary and pharmacologic interventions, important effects on the rates of progression of the advanced underlying atherosclerotic process and/or actual regression can be achieved in treated individuals through favorable alterations in lipid and lipoprotein parameters (75). Deposition of lipid, particularly cholesterol, and ingestion of modified low-density lipoproteins by macrophages with ultimate transformation to foam cells are hallmark events in the evolution of the atherosclerotic lesions, from the earliest fatty streaks to the clinically important fibrous plaques and complicated lesions.

In terms of the relation between the various lipoprotein classes that transport cholesterol throughout the blood and CHD, low-density lipoprotein (LDL) cholesterol and high-density lipoprotein (HDL) cholesterol have emerged as the most important lipoprotein complexes related to the risk of CHD. Information obtained from numerous epidemiologic studies has shown LDL to be the atherogenic component of the serum total cholesterol that is positively related to the incidence rates of CHD. The other important lipoprotein related to the development of CHD is HDL cholesterol. Levels of HDL cholesterol are inversely related to the incidence rates of CHD, given the key role of this lipoprotein fraction in cholesterol clearance. Based on the evidence linking levels of lipids and lipoproteins to the incidence rates of CHD, use of either total serum cholesterol levels, or of ratios of LDL to HDL or total cholesterol to HDL, has been advocated as a useful methodology for judging an individual's future risk of CHD, and as a gauge for the efficacy of dietary or pharmacologic interventions.

With regard to the apoproteins, CHD has been shown to be positively associated with apolipoprotein B, the principal protein moiety of LDL cholesterol, and inversely associated with apolipoprotein A, the principal apolipoprotein of HDL cholesterol (76–78).

High concentrations of Lp(a) have been associated with an increased risk for CHD in most but not all studies (79–82). Considerable recent attention has focused on the mechanisms of LDL oxidation and the potential role of oxidized lipoproteins in the development of coronary atherosclerosis. Focal accumulation in the arterial intima of excessive amounts of LDL is thought to lead to the migration of monocytes, which may then differentiate into macrophages after taking up large amounts of oxidatively modified LDL; in turn, these macrophages become transformed to lipid-rich foam cells within the subendothelial space. These events have been postulated to lead to pathophysiologic disturbances in vascular relaxation and to the development of atherosclerotic plaques (83). Considerable investigative work is being devoted to studying the atherogenic properties of oxidized LDL and how intervention approaches, such as the use of antioxidants and other measures, may reduce the susceptibility of LDL to oxidation and attenuation of the atherosclerotic process.

Debate continues with regard to the role of triglycerides as an independent risk factor for CHD. Some studies have, whereas others have not, found triglycerides to correlate with the subsequent risk of CHD (84–90). When multivariate analyses, however, are carried out in which the other lipoprotein fractions and principal coronary risk factors are simultaneously controlled for, triglycerides appear to exert little, if any, independent influence on the risk of CHD. Questions concerning the independent role of triglycerides have nonetheless remained rekindled based on findings from the Framingham and Honolulu heart studies that have shown higher levels of triglycerides to be related to CHD.

Whereas the relation between elevated blood lipids and specific lipoprotein fractions to risk of CHD has been consistently demonstrated and is well established, concerns continue regarding the relationship of dietary habits to CHD. In the Seven Countries Study, a significant and independent association was seen between the population percentage of calories coming from saturated fat, amount of cholesterol in the diet, and occurrence of CHD (91); longitudinal studies have also suggested an independent association between selected dietary variables, primarily saturated fat and cholesterol, and risk of, and mortality from, CHD (92–94). As a means to, in part, explain these relationships, international comparisons in varying population samples have shown associations between diet and serum cholesterol levels. Human metabolic studies and feeding experiments in animals have also implicated the habitual consumption of diets high in saturated fats and dietary cholesterol as causing increased levels of cholesterol in the blood (95–98). On the other hand, most likely as a consequence of the limited variation within the atherogenic diet consumed among the populations studied and/or because of the dietary assessment utilized, within-country studies of dietary intake have not been persuasive in correlating diet to the level of serum cholesterol and CHD.

Fish consumption (99,100), diets rich in fiber, fruits and vegetables, and complex carbohydrates (101,102), features of a Mediterranean diet (103), and intake of supplemental antioxidants and other nutrients (104,105) also may be important in reducing the risk of CHD.

Physical Inactivity

Beginning with such landmark studies as those of bus drivers and conductors in the London transport system (106) and San Francisco longshoremen, showing a protective effect of high-level energy expenditure (107), considerable evidence has accumulated for an independent role of increased physical activity in the primary prevention of CHD. This subject has been the focus of several extensive reviews in the past decade (108–110). The consensus of these studies is that individuals engaged in regular physical activity are at reduced risk for CHD when compared to their more sedentary counterparts. Physical inactivity is presently considered by a number of scientific advisory committees to be a major modifiable risk factor for the development of CHD.

A meta-analysis of the available literature has assessed the role of physical activity in the prevention of CHD (110). Such an analysis has to deal with methodologic considerations as to the varying definitions of physical activity used, measurement of activity levels either at work or during leisure time, and potential confounding of the apparent association between physical activity and CHD by the influence of changes in physical activity on the prevalence as well as severity of accompanying coronary risk factors. This review of the findings from 27 cohort studies suggested a beneficial effect of physical activity on reduced risk for CHD; this association was shown to be strongest in contrasting highly physically active groups with sedentary ones and in the more methodologically rigorous studies.

Few investigations, however, have examined the relation between physical fitness, as assessed through objective quantifiable measures, and future risk of CHD morbidity and/or mortality (111,112). Utilizing data obtained from submaximal exercise treadmill testing of over 3000 men between the ages of 30 and 69 years enrolled in the Lipid Research Clinics Prevalence Survey, the risk of dying from CHD was significantly greater among men with low levels of physical fitness (111). Consistent with prior work in this area, persons at the highest levels of fitness also tended to have a more favorable risk factor profile; however, the beneficial effect of fitness remained after multivariate adjustment for age and accompanying cardiovascular risk factors.

A more physically active lifestyle is being increasingly viewed as an integral component of a comprehensive coronary risk reduction program given documented benefits on HDL cholesterol, blood pressure, body weight, and insulin resistance. Maintenance of regular physical activity may also be associated with beneficial effects on the precipitation of acute coronary disease, particularly in the setting of an extreme physical stressor (42).

Obesity

The association between obesity and illness was initially alluded to by Hippocrates, who observed that "When more food than is proper has been taken, it occasions disease." Substantial evidence indeed exists to confirm this impression; increased body weight for height is associated with various risk factors for CHD as well as more directly influencing the risk of CHD, although the latter association remains less evident and inconsistent between studies.

Based on studies utilizing either comparisons of weight relative to a desirable standard compiled by the Metropolitan Life Insurance company tables or body mass index as proxy measures for obesity, obesity has been shown to be positively related to the levels of serum cholesterol and to blood pressure in a continuous and graded manner (113–115). Although a consistent association of obesity with an unfavorable coronary risk factor profile has been repeatedly observed in cross-sectional and prospective epidemiologic studies, an apparent paradox exists with regard to the association of obesity to the incidence of CHD. Data from the Pooling Project suggest that there was either a lack of, a U-shaped, or a positive association between obesity and CHD depending on the cohort under study. A review of the major longitudinal studies from North America, carried out primarily among men, that utilized multivariable analyses to control for other potentially confounding factors, found a significant independent relation between obesity and the incidence of CHD, primarily in the younger cohorts studied. On the other hand, in reviewing data from cross-cultural and population-based studies, divergent results were observed in terms of the association of obesity with subsequent risk of CHD as well as with the CHD endpoint examined (115). The few prospective studies of obesity and CHD in women have found either a lack of association (116,117) or strong positive association between relative weight and the incidence of CHD (118,119). Extending and refining work in this area, studies carried out in the past decade suggest that the distribution of adipose tissue ("pears" versus "apples"), namely central or abdominal obesity, is an independent risk factor for CHD.

Diabetes Mellitus

CHD is the most common underlying cause of death in diabetic adults in the United States, accounting for more than one third of all deaths in diabetic adults 40 years of age and older (120,121). Additional macrovascular sequelae, including cerebrovascular disease, congestive heart failure, and peripheral vascular disease, occur more frequently in diabetics than in nondiabetics. Insulin resistance, hyperinsulinemia, and glucose intolerance have been found to be atherogenic.

Adult-onset diabetics commonly have the risk factors of obesity, an adverse serum lipid profile, and elevated blood pressure contributing to an insulin resistance syndrome and accelerated risk of atherosclerosis (122,123). Substantial evidence exists to show that diabetes exerts an independent influence on the risk of developing as well as dying from CHD, irrespective of serum insulin levels. Although controversy continues concerning the independent role of plasma insulin levels in the development of CHD (124,125), several lines of evidence suggest that hyperinsulinemia is an important risk factor for coronary atherosclerosis, contributing directly to adverse effects on the arterial wall and to the development of hyperlipidemia. The increased atherogenicity associated with the prediabetic state may be a significant contributor to the subsequent risk of CHD even before clinically apparent diabetes develops. As opposed to the usual disproportionate burden that CHD places on men, the effect of diabetes appears to be relatively stronger in women. Data from the Framingham Heart Study, for example, have shown an approximate threefold increased risk of selected coronary events in diabetic women relative to nondiabetic women, and an approximate twofold increase among diabetic as compared to nondiabetic men (126). The impact of diabetes on CHD was also seen to diminish with advancing age in women, with less apparent trends seen in men. Results from the Framingham study suggest that adult-onset diabetes mellitus appears to exact its greatest relative toll on intermittent claudication and congestive heart failure. However, the greatest absolute risk of diabetes is seen on coronary disease, given its far higher incidence rates.

Alcohol

Consumption of alcohol has not been shown to lead to an increased risk of CHD, and a substantial body of evidence indicates that moderate alcohol intake is associated with a reduced risk of developing and dying from CHD. The majority of studies examining the association between alcohol use and CHD have either suggested a negative or a U-shaped relation between alcohol consumption and CHD (127–131). In the Framingham study, a negative effect of moderate alcohol consumption on mortality from CHD as well as on deaths from all causes was seen, particularly in men, with inconsistent patterns seen for women (132). Although the majority of studies examining the association of alcohol consumption patterns and cardiovascular disease have been carried out among men, data from the Nurses Health Study have shown essentially similar results; when compared with nondrinkers and after adjusting for additional coronary risk factors, an approximately 50% lower risk of nonfatal myocardial infarction or death due to coronary disease was observed among women consuming approximately one alcoholic drink per day (133). The consensus of findings supports an association for moderate alcohol consumption with decreased mortality rates from CHD, irrespective of the type of alcoholic beverage consumed; all alcoholic drinks are associated with a lowered risk for CHD, suggesting beneficial effects of alcohol rather than from the components of each type of drink. Alcohol may reduce the risk of CHD, in part, through mechanisms such as increases in HDL cholesterol levels, increased fibrinolysis, or through its peripheral vasodilating effects. Although appropriate concerns have been expressed over broad-based public health recommendations for alcohol consumption, given the well-documented deleterious effects of excessive alcohol intake and abuse, the abundance of data in this area suggest, on balance, a protective benefit of small daily amounts of alcohol on morbidity and mortality from CHD (131,134).

Psychosocial Factors

The type A, or coronary-prone behavior, as described by Osler as a "keen and ambitious man, the indicator of whose engine is always set at full speed ahead" (135) and measured by Friedman and Rosenman (136), has been actively investigated over the past several decades in relation to CHD and summarized in detail (137,138).

Early case-control and prospective investigations of the relation between the type A behavior pattern and risk of CHD found a positive association, independent of the major coronary risk factors (139). On the other hand, findings from the Multiple Risk Factor Intervention Trial (MRFIT), the Aspirin Myocardial Infarction Study, and the Western

Collaborative Group Study have shown no association between type A behavior pattern and CHD (140–142), findings consistent with a review of studies carried out over the past decade (137). Life stress, social isolation and lack of social support, and behavioral coping styles have also been associated with an increased risk of dying from CHD, with inconsistent results obtained with regard to the influence of these factors on the development of initial CHD events. Adverse psychosocial characteristics associated with employment, such as low job control in the workplace, have been associated with an increased risk for CHD.

Recent attention has focused on the role of hostile and suspicious anger and aggressiveness in relation to elevated serum cholesterol levels as well as to risk of CHD and total mortality (143–146). Consistent suppressed anger may be related to an overactive "fight or flight" response in predisposed individuals that may have an adverse effect on catecholamines as well as clotting factors. Episodes of anger have been associated with a transient doubling of the risk of onset of AMI (43), providing novel insights into the ways in which the acute coronary process may be precipitated.

Accumulating evidence suggests that depression among individuals with existing CHD is associated with an increased risk of fatal and nonfatal coronary events (147,148). Several recent studies also suggest that depression may increase the risk for incident CHD events (149,150), although supportive evidence remains lacking in the elderly (151).

Family History and Genetics

Familial as well as environmental risk factors are intimately involved in the pathogenesis of coronary artery disease (152–154).

Early studies assessing the role of genetic factors in the etiology of CHD demonstrated familial aggregation of this disease among the relatives of those with CHD when compared to the relatives of those without CHD (155,156). Studies of separated monozygotic twins and dizygotic twins have also provided supportive evidence for the heritability of CHD through comparison of concordance rates of myocardial infarction and risk factors for CHD (157). Studies of the offspring of patients with premature myocardial infarction have reported higher serum cholesterol levels when compared to the total serum cholesterol levels of children without CHD, and significant clustering of the lipoprotein profile among siblings (158,159). Familial combined hyperlipidemia is one of the major genetic causes of CHD, and this disorder is characterized by elevated levels of plasma cholesterol and/or triglycerides within families.

A limited number of studies have examined the predictive utility of a positive family history of coronary disease to the risk of CHD while simultaneously adjusting for the role of concomitant risk factors. Among men followed longitudinally in the Western Collaborative Group Study, a parental history of CHD was shown to be predictive of CHD, primarily in younger men (160); findings from the Framingham study of an older brother's positive history for CHD (161) and a positive paternal history of CHD (162) in the Paris Prospective Study were also shown to be independently predictive of CHD. The Nurses Health Study has shown that a parental history of premature myocardial infarction in women was independently associated with CHD (163).

These studies suggest that family history is an important predictor for the risk of subsequent CHD, particularly in men, with an approximate 1.5- to 2-fold increased risk for those with a positive parental history of CHD. Limited evidence also suggests a possible etiologic link between DNA polymorphisms at candidate loci to the occurrence rates of CHD as well as to variations in serum lipoproteins. An apoliprotein allele has been linked to an increased risk of CHD in middle-aged men and women, as have the angiotensinogen gene and polymorphism of the angiotensin-converting enzyme gene (DD genotype) (164–166). Limited data also exist to suggest that death from CHD at a comparatively young age may be more influenced by genetic rather than environmental factors, with the influence of genetics declining with advancing age.

Oral Contraceptives and Hormone Replacement Therapy

Several case reports published in the British literature in the early to mid-1960s suggested that the use of oral contraceptives might be associated with increased risk of myocardial infarction in young women. Subsequent case-control and longitudinal studies confirmed that current use of oral contraceptives was associated with an increased risk of fatal and nonfatal myocardial infarctions, being approximately three to four times greater among current users than among women who had never used oral contraceptives (167–169). This risk was shown to increase in a multiplicative fashion with age in individuals who smoked and were hypertensive and in those with underlying coronary atherosclerosis (170). Although current use of oral contraceptives has been shown to place women at increased risk for CHD, this risk diminishes relatively soon after discontinuation of use (171).

On the other hand, use of low-dose exogenous estrogen replacement therapy following the menopause has consistently been associated with a beneficial cardioprotective effect although treatment of postmenopausal women with established CHD with estrogen plus progestin may not be associated with a reduced risk of CHD (172,173). Using decision analysis, the benefits of hormone replacement therapy have been shown to increase life expectancy in the majority of postmenopausal women, with the gains dependent on the individual's profile of risk factors for CHD and breast cancer (174). These gains in life expectancy compared favorably to those predicated from other coronary lifestyle interventions.

Coffee

Case-control as well as prospective observational studies have found either a weak or no relationship between consumption of coffee and development of CHD, with numerous conflicting reports (175–177). Interpretation of these studies, however, is clouded by methodologic difficulties in accurately measuring the intake of coffee as well as the intake of caffeine obtained through other beverages or foods; in assessing dietary intake that may vary with coffee intake; in adjustment, or lack thereof, for the role of potentially confounding factors (e.g., cigarette smoking); and by the diverse design approaches utilized. Interpretation of data relating coffee consumption to the risk of CHD from an international perspective is made

even more difficult by differences in methods of preparation and strength of coffee.

Two prospective epidemiologic investigations serve to highlight the conflicting findings related to coffee consumption and CHD and the difficulties in extrapolating from these data (178,179). In a study of white male medical students enrolled in the Johns Hopkins University Precursors Study, various measures of coffee intake were shown to be associated with an increased risk of CHD, with the greatest risks observed among heavy (five or more cups per day) coffee drinkers over the 35-year follow-up period. Conversely, using data from over 45,000 middle-aged to elderly men participating in the Health Professionals Follow-up Study, no significant association was observed between coffee or caffeine consumption and risk of CHD over a 2-year follow-up period (178). A meta-analysis of 8 case-control studies and 15 cohort studies suggested no increased risk of CHD and heavy (five cups/day) daily coffee consumption in the longitudinal studies reviewed, whereas the results of case-control studies could not rule out an increased risk of CHD associated with high levels of coffee intake (179). Based on the evidence collected to date, it would appear that moderate coffee consumption is not harmful in and of itself to the myocardium but that consumption of coffee in excess of five cups per day may place these persons at increased risk for CHD.

Hemostatic Factors

Given the recent rediscovery of the role of the thrombus in the onset of acute coronary disease and the significant benefits associated with use of clot-lysing agents in patients with evolving myocardial infarction, interest in the role of plasma fibrinogen in the pathogenesis of CHD has been rekindled. Data from the Northwick Park Heart Study and Framingham Heart Study have identified raised fibrinogen levels with an increased risk for CHD (180,181). Support for this hypothesis has come from several case-control and cross-sectional studies that have demonstrated an association of increased fibrinogen levels with either clinical or angiographically confirmed coronary artery disease (182–184). In a large prospective study, baseline fibrinogen level was shown to be predictive of subsequent myocardial infarction in univariate analyses, but the strength of this potential predictor diminished when the other well-established risk factors for CHD were adjusted for (185). An elevated leukocyte count may also be independently associated with CHD in addition to its documented association with other established CHD risk factors (184). Factor VII, fibrinolytic potential, and platelet reactivity have been associated with an increased risk for CHD (186). Hemostatic factors may also be involved in the triggering of acute coronary events, suggesting a biologically plausible mechanism by which coagulation factors may be intimately involved in the expression of CHD.

Inflammation

Several lines of evidence from recently completed prospective epidemiologic studies suggest that markers of the inflammatory response, such as C-reactive protein, are associated with risk of initial AMI and other atherosclerotic events among apparently healthy middle-aged men (187–192). C-reactive protein, which is an acute phase reactant, has also been associated with risk of infarction among high-risk coronary patients as well as with increased risk of recurrent coronary events in persons with prior MIs. These and additional data suggest that markers of low-level inflammation may be associated with increased risk of AMI and other vascular events in healthy individuals. These findings have opened up new lines of investigation for assessment of coronary risk and proper management of patients at increased risk for an initial or recurrent coronary event (193).

Homocysteine

Homocysteine is a metabolite of methionine, an essential amino acid present in large amounts in protein from animal sources. Elevated homocysteine levels are thought to be a result of deficiencies in vitamins B_6, and B_{12} and folic acid and a high dietary intake of animal protein. Observational studies, conducted primarily in young to middle-aged men, suggest that mildly elevated serum levels of homocysteine are associated with an increased risk for vascular disease (194,195). A recent case-control study extends these observations to young women (196). Although additional epidemiologic research needs to be carried out on this potentially important and modifiable risk factor, these findings provide potential encouragement for dietary supplementation of select B vitamins and folic acid. These observations provide further insights to the ways in which unfavorable diets high in animal protein and low in fresh fruits and vegetables might contribute to the underlying atherosclerotic process.

Infectious Agents

Interest has recently focused on the possible role that infectious agents might play in the development of CHD since it is hypothesized that chronic infections may be associated with vascular endothelial damage (197–199). A limited number of observational studies have suggested a possible association of prior infection with chlamydial pneumonia and angiographically confirmed coronary artery disease as well as with clinically evident CHD (200). Pathologic studies have extended these epidemiologic findings identifying chlamydial pneumonia in atherosclerotic lesions (201), although the clinical significance of these observations is unclear. In accord with these findings, male survivors of myocardial infarction seropositive for chlamydia were at reduced risk for adverse CVD events over an average follow-up of 18 months after a short course of antibiotic treatment (202). These observations provide new insights into the pathologic mechanisms involved in CAD and the potential importance of chronic infectious illnesses in plaque vulnerability, rupture, and development of acute clinical events.

Body Iron Stores

Several lines of investigation have suggested that increased iron intake or body iron stores may promote atherogenesis by increasing free radical formation and associated oxidative stress (203). A prospective epidemiologic study of CHD in Finnish men provided early support for this hypothesis, noting an increased risk of AMI with increasing serum ferritin levels (204). However, the majority of published reports since this initial publication have failed to confirm the hypothesis that iron overload states are associated with an increased risk of coronary atherosclerosis. Given this intriguing hypothesis, however, and the novel insights that this possible association may provide to the pathogenesis of CHD and need for change in dietary recommendations, further research efforts are needed to more fully explore the association between iron status and risk of CHD.

Sleep Disturbances

Several prospective studies have shown an association between disturbances of sleep and occurrence of CHD. This excess risk has been seen in various types of sleep disturbances and may be particularly problematic in the elderly. Snoring has been associated with an increased risk of high blood pressure, stroke, and coronary disease, reflecting an altered breathing pattern during sleep.

Fetal Origins of CHD

An extensive array of data collected in clinical and epidemiologic studies suggests that CHD has its roots of development in the early childhood years extending into young adulthood. Some intriguing data suggest that the pathologic substrate for CHD may originate developmentally as early as in utero. In a large cohort of men born between 1911 and 1930, there was a progressive decline in CHD death rates between those with the lowest and highest birth weights (205). Several studies suggest that growth in utero and during infancy may be related to risk factors for cardiovascular disease (206). A prevailing hypothesis is that CHD is associated with specific patterns of disproportionate fetal growth that may result from fetal undernutrition in middle to late gestation (207). These and additional data provide support for the hypothesis that CHD may have its origins in impaired development in utero and during early infancy. This phenomenon has been referred to as *programming*, in which the structure and physiology of the body's tissue may be adversely affected during sensitive periods of early life, and it may suggest areas for further research and application of intervention strategies.

Miscellaneous Risk Factors

A number of other potential risk factors have been examined in relation to CHD. Although varying degrees of association, or absence of association, with either the risk of developing or dying from CHD have been observed with regard to these factors, they will only be mentioned because of a relative lack of supportive and/or definitive information. These factors include antioxidant vitamins, gout and uric acid, sexual activity, vasectomy, hardness of drinking water, environmental and air pollutants, and sucrose consumption (208,209).

MULTIFACTORIAL NATURE OF CORONARY HEART DISEASE

It is clear that CHD is a chronic disease of multifactorial origin with its pathogenic roots beginning in the first and second decades of life (210–212). The clinical manifestations of the atherosclerotic process reflect the interaction of host and environmental factors. A number of risk factors for CHD also have been associated with all-cause mortality in both middle-aged men and women, emphasizing the continued understanding of the manner by which these risk factors may contribute to chronic disease and total mortality and need for devising novel and acceptable intervention strategies (213).

A variety of formulations using stratified and multivariate analytic techniques have been used to identify persons at moderate to markedly increased risk for CHD through various combinations of the primary and secondary risk factors for coronary disease. These estimates have provided not only analytic rigor in showing the independence of the well-established risk factors associated with the development of CHD but also have shown how the risk factors interact in an additive as well as multiplicative fashion (21,214,215). These risk estimates have allowed for the characterization of those asymptomatic persons among whom approximately one half of all incident cases of CHD will appear and in whom these risk factors may be readily assessed in a clinician's office. Although the risk factors for CHD relate to the different clinical manifestations of coronary atherosclerosis in slightly different ways, and with varying degrees of predictive utility depending on the endpoint examined and the interaction of other risk factors, practicing clinicians are armed with considerable information by which reliable estimates of an individual's future risk of CHD may be assessed.

TEMPORAL TRENDS IN CORONARY HEART DISEASE MORTALITY RATES

Beginning at the turn of the twentieth century, death rates from CHD in the United States increased dramatically, reaching epidemic proportions by the mid-1960s (216–219). Since that time, the age-adjusted mortality attributed to CHD has leveled off and then turned markedly downwards, declining by approximately 2% to 3% annually (Figure 1-3). All-cause mortality as well as mortality from cardiovascular disease and stroke also have declined over time. The annual number of deaths and crude death rate from CHD and AMI have exhibited consistent declines over the past nearly 2½ decades; there were approximately 70,000 less deaths due to CHD annually in the early 1990s than during the late 1970s. Although this significant and encouraging decline appears real, being seen in all age groups, in men and women, and in the major race/ethnic groups examined, and not due to artifactual changes in death certification or recording practices, the reasons for this decrease remain unknown. Lest complacency set in that the problem of CHD has been sent into permanent retreat based on these encouraging mortality trends, in 1992 and 1993 there was an upturn in the absolute number of deaths attributed to CHD in the United States (2). In 1992, there were 480,000 deaths attributed to CHD, whereas 481,000 persons died from CHD in 1995; these trends may reflect the aging of the population, population shifts in coronary risk factors, or changes in other related determinants of CHD.

The decline in mortality rates attributed to CHD has been observed not only in the United States but also in a number of other countries (Figure 1-4) (219,220). Nonetheless, reasons for the dramatic decline in CHD death rates remain uncertain and a paucity of population-based data exists to determine whether or not the observed temporal trends are due to changes in the incidence rates of new coronary events, changes in survival after an acute coronary episode, or combinations thereof. Declines in the incidence rates of CHD would suggest that the mortality decline may be due to a decrease in the occurrence rates of AMI and sudden cardiac death (SCD) secondary to modification of lifestyle characteristics and changes in the prevalence and/or levels of the major coronary risk factors. If, however, the reported incidence rates of AMI and out-of-hospital SCD have stabilized or even increased, a likely explanation for the observed downward trend in CHD would be attributed to improvements in medical care.

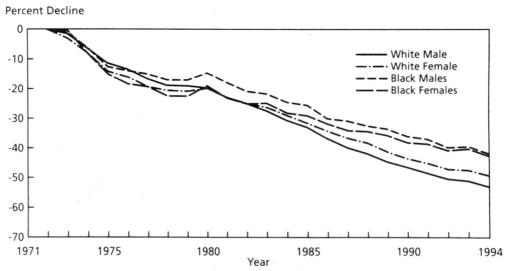

Figure 1-3 Percentage decline in age-adjusted mortality rates for coronary heart disease by sex and race: United States, 1972–1994.

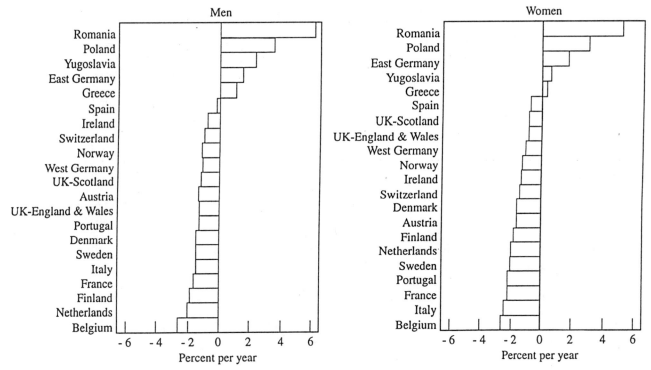

Figure 1-4 Annual percentage change in mortality rates from coronary heart disease in European countries (1970–1972).

TEMPORAL TRENDS IN THE PRIMARY CORONARY RISK FACTORS

Cigarette Smoking

Since the release of the first Surgeon General's report on smoking and health in 1964, the prevalence of cigarette smoking has declined over the past nearly 3 decades in the United States. While the two sexes have exhibited consistent decreases in the prevalence of current cigarette smoking over time, more marked declines have been observed among men over the periods examined. Overall population rates of cigarette smoking have declined from approximately 42% of the adult population being current smokers in 1965 to approximately 26% in 1995 (2). A slightly greater proportion of men (28%) as compared to women (23%) currently smoke. Prevalence rates of current smoking are highest in African-American men (34%) and comparatively low in Hispanic (15%) and Asian (8%) women (2). The prevalence of current pipe smoking in men has declined over the period of declining CHD death rates, with pipe smoking remaining very uncommon in women. Despite the encouraging decline in the national and selected population sample prevalence estimates of current cigarette smoking, the proportion of heavy smokers among current cigarette smokers has increased, particularly in women.

Elevated Blood Pressure and Hypertension

Data compiled from several nationally based representative population surveys have shown marked increases in awareness and control of hypertension over time. In the early 1970s, nearly half of the hypertensive population was unaware of their hypertensive status; this proportion declined to 27% in

1976 to 1980 and to 16% in 1988 to 1991. The proportion of hypertensives on medication and in whom blood pressure was controlled increased from 16% in the early 1970s to nearly double that rate in the late 1980s (2). Although there have been significant improvements over time in the percentage of hypertensives whose blood pressure has been controlled, sizeable African-American–white and man-woman gaps continue to exist.

Serum Cholesterol Levels

Declines in the overall as well as age-specific average population cholesterol levels have been observed in the United States since the beginning of declining CHD mortality rates. Utilizing data from nationally based health surveys of the noninstitutionalized population of the United States, namely the Health and Examination Survey (HES-1) in 1960 to 1962, National Health and Nutrition Examination Survey (NHANES) I carried out between 1971 and 1974, and NHANES II conducted between 1976 and 1980, the average age-adjusted race and sex-specific serum cholesterol levels declined slightly over the periods under study among each of the population groups examined (2). On average, these serum cholesterol levels decreased by 3% to 4% among the surveyed sample with a significant decline observed in men (217 to 211 mg/dL) and women (223 to 215 mg/dL) from the time of the initial cross-sectional survey in 1960 to 1962 to the time of the later survey in the mid to late 1970s.

Despite the relatively large population burden from elevated lipid levels, slight declines in the proportion of men (3%) or women (5%) considered at high risk for CHD have been observed between 1960 and 1962 and 1976 and 1980. Slight decreases were also observed in the age-adjusted percentage of men and women considered at moderate risk for CHD based on the observed cholesterol distribution. Despite these encouraging declines, surveys conducted between 1988 and 1994 suggest that approximately 20% of American adults have serum cholesterol levels that are considered high and in need of potential intervention (2).

Dietary Changes

Although total fat intake increased in the United States between 1910 and the mid-1960s, the composition of available fats changed significantly. Between 1910 and 1965 per capita availability of animal fats decreased slightly, whereas there was a more than twofold increase in the intake of vegetable or polyunsaturated fats (219). More recent changes over time in the annual per capita availability of selected foods have been examined since the beginning of the decline in CHD mortality rates in the late 1960s (219). Although the availability of meat, poultry, and fish has increased in the aggregate by approximately 4% over the periods examined (1968 to 1985), consumption of meat has slightly decreased, whereas consumption of fish, shellfish, and poultry has markedly increased. Availability of eggs and whole milk declined by 17% and 43%, respectively, whereas use of low-fat milk approximately doubled between the late 1960s and mid-1980s. Availability of animal fat and oils declined by 16%, whereas use of vegetable fats and oils increased by 30%; the majority of the latter increase was accounted for by a large increase over time in the use of salad and cooking oils. An analysis of studies carried out in the United States since the 1920s assessing actual individual dietary intake has shown relatively similar results (221). The percentage of fat, as a proportion of total energy, increased from the 1920s (36%) to the 1960s (40%), after which time a small decline in the percentage of energy ingested as fat was seen between 1970 and 1979 and 1980 and 1985 (38%). In addition, the percentage of saturated fat in relation to total energy declined over time with a concomitant increase in polyunsaturated fatty acids. Recent U.S. population data suggest that fat consumption as a percentage of total calories may have decreased even further (222).

Obesity

The prevalence of obesity, as expressed in terms of body mass index (kg/m^2), has increased over time based on data obtained from selected national health examination surveys and remains a national problem given its adverse health effects. Between 1960 and 1962 and 1988 and 1991, the frequency of obesity among white men increased from 23% to 32%; the prevalence of obesity similarly increased in white women (24% in 1960 to 1962; 34% in 1988 to 1991). In African-American men, the prevalence of overweight increased from 22% in 1960 to 1962 to 32% in 1988 to 1991, whereas increases from 42% to 50% were observed among African-American women over this period, emphasizing the high prevalence of obesity in this high-risk group of women. Among adults in the United States over the period between 1988 and 1994, slightly more than one fifth of the U.S. population was considered obese (body mass index of ≥30) with disturbingly high rates of obesity observed in African-American and Mexican-American women (2).

Physical Inactivity

Despite interest in examining changes over time in physical activity levels of the U.S. population and an apparent national obsession with physical fitness, only limited data exist to assess temporal trends in physical activity, and methodologic concerns limit extrapolation and comparability. Although appropriate caveats must be placed on the interpretation of temporal trends in physical activity, the sex-specific prevalence rates of adult participation in no physical activity have shown increases between 1985 and 1990 (223). The proportion of the population engaged in regular sustained activity has not changed during recent years, whereas participation in regular vigorous activity declined in both men and women between 1985 and 1990. Approximately 25% of American adults presently report no leisure time physical activity (2). These disturbing trends have led to policy statements by various health agencies in an attempt to increase the proportion of the U.S. adult, as well as adolescent, populations engaged in regular sustained physical activity (5).

TEMPORAL TRENDS IN INCIDENCE RATES OF ACUTE MYOCARDIAL INFARCTION

Over the last 2 decades, several community-based studies in Rochester (224) and Minneapolis-St. Paul, Minn (225), Worcester, Mass (226,227), and Pee Dee and Columbia, SC (228), have examined temporal trends in the incidence rates of AMI. Appropriate caution should be exercised in the interpretation of these data, given that the sociodemographic characteristics of the populations under study and diagnostic criteria for AMI may have differed; the size of the populations may have varied; and the periods of investigation were limited, thus making estimates of temporal trends tenuous. Nonetheless, each of these population-based investigations has shown a decline in the incidence rates of acute coronary events over the various periods examined (219).

TEMPORAL TRENDS IN CASE FATALITY RATES OF ACUTE MYOCARDIAL INFARCTION

Several population-based studies have examined changes over time in the in-hospital case fatality rates associated with AMI (219). As with the examination of hospital-based incidence data of AMI, appropriate reservation should be exercised in the interpretation of the case fatality data. Factors such as the sample sizes of the populations under consideration, diagnostic criteria for AMI utilized, length of hospital stay, and differing characteristics of the populations compared, particularly with regard to those factors that might affect short-term prognosis as well as therapeutic interventions employed, make interpretation of the findings across studies difficult. Despite these caveats, an improvement in in-hospital survival is seen in the majority of studies examined. Recent data from the multisite Atherosclerosis Risk in Communities Study suggest declines in mortality from CHD between 1987 and 1994 in a number of racially diverse communities throughout the United States (229).

Despite the use of different criteria to define out-of-hospital deaths due to CHD, each of the major population-based studies of CHD in the United States has shown consistent declines in the incidence rates of out-of-hospital deaths due to CHD, particularly SCD (219).

CONTRIBUTIONS OF PREVENTIVE AND THERAPEUTIC EFFORTS TO DECLINING CHD MORTALITY RATES

Despite the lack of adequate and systematically collected sources of data to distinguish effects of primary from those of secondary prevention on declining CHD mortality trends, several investigators have thoughtfully attempted to sort out the contributions of changes in lifestyle characteristics from those of secondary prevention during periods of declining CHD mortality rates (230–232). Based on data, albeit limited, from a multiplicity of published sources, it has been estimated that favorable reductions in the examined lifestyle factors may have accounted for slightly more than one half of the observed decline in CHD mortality rates between 1968 and 1976, whereas medical care interventions may have contributed to approximately 40% of the decline. The results of a more recent computer-simulated model suggest contributions of both primary and secondary prevention to declining rates of CHD observed in the 1980s (230). Given the magnitude of CHD, the impaired, albeit improving, prognosis of those with established CHD, and the availability of primary and secondary preventive efforts, it remains of importance to continue to monitor trends in the incidence and case fatality rates of CHD and its specific clinical manifestations.

REFERENCES

1. National Heart, Lung, and Blood Institute. Chartbook on cardiovascular, lung, and blood diseases. Bethesda, MD: U.S. Department of Health and Human Services, Public Health Service, National Institutes of Health, 1994.

2. American Heart Association. 1998 Heart and stroke statistical update. Dallas: American Heart Association, 1997.

3. Inter-Society Commission for Heart Disease Resources. Atherosclerosis Study Group and Epidemiology Study Group. Primary prevention of the atherosclerotic diseases. Circulation 1970; 42:A55–A94.

4. American Heart Association Committee Report. Risk factors and coronary disease: a statement for physicians. Circulation 1980; 62:449A–455A.

5. Fletcher GF, Blair SN, Blumenthal J, et al. Statement on exercise: benefits and recommendations for physical activity programs for all Americans: a statement for health professionals by the Committee on Exercise and Cardiac Rehabilitation of the Council on Clinical Cardiology, American Heart Assocation. Circulation 1992;86:340–344.

6. Eckel RH. Obesity and heart disease: a statement for health-care professionals from the nutrition committee, American Heart Association. Circulation 1997; 96:3248–3250.

7. Krauss RM, Winston M. Obesity: impact on cardiovascular disease. Circulation 1998;1472–1476.

8. Omran AR. Epidemiologic transition in the United States: the health factor in population change. Popul Bull 1997;32: 1–42.

9. Omran AR. The epidemiological transition: a theory of the epidemiology of population change. Milbank Q 1971;49:509–538.

10. Reddy KR, Yusuf S. Emerging epidemic of cardiovascular disease in developing countries. Circulation 1997;97:596–601.

11. Lopez AD. Assessing the burden of mortality from cardiovascular disease. World Health Stat Q 1993;46:91–96.

12. Dawber TR, Meadors GF, Moore FE Jr. Epidemiological approaches to heart disease: the Framingham Study. Am J Public Health 1951;41:279–286.

13. Gordon T, Kannel WB. Premature mortality from coronary heart disease: the Framingham Study. JAMA 1971;215:1617–1625.

14. Stamler J, Lindberg HA, Berkson DM, et al. Prevalence and incidence of coronary heart disease in strata of the labor force of a Chicago industrial corporation. J Chron Dis 1960;11:405–420.

15. Paul O, Lepper MH, Phelan WH, et al. A longitudinal study of heart disease. Circulation 1963;28:20–31.

16. Epstein FH, Ostrander LD Jr, Johnson BC, et al. Epidemiological studies of cardiovascular disease in a total community—Tecumseh, Michigan. Ann Intern Med 1965;62:1170–1187.

17. Doyle JT, Heslin AS, Hilleboe HE, et al. A prospective study of degenerative cardiovascular disease in Albany: report of three years' experience—I. ischemic heart disease. Am J Public Health 1957;47:25–32.

18. Chapman JM, Goerke LS, Dixon W, et al. The clinical status of a population group in Los Angeles under observation for two to three years. Am J Public Health 1957; 47:33–42.

19. Keys A, Taylor HL, Blackburn H, et al. Coronary heart disease among Minnesota business and professional men followed 15 years. Circulation 1963;28: 381–395.

20. Rosenman RH, Friedman M, Straus R, et al. A predictive study of coronary heart disease: the Western Collaborative Group Study. JAMA 1964;189:15–22.

21. Wilson PW, D'Agostino RB, Levy D, et al. Prediction of coronary heart disease using risk factor categories. Circulation 1998; 18:1837–1847.

22. Reid DD, Hamilton PJS, McCartney P, Rose G. Smoking

and other risk factors for coronary heart disease in British civil servants. Lancet 1976;2:979–983.

23. Kagan A, Gordon T, Rhoads GG, Schiffman JC. Some factors related to coronary heart disease incidence in Honolulu Japanese men: the Honolulu Heart Study. Int J Epidemiol 1975;4: 271–279.

24. Groen JJ, Medalie JH, Neufeld HN, et al. An epidemiologic investigation of hypertension and ischemic heart disease within a defined segment of the adult male population of Israel. Isr J Med Sci 1968;4:177–194.

25. Johnson KG, Yano K, Kato H. Coronary heart disease in Hiroshima, Japan: a report of a six-year period of surveillance, 1958–1964. Am J Public Health 1968;58:1355–1367.

26. Carlson LA, Bottiger LE. Ischemic heart disease in relation to fasting values of plasma triglygerides and cholesterol. Stockholm Prospective Study. Lancet 1972;1:865–868.

27. Keys A, Aravanis C, Blackburn H, et al. Epidemiological studies related to coronary heart disease: characteristics of men aged 40–59 in seven countries. Acta Med Scand 1967;180(suppl 460):1–392.

28. Worth RM, Kato H, Rhoads GG, et al. Epidemiologic studies of coronary heart disease and stroke in Japanese men living in Japan, Hawaii and California: Mortality. Am J Epidemiol 1975;102: 481–490.

29. Ockene IS. Primary prevention of triggering of coronary heart disease. In: Willich SN, Muller JE, eds. Triggering of acute coronary syndromes: implications for prevention. Dordrecht: Kluwer, 1996:285–294.

30. Steinberg D, Witztum JL. Lipoproteins and atherogenesis: current concepts. JAMA 1990; 264:3047–3052.

31. McGill HC, ed. The geographic pathology of atherosclerosis. Baltimore: Williams & Wilkins, 1968.

32. Ross R, Glomset JA. The pathogenesis of atherosclerosis. N Engl J Med 1976;295:369–377, 420–425.

33. Ross R. The pathogenesis of atherosclerosis—an update. N Engl J Med 1986;314:488–500.

34. Davies MJ. A macro and micro view of coronary vascular insult in ischemic heart disease. Circulation 1990;82(suppl): 38–46.

35. Fuster V, Badimon L, Badimon JJ, Chesebro JH. The pathogenesis of coronary artery disease and the acute coronary syndromes. N Engl J Med 1992;326:242–250, 310–318.

36. Muller JE, Tofler GH, Stone PH. Circadian variation and triggers of onset of acute cardiovascular disease. Circulation 1989; 79:733–743.

37. Tofler GH, Stone PH, Maclure M, et al. Modifiers of timing and possible triggers of acute myocardial infarction in the Thrombolysis in Myocardial Infarction Phase II (TIMI-II) Study Group. J Am Coll Cardiol 1992;20: 1049–1055.

38. Muller JE, Stone PH, Turi ZG, et al. Circadian variation in the frequency of onset of AMI. N Engl J Med 1985;313: 1315–1322.

39. Hjalmarson A, Gilpin E, Nicod P, et al. Differing circadian patterns of symptom onset in subgroups of patients with AMI. Circulation 1989;80:267–275.

40. Willich SN, Levy D, Rocco MB, et al. Circadian variation in the incidence of sudden cardiac death in the Framingham Heart Study population. Am J Cardiol 1987;60:801–806.

41. Goldberg RJ, Brady P, Muller JE, et al. Time of onset of symptoms of AMI. Am J Cardiol 1990; 66:140–144.

42. Mittleman MA, Maclure M, Tofler GH, et al. Triggering of acute myocardial infarction by heavy physical exertion: protection by regular exertion. N Engl J Med 1993;326:1677–1683.

43. Mittleman MA, Maclure M, Sherwood JB, et al. Triggering of acute myocardial infarction onset by episodes of anger: determinants of myocardial infarction onset study investigators. Circulation 1995;92:1720–1725.

44. Maclure M. The case-crossover design: a method for studying transient effects on the risk of acute events. Am J Epidemiol 1991;133:144–153.

45. Castelli W, Leaf A. Identification and assessment of cardiac risk—an overview. Cardiol Clin 1985; 3:171–178.

46. Kannel WB. Metabolic risk factors for coronary heart disease in women: perspective from the Framingham Study. Am Heart J 1987;114:413–419.

47. Eaker ED, Castelli WP. Coronary heart disease and risk factors among women in the Framingham Study. In: Eaker ED, Packard B, Wenger NK, et al, eds. Coronary heart disease in women: proceedings of an NIH Workshop. New York: Haymarket Doyma, 1987:22–28.

48. Gillum RF. Coronary heart disease in black populations. I. Mortality and morbidity. Am Heart J 1982; 104:839–850.

49. Report of National Heart Lung and Blood Institute working conference on coronary heart disease in black populations and proceedings of a symposium on coronary heart disease in black populations. Am Heart J 1984; 108:633–662.

50. Gillum RF, Grant CT. Coronary heart disease in black populations. II. risk factors. Am Heart J 1982;104:852–864.

51. Rowland ML, Fulwood R. Coronary heart disease risk factor trends in blacks between the first and second National Health and Nutrition Examination Surveys, United States, 1971–1980. Am Heart J 1984;108:771–779.

52. Hutchinson RG, Watson RL, Davis CE, et al. Racial differences in risk factors for atherosclerosis: the ARIC study. Angiology 1997;48:279–290.

53. Maynard C, Fisher LD, Passamani ER, Pullum T. Blacks in the coronary artery surgery study: risk factors and coronary artery disease. Circulation 1986;74: 64–71.

54. Kaplan GA, Keil JE. Socioeconomic factors and cardiovascular disease: a review of the literature. Circulation 1993;88: 1973–1998.

55. U.S. Department of Health and Human Services. The health consequences of smoking: cardiovascular disease. A report of the Surgeon General. Publ. No. USDHHS (PHS) 84-50204. Washington, DC: USDHHS, 1983.

56. Bartecchi CE, MacKenzie TD, Schrier RW. The human costs of tobacco use. N Engl J Med 1994;330:907–912.

57. MacKenzie TD, Bartecchi CE, Schrier RW. The human costs of tobacco use. N Engl J Med 1994;330:975–980.

58. Ockene IS, Miller NH. Cigarette smoking, cardiovascular disease, and stroke: a statement for healthcare professionals from the American Heart Association. Circulation 1997;96:3243–3247.

59. Ockene JK, Kuller LH, Svendsen KH, Meilahn E. The relationship of smoking cessation to coronary heart disease and lung cancer in the Multiple Risk Factor Intervention Trial (MRFIT). Am J Public Health 1990;80:954–958.

60. Wilhelmsson C, Elmfeldt D, Vedin JA, et al. Smoking and myocardial infarction. Lancet 1975; 1:415–420.

61. Sparrow D, Dawber TR, Colton T. The influence of cigarette smoking on prognosis after a first myocardial infarction. J Chron Dis 1978;31:425–432.

62. Diex-Roux AV, Nieto FJ, Comstock GW, et al. The relationship of active and passive smoking to carotid atherosclerosis 12–14 years later. Prev Med 1995;24:48–55.

63. Howard G, Wagenknecht HG, Burke GL, et al. Cigarette smoking and progression of atherosclerosis: the Atherosclerosis Risk in Communities (ARIC) Study. JAMA 1998;279:119–124.

64. MacMahon S, Peto R, Cutler J, et al. Blood pressure, stroke, and coronary heart disease, I: prolonged differences in blood pressure: prospective observational studies corrected for the regression dilution bias. Lancet 1990;335:765–774.

65. MacMahon SW, Cutler JA, Furberg CD, Payne GH. The effects of drug treatment for hypertension on morbidity and mortality from cardiovascular disease: a review of randomized controlled trials. Prog Cardiovasc Dis 1986;29(suppl I):99–118.

66. Stamler J, Wentworth D, Neaton JD for the MRFIT Research Group. Is relationship between serum cholesterol and risk of premature death from coronary heart disease continuous and graded? Findings in 356,222 primary screenees of the Multiple Risk Factor Intervention Trial (MRFIT). JAMA 1986;256:2823–2828.

67. Kannel WB, Castelli WP, Gordon T. Cholesterol in the prediction of atherosclerotic disease: new perspectives based on the Framingham Study. Ann Intern Med 1979;90:85–91.

68. Pekkanen J, Linn S, Heiss G, et al. Ten-year mortality from cardiovascular disease in relation to cholesterol level among men with and without pre-existing cardiovascular disease. N Engl J Med 1990;322:1700–1707.

69. Grundy SM, Balady GJ, Criqui MH, et al. When to start cholesterol-lowering therapy in patients with coronary heart disease: a statement for healthcare professionals from the American Heart Association task force on risk reduction. Circulation 1997;95:1683–1685.

70. The Lipid Research Clinics Program. The Lipid Research Clinics Coronary Primary Prevention Trial Results. I: reduction in incidence of coronary heart disease. JAMA 1984;251:351–364.

71. Frick MH, Elo O, Haapa K, et al. Helsinki Heart Study: Primary-prevention trial with gemfibrozil in middle-aged men with dyslipidemia: safety of treatment, changes in risk factors, and incidence of coronary heart disease. N Engl J Med 1987;317: 1237–1245.

72. Brensike JF, Levy RI, Kelsay SF, et al. Effects of therapy with cholestyramine on progression of coronary arteriosclerosis: results of the NHLBI type II Coronary Intervention Study. Circulation 1984;69:313–324.

73. Blankenhorn DH, Nessim SA, Johnson RL, et al. Beneficial effects of combined colestipol-niacin therapy on coronary atherosclerosis and coronary venous bypass grafts. JAMA 1987;257: 3233–3240.

74. Downs JR, Clearfield M, Weis S, et al. Primary prevention of acute coronary events with lovastatin in men and women with average cholesterol levels: results of AFCAPS/TexCAPS. JAMA 1998; 279:1615–1622.

75. Cashin-Hemphill L, Mack WJ, Pogoda JM, et al. Beneficial effects of colestipol-niacin on coronary atherosclerosis: a 4 year follow-up. JAMA 1990;264: 3013–3017.

76. De Backer G, Rosseneu M, Deslypere JP. Discriminative value of lipids and apoproteins in coronary heart disease. Atherosclerosis 1982;42:197–203.

77. Maciejko JJ, Holmes DR, Kottke BA, et al. Apolipoprotein A-I as a marker of angiographically assessed coronary artery disease. N Engl J Med 1983;309: 385–389.

78. Brunzell JD, Sniderman AD, Albers JJ, Kwiterovich PO Jr. Apoproteins B and A–I and coronary artery disease in humans. Arteriosclerosis 1984;4:79–83.

79. Nguyen TT, Ellefson RD, Hodge DO, et al. Predictive value of electrophoretically detected lipoprotein (a) for coronary heart disease and cerebrovascular disease in a community-based cohort of 9936 men and women.

Circulation 1997;96:1390–1397.

80. Bostom AG, Cupples LA, Jenner JL, et al. Elevated plasma lipoprotein (a) and coronary heart disease in men aged 55 years and younger: a prospective study. JAMA 1996;276:544–548.

81. Stein JH, Rosenson RS. Lipoprotein Lp(a) excess and coronary heart disease. Arch Intern Med 1997;157:1170–1176.

82. Bostom AG, Gagnon DR, Cupples LA, et al. A prospective investigation of elevated lipoprotein (a) detected by electrophoresis and cardiovascular disease in women: the Framingham Heart Study. Circulation 1994;90:1688–1695.

83. Davies MJ, Thomas AC. Plaque fissuring—the cause of acute myocardial infarction, sudden ischaemic death, and crescendo angina. Br Heart J 1985;53: 363–373.

84. Albrink MJ, Mann EB. Serum triglycerides in coronary artery disease. Arch Intern Med 1959;103:4–8.

85. Brunzell JD, Austin MA. Plasma triglyceride levels and coronary disease. N Engl J Med 1989; 320:1273–1275.

86. Hulley SB, Rosenman RH, Bawol RD, Brand RJ. Epidemiology as a guide to clinical decisions: the association between triglyceride and coronary heart disease. N Engl J Med 1980;302: 1383–1389.

87. Castelli WP. The triglyceride issue: a view from Framingham. Am Heart J 1986;112:432–437.

88. Burchfiel CM, Laws A, Benfante R, et al. Combined effects of HDL cholesterol, triglyceride, and total cholesterol concentrations on 18-year risk of atherosclerotic disease. Circulation 1995;92: 1430–1436.

89. Gotto AM. Triglyceride: the forgotten risk factor. Circulation 1998;97:1027–1028.

90. Gaziano JM, Hennekens CH, O'Donnell CJ, et al. Fasting triglycerides, high-density lipoprotein, and risk of myocardial infarction. Circulation 1997;96: 2520–2525.

91. Keys A. Seven Countries. A multivariate analysis of death and coronary heart disease. Cambridge, MA: Harvard University Press, 1980.

92. Shekelle RB, Shryock AM, Paul O, et al. Diet, serum cholesterol, and death from coronary heart disease: the Western Electric Study. N Engl J Med 1981; 304:65–70.

93. Kushi LH, Lew RA, Stare FJ, et al. Diet and 20-year mortality from coronary heart disease: the Ireland-Boston diet-heart study. N Engl J Med 1985;312: 811–818.

94. Lapidus L, Anderson H, Bengtsson C, Bosaeus I. Dietary habits in relation to incidence of cardiovascular disease and death in women: a 12-year followup of participants in the population study of women in Gothenburg, Sweden. Am J Clin Nutr 1986; 44:444–448.

95. Hegsted DM, McGandy RB, Meyers ML, Stare FJ. Quantitative effects of dietary fat on serum cholesterol in man. Am J Clin Nutr 1965;17:281–295.

96. Mattson FH, Grundy SM. Comparisons of effects of dietary saturated, monounsaturated and polyunsaturated fatty acids on plasma lipid and lipoproteins in man. J Lipid Res 1985;26: 194–202.

97. Bonanome A, Grundy SM. Effect of dietary stearic acid on plasma cholesterol and lipoprotein levels. N Engl J Med 1988;318: 1244–1248.

98. Kris-Etherton PM, Krummel D, Russell ME, et al. The effect of diet on plasma lipids, lipoproteins, and coronary heart disease. J Am Diet Assoc 1988;88: 1373–1400.

99. Daviglus ML, Stamler J, Orencia AJ, et al. Fish consumption and the 30-year risk of fatal myocardial infarction. N Engl J Med 1997;336:1046–1053.

100. Ascherio A, Rimm EB, Stampfer MJ, et al. Dietary intake of marine n-3 fatty acids, fish intake, and the risk of coronary disease among men. N Engl J Med 1995;332:977–982.

101. Rimm EB, Ascherio A, Giovannucci E, et al. Vegetable, fruit, and cereal fiber intake and risk of coronary heart disease among men. JAMA 1996;275:447–451.

102. Rimm EB, Willett WC, Hu FB, et al. Folate and vitamin B_6 from diet and supplements in relation to risk of coronary heart disease among women. JAMA 1998;279:359–364.

103. de Lorgeril M, Salen P, Martin JL, et al. Mediterranean dietary pattern in a randomized trial: prolonged survival and possible reduced cancer rate. Arch Intern Med 1998;158:1181–1187.

104. Rimm EB, Katan MB, Ascherio A, et al. Relation between intake of flavonoids and risk for coronary heart disease in male health professionals. Ann Intern Med 1996;125:384–389.

105. Hoffman RM, Garewal HS. Antioxidants and the prevention of coronary heart disease. Arch Intern Med 1995;155:241–246.

106. Morris JN, Heady JA, Raffle PAB, et al. Coronary heart disease and physical activity of work. Lancet 1953;2:1053–1057, 1111–1120.

107. Paffenbarger RS, Hale WE. Work activity and coronary heart mortality. N Engl J Med 1975;292: 545–550.

108. Powell KE, Thompson PD, Caspersen CJ, Kendrick JS. Physical activity and the incidence of coronary heart disease. Annu Rev Public Health 1987;8: 253–287.

109. Oberman A. Exercise and the primary prevention of cardiovascular disease. Am J Cardiol 1985;55:10D–20D.

110. Berlin JA, Colditz GA. A meta-analysis of physical activity in the prevention of coronary heart disease. Am J Epidemiol 1990;132:612–628.

111. Ekelund LG, Haskell WL, Johnson JL, et al. Physical fitness as a predictor of cardiovascular mortality in asymptomatic North American men: the Lipid Research Clinics Mortality Follow-up Study. N Engl J Med 1988;319:1379–1384.

112. Blair SN, Kohn HW, Paffenbarger RS Jr, et al. Physical fitness and all-cause mortality: a prospective study of healthy men and women. JAMA 1989;262:2395–2401.

113. National Institutes of Health Consensus Development Panel on the Health Implications of Obesity. Health implications of obesity. Ann Intern Med 1985;103:1073–1077.

114. Hubert HB. The importance of obesity in the development of coronary risk factors and disease: the epidemiologic evidence. Annu Rev Public Health 1986;7:493–502.

115. Barrett-Connor EL. Obesity, atherosclerosis, and coronary artery disease. Ann Intern Med 1985;103:1010–1019.

116. Noppa H, Bengtsson C, Wedel H, Wilhelmsen L. Obesity in relation to morbidity and mortality from cardiovascular disease. Am J Epidemiol 1980;111:682–692.

117. Tuomilehto J, Salonen JT, Marti B, et al. Body weight and risk of myocardial infarction and death in the adult population of eastern Finland. Br Med J 1987;295:623–627.

118. Hubert HB, Feinleib M, McNamara PM, Castelli WP. Obesity as an independent risk factor for cardiovascular disease: a 26-year follow-up of participants in the Framingham Heart Study. Circulation 1983;67:968–977.

119. Manson JE, Colditz GA, Stampfer MJ, et al. A prospective study of obesity and risk of coronary heart disease in women. N Engl J Med 1990;322:882–889.

120. Kleinman JC, Donahue RP, Harris MI, et al. Mortality among diabetics in a national sample. Am J Epidemiol 1988;128:389–401.

121. Barrett-Connor E, Orchard T. Diabetes and heart disease. In: National Diabetes Data Group. Diabetes in America: diabetes data compiled 1984. Washington, DC: U.S. Department of Health and Human Services, NIH Publication No. 85–1468, 1985.

122. Wingard DL, Barrett-Connor E, Criqui MH, Suarez L. Clustering of heart disease risk factors in diabetic compared to nondiabetic adults. Am J Epidemiol 1983;117:19–26.

123. Kannel WB, McGee DL. Diabetes and cardiovascular disease: the Framingham Study. JAMA 1979;241:2035–2038.

124. Reaven GM. Role of insulin resistance in human disease. Diabetes 1988;37:1595–1607.

125. Jarrett RJ. Is insulin atherogenic? Diabetologia 1988;31:71–75.

126. Kannel WB, Hjortland M, Castelli WP. Role of diabetes in congestive heart failure: the Framingham Study. Am J Cardiol 1974;34:29–34.

127. LaPorte RE, Cresanta JL, Kuller LH. The relationship of alcohol consumption to atherosclerotic heart disease. Prev Med 1980;9:22–40.

128. Moore RD, Pearson TA. Moderate alcohol consumption and coronary artery disease. Medicine 1986;65:242–267.

129. Klatsky A, Friedman GD, Siegelaub AB. Alcohol and mortality: a ten year Kaiser-Permanente experience. Ann Intern Med 1981;95:139–145.

130. Goldberg RJ, Burchfiel CM, Reed DM, et al. A prospective study of the health effects of alcohol consumption in middle-aged and elderly men: the Honolulu Heart Program. Circulation 1994;89:651–659.

131. Thun MJ, Peto R, Lopez AD, et al. Alcohol consumption and mortality among middle-aged and elderly U.S. adults. N Engl J Med 1997;337:1705–1714.

132. Aronson Friedman L, Kimball AW. Coronary heart disease mortality and alcohol consumption in Framingham. Am J Epidemiol 1986;124:481–489.

133. Stampfer MJ, Colditz GA, Willett WC, et al. A prospective study of moderate alcohol consumption and the risk of coronary disease and stroke in women. N Engl J Med 1988;319:267–273.

134. Ellison RC. Cheers! Epidemiology 1990;1:337–339.

135. Osler W. Lecture on angina pectoris and allied states. NY Med J 1896;64:177–183.

136. Friedman M, Rosenman RH. Association of a specific overt behavior pattern with increases in blood cholesterol, blood clotting time, incidence of arcus senilis and clinical coronary heart disease. JAMA 1959;169:1286–1296.

137. Krantz DS, Contrada RJ, Hill DR, Friedler E. Environmental stress and biobehavioral antecedents of coronary heart disease. J Consult Clin Psychol 1988;56:333–341.

138. Matthews KA, Haynes SG. Type A behavior pattern and coronary disease risk: update and critical evaluation. Am J Epidemiol 1986;123:923–960.

139. Jenkins CD, Rosenman RH, Zyzanski SJ. Prediction of clinical coronary heart disease by a test for the coronary-prone behavior pattern. N Engl J Med 1974;290:1271–1275.

140. Shekelle RB, Gale M, Norusis M. Type A score (Jenkins Activity Survey) and risk of recurrent coronary heart disease in the Aspirin Myocardial Infarction Study. Am J Cardiol 1985;56:221–225.

141. Shekelle RB, Hulley SB, Neaton JD, et al. The MRFIT Behavioral Pattern Study: II. type A behavior and incidence of coronary heart disease. Am J Epidemiol 1985;122:559–570.

142. Ragland DR, Brand RJ. Type A behavior and mortality from coronary heart disease. N Engl J Med 1988;318:65–69.

143. Williams RB Jr, Haney TL, Lee KL, et al. Type A behavior, hostility, and coronary atherosclerosis. Psychosom Med 1980;42:539–549.

144. Shekelle RB, Gale M, Ostfeld AM, Paul O. Hostility, risk of coronary heart disease, and mortality. Psychosom Med 1983;45:109–114.

145. Helmer DC, Ragland DR, Syme SL. Hostility and coronary artery disease. Am J Epidemiol 1991;133:112–122.

146. Everson SA, Kauhanen J, Kaplan GA, et al. Hostility and increased risk of mortality and acute myocardial infarction: the mediating role of behavioral risk factors. Am J Epidemiol 1997;146:142–152.

147. Frasure-Smith N, Lesperance F, Talajic M. Depression following myocardial infarction: impact on 6-month survival. JAMA 1993;270:1819–1825.

148. Silverstone PH. Depression and outcome in acute myocardial infarction. BMJ 1987;294:219–220.

149. Anda R, Williamson D, Jones D, et al. Depressed affect, hopelessness, and the risk of ischemic heart disease in a cohort of U.S. adults. Epidemiology 1993;4:285–294.

150. Barefoot JC, Schroll M. Symptoms of depression, acute myocardial infarction, and total mortality in a community sample. Circulation 1996;93:1976–1980.

151. Mendes de Leon CF, Krumholz HM, Seeman TS, et al. Depression and risk of coronary heart disease in elderly men and women. Arch Intern Med 1998;158:2341–2348.

152. Goldbourt U, Neufeld HN. Genetic aspects of arteriosclerosis. Arteriosclerosis 1986;6:357–377.

153. Robertson FW. The genetic component in coronary heart disease—a review. Genet Res 1981;37:1–16.

154. Wilson PWF, Myers RH, Larson MG, et al. Apolipoprotein E alleles, dyslipidemia, and coronary heart disease: the Framingham Offspring Study. JAMA 1994;272:1666–1671.

155. Thomas CB, Cohen BH. The familial occurrence of hypertension and coronary artery disease, with observations concerning obesity and diabetes. Ann Intern Med 1955;42:90–127.

156. Slack J, Evans KA. The increased risk of death from ischaemic heart disease in the first degree relatives of 121 men and 96 women with ischemic heart disease. J Med Genet 1966;3:239–257.

157. Feinleib M, Garrison RJ, Fabsitz R, et al. The NHLBI twin study of cardiovascular disease risk factors: methodology and summary of results. Am J Epidemiol 1977;106:284–295.

158. Shear CL, Frerichs RR, Weinberg R, Berenson GS. Childhood sibling aggregation of coronary artery disease risk factor variables in a biracial community. Am J Epidemiol 1978;107:522–528.

159. Morrison JA, Khoury P, Laskarzewski PM, et al. Familial associations of lipids and lipoproteins in families of hypercholesterolemic probands. Arteriosclerosis 1982;2:151–159.

160. Sholtz RI, Rosenman RH, Brand RJ. The relationship of reported parental history to the incidence of coronary heart disease in the Western Collaborative Group Study. Am J Epidemiol 1975;102:350–356.

161. Snowden CB, McNamara PM, Garrison RJ, et al. Predicting coronary heart disease in siblings—a multivariate assessment: the Framingham Heart Study. Am J Epidemiol 1982;115:217–222.

162. Cambien F, Richard JL, Ducimetiere P. Familial history of coronary heart diseases and high blood pressure in relation to the prevalence of risk factors, and the incidence of coronary heart disease. Rev Epidemiol Sante Publique 1980;28:21–37.

163. Colditz GA, Stampfer M, Willett WC, et al. A prospective study of parental history of myocardial infarction and coronary heart disease in women. Am J Epidemiol 1986;123:48–58.

164. Wilson PWF, Myers RH, Larson MG, et al. Apolipoprotein E alleles, dyslipidemia, and coronary heart disease: the Framingham Offspring Study. JAMA 1994;272:1666–1671.

165. Iacoviello L, Di Castelnuovo A, De Knijff P, et al. Polymorphisms in the coagulation factor VII gene and the risk of myocardial infarction. N Engl J Med 1998;338:79–85.

166. Keating M. Risk, genotype, and cardiovascular disease. Circulation 1992;86:688–690.

167. Stadel BV. Oral contraceptives and cardiovascular disease. N Engl J Med 1981;305:672–677.

168. Mann JI, Doll R, Thorogood M, et al. Risk factors for myocardial infarction in young women. Br J Prev Soc Med 1976;30:94–100.

169. Jick H, Dinan B, Rothman KJ. Oral contraceptives and nonfatal myocardial infarction. JAMA 1978;239:1403–1406.

170. Dalen JE, Hickler RB. Oral contraceptives and cardiovascular disease. Am Heart J 1981;101:626–639.

171. Rosenberg L, Hennekens CH, Rosner B, et al. Oral contraceptive use in relation to nonfatal myocardial infarction. Am J Epidemiol 1980;111:59–66.

172. Stampfer MF, Colditz GA. Estrogen replacement therapy and coronary heart disease: a quantitative assessment of the epidemiologic evidence. Prev Med 1991;20:47–63.

173. Petitti DB. Hormone replacement therapy and heart disease prevention: experimentation trumps observation. JAMA 1998;280:650–651.

174. Col NF, Eckman MH, Karas RH, et al. Patient-specific decisions about hormone replacement therapy in postmenopausal women. JAMA 1997;277: 1140–1147.

175. Jick H, Miettinen OS, Neff RK, et al. Coffee and myocardial infarction. N Engl J Med 1973;289:63–67.

176. Dawber TR, Kannel WB, Gordon T. Coffee and cardiovascular disease: observations from the Framingham Study. N Engl J Med 1974;291:871–874.

177. Hennekens CH, Drolette ME, Jesse MJ, et al. Coffee drinking and death due to coronary heart disease. N Engl J Med 1976; 294:633–636.

178. LaCroix AZ, Mead LA, Liang KY, et al. Coffee consumption and the incidence of coronary heart disease. N Engl J Med 1986; 315:977–982.

179. Grobbee DE, Rimm EB, Giovannucci E, et al. Coffee, caffeine, and cardiovascular disease in men. N Engl J Med 1990;323: 1026–1032.

180. Meade TW, Mellows S, Brozovic M, et al. Haemostatic function and ischaemic heart disease: principal results of the Northwick Park Heart Study. Lancet 1986;2:533–537.

181. Kannel WB, Wolf PA, Castelli WP, D'Agostino RB. Fibrinogen and risk of cardiovascular disease: the Framingham Study. JAMA 1987;258:1183–1186.

182. Yarnell JWG, Sweetnam PM, Elwood PC, et al. Haemostatic factors and ischaemic heart disease: the Caerphilly Study. Br Heart J 1985;53:483–487.

183. Lowe GDO, Drummond MM, Lorimer AR, et al. Relation between extent of coronary artery disease and blood viscosity. Br Med J 1980;1:673–674.

184. Danesh J, Collins R, Appleby P, Peto R. Association of fibrinogen, C-reactive protein, albumin, or leukocyte count with coronary heart disease. JAMA 1998;279:1477–1482.

185. Wilhelmsen L, Svardsudd K, Korsan-Bengtsen K, et al. Fibrinogen as a risk factor for stroke and myocardial infarction. N Engl J Med 1984;311:501–505.

186. Folsom AR, Wu KK, Rosamond WD, et al. Prospective study of hemostatic factors and incidence of coronary heart disease: the Atherosclerosis Risk in Communities (ARIC) Study. Circulation 1997;96:1102–1108.

187. Ridker PM, Cushman M, Stampfer MJ, et al. Inflammation, aspirin, and the risk of cardiovascular disease in apparently healthy men. N Engl J Med 1997;336:973–979.

188. Ridker PM, Glynn RJ, Hennekens CH. C-Reactive protein adds to the predictive value of total and HDL cholesterol in determining risk of first myocardial infarction. Circulation 1998;97:2007–2011.

189. Kovanen PT, Manttari M, Palosuo T, Manninen V, Aho K. Prediction of myocardial infarction in dyslipidemic men by elevated levels of immunoglobulin classes A, E, and G, but not M. Arch Intern Med 1998;158:1434–1439.

190. Bittner V. Atherosclerosis and the immune system. Arch Intern Med 1998;158:1395–1396.

191. Ridker PM, Rifai N, Pfeffer MC, et al. Inflammation, pravastatin, and the risk of coronary events after myocardial infarction in patients with average cholesterol levels. Circulation 1998;98: 839–844.

192. Hwang SJ, Ballantyne CM, Sharrett AR, et al. Circulating adhesion molecules VCAM-1, ICAM-1, and E-selectin in carotid atherosclerosis and incident coronary heart disease cases: the Atherosclerosis Risk in Communities (ARIC) Study. Circulation 1997;96:4219–4225.

193. Tracy RP. Inflammation in cardiovascular disease: cart, horse, or both? Circulation 1998;97: 2000–2002.

194. Wald NJ, Watt HC, Law MR, et al. Homocysteine and ischemic heart disease: results of a prospective study with implications regarding prevention. Arch Intern Med 1998;158:862–867.

195. Kuller LH, Evans RW. Homocysteine, vitamins and cardiovascular disease. Circulation 1998;98:196–199.

196. Moghadasian MH, McManus BM, Frohlich JJ. Homocyst(e)ine and coronary artery disease: clinical evidence and genetic and metabolic background. Arch Intern Med 1997;157:2299–2308.

197. Saikku P, Leinonen M, Mattila KJ, et al. Serological evidence of an association of a novel chlamydia, TWAR, with chronic coronary heart disease and AMI. Lancet 1988;2:986.

198. Thom DH, Grayston JT, Siscovick DS, et al. Association of prior infection with Chlamydia pneumoniae and angiographically demonstrated coronary artery disease. JAMA 1992;268:68–72.

199. Libby P, Egan D, Skarlatos S. Roles of infectious agents in atherosclerosis and restenosis: an assessment of the evidence and need for future research. Circulation 1997;96:4095–4103.

200. Kur CC, Shor A, Campbell LA, et al. Demonstration of Chlamydia pneumoniae in atherosclerotic lesions of coronary arteries. J Infect Dis 1993;167:841–849.

201. Muhlestein JB, Hammond EH, Carlquist JF, et al. Increased incidence of Chlamydia species within the coronary arteries of patients with symptomatic atherosclerotic versus other forms of cardiovascular disease. J Am Coll Cardiol 1996;27:1555–1561.

202. Sandeep G, Leatham EW, Carrington D, et al. Elevated Chlamydia pneumoniae antibodies, cardiovascular events, and azithromycin in male survivors of myocardial infarction. Circulation 1997;96:404–407.

203. Keichl S, Willeit J, Egger G, et al, for the Bruneck Study Group. Body iron stores and the risk of carotid atherosclerosis: prospective results from the Bruneck Study. Circulation 1997;96: 3300–3307.

204. Salonen JT, Nyyssonen K, Korpela H, et al. High stored iron levels are associated with excess risk of myocardial infarction in eastern Finnish men. Circulation 1992;86: 803–811.

205. Barker DJP, Winter PD, Osmond C, et al. Weight in infancy and death from ischemic heart disease. Lancet 1989;ii: 577–580.

206. Osmond C, Barker DJP, Winter PD, et al. Early growth and death from cardiovascular disease in women. BMJ 1995;311: 171–174.

207. Barker DJP, Gluckman PD, Godfrey KM, et al. Fetal nutrition and cardiovascular disease in adult life. Lancet 1993;334: 938–941.

208. Smith GD, Frankel S, Yarnell J. Sex and death: are they related? Findings from the Caerphilly cohort study. BMJ 1997;315: 20–27.

209. Goldberg RJ. Coronary heart disease: Epidemiology and risk factors. In: Ockene IS, Ockene JK, eds. Prevention of coronary heart disease. Boston: Little, Brown, 1992:3–39.

210. Bao W, Srinivasan SR, Valdez R, et al. Longitudinal changes in cardiovascular risk from childhood to young adulthood in offspring of parents with coronary artery disease: the Bogalusa Heart Study. JAMA 1997;278: 1749–1754.

211. Van Horn L, Greenland P. Prevention of coronary artery disease is a pediatric problem. JAMA 1997;278:1779–1789.

212. Berenson GS, Srinivasan SR, Bao W, et al. Association between multiple cardiovascular risk factors and atherosclerosis in children and young adults. N Engl J Med 1998;338: 1650–1656.

213. Hennekens CH. Increasing burden of cardiovascular disease: current knowledge and future directions for research on risk factors. Circulation 1998;97: 1095–1102.

214. Yusuf HR, Giles WH, Croft JB, et al. Impact of multiple risk factor profiles on determining cardiovascular disease risk. Prev Med 1998;27:1–9.

215. Grover SA, Paquet S, Levinton C, et al. Estimating the benefits of modifying risk factors of cardiovascular disease: a comparison of primary vs secondary prevention. Arch Intern Med 1998;158: 655–662.

216. Stern MP. The recent decline in ischemic heart disease mortality. Ann Intern Med 1979;91: 630–640.

217. Stallones RA. The rise and fall of ischemic heart disease. Sci Am 1980;243:53–59.

218. Luepker RV, Higgins MH, eds. Trends in coronary heart disease mortality. Oxford University Press, 1988.

219. Goldberg RJ: Temporal trends and declining mortality rates from coronary heart disease in the United States. In: Ockene IS, Ockene JK, eds. Prevention of coronary heart disease. Boston: Little, Brown, 1992:41–68.

220. Sans S, Kesteloot H, Kromhout D. The burden of cardiovascular diseases mortality in Europe: task force of the European Society of Cardiology on cardiovascular mortality and morbidity statistics in Europe. Eur Heart J 1997;18:1231–1248.

221. Stephen AM, Wald NJ. Trends in individual consumption of dietary fat in the United States, 1920–1984. Am J Clin Nutr 1990;42:457–469.

222. Popkin BM, Siega-Riz AM, Haines PS. A comparison of dietary trends among racial and socioeconomic groups in the United States. N Engl J Med 1996;335:716–720.

223. Stephens T. Secular trends in adult physical activity: exercise boom or bust? Res Quart Exerc Sport 1987;58:94–99.

224. Elveback LR, Connolly DC, Melton LJ. Coronary heart disease in residents of Rochester, Minnesota. VII. Incidence, 1950

through 1982. Mayo Clin Proc 1986;61:896–900.

225. McGovern PG, Pankow JS, Shahar E, et al. Recent trends in acute coronary heart disease: mortality, morbidity, medical care and risk factors. N Engl J Med 1996;334:884–890.

226. Goldberg RJ, Gore JM, Alpert JS, Dalen JE. Recent changes in attack and survival rates of acute myocardial infarction (1975 through 1981): the Worcester Heart Attack Study. JAMA 1986;255:2774–2779.

227. Goldberg RJ, Gorak EJ, Yarzebski J, et al. A community-wide perspective of gender differences and temporal trends in the incidence and survival rates following acute myocardial infarction and out-of-hospital deaths due to coronary heart disease. Circulation 1993;87:1947–1953.

228. Keil JE, Saunders DE, Lackland DT, et al. AMI: period prevalence, case fatality, and comparison of black and white cases in urban and rural areas of South Carolina. Am Heart J 1985;109:776–784.

229. Rosamond W, Chambless L, Folsom A, et al. Trends in the incidence of myocardial infarction and in mortality due to coronary heart disease, 1987 to 1994. N Engl J Med 1998;339: 861–867.

230. Hunink MG, Goldman L, Tosteson AN, et al. The recent decline in mortality from coronary heart disease, 1980–1990: the effect of secular trends in risk factors and treatment. JAMA 1997;277: 535–542.

231. Goldman L, Cook EF. The decline in ischemic heart disease mortality rates: an analysis of the comparative effects of medical interventions and changes in lifestyle. Ann Intern Med 1984;101:825–836.

232. Kaplan GA, Cohn BA, Cohen RD, Guralnik J. The decline in ischemic heart disease mortality: prospective evidences from the Alameda County Study. Am J Epidemiol 1988;127: 1131–1142.

Chapter 2

The Pathobiology of Hypercholesterolemia and Atherosclerosis

Robert J. Nicolosi
David Kritchevsky
Thomas A. Wilson

PLASMA LIPIDS, LIPOPROTEIN CLASSES, AND APOLIPOPROTEINS

Normal blood serum is a clear, straw-colored liquid, which contains an appreciable amount of fat. The fat is kept in solution by being complexed to protein in large agglomerates called *lipoproteins*.

The major circulating lipid classes in plasma are cholesterol, as either free cholesterol (FC) or cholesterol ester (CE), phospholipid (PL), triglycerides (TG) and unesterified or free fatty acids (FFAs). The FFAs circulate in the bloodstream in association with albumin. All other lipids, because of their hydrophobic nature (i.e., insolubility in water), are packaged with proteins into large molecular weight molecules (lipoproteins). The densities of individual plasma lipoproteins are determined by their relative content of protein and lipid. Differences in density, composition, and electrophoretic mobility have been used to divide lipoproteins into five major classes, which have been described in Table 2-1. Chylomicrons are triglyceride-rich lipoproteins produced by the intestine and have a density (d) of approximately 0.95 g/mL. Triglyceride-rich very-low-density lipoproteins (VLDL) ($d < 1.006$ g/mL) are made by the liver and have pre-beta mobility upon electrophoresis. Intermediate-density lipoproteins (IDL) ($d = 1.006$ to 1.019 g/mL) are produced by the catabolism of VLDL and have electrophoretic mobility between pre-beta and beta. Low-density lipoproteins (LDL) ($d = 1.019$ to 1.063 g/mL) are derived from the catabolism of both VLDL and IDL and are the major cholesterol-carrying lipoproteins of plasma in humans. They have beta mobility on electrophoresis. LDL has been further subdivided by ultracentrifugation into LDL-1 ($d = 1.019$ to 1.035 g/mL) and LDL-2 ($d = 1.035$ to 1.065

g/mL), although these densities may vary. It is the larger LDL particle (LDL-1) that generally fluctuates in response to environmental factors such as diet, drug, or hormonal intervention. High-density lipoproteins (HDL) ($d = 1.063$ to 1.21 g/mL) have alpha mobility and are derived from a variety of sources, including liver, intestine, other lipoproteins, and other tissue. HDL has been further subfractionated by ultracentrifugation into HDL_2 ($d = 1.063$ to 1.125 g/mL) and HDL_3 ($d = 1.125$ to 1.21 g/mL). Changes in HDL levels by environmental factors are usually associated with the larger HDL_2 fraction.

The lipoproteins are not chemical compounds in the usual sense but are described by their hydrated densities. As separation techniques improve and become more sophisticated, one can expect refinement in the classification of lipoproteins, as has occurred in the gradient gel electrophoresis technique, which results in at least six subfractions of LDL. The small, dense particles are associated with increased risk of cardiovascular disease, whereas the larger, triglyceride-rich particles are not.

Lp(a) lipoprotein, recently reviewed by several investigators (1,2), was first described as early as 1963 but recently has received considerable attention because high circulating levels are significantly correlated with the incidence of coronary heart disease (3,4) and predilection to vein graft occlusion following coronary bypass surgery (5). Lp(a) resembles an LDL particle in which the major apoprotein of LDL, apo B-100, is disulfide-linked to a specific apolipoprotein designated apo(a) that has a striking homology to plasminogen, a protein involved in the regulation of fibrinolysis (1). Apo(a) is heterogeneous in size and density with a molecular weight of approximately 600,000. At least seven apo(a) isoforms have

Table 2-1 Classification of Plasma Lipoproteins

Lipoprotein Class	Density (g/mL)	Electrophoretic Mobility	Sources	Composition (Wt%)				
				FC	CE	TG	PL	PROT
Chylomicron	<0.95	Origin	Intestine	1	3	90	4	2
Very-Low-Density Lipoproteins (VLDL)	0.95–1.006	Pre-beta	Liver	7	14	55	16	8
Intermediate-Density Lipoproteins (IDL)	1.006–1.019	Between beta and pre-beta	Catabolism of VLDL	6	22	30	24	18
Low-Density Lipoproteins (LDL)	1.019–1.063	Beta	Catabolism of VLDL and IDL	7	48	5	20	20
High-Density Lipoproteins (HDL)	1.063–1.210	Alpha	Liver, intestine, other	4	15	4	27	50

CE = cholesterol ester; FC = free cholesterol; PL = phospholipids; PROT = protein; TG = triglycerides.

Table 2-2 Characteristics and Functions of Major Apolipoproteins

Apolipoprotein	Lipoproteins	Approximate Molecular Weight (Daltons)	Sources	Average Plasma Concentration (mg/dL)	Physiologic Function
B48	Chylomicrons	264,000	Intestine	Trace	Major structural apoprotein; secretion and clearance of chylomicrons
B-100	VLDL, LDL	550,000	Liver	100–125	Ligand for LDL receptor, structural apoprotein of VLDL and LDL
A-I	HDL, chylomicrons	28,000	Liver, intestine	100–120	Structural apoprotein of HDL, cofactor for LCAT
A-II	HDL, chylomicrons	17,000	Intestine, liver	35–45	Structural apoprotein of HDL, cofactor for hepatic lipase
A-IV	HDL, chylomicrons	46,000	Liver, intestine	10–20	Unknown
Apo (a)	Lp (a)	600,000	Liver	1–10	Unknown
C-I	Chylomicrons, VLDL, HDL	5,800	Liver	6–8	Cofactor for LCAT
C-II	Chylomicrons, VLDL, HDL	9,100	Liver	3–5	Cofactor for LPL
C-III	Chylomicrons, VLDL, HDL	8,750	Liver	12–15	Inhibitor of LPL, involved in lipoprotein remnant uptake
E-2	Chylomicrons, VLDL, HDL	35,000	Liver, peripheral tissues	4–5	Ligand for cell receptor
E-3	Chylomicrons, VLDL, HDL	35,000	Liver, peripheral tissues	4–5	Ligand for cell receptor
E-4	Chylomicrons, VLDL, HDL	35,000	Liver, peripheral tissues	4–5	Ligand for cell receptor

been described, and their size appears to be inversely correlated with Lp(a) concentration.

Lipoproteins can also be classified according to their apolipoprotein (apo) composition, whose major function is lipid transport (Table 2-2). The differences in apolipoprotein composition between and within apolipoprotein classes often determines their metabolic fate. The apolipoproteins classified as the major apo Bs are B-48, synthesized in the intestine and carried by chylomicrons, and B-100, produced by the liver and carried on the surface of VLDL, IDL, and LDL. The apo As (i.e., A-I, A-II, and A-IV) are made by both the intestine and liver and are transported in both chylomicron and HDL particles. The apo Cs (i.e., C-I, C-II, and C-III) are made by the liver and are found in chylomicrons, VLDL,

IDL, and HDL. Apolipoprotein E (apo E) is transported as a constituent of chylomicrons, VLDL, IDL, and HDL. It exists in several polymorphic forms because of the presence of multiple, genetically determined alleles at a single gene locus. Three homozygous (E4/4, E3/3, and E2/2) and three heterozygous (E4/3, E4/2, and E3/2) phenotypes have been detected with E3/3, present in 60% of the population, being the most common (6).

OVERVIEW OF CHOLESTEROL METABOLISM

Cholesterol is an essential steroid molecule in cell membranes and lipoproteins, having particularly important functions for permeability and enzyme activities in membranes. Cholesterol and/or its derivatives are precursors of adrenal steroids (hydrocortisone and aldosterone), sex hormones (estrogens and androgens), bile acids (which facilitate the absorption of intestinal fat), and vitamin D. Although all nucleated mammalian cells can produce cholesterol, the major organs of synthesis are the intestine and liver. Since the liver is the major organ capable of metabolizing cholesterol, an elaborate system of cholesterol transport via lipoproteins from peripheral tissues back to the liver has evolved (see Figure 2-1).

Sources of Cholesterol

Cholesterol in the intestinal lumen originates from two major sources, the diet and bile, although some cholesterol is also derived from the desquamation of intestinal mucosal cells.

In humans, the amount of dietary cholesterol can vary from virtually zero, as in the case of true vegetarians, to 2000 mg/day in people consuming large quantities of animal fats. The average intake of adult men and women is 450 mg/day. All dietary cholesterol is from animal sources. Plants do not contain cholesterol but instead have other cell membrane sterols such as β-sitosterol.

Absorption of Cholesterol

Cholesterol entering the lumen of the intestine is absorbed (approximately 50%) and the remainder excreted in the feces. Because of the insoluble nature of cholesterol, it is first solubilized into micelles that contain bile acids and more polar lipids such as fatty acids, monoglycerides, and lecithin. In the intestinal lumen, the detergent nature of these more polar lipids facilitates the solubilization of cholesterol, which, upon incorporation into the intestinal mucosal cell, is packaged along with more nonpolar lipids (triglycerides and cholesterol ester) and protein into chylomicrons for secretion into the bloodstream.

Hepatic Synthesis and Catabolism of Cholesterol

As previously mentioned, the liver is the major site of cholesterol synthesis. Briefly, the synthesis of cholesterol is initiated from the conversion of the 2-carbon fragment, acetate, to 3-hydroxy-3-methylglutaryl coenzyme A (HMG-CoA). The conversion of HMG-CoA to mevalonic acid is mediated via the enzyme HMG-CoA reductase and is the rate-limiting step in cholesterol biosynthesis. Approximately 600 to 800 mg of cholesterol is synthesized per day. The cholesterol that accumulates in the liver may have one of three fates: 1) It can be

re-packaged as VLDL and enter the circulation, 2) it may be converted to the primary bile acids, cholate and chenodeoxycholate, by the regulatory enzyme 7alpha-hydroxylase, or 3) it may be secreted into the bile and therefore the intestine, as biliary cholesterol along with bile acids. The principal catabolic pathway of cholesterol is to bile acids (about 75% to 90% of synthesized cholesterol is converted to bile acids).

Enterohepatic Circulation

The process of continuous transport of cholesterol and bile acids between the liver and intestine is referred to as the *enterohepatic circulation*. During this process, approximately one half of the dietary cholesterol entering the intestine is reabsorbed and returns to the liver. The amount of cholesterol that returns to the liver can regulate the degree of hepatic synthesis of cholesterol by feedback inhibition of HMG-CoA reductase. Thus, the more cholesterol reabsorbed by the liver, the greater is the inhibition of cholesterol synthesis. The hepatic synthesis of bile acids is also regulated by feedback inhibition through their return to the liver via the enterohepatic circulation. Approximately 95% of the bile acids synthesized by the liver and secreted into the bile and eventually the intestine are returned to the liver in this process.

OVERVIEW OF LIPOPROTEIN METABOLISM
Chylomicrons

The metabolism of lipoproteins has been reviewed by several investigators, including Schaefer et al (7). In humans and most subhuman species, lipoproteins are produced by the intestine and the liver. The intestine secretes chylomicrons containing several apoproteins, the most essential one for chylomicron secretion being apo B-48, the intestinal form of apo B. This large, triglyceride-rich particle originates in the intestine in response to such dietary factors as fat. Once these chylomicrons are secreted from the intestine into the circulation, they are acted on by the enzyme lipoprotein lipase (LPL), which after activation by apo C-II, results in hydrolysis of triglycerides and formation of chylomicron remnants. The enzyme hepatic lipase (HL) is also active in the formation of chylomicron remnants from chylomicrons. During the process of lipolysis, triglycerides are catabolized to form free fatty acids and glycerol. As the core of chylomicrons is depleted of triglycerides, surface components such as apo A-I, apo A-II, apo Cs, and phospholipids are released to form nascent HDL, which goes on to form mature HDL. During the process of HDL metabolism, certain of its surface components such as apo E are transferred to chylomicron remnants. The TG-poor chylomicron remnants, enriched in apo E, are then taken up by the apo E receptor in the liver. The apo E receptor is not regulated by environmental factors.

Very-Low-Density Lipoproteins (VLDL)

The liver also secretes VLDL and, in particular, apo B-100 (see Figure 2-1). The secretion and synthesis of VLDL is increased in obese individuals and is also responsive to dietary variables, such as high carbohydrate intake and increases in dietary fatty acids. The catabolism of VLDL triglycerides (VLDL-TG) is similar to chylomicron degradation, involving

A: Overproduction of lipoproteins----------------

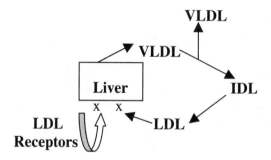

> *Obesity*
> *Excess Calories*
> *Excess Alcohol*

B: Decreased LDL Catabolism----------

> **LDL receptor activity decreased by:**
> *Excess saturated fatty acids*
> *Excess dietary cholesterol*

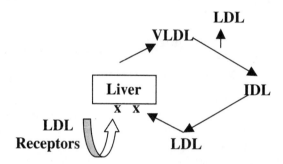

C: Production of abnormal LDL enriched in cholesterol

> 1. *Secretion of cholesterol-rich VLDL (B-VLDL) by the liver*
> 2. *Transfer of cholesterol ester from HDL to LDL by CETP*
> 3. *Esterification of LDL cholesterol by LCAT*

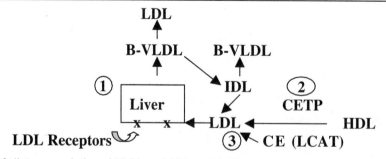

Figure 2-1 Overview of dietary regulation of VLDL and LDL metabolism.

both lipoprotein lipase and hepatic lipase. During the formation of VLDL remnants (IDL) from the catabolism of VLDL, certain consituents such as apo E and apo C are also transferred to HDL while apo B-100 remains with the IDL parti-cle. The major products of VLDL and IDL catabolism are low-density lipoproteins (LDL), although some VLDL may be removed from plasma prior to LDL formation, especially in individuals with severe hypertriglyceridemia.

Low-Density Lipoproteins (LDL)

LDL, the major cholesterol-transporting lipoprotein in humans, is derived predominantly via the catabolism of VLDL and IDL, although in certain individuals with familial hypercholesterolemia (8,9) and in some animal models, such as the pig (10,11), there is some direct LDL synthesis. LDL can be catabolized by both hepatic and extrahepatic tissues with approximately 75% of LDL being catabolized by the liver and the remaining 25% by extrahepatic tissue (12,13). The clearance of LDL by these tissues involves both receptor-mediated and non–receptor-mediated pathways. The predominant pathway of clearance is receptor-mediated via the B-E receptor (LDL receptor), accounting for nearly 75% of the clearance of LDL, whereas approximately 25% is cleared by nonreceptor pathways (14,15) (see Figure 2-1). During catabolism of LDL via the B-E receptor, LDL binds to the receptor and becomes internalized in association with cytoplasmic lysozomes. Once internalized, the receptors disassociate themselves from LDL and return to the cell surface to be used again. The cholesterol esters and apo B of LDL are hydrolyzed by enzymes within the lysozome to unesterified cholesterol and amino acids, respectively. The unesterified cholesterol can 1) be used for cell membrane components, 2) be re-esterified as cholesterol ester for storage, or 3) leave the cell, as in the case of the liver, where it can become incorporated into bile for final fecal excretion. The B-E receptor appears to be influenced by 1) changes in the levels of dietary cholesterol (16,17), 2) the type of dietary fat (18–20), 3) hormones (21), and 4) increasing age (22,23). The amount of cholesterol entering the cell can regulate the synthesis of cholesterol and the rate of LDL receptor synthesis by influencing HMG-CoA reductase activity (24), the major enzyme that controls cholesterol synthesis. Environmental factors that regulate LDL receptor synthesis and activity will be discussed in a later section.

Lp(a) Lipoprotein

Very little information is currently available on Lp(a) metabolism. The liver is the primary site of synthesis of Lp(a) and, although its catabolic site has not been determined with certainty, the LDL receptor pathway has emerged as a major route, although possibly not as effective as it is for LDL (25,26). Levels of Lp(a) seem to be regulated by rates of synthesis (25). Its value as a predictor of coronary heart disease risk probably resides in its striking homology with plasminogen (27). Plasminogen is converted to plasmin, which normally dissolves clots. Lp(a) at high concentrations competes with plasminogen, counteracting the fibrinolytic system and thereby increasing the risk of thrombosis.

High-Density Lipoproteins (HDL)

HDL is a heterogeneous group of particles that can be divided into several subfractions depending upon the method of separation used. In general, the mature HDL particle is spherical in shape, whereas the precursor or nascent HDL particles are usually viewed as disks consisting of phospholipid bilayers enriched with either apo A-I and/or apo E molecules. Nascent HDL (sometimes referred to as HDL$_3$) can originate from the catabolism of VLDL and chylomicrons. Nascent HDL can also be secreted directly by the liver and the intestine. These nascent forms of HDL may associate with cholesterol and phospholipid originating from the degradation of cell membranes. Nascent HDL particles also provide excellent substrates for lecithin-cholesterol acyl-transferase (LCAT), the major plasma cholesterol-esterifying enzyme. By acquiring cholesterol esters generated during the LCAT reaction, these disk-shaped nascent HDLs (HDL$_3$) are converted to mature, spherical HDL (HDL$_2$ particles) in plasma, upon movement of cholesterol ester into the hydrophobic core regions of HDL. The cholesterol esters from the core of HDL can be exchanged or transferred to chylomicrons or VLDL in exchange for triglyceride molecules by a cholesterol ester transfer protein (CETP). These cholesterol esters transferred to triglyceride-rich lipoproteins may then be cleared from circulation via the LDL receptor or remnant pathway. Some HDL particles may be directly cleared from plasma by the liver through a putative HDL receptor (28), although probably not as intact particles since the rates of removal of the HDL lipid and apoproteins differ (29).

Reverse Cholesterol Transport

Since cholesterol can only be degraded and excreted by the liver, any removal of excess cholesterol from peripheral tissues, such as blood vessel walls, must involve the transport of cholesterol back to the liver. In this scenario, unesterified cholesterol, a normal constituent of cellular membranes but also found in atherosclerotic plaques, is transferred to HDL and through the action of the enzyme LCAT becomes esterified cholesterol. Some of the HDL cholesterol ester is transferred to VLDL by CETP. The cholesterol ester in VLDL can then be returned to the liver by direct incorporation of VLDL remnants (IDL) through the apo E receptor or be taken up by the B-E receptor subsequent to conversion of VLDL to LDL.

DEFINITION OF DYSLIPOPROTEINEMIAS

Dyslipoproteinemias are disorders of plasma lipid transport that can be associated with deficiencies of apolipoproteins, enzymes, lipid transfer proteins, and cellular receptors. Because the end result includes alterations in the synthesis and/or removal of lipoproteins from the bloodstream, the critical significance of the dyslipoproteinemias is therefore attributable to their involvement in enhanced risk of atherosclerosis and coronary artery disease.

However, it is important to understand that the true familial hyperlipidemias make up only a minor portion of individuals with elevated serum cholesterol levels, and are thus only briefly described in Tables 2-3 and 2-4.

Basic Mechanisms of Diet-Induced Hypercholesterolemia

The three basic mechanisms that lead to elevations in LDL cholesterol, especially in response to dietary cholesterol and the type of dietary fat, are: 1) reduced catabolism of LDL; 2) overproduction of LDL and/or its precursors, VLDL and IDL; and 3) production of abnormal LDL enriched in cholesterol.

In Tables 2-3 and 2-4 genetic dyslipoproteinemias, abnormalities in the LDL receptor gene (as in type IIa dys-

Table 2-3 Primary Dyslipoproteinemias

Type	Plasma Lipid Changes	Plasma Lipoprotein Changes	Genetic Disorder	Apparent Biochemical Defect	Clinical Manifestations
I	Triglycerides ↑	Chylomicrons ↑	Familial lipoprotein lipase (LPL) deficiency	Loss of LPL activity	Acute pancreatitis, eruptive xanthomas, hepatosplenomegaly, lipemia retinalis
			Familial apo CII deficiency	Abnormal CII structure or levels	
IIA	Cholesterol ↑	LDL ↑	Familial hypercholesterolemia	Deficiency of LDL receptor number and/or activity	Premature atherosclerosis, tendon xanthomas, corneal arcus
IIB	Cholesterol, ↑ triglycerides	LDL and ↑ VLDL	Familial combined hyperlipidemia	Unknown	Increased risk of premature coronary artery disease
III	Cholesterol, ↑ triglycerides	beta-VLDL ↑	Familial type III hyperlipoproteinemia homozygous for apo E-2	Defective clearance of triglyceride-rich remnants, hepatic lipase deficiency	Premature coronary artery and peripheral vascular disease, tuberous xanthomas, hyperuricemia, glucose intolerance
IV	Triglycerides ↑	VLDL ↑	Familial hypertriglyceridemia	Increased synthesis and decreased catabolism of VLDL	Acute pancreatitis, glucose intolerance, hyperuricemia
V	Triglycerides, ↑ cholesterol	VLDL, ↑ chylomicrons	Familial type V hyperlipoproteinemia	Defective lipolysis of triglyceride-rich lipoproteins and overproduction of VLDL triglycerides	Acute pancreatitis, eruptive xanthomas, glucose intolerance, hyperuricemia, peripheral neuropathy
Hyper Lp (a)	Cholesterol ↑	Lp (a) ↑	Familial hyper apo (a)	Resemblance to plasminogen causes competitive inhibition lowering fibrinolytic activity in plasma	Increased coronary artery disease, xanthomatosis
Hyperapobeta lipoproteinemia	Triglycerides ↑	VLDL and ↑ LDL	Familial hyper apo B, familial Type IV	Increased VLDL apo B synthesis	Predisposition to coronary, cerebral and peripheral atherosclerosis
Hyperalpha lipoproteinemia	Cholesterol ↑	HDL ↑	Familial hyperalpha lipoproteinemia	CETP deficiency	Decreased frequency of CHD, increased longevity
Familial hypobeta lipoproteinemia	Cholesterol, ↓ triglycerides	Chylomicrons, ↓ VLDL, LDL	Unknown	Inability to synthesiize apo B-100 and apo B-48	Development of neurological or eye complications, abnormal clotting function
Abetalipo proteinemia	Cholesterol, ↓ triglycerides	Chylomicrons, ↓ VLDL, LDL	Unknown	Apo B-100 and apo B-48 not secreted into plasma	Fat malabsorption, acanthocytosis, retinitis pigmentosa
Hypoalpha lipoproteinemia (Tangier Disease, Fish Eye Disease)	Triglycerides, ↓ cholesterol	HDL ↓	Unknown	LCAT deficiency, combined apo A-I, CIII deficiency, apo A-I defects may all lead to abnormal metabolism of apo A-I and apo A-II	Premature coronary artery disease

lipoproteinemia), were outlined that lead to decreases in LDL receptor number and/or activity. However, several environmental factors can regulate LDL receptor synthesis and/or activity.

Dietary Cholesterol

We previously mentioned that dietary cholesterol can influence LDL receptor activity and/or synthesis (16,17). For example, perturbations, which increase a regulatory pool of hepatic cellular cholesterol, can decrease LDL receptor synthesis. Thus, increases in absorption of dietary cholesterol (30–32), inability to down-regulate cholesterol synthesis (33), and decreases in cholesterol catabolism or conversion to bile acids or neutral sterols (34) could lead to accumulation of cellular cholesterol, thereby decreasing LDL receptor synthesis and/or activity.

Dietary cholesterol per se has little effect on levels of blood cholesterol. A recent meta-analysis by Howell et al (35) indicates that for every 100 mg of dietary cholesterol blood cholesterol is increased between 2 and 3 mg/dL.

Saturated Fatty Acids

LDL receptor activity is also influenced by the type of dietary fatty acids. There is considerable evidence that saturated fatty acids, in general, raise serum cholesterol and, in particular, LDL cholesterol levels. Several epidemiologic studies have shown that populations consuming large amounts of saturated fatty acids, particularly of animal fat origin, have elevated levels of circulating cholesterol. In contrast, those populations that consume lower levels of saturated fatty acids have lower serum cholesterol levels. Studies performed by Keys et al (36) and Hegsted et al (37) support the notion that saturated fatty acids are the major nutrients that influence cholesterol levels. Both of these investigators developed predictive equations that

Table 2-4 Secondary Dyslipoproteinemias			
TYPE	ASSOCIATED DISEASE	LIPOPROTEINS ELEVATED	UNDERLYING DEFECT
I	Lupus erythematosus	Chylomicrons	Circulating LPL inhibitor
II	Nephrotic syndrome, Cushings syndrome	VLDL and LDL	Overproduction of VLDL particles, defective lipolysis of VLDL triglycerides
III	Hypothyroidism, dysglobulinemia	VLDL and LDL	Suppression of LDL receptor activity, overproduction of VLDL triglycerides
IV	Renal failure, diabetes mellitus, acute hepatitis	VLDL	Defective lipolysis of triglyceride-rich VLDL due to inhibition of LPL and HL
V	Non-insulin-dependent diabetes	VLDL	Overproduction and defective lipolysis of VLDL triglycerides

relate the degree of serum cholesterol increase to saturated fatty acid intake. These equations indicate that for every 1% of calories consumed from saturated fatty acid there is an approximately 2.7-mg/dL increase in serum cholesterol. In addition, several studies indicate that saturated fatty acids also increase LDL cholesterol (38–40). Although the cholesterol-raising action of dietary saturated fatty acids, as a lipid class, is well established, the mechanisms whereby these saturated fatty acids raise LDL is not well understood. Although many mechanisms have been postulated, the most probable explanation is that saturated fatty acids interfere with normal LDL receptor-mediated clearance of LDL (12,20) (see Figure 2-1B). However, the precise mechanism of down-regulation of the LDL receptor is not known. One possibility is that increased saturated fatty acid intake enlarges a hepatic pool of cholesterol that can suppress the expression (messenger RNA levels) of the LDL receptor protein, an explanation supported by a study in animals fed saturated fatty acids and cholesterol (41). Another mechanism postulated from both in vivo (20) and in vitro studies (42,43) suggests that enrichment of phospholipid membranes of various cells by saturated fatty acids interferes with the normal function of LDL receptors, possibly through alterations in the binding and/or internalization of circulating LDL. It is also possible that newly secreted lipoproteins from cholesterol-fed animals, abnormally enriched in cholesterol or having altered apoproteins (44,45), may be less avidly bound to the LDL receptor (see Figure 2-1C).

Although dietary saturated fatty acids, in general, can raise serum cholesterol and LDL cholesterol levels, earlier studies (36,37) as well as more recent evidence (40) suggest that the various saturated fatty acids have different serum cholesterol–raising effects. For example, saturated fatty acids with chain lengths less than 10 carbons (i.e., medium chain fatty acids) are thought to have little or no cholesterol–raising capabilities (46,47). To what extent lauric acid, a 12-carbon chain fatty acid, will raise serum cholesterol levels is not known at this time with any certainty. There is substantial evidence that myristic acid, a 14-carbon chain fatty acid, and palmitic acid, a 16-carbon chain fatty acid, increase both total and LDL serum cholesterol levels. Earlier studies by both Keys et al (36) and Hegsted et al (37) and the more recent investigations from the laboratory of Grundy et al (38–40) have clearly shown that palmitic acid increases total serum and LDL cholesterol levels when substituted for carbohydrates or monounsaturated fat in the diet. Another saturated fatty acid found in animal fats and cocoa butter is stearic acid, an 18-carbon chain fatty acid. Previous studies by Keys et al (36) and Hegsted et al (37) and more recent studies by Bononome et al (40) suggest that stearic acid may be neutral in its cholesterol-raising capabilities, thus leaving palmitic, myristic, and possibly lauric acid as the major cholesterol-raising saturated fatty acids in the diet.

The source of saturated fatty acids in the diet is typically animal fats, although certain vegetable oils such as coconut oil, palm oil, palm kernel oil, and cocoa butter are rich in saturated fatty acids. Coconut oil and palm kernel oil have similar compositions and are particularly rich in the medium chain fatty acids of 8- to 12-carbon chain length. Animal fat is relatively rich in myristic acid but can also contain substantial quantities of the medium chain fatty acids. Palm oil can contain almost 50% of its fatty acids in the form of saturates, with the major one being palmitic acid. Although cocoa butter also contains a percentage of total saturated fatty acid similar to that of palm oil, it is predominantly made up of stearic acid, which, as just mentioned, is thought to be neutral in its cholesterol-raising ability. Beef fat is high in total saturated fatty acids and is rich in both palmitic acid and stearic acid. Fat from both pork and chicken, in general, has relatively high amounts of palmitic acid and lesser amounts of stearic acid. The major nonsaturated fatty acid in palm oil and beef is oleic acid.

Thus, the type of saturated fat present in various foods is of considerable importance in determining the atherogenic potential of such foods, and it may be possible, as suggested by St. John et al (48), to "engineer" various foods (i.e., beef) to contain greater amounts of stearic and lesser amounts of palmitic acid, and thus make them more "heart-healthy."

Polyunsaturated Fatty Acids (n-6) from Vegetable Oils

In contrast to saturated fatty acids, which in general raise cholesterol levels, unsaturated fatty acids, which include monounsaturated fatty acids such as oleic acid and polyunsaturated fatty acids such as linoleic acid, have a cholesterol-lowering effect when replacing saturated fat in the diet. Two types of polyunsaturated fatty acids have been identified. The predominant n-6 fatty acid (first double bond starts at the sixth carbon from the methyl end) is linoleic acid, derived from plant oils, whereas the n-3 fatty acids (first double bond starts at the third carbon from the methyl end) eicosapentaenoic (EPA) and docosahexaenoic (DHA) are largely derived from fish oils. The action of these fish oil fatty acids will be discussed later. Very early studies of Kinsell et al (49,50) and Ahrens et al (51) clearly demonstrated that vegetable oils enriched in linoleic acid lowered serum cholesterol levels when substituted for saturated fatty acids. These observations led Keys et al (36) and Hegsted et al (37) to establish equations that quantified the cholesterol-lowering activity of linoleic acid.

The mechanisms by which polyunsaturated fatty acids, such as linoleic acid, lower serum cholesterol and LDL cholesterol levels have been investigated for many years. These mechanisms include: 1) enhanced fecal excretion of cholesterol from the body and 2) reduced synthesis of apo B–containing lipoproteins. More recent evidence from both human and animal studies suggests that substitution of linoleic acid for saturated fatty acids increases the fractional clearance of LDL from the bloodstream by up-regulation of LDL receptor activity (19,20). Although the exact mechanism by which polyunsaturated fatty acids increase LDL receptor activity is not known, hypotheses put forth include: 1) a reduction in hepatic pools of cholesterol that would normally down-regulate the receptor (24) and 2) an increase in membrane fluidity associated with enhanced polyunsaturated fatty acid incorporation into membrane phospholipids resulting in up-regulation of the LDL receptor by increasing binding and internalization of the LDL particle by the LDL receptor (42,43). All of these proposed mechanisms remain to be further established.

Monounsaturated Fatty Acids

More recently, monounsaturated fatty acids, and oleic acid in particular, have been shown to lower total plasma and LDL cholesterol levels when substituted for saturated fatty acids (38,52,53). Although the mechanism is not known with certainty, there are reports indicating that monounsaturates may decrease the suppression of LDL receptor activity that is produced by saturated fatty acids (54).

Although recent investigations have indicated that monounsaturated fatty acids can lower serum LDL levels, these studies have focused on oleic acid, a monounsaturate with the *cis* configuration (the carbon moieties on the two sides of a double bond lie on the same side) as occurs in most natural fats and oils. However, during the process of hydrogenation of polyunsaturated vegetable and fish oils to produce fats that have more firmness and resist rancidity, *trans* fatty acids are formed (unsaturated fatty acids in which the carbon atoms on the two sides of the double bond point in opposite directions). The estimated daily intake of *trans* fatty acids in the United States is 8 to 10 g or 6% to 8% of total fat calories. The most abundant *trans* fatty acids are elaidic acid and its isomers, which are 18-carbon fatty acids with one double bond. Studies to determine whether the *trans* form of oleic acid (elaidic) influences serum cholesterol levels have been inconsistent; one earlier study demonstrated that *trans* unsaturated fatty acids elevated serum cholesterol levels (55), whereas several others (56–60) did not demonstrate an effect. However, a more recent study (61) demonstrated that consumption of a diet enriched in *trans* fatty acids (11% of total fat calories) was associated with increased serum LDL and decreased HDL levels. Additional studies utilizing more reasonable intakes of

trans fatty acid will need to be conducted before any conclusions can be drawn. Since 1972 the amount of *trans* fatty acid available in the American diet has changed very little (7 to 8 g/day), but death from heart disease has fallen markedly during this period. Concern about *trans* fat has been with us since the 1940s. *Trans* fats are absorbed and deposited and also turned over. It has been suggested that *trans* fatty acids be regarded as saturated fatty acids.

Polyunsaturated Fatty Acids (n-3) from Fish Oil

Dietary fish oil studies in animals have been inconsistent, with increases and/or decreases in receptor clearance of LDL being reported. Dietary fish oils enriched in omega-3 fatty acids can influence lipoprotein metabolism by altering key lipolytic and transfer enzymes. The activity of lecithin-cholesterol acyl-transferase (LCAT), the enzyme largely responsible for formation of plasma cholesteryl ester, is significantly increased in rats (62) and cardiac patients (63) fed fish oil. In contrast, fish oil consumption by monkeys (64) and normolipidemic patients (63) reduced LCAT activity.

The effect of fish oil consumption on lipoprotein lipase (LPL) activity, the enzyme which catabolizes TG-rich lipoproteins such as intestinal chylomicrons and hepatic VLDL, has been equivocal, with reports of no effect (62) or striking decreases in activity in rats (65). A decrease in VLDL-TG and apo B production and secretion seems to be the predominant mechanism explaining the striking hypotriglyceridemic effect seen with fish oil consumption. Although the hypotriglyceridemic action of fish oils has been consistently observed, their effect on serum cholesterol levels is less reproducible, for reasons which may include variability in populations studied, dosages and composition of fish oil, and duration of study.

Human studies of the effect of dietary fish oils rich in EPA and DHA on total plasma and LDL cholesterol levels have also been equivocal. Although early studies using pharmacologic doses of fish oil lowered total plasma and LDL cholesterol levels, more recent studies of fish oil consumption have shown small but significant increases in LDL cholesterol (66).

Structured Triglycerides

It has been shown recently that the structure of a triglyceride may influence its atherogenicity for rabbits. The presence of palmitic acid at the SN2, position confers greater atherogenic potential. Tallow and lard both contain about 24% palmitic acid. In tallow about 15% of the palmitic acid is at SN2, whereas in lard 99% is. Lard is significantly more atherogenic than tallow. When the fats are subjected to randomization, which results in 8% of the total palmitic acid being at SN2, they become equivalent in atherogenicity. Cottonseed oil also contains 24% palmitic acid, mostly at SN1 and SN3. Randomization of cottonseed oil results in a fat with 8% palmitic acid at SN2, and that fat is more atherogenic than native cottonseed oil. Randomized fats are no more cholesterolemic than their native counterparts.

High-Carbohydrate Diets

High-carbohydrate diets enriched in monosaccharides, disaccharides, and polysaccharides can also lower LDL cholesterol levels when replacing dietary fat, although the mechanism(s) are not well established. A recent review article by Grundy et al (54) suggests that there may be a reduction in the suppression of LDL receptor activity by saturated fat.

Overproduction of Lipoproteins

Increases in apo B–containing lipoproteins, and LDL cholesterol in particular, may also result from the overproduction of lipoproteins. For example, in obesity associated with excessive caloric intake, an increased production of both VLDL and LDL apo B has been reported (67–69) (see Figure 2-1A). This overproduction of lipoproteins is further augmented if the excessive caloric intake is in the form of saturated fatty acids, which would, in addition, suppress LDL receptor activity (70) (see Figure 2-1B). Excessive alcohol consumption can also enhance VLDL production. Plasma LDL cholesterol can also be increased if a disproportionate increase in the cholesterol moiety occurs relative to LDL apo B. For example, VLDL enriched in cholesterol, as occurs in animals fed excess cholesterol (44,45), can lead to LDL particles also enriched in cholesterol. In humans, LDL can also be enriched in cholesterol by the action of CETP, which can transfer cholesterol from HDL to LDL, and by the LCAT enzyme, which can enrich the LDL particle in cholesterol ester (see Figure 2-1C).

Regulation of HDL

The regulation of HDL levels by environmental factors is only beginning to be understood. Dietary factors that have been demonstrated to influence HDL levels include the type of dietary fat and the level of dietary cholesterol and carbohydrates consumed. For example, human studies have demonstrated that a high-carbohydrate diet decreases levels of HDL by increasing the rate of catabolism of HDL with no effect on HDL synthesis (71). Changing the polyunsaturated-saturated (P/S) fatty acid ratio in the diet from 0.25 to 4.0 in men resulted in significant decreases in HDL cholesterol, which were associated with a decrease in apo A-I production rate with no effect on fractional catabolic rate (72). Similarly, studies in humans demonstrated that changing the diet from a high saturated fat to a low fat intake caused significant reductions in both HDL cholesterol and apo A-I levels, which were significantly correlated with a decrease in apo A-I production rate (73). Animal studies in which the P/S ratio of dietary fat was increased several-fold have also shown reductions in HDL cholesterol and apo A-I that were associated with increases in apo A-I fractional catabolic rate (74,75) and decreases in apo A-I production rate, the latter also associated with a decrease in hepatic mRNA levels of apo A-I (76). It should be mentioned that more modest increases in P/S ratios are not accompanied by decreases in HDL. It is also worth noting that, in most cases, LDL levels fall to a greater extent than HDL levels, giving rise to a favorable LDL/HDL ratio.

Finally, there are no intervention studies that have shown that diet or drug-induced reduction of HDL levels increases the risk of CHD. Other environmental factors that influence HDL levels include certain hormones, increased alcohol consumption, and aerobic exercise. HDL cholesterol and apo A-I levels in women are generally higher than in men, and this observation has been associated with increased apo A-I synthesis in women as compared to men. Estrogen treatment raises HDL levels by prolonging the residence time of apo A-I in women (77). The increase in HDL cholesterol

seen with aerobic exercise is associated with enhanced catabolism of certain components of VLDL remnants and transfer to HDL, as well as prolonged residence time of HDL (78). Alcohol-induced increases in HDL have been reported to result from both decreased HDL catabolism (79) and increased HDL production (80).

Diet and Hemostasis

The mechanisms that explain the effects of diet, and unsaturated fatty acids in particular, on parameters of hemostasis such as platelet function are not well established. However, there is a considerable body of knowledge that indicates that unsaturated fatty acids derived from vegetable oils, i.e., omega-6 fatty acids such as linoleic acid (C18:2) and arachidonic acid (C20:4), induce alterations in platelet function and in endothelial cells distinct from those observed with the omega-3 fatty acids of fish oil (Figure 2-2). Platelets function in hemostasis by aggregating on the exposed surface of collagen of a blood vessel wall in response to injury. The degree of platelet aggregation and vasoconstriction is modulated by the release of prostanoids, whose properties and function can be influenced by the source of unsaturated fatty acids. The prostanoid thromboxane A_2 (TXA_2), produced by platelets in response to the consumption of omega-6 fatty acids, especially linoleic (C18:2) and arachidonic acid (C20:4) derived from vegetable oils, has vasoconstrictor and proaggregatory effects, thereby increasing platelet aggregation (see Figure 2-2). The proaggregatory effects of TXA_2 are normally balanced by the vasodilating, antiaggregatory properties of PGI_2, a prostanoid secreted by endothelial cells of blood vessel walls. However, if the effects of TXA_2 released by the platelet exceed those of PGI_2 released by the endothelium, a shift in favor of thrombus formation results. In response to fish oil consumption, the omega-3 fatty acids (EPA and DHA) are incorporated into platelet phospholipids, reducing the synthesis of the proaggregatory TXA_2 in favor of TXA_3, which has little biologic activity. In addition, consumption of fish oil enhances the antithrombotic environment by inducing endothelial cells to produce PGI_3, which acts in concert with PGI_2 to maintain the antiaggregatory property of the latter.

PATHOBIOLOGY OF ATHEROSCLEROSIS: ROLE OF HYPERCHOLESTEROLEMIA AND ALTERED HEMOSTASIS

The role of hypercholesterolemia and hemostasis in the development of atherosclerosis as described in the following section represents a synthesis of information derived from the reviews by Ross (81), Steinberg et al (82), and Nicolosi et al (83). Elevated serum cholesterol levels associated with the uptake by arteries of atherogenic lipoproteins such as LDL, VLDL remnants, and/or beta-VLDL appear to be a necessary prerequisite for initiating atherogenesis (Figure 2-3). The enhanced uptake of these atherogenic lipoproteins may be associated with nonspecific endothelial dysfunction or with endothelial injury resulting from risk factors such as hypertension, smoking, or diabetes. If endothelial dysfunction exists, once these lipoproteins move into the subintimal space, their residence time may be extended by their interaction with

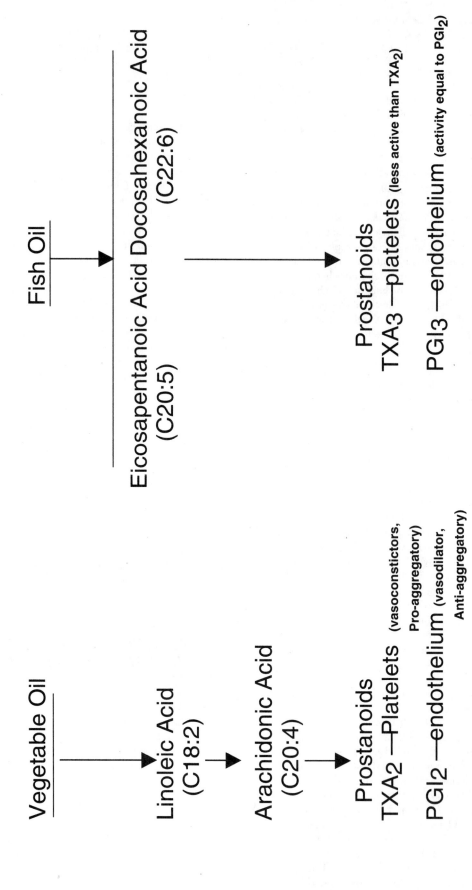

Figure 2-2 Abbreviated flowchart of prostanoid formation.

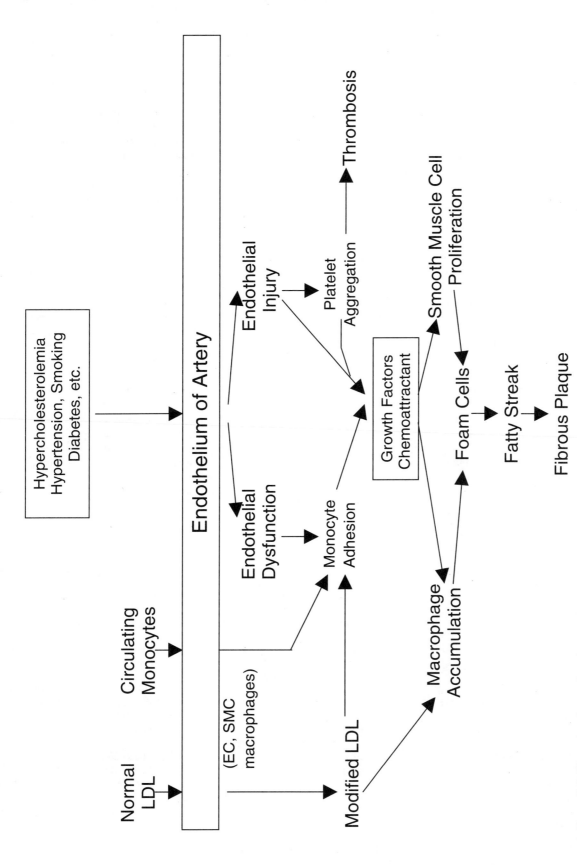

Figure 2-3 Steps in atherosclerosis.

proteoglycans, substances that make up the connective tissue matrix of the blood vessel wall and bind avidly to apo B–containing lipoproteins such as LDL and VLDL remnants. This increase in the residence time of these lipoproteins provides a greater opportunity for oxidative modification of LDL. Oxidized LDL acts as a chemoattractant, causing more monocytes to adhere to and penetrate the endothelium. In the presence of endothelial dysfunction, the increased adhesion of monocytes to the endothelial surface results in their release of growth factors and chemoattractants. As more monocytes penetrate the endothelium and move into the subendothelial space, they are converted to macrophages. Macrophages, having receptors for modified LDL, can take up more of the modified LDL, forming many intracellular cholesterol ester–laden lipid droplets, ultimately resulting in conversion of the macrophage into a foam cell. These foam cells, engorged with oxidized lipid and apoproteins, may lyse, releasing their content into the extracellular space. This oxidized material is cytotoxic and causes further endothelial injury.

Thus a vicious cycle develops, in which progressive endothelial injury and foam cell production occurs, accelerated by the presence of other risk factors. Ultimately, in response to progressive endothelial injury platelets begin to adhere to the exposed underlying connective tissue and become activated, leading to the release of TXA_2, a vasoconstrictor that further enhances platelet aggregation. In response to increased platelet aggregation, platelet-derived growth factor (PDGF) and similar growth factors released by monocytes, smooth muscle cells, and altered endothelial cells stimulate smooth muscle cell migration and proliferation at the site of injury. These steps initiate the conversion of smooth muscle cell–derived foam cells to fatty streaks. With the con-

comitant increase in connective tissue formation and adhering thrombi, these fatty streaks can be converted to fibrous plaques, and further narrowing of the lumen of the artery results, eventually leading to thrombosis, luminal occlusion, and myocardial infarction.

The exact mechanisms by which risk factors directly affect the development of atherosclerosis is not well understood, but there are some general principles that are operative. As already mentioned, it is likely that hypercholesterolemia, associated in particular with elevations of atherogenic lipoproteins, increases the infiltration of lipoproteins into the arterial wall, thereby enhancing the accumulation of intramural cholesterol. In response to the uptake of cholesterol by macrophages and smooth muscle cells, foam cells are formed, leading to a cascade of events that ultimately transforms the fatty streak into the advanced lesion and the fibrous plaque. Hypertension contributes to the increased risk of atherosclerosis by enhancing the uptake of lipoproteins into the blood vessel wall and also by causing subsequent endothelial damage from the increased shear forces that result from the increase in blood pressure. Cigarette smoking probably increases the risk of atherosclerosis by multiple mechanisms, but many of the toxic products of cigarette smoke can induce hypoxia of the arterial wall, which can reduce circulating antioxidant levels so that more oxidized LDL is produced, leading to increased macrophage-derived foam cell formation and the development of subsequent fatty streaks and fibrous plaques. Diabetes may promote the development of atherosclerosis by a combination of increases in serum lipid levels, modifications of lipoproteins, and enhanced production of growth factors and chemoattractants that may act together to accelerate the development of atherosclerosis.

REFERENCES

1. Utermann G. Lipoprotein (a): a genetic risk factor for premature coronary heart disease. Curr Opin Lipidol 1990;1:404–410.

2. Loscalzo J. Lipoprotein (a): a unique risk factor for atherothrombotic disease. Arteriosclerosis 1990;10:672–679.

3. Armstrong VW, Cremer P, Eberle E, et al. The association between Lp(a) concentrations and angiographically assessed coronary atherosclerosis—dependence on serum LDL levels. Atherosclerosis 1986;62:249–257.

4. Rath M, Niendorf A, Reblin T, et al. Detection and quantification of lipoprotein (a) in the arterial wall of 107 coronary bypass patients. Arteriosclerosis 1989;9:579–592.

5. Cushing GL, Ganbatz JW, Nava ML, et al. Quantitation and localization of apolipoprotein (a) and B

in coronary artery bypass vein grafts resected at re-operation. Arteriosclerosis 1989;9:593–603.

6. Utermann G, Steinmetz A, Weber W. Genetic control of human apolipoprotein e polymorphism: comparison of one- and two-dimensional techniques of isoprotein analysis. Hum Genet 1982;60:344–351.

7. Schaefer EJ, Levy RI. Pathogenesis and management of lipoprotein disorders. N Engl J Med 1985;312:1300–1310.

8. Reardon MD, Poapst ME, Steiner G. The independent synthesis of intermediate density lipoproteins in Type III hyperlipoproteinemia. Metabolism 1982;31:421–427.

9. Soutar AK, Myant NB, Thompson GR. Simultaneous measurement of apolipoprotein B turnover in very low and low density lipoproteins in

familial hypercholesterolemia. Atherosclerosis 1977;28:247–256.

10. Naraya N, Chung BH, Tauntin OD. Synthesis of plasma lipoproteins by the isolated perfused liver from the fasted and fed pig. J Biol Chem 1977;252:5258–5261.

11. Huff MW, Telford DE. Direct synthesis of low density lipoprotein apoprotein B in the miniature pig. Metabolism 1985;34:36–42.

12. Spady DK, Dietschy JM. Interaction of dietary cholesterol and triglycerides in the regulation of hepatic low density lipoprotein transport in the hamster. J Clin Invest 1988;81:300–309.

13. Spady DK, Turley SD, Dietschy JM. Rates of low density lipoprotein uptake and cholesterol synthesis are regulated independently in the liver. J Lipid Res 1985;26:465–472.

14. Kesaniemi YA, Witzum JL, Steinbrecher UP. Receptor mediated catabolism of low density lipoprotein in man: quantitation using glycosolated low density lipoprotein. J Clin Invest 1983;71: 950–959.

15. Bilheimer DW, Watanabe Y, Kita T. Impaired receptor-mediated catabolism of low density lipoprotein in the WHHL rabbit, an animal model of familial hypercholesterolemia. Proc Natl Acad Sci USA 1982;79: 3305–3309.

16. Kovanen PT, Brown MS, Basu SK, et al. Saturation and suppression of hepatic lipoprotein receptors: a mechanism for the hypercholesterolemia of cholesterol-fed rabbits. Proc Natl Acad Sci USA 1981;78:1396–1400.

17. Packard CJ, McKinney L, Carr K, et al. Cholesterol feeding increases low density lipoprotein synthesis. J Clin Invest 1983;72:45–51.

18. Shepherd J, Packard CJ, Grundy SM, et al. Effects of saturated and polyunsaturated fat diets on the chemical composition and metabolism of low density lipoproteins in man. J Lipid Res 1980;21:91–99.

19. Spady DK, Dietschy JM. Dietary saturated triacylglycerols suppress hepatic low density lipoprotein receptors in the hamster. Proc Soc Natl Acad Sci USA 1985;82: 4526–4530.

20. Nicolosi RJ, Stucchi AF, Kowala MC, et al. Effect of dietary fat saturation and cholesterol on LDL composition and metabolism. Arteriosclerosis 1990;10:119–128.

21. Windler EE, Kovanen PT, Chao YS, et al. The estradiol-stimulated lipoprotein receptor of rat liver: a binding site that membrane mediates the uptake of rat lipoproteins containing apoproteins B and E. J Biol Chem 1980;255:10464–10471.

22. Miller NE. Why does plasma low density lipoprotein concentration in adults increase with age? Lancet 1984;1:263–266.

23. Grundy SM, Vega GL, Bilheimer DW. Kinetic mechanisms determining variability in low density lipoprotein levels and their rise with age. Arteriosclerosis 1985;5: 623–630.

24. Brown MS, Goldstein JL. A receptor-mediated pathway for cholesterol homeostasis. Science 1986;232:34–47.

25. Krempler F, Kostner GM, Rascher A, et al. Studies on the role of specific cell surface receptors in the removal of lipoprotein (a) in man. J Clin Invest 1983;71: 1431–1441.

26. Hackes L, Jurgens G, Holasek A, et al. In vivo studies on the binding sites for lipoprotein (a) in parenchymal and nonparenchymal rat liver cells. FEBS Lett 1988; 227:27–31.

27. Karadi I, Kostner GM, Gries A, et al. Lipoprotein (a) and plasminogen are immunochemically related. Biochim Biophys Acta 1988;960: 91–97.

28. Oram JF. Cholesterol trafficking in cells. Curr Opin Lipidol 1990;1: 416–421.

29. Rifai N. Lipoproteins and apolipoproteins—composition, metabolism and association with coronary heart disease. Arch Pathol Lab Med 1986;110:694–701.

30. Kesaniemi YA, Miettinen TA. Cholesterol absorption efficiency regulates plasma cholesterol level in the Finnish population. Eur J Clin Invest 1987;17:391–395.

31. Kesaniemi YA, Ehnholm C, Miettinen TA. Intestinal cholesterol absorption efficiency in man is related to apoprotein E phenotype. J Clin Invest 1987;80:578–581.

32. Miettinen TA, Kesaniemi YA. Cholesterol absorption: regulation of cholesterol synthesis and elimination and within population variations of serum cholesterol levels. Am J Clin Nutr 1989;49: 629–635.

33. McNamara DJ, Kolb R, Parker TS, et al. Heterogeneity of cholesterol homeostasis in man. J Clin Invest 1987;79:1729–1739.

34. Miettenen TA. Fecal fat bile acid excretion, and body height in familial hypercholesterolemia and hypertriglyceridemia. Scand J Clin Lab Invest 1972;30:85–88.

35. Howell WH, McNamara DJ, Tosca MA, et al. Plasma lipid and lipoprotein responses to dietary fat and cholesterol: a meta-analysis. Am J Clin Nutr 1997;65: 1747–1764.

36. Keys A, Anderson JT, Frande F. Serum cholesterol response to changes in the diet. IV. Particular saturated fatty acids in the diet. Metabolism 1965;14: 776–787.

37. Hegsted DM, McGandy RB, Myers ML, et al. Quantitative effects of dietary fat on serum cholesterol in man. Am J Clin Nutr 1965;17: 281–295.

38. Mattson FH, Grundy SM. Comparison of effects of dietary saturated, monounsaturated and polyunsaturated fatty acids on plasma lipids and lipoproteins in man. J Lipid Res 1985;26:194–202.

39. Grundy SM, Vega GL. Plasma cholesterol responsiveness to saturated fatty acids. Am J Clin Nutr 1988;47:822–824.

40. Bonanome A, Grundy SM. Effect of dietary stearic acid on plasma cholesterol and lipoprotein levels. N Eng J Med 1988;318:1244–1248.

41. Fox JC, McGill Jr HC, Carey KD, et al. In vivo regulation of hepatic LDL receptor mRNA in the baboon: differential effects of saturated and unsaturated fat. J Biol Chem 1987;262:7014–7020.

42. Kuo PC, Rudd MA, Nicolosi RJ, et al. Effect of dietary fat saturation and cholesterol on low density lipoprotein degradation by mononuclear cells of cebus monkeys. Arteriosclerosis 1989;9:919–927.

43. Loscalzo JL, Freedman J, Rudd MA, et al. Unsaturated fatty acids enhance low density lipoprotein uptake and degradation by peripheral blood mononuclear cells. Arteriosclerosis 1987;7:450–455.

44. Noel S-P, Wong L, Dolphin PJ, et al. Secretion of cholesterol-rich

lipoproteins by perfused livers of hypercholesterolemic rats. J Clin Invest 1979;64:674–683.

45. Swift LL, Manowitz NR, Dun GD, et al. Cholesterol and saturated fat diet induces hepatic synthesis of cholesterol-rich lipoproteins. Clin Res 1979;27:378A.

46. Grande F. Dog serum lipid responses to dietary fats differing in the chain length of the saturated fatty acids. J Nutr 1962;76:255–264.

47. Hashim SA, Arteaga A, van Itallie TB. Effect of a saturated medium-chain triglyceride on serum lipids in man. Lancet 1960;1:1105–1108.

48. St. John LC, Young CR, Knabe DA, et al. Fatty acid profiles and sensory and carcass traits of tissues from steers and swine fed an elevated monounsaturated fat diet. J Anim Sci 1987;64:1441–1447.

49. Kinsell LW, Partridge WJ, Boling L, et al. Dietary modification of serum cholesterol and phospholipid levels. J Clin Endocrinol 1952;12:909–913.

50. Kinsell LW, Michaels GD, Partridge JW, et al. Effect upon serum cholesterol and phospholipids of diets containing large amounts of vegetable fat. J Clin Nutr 1953;1:231–244.

51. Ahrens EH, Hirsch J, Insull W, et al. The influence of dietary fats on serum-lipid levels in man. Lancet 1957;1:943–953.

52. Mensink RP, Katan MB. Effect of a diet enriched with monounsaturated or polyunsaturated fatty acids on levels of low density and high density lipoprotein cholesterol in healthy women and men. N Engl J Med 1989;321:436–441.

53. Dreon DM, Vranizan KM, Krauss RM, et al. The effects of polyunsaturated fat vs monounsaturated fat on plasma lipoproteins. JAMA 1990;263:2462–2466.

54. Grundy SM, Denke MA. Dietary influences on serum lipids and lipoproteins. J Lipid Res 1990;31:1149–1172.

55. Vergroesen AJ. Dietary fat and cardiovascular disease: possible modes of action of linoleic acid. Proc Nutr Soc 1972;31:323–329.

56. Grasso S, Gunning B, Imaichi K, et al. Effects of natural and hydrogenated fats of approximately equal dienoic acid content upon plasma lipids. Metabolism 1962;11:920–924.

57. McOsker DE, Mattson FH, Swerningen HB, et al. The influence of partially hydrogenated dietary fats on serum cholesterol levels. JAMA 1962;180:380–385.

58. Erickson BA, Coots RH, Mattson FH, et al. The effect of partial hydrogenation of dietary fats, of the ratio of polyunsaturated to saturated fatty acids and of dietary cholesterol upon plasma lipids in man. J Clin Invest 1964;43:2017–2025.

59. Mattson FH, Hollenback EJ, Kligman AM. Effect of hydrogenated fat on plasma cholesterol and triglyceride levels of man. Am J Clin Nutr 1975;28:726–731.

60. Laine DC, Snodgrass CM, Dawson EA, et al. Lightly hydrogenated soy oil versus other vegetable oils as a lipid lowering dietary constituent. Am J Clin Nutr 1982;35:583–590.

61. Mensink RP, Katan MB. Effect of dietary trans fatty acids on high density and low density lipoprotein cholesterol levels in healthy subjects. N Eng J Med 1990;323:439–445.

62. David JSK, Bazzan A, Weaver J, et al. Cholesterol lowering mechanism by omega 3 fatty acids in rat models. Arteriosclerosis 1987;7:535a.

63. Davis JSK, de Pace N, Noval J, et al. Cholesterol-lowering mechanism of fish oil rich in omega 3 fatty acids in cardiac patients. Arteriosclerosis 1987;7:512b.

64. Parks JS, Bullock BC, Rudel LL. The reactivity of plasma phospholipids with lecithin: cholesterol acyl transferase is decreased in fish oil-fed monkeys. J Biol Chem 1989;264:2545–2551.

65. Haug A, Hostmark AT. Lipoprotein lipases, lipoproteins and tissue lipids in rats fed fish oil or coconut oil. J Nutr 1987;117:1011–1016.

66. Failor RA, Childs MT, Bierman E. The effects of omega-3 and omega-6 fatty acid enriched diets on plasma lipoprotein and apoproteins in familial combined hyperlipidemia. Metabolism 1988;37:1021–1027.

67. Kesaniemi YA, Grundy SM. Increased low density lipoprotein production associated with obesity. Arteriosclerosis 1983;3:170–177.

68. Kesaniemi YA, Beltz WF, Grundy SM. Comparisons of metabolism of apolipoprotein B in normal subjects, obese patients and patients with coronary heart disease. J Clin Invest 1985;76:586–595.

69. Egusa G, Beltz WF, Grundy SM, et al. The influence of obesity on the metabolism of apolipoprotein B in man. J Clin Invest 1985;76:596–603.

70. Cagguila AW, Christakis G, Ferrand M, et al. The multiple risk factor intervention trial (MRFIT) IV: intervention on blood lipids. Prev Med 1981;10:443–475.

71. Blum CB, Levy RI, Eisenberg S, et al. High density lipoprotein metabolism in man. J Clin Invest 1977;60:795–807.

72. Shepherd J, Packard CJ, Patsch JR, et al. Effects of dietary polyunsaturated and saturated fat on the properties of high density lipoprotein and metabolism of apolipoprotein A-I. J Clin Invest 1978;61:1582–1592.

73. Brinton EA, Eisenberg S, Breslow JL. Elevated high density lipoprotein cholesterol levels correlate with decreased apolipoprotein A-I and A-II fractional catabolism rate in women. J Clin Invest 1989;84:262–269.

74. Chong KS, Nicolosi RJ, Rodger RF, et al. Effect of dietary fat saturation on plasma lipoproteins and high density lipoprotein metabolism of the rhesus monkey. J Clin Invest 1987;79:675–683.

75. Parks JS, Rudel LL. Different kinetic fates of apolipoproteins A-I and A-II from lymph chylomicra of nonhuman primates: effect of saturated vs polyunsaturated dietary fat. J Lipid Res 1982;23:410–421.

76. Sorci-Thomas M, Prack MM, Dashti N, et al. Differential effects of dietary fat on the tissue-specific expression of the apolipoprotein A-I gene: relationship to plasma concentration of high density lipoproteins. J Lipid Res 1989;30:1397–1403.

77. Hazzard WR, Haffner SM, Kushwaha RS, et al. Preliminary report: kinetic studies on the modulation of high density lipoprotein, apolipoprotein, and subfraction metabolism by sex steroids in a post-menopausal woman. Metabolism 1984;33:779–784.

78. Herbert PN, Bernier DN, Cullinane EM, et al. High density lipoprotein metabolism in runners and sedentary men. JAMA 1984;252:1034–1037.

79. Cluett-Brown J, Mullitan J, Igoe F, et al. Ethanol induced alterations in low and high density lipoproteins. Proc Soc Exp Biol Med 1985;178:495–500.

80. Baraona E, Lieber CS. Effects of chronic ethanol feeding on serum lipoprotein metabolism in the rat. J Clin Invest 1970;49:769–777.

81. Ross R. The pathogenesis of atherosclerosis—an update. N Engl J Med 1986;314:488–500.

82. Steinberg D, Parthasarathy S, Carew TE, et al. Modifications of low-density lipoprotein that increase its atherogenicity. N Engl J Med 1989;320:915–924.

83. Nicolosi RJ, Stucchi AF. n-3 Fatty acids and atherosclerosis. Curr Opin Lipidol 1990;1:442–448.

Chapter 3

The Rationale for Intervention to Reduce the Risk of Coronary Artery Disease

James M. Rippe
Diane O'Brien

Coronary artery disease (CAD) is the leading cause of both morbidity and mortality in the United States and many other industrialized nations. Each year in the United States CAD is the leading cause of death for both men and women and results in one half of the approximately one million deaths each year from all forms of cardiovascular disease (1). Each year over 1.4 million individuals in the United States suffer acute myocardial infarction, causing enormous health and economic burdens. It is estimated that coronary artery disease alone results in between $50 and $100 billion dollars per year in direct medical expenses and other associated costs (2,3).

There has been a significant and encouraging downward trend in death rates from coronary artery disease in the United States since the 1960s. Between 1963 and 1990, mortality from coronary artery disease fell over 50% and accounted for half of the decline in total mortality rates in the United States during this period of time (4). Importantly, these decreases have coincided with the identification of risk factors for CAD and a national effort to reduce these risks, which began in the late 1960s and has continued since that time. Major national campaigns have been launched to reduce major risk factors for coronary artery disease such as hypercholesterolemia, hypertension, and smoking. In addition, advances have occurred in the treatment of acute myocardial infarction, unstable angina, and angina, further contributing to declines in mortality from CAD.

In the 1990s, efforts to identify and lower risk factors have continued and expanded. The increasingly sedentary lifestyle in the United States has now been recognized as a major risk factor for coronary artery disease. In a statement published in 1995, the American Heart Association listed an inactive lifestyle as a major risk factor for CAD (5). In 1998, the AHA upgraded obesity from a contributing to "major" risk factor for coronary artery disease.

Despite the heightened awareness of the desirability of lowering risk factors for coronary artery disease the record has been somewhat inconsistent, particularly in the areas of lifestyle management for risk factor reduction. On the positive side, the percentage of Americans who smoke has decreased by 37% since the mid-1960s (1). However, recent evidence suggests that there has now been a leveling off in the decline of cigarette smoking and this dangerous habit may have actually increased in some groups, such as young women (6).

The annual death rate from hypertension has declined dramatically between 1950 and 1991 from 56.0 per 100,000 to 6.5 per 100,000 in 1991 (1). However, despite years of effort, hypertension remains poorly controlled on a population basis in the United States (7,8). Approximately one half of individuals who have high blood pressure are unaware of this condition (9). Of those individuals who are aware of their high blood pressure less than 20% are adequately controlled (7).

The average cholesterol levels in the United States have declined from 220 mg/dL in 1960 to 205 mg/dL in 1991 (4). Nevertheless, it is estimated that over 30% of women and over 25% of men in the United States still have elevated blood cholesterol (10).

Physical activity levels remain far too low in the United States. It has been estimated that less than 25% of individuals achieve appropriate levels of physical activity in the United States (11). Slightly over 50% of individuals achieve some intermittent physical activity, and 25% of individuals are entirely sedentary people. These numbers are far below the desired levels of at least 30% of individuals achieving adequate levels of physical activity hoped for in the Healthy People 2000 initiative (12).

Perhaps in the area of obesity the most serious problem related to cardiovascular disease has emerged and is growing at an alarming pace. In the period between 1980 and 1990 the percentage of individuals considered overweight or obese increased from 25% of the population to 35% of the population (13,14). This represents a shocking 40% relative increase in the prevalence of overweight and obesity in the United States. Obesity has been clearly associated with other risk factors for coronary artery disease such as hypertension (15–17), dyslipidemias (18–20), and diabetes (21–23). Moreover, obesity is independently associated with an increased risk of coronary artery disease (24–27).

The primary clinical modality to lower CAD morbidity and mortality is risk factor reduction. Numerous population-based studies have shown that lowering risk factors such as cigarette smoking, elevated cholesterol, and high blood pressure can significantly reduce the burden of coronary artery disease on the population (28–30).

The purpose of this chapter is to provide an overall rationale for risk factor reduction, with a particular emphasis on lifestyle measures that have been shown to be effective in reducing risk factors for CAD. The next chapter in this section will focus more specifically on clinical strategies for incorporating these risk factor reduction strategies into everyday medical practice.

THE CONCEPT OF RISK FACTORS

The concept of risk factors for coronary artery disease represented a major advance in strategies designed to prevent CAD. A variety of studies, perhaps most prominently the Framingham study (31), showed that certain factors such as high blood pressure (32–35), cigarette smoking (36–39), dyslipidemia (40–44), and diabetes mellitus (45–48) all independently significantly increase the risk of CAD. Recently, both physical inactivity (5) and obesity (6) have been added to the category of "major" risk factors for coronary artery disease. Although the presence of any one of the major risk factors for heart disease significantly increases the risk of CAD, Framingham study data also clearly established that risk factors tend to act synergistically with each other (49). Thus, the presence of two or more risk factors quadrupled the risk of CAD, whereas the presence of three risk factors increased the risk of CAD from eightfold to twentyfold compared to individuals who had no risk factors (50). Other risk factors for CAD, as established by the Framingham study and other studies, include age, gender, family history of CAD, certain hemostatic factors, hypertriglyceridemia, excessive alcohol consumption, elevated homocystine levels, and perhaps stress and certain psychological factors (1).

Identification of risk factors provides a potent mechanism for decreasing coronary artery disease through the reduction of those factors that are modifiable. Numerous studies have shown that reduction of major risk factors for CAD can significantly lower its likelihood (51,52). The advantage of utilizing lifestyle measures as part of the treatment plan to lower risk factors for CAD resides not only in the independent effect of these lifestyle measures on specific risk factors but also the fact that such lifestyle measures as proper nutrition, increased physical activity, and proper management of body weight can synergistically affect multiple other risk factors for CAD, in addition to removing or diminishing the specific risk factor that they are designed for (15,50,53).

RELATIVE RISK VERSUS ABSOLUTE RISK

There is a critical difference between the concept of "relative" risk and "absolute" risk that underlies treatment strategies for risk factor reduction. Relative risk represents the ratio of the chance that an individual with a specific risk factor for CHD will develop CHD compared to the chance of an individual without the specific risk factor. Absolute risk represents the probability of developing CAD over a finite period of time, such as over the next 10 years.

A young adult with either high serum cholesterol or hypertension provides a good example of how the difference between relative and absolute risk is applied to clinical decision making. A young individual with either of these risk factors for CAD is unlikely to develop this condition over the next 10 years, but his or her chances of developing CAD over an extended period of time (such as before the age of 70) are high.

In a sense, relative risk indicates how rapidly a person acquires absolute risk. Numerous studies have shown that individuals and young adults who have high relative risk ultimately develop high absolute risk (54–56). Thus, the goal for reducing either high blood pressure or elevated cholesterol in young adults is to slow the process of developing coronary artery disease over an extended period rather than lowering the absolute risk of CAD or its manifestations over the next 10 years (57).

This concept is particularly relevant to lifestyle measures, which carry little expense or risk and can significantly alter both relative and absolute risk of CAD. In contrast, extensive pharmaceutical therapy may not be appropriate in young adults. Treatment strategies must be based on both the concepts of relative risk and absolute risk.

PRIMARY VERSUS SECONDARY PREVENTION

The distinction between primary and secondary prevention also carries important clinical ramifications. The same level of aggressive therapy that has been demonstrated to be efficacious in secondary prevention is typically often not warranted in primary prevention (52,58).

Primary prevention refers to efforts to modify risk factors or, in the best-case scenario, prevent their development with the goal of delaying or preventing new onset of coronary artery disease. *Secondary prevention* refers to therapeutic measures designed to reduce the likelihood of current cardiovascular events and mortality in patients in whom CAD is already established (59). Secondary prevention is thus focused both on lowering risk factors and on measures designed to prevent plaque eruption in coronary arteries that are already diseased. In a sense, this expanded view of secondary prevention should also be viewed as treatment of coronary artery disease. This approach is justified because once individuals have manifestations of coronary artery disease, they are at much higher risk for developing acute coronary syndromes. Those entities that would qualify for secondary prevention include a variety of manifestations of CAD such as a history of documented myocardial infarction, angina pectoris, previous coronary artery procedures (angioplasty or coronary artery bypass grafting), symptomatic coronary artery disease, peripheral vascular disease, or aortic aneurysm. In individuals with these conditions, the American Heart Association has established guidelines for secondary prevention (60).

A variety of frameworks are available in the area of primary prevention of CAD. Perhaps the most widely used is the Framingham Risk Scoring System, which was updated and expanded in 1998 (31). These scores reflect absolute risk predictions and do not apply to individuals who have already established coronary artery disease.

ANIMAL STUDIES

A detailed discussion of the pathobiology of atherosclerosis is found in Chapter 2. Much of the early information related to the development of atherosclerosis came from animal models. Although a detailed discussion of this literature is beyond the scope of this chapter, key studies will be briefly highlighted.

It has been demonstrated that atherosclerosis in animal models, particularly monkeys and swine, resembles that seen in humans although it develops over a shorter period of time (61–65). In one early experiment, Taylor et al fed rhesus monkeys a highly atherogenic diet, causing their cholesterol to rise from 150 mg/dL (on control) to an average of 382 mg/dL on the high-fat diet (62). This investigation demonstrated that when serum cholesterol levels remain below 200 mg/dL atherosclerotic lesions did not develop. Manifestations of atherosclerotic disease in both coronary arteries and peripheral arteries were observed that resembled those in humans, both in terms of distribution and characteristics. The nature of the atherosclerotic plaque, including necrotic core, cholesterol clefts, and fibrous cap, found in these animals was similar to that found in humans. Subsequent animal studies have shown that lowering cholesterol into the 130- to 145-mg/dL range can result in regression of lesions (66,67). These studies paved the way for modern trials of both lifestyle therapy and pharmaceutical therapy showing regression of atherosclerotic plaque in human beings following significant reductions in cholesterol levels.

In one animal model, Kaplan et al investigated the effect of social environment and social status on coronary artery disease and other manifestations of atherosclerosis in male monkeys (68). This study is useful since it provides an example of how complex behavior applicable to human beings may interact with risk factors to potentially stimulate the development of coronary atherosclerosis. Experimental animals were divided into six groups, and all animals were fed a moderately atherogenic diet containing 43% of calories from fat and high levels of cholesterol for 22 months. On this diet their mean serum cholesterol rose to 471 ± 83 mg/dL. The monkeys were then assigned to different social groups. Those monkeys considered "dominant" and put in an unstable social condition developed significantly higher levels of

atherosclerosis than did either subordinate monkeys who were in a stable social condition or dominant monkeys in such a stable condition. This type of experiment has shown that factors other than simply cholesterol levels can contribute to atherosclerosis.

HUMAN STUDIES

A wide variety of human studies conducted in the last 25 years have provided strong evidence for the link between risk factors and development of coronary artery disease. Other studies have shown modification of risk factors can result in substantial reduction in the likelihood of developing coronary artery disease. These studies can be conveniently divided into observational studies involving large population groups and interventional studies.

Observational Studies

Important information concerning the link between individual risk factors and combinations of risk factors has come from observational studies such as the Framingham study (27), the Nurses' Health Study (35), the U.S. Male Professional Health Study (26), and the Multiple Risk Factor Intervention Trial (MRFIT) (69). In all of these studies elevations of individual risk factors for coronary artery disease have been associated with significant increases in the likelihood of developing this entity.

Interventional Studies

A variety of interventional studies have shown that reduction of risk factors is an effective tool, both in primary prevention and secondary prevention of coronary artery disease. Most of these studies have focused on individual risk factors and will be handled in sections on each respective factor later in this chapter.

RISK FACTORS THAT CAN BE MODIFIED

Numerous studies have focused on the relationship between risk factors that can be modified and the development of coronary artery disease. These studies have provided important information related to linkages between a specific risk factor and coronary artery disease as well as the response to interventions designed to reduce this risk factor. Those modifiable risk factors that have been studied in detail include dyslipidemias, hypertension, tobacco use, physical inactivity, and obesity.

Dyslipidemias

A variety of dyslipidemias have been demonstrated to increase the risk of coronary artery disease. Lipids are carried through the blood plasma combined in complex water-soluble molecules containing cholesterol and triglycerides covered by a layer of phospholipids, cholesterol, and apolipoproteins. Various plasma lipoproteins can be distinguished by size, density, and proteins on their surface. A variety of lipid fractions and lipoproteins have been demonstrated to be atherogenic (see Chapter 2).

Hypercholesterolemia

Of all the dyslipidemias, hypercholesterolemia has been most clearly associated with the increased risk of coronary artery disease. Elevated plasma levels of LDL have been particularly associated with elevated incidences of CAD. Approximately 70% of the cholesterol in the blood is carried in LDL. Reduction of LDL is a primary target for intervention in the guidelines established by the National Cholesterol Education Program (52) (see Chapter 4). The association between elevated blood cholesterol and coronary artery disease has been established by both observational studies and interventional studies. The MRFIT study, the Nurses' Health Study, and the U.S. Male Health Professional Study have all demonstrated that elevated blood cholesterol increases risk of coronary artery disease (52).

A variety of interventional studies have demonstrated both that elevated blood cholesterol is associated with coronary artery disease and that reduction of blood cholesterol will reduce the incidence of CAD. The Lipid Clinic's Research Coronary Primary Prevention Trial (LRC-CPPT) randomized over 3800 hypercholesterolemic men (total cholesterol ≥ 265 mg/dL, LDL cholesterol ≥ 190 mg/dL, triglyceride ≤ 300 mg/dL) aged 35 to 59 years, half of whom received cholestyramine to lower cholesterol and the other half of whom received a placebo (70). Those who received cholestyramine reduced their blood cholesterol levels an average of 13% from baseline, whereas the placebo group on diet alone reduced cholesterol 5% on average. In the cholestyramine group, nonfatal myocardial infarction was reduced 19% and development of new onset angina was reduced 20%. Other trials of primary prevention have consistently demonstrated that lowering cholesterol will lower the likelihood of new onset coronary artery disease. Trials that have demonstrated this include the Helsinki Heart Study (71), the Oslo Study Diet and Antismoking Trial (72), the World Health Organization Cooperative Trial (73), and the West of Scotland Coronary Prevention Study (74).

A variety of studies have also shown that lowering cholesterol is highly effective in secondary prevention. Individuals who already have coronary artery disease are at highest short-term risk for a CAD event. Aggressive intervention to lower cholesterol has been repeatedly shown to lower that risk. Although a detailed description of the numerous trials to demonstrate the effectiveness of lowering cholesterol to lower the risk of CAD is beyond the scope of this chapter, some of the trials will be listed in this section and are summarized in Table 3-1.

Major interventional trials that have demonstrated lowering risk of CAD with aggressive secondary intervention include the Coronary Drug Project (75), The National Heart, Lung, and Blood Institute Type II Coronary Artery Intervention Study (76), the Cholesterol Lowering Atherosclerosis Study (CLAS) (77), the Familial Atherosclerosis Treatment Study (FATS) (78), the St. Thomas Atherosclerosis Regression Study (STARS) (79), the Program for the Surgical Control of Hyperlipidemias (POSCH) (80), and others as summarized in Table 3-1. These studies have been remarkably consistent in demonstrating that lowering cholesterol levels in individuals with established coronary artery disease significantly reduces the risk of complications of this entity.

It is worth pointing out that several epidemiologic studies have found an increased mortality at very low cholesterol levels (81–83). Although the exact definition of low cholesterol has not been firmly established, many experts consider total cholesterol levels below 160 mg/dL to be low. Studies that have shown an association between very low levels of cholesterol and increased mortality may have been confounded by diseases that cause a decrease in cholesterol. In both the LRC-CPP Trial and Helsinki Heart Study, increases in accidental and violent deaths were reported in individuals with low cholesterol levels; however, when these data were reanalyzed, it appeared that these deaths were unrelated to cholesterol levels (84). At this juncture it appears that although this may represent a clinically relevant consideration, conclusive evidence is lacking to establish a cause-and-effect relationship between low cholesterol levels and cardiac deaths.

Low High-Density Lipoprotein Cholesterol

Low HDL cholesterol increases the risk of CAD. Conversely, elevated HDL appears to have the protective effect of lowering the risk of CAD (85,86). The exact mechanism by which HDL lowers the risk of CAD is not well understood. It has been proposed that HDL is a possible vehicle for reverse cholesterol transport, which may decrease atherosclerosis.

Low HDL cholesterol has been defined as HDL lower than 35 mg/dL and is considered an independent risk for CAD in the most recent National Cholesterol Education Guidelines (52). The major therapy for low HDL cholesterol involves regular exercise, smoking cessation, and weight reduction. Thus, lifestyle management plays an important role in treating low HDL cholesterol.

Hypertriglyceridemia

There is a clear linkage between elevated plasma triglycerides and CAD, although this relationship is not as well established as the relationship between elevated cholesterol and CAD (87). According to NCEP guidelines, a triglyceride of less than 200 mg/dL is considered normal, 200 to 400 mg/dL is borderline high, and 400 to 1000 mg/dL is high. A triglyceride level greater than 1000 mg/dL is considered very high (52). As in the case of low HDL cholesterol, primary therapy for hypertriglyceridemia includes a variety of lifestyle modifications, including dietary modifications, weight control, regular exercise, and smoking cessation and, in some patients, alcohol restriction.

Elevated Lipoprotein (a)

Elevated Lp(a) level has been shown to be an independent risk factor for coronary artery disease (88). From a structural standpoint, Lp(a) is very similar to LDL. The primary determinant of elevated LDL levels is genetic. The exact mechanism by which Lp(a) may cause an increase in CAD is complex and poorly understood.

Hypertension

Systemic hypertension represents a significant risk factor for coronary artery disease (58). In the United States and other industrialized countries there is a high prevalence of hypertension, which increases with age (89). It has been estimated that the overall prevalence of hypertension in American

Table 3-1 Major Angiographically Monitored Lipid-Lowering Trials in Patients with Coronary Atherosclerosis: Lipid and Angiographic Results

Trial*	Subjects†	Trial Period (YR)	Intervention‡	Percent Lipid Response (Rx/Control)		Assessment§	Percent Patients with Coronary Lesion		Events (Rx/Control)‖
				TC	LDL-C		Progression (Rx/Control)	Regression (Rx/Control)	
NHLBI	143 M + F	5	Ch	−17/−1	−26/−5	P	32/49	7/7	8/12
CLAS I	188 M	2	C + N	−26/−4	−43/−5	P	39/61	16/4	25/25
CLAS II	103 M	4	C + N	−25/−6	−40/−6	P	48/85	18/6	15/14
FATS	120 M	2.5	C + N	−23/−3	−32/−7	Q	25/46	39/11	2/10
			C + L	−34/−3	−46/−7	Q	21/46	32/11	3/10
UCSF-SCOR	72 M + F	2	C/N/L¶	−31/−9	−39/−12	Q	20/41	32/13	0/1
STARS	90 M	3	Ch	−25/−2	−36/−3	Q	12/46	33/4	1/10
			Diet alone	−14/−2	−16/−3	Q	15/46	38/4	3/10
POSCH	838 M + F	5**	PIB	−28/−5	−42/−7	P	37/65	13/5	
		10**		−22/−4	−39/−6	P	55/85	6/4	82/125
LHT	48 M + F	1	Life style	−24/−5	−37/−6	Q	18/53	82/42	Not available
						Q	29/41	23/12	22/31
MARS	270 M + F	2	L	−32/−2	−45/−3	P	47/65	23/11	
CCAIT	331 M + F	2	L	−21/−1	−29/−2	Q	33/50	10/7	15/20
REGRESS	885 M	2	P	−20/+2	−29/+2	Q	45/55	17/9	59/93
MAAS	381 M + F	4	S	−22/+3	31/+7	Q	41/54	33/20	53/74

TC = total cholesterol; LDL-C = low-density lipoprotein cholesterol.
* NHLBI: National Heart, Lung, and Blood Institute Type II Coronary Intervention Study[30]; CLAS I: Cholesterol Lowering Atherosclerosis Study I[33]; CLAS II[35]; FATS: Familial Atherosclerosis Treatment Study[36]; UCSF-SCOR: University of California, San Francisco, Arteriosclerosis Specialized Center of Research Intervention Trial[37]; STARS: St. Thomas' Atherosclerosis Regression Study[38]; POSCH: Program on the Surgical Control of the Hyperlipidemias[39]; LHT: Lifestyle Heart Trial[41]; MARS: Monitored Atherosclerosis Regression Study[42]; CCAIT: Canadian Coronary Atherosclerosis Intervention Trial[44]; REGRESS: Regression Growth Evaluation Statin Study[46]; MAAS: Multicentre Anti-Atheroma Study.[47]
† M = male; F = female.
‡ All interventions included diet. C = colestipol; Ch = cholestyramine; L = lovastatin; N = nicotinic acid; P = pravastatin; PIB = partial ileal bypass; S = simvastatin.
§ P = panel assessment of lesion change (viewer estimation); Q = assessment by quantitative coronary angiography.
‖ Events variably defined among trials; generally, coronary death, myocardial infarction, unstable ischemia requiring revascularization.
¶ Various binary and ternary drug combinations.
** Follow-up rather than trial period (intervention was surgery).
Adapted from Jones PH, Gotto AM Jr. Prevention of coronary heart disease in 1994: evidence for intervention. Heart Dis Stroke 1994;3:290. Reproduced by permission from Farmer JA, Gotto AM. Dyslipidemia and other risk factors for coronary artery disease. In: Braunwald E, ed. Heart disease: a textbook of cardiovascular medicine. 5th ed. Philadelphia: W.B. Saunders, 1997.

adults is approximately 25%, representing 43 million individuals. Approximately 15% of individuals in their thirties have hypertension; however, by the time an individual in the United States reaches the age of 70 years of age, he or she has a greater than 60% chance of having high blood pressure (89).

Although a systolic blood pressure reading of greater than 150 mm Hg and a diastolic blood pressure reading of greater than or equal to 90 mm Hg have traditionally been regarded as defining hypertension, recent data have suggested that even somewhat lower blood pressures carry an increased risk of cardiovascular disease (58). It is important to understand that the relationship between blood pressure and coronary artery disease follows a bell-shaped curve, as illustrated in Figure 3-1.

Data such as these have influenced recommendations to encourage people to maintain blood pressures significantly lower than 140/90 mm Hg. In the most recent report of the Joint National Commission on the Evaluation and Detection of High Blood Pressure, the concept of "high normal" blood pressure is emphasized (58). Individuals with a systolic blood pressure between 130 and 190 mm Hg and a diastolic

blood pressure between 85 and 89 mm Hg are considered to have high normal blood pressure.

Importantly, in the JNC-VI Guidelines, the new category "optimal" blood pressure is established. This is defined as blood pressure of 120/70 mm Hg. The new classifications for blood pressure categories established in JNC-VI are found in Table 3-2 (58).

Recognition that blood pressures of 130/80 mm Hg or higher start to carry increased risk of CAD is particularly important in terms of lifestyle interventions. The first line of defense to control blood pressure, particularly for people with high normal and stage 1 high blood pressure, involves lifestyle change. Such interventions as increased aerobic activity (90), weight management (91), and proper nutritional practices all have important implications for blood pressure control. These are handled in more detail in Chapter 9.

Numerous observational studies have found that high blood pressure increases the risk of CAD and stroke. Several recent meta-analyses have demonstrated both a clear association with high blood pressure and these complications, as well as a reduction in the risk of CAD when blood pressure is lowered (92,93).

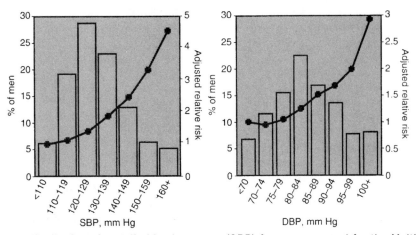

Figure 3-1 Left, percentage distribution of systolic blood pressure (SBP) for men screened for the Multiple Risk Factor Intervention Trial who were aged 35 to 57 years and had no history of myocardial infarction (n = 347,978) (shaded bars) and corresponding 12 year rates of cardiovascular mortality by SBP level adjusted for age, race, total serum cholesterol level, cigarettes smoked per day, reported use of medication for diabetes mellitus, and imputed household income (using census tract of residence). Right, same as at left but for diastolic blood pressure (DBP) (n = 356,222). (From National High Blood Pressure Education Program Working Group report on primary prevention of hypertension. Arch Inter Med 153:186:1993. Copyright 1993 American Heart Association. In Kaplan NM. Systemic hypertension: Mechanisms and diagnosis. In: Braunwald E, ed. Heart disease, 5th ed. Philadelphia: WB Saunders, 1997.)

Table 3-2 Classification of Blood Pressure for Adults Age 18 and Older*

CATEGORY	SYSTOLIC (mm Hg)		DIASTOLIC (mm Hg)
Optimal†	<120	and	<80
Normal	<130	and	<85
High Normal	130–139	or	85–89
Hypertension‡			
Stage 1	140–159	or	90–99
Stage 2	160–179	or	100–109
Stage 3	≥180	or	≥110

- Not taking antihypertensive drugs and not acutely ill. When systolic and diastolic blood pressures fall into different categories, the higher category should be selected to classify the individuals' blood pressure status. For example. 160/92 mm Hg should be classified as stage 2 hypertension, and 174/120 mm Hg should be classified as stage 3 hypertension. Isolated systolic hypertension is defined as SBP of 140 mm Hg or greater and DBP below 90 mm Hg and staged appropriately (e.g., 170/82 mm Hg is defined as stage 2 isolated systolic hypertension). In addition to classifying stages of hypertension on the basis of average blood pressure levels, clinicians should specify presence or absence of target organ disease and additional risk factors. This specificity is important for risk classification and treatment.
† Optimal blood pressure with respect to cardiovascular risk is below 120/80 mm Hg. However, unusually low readings should be evaluated for clinical significance.
‡ Based on the average of two or more readings taken at each of two or more visits after an initial screening.
From National Institutes of Health. National Heart, Lung and Blood Institute. National Cholesterol Education Program. The Sixth Report of the Joint National Committee on Prevention, Detection, Evaluation, and Treatment of High Blood Pressure in Adults. NIH Publication No. 93-3095. Washington, DC: NIH, 1993.

It is also important to recognize that hypertension frequently coexists with other risk factors for CAD. In fact, if an individual has hypertension (as defined as a blood pressure of greater than 140/90 mm Hg), he or she has a 46% chance of having a blood cholesterol of greater than 240 mg/dL (94). The coexistence of multiple risk factors for CAD carries important implications for treatment of high blood pressure since certain antihypertensive medications may exacerbate other risk factors for CAD. This issue is discussed in a subsequent section of this chapter, as well as in Chapter 9.

Tobacco Use

Use of tobacco products remains a major risk for coronary artery disease and a major public health hazard in the United States. In the United States 25% of the adult population, or approximately 46 million adults, smoke cigarettes (5). Cigarette smoking is the leading cause of premature death in the United States. It is estimated that over 400,000 Americans die from smoking-related diseases every year (1). Smoking acts synergistically with other risk factors for coronary artery disease and is estimated to be the cause of one fifth of all deaths from cardiovascular disease in the United States (95).

Multiple observational studies have linked cigarette smoking to increased risk of coronary artery disease. Framingham data demonstrated an increase of cardiovascular mortality of 18% in men and 31% in women for each 10 cigarettes smoked per day (96). Smokeless tobacco and low-tar cigarettes do not reduce the risk of CAD. Multiple epidemiologic studies have shown significant increased risk of CAD in individuals utilizing these products (97,98). Individuals who are exposed to the smoke of others on a regular basis (so-called "passive smoke") have also been shown to have an increased relative risk for heart disease (99).

There are multiple possible pathways through which the use of tobacco products may increase risk of coronary artery disease. Use of tobacco products increases HDL cholesterol (100) and decreases coronary flow through a variety of mechanisms, most prominently through spasm of the coronary arteries.

Smoking cessation has been shown to improve longevity and reduce the risk of coronary artery disease. It has been estimated that smoking cessation would increase the life expectancy of male cigarette smokers by 2.3 years and female cigarette smokers by 2.8 years (101). In recent studies, HDL cholesterol has been shown to increase by approximately 3% and LDL cholesterol lowered by over 5% in cigarette smokers who stopped smoking (102). Smoking cessation results in clinically significant benefits in short periods of time. In one recent case-control study comparing 1282 cigarette smokers to 2068 controls, the risk of coronary artery disease declined quickly when individuals stopped smoking cigarettes (103). At 3 years following smoking cessation, risk among former smokers was similar to subjects who had never smoked.

Despite the fact that approximately 70% of chronic smokers report a desire to stop cigarette smoking, the medical community has not been active enough in encouraging efforts to stop the smoking of cigarettes (5). Recent data from the Centers for Disease Control indicate that only slightly more than half of smokers who have had at least one physician visit within the past year reported being advised to quit smoking cigarettes (104). Further information concerning cigarette smoking cessation and available therapies is found in Chapter 5.

Physical Inactivity

Adults in the United States have become increasingly inactive. Physical inactivity has been regularly and reliably demonstrated to increase the risk of CAD (11). Recently, the American Heart Association listed lack of physical activity as a major risk factor for CAD (5).

In the Healthy People 2000 Initiative, physical activity recommendations included that at least 30% of the population over the age of 6 should engage in regular daily light-to-moderate physical activity of at least 30 minutes per day (13). However, recent surveys have shown that only 22% of adults are active at this level; 54% are somewhat active but do not meet this criteria; and 24% or more are completely sedentary, reporting no recent physical activity during the past month (11). Although participation in regular physical activity increased in the 1960s through the 1980s, recently there has been a leveling off and perhaps even a slight decline in physical activity.

Multiple observational studies have concluded that inactivity increases the risk of CAD. In one meta-analysis, conducted by the Centers for Disease Control, individuals who were classified as inactive (representing 60% of the adult population in the United States by CDC criteria) increased their risk of CAD by 1.9 times compared to active individuals (105). Thus, these individuals increased their relative risk of CAD by the same amount as if they had smoked a pack of cigarettes a day.

Recently, an expert panel convened by the American College of Sports Medicine and the Centers for Disease Control issued guidelines recommending increased physical activity as a means of lowering the risk of chronic disease (106). These recommendations, which apply to coronary artery disease as well as other chronic diseases, recommend that adults be encouraged to accumulate a minimum of 30 minutes of moderate-level physical activity on most if not all days.

The dose-response curve between physical activity and reduction in risk of chronic disease has been estimated to follow that shown in Figure 3-2.

From a practical standpoint, it has been demonstrated that over 90% of physicians feel most comfortable with prescribing walking exercise for their patients (107). Walking qualifies as moderate-intensity aerobic activity as recommended by the CDC and ACSM expert panel. Walking has often been shown to confer a wide variety of health benefits. Specific recommendations for how healthcare professionals can encourage patients to walk are found in Chapter 4.

Obesity

Obesity has long been recognized to carry an increased risk of coronary artery disease (15). In the past it was thought that this interaction was through the known association between obesity and other risk factors for coronary artery disease such as hypertension, type 2 diabetes, and dyslipidemias. However, recent epidemiologic studies have demonstrated that obesity carries an independent risk of CAD over and above its known association with other risk factors (25–27). For this reason, the American Heart Association has recently upgraded obesity to the classification of a "major" risk factor for CAD (6).

Perhaps the most practical way for assessing obesity in clinical practice is to obtain the body mass index (BMI). This is the weight in kilograms divided by the height in meters squared, or BMI = weight (kg) / height (meter)^2.

Recently, the National Institutes of Health have recommended that a BMI between 25 and 30 be considered

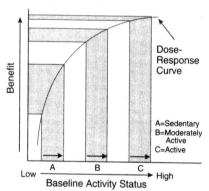

Figure 3-2 The dose-response curve represents the best estimate of the relationship between physical activity (dose) and health benefits (response). The lower the baseline physical activity status, the greater will be the health benefit associated with a given increase in physical activity (arrows A, B, and C). (Reproduced by permission from Pate R, Pratt M, Blair S, et al. Physical activity and public health: A recommendation from the Centers for Disease Control and Prevention and the American College of Sports Medicine. JAMA 1995;273:402–407. Copyright 1995, American Medical Association.)

"overweight", and that a BMI of greater than 30 be considered to be "obese" (108). By these criteria over half of the adult population in the United States is overweight. Unfortunately, the prevalence of both overweight and obesity have risen dramatically in the United States.

In addition to the increased risk of CAD carried by obesity, there is an independent increased risk of CAD associated with predominant abdominal distribution of body fat. Waist circumference of greater than 35 in. in women and greater than 39 in. in men has been shown to significantly increase the risk of coronary artery disease (108,109). It has been postulated that the mechanism underlying this increased risk of CAD carried by abdominal obesity is related to particular properties of visceral adiposites (109,110). It has been postulated that metabolic properties of these visceral adiposites stimulate abnormalities in glucose handling.

Adult weight gain also confers an additional risk of both CAD and type 2 diabetes. Both the Nurses' Health Study (111) and the U.S. Male Health Professional Trial showed that individuals who gained as little as 20 pounds as adults significantly increased their risk of CAD and type 2 diabetes (112).

The implications of the increased risk of CAD carried by obesity, abdominal distribution of body fat, and adult weight gain mandate that physicians be more alert to treating these conditions. Numerous studies have shown that a weight loss of 5% to 10% can substantially reduce the risk of CAD (113). Details about treatment of obesity in clinical practice are found in Section XVI.

MULTIPLE RISK FACTORS

Recently, there has been increased recognition that risk factors tend to cluster in individuals (114,115). One form of this clustering has been described as the *insulin resistance syndrome* (also called the *metabolic syndrome* or *syndrome X*) (116). This syndrome is characterized by resistance to insulin mediation of glucose uptake, glucose intolerance, hypertension, and dyslipidemia.

It appears that individuals who are obese are particularly prone to clustering of risk factors for CAD. In the Framingham study, obese individuals had an approximately 50% chance of having at least two other risk factors for coronary artery disease. Individuals whose weight is greater than 20% over normal are at risk of having at least three other risk factors for coronary artery disease (50).

This high incidence of clustering of risk factors for CAD, particularly in obese individuals, carries important clinical implications. Over 60% of all coronary artery disease is found in individuals with two or more risk factors (50). Thus, individuals who are found to have at least one risk factor, and particularly individuals who are obese, should be investigated for other risk factors for coronary artery disease.

NONMODIFIABLE RISK FACTORS

All of the risk factors described in the previous section can be modified through positive practices and habits in patients' daily lives. In this section, nonmodifiable risk factors for coronary artery disease will be discussed. Although these risk factors cannot be changed, it is important that they be identified in order to help assess a patient's risk of CAD. Individuals who have increased risk by virtue of one or more nonmodifiable risk factors should be counseled to pay particular attention to control of modifiable risk factors for CAD.

Age

Increased age is a clear risk for coronary artery disease (1). Approximately 80% of all fatal myocardial infarctions occur in individuals over the age of 65 (1). These individuals are at particular risk for events related to CAD. Reduction of modifiable risk factors in the elderly population is particularly efficacious in terms of decreased CAD events. In the Systolic Hypertension in the Elderly Program (SHEP) major cardiovascular events were reduced by 32% with antihypertensive therapy in individuals over the age of 60 (117). In elderly patients it is particularly important to assess overall risk factors and health status as well as othercurrent illnesses when devising a program for risk factor reduction.

Gender

It has been well established that heart disease is more prevalent in men and occurs at a younger age in men than it does in women. In the Framingham study in a 26-year follow-up of individuals aged 35 to 84, men accounted for 60% of all coronary events and had twice as much morbidity from CAD as did women (118). Men typically have an onset of symptomatic CAD 10 years earlier than women. CAD incidence in women increases rapidly following menopause. In general, women have the same modifiable risk factors as men, although type 2 diabetes appears to confer greater risk in women than in men.

Family History

A positive family history for coronary artery disease has been demonstrated to be a strong and independent risk factor for CAD. In one study of over 45,000 men aged 40 to 75 years without known coronary artery disease at baseline, for individuals who had a parent with myocardial infarction before the age of 70, the relative risk of myocardial infarction was 2.2 (119). The mechanism for the aggregation of coronary atherosclerosis in families is not completely understood. It may be mediated through genetic effects or other risk factors that appear to have a lifestyle component, such as obesity and dyslipidemia.

OTHER RISK FACTORS

A variety of other risk factors for coronary artery disease have either been identified or postulated to potentially influence the risk of CAD.

Alcohol

There is a complex interplay between alcohol consumption and risk of CAD. Moderate alcohol consumption has been shown in a number of studies to reduce coronary risk (120). Moderate alcohol consumption is typically defined as no more than one to two "shots" of distilled spirits a day or one to two glasses of wine or one to two beers. However, heavier alcohol consumption (three alcoholic drinks per day or more) has been associated with the increased risk of hypertension and may increase the risk of various forms of heart disease as well as motor vehicle accidents.

The mechanism through which moderate alcohol consumption may lower the risk of heart disease has been postulated to involve either increased HDL and/or increased thrombolysis (121).

Homocysteine

Elevated homocysteine levels have been associated with an increased incidence of coronary artery disease (122,123). In the Physicians' Health Study, individuals who had myocardial infarctions during the 5-year follow-up had significantly higher homocysteine levels than individuals in controls matched for age and smoking habits (123). Recent studies have suggested that intake of folate of 400 μg a day or more may result in significant declines in blood homocysteine levels (124).

Hemostatic Factors

Factors that contribute to thrombogenesis have been associated with increased events from coronary artery disease. Although such factors are typically not measured in clinical practice, this area represents one of increasing research interest. Factors that are currently under investigation that may contribute to thrombogenesis include fibrinogen (125), coagulation factor VII (126), and plasminogen activator inhibitor 1 (127).

Levels of Antioxidants

Low levels of antioxidants may contribute to increased risk of coronary artery disease by increasing the susceptibility of LDL and Lp(a) to oxidation. Oxidation of these lipids has been thought to play a role in athrogenesis. Observational studies such as the U.S. Male Health Professional Follow-up Study (128) and the Nurses' Health Trial have shown associations with high levels of intake of vitamin E with lowered risk of coronary artery disease (129). However, recent evidence

from interventional trials has been disappointing concerning the ability to influence risk of coronary artery disease by increasing antioxidants in the diet. The Alpha-Tocopherol Beta Carotene Cancer Prevention Study enrolled over 29,000 Finnish men smokers between the ages of 50 and 69 years (130). Those who were randomized to receive antioxidants showed no significant reduction in CAD mortality. At the current time, the American Heart Association does not recommend antioxidant supplementation as a means of reducing CAD risk because of insufficient data and lack of knowledge about the long-term consequences of this type of supplementation.

Stress and Type A Personality

Whether levels of stress and personality types contribute to risk of coronary artery disease remains controversial (131,132). The Type A personality has been defined as individuals who are in constant struggle with their environment and are highly competitive and ambitious. There is also an anger element to the Type A personality. Several studies have suggested that individuals who possess these personality types may have increased risk of CAD (133,134). Those studies have suggested that the component of anger in these individuals may be particularly associated with CAD. The literature on lowering the risk of CAD through mechanisms to lower stress has been inconclusive.

CONCLUSIONS

Identification of risk factors for coronary artery disease has represented a major breakthrough of great clinical relevance. Numerous lifestyle treatment modalities such as increased physical activity, maintenance of proper weight, proper nutrition, and avoidance of tobacco use have all been demonstrated to have a profound impact in terms of lowering the risk of CAD. Specific techniques and recommendations for how to incorporate these lifestyle measures to clinical practice are found in Chapter 4.

REFERENCES

1. American Heart Association. Heart and stroke facts: 1995 statistical supplement. Dallas: American Heart Association, 1994.

2. Expert Panel on Detection, Evaluation, and Treatment of High Blood Cholesterol in Adults. Summary of the second report of the National Cholesterol Education Program (NECP) Expert Panel on Detection, Evaluation and Treatment of High Blood Cholesterol in Adults (Adult Treatment Panel II). JAMA 1993;269:3015.

3. National Cholesterol Education Program: Second report of the Expert Panel on Detection, Evaluation, and Treatment of High Blood Cholesterol in Adults (Adult Treatment Panel II). Circulation 1994;89:1329.

4. Johnson CL, Rifkind BM, Sempos CT, et al. Declining serum total cholesterol levels among US adults: the National Health and Nutrition Examination Surveys. JAMA 1993;269:3002.

5. Cigarette smoking among adults—United States. MMWR 1993;43:925.

6. Fletcher G, Blair S, Blumenthal J, et al. AHA Medical/Scientific Statement. Statement on Exercise. Benefits and recommendations for physical activity programs for all americans. Circulation 1992;86:340–344.

7. Kaplan NM. Systemic hypertension: Mechanisms and diagnosis. In: Braunwald, E. Heart disease, 5th ed. Philadelphia: W.B. Saunders, 1997.

8. Heyka RJ. Obesity and hypertension. Nutr Clin Care 1998;1: 30–37.

9. Schappert SM. National ambulatory medical survey: 1991 summary. NCHS Advance Data, No. 230, Vital and Health Statistics of the National Center for Health Statistics. USDHHS Publication (PHS) 93-1250. Hyattsville, MD: U.S. Department of Health and Human Services, 1993.

10. Sempos CT, Cleeman JI, Carroll MD, et al. Prevalence of high blood cholesterol among US adults: an update based on guidelines from the second report of the National Cholesterol Education Program Adult Treatment Panel. JAMA 1993;269:3009.

11. U.S. Department of Health and Human Services. Physical activity and health: a report of the Surgeon General. Atlanta, GA: USDHSS, 1996.

12. Public Health Service. Healthy People 2000: National Health Promotion and Disease Preventive Objectives. U.S. Dept. of Health and Human Services Publication PHS 90-50212. Washington, DC: USDHHS, 1990.

13. Kuczmarski RJ, Flegal KM, Campbell SM, Johnson CL. Increasing prevalence of overweight among US adults: the National Health and Nutrition Examination surveys, 1960–1991. JAMA 1994;272: 205–211.

14. Update: Prevalence of overweight among children, adolescents, and adults—United States, 1988–1994. MMWR 1997;46: 99–202.

15. Rippe JM. Obesity as a risk factor for heart disease: an overview. Nutr Clin Care 1998;1: 3–14.

16. Stamler J. Epidemiologic findings on body mass and blood pressure in adults. Ann Epidemiol 1991;4:347–362.

17. MacMahon S, Cutler J, Brittain E, Higgins M. Obesity and hypertension: epidemiological and clinical issues. Eur Heart J 1987;8: 57–70.

18. Denke MA, Sempos CT, Grundy SM. Excess body weight: an unrecognized contributor to high blood cholesterol levels in white American men. Arch Intern Med 1993;153:1093–1103.

19. Denke MA, Seppos CT, Grundy SM. Excess body weight: an unrecognized contributor to high blood cholesterol levels in white American women. Arch Intern Med 1994;154:401–410.

20. Ebbeling CB, Ockene IS. Obesity and dyslipidemia. Nutr Clin Care 1998;1:15–29.

21. Wing RR, Bunker CH, Kuller LH, Matthews KA. Weight gain as a risk factor for clinical diabetes mellitus in women. Ann Intern Med 1995;122:481–486.

22. Colditz GA, Willett WC, Rotnizky A, Manson JE. Weight gain as a risk factor for clinical diabetes mellitus in women. Ann Intern Med 1995;122:481–486.

23. Kelley DE. Managing obesity as first-line therapy for diabetes mellitus. Nutr Clin Care 1998;1:38–43.

24. Rippe JM. Obesity and heart disease: the last great risk factor? Nutr Clin Care 1998;1: 1–2.

25. Manson JE, Willett WC, Stampler MJ, et al. Body weight and mortality among women. N Engl J Med 1995;333:677–685.

26. Rimm EB, Stampler MJ, Giovannucci B, et al. Body size and fat distribution as predictors of coronary heart disease among middle-aged and older US men. Am J Epidemiol 1995;141:1117–1127.

27. Garrison RJ, Castelli WP. Weight and thirty-year mortality of men in the Framingham Study. Ann Int Med 1985;103:1006–1009.

28. Anderson KM, Wilson PWF, Odell PM, Kannel WB. An updated coronary risk profile: a statement for health professionals. Circulation 1991;83:356.

29. Stamler J. Epidemiology, established major risk factors and the primary prevention of coronary heart disease. In: Chatterjee K, Cheitlin MP, Karlines J, et al, eds. Cardiology: an illustrated text/reference, vol. 2. Philadelphia: J.B. Lippincott, 1991:1.

30. Eckel R. Obesity and heart disease: a statement for the healthcare professionals from the Nutrition Committee, American Heart Association. Circulation 1997;96:3248–3250.

31. Wilson P, D'Agostino R, Levy D, et al. Prediction of coronary heart disease using risk factor categories. Circulation 1998;97: 1837–1847.

32. Shea S, Cook EF, Kannel WB, Goldman L. Treatment of hypertension and its effect on cardiovascular risk factors: data from the Framingham Heart Study. Circulation 1985;71:22–30.

33. Kannel WB, Danneberg AL, Abbott RD. Unrecognized myocardial infarction and hypertension: the Framingham Study. Am Heart J 1985;109:581–585.

34. Harris T, Cook EF, Kannel W, et al. Blood pressure experience and risk of cardiovascular disease in the elderly. Hypertension 1985;7:118–124.

35. Castelli WP, Anderson K. A population at risk: prevalence of high cholesterol levels in hypertensive patients in the Framingham Study. Am J Med 1986;80:23–32.

36. Kannel WB. Cigarette smoking and coronary heart disease. Ann Intern Med 1964;60:1103–1106.

37. Wilson PW, Garrison RJ, Castelli WP. Postmenopausal estrogen use, cigarette smoking, and cardiovascular morbidity in women over 50: the Framingham Study. N Engl J Med 1985;313: 1038–1043.

38. Kannel WB, McGee DL, Castelli WP. Latest perspectives on cigarette smoking and cardiovascular disease: the Framingham Study. J Card Rehabil 1984;4:267–277.

39. Kannel WB, D'Agostino RB, Belanger AJ. Fibrinogen, cigarette smoking and risk of cardiovascular disease: insights from the

Framingham Study. Am Heart J 1987;113:1006–1010.

40. Kannel WB, Castelli WP, Gordon T, McNamara PM. Serum cholesterol, liproproteins, and the risk of coronary heart disease: the Framingham Study. Ann Intern Med 1971;74:1–12.

41. Wilson PW, Garrison RJ, Castelli WP, et al. Prevalence of coronary heart disease in the Framingham Offspring Study: role of lipoprotein cholesterols. Am J Cardiol 1980;46:649–654.

42. Castelli WP, Abbott RD, McNamara PM. Summary estimates of cholesterol used to predict coronary heart disease. Circulation 1983;67:730–734.

43. McNamara JR, Cohn JS, Wilson PW, Schaefer EJ. Calculated values for low-density lipoprotein cholesterol in the assessment of lipid abnormalities and coronary disease risk. Clin Chem 1990;36:36–42.

44. Gordon DL, Probstfield JL, Garrison RJ, et al. High-density lipoprotein cholesterol and cardiovascular disease: four prospective American studies. Circulation 1989;79:8–15.

45. Garcia MJ, McNamara P, Gordon T, Kannel WB. Morbidity and mortality in diabetics in the Framingham population 16-year follow-up study. Diabetes 1974; 23:105–111.

46. Kannel WB, McGee DL. Diabetes and cardiovascular risk factors: the Framingham Study. Circulation 1979;59:8–13.

47. Abbott RD, Donahue RP, Kannel WB, Wilson PW. The impact of diabetes on survival following myocardial infarction in men vs women: the Framingham Study. JAMA 1988;260:3456–3460.

48. Kannel WB, D'Agostino RB, Wilson PW, et al. Diabetes, fibrinogen, and risk of cardiovascular disease: the Framingham experience. Am Heart J 1990;120:672–676.

49. Kannel WB. Contributions of the Framingham Study to the conquest of coronary artery disease.

Am J Cardiol 1988;62:1109–1112.

50. Wilson P. Clustering of risk factors, obesity, and Syndrome X. Nutr Clin Care 1998;1(suppl): 44–50.

51. Farmer JA, Gotto AM. Dyslipidemia and other risk factors for coronary artery disease. In: Braunwald E. Heart disease: a textbook of cardiovascular medicine, 5th ed. Philadelphia: W.B. Saunders, 1997.

52. Grundy SM, Balady GJ, Criqui MH, et al. Primary prevention of coronary heart disease: guidance from Framingham. A statement for healthcare professionals from the AHA Task Force on Risk Reduction. Circulation 1998;97: 1876–1887.

53. Rippe JM. The case for medical management of obesity: a call for increased physician involvement. Obesity Res 1998;6:23S–33S.

54. Klag MJ, Ford DE, Mead LA, et al. Serum cholesterol in young men and subsequent cardiovascular disease. N Engl J Med 1993;308:363–366.

55. Law MR, Wald NJ, Wu T, et al. Systematic underestimation of association between serum cholesterol concentration and ischemic heart disease in observational studies: data from the BUPA study. Br Med J 1994;308:363–366.

56. Law MR, Wald NJ, Thompson SG. By how much and how quickly does reduction in serum cholesterol concentration lower risk of ischemic heart disease? Br Med J 1994;308:367–373.

57. Cleeman JI, Grundy SM. National Cholesterol Education Program recommendations for cholesterol testing in young adults: a science-based approach. Circulation 1997;95:1646–1650.

58. National Institutes of Health, National Heart, Lung, and Blood Institute, National Cholesterol Education Program. The sixth report of the Joint National Committee on Prevention, Detection, Evaluation, and Treatment of High Blood Pressure in Adults.

NIH Publication No. 93-3095. Washington, DC: NIH, 1993.

59. U.S. Department of Health and Human Service. Public Health Service. Cardiac rehabilitation as a secondary prevention. AHCPR Publication No. 96-0673. Washington, DC: USDHSS.

60. Smith SC, Blair SN, Criqui MH, et al. Preventing heart attack and death in patients with coronary disease. Circulation 1995; 92:2–4.

61. Taylor CB. Experimentally induced arteriosclerosis in nonhuman primates. In: Roberts JC, Straus R, eds. Comparative atherosclerosis. New York: Harper & Row, 1965:215.

62. Taylor CB, Cox GE, Manalo-Estrella P, et al. Atherosclerosis in rhesus monkeys. II. Arterial lesions associated with hypercholesterolemia induced by dietary fat and cholesterol. Arch Pathol 1962;74:16–34.

63. Wissler RW, Vesselinovitch D. Differences between human and animal atherosclerosis. In: Schettler G, Wiezel A, eds. Atherosclerosis III. Proceedings of the 3rd International Symposium. New York: Springer, 1974:319–325.

64. Wissler RW, Vesselinovitch D. Atherosclerosis in non-human primates. In: Brandly CA, Cornelius CE, Simpson CF, eds. Advances in veterinary science and comparative medicine, vol. 21. New York: Academic Press, 1977: 351–420.

65. Weiner BH, Ockene IS, Jarmolych J, et al. Comparison of pathology and angiography in swine model of coronary atherosclerosis. Circulation 1985;72:1081–1086.

66. Wissler RW, Vesselinovitch D, Schaffner TJ, et al. Quantitating rhesus monkey atherosclerosis programs and regression with time. In: Gotto AM, Smith LC, Allen B, eds. Atherosclerosis V. Proceedings of the 5th International Symposium. New York: Springer, 1980:757–761.

67. Wissler RW, Vesselinovitch D. Can atherosclerotic plaques regress—Anatomic and biochemi-

cal evidence from nonhuman animal models. Am J Cardiol 1990;65:F33–F40.

68. Kaplan JR, Manuck SB, Clarkson TB, et al. Social status, environment, and atherosclerosis in cynomolgus monkeys. Arteriosclerosis 1982;2:359–368.

69. Stamler J, Wentworth D, Naton JD. For the MRFIT Research Group: Is relationship between serum cholesterol and risk of premature death from coronary heart disease continuous and graded? finding in 356,222 primary screenees of the Multiple Risk Factor Intervention Trial (MRFIT). JAMA 1986;256:2823.

70. Lipid Research Clinics Program. The Lipid Research Clinics Coronary Primary Prevention Trial results I. Reduction in incidence of coronary heart disease. JAMA 1984;251:351.

71. Huttunen JK, Manninen V, Manttair M, et al. The Helsinki Heart Study: central findings and clinical implications. Ann Med 1991; 23:155.

72. Hjermann I, Velve Byre K, Holme I, Leren P. Effect of diet and smoking intervention on the incidence of coronary heart disease: report from the Oslo Study Group of a randomized trial in healthy men. Lancet 1991;2: 1303.

73. Committee of Principal Investigators. A co-operative trial in the primary prevention of ischemic heart disease using clofibrate. Br Heart J 1978;40:1069.

74. Shepherd J, Cobbe SM, Ford I, et al for the West of Scotland Coronary Prevention Study Group. Prevention of coronary heart disease with provastatin in men with hypercholesterolemia. N Engl J Med 1995;333:1301.

75. Coronary Drug Project Research Group. Clofibrate and niacin in coronary heart disease. JAMA 1995;231:360.

76. Brensike JF, Levy RI, Kelsy SF, et al. Effects of therapy with cholestryamine on progression of coronary ateriosclerosis: results of NHLBI Type II Coronary Interven-

tion Study. Circulation 1984; 69:313.

77. Blankenhorn DH, Nessim SA, Johnson RL, et al. Beneficial effects of combined colestipolniacin therapy on coronary atherosclerosis and coronary venous bypass grafts. JAMA 1987;257: 3233.

78. Brown G, Albers J, Fisher L, et al. Regression of coronary artery disease as a result of intensive lipid-lowering therapy in men with high levels of apoliporotein B. N Engl J Med 1990;323:1289.

79. Watts GF, Lewis B, Brunt JNH, et al. Effects on coronary artery disease of lipid-lowering diet or diet plus cholestyramine in the St. Thomas' Atherosclerosis Regress Study (STARS). Lancet 1992;339:563.

80. Buchwald H, Varco RL, Matts JP, et al. Effect of partial ileal bypass surgery on mortality and morbidity from coronary heart disease in patients with hypercholesterolemia: report of the Program on the Surgical Control of the Hyperlipidemias (POSCH). N Engl J Med 1990;323:946.

81. Neaton JD, Blackburn H, Jacobs D, et al. Serum cholesterol level and mortality findings for men screened in the Multiple Risk Factor Intervention Trial. Arch Intern Med 1992;152:1490.

82. Lewis B, Paoletti R, Tikkanen MJ, eds. Low blood cholesterol: health implications: proceedings of a workshop held in Milan, July 1993, under the auspices of the International Task Force for the Prevention of Coronary Heart Disease, International Society and Federation of Cardiology, Giovanni Lorenzini Foundation. London: Current Medical Literature, 1993.

83. Rossouw JE, Gotto AM. Does low cholesterol cause death? Cardiovasc Drugs Ther 1993;7:789. Editorial.

84. Wysowski DK, Gross TP. Deaths due to accidents and violence in two recent trials of cholesterol-lowering drugs. Arch Intern Med 1990;150:2169.

85. Gordon T, Castelli WP, Hjortland MC, et al. High-density lipoprotein as a protective factor against coronary heart disease: the Framingham Study. Am J Med 1977;62:707.

86. Gordon DJ, Probstfield JL, Garrison RJ, et al. High-density lipoprotein cholesterol and cardiovascular disease: four prospective American studies. Circulation 1989;79:8.

87. Austin MA. Plasma triglyceride and coronary heart disease. Arterioscler Thromb 1991;11:2.

88. Loscalzo J. Lipoprotein (a): a unique risk factor for atherothrombotic disease. Arteriosclerosis 1990;10:672.

89. National High Blood Pressure Education Program Working Group. Report on primary prevention of hypertension. Arch Intern Med 1993;153:186.

90. American College of Sports Medicine. Physical activity, physical fitness, and hypertension. Med Sci Sports Exerc 1993;25:i–x.

91. Appel LJ, Moore JT, Obarzanek E, et al for the DASH Collaborative Research Group. A clinical trial on the effects of dietary patterns on blood pressure. N Engl J Med 1997;336:1117–1124.

92. MacMahon S, Peto R, Cutler J, et al. Blood pressure, stroke, and coronary heart disease. Part 1. Prolonged differences in blood pressure: prospective observational studies corrected for the regression dilution bias. Lancet 1990;335:765.

93. Collins R, Peto R, MacMahon S, et al. Blood pressure, stroke, and coronary heart disease. Part 2. Short-term reductions in blood pressure: overview of randomized drug trials in their epidemiological context. Lancet 1990;335: 827.

94. Working Group on Management of Patients with Hypertension and High Blood Cholesterol. National Education Programs Working Group report on the management of hypertension and high blood cholesterol. Ann Intern Med 1991;114:224–237.

95. Office of Technology Assessment. Smoking-related deaths and financial costs: estimates for 1990, rev. ed. Washington, DC: Office of Technology Assessment, 1993.

96. Kannel WB, Higgins M. Smoking and hypertension as predictors of cardiovascular risk in population studies. J Hypertens 1990;8(suppl):S3.

97. Negri E, Franzosi MG, LaVecchia C, et al. Tar yield of cigarettes and risk of acute myocardial infarction. BMJ 1993;306:1567.

98. Bolinder G, Alfredsson L, Englund A, deFaire U. Smokeless tobacco use and increased cardiovascular mortality among Swedish construction workers. Am J Public Health 1994;84:399.

99. Steenland K. Passive smoking and the risk of heart disease. JAMA 1992;267:94.

100. Sigurdsson G Jr, Gudnason V, Sigurdsson G, Humphries SE. Interaction between a polymorphism of the apo A-I promoter region and smoking determines plasma levels of HDL and apo A-I. Arterioscler Thromb 1992;12:1017.

101. Tsevat J, Weinstein MC, Williams LW, et al. Expected gains in life expectancy from various coronary heart disease risk factors modifications. Circulation 1991;83:1194.

102. Terres W, Becker P, Rosenberg A. Changes in cardiovascular risk profile during the cessation of smoking. Am J Med 1994;97:242.

103. Dobvson AJ, Alexander HM, Heller RF, Lloyd DM. How soon after quitting smoking does risk of heart attack decline? J Clin Epidemiol 1991;44:1247.

104. Physician and other health-care professional counseling of smokers to quit—United States, 1991. MMWR 1993;42:854.

105. Powell K, Thompson P, Caspersen C, Kendrick J. Physical activity and the incidence of coronary heart disease. Annu Rev Public Health 1987;8:253–287.

106. Pate R, Pratt M, Blair S, et al. Physical activity and public health: a recommendation from the Centers for Disease Control and Prevention and the American College of Sports Medicine. JAMA 1995;273:402–407.

107. Goldfine H, Ward A, Taylor P, et al. Exercising to health: what's really in it for your patients? Part I: The health benefits of exercise. Phys Sports Med 1991;19(6):81.

108. Committee of Principal Investigators. WHO Cooperative Trial on Primary Prevention of Ischemic Heart Disease with Clofibrate to Lower Serum Cholesterol: final mortality follow-up. Lancet 1984;2:600.

109. Despres JP. Abdominal obesity as important component of insulin-resistance syndrome. Nutrition 1993;4:452–459.

110. Despres JP. Dyslipidaemia and obesity. Baillieres Clin Endocrinol Metab 1994:8:629,660.

111. Willett W, Manson J, Stampfer M, et al. Weight, weight change, and coronary heart disease in women. JAMA 1995;273:461–465.

112. Chan JM, Rimm EB, Colditz GA, et al. Obesity, fat distribution, and weight gain as risk factors for clinical diabetes in men. Diabetes Care 1994;17:961–969.

113. Institute of Medicine. Weighing the options: criteria for evaluating weight-management programs. Washington, DC: National Academy Press, 1994.

114. Williams RR, Hunt SC, Hopkins PN, et al. Familial dyslipidemic hypertension: evidence from 58 Utah families for a syndrome present in approximately 12% of patients with essential hypertension. JAMA 1988;259:3579–3586.

115. National Heart, Lung, and Blood Institute. Working Group Report on Management of Patients with Hypertension and High Blood Cholesterol. NIH publication No. 90-2361. Bethesda, MD: U.S. Dept. of Health and Human Services, 1990.

116. Grundy SM, Small LDL. Atherogenic dyslipidemia and the metabolic syndrome. Circulation 1997;95:1–4.

117. SHEP Cooperative Research Group. Prevention of stroke by antihypertensive drug treatment in older persons with isolated systolic hypertension: final results of the Systolic Hypertension in the Elderly Program (SHEP). JAMA 1991;265:3255.

118. Lerner DJ, Kannel WB. Patterns of coronary heart disease morbidity and mortality in the sexes: a 26-year old follow-up of the Framingham population. Am Heart J 1994;15:1571.

119. Colditz GA, Rimm EB, Giovannucci E, et al. A prospective study of parental history of myocardial infarction and coronary artery disease in men. Am J Cardiol 1991;67:993.

120. Pohorecky LA. Interaction of alcohol and stress at the cardiovascular level. Alcohol 1990;7:537.

121. Gaziano JM, Buring JE, Breslow JL, et al. Moderate alcohol intake, increased levels of high-density lipoprotein and its sub-fractions and decreased risk of myocardial infarction. N Engl J Med 1993;329:1829.

122. Glueck CJ, Shaw P, Lang JE, et al. Evidence that homocysteine is an independent risk factor for atherosclerosis in hyperlipidemic patients. Am J Cardiol 1995;75:132.

123. Stampfer MJ, Malinow MR, Willett WC, et al. A prospective study of plasma homocyst(e)ine and risk of myocardial infarction in US physicians. JAMA 1992;268:877.

124. Malinow MR, Duell PB, Hess DL, et al. Reduction of plasma homocysteine levels by breakfast cereal fortified with folic acid in patients with coronary heart disease. N Engl J Med 1998;338:1009.

125. Iso H, Folsom AR, Sato S, et al. Plasma fibrinogen and its correlates in Japanese and US population samples. Arterioscler Thromb 1993;783:13.

126. Miller GJ. Hemostasis and cardiovascular risk: the British and European experience. Arch Pathol Lab Med 1992;116:1318.

127. Juhan-Vague I, Aless MC. Plasminogen activatory inhibitor 1 and atherothrombosis. Thromb Haemost 1993;70:138.

128. Rimm EB, Stampfer MD, Ascherio A, et al. Vitamin E consumption and the risk of coronary heart disease in men. N Engl J Med 1993;328:1450.

129. Stampfer MJ, Hennekens CH, Manson JE, et al. Vitamin E consumption and the risk of coronary heart disease in women. N Engl J Med 1993;328;1444.

130. Alpha-Tocopherol, Beta Carotene Cancer Prevention Study Group. The effect of vitamin E and beta carotene on the incidence of lung cancer and other cancers in male smokers. N Engl J Med 1994;330:1029.

131. Lachar BL. Coronary-prone behavior: type A behavior revisited. Tex Heart Inst J 1993;20:143.

132. Littman AB. Review of psychosomatic aspects of cardiovascular disease. Psychother Psychosom 1993;60:148.

133. Rosenman RH, Brand RJ, Jenkins CD, et al. Coronary heart disease in the Western Collaborative Group Study: final follow-up experience of 8½ years. JAMA 1975;233:872.

134. Shekelle RB, Hulley SB, Neaton JD, et al. The MRFIT Behavior Patterns Study II: type A behavior and incidence of coronary heart disease. Am J Epidemiol 1985;122:559.

Chapter 4

Lifestyle Strategies for Risk Factor Reduction and Treatment of Coronary Artery Disease: An Overview

James M. Rippe
Diane O'Brien
Kathleen Taylor

Various lifestyle strategies play a major role, not only in risk factor reduction, but also the effective treatment of coronary artery disease. The previous chapter focused on "why" to utilize various lifestyle strategies for risk factor reduction and treatment. This chapter will focus on the practical considerations of "how" to employ these strategies in the treatment of coronary artery disease (CAD).

Other chapters in this section provide an in-depth treatment of lifestyle measures as they relate to such risk factors for coronary artery disease as smoking, poor nutrition, sedentary lifestyle, hypertension, and dyslipidemias. In this chapter, an overview will be provided for lifestyle strategies both for risk factor reduction and treatment of CAD, as well as an overall rationale for why physicians and other healthcare workers should be involved in this important area.

Lifestyle measures such as increased physical activity (1,2), proper nutrition (3,4), and weight management (5–10) are critically important in the reduction in the risk of developing CAD, as well as in the treatment of established CAD. Not only are these measures typically the first line of intervention but, in addition, many of these lifestyle measures are highly effective in the reduction of multiple risk factors for CAD. Thus, lifestyle measures provide a very important tool for physicians and other healthcare workers in their goal of advising patients about ways to lower risk factors, as well as helping to treat patients who have established CAD.

Recently, a number of national guidelines have been developed to help healthcare professionals counsel their patients about lowering the risk of CAD. Many of these guidelines have focused on the important role of positive lifestyle behaviors in risk factor reduction for CAD. Unfortunately, many healthcare workers still under-emphasize the role of lifestyle interventions in their daily clinical practices.

Guidelines from the National Cholesterol Education Program (3) emphasize the important role of proper nutrition as a first-line treatment for elevated blood cholesterol and other dyslipidemias. The recently released report of the Joint National Committee on the Prevention, Detection, Evaluation and Treatment of High Blood Pressure (JNC-VI) has highlighted the important role of lifestyle measures such as regular physical activity, proper nutrition, and weight management as key first-line therapies in the treatment of hypertension (11). The Surgeon General's report on physical activity and health (1) and the consensus statement on physical activity and health from the American College of Sports Medicine and Centers for Disease Control (2) both emphasize the role of increased physical activity in the reduction of coronary artery disease and other chronic diseases. A number of recently released publications from the Institute of Medicine (12), National Institutes of Health (10), and American Heart Association (9) have all emphasized lifestyle measures in the treatment and prevention of obesity as important interventions for lowering the risk of CAD, type 2 diabetes, and other comorbidities of obesity.

This chapter provides an overview on how this important body of literature can be employed in a clinical practice setting to help patients lower their risk of CAD (primary prevention) as well as to help in the treatment of individuals who have already established chronic CAD (secondary prevention).

THE ROLE OF THE PHYSICIAN AND OTHER HEALTHCARE WORKERS IN LIFESTYLE CHANGE

Physicians occupy a crucial position in helping patients make positive lifestyle changes to lower their risk of CAD (13–17). Physician recommendation has been demonstrated to significantly improve patients' efforts to change behaviors such as diet (14,18,19), smoking (13), and adherence to medical regimens (15–17).

There are a variety of reasons why physicians, in particular, play a critical role in helping patients adopt positive lifestyle changes. First, a number of studies have shown that the general public perceives physicians as the most reliable and credible source of advice and information concerning health matters (20,21). Unfortunately, physicians often underestimate how much health-related information patients actually desire. It has been estimated that the average adult in the United States visits a physician's office over five times a year (22). Thus, it is likely that physicians and other healthcare workers come in contact with over 75% of adults in the United States over any given year. Physicians are also uniquely placed to provide continuity of care in the primary care setting. Furthermore, when patients come to a physician's office, they are typically seeking improvement in their health. This provides further motivation for the patient to adopt lifestyle changes recommended by physicians.

It should also be noted that the majority of individuals who change lifestyle behaviors make this change without formal participation in an organized program. For example, over 90% of individuals who have stopped smoking have done this without a formal smoking cessation program (23). Thus, physician recommendations and the provision of information are particularly important to the majority of individuals who are seeking behavioral change.

Given the powerful position occupied by physicians and healthcare workers for the recommendation of positive lifestyle behaviors, it is unfortunate that physicians have not been more proactive in this area. For example, a recent survey indicated that less than 50% of smokers had been counseled by their physicians in the past year about the importance of stopping this habit (24). Another survey revealed that less than 40% of obese women and less than 25% of obese men received any counseling from their physician concerning their weight in the previous year (25). The medical community needs to approach the task of lifestyle recommendation with more concerted effort and energy. The health-related benefits to a large number of patients should provide impetus for physicians to become more involved in this critically important area.

LIFESTYLE MEASURES TO TREAT DYSLIPIDEMIAS

The National Cholesterol Education Program (NCEP) guidelines emphasize the importance of treating various dyslipidemias (particularly of elevated cholesterol and LDL) in the context of overall cardiac risk (3). This framework allows for the most intense intervention to be reserved for individuals who are at highest risk, whereas less intense therapy is utilized for individuals who are at lower risk. An outline of risk status as defined in the NCEP is found in Table 4-1.

In the NCEP guidelines, nutritional therapy is viewed as the first line of intervention (3). For individuals who are at

---

Table 4-1 Risk Status Based on Presence of CHD Risk Factors Other Than LDL-Cholesterol

Positive Risk Factors
- ❏ Age
  - Male: ≥45 years
  - Female: ≥55 years, or premature menopause without estrogen replacement therapy
- ❏ Family history of premature CHD (definite myocardial infarction or sudden death before 55 years of age in father or other male first-degree relative, or before 65 years of age in mother or other female first-degree relative)
- ❏ Current cigarette smoking
- ❏ Hypertension (≥140/90 mm Hg,* or on antihypertensive medication)
- ❏ Low HDL-cholesterol (<35 mg/dL*)
- ❏ Diabetes mellitus

Negative Risk Factor**
- ❏ High HDL-cholesterol (≥60 mg/dL)

High risk, defined as a net of two or more CHD risk factors, leads to more vigorous intervention. Age (defined differently for men and for women) is treated as a risk factor because rates of CHD are higher in the elderly than in the young, and in men than in women of the same age. Obesity is not listed as a risk factor because it operates through other risk factors that are included (hypertension, hyperlipidemia, decreased HDL-cholesterol, and diabetes mellitus), but it should be considered a target for intervention. Physical inactivity is similarly not listed as a risk factor, but it too should be considered a target for intervention, and physical activity is recommended as desirable for everyone.

* Confirmed by measurements on several occasions.
** If the HDL-cholesterol level is ≥60 mg/dL, subtract one risk factor (because high HDL-cholesterol levels decrease CHD risk).
Reproduced by permission from Expert Panel on Detection, Evaluation, and Treatment of High Blood Cholesterol in Adults. Summary of the second report of the National Cholesterol Education Program (NECP) Expert Panel on Detection, Evaluation and Treatment of High Blood Cholesterol in Adults. (Adult Treatment Panel II). JAMA 1993;269:3015.

low risk, nutritional therapy alone may suffice for the control of elevated blood cholesterol. In individuals who are at higher risk, nutritional therapy coupled with pharmacologic intervention may be required. Other lifestyle interventions, such as increased physical activity and weight management, also represent key components of the overall lifestyle approach to controlling blood cholesterol.

Nutritional Intervention to Lower Cholesterol

The general goal of proper nutrition in individuals with elevated blood cholesterol is to help lower cholesterol (and correct other dyslipidemias) while maintaining a balanced and nutritionally adequate eating pattern. The American Heart Association has developed two diets to help individuals lower their blood cholesterol. These are called the Step 1 diet and the Step 2 diet. The overall structure of the Step 1 and Step 2 diets is found in Table 4-2.

Many of the principles of the Step 1 diet follow general nutritional patterns for good health recommended by virtually every health organization in America. Saturated fat in the Step 1 diet (usually fat coming from animal sources, although some plant oils also contain saturated fat) should be reduced to 8% to 10% of calories. Calories from all fats are reduced to 30% or less of total calories. Daily intake of cholesterol should be reduced to 300 mg/day or less while following the Step 1 diet. Although many physicians are comfortable explaining the Step 1 diet to patients, the assistance of a registered dietician will often be helpful for practical issues such as menu planning. If the Step 1 diet does not lower blood cholesterol below 200 mg dL, the next step is to move to the Step 2 diet. This diet calls for further reduction of saturated fat to no more than 7% of calories and the reduction of dietary cholesterol to less than 200 mg/day. Since the Step 2 diet is somewhat more restrictive than the Step 1 diet, advice from a nutritionist is often invaluable in helping patients determine proper eating patterns and food choices.

Both the American Heart Association and the National Cholesterol Education Program have developed a variety of specific dietary plans and recipes that conform to both the Step 1 and Step 2 dietary guidelines. These recipes and dietary plans will help patients understand that the lower fat and cholesterol recommendations from these plans do not require sacrifice of good taste and enjoyment of eating.

Physical Activity

Physical activity can help with the control of cholesterol (26–28). Regular aerobic activity has been demonstrated to yield increases in HDL cholesterol, which are associated with decreased risk of heart disease. Even moderately intense physical activity, such as brisk walking, can raise HDL cholesterol (29). In a recent study of individuals following a low-fat diet, individuals who also engaged in regular physical activity achieved significant reductions in LDL, whereas those who only followed the low-fat eating plan without exercise did not (30).

Weight Management

Obesity is associated with a particularly dangerous constellation of dyslipidemias. Obesity is associated with modest elevations of total cholesterol and LDL, a reduction of HDL, and an increase in triglycerides (31). Weight reduction can result in improvement of all of these dyslipidemias and should be included as part of lifestyle management of cholesterol in every patient with a dyslipidemia.

Special Issues in Lifestyle Management of Dyslipidemias

Low HDL

Low HDL cholesterol has been shown to be an independent risk factor for CAD (32). Lifestyle measures that may be helpful in elevating HDL include regular aerobic exercise and weight reduction.

Elevated Blood Triglycerides

Elevated blood triglycerides have also been shown to increase the risk of coronary artery disease (33). Lifestyle measures

NUTRIENT*	RECOMMENDED INTAKE		
	Step I Diet		Step II Diet
Total Fat		30% or less of total calories	
Saturated Fatty Acids	8–10% of total calories		Less than 7% of total calories
Polyunsaturated Fatty Acids		Up to 10% of total calories	
Monounsaturated Fatty Acids		Up to 15% of total calories	
Carbohydrates		55% or more of total calories	
Protein		Approximately 15% of total calories	
Cholesterol	Less than 300 mg/day		Less than 200 mg/day
Total Calories		To achieve and maintain desirable weight	

Table 4-2 Dietary Therapy of High Blood Pressure

* Calories from alcohol not included.
Reproduced by permission from Expert Panel on Detection, Evaluation, and Treatment of High Blood Cholesterol in Adults. Summary of the second report of the National Cholesterol Education Program (NECP) Expert Panel on Detection, Evaluation and Treatment of High Blood Cholesterol in Adults (Adult Treatment Panel II) JAMA 1993;269:3015.

that are effective in lowering blood triglycerides include weight reduction for overweight patients, restricting alcohol consumption, and increasing physical activity.

LIFESTYLE TREATMENT OF HYPERTENSION

A variety of lifestyle measures can play significant roles in reducing the likelihood of hypertension or treating existing hypertension (11,34). The JNC-VI guidelines include such lifestyle measures as weight management, proper nutrition, regular physical activity, cessation of cigarette smoking, and moderation of alcohol intake as important first-line measures in the treatment of hypertension (11).

Weight Management

Increased body weight has been reliably associated with increased risk of high blood pressure (35). Weight reduction in individuals who are overweight represents a reliable way of lowering blood pressure. In fact, of all of the lifestyle measures to control blood pressure in overweight individuals, weight loss appears to be the most effective (11,35).

In most studies, individuals lose over 1 mm Hg from both their systolic and diastolic blood pressures for every 2 lb of weight loss (36). There does not appear to be either a "ceiling" or "floor" effect on the relationship between weight loss and lowered blood pressure. Thus, even small amounts of weight loss can make a significant difference in control of blood pressure, and the more weight loss accomplished, the more profound the lowering of blood pressure.

An overweight individual who loses even 10 lb can anticipate a 5 to 7 mm Hg reduction in both systolic and diastolic blood pressure. Although the exact mechanism of blood pressure lowering resulting from weight loss is not fully understood, an initial diuresis and decrease in blood volume are thought to play major roles (37,38).

Proper Nutrition

Many aspects of proper nutrition play important roles in blood pressure control. Both the JNC-VI guidelines and the American Heart Association (38) recommend consuming a diet that is low in sodium for individuals who have high blood pressure. Both JNC-VI and AHA guidelines emphasize that individuals with hypertension should consume no more than 2 g of sodium per day. This is about one fourth the amount of sodium that the average American consumes in the daily diet. The most reliable way to encourage patients to lower sodium in their diet is to ask them to remove the salt shaker from the table and also to emphasize fresh fruits, vegetables, and grains in their diet rather than processed foods, which are typically high in salt.

A variety of other nutritional practices may also help lower blood pressure. A recent study showed that a diet emphasizing low-fat dairy products and whole grains, fruits, and vegetables significantly lowered blood pressure (39). There may also be a role for increasing potassium intake for lowering blood pressure. Other dietary factors, including adequate intake of calcium and magnesium, lowering dietary fats, and possibly lowering caffeine consumption, have all been hypothesized to contribute to lowering blood pressure (40). The evidence for these factors is less compelling than for sodium reduction.

Regular Physical Activity

Regular, moderate-intensity physical activity carries a multitude of health benefits (see Chapter 7). One of the most important benefits of regular physical activity is to help prevent hypertension or lower blood pressure in individuals who have existing high blood pressure (41,42).

Individuals who are physically active reduce their risk of developing hypertension by 20% to 50%. Individuals who already have established hypertension can often lower blood pressure by 5 to 10 mm Hg simply by participating in moderately intense aerobic activity 30 to 45 minutes on most days of the week (43). An exercise prescription needs to be modified somewhat for individuals with hypertension. It is important that physical activity be conducted at a moderate level. Individuals should be instructed to conduct their aerobic exercise at 50% to 60% of their predicted maximum heart rate (44).

The reduction in blood pressure that comes from physical activity occurs in addition to the blood pressure reduction that comes from weight loss. Moreover, regular physical activity may be particularly beneficial for abdominal weight loss (45).

Moderation of Alcohol Intake

Excessive alcohol consumption constitutes an important risk factor for hypertension and can also contribute to difficulty in controlling blood pressure (46). Excessive alcohol consumption is also an established risk factor for stroke. Patients should be encouraged to drink no more than 2 oz of distilled spirits, one to two beers a day, or one to two glasses of wine a day if they consume alcoholic beverages. Women should limit their alcohol consumption to about half of this amount.

Avoiding Tobacco

Smoking and the use of other tobacco products such as chewing tobacco have been repeatedly shown to raise blood pressure (47). Cigarette smoking, of course, carries multiple other risk factors but also represents a significant risk for elevated blood pressure. Cigarette smoking not only raises blood pressure chronically but also acutely after each cigarette (48). This is presumably due to vascular spasm and other effects of nicotine and other components of cigarette smoke on the cardiovascular system.

Stress Reduction

As a mechanism for lowering blood pressure, stress reduction has been found to be less important than many of the other lifestyle factors already described in this section (49). However, individuals who are experiencing high amounts of stress in their life may benefit from adopting such strategies as meditation, the relaxation response, or visualization.

STRATEGIES TO INCREASE PHYSICAL ACTIVITY

An overwhelming body of literature supports the concept that regular physical activity reduces the risk of coronary

Table 4-3 Examples of Common Physical Activities for Healthy U.S. Adults by Intensity of Effort Required in MET Scores and Kilocalories per Minute*

LIGHT (<3.0 METs OR <4 kcal·min⁻¹)	MODERATE (3.0–6.0 METs OR 4–7 kcal·min⁻¹)	HARD/VIGOROUS (>6.0 METs OR >7 kcal·min⁻¹)
Walking, slowly (strolling) (1–2 mph)	Walking, briskly (3–4 mph)	Walking, briskly uphill or with a load
Cycling, stationary (<50 W)	Cycling for pleasure or transportation (≤10 mph)	Cycling, fast or racing (>10 mph)
Swimming, slow treading	Swimming, moderate effort	Swimming, fast treading or crawl
Conditioning exercise, light stretching	Conditioning exercise, general calisthenics	Conditioning exercise, stair ergometer, ski machine
...	Racket sports, table tennis	Racket sports, singles tennis, racketball
Golf, power cart	Golf, pulling cart or carrying clubs	...
		...
Bowling	...	
Fishing, sitting	Fishing, standing/casting	Fishing in stream
Boating, power	Canoeing, leisurely (2.0–3.9 mph)	Canoeing, rapidly (≥4 mph)
Home care, carpet sweeping	Home care, general cleaning	Moving furniture
Mowing lawn, riding mower	Mowing lawn, power mower	Mowing lawn, hand mover
Home repair, carpentry	Home repair, painting	...

* The METs (work metabolic rate/resting metabolic rate) are multiples of the resting rate of oxygen consumption during physical activity. One MET represents the approximate rate of oxygen consumption of a seated adult at rest, or about 3.5 mL·min⁻¹·kg⁻¹. The equivalent energy cost of 1 MET in kilocalories·min⁻¹ is about 12 for a 70-kg person, or approximately 1 kcal·kg⁻¹·hr⁻¹.
Reproduced by permission from Pate R, Pratt M, Blair S, et al. Physical activity and public health: a recommendation from the Centers for Disease Control and Prevention and the American College of Sports Medicine. JAMA 1995;273:402–407.

artery disease (1,2,50–55). In addition, physical activity is an important component of secondary prevention. Increased physical activity is a cornerstone for virtually every cardiac rehabilitation program in the United States and around the world (56). A detailed description of the linkage between physical activity and reduction of CAD is found in Chapters 7 and 68.

Recent recommendations from the American College of Sports Medicine and The Centers for Disease Control encourage adults to accumulate at least 30 minutes of moderate intensity physical activity on most, if not all, days (2). Examples of the types of physical activity that fit the classification of "moderate" are found on Table 4-3.

As a practical matter, most patients will be well advised to adopt walking as the cornerstone of their program of increased physical activity (57). Walking carries the advantages of being flexible, convenient, and low cost. Regular walking has also been clearly shown to lower the risk of CAD and results in a variety of other benefits including increased HDL, lowered blood pressure, and helping to maintain proper body weight (58,59).

Medical Evaluation Prior to Prescription of Physical Activity

For moderate-intensity activities such as walking, often all that is required is physician consultation with medical history and brief physical examination. The American College of Sports Medicine recommends that for individuals over the age of 45 or individuals with significant risk factors for CAD, a graded exercise tolerance test be performed before prescribing increased physical activity (60). Criteria utilized by the Ameri-

can College of Sports Medicine for obtaining an exercise tolerance test prior to exercise prescription are found in Table 4-4.

Exercise Prescription

Physicians and other healthcare workers should be encouraged to make the exercise prescription as specific as possible, based on patient background, previous exercise history, and needs.

The exercise prescription is commonly based on the principles of frequency, intensity, and duration of exercise. Multiple frameworks have been established to help guide patient selection of the proper exercise program. One such framework is presented in Table 4-5.

TREATMENT STRATEGIES FOR PREVENTION AND TREATMENT OF OBESITY

Adult obesity (5–10), adult weight gain (61), and abdominal distribution of body fat (62) are all independent risk factors for coronary artery disease. Obesity not only contributes to other risk factors for CAD such as type 2 diabetes, dyslipidemias, and hypertension, but also represents an independent risk factor for CAD (9). Moreover, obese individuals are particularly likely to present with multiple risk factors for coronary artery disease (63).

For all of these reasons, it is incumbent upon physicians to aggressively treat obesity both as a means of reducing CAD and also as a powerful means of secondary prevention in individuals who already have established CAD. A struc-

Table 4-4 Recommendations from the American College of Sports Medicine for (A) Medical Examination and Exercise Testing Prior to Participation in Exercise Programs and (B) Physician Supervision of Exercise Tests

A. Medical examination and clinical exercise test recommended prior to:

| | APPARENTLY HEALTHY | | INCREASED RISK* | | |
	YOUNGER[‡]	OLDER	NO SYMPTOMS	SYMPTOMS	KNOWN DISEASE[†]
Moderate Exercise[§]	No[‖]	No	No	Yes	Yes
Vigorous Exercise[¶]	No	Yes[#]	Yes	Yes	Yes

B. Physician supervision recommended during exercise test:

| | APPARENTLY HEALTHY | | INCREASED RISK* | | |
	YOUNGER[‡]	OLDER	NO SYMPTOMS	SYMPTOMS	KNOWN DISEASE[†]
Submaximal Testing	No[‖]	No	No	Yes	Yes
Maximal Testing	No	Yes[#]	Yes	Yes	Yes

* Persons with two or more risk factors or one or more signs or symptoms.

[†] Persons with known cardiac, pulmonary, or metabolic disease.

[‡] Younger implies ≤40 yeas for men, ≤50 years for women.

[§] Moderate exercise as defined by an intensity of 40% to 60% $\dot{V}o_{2max}$; if intensity is uncertain, moderate exercise may alternately be defined as an intensity well within the individual's current capacity, one which can be comfortably sustained for a prolonged period of time that is, 60 minutes, which has a gradual initiation and progression, and is generally noncompetitive.

[‖] A "No" response means that an item is deemed "not necessary." The "No" response does not mean that the item should not be done.

[¶] Vigorous exercise is defined by an exercise intensity >60% $\dot{V}o_{2max}$; if intensity is uncertain, moderate exercise may alternately be defined is exercise intense enough to represent a substantial cardiorespiratory challenge or if it results in fatigue within 20 minutes.

[#] A "Yes" response means that an item is recommended. For physician supervision, this suggests that a physician is in close proximity and readily available should there be an emergent need.

Reproduced by permission from American College of Sports Medicine. Guidelines for exercise testing and prescription. 5th ed. Philadelphia: Lippincott Williams & Wilkins, 1995.

tured approach to treatment of obesity will enhance the likelihood of therapeutic success.

Obtain the "Vital Signs" of Obesity

An initial step in the clinical management of obesity is to gather appropriate baseline information. Weight, body mass index (BMI), and waist circumference all carry relevant information related to the health risk of obesity and should be routinely recorded during physician encounters. These have been called the "vital signs" of obesity and constitute an appropriate database for all patients whether or not they are obese at baseline (64).

Lifestyle Measures

Proper nutrition, increased physical activity, and other aspects of behavior modification are important components of an overall approach to the treatment of obesity. Patients should be routinely counseled on these lifestyle issues.

Physical Activity

Regular physical activity is a key component both for short-term weight loss and, even more importantly, for long-term maintenance of weight loss (65). Although increased physical activity alone is unlikely to result in substantial weight loss, it remains an important component of an overall approach. Physical activity helps preserve lean muscle tissue and results in a variety of psychological enhancements and improved quality of life during weight loss. In recent study of over 600 individuals who had lost at least 12 kg and kept weight off for at least 5 years, physical activity was invariably a component of the successful program adopted by these individuals (66). As a practical matter, the vast majority of individuals who are overweight will find that the most appropriate form of physical activity for weight loss and maintenance of weight loss is walking.

Physical activity appears to be particularly important in the maintenance of weight loss. A variety of studies have suggested that expending between 1500 kcal and 2000 kcal per week is most likely to help people successfully maintain weight loss (67,68).

Proper Nutrition

Proper nutrition is a cornerstone of both short-term weight loss and long-term maintenance of weight loss (69,70). Reduction in calories from fat as well as overall reduction of calories are both highly relevant. Although nutritional plans need to be customized to individual patients, the Step 1 American Heart Association diet, which is recommended for cholesterol control, is also a good starting point for weight loss recommendations (see Table 4-3). Most weight loss diets attempt to create a caloric deficit of 500 to 600 kcal per day.

Nutritional counseling from a registered dietician is particularly important in weight loss. Such counseling assumes even more importance when individuals present with comorbidities such as dyslipidemia, CAD, or type 2 diabetes.

Pharmacologic Therapy

Few pharmacologic therapies are currently available to assist in weight loss. Despite the recent withdrawal of fenfluramine and dexfenfluramine from the market, patients may benefit from the adjunctive use of pharmacologic therapy in addition to lifestyle measures. Sibutramine, which is a serotonin-norepinephrine reuptake inhibitor that decreases hunger, was approved by the FDA in 1997 to assist in weight loss (71). Orlistat, a partial pancreatic lipase inhibitor that acts at the

Table 4-5 Example of a Framework

PROGRAM A

Week#	1–2	3–4	5–6	7–8	9–10	11–12	Maintenance
Warm-Up (min)*	5	5	5	5	5	5	5
Duration (min)	15	20	25	30	30	30	30–40
Approx. Pace (min/mi)†	30	30	30	30	27	25	25
Suggested Mileage	0.5	0.7	0.83	1.0	1.1	1.2	1.2–1.6
Cool-Down (min)*	5	5	5	5	5	5	5
Total Time (min)	25	30	35	40	40	40	40–50
Frequency (days/wk)	3–4	3–4	3–4	3–4	3–4	3–4	3–4

PROGRAM B

Week#	1	2	3–4	5–6	7–8	9–10	11–12	Maintenance
Warm-Up (min)*	5	5	5	5	5	5	5	5
Duration (min)	20	25	30	35	40	40	40	40–50
Approx. Pace (min/mi)†	20	18	18	18	18	17	16	16
Suggested Mileage	1.0	1.4	1.7	1.9	2.2	2.4	2.5	2.5–3.1
Cool-Down (min)*	5	5	5	5	5	10	10	10
Total Time (min)	30	35	40	45	50	55	55	55–65
Frequency (days/wk)	4–7	4–7	4–7	4–7	4–7	4–7	40–7	4–7

PROGRAM C

Week#	1–2	3–4	5–6	7–8	9–10	11–12	Maintenance
Warm-Up (min)*	5	5	5	5	5	5	5
Duration (min)	30	40	40	40	45	45	45–55
Approx. Pace (min/mi)†	17	17	16	15	15	14	14
Suggested Mileage	1.8	2.4	2.5	2.7	3.0	3.2	3.2–3.9
Cool-Down (min)*	10	10	10	10	10	10	10
Total Time (min)	45	55	55	55	60	60	60–70
Frequency (days/wk)	4–7	4–7	4–7	4–7	4–7	4–7	4–7

* Warm-up and cool-down should be slow walking which gradually increases to the training pace.
† The pace listed is only an approximation. The actual pace which should be used is the one that keeps the heart rate at the recommended level.
Reproduced by permission from Ward A, Rippe J. W.A.L.K. Walking with angina/learning is key, just for the health of it program guide. Kenilworth, NJ: Key Pharmaceuticals, Inc., 1992.

gut level to inhibit absorption of approximately one third of fat consumed, is currently under consideration by the FDA (72). A decision concerning this compound is likely by the end of 1998 or early 1999. This medication has particular potential to benefit patients at risk for CAD or with established CAD. As a partial fat blocker, Orlistat has an independent and strong effect on lowering LDL cholesterol (73). Decreases of 10% to 15% of LDL are common on this medication.

Adopting a Chronic Disease Treatment Model

Effective medical treatment of obesity hinges on adopting an appropriate chronic disease treatment model (64). This is the same type of approach that has worked well for coronary artery disease, hypertension, and dyslipidemias. By adopting a chronic disease treatment model, physicians and other health-care workers can recognize that obesity represents a chronic disease, carrying significant morbidity and mortality. This treatment model is helpful in terms of combating unwarranted stereotypes of obese individuals as guilty of "willful misconduct" or "laziness."

Prevention

One of the most important clinical aspects of obesity management is its prevention. It is clear that any significant weight gain in adults (any weight gain over 10 lb during adult years) begins to increase the risk for CAD (61). Thus, physicians should counsel any patient who experiences his or her first significant weight gain during adult years to control this problem before it becomes an established risk factor for CAD.

LIFESTYLE TREATMENT OF INDIVIDUALS WITH MULTIPLE RISK FACTORS FOR CAD

Recent evidence has suggested that a higher incidence of "clustering" of risk factors for CAD occurs than had been previously estimated (63,74). This clustering of risk factors has been identified as the "metabolic syndrome" or "syndrome X" when seen in its full manifestation (74). Clustering of risk factors for CAD has been particularly associated with abdominal obesity, in which insulin resistance, hyperinsulinemia, rela-

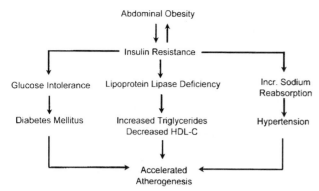

Figure 4-1 Insulin resistance syndrome potential relations. (Reproduced by permission from Wilson PWF, Kannel WB. Clustering of risk factors, obesity and syndrome X. Nutr Clin Care 1998;1:44–50. Reprinted by permission of Blackwell Science.)

tive deficiency of lipoprotein lipase, elevated triglycerides, reduced HDL cholesterol, and small dense LDL particles may form the metabolic cluster of abnormalities. Insulin resistance also contributes to glucose intolerance and diabetes. The mechanism of how all of these interrelated metabolic abnormalities contribute to increased coronary artery disease is not fully understood. One potential mechanism by which insulin resistance syndrome may contribute to increased atherogenesis is found in Figure 4-1.

Even in the absence of the complete metabolic syndrome there is an increased incidence of multiple risk factors in individuals who are obese. According to data from the Framingham study, there was a greater than 20% likelihood of obese men having at least three other risk factors and a greater than 25% likelihood of obese women having at least three other risk factors for CAD. In this population, 38% of obese men and 54% of obese women had at least two additional risk factors for CAD (63). Clustering of risk factors is clinically important since more than half of all coronary disease in the United States is found in individuals with two or more risk factors for CAD.

Fortunately, many of the lifestyle measures already discussed in this chapter are beneficial in treatment of multiple risk factors. Such lifestyle measures as maintaining proper weight, participation in regular physical activity, and maintenance of proper nutritional habits all contribute to successful management of individuals with multiple risk factors for CAD.

LIFESTYLE MANAGEMENT OF OTHER RISK FACTORS FOR CAD

Several other risk factors for CAD are amenable to lifestyle interventions and should be addressed with appropriate patients.

Alcohol

There is a complex relationship between alcohol and the risk of CAD. Moderate consumption of alcohol has been shown to reduce the risk of CAD (75,76). However, at higher levels of alcohol consumption (three or more alcoholic drinks per day) there is an increased risk of hypertension and cardiomyopathy. Counseling about alcohol consumption should be a part of the discussion of lifestyle factors related to CAD for all patients. Individuals who do not consume alcohol should not be advised to start consumption of alcohol; however, individuals who exceed moderate alcohol consumption should be advised about the increased risk of CAD associated with this habit.

Homocysteine

Elevated homocysteine levels have been associated with increased risk of CAD in a number of studies (77–79). In at least one study, this association has not been found. Since the treatment of elevated homocysteine is very simple, it seems appropriate to include it in the counseling of all patients who are at increased risk. Daily consumption of 400 µg of folate has been shown to significantly reduce homocysteine levels (80). Although folate is found in a variety of fruits and vegetables (particularly green vegetables), the consumption of 400 µg of folate on a daily basis is beyond the capacity of the normal diet for most people. Therefore, it seems reasonable to recommend that individuals at risk for CAD take a multivitamin with 400 µg of folate on a daily basis or consume a bowl of cereal fortified with 400 µg on a daily basis. In the future, this recommendation will become more precise as more information becomes available.

Stress/Type A Personality

The role of stress and personality type as risk factors for CAD remains controversial (81–84). Some studies have supported this association whereas others have not. For individuals who are either highly anxious or for whom emotional disorders are hindering other treatments for CAD, it may be prudent to recommend therapy for stress. Such modalities as biofeedback, meditation, visualization, and the relaxation response may be valuable in selected patients to help lower stress.

Lifestyle Measures for the Treatment of Established Coronary Artery Disease

Lifestyle measures have been demonstrated in a wide variety of studies to be highly effective as secondary prevention modalities in individuals with established coronary artery disease (56). Effective lifestyle measures as part of overall treatment for patients with CAD include regular physical activity, smoking cessation, stress reduction, nutritional counseling, and blood pressure control. These modalities are discussed in detail in Chapter 68.

Despite the abundant literature supporting the efficacy of lifestyle measures in reducing subsequent cardiac morbidity and mortality in patients with established CAD, only a distinct minority of eligible patients in the United States receive cardiac rehabilitation. A recent report from The Agency for Healthcare Policy Research estimated that less than 25% of the 11 million individuals eligible for cardiac rehabilitation currently receive it (56). Physicians should be aware of the value of comprehensive lifestyle measures in secondary prevention in individuals with CAD and actively recruit such patients into appropriate cardiac rehabilitation programs.

NEW APPROACHES TO LIFESTYLE THERAPY IN INDIVIDUALS WITH ESTABLISHED CORONARY ARTERY DISEASE

In a climate of managed care and increased cost consciousness, new approaches have been proposed to deliver lifestyle measures to patients in cost-effective ways. One such approach is the delivery of information and services to patients via telephonic contact. One such program, initiated by The Center for Clinical and Lifestyle Research in Shrewsbury, Mass, involves a series of educational brochures and telephonic support by cardiac rehabilitation nurses (85). This program features the delivery of information about physical activity, control of blood pressure, proper nutritional choices, compliance with medical regimen, and stress reduction in patients with established coronary artery disease or at high risk for CAD. In preliminary studies, this approach has been demonstrated to help in lowering fat intake and increasing physical activity among participants (85).

DETERMINANTS OF BEHAVIOR CHANGE

The concept of intervening to help patients adopt positive lifestyle behaviors to lower their risk of CAD or to help in the treatment of established CAD is based on the belief that it is possible to change patient behavior. There is a large literature related to the determinants of health behaviors and change in these behaviors. This literature has recently been reviewed by Ockene et al (86). As summarized by these authors, there are four theoretical constructs related to health behaviors and change in these behaviors:

- Consumer information processing theory
- Social learning theory
- The health belief model
- Stages of change model

Although it is not anticipated that physicians will become deeply familiar with this literature, it is valuable to at least summarize key issues related to each of these theoretical models.

Consumer Information Processing Theory

This model posits that appropriate information is acquired for rational decision making and that this information has an important influence on human behavior. In this model it is important for the clinician to make information available and to present it in a fashion that the patient can comprehend and act upon.

Social Learning Theory

This theory is based on the assumption that behaviors can be learned and therefore unlearned or altered. The components of this theory involve reaching small goals, monitoring progress, and self-reward.

Health Belief Model

This model focuses on attitudes and beliefs as a way of understanding what motivates a patient to change. Individuals who do not believe that their own actions or habits will impact on their health are unlikely to make changes.

Stages of Change Model

This model starts from the assumption that change is a dynamic concept. Both physician and patient can develop more realistic expectations of the potential for change by recognizing where the patient is on a spectrum of stages of change. Five stages of change and strategies to help individuals move to the next stage are found in Table 4-6.

Having at least a working knowledge of the theoretical models supporting behavior change theory is important for every physician who counsels patients on lifestyle management and prevention of CAD.

Table 4-6 Stages of Behavior Change and Strategies to Help the Patient Move to the Next Stage

STAGE	STRATEGIES
Precontemplation: Patient Not Yet Considering Change	• Provide more information. • Help patient develop belief in ability to change (self-efficacy). • Personalize assessment/feedback.
Contemplation: Patient Thinking about and Making Plans to Change Behavior	• Help patient develop skills for behavior change. • Provide support. • Help patient develop plan for behavior change. • Provide self-help materials.
Action: Patient Changing Behavior	• Provide support. • Help patient prepare for possible problems.
Maintenance: Patient Maintaining Behavioral Change Relapse: Patient Returning to Old Behavior	• Help patient prepare for possible problems. • Help patient understand reasons for relapse. • Provide information about process of change. • Help patient make plans for next attempt. • Faciliate patient's belief in ability to change again. • Provide unconditional support.

Reproduced by permission from Ockene IS, Ockene JK. Helping patients to reduce their risk of coronary heart disease. In: Ockene IS, Ockene JK. Prevention of coronary heart disease. Boston: Little, Brown, 1992.

Table 4-7 Steps to Clinical Preventive Cardiology	
STEP	PHYSICIAN'S ROLE
Step 1: Disagnosis/ Assessment	Assess health and risks using: Medical interview Questionnaires Laboratory tests
Step 2: Treatment/ Intervention	Advise need for behavioral change. Provide information/personalize risk. Help patient to establish motivation, understand strengths, and deal with barriers.
Step 3: Plan for Change	Negotiate goals with patient and plan strategies to achieve them.
Step 4: Follow-up/ Maintenance	Schedule follow-up visits. Provide support.

Reproduced by permission from Ockene IS, Ockene JK. Helping patients to reduce their risk of coronary heart disease. In: Ockene IS, Ockene JK. Prevention of coronary heart disease. Boston: Little, Brown 1992.

ESTABLISHING A LIFESTYLE EMPHASIS IN CLINICAL PRACTICE

As already indicated, the physician plays a critical role along with other members of the healthcare team in helping patients to adopt positive lifestyle strategies, both to prevent CAD and to help in the treatment of established CAD. A theoretical model established by Ockene et al (86) involves four steps as outlined in Table 4-7.

This model, which provides for a specific sequence of steps to help the physician guide patients through lifestyle change, focuses on the concept of "patient-centered counseling." This type of counseling adopts the patient's point of view and requires the physician to ask a series of open-ended questions to help the patient deal with the realities and barriers that may either encourage or discourage the patient from adopting positive lifestyle behaviors. It has been demonstrated that provision of such patient-centered counseling in 3- to 5-minute sessions included in normal doctor-patient encounters can significantly enhance the likelihood of the patient adopting positive lifestyle behaviors to either reduce the risk of coronary artery disease or help in its treatment.

SUMMARY

A wide body of literature supports that lifestyle strategies are highly effective, both for lowering risk factors and as an adjunctive part of therapy for individuals with coronary artery disease. These lifestyle interventions carry the significant advantages of being low cost, carrying virtually no adverse side effects, and often treating multiple risk factors for CAD simultaneously. The key issue for most physicians and other healthcare workers is to make a commitment to learning how to implement these lifestyle measures and establishing procedures in clinical practice to bring this valuable information to individual patients.

REFERENCES

1. U.S. Department of Health and Human Services. Physical activity and health: A report of the Surgeon General. Atlanta: USDHHS, 1996.

2. Pate R, Pratt M, Blair S, et al. Physical activity and public health: A recommendation from the Centers for Disease Control and Prevention and the American College of Sports Medicine. JAMA 1995;273:402–407.

3. Expert Panel on Detection, Evaluation, and Treatment of High Blood Cholesterol in Adults. Summary of the second report of the National Cholesterol Education Program (NECP) Expert Panel on Detection, Evaluation and Treatment of High Blood Cholesterol in Adults (Adult Treatment Panel II) JAMA 1993;269:3015.

4. U.S. Department of Agriculture, Agricultural Research Service, Dietary Guidelines Advisory Committee. Report of the Dietary Guidelines Advisory Committee on the Dietary Guidelines for Americans. Dietary Guidelines for America 1995. Washington, DC: USDA, 1995.

5. Rippe JM. Obesity as a risk factor for heart disease: An overview. Nutr Clin Care. 1998;1:3–14.

6. Manson JE, Willett WC, Stampler MJ, et al. Body weight and mortality among women. N Engl J Med 1995;333:677–685.

7. Rimm EB, Stampler MJ, Giovannucci B, et al. Body size and fat distribution as predictors of coronary heart disease among middle-aged and older US men. Am J Epidemiol 1995;141:1117–1127.

8. Garrison RJ, Castelli WP. Weight and thirty-year mortality of men in the Framingham Study. Ann Int Med 1985;103:1006–1009.

9. Eckel R. Obesity and heart disease: a statement for the healthcare professionals from the Nutrition Committee, American Heart Association. Circulation 1997;96:3248–3250.

10. World Health Organization. Prevention and management of the global epidemic of obesity. Report of the WHO Consultation on Obesity, No. 10. Geneva: WHO, 1997.

11. National Institutes of Health. National Heart, Lung, and Blood Institute. National High Blood Pressure Education Program. The Sixth Report of the Joint National Committee on Prevention, Detection, Evaluation, and Treatment of High Blood Pressure. NIH Publication No. 98-4080. Washington, DC: NIH, 1997.

12. Institute of Medicine. Weighing the options: Criteria for evaluating weight-management programs.

Washington, DC: National Academy Press, 1994.

13. Ockene JK, Quirk ME, Goldberg RJ, et al. A resident's training program for the development of smoking intervention skills. Arch Intern Med 1988;148: 1039–1045.

14. Mojonnier ML, Hall Y, Berkson DM, et al. Experience in changing food habits of hyperlipidemic men and women. J Am Diet Assoc 1988;77:140–148.

15. Dunbar J. Assessment of medication compliance: a review. In: Haynes RB, Mattson ME, Engebretson TO, eds. Patient compliance to prescribed antihypertensive medication regimen. USDHHS Pub No. (NIH) 81-2101. Washington, DC: USDHHS, 1988.

16. Greenfield S, Kaplan SH, Ware JE, et al. Patients' participation in medical care: effects on blood sugar control and quality of life in diabetes. J Gen Intern Med 1988;3:448–457.

17. Schulman BA. Active patient orientation and outcomes in hypertensive treatment: application of a socio-organizational perspective. Med Care 1979;17:267–280.

18. Harris SS, Caspersen CJ, DeFriese GH, Estes GH Jr. Physical activity counseling for healthy adults as a primary prevention intervention in the clinical setting: report for the U.S. Preventive Services Task Force. JAMA 1989;261:3590–3598.

19. Campbell MK, DeVellis BM, Strecher VJ, Ammerman AS, DeVellis RF, Sandles RS. Improving dietary behavior: the effectiveness of tailored messages in primary care settings. Am J Public Health 1984;84:783–787.

20. Glynn TJ, Manley MW, Cullen JW, Mayer JW. Cancer prevention through physician interventions. Semin Oncol 1990;17:391–401.

21. Ford AS, Ford WS. Health education and the primary care physician: the practitioner's perspective. Soc Sci Med 1983;17: 1505–1512.

22. National Center for Health Statistics. Health, United States 1987 USDHHS Pub No. (PHS) 88-1232. Washington, DC: U.S. Department of Health and Human Services, Public Health Service, 1988.

23. Fiore M, Novotny T, Lynn W, et al. Methods used to quit smoking in the United States: do cessation programs help? JAMA 1990;263: 2760–2765.

24. Ockene JK. Physician-delivered interventions for smoking cessation: strategies for increasing effectiveness. Prev Med 1987;16:723–737.

25. Rippe J, Aronne L, Gilligan, V, et al. Public policy statement on obesity and health. Nutr Clin Care 1998, 1(1).

26. Ebbeling CB, Ockene IS. Obesity and dyslipidemia. Nutr Clin Care 1998;1:15–29.

27. Wood P, Stefanick M, Dreon D, et al. Changes in plasma lipids and lipoproteins in overweight men during weight loss through dieting as compared with exercise. N Engl J Med 1988;319:1173–1179.

28. Stein R, Michielli D, Glantz M, et al. Effects of different exercise training intensities on lipoprotein cholesterol fractions in healthy middle-aged men. Am Heart J 1990;119:277–283.

29. Ward A, Morris DH, Porcari JP, et al. Effects of walking and/or low fat diet on total and HDL cholesterol and risk ratio (accepted national meeting, American Heart Association, 1989).

30. Stefanick ML, Mackey S, Sheehan M, et al. Effects of diet and exercise in men and postmenopausal women with low levels of HDL cholesterol and high levels of LDL cholesterol. N Engl J Med 1998;339:12–20.

31. Despres JP. Abdominal obesity as important component of insulin-resistance syndrome. Nutrition 1993;4:452–459.

32. Gordon DJ, Probstfield JL, Garrison RJ, et al. High-density lipoprotein cholesterol and cardiovascular disease: four prospective American studies. Circulation 1989;79:8.

33. Austin MA. Plasma triglyceride and coronary heart disease. Arterioscler Thromb 1991;11:2.

34. American College of Sports Medicine. Position stand on the recommended quantity and quality of exercise for developing and maintaining cardiorespiratory and muscular fitness in healthy adults. Med Sci Sports Exerc 1990;22: 265–274.

35. Heyka R. Obesity and hypertension. Nutr Clin Care 1998; 1(suppl):30–37.

36. Stevens V, Corrigan S, Obarzanke E, et al. Weight loss intervention in phase I of the trials of hypertension prevention. Arch Intern Med 1993;153:849–858.

37. National High Blood Pressure Education Program Work Group. National High Blood Pressure Education Program Working Group report on primary prevention of hypertension. Arch Intern Med 1993;153:186–208.

38. Stepniakowski K, Egan BM. Additive effects of obesity and hypertension to limit venous volume. Am J Physiol 1995;268: R562–R568.

39. Appel LJ, Moore JT, Obarzanek E, et al for the DASH Collaborative Research Group. A clinical trial on the effects of dietary patterns on blood pressure. N Engl J Med 1997;336:1117–1124.

40. Kaplan NM. Clinical hypertension. 6th ed. Baltimore: Williams and Wilkins, 1994.

41. Arroll B, Beaglehold R. Does physical activity lower blood pressure? a critical review of the clinical trials. J Clin Epidemiol 1992;45: 439–447.

42. Rippe JM. Hypertension. In: Alpert JS, Rippe JM. Manual of cardiovascular diagnosis and therapy. 4th ed. Boston: Little, Brown, 1996.

43. ACSM Position Stand. Physical activity, physical fitness, and hypertension. Med Sci Sports Exerc 1993;25:i–x.

44. Matsusaki M, Ikeda M, Tashiro E, et al. Influence of workload on the antihypertensive effect of exercise. Clin Exp Pharmacol Physiol 1992;19:471–479.

45. Wing RR, Matthews KA, Kuller LH, et al. Waist to hip ratio in middle aged women: association with behavioral and psychosocial factors and with changes in cardiovascular risk factors. Arterioscler Thromb 1991;11:1250–1257.

46. Marmot MG, Elliott P, Shipley MJ, et al. Alcohol and blood pressure: the INTERSALT Study. Br Med J 1994;308:1263.

47. Kaplan NM. Systemic hypertension:therapy. In: Braunwald E, ed. Heart disease. 5th ed. Philadelphia: W.B. Saunders, 1997.

48. Giannattasio C, Mangoni AA, Stella ML, et al. Acute effects of smoking on radial artery compliances in humans. J Hypertens. 1994;12:691.

49. Eisenberg DM, Delbanco TL, Berkey CS, et al. Cognitive behavioral techniques for hypertension: are they effective? Am J Hypertens 1993;4:416.

50. Powell KE, Thompson PD, Casperson CJ, et al. Physical activity and the incidence of coronary heart disease. Annu Rev Public Health 1987;8:253.

51. Berlin JA, Colditz, GA. A meta-analysis of physical activity in the prevention of coronary heart disease. Am J Epidemiol 1990;132:612.

52. Leon AS, Connett J for the MRFIT Research Group Physical activity and 10.5 year mortality in the Multiple Risk Factor Intervention Trial (MRFIT). Int J Epidemiol 1991;20:690.

53. Ekelunch L-G, Haskell WL, Johnson JL, et al. Physical fitness as a predictor of cardiovascular mortality in asymptomatic North American men: the Lipid Research Clinics Mortality Follow-up Study. N Engl J Med 1988;319:1379.

54. Sandvik L, Erikssen J, Thaulow E, et al. Physical Fitness as a predictor of cardiovascular mortality among healthy, middle-aged Norwegian men. N Engl J Med 1993;328:533.

55. Lakka TA, Venalainen JM, Rauramaa R, et al. Relation of leisure-time physical activity and cardiorespiratory fitness to the risk of acute myocardial infarction. N Engl J Med 1994;330:1549.

56. U.S. Department of Health and Human Service. Public Health Service. Cardiac rehabilitation as a secondary prevention. AHCPR Publication No. 96-0673. Washington, DC: USDHHS, 1995.

57. Rippe JM, Ward A, Porcari J, Freedson PS. Walking for health and fitness. JAMA 1988;259:272.

58. Rippe JM, Ward A. The complete book of fitness walking. New York: Prentice Hall, 1990.

59. Goldfine H, Ward A, Taylor P, et al. Exercising to health: what's really in it for your patients? Part I: the health benefits of exercise. Phys Sports Med 1991;19(6):81.

60. Kenney WL, Humphrey RH, Bryant CX, eds. American College of Sports Medicine's guidelines for exercise testing and prescription. 5th ed. Baltimore: William and Wilkins, 1995.

61. Chan JM, Rimm EB, Colditz GA, et al. Obesity, fat distribution, and weight gain as a risk factor for clinical diabetes in men. Diabetes CARE 1994;17:961–969.

62. Pouliot MC, Despres JP, Lemieux S, et al. Waist circumference and abdominal sagittal diameter: best simple anthropometric indexes of abdominal visceral adipose tissue accumulation and related cardiovascular risk in men. Am J Cardiol 1994;73:460–468.

63. Wilson P. Clustering of risk factors, obesity, and Syndrome X. Nutr Clin Care 1998;1(suppl):44–50.

64. Rippe JM. The case for medical management of obesity: a call for increased physician involvement. Obes Res 1998;6:23S–33S.

65. Rippe JM, Hess S. The role of physical activity in the prevention and management of obesity. J Am Diet Assoc 1998;S31–S38.

66. Klem M, Wing R, McGuire M, et al. A descriptive study of individuals successful at long-term maintenance of substantial weight loss. Am J Clin Nutr 1997;66:239–246.

67. Ewbank P, Darga K, Lucas C. Physical activity as a predictor of weight maintenance in previously obese subjects. Obes Res 1995;3:257–263.

68. Schoeller D, Shay K, Kushner R. How much physical activity is needed to minimize weight gain in previously obese women. Am J Clin Nutr 1997:66:551–556.

69. Rippe JM, Crossley S, Ringer R. Obesity as a chronic disease: modern medical and lifestyle management. J Am Diet Assoc 1998:S9-S15.

70. Nonas CA. A model for chronic care of obesity through dietary treatment. J Am Diet Assoc 1998;98:S16-S22.

71. Silverstone T. Appetite suppressants: a review. Drugs 1992;43:820–836.

72. Guercioloini R. Mode of action of Orlistat. Int J Obes 1997;21(suppl 13):S12–S23.

73. Sjostrom L, Rissanen A, Andersen T, et al for the European Multicentre Orlistat Study Group. Lancet 1998;352:167–172.

74. Grundy SM, Small IDL. Atherogenic dyslipidemia and the metabolic syndrome. Circulation 1997;95:1–4.

75. Pohorecky LA. Interaction of alcohol and stress at the cardiovascular level. Alcohol 1990;7:537.

76. Gaziano JM, Buring JE, Breslow JL, et al. Moderate alcohol intake, increased levels of high-density lipoprotein and its subfractions and decreased risk of myocardial infarction. N Engl J Med 1993;329:1829.

77. Glueck CJ, Shaw P, Lang JE, et al. Evidence that homocysteine is an independent risk factor for atherosclerosis in hyperlipidemic patients. Am J Cardiol 1995;75:132.

78. Stampfer MJ, Malinow MR, Willett WC, et al. A prospective study of plasma homocysteine and risk of myocardial infarction in US physicians. 1992;268:877.

79. Rimm EB, Willett WC, Hu FB, et al. Folate and vitamin B_6 from diet and supplements in relation to risk of coronary heart disease among women. JAMA 1998;279: 359–364.

80. Malinow MR, Duell PB, Hess DL, et al. Reduction of plasma homocysteine levels by breakfast cereal fortified with folic acid in patients with coronary heart disease. N Engl J Med 1998;338:1009.

81. Lachar BL. Coronary-prone behavior: type A behavior revisited. Tex Heart Inst J 1993;20:143.

82. Littman AB. Review of psychosomatic aspects of cardiovascular disease. Psychother Psychosom 1993;60:148.

83. Rosenman RH, Brand RJ, Jenkins CD, et al. Coronary heart disease in the Western Collaborative Group Study: final follow-up experience of 8 1/2 years. JAMA 1975;233:872.

84. Matthews KA, Haynes SG. Type A behavior pattern and coronary disease risk: an update and critical evaluation. Am J Epidemiol 1986;123:923.

85. Hess S, Taylor K, Partsch D, et al. Effectiveness of cardiovascular disease management program in promoting physical activity. J Card Rehab 1998;118:374.

86. Ockene IS, Ockene JK. Prevention of coronary heart disease. Boston: Little, Brown, 1992.

Chapter 5

Managing Smoking as a Risk Factor in Cardiac Disease: An Educational, Behavioral, and Pharmacologic Perspective

Jean L. Kristeller

The relationship between smoking and cardiovascular disease is now as well established as the link between smoking and lung disease (1,2). Although smoking accounts for only about 50% of the attributable risk for cardiac disease, as compared to 80% to 90% for chronic obstructive pulmonary disease (COPD) and lung cancer, over 100,000 smokers die annually from cardiac disease, more than from lung cancer (3). In addition, it is now estimated that as many as 37,000 heart disease deaths can be attributed annually to exposure to environmental smoke (passive smoking) (4).

Smokers experience a first myocardial infarction (MI) at a younger age, may be more likely to have an MI in the absence of coronary artery disease, and may experience different patterns of infarct than a nonsmoker, both in location and size (5). Smokers are much more likely to experience angina pectoris (6). The Nurses' Health Study recently found that smoking doubles the likelihood of a pulmonary embolism for lighter (25–34 cigarettes per day) smokers and triples it for heavier smokers (35 or more cigarettes per day) (7). Recent evidence suggests that the long-term benefits of angioplasty are greatly decreased for patients who continue to smoke (8); the same may be true for coronary bypass surgery (9). The risk of peripheral vascular disease is also greatly increased, particularly for diabetics (2).

Smoking affects the cardiovascular system through several pathways. Nicotine and other toxic components appear to accelerate the development of atherosclerosis, both by damaging the arterial walls and by facilitating aggregation of platelets to endothelium; smoking may also promote development of the clots that block narrowed arteries, thereby causing infarctions. Nicotine activates the sympathetic nervous system and may cause arterial spasming, promote arrythmias,

and increase cardiac load by leading to peripheral vascular constriction (10). Nicotine reduces the blood's ability to deliver oxygen to the myocardium and reduces the ability of the myocardium to effectively use the oxygen it receives. Smoking is of particular risk for sudden cardiac death; data suggests that this is due to acute thrombosis related to increased platelet aggregation and increased plasma epinephrine (11,12). Smoking increases blood pressure, both during the day and transiently, and acutely increases stiffness in arterial walls. Even low exposure to nicotine and other cigarette constituents can increase free radicals that increase reperfusion injury; these effects may be even greater for passive smoke inhalation (4). Benowitz et al (13) provide an excellent review of the cardiovascular toxicity effects of nicotine.

CARDIAC-RELATED BENEFITS OF QUITTING

Because smokers who experience an MI generally have lower levels of other cardiopathology, stopping smoking is particularly important in reducing future risk. Prospective studies (6,14) have shown that patients who stop smoking reduce the likelihood of a second MI by as much as 50%, reduce the likelihood of future events after bypass surgery (9), and greatly reduce the likelihood of death during long-term follow-up after angioplasty (8). Some of the effects of smoking, in particular arterial spasming, platelet aggregation, increased arrythmias, and effect on oxygenation, are rapidly reversible. Effects on artherosclerotic processes make take much longer to reverse.

Although the majority of patients stop smoking at the time of an MI, if only because of the trauma of the event and restrictions on smoking imposed by hospitalization, fewer remain abstinent than might be expected. After about 3 months, the proportion of post-MI patients reporting abstinence is approximately one half (15,16), but this proportion may be lower when biochemical validation techniques are employed. Seriousness of the disease also affects the likelihood of smoking cessation in cardiovascular disease, both among post-MI patients and among patients with documented coronary artery disease (17). Cutter (18) reported a range of abstinence from only 7% in individuals with no disease, to 30% in patients with one-or two-vessel disease, to 47% in those with three-vessel disease. Hasdai (8) found that 37% of smokers receiving percutaneous transluminal coronary angioplasty (PTCA) were abstinent approximately 5 years later. These proportions are similar to relapse rates observed with other addictions (19).

A BIOPSYCHOSOCIAL MODEL OF SMOKING AND SMOKING CESSATION

Social influence, psychological needs, and physiologic dependence are all recognized as playing significant roles in initiating and maintaining smoking and contributing to relapse. Although a medical problem or hospitalization may both increase motivation to quit and provide environmental support to do so, many of the same psychobiologic barriers and challenges to successful smoking cessation exist for medical inpatients as for the general population (20,21).

Social Influences

Social influence is important in both initiating and maintaining smoking. Teenagers are far more likely to start smoking if friends or family members smoke; smoking also contributes to development of self-image, an aspect exploited aggressively by tobacco advertising. For example, smoking initiation among young women appeals to images of independence and attractiveness, with a strong overt play to social concerns about weight management and remaining thin (22); such issues can remain important motivating factors far into adult life. Social influence is also highly relevant to smoking cessation. Whether a spouse smokes and is supportive of efforts to quit affects likelihood of quitting; for example, supportive behaviors from a spouse facilitates quitting (23–25), while the presence of other smokers in the household predicts less success (26).

Considering social influence is important when addressing smoking cessation. If the immediate social environment contains many other smokers, whether the spouse or close friends, a smoker may find it more difficult to resist temptations to smoke, and exploring the issues related to this social pressure may be helpful. Smokers in sociodemographic groups with high prevalence of smoking may be perceived as "hard core" and therefore resistant to intervention. Conversely, the real hard-core smoker may be the individual from a social group with very low rates of smoking, whose high level of physiologic or psychological dependence leads them to continue smoking regardless of the social pressures to quit (27). Therefore, regardless of the sociodemographic background of the smoker, it is important to consider what the social context

of smoking means to that person and to facilitate their ability to abstain in the face of the social influence involved. Finally, the impact of the physician and the health-care team in encouraging patients to smoke reflects the role of social influence in promoting smoking cessation. Evidence is quite clear that the more assistance offered by the physician, the higher the likelihood of quitting among medical patients (28) and the more helpful patients perceive the physician to be in their efforts to stop smoking (29).

Behavioral and Psychological Dependence

It usually takes 1 to 2 years for smoking to move from an occasional activity to a daily addicted pattern; during this time, both behavioral and physiologic patterns of dependence gradually develop. A one-pack-per-day smoker engages in the behavior of smoking over 7000 times in a year, and develops highly individual patterns of smoking associated with particular places, behaviors, thoughts, and feelings. Smoking becomes a very strong habit, and many types of situations and experiences will trigger a desire for a cigarette. According to behavioral principles, one of the values of cutting back gradually on amount smoked ("tapering") to about half a pack a day before quitting "cold turkey" is that less desired cigarettes can be cut out first, not only decreasing amount of nicotine but also decreasing the number of situations in which a cigarette is desired and increasing a sense of confidence (self-efficacy) in resisting such desires. Even heavy smokers who cut down to at least 15 cigarettes per day are twice as likely to be abstinent at follow-up than those who quit from heavier levels (30). The higher the level of self-efficacy, the greater the likelihood of success in remaining abstinent. It is also well recognized that relapse risk continues long after actual nicotine withdrawal has occurred; most relapse occurs under one of three general situations: under stress; in a social setting; or when alcohol has lowered inhibitions (31). Anticipating and guarding against these situations and others that a smoker has identified as a high-risk situation for him- or herself is an important part of relapse prevention. Using positive cognitive coping techniques will decrease the chance of a temptation turning into a lapse (32).

Nicotine Addiction and Physiologic Dependence

There is no longer any question that nicotine is a highly addicting substance (33). With some exceptions, anyone smoking more than five cigarettes per day (34) is taking in enough nicotine to show characteristics of addiction. Two factors contribute to the regular intake of tobacco: the positive drug effects, and the difficulty in quitting due to the discomfort of withdrawal symptoms. Unlike such drugs as alcohol, cocaine, or marijuana, the drug effects of nicotine are generally milder, and it is not an intoxicant; therefore, the addictive potential of nicotine is often misunderstood. The Surgeon General's 1988 Report on Nicotine Addiction (33) defined addiction as the compulsive use of a drug that has psychoactive value and that is associated with tolerance and withdrawal symptoms if intake is decreased or interrupted. In these terms, nicotine is one of the most addicting substances available, with about 90% of daily smokers developing dependence.

As a psychoactive drug, nicotine appears to have multiple effects, the appeal of which may vary across individuals. It is a mild relaxant and a peripheral nervous system stimulant; it may act as a mood elevator; and it can be an effective anorexant. Seeking out nicotine use for one of these reasons is also a basis for relapse, even many months after quitting. Hughes et al (35) have identified a core set of nicotine withdrawal symptoms that form the basis for the American Psychiatric Association's (36) definition of nicotine withdrawal. Nicotine withdrawal involves the occurrence of at least four (or more) of the following symptoms, which cause impairment or significant distress: depressed mood, insomnia, irritability or anger, anxiety, difficulty concentrating, restlessness, decreased heart rate, and increased appetite/weight gain. These symptoms appear at various stages, from several hours to several days after stopping smoking; although maximal discomfort usually occurs between 2 to 5 days, some withdrawal symptoms, such as difficulty concentrating and change in appetite, may persist for several weeks. Others, such as depressed mood, anxiety, irritability, or continued binge eating, may indicate a comorbid condition that had been masked or ameliorated by the biologic or behavioral value of smoking.

Comorbidity with Depression, Alcohol Intake, and Other Psychiatric Disorders

For reasons that are likely related to the psychoactive effects of nicotine, individuals with current or past history of significant psychiatric problems, including depression, schizophrenia, and alcoholism, are much more likely to be smokers than are people in the general population, and may have a particularly difficult time stopping smoking (37–39). Smokers who are depressed may be more nicotine dependent and be more likely to "self-medicate," using smoking to deal with negative affect and to provide stimulation (40). Smokers with psychiatric comorbidities may be at greater risk of premature death from medical problems related to smoking than from their other addictions or psychiatric problems. For example, a study of patients treated initially for alcoholism found that after an average of 10 years, half of the subsequent deaths were attributable to smoking-related diseases as compared to 34% from alcohol (41). Individuals with a history of these issues may need more intensive or specialized assistance in stopping smoking (42), to support abstinence or to prevent worsening of depression (43), but may nevertheless be successful, even without full remission of the comorbid disorder. Many of these issues have been reviewed and practice guidelines for smoking intervention developed under the direction of the American Psychiatric Association (44,45).

SMOKING INTERVENTION AND CARDIAC DISEASE: RESEARCH

As smoking becomes more clearly recognized as a medical risk factor, the concern with providing both primary and secondary prevention within the medical context has increased. A number of studies (28,29,46,47) have demonstrated that providing patients with brief counseling during the course of

an outpatient visit increases the likelihood of subsequent quitting, and the medical visit or inpatient hospitalization has been recognized as a "window of opportunity" for providing advice, quit-smoking materials, and brief counseling (21).

Primary prevention, within this context, means addressing smoking prior to any evidence of heart disease, through increased public awareness, in the primary care population, and particularly in individuals with familial risk for cardiac disease. Providing such intervention to patients with documented cardiac disease, either at the point when symptoms first occur, or after a myocardial infarction, is secondary prevention. The impetus to provide intervention at this point has increased with the growth of the cardiac rehabilitation movement and with evidence that the likelihood of a subsequent MI was reduced as much as 50% in people who stopped smoking (48,49).

Prevention in High-Risk Populations

Both community interventions, largely educational in focus, e.g., the WHO European Collaborative Trial (50), and individually-focused interventions, such as the Multiple Risk Factor Intervention Trial (MRFIT) (3,51,52) and the Stanford Three Community Study (53), demonstrated early that smoking intervention can be effectively targeted at individuals at risk for heart disease (1). These studies have shown changes in smoking rates in the range of 15% to 50% (54) in individuals at high risk for coronary heart disease, depending on intensity of the intervention, length of follow-up, and study participants. Another appropriate target for smoking intervention may be relatives of cardiac patients (55).

Intervention with Cardiac Patients: Outpatient

Although a number of early intervention trials focused on patients at high risk for cardiac disease (1), only limited research has focused specifically on treatment of the cardiac patient in the outpatient setting. Joseph (56) conducted a large multisite study of VA patients with cardiovascular disease, with a primary goal of examining the safety of the nicotine patch. Patients also received brief behavioral counseling for a total of about 35 minutes. Initial abstinence rates were higher in the nicotine group, although no higher than might be expected in the general population (21%), but after 6 months the rates had dropped in that group to only 14%, not significantly different from those receiving placebo (11%). The authors point out that these rates may be low because of a high prevalence of psychiatric disorders in this population.

Some evidence suggests that physicians are more likely to address smoking in patients already diagnosed with smoking-related diseases than in health patients. Ockene (29) conducted exit interviews with smokers who had just had an outpatient visit; approximately 40% of healthy patients and 40% of those with smoking-related symptoms reported that their physician mentioned smoking, as compared to 80% of those with a smoking-related diagnosis, including cardiac disease.

Intervention with Cardiac Patients: Inpatient

When smokers are hospitalized, the admission to the hospital may serve as a trigger to stop smoking (16,57), particularly as hospitals have become smokefree, consistent with the JCAHO accreditation guidelines. Because of the immediate and long-term health benefits of quitting smoking and remaining abstinent (2), there is considerable individual and public health value to be gained by identifying how the hospital environment can be optimally utilized to promote smoking cessation.

Ockene et al (15) investigated the effect of an individually-delivered behavioral intervention on smoking in hospitalized patients with a range of underlying disease who had just undergone coronary arteriography. Treatment, delivered by health educators, consisted of bedside counseling oriented toward self-management and relapse prevention, an outpatient visit (attended by approximately half of the eligible patients), telephone counseling at weekly and then monthly intervals, and self-help materials, including a relaxation tape, geared toward the needs of an older, more disabled population. After 6 months, validated cessation rates were 34% for the control group versus 45% for the intervention group, and at 12 months the rates were 28% and 35% for the two groups. Level of disease greatly affected quit rates; of those with no disease, only 21% were abstinent; with one vessel, 47% were abstinent, increasing to 56% for two vessels and 76% for three vessels. Patients with less serious disease (only one occluded vessel or no history of MI) also showed little response to the intervention, whereas patients with more substantial disease were far more likely to quit if they received intervention. This finding suggests that the intervention was more successful in increasing behavioral management skills, providing support, and preventing relapse than in changing underlying attitudes.

Taylor et al (16) provided a similar intervention approach, but it was delivered by a nurse who had received approximately 12 hours of training. Patients who continued or returned to smoking were asked to return for outpatient visits. The total average contact time for the intervention was approximately 2 hours. Probably because these patients were all immediately post-MI, the smoking cessation rate at one year was 71%, as compared to 45% in the usual care condition. Intervention had the least impact for patients reporting less motivation initially, and increased effort directed toward less motivated patients did not appear to improve likelihood of abstinence.

A more recent study by this same group (57) included less seriously ill cardiac patients and varied whether patients received one or four follow-up calls after the nurse-managed inpatient counseling contact. In addition to the bedside counseling, a 16-minute videotape about smoking relapse was played for the patient. Nicotine replacement therapy was offered as appropriate, resulting in 44% of the intensive care patients, 39% of the minimal follow-up patients, and 29% of the usual care patients receiving a prescription. The more intensive follow-up produced 1-year abstinence rates of 34% as compared to the minimal (28%) or usual care situation (24%). Quit rates between the intensive and minimal follow-up groups two days after discharge were very similar (74% and 79% respectively); therefore, the differences at 12 months are likely due to the more intensive follow-up. A cost analysis found that the intensive condition cost $58.00 (nursing time and materials) per patient to deliver.

EVIDENCE-BASED GUIDELINES FOR SMOKING INTERVENTION FOR MEDICAL PATIENTS

The Agency for Health Care Policy and Research (AHCPR), after reviewing the smoking and tobacco literature in depth, has developed guidelines for smoking intervention in medical settings (28). The major recommendations for primary care clinicians are to use office-wide systems to identify smokers, to treat every smoker with a cessation or motivational intervention, to offer nicotine replacement (or other medication) unless inappropriate, and to schedule follow-up contact after cessation. The HEDIS "report card" for medical standards of care, developed jointly by the National Committee on Quality Assurance (which accredits HMOs) and Medicare/Medicaid, also now includes basic screening for smoking status and for the occurrence of "advice to quit" (58). Although the primary focus of these smoking guidelines is on the primary care setting, they can readily be applied to a cardiac clinic setting. Patients may be particularly motivated by a message coming from their cardiologist; furthermore, the absence of such a message may be interpreted as tacit approval of continued smoking. Given the lower quit rates among patients with milder cardiac disease, a strong message from the cardiologist may be particularly important to encourage quitting.

The four "As" outlined in the National Cancer Institute manual "How to Help Your Patient Stop Smoking" (59) remain the core of the intervention of the AHCPR recommendations: Ask, Advise, Assist, Arrange. See Table 5-1 for an outline of these key areas and the elements involved. *Ask* refers to screening; *advise* refers to simple recommendations to stop smoking; *assist* entails more extended help, such as brief counseling and pharmacological assistance; and *arrange* implies providing active referrals for further assistance and provision of followup. While all of these steps can be performed minimally in a minute or two, the data strongly suggest that a somewhat more extensive interaction has substantially more impact. Therefore, the material below will discuss ways to develop brief assessment, intervention, and follow-up protocols that can be adapted to fit into an office visit or bedside contact, and that are consistent with the intent of providing meaningful intervention to all smokers in a medical setting.

A short standard assessment procedure is recommended. For efficient brief counseling, a patient-centered individual counseling approach (29), which is well-suited for a medical environment and easily taught to physicians (60), is recommended as part of the "assist" component. This approach combines brief motivational interviewing with behavioral and social support components, and can be adapted to as little time as 5 minutes or expanded to 30 or more minutes. Many of these elements can be initiated or augmented by members of the health care team other than the physician. For smokers ready to quit smoking, pharmacologic aids should be strongly considered for recommendation. Finally, follow-up, either in person or by telephone, is very important. While there is some truth to the perception that the more intensive the intervention, the more effective it is, the health care provider must keep in mind that his or her task is not to "make" the patient stop smoking, but rather to empower the person to change—the desire and efforts for changes in behavior rest with the patient.

Table 5-1 Ask, Advise, Assist, Arrange: Key Elements

A. Ask/Assessment

Minimal Assessment: Screen for smoking status at every visit or admission.

Augmented Assessment: Assess characteristics of smoking history and patterns.
- Amount smoked.
- Quit history.
- Nicotine addiction: Fagerstrom Test for Nicotine Dependence.
- Behavioral patterns: "Why Do You Smoke?" Scale.

B. Advise

Minimal Advice: "As your physician, I must advise you that smoking is bad for you health, and it would be important for you to stop."

Augmented Advice: "Because of your [_____] condition, it is particularly important for you to stop. If you stop now, [briefly educate patient about basic health benefits from quitting]."

C. Assist/Counsel

Minimal Assistance: Provide self-help materials; assess interest in quitting; assess interest in and appropriateness of pharmacologic aids.

Augmented Assistance: For outpatients, provide brief 5–7 minute patient-centered counseling. For medical inpatients, provide 15–30 minute counseling session. See Table 5-3 for outline of counseling content.

D. Arrange Follow-up Support

Minimal Follow-up Support: Arrange for single follow-up contact by visit or by telephone in about 2 weeks; provide referral to a smoking counselor or group.

Extended Follow-up Support: Establish "quit smoking" contract with quit date. Arrange for 3 or more follow-up contacts by visit or by telephone.

Standard Assessment

Before intervention is initiated, a brief standard assessment of individual patterns of smoking and concerns about quitting can increase efficiency by providing the physician/provider with enough information to focus intervention. The patient can complete self-rating scales in the waiting or exam room, or at the bedside. For an older or more incapacitated patient, assessment may need to be incorporated into the counseling interview. More extensive assessment tools are available and are reviewed in Chapter 47.

Basic standard assessment should cover motivation ("stage of change"), a brief smoking and quit history, nicotine addiction, and current social environment in regard to smoking. Individual behavioral patterns are also useful to assess. Stage of change (61) can be assessed with one or two questions (see discussion below, Figure 5-1 and Table 5-2); the Fagerstrom Test for Nicotine Dependence (FTND) assesses nicotine addiction; and brief questions can cover smoking and quit history, and social support. Another useful tool, if time allows, is the "Why Do You Smoke?" Scale (62) that allows self-scoring of six common behavioral motives for smoking: for relaxation, pleasure, addiction, "handling," stimulation, and habit. While the validity of this and similar scales in regard to actual strength of motives has been questioned (63), it remains useful to initiate discussion of individual patterns of smoking, and to encourage the smoker to think about specific strategies for dealing with each type of typical smoking situation.

A brief smoking history most usefully includes number of cigarettes smoked (and any other regular tobacco usage), number of quit attempts, date of most recent quit (of at least 24 hours), and length of longest quit. In addition, the smoking status of close family (especially the spouse) and friends should be identified.

Nicotine Dependence/Withdrawal

A high score on the six-item Fagerstrom Test for Nicotine Dependence (64) indicates more difficulty in quitting or higher rates of relapse. In addition to taking into account number of cigarettes, the FTND includes how soon a person smokes in the morning (a measure of discomfort due to night-time abstinence), ease of not smoking in social settings where smoking is not allowed, and smoking while ill. If time is limited, the number of cigarettes habitually smoked, and how soon after waking the first is smoked, will give a good indication of nicotine dependence and withdrawal potential. As withdrawal is a very common concern, smokers should also be asked about their past experience with withdrawal symptoms and the length of time of their longest previous quit. A history of relapsing within several days suggests that withdrawal symptoms play an important role, as nicotine withdrawal is most intense at about the fourth day of abstinence. In the hospitalized patient, discomfort from enforced withdrawal, due to hospital policy, may be an indicator of the need for considering pharmacologic treatment; however, withdrawal symptoms in hospitalized patients may be masked by medication or may appear as agitation or reports of anxiety. A patient discharged during peak periods of withdrawal may be at particular risk for relapse, if no assistance is provided in coping with the discomfort.

Personal Motivation for Quitting: Stages of Change

Extensive research by Prochaska et al (61) has identified predictable stages that smokers go through in the process of stopping smoking: precontemplation, contemplation, preparation, action, relapse, and maintenance. Each stage is accompanied by a characteristic balance of positive and negative perceptions of smoking and by different types of cognitive and

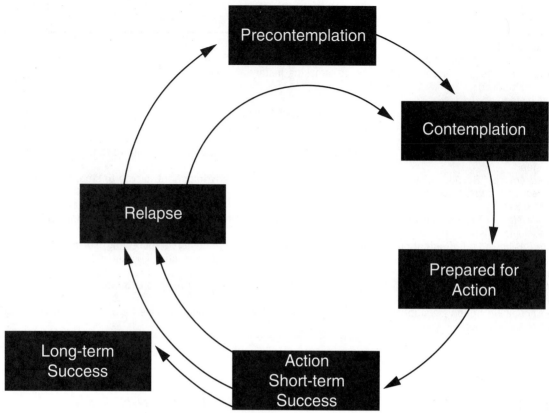

Figure 5-1 Stages of change. (Adapted with permission from Prochaska JO, DiClemente CC. NIH Pub No. 92–3316. 1986).

Table 5-2 Comparison of Stage Definitions for Outpatient and Inpatient Smokers		
STAGE	**OUTPATIENT**	**INPATIENT**
Precontemplation	Is not thinking about quitting in the next 6 months.	Intends to return to smoking after discharge.
Contemplation	Is seriously thinking about quitting in the next 6 months.	Is uncertain about remaining abstinent after discharge.
Prepared for Action	Is seriously thinking about quitting in the next month.	Intends to remain abstinent after discharge but expresses some uncertainty.
Action	Has quit smoking within the last 6 months.	Expresses strong commitment about remaining abstinent after discharge.
Relapse	Current smoker who has quit for at least 24 hours in the last 6 months.	Had quit within 6 months but was smoking at time of admission.
Maintenance/success	Has been abstinent for the last 6 months.	Has been abstinent for the last 6 months.

behavioral processes (65) involved in smoking cessation. Figure 5-1 and Table 5-2 shows the cycle of these stages and definitions of each stage for outpatient smokers, and as adapted to inpatient use. Smokers, on the average, move through these stages three or more times before long-term maintenance occurs. It is particularly important to keep these stages in mind in a health care setting committed to providing assistance to all smokers. It is much less frustrating to the health care staff if they realize that a smoker is likely to move no more than one stage at any given time—and that relapse is part of the quitting process. Furthermore, smokers at different stages will benefit from different types of intervention. For example, a precontemplator may need encouragement to even start thinking about quitting smoking, while someone in the preparation stage may be ready to set a quit date.

A medical crisis, such as a heart attack, may move a smoker through the stages more rapidly, but because hospitalization enforces abstinence on a smoker, the questions must be adapted slightly, as indicated in Table 5-2 to ask about intention to quit or remain abstinent after discharge. However, the types of processes and decision making that accompany each stage remain similar even in seriously ill patients (20).

Individualized Assessment and Patient-Centered Counseling

All smokers, despite similarities in experience and background, have unique patterns to their smoking. Brief patient-centered counseling uses open-ended questions to both assess individual differences and to encourage (empower) the smoker to give more thought to their own motivation, problems they anticipate, strategies they might use to deal with these problems, and specific steps toward quitting or maintaining abstinence that best fits their own situation. While the patient-centered counseling approach described below may appear excessively time consuming or difficult, it has formed the basis for a highly effective smoking intervention program tested by primary care physicians that took approximately 5 to 7 minutes to carry out with the average clinic patient (29,60). The approach is summarized in Table 5-3. Patients receiving counseling were also much more likely to perceive their physician as having been helpful when this approach, rather than just simple advice to quit, was offered. Exploring each area can of course be expanded and adapted to other settings and for use by other health care professionals.

Motivation

A basic question to assess motivation is "How do you feel about your smoking?" followed by "How do you feel about stopping smoking?" While medical concerns are foremost in the mind of the health care provider, other reasons for quitting may be more salient for the smoker, either because of an inadequate understanding of how smoking is affecting health, or because they are more concerned about issues such as cost or social disapproval. Inquiring as to why the smoker might like to quit will uncover such issues, and is likely to make him or her feel better understood and less defensive about receiving assistance.

As noted above, it is also usual for smokers to have mixed feelings about their smoking. Prochaska and his colleagues (65) found that each stage of change is characterized by a different "balance" between the "pros" and "cons" of smoking. As might be expected, precontemplators are characterized by a very strong preponderance of pros with very little acknowledgment of the cons; as contemplators move into the preparation stage, the strength of the cons increase over the pros, but positive feelings about smoking still remain even for successful quitters for many months after quitting. This process in quitting holds for both healthy individuals and for cardiac patients (20). Therefore, another excellent open-ended question is, "What do you like about smoking?" This is a particularly good question for a precontemplator or other indi-

---

Table 5-3 Patient-Centered Counseling: Key Elements

A. Motivation
Basic Question:
  "How do you feel about your smoking?"
Follow-up Questions:
  "How do you feel about stopping smoking?"
  "Have you ever tried to stop before?"/"What happened?"
  "What do you like about smoking?"
  "What do you not like about smoking?"

B. Anticipated Problems
Basic Question:
  "What do you think will be the problems if you stop smoking?"
Follow-up Questions:
  "Anything else?"
  "On the "Why Do You Smoke?" you scored high on [_____]. How do you think you can handle that type of situation?"

C. Resources for Dealing with Problems
Basic Question:
  "How do you think you can handle that?"
Follow-up Questions:
  "What else could you do?"
  "How do you expect your [family/spouse/friends] to help you?"

D. Creating a Plan for Change
Basic Questions:
  "What would you like to do next?"
  "What can I do to help?"
Follow-up Questions:
  "Can we set a quit date?"
  "Would you like to try nicotine patch or gum or (another approved aid)?"
  (if not ready to quit): "Would you like to try to cut back in some way?"
  Can we set a follow-up date [for visit or telephone contact]?"

vidual who seems defensive about discussing their smoking. It can also be helpful to reassure the smoker that continuing to have positive associations with smoking is normal and not a sign of inadequate willpower or likelihood of relapse.

Another question that often taps motivational issues is "Have you ever tried to stop before?" followed by ". . . and what happened?" if the smoker has made previous attempts. Past experience is one of the best predictors of future issues. This type of concrete question also decreases defensiveness, encourages the patient to open up, and leads directly into the next area to explore: anticipated problems.

Anticipated Problems

Asking "What do you think will be the problems if you stop smoking?" will uncover individual concerns or past problems. In addition to information provided by the "Why Do You Smoke?" Scale, this question allows exploration of concerns related to nicotine addiction and to specific behavioral problems. For example, some smokers may be more concerned with social pressures on them to continue smoking, while other smokers may have developed few alternative ways of coping with the minor stressors of the day.

One of the most consistently identified problems interfering with success in maintaining abstinence is low self-confidence or self-efficacy in handing tempting or "high-risk" situations. Repeated attempts and failures at quitting are one reason why someone may develop a sense of poor self-efficacy. Such individuals also often describe themselves as having little willpower, as they see the task of becoming a non-smoker in terms of resisting the urge to smoke, rather than as learning new skills. These individuals may indeed have poor self-management skills, either in general or in one specific area, such as finding ways other than smoking to relax or handle stress. Asking about what the person perceives as their specific problem areas is part of brief counseling because it allows for more efficient assistance specific to that area, rather than covering a full range of problems and possible solutions, as happens in intensive group smoking intervention programs.

Resources for Dealing with Problems

When prompted, most smokers are quite good at coming up with various solutions to the problems that they pose. The question "How do you think you could handle that problem?" is more likely to empower the person than is providing a readymade solution. On the other hand, sometimes a smoker has tried ineffective strategies that need to be explored further. For example, a smoker who repeatedly has tried to cut out the first cigarette of the day (usually the hardest one to cut out due to overnight nicotine withdrawal) is less likely to feel successful than someone who cuts out a low-need cigarette. Asking the question "Which cigarettes do you think you would miss least?" would redirect their efforts at cutting back in a more useful direction. Smokers also often report "trying to keep busy" to avoid reaching for a cigarette, and may then fail because they have not developed other ways to relax than smoking. While exploring resources is also a good time to provide encouragement and to reinforce the idea that most people need time to learn to become a nonsmoker, but are usually successful in the long run.

While addressing anticipated problems is also the time at which to address the issue of social support in the environment. If formal assessment indicated that the spouse or other immediate family members still smoke, this will virtually always pose a problem, even if the smoker does not mention it as a concern. How does the smoker plan to handle this? Will the person agree not to smoke in front of them? Will they be supportive or tend to sabotage efforts? Would it help if the physician or other health care provider spoke to them about the need for the patient to stop? If the smoker is an inpatient, it may be easier—and particularly important—to meet briefly with the spouse to assess their situation and perspective. If the spouse does not smoke, he or she may need to know how to best support the smoker in making and maintaining changes. Research (23) suggests that negative support—i.e., nagging—can be harmful to the patient's efforts, but the spouse may need assistance in learning how to be supportive and understanding in a more positive way. If the spouse smokes, he or she may feel pressured to stop, or may be interested in getting assistance as well. Again, empowering the patient to maintain his or her efforts, regardless of the influence of the spouse, is probably more important than expecting both partners to quit together.

Creating and Facilitating a Plan for Change

The final step in brief patient-centered counseling is helping the patient identify a specific plan for change. Asking "What would you like to do next?" emphasizes the importance placed by the health care provider on making at least some change. Even if the person is not ready to quit, he or she may be ready to cut back on the amount smoked. Cutting back or tapering is very useful to reduce a heavier smoker to a level more likely to lead to successful quitting, both to reduce nicotine dependence and to increase sense of efficacy in handling behavioral triggers to smoke. Identifying and then cutting out lower-need cigarettes may enable a smoker to gradually cut back to a lower level.

For the person ready to quit, asking "Can we set a quit date?" has been identified as a very important question for health care providers to ask smokers in a primary care setting (29). For the hospitalized smoker who has not smoked for several days, asking what they plan to do after discharge is critical. The next question is "What can I do to help?" Creating a "contract" with a quit date on it may be helpful; in addition, providing self-help materials reinforces the importance placed by the health care provider on the stopping smoking. For the smoker ready to quit, this is also the time to discuss the use of medication, either a nicotine replacement therapy and/or antidepressant medication (see below). Finally, the AHCPR guidelines strongly recommend setting a follow-up appointment. This not only reinforces the importance of quitting but also allows reevaluation of medication use and problems encountered in quitting. Offering the follow-up, regardless of whether the appointment is kept, may increase likelihood of successful abstinence. For the patient involved in ongoing care for a smoking-related health problem, inquiring into smoking at every visit should be part of ongoing care. Obviously, this should be done sensitively so that the person is not intimidated or embarrassed by lack of success.

Referral to a more intensive or more specialized formal treatment programs is indicated for patients who lack confidence that they can quit without such help. Such clinics can be customized for the cardiac patient to bolster quitting motivation and success, or may exist as part of a cardiac rehabilitation program. However, the majority of smokers, even if motivated to quit, are unlikely to attend a group program. An alternative is referral to a professional who specializes in smoking intervention, for individual treatment; this may be particularly indicated if other comorbid psychiatric conditions exist, such as depression, an anxiety disorder, or an eating disorder, and when there is a medical urgency for the individual to stop smoking.

PHARMACOLOGIC TREATMENTS

Nicotine Replacement Therapy (NRT)

The AHCPR guidelines strongly recommend use of FDA-approved nicotine replacement therapy (e.g., nicotine gum or patch) in a smoking intervention program with any smoker. Even lighter smokers (10 to 20 cigarettes/day) have been found to benefit from NRT. Nicotine replacement therapy has been clearly identified as an effective adjunct to behavioral smoking intervention that significantly reduces tobacco withdrawal symptoms and enhances smoking cessation rates (35,66). While the evidence supporting the value of the patch, in combination with behavioral intervention, is extensive and compelling (67–69), each of the four types of FDA-approved NRTs (gum, patch, nasal spray, and inhaler) have received substantial testing and each have somewhat different characteristics in terms of nicotine delivery and patient preference (28,70–74). The nasal spray delivers a strong dose of nicotine very quickly and appears to mimic most closely the effects of nicotine delivery from cigarettes, but because a substantial amount of nicotine is delivered in a single spray-dose, it has the potential for providing too much nicotine. The inhaler provides smaller dosages and is designed to be used repeatedly, more similar to taking multiple draws on a cigarette. While combinations of these products have not been systematically evaluated, use of one of the short-term products, especially the gum, in combination with the steadier release of the patch, may be useful for some individuals to help them respond to more intense periods of nicotine craving or to use intermittently once the patch has been discontinued (66).

The safety of NRTs for cardiac patients has received considerable attention (13), particularly after several reports of MIs during patch use. However, a major clinical trial which examined the safety of the transdermal patch in over 500 patients with cardiac disease (56) found no higher rates of cardiovascular events in patients using NRT than patients on placebo. There is now general consensus (75) that the patch, for those patients who will benefit from it, is likely to deliver nicotine in a safer manner than nicotine from smoking. This is because the nicotine level is generally lower and is delivered in even doses throughout the day, rather than reaching peak levels with each cigarette smoked.

Antidepressant Medication

Two roads led toward the examination of antidepressant medication as a possible means to facilitate smoking cessation: the identification of high levels of comorbidity between smoking and depression, and the realization that the new class of serotonin-uptake inhibitors might have more general applications in treating addictive patterns such as bulimia. Fluoxetine has been examined in one major clinical trial (76) that compared 30-mg and 60-mg dosages to placebo, in combination with individual counseling; while the results of that trial did not lead to FDA approval for its use, long-term cessation rates were significantly higher in the medication groups, with a dose-response pattern evident. However, another antidepressant, bupropion, has recently received FDA approval (77); both 150-mg and 300-mg doses showed somewhat comparable effects, with higher abstinence rates after both 7 weeks of treatment (placebo: 19%; 150 mg: 38.6%; 300 mg: 44.2%) and at 1 year (placebo: 12.4%; 150 mg: 22.9%; 300 mg: 23.1%). The most substantial side effects included insomnia in about 30% of smokers and dry mouth in about 13%. Of note, neither of these trials have examined the use of these drugs in depressed patients; therefore, the results are applicable to the general population of smokers. Bupropion, unlike fluoxetine, does not effect serotonin; the effects on smoking cessation may be mediated through its noradrenergic and dopaminergic pathways. These pathways are also involved in nicotine activity. While there are no published trials combining bupropion with the nicotine patch or with nicotine gum, investigation of the combination therapy is underway.

Other Tools in the Medical Environment

Spirometry findings are sometimes considered of value to motivate patients (78), but because even with significant lung disease the findings often do not improve after smoking cessation, they have limited value in following progress. A more useful tool is a carbon monoxide meter, which is highly sensitive to smoking levels, is easy to use, relatively inexpensive to purchase, and has been reported to enhance efficacy of physician advice (79,80). It therefore should be considered as standard equipment when smoking intervention is being offered on a regular basis (81).

SMOKING INTERVENTION IN PATIENTS WITH CARDIOVASCULAR DISEASE: SPECIAL ISSUES

Addressing Smoking with Cardiac Outpatients

All of the counseling approaches outlined above can be provided within either outpatient or inpatient environments. In the study of cardiac patients in a VA setting who received the nicotine patch (56), all patients also received about 15 minutes of behavioral counseling initially and then another 10 minutes at 1 and 6 week follow-up visits. About 40% of these patients had had a previous MI. Quit rates were surprisingly low, about 10% in the placebo group at both 14 weeks after baseline and at 6 months, and 21% in the group using the patch at 14 weeks, decreasing to 14% at 6 months. While low, they are likely to be higher than had no systematic intervention occurred. The challenge of providing intervention in any outpatient setting is to develop a system that screens patients systematically, provides intervention, and includes follow-up. However, because of the increased clinical need for cardiac patients to stop smoking, more intensive intervention and more systematic follow-up is indicated. As noted above, group treatment may play a role but appeals to only a very small proportion of smokers, often less than 10% to 15% of motivated quitters (82). Therefore, providing groups should be seen as only one component of a comprehensive intervention plan for cardiac patients. For the more motivated smoker, intensive individual treatment is indicated and is recommended by the AHCPR guidelines. This should be provided by a smoking specialist who has a counseling background. For the contemplator, reinforcing the need to consider quitting at every office visit, both with primary care physicians and with the cardiologist, is extremely important.

Addressing Smoking with Cardiac Inpatients

Quit rates immediately following an MI, as discussed above, tend to be much higher, and as discussed above, can be increased substantially with a counseling intervention. The medical setting also presents unique challenges to providing behavioral components of smoking intervention. While the medical setting has been shown to be quite conducive to smoking intervention (16,19,21) when initiated and delivered in a structured manner, many characteristics of the inpatient setting can interfere with provision of effective smoking intervention. These include diffusion of responsibility across multiple caregivers for screening, referral, and intervention, inconsistent messages, viewing prescription of the patch as a purely medical intervention, and unfamiliarity among the available caregivers with delivery of even simple behavioral smoking cessation techniques. Current practice, based on a consultation model in which only selected smokers receive any intervention, whether a patch or counseling, is inadequate from either a public health or secondary prevention perspective. Evidence (83,84) suggests that only a very small proportion of smokers are identified to receive intervention; furthermore, with decreasing lengths of stay, consult requests may be called too late to see the patient before discharge. A systematic screening of all admissions for smoking status is the first step; however, even if documentation occurs, a referral system may be necessary to initiate smoking counseling. In a recent study (84), less than 5% of smokers were referred to a "free smoking counseling program" that had been well promoted and for which referral procedures were prominently displayed in the nurses' station on a general medical service. When all charts were flagged with a reminder sheet to assess smoking status and make referrals, the rate increased to over 30%, returning again to less than 5% when the reminder sheets were removed. A more effective model is to avoid the need for consults by having screening information trigger a counseling contact, a system more comparable to the high levels of dietary care provided diabetic patients or respiratory care provided COPD patients. Another alternative is to provide smoking intervention training to nursing staff. However, all these models entail changes in expectations for standard care, support by the medical environment for doing so, and involvement by quality assurance staff to review the level of compliance.

Nicotine replacement therapy should also be considered for medical inpatients. The hospital environment may be particularly suited to use of NRT due to the enforced quit. During a 3 to 4 day hospitalization, withdrawal symptoms are likely to be at their peak (35), so that even patients motivated by the hospitalization to remain abstinent may have difficulty doing so. Although nicotine gum and the patch are now available over the counter, the hospital pharmacy should be encouraged to stock all the NRT formats in order to help alleviate withdrawal symptoms during hospitalization and to start patients on the patch while in the hospital. However, as there have not yet been clinical trials accessing efficacy or safety in a more seriously ill population, clinical judgement must weigh possible risk for nicotine effects from NRT against the possibility of relapse to smoking upon hospital discharge. On the inpatient service, medical staff, including residents, nurses, and attending physicians, can benefit from training in appropriate use and prescribing practices. The nicotine patch has the potential to be of use to patients at different stages of quitting, yet in an unpublished study (83) less than 5% of hospitalized smokers were estimated to have been prescribed a patch. Of those prescribed it, 59% stated that their goal after discharge was to remain abstinent, but only 6% reported receiving any information at all regarding smoking cessation. For all smokers admitted to the hospital, the patch has the potential to reduce withdrawal and craving, in a situation of enforced abstinence. For the smoker ready to quit, using the patch in the context of behavioral intervention during hospitalization and continuing its use after discharge may increase the likelihood for sustained abstinence. For the less motivated smoker, use of the patch may provide an experience of abstinence with less discomfort from withdrawal, helping the patient gain more confidence in quitting in the future.

Severity of Disease

Severity of disease affects response to intervention (17). Given the value of smoking cessation, this pattern deserves further exploration, as it may result from several factors. One possibility is that healthier patients are given reassuring messages that their heart disease is relatively less serious; although such a message is consistent with encouraging cardiac patients to return to as active a lifestyle as is feasible, it may translate into denial of risk for some individuals. Conversely, patients with more serious disease may be receiving stronger medical advice to quit. Another possibility is that patients with more serious disease experience greater disability and therefore find it less physically comfortable to continue smoking. Scott et al (85) found that regardless of disease severity, continued smokers were less likely to believe that smoking was related to their heart disease. In any case, stronger messages from health care professionals concerning the dangers of smoking may be needed. Epstein et al (86) posit several other intervening factors, particularly increased social support for sustained abstinence, in the more seriously ill patient. It may be that the physician needs to be more confident in his or her role in motivating the patient with less severe disease to quit, communicating strongly the benefit to future health of remaining abstinent, while nevertheless conveying the good news that the cardiac disease is still relatively limited.

Follow-up after Hospitalization

Both clinical and cost effectiveness appears to be improved by providing follow-up by telephone. Although group treatment programs are effective and have an important role for treatment of smokers in the general population, they are less appropriate for providing treatment to the post-MI patient. This is because of both clinical and logistic reasons. Clinically, most post-MI patients who are going to benefit from intervention have already stopped smoking at the time of hospital discharge and are unlikely, in our experience, to be interested in a group (82). Those for whom the MI or hospitalization was not sufficient motivation to quit are also unlikely to find a group appealing. Furthermore, the effectiveness of group intervention has only been evaluated for current smokers, not for those who have already been abstinent for some time. Logistically, groups require substantial staff time to organize and lead, and are unlikely to attract sufficient participants at any given time, even in a large medical setting, to offset the benefits from providing group intervention. However, continued outpatient contact in the context of a cardiac rehabilitation program might be efficient, as these programs often attract the more motivated patient (87). Taylor (16) estimates that at a time commitment of 2 hours per patient (the average time provided to most patients in his study), a single nurse working quarter-time could provide effective intervention for 120 post-MI patients in a 6-month period. This time commitment is similar to that required for post-cardiac patients in our program at the University of Massachusetts Medical Center (15).

Cost Effectiveness

Cost effectiveness has been raised as a somewhat controversial issue related to smoking intervention in the medical environment (88,89). Far more expensive primary and secondary prevention interventions, from mammography to hypertension screening to angioplasty, are readily covered under current standards of health care. The argument both for and against covering smoking intervention is usually framed in terms of primary prevention, with health care insurers pointing out the long-term cost savings in decreased health risks are unlikely to accrue to them due to frequent movement of policy holders. Yet even under those conditions, cost analysis of the AHCPR

guidelines (90) suggest that costs per quality-adjusted-life-years (QALY) saved are substantial, and increase with the intensiveness of the intervention provided. Interventions offered to individuals who already have smoking-related disease may be even more cost effective. For example, an analysis (91) of the type of intervention provided by Taylor et al (16) estimated that it costs only $220 per year of life saved, far lower than other well-accepted medical interventions for post-MI patients, such as beta-adrenergic antagonist therapy at $4700 or more per year of life saved. As cost analyses are incorporated increasingly into research with health policy implications, better estimates can be provided. However, use of these figures as a primary rationale for providing intervention should not occur without considering the same justification for other, more standard, interventions.

SUMMARY

In summary, the evidence now strongly supports the medical value of smoking cessation for cardiac patients. Smoking intervention is both clinically valuable and cost effective in terms of continued medical problems. Although there are no "magic bullets" leading to guaranteed abstinence, numerous tools now exist for assisting the individual who is motivated to be more successful in his or her attempts. Counseling and consistent follow-up also appear to help less motivated patients to move across "stages" toward an attempt in future. Nevertheless, most health care settings do not yet consistently address smoking, even in these high-risk patients, in an effective way, although that is now more likely within outpatient settings than with inpatient settings. Increased training of staff in the value of smoking intervention, increased availability of smoking intervention experts, and increased awareness among policy makers are areas that would help deliver these services more effectively to the patients in need.

REFERENCES

1. U.S. Dept. of Health and Human Services. The health consequences of smoking: cardiovascular disease. A report of the Surgeon General. Rockville, MD: U.S. Dept. of Health and Human Services, Public Health Service, Centers for Disease Control, Office on Smoking and Health, 1983. DHHS pub. no. (PHS) 84-50204.

2. U.S. Dept. of Health and Human Services. Reducing the health consequences of smoking: 25 years of progress. A report of the Surgeon General. Rockville, MD: U.S. Dept. of Health and Human Services, Public Health Service, Centers for Disease Control, Office on Smoking and Health. DHHS pub. no. (CDC) 89-8411.

3. Shopland DR, Burns DM. Medical and public health implications of tobacco addiction. In: Orleans CT, Slade J, eds. Nicotine addiction: principles and management. New York: Oxford University Press, 1993.

4. Glantz SA, Parmley WW. Passive smoking and heart disease: mechanisms and risk. JAMA 1995;273:1047–1053.

5. Robinson K, Conroy RM, Mulcahy R. Smoking and acute coronary heart disease: a comparative study. Br Heart J 1988;60:465–469.

6. U.S. Dept. of Health and Human Services. The health benefits of smoking cessation: a report of the Surgeon General. Rockville, MD:

U.S. Dept. of Health and Human Services, Public Health Service, Centers for Disease Control, Office on Smoking and Health, 1990. DHHS pub. no. (CDC) 90-8416.

7. Goldhaber SZ, Grodstein F, Stampfer MJ, et al. A prospective study of risk factors for pulmonary embolism in women. JAMA 1997;277:642–645.

8. Hasdai D, Garratt KN, Grill DE, et al. Effect of smoking status on the long-term outcome after successful percutaneous coronary revascularization. N Engl J Med 1997;336:755–761.

9. Voors AA, van Brussel BL, Plokker HW, et al. Smoking and cardiac events after venous

coronary bypass surgery: a 15-year follow-up study. Circulation 1996;93:42–47.

10. Benowitz NL. The role of nicotine in smoking-related cardiovascular disease. Prev Med 1997;26:412–417.

11. Burke AP, Farb A, Malcom GT, et al. Coronary risk factors and plaque morphology in men with coronary disease who died suddenly [see comments]. N Engl J Med 1997;336:1276–1282.

12. Hung J, Lam JY, Lacoste L, Letchacovski G. Cigarette smoking acutely increases platelet thrombus formation in patients with coronary artery disease taking aspirin. Circulation 1995;92:2432–2436.

13. Benowitz NL, Gourlay SG. Cardiovascular toxicity of nicotine: implications for nicotine replacement therapy. J Am Coll Cardiol 1997;29:1422–1431.

14. Hallstrom AP, Cobb LA, Ray R. Smoking as a risk factor for recurrence of sudden cardiac arrest. N Engl J Med 1986;314:271–275.

15. Ockene J, Kristeller JL, Goldberg R, et al. Smoking cessation and severity of disease: the Coronary Artery Smoking Intervention Study. Health Psychol 1992;11:119–126.

16. Taylor CB, Houston-Miller N, Killen JD, DeBusk RF. Smoking cessation after acute myocardial infarction: effects of a nurse-managed intervention. Ann Intern Med 1990;113:118–123.

17. Frid D, Ockene IS, Ockene JK, et al. Severity of angiographically proven coronary artery disease predicts smoking cessation. Am J Prev Med 1991;7:131–135.

18. Cutter G, Oberman MK, Kimmerling R, Oberman A. The natural history of smoking cessation among patients undergoing coronary angiography. J Card Rehab 1985;5:332–340.

19. Brownell K, Marlatt GA, Lichtenstein E, Wilson GT. Understanding and preventing relapse. Am J Psychol 1986;41:765–782.

20. Kristeller JL, Rossi JS, Ockene JK, et al. Processes of change in smoking cessation: a cross-validation study in cardiac patients. J Subst Abuse 1992;4:263–276.

21. Orleans CT, Kristeller JL, Gritz ER. Helping hospitalized smokers quit: new directions for treatment and research. J Consult Clin Psychol 1993;61:778–789.

22. Kaufman NJ. Smoking and young women: the physician's role in stopping an equal opportunity killer. JAMA 1994;271:629–630. Editorial; comment.

23. Roski J, Schmid LA, Lando HA. Long-term associations of helpful and harmful spousal behaviors with smoking cessation. Addict Behav; 1996:21:173–185.

24. Murray RP, Johnston JJ, Dolce JJ, et al. Social support for smoking cessation and abstinence: the Lung Health Study. Lung Health Study Research Group. Addict Behav 1995;20:159–170.

25. Venters MH, Kottke TE, Solberg LI, et al. Dependency, social factors, and the smoking cessation process: the doctors helping smokers study. Am J Prev Med 1990;6:185–193.

26. Gourlay SG, Forbes A, Marriner T. et al. Prospective study of factors predicting outcome of transdermal nicotine treatment in smoking cessation. BMJ 1994;309:842–846.

27. Kristeller JL. The hard-core smoker: finding a definition to guide intervention. Health Values 1994;18:25–32.

28. Sachs DL, Fagerstrom KO. Medical management of tobacco dependence: practical office considerations. In: Tierney DF, ed. Current pulmonology, vol. 16. St. Louis: Mosby; 1995:239–249.

29. Ockene JK, Kristeller J, Goldberg R, et al. Increasing the efficacy of physician-delivered smoking interventions: a randomized clinical trial [see comments]. J Gen Intern Med 1991;6:1–8.

30. Farkas AJ. Does cigarette fading increase the likelihood of future cessation? Ann Behav Med 1999;2:1–7.

31. Shiffman S, Hickcox M, Paty JA, et al. Progression from a smoking lapse to relapse: prediction from abstinence violation effects, nicotine dependence, and lapse characteristics. J Consult Clin Psychol 1996;64:993–1002.

32. Shiffman S, Paty JA, Gnys M, et al. First lapses to smoking: within-subjects analysis of real-time reports. J Consult Clin Psychol 1996;64:366–379.

33. U.S. Dept. of Health and Human Services. The health consequences of smoking: nicotine addiction. A report of the Surgeon General. Rockville, MD: U.S. Dept. of Health and Human Services, Public Health Service, Centers for Disease Control, Office on Smoking and Health, 1988. DHHS pub. no. (CDC) 88-8406.

34. Benowitz NL, Henningfield JE. Establishing a nicotine threshold for addiction: the implications for tobacco regulation. N Engl J Med 1994;331:123–125.

35. Hughes JR, Gust SW, Skoog K, et al. Symptoms of tobacco withdrawal: a replication and extension. Arch Gen Psychiatry 1991;48:52–59.

36. American Psychiatric Association. Diagnostic and statistical manual of mental disorders. 4th ed. Washington, DC: American Psychiatric Association, 1994.

37. Breslau N, Kilbey MM, Andreski P. Vulnerability to psychopathology in nicotine-dependent smokers: an epidemiologic study of young adults. Am J Psychiatry 1993;150:941–946.

38. Breslau N, Kilbey MM, Andreski P. DSM-III-R nicotine dependence in young adults: prevalence, correlates and associated psychiatric disorders. Addiction 1994;89:743–754.

39. Glassman AH. Cigarette smoking: implications for psychiatric illness [see comments]. Am J Psychiatry 1993;150:546–553.

40. Lerman C, Audrain J, Orleans CT, et al. Investigation of mechanisms linking depressed mood to nicotine dependence. Addict Behav 1996;21:9–19.

41. Hurt RD, Offord KP, Croghan IT, et al. Mortality following inpatient addictions treatment: role of tobacco use in a community-based cohort. JAMA 1996;275:1097–1103.

42. Covey LS, Glassman AH, Stetner F, Becker J. Effect of history of alcoholism or major depression on smoking cessation. Am J Psychiatry 1993;150:1546–1547.

43. Covey LS, Glassman AH, Stetner F. Major depression following smoking cessation. Am J Psychiatry 1997;154:263–265.

44. American Psychiatric Association. Practice guideline for the treatment of patients with nicotine dependence. Am J Psychiatry 1996;153(suppl):1–31.

45. Ockene JK, Kristeller JL. Tobacco. In: Galanter M, Kleber HD, eds. Textbook of substance abuse treatment. 2nd ed. Washington, DC: National Academy Press 1999:215–238.

46. Wilson D, Taylor W, Glibert R, et al. A randomized trial of a family physician intervention for smoking cessation. JAMA 1988;260:1570–1574.

47. Kottke TE, Battista RN, DeFriece GH, Brekke ML. Attributes of successful smoking cessation interventions in medical practice: a meta-analysis of 39 controlled trials. JAMA 1988;259:2883–2889.

48. Mulcahy R, Hickey N, Graham IM, Macairt J. Factors affecting the 5-year survival rate of men following acute coronary heart disease. Am Heart J 1977;93:556–559.

49. Mulcahy R. Influence of cigarette smoking on morbidity and mortality after myocardial infarction. Br Heart J 1983;49:410–415.

50. World Health Organization European Collaborative Group. Multifactorial trial in the prevention of coronary heart disease: 2. risk factor changes at two and four years. Eur Heart J 1982;3:184–190.

51. Multiple Risk Factor Trial Research Group. Multiple risk intervention trial—risk factor changes and mortality results. JAMA 1982;248:1465–1467.

52. Jarvis M, West R, Tunstall-Perdoe H, Vesey C. An evaluation of the intervention against smoking in the Multiple Risk Factor Intervention Trial. Prev Med 1984;13:501–509.

53. Farquhar JW, Maccoby N, Wood PD, et al. Community education for cardiovascular health. Lancet 1977;1:1192–1195.

54. Langeluddecke P. The role of behavioral change procedures in multifactorial coronary heart disease prevention programs. Prog Behav Modif 1986;20:199–225.

55. Becker DM, Levine DM. Risk perception, knowledge, and lifestyles in siblings of people with premature coronary artery disease. Am J Prev Med 1987;3:45–50.

56. Joseph AM, Norman SM, Ferry LH, et al. The safety of transdermal nicotine as an aid to smoking cessation in patients with cardiac disease. N Engl J Med 1996;335:1792–1798.

57. Miller NH, Smith PM, DeBusk RF, et al. Smoking cessation in hospitalized patients: results of a randomized trial. Arch Intern Med 1997;157:409–415.

58. Davis RM. Healthcare report cards and tobacco measures. Tob Control 1997;6(suppl):S70–S70.

59. Glynn TJ, Manley MW. How to help your patients stop smoking: a National Cancer Institute manual for physicians. Bethesda, MD: U.S. Department of Health and Human Services, Public Health Service, National Institutes of Health, National Cancer Institute, 1990. NIH pub. no. 90-3064.

60. Quirk M, Ockene J, Kristeller J, et al. Training family practice and internal medicine residents to counsel patients who smoke: improvement and retention of counseling skills. Fam Med 1991;23:108–111.

61. DiClemente CC, Prochaska JO, Fairhurst SK, et al. The process of smoking cessation: an analysis of precontemplation, contemplation, and preparation stages of change. J Consult Clin Psychol 1991;59:295–304.

62. U.S. Dept. Of Health and Human Services. "Why Do You Smoke?" Bethesda, MD: U.S. Dept. of Health and Human Services, Public Health Service, National Cancer Institute, 1994. NIH pub. no. 94-1822.

63. Shiffman S. Assessing smoking patterns and motives. J Consult Clin Psychol 1993;61:732–742.

64. Heatherton TF, Kozlowski LT, Frecker RC, Fagerstrom KO. The Fagerstrom Test for Nicotine Dependence: a revision of the Fagerstrom Tolerance Questionnaire. Br J Addict 1991;86:1119–1127.

65. Prochaska JO, Velicer WF, DiClemente CC, Fava JS. Measuring processes of change: applications to the cessation of smoking. J Consult Clin Psychol 1988;56:520–528.

66. Henningfield JE. Nicotine medications for smoking cessation. N Engl J Med 1995;333:1196–1203.

67. Tonnesen P, Norregaard J, Simonsen K, Sawe U. A double-blind trial of a 16-hour transdermal nicotine patch in smoking cessation. N Engl J Med 1991;325:311–315.

68. Rose JE, Levin ED, Behm FM, et al. Transdermal nicotine facilitates smoking cessation. Clin Pharmacol Ther 1990;47:323–330.

69. Daughton DM, Heatley SA, Prendergast JJ, et al. Effect of

transdermal nicotine delivery as an adjunct to low-intervention smoking cessation therapy: a randomized, placebo-controlled, double-blind study. Arch Intern Med 1991;151:749–752.

70. Hjalmarson A, Franzon M, Westin A, Wiklund O. Effect of nicotine nasal spray on smoking cessation: a randomized, placebo-controlled, double-blind study. Arch Intern Med 1994;154:2567–2572.

71. Schneider NG, Olmstead R, Mody FV, et al. Efficacy of a nicotine nasal spray in smoking cessation: a placebo-controlled, double-blind trial. Addiction 1995;90: 1671–1682.

72. Hjalmarson A, Nilsson F, Sjostrom L, Wiklund O. The nicotine inhaler in smoking cessation. Arch Intern Med 1997;157:1721–1728.

73. Schneider NG, Olmstead R, Nilsson F, et al. Efficacy of a nicotine inhaler in smoking cessation: a double-blind, placebo-controlled trial. Addiction 1996; 91:1293–1306.

74. Leischow SJ, Nilsson F, Franzon M, et al. Efficacy of the nicotine inhaler as an adjunct to smoking cessation. Am J Health Behav 1996;20:364–371.

75. Working Group for the Study of Transdermal Nicotine in Patients with Coronary Artery Disease. Nicotine-replacement therapy for patients with coronary artery disease. Arch Intern Med 1994;154:989–995.

76. Niaura R, Goldstein MG, Depue J. Fluoxetine, symptoms of depression, and smoking cessation. Poster presented at the Society of Behavioral Medicine meeting, San Diego, March 1995.

77. Hurt RD, Sachs DP, Glover ED, et al. A comparison of sustained-release bupropion and placebo for smoking cessation [see comments]. N Engl J Med 1997; 337:1195–1202.

78. Risser NL, Belcher DW. Adding spirometry, carbon monoxide, and pulmonary symptom results to smoking cessation counseling: a randomized trial. Gen Intern Med 1990;5:16–22.

79. Jarvis MJ, Belcher M, Vesey C, Hutchinson DCS. Low cost carbon monoxide monitors in smoking assessment. Thorax 1986;41: 886–887.

80. Jamrozik K, Vessey M, Fowler G, et al. Controlled trial of three different antismoking interventions in general practice. BMJ 1984; 288:1499–1502.

81. Sirota AD, Curran JP, Habif V. Smoking cessation in chronically ill medical patients. J Clin Psychol 1985;41:575–579.

82. Kristeller JL, Merriam PA, Ockene JK, et al. Smoking intervention for cardiac patients: in search of more effective strategies. Cardiology 1993;82:317–324.

83. Kristeller JL. Use of the nicotine transdermal patch in hospitalized patients: a lost opportunity. Poster presented at the Society for Research on Nicotine and Tobacco, San Diego, March 1995.

84. McDaniel AM, Kristeller JL, Hudson D. Chart reminders increase referrals for inpatient smoking cessation. Nicotine Tob Res. In press.

85. Scott RR, Lamparski D. Variables related to long-term smoking status following cardiac events. Addict Behav 10:257–264.

86. Epstein LH, Perkins KA. Smoking, stress, and coronary heart disease. J Consult Clin Psychol 1988;56:342–349.

87. Comoss PM. Nursing strategies to improve compliance with life-style changes in a cardiac rehabilitation population. J Cardiovasc Nurs 1988;2:23–36.

88. Barendregt JJ, Bonneux L, van der Maas PJ. The health care costs of smoking. N Engl J Med 1997;337:1052–1057.

89. Warner KE. Cost-effectiveness of smoking-cessation therapies. Pharmacoeconomics 1997; 11:538–549.

90. Cromwell J, Bartosch WJ, Fiore MC, et al. Cost-effectiveness of the clinical practice recommendations in the AHCPR guideline for smoking cessation. JAMA 1997;278:1759–1766.

91. Krumholz HM, Cohen BJ, Tsevat J, et al. Cost-effectiveness of a smoking cessation program after myocardial infarction. J Am Coll Cardiol 1993;22:1697–1702.

Chapter 6

Nutrition Intervention: Behavioral and Educational Considerations

Karen Glanz

NUTRITION IN PREVENTION AND RISK REDUCTION

Nutrition plays an important role in the etiology, progression, and sequelae of cardiovascular disease (CVD) risk factors, coronary artery disease, and other widespread chronic illnesses (1–4). Dietary change is central to reducing CVD risk due to obesity, dyslipidemias, and hypertension (5–7). Until recently, nutrition intervention to prevent and manage CVD focused primarily on restricting intake of dietary fat (especially saturated fat and cholesterol), avoiding excess caloric intake, and restricting sodium intake (8). However, recent controlled trials, combined with accumulating epidemiologic evidence, point to the role of a total healthy diet for controlling lipids (9), blood pressure (10,11), and body weight (12).

The "total healthy diet" is one that is high in fruits and vegetables and includes low-fat dairy products or plant sources of fat (9,11). Such an eating pattern is consistent with CVD risk reduction and disease prevention more generally. In fact, this type of eating pattern fits population-wide dietary guidelines for good health (13) and cancer prevention (14,15). Although individuals with clinical CVD risk factors may need to adhere more strictly to specific guidelines to achieve risk reduction, today more than ever before they should be consuming diets similar to those recommended for good overall health maintenance.

This chapter discusses behavioral and educational considerations in nutrition intervention for cardiovascular disease prevention and management. Chapter 8 (Clinical Strategy for Managing Dyslipidemias) and Chapter 9 (Lifestyle Management and Prevention of Hypertension), as well as chapters in later sections of this text on obesity and weight management, will provide specific recommendations for nutritional management of patients. In this chapter, we 1) introduce issues related to the role of health providers in dietary intervention; 2) review behavioral issues related to healthful diets; 3) provide a summary of current thinking about the determinants of dietary behavior and change processes; and 4) briefly review clinical nutrition intervention opportunities and their relation to healthcare delivery and public health nutrition.

THE ROLE OF HEALTH PROVIDERS IN DIETARY INTERVENTION

Nutritional intervention is a central component of CVD prevention and management. Physicians' roles in nutritional intervention are pivotal because of their centrality in healthcare and their credibility as patient educators (16). Current public health recommendations in the United States give high priority to including nutrition education in all routine healthcare contacts (17). People who report receiving advice about dietary change from their physicians report more health-enhancing diet changes than those who received no such advice (18). Also, most respondents to a nation-wide survey of family physicians were supportive of the U.S. Preventive Services Task Force recommendations on nutrition counseling (19).

Although there has been an increase in attention to nutritional management in primary healthcare, the educational opportunities and practices of physicians have shown only modest increases over the past decade (16,20,21). Key barriers include lack of training, lack of confidence, and organizational barriers such as limited time, inadequate education materials, and inadequate reimbursement (20,22–26). These issues continue to be important challenges for continuing medical education and healthcare administration. In addition, coordination with other health professionals should be expanded. Physicians' referral of patients with hypercholesterolemia, hypertension, and obesity to dietitians can expand the delivery of quality nutrition counseling (27,28). Nonetheless, physicians retain a critical responsibility—communicating the importance of nutrition to patients' health, providing credible nutrition advice, and understanding the challenges of adherence to long-term nutritional changes.

CHARACTERISTICS OF HEALTHFUL DIETS: BEHAVIORAL ISSUES

Dietary behavior changes can only be effective for preventing cardiovascular disease when they are sustained over the long term and in people's natural environments, outside the clinical setting. To be effective in nutritional intervention, healthcare providers need to understand both the principles of clinical nutrition management and a variety of behavioral and educational issues (8).

There are several core issues about nutritional change that should be recognized. First, most diet-related CVD risk factors are asymptomatic and do not present immediate or dramatic symptoms. Second, health-enhancing dietary changes require qualitative change, not just modification of the amount of food consumed, and cessation is not a viable option (as with smoking or other addictive behaviors). Third, both the act of making changes and self-monitoring require accurate knowledge about the nutrient composition of foods. Thus, information acquisition and processing may be more complex for dietary change than for changes in some other health behaviors, such as smoking and exercise (29). Other important issues include long-term maintenance, the format of dietary advice, nutritional adequacy, options for initiating the change process, the changing food supply, fad diets, and special populations.

Long-Term Dietary Change

Because nutritional intervention leads to meaningful improvements in cardiovascular health only when long-term change is achieved, physicians and patients both need to "look down the road" when formulating expectations and setting goals (30). For example, for most patients who follow recommended dietary changes for cholesterol reduction, significant reductions are seen within 4 to 6 weeks, and cholesterol reduction goals can be reached within 3 to 6 months (31). Even after goals are achieved, new dietary habits must be maintained. Thus, if it takes several weeks or even months to adjust to the new dietary regimen, patience and persistence by both physician and patient may be worthwhile in the long run. And different skills are required to make initial changes and to maintain them over the long term, so follow-up consultations and advice should address new issues, not merely repeat or rehash old information.

Restrictive and Additive Recommendations: Typical Reactions

Traditionally, nutrition intervention has focused on advice to *restrict* intake of certain foods or nutrients (e.g., reducing fat and saturated fat intake, limiting calorie intake, limiting sodium/salt). Yet the most often-mentioned obstacle to achieving a healthful diet is not wanting to give up the foods we like (32). Basic psychological principles hold that when people are faced with a restriction, or loss of a choice, that choice or commodity becomes more attractive. In other words, focusing mainly on what *not* to eat, or on eating less of some types of foods, may evoke conscious or unconscious negativism in some people. As an alternative, emphasizing *additive* recommendations, such as increasing intake of fruits and vegetables, or eating more fiber-rich foods, often appeals to people because it sanctions their doing more of something. The challenge is to make these recommendations attractive to patients, and to ensure that they are presented in the context of an overall healthful diet—so there is no mistake that "eating more vegetables" does not suggest adopting a steady diet of deep-fried zucchini and mushrooms!

Gradual Change or Very Strict Diets: Choices and Implications

Common wisdom holds that the chances of long-term dietary compliance are greater when efforts to change are guided in a gradual, stepwise manner. This might involve attempting changes within specific food groups one at a time, until the total diet comes close to recommendations. A basic principle involved is that small successes (i.e., recognition of each successful behavioral change) increase confidence and motivation for each successive change. Although this is effective for many people, others become impatient or even lose their enthusiasm for changes that are minimally recognizable. An alternative is to begin with a highly restrictive diet such as the Pritikin program (33), Dr. Dean Ornish's Lifestyle Heart Diet (34), or a very-low-calorie diet for weight loss. These types of programs, with very strict dietary regimens, may be useful for patients who are highly motivated, postsurgically, after a coronary incident, or for those who have not been successful in making gradual changes. In some cases, a strict diet for an initial short time period will yield visible and/or clinical changes that help motivate patients to continue adhering to a less extreme regimen. Such diets require careful supervision and may work best in residential settings for those who can afford them or whose health insurance will provide reimbursement.

New and Modified Foods in the Marketplace, and Prepared Meal Diet Plans

The past decade has brought a virtual explosion in the availability of fat- and calorie-modified foods. A recent review of the data shows that fat-modified foods make a more significant contribution to diets of consumers with low-fat intakes (35). Indeed, these foods, and the availability of nutrition labeling, should make dietary change easier to achieve. However, many low-fat foods are not low in calories, so if energy restriction for weight loss is indicated, patients must be aware that fat content alone should not determine food choice. At the same time, many modified foods are portion-controlled. Thus, they may be important parts of a CVD risk-reducing eating pattern, especially for busy people who have limited time or skills for food preparation. One controlled trial recently found that a prepared meal plan, when compared with a nutritionally similar self-selected diet, yielded greater compliance and CVD risk factor response (36). Diets based on packaged prepared foods, although generally considered useful, should not be considered as sole long-term replacements for learning basic skills of food choice and preparation.

Nutritional Adequacy

A prudent diet that is low in calories and fat, especially animal fat, and high in fruits, vegetables, and whole grains is consistent with overall good nutrition (13). Such diets, when prescribed for cardiovascular risk reduction, should not lead to clinical nutritional deficiencies. However, some patients may alter their eating patterns to the extent that they consume too little calcium and iron, or ingest complex carbohydrates in quantities so great that they interfere with nutrient absorption. Patients should be encouraged to eat a variety of foods, which will help ensure dietary adequacy (8). Those with increased nutritional needs, such as adolescents and pregnant and lactating women, should be supervised more closely and/or referred to a qualified registered dietitian for additional counseling.

Fad Diets

Bookstores and best-seller lists are seldom without several books touting the latest fad diets. Although most fad diets promise rapid and painless weight loss, more books have emerged recently that promise cholesterol reduction, blood pressure control, cancer prevention, and greater longevity. Some "fad diets" are simply healthful diets in slick packaging. Others, however, may be frankly dangerous for patients with cardiovascular risk factors. Because your patients may be drawn to these books, it is helpful to become educated about them and to encourage your patients to ask questions. If you do not devote enough time to nutrition intervention to keep up-to-date on the latest diet fads, you may want to obtain current critical reviews or consultation from a registered dietitian in your practice, hospital, or community.

Special Populations

Ideally, each patient should be treated as an individual with unique circumstances and health history. Still, epidemiologic research indicates that certain demographic subgroups differ in terms of cardiovascular risk factors and diet. Understanding these population trends can help prepare a physician to work with various types of patients. Data from the National Health and Nutrition Examination Survey show that most CVD risk factors are higher among ethnic minority women (African-American and Mexican-American) than among white women (37). Women of lower socioeconomic status tend to have a higher body mass index (BMI) than more affluent women, across all ethnic groups (37). White women also tend to have more positive attitudes toward the impact of diet on health than African-American women, even when accounting for differences in age, education, and income (38). Women experience gender-specific differences in cardiovascular risks

related to hormones, contraceptives, and hormone replacement therapy (39). Younger persons may feel invulnerable to coronary events, and older adults may be managing multiple chronic conditions and using both prescribed and over-the-counter medications that could interact with foods. These are just a few examples of how population subgroups may differ, and they serve as a reminder to be sensitive to group patterns, but to avoid stereotyping in the absence of first-hand evidence about an individual.

DIETARY BEHAVIOR: DETERMINANTS AND CHANGE PROCESSES

Multiple Levels of Influence

For nutrition interventions to be effective, they must be targeted not only at individuals, but must also affect the interpersonal, organizational, marketplace, and community factors that affect food choice (40). This is most clearly illustrated when one thinks of the context of selecting and purchasing food. Consumers learn about foods through advertising and promotion in the media, by labels on food packages, and via product information in grocery stores, cafeterias, and restaurants (41). Their actual purchases are influenced by personal preferences, family habits, medical advice, availability, cost, packaging, placement, and intentional meal planning. The foods they consume may be further changed in the preparation process, either at home or while eating out. The process is complex and clearly determined not only by multiple factors but by factors at multiple *levels*. Still, much food choice can be represented by routines and simple, internalized rules.

Multiple Determinants of Food Choice

Many social, cultural, and economic factors contribute to the development, maintenance, and change of dietary patterns. No single factor or set of factors has been found to adequately account for why people eat as they do. Physiologic and psychological factors, acquired food preferences, and knowledge about foods are important individual determinants of food intake. Families, social relationships, socioeconomic status, culture, and geography are also important influences on food choices. Five factors that have been examined as important in food selection through the past decade are: taste, nutrition, cost, convenience, and weight control (42). For the general public, taste has been reported to be the most important influence on food choice, followed by cost (43). A broad understanding of some of the key factors and models for understanding food choice can provide a foundation for well-informed clinical nutrition intervention, help identify the most influential factors for a particular patient, and enable clinicians to focus on issues that are most salient for their patients.

Knowledge, Information, and Skills

Knowledge about which foods to choose and how much to consume on a therapeutic diet is the *sine qua non* of dietary adherence. However, knowledge that supports the application of nutrition information, and the skills to choose or prepare healthful foods, is not enough without motivation and support. The availability of widespread nutrition labeling on packaged foods has greatly increased the amount of practical nutrition information available, but its actual usefulness and use are not yet well understood. Patients with low literacy skills may require more explanations and fewer printed materials, thus posing important challenges (44). One community-based dietary fat intervention that used few print materials, emphasized interactive experiences, and was targeted to the cultural backgrounds of participants was successful in promoting desirable dietary changes (45).

The Motivational Role of Concern About Health

Effective nutritional intervention with patients requires their understanding of how to apply specific knowledge to their personal dietary behavior. Although the general public tends to place taste and cost at the top of its list of important factors in food choice (43), persons with clinical cardiovascular risk factors are faced with the important and often overriding concern about health. Health concerns are most likely to be influential when they are emphasized in a clear and specific manner, placed in the context of overall risk for CVD and other chronic diseases, and when dietary change recommendations can be linked prospectively to tangible risk reduction (8). Symptomatic patients also tend to be more motivated (5).

Social Cognitive Factors and Self-Efficacy

Social cognitive theory (SCT), the cognitive formulation of social learning theory that has been best articulated by Bandura (46,47), explains human behavior in terms of a three-way, dynamic, reciprocal model in which personal factors, environmental influences, and behavior continually interact. SCT synthesizes concepts and processes from cognitive, behavioristic, and emotional models of behavior change, so it can be readily applied to nutritional intervention for CVD prevention and management. A basic premise of SCT is that people learn not only through their own experiences, but also by observing the actions of others and the results of those actions (48). Key constructs of social cognitive theory that are relevant to nutritional intervention include observational learning, reinforcement, self-control, and self-efficacy (40).

Principles of behavior modification, which have often been used to promote dietary change, are derived from SCT. Some elements of behavioral dietary interventions based on SCT constructs of self-control, reinforcement, and self-efficacy include goal setting, self-monitoring, and behavioral contracting (8,40).

Self-efficacy, or a person's confidence in his or her ability to take action and to persist in that action despite obstacles or challenges, seems to be especially important for influencing health behavior and dietary change efforts (47). Health providers can make deliberate efforts to increase patients' self-efficacy using three types of strategies: 1) setting, small, incremental, and achievable goals; 2) using formalized behavioral contracting to establish goals and specify rewards; and 3) monitoring and reinforcement, including patient self-monitoring by keeping records (48).

Readiness to Change: Stages of Change as Mediators to Change

Long-term dietary change for CVD risk reduction involves multiple actions and adaptations over time. Some people may not be ready to attempt changes, whereas others may have already begun implementing diet modifications. The construct of "stage of change" is a key element of the transtheoretical model of behavior change, and proposes that people are at different stages of readiness to adopt healthful behaviors (49,50). The notion of readiness to change, or stage of change, has been examined in dietary behavior research and found useful in explaining and predicting eating habits (29,51–55).

Five distinct stages are identified in the stages of change model: precontemplation (unaware, not interested in change), contemplation (thinking about change in the near future), preparation (making plans to change), action (actively modifying behavior or environment), and maintenance (continuation of new, healthier behaviors) (48,50). People are not thought to move through the stages of change in a linear manner—they often recycle and repeat certain stages; for example, individuals may relapse and go back to an earlier stage depending on their level of motivation and self-efficacy.

The stages of change model can be used both to help understand why patients might not be ready to undertake dietary change, and to improve the success of nutritional intervention (8,48). Patients can be classified according to their stage of change by asking a few simple questions—Are they interested in trying to change their eating patterns, thinking about changing their diet, ready to begin a new eating plan, already making dietary changes, or trying to sustain changes they have been following for some time? By knowing their current stage, you can help determine how much time to spend with the patient, whether to wait until he or she is more ready to attempt active changes, whether referral for in-depth nutritional counseling is warranted, and so on. Knowledge of the patient's current stage of change can also lead to appropriate follow-up questions about past efforts to change, obstacles and challenges, and available strategies for overcoming barriers or obstacles to change (8).

Applying an Understanding of Determinants of Dietary Behavior to Clinical Nutritional Intervention

A central premise in applying an understanding of the influences on dietary behavior to clinical nutritional intervention is that you can gain an understanding of a patient through an interview or written assessment, and better focus on that individual's readiness, self-efficacy, knowledge level, and so on. Clearly, it is necessary to select a "short list" of factors to evaluate, and this may differ depending on clinical risk factors or a patient's history. Once there is a good understanding of that person's cognitive and/or behavioral situation, the intervention can be personalized, or "tailored." Tailored messages and feedback have been found to be promising strategies for encouraging healthful dietary changes in primary care settings (56,57) and in community- or home-based settings (58). Also, people's initial stage of change may influence their participation in nutritional intervention. People who are initially in the later stages of change (preparation, action, and maintenance) tend to spend more time on dietary change (55) and to report making more healthful changes in their food choices (57).

CLINICAL NUTRITION INTERVENTION

Does Nutrition Intervention Work?

Recently, several review articles have examined the question of whether dietary interventions change diet and cardiovascular risk factors. Reviews by Brunner et al (59) and by Burke et al (60) concluded that individual dietary interventions in primary prevention can achieve modest improvements in diet and cardiovascular disease that are maintained for more than a year. Another meta-analysis of randomized controlled trials of multiple risk factor interventions for preventing coronary heart disease examined the effectiveness of intervention on reducing CVD risk and mortality from coronary heart disease (CHD) (61) and was less conclusive about the use of preventive interventions for the general population. One other review, examining dietary change interventions, focused on understanding the varying conditions under which nutrition intervention research has been conducted. That review concluded that there is clear evidence for the efficacy of intensive educational and behavioral interventions for promoting lower-fat diets, and that less intensive clinical and community-based interventions have achieved significant, though smaller, changes across large populations (62). Clinical nutrition interventions might be most successful if they attempt to emulate the more intensive interventions that have been studied in large clinical trials such as the Multiple Risk Factor Intervention Trial (MRFIT) and the Women's Health Initiative Vanguard Study.

Physician-based cardiovascular nutrition intervention models have been developed (63) and tested empirically (64) in primary care practices since the early 1990s. These programs have included training for clinicians and model intervention strategies, often targeted for special high-need populations (e.g., low-income persons, ethnic minorities). Such programs have been shown to successfully increase physician self-confidence and practice of nutrition counseling intervention steps (65–67). Those that have reported risk factor effects have found modest total cholesterol and LDL-C reductions (67–69), and in one Dutch study, an association between being in a maintenance stage of change and lower saturated fat intake (70). In interpreting these recent findings, it is possible to conclude that more intensive interventions might have been more efficacious, as suggested above.

Overview of Nutrition Intervention

Comprehensive nutrition intervention for cardiovascular risk reduction involves a cyclical sequence of assessment, treatment, evaluation, and monitoring and follow-up (8,71–74). Thorough *assessment* should include diagnostic evaluation of lipids, blood pressure, BMI, and other CVD risk factors; dietary evaluation; and assessment of other relevant psychosocial, behavioral, and educational factors, including physical activity. *Treatment* includes nutrition counseling, dietary advice, referral if necessary, and provision of supporting materials. If necessary, pharmacologic agents may complement nutritional intervention. *Evaluation, monitoring, and follow-up* are the cornerstones of long-term change. They include assessment of adherence and treatment efficacy, negotiating new goals, and periodic monitoring once risk factor control is achieved.

Although these steps may sound very time-consuming, the relevant intervention components can be accomplished in as little as 5 minutes at an office visit. More in-depth counseling can require a half-hour or more, but can be completed by auxiliary providers and need not be done entirely by a physician. Also, some of the activities can be done efficiently by having patients complete written assessments before meeting with the physician, completing some activities by telephone or mail, and using computer or other multimedia technologies.

Dietary, Behavioral, and Educational Assessment

Measurement of dietary intake is a mainstay of nutritional management and helps to focus initial dietary advice and evaluation of adherence (75). In clinical settings dietary assessment may differ from measurement for research purposes, since it aims mainly to identify areas requiring emphasis for individual patients and to facilitate evaluation of progress. Although no dietary assessment method is perfect, clinicians should use approaches that are both feasible and elicit valid data representing patients' usual diets over time. Brief measures such as the Dietary Risk Assessment (DRA) (76) are increasingly available and can be quite useful. Special care should be taken to encourage patients to disclose what they are eating honestly and openly.

Behavioral and educational assessment should emphasize the issues discussed in the preceding section (8), particularly readiness to change (or stage of change), self-efficacy, knowledge level, prior experience with dietary change, barriers to change, and the most important factors in food choice. Asking about these matters helps identify and overcome barriers to change in a manner that is personally relevant to the patient.

Intervention: Dietary Advice, Counseling, Education Materials, and Innovative Strategies

Assessment, however brief it may be, should be used to establish viable treatment goals and identify motivational opportunities and obstacles. When giving *brief dietary advice*, it is essential to focus on a small number of core concepts. *Brief counseling* expands on dietary advice by incorporating motivational strategies based on the behavioral assessment. For example, the physician might emphasize the importance of CVD risk reduction to one's family life, or suggest ways to overcome barriers such as time constraints and the inconvenience of preparing fresh foods. *Nutrition counseling by an ancillary provider*, usually a registered dietitian but sometimes a nurse educator or other patient educator, can extend counseling sessions and build on physician guidance. Ongoing communication between the physician and the nutrition counselor is essential, to send a strong message and support the credibility of the nonphysician provider.

Written educational materials are important adjuncts to nutritional intervention, since even the best oral communication with a patient can be misunderstood or forgotten over time. Many high-quality off-the-shelf materials are available from federal and state government agencies, local American Heart Association affiliates, and professional associations including the American Dietetic Association. Providers should pay close attention to selecting these materials, and develop new materials only when they identify gaps in what is available. Desktop publishing software makes it easier than ever before to create attractive new educational materials. It often helps to have a nutritionist review materials for technical accuracy and clarity, and to ask a few patients to "pretest" any new materials and provide feedback about their appropriateness, motivational value, and understandability.

New communication and information management technologies are opening the door to exciting *innovative and adjunct technologies* that physicians can incorporate into their ongoing practices. Interactive computer programs and Internet- and Web-based resources are rapidly emerging. An important caveat is to check the credibility of any such sources that are recommended, or to provide patients with guidelines to evaluate possible conflicts of interest (e.g., advertisements disguised as educational resources). Videos to support nutritional intervention are also increasingly available, and reviews of these materials may be found in journals such as the *Journal of the American Dietetic Association* and the *Journal of Nutrition Education*. Telephone counseling can be a convenient and low-cost extension of physician time, and can be done by trained nonphysician office staff as well. Automated telephone counseling techniques for nutrition intervention in cholesterol reduction are now being tested in a randomized controlled trial (77). All these techniques offer new, viable, and engaging supports to traditional office-based nutrition education and counseling.

Follow-Up

Assessment of adherence and risk factor control is the basis for ongoing treatment decisions. Expectations about when clinical changes will be achieved should be tied to the dietary change approach selected by the patient and physician. Strict diet adherence will produce fairly rapid change, whereas gradual change may result in much slower progress. Bear in mind that sustained long-term change is the most important change, not merely an initial indication of risk reduction. Long-term change requires long-term intervention. Follow-up should include medical monitoring and problem solving, with a gradual shift to patient self-monitoring and self-management techniques. Support groups, buddy systems, and engaging family members' cooperation are often most important at this point in treatment (5,8).

ORGANIZATIONAL CONSIDERATIONS

In the practice setting the responsibility for nutritional intervention for cardiovascular disease is divided among physicians, nurses, dietitians, and other health professionals and ancillary personnel. Effective practice management for nutritional intervention includes designation of roles among office staff, identification of referral sources, organizing protocols for patient management and follow-up, and developing informa-

tion systems (8). The opportunities are great, but contemporary health care has not yet fully embraced lifestyle management systems. Model office management systems have been suggested (78), but the realities of office management often deter full implementation of these models (79). Practitioners who are dedicated to clinical cardiovascular disease prevention and management need to take on the role of advocate and organizer in order to more fully implement components of prevention systems at the local level. Nationally and internationally, there are continuing needs for leadership and innovations in medical education and health policy.

A public health view of clinical nutritional intervention is fundamental to further long-term improvements in cardiovascular health. As noted at the beginning of this chapter, dietary guidelines to reduce CVD risk are consistent with dietary guidelines for chronic disease prevention in the United States and internationally. Thus, adoption of healthful diets and prevention of obesity are population-wide goals, not just goals for individual patients. Patient-based approaches should complement population-based approaches to promoting healthful eating through environmental change and public policy (80,81). Physicians and other health professionals can and should work with community health organizations, government agencies, the food industry, and in research and surveillance to help reduce diet-related risk in the population at large.

LIFESTYLE MANAGEMENT AND PREVENTION: ACCEPTING THE CHALLENGE

Our understanding of behavior and educational factors influencing the success of nutrition intervention has become more sophisticated in the past decade, and behavioral research that attempts to explain and evaluate interventions has advanced markedly (82). We have seen evidence of successful interventions, but they have been those that are most intensive. Some low-intensity interventions have been found effective, and these should be disseminated more widely (82).

Many challenges remain for developing practical and effective nutrition interventions that can be adopted in healthcare practice. The accumulated knowledge suggests that frequent patient monitoring, family involvement, group support, and providing prepared foods and/or acceptable products are likely to help improve adherence (5). Further, research to date indicates that successful interventions with patients should include baseline assessment, individualized dietary recommendations, goal setting, assessing stage of change, self-monitoring, and self-management strategies for maintaining behavior change (5). Motivating and guiding adult patients to change remain a multidisciplinary challenge, a healthcare goal, and an important public health challenge for the twenty-first century.

REFERENCES

1. National Research Council, National Academy of Sciences. Diet and health: implications for reducing chronic disease risk. Washington, DC: National Academy Press, 1989.

2. Thomas P, ed. Improving America's diet and health: from recommendations to action. Washington, DC: National Academy Press, 1991.

3. Department of Health and Human Services. The Surgeon General's report on nutrition and health. Washington, DC: U.S. Government Printing Office, 1988.

4. Doll R, Peto R. The causes of cancer: quantitative estimates of avoidable risks of cancer in the United States today. J Natl Cancer Inst 1981;66:1191–1308.

5. Van Horn L, Kavey RE. Diet and cardiovascular disease prevention: what works? Ann Behav Med 1997;19:197–212.

6. Masley SC. Dietary therapy for preventing and treating coronary artery disease. Am Fam Physician 1998;57:1299–1306.

7. Kendler BS. Recent nutritional approaches to the prevention and therapy of cardiovascular disease. Prog Cardiovasc Nurs 1997;12:3–23.

8. Glanz K. Nutritional intervention: A behavioral and educational perspective. In: Ockene IS, Ockene JK, eds. Prevention of coronary heart disease. Boston: Little, Brown, 1992:231–265.

9. Jenkins DJ, Popovich D, Kendall C, et al. Effect of a diet high in vegetables, fruit, and nuts on serum lipids. Metabolism 1997;46:530–537.

10. Appel LJ, Moore TJ, Obarzanek E, et al. A clinical trial of the effects of dietary patterns on blood pressure: DASH Collaborative Research Group. N Engl J Med 1997;336:1117–1124.

11. Sacks FM, Obarzanek E, Windhauser MM, et al. Rationale and design of the Dietary Approaches to Stop Hypertension trial (DASH): a multicenter controlled-feeding study of dietary patterns to lower blood pressure. Ann Epidemiol 1995;5:108–118.

12. McCarron DA, Oparil S, Resnick LM, et al. Comprehensive nutrition play improves cardiovascular risk factors in essential hypertension. Am J Hypertens 1998;11:31–40.

13. Kennedy E, Meyers L, Layden W. The 1995 Dietary Guidelines for Americans: an overview. J Amer Diet Assoc 1996;96:234–237.

14. Butrum R, Clifford CK, Lanza E. NCI dietary guidelines rationale. Am J Clin Nutr 1988;48:888–895.

15. American Institute for Cancer Research. Diet and health recommendations for cancer prevention. Washington, DC: American Institute for Cancer Research, 1998.

16. Glanz K, Gilboy MB. Physicians, preventive care, and applied nutrition: selected literature. Acad Med 1992;67:776–781.

17. U.S. Preventive Services Task Force. Guide to clinical preventive services. 2nd ed. U.S. Department of Health and Human Services, Office of Disease Prevention and Health Promotion. Washington, DC: U.S. Government Printing Office, 1996.

18. Hunt JR, Kristal AR, White E, et al. Physician recommendations for dietary change: their prevalence and impact in a population-based sample. Am J Public Health 1995;85:722–726.

19. Soltesz KS, Price JH, Johnson LW, Tellijohann SK. Family physicians' views of the preventive services task force recommendations regarding nutritional counseling. Arch Fam Med 1995;4:589–593.

20. Ammerman AS, DeVellis RF, Carey TS, et al. Physician-based diet counseling for cholesterol reduction: current practices, determinants, and strategies for improvement. Prev Med 1993;22:96–109.

21. Glanz K. A review of nutritional attitudes and counseling practices of primary care physicians. Am J Clin Nutr 1997;65:2016S–2019S.

22. Hiddink GS, Hautvast JG, van Woerkum CM, et al. Nutrition guidance by primary-care physicians: perceived barriers and low involvement. Eur J Clin Nutr 1995;49:842–851.

23. Kushner RF. Barriers to providing nutrition counseling by physicians: a survey of primary care practitioners. Prev Med 1995;24:546–552.

24. Levine MA, Grossman RS, Darden PM, et al. Dietary counseling of hypercholesterolemic patients by internal medicine residents. J Gen Intern Med 1992;7:511–516.

25. Glanz K, Tziraki C, Albright C, Fernandes J. Nutritional assessment and counseling practices: attitudes and interests of primary care physicians. J Genl Intern Med 1995;10:89–92.

26. Bruer RA, Schmidt RE, Davis H. Nutrition counseling—Should physicians guide their patients? Am J Prev Med 1994;10:308–311.

27. Elson RB, Splett PL, Bostick RM, et al. Dietitian practices for adult outpatients with hypercholesterolemia referred by physicians: the Minnesota Dietitian Survey. Arch Fam Med 1994;3:1073–1080.

28. Boyhtari ME, Cardinal BJ. The role of clinical dietitians as perceived by dietitians and physicians. J Am Diet Assoc 1997;97:851–855.

29. Glanz K, Patterson RE, Kristal AR, et al. Stages of change in adopting healthy diets: fat, fiber, and correlates of nutrient intake. Health Educ Q 1994;21:499–519.

30. Glanz K. Patient and public education for cholesterol reduction: A review of strategies and issues. Patient Educ Couns 1988;12:235–257.

31. Report of the National Cholesterol Education Program Expert Panel on Detection, Evaluation and Treatment of High Blood Cholesterol in Adults. Arch Intern Med 1988;148:36–69.

32. Morreale SJ, Schwartz NE. Helping Americans eat right: Developing practical and actionable public nutrition education messages based on the ADA Survey of American Dietary Habits. J Amer Diet Assoc 1995;95:305–308.

33. Barnard RJ. Effects of life-style modification on serum lipids. Arch Intern Med 1991;151:1389–1394.

34. Ornish DM. Dr. Dean Ornish's program for reversing heart disease. New York: Random House, 1990.

35. Lichtenstein AH, Kennedy E, Barrier P, et al. Dietary fat consumption and health. Nutr Rev 1998;56:S3–S19.

36. Metz JA, Kris-Etherton PM, Morris CD, et al. Dietary compliance and cardiovascular risk reduction with a prepared meal plan compared with a self-selected diet. Am J Clin Nutr 1997;66:373–385.

37. Winkleby MA, Kraemer HC, Ahn DK, Varady AN. Ethnic and socioeconomic differences in cardiovascular risk factors: findings for women from the Third National Health and Nutrition Examination Survey, 1988–1994. JAMA 1998;280:356–362.

38. Gates G, McDonald M. Comparison of dietary risk factors for cardiovascular disease in African-American and white women. J Am Diet Assoc 1997;97:1394–1400.

39. Rao AV. Coronary heart disease risk factors in women: focus on gender differences. J La State Med Soc 1998;150:67–72.

40. Glanz K, Eriksen MP. Individual and community models for dietary behavior change. J Nutr Educ 1993;25;80–86.

41. Glanz K, Hewitt AM, Rudd J. Consumer behavior and nutrition education: an integrative review. J Nutr Educ 1992;24:267–277.

42. Food Marketing Institute. Trends in the United States: consumer attitudes and the supermarket. Washington, DC: Food Marketing Institute, 1996.

43. Glanz K, Basil M, Maibach E, et al. Why Americans eat what they do: Taste, nutrition, cost, convenience, and weight control concerns as influences on food consumption. J Amer Diet Assoc 1998;98:1118–1126.

44. Macario E, Emmons KM, Sorensen G, et al. Factors influencing nutrition education for patients with low literacy skills. J Amer Diet Assoc 1998;98:559–564.

45. Howard-Pitney B, Winkleby M, Albright CL, et al. The Stanford Nutrition Action Program: a dietary fat intervention for low-literacy adults. Am J Public Health 1997;87:1971–1976.

46. Bandura A. Social foundations of thought and action: a social cognitive theory. Englewood Cliffs, NJ: Prentice-Hall, 1986.

47. Bandura A. Self-efficacy: the exercise of control. New York: W.H. Freeman, 1997.

48. Glanz K, Rimer BK. Theory at a glance: a guide for health promotion practice. NIH Publication No. 95-3896. Bethesda, MD: National Cancer Institute, 1995.

49. Prochaska JO, DiClemente CC, Norcross JC. In search of how people change: applications to addictive behaviors. Am Psychol 1992;47:1102–1114.

50. Prochaska JO, Redding C, Evers K. The transtheoretical model of behavior change. In: Glanz K, Lewis FM, Rimer BK, eds. Health behavior and health education: theory, research, and practice. 2nd ed. San Francisco: Jossey-Bass, 1997:60–84.

51. Curry SJ, Kristal AR, Bowen DJ. An application of the stage model of behavior change to dietary fat reduction. Health Educ Res 1992;7:97–105.

52. Greene GW, Rossi SR, Reed GR, et al. Stage of change for reducing dietary fat to 30% of energy or less. J Amer Diet Assoc 1994;94: 1105–1110.

53. Brug J, Glanz K, Kok G. The relationship between self-efficacy, attitudes, intake compared to others, consumption, and stages of change related to fruits and vegetables. Am J Health Promot 1997;12:25–30.

54. Glanz K, Kristal AR, Tilley BC, Hirst K. Psychosocial correlates of healthful diets among male auto workers. Cancer Epidemiol Biomarkers Prev 1998;7:119–126.

55. Glanz K, Patterson RE, Kristal AR, et al. Impact of work site health promotion on stages of dietary change: the Working Well Trial. Health Educ Behav 1998;25:448–463.

56. Campbell MK, DeVellis BM, Strecher VJ, et al. Improving dietary behavior: the effectiveness of tailored messages in primary care settings. Amer J Publ Health 1994;84:783–787.

57. Beresford SA, Curry SJ, Kristal AR, et al. A dietary intervention in primary care practice: the Eating Patterns Study. Am J Publ Health 1997;87:610–616.

58. Brug J, Glanz K, Van Assema P, et al. The impact of computer-tailored feedback and iterative feedback on fat, fruit, and vegetable intake. Health Educ Behav 1998;25:517–531.

59. Brunner E, White I, Thorogood M, et al. Can dietary interventions change diet and cardiovascular risk factors? a meta-analysis of randomized controlled trials. Am J Publ Health 1997;87:1415–1422.

60. Burke LE, Dunbar-Jacob JM, Hill MN. Compliance with cardiovascular disease prevention strategies: a review of the research. Ann Behav Med 1997;19:239–263.

61. Ebrahim S, Smith GD. Systematic review of randomised controlled trials of multiple risk factor interventions for preventing coronary heart disease. Br Med J 1997;314:1666–1674.

62. Glanz K. Reducing breast cancer risk through changes in diet and alcohol intake: from clinic to community. Ann Behav Med 1994;16:334–346.

63. Ammerman A, DeVellis B, Haines P, et al. Nutrition education for cardiovascular disease prevention among low income populations— description and pilot evaluation of a physician-based model. Patient Educ Couns 1992;19:5–18.

64. Ammerman A, Caggiula A, Elmer P, et al. Putting medical practice guidelines into practice: the cholesterol model. Am J Prev Med 1994;10:209–216.

65. Ockene JK, Ockene IS, Quirk ME, et al. Physician training for patient-centered nutrition counseling in a lipid intervention trial. Prev Med 1995;24:563–570.

66. Ockene IS, Hebert JR, Ockene JK, et al. Effect of training and a structured office practice on physician-delivered nutrition coun-

seling: the Worcester-Area Trial for Counseling in Hypertension (WATCH). Am J Prev Med 1996; 12:252–258.

67. Evans A, Rogers L, Peden J, et al. Teaching dietary counseling skills to residents: patient and physician outcomes. The CADRE Study Group. Am J Prev Med 1996;12: 259–265.

68. Keyserling T, Ammerman A, Davis C, et al. A randomized, controlled trial of a physician-directed treatment program for low income patients with high blood cholesterol: the Southeast Cholesterol Project. Arch Fam Med 1997;6: 135–145.

69. Caggiula A, Watson J, Kuller L, et al. Cholesterol-lowering intervention program: effect of the step I diet in community office practices. Arch Intern Med 1996;156:1205–1213.

70. Bakx JC, Stafleu A, van Staveren W, et al. Long-term effect of nutritional counseling: a study in family medicine. Am J Clin Nutr 1997; 65:1946S–1950S.

71. Raab C, Tillotson J, eds. Heart to heart: a manual on nutrition coun-seling for the reduction of cardio-vascular disease risk factors. USDHHS Publ. No. (NIH) 83-1528. Bethesda, MD: USDHHS, 1983.

72. Glanz K. Nutrition education for risk factor reduction and patient education: a review. Prev Med 1985;14:721–752.

73. Snetselaar LG. Nutrition counseling skills: assessment, treatment, and evaluation. 2nd ed. Rockville, MD: Aspen Publishers, 1989.

74. Kris-Etherton PM, ed. Cardiovascular disease: nutrition for prevention and treatment. Chicago: The American Dietetic Association, 1990.

75. Glanz K. Compliance with dietary regimens: its magnitude, measurement and determinants. Prev Med 1980;9:787–904.

76. Ammerman A, Haines P, DeVellis R, et al. A brief dietary assessment to guide cholesterol reduction in low income individuals: design and validation. J Am Diet Assoc 1991;91:1385–1390.

77. Friedman RH. DietAid: Computer-automated telephone counseling for dyslipidemia management. R01 supported by National Heart, Lung, and Blood Institute, NIH, 1998–2002.

78. Solberg LI, Kottke TE. The prevention-oriented practice. In: Ockene IS, Ockene JK, eds. Prevention of coronary heart disease. Boston: Little, Brown, 1992: 468–490.

79. Solberg LI, Kottke TE, Conn SA, et al. Delivering clinical preventive services is a systems problem. Ann Behav Med 1997;19:271–278.

80. Glanz K, Mullis RM. Environmental interventions to promote healthy eating: a review of models, programs, and evidence. Health Educ Q 1988;15:395–415.

81. Glanz K, Lankenau B, Foerster S, et al. Environmental and policy approaches to cardiovascular disease prevention through nutrition: opportunities for state and local action. Health Educ Q 1995;22:512-527.

82. Glanz K. Behavioral research contributions and needs in cancer prevention and control: dietary change. Prev Med 1997;26: S43–S55.

Chapter 7

Exercise and Exercise Intervention in the Prevention of Coronary Artery Disease

Ann Ward

Although age-adjusted cardiovascular disease mortality in the United States has decreased in the past 3 decades, coronary artery disease (CAD) is still the leading cause of mortality. Regular, dynamic physical activity can be beneficial in the primary and secondary prevention of CAD by improving cardiovascular function and reducing risk factors associated with cardiovascular disease. Although most people realize that exercise is important for health, over 60% of adults in the United States do not get enough exercise to attain health benefits and 25% are totally inactive. Less than 20% of adults report exercise at a level approximating recommended levels for cardiovascular fitness (1). The 60% prevalence of physical inactivity as a risk factor for CAD compares to 10% of adults with a systolic pressure greater than 150 mm Hg, 30% who smoke cigarettes, or 50% who have a cholesterol level greater than 200 mg/dL (2). Furthermore, the prevalence of physical activity decreases with age and is lower in women and certain ethnic groups (1). It is particularly important to note that small increases in physical activity among the most inactive persons are associated with large reductions in risk for developing CAD (3).

Based on all the evidence linking exercise and health, a U.S. Preventive Services Task Force recommended that physicians counsel all patients to "engage in a program of regular physical activity tailored to meet their health and personal lifestyle" (4). Physicians have an opportunity to play a major role in increasing the activity level of their patients. A majority of individuals have contact with their physicians each year and adult patients visit a physician an average of three times per year (5). Physicians and other healthcare providers are identified by patients as an important source for motivating lifestyle change (6). Patients report that they want and expect their physicians to counsel them about physical activity (7,8) and physician advice has been proven to be effective in health promotion (5,9) including exercise (10,11). Yet, one survey found that only 15% of internists in the United States counseled patients regarding exercise in primary prevention (12).

Healthcare professionals can help their patients increase their physical activity in several ways. First, they can encourage patients to exercise by discussing the health benefits of exercise and the patient's perceived health and ability to exercise. They can determine which patients need a physical examination and exercise testing before beginning an exercise program and provide medical clearance for patients wishing to start an exercise program. They can prescribe exercise for patients with chronic medical problems or refer them to appropriate exercise professionals for counseling.

For all healthcare professionals, an understanding of the health benefits of exercise is important. This chapter reviews the evidence linking exercise and physical activity with improved cardiovascular health and the primary prevention of CAD.

DEFINITION OF TERMS

Physical activity is defined as "bodily movement that is produced by the contraction of skeletal muscle and that substantially increases energy expenditure" (1). Common categories of physical activity include occupational, household, leisure time, and transportation. Exercise or exercise training is a subset of physical activity and is defined as "planned, structured, and repetitive bodily movement done to improve or maintain one or more components of physical fitness" (1).

The generally accepted definition of physical fitness is "a set of attributes that people have or achieve that relates to the ability to perform physical activity" (1). The components of health-related physical fitness includes cardiorespiratory endurance, muscular endurance and strength, and flexibility and body composition.

RECOMMENDATIONS FOR PHYSICAL ACTIVITY AND EXERCISE FOR HEALTH AND FITNESS

Since 1965, many health and fitness–oriented organizations have developed recommendations for physical activity and exercise. In 1978, the American College of Sports Medicine (ACSM) published its first position statement on the Recommended Quantity and Quality of Exercise for Developing and Maintaining Fitness in Healthy Adults (13). This statement recommended aerobic exercise training for 15 to 60 minutes 3 to 5 days per week at an intensity of 50% to 85% of maximal oxygen uptake. Subsequent position statements by ACSM (14,15) and recommendations of other organizations began to recognize the health benefits of more moderate-intensity exercise as well as vigorous exercise. In other words, health-related benefits may accrue from levels of physical activity that may not be of sufficient quantity and quality to improve maximal oxygen uptake.

In 1995, The Centers for Disease Control and Prevention (CDC) and the ACSM developed a statement on Physical Activity and Public Health (3). This statement published by the CDC/ACSM recommended that "Every U.S. adult accumulate 30 minutes or more of moderate intensity physical activity on most, preferably all, days of the week." Moderate intensity activities are those requiring 3 to 6 METs or 4 to 7 kcal per minute, such as brisk walking. (1 MET is the resting metabolic rate, and is approximately equal to 3.5 mL of oxygen uptake per kg of body weight per minute.) The recommended 30 minutes of activity can be performed in a single session or accumulated in multiple bouts, each lasting at least 8 to 10 minutes. The NIH Consensus Conference on Physical Activity and Cardiovascular Health adopted a similar recommendation in 1996 (16).

In July 1996, the Surgeon General's Report on Physical Activity and Health was published (1). This report states that "Americans can substantially improve their health and quality of life by including moderate amounts of physical activity in their daily lives. For those already achieving regular moderate amounts of activity, additional benefits can be gained by further increases in activity level by increasing either intensity and/or duration." A "moderate amount" of physical activity in this report was defined as attaining an energy expenditure of 150 kcal per day. Duration of exercise would vary inversely with intensity. Higher-intensity activities such as jogging could be performed for 15 minutes to achieve the 150 kcal of energy expenditure, whereas lower intensity activities such as gardening would need to be performed for longer duration.

These landmark statements and recommendations are based on the accumulating evidence relating the level of habitual physical activity to the risk of CAD. This evidence comes from a variety of sources including epidemiologic studies, animal studies, and experimental studies on the effects of exercise on specific risk factors. No randomized controlled

trial of the effects of exercise or physical activity on the primary prevention of CAD has been performed and is unlikely to be done because of the size, cost, and adherence problems associated with such a study. However, multiple epidemiologic studies have linked physical activity to a decreased incidence of all-cause mortality, cardiovascular disease mortality, and myocardial infarction. These epidemiologic studies, taken together, meet the criteria for causality: consistency, strength, temporal sequencing, dose-response, and plausibility.

EFFECTS OF PHYSICAL ACTIVITY ON CARDIOVASCULAR HEALTH: EPIDEMIOLOGIC EVIDENCE

The early epidemiologic studies had serious limitations, including job and leisure activity changes by participants because of changes in health status; confounding independent variables such as hypertension, obesity, and hypercholesterolemia; difficulty assessing physical activity levels; and lack of standardization and confirmation of the diagnosis of CAD (17). The populations in these studies have consisted primarily of middle-aged and older white men. Only a small number of studies have included women and racial minorities.

The Surgeon General's Report on Physical Activity and Health (1) provides a detailed review of the epidemiologic data supporting a relationship between physical activity and cardiovascular health. Compared with people who are most active, sedentary people have a 1.2- to 2-fold increased risk of dying prematurely. It is important to note that in the many cohort studies performed, the protective effect of physical activity is a consistent finding. In the Harvard Alumni Study (18), men who regularly expended between 500 and 3500 kcal per week in leisure time physical activity had significant reductions in risk of premature mortality from CAD. The Multiple Risk Factor Intervention Trial (MRFIT) (19) demonstrated reduced risk of premature mortality in men with cardiovascular disease risk factors who pursued physical activities during their leisure time. Men who averaged more than 30 minutes per day year round of moderate-intensity physical activity had one third fewer deaths from CAD and a 20% lower overall mortality rate compared to inactive men.

In the studies that measured cardiorespiratory fitness, a somewhat stronger relationship has been found. In the Aerobics Center Longitudinal Study (20), men in the lowest fitness quintile compared to the upper 40% had a relative risk for all-cause mortality of 3.16 (95% CI, 1.92-5.2) and women in the lowest fitness quintile had a relative risk of 5.35 (95% CI, 2.44-11.73). The relative risk of death due to cardiovascular disease in this study was 7.9 for men and 9.2 for women. The Lipid Research Clinics Prevalence Study found a relative risk of 3.6 (95% CI, 1.6-5.6) for death due to cardiovascular diseases and 2.8 (95% CI, 1.3-6.1) for death due to CAD for the least fit men compared to the most fit men (21).

The health-promoting aspects of physical activity appear to be related in a dose-response fashion. In the College Alumni Study a reduced risk of CAD was demonstrated at energy expenditure levels as low as 500 kcal per week (18). Risk levels became lower as the volume of exercise increased up to 2000 kcal per week. In the Aerobics

Longitudinal Study the reduction in risk was graded from the lowest fitness quintile to the highest fitness quintile (20). The greatest difference in risk was achieved between those individuals in the lowest fitness quintile and those in the moderate fitness level. Much smaller differences were observed between the moderate- and high-fitness categories. Thus, moderate amounts of physical activity or moderate levels of physical fitness may be protective.

Most of the epidemiology studies on physical activity or fitness and mortality have relied on a single baseline assessment of physical activity or fitness, with subsequent follow-up for mortality or disease occurrence. With single-exposure assessments, evaluation of the effects of genetics and changes in physical activity or fitness is difficult. Three studies have assessed physical activity or cardiorespiratory fitness at two time points. Men in the Harvard Alumni Study who were 45 to 84 years of age completed questionnaires in 1962 or 1966 and again in 1977 and then were followed until 1988 or age 90. Men initially classified as sedentary who increased their physical activity through walking, stair climbing, and sports or recreational activities to 1500 kcal or more per week had a relative risk of 0.72 (95% CI, 0.64-0.82) compared to 1.00 for men who remained less active (22). Men in the British Regional Heart Study (23) who were assessed in 1978 to 1980 (Q1) and again in 1992 (Q92) were followed for 4 years. Men who were sedentary at Q1 and who began at least light activity by Q92 had significantly lower all-cause mortality than those who remained sedentary, even after adjustment for potential confounders. In the Aerobics Longitudinal Study, 9777 men completed two examinations with assessment of physical fitness by maximal exercise tests (mean interval between examinations, 4.9 years) and followed for an average of 5.1 years. Men who improved from the lowest fitness quintile to a fit category between the first and subsequent examinations had a reduction in mortality risk of 44% compared to men who remained unfit at both examinations (24). Based on these studies we can conclude that middle-aged men who maintain or increase their level of physical activity or fitness can achieve significant reductions in mortality.

Evaluation of Risk Subgroups

Blair et al (25) quantified the relation of fitness to risk of cardiovascular and all-cause mortality in the Aerobics Center Longitudinal Study within strata of other predictors of early mortality (smoking, cholesterol, systolic blood pressure, and health status). An inverse gradient of risk was seen across fitness groups within each stratum of the other predictors, a lower death rate in both strata of each of the other predictors for moderately fit men when compared with low-fit men, and an even lower rate for high-fit men. The reduced risk for all-cause mortality in the high-fit men compared with the low-fit men ranged from 32% for elevated systolic blood pressure to 50% for elevated cholesterol level and poor health status. The results for women were consistent with those observed in men. Data were also analyzed across the three fitness categories by the presence or absence of the three other major risk factors (cigarette smoking, elevated systolic blood pressure >140 mm Hg, and elevated cholesterol >240 mg/dL). Participants were grouped in three risk categories based on the total number of the other predictors that were present (none, any one, or any two or all three). A graded inverse trend of death rates was seen from low to high fitness within strata of the number of other risk factors.

Intensity of Exercise Required to Achieve Health Benefits

The relative importance of the intensity as compared with the quantity of exercise for optimal health benefit is not easily determined. In the analysis of the Harvard Alumni Study, men who engaged in moderately vigorous sports activity had a lower risk of death than those who were physically active but did not participate in moderately vigorous sports activities (26). In a subsequent analysis of data from the Harvard Alumni Study, Lee et al (27) evaluated all-cause mortality in men who performed vigorous exercise (defined as ≥ 6 METs) compared to men involved in nonvigorous activity (<6 METs). In this study, only vigorous physical activity predicted lower all-cause mortality rates. In contrast, in MRFIT (19), significant reductions in mortality were observed with increasing duration of physical activity, although very few men performed vigorous exercise.

Although the optimal level of exercise to achieve improved cardiovascular health has not been precisely defined, the results of these studies suggest that physical activity should be consistent and life-long and that moderate levels of exercise and physical fitness, which are attainable by most adults, appear to protect against early mortality.

Mechanisms of Action by Physical Activity to Decrease CAD Risk

The exact mechanisms for the decrease in morbidity and mortality are unclear. There are, however, changes associated with exercise that may exert a favorable effect on CAD, such as decreased blood pressure (28), decreased obesity (29), increased high-density lipoprotein HDL cholesterol (30), increased fibrinolytic activity in response to thrombotic stimuli (31), increased insulin sensitivity (32), and altered baroreflex function resulting in reduced susceptibility to serious ventricular arrhythmias (33). The results of animal studies have shown increased size of coronary arteries, enhancement of coronary collateral circulation, and decreased vasospasm following exercise training (34,35).

EFFECTS OF PHYSICAL ACTIVITY OR EXERCISE ON RISK FACTORS FOR CAD

Effects of Physical Activity or Exercise on Obesity and Fat Distribution

The prevalence of obesity has increased in the last decade from 25% of the adult population to 34% (36). Using a body mass index (BMI) ≥ 25 kg/m^2 as the criterion, 55% of the adult population is overweight or obese (37). Obesity is associated with a higher prevalence of hypertension, non-insulin-dependent diabetes (NIDDM), hypertriglyceridemia, reduced HDL cholesterol, elevated low-density lipoprotein (LDL) cholesterol, and increased risk of developing CAD (38). Recently, the American Heart Association reclassified obesity as a major modifiable risk factor for CAD. Body fat distribution may be a more critical factor in medical complications than body fat. In particular, the amount of abdominal fat is correlated with insulin resistance, diabetes, hypertension, and hyperlipidemia (39) and reduction of abdominal adiposity is associated with improvement in insulin, glucose, and lipid metabolism (40).

Exercise can be beneficial in both the prevention and treatment of obesity. Theoretically, small increases in physical activity (50 to 100 kcal per day) could offset the 0.5 kg per year increase in body weight observed with aging. Cross-sectional studies have generally shown that physical activity is inversely related to body weight and rate of weight gain (37). Exercise can contribute to weight management and cardiovascular health by burning calories, decreasing abdominal fat, and increasing cardiorespiratory fitness and may contribute to the long-term maintenance of weight loss (37).

Aerobic exercise without diet results in modest weight loss. A meta-analysis of 28 publications on the effect on weight loss of exercise compared to diet or control groups showed that aerobic exercise alone produced a modest weight loss of 3 kg in men and 1.4 kg in women compared to controls (41). When exercise is combined with diet, a greater proportion of the weight loss is fat weight compared to diet only (42). Addition of resistance training to diet and aerobic exercise may result in a more favorable effect on preservation of lean body mass and increased fat loss (43).

Schwartz et al (44) observed significant reductions in abdominal fat in both young and older men in response to 6 months of endurance exercise associated with a small weight reduction (~2 kg). In contrast, Depres et al (45) observed no significant reductions in abdominal fat in a group of pre-menopausal women with low levels of abdominal fat undergoing endurance exercise.

In summary, exercise alone and in combination with a calorie-restricted diet can lead to reductions in body weight and abdominal fat. For most persons, the optimal approach to weight loss combines a mild calorie restriction with regular endurance exercise and avoids nutritional deficiencies. In designing the exercise component of a weight loss program, the balance between intensity, duration, and frequency can be manipulated to promote a total caloric expenditure of 1000 to 2000 kcal per week. Obese individuals are at greater relative risk for orthopedic injuries, so lower-intensity (40% to 70% Vo_2max) activities performed for a longer duration (30 to 60 minutes) and/or greater frequency (5 to 7 days per week) are recommended.

Effects of Physical Activity or Exercise on Hypertension

Epidemiologic data (46,47) suggest that physically inactive individuals have a 35% to 52% greater risk of developing hypertension than active individuals. Reaven et al (48) reported that active older women (aged 50 to 89 years) had systolic and diastolic blood pressures (BP) 9 to 24 mm Hg and 3 to 13 mm Hg lower, respectively, than the least active women. The inverse relationship persisted even after correction for differences in BMI. In a primary prevention trial involving diet and exercise (49), 201 men and women with high normal blood pressure at baseline were randomized to

either intervention or control. The incidence of hypertension in the 5-year follow-up was 8.8% in the intervention group and 19.2% in the control group.

Data from longitudinal studies suggest that exercise training is effective in reducing blood pressure by approximately 5 to 10 mm Hg in patients with mild essential hypertension (140–180/90–105 mm Hg) (28,50,51). However, many of the studies of the effects of exercise on hypertension had serious methodological problems, including absence of a control group and presence of confounding variables such as weight loss (50). When results from studies published since 1984, which appear to have corrected many methodological flaws of earlier work, are averaged, the decreases in BP were 11 mm Hg systolic and 7.7 mm Hg diastolic pressure (pretraining: 149.6 ± 8.5/97.3 ± 4.4; posttraining: 138.6 ± 8.5/89 ± 4.0) (52). A recent meta-analysis (53) combining nine studies with hypertensive patients found effect sizes corresponding with decreases of approximately 7 ± 5 and 6 ± 5 mm Hg for resting systolic and diastolic pressure, respectively. No changes were noted in the control groups. In a study by Hagberg et al (54) with hypertensive patients, a 1-hour walk three times a week was associated with a significant reduction in both systolic and diastolic blood pressure indicating that lower-intensity exercise may be as or more effective than vigorous exercise in lowering BP. Further evidence for the blood pressure–lowering effect of exercise was provided in a crossover study by Roman et al (55). In this study resting BP fell significantly with training but returned to baseline levels when training was discontinued.

The effects of exercise on ambulatory BP are less consistent and smaller than those for resting BP (56–58). The reductions in 24-hour ambulatory BP are due primarily to reductions in daytime systolic pressure with little effect on nighttime pressures or diastolic pressure. Exercise in sedentary hypertensive patients also has an acute BP-lowering effect that persists for up to 8 to 12 hours after a single exercise session and results in a significant 6-mm Hg reduction in average 24-hour systolic BP (59,60).

Very little data are available on the effects of exercise training on BP in African-Americans. In a recent study by Kokkinos et al (61) hypertensive African-American men with initial BP values greater than 180/110 mm Hg were randomized to an exercise or a control group for 16 weeks. The exercise group had a significantly lower diastolic BP and a trend toward a lower systolic BP compared to the control group.

The mechanism for the BP-lowering effect of exercise is unclear. The most likely explanation is the attenuation of sympathetic nervous system activity, which may result in reduced renin-angiotensin activity, resetting of arterial baroreflexes, arterial vasodilation, and reduction in elevated peripheral vascular resistance (28,51).

For individuals with mild hypertension, ACSM recommends endurance exercise 3 to 5 days per week for 20 to 60 minutes per session at an intensity of 50% to 85% Vo_2max (51). Lower intensities (40% to 70% Vo_2max) may lower BP as much or more than higher-intensity exercise. Resistance or strength training is not recommended as the only form of exercise training for hypertensive individuals with the exception of circuit weight training. However, resistance training can be performed as one component of a well-rounded fitness program. A resistance program consisting of low resistance and high repetitions is recommended to minimize the pressor response.

Effects of Physical Activity and Exercise on Blood Lipids

Exercise may reduce the risk for CAD through effects on blood lipids. However, studies evaluating blood lipid responses to exercise are confounded by changes in body mass and diet, so results are somewhat conflicting. Early cross-sectional studies indicated that habitually active individuals had lower total cholesterol levels than sedentary individuals (62). However, when habitually active men and women are matched for age and weight with sedentary individuals, total cholesterol is not different. Cross-sectional studies have also shown that active men and women have HDL cholesterol values that are 20% to 30% higher than sedentary individuals (30).

Training studies have generally failed to show changes in total cholesterol or LDL cholesterol (30); however, modest increases in HDL cholesterol (3 to 8 mg/dL) have been demonstrated with exercise training in men (62–66). The amount and intensity of exercise needed to raise HDL cholesterol is unclear. Kokkinos et al (66) found a dose-response relationship between running mileage and HDL cholesterol. In this study, HDL cholesterol was significantly elevated in men who ran about 10 miles per week. Cook et al (64) reported a significant correlation between miles walked per day by postal carriers and HDL_2 cholesterol. A study comparing men training 3 days per week at either 65%, 75%, or 85% of maximal heart rate suggests that exercise at 75% of maximal heart rate is required to increase HDL cholesterol (67). In contrast, Duncan et al (68) reported similar increases in HDL cholesterol in middle-aged women after 24 weeks of training consisting of strolling (4.8 km/hr), brisk walking (6.4 km/hr), or aerobic walking (8 km/hr).

For women, fewer well-designed studies have evaluated the effects of exercise on HDL cholesterol while also controlling for confounding factors such as menstrual status, cigarette smoking, and use of female hormones (69). Two exercise intervention studies suggested that very high levels of exercise were necessary to increase HDL cholesterol in premenopausal women (70,71). However, Duncan et al (68) found significant improvements in HDL cholesterol in women who walked 24 km per week. In postmenopausal women, epidemiologic studies show a relationship between physical activity and HDL cholesterol (72,73).

The increase in HDL cholesterol is usually associated with significant fat loss (74), although increases have been demonstrated without weight loss (75,76). Wood et al (74) compared the effects on HDL cholesterol of weight loss achieved through either dieting or exercise. Both groups had a weight loss of 7.8 kg and similar increases in HDL cholesterol. Sopko et al (75) compared three groups: an exercise group that maintained weight by increasing caloric intake, an exercise group that was not provided additional caloric intake and lost weight, and a nonexercise group that lost weight by dieting. All three groups had significant increases in HDL cholesterol with the exercise plus weight loss group attaining almost twice the increase found in the other two groups, sug-

gesting an additive effect of exercise and weight reduction. More recently, Thompson et al (76) found a 10% increase in HDL cholesterol and a 7% reduction in triglycerides in overweight men following a 1-year endurance exercise program without weight loss. Consequently, weight loss is not required to increase HDL cholesterol with endurance exercise training in overweight men, but without weight loss the change in HDL cholesterol is very modest.

Effects of Physical Activity and Exercise on Diabetes

Diabetes is commonly classified into two major categories: insulin-dependent diabetes (IDDM or type I) and non-insulin-dependent diabetes (NIDDM or type II). IDDM is caused by a lack of insulin production, whereas NIDDM is related to cellular resistance to insulin caused by either decreased insulin binding to cell receptors or to a postreceptor defect (77). Obesity and fat distribution are contributing factors to insulin resistance (78). A sedentary lifestyle appears to be another important risk factor for NIDDM because of its relationship to obesity and has an independent effect on insulin sensitivity (77). An increased incidence of NIDDM also occurs with aging, possibly as a result of decreased physical activity and weight gain that occur as adults age.

Several recent prospective studies in men and women (79–82) show an inverse dose-response relationship between physical activity and incidence of NIDDM. Data from the College Alumni Study indicate that increased physical activity is effective in preventing NIDDM. This protective effect was especially pronounced in the men at the highest risk for the disease (79). Each 500-kcal increment in leisure time physical activity was associated with a 6% decrease in risk of developing NIDDM after adjusting for confounding variables. In the Nurses' Health Study, women who reported engaging in vigorous physical activity at least once a week had a 16% lower adjusted relative risk of self-reported NIDDM during the 8-year follow-up than women who reported no vigorous physical activity (80).

Acute endurance exercise in both diabetic and nondiabetic individuals is associated with an increase in glucose uptake by skeletal muscle and increased insulin sensitivity that may persist up to 48 hours after exercise (83). Improvement in glucose-insulin dynamics can be attained even in moderate-intensity (50% to 65% of functional capacity) dynamic exercise if exercise is performed 30 to 60 minutes per session. Travoti et al (84) exercised five patients with NIDDM on a cycle ergometer for 1 hour a day, 7 days a week, for 6 weeks at 50% to 60% VO_2max. All subjects had improved glucose tolerance and insulin sensitivity 48 hours after their last exercise session. A recent study has found improvements in glucose tolerance with strength training in men with abnormal glucose regulation (85). Regular exercise may also benefit the diabetic patient through improved weight management, body fat distribution, blood lipid profile, psychosocial profile, and reduction in BP.

In IDDM patients, the ACSM (86) recommends daily aerobic exercise for 20 to 30 minutes per session at 40% to 85% VO_2max. For NIDDM the goal is to maximize caloric expenditure for weight control. A moderate-intensity (40% to 70% VO_2max) program performed 5 to 7 days per week for 30 to 60 minutes is recommended.

SUMMARY

Physical activity has been shown to have a protective effect against the development of CAD in both epidemiologic and intervention studies. The protective effect may be due to a direct effect of physical activity or the beneficial effects of exercise on risk factors such as hypertension, blood lipids, obesity, and glucose tolerance. Recommendations have been made based on available research for the amount of physical activity or exercise to decrease CAD risk or improve CAD risk factors.

REFERENCES

1. U.S. Department of Health and Human Services. Physical activity and health: a report of the Surgeon General. Atlanta, GA: U.S. Department of Health and Human Services, Centers for Disease Control and Prevention, National Center for Chronic Disease Prevention and Health Promotion, 1996.

2. Casperson CJ, Christenson GM, Pollard RA. Status of the 1990 physical fitness and exercise objectives evidence from NHIS 1985. Public Health Rep 1986;101:587–592.

3. Pate RR, Pratt M, Blair SN, et al. Physical activity and public health. JAMA 1995;273:402–407.

4. Harris SS, Casperson CJ, DeFriese GH, et al. Physical activity counseling for healthy adults as a primary preventive intervention in the clinical setting. Report for the U.S. Preventive Services Task Force. JAMA 1989;261:3590–3598.

5. Belcher DW, Berg AO, Inui TS. Practical approaches to providing better preventive care: are physicians a problem or solution? Am J Prev Med 1988;4:27–48.

6. Anda RF, Remmington PL, Sienko DG, et al. Are physicians advising smokers to quit? the patient's perspective. JAMA 1987;257:1916–1919.

7. Lomas J, Haynes RB. A taxonomy and critical review of tested strategies for the application of clinical practice recommendations: from "official" to "individual" clinical policy. Am J Prev Med 1988;4:77–94.

8. Long B, Calfas KJ, Wooten W, et al. A multi-site field test of the acceptability of physical activity counseling in primary care: Project PACE. Am J Prev Med 1996;12:73–81.

9. Inui TS, Yourtree EL, Williamson JW. Improved outcomes in hypertension after physician tutorials: a controlled trial. Ann Intern Med 1976;84:646–664.

10. Lewis BS, Lynch WD. The effect of physician advice on exercise behavior. Prev Med 1993;22:110–121.

11. Calfas KJ, Long BJ, Sallis JF, et al. A controlled trial of physician counseling to promote the adoption of physical activity. Prev Med 1996;25:225–233.

12. Wells KB, Lewis CE, Leake B, et al. The practices of general and subspecialty internist in counseling about smoking and exercise. Am J Public Health 1986;76:1009–1013.

13. American College of Sports Medicine. Position stand on the recommended quantity and quality of exercise for developing and maintaining fitness in healthy adults. Med Sci Sports Exerc 1978;10:vii–x.

14. American College of Sports Medicine. Position stand on the recommended quantity and quality of exercise for developing and maintaining cardiorespiratory and muscular fitness in healthy adults. Med Sci Sports Exerc 1990;22:265–274.

15. American College of Sports Medicine. Position stand on the recommended quantity and quality of exercise for developing and maintaining cardiorespiratory and muscular fitness, and flexibility in healthy adults. Med Sci Sports Exerc 1998;30:975–991.

16. Leon AS, ed. Physical activity and cardiovascular health: a national consensus. Champaign, IL: Human Kinetics, 1997.

17. Leon AS, Blackburn H. The relationship of physical activity to coronary heart disease and life expectancy. Ann NY Acad Sci 1977;301:561–578.

18. Paffenbarger RS, Hyde RT, Wing AL, et al. Physical activity, all-cause mortality and longevity of college alumni. N Engl J Med 1986;314:605–613.

19. Leon AS, Connett J, Jacobs DR, et al. Leisure-time physical activity levels and risk of coronary heart disease and death: the Multiple Risk Factor Intervention Trial. JAMA 1987;258:2388–2395.

20. Blair SN, Kohl HW, Paffenbarger RS, et al. Physical fitness and all-cause mortality—a prospective study of healthy men and women. JAMA 1989;262:2395–2401.

21. Ekelund LG, Haskell WL, Johnson JL, et al. Physical fitness as a prevention of cardiovascular mortality in asymptomatic North American men. N Engl J Med 1988;319:1379–1384.

22. Paffenbarger RS Jr, Kambert JB, Lee I-M, et al. Changes in physical activity and other lifeway patterns influencing longevity. Med Sci Sports Exerc 1994;26:857–865.

23. Wannamethee SG, Shaper AG, Walker M. Changes in physical activity, mortality, and incidence of coronary heart disease in older men. Lancet 1998;351:1603–1608.

24. Blair SN, Kohl HW III, Barlow CE, et al. Changes in physical fitness and all-cause mortality: a prospective study of healthy and unhealthy men. JAMA 1995;273:1093–1098.

25. Blair SN, Kampert JB, Kohl HW III, et al. Influences of cardiorespiratory fitness and other precursors on cardiovascular disease and all-

cause mortality in men and women. JAMA 1996;276: 205–210.

26. Paffenbarger RS Jr, Wing AI, Hyde RT. Physical activity as an index of heart attack risk in college alumni. Am J Epidemiol 1978;108:161–175.

27. Lee I-M, Hsish CC, Paffenbarger RS Jr. Exercise intensity and longevity in men: the Harvard Alumni Study. JAMA 1995;273:1179–1184.

28. Hagberg JM. Physical activity, physical fitness and blood pressure. In: Leon AS, ed. Physical activity and cardiovascular health: a national consensus. Champaign, IL: Human Kinetics, 1997:112–119.

29. MacMahon SW, Wilcken DEL, MacDonald GJ. The effect of weight reduction on left ventricular mass: a randomized controlled trial in young, overweight, hypertensive patients. N Engl J Med 1986;314:334–339.

30. Stefanick ML. Physical activity and lipid metabolism. In: Leon AS, ed. Physical activity and cardiovascular health: a national consensus. Champaign, IL: Human Kinetics, 1997:98–104.

31. Williams RS, Logue EE, Lewis J, et al. Physical conditioning augments the fibrinolytic response to venous occlusion in healthy adults. N Engl J Med 1980;302:987–991.

32. Jennings G, Nelson L, Nestel P, et al. The effects of changes in physical activity on major cardiovascular risk factors, hemodynamics, sympathetic function, and glucose utilization in man: a controlled study of four levels of activity. Circulation 1986;73:30–40.

33. Schwartz PJ, Stone HL. The analysis and modulation of autonomic reflexes in the prediction and prevention of sudden death. In: Zipes K, Jalif D, eds. Cardiac electrophysiology and arrythmias. New York: Grune and Stratton, 1985.

34. Roth DM, White FC, Nichols ML, et al. Effect of long-term exercise on regional myocardial function and coronary collateral develop-

ment after gradual coronary artery occlusion in pigs. Circulation 1990;82:1778–1779.

35. Bove AA, Dewey JD. Proximal coronary vasomotor reactivity after exercise training in dogs. Circulation 1985;71:620–625.

36. Kuczmarski RF, Flegal KM, Campbell SM, et al. Increasing prevalence of overweight among US adults. JAMA 1994;272:205–211.

37. National Heart, Lung, and Blood Institute. Clinical guidelines on the identification, evaluation, and treatment of overweight and obesity in adults, 1998. Washington, DC: NIH.

38. Pi-Sunyer FX. Medical hazards of obesity. Ann Intern Med 1993;119:655–665.

39. Bjorntorp P. Metabolic implications of body fat distribution. Diabetes Care 1991;14:1132–1143.

40. Bouchard C. Physical activity and prevention of cardiovascular diseases: potential mechanisms. In: Leon AS, ed. Physical activity and health: a national consensus. Champaign, IL: Human Kinetics, 1997:48–56.

41. Garrow JS, Summerbell CD. Meta-analysis: effect of exercise, with or without dieting, on body composition of overweight subjects. Eur J Clin Nutr 1995;49:1–10.

42. Hammer RL, Barrier CA, Roundy ES, et al. Calorie-restricted low-fat diet and exercise in obese women. Am J Clin Nutr 1989;49:77–85.

43. Marks BL, Ward A, Morris DH, et al. Fat-free mass is maintained in women following a moderate diet and exercise program. Med Sci Sports Exerc 1995;27:1243–1251.

44. Schwartz RS, Sherman WP, Larson V, et al. The effect of intensive endurance exercise training on body fat distribution in young and older men. Metabolism 1991;40:545–551.

45. Depres JP, Pouliot MC, Moorjani S, et al. Loss of abdominal fat and metabolic response to exercise training in obese women. Am J Physiol 1991;261:E159–E167.

46. Paffenbarger RS Jr, Wing A, Hyde R, et al. Physical activity and incidence of hypertension in college alumni. Am J Epidemiol 1983;117:245–256.

47. Blair S, Goodyear N, Gibbons L, et al. Physical fitness and incidence of hypertension in healthy normotensive men and women. JAMA 1984;252:487–490.

48. Reaven PD, Barrett-Connor E, Edelstein S. Relation between leisure-time physical activity and blood pressure in older women. Circulation 1991;83:559–565.

49. Stamler R, Stamler J, Gosch FC, et al. Primary prevention of hypertension by nutritional-hygienic means: final report of a randomized, controlled trial. JAMA 1989;262:1801–1807.

50. Seals DR, Hagberg JM. The effect of exercise training on human hypertension: a review. Med Sci Sports Exerc 1984;16:207–225.

51. American College of Sports Medicine. Position stand on physical activity, physical fitness, and hypertension. Med Sci Sports Exerc 1993;25:i–x.

52. Dunbar CC. The antihypertensive effects of exercise. NY State J Med 1992;92:250–255.

53. Kelly G, McClelland P. Antihypertensive effects of aerobic exercise. Am J Hypertens 1994;7:115–119.

54. Hagberg JM, Montain SJ, Martin WH, et al. Effect of exercise training on 60–69 year old persons with essential hypertension. Am J Cardiol 1989;64:348–353.

55. Roman O, Camuzzi AL, Villalon E, et al. Physical training program in arterial hypertension: a long-term prospective follow-up. Cardiology 1981;67:230–243.

56. Van Hoof R, Hespel P, Fagard R, et al. Effects of endurance training on blood pressure at rest, during exercise and during 24 hours in sedentary men. Am J Cardiol 1989;63:945–949.

57. Gilders RM, Voner C, Dudley GA. Endurance training and blood pressure in normotensive and

hypertensive adults. Med Sci Sports Exerc 1989;21:629–636.

58. Seals DR, Reiling MJ. Effect of regular exercise on 24-hour arterial pressure in older hypertensive humans. Hypertension 1991;18:583–592.

59. Pescatello LS, Fargo AE, Leach CN, et al. Short-term effect of dynamic exercise on arterial blood pressure. Circulation 1991;83:1557–1561.

60. Hagberg JM, Montain SJ, Martin WH. Blood pressure and hemodynamic responses after exercise in older adults. J Appl Physiol 1987;62:270–276.

61. Kokkinos PF, Narayan P, Colleran JA, et al. Effects of regular exercise on blood pressure and left ventricular hypertrophy in African-American men with severe hypertension. N Engl J Med 1995;333:1462–1467.

62. Haskell WL. The influence of exercise training on plasma lipids and lipoproteins in health and disease. Acta Med Scand 1986;711(suppl):25–37.

63. Superko HR, Haskell WL. The role of exercise training in the therapy of hyperlipoproteinemia. Cardiol Clin 1987;5:285–310.

64. Cook TC, Laporte RE, Washburn RA, et al. Chronic low level physical activity as a determinant of high density lipoprotein cholesterol and subfractions. Med Sci Sports Exerc 1986;18:653–657.

65. Leon AS, Conrad J, Hunninghake DB, et al. Effects of a vigorous walking program on body composition, carbohydrate and lipid metabolism of obese young men. Am J Clin Nutr 1979;32:1776–1779.

66. Kokkinos PF, Holland JC, Narayan P, et al. Miles run per week and high-density lipoprotein cholesterol levels in healthy middle-aged men. Arch Intern Med 1995;155:415–420.

67. Stein RA, Michielli DW, Glantz MD, et al. Effects of different exercise intensities on lipoprotein cholesterol fractions in healthy middle-aged men. Am Heart J 1990;119:277–283.

68. Duncan JJ, Gordon NF, Scott CB. Women walking for health and fitness: how much is enough? JAMA 1991;266:3295–3299.

69. Taylor PA, Ward A. Women, high-density lipoprotein cholesterol, and exercise. Arch Intern Med 1993;153:1178–1184.

70. Rotkis TC, Boyden TW, Stanforth PR, et al. Increased high-density lipoprotein cholesterol and lean body weight in endurance-trained women runners. J Card Rehabil 1984;4:62–66.

71. Goodyear LJ, Fronsoe MS, Van Houten DR, et al. Increased HDL-cholesterol following eight weeks of progressive endurance training in female runners. Ann Sports Med 1986;3:33–38.

72. Cauley JA, Laporte RE, Kuller LH, et al. The epidemiology of high-density lipoprotein cholesterol levels in postmenopausal women. J Gerontol 1982;37:10–15.

73. Cauley JA, Laporte RE, Sandler RB, et al. The relationship of physical activity to high-density lipoprotein cholesterol in postmenopausal women. J Chron Dis 1986;39:687–697.

74. Wood PD, Stefanick ML, Dreone D, et al. Changes in plasma lipids and lipoproteins in overweight men during weight loss through dieting compared with exercise. N Engl J Med 1988;319:1173–1179.

75. Sopko G, Leon AS, Jacobs DR Jr, et al. The effects of exercise and weight loss on plasma lipids in young obese men. Metabolism 1985;39:227–236.

76. Thompson PD, Yurgalevitch SM, Flynn MM, et al. Effect of prolonged exercise training without weight loss on high-density lipoprotein metabolism in overweight men. Metabolism 1997;46:217–223.

77. Leon AS. Patients with diabetes mellitus. In: Franklin BA, Gordon S, Timmis GC, eds. Exercise in modern medicine. Baltimore: Williams and Wilkins, 1989:118–145.

78. Bjorntorp P. Metabolic implications of body fat distribution. Diabetes Care 1991;14:1132–1143.

79. Helmrich SP, Ragland DR, Leung RN, et al. Physical activity and reduced occurrence of non-insulin-dependent diabetes mellitus. N Engl J Med 1991;325:147–152.

80. Manson JE, Rimm EB, Stampfer MJ, et al. Physical activity and incidence of non-insulin-dependent diabetes mellitus in women. Lancet 1991;338:774–778.

81. Manson JE, Nathan DM, Krolewski AS, et al. A prospective study of exercise and incidence of diabetes among U.S. male physicians. JAMA 1992;268:63–67.

82. Perry I, Wannamethee S, Walker M, et al. Prospective study of risk factors for development of non-insulin-dependent diabetes in middle-aged British men. BMJ 1995;310:560–564.

83. Vranic M, Wasserman D. Exercise, fitness, and diabetes. In: Bouchard C, Shephard RJ, Stephens T, et al, eds. Exercise, fitness, and habits: a consensus of current knowledge. Champaign, IL: Human Kinetics, 1990:467–490.

84. Travoti M, Carta Q, Cavalot F, et al. Influence of physical training on blood glucose control, glucose intolerance, insulin secretion, and insulin activity in non-insulin dependent diabetic patients. Diabetes Care 1985;17:416–420.

85. Smutok M, Reece C, Kokkinos P, et al. Effects of exercise training modality on glucose tolerance in men with abnormal glucose regulation. Int J Sports Med 1994;15:283–289.

86. American College of Sports Medicine. ACSM's guidelines for exercise testing and prescription. 5th ed. Baltimore: Williams and Wilkins, 1995.

Chapter 8

Clinical Strategy for Managing Dyslipidemias

Mary P. McGowan

Heart disease is the leading cause of death in the United States in both men and women. In 1994, there were 487,490 deaths secondary to coronary heart disease (CHD) and there are 13.7 million Americans alive today who have a history of myocardial infarction, angina, or both. The cost of treating CHD in the United States is astronomical, on the order of $150 billion per year. A full 60% of the money spent on CHD is used to pay for hospitalizations and cardiovascular interventions, such as percutaneous transluminal coronary angioplasty (PTCA) and coronary artery bypass grafting (CABG) (1).

If we are to reduce both the economic and social burden of cardiovascular disease in the United States, it is imperative that we address all cardiovascular risk factors. This chapter focuses on the impact of cholesterol as a cardiac risk factor and through a series of case discussions highlights the importance of aggressively managing dyslipidemias in persons with or at high risk for the development of cardiac disease.

At the present time it is estimated, based on the National Cholesterol Education Program (NCEP) guidelines (discussed later in this chapter), that 52 million U.S. adults qualify for lipid-lowering therapy (i.e., diet and or medication) (2). Unfortunately, recent studies also reveal that only between 4% and 9% of people with hyperlipidemia are achieving the lipid goals set by the NCEP guidelines (3–5).

Although this chapter focuses on hyperlipidemia, it should be noted that most patients with cardiac disease have multiple risk factors. Diet and exercise are the first lines of therapy in treating hyperlipidemia; since these therapies can improve blood pressure and diabetes as well as lower lipids, their importance cannot be overstated. If diet and exercise fail to fully normalize lipid levels, cholesterol-altering medications should be added.

BLOOD CHOLESTEROL AND CORONARY ARTERY DISEASE

Data from multiple epidemiologic studies have given conclusive evidence regarding the causal link between elevated cholesterol levels and the subsequent development of coronary artery disease (CAD). The published regression trials have provided evidence that aggressive cholesterol reduction could lead to regression of existing cardiac disease. The studies also found that significant cholesterol reductions in persons with existing cardiac disease also resulted in dramatic reductions in clinical cardiac events.

Although the regression studies contributed to our overall understanding of the vascular biology of atherosclerosis and provided proof that cholesterol reduction is associated with a substantial reduction in clinical cardiac events, they were not powered to show a reduction in all-cause mortality.

MORTALITY STUDIES

In order to confirm what had long been suspected (i.e., that aggressive cholesterol reduction would reduce all-cause mortality), large primary and secondary prevention studies were carried out. The first of these studies was the Scandinavian Simvastatin Survival Study (4S) (6). In this trial 4444 men and women, all with documented cardiac disease, were randomized to receive either 20 or 40 mg of simvastatin per day (n =

98

2221) or a placebo (n = 2223). At the conclusion of this 5.4-year trial, the participants treated with simvastatin had lowered their LDL level by 35%, whereas those receiving a placebo experienced a 1% increase in LDL levels. Overall, participants treated with simvastatin enjoyed a 30% reduction in all-cause mortality ($p = .0003$), a 42% reduction in the risk of definite or suspected cardiac death ($p = .00001$), and a 37% reduction in revascularization procedures ($p < .00001$) as compared to individuals receiving placebo.

In addition to conclusively proving that all-cause mortality could be positively affected with aggressive cholesterol reduction, the 4S study also demonstrated that cholesterol reduction with simvastatin was not accompanied by any increased risk of noncardiac mortality, including deaths due to violence or cancer.

Recently the findings of the 4S study were confirmed by the Long-Term Intervention with Pravastatin in Ischemic Disease (LIPID) Study (7). This study included over 9000 men and women with existing cardiac disease. Participants received either pravastatin 40 mg or placebo. At the conclusion of this 7-year trial, patients receiving pravastatin enjoyed a 23% reduction in all-cause mortality ($p = .00002$), a 24% reduction in coronary mortality ($p = .0004$), a 20% reduction in stroke ($p = .022$), a 29% reduction in fatal and nonfatal myocardial infarctions ($p = .00001$), and a 24% reduction in the need for CABG procedures ($p = .0001$).

The 4S and LIPID studies included only persons with documented cardiac disease. In order to determine whether the all-cause mortality benefits might be extended to include persons without a history of cardiac disease, the West of Scotland Study was undertaken (8).

In the study (also known as The Pravastatin Primary Prevention Study) 6595 hypercholesterolemic men were randomized to either pravastatin (40 mg/day) or placebo and followed for 5 years. Pravastatin resulted in a 22% reduction in total mortality ($p = .051$). In addition it reduced the risk of first myocardial infarction by 31% ($p = .0001$). Likewise it reduced the need for PTCA or CABG by 37% ($p = .0009$). Finally, pravastatin reduced the risk of cardiovascular mortality by 32% ($p = .033$).

CLINICAL PRACTICE

Now that the causal relationship between cholesterol and cardiac disease has been firmly established, clinicians must incorporate cholesterol screening and therapy into their practices. The National Cholesterol Education Program (NCEP) has issued guidelines for the detection and treatment of hypercholesterolemia in adults (9). Since their publication in 1993, these guidelines have been widely publicized and will not be reviewed in detail here. Briefly, they recommend screening all Americans over age 20 for hypercholesterolemia. The initial screen may be performed in the nonfasting state and should measure total and high-density lipoprotein (HDL) cholesterol levels.

The guidelines separate lipid levels into categories (Table 8-1) that are used to determine if there is a need for a more detailed lipoprotein analysis. Once an initial total and HDL screen has been performed, the need for a complete fasting lipid profile is determined, based on both the lipid

Table 8-1 Total and HDL Cholesterol Levels: Relationship to Classification of Individuals

TOTAL CHOLESTEROL LEVEL	CLASSIFICATION	HDL CHOLESTEROL LEVEL	CLASSIFICATION
<200 mg/dL	Desirable	<35 mg/dL	Low
200–239 mg/dL	Borderline high	≥60 mg/dL	High
>240 mg/dL	High		

SOURCE: Modified from Expert Panel on Detection, Evaluation and Treatment of High Blood Cholesterol in Adults. Summary of the second report of the National Cholesterol Education Program (NCEP) Expert Panel on Detection, Evaluation, and Treatment of High Blood Cholesterol in Adults (Adult Treatment Panel II). JAMA 1993;269:3015–3023.

Table 8-2 Classification of Triglycerides

TRIGLYCERIDE LEVEL	CLASSIFICATION
<200 mg/dL	Normal
200–400 mg/dL	Borderline high
400–1000 mg/dL	High
>1000 mg/dL	Very high

levels and the number of additional cardiac risk factors a person has (see Chapter 1 for a discussion of risk factors).

Regardless of the number of risk factors, a full lipid profile is recommended for any person with the diagnosis of vascular disease (peripheral, cerebral, or coronary). Once a full lipid profile is obtained, most treatment decisions are based on the low-density lipoprotein (LDL) cholesterol level (Table 8-2).

The complete lipid profile also assesses triglyceride and HDL levels. According to the NCEP (Table 8-2), triglycerides are considered in the normal range if they are below 200 mg/dL. Any HDL below 35 mg/dL is considered low.

In the cases that follow it can be seen that in this author's clinical practice more rigorous goals for both HDL and triglycerides are set forth. This is based on evidence that triglycerides are an independent predictor of cardiac risk in both men and women (10,11) and HDL likewise strongly predicts cardiac risk (12,13).

The following cases reflect the challenges faced in treating patients with dyslipidemias. As you review these cases, I encourage you to decide how you would approach each patient's therapy. From my point of view, as a lipid specialist, the most important aspect of cholesterol management is helping one's patients to appreciate the importance of cholesterol reduction. If your patients perceive something as important, they are much more likely to understand the need for both lifestyle changes and the use of lipid-altering agents. Likewise, it is important to enlist the help of family members, since they can either reinforce or undermine all your efforts.

CASE 1

S.C. is a 40-year-old woman with a strong family history of CAD. Her father died at age 45 of a myocardial infarction. At the age of 25 she was told she had an elevated cholesterol and a reduced-fat diet was recommended.

At the age of 35 her lipids were reevaluated by her primary care doctor. Her total cholesterol was 360 mg/dL and she was started on a bile acid resin but was unable to tolerate it. Over the next 4 years she was on and off lovastatin with only modest success. A repeat lipid profile in February 1997 revealed the following:

	S.C.'s level	Desirable level
Total cholesterol	412 mg/dL	<200 mg/dL
Triglycerides	139 mg/dL	<150 mg/dL
HDL cholesterol	49 mg/dL	>45 mg/dL
LDL cholesterol	335 mg/dL	<130 mg/dL
Lp (a)	126 mg/dL	<20 mg/dL

On physical examination, S.C. was a 40-year-old woman who looked her stated age. She was 67 in. tall and weighed 155 lb (ideal body weight 135 lb). The rest of her examination was remarkable for xanthelasmas (lipid accumulations around the eyes), corneal arcus (white circles around the iris of the eye), and multiple tendon xanthomas (cholesterol depositions within the tendons of the hands or feet or the Achilles tendon).

Her social history was significant for a very sedentary, high-stress job. She was an ex-smoker with no regular exercise program, and she ate the typical American diet, deriving about 34% to 36% of her calories from fat.

The first question to ask yourself is: What is this woman's diagnosis? The combination of a total cholesterol level above 340 mg/dL in an adult with a normal triglyceride level, a family history of early cardiac disease, and tendon xanthomas make the diagnosis of familial hypercholesterolemia (FH) virtually certain (14).

FH is a common genetic cholesterol abnormality, striking 1 in 500 persons in the general population. It can be found in 5% of persons who suffer a heart attack before the age of 65, and FH tends to occur more frequently in certain populations; French-Canadians, Afrikaners in South Africa, the Finnish, the Lebanese, and Ashkenazi Jews all run about a 1 in 100 chance of inheriting this disorder (14). In the United States alone it is estimated that there are 500,000 FH heterozygotes. Unfortunately, most of them are unaware of their diagnosis. A recent study of 502 FH heterozygotes in Utah found only 31% were diagnosed, only 42% were taking any medication to reduce their cholesterol, and only 25% had treated cholesterol levels below the 90th percentile (15).

FH causes very high cholesterol levels (in adults FH should be suspected when total cholesterol is 340 mg/dL or higher, and in children at a level of 270 mg/dL) and greatly inceases the chance of having an early heart attack, even as early as age 20. In general, however, most men with untreated FH have had at least one heart attack by age 55 and most women with this disorder have had the same experience by age 65.

FH is caused by mutations at the LDL receptor locus on the short arm of chromosome 19. To date, at least 150 dif-

ferent mutations of the LDL receptor gene have been identified as causing FH (16). The gene for FH is inherited in an autosomal dominant fashion; therefore, if a person has FH, on average, half of his or her first-degree relatives will also have FH and likewise be at risk for early heart disease (14).

My diagnosis of FH was a shock to S.C. She had never heard the term before and the thought of having a genetic disease was, in her words, "very frightening." At the same time, however, she had a curious sense of liberation. As she got used to the idea that she actually carried an abnormal gene that prevented her body from processing cholesterol properly, she began to realize that her unsatisfactory levels were not her fault. Previously, she had always felt vaguely guilty about her lipid levels, believing that if she were only more rigid about her diet or more vigorous about her exercise program, her levels would be normal.

I explained to S.C. that although diet and exercise were extremely important in the treatment of FH, they were not the entire answer. All persons with FH require cholesterol-lowering medications in conjunction with a strict diet and exercise program.

At her first visit she was started on a 1200-calorie, 27-g fat diet and atorvastatin, 10 mg/day. She was asked to initiate a daily walking program (3 miles/day). Six weeks later she had lost 8 lb, was walking 3 miles/day, and had the following lipid profile:

	S.C.'s level	Desirable level
Total cholesterol	219 mg/dL	<200 mg/dL
Triglycerides	71 mg/dL	<150 mg/dL
HDL cholesterol	37 mg/dL	>45 mg/dL
LDL cholesterol	167 mg/dL	<130 mg/dL
Lp (a)	126 mg/dL	<20 mg/dL

At this point S.C. was thrilled with her overall results but wanted more information regarding the importance of her elevated lipoprotein (a) [Lp(a)]. She was also wondering why her HDL had fallen.

Lp(a) is an LDL-like particle consisting of a characteristic polymorphic glycoprotein called apoprotein (a), which is linked to the apolipoprotein B moiety of the LDL particle by a disulfide bridge (17). Lp(a) is important because, like LDL, it is an atherogenic lipoprotein. Lp(a) has been found to be a constituent of the atherosclerotic plaque (18). In addition to its atherogenic qualities, because of its structural similarities to plasminogen, Lp(a) can interfere with the fibrinolytic system. Individuals with high levels of Lp(a) are at increased risk for clotting (17).

Lp(a) is a very good independent predictor of atherosclerotic risk. The average Lp(a) in the white population is approximately 4 mg/dL, with levels somewhat higher in the African-American population. Lp(a) levels above 25 to 30 mg/dL increase the risk of developing cardiac disease (19). Elevated Lp(a) levels seem to predict not only the development of cardiac disease but also an increased risk of restenosis after bypass and angioplasty (20,21). Diet and exercise have little effect on this highly heritable atherogenic lipoprotein. To date only estrogen and niacin have been conclusively shown to lower Lp(a) levels (22,23).

It is worthwhile to measure Lp(a) in all cardiac patients. Since it has been shown that up to 50% of persons with FH will also have an elevated Lp(a) (24), and that this elevation predicts high risk for very early heart disease (earlier than if a person had FH alone), all persons with FH should be evaluated for Lp(a).

There is little information on the effect of Lp(a) reduction on arteriographically defined CAD. However, recently lipoprotein apheresis was used in an attempt to reduce the rate of restenosis following PTCA, and it was reported that the restenosis rate was 21% for subjects in whom Lp(a) was reduced more than 50%, compared with a 50% restenosis rate for subjects in whom less than a 50% reduction in Lp(a) was achieved (25). We agreed with S.C. that if at all possible, her Lp(a) should be lowered.

Regarding the drop in S.C.'s HDL, we explained that sometimes with active weight loss a transient decline in HDL is observed (26); also, a very low fat diet can also contribute to a slight decline in HDL. We planned to monitor this closely.

At her second visit, S.C. saw our dietitian, who fine-tuned her diet. Together they decided to try a 15% fat diet (1200 calories, 20 g of fat) and, in order to lower her Lp(a), niacin at 500 mg three times a day was added (niacin at this level would also raise HDL and lower LDL). All side effects of the atorvastatin-niacin combination, including an increased risk of hepatotoxicity and myositis, were reviewed with S.C. We made the decision that the benefits of therapy outweighed the risks. Three months later this was her lipid profile:

	S.C.'s level	Desirable level
Total cholesterol	195 mg/dL	<200 mg/dL
Triglycerides	62 mg/dL	<150 mg/dL
HDL cholesterol	56 mg/dL	>45 mg/dL
LDL cholesterol	128 mg/dL	<130 mg/dL
Lp (a)	95 mg/dL	<20 mg/dL

At this point S.C. asked me if we should increase her niacin dose in hopes of a further reduction in her Lp(a). I explained that a recent study had found that Lp(a) becomes a less significant cardiac risk factor when LDL is dramatically reduced (27).

With this in mind and given the fact that higher doses of niacin in combination with atorvastatin can significantly increase the risk of toxicity, I suggested that we continue her current program. I did, however, point out that she should strongly consider estrogen replacement at the time of menopause.

Now, 10 months after our initial meeting, S.C. has lost 20 lb, is following a 15% fat diet, is walking 3 miles a day and attends a weekly yoga class. Her risk for a cardiac event has been dramatically reduced, and her understanding of the genetic basis of her cholesterol abnormality has resulted in many of her family members also being diagnosed with FH.

CASE 2

F.P. is a 56-year-old nun with the following lipid profile:

	F.P.'s level	Desirable level
Total cholesterol	311 mg/dL	<200 mg/dL
HDL cholesterol	33 mg/dL	>45 mg/dL
Triglycerides	532 mg/dL	<150 mg/dL
LDL cholesterol	Invalid	<130 mg/dL
Lp (a)	8 mg/dL	<20 mg/dL

Note that if triglycerides are above 400 mg/dL, LDL cannot be accurately calculated. In addition F.P. was noted to have the following cardiac risk factors:

- She is postmenopausal without estrogen replacement.
- She has diabetic range fasting blood sugar (136 mg/dL).
- She has a positive family history. Her mother died of an myocardial infarction at the age of 39. Her brother died of a myocardial infarction at the age of 66. He had been known to have elevated triglyceride and LDL levels.
- She has two younger sisters with breast cancer (ages 50 and 53). Although neither sister has had a cardiac event, both have isolated elevated triglycerides.
- She has hypertension and is on Lopressor 25 mg twice a day (on therapy her blood pressure was 160/70 mm/Hg).
- At 65 ins she weighs 173 lb. Her ideal body weight is 125 lb.

Her diet is as follows:

Breakfast: cereal with skim milk, orange juice (8 to 10 oz), an apple, and coffee with Half-and-Half
Lunch: chicken with sauce or beef with gravy, potato, vegetables, and fruit; uses stick margarine on the potato
Supper: cereal with skim milk or soup
Snacks: peanuts, popcorn, and prunes; admits to a weakness for chocolate

For exercise she walks 15 minutes on fair weather days; if it is raining or cold, she will bike indoors for 10 minutes.

The first question to ask yourself is: Does this woman have a genetic dyslipidemia? Because she has diabetes, which can cause a secondary dyslipidemia, one cannot say conclusively that she has a genetic dyslipidemia. But based on her family history of cardiac disease and hyperlipidemia, it is likely that she has familial combined hyperlipidemia (FCH).

FCH was first described at the University of Washington in 1973 by Goldstein et al (28). To date, however, its genetics have not been fully worked out. It appears that individuals with FCH overproduce very low density lipoprotein (VLDL). VLDL is a triglyceride-rich lipoprotein, produced by the liver and other cells, which is converted in the bloodstream by the action of lipoprotein lipase to intermediate-density lipoprotein (IDL).

IDL contains a significant amount of both triglycerides and cholesterol and is felt to be an atherogenic lipoprotein. Finally, by the action of hepatic triglyceride lipase, IDL is converted to LDL, a highly atherogenic cholesterol-rich lipoprotein. Persons with FCH, depending on how rapidly they metabolize their VLDL, may have a number of different lipoprotein abnormalities including: 1) elevated triglycerides alone, 2) elevated triglycerides and LDL, or 3) elevated LDL alone. The diagnosis of FCH depends on finding several different cholesterol abnormalities in a family with cardiac disease (29).

In approaching this woman's therapy we first pointed out to her that a low-fat, low-sugar, calorie-restricted diet and exercise would dramatically improve her lipids (persons with FCH often respond very briskly to diet), her blood pressure, and her diabetes. Although it was likely that Lopressor was contributing slightly to her blood sugar elevation and her hypertriglyceridemia (30), we decided not to change this initially.

Given the degree of her hypertriglyceridemia, we decided to use gemfibrozil, a fibric acid derivative that can lower triglycerides as much as 45%. The decision to use gemfibrozil was really a judgment call; it would have been perfectly reasonable to give FP a 3-month trial of diet before initiating medications.

Three months later she returned 12 lb lighter, with the following lipid profile, blood pressure, and blood sugar level:

	F.P.'s level	Desirable level
Total cholesterol	297 mg/dL	<200 mg/dL
HDL cholesterol	48 mg/dL	>45 mg/dL
Triglycerides	219 mg/dL	<150 mg/dL
LDL cholesterol	205 mg/dL	<130 mg/dL
Blood pressure	120/80 mm Hg	<140/80 mm Hg
Blood glucose	89 mg/dL	<126 mg/dL

She was biking or walking 15 minutes/day, following a 1200-calorie, fat (<27 g/day)- and sugar (<35 g/day)-restricted diet.

At this point, the major questions are: Should you add a second medication at this visit, and what additional lifestyle changes might you suggest?

In a postmenopausal woman who is not on estrogen replacement therapy, one must consider the use of estrogen (in F.P.'s case it would be estrogen and progesterone since she has not had a hysterectomy), which appears to reduce the risk of an initial cardiac event by between 35% and 50% (31).

The fact that F.P. has two sisters with breast cancer makes this a more difficult decision, but it was made easier by her absolute refusal even to consider estrogen. Some battles are not worth fighting—and this was one of them. It is my opinion that people have to feel comfortable with their medications, and must feel that they are doing them more good than harm; otherwise, compliance becomes a major issue.

Nonetheless, I felt F.P. needed a second medicine to lower her LDL. There is good evidence that the 3-hydroxyl-3 methylglutaryl coenzyme A reductase inhibitors (HMGs) reduce cardiac risk in women as well as men (32). With regard to the combination of gemfibrozil and an HMG, until recently there was much more literature on the combination of pravastatin and gemfibrozil than on any other HMG (33,34). Very recently good safety data have become available on the use of simvastatin and gemfibrozil as well (35). Because the data on the simvastatin—gemfibrozil combination were not available when I was considering dual therapy for F.P., I chose the pravastatin—gemfibrozil combination. Because there is an increased risk of hepatotoxicity and an increased risk of rhabdomyolysis with the combination of a fibric acid derivative and an HMG, I felt it was best to begin with the combination that was most well studied and had the greatest amount of safety data to back up such a choice. The risks and benefits of combination therapy were discussed with F.P. and ultimately pravstatin at 40 mg/day (taken at night) was prescribed.

In addition she was asked to increase her daily aerobic activity to 30 minutes/day. Reluctantly she agreed to work harder at exercise.

Six weeks later she returned with the following lipid profile:

	F.P.'s level	Desirable level
Total cholesterol	192 mg/dL	<200 mg/dL
HDL cholesterol	54 mg/dL	>45 mg/dL
Triglycerides	178 mg/dL	<150 mg/dL
LDL cholesterol	102 mg/dL	<130 mg/dL

At this point she had lost another 4 lb and her blood pressure and blood sugar were under excellent control. She was biking or walking 25 to 30 minutes/day. Her only complaint on the combination of gemfibrozil and pravastatin was constipation. Her pravastatin was reduced to 20 mg/day, her symptoms improved, and her LDL remained acceptable at 112.

Over the past 18 months F.P. has maintained her program and has actually lost an additional 6 lb. Her lipids, blood chemistries, and blood pressure are under excellent control.

Her case illustrates the impact diet and exercise can have on cardiac risk factors other than lipids (i.e., blood pressure and diabetes) and the role of cholesterol-lowering medications in the treatment of genetic dyslipidemias.

CASE 3

C.G. is a 48-year-old man with documented CAD. In 1993 he presented to his primary care doctor with exercise-induced chest pain. After an abnormal exercise tolerance test (ETT), he underwent a cardiac catheterization that demonstrated the following:

- Left anterior descending (LAD) with a 60% proximal occlusion
- Dominant right coronary artery (RCA) with a proximal 90% occlusion
- Multiple additional 40% to 50% lesions
- Good LV function

He underwent an angioplasty of the right coronary lesion and was placed on an antianginal regimen, including a beta blocker, long-acting nitrates, and an aspirin.

His cardiac risk factors included:

- Smoking: smoked five cigars a day
- Diabetes: poorly controlled with diet (fasting blood sugar 140 to 190 mg/dL)
- Family history: father myocardial infarction (MI) age 60, CABG age 66
- Sedentary lifestyle
- Overweight (70.5 in. tall, weight 211 lb, ideal body weight (IBW): 170)
- Hyperlipidemia:

	C.G.'s level	Desirable level
Total cholesterol	304 mg/dL	<200 mg/dL
HDL cholesterol	31 mg/dL	>45 mg/dL
Triglycerides	230 mg/dL	<150 mg/dL
LDL cholesterol	227 mg/dL	<100 mg/dL
Lp (a)	15 mg/dL	<20 mg/dL

In order to achieve his LDL goal, he required a 59% LDL reduction. His diet was as follows:

Breakfast: low-fat muffin, 10 oz of orange juice, coffee with cream and sugar
Lunch: tuna sandwich or ham and cheese sandwich, apple
Supper: burger or chicken with skin, potato, vegetables with stick margarine, coffee with cream and sugar
Snacks: ice cream, cupcakes (rare alcohol)

At the time of his referral to our cholesterol management center, C.G. continued to experience angina with vigorous exertion, especially while mowing his lawn.

C.G.'s care was made more complex because despite his obvious intelligence (he is a master plumber), he was completely illiterate. Fortunately, he had a very supportive wife who was more than willing to make dietary changes and to learn to read food labels.

Although somewhat skeptical about the possibility of dramatically reducing his risk for a future cardiac event, C.G. agreed to give our program an 8-week trial.

Even though it was clear that his diabetes, triglycerides, and HDL level were being adversely effected by the use of a beta blocker (30), we recognized the importance of this cardioprotective agent and explained that he would have to work event harder on our diet and exercise program. We asked C.G. to do four things:

1. We explained that giving up cigar smoking would result in an increase in his HDL (typically 5.0 to 8.0 mg/dL over the course of about 6 months) (36,37). In addition, quitting cigars would reduce his burden of oxidized LDL (38). We explained that oxidized LDL is the most atherogenic form of LDL.

2. We asked him to follow a 20% fat diet, which restricted calories to 1500/day and fat to 33 g/day. We also suggested that he restrict the sugar in his diet to no more than 35 g/day. We explained that this suggestion would improve his blood sugar and also result in an improvement in his triglycerides. Rather than simply give him a fat, sugar, and calorie allowance, we provided him with substitutions for his current food choices. Our dietitian explained why each change was necessary.

At breakfast we asked him to eliminate his muffin and choose instead a small bagel (for example, a frozen bagel as opposed to the typical deli bagels, which contain about 450 calories, the equivalent of four slices of bread). This could be topped with with either a small amount (1 to 2 teaspoons) of lite cream cheese or a reduced-fat tub margarine.

We told C.G. that muffins are loaded with sugar and contain about 400 calories. Instead of orange juice, he was encouraged to eat an entire orange. Orange juice provides a large number of calories and simple sugars; the whole orange has fewer calories and provides water-soluble fiber. In general, in our clinic we limit fruit for persons with hypertriglyceridemia to four pieces per day, with a 4-oz glass of juice constituting one fruit serving.

Finally, based on his history, he was getting about 12 g of fat (mostly saturated) from the cream in his coffee. We asked him to switch to whole milk. Although the ultimate goal is skim or 1% milk in his

coffee, this is a good first step. We also encouraged elimination of sugar in his coffee. Although he would be best served by eliminating any type of sweetener, we do allow small amounts (two servings per day) of a sugar substitute.

As for lunch, we pointed out that a typical deli tuna sandwich contains about 36 g of fat and we recommended that he begin packing his own lunch. We suggested a tuna or turkey sandwich made with a small amount (1 to 2 teaspoons) of lite mayonnaise. We brought to his attention that there are good low-fat or nonfat cheeses available. He was asked to continue his practice of having a piece of fruit with lunch, and pretzels or another piece of fruit were suggested as a midafternoon snack.

For supper, we suggested small portions (4 to 6 oz.) of red meat be used only once a week. We explained that pork counts as a red meat (this is a popular misconception). He was encouraged to have skinless chicken or broiled or baked fish three to four times a week and a meatless meal once or twice a week. A variety of vegetables and potato or rice were suggested. Instead of stick margarine, which provides a fair amount of transfatty acids, we suggested diet or spray margarine.

Finally, he was advised to try low-fat popcorn (one third of a bag of low-fat microwave popcorn), graham crackers (two crackers), two rice cakes (any flavor), baked tortilla chips (13 chips), or sugar-free fat-free frozen yogurt (one half cup) as evening snacks.

We explained that in our experience this type of diet tends to reduce LDL cholesterol by about 20%. Since C.G. required almost a 60% reduction in LDL, we explained that cholesterol-lowering medications would also be necessary.

3. Before discussing cholesterol-lowering medications, we moved on to our third request, which was for daily exercise. We provided C.G. with an exercise prescription. As a rule, we prefer to initiate exercise with enrollment in cardiac rehabilitation, as we feel strongly that it provides patients with the confidence they need to maintain exercise for the long term. In fact, participation in a cardiac rehabilitation program following a myocardial infarction has been shown to result in a 20% reduction in all-cause mortality (39). Unfortunately, since C.G. was now 4 months postangioplasty, his insurance program failed to cover cardiac rehabilitation. We asked him to initiate a daily walking program.

Based on his postangioplasty exercise tolerance test, it appeared that he could exercise at 70% of his maximum heart rate without becoming ischemic; thus, following the American Heart Association Scientific Statement on Exercise, we recommended that he work up to walking 3 miles a day 6 days a week and 2 miles on the seventh day, for a total of 20 miles a week (40). Using the formula (220 − age = maximum heart rate and multiplying this by 0.7 (C.G.'s ischemic threshold)), we asked him to keep his heart rate below 130 beats per minute (bpm) during exercise. We recommended 120 as a good target heart rate. We told him that exercise does not tend to result in a reduction in LDL, but that we could reasonably expect an increase in HDL by as much as 4.5 mg/dL (41) and a drop in triglycerides of about 20% to 30% (42).

4. Finally, we discussed the need for an LDL-lowering medication. We explained that there have now been many published regression trials, which have proven that coronary artery disease can be reversed with aggressive cholesterol reduction. We further explained that much more important than the angiographic appearance of the cholesterol deposits is the fact that aggressive cholesterol reduction could reduce C.G.'s risk of another cardiac event by as much as 72% (43). (We think it is important to provide patients with hard data to support the difficult program we are asking them to adhere to.)

Since C.G. required approximately a 60% reduction in his LDL to achieve his NCEP goal of 100 mg/dL, and we estimated diet would lower his LDL by about 20%, our only choices for an additional 40% reduction in LDL were lovastatin or simvastatin (atorvastatin was not available when we first saw C.G.).

At maximum doses (lovastatin = 80 mg/day, simvastatin = 80 mg/day), both these drugs can achieve LDL reductions of up to 40%. Because there is some variation in response to lipid-lowering therapy, we initially started C.G. on 20 mg/day of simvastatin. I prefer simvastatin to lovastatin because simvastatin is a once-a-day drug, whereas at high doses lovastatin is a twice-a-day drug.

Eight weeks later C.G. returned weighing 177 lbs. He had a fasting blood sugar level of 102 mg/dL and the following lipid profile:

	C.G.'s level	Desirable level
Total cholesterol	152 mg/dL	<200 mg/dL
HDL cholesterol	47 mg/dL	>45 mg/dL
Triglycerides	98 mg/dL	<150 mg/dL
LDL cholesterol	85 mg/dL	<100 mg/dL

At this point his lipid-lowering program consisted of the following:

*   Riding his exercise bike daily for 30 minutes
*   Following a 1500-calorie, 33-g fat, 35-g sugar diet
*   Simvastatin 20 mg/day at bedtime
*   Quitting smoking

When asked how he felt, his answer was, "Better than I have felt in years!" He had not experienced angina in the previous 6 weeks, even when mowing the lawn. He commented that his weight loss had served to make moving around in tight spots (a situation frequently encountered in his job as a plumber) much easier. He also liked being able to look down and actually see his cowboy boots. The diet, he said, was easy to stick with and the exercise had become part of his daily

routine. He had not experienced any side effects from the simvastatin. We suggested that he continue with his current diet and exercise program and asked him to return for a follow-up evaluation in 3 months.

At his follow-up visit he was 7 lbs lighter and his fasting blood sugar and lipid profile were essentially the same. We scheduled him to return for a final lipid clinic visit in 3 months. (With the exception of patients with genetic cholesterol abnormalities whom we see on a long-term basis, we usually see patients referred to us for three or four visits, at which point they return to their own primary care providers for routine follow-up.)

Three months later his weight was stable at 170 lbs. Although he continued with his daily exercise program and simvastatin, he freely admitted he was not as religious with his diet. He had just returned from a 3-week vacation in Key West, Florida. Although he and his wife made some of their own meals, they ate out every evening and by his own report, "I didn't worry about the fat content and I ate everything from appetizers to dessert." This was his lipid profile:

	C.G.'s level	Desirable level
Total cholesterol	238 mg/dL	<200 mg/dL
HDL cholesterol	50 mg/dL	>45 mg/dL
Triglycerides	142 mg/dL	<150 mg/dL
LDL cholesterol	160 mg/dL	<100 mg/dL
Blood sugar:	135 mg/dL	<126 mg/dL

Had he forgotten to take his simvastatin while on vacation? The answer was no. His levels were the consequence of his dietary indiscretions. He resolved to improve his diet, but just to hedge our bets, I also increased his simvastatin to 40 mg/day at bedtime. I explained that the dose increase would likely result in a 6% to 10% reduction in his LDL, but since this would not totally correct the situation, that is, reduce his LDL to the 100-mg/dL range, he really needed to get his diet back on track. And since Key West was a yearly trip for him, we discussed the need to plan for next year.

Three months later, on simvastatin 40 mg/day at bedtime and a 20% fat diet and continued daily exercise, he had the following lipid profile:

	C.G.'s level	Desirable level
Total cholesterol	166 mg/dL	<200 mg/dL
HDL cholesterol	47 mg/dL	>45 mg/dL
Triglycerides	138 mg/dL	<150 mg/dL
LDL cholesterol	91 mg/dL	<100 mg/dL
Blood sugar	112 mg/dL	<126 mg/dL
Weight	170.5 lb	

Over the past year he has followed up regularly in the lipid clinic and has maintained these levels. He has remained on simvastatin 40 mg/day at bedtime and been faithful to both diet and exercise. This past year in Key West, knowing the consequences of a high-fat diet, he was much more compliant with his restrictions.

This case illustrates the importance of lifestyle modification and how failure to follow a low-fat diet, regardless of a person's weight, can result in a deterioration in lipid status. Allowing a patient to see the consequences of his or her actions is a powerful teaching tool. I feel strongly that at least for the first year on a lipid-lowering program, patients should be followed up every 2 to 3 months.

CASE 4

For S.W. the idea that she might be at risk for a cardiac event was about as ridiculous as telling her she was from Mars. At 54 she was postmenopausal, having had her last menses at age 50. She had declined estrogen replacement therapy, feeling it was "unnatural." At 5 ft 8 in. tall she weighed 150 lbs (ideal body weight 140 lbs), she had quit smoking 5 years ago, her blood pressure was never high, and her only family history was a male cousin who died at age 40 of a myocardial infarction. She was sedentary and had the following lipid profile:

	S.W.'s level	Desirable level
Total cholesterol	200 mg/dL	<200 mg/dL
HDL cholesterol	30 mg/dL	>45 mg/dL
Triglycerides	248 mg/dL	<150 mg/dL
LDL cholesterol	120 mg/dL	<100 mg/dL
Total/HDL ratio	6.6	≤4.0

On January 8, 1996, while shoveling snow, she developed substernal chest pressure that failed to resolve with rest. One hour later she presented to her local emergency room where an electrocardiogram revealed an evolving anterior wall myocardial infarction. She was immediately taken to the catheterization laboratory where she underwent a successful angioplasty of a 90% mid-left anterior descending (LAD) artery lesion. Although she had multiple other 30% to 40% percent lesions, she had no other lesions requiring angioplasty.

When S.W. was referred to our cholesterol management center (10 weeks after her MI), she was already attending cardiac rehabilitation and was exercising three times a week. She had made significant dietary changes, which had resulted in a weight loss of 6 pounds. Her lipid profile looked like this:

	S.W.'s level	Desirable level
Total cholesterol	201 mg/dL	<200 mg/dL
HDL cholesterol	35 mg/dL	>45 mg/dL
Triglycerides	194 mg/dL	<150 mg/dL
LDL cholesterol	127 mg/dL	<100 mg/dL
Lp(a)	0 mg/dL	<20 mg/dL
Total/HDL ratio	5.7	<4

When SW saw these results she was quite upset, noting that her LDL cholesterol had not fallen as a result of her dietary modifications. Although I could not give her a definite answer as to why her LDL had not fallen, I did point out that often when triglycerides fall LDL will increase slightly (this may be the result of increased conversion of VLDL to LDL).

We pointed out that her exercise and diet efforts had resulted in improved HDL and triglyceride levels and since these are the strongest lipid predictors of cardiac risk in women (44), we were very pleased with this change. But her lipid profile was not yet perfect. While her Lp(a) was in the normal range, all the rest of her lipoproteins could be improved upon.

We questioned her regarding lifestyle factors that influence triglyceride level, including alcohol ingestion, sugar intake, and inadequate exercise. On average, S.W. consumed one glass of wine per week and ate virtually no sweets. She was exercising 3 days a week at her cardiac rehabilitation program. I suggested that she increase her exercise to 6 to 7 days a week. I explained that the American Heart Association had recently revised its scientific statement on exercise and that the current recommendation was to burn 2000 calories/week exercising (40). I told her that if she added a 3-mile walk on her nonrehabilitation program days, she should be able to improve both her triglycerides and HDL further. In order to lower her LDL to below 100 mg/dL, I also suggested that she add estrogen replacement therapy (ERT).

Given her feeling that ERT was "not natural" and her reasonable concern regarding the link between estrogen and breast cancer, I felt that it was important to spend a little time discussing the basis for my recommendation. I explained that there was a substantial body of data indicating that estrogen use could decrease her risk of another cardiac event by as much as 80% (45).

Given that she had already had one heart attack and that 250,000 women die per year of CAD and only 43,000 of breast cancer (1), it would appear that in her situation the benefits of estrogen would far outweigh the risks of its use.

S.W. had recently had both a mammogram and Pap smear, both were normal, and she had no family history of breast cancer. I suggested that she go home and give some thought to the issue of ERT. Because as many as 60% of women discontinue estrogen within 1 year of initiation (46), I wanted her to come on her own to the conclusion that ERT was the right choice for her.

I gave her some materials to read and asked her to call me in 1 week with her decision. When she called, she had decided that ERT was the way to go. Since she had not had a hysterectomy, she required both estrogen and progesterone (progesterone to protect her uterus).

I prescribed Prempro, which provides 0.625 mg/day of conjugated estrogen and 2.5 mg/day of medroxyprogesterone acetate. Using this combination preparation, most postmenopausal women are completely amenorrheic within 3 months. Spotting can be expected for a couple of months, but bleeding after 3 months should be evaluated.

Three months later, S.W. returned with the following lipid profile:

	S.W.'s level	Desirable level
Total cholesterol	198 mg/dL	<200 mg/dL
HDL cholesterol	42 mg/dL	>45 mg/dL
Triglycerides	195 mg/dL	<150 mg/dL
LDL cholesterol	117 mg/dL	<100 mg/dL
Total/HDL ratio	4.7	<4

Although this was a big improvement, her lipids were not yet perfect; thus I suggested consideration of niacin, a B vitamin that can improve HDL, triglycerides, LDL, and Lp(a). It has been my experience that, if given proper coaching, most patients can get through the first month of niacin therapy. Once a person makes it through this first critical month, most of niacin's unpleasant side effects (primarily flushing and itching) have subsided. I give patients the following advice:

1. Always take niacin with food or skim milk.

2. Take an aspirin (325 mg) or a nonprescription dose of ibuprofen (200 mg) about half an hour prior to niacin. This will minimize the flushing.

3. Avoid hot showers and hot beverages immediately following niacin. This too will minimize flushing.

4. Take niacin as prescribed; skipping doses tends to accentuate flushing.

Niacin is available in either an immediate-release or slow-release form. Until recently I recommended only immediate-release niacin because although immediate-release preparations cause more flushing and itching, they are less likely to occasion hepatic toxicity. Recently, however, a new once-a-day (bedtime dosing) niacin has become available. When taken in doses as high as 2000 mg/day, Niaspan (marketed by Kos pharmaceuticals) did not increase the risk of liver toxicity beyond what would be seen with the standard immediate-release preparations (47).

After some initial difficulties (mainly nausea) with the niacin, S.W. was able to take 1500 mg without any significant side effects. Three months later she returned with the following lipid profile:

	S.W.'s level	Desirable level
Total cholesterol	157 mg/dL	<200 mg/dL
HDL cholesterol	52 mg/dL	>45 mg/dL
Triglycerides	98 mg/dL	<150 mg/dL
LDL cholesterol	85 mg/dL	<100 mg/dL
Total/HDL ratio	3.0	<4.0

For the past year S.W. has maintained these levels and has continued her daily exercise and low-fat diet.

SUMMARY

The previous four cases illustrate some common problems encountered in our lipid management center. The field of lipid metabolism and cardiovascular care continues to evolve and change. As this chapter goes to press, the Heart and Estrogen/progestin Replacement Study (HERS) has just been published (48). This trial has called into question the use of hormone replacement as a means of reducing cardiac risk in women with existing cardiac disease. While it is unlikely that we have heard the end of the estrogen story, the HERS trial has taught us a very important lesson: estrogen is not a replacement for cholesterol reduction. In high-risk women (and men) we must be vigorous in the treatment of hyperlipidemia. Diet, exercise, and, when necessary, lipid-lowering medications should be used to achieve NCEP lipid goals. It is clear that cholesterol reduction has the potential to dramatically reduce both cardiac and all-cause mortality.

REFERENCES

1. American Heart Association. 1997 Heart and stroke facts statistical update. Dallas, TX: American Heart Association, 1997:1–28.

2. Sempos CT, Cleeman JI, Carroll MD, et al. Prevalence of high blood cholesterol among US adults: an update based on guidelines from the second report of the National Cholesterol Education Program Adult Treatment Panel. JAMA 1993;269:3009–3014.

3. Nieto FJ, Alonso J, Chambless LE, et al. Population awareness and control of hypertension and hypercholesterolemia: the Atherosclerosis Risk in Communities Study. Arch Intern Med 1995;155:677–684.

4. Schrott HL, Bittner V, Vittinghoff E, et al for HERS Research Group. Adherence to National Cholesterol Education Program treatment goals in postmenopausal women with heart disease: the Heart and Estrogen/Progestin Replacement Study (HERS). JAMA 1997;277:1281–1286.

5. Goldberg RJ, Ockene IS, Yarzebski J, et al. Use of lipid-lowering medication in patients with acute myocardial infarction (Worcester Heart Attack Study). Am J Cardiol 1997;79:1095–1097.

6. Scandinavian Simvastatin Survival Study Group. Randomized trial of cholesterol lowering in 4444 patients with coronary heart disease: the Scandinavian Simvastatin Survival Study. Lancet 1994;344:1383–1389.

7. Lipid Study Group. Long-term intervention with pravastatin in ischemic disease (LIPID). N Engl J Med 1998;339:1349–1357.

8. Shepherd J, Cobbe SM, Ford I, et al. Prevention of coronary heart disease with pravastatin in men with hypercholesterolemia. N Engl J Med 1995;333:1301–1307.

9. Expert Panel on Detection, Evaluation and Treatment of High Blood Cholesterol in Adults. Summary of the second report of the National Cholesterol Education Program (NCEP) Expert Panel on Detection, Evaluation, and Treatment of High Blood Cholesterol in Adults (Adult Treatment Panel II). JAMA 1993;269:3015–3023.

10. Hypertriglyceridaemia and vascular risk: report of a meeting of physicians and scientists, University College London Medical School. Lancet 1993;342:781–787.

11. Assmann G, Schulte H, von Eckardstein A. Hypertriglyceridemia and elevated $L_p(a)$ are risk factors for major coronary events in middle-aged men. Am J Cardiol 1996;77:1179–1184.

12. Miller M, Seidler A, Kwiterovich PO, Pearson TA. Long-term predictors of subsequent cardiovascular events with coronary artery disease and "desirable" levels of plasma total cholesterol. Circulation 1992;86:1165–1170.

13. Kreisberg RA. Low high-density lipoprotein cholesterol: what does it mean, what can we do about it, and what should we do about it? Am J Med 1993;94:1–5.

14. Bild DE, Williams RR, Brewer HB, et al. Identification and management of heterozygous familial hypercholesterolemia: summary and recommendations from an NHLBI workshop. Am J Cardiol 1993;72:1D–5D.

15. Williams RR, Schumacher MC, Barlow GK, et al. Documented need for more effective diagnosis and treatment of familial hypercholesterolemia according to data from 502 heterozygotes in Utah. Am J Cardiol 1993;72:18D–24D.

16. Hobbs HH, Russell DW, Brown MS, Goldstein JL. The LDL receptor locus in familial hypercholesterolemia. Annu Rev Genet 1990;24:133–170.

17. Scanu AM, Lawn RM, Berg K. Lipoprotein (a) and atherosclerosis. Ann Intern Med 1991;115:209–218.

18. Rath M, Niendorf A, Reblin T, et al. Detection and quantification of lipoprotein (a) in the arterial wall of 107 coronary bypass patients. Arteriosclerosis 1989;9:579–592.

19. Scanu AM. Lipoprotein (a): A genetic risk factor for premature coronary heart disease. JAMA 1992;267:3326–3329.

20. Desmarais RL, Sarembock IJ, Ayers CR, et al. Elevated serum lipoprotein (a) is a risk factor for clinical recurrence after coronary balloon angioplasty. Circulation 1995;91:1403–1409.

21. Hoff HF, Beck GJ, Skibinski MS, et al. Serum Lp(a) level as a predictor of vein graft stenosis after coronary artery bypass surgery in patients. Circulation 1988;77:1238–1244.

22. Kim CJ, Jang HC, Cho DH, Min Yk. Effects of hormone replacement therapy on lipoprotein (a) and lipids in postmenopausal women. Arterioscler Thromb 1994;14:275–281.

23. Lepre F, Campbell B, Crane S, Hickman P. Low-dose sustained release nicotinic acid (Tri-B3) and Lipoprotein (a). Am J Cardiol 1992;70:133.

24. Seed M, Hoppichler F, Reaveley D, et al. Relations of serum lipoprotein (a) concentration and apolipoprotein (a) phenotype to coronary heart disease in patients with familial hypercholesterolemia. N Engl J Med 1990;322:1494–1499.

25. Daida H, Young JL, Yokoi H, et al. Prevention of restenosis after percutaneous transluminal coronary angioplasty by reducing lipoprotein (a) levels with low-density lipoprotein apheresis. Am J Cardiol 1994;73:1037–1040.

26. Dattilo AM, Kris-Etherton PM. Effects of weight reduction on blood lipids and lipoproteins: A meta-analysis. Am J Clin Nutr 1992;56:320–328.

27. Maher VM, Brown GB, Marcovina SM, et al. Effects of lowering elevated LDL cholesterol on the cardiovascular risk of lipoprotein (a). JAMA 1995;274:1771–1774.

28. Goldstein JL, Schrott HG, Hazzard WR, et al. Hyperlipidemia in coronary heart disease, II: genetic analysis of lipid levels in 176 families and delineation of a new inherited disorder, combined hyperlipidemia. J Clin Invest 1973;52:1544–1568.

29. Brunzell JD, Austin MA, Deeb SS, et al. Familial combined hyperlipidemia and genetic risk of atherosclerosis. In: Woodford FP, Davignon J, Sniderman A, eds. Atherosclerosis X. Amsterdam: Elsevier Science, 1995.

30. Rohlfing JJ, Brunzell JD. The effects of diuretics and adrenergic-blocking agents on plasma lipids. West J Med 1986;145:210–218.

31. Grodstein F, Stampfer MJ, Manson JE, et al. Postmenopausal estrogen and progestin use and the risk of cardiovascular disease. N Engl J Med 1996;335:453–461.

32. Downs JR, Clearfield M, Weis S, et al for the AFCAPS/Tex CAPS Research Group. Primary preventim of acute coronary events with lovastatin in men and women with average cholesterol levels. JAMA 1998;279:1615–1622.

33. Athyros V, Papageorgiou A, Avramidis M, et al. Combined treatment with pravastatin and gemfibrozil in patients with refractory familial combined hyperlipidemia. Drug Invest 1994;7:134–142.

34. Wiklund O, Angelin B, Bergman M, et al. Pravastatin and gemfibrozil alone and in combination for the treatment of hypercholesterolemia. Am J Med 1993;94:13–20.

35. Athyros V, Papageorgiou A, Hatzikonstandinou H, et al. Safety and efficacy of long-term statin-fibrate combinations in patients with refractory familial combined hyperlipidemia. Am J Cardiol 1997;80:608–613.

36. Criqui MH. Cigarette smoking and plasma high-density lipoprotein cholesterol. Circulation 1980;62(suppl II):70.

37. Stubbs I. High-density lipoprotein concentrations increase after stopping smoking. Br Med J 1982;284:1511–1514.

38. Kita T, Yokode M, Arai H, et al. Cigarette smoke, LDL and cholesterol ester accumulation in macrophages. Ann NY Acad Sci 1993;686:91–97.

39. O'Connor GT, Buring JE, Yusuf S, et al. An overview of randomized trials of rehabilitation with exercise after myocardial infarction. Circulation 1989;80:234–244.

40. Fletcher GF, Balady G, Froelicher VF, et al. Exercise standards: a statement for healthcare professionals from the American Heart Association. Circulation 1995;91:580–615.

41. Wood PD. Haskell WL, Blair SN, et al. Increased exercise level and plasma lipoprotein concentrations: a one-year randomized controlled study in sedentary middle-aged men. Metabolism 1983;32:31–39.

42. Lampman RM, Santinga JT, Hodge MF, et al. Comparative effects of physical training and diet in normalizing serum lipids in men with type IV hyperlipoproteinemia. Circulation 1977;55:652–659.

43. Brown G, Albers JJ, Fisher LD, et al. Regression of coronary artery disease as a result of intensive lipid lowering therapy in men with high levels of apolipoprotein B. N Engl J Med 1990;323:1289–1298.

44. Eaker ED, Castelli WP. Coronary heart disease and its risk factors among women in the Framingham Study. In: Eaker ED, Packard B, Wenger N, et al. Coronary heart

disease in women. New York: Hay-market Doyma, 1987:122–130.

45. Sullivan JM, Vander Zwang R, Maddock V, et al. Estrogen replacement and coronary disease: effect on survival in post-menopausal women. Arch Intern Med 1990;150:2557–2562.

46. Wren BG, Brown I. Compliance with hormonal replacement. Maturitas 1991;13:17–21.

47. Niaspan dosing data: Data on file. Miami: Kos Pharmaceuticals.

48. Hulley S, Grady D, Bush T, et al. for the Heart and Estrogen/prog-estin Replacement (HERS) Research Group. Randomized trial of estrogen plus progestin for secondary prevention of coronary heart disease in postmenopausal women. JAMA 1998;280:605–613.

Chapter 9

Lifestyle Management and Prevention of Hypertension

Robert J. Heyka

During the last 20 years there has been a dramatic decrease in morbidity and mortality related to hypertension. Age-adjusted, stroke-related death rates have decreased 60%, and coronary heart disease (CHD) death rates have decreased by 30% (1). The improved survival has been seen regardless of gender or ethnicity. However, since 1993, age-adjusted cerebrovascular accident (CVA) rates have risen and the rate of decline in CHD has flattened. CHD and CVA remain the first and third most common causes of death in the USA, respectively. The prevalence of both congestive heart failure (CHF) and end-stage renal disease (ESRD) continues to increase and has never shown any tendency toward decline (1).

Hypertension remains the most common cardiovascular risk factor in the U.S. population. An estimated 50 million Americans have hypertension, with higher prevalence in men and the African-American population, but a rapidly increasing prevalence in women with increasing age (2). The awareness, treatment, and control of hypertension have not improved, as reported in the National Health and Nutrition Examination Survey (NHANES III) (2), and up to 75% of patients have inadequately controlled hypertension (Table 9-1). It is particularly disturbing that these trends are apparent with hypertension defined as blood pressure above 140/90 mm Hg, a level that is too high for maximum cardiovascular disease (CVD) risk reduction (3). Recent epidemiologic data have shown risks for cardiovascular, renal, and all-cause mortality begin with systolic blood pressure (SBP) greater than 120 mm Hg and diastolic blood pressure (DBP) greater than 80 mm Hg, regardless of gender or ethnicity (4). Thus current recommendations are to define "optimal" blood pressure at this level (5) (Table 9-2). It is widely assumed that a rise in

blood pressure is an inevitable and natural consequence of aging. In the International Cooperative INTERSALT trial of more than 10,000 men and women at 52 centers in 32 countries, the slopes of both SBP and DBP were positively and significantly related to age in the participants from 20 to 59 years. On average, participants more than 55 years of age had SBP/DBP levels that were higher by 15/11 mm Hg compared to 25-year-olds (6). However, this finding is limited to industrialized societies and is probably not an inevitable consequence of aging but a reflection of an unhealthy lifestyle (7). The *usual* blood pressure patterns in the United States and other developed countries are certainly not *normal* or inevitable. From both an individual and population perspective, attempts to control hypertension and prevent its consequences must begin with the primary prevention of hypertension. Without effective primary prevention, the problem of hypertension can never be solved (7).

ADVANTAGES OF LIFESTYLE MODIFICATION

The most recent report of the Joint National Committee on the Prevention, Detection, Evaluation, and Treatment of High Blood Pressure (JNC-VI) states that "The goal of prevention and management of hypertension is to reduce morbidity and mortality by the least intrusive means possible." (1). Within this paradigm nonpharmacologic treatment by lifestyle modification (LM) offers several advantages: 1) LM plays a role in the primary prevention of hypertension (7). 2) Once hypertension is diagnosed, LM offers the potential for control without the use of medication. After stratification of patients based on overall cardiovascular risk, a trial of 6 to 12 months may be attempted to lower blood pressure (Table 9-3). 3) Even if medication is necessary to control blood pressure, continued attention to LM can lead to a lower dosage or number of medications needed and lower risk of side effects, especially in the large percentage of the hypertensive population with stage 1 and 2 hypertension. 4) Cardiovascular risk

Table 9-1 Trends in the Awareness, Treatment, and Control of High Blood Pressure in Adults: United States, 1976–1994*

	NHANES II (1976–1980) (%)	NHANES III (PHASE I) 1988–1991 (%)	NHANES III (PHASE 2) 1991–1994 (%)
Awareness	51	73	68.4
Treated	31	55	53.6
Controlled[†]	10	29	27.4

* Adults aged 18 to 74 years with SBP ↓140 mm Hg or DBP ↓90 mm Hg or taking antihypertensive medication.
† SBP < 140 mm Hg and DBP < 90 mm Hg.
SOURCE: Adapted from Burt et al. Prevalence of hypertension in the US adult population: results from the Third National Health and Examination Survey, 1998–1991. Hypertension 1995;25:305–313. Unpublished data from the National Center for Health Statistics, 1997 (NHANES III, Phase 2), cited in Joint National Committee on the Detection, Evaluation and Treatment of High Blood Pressure (JNC-VI). Arch Intern Med 1997;157:2413–2446.

Table 9-2 Classification of Blood Pressure for Adults Age 18 Years and Older*

CATEGORY	SYSTOLIC (mm Hg)		DIASTOLIC (mm Hg)
Optimal[†]	<120	and	<80
Normal	<130	and	<85
High normal	130–139	or	85–89
HYPERTENSION[‡]			
Stage 1	140–159	or	90–99
Stage 2	160–179	or	100–109
Stage 3	↓180	or	↓110

* Not taking antihypertensive drugs and not acutely ill. When systolic and diastolic blood pressures fall into different categories, the higher category should be selected to classify the individual's blood pressure status. For example, 160/92 mm Hg should be classified as stage 2 hypertension, and 174 ≠ 120 mm Hg should be classified as stage 3 hypertension. Isolated systolic hypertension is defined as SBP ↓140 mm Hg and DBP < 90 mm Hg and staged appropriately (e.g., 170/82 mm Hg is defined as stage 2 isolated systolic hypertension). In addition to classifying stages of hypertension on the basis of average blood pressure levels, clinicians should specify presence or absence of target organ disease and additional risk factors. This specificity is important for risk classification and treatment (see Table 9-3).
† Optimal blood pressure with respect to cardiovascular risk is <120/80 mm Hg. However, unusually low readings should be evaluated for clinical significance.
‡ Based on the average of two or more readings taken at each of two or more visits after initial screening.
SOURCE: Joint National Committee. Sixth report of the Joint National Committee on the Prevention, Detection,Evaluation, and Treatment of High Blood Pressure. Arch Int Med 1997;157:2413–2446.

Table 9-3 Risk Stratification and Treatment*

BLOOD PRESSURE STAGES (mm Hg)	RISK GROUP		
	A: NO RISK FACTORS NO TOD/CCD[†] (SEE TABLE 9-4)	B: AT LEAST ONE RISK FACTOR, NOT INCLUDING DIABETES MELLITUS; NO TOD/CCD[†] (SEE TABLE 9-4)	C: TOD/CCD[†] AND/OR DIABETES, WITH OR WITHOUT OTHER RISK FACTORS (SEE TABLE 9-4)
High normal (130–139/85–89)	Lifestyle modification	Lifestyle modification	Drug therapy[§]
Stage 1 (140–159/90–99)	Lifestyle modification (up to 12 months)	Lifestyle modification[‡] (up to 6 months)	Drug therapy
Stage 2 and 3 (↓160/↓100)	Drug therapy	Drug therapy	Drug therapy

For example: A patient with diabetes and a BP of 142/94 mm Hg plus LVH should be classified as having stage 1 hypertension with TOD (LVH) and with another major risk factor (diabetes). This patient would be categorized as stage 1, risk group C, and recommended for immediate initiation of pharmacologic treatment.
* Lifestyle modification should be adjunctive therapy for all patients recommended for pharmacologic therapy.
† TOD/CCD = target organ disease/clinical cardiovascular disease.
‡ For patients with multiple risk factors, clinicians should consider drugs as initial therapy plus lifestyle modifications.
§ For those with heart failure or renal disease or those with diabetes mellitus.
SOURCE: Joint National Committee. Sixth report of the Joint National Committee on the Prevention, Detection, Evaluation, and Treatment of High Blood Pressure. Arch Int Med 1997;157:2413–2446.

Table 9-4 Components for Cardiovascular Risk Stratification in Patients with Hypertension

MAJOR RISK FACTORS	TARGET ORGAN DAMAGE/CLINICAL CARDIOVASCULAR DISEASE

Smoking
Dyslipidemia
Diabetes mellitus
Age older than 60 years
Gender (men and postmenopausal women)
Family history of cardiovascular disease: women under age 65 or men under age 55
	Heart disease
	    Left ventricular hypertrophy
	    Angina/prior myocardial infarction
	    Prior coronary revascularization
	    Heart failure
	Stroke or transient ischemic attack
	Nephropathy
	Peripheral arterial disease
	Retinopathy

SOURCE: Joint National Committee. Sixth report of the Joint National Committee on the Prevention, Detection, Evaluation, and Treatment of High Blood Pressure. Arch Int Med 1997;157:2413–2446

Table 9-5 Lifestyle Modification Useful for Hypertension Prevention and Management

- ⇨ Lose weight if overweight
- ⇨ Limit alcohol intake to no more than 1 oz (30 mL) ethanol [e.g., 24 oz (720 mL) beer, 10 oz (300 mL) wine, or 2 oz (60 mL) 100-proof whiskey [per day or 0.5 oz (15 mL) ethanol per day for women and lighter weight people
- ⇨ Increase aerobic physical activity (30 to 45 minutes most days of the week)
- ⇨ Reduce sodium intake to less than 100 mmol per day (2.4 g sodium or 6 g sodium chloride)
- ⇨ Maintain adequate intake of dietary potassium (approximately 90 mmol per day)
- ⇨ Maintain adequate intake of dietary calcium and magnesium for general health
- ⇨ Stop smoking and reduce intake of dietary saturated fat and cholesterol for overall cardiovascular health

SOURCE: Joint National Committee. Sixth report of the Joint National Committee on the Prevention, Detection, Evaluation, and Treatment of High Blood Pressure. Arch Int Med 1997; 157:2413–2446.

factors often cluster in patients with hypertension, and LM can lower both BP and other CVD risks (8). 5) LM is usually achieved with little or no long-term additional costs or personal risk to the patient, neither of which can be said for pharmacologic therapy. Current recommendations for treatment of hypertension are based on an individual patient's risk of CVD. The level of blood pressure is important, but a better assessment can be made if the office or home blood pressure levels are supplemented with information about the presence of target organ damage (TOD) and other cardiovascular risk factors (Table 9-4). "Lifestyle modification . . . could have an additional and even greater impact on CVD prevention and should be recommended to the entire population. Patients should be strongly encouraged to adopt these LMs,

particularly if they have additional risk factors for CVD such as diabetes or dyslipidemias" (1).

SPECIFIC LIFESTYLE MODIFICATIONS
The Big Four

Many LMs have been proposed in patients with or at risk for hypertension. However, JNC-VI specifically mentions nine LMs (Table 9-5), for which there is some support. The "Big Four" LMs include moderation of sodium intake, increased physical activity, weight loss and avoidance of excess weight, and limited alcohol use. A recent report on the primary prevention of hypertension stated that these four interventions are of "documented efficacy" (7).

Moderation of Sodium Intake

The average sodium intake in the United States is around 150 mmol/day (3.6 g Na, 9 g NaCl) with 75% of the intake from processed and fast foods (7). The risks with excess salt, i.e., sodium chloride, intake are manifest on both a population-wide and an individual level. The INTERSALT study of more than 10,000 people showed a clear association between the percentage of hypertensive patients in a population and its median sodium intake (Figure 9-1). Populations with low salt intakes, low sodium to potassium dietary intake, leanness, daily physical activity, and limited alcohol use experienced little rise in blood pressure with aging (9). Across populations, there was a significant relationship between sodium intake and SBP. The correlation held independent of body mass index (BMI), although a higher BMI was associated with increased 24-hour sodium excretion in across-population analyses. In the INTERSALT study the decrease in SBP/DBP per 100 mmol/day less sodium intake was modest at 5/2 mm Hg. For older patients (55 vs. 25 years), the decrease was greater at 10 to 12 / 6 to 7 mm Hg. Habitual low salt intake was associated with low normal SBP/DBP, little or no increase in BP with age, and little or no development of hypertension (9). Individual responses to sodium intake are heterogenous. A subset of the population may be more "salt-sensitive." Definitions vary, but most reflect a short-

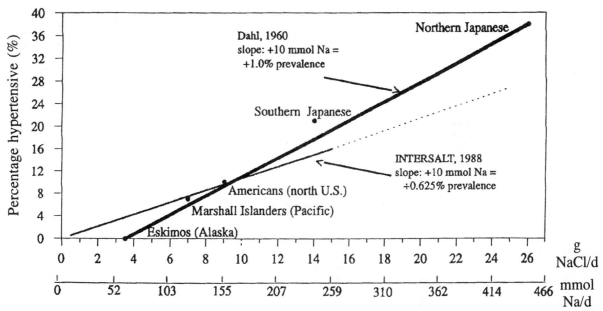

Figure 9-1 Average daily salt intake of population samples and prevalence of high blood pressure in studies by Dahl (67) and in the INTERSALT Cooperative Research Group (68). INTERSALT criteria for high blood pressure were systolic blood pressure ↓140 mm Hg, diastolic blood pressure ↓90 mm Hg, or use of antihypertensive medication, n = 52 in the INTERSALT Study; values are adjusted for age and sex. (Reproduced by permission from Stamler J. The INTERSALT study: background, methods, findings and implications. Am J Clin Nutr 1997;65:6295. © American Society for Clinical Nutrition. A portion is reproduced with permission from Dahl L. Possible role of salt intake in the development of hypertension. In: Cottier P, Bock KD, eds. Essential hypertension: an international symposium. Berlin: Springer-Verlag, 1960:53–65.)

term rise in blood pressure with normal or high salt intake, and fall in blood pressure with low, at times artificially low, salt intake (10). The definition does not imply etiology as multiple, and different mechanisms may be operative. Salt sensitivity is thought to be more prevalent in hypertensive patients who are African-American, female, elderly, or obese or who have more severe hypertension (10).

In the Trials of Hypertension Prevention (TOHP I), 2100 younger patients with high normal BP were studied over 6 months to compare seven different nutritional health interventions: Three were lifestyle related—weight reduction (WR), sodium restriction (Na), and stress management (SM); four involved nutritional supplementation—with calcium (Ca), magnesium (Mg), potassium (K), or fish oil (FO). Figure 9-2 shows that sodium restriction (decreased intake by an average of 44 mmol/day) and weight loss were the only two interventions that were effective (11). The recent report of the Trial of Nonpharmacologic Interventions in the Elderly (TONE) also found that sodium restriction and weight loss were effective in controlling borderline hypertension and allowed the discontinuation of medication in a significant percentage of the study population (12). Meta-analysis of the effects of reduced salt intake on blood pressure in randomized controlled trials (RCTs) showed a modest effect of salt restriction. A recent review of 56 trials of sodium restriction (28 in normotensive patients) recommended that sodium restriction be considered only for older patients with hypertension, but not in the normotensive population (13). A second meta-analysis of 32 RCTs found a significant decrease in SBP/DBP among hyper-

tensive and normotensive patients and advocated a population-wide program to decrease sodium intake (14).

Recently, concerns about the safety of sodium restriction have been raised. A retrospective trial found an increased risk of myocardial infarction among patients with the lowest quartile of urinary sodium excretion (15). Concerns with these findings include a small number of events to evaluate, a number of potential confounding factors, and dependence on a single urine collection without serial measurements of actual sodium intake (16). No significant safety issues were identified in the meta-analyses mentioned above or in TOHP-I or TONE.

The recommended sodium intake by JNC-VI is 100 mmol of sodium per day (2.4 g sodium, 6 g NaCl) (1). This degree of sodium intake is associated with lower blood pressure especially in African-Americans, older patients, diabetics, obese patients, and those with more severe hypertension and should decrease both the incidence of hypertension and the amount of medication taken. Other benefits include a decreased risk of diuretic-associated potassium wasting, regression of left ventricular hypertrophy (LVH), and protection against renal stones and osteoporosis (1). Practically, the recommendations mean no salt at table, no salt with cooking, and the avoidance of processed and fast foods. Some in the population are at higher risk for continued, hidden high salt intake such as younger patients and others who eat out more often, including travelers and retirees. Whether sodium restriction is warranted on a population-wide basis remains controversial (13,14,16).

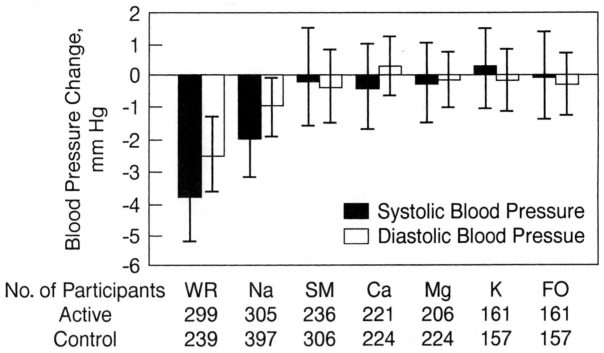

No. of Participants	WR	Na	SM	Ca	Mg	K	FO
Active	299	305	236	221	206	161	161
Control	239	397	306	224	224	157	157

Figure 9-2 Net mean changes in systolic and diastolic blood pressure (baseline minus follow-up) with 95% confidence intervals. WR = weight reduction; Na = sodium reduction; SM = stress management; Ca = calcium supplementation; Mg = magnesium supplementation; K = potassium supplementation; and FO = fish oil supplementation. (Reproduced by permission from Trials of Hypertension Prevention Collaborative Research Group. The effects of nonpharmacologic interventions on blood pressure of persons with high normal levels: results of the trials of hypertension prevention, phase I. JAMA 1992;267:1213–1220.)

Increased Physical Activity

The importance of increased physical activity is highlighted by several recent position statements. The American Heart Association recognizes physical inactivity as a risk factor for coronary heart disease (17). The NIH Consensus Development Panel on Physical Activity and Cardiovascular Health (18), and the Centers for Disease Control and Prevention and the American College of Sports Medicine's statement (19) all reach similar conclusions. The recommendations center on either a more structured approach with specific guidelines for type, frequency, intensity, and duration of activity, or a general approach with calls for a daily increase in physical activity. In summary these recommendations state: 1) All people over 2 years of age should accumulate at least 30 minutes of endurance-type physical activity of at least moderate intensity on most (preferably all) days of the week; 2) additional health and functional benefits can accrue with increased time and moderately intense activity, or with more vigorous activity; 3) people with symptomatic CHD, diabetes mellitus, or other chronic health problems should be evaluated by a physician and given an exercise program appropriate for their situation; 4) inactive men over 40 years of age, women over 50, or patients at high risk for CHD should see their physician before starting a program of vigorous physical activity; and 5) resistance or strength-developing activities should be added at least two times a week, and should involve the major muscle groups (20). It remains an "American paradox"

(21) that despite this increased public awareness of the benefits of various LMs, the implementation of these recommendations lags far behind (22). Longitudinal studies, most notably the Harvard Alumni Study of 15,000 male alumni, have shown the benefits of physical activity in the primary prevention of hypertension. This cohort included alumni who were initially normotensive (defined as BP <160/95 mm Hg) in 1962 and 1966, but who developed hypertension (defined as BP >160/95 mm Hg) on a second survey in 1977. Alumni who were inactive—as measured by step-climbing, walking, participation in sports, and a total kcal expenditure less than 2000/week—were at 35% greater risk to develop hypertension than those who were active. Risk was also influenced by BMI greater than 36, weight gain of more than 25 lb since graduation, and family history of hypertension. Participation in varsity sports during college years was not protective (23). A follow-up report found not only decreased risk for hypertension, but for all-cause mortality among the most physically active members of the cohort (24). Among alumni who were initially sedentary, those who became more physically active between the first and second follow-up had a decreased risk of developing hypertension and a decreased risk ratio of all-cause mortality. Obesity and cigarette smoking were also associated with increased CVD risk (25).

A similar study among 40,000 women (aged 55 to 69 years) followed for an average of 7 years showed a graded, inverse relationship between physical activity and risk of hypertension as well as all-cause mortality, an effect seen in all age categories and not affected by BMI or waist-to-hip ratio (26). The only randomized controlled trial on primary prevention of hypertension used interventions to decrease weight, salt intake and alcohol intake and increase physical activity (with a goal of 30 minutes, three times a week) versus a control group. In male and female participants aged 30 to 45 with a baseline high normal blood pressure (DBP 80 to 99 mm Hg), the intervention group had an incidence of established hypertension of 8.8% versus 19.2% among control patients. Since patients in the intervention group were advised on all four LMs, it is difficult to separate out the independent effects of each (27). Among patients with preexistent hypertension, a meta-analysis of nine RCTs showed that patients who initiated an aerobic exercise program of the lower extremities (walking, jogging, cycling, or combination) had an average decrease in SBP/DBP of $7 \pm 5 / 6 \pm 2$ mm Hg. Most of these studies used regimens of 3 to 4 days per week, to 50% to 75% of maximum O_2 consumption (Vo_2 max), and lasting 30 to 60 minutes per session. The majority of patients in these studies had stage one or two hypertension (28).

Although African-Americans are at increased risk of developing hypertension, their participation in the above-mentioned studies has been limited. A study of 46 African-American men with stage 3 hypertension and LVH showed a decrease in DBP, medication usage, and LVH with increased physical activity (cycling three times a week) over a 32-week study period (29).

Amount of Exercise

The current recommendations for physical activity in the prevention and control of hypertension are based on the summary statements quoted above; that is, moderately increased physical activity aimed at moving sedentary patients to a more active lifestyle (1,20). Whether additional benefits for hypertension and CVD risk accrue from increased intensity of exercise (measured as a percentage of Vo_2 max) or duration of exercise (measured as energy costs) remains unclear and debated (30). The National Runners' Health Study was a cross-sectional survey of approximately 8000 men recreational runners solicited through a running magazine. Among the runners with self-reported distance of more than 48 miles per week, there was a 50% lower prevalence of hypertension compared with runners who reported 0 to 10 miles per week, and a 70% lower use of blood pressure medications (31). A more recent report of the same database suggests that exercise intensity measured as Vo_2 max (determined by reported race times) may have more of an effect on SBP and DBP than energy expenditure, i.e., miles run per week (32). Patients must be evaluated and counseled on the small but definite risks of sudden death. In younger patients risk is related to congenital cardiac abnormalities. In older patients the risk of sudden death is overwhelmingly linked with the presence of CHD. The risk is greater for sedentary patients with CHD who start a strenuous exercise program (33). Comprehensive information on the evaluation of patients at risk and any patient initiating an exercise program is provided in the summary statements and in the Surgeon General's Report on Physical Activity and Health (17–20).

Weight Loss and Avoidance of Excess Weight/Obesity

Obesity may be most important and controllable LM. Obesity is associated with an increased risk of developing hypertension, with onset at an earlier age, and with more severe hypertension (34). An estimated 33 million Americans are overweight. Importantly, once hypertension develops with obesity, it is likely that other cardiovascular risk factors are also present. As with physical inactivity, obesity has become increasingly prevalent and has reached levels considered "epidemic" (35). Obesity represents a profound risk factor not only for hypertension but for type 2 diabetes mellitus, LVH independent of age and blood pressure, ischemic and total CVA risk in women, major CHD events, and total mortality in men (36). A nationwide screening of more than 1 million people aged 20 to 64 was done in the Community Hypertension Evaluation Clinic report (37). The prevalence of DBP greater than 95 mm Hg was strongly correlated with increased weight for all age, gender, and ethnic groups. For screenees between 20 and 39 years of age, the prevalence of hypertension was more than double that of normal weight screenees and more than triple that of underweight screenees. Overweight screenees were more likely to have elevated DBP, develop hypertension at an early age, and have more severe hypertension. The Nurses' Health Study, a prospective cohort of over 51,000 American women nurses, found that body weight, alcohol consumption, and age were strong predictors of incident and prevalent hypertension (38).

Figure 9-2 shows that weight reduction was the most effective nutritional-hygienic intervention in the TOHP-I study with a mean decrease in SBP/DBP of 2.9/2.3 mm Hg after an average weight loss of 3.9 kg. Blood pressure reduction was greater with greater weight loss (11). TOHP-II, a longer follow-up study looking at sodium restriction and weight loss, reported the same findings (39). In TONE there was a synergistic benefit to weight loss and sodium restriction in an older population (12). Controversy exists whether obesity-related hypertension is a more benign entity than hypertension with leanness. The Framingham study (40) found no evidence that obesity-related hypertension was more benign. Review of data from the Hypertension Detection and Follow-up Program (HDFP) likewise showed no decrease in cardiovascular risk with obesity. There was a large relative risk of death from noncardiac disease in the leanest men and women from neoplasia, other respiratory disorders, and cirrhosis. The authors hypothesize that the excess mortality of lean hypertension was not from leanness per se, but from other factors associated with their lifestyles, especially cigarette smoking and alcohol intake (41). In the Harvard Alumni Study (42), the lowest mortality rates were observed among men with weights below the U.S. average.

Obesity plays a large role in the development of hypertension. In the Framingham Offspring Study of young to middle-age adults, obesity was a major controllable contributor to new-onset hypertension; between 64% and 78% of newly developed hypertension among offspring was associated with obesity or excess weight gain (43). It has been estimated that 80% of obese adolescents have elevated blood pressures and 97% have at least one increased cardiovascular risk factor (44). Follow-up of children and adolescents showed an increased risk for adult hypertension with initially high blood pressure readings (especially SBP), higher BMI or weight at any age, and increased interim weight gain. The Dormont High School Study followed students from adolescence into adulthood and middle age. The greatest risk for elevated blood pressure was weight gain. For men, weight gain occurred in early adulthood, whereas for women the greatest weight gain and increase in blood pressure were in later adulthood (45), mirroring the data from NHANES III (2). The problem of obesity-related hypertension and increased cardiovascular risk in the population in general will not be solved without major efforts to improve the lifestyles of the young.

Weight loss for obesity-related hypertension is recommended for all patients with hypertension at all levels of blood pressure (1). A rapid reduction in blood pressure is seen over 8 to 10 weeks, probably related to diuresis and natriuresis (46). The decrease in blood pressure occurs before ideal body weight is attained. Although a "floor effect" for blood pressure reduction may exist, most patients experience a continued drop in blood pressure with continued weight loss (47). The effects of weight loss on blood pressure are maintained as long as weight does not increase (46). In an individual patient there is only a weak correlation between weight and level of blood pressure. Patients often have different blood pressures at identical degrees of overweight. A better correlation exists between the reduction in weight and the reduction of blood pressure independent of the patient's starting weight. Reduction in blood pressure with weight loss is proportional to the initial blood pressure, not the initial weight (48). The hypotensive response to weight loss can occur even with continued high sodium intake (49).

Attempts at weight reduction are probably more effective when combined with increased physical activity. For example, if a patient walked 15 minutes a day and kept the same caloric intake, the weight loss in 1 year would be 10 lb (20).

Alcohol Ingestion

Excessive alcohol intake is the fourth of the Big Four LMs. Precisely how alcohol raises blood pressure is unknown. Several hypotheses have been advanced: 1) Alcohol may have a direct pressor effect on vessel walls; 2) a sensitization of the vessels may occur for other pressors; 3) alcohol may directly stimulate the sympathetic nervous system; 4) alcohol may have an effect mediated by metabolites such as acetaldehyde (50); or 5) alcohol's effect may be mediated by humoral substances—specifically corticotropin-releasing hormone (CRH) via an effect on central efferent sympathetic activity (51). Men with normal blood pressure who decrease their alcohol intake experience a decrease in SBP of approximately 3 mm Hg (52), and men with hypertension have decreases in SBP/DBP of approximately 5/3 mm Hg with decreased alcohol ingestion (53). The hypotensive effects occur independent of weight loss; in fact, they can be confounded by changes in other lifestyle factors at the same time (27). There may be a J-shaped risk profile for alcohol intake, where small amounts of alcohol are actually cardioprotective, causing an increase in HDL cholesterol levels, or coronary artery vasodilation (16,50). Thus, the recommendations of JNC-VI (see Table 9-5) for a limited alcohol intake rather than total abstinence

seemed prudent. Patients with a higher intake of alcohol, particularly binge drinking patterns, should be strongly encouraged to decrease their alcohol intake to these acceptable levels.

Dietary Nutritional Factors

Most studies on various nutritional factors, including fish oil, fiber, fat, caffeine, protein, or vitamin C, yield equivocal results (54). However, this may not be the entire story. The effects of individual nutrients may be too small to detect in trials, whereas a cumulative effect may be large enough for detection. Nutrients not studied may be the important factors. Lastly, supplements used in trials may not affect blood pressure the same way as nutrients contained in food (55). The recent Dietary Approaches to Stop Hypertension (DASH) study tested 1) a controlled, typical diet with 2) one high in fruits and vegetables (fruit/veg) and 3) a diet high in fruits and vegetables with reduced fat and cholesterol intake (combin). Over an 8-week study period, the combin diet lowered SBP/DBP by 5.5/3.0 mm Hg, whereas the fruit/veg diet lowered SBP/DBP by 2.8/1.1 mm Hg, compared with the control diet. The effect was evident in patients with or without hypertension, in men and women of all ethnic groups, and occurred with the usual sodium intake of 3 g/day and without weight loss. Among patients with hypertension the drop in SBP/DBP was even greater—up to 11.4/5.5 mm Hg versus the control diet (55). Thus, prescribing a generally healthy diet with fruits, vegetables, and decreased saturated fat intake for its effect on blood pressure and overall cardiovascular risk may be more beneficial than focusing on individual nutrients.

Potassium

Data from the INTERSALT study showed that a habitually low intake of potassium was associated with an increased risk of high SBP and DBP (5). A recent meta-analysis of RCTs showed that potassium (K) supplementation was associated with a decrease in SBP/DBP in the range of 3/2 mm Hg (56). In the Nurses' Health Study cohort, normotensive women at the lowest percentage of K intake, based on food questionnaires, had a modest decrease in SBP/DBP of 2.0/1.7 mm Hg with K supplementation (57). Among the entire study population, however, there was no correlation of dietary K intake and risk of developing hypertension after adjustment for age, weight, and alcohol consumption (38). Similarly in an RCT of hypertension prevention (TOHP-I), there was no effect from K supplementation on blood pressure over a 6-month period (11). The overall effect of K supplementation on blood pressure is probably mild and seems to be limited to those with low K intake. Thus, all patients should be advised to maintain adequate K in the diet—especially through the addition of fruits and vegetables (see Table 9-5). Caution must be exercised in patients at risk for hyperkalemia from renal disease or use of angiotensin-converting enzyme inhibitors or angiotensin receptor blockers.

Calcium

In the Nurses' Health Study cohort there was no relationship of calcium (Ca) intake with subsequent development of hypertension and supplementation of women with low Ca intake did not lower blood pressure (38,57). A recent meta-analysis of observational reports from 1983 to 1993 found no effect on blood pressure with Ca supplementation (58). A further meta-analysis of 50 RCTs by some of the same authors found a small effect of Ca supplementation in the range of lowering SBP/DBP by 0.9/0.2 mm Hg. Their conclusion was that the effect was too small to justify routine use of Ca supplements specifically for preventing hypertension (59). Reasonable recommendations are that calcium intake should be maintained at recommended levels especially in patients at risk for osteoporosis, but Ca supplementation seems to have no significant effect on hypertension prevention or treatment (Table 9-5).

Tobacco Use

Each smoked cigarette raises blood pressure even in chronic tobacco users (60). Ambulatory blood pressure monitoring has shown that patients who are frequent smokers can have a sustained rise in blood pressure due to regular nicotine infusions (61). These effects seem to occur with cigars and smokeless tobacco, but not with transdermal nicotine patches (16). However, the specific long-term contribution of tobacco use to development and maintenance of hypertension is also confounded by other lifestyle factors. For example, smokers tend to drink more alcohol, eat fewer fruits and vegetables, and have a lower BMI when compared to nonsmokers (62). Since the cardiovascular risk associated with tobacco use eclipses the risk of hypertension alone, there are independent overwhelming reasons to urge patients to discontinue tobacco use even if the use of transdermal nicotine patches is necessary.

Biofeedback and Stress Reduction

The contribution of stress—especially job-related stress—to the development and maintenance of hypertension is controversial (63). Evidence is accumulating that job-related stress may be persistent enough to alter long-term blood pressure (16). Although numerous short-term studies of applied stress have been associated with short-term increases in blood pressure, a recent consensus statement on primary prevention of hypertension stated that "on balance the available results provide insufficient evidence to advocate stress management as a useful strategy for the prevention of hypertension." (7). Similarly, the JNC-VI report found no support for the use of relaxation techniques in the prevention or control of hypertension. In the TOPH-I trial no benefit was shown from stress reduction strategies over the 6-month study period (Figure 9-2). A recent meta-analysis also showed no sustained effect from stress reduction, biofeedback, or meditation for control of blood pressure (64). Rather, factors such as dietary patterns, alcohol intake, lack of physical activity, or obesity that can be coping mechanisms and may be present with stress should be addressed (65).

IMPLEMENTATION OF LIFESTYLE MODIFICATIONS

The maintenance of LM is difficult and recidivism is high, even in RCTs. Since multiple changes are often necessary to control blood pressure, the best approach is with a multidisciplinary team that includes physicians, physician-extenders, dieticians, and exercise medicine specialists. NHANES III reported that 76% of Americans diagnosed with hypertension had received an LM prescription. Over two thirds of interviewees were using one or more of the Big Four LMs with decreased sodium intake the most common LM (2). Data from RCTs, especially the TOHP-I and TONE, support weight and maintenance of leanness as the most effective LM. The benefits of sodium restriction to around 100 mmol/day differ among patients with one third "salt-sensitive." It is difficult to separate the role of individual LMs, and there are advantages from a more holistic application of LM. For example, weight loss is easier and more likely to persist with the addition of exercise to caloric reduction and is synergistic with sodium restriction (12). All patients should be counseled on incorporation of multiple risk-reducing behaviors into their lifestyle with special attention to evident CVD risk factors. No demonstrable adverse effect has been found with any LM. The LM recommendations should be addressed on at least two levels. A community-based approach must have broad objectives for the simultaneous decrease in several cardiovascular risk factors including hypertension (7). Interventions such as control of salt content of food, national guidelines for physical activity and desirable weight, and national cholesterol targets are examples of this strategy. Mass media education, community-based activities, physician education, school-based initiatives, senior centers, and retirement communities are the arenas for such health-promoting activities. Clinic and office-based recommendations for individual patients are the second venue. Here attention is focused on the cardiovascular risk factors of the individual patient. The active involvement of the patient in his or her own care, the process of setting goals, and specific recommendations based on the patient's cardiovascular risk profile and target organ damage is the goal here (7). It is also wise to remember the saying, "Physician, heal thyself." In the matter of lifestyle modifications, it is important that the physician act not only as caregiver, but also as role model (66).

REFERENCES

1. Joint National Committee. The sixth report of the Joint National Committee on the Prevention, Detection, Evaluation and Treatment of High Blood Pressure (JNC-VI). Arch Intern Med 1997;157: 2413–2446.

2. Burt VL, Whelton P, Roccella EJ, et al. Prevalence of hypertension in the US adult population: results from the Third National Health and Nutrition Examination Survey, 1988–1991. Hypertension 1995;25:305–313.

3. Stamler J, Stamler R, Neaton JD. Blood pressure, systolic and diastolic, and cardiovascular risks. US Population Data. Arch Intern Med 1993;153:598–615.

4. Neaton JD, Wentworth D, for the Multiple Risk Factor Intervention Trial Research Group. Serum cholesterol, blood pressure, cigarette smoking, and death from coronary heart disease: overall findings and differences by age for 316,099 white men. Arch Intern Med 1992;152:56–64.

5. Stamler J. Blood pressure and high blood pressure: Aspects of risk. Hypertension 1991;18(suppl I): I-95–I-107.

6. Stamler J, Rose G, Elliott P, et al. Findings of the International Cooperative INTERSALT Study. Hypertension 1991;17:I-9–I-15.

7. National High Blood Pressure Education Program (NHBPEP) Working Group. National High Blood Pressure Education Program Working Group report on primary prevention of hypertension. Arch Intern Med 1993;153:186–208.

8. Grundy SM, Balaby GJ, Criqui MH, et al. Guide to primary prevention of cardiovascular diseases: a statement for health care professionals from the Task Force on Risk Reduction. American Heart Association Science Advisory and Coordinating Committee. Circulation 1997;95:2329–2331.

9. Stamler J. The INTERSALT Study: background, methods, findings and implications. Am J Clin Nutr 1997;65:626S–642S.

10. Dustan HP. A perspective on the salt-blood pressure relation. Hypertension 1991;17:I-166–I-169.

11. Trials of Hypertension Prevention Collaborative Research Group. The effects of nonpharmacologic interventions on blood pressure of persons with high normal levels: results of the trials of hypertension prevention, phase I. JAMA 1992;267:1213–1220.

12. Whelton PK, Appel LJ. Espeland MA, et al. Sodium restriction and weight loss in the treatment of hypertension in older persons: a randomized controlled trial of non-pharmacologic interventions on the elderly (TONE). JAMA 1998;279: 839–846.

13. Midgley JP, Matthew AG, Greenwood CM, Logan AG. Effect of reduced dietary sodium on blood pressure: a meta-analysis of randomized controlled trials. JAMA 1996;275:1590–1597.

14. Cutler JA, Follmann D, Allender PS. Randomized trials of sodium restriction: an overview. Am J Clin Nutr 1997;65:643S–651S.

15. Alderman MH, Madhavan S, Cohen H, et al. Low urinary sodium is associated with greater risk of myocardial infarction among treated hypertensive men. Hypertension 1995;25:1144–1152.

16. Kaplan NM. Clinical hypertension. 7th ed. New York: Williams and Wilkins, 1997.

17. Fletcher GF, Balady G, Blair SN, et al. Statement on exercise: benefits and recommendations for physical activity programs for all Americans. A statement for health professionals by the Committee on Exercise and Cardiac Rehabilitation of the Council on Clinical Cardiology, American Heart Association. Circulation 1996;94:857–862.

18. NIH Consensus Development Panel on Physical Activity and Cardiovascular Health. Physical activity and cardiovascular health. JAMA 1996;273:241–246.

19. Pate RR, Pratt M, Blair SN, et al. Physical activity and public health: a recommendation from the Centers for Disease Control and Prevention and the American College of Sports Medicine. JAMA 1995;273:402–407.

20. U.S. Department of Health and Human Services. Physical activity and health: A report of the Surgeon General. Atlanta GA: Centers for Disease Control and Prevention, National Center for Chronic Disease Prevention and Health Promotion, 1996.

21. Heini AF, Weinsier RL. Divergent trends in obesity and fat intake patterns: the American paradox. Am J Med 1997;102: 259–264.

22. Crespo CJ, Keteyian SJ, Heath GW, Sempos CT. Leisure-time physical activity among US adults: results from the Third National Health and Nutrition Examination Survey. Arch Intern Med 1996; 156:93–98.

23. Paffenbarger RS Jr, Wing AL, Hyde RT, Jung DL. Physical activity and incidence of hypertension in college alumni. Am J Epidemiol 1983;117:245–257.

24. Lee IM, Hsieh CC, Paffenbarger RS Jr. Exercise intensity and longevity in men. The Harvard Alumni Health Study. JAMA 1995;273:1179–1184.

25. Paffenbarger RS Jr, Hyde RT, Wing AL, et al. The association of changes in physical-activity level and other lifestyle characteristics with mortality among men. N Engl J Med 1993;328:538–545.

26. Kushi LH, Fee RM, Folsom AR, et al. Physical activity and mortality in postmenopausal women. JAMA 1997;277:1287–1292.

27. Stamler R, Stamler J, Gosch F, et al. Primary prevention of hypertension by nutritional-hygienic means: final report of a randomized, controlled trial [published erratum appears in JAMA 1989; 262(22):3132]. JAMA 1989;262: 1801–1807.

28. Kelley G, McClellan P. Antihypertensive effects of aerobic exercise: a brief meta-analytic review of randomized controlled trials. Am J Hypertens 1994;7: 115–119.

29. Kokkinos PF, Narayan P, Colleran JA, et al. Effects of regular exercise on blood pressure and left ventricular hypertrophy in African-American men with severe hypertension. N Engl J Med 1995;333: 1462–1467.

30. Blair SN, Cooper KH. Dose of exercise and health benefits [editorial; comment] [published erratum appears in Arch Intern Med 1997;157(5):486]. Arch Intern Med 1997;157:153–154.

31. Williams PT. Relationship of distance run per week to coronary heart disease risk factors in 8283 male runners: the National Runners' Health Study. Arch Intern Med 1997;157:191–198.

32. Williams PT. Relationships of heart disease risk factors to exercise quantity and intensity. Arch Intern Med 1998;158:237–245.

33. Thompson Paul D. The cardiovascular complications of vigorous physical activity. Arch Intern Med 1996;156:2297–2302.

34. Heyka P. Obesity and hypertension. Nutr Clin Care 1998;1(suppl 1):30–37.

35. Stamler R. Epidemic obesity in the United States. Arch Intern Med 1993;153:1040–1044.

36. Rosenbaum M, Leibel RL, Hirsch J. Obesity. N Engl J Med 1997;337:396–407.

37. Stamler R, Stamler J, Riedlinger WF, et al. Weight and blood pressure: findings in hypertension screening of 1 million Americans. JAMA 1978;240:1607–1610.

38. Ascherio A, Hennekens C, Willett WC, et al. Prospective study of nutritional factors, blood pressure, and hypertension among US women. Hypertension 1996;27:1065–1072.

39. The Trials of the Hypertension Prevention Collaborative Research Group. Effects of weight loss and sodium restriction on blood pressure and hypertension incidence on overweight people with high-normal blood pressure: the trials of hypertension prevention, phase II. Arch Intern Med 1997;157:657–667.

40. Kannel WB, Zhang T, Garrison RJ. Is obesity-related hypertension less of a cardiovascular risk? the Framingham Study. Am Heart J 1990;120:1195–1201.

41. Stamler R, Ford CE, Stamler J. Why do lean hypertensives have higher mortality rates than other hypertensives? findings of the Hypertension Detection and Follow-up Program. Hypertension 1991;17:553–564.

42. Lee IM, Manson JE, Hennekens CH, Paffenbarger RS Jr. Body weight and mortality: a 27-year follow-up of middle-aged men. JAMA 1993;270:2823–2828.

43. Garrison RJ, Kannel WB, Stokes J 3d, Castelli WP. Incidence and precursors of hypertension in young adults: the Framingham Offspring Study. Prev Med 1987;16:235–251.

44. Rocchini AP. Cardiovascular causes of systemic hypertension. Pediatr Clin North Am 1993;40:141–147.

45. Yong LC, Kuller LH, Rutan G, Bunker C. Longitudinal study of blood pressure: changes and determinants from adolescence to middle age. The Dormont High School follow-up study, 1957–1963 to 1989–1990. Am J Epidemiol 1993;138:973–983.

46. Dustan HP, Weinsier RL. Treatment of obesity-associated hypertension. Ann Epidemiol 1991;1:371–379.

47. Cohen N, Flamenbaum W. Obesity and hypertension: demonstration of a "floor effect." Am J Med 1986;80:177–181.

48. Eliahou HE, Iaina A, Gaon T, et al. Body weight reduction necessary to attain normotension in the overweight hypertensive patient. Int J Obes 1981;5(suppl 1):157–163.

49. Reisin E, Abel R, Modan M, et al. Effect to weight loss without salt restriction on the reduction of blood pressure in overweight hypertensive patients. N Engl J Med 1978;298:1–6.

50. Victor RG, Hansen J. Alcohol and blood pressure—a drink a day . . . [editorial; comment]. N Engl J Med 1995;332:1782–1783.

51. Randin D, Vollenweider P, Tappy L, et al. Suppression of alcohol-induced hypertension by dexamethasone. N Engl J Med 1995;332:1733–1737.

52. Puddey IB, Beilin LJ, Vandongen R, et al. Evidence for a direct effect of alcohol consumption on blood pressure in normotensive men: a randomized controlled trial. Hypertension 1985;7:707–713.

53. Puddey IB, Beilin LJ, Vandongen R. Regular alcohol use raises blood pressure in treated hypertensive subjects: a randomised controlled trial. Lancet 1987;1:647–651.

54. Stamler J, Caggiula AW, Grandits A. Relation of body mass and alcohol, nutrient, fiber, and caffeine intakes to blood pressure in the special intervention and usual care groups in the Multiple Risk Factor Intervention Trial. Am J Clin Nutr 1997;65:338S–365S.

55. Appel LJ, Moore, TJ, Obarzanek E, et al. A clinical trial of the effects of dietary patterns on blood pressure. DASH Collaborative Research Group. N Engl J Med 1997;336:1117–1124.

56. Whelton PK, He J, Cutler JA, et al. Effects of oral potassium on blood pressure: meta-analysis of randomized controlled clinical trials. JAMA 1997;277:1624–1632.

57. Sacks FM, Willett WC, Smith A, et al. Effect on blood pressure of potassium, calcium, and magnesium in women with low habitual intake. Hypertension 1998;31:131–138.

58. Pryer, J, Cappuccio FP, Elliott P. Dietary calcium and blood pressure: a review of the observational studies. J Hum Hypertens 1995;9:597–604.

59. Allender PS, Cutler JA, Follmann D, et al. Dietary calcium and blood pressure: a meta-analysis of randomized clinical trials. Ann Intern Med 1996;124:825–831.

60. Groppelli A, Giorgi DM, Omboni S, et al. Persistent blood pressure increase induced by heavy smoking. J Hypertens 1992;10:495–499.

61. Verdecchia P, Schillaci G, Borgioni C, et al. Cigarette smoking, ambulatory blood pressure and cardiac hypertrophy in essential hypertension. J Hypertens 1995;13:1209–1215.

62. Sleight P. Smoking and hypertension. Clin Exp Hypertens 1993;15:1181–1192.

63. Markovitz JH, Matthews KA, Kannel WB, et al. Psychological predictors of hypertension in the

Framingham Study: is there tension in hypertension? JAMA 1993;270:2439–2443.

64. Eisenberg DM, Delbanco TL, Berkey CS, et al. Cognitive behavioral techniques for hypertension: are they effective? Ann Intern Med 1993;118:964–972.

65. Lindquist TL, Beilin LJ, Knuiman MW. Influence of lifestyle, coping, and job stress on blood pressure in men and women. Hypertension 1997;29:1–7.

66. Andersen RE, Blair SN, Cheskin LJ, Bartlett SJ. Encouraging patients to become more physically active: the physician's role. Ann Intern Med 1997;127:395–400.

67. Dahl L. Possible role of salt intake in the development of hypertension. In: Cottier P, Bock KD, eds. Essential hypertension: an international symposium. Berlin: Springer-Verlag, 1960:53–65.

68. Intersalt Cooperative Research Group. Intersalt: an international study of electrolyte excretion and blood pressure: results for 24 hour urinary sodium and potassium excretion. Br Med J 1988;297:319–328.

Chapter 10

Community Approaches to Reduce the Risks of Cardiovascular Disease

Beti Thompson

In the past century, dramatic decreases have occurred in the rates of infectious diseases as a result of intensive public health efforts (36,51). The decline in those diseases, however, has not been paralleled in chronic diseases, in which the incident rates are increasing (21,44,80). The case of coronary heart disease is illustrative. In 1930, coronary heart disease became the major cause of death in the United States, overtaking infectious diseases (4). Although cardiovascular mortality has declined since 1950 and is continuing to decline, it still accounts for almost 1 million of all deaths annually (41.5% of all deaths) in the United States, with 50% of those deaths due to coronary heart disease (4).

Much of the risk for chronic diseases such as cardiovascular disease is behavioral and can be controlled (13). For cardiovascular disease, the most frequently mentioned risk factors include smoking, lack of exercise, poor dietary patterns, obesity, and high sodium intake (30,38). Basic lifestyle changes can greatly reduce the risk factors; for example, smoking cessation has been demonstrated to produce an almost immediate reduction of cardiovascular disease risk (39). Similarly the management of diet to include a low intake of saturated fat and a high intake of fruits and vegetables appears to reduce risk (4,54,59). Regular physical exercise also reduces risk (42,71). Only a few of the contributing factors to heart disease, such as age, gender, socioeconomic status, and hereditary characteristics, cannot be controlled.

The remarkable decrease in cardiovascular disease since 1950 coincided with substantial developments in treatment technology. More aggressive medical treatment of myocardial infarction (MI), surgical management, specialized hospital units for cardiac patients, and the availability of immediate assistance through emergency medical services and individuals trained in cardiopulmonary resuscitation (CPR) developed in concert with the recognition that lifestyle behaviors were associated with cardiovascular disease (31,33,87). Although few studies have documented the relative contribution of medical management versus lifestyle behavior changes to cardiovascular disease mortality, studies have estimated that more than half of the reduction could be attributed to modification of lifestyle behaviors (32,44,45).

A long history exists of experimental studies designed to modify selected health-risk behaviors. For the most part, the emphasis has been on the individual model, in which individuals have been targeted for behavior change. Although some of these experiments have focused on compliance with medical regimens (e.g., taking hypertension medication) (10,56), others have emphasized changes in lifestyle behaviors (e.g., diet, weight control, and regular exercise) (23,52,59,88). A good example of such interventions is smoking cessation. In the more than 25 years since smoking has been recognized as a primary preventable cause of disease and death, numerous studies have been conducted on the best methods of assisting individual smokers in stopping their habit (46,67,83).

Smoking cessation success rates have generally been established in randomized, controlled trials where individuals are assigned to various conditions. Until recently, individuals were the focus of both the intervention and the evaluation (67). Unfortunately, the programs that fared the best in achieving individual change were not very effective when applied across a large spectrum of people and have not been able to reach large numbers of people (22,58,83). This may be because such programs have relied on volunteers to participate in small group sessions or to attempt to achieve cessation with the help of written self-help materials. Small group or clinical programs are limited in the numbers of people that can be reached (83). Self-help programs appear to have relatively low success rates (11).

Recently, a change has been occurring in the way in which smoking and other lifestyle behaviors are viewed. Increasingly, smoking and other behaviors are being perceived not as individual problems, but as public health problems (81,83). The effects of smoking, for example, are now seen as problems that extend beyond the smoker and have implications for nonsmokers as well (12,79,86). As a result, smoking control policies have been implemented in a variety of public and private places, including hospitals, worksites, schools, and restaurants. Smoking control is no longer an individual matter, but one that is the focus of many agencies and groups, including various government sectors (83).

Dietary patterns are also becoming a matter of public health. The Food and Drug Administration and the United States Department of Agriculture now require labeling of food to provide the consumer with accurate information on nutrition components (15). The new, revised food pyramid has found its way into schools and other places where individuals are taught about appropriate dietary patterns. Numerous eating establishments offer "heart healthy choices." Grocery stores may have areas devoted to "healthy products." Even some fast food restaurants provide healthy alternatives to their typical fare.

In an attempt to achieve large-scale, widespread lifestyle behavior change, in the past 3 decades individual change efforts have been supplemented with community intervention trials for change. Community approaches typically involve numerous community individuals, groups, organizations, and institutions, providing a greater base of support for behavior change. In this chapter, a brief overview of the theories behind community approaches and community change is followed by a discussion of various community-based cardiovascular disease intervention projects, their findings, and their implications for interventions for the future. A brief description is provided for the role of the physician in community-based cardiovascular disease prevention.

COMMUNITY APPROACHES TO LIFESTYLE BEHAVIOR CHANGE

Individual behavior is shaped by many factors, some of which are internal (3,60,73) and some external (5,74,78,89). Almost all theories of behavior change take into account the importance of the social environment within which the individual lives. Primarily, this is because individuals do not behave in a vacuum; thoughts of smoking or not smoking and access or lack thereof to healthy foods are examples of how behavior may be encouraged or constrained by the social environment.

The social environment contains many rules for behaviors. These rules and expectations are called *social norms* and every community, no matter how small, has a complex system of formal and informal norms that provides guidance for appropriate behavior in specific situations (62). All individuals within a community are greatly influenced by norms. As an example of a formal norm, employees in worksites (small communities) may restrict their smoking only to regular breaks because smoking at one's workstation is in violation of company policy. An informal norm, however, might be participation in a worksite's lunchtime "walking club" because the supervisor looks favorably upon employees who participate.

Norms are dynamic and change by time and place. Again, smoking provides an excellent example. Although the causal agent is not clear, as smoking prevalence decreases, the number of places in which smoking is restricted increases (81,83). As it becomes increasingly difficult to find places to smoke, more and more smokers give up the habit (83). Should such a trend continue over time, smoking will eventually become a genuinely deviant behavior.

The community approach to lifestyle behavior change is based on the premise that long-term and widespread behavior change is best achieved by changing norms about the behavior. It recognizes that norms are among the most important determinants of behavior. Advocates of the community approaches perceive that targeting an individual for a specific health-risk behavior without changing the environment within which that individual operates may result in difficulty in maintaining behavior change; individuals are likely to revert back to the undesired behavior when reentering social environments that are conducive to specific behaviors.

The recognition of the importance of the environment in social change led to community approaches to health promotion as a means of achieving large-scale change in both primary prevention and treatment of chronic health problems. Experts argued that community organization could change the community setting to support healthier lifestyles (6,18,34). That change would be translated to reductions in individuals' health-risk behavior, which would in turn lead to decreases in chronic disease morbidity and mortality. A number of community intervention studies have been conducted to reduce cardiovascular risk factors.

COMMUNITY CARDIOVASCULAR PROJECTS
Multiple Risk Factor Approaches

Since the 1970s numerous public health proponents accepted the importance of changing the social environment and embarked on a number of studies to reduce cardiovascular morbidity and mortality by changing behavioral risk factors related to cardiovascular diseases. Some of the community studies that addressed cardiovascular disease prevention and their essential intervention strategies are summarized in Table 10-1, while Table 10-2 provides an overall picture of the results. Because of the complexity of the various comparisons among communities, the results are presented in detail in the following section.

The CHAD Program

The Community, Hypertension, Atherosclerosis and Diabetes (CHAD) Program, initiated in 1971, was a forerunner of the first generation of community cardiovascular programs. The "communities" were housing projects in western Jerusalem. A multiple risk factor program, CHAD was aimed at reducing cardiovascular risk factors among adults living in four adjacent housing projects (2). Using primary care practices, physicians and nurses met with individuals, couples, and families to educate them on ways to reduce cardiovascular risk. In addition to one-on-one counseling, small group classes were held to discuss lifestyle changes and to provide support for such changes. The control group, families and individuals in an adjacent neighborhood, received usual clinical care. Assessment of a population cross section at baseline (1970) and another 5 years later (1975) showed a significant mean net reduction, standardized by age and gender, in systolic blood pressure (3.1 mm Hg), diastolic pressure (2.0 mm Hg), and weight (0.6 lb) in the intervention practices (2). Reductions in smoking prevalence were significant for men (5.9%), but not for women (0.5%). Significant changes were not observed for serum cholesterol. After an additional 5 years of intervention (1976 to 1981), study investigators went back to all individuals who had been involved in CHAD and still lived in the neighborhood (the cohort). For this group, reductions increased or held for diastolic blood pressure (−3.6 mm Hg) and smoking

prevalence (−12.8%) compared to the 1976 data despite the aging of the population. There was no change in weight or serum cholesterol, and systolic pressure was not significantly different (29).

The Stanford Three-Community Study

Two landmark true community studies commenced in 1972: the Stanford Three-Community Study and the Finnish North Karelia study (see Table 10-1). Both projects used mass media; in addition, Stanford used intensive face-to-face intervention for a sample of high-risk individuals (20,49), whereas North Karelia used community organization, environmental modification, and educational programs (50,61,66). The Stanford study had an elaborate design involving three communities. One community was designated as control. Another

Table 10-1 Community Studies for Cardiovascular Disease Prevention with Targeted Risk Factors and Intervention Modalities

PROJECT	COMMUNITIES		RISK FACTORS	INTERVENTIONS
	INTERVENTION	COMPARISON		
CHAD Program (Israel) (1971–1981)	Four housing projects	Adjacent community	• Hypertension • Hypercholesterolemia • Obesity • Smoking	• Screening • Individual face-to-face counseling • Small discussion groups
Stanford Three-Community Study (1972–1975)	One media, one media plus intensive	One no treatment community	• Hypertension • Hypercholesterolemia • Obesity • Physical activity • Smoking	• Mass media • Face-to-face counseling for high-risk individuals in one community
North Karelia Study (1973–1983)	One rural county	One matched neighboring county	• Hypercholesterolemia • Smoking • Hypertension	• Community organization • Environmental modification (e.g., availability of healthful foods, restriction of smoking in places) • Educational programs (e.g., food preparation groups)
Switzerland National Research Program	Two	Two	• Smoking • Hypertension • Weight • Body mass index • Hypercholesterolemia	• Community mobilization • Mass media • Environmental changes • Telephone hotline • Integration with health service
CORIS (Coronary Risk Factor Study)	One low-intensity, one high-intensity	One control	• Smoking • Hypertension • Hypercholesterolemia	• Small media (e.g., posters, billboards, mailings, local newspapers) • Small media plus interpersonal intervention
Stanford Five-City Project	Two	Three	• Hypercholesterolemia • Hypertension • Body mass index • Smoking • Physical activity	• Community organization • General education • Separate risk factor campaigns per year • Media
Minnesota Heart Health Program	Three	Three	• Hypercholesterolemia • Hypertension • Body mass index • Smoking • Physical activity	• Community organization • Mass media • Integrated health services • Screening activities • Community-wide events • School programs
Pawtucket Heart Health Program	One	One	• Hypercholesterolemia • Smoking • Hypertension • Body mass index	• Community mobilization • Direct education through community organizations involved in all intervention activities (e.g., schools, worksites, grocery stores, restaurants)

Table 10-1 continues

Table 10-1 (*Continued*)

| PROJECT | COMMUNITIES | | RISK FACTORS | INTERVENTIONS |
	INTERVENTION	COMPARISON		
Australian North Coast	One media only, one media plus community programs	One control	• Smoking	• Mass media • Community programs (e.g., skills training, quit aids, quit tips)
Sydney	One	Remainder of Australia	• Smoking	• Mass media • Counseling available for those who desired it
COMMIT (Community Intervention Trial for Smoking Cessation)	11	11	• Smoking	• Community mobilization of health care settings, worksites, schools, media, etc., to provide regular opportunities for smoking cessation
Working Well Trial	56 worksites	56 worksites	• Smoking • Dietary patterns (fat, fiber)	• Participation of employees in planning intervention activities • Direct education • Contests, campaigns • Small media
Take Heart Program	13	13	• Smoking • Dietary patterns (fat) • Serum cholesterol	• Participation of employees in planning • "Kick-off" event to introduce project to worksite employees • Motivational sessions • Direct education • Environmental changes

received media intervention only. A third received the media intervention, plus two thirds of an identified cohort of high-risk individuals in the community received an intensive intervention (49). Evaluation was presented in terms of five groups: 1) the control community; 2) the media only community; 3) the media plus intensive intervention community, including only the individuals who were randomized to receive the intensive care; 4) the media plus intensive intervention community, including only the individuals who were randomized *not* to receive the intensive care; and 5) a "reconstituted sample" that combined the high-risk individuals in the media only community.

After 2 years of follow-up, the study produced mixed results. Cohort analyses indicated significant increases in cardiovascular risk knowledge in all intervention communities (53). Significant reductions in dietary cholesterol were seen in all communities relative to the control community [media only community, −38.6 mg/day; media plus intensive (intensive instruction group only), −42.3 mg/day; media plus intensive (media sample only), −27.2 mg/day]. Only among the media plus intensive (intensive instruction group), however, was there a corresponding decrease in serum cholesterol (−3.1 mg/100 mL). Changes in systolic blood pressure were significant for all intervention communities (and ranged from a reduction of 6.6 to 8.9 mm Hg). Diastolic blood pressure results were mixed; in the media only community, there was an increase in diastolic pressure (+2.5 mm Hg). The media plus intensive group decreased whether examining the intensive instruction cohort alone in that group (−3.9 mm Hg) or the media cohort alone in the group (−6.2 mm Hg), but the control community also decreased (−5.4 mm Hg), resulting in

no significant difference. A similar pattern was seen for weight with the control community showing a decrease (−0.8 lb), which was about as great as the media plus intensive community, both cohorts. In the media plus intensive intervention group, there was a significant decrease in smoking prevalence; this was not seen in the other communities. No significant change was seen in physical activity in any of the communities (20,49,53).

The North Karelia Study

The North Karelia project emerged as a result of identifying very high cardiovascular disease rates in a specific area in Finland (50). The program objectives were to provide preventive services to persons at high risk, to educate people about their health, to persuade people to take action for health change, to train individuals in skills of change, to create social support for change, and to change the environment for health (50). Using a neighboring county as a reference area, 5-year cross-sectional results showed significant net reductions in serum cholesterol for men (−11.1 mg/100 mL) but not for women (−3.0 mg/100 mL); significant net reductions in both systolic and diastolic blood pressure for both men and women (systolic: 5.3 mm Hg, 7.2 mm Hg; diastolic: 2.6 mm Hg, 3.7 mm Hg, respectively), and a nonsignificant reduction in smoking prevalence for both men and women (2.5% and 6.1%, respectively). There were no differences in the body mass index for either men or women. A 10-year follow-up of the North Karelia study indicated that significant differences remained for both systolic and diastolic blood pressure. For men, daily smoking and serum cholesterol were still significantly lower

Table 10-2 Change in Cardiovascular Risk Factors as a Result of Community Intervention*

PROJECT	CHOLESTEROL		BLOOD PRESSURE		WEIGHT	BMI	SMOKING		EXERCISE
	DIETARY	SERUM	SYSTOLIC	DIASTOLIC			PREVALENCE	CESSATION	
Multifacor Intervention									
CHAD Program									
Cross-sectional at 5 years	NS	NA	Decrease	Decrease	Decrease	NA	Decrease for men only	NR	NR
Cohort after 10 years	NS	NS	NS	Decrease	NS	NA	Decrease	NR	NR
Stanford Three-Community study									
Media only vs. control	Decrease	NS	Decrease	Increase	Increase	NA	Decrease		Decrease
Media plus intensive vs. control						NA			
Media cohort only	Decrease	NS	Decrease	NS	Decrease		NS		Decrease
Media and intensive	Decrease	Decrease	Decrease	NS	Decrease		Decrease		Increase
Reconstituted	Decrease	NS	Decrease	NS	Decrease		NR		NR
North Karelia study									
After 5 years	NR	Men only	Decrease	Decrease	NR	NS	Men only	NR	NR
After 10 years	NR	Men only	Decrease	Decrease	NR	NR	Men only	NR	NR
Switzerland National Research Program	NR	NS	NS	NS	NS	Decrease	Decrease	NR	NR
CORIS Coronary Risk Factor Study									
High-intensity over control	NR	NS	Decrease	Decrease			Women only	Women only	
Low-intensity over control	NR	NS	Decrease	Decrease	NR	NR	NS	Women only	NR
Stanford Five-city Project (FCP)									
Cohort	NR	NS	Decrease	Decrease	NR	NS	NS	NS	NS
Cross-sectional	NR	NS	NS	NS	NR	Decrease	Men only	NS	Increase
Minnesota Heart Health Program (MHHP)									
Cohort	NR	NS	NS	NS	NR	NS	NS	NS	Increase
Cross-sectional	NR	NS	NS	NS	NR	NS	Women only	NS	Increase
Pawtucket Heart Health Program (PHHP)									
Cohort	NR	NS	NS	NS	NR	NS	NA	NS	NA
Cross-sectional	NR	NS	NS	NS	NR	Decrease	NS	NA	NA
Single Factor Intervention									
Smoking Studies									
Australian "North Coast"									
One media over control	NA	NA	NA	NA	NA	NA	Decrease	NR	NA
One media plus community programs over control	NA	NA	NA	NA	NA	NA	Decrease	NR	NA
Sydney (vs. Australia)	NA	NA	NA	NA	NA	NA	NS	NR	NA
COMMIT (Community Intervention Trial for Smoking Cessation)	NA	NA	NA	NA	NA	NA	NS	Decrease	NA
Worksite Studies									
The Working Well Trial	Decrease	NA	NA	NA	NA	NA	NS	NS	NA
Take Heart	NA	NS	NA	NA	NA	NA	NA	NA	NA

NA = not applicable; NR = data not reported; NS = change not significant.
* Table gives only whether significant changes were reported and direction of change; see text for specific changes.

than at the beginning of the study; however, any net reductions in those areas for women disappeared (61).

The Switzerland National Research Program

In 1977, the Switzerland National Research Program (NRP 1A) undertook a community intervention to reduce cardiovascular risk. Four communities were randomized to intervention or control (35). Intervention focused on participation of the entire population, mobilization of the community, and integration of the program into existing health services. Media, environmental changes (e.g., distributors of food products, restaurants), and a telephone hotline were among the services offered. Smoking prevalence decreased significantly (−3.6%) as did body mass index. No change was observed in serum cholesterol. Neither systolic nor diastolic blood pressure showed significant changes between communities. Body weight increased slightly in both communities.

The Coronary Risk Factor Study

The Coronary Risk Factor Study (CORIS) in three South African communities used small media to encourage individuals to lower coronary heart disease risk factors. Small media are localized, specific ways of transmitting messages within a community and can include posters, billboards, newspapers, and direct mailing. The media campaign was supplemented with an interpersonal intervention for high-risk individuals in one of the communities. Significant net reductions were found in both systolic and diastolic blood pressure for men and women alike in both towns receiving high- and low-intensity interventions. Net decreases in the prevalence of smoking for women ranged from 19.2% to 30.6% in the two intervention communities compared to an increase of 0.9% and a decrease of 3.7% for men in the two intervention communities. Quit rates for women were significantly higher in the intervention communities over the control community. The quit rates for men did not differ among communities. Although total lipid cholesterol fell in the intervention communities, the difference was not statistically significant from the control community. Except for a net reduction of 0.5 mm Hg for men in the low-intensity town (not significant), significant decreases were seen in both systolic and diastolic blood pressure among hypertensives in the three communities (systolic: 4.5 to 7.5 mm Hg; diastolic: 3.4 to 6.1 mm Hg). Similar changes were found in the total population in the three communities (64,70,72).

The results of the first-generation community cardiovascular disease prevention studies were perceived as very positive and intervention activities were seen as feasible. Public health proponents saw the projects as demonstrating the unique contribution of population-based health interventions with epidemiology and medical science (17). Communities saw the projects as providing important and valuable resources for community members. By the early to middle 1980s, three very large, heavily research-oriented community cardiovascular disease prevention projects in the United States were funded by the National Heart, Lung, and Blood Institute: the Stanford Five-City Project (FCP); the Minnesota Heart Health Program (MHHP); and the Pawtucket Heart Health Program (PHHP). Although each project had somewhat different theoretical frameworks and intervention plans, they also shared many commonalities. Each of the three

studies attempted to maximize the research rigor of its project.

The Stanford Five-City Project

The Stanford study had five cities, two treatment cities and three control. The intervention consisted of widespread community education through mass media and interpersonal contacts. Intermediary agents such as health professionals were trained to provide lifestyle behavior change advice and education to individuals. Community groups and organizations helped support the change agenda. Activities were conducted in schools, workshops, conferences, and other community forums. The intervention lasted approximately 6 years (25).

Evaluation strategies for trial assessment were ambitious. Four independent cross-sectional surveys of randomly selected households were conducted in the five communities. In addition, four repeated surveys were conducted of a cohort in four of the communities (one control community was not included in the cohort surveying). Blood pressure among normotensives decreased significantly in the treatment communities (−4.3 mm Hg systolic and −2.3 diastolic in the cohort survey). In the cross-sectional surveys, differences peaked in year 3 but were no longer significant by the final cross-sectional survey. A difference in smoking prevalence in the cohort surveys was noted at baseline ($p = .10$, two-tailed), but subsequent data showed no significant decline between communities. None of the other risk factors were significantly reduced in the treatment communities (19,24,25).

The Minnesota Heart Health Program

The Minnesota Heart Health Program (MHHP) had the strongest statistical design of the three second-generation community cardiovascular studies. Three pairs of communities, matched on size, community type, and distance from the university researchers, were assigned to either an educational intervention or control condition. Community organization strategies were used to involve community groups and organizations in promoting cardiovascular disease risk factor reduction. Accepted behavior change theories were used to plan intervention activities. All aspects of the communities were involved including healthcare professionals, schools, adult education, mass media, and environmental arenas such as grocery stores and restaurants (37,55).

Evaluation of the MHHP was comprehensive. Regular cross-sectional surveys were conducted of independent samples of residents. Surveys were conducted of cohorts selected at random from the initial cross-sectional survey. To reduce the risk of remeasurement bias, half the cohort was surveyed 2 years after intervention and the other half 4 years after intervention. The entire cohort was surveyed at the end of the study. Study results overall were disappointing. Although there appeared to be some trends toward risk reduction in specific areas in either the cohort or cross-sectional surveys early in the intervention (e.g., decrease in cholesterol, decrease in smoking prevalence among women reported in the cross-sectional survey, and decrease in diastolic blood pressure), all of those trends except the lower prevalence of female smokers in the cross-sectional survey and increased physical activity in the intervention communities disappeared by the end of the study (41,48).

The Pawtucket Heart Health Program

The Pawtucket Heart Health Program (PHHP) used a two-community design. A community with similar sociodemographic characteristics was selected to be the comparison community for Pawtucket. The PHHP used an intervention framework that was similar to that of the FCP and MHHP. It differed in that it was more closely focused on enrolling individuals in the program so that their use of program activities could be tracked throughout the trial. In addition to established behavior change theories, the PHHP phased in intervention activities in a way designed to first promote awareness of the project, then develop simple skills, and then increase social support for maintenance of behavior change. The program also had a community activation component that recruited individuals and organizations to participate in some part of the project (8,43).

Evaluation of the PHHP was somewhat different because it utilized a comprehensive database of individuals who had participated in some level of the program. Over 42,000 individuals participated in more than 110,000 contacts. In addition to the tracking system of contact, a total of six cross-sectional surveys were conducted over the course of the trial years. By the end of the trial, body mass index was approximately the same in the intervention community as it had been when the trial commenced, but had increased significantly in the control community. There were no significant differences in other cardiovascular risk factor behaviors between the intervention or control community (9).

Single Risk Factor Approaches

Some researchers have wondered whether a focus on changing multiple risk factors might be overly daunting for the public. A number of single risk factor community studies have been conducted with the majority of them focusing on smoking cessation. A few examples follow.

The Australian Studies

A series of community-based antismoking campaigns in Australia commenced in 1978 and used mass media and community programs to encourage smoking cessation. In the "North Coast" study, two test towns, one media only and one media plus community intervention, were compared to a third town (no intervention). The investigators used mass media and focused on behavioral change (i.e., smoking cessation) rather than health outcomes. Media messages were complemented with community programs that distributed smoking cessation kits, aids to assist smokers in quitting, tip sheets, and community-wide events. A baseline survey was followed with a survey from an independent sample 2 years later. Smoking prevalence decreased in both treatment communities; the media plus intervention community decreased its prevalence from 6% to 15% (depending on age and gender), whereas the media only community decreased from 6% to 11%. The control community showed only a 2% to 5% decrease (16).

Another smoking cessation study used Sydney as the intervention community with the rest of Australia as the comparison community. The study intervention was similar to that described for the North Coast study. Change in prevalence was assessed by comparing a preintervention survey with a postintervention survey 1 year later. Although the differences were not statistically significant, Sydney showed a 2.8% decrease in prevalence compared to 1.2% for the rest of Australia (14).

The Community Intervention Trial for Smoking Cessation (COMMIT)

COMMIT has been the only community study with a sufficient number of communities to have good power to detect differences. This study of 11 pairs of communities randomized one community within each pair to an intervention and one to a comparison condition. Within intervention communities, community organization techniques were used to establish a community board and affiliated task forces that would be responsible for implementing the project in the community. Intervention activities were intended to have an impact on every aspect of the community and were organized around public education, healthcare providers, worksites, cessation resources and services, media, and public events. Cohorts of heavy smokers (25 or more cigarettes per day) and light and moderate smokers (less than 25 cigarettes per day) were followed annually, with end-of-study smoking cessation the final outcome. A cross-sectional survey was conducted at baseline and again at the end of the study to assess changes in prevalence (75). In the heavy smoker cohort, there was no intervention effect in cessation. In the cohort of light and moderate smokers, however, smokers in the intervention communities quit at significantly higher rates than comparison communities. The cross-sectional surveys showed a slightly higher decrease in smoking prevalence in the intervention over comparison communities; however, the difference was not significant (76,77).

WORKSITE CARDIOVASCULAR PROJECTS

Worksites may be considered small communities in that groups of people interact regularly in settings that have intensive interrelationships and interdependence. Numerous worksites offer health promotion programs (84), with both employees and employers perceiving benefits of such programs. Many of these programs address one or more cardiovascular disease risk factors (e.g., smoking cessation, blood pressure control, exercise, weight control). Worksites are convenient places for interventions since approximately 60% of adults in the United States work away from home (85).

Many worksite health promotion programs suffer methodological problems as effectiveness studies (e.g., evaluating only those individual employees who volunteer to participate, not randomizing worksites) (26). In recent years, a few worksite studies following the methodology of community studies have been conducted. Two of these will be presented.

The Working Well Trial was the largest randomized, controlled worksite trial conducted in the United States. Although it was focused on cancer prevention, its primary intervention targets were dietary change (reduce fat, increase fiber, increase fruit and vegetable consumption) and smoking cessation—areas that are also important for cardiovascular risk reduction. In the trial, 114 worksites spread throughout Texas and its proximate states, Florida, Massachusetts, and

Rhode Island participated. The worksites employed an average of 316 workers. Intervention activities began with "participatory strategies," which may be considered similar to community organization strategies; various members of the worksite were recruited to serve on an employee advisory board and the advisory board helped plan and implement intervention activities. The activities themselves focused on changes at the environmental (e.g., changes in company cafeterias) and individual levels (e.g., providing self-help materials for change, offering classes) (1). After 2 years of intervention, a cross-sectional survey of employees showed a significant net reduction in fat consumption (−0.37% in calories from fat), significant increases in fiber (0.13 g/1000 kcal) and in fruit and vegetable consumption (0.18 of a serving). Changes in tobacco use were in the desired direction, but were not significant (69).

The Take Heart Program randomized 26 worksites in Oregon to an early or delayed intervention condition (27). The worksites averaged 247 employees each. As with The Working Well Trial, participatory strategies were used for employee input into intervention activities. Cardiovascular risk reduction intervention activities addressed smoking, diet, knowledge of cholesterol level, and physical activity. After 2 years of intervention, there were no significant differences between the early intervention group and the delayed treatment group (which had not yet received intervention) (27). After continued intervention, however, the project showed significant effects on eating behavior in the cohort, but not on cholesterol levels (28).

CONCLUSIONS FROM THE COMMUNITY AND WORKSITE STUDIES

Although community studies that target the reduction of cardiovascular diseases have had mixed results, there are some compelling reasons to continue such efforts at the community and worksite levels. Process measures have indicated that community programs are well utilized (9). It may be that community-based programs have themselves increased the secular trend for change by convincing media and consumer product industries to promulgate messages and products for health behavior change in other communities before trial results were known, thereby accelerating secular trends. Community activities, by providing ongoing intervention messages and activities, enable all individuals in a community to have ongoing access to assistance in behavior change as opposed to the occasional program aimed at those who voluntarily attend a clinic (17,90). Further, evidence is increasing that community interventions lead to sustained community activity when the research study external funding ends (7,47).

IMPLICATIONS FOR HEALTHCARE PROVIDERS

Healthcare providers can have profound effects on the lives of their patients, both in their practices and outside of them. Research indicates that physicians can be influential in smoking cessation, dietary change, diabetes control, hypertension control, and other lifestyle behavior change (40,57,65). Patients tend to see physicians as extremely credible sources of

information and are likely to heed physician advice. Physician advice in the context of an office setting that also promotes health behavior change is especially effective in promoting change (68). Physicians, on the other hand, may be reluctant to provide counsel about behavior change (65).

The influence of the healthcare provider is not limited to the office setting. Because of the high esteem in which the public holds healthcare providers, they can be influential policy makers and advocates in the promotion of cardiovascular health. At the local level, healthcare providers can provide expert testimony for legislative efforts to improve health (e.g., testifying about the harmful effects of exposure to environmental tobacco smoke, urging medicare and medicaid reimbursement for regular cholesterol screening).

Healthcare providers can become involved in media advocacy in communities. Using media advocacy approaches (82), healthcare providers can become involved in advancing a public health initiative (e.g., dietary change, hypertension screening, cholesterol screening). Healthcare providers can also contribute time to follow up on suspicious results of such screening. Collaboration with health voluntary groups, such as the American Heart Association, can take the form of making presentations to groups at worksites or other organizations, sponsoring contests that promote good cardiovascular health, and talking to school children about the importance of their lifestyle in fostering good cardiovascular health. Table 10-3 summarizes a few of the activities that healthcare providers can participate in to become part of community intervention for cadiovascular health.

Table 10-3 Strategies for Physicians to Become Involved in Community-wide Cardiovascular Risk Factor Reduction	
STRATEGY AREAS	**SPECIFIC ACTIVITIES**
Office Practice	• Establish systems to identify patients with cardiovascular risk factors. • Establish systems to discuss cardiovascular risk factors with patients. • Provide plans to patients for behavior change. • Establish reminder systems to follow-up patients at risk.
Advocacy	• Provide expert testimony regarding the need for cardiovascular risk reduction. • Lobby for health promotion. • Join voluntary health groups that are active in health promotion.
Education	• Provide presentations for colleagues and peers. • Provide presentations for students at all levels of education.

SUMMARY

The theoretical underpinnings of community approaches to behavior change go back to the beginnings of sociology and anthropology. A basic premise of the community approach is that large-scale, widespread behavior change is most likely to occur when norms about the behaviors are changed. In an attempt to change those norms, numerous community interventions for cardiovascular risk factor reduction have been conducted in the past 30 years. The results of those studies have been mixed. It remains unclear how much effect can be realized from a large community intervention for change. Despite the mixed results in terms of behavioral outcomes, process evaluation strongly suggests that some people are making changes. Similarly, an overall secular trend for reduced risk factors is strong.

Healthcare providers should take advantage of their influential positions in society by promoting behavior change for good cardiovascular health. This should be done on many levels, including the office practice, office and hospital settings, and in the community. In the case of the community, health care providers can be powerful advocates for behavior change that, in combination with the efforts of other community groups and organizations, can have significant effects of cardiovascular risk factors and cardiovascular disease.

REFERENCES

1. Abrams DB, Boutwell BW, Grizzle J, et al. Cancer control at the workplace: the Working Well Trial. Prev Med 1994;23:15–27.

2. Abramson JH, Gofin R, Hopp C, et al. Evaluation of a community program for the control of cardiovascular risk factors: the CHAD program in Jerusalem. Isr J Med Sci 1981;17:201–212.

3. Ajzen, I. The theory of planned behavior. Organiz Behav Hum Decision Processes 1991;50:179–211.

4. American Heart Association. Http://www.amhrt.org/Scientific/Hsstats98/03cardio.html., 1998.

5. Bandura, A. Principles of behavior modification. New York: Holt, 1969.

6. Blackburn, H. Research and demonstration projects in community cardiovascular disease prevention. J Public Health Policy 1983;4:398–421.

7. Bracht N, Finnegan JR, Rissel C, et al. Community ownership and program continuation following a health demonstration project. Health Educ Res 1994;9:243–255.

8. Carleton RA, Lasater TM, Assaf A, et al. The Pawtucket Heart Health Program, I: an experiment in population-based disease prevention. Rhode Island Med J 1987;70:533–538.

9. Carleton RA, Lasater TM, Assaf AR, et al. The Pawtucket Heart Health Program: community changes in cardiovascular risk factors and projected disease risk. Am J Public Health 1995;85:777–785.

10. Christensen DB, Williams B, Goldberg HI, et al. Assessing compliance to antihypertensive medications using computer-based pharmacy records. Med Care 1997;35:1164–1170.

11. Cohen S, Lichtenstein E, Prochaska JO, et al. Debunking myths about self-quitting: evidence from 10 prospective studies of persons who attempt to quit by themselves. Am Psychologist 1980;44:1355–1365.

12. Committee on Substance Abuse. Tobacco-free environment: an imperative for the health of children and adolescents. Pediatrics 1994;93:866–868.

13. Doll R, Peto R. The causes of cancer: quantitative estimates of avoidable risks of cancer in the United States today. J Natl Cancer Ins 1981;66:1191–1303.

14. Dwyer T, Pierce JP, Hannam CD, et al. Evaluation of the Sydney "Quit for Life" anti-smoking campaign. Part 2. Changes in smoking prevalence. Med J Aust 1986;144:344–347.

15. Earl R, Porter DV, Wellman NS. Nutrition labeling: issues and directions for the 1990s. J Am Diet Assoc 1990;90:1599–1601.

16. Egger G, Fitzgerald W, Frape G, et al. Results of large scale media antismoking campaign in Australia: North Coast "Quit for Life" programme. Br Med J 1983;287:1125–1128.

17. Elder JP, Schmid TL, Dower P, et al. Community heart health programs: components, rationale, and strategies for effective interventions. J Public Health Policy 1993;14:463–479.

18. Farquhar J. The community-based model of life style intervention trials. Am J Epidemiol 1978;108:103–111.

19. Farquhar JW, Fortmann SP, Flora JA, et al. Effects of community-wide education on cardiovascular disease risk factors: the Stanford Five-City Study. JAMA 1990;264:359–365.

20. Farquhar JW, Maccoby N, Wood PD, et al. Community education for cardiovascular health. Lancet 1977;1:1192–1195.

21. Feinleib M. The magnitude and nature of the decrease in coronary heart disease mortality rate. Am J Cardiol 1984;54:2C–6C.

22. Fiore MC, Novotny TE, Pierce JP, et al. Methods used to quit smoking in the United States: do cessation programs help? JAMA 1990;263:2760–2769.

23. Folsom AR, French SA, Zheng W, et al. Weight variability and mortality: the Iowa Women's Health Study. Int J Obes Rela Metab Disord 1996;20:704–709.

24. Fortmann SP, Taylor CB, Flora JA, et al. Changes in adult cigarette smoking prevalence after 5 years of community health education: the Stanford Five-City Project. Am J Epidemiol 1993;137:82–96.

25. Fortmann SP, Winkleby MA, Flora JA, et al. Effect of long-term community health education on blood pressure and hypertension control. Am J Epidemiol 1990;132: 629–646.

26. Glasgow RE, McCaul KD, Fisher KJ. Participation in worksite health promotion: a critique of the literature and recommendations for future practice. Health Educ Q 1991;20;391–408.

27. Glasgow RE, Terborg JR, Hollis JF, et al. Take Heart: results from the initial phase of a worksite wellness project. Am J Public Health 1995;85:209–216.

28. Glasgow RE, Terborg JR, Strycker LA, et al. Take Heart II: replication of a worksite health promotion trial. J Behav Med 1997;20: 143–161.

29. Gofin J, Gofin R, Abramson JH, et al. Ten-year evaluation of hypertension, overweight, cholesterol, and smoking control: the CHAD Program in Jerusalem. Prev Med 1986;15;304–312.

30. Goldberg RJ. Coronary heart disease: epidemiology and risk factor. In: Ockene IS, Ockene JK, eds. Prevention of coronary heart disease. Boston: Little, Brown, 1992:3–39.

31. Goldberg RJ. Temporal trends and declining mortality rates from coronary heart disease in the United States. In: Ockene IS, Ockene JK, eds. Prevention of coronary heart disease. Boston: Little, Brown, 1992:41–68.

32. Goldman L, Cook EF. The decline in ischemic heart disease mortality rates: an analysis of the comparative effects of medical intervention and changes in lifestyle. Ann Intern Med 1984;101:825–836.

33. Gore JM, Dalen JE. Cardiovascular disease. JAMA 1989;261: 2829–2831.

34. Green LW. The theory of participation: a qualitative analysis of its expression in national and international health politics. In: Advances in health education and promotion: Vol 1. Greenwich, CT: JAI Press, 1978:211–236.

35. Gutzwiller F, Nater B, Martin J. Community-based primary prevention of cardiovascular disease in Switzerland: methods and results of the National Research Program (NRP 1A). Prev Med 1985;14: 482–491.

36. Hennekens C, Burring J. Epidemiology in medicine. Boston: Little, Brown, 1987.

37. Jacobs DR, Luepker RV, Mittelmark MB, et al. Community-wide prevention strategies: evaluation design of the Minnesota Heart Health Program. J Chronic Dis 1986;39:775–788.

38. Kaplan NM. The challenge of managing multiple cardiovascular risk factors. Am J Hypertens 1997;10(7 Pt 2):167S–169S.

39. Kawachi I, Colditz GA, Stampher MJ, et al. Smoking cessation and time course of decreased risks of coronary heart disease in middle-aged women. Arch Intern Med 1994;154:169–175.

40. Kottke TE, Battista RN, DiFriese GH, et al. Attributes of successful smoking cessation interventions in medical practice. JAMA 1988; 259:2883–2889.

41. Lando HA, Pechacek TF, Pirie PL, et al. Changes in adult cigarette smoking in the Minnesota Heart Health Program. Am J Public Health 1995;85(2):201–208.

42. Lee IM, Paffenbarger RS, Hennekens CH. Physical activity, physical fitness, and longevity. Aging 1997;9:2–11.

43. Lefebvre RC, Lasater TM, Carleton RA, et al. Theory and delivery of health programming in the community: the Pawtucket Heart Health Program. Prev Med 1987; 16:80–95.

44. Levy RI. Causes of the decrease in cardiovascular mortality. Am J Cardiol 1984;54:7C–13C.

45. Levy RI, Moskowitz J. Cardiovascular research: decades of progress, a decade of promise. Science 1982;217:121–129.

46. Lichtenstein E, Mermelstein R. Review of approaches to smoking treatment: behavior modification strategies. In: Matarazzo JD, Herd JA, Miller NE, et al, eds. Behavioral health: A handbook of health enhancement and disease prevention. New York: John Wiley, 1984:695–712.

47. Lichtenstein E, Thompson B, Nettekoven L, et al. Durability of tobacco control activities in eleven North American communities. Health Ed Res 1996;11(4): 527–534.

48. Luepker RV, Murray DM, Jacobs DR, et al. Community education for cardiovascular disease prevention: risk factor changes in the Minnesota Heart Health Program. Am J Public Health 1994;84: 1383–1393.

49. Maccoby N, Farquhar JW, Wood PD, et al. Reducing the risk of cardiovascular disease: effects of a community-based campaign on knowledge and behavior. J Community Health 1977;3:100–114.

50. McAlister A, Puska P, Salonen JT, et al. Theory and action for health promotion: illustrations from the North Karelia Project. Am J Public Health 1982;72:43–50.

51. McKeown T. The role of medicine: Dream, mirage, or nemesis? Princeton, NJ: Princeton University Press, 1979.

52. Metz JA, Kris-Etherton PM, Morris CD, et al. Dietary compliance and cardiovascular risk reduction with a prepared meal plan compared with a self-selected diet. Am J Clin Nutr 1997;66:373–385.

53. Meyer AJ, Nash JD, McAllister AL, et al. Skills training in cardiovascular health education campaign. J Consult Clin Psychol 1980;48: 129–142.

54. Midgette AS, Baron JA, Rohan TE. Do cigarette smokers have diets that increase their risks of coronary heart disease and cancer? Am J Epidemiol 1993;137:521–529.

55. Mittelmark M, Luepker RV, Jacobs D, et al. Education strategies of the MHHP. Prev Med 1986;15: 1–17.

56. Morrell RW, Park DC, Kidder DP, et al. Adherence to antihypertensive medications across the life

span. Gerontolgoist 1997;37: 609–619.

57. Ockene, JK. Physician-delivered interventions for smoking cessation: strategies for increasing effectiveness. Prev Med 1987;16:723–737.

58. Omenn GS, Thompson B, Sexton M, et al. A randomized comparison of worksite-sponsored smoking cessation programs. Am J Prev Med 1988;4:261–267.

59. Omura Y, Lee AY, Beckman SL, et al. 177 cardiovascular risk factors, classified in 10 categories, to be considered in the prevention of cardiovascular diseases: an update of the original 1982 article containing 96 risk factors. Acupunct Electrother Res 1996;21:21–76.

60. Prochaska JO, Norcross JC, DiClemente CC. Changing for good. New York: Morrow, 1994.

61. Puska P, Salonen JT, Nissinen A, et al. Change in risk factors for coronary heart disease during 10 years of a community intervention programme (North Karelia project). Br Med J 1983;287:1840–1844.

62. Robertson, I. Sociology. New York: Worth Publishers, 1977.

63. Rose G. Sick individuals and sick populations. Br Med J 1981;14: 32–38.

64. Rossouw JE, Jooste PL, Chalton DO, et al. Community-based intervention: the Coronary Risk Factor Study (CORIS). Int J Epidemiol 1993;22:428–438.

65. Roter DL, Hall JA. Patient-provider communication. In: Glanz K, Lewis FM, Rimer B, eds. Health behavior and health education: Theory, research, and practice. 2nd ed. San Francisco: Jossey-Bass, 1997.

66. Salonen JT, Puska P, Kottke TE, et al. Changes in smoking, serum cholesterol and blood pressure levels during a community-based cardiovascular disease prevention program—the North Karelia Project. Am J Epidemiol 1981;114(1):81–94.

67. Schwartz, JL. Review and evaluation of smoking cessation

methods: the United States and Canada. NIH Publication No. 87-2940. Washington, D.C.: U.S. Department of Health and Human Services, 1987.

68. Solberg LI, Kottke TE, Brekke ML. The prevention-oriented practice. In: Ockene IS, Ockene JK, eds. Prevention of coronary heart disease. Boston: Little, Brown, 1992:469–490.

69. Sorensen G, Thompson B, Glanz K, et al. Working Well: Results from a worksite-based cancer prevention trial. Am J Public Health 1996;86:939–947.

70. Steenkamp HJ, Jooste PL, Jordaan PC, et al. Changes in smoking during a community-based cardiovascular disease intervention programme: the Coronary Risk Factor Study. S Afr Med J 1991;79: 250–253.

71. Steenland K. Epidemiology of occupation and coronary heart disease: research agenda. Am J Ind Med 1996;30:495–499.

72. Steyn K, Rossouw JE, Jooste PL, et al. The intervention effects of a community-based hypertension control programme in two rural South African towns: The CORIS Study. S Afr Med J 1993;83; 885–891.

73. Strecker VJ, Rosenstock IM. The health belief model. In: Glanz K, Lewis FM, Rimer BK, eds. Health behavior and health education: theory, research, and practice 2nd ed. San Francisco: Jossey-Bass, 1997:41–59.

74. Syme LS, Alcalay R. Control of cigarette smoking from a social perspective. Annu Rev Public Health 1982;3:179–199.

75. The COMMIT Research Group. Community Intervention Trial for Smoking Cessation (COMMIT): summary of design and intervention. J Natl Cancer Inst 1991;83:1620–1628.

76. The COMMIT Research Group. Community Intervention Trial for Smoking Cessation (COMMIT): I. cohort results from a four-year community intervention. Am J Public Health 1995;85: 183–192.

77. The COMMIT Research Group. Community Intervention Trial for Smoking Cessation (COMMIT): II. changes in adult cigarette smoking prevalence. Am J Public Health 1995;85:193–200.

78. Thompson B, Lichtenstein E, Wallack L, et al. Principles of community organization and partnership for smoking cessation in the Community Intervention Trial for Smoking Cessation (COMMIT). Int Q Community Health Educ 1990–1991;11:187–203.

79. U.S. Department of Health and Human Services. The health consequences of involuntary smoking: a report of the Surgeon General. DHHS Publication No. (CDC) 87-8398. Washington, D.C.: U.S. Department of Health and Human Services, Public Health Service, 1986.

80. U.S. Department of Health and Human Services. Cancer statistics review 1973–1986. NIH Publication No. 89-2789. Washington, D.C.: U.S. Department of Health and Human Services, Public Health Service, National Institutes of Health, National Cancer Institute, 1989.

81. U.S. Department of Health and Human Services. Reducing the health consequences of smoking: 25 Years of progress. A report of the Surgeon General. DHHS Publication No. (CDC) 89-8411. Washington, D.C.: U.S. Department of Health and Human Services, Public Health Service, Centers for Disease Control, Center for Chronic Disease Prevention and Health Promotion, Office on Smoking and Health, 1989.

82. U.S. Department of Health and Human Services. Media strategies for smoking control: guidelines. Publication No. 89-3013. Washington, D.C.: U.S. Department of Health and Human Services, Public Health Service, National Institutes of Health, 1989.

83. U.S. Department of Health and Human Services. The health benefits of smoking cessation: a report of the Surgeon General. DHHS Publication No. (CDC) 90-8416. Washington, D.C.: U.S. Department of Health and Human Services, Public Health Service,

Centers for Disease Control, Center for Chronic Disease Prevention and Health Promotion, Office on Smoking and Health, 1990.

84. U.S. Department of Health and Human Services. 1992 National survey of worksite health promotion activities: summary. Am J Health Promotion 1993;7: 452–464.

85. U.S. Department of Labor. Employment and earnings. Washington, D.C.: Bureau of Labor Statistics, 1992.

86. U.S. Environmental Protection Agency Report. Respiratory health effects of passive smoking: lung cancer and chronic disorders. Washington, D.C.: U.S. Environmental Protection Agency, Office of Research and Development, 1992.

87. Yusuf S, Wittes J, Friedman L. Overview of results of randomized clinical trials in heart disease: I. treatments following myocardial infarction. JAMA 1998;260: 2088–2093.

88. Wenger NK. Physical inactivity and coronary heart disease in elderly patients. Clin Geriatr Med, 1996;12:79–88.

89. Wallach L, Wallerstein N. Health education and prevention: designing community initiatives. Int Q Health Educ 1986;7:319–342.

90. Lichtenstein E, Glasgow RE. Smoking cessation: what have we learned over the past decade? J Consult Clin Psychol 1992;60: 518–527.

Part II.

NUTRITION

Edited by
Johanna T. Dwyer

Introduction to Nutrition

Johanna T. Dwyer

The great physiologist and nutrition scientist Jean Mayer always regarded nutrition as a set of problems to be solved, not as a separate scientific discipline. Nutrition is essentially a way of looking at problems relating to human health and well-being. In order to do that, it must draw on many disciplines, including physiology, medicine, biochemistry, the food sciences, and many of the social sciences. Nutrition-related lifestyle decisions have an impact on both short- and long-term health, quality of life, and disease risk. This section focuses on critical issues that are of special importance in a textbook that is addressed to medicine, exercise, nutrition, and health and provides guidance on how to communicate about them.

The section begins with an overview of our nation's preventively oriented nutrition-related objectives and our progress toward meeting them over the past decade. It discusses some short-term objectives and some longer term trends that will drive the future of nutrition far into the next century and beyond.

The concept of dietary standards and of nutritional status is vital for providing benchmarks against which dietary intakes can be evaluated. This chapter describes the new Dietary Reference Intakes, which have just been issued by the Food and Nutrition Board of the National Academy of Sciences. A brief review of the elements of nutritional status and how it is measured follows. The chapter concludes with a brief overview of various food-based dietary guidance and other nutrition education tools in use in the United States today.

Nutritional needs change over the life cycle. We select two especially vulnerable groups to provide the reader with a sample of why such considerations are relevant. Priscilla M. Clarkson discusses nutritional considerations for the active adolescent. The chapter begins with a brief discussion of body composition in the second decade of life and young adulthood. The influence of dietary intakes and other lifestyle-related factors on body composition, nutrition, and health are discussed. Alice Lichtenstein reviews nutrient needs for aging Americans with an emphasis on nutrition and physical activity. Specific suggestions for well and frail elders in their 60s and beyond are provided.

Nutritional needs also change with physical activity. Joan E. Benson and E. Wayne Askew discuss the special problems of elite athletes. Elite athletes look for any way they can find to get an edge in performance, and their thoughts often turn to special diets and dietary aids. The unique nutritional needs of elite athletes are often neglected, because most recommendations concentrate on recreational athletes. The chapter addresses whether they need to modify their diets and if so, how, and why such modifications are necessary. It includes an examination of various questions athletes often have and some practical advice to optimize performance and health.

In the real world, many experts encounter pitfalls in communicating what they have to tell people about good nutrition. Barbara Moore and Idamarie Laquatra focus on communicating the message about sound nutrition and other lifestyle practices, drawing on their extensive experience working with Dr. Everett Koop, former Surgeon General of the United States, on the "Shape Up! America" campaign. Dr. Moore also draws on her experience working with Weight Watchers to describe what the problems and opportunities are for getting messages out to the public on these important issues. These authors provide some tips for readers who wish to communicate more effectively in the future.

Chapter 11

Healthy People 2010: Nutrition Objectives for the Nation as It Reaches the Third Millennium

Johanna T. Dwyer

Since the beginning of recorded history, human beings have recognized the importance of nutrition as one of the pleasures of life and as necessary to sustaining health and quality of life. However, only within the past 200 years, as the biologic and social sciences grew and flourished, could the relationships between food composition, nutritional status, and health be described and quantified more precisely. During the twentieth century, nutrition and health concerns first focused somewhat narrowly on the classic dietary deficiency diseases, such as protein-calorie malnutrition, rickets, pellagra, scurvy, and the nutritional anemias. With progress in preventing or controlling these dietary deficiency diseases and the infectious diseases, other diseases of more complex etiology became more prevalent. Public health and nutritional science advances since then have permitted the development of better understanding and broader views on the role of dietary factors in these disorders. Today nutrition is recognized as key in promoting health and reducing chronic disease risk, disease progression, debility, and premature death. Dietary factors influence the risks for many of the chronic degenerative diseases that plague our nation. These include coronary heart disease, some types of cancer (e.g., breast, colon, prostate, stomach, and cancers of the head and neck), alcohol-related diseases, type 2 diabetes, and osteoporosis. The latest analyses show that dietary factors are associated with four of the leading causes of death and that the medical costs and other burdens these impose on society are enormous (1). These facts have led medical and public health experts to develop explicit plans for decreasing dietary factors that increase risk and for fostering the health-promoting qualities of diet. For maximal effectiveness, other related preventive and curative health measures must also be implemented in concert with nutritional measures.

This chapter focuses on health planning for prevention in the United States today. The section begins with an overview of our nation's preventively oriented nutrition-related objectives and our progress toward meeting them over the past decade. It then discusses some short-term objectives and some longer term trends that will drive the future of nutrition into the next century and beyond.

FOUNDATIONS OF PROGRESS IN PREVENTION

Progress in prevention, whether it be in nutrition or in some other area, must build on a strong foundation. There are six essential elements that provide the solid ground upon which preventive health services structures can be erected.

First, any preventively oriented program must have a sound scientific basis, including both basic and applied facets. From such a base of evidence, sound dietary recommendations and effective interventions spring.

A second prerequisite to implementing preventively oriented strategies is monitoring and surveillance. A national nutrition monitoring program provides vital information on which status is assessed and progress is measured. In addition, community data collection and surveillance systems must be in place.

The third vital component to effect prevention planning is ensuring access to nutrition information, education, services, and a healthful food supply.

The fourth component is distributive justice, to ensure that persons in all circumstances have access to preventive programs.

Fifth, training and technical assistance to individuals or

groups is vital. Help in implementing interventions from various social institutions is necessary since the very parts of the population most in need, or communities most afflicted with problems, are the least likely to have the resources to implement programs without help.

Sixth, political will is essential. Large-scale programs cost money and demand a degree of societal consensus on the merit of the ultimate goals and objectives.

A seventh essential element, which applies only to nutrition, is that a safe, wholesome, and affordable food supply must be present.

Over the past century, the United States has achieved much in building a preventive services infrastructure. But further strengthening is needed. As we review goals and objectives for the nation, this reality must be kept in mind.

PROMOTING HEALTH, PREVENTING DISEASE: OBJECTIVES FOR THE NATION

In the mid-1970s the need for explicit, measurable prevention objectives for government, private, and voluntary groups became increasingly apparent. The office of the Assistant Secretary for Health in the Department of Health, Education, and Welfare began the process of developing a consensus on some national goals that could guide prevention efforts in the future. The first effort was a slim volume stating general goals and objectives in various areas of public health and preventive medicine and ways to measure progress in achieving them. In the late 1970s, Surgeon General Julius Richmond, who was also Assistant Secretary for Health, commissioned a much larger effort, entitled Healthy People (2). It set forth an ambitious prevention plan, entitled Promoting Health, Preventing Disease: Objectives for the Nation (3). Using a management-by-objectives planning process, the U.S. Public Health Service set out objectives focusing on improving health status, risk reduction, public and professional awareness of prevention, health services and protective measures, surveillance, and evaluation. The objectives were organized into 15 priority areas under the general headings of preventive services, health protection, and health promotion. Targets for achieving the objectives were set; usually with a 10-year time frame. To achieve the objectives, a health system reaching all Americans, integrating personal health care and public health measures, and focusing on the entire population (i.e., population-based measures), was necessary. Most prevention does not occur only within the health system but in community institutions as well, including schools, workplaces, families, and neighborhoods. Therefore, these environments as well as the traditional health care system were included as a focus for the preventive efforts.

Starting in 1980 and at the beginning of every decade thereafter, the Department of Health and Human Services has convened public, private, and voluntary groups to update the plan and assess progress toward achieving goals. It is now customary to issue a "mid-course review" halfway through the decade to make mid-term corrections and to redirect resources, if this should prove to be necessary.

The current prevention plan is entitled "Healthy People 2000." The overall goals are general ones. They are to increase the span of healthy life, reduce health disparities among Americans, and to achieve access to preventive services for all Americans. For each life stage, there are specific objectives stated in terms of reducing mortality. Goals are also set for each priority area. Nutrition is considered as one of these priority areas. In the "Healthy People 2000" document there are 27 nutrition-related objectives. They deal with health status, risk reduction, and service-related issues and set measurable objectives in each area. The latest review of progress was done in 1995 (4). For about two-thirds of all the goals, including many nutrition-related goals, satisfactory progress has been made, and for some the target has been met. For other objectives, little progress has been made, or the trend has been in the wrong direction. These are the areas where particular attention needs to be paid in setting objectives for the future.

Table 11-1 presents the year 2000 goals and progress to date.

Challenges: Unmet Goals

Although substantial progress has been made in reaching the year 2000 goals, there is much remaining to do (Table 11-2). Some of the nutrition challenges that remain are summarized in the tentative nutrition goals for the year 2010, which are listed in Table 11-3.

Next Steps: Goals in Nutrition for 2010

The goals for the year 2010 build on progress to date and include attention to new problems that confront public health in the United States. Drafted objectives are listed in Table 11-3. In the coming years, we can hope that progress toward reaching these working goals will accelerate and reach fruition. The factors that will influence the environment in which these events play out are described in the next sections.

TRENDS THAT WILL SHAPE NUTRITION IN THE THIRD MILLENNIUM

Key trends in science, policy, and politics are shaping new views of the role of diet and its potential contributions to health and will continue to do so in the next century. Many scientific, methodologic, and political issues that these views engender must be addressed by decision makers before public health gains can become reality. As we begin the new millennium, we can further improve health, longevity, and quality of life. Food and nutrition are two fields that can contribute to these efforts.

REVOLUTION IN HUMAN GENETICS
Scientific Basis

Our limited understanding of genetic influences on the risk of human disease is expanding rapidly. The National Institutes of Health's Human Genome Project is now in the process of identifying 80,000 human genes. In the next decades, gene functions will become increasingly clear, but even today, it is obvious that genetic differences are many and that they are more significant to human health than was previously imagined. Epidemiologic studies reveal that common, complex, prevalent chronic diseases as well as rare conditions share

Table 11-1 Status of Sentinel Nutrition Objectives for "Healthy People 2000": Mid-course Review, 1995

OBJECTIVE	FAILED	SUCCEEDED	COMMENTS
Decrease coronary heart disease deaths		×	Achieved over 60% of goal
Decrease overweight prevalence in adults aged 20–74	×		−133% of goal; −200% in men, −114% in women
Decrease growth retardation in low income children under age 5		×	Achieved 300% of goal
Decrease average dietary fat intake in persons over age 2 and decrease percentage of total calories from fat		×	Achieved 40% of goal
Improve weight loss practices among overweight persons, age 18 and over	×		Achieved 40% of goal in women, 60% in men
Increase consumption of foods rich in calcium: pregnant and lactating women should receive 3 or more servings daily	×		Achieved 70% of goal in pregnant and lactating women, and achieved little progress in either women or men aged 19–24 (3 servings or more daily for either sex; men aged 25–50, 2 or more servings daily)
Encourage breastfeeding in early postpartum period, and at 5–6 mo		×?	Slight success (10%) in early postpartum period; no success through 5–6 mo
Encourage use of food labels		×	Achieved 30% of goal
Increase informative nutritional labeling of processed and packaged foods		×	Achieved 20% of goal
Increase availability of reduced-fat processed foods		×	Achieved 125% of goal
Encourage low-fat, low-calorie restaurant food choices		×	Achieved 30% of goal
Increase worksite nutrition and weight management programs, nutrition education		×	Achieved 50% of goal
Encourage weight control		×	Achieved 30% of goal

potent genetic determinants. Genetic influences on risk of these diseases are considerable, and groups at risk can be identified. These diseases include obesity, atherosclerosis, diabetes, hypertension, kidney disease, and many cancers (e.g., breast, colon, and prostate cancer). Epidemiologic studies will be important in evaluating the prevalence of these genetic risk factors and the influences of environmental factors, including diet, on the phenotypic expression of these genotypes.

Genetic makeup imparts individuality in nutritional needs. For some conditions, drugs to alter gene expression or gene therapy may soon be possible. Nutrient-gene interactions may also have great health significance. Clinical trials will provide information on the beneficial roles of nutrients or other food constituents on influencing genetic expression and in preventing or controlling resulting disease. Dietary measures, such as diets high in fiber or fruits and vegetables, are now being tested for their ability to decrease cancer risk in persons with familial hereditary polyposis. In the future, early identification of genetic risks may lead to the development of special foods and dietary measures, just as low-phenylalanine formulas for persons with phenylketonuria or lactose-free formulas and lactose-treated milk for persons with lactase deficiency are now used.

Policy and Politics

While human genetics has made spectacular advances as a science, it has made few strides in harnessing this knowledge to prevent or treat common diseases. At present, the ability to identify genetic influences on disease incidence has unfortunately outstripped the ability to take action to lessen risks or to better the condition of affected individuals. Public confusion is rife about genetics and the appropriate use of human genetic information. This has given rise to justifiable public concerns, including uncertainty about the confidentiality and privacy of genetic testing and fears that results will be used to trigger rejections for health insurance or to fix liability for the costs of care for genetic disease on its victims.

FOOD AND NUTRITION SCIENCE REVOLUTION
Scientific Basis
Biotechnology

Knowledge of the genetics of plants and animals is expanding rapidly. "Designer gene" applications for plants and food animals are much farther along than they are for human genetic engineering. "Biotech" products are present in every supermarket. They include milk from cows treated with bovine somatotrophin to increase milk yields, tomatoes with genes introduced to keep peak flavor, and recombinant enzymes used for manufacturing cheeses. Although the quantity and quality of the food supply may have benefited as a result of these applications, there are as yet few examples of

Table 11-2 Areas Failing to Achieve Goals for the Year 2000

OVERWEIGHT

- The prevalence of overweight has increased substantially since 1976–1980. Americans of all ages are becoming fatter and heavier. A major challenge is to reverse this trend.
- The proportion of self-defined overweight adults who reported that they were consuming fewer calories and exercising more has decreased.
- Worksite nutrition and weight management programs: The proportion of worksites (with 50 or more employees) that offer programs for employees increased from 17% in 1985 to 35% in 1992. But more efforts are needed.

GROWTH RETARDATION AMONG LOW INCOME CHILDREN

- Substantial progress was made for most groups, but the target for black children under age 1 has still not been met, and it needs to be.

NUTRITION ASSESSMENT, COUNSELING, AND REFERRAL BY CLINICIANS

- No data are available in measuring progress toward this objective.

DIETARY FAT INTAKE AMONG CITIZENS AGE 2 AND OLDER

- Average fat and saturated fat intake as percentage of total calories among this group has decreased, and the proportion of the population meeting these goals has increased.
- However, 66% (the majority of the population) still do not meet these goals, and they need to.

AVERAGE INTAKE OF FRUITS, VEGETABLES, AND GRAIN PRODUCTS AMONG PERSONS AGED 2 AND OLDER

- Average intake has increased since 1990, and the proportion of the population meeting the average daily goal has also increased.
- However, 65% (the majority) still do not meet the goals.

CONSUMPTION OF FOODS RICH IN CALCIUM

- Unfortunately, since 1990, the proportion of those in the population who meet recommendations for consumption of calcium-rich foods has changed little or decreased, with consumption still falling short of recommendations for most of the population.
- In 1996, less than 10% of females aged 11 to 24 consumed an average of three or more servings of milk and milk products daily.

SALT AND SODIUM INTAKE

- Here too, there has been little change since the late 1980s in behaviors to reduce salt and sodium intakes, such as purchasing foods with reduced sodium or the avoidance of salt use at the table.

PREVALENCE OF IRON DEFICIENCY

- The prevalence of iron deficiency decreased for low-income children from 1976–80 to 1988–1994.
- However, prevalence has remained essentially constant for all children and for women aged 20–44.

LOW-FAT, LOW-CALORIE FOOD CHOICES IN RESTAURANTS

- Progress is not clear and more efforts are needed.

NUTRITIOUS SCHOOL AND CHILD CARE FOOD SERVICES

- Progress in meeting this objective is not clear, especially with respect to "a la carte" items in school food services.

NUTRITION EDUCATION IN SCHOOLS

- The proportion of states requiring nutrition education has increased since 1990. The percentage of states having such curricula has increased from 60% to 69%. More progress is warranted.

RECEIPT OF HOME-DELIVERED MEALS FOR PEOPLE AGE 65 AND OVER

- In spite of more persons in this age group needing help, there is little change evident since the early 1990s in achieving this goal.

Table 11-3 Nutrition Objectives for "Healthy People 2010" (Draft 1998)

OBJECTIVE	BASELINE	TARGET	COMMENTS
Body Weight Status			
Increase the prevalence of healthy body weight (BMI 19–25) among persons aged 20 and older to 65%	41%	65%	In 1988–1994, only 39% of males and 44% of females were at their healthy weights
Reduce the prevalence of overweight and obesity (BMI > 30) among persons aged 20 and older to no more than 15%	22%	15%	In 1988–1994, 20% of men and 25% of women were overweight or obese
Reduce the prevalence of overweight and obesity (i.e., those over the sex- and age-specific ninety-fifth percentile of BMI) in children aged 6–11 and adolescents aged 12–19 to 5% or less	10–11%	5%	In 1988–1994, 11% of all children and 10% of all adolescents were overweight or obese (using newly revised National Center for Health Statistics, Centers for Disease Control and Prevention [NCHS/CDC] growth charts as the criterion)
Reduce growth retardation among low-income children aged 5 and under to 5% or less	8%	5%	Growth retardation is defined as height-for-age below the fifth percentile of children in the NCHS reference population
Total Fat and Saturated Fat Intake			
Increase the percentage of people aged 2 and older who meet the dietary guidelines' average daily goal of no more than 30% of total calories from fat to at least 75%	33%	75%	
Increase the percentage of people aged 2 and older who meet the dietary guidelines' average daily goal of less than 10% of total calories from saturated fat to at least 75%	35%	75%	In 1994–1996, 35% of people aged 2 and older met the goal
Fruit, Vegetable, and Grain Product Intake			
Increase the proportion of people aged 2 and older who meet the dietary guidelines' minimum average daily goal of at least five servings of vegetables and fruits	40%	75%	In 1994–1996, 40% of people met the goal
Increase the percentage of people aged 2 and older who meet the dietary guidelines' minimum average daily intake of at least six servings of grain products to at least 75%	52%	75%	In 1994–1996, 52% of people met the goal
Calcium Intake			
Increase the proportion of people aged 2 and older who meet dietary recommendations for calcium	45%	Not yet set	In 1988–1994, 45% of people were at or above approximated mean calcium requirements
Sodium			
Increase the proportion of people aged 2 and older who meet the daily value of 2400 mg or less of sodium, consistent with the	30%	Not yet set	In 1988–1994, 45% of people were at or above approximated mean calcium requirements

Table 11-3 continues

Table 11-3 (*Continued*)

OBJECTIVE	BASELINE	TARGET	COMMENTS
Iron Deficiency and Anemia Reduce iron deficiency to 5% or less among children aged 1 and 2, to less than 1% among children aged 3 and 4, and to 7% or less among females of childbearing age Reduce anemia among low-income pregnant women in their third trimester to 23%	Children, aged 1–2, 9% Children, aged 3–4, 4% Nonpregnant females, 11% 29%	Children, aged 1–2, 5% Children, aged 3–4, <1% Nonpregnant females, 7% 23%	Iron deficiency is defined as having abnormal levels of two or more of the following: serum ferritin, free erythrocyte protoporphyrin, and transferrin saturation Anemia is defined according to CDC criteria
Food Habits in Children Increase the proportion of children and adolescents aged 6–19 whose intake of meals and snacks at school from all sources contributes proportionally to good overall dietary quality	Not yet set	Not yet set	The energy-adjusted Healthy Eating Index will be used (see Chapter 14)
Nutrition Education in Public and Private Schools Increase the proportion of the nation's schools that teach all essential nutrition education topics to their students in at least three different grades	Not yet set	Not yet set	Essential nutrition education topics include: the food guide pyramid; benefits of healthy eating; making healthy food choices for meals and snacks; using food labels; eating more fruits, vegetables, and grains; balancing food intake and physical activity; accepting body size differences; and following food safety practices
Increase the proportion of the nation's middle and junior high schools that teach all essential nutrition education topics in at least one required course	Not yet set	Not yet set	Topics to include at the middle school and junior and senior high levels include: dietary guidelines for Americans; eating disorders; healthy weight control; understanding influences on food choices, such as advertising, culture, and emotions; and setting goals for dietary improvement
Increase the proportion of the nation's senior high schools that teach all essential nutrition education topics in at least one required course	Not yet set	Not yet set	
Worksites Increase to at least 50% the percentage of worksites that offer nutrition education and weight management programs for employees	Nutrition education, 18% Weight management, 14%	Nutrition education, 50% Weight management, 50%	Programs should include nutrition or blood cholesterol–lowering groups, workshops, or lectures; and weight management groups, workshops, and lectures

	Table 11-3 (*Continued*)		
OBJECTIVE	**BASELINE**	**TARGET**	**COMMENTS**
Nutrition Services in Primary Care			
Increase to at least 75% the percentage of primary care providers who provide nutritional assessment when appropriate and to at least 75% the percentage that formulate a diet and nutrition plan for patients who need the intervention	(see comments)	75%	In 1992, 53% of pediatricians, 46% of nurses, 15% of obstetricians and gynecologists, 36% of internists, and 19% of family physicians inquired about diet and nutrition. In 1992, 31% of pediatricians, 31% of nurses, 19% of obstetricians and gynecologists, 33% of internists, and 24% of family physicians formulated a diet and nutrition plan
Increase to at least 75% the percentage of physician office visits with patients who have cardiovascular disease at which counseling and educational services are ordered or provided for diet, weight reduction, and cholesterol reduction	(see comments above)	75%	
Increase the proportion of office visits with patients who have diabetes mellitus at which counseling and education services are ordered or provided for diet or weight reduction	(see comments above)		

BMI, body mass index.

recombinant products on the market that confer distinct advantages in terms of a nutrient profile.

Food Composition

Great advances in knowledge of food composition have occurred over the past 25 years. It defies the imagination to remember that 40 years ago, the prevailing dogma was that all the important letters in the nutritional alphabet were known and all that was necessary was to fill in the blanks in tables of food composition with analyses for a few vitamins.

There are many causes for consumer excitement today. Some are negative and involve concerns about disease risk. Government first became involved in food regulation to protect against misrepresentation, adulteration, and damage to health that might occur as the result of food processing. Today, consumers are concerned that old hazards are reappearing. There are concerns about the health risks of both conventional and new, emerging types of foodborne disease. Examples include bovine spongiform encephalopathy (BSE), some of the foodborne pathogenic *Escherichia coli* strains, toxoplasmosis from eating poorly cooked meat, the risks of hepatitis from contaminated food and of HIV infection (albeit rare) from human breast milk, and foodborne *Helicobacter pylori* infection. Some consumers are upset because they have no way of knowing if they are eating foods produced using biotechnology and genetic modification. Irradiated foods continue to be negatively regarded by consumers, even though

numerous scientific bodies have declared them to be safe. The detrimental effects on health of previously poorly characterized constituents, such as trans-fatty acids, that result from processing, concern consumers. The effects of processing on removing or inactivating beneficial substances that were present in the food in its unprocessed form are also worrisome to some.

On the other hand, many consumers see the promise of food as a vehicle for enhancing health in previously unrecognized ways. New functions in health are becoming apparent for such nutrients as folic acid, vitamins B_6, B_{12}, and E, and carotenoids, for example. Food fortification and supplementation with some of these nutrients is now being considered (5). Some food additives, such as butylated hydroxyanisole (BHA) and butylated hydroxytoluene (BHT), are also receiving interest for their antioxidant properties. Other nutrients, such as short-chain fatty acids and stearic acid, are recognized as having different and more beneficial metabolic effects than their more saturated peers.

Hundreds, perhaps thousands, of food constituents with potentially beneficial health effects exist. They include the flavonoids, alpha linoleic acid, and many other classes of complex chemicals found in natural products. The phrase "functional foods" encompasses all of these materials, which, by virtue of their content of physiologically active constituents, might provide health benefits beyond basic nutrition (6). Natural product chemists have only begun the task of filling in the analytical blanks on food composition tables. Much work remains to be done in elucidating the metabolism and effects on health of these substances, however. Until recently, many were not available in purified forms, and their health effects were inferred from studies of populations or groups consuming them as they occurred naturally in foods. Standardized, highly concentrated constituents are available in food products today. This means that individuals can eat very much larger amounts of them than it was possible to do on usual diets in the past (7). However, knowledge about the health effects of high levels of these individual constituents is only now emerging.

Finally, macronutrient replacers and new food ingredients that act as replacements for macronutrients are now either in the regulatory process or already approved (8). They include fat substitutes such as olestra and salatrim, sugar substitutes such as sucralose and acesulfame K, and others.

Lack of Information in Food Composition Databases

Food composition databases are not up to date with respect to many food constituents. Government food analysis efforts are underfunded. Federally produced databases lack product-specific identifying information, which is often critical in distinguishing one product from another, especially with respect to positive attributes. The analyses of individual scientists sometimes provide insufficient identifying or sampling information on the foods studied to link them with federally sponsored efforts. Industry's focus is chiefly on generating food analysis efforts for proprietary products. Trade association efforts to find better analyses of proprietary ingredients as well as whole groups of foods, such as fruits and vegetables, would be helpful.

Policy and Politics
Concerns About Biotechnology

Public attitudes toward genetics and biotechnology, especially toward applications that involve human beings or other animals, are fraught with suspicion.

Food Safety Concerns and Public Trust

The safety of the food supply is perceived by some experts and many in the public at large as lagging behind the health risks posed by new and emerging foodborne diseases and changes in the food supply. The economic and public health consequences of major incidents involving failures of food safety and public confidence are enormous. They go far beyond economic considerations. Such incidents are the nutritional equivalent of land mines, which cost less than a dollar to lay, but $1000 to inactivate. Food safety lapses are viewed as serious failures of whole sectors of society in keeping the trust of the public. They also may incur additional costs later as a result of governmental actions taken in the heat of crisis to counteract what is perceived as a failure of the public's trust. For example, in the late 1970s, an infant formula that was marketed as having a health advantage of being low in sodium was found to be deficient in chloride and associated with potential mental retardation in the infants who were fed it as their sole source of food. This event led to the passage of the U.S. Infant Formula Act and a great deal of regulation of the infant formula indus-

try. Currently, the faith of British consumers has been shaken by fears of "mad cow disease" (BSE). A major restructuring of the animal industry in Britain has resulted.

Confusion About What's What in the Food Regulatory System

The food regulatory framework is currently experiencing growing pains, especially with respect to health claims and "functional foods" (9,10). Often the scientific data to support the putative functional benefit is lacking, and more research will be needed to support these claims. However, regulations also need elaboration. Legal definitions of what constitutes a functional food do not yet exist, nor do current drug, nutrient supplement, and medical food definitions easily encompass these new types of food. Neither lawyers, nor doctors, nor food manufacturers, nor policy makers appear to be certain about what is and is not allowed under current law. All agree that the "rules of the game" and a "level playing field" for all contenders must be established, but the complexity of the food science and concepts involved is considerable. Scientists, lawyers, and manufacturers must work together from early on to make sure that food regulatory changes are made that will benefit public health.

REALITIES OF HEALTH AND DISEASE
Scientific Basis
Greater Understanding of Mechanisms of Disease

Research that provides a basic understanding of the mechanisms of disease causation is essential to developing the means to prevent it. Insights are necessary in molecular and cellular biology as well as at the organ and whole body level. To protect and promote the public health and prevent disease, applied public health research is also necessary. Epidemiology and the other public health sciences can help to provide information on genetic influences and permit assessment of the effects on humans of different doses and exposures to various environmental influences.

Advances in Disease Treatment: Two Steps Forward, One Step Back

As we go forward in conquering disease and people live longer, new diseases and conditions emerge: Thus, we take two steps forward and one step back. Advances in pharmacological and dietary therapy for many acute and chronic diseases continue, but much remains to be done, especially in controlling chronic degenerative diseases. Infectious and foodborne disease problems are still prevalent in some parts of the world, and as the world becomes smaller owing to the ease of international travel, these problems become everyone's problems. Also, new diseases are constantly emerging, as recent epidemics of human immunodeficiency virus (HIV) infection, Legionnaires' disease, and Ebola virus illustrate. In an increasingly global world, all of these health problems are easily exported and leap easily over national borders. The process is facilitated if the countries involved differ greatly in the adequacy of their public and personal health systems and citizens, in their health status. For example, the North American Free Trade Accord (NAFTA) countries (Canada, the USA, and Mexico) differ greatly in the economic status of their populations. As trade barriers fall and population mobility across national borders increases, diseases that were thought to have been vanquished may appear in new locales, including highly industrialized countries.

The development of medical and surgical therapies for both risk factors for and development of overt chronic degenerative diseases is also continuing. But as individuals who formerly perished survive, they may do so with impaired health. Thus, they are victims of medical successes—keeping sick people alive longer. Even if such persons are healthier, this means that the chronic degenerative disease burden of society will also rise, at least in the most advanced age groups.

Shifts from Medical Models to Prevention and Public Health Models

Since the publication of the first volume of the nation's prevention plan in 1976, *Promoting Health, Preventing Disease: Objectives for the Nation*, each successive edition has doubled in size (11). The shift in emphasis from medical model to an integrated prevention and public health model has also proceeded rapidly. The current year 2000 goals stated in Healthy People 2000 encompass thousands of specific, actionable public health objectives for the population as a whole and for various subgroups (12). The goals for the year 2010 will no doubt be even more complete.

The impetus for this rapid expansion of a preventively oriented approach has been both the inherent appeal of primary prevention and fears about the enormous health burdens and costs that are involved in disease treatment if preventable ills are not averted. For example, dietary treatments are usually adjunctive and of only moderate efficacy. Diet is most effective as preventive medicine or early on in the disease process. However, it is also folly to neglect nutritional care of the ill—such a stance is penny-wise and pound-foolish.

Recognition of the Importance of Prevention and Health Promotion

The role of preventive medicine is a key to further advances in health and quality of life. Diet is now recognized as important in health promotion and in the prevention and control of nutritional deficiencies, chronic degenerative diseases, and obesity. Food fortification has been expanded to play new roles, as in fortification of cereal products with folic acid to reduce risks of neural tube defects. The avoidance of dietary excess has potential in helping to control chronic degenerative diseases. The interactions of diet and other environmental factors, such as sedentary lifestyles, cigarette smoking, and use of medication, on disease risk exist. For certain conditions, such as neural tube defects, nutrient supplements may also be important in disease risk reduction.

The Rise of Public Health Approaches

Preventively oriented public health approaches are more palatable than efforts based solely on disease treatment. "Healthy People 2000" (12) is an integrated national prevention plan that includes actionable objectives in over a dozen health areas, including dietary measures. It is updated approximately every 5 years and totally revised each decade. Several models for implementing the objectives are available. For individual diseases or conditions, The National Cholesterol Education Program (NCEP) (13) and the National High Blood Pressure Education Program (NHBP) (14) are two examples of disease-specific comprehensive programs that combine both the high-risk and population approaches to improve the health of the public. These integrated approaches focus efforts on those persons at high risk of coronary artery disease (NCEP) or hypertension (NHBP) who need medical treatment. Both NCEP and NHBP also have educational and public health components that focus on primary prevention. Public health and educational approaches are provided for those in the general population who are at lower risk and who need primary preventive efforts. Population approaches are useful when the health problem or risk factors are very widespread or when risks cannot be easily identified in individuals. Educational efforts include consensus conference documents with care guidelines and training for health professionals and health promotion materials for the public (15).

Another approach to diet-related guidance is to suggest dietary patterns that cut across diseases, rather than dietary and other measures that focus on a single disease. The Food and Nutrition Board of the National Academy of Sciences recently recommended dietary patterns to reduce risks of chronic diseases as a group, rather than focusing on a specific disease (16).

There is also a trend toward the incorporation of preventive measures in individual health services. Those measures thought worthy of such incorporation are described in the Guide to Clinical Preventive Services (15), which emphasizes prevention in medical settings.

Together, these programs and documents provide a solid basis for preventive efforts.

Rise of Spending in Other Sectors to Promote Health: Societies That Promote Health

The health care system today is largely a hospital-based, curatively oriented system, and most "health care" costs are actually spent on the treatment of symptomatic acute conditions. Of course, it is important for all Americans to have access to both preventive and curative medical care. But prevention goes far beyond this. Health insurance is simply a way of ensuring access and controlling costs of medical care services; as such, it does not guarantee that health will result. A newer, more radical view with respect to promoting health is that the broader determinants of health, including food, may be just as, if not more, important than more health care. Health and medical *care* and the development of societal systems that operate for the improvement of health are two very different concepts. Often investments in non–health care sectors (e.g., education, the environment) foster health in a more cost-effective manner than more input directly into the health sector (17). This discovery affords an opportunity for those who are able to demonstrate that what they do, or what they sell, really makes a difference in health outcomes even if they are not traditional health services providers. But these innovations must be truly efficacious, and they must demonstrate efficacy in the same manner that is required to demonstrate efficacy of other health measures.

Policy and Politics

Improved Nutrition Knowledge

Americans are growing increasingly sophisticated in their understanding of food and health connections. They have long understood that foods may contain constituents and toxins that cause disease. They are also aware that foods may be deficient in nutrients or constituents and that these lacks may also cause ill health. Now they also know that it is possible to eat or drink so much excess food and supplements that it makes them sick. The notion that food provides positive health benefits is an old one. It is not clear if people understand what "nutraceuticals" and "functional foods" can and cannot do (18,19).

Nutrition Monitoring and Surveillance Advances

The scientific basis to justify and better target primary and secondary prevention is now available. Integrated health and nutrition monitoring and surveillance efforts at the federal level have greatly improved. It is now possible to measure the burdens of disease and disability on various subgroups in the population and to monitor changes in them over time. Information is also increasingly available on the associations of demographic shifts with disease burdens, and the costs of such illnesses to society (16). With better targeting in the future it may be possible to prevent ills that are prevalent today among those who have the disadvantages of extreme youth, advanced age, low socioeconomic status, minority status, and chronic illnesses. Failure to do so will further increase health care costs.

Confusion About How Best to Modify the Food Supply

Advances in food science and technology have come so fast that there is currently a lack of consensus about how best to modify the food supply to take advantage of new scientific developments for improving the public health. One school favors *traditional food-based approaches*. Federal nutrition education materials, such as the US Department of Agriculture (USDA) food guide pyramid and the USDA-US Department of Health and Human Services (USDHHS) dietary guidelines for Americans, favor such approaches (20,21). The Diet and Health Report of the National Academy of Sciences also advocates modifications in dietary patterns using foods (16). Most of the professional and voluntary associations, such as the American Heart Association, the American Cancer Society and the American Dietetic Association, also favor food-based approaches. Some groups, such as "Oldways," favor a return to various traditional ethnic cuisines, and they have popularized various food guide pyramids that encourage this. Vegetarians favor food guides that emphasize lacto-ovo-vegetarian or lacto-vegetarian patterns. Other groups, including many in the food industry, advocate greater use of fortified, designer, bioengineered, functional, and medical foods within such food-based approaches.

A second school of thought favors reliance on *dietary supplements*, both of nutrients and botanicals. There is good evidence on the efficacy of nutrient supplements for some purposes, such as preventing deficiency disease. However, with a few exceptions (such as folic acid and neural tube defects), there is little agreement on the role of supplements in decreasing risks of chronic degenerative diseases, the aging process, or other illnesses. Evidence is also lacking on whether many "nutraceuticals" or "functional foods" actually have any beneficial effects on health or performance. Concerns center on whether the purported benefits of nutrient supplements have been substantiated, whether the preparations on the market are standardized and truly efficacious, and their costs. Opinions are even farther apart on the efficacy on the use of botanicals and herbal preparations and concentrates of these substances. There is uncertainty about the uniformity of such substances, whether they are safe at high levels rather than the relatively low levels that are usually found in nature, about their efficacy in improving health, and about the hazards that are involved when they are used by individuals in place of more efficacious therapies to treat disease.

Citizens Need Help in Making Behavior Changes to Optimize Diets

People are confused about what they need to eat, drink, or swallow to achieve optimal health. They do not know where to turn for objective, practical advice. If and when consumers *do* decide to modify their diets, they will need help in doing so. Health professionals need to develop the tools that will help consumers.

Most of the adjustments in diet and health that are needed today to lessen chronic degenerative disease involve multiple changes in eating behavior and dietary patterns over the long term. But these changes are more difficult to achieve than modifying a single behavior, such as smoking. Any means that can be found to make the process easier for people should be investigated. Sound nutrition education is key, and much progress has been made, but much remains to be done.

Rise of Health Self-Care and Self-Treatment

There has been a decline in the public's trust of traditional health care providers that has made self-care appealing to consumers. Also, one result of health care rationing and spiraling health care costs is that people are looking for ways to treat their illnesses that do not involve paying a doctor out of pocket. Also health information is readily available to everyone. All of these factors have contributed to the rise in self-diagnosis, self-treatment, and self-care. This trend is not confined to the poor or those who lack education; it extends to individuals of all ages and incomes. Self-directed health improvement approaches, including interactive computerized dietary analysis and behavior change programs, classes, "virtual" self-help groups on computer or over the Internet, and 1–800 or 1–900 numbers to reach nutrition resource centers staffed by knowledgeable health professionals, are in the offing or already available.

Over the past few years, more and more drugs formerly available only by prescription have become available over the counter. In a society that is increasingly turning to self-treatment with these and other medications, the likelihood of drug-drug and drug-nutrient interactions increases along with these developments.

Self-diagnosis and self-medication have both economic and health risks. The markets for self-prescribed medications and alternative therapies are growing rapidly, even as efforts to tame health care costs continue unabated. If the medications are not efficacious, much money and time are wasted. The problem with many of the dietary self-care measures that people currently use (such as natural and organic foods and alternative herbal, botanical, and other therapies) is that their efficacy in really improving health outcomes is questionable. The health risks involved chiefly result from lack of information about when self-treatment efforts should cease and professional help should be sought. Fortunately most self-treatment efforts appear to be complementary to conventional medical treatment. However, some people substitute self-treatment for medical care, and this may be dangerous. It is essential that self-care information be sound, reasonable, and actionable.

COMMUNICATIONS REVOLUTION

Fifty years ago, the print media and radio were the dominant mass media. Today, television and radio have supplanted other sources for information; very few people are readers, and print media are no longer the major source of information. Television is king. Another development is the growth of the Internet and other computer networks that benefit from the low costs of local phone calls. Computerized information networks now broker information and have created new, decentralized worldwide information networks.

The communications revolution has immensely increased the quantity of information available to the public on scientific developments that involve diet and health. However, the quality of information provided over all of these channels is highly variable. It ranges from legitimate science-based, objective reports to incomplete and distorted views, but all of it influences consumers. Consumers in a sense are more "nutrition savvy" than ever before, but in another sense they are pitifully trusting and naive about media sources. Apparently, they assume more regulation over the quality of information exists than is actually the case.

There is no doubt that improved consumer communication and education about healthy living, including diet, are essential. In the past 20 years, federal information efforts, including the Dietary Guidelines for Americans, the USDA food guide pyramid, and nutrient labeling of processed foods, have greatly increased the availability of objective dietary recommendations and information about food. A more proactive role from government is unlikely in the future, given current downsizing of government and the anti-government and anti-regulatory views of much of the public. Actionable, objective, diet and food–related information and messages still need to come from somewhere. One recent development is the growth of third party endorsements by professional associations. These include endorsements of grapefruit (American Cancer Society), many low saturated fat, low-fat products (American Heart Association), and nutrition education messages (McDonalds and the Society for Nutrition Education). These sorts of arrangements have both benefits and risks which have been discussed elsewhere (22).

DEMOGRAPHIC REVOLUTION

The demographic revolution must also be considered. The aging of America and Western Europe, as well as other industrialized countries in Asia, and the growth of the number of elders mean that patterns of disease and disability have also changed. The growth of poor minority populations has increased the incidence of some diseases. In most countries, the gaps between rich and poor are also growing. Changes in the status of women and their role in the work force are also apparent. Women have less time and perhaps less desire to cook and perform other household chores. All Americans, including women, eat more meals outside of the home than ever before. All of these trends mean consumer demands for food are changing.

GOVERNANCE REVOLUTION

Decline of the Nation-State

Throughout the world, the role of nation-states and the power of national governments are declining in importance. In many countries, including the U.S., anti-government, anti-regulatory sentiments go beyond concerns about budgets and the costs of publicly funded programs. They also involve often deep public mistrust of government actions and a lack of consensus on the proper role of government in society. The power gap has been partially filled at the national level by nongovernmental organizations, including voluntary, private, and nongovernmental networks or groups. But many functions have not been picked up by any sector. This has left a power vacuum. Within this country, budgetary concerns and problems, such as health care for the poor or public welfare programs, are passed along from one level of government to another without being resolved either by government or nongovernmental groups. The public health and regulatory infrastructures are increasingly underfunded and ill-prepared to play a role. These developments have potent implications for public health and food safety. Both public health services and regulation have traditionally been considered functions of national and local governments. As states do less and less, less is likely to be done. Unless new roles and new structures are developed for dealing with problems by voluntary and private sector nongovernmental organizations, the public health system could deteriorate.

At the international level, international organizations, nongovernmental networks, and multinational organizations are partially filling the gaps created by the decline of the nation-state. Nongovernmental organizations are playing an increasing role in influencing regulations. These include not only multinational companies but professional and trade organizations. The International Life Sciences Institute (ILSI) is one relevant example of such an institution, which funds scientific studies on issues related to food and nutrition. The most effective private companies and associations in the future are likely to be those that use informational and communications technology networks to their advantage. So equipped, they will be in a good position to forge strong links and working relationships between nongovernmental organizations, others in the private sector, and governments.

Globalization

Global markets and regional economic integration are increasing in importance. These supranational bodies, rather than national governments, are increasingly setting the economic and health rules of the food marketplace. The public has continuing concerns about food safety and "wholesomeness" in the face of regional and international economic integration. For example, the advent of NAFTA has stimulated the fears of many Americans that industries are moving south to "get away with" lower labor costs and environmental standards.

Regional and international regulatory bodies have the potential for rationalizing health and safety regulations at the same time that they facilitate international trade. But they are not free of politics either. These entities occasionally promulgate health and food safety regulations that are based not on science and health protection criteria but rather on economic or other considerations. They may extend local or regional preferences for a domestic trade advantage by creating artificial trade barriers.

Global multinational companies are no longer feared as representing a specific country's interests. Current worries about multinational companies are that they are not firmly connected to *any* country. Critics view multinationals as having narrow special interests involving only a few issues with potential impacts on their businesses. Critics say that the companies show little concern for any population in any country. Corporate management is accused of exhibiting no sense of responsibility or having no reason for investing in societal infrastructures that foster the general public welfare. Whether these perceptions are true or false is debatable. What is clear is that these perceptions must be dealt with by the companies.

Globalization of Food Regulations

The trend toward the globalization of food safety regulations is proceeding rapidly. Although there do not appear to be insurmountable problems or obstacles in the way of global harmonization of regulations, experience with the General Agreement on Tariffs and Trade (GATT) and NAFTA suggests that the process will be slow. The various actors come with very different views of the adequacy of proof of efficacy and with varying regulatory perspectives. For example, Europeans and Asians permit merchandising of dietary supplements and alternative medicines with far more latitude for making health claims than has been traditional in this country. The public health benefits of such laissez-faire approaches are not apparent, although the marketing advantages are evident.

Globalization of Dietary Standards

Dietary standards in industrialized countries are being reformulated, and increasingly, this is being done collaboratively. For example, Canada and the U.S. have issued their next Dietary Reference Intakes conjointly, and in the future Mexico is likely to join as well (23). The European Union countries are also working more closely together. The United Nations agencies have also been active; the World Health Organization has published nutrient reference standards that apply to all countries; and the Food and Agricultural Organization provides international standards for food ingredients in the Codex Alimentarius. In the future, the range of "accept-able" upper and lower nutrient values that are safe will probably be increasingly endorsed by many countries. The same approach may extend to regulations on safe intake levels of ingredients in functional foods and to regulations governing these and other food products.

SUMMARY

The future cannot be predicted. It must be invented. To ensure that the impact of diet on health is positive, action is required to make the vision of better health and nutrition for all a reality. Government; the food, pharmaceutical, and health industries; and the other private sector groups must be key players in these efforts. To the extent that all actors in society attempt to steer their organizations responsibly with the same common ultimate objectives of improving human health in view, the goal of health for all is more attainable than ever before.

Research to Expand Fundamental and Applied Knowledge

Research must continue. Since 1900, biologic science in general and the food and nutritional sciences in particular have made astonishing discoveries that can improve human health and welfare. We do not know enough. We must continue to expand our fundamental understandings of biology involving health, disease, and their genetic and environmental causes, including those that involve food and nutrition. Food and health–related industries need to help support this research to a much greater extent than they have lately.

Wise Food and Nutritional Policies with Health Goals

We must articulate these new understandings of the biology of food and nutrition in wise policies. Scientific knowledge itself and the development of technologies to apply it are two critical substrates necessary for ensuring that advances in biology will be applied for human benefit. However, the facilitating roles of the larger economy, social well-being, political will, and distributive justice are also important. History suggests that to speed application of biologic science advances to better human health, attention must be paid to distributive justice, access to health care, healthier environments, and preventively oriented strategies without neglecting access to disease treatment. The application of preventive and curative medical measures delivered by the health sector is critical in achieving health goals, but other institutions in society must also play increasingly important roles if we are to have societies that truly promote health in the third millennium.

The American food industry and its trade associations have a long and proud record of enhancing food safety that dates from the efforts of Harvey Wiley (the first director of the Food and Drug Administration) early in this century. They have also played a generally positive role in improving nutritional status and the public health by creating a safe, wholesome, and affordable food supply with options that can accommodate many dietary choices. Now they must meet the new challenges by developing safe products that are truly efficacious in enhancing the health of the public.

Programs That Involve New Collaborations Between Sectors

Policies must be put into practice in programs that enhance health and quality of life for all Americans. This will involve rethinking how best to ensure the conjoint application of new scientific advances in preventive and curative medicine at both the individual and societal level to realize the potential of the new biology. Policies inevitably also involve politics. Government has a legitimate role in determining and enforcing the rules of the game so that the social good that can result from sound food, nutrition, and health policies is realized. In this era of downsizing of governmental efforts, public health and curative medicine efforts must be joined in new ways that include all societal institutions, not only government, as responsible participants in reaching solutions on questions involving food, nutrition, and health.

Responsible Food, Drug, and Health Care Industries with Public Health Goals

Food production, pharmaceutical marketing, and health care are not simply economic activities; they also involve social values. Therefore, the leaders of these industries must base their actions on a sense of responsible stewardship of the public's health as well as on economic objectives.

There is a danger that, if specific companies within these industries or whole industries adopt more limited objectives that focus solely on private gain or market share with little concern for positive consequences on health, society as a whole may suffer. The public may view the entire industry as irresponsible and as part of the problem rather than part of the solution, and unfortunate political consequences may result. Also, the immense positive contributions that these industries might otherwise make are unlikely to be realized.

In conclusion, enlightened public, private, and voluntary sectors' efforts and collaborations, based on a sense of responsible stewardship, must be put into action for public health benefit if the potential of functional foods is to become a reality in improving diet and health.

Note: The project has been funded at least in part with federal funds from the U.S. Department of Agriculture, Agricultural Research Service, under contract 53/3-K06-5-10. The contents of the article do not necessarily reflect the views or policies of the U.S. Department of Agriculture.

REFERENCES

1. Frazao E. The American diet: a costly problem. Food Review 1996;19:2–6. Washington, DC: U.S. Department of Agriculture, Economic Research Service.

2. U.S. Department of Health and Human Services. Healthy people: The Surgeon General's report on health promotion and disease prevention. Washington, DC: U.S. Department of Health and Human Services, 1979.

3. Office of the Assistant Secretary for Health, U.S. Department of Health and Human Services. Promoting health, preventing disease: objectives for the nation. Washington, DC, 1980.

4. U.S. Department of Health, Education, and Welfare, Public Health Service. Healthy people 2000: midcourse review and 1995 revisions. Washington, DC: U.S. Department of Health and Human Services, 1995.

5. Finlay JW. Designer foods: is there a role for supplementation/fortification? In: American Institute for Cancer Research. Phytochemicals in cancer prevention and treatment. New York and London: Plenum Press, 1996:213–226.

6. Clydesdale FM. What scientific data are necessary? In: Clydesdale FM, Chan Soh Ha, eds. First International Conference on East-West Perspectives on Functional Foods. Nutrition Reviews 1995;(suppl): 195–198.

7. Dwyer J. Is there a need to change the American diet? In: American Institute for Cancer Research. Phytochemicals in cancer prevention and treatment. New York and London: Plenum Press, 1996:189–197.

8. Runhel A, Race J. Regulatory and legal aspects of functional foods. S 156–161 In: Clydesdale FM, Chan Soh Ha, eds. First International Conference on East West Perspectives on Functional Foods. Nutrition Reviews 1997;54(suppl):S1–S202.

9. Tillotson JE. America's foods: health messages and claims: scientific, regulatory, and legal issues. Boca Raton, Florida: CRC Press, 1993.

10. Glinsmann WH. Functional foods in North America. In: Clydesdale FM, Chan Soh Ha, eds. First International Conference on East-West Perspectives on Functional Foods. Nutrition Reviews 1997;54(suppl): S1–S202.

11. U.S. Department of Health, Education, and Welfare. Promoting health, Preventing disease: objectives for the nation. Washington, DC, 1976.

12. U.S. Department of Health and Human Services. Healthy people 2000. Washington, DC, 1990.

13. National Cholesterol Education Program. Bethesda, MD: National Institutes of Health, U.S. Department of Health and Human Services, 1990.

14. National High Blood Pressure Education Program. Bethesda, MD: National Institutes of Health, U.S. Department of Health Human Services, 1990.

15. U.S. Preventive Health Services Task Force Guide to Clinical Preventive Services. Philadelphia: Williams and Wilkins, 1995.

16. Committee on Diet and Health. Diet and health: recommendations to reduce chronic disease risk. Food and Nutrition Board. Washington, DC: National Academy Press, 1989.

17. Beaglehole R, Bonita R. Public health at the crossroads. Cambridge: Cambridge University Press, 1997.

18. Hillian M. Functional foods: the Western consumer viewpoint. S189–194 In: Clydesdale FM, Chan Soh Ha, eds. First International Conference on East-West Perspectives on Functional Foods. Nutrition Reviews 1997; 54:(suppl):S1–S202.

19. Hillian M. The coming boom(er) market. Food Insight 1997;

(March–April): Washington, DC: IFIC Foundation, 1997.

20. U.S. Department of Agriculture. Food guide pyramid. Washington, DC, 1992.

21. U.S. Department of Agriculture, U.S. Department of Health and Human Services. Dietary guidelines for Americans. Washington, DC: U.S. Government Printing Office, 1995.

22. Tobin DS, Dwyer JT, Gussow D. Cooperative relationships between

professional societies and the food industry: opportunities or problems? Nutrition Reviews 1992;50: 1–8.

23. Committee on Dietary Reference Intake, Food and Nutrition Board. Dietary reference intakes: calcium and related nutrients. Washington, DC: National Academy Press, 1997.

Chapter 12

Nutritional Considerations for the Active Adolescent

Priscilla M. Clarkson

INTRODUCTION

Adolescence is a period of great change. Starting with the onset of sexual maturation, these individuals undergo the second highest peak growth velocity of their lives, endure dramatic alterations in body composition, and then end as a mature adult. Both height (stature) and weight increase during adolescence. Fat free mass (FFM) increases linearly in childhood with little difference between boys and girls up to adolescence (1). At adolescence, there is a growth spurt in muscle mass for boys, and at the end of adolescence, males have 1.5 times more FFM than females. Males also have a greater increase in stature. For females, there is an increase in fat mass that continues during adolescence, while males show a plateau during this time. FFM per unit height at the end of adolescence is about 0.36 kg/cm of body height for males and 0.26 kg/cm of body height for females (1). This growth from puberty to young adulthood must be supported by adequate nutrition.

Providing recommendations regarding nutrition for adolescents is problematic because the changes that occur happen at different ages in different individuals. The recommended dietary allowances (RDA) established by the Food and Nutrition Board provide some guidelines for requirements but these are stated by chronological, rather than matura-tional, age: 11 to 14, 15 to 18, and 19 to 24 years (2). Moreover, these recommendations are based on few actual studies of adolescents, and often information is interpolated from data on adults and children.

Little is also known about nutritional requirements for those adolescents who participate in vigorous exercise, especially those involved in competitive sports. Because the stress of vigorous exercise is superimposed on that of growth, it is especially important that adolescent athletes meet nutritional requirements. This chapter will review the nutritional require-ments of adolescents, examine the extent to which adolescents meet these requirements, provide information on dietary habits of adolescent athletes, and discuss factors influencing nutrition behaviors.

ENERGY INTAKE

Before reviewing studies that examined nutritional intake of adolescents, it is necessary to briefly discuss errors associ-ated with measurement techniques. Most studies assessing eating patterns and nutrient intake have used surveys of large populations or have assessed diets in selected populations by using food records or diaries and food frequency question-naires (3). For a detailed review of the strengths and weak-nesses of these assessment techniques, see Pao and Cypel (4). There can be many sources of error in examining nutritional intake (3,5). Factors that contribute to measurement errors are 1) respondent biases, 2) interviewer biases, 3) respondent memory lapses, 4) incorrect estimation of portion sizes and tendencies to overestimate low intake and underestimate high intakes, 5) supplement use that is not always taken into account, 6) coding and computation errors, and 7) errors associated with computer programs and associated databases (2).

Subjects underreport what they have eaten, so that all diet surveys tend to underestimate dietary intake (2,5). Studies assessing energy expenditure by doubly labeled water assess-ment and self-reported energy intake found that reported intakes tended to be lower than expenditure, thus underestimating true energy intake (6). Because of the errors described above, deviations of 25% or less from the RDA are acceptable. Little information exists on assessment errors specifically in adolescents.

There is a large variability in the timing and degree of the growth spurt, which lasts about 24 to 36 months, differing among individuals (7). Also the physical activity patterns of adolescents vary widely. These differences make it difficult to estimate nutritional needs of adolescents. Recommendations for energy intake should be viewed with caution, and adjustments made for maturation level, growth spurt timing, and physical activity level. Table 12-1 provides equations to estimate energy needs for males and females. These values are adjusted for weight and activity level as described in the table. However, expressing energy intake by height has also been used (8).

The Third National Health and Nutrition Examination Survey (NHANES III) assessed nutritional intake of 711 adolescents, aged 12 to 15, and 765 adolescents, aged 16 to 19 (9). Table 12-2 presents the NHANES III results for these adolescents. Males of all ethnicities had higher caloric intakes than females, but all values for males and females were similar or slightly lower than the RDA estimated requirements. This is interesting in light of the fact that the incidence of obesity is on the rise, suggesting that these values are likely underestimated (10). There was an increase in energy intake, by about 100 to 200 kcal, reported in the NHANES III compared with NHANES II for adolescents. Also, although mean values may indicate adequate nutrition, there will always be those individuals who fall considerably below (or above) the mean level. For example, there is a growing number of adolescents, especially females, who are restricting caloric (energy) intake to achieve a slim appearance.

Several studies are available that have assessed nutritional intake of adolescent athletes, and it appears that some adolescent athletes are ingesting sufficient calories, while others are not. Berning et al (11) reported that adolescent male and female swimmers (14 to 18 years of age) were ingesting 5222 and 3572 kcal/day, respectively, and Hawley et al (12) reported that male and female swimmers ingested 3072 and 2130 kcal/day, respectively. Rankinen et al (13) found that male ice hockey players (mean age, 12) ingested 2429 kcal/day. These values generally reflect marginal to adequate energy consumption.

Athletes who participate in sports where leanness is emphasized for performance, such as running, or for aesthetic reasons, such as gymnastics and dance, are often restricting caloric intake to maintain low body weights (1). From the recommendations provided in Table 12-1, a 12-year-old girl who weighs 40 kg and is engaged in strenuous physical activity should ingest about 2345 kcal. However, many adolescent athletes ingest less than 1500 calories per day. Benson et al (14) reported that 92 female ballet dancers, ranging in age from 12 to 17 years, who were enrolled in professional schools had an average caloric intake of 1890 kcal/day. However, 44 (48.1%) of the dancers ingested less than 1800 kcal/day, 27 (28.9%) ingested less than 1500 kcal/day, and 10 (10.8%) consumed less than 1200 kcal/day. For a group of 14 ballet dancers ranging in age from 12 to 17, Clarkson et al (15) reported an average

caloric intake of 1776 kcal/day. Another study (16) of young dancers (mean age, 16.4) found that the average caloric intake was 1584 kcal/day with 13 (42%) of the 32 dancers ingesting less than 70% of the RDA for calories.

Table 12-1 Estimates for Recommended Energy Intake for Adolescents Based on Body Weight and Activity Level

	Equation to Derive REE (kcal/day)	Multiples of REE Recommended for Light to Moderate Activity*
Boys (age)		
11–14 yr	17.5 × body weight	1.70
15–18 yr	(kg) + 651	1.67
Girls (age)		
11–14 yr	12.2 × body weight	1.67
15–18 yr	(kg) + 746	1.60

REE, resting energy expenditure.
* For adolescent athletes, the adjustment factor should be about 2.1 for males and about 1.9 for females, which reflects heavy exercise/training.
An example of calculations for a 40-kg, female, age 13:
REE = (12.2 × 40) + 746 = 1234 kcal
To adjust for light to moderate activity, multiply by 1.67:
1234 × 1.67 = 2060 kcal
source: Food and Nutrition Board. Recommended dietary allowances. 10th ed. Washington DC: National Academy Press, 1989.

Table 12-2 Energy Intake (kcal) and Protein, Carbohydrate, and Fat (% of Total Energy) of Adolescents

	Males		Females	
	Mean	SE	Mean	SE
Energy				
12–15 yr	2578	87	1838	46
16–19 yr	3097	96	1958	57
Protein				
12–15 yr	14.2	0.3	13.5	0.3
16–19 yr	14.4	0.3	14.1	0.3
Carbohydrate				
12–15 yr	54.0	0.8	54.4	0.8
16–19 yr	49.6	0.9	52.4	0.9
Fat				
12–15 yr	33.1	0.6	33.7	0.7
16–19 yr	34.6	0.6	34.4	0.7

SE, standard error.
source: Centers for Disease Control and Prevention, National Center for Health Statistics, Advance Data 255, 1994.

Loosli et al (17) reported that a group of 97 adolescent gymnasts averaged only 1838 kcal/day. This latter study was published in 1985, and the body weights of gymnasts have dropped since that time. In a more recent study, Benson et al (18) found that Swiss gymnasts ingested 1544 kcal/day. When expressing the results as a ratio of body weight, Loosli et al (17) in 1986 found that gymnasts were ingesting 42.6 kcal/kg of body weight, while in 1990, Benson et al (18) reported that the gymnasts were ingesting 39.5 kcal/kg, showing a trend for lower food intake over time.

Adolescent female runners were found to consume an average of 1912 kcal/day for those who were amenorrheic and 1644 kcal/day for those who were eumenorrheic, a nonsignificant difference (19). Junior high and high school female cross-country runners had an average energy intake of 2488 kcal, which was slightly below the calculated energy needs (20). Wiita et al (21) reported that adolescent female runners (mean age, 16) had an average caloric intake of 2150 kcal, and when assessed 3 years later, the intake significantly decreased to 1647 kcal. The runners at age 19 were significantly heavier and taller but had lower energy intake.

To what extent these findings for athletes may be the result of underreporting is not known. Even taking this into account, there is still an alarming number of young girls who may not be ingesting sufficient energy. Insufficient intake of calories during the growth spurt can negatively affect growth (7). Pugliese et al (22,23) reported that caloric restriction during adolescence resulted in growth retardation. In one study, 24 swimmers and 22 gymnasts were followed for a little over 2 years to assess whether intense physical activity during puberty could alter growth potential (24). At the start of the study, only 1 (5%) of the gymnasts and 6 (25%) of the swimmers had achieved menarche, and during the course of the study, 11 (50%) of the gymnasts (mean age, 14.5) and 17 (71.4%) of the swimmers (mean age, 12.9) achieved menarche. Gymnasts showed reduced stature caused mainly by a marked stunting of lower limb growth. Theintz et al (25) also found that fathers and mothers of gymnasts were significantly shorter and lighter than parents of swimmers and controls. Thus it is difficult to attribute short stature of athletes to nutrition or physical activity alone, as there may be selection for body type in the sport.

MACRONUTRIENTS

The recommended proportions of protein, carbohydrate, and fat in a diet that is sufficient in energy are 15%, 55%, and 30% of total calories, respectively. The results of protein, carbohydrate (CHO), and fat intake for adolescents from the NHANES data are presented in Table 12-2. These values are similar to other reports (7).

Most surveys found that 12% to 15% of energy intake is from protein, which appears to be adequate for most adolescents (7,10). One study of adolescent females found that about a third of vegetarian (lacto-ovo) and semi-vegetarians had protein intakes below their own requirements, while only a quarter of the nonvegetarians did (26). The percent of energy intake from carbohydrate has been found to be about 48% to 52%, which is slightly lower than the recommended levels (7,10). However, fat intake is somewhat higher than

desirable (34% to 39%), although fat intake has been declining over the years (10).

It is recommended that athletes also achieve 55% of their total calories from CHO, since it is the major fuel for physical activity. For adolescent female cross-country runners, the percent of energy from protein, CHO, and fat of total energy intake was 15.5%, 49.5%, and 34.5%, respectively (20). Baer et al (19) reported that adolescent female runners ingested 13.6% protein, 50% CHO, and 36.9% fat. Berning et al (11) found that male adolescent swimmers ingested 12.6% protein, 45.6% CHO, and 42.8% fat. The corresponding percentages for the female adolescent swimmers were 12.0%, 47.9%, and 41.4%, respectively. Adolescent male ice hockey players ingested 16% protein, 48.7% CHO, and 35.3% fat (13).

Adolescent ballet dancers were ingesting adequate amounts of protein, but fat intake was high for some dancers, with one-quarter of the dancers ingesting more that 40% of their calories as fat (14). Also, carbohydrate intake for the group averaged 49.8% of total calories. Similar results were found for the gymnasts, in whom the percent of energy from protein, CHO, and fat was 15%, 49%, and 36%, respectively (17). A later study of gymnasts showed a lower fat intake, with percent energy from protein, CHO, and fat averaging 17%, 53.1%, and 30.7%, respectively (18). These data were similar to those for groups of adolescent swimmers and nonathletes (18).

Intakes of 1.2 to 1.8 g of protein/kg of body weight are recommended for adult athletes (27), and these values should be the same for adolescent athletes (28). Those athletes ingesting sufficient calories generally consumed sufficient protein (about 1.6 g/kg of body weight) (28). For athletes not ingesting sufficient calories, even if a correct percentage of total calories from protein is achieved, the absolute amount may not be sufficient. For example, a young dancer weighing 40.9 kg who ingests 1200 kcal with 15% protein would be ingesting 1.1 g of protein/kg of body weight. Moreover, if energy, and especially carbohydrate, intake is inadequate, there will be an increased reliance on protein for energy, which will increase protein requirements.

Many studies cited above were done before the nationwide awareness of the need for lowering fat in the diet. In a recent study of female adolescent runners (21), it was found that they ingested 15.2%, 53.1%, and 31.7% of total caloric intake of protein, CHO, and fat, respectively. In a 3-year follow up, the diets were higher in CHO (59.6%) and lower in fat (26.4%). It is probably safe to assume that most young athletes and nonathletes, who are not trying to restrict caloric intake, are ingesting sufficient amounts of protein. Adolescents should be careful to ingest adequate amounts of CHO and reduce fat intake to 30% of calories consumed.

FIBER

Williams et al (29) recommended that dietary fiber for children older that 2 years of age be equivalent to age-plus-5 g/day, with a safety range of age-plus-5 g/day to age-plus-10 g/day, and this recommendation is also supported by Dwyer (30). Several dietary surveys found that adolescents are not ingesting sufficient fiber, which could lead to impaired health in later years (31). Fifty-five percent to 90% of children are not meeting minimum fiber intake recommendations. Increasing consumption of a variety of fruits, vegetables, cereals, and other whole grain products is recommended to increase fiber intake, and because dietary fiber increases water retention in the colon, producing bulkier, softer stools, water intake should also be increased (29). Children with low-fiber diets were found to consume foods that were higher in fats (32). A decline in fruit and vegetable consumption is largely responsible for the low-fiber diets (31).

Krebs-Smith et al (33) examined dietary data from 3148 children aged 2 to 18 years. They found that nearly one-quarter of all vegetables consumed by children and adolescents were french fries. Intake of fruits and dark green or deep yellow vegetables was low. Only one in five children ingested the recommended five or more fruits and vegetables per day. Data from the Minnesota Adolescent Health Survey showed that inadequate consumption of fruits and vegetables was reported by 37.9% of the adolescents from low socioeconomic backgrounds compared to 19.6% from upper and 29.8% from middle socioeconomic levels (34). Health-compromising behaviors, such as binge eating, substance abuse, and suicide attempts, demonstrated a modest correlation with inadequate intake of fruits and vegetables.

Few data are available on fiber content of adolescent athletes' diets. Wiita et al (21) found that female adolescent runners ingested 9.7 grams of fiber per day, and in a 3-year follow-up, they ingested 11.9 g/day. These values are far below the recommended value of about 22 to 25 g. On the other hand, adolescent ice hockey players ingested 20.5 g of fiber, and a mixed group of adolescent female athletes (gymnasts, track and field athletes, figure skaters) ingested 17.1 g of fiber (13). Although in most cases the amount of fiber was somewhat lower than recommended, the corresponding control groups of nonathletes ingested even less fiber, 19.2 g and 15.9 g, respectively.

MICRONUTRIENTS

Data from the NHANES survey show that most male adolescents are ingesting sufficient micronutrients, which is consistent with their higher energy intake. However, female adolescents had low or marginal intake of some micronutrients, especially iron and calcium. Other surveys and studies found that adolescents in general and adolescent athletes had insufficient intake of several micronutrients (7,10,35,36). The RDAs for adolescents are found in Table 12-3.

Iron

Iron intake from the NHANES data was 19.51 mg/day and 18.64 mg/day for males, ages 12 to 15 and ages 16 to 19 yrs, respectively, and the corresponding values for females were 12.26 mg/day and 12.52 mg/day (37). These values were adequate for males but low for females. Looker et al (38) estimated iron deficiency based on the NHANES data from laboratory tests of iron status. They found that for male adolescents, less than 1% would be classified as iron-deficient. However, for female adolescents the estimated incidence of

Table 12-3 Recommended Dietary Allowances of Selected Micronutrients for Adolescents

	Boys		Girls	
	11–14 yr	15–18 yr	11–14 yr	15–18 yr
Minerals				
Calcium (mg)	1200	1200	1200	1200
Phosphorus (mg)	1200	1200	1200	1200
Magnesium (mg)	270	400	280	300
Iron (mg)	12	12	15	15
Zinc (mg)	15	15	12	12
Selenium (μg)	40	50	45	50
Copper (mg)	1.5–2.5	1.5–2.5	1.5–2.5	1.5–2.5
Chromium (μg)	50–200	50–200	50–200	50–200
Vitamins				
Vitamin A (μg)	1000	1000	800	800
Vitamin D (μg)	10	10	10	10
Vitamin E (mg)	10	10	8	8
Vitamin C (mg)	50	60	50	60
Thiamin (mg)	1.3	1.5	1.1	1.1
Riboflavin (mg)	1.5	1.8	1.3	1.3
Niacin (mg)	17	20	15	15
Vitamin B_6 (mg)	1.7	2.0	1.4	1.5
Folate (μg)	150	200	150	180
Vitamin B_{12} (μg)	2.0	2.0	2.0	2.0

SOURCE: Food and Nutrition Board. Recommended dietary allowances. 10th ed. Washington DC: National Academy Press, 1989.

iron deficiency was 9% to 11% and of iron deficiency anemia was 2% to 3%. Losses of iron during menstruation, coupled with the need during rapid growth, increase iron requirements in adolescents (8). In a study of lacto-ovo-vegetarians (LAC), semi-vegetarian (SV), and omnivorous (OM) adolescent females, it was found that based on a normal level of plasma ferritin of less than 12 μg/L, 29% of LAC, 44% of SV, and 17% of OM had low iron stores (39). Willows et al (40) examined iron status in 26 female and 23 male adolescent athletes and found that the overall incidence of marginal iron stores (more than 12 μg/L and less than 20 μg/L) was 29% and 43% for boys and girls, respectively, and the incidence of iron deficiency (less than 12 μg/L) was 5% and 11%, respectively. Although these values are slightly higher than those reported by Looker et al (38), the authors did not attribute this to increased physical activity, although they did not include a control group for comparison.

Iron intake among female adolescent athletes showed that gymnasts, ballet dancers, and runners consumed considerably less iron than the RDA (14,17,18,41, 42). For swimmers, although the average value was slightly above the RDA, about 50% of the female swimmers did not meet the RDA (11). Rankinen et al (13) reported that male adolescent athletes ingested sufficient iron (16 mg), but females had somewhat lower ingestion levels (13 mg), although these values were higher than the controls (14 mg and 12 mg, respectively). Willows et al (40) reported adequate iron intake for the athletes examined, but Hawley and

Williams reported that 65% of adolescent swimmers had iron intakes lower that the RDA. The groups most at risk are adolescent female vegetarians, and low iron intakes are attributed to consumption of foods that are poor sources of available iron (26,39).

Adolescents, especially females, should increase their intake of heme iron (in meat, fish, and poultry), because heme iron is more absorbable than non-heme iron (in vegetables and grains). Vegetarians can increase the absorption of nonheme iron by increasing "enhancing" factors and decreasing "inhibitory" factors in the diet. Vitamin C will enhance absorption of iron while tea, coffee, antacids, and additives such as EDTA, used in fats and soft drinks, will inhibit absorption (8). Therefore, drinking a glass of orange juice with cereal is helpful, but drinking tea or coffee is counterproductive. Iron supplements should not be used indiscriminately, and iron deficiency should be documented from blood samples before taking iron supplements. However, the amount of iron in a multivitamin and mineral supplement is not considered harmful.

Calcium

The average calcium intake for adolescent girls in the NHANES survey was 900 mg/day, considerably below the recommended level of 1200 mg/day (37). Albertson et al (43) examined dietary calcium consumption from 1980 to 1992 and found a significant decline for the age 15 to 18 group. Over 90% of all adolescent females consumed less that 100% of the RDA for calcium and 77% of the 15 to 18-year-olds consumed less that 67% of the RDA. The authors attributed their finding in part to a decrease in milk and milk product consumption, especially fluid milk. In 1980 to 1982, 58.7% of the dietary sources of calcium were from milk and milk products, but in 1990 to 1992, this percentage had decreased to 47.7%.

The decline in calcium ingestion in adolescents is of concern because adequate calcium is needed to achieve peak bone mass and support the longitudinal growth of bones (44). Moreover, the RDA of 1200 mg has been questioned, because young adolescent girls are thought to need more than the RDA to achieve maximum calcium balance (8). Theintz et al (45) found that the increase in bone mineral density and content was particularly pronounced from ages 11 to 14 in females and ages 13 to 17 in males. After 16 years of age, girls had a dramatic fall in the rate of increase in bone mass accumulation, even though they had an apparently adequate intake of energy and calcium. For a detailed review of changes in bone during adolescence, see Blimkie et al (46).

Barr (47) examined 785 food frequency questionnaires from high school students and found that boys ingested 1146 mg of calcium per day, but girls ingested only 676 mg/day. More than half of the students' intakes were below current recommendations. The authors concluded that educational programs focusing on taste enjoyment of dairy products and building on the influence of peer and family members may have a positive influence on calcium ingestion in adolescents.

Similar to the groups studied regarding iron, the groups most at risk for not ingesting sufficient calcium are adolescent female vegetarians (26). Also, many adolescents have replaced

drinking milk with drinking sodas. No only does this lower the amount of calcium they ingest but also the amount of vitamin D. Vitamin D plays a major role in calcium metabolism. Although the adolescent may achieve adequate calcium intake from cheese and yogurt, the lower amount of milk consumption will mean less vitamin D intake (8).

Adolescent female gymnasts (42), ballet dancers (14), and distance runners (41) have been found to have low calcium intakes. Even though swimmers had an average calcium intake slightly above the RDA, 52% of the female swimmers were below the RDA (compared with only 14% of male swimmers) (11). Hawley and William (12) reported that 55% of adolescent swimmers ingested less than the RDA.

Calcium metabolism in adolescents is not fully understood. Recently, Weaver et al (48) examined calcium balance in adolescent girls and young adult women in a 3-week metabolic study. They found that the growth demands of girls were met by a more effective net absorption and retention of calcium compared with the young adult women, suggesting that the body is able to respond appropriately to increased need. Moreover, during short periods (10 days) of inadequate calcium intake, there was an increase in efficiency of calcium absorption and a decrease in urinary calcium losses (49). What is not known is whether this defense against low calcium intakes can continue over a long period of time or whether the low calcium intake will ultimately result in compromised health. At present it is thought that reduced calcium intake will impair bone accretion. In fact, the NIH Consensus Development Conference on Optimal Calcium Intake suggested that calcium intake among adolescents be increased from 1200 mg/day to 1500 mg/day (50).

Adequate calcium should be obtained through ingesting calcium-rich foods. However, if adequate amounts of calcium cannot be achieved through the diet, then, of the commercially available supplements, calcium carbonate is recommended because it contains the highest proportion of elemental calcium by weight and is least expensive (7). Absorption of calcium can be enhanced by ingesting no more that 400–500 mg at a time, taking the supplement with a meal, and avoiding co-ingestion of inhibiting substances, which include spinach, beet greens, and phytates. High amounts of phosphorus, protein, and sodium in the diet may also adversely affect calcium metabolism (7).

Other Vitamins and Minerals

The NHANES data found that adolescents were ingesting sufficient amounts of vitamin A, vitamin C, thiamin, riboflavin, niacin, vitamin B_6, folic acid, and vitamin B_{12} (37). Intakes of iron and calcium were low, and intakes of magnesium and zinc were marginal. Data from the Nationwide Food Consumption Survey (51) found that, in addition to iron and calcium, vitamins A and E and magnesium and zinc were consumed below recommended levels. Donovan et al (39) reported that 18% to 33% of adolescent females had serum zinc levels below normal, and 14% to 17% had low levels of zinc in hair samples.

Data from the Bogalusa Heart Study showed that intakes of several vitamins and minerals (vitamins A, B_6, E, D, and C, folic acid, magnesium, iron, zinc, and calcium) were not adequate for adolescents and that females tended to have a greater chance of not ingesting sufficient micronutrients

(52). Underingestion of various micronutrients does not always lead to lower nutritional status. For example, Rankinen et al (13) reported that about 40% to 45% of nonathletic adolescents had inadequate intake of zinc, but the number of those with suboptimal status was very low.

In a study of adolescent nonathletes and athletes representing several sports, it was found that the athletes generally ingested sufficient vitamins and minerals compared with the controls (13). However, low intake of vitamins and minerals is especially prevalent for those athletes maintaining low body weights. Of adolescent gymnasts and ballet dancers, more than 30% consumed less than two-thirds of the RDA for vitamin B_6, folic acid, and vitamin E; 7% to 20% consumed less than two-thirds of the RDA for thiamin, niacin, vitamin B_{12}, vitamin C, and vitamin A; about 40% did not consume two-thirds of the RDA for magnesium; and more than 70% ingested less than two-thirds of the RDA for zinc (14,17). For Swiss adolescent athletes (12 members of the Swiss national gymnastics team and 18 highly trained swimmers), the mean micronutrient intake was less than 75% of the RDA for folic acid and iron. Additionally, for the swimmers, the mean micronutrient intake was less than 75% of the RDA for calcium and vitamin B_6 (18).

In sports that emphasize leanness and for which caloric intake is low, female adolescents do not appear to meet the micronutrient needs. Although sufficient data are not available for adolescent nonathletic females who are dieting to achieve a lean appearance, it can probably be assumed that they too have compromised micronutrient status. This could have serious implications for growth and health in later years. It must be determined to what extent these data result from underreporting before firm conclusions can be made regarding the inadequacy of the diets for these adolescents. Moreover, it is not known to what extent adolescents can defend against low intakes by increasing absorption or retention of a micronutrient consumed in lower-than-recommended amounts. More studies are needed on the micronutrient status of adolescents, because a low ingestion does not always result in compromised status.

Although it is a common belief that supplements will correct deficiencies, data have shown that suboptimal intake is improved but not fully corrected by supplements. Zive et al (52) found that, of adolescents who reported that they took vitamin and mineral supplements, the percentage of those not meeting two-thirds of the RDA for selected vitamins and minerals ranged from 2% (vitamins A and E) to 38% (magnesium), while the range for those not taking supplements was 20% (vitamin B_{12}) to 70% (vitamin D). Rather than taking supplements, adolescents should obtain their micronutrient requirements from food. A diet sufficient in energy and comprising a wide variety of foods, including fruits, vegetables, dairy products, lean red meat, and whole grains, should provide the necessary amounts of micronutrients.

FLUID INGESTION

Adequate fluid intake is necessary for thermoregulation during exercise (53,54). Children have thermoregulatory systems that are less effective than adults have, which makes them more susceptible to heat illness (54). They have lower sweat rates than adults and have a faster increase in rectal temperature in response to hypohydration. During adolescence, the adult ability to thermoregulate develops, but when and how this happens is not known.

Most studies examining the effects of hydration and rehydration after exercise in children have been in children less than 13 years of age, so data for adolescents are scant. During exercise, children are not able to replenish the fluid lost and become dehydrated unless forced to drink (55,56). After exercise, if given free access to fluids, they can replenish what was lost (57).

Because it is important to maintain hydration, adolescents should be encouraged to drink fluids before, during (if possible), and after recreational physical activity, training, or competition. A simple method to determine whether dehydration has occurred after exercise is to check body weight before and after. Any loss in body weight results from water loss. It is recommended that children drink 300 to 420 mL of cold water 1 to 2 hours before exercise, 90 to 120 mL of water every 25 minutes during exercise, and 480 mL of water after exercise for every 0.5 kg of body weight that is lost (54). While water is sufficient, children may drink more if the water is flavored (58). The most important goal during rehydration is to ingest sufficient fluids, and with that in mind, the drink that tastes better will likely be consumed to a greater extent. Glucose and electrolytes improve taste. The recommended "sport" drink for adults is a dilute glucose-electrolyte solution containing about 2% to 8% of CHO and about 20 to 25 mmol/L of sodium, which describes several sport drinks commercially available (57,59).

There is not sufficient information on the composition of sport beverages specifically for adolescents, but commercially available sport drinks should be adequate for this group as well. Frequent ingestion of small volumes will prevent a bloating feeling. Drinks containing caffeine are not effective re-hydrators because the caffeine can act as a diuretic. Soda and undiluted fruit juice have high amounts of carbohydrate, which can cause stomach cramps, nausea, and diarrhea.

DIETARY BEHAVIORS

Clavien et al (60) assessed whether modifications in food habits occur during puberty. They examined 5-day dietary diaries of 193 adolescents, aged 9 to 19 years, and determined pubertal stage (P1, prepubertal, to P5, adult). There appeared to be no difference in dietary patterns over the stages. All groups were ingesting sufficient energy but had an excessive quantity of dietary fat, especially saturated fatty acids, and an insufficient ingestion of fiber. The high-fat diets of adolescents are most likely related to snacking and fast food (61).

During puberty and through adolescence, there is an excessive degree of "dieting" or trying to lose weight. The societal value of thinness prompts these behaviors, especially in young girls who are experiencing a normal increase in fat mass after puberty. An increase in unhealthy weight loss behaviors occurs from the 6th to the 9th grade in girls of all ethnicities (62). Contento et al (63) reported that, in high school students, body weight was not related to dieting behavior. The authors concluded that a "psychology of dieting" was more relevant than "psychology of being fat versus thin." A study of 141 high school students found that 62 (44%) felt themselves to be overweight, 77 (53.4%) wanted to be thinner, and about 71 (50%) were on "diets" (64). The major sources of information on diet and nutrition were the media.

Important factors that influence food choices in adolescents are family, the communications media, and peers (8). As children move into adolescence, they eat fewer meals at home. Also, with both parents working or in single-parent families, many adolescents eat more fast food and processed food, often high in fat. Adolescents spend several hours watching television, where many of the commercials are for food. Items targeted to a young audience are sweetened cereals, fast food, snack foods, and candy (8). During adolescence, snacking and eating become more of a social event, and peer groups often influence the types of food eaten.

Many adolescent athletes believe that supplements are the key to good nutrition (65). In one study of 742 adolescent athletes, it was found that 282 (38%) used supplements. Krowchuk et al (66) reported that 97 (33%) of 295 high school athletes used vitamin and mineral supplements and 103 (35%) used protein supplements. Massad et al (67) examined supplement use by 509 high school athletes, and of these athletes, 218 (42.8%) reported weekly to daily use of fluid replacement drinks, 212 (41.7%) took multivitamin or multimineral supplements regularly, and 151 (29.7%) took vitamin C regularly. Less than 127 (25%) took other supplements, 110 (21.7%) ingested protein drinks, and 109 (21.46%) consumed carbohydrate-loading drinks. Athletes who participated in contact sports such as football, boxing, and wrestling used more supplements than other athletes, which is likely owing to their attempt to increase muscle mass by protein and "muscle building" supplements. The authors also examined nutritional knowledge of these adolescents. The mean knowledge score was 13.56 correct responses out of 21 questions, which was quite low, although females scored higher than males. The finding that greater knowledge about supplements was associated with less use strongly suggests that adolescents are an important target for education on general and sport nutrition.

DISORDERED EATING

While the term "eating disorder" typically refers to labels and criteria set forth by the American Psychiatric Association's Diagnostic and Statistical Manual, fourth edition (DSM-IV), disordered eating could also include restrained eating, insufficient caloric intake, or inappropriate behaviors such as bingeing and purging only once a week, none of which meet the DSM-IV criteria but may have serious implications for the adolescent. The Eating Aptitude test (EAT) and the Eating Disorder Inventory (EDI) commonly are used to assess the presence of an eating disorder (68,69). The most recent EAT test (EAT-26) requires an individual to respond to 26 statements concerning abnormal weight and eating conditions and emotional disturbances of anorexia nervosa (69). The EDI tests for psychological characteristics of anorexia and bulimia nervosa and indicates disturbed attitudes towards eating and body image (68). Other tests of disordered eating have been developed, such as the Michigan State University (MSU) Weight Control Survey (70,71). This survey is not

primarily concerned with diagnosing anorexia and bulimia but attempts to identify pathogenic weight control methods (72). Also, the EAT ad EDI tests are often modified or abbreviated (73).

Although the EAT and EDI have been shown to be reliable and valid for the general public (68,69), they may be less valid for adolescents. Fear of intervention and control by parents or teachers may result in inaccurate reporting. Validity for athletes is also problematic. Athletes may not respond accurately for fear that their coach will discover who might have disordered eating, despite assurance of anonymity. They may try to cover up their problem to avoid jeopardizing their position on a team (74).

Using a 71-item questionnaire, Kagan et al (75) assessed the prevalence of eating disorders in 2004 students enrolled in grades 9 through 12. Disordered eating was defined as bingeing and purging or emotional eating. Binge-purge disorders and borderline values were found in 2% of male and 3% of female students, and 5% of males and 17% of females were classified as emotional eaters or borderline emotional eaters. Winkler and Vacc (76) compared results of the Adapted Eating Attitudes Test (AEAT) in 265 girls in grades 4, 6, and 8. The AEAT is a modification of language used in the EAT, so that it can be better used for adolescents. Nineteen percent scored above 20/21 on the AEAT test, which is considered to be symptomatic of eating disorder behavior, and there was no difference among the grades.

Killen et al (77) suggested that puberty may be a risk factor for development of eating disorders. They found that females manifesting eating disorder symptoms were more developed (determined by Tanner self-staging) than those who were asymptomatic. Attie and Brooks-Gunn (78) found that girls during early adolescence who felt more negative about their bodies were more likely to develop eating problems. In one study, only 4% of young girls (ages 11 to 13) were actually overweight, but more than 40% considered themselves overweight, and by age 18, 80% of females had dieted to lose weight and 60% had begun dieting practices by age 13 (79). Girls as young as age 5 reported restricted food intake to prevent weight gain (80). Even though black female adolescents appear to diet to lose weight less than white female adolescents, they are more likely to use fasting, laxatives, and diuretics (81).

Based on hospitalized patients and psychiatric case registers from 1935 to 1984, prevalence rates for anorexia nervosa were reported to be highest for females aged 15 to 19 years (82). There was a linear increase over time in the incidence rate for the 15 to 24-year-olds. From 1935 to 1939, the incidence was 13.4 per 100,000 and from 1980 to 1984, the rate had grown to 76.1 per 100,000.

Female adolescent athletes in sports emphasizing leanness are likely to be restricting calories, and these female athletes tend to have a greater frequency of disordered eating when compared either with males or female nonathletes (74,83–87). Dummer and others (70) studied 487 girls and 468 boys, aged 9 to 18 years, who were attending a competitive swimming camp and completed the MSU Weight Control Survey. Pathogenic weight control methods were used by 75 (15.4%) girls and 17 (3.6%) boys.

Although one study of high school girls, 100 athletes and 112 nonathletes, found little difference in the risk for developing an eating disorder between groups, the athletes mostly represented sports that did not emphasize leanness, such as volleyball, basketball, tennis, softball, and track (88). In another study (18), a small but significant risk for an eating disorder, based on the EDI, was found for Swiss adolescent athletes (N = 30) (gymnasts, n = 12, and swimmers, n = 18). Significantly more swimmers (38%) scored high on body dissatisfaction than controls (9%) or gymnasts (1%). Although swimmers compete in a sport where leanness is not particularly emphasized for performance, their distress over body weight may be due to concern with personal appearance since they must train and compete in swimsuits.

In 1985, Braisted et al (89) found that adolescent ballet dancers reported characteristics of anorexia nervosa significantly more often than controls. Garner et al (90) studied adolescent ballet dancers aged 11 to 14 for 2 to 4 years to determine the persistence of eating disorders and to identify factors that could predict an eating disorder. From the EDI test, it was found at follow-up that 25.7% met the criteria for anorexia nervosa and 14.2% had bulimia nervosa or a "partial syndrome." "Drive for thinness" and "body dissatisfaction" from the EDI scales predicted the development of eating disorders at follow-up. In a study of high school cheerleaders who completed the Desire for Thinness, Restrained Eating, EDI, and EAT scales, it was found that the cheerleaders who expressed a strong desire for thinness generally had significantly higher scores on the eating disorder scales (91).

SUMMARY

The growth spurt and changes in body composition during adolescence present a substantial challenge to the body that must be supported by adequate nutrition. Large surveys of adolescents have found that most are ingesting sufficient energy. However, those individuals who are restricting energy intake to maintain a lean body type either for aesthetic reasons or to improve athletic performance may not consume adequate energy. The macronutrient composition of adolescents' diets appears to be higher in fat than is desirable, but the trend in fat intake is declining. Fiber intake is low for adolescents, as a result of underingestion of fruits and vegetables. Micronutrient intake appears adequate or marginal for most males, but female adolescents have marked deficiencies in iron and calcium intake and marginal intakes of several other micronutrients. The low intake of calcium is of particular concern because calcium is needed to support the dramatic bone growth that occurs during adolescence. Those adolescents, especially athletes, who are restricting caloric intake may not obtain recommended levels of other vitamins and minerals, as well. It is not known to what extent adolescents can defend against marginal to low intakes of micronutrients before health is impaired. Adolescents should increase fluid consumption, especially during exercise, when they can become dehydrated unless forced or reminded to drink. Adequate hydration is necessary to maintain thermoregulation and prevent heat illness during exercise.

Important influences on food choices during adolescence are family, the communications media, and peers. The high-fat diets of adolescents are most likely related to snacking and fast food, especially outside the home. Television commercials target young audiences with advertisements for sweet and high-fat foods. Young athletes are lured by magazine ads for muscle-building products and energy boosters, but most such products have not been proven effective. The desire to be thin has made adolescents, especially females who begin to increase fat mass, particularly susceptible to disordered eating. Adolescents should be an important target for nutrition education because inadequate nutrition during this period could have a profound impact on health.

REFERENCES

1. Clarkson PM, Going S. Body composition and weight control: a perspective on females. In: Bar-Or O, Lamb DR, Clarkson PM, eds. Exercise and the female: a life span approach, perspectives in exercise science and sports medicine. vol. 9. Carmel, IN: Cooper, 1996:147–214.

2. Food and Nutrition Board. Recommended dietary allowances. 10th ed. Washington DC: National Academy Press, 1989.

3. Gibson RS. Principles of nutritional assessment. New York: Oxford University Press, 1990: 37–136.

4. Pao EM, Cypel YS. Estimation of dietary intake. In: Ziegler EE, Filer Jr LJ, eds. Present knowledge in nutrition. Washington, DC: International Life Sciences Institute, 1996:498–507.

5. Garry PJ, Koehler KM. Problems in interpretation of dietary and biochemical data from population studies. In: Brown ML, ed. Present knowledge in nutrition. Washington, DC: International Life Sciences Institute, 1990:407 –414.

6. Schoeller DA. How accurate is self-reported dietary energy intake? Nutr Rev 1990;48:373–379.

7. Story M, Alton I. Becoming a woman: nutrition in adolescence. In: Krummel DA, Kris-Etherton PM, eds. Nutrition in women's health. Gaithersburg, MD: Aspen Publishers, 1996:1–34.

8. Lucas B. Normal nutrition from infancy through adolescence. In: Queen PM, Lang CE, eds. Handbook of pediatric nutrition. Gaithersburg, MD: Aspen Publishers, 1993:145–170.

9. McDowell MA, Briefel RR, Alaimo K, et al. Energy and macronutrient intakes of persons ages 2 months and over in the United States: third national health and nutrition examination survey, phase 1, 1988–91. In: Vital and health statistics of the Centers for Disease Control and Prevention, National Center for Health Statistics. Advance Data #255, 1994.

10. Dwyer JT. Adolescence. In: Ziegler EE, Filer Jr LJ, eds. Present knowledge in nutrition.

Washington, DC: International Life Sciences Institute, 1996: 404–413.

11. Berning JR, Troup JP, VanHandel PJ, et al. The nutrition habits of young adolescent swimmers. Int J Sport Nutr 1991;1:240–248.

12. Hawley JA, Williams MM. Dietary intakes of age-group swimmers. Br J Sports Med 1991;25:154–158.

13. Rankinen T, Fogelholm M, Kujala U, et al. Dietary intake and nutritional status of athletic and nonathletic children in early puberty. Int J Sport Nutr 1995; 5:136–150.

14. Benson J, Gillien DM, Bourdet K, Loosli AR. Inadequate nutrition and chronic calorie restriction in adolescent ballerinas. Phys Sportsmed 1985;13:79–90.

15. Clarkson PM, Freedson PS, Keller B, et al. Maximal oxygen uptake, nutritional patterns, and body composition of adolescent female ballet dancers. Res Quart Exerc Sport 1985;56:180–184.

16. Bonbright JM. The nutritional status of female ballet dancers 15 to 18 years of age. Dance Res J 1989;21:9–14.

17. Loosli AR, Benson J, Gillien DM, Bourdet K. Nutrition habits and knowledge in competitive adolescent female gymnasts. Phys Sportsmed 1986;14:118–130.

18. Benson JE, Allemann Y, Theintz GE, Howald H. Eating problems and calorie intake levels in Swiss adolescent athletes. Int J Sports Med 1990;11:249–252.

19. Baer JT, Taper LJ. Amenorrheic and eumenorrheic adolescent runners: dietary intake and exercise training status. J Am Diet Assoc 1992;92:89–91.

20. Bergen-Cico DK, Short SH. Dietary intakes, energy expenditures, and anthropometric characteristics of adolescent female cross-country runners. J Am Diet Assoc 1992;92:611–612.

21. Wiita BG, Stombaugh IA. Nutrition knowledge, eating practices, and health of adolescent female runners: a 3-year longitudinal study. Int J Sport Nutr 1996;6: 414–425.

22. Pugliese MT, Lifshitz F, Grad G, et al. Fear of obesity: a cause of short stature and delayed puberty. N Engl J Med 1983;309:513–518.

23. Pugliese MT, Recker B, Lifshitz F. A survey to determine the prevalence of abnormal growth patterns in adolescents from a suburban school district. J Adolesc Health Care 1988;9:181–187.

24. Theintz GE, Howald H, Weiss U, Sizonenko PC. Evidence for a reduction of growth potential in adolescent female gymnasts. J Pediatr 1993;122:306–313.

25. Theintz GE, Howald H, Allemann Y, Sizonenko PC. Growth and pubertal development of young female gymnasts and swimmers: a correlation with parental data. Int J Sports Med 1989;10:87–91.

26. Donovan UM, Gibson RS. Dietary intakes of adolescent females consuming vegetarian, semi-vegetarian, and omnivorous diets. J Adolesc Health 1996;18:292–300.

27. Lemon PWR. Do athletes need more dietary protein and amino acids? Int J Sport Nutr 1995; 5(suppl):S39–S61.

28. Maughan RJ, Shirreffs SM. Nutrition for young athletes. In: Rogozkin VA, Maughan RJ, eds. Current research in sports science. New York: Plenum 1996:41–46.

29. Williams CL, Bollella M, Wynder EL. A new recommendation for dietary fiber. Childhood Pediatr 1995;96:985–994.

30. Dwyer JT. Dietary fiber for children: how much? Pediatrics 1995;96:1019–1022.

31. Saldanha LG. Fiber in the diet of US children: results of national surveys. Pediatrics 1995;96: 994–997.

32. Nicklas TA, Myers L, Berenson GS. Dietary fiber intake of children: the Bogalusa Heart Study. Pediatrics 1995;96:988–994.

33. Krebs-Smith SM, Cook A, Subar AF, et al. Fruit and vegetable intakes of children and adolescents in the United States. Arch Pediatr Adolesc Med 1996;150: 81–86.

34. Neumark-Sztainer D, Story M, Resnick MD, Blum RW. Correlates of inadequate fruit and vegetable consumption among adolescents. Prev Med 1996;25:497–505.

35. Clarkson PM, Haymes EM. Trace mineral requirements for athletes. Int J Sport Nutr 1994;4:104–119.

36. Clarkson PM, Haymes EM. Exercise and mineral status of athletes: calcium, magnesium, phosphorus, and iron. Med Sci Sport Exerc 1995;27:831–843.

37. Alaimo K, McDowell MA, Briefel RR, et al. Dietary intake of vitamins, minerals, and fiber of persons ages 2 months and over in the United States: third national health and nutrition examination survey, phase 1, 1988–1991. In: Vital and health statistics of the Centers for Disease Control and Prevention/National Center for Health Statistics. Advance Data #258, 1994.

38. Looker AC, Dallman PR, Carroll M, et al. Prevalence of iron deficiency in the United States. JAMA 1997;277:973–976.

39. Willows ND, Grimston SK, Smith DJ, Hanley DA. Iron and hematological status among adolescent athletes tracked through puberty. Pediatr Exerc Sci 1995;7:253–262.

40. Moen SM, Sanborn CF, DiMarco N. Dietary habits and body composition in adolescent female runners. Women Sport Phys Activ J 1992;1:85–95.

41. Moffatt RJ. Dietary status of elite female high school gymnasts: inadequacy of vitamin and mineral intake. J Am Diet Assoc 1984;84:1361–1363.

42. Donovan UM, Gibson RS. Iron and zinc status of young women aged 14 to 19 years consuming vegetarian and omnivorous diets. J Am Coll Nutr 1995;14:463–472.

43. Albertson AM, Tobelmann RC, Marquart L. Estimated dietary

calcium intake and food sources for adolescent females: 1980–1992. J Adolesc Health 1997;20:20–26.

44. Gallo AM. Building strong bones in childhood and adolescence: reducing the risk of fractures in later life. Pediatr Nurs 1996;22: 369–374.

45. Theintz G, Buchs B, Rizzoli R, et al. Longitudinal monitoring of bone mass accumulation in healthy adolescents: evidence for a marked reduction after 16 years of age at the levels of lumbar spine and femoral neck in female subjects. J Clin Endocrinol Metab 1992;75: 1060–1065.

46. Blimkie JR, Chilbeck PD, Davison KS. Bone mineralization patterns: reproductive endocrine, calcium, and physical activity influences during the life span. In: Bar-Or O, Lamb DR, Clarkson PM, eds. Exercise and the female: a life span approach, perspectives in exercise science and sports medicine. vol. 9. Carmel, IN: Cooper, 1996: 73–146.

47. Barr SI. Associations of social and demographic variables with calcium intakes of high school students. J Am Diet Assoc 1994;94: 260–269.

48. Weaver CM, Martin BR, Plawecki KL, et al. Differences in calcium metabolism between adolescent and adult females. Am J Clin Nutr 1995;61:577–581.

49. O'Brien KO, Abrams SA, Liang LK, et al. Increased efficiency of calcium absorption during short periods of inadequate calcium intake in girls. Am J Clin Nutr 1996;63:579–583.

50. Porter D. Washington update: NIH consensus development conference statement: Optimal calcium intake. Nutr Today 1994; 29:37–49.

51. Johnson RK, Johnson DG, Wang MQ, et al. Characterizing nutrient intakes of adolescents by sociodemographic factors. J Adolesc Health 1994;15:149–54.

52. Zive MM, Nicklas TA, Busch EC, et al. Marginal vitamin and mineral intakes of young adults: the Bogalusa Heart Study. J Adolesc Health 1996;19:39–47.

53. Meyer F, Bar-Or O. Fluid and electrolyte loss during exercise: the paediatric angle. Sport Med 1994; 18:4–9.

54. Steen SN. Nutrition for young athletes: special considerations. Sports Med 1994;17:152–162.

55. Bar-Or O, Dotan R, Inbar O, et al. Voluntary hypohydration in 10- to 12-year-old boys. J Appl Physiol 1980;48:104–108.

56. Bar-Or O, Wilk B. Water and electrolyte replenishment in the exercising child. Int J Sport Nutr 1996;6:93–96.

57. Meyer F, Bar-Or O, Salsberg A, Passe D. Hypohydration during exercise in children: effect on thirst, drink preferences, and rehydration. Int J Sport Nutr 1994;4: 22–35.

58. Bar-Or O. The young athlete: some physiological considerations. J Sport Sci 1995;13(suppl):S31–33.

59. Maughan R. Optimizing hydration for competitive sport. In: Lamb DR, Murray R, eds. Optimizing sport performance: perspectives in exercise science and sports medicine. vol. 10. Carmel, IN: Cooper, 1997:139–177.

60. Clavien H, Theintz G, Rizzoli R, Bonjour JP. Does puberty alter dietary habits in adolescents living in a Western society? J Adolesc Health 1996;19:68–75.

61. Cusatis DC, Shannon BM. Influences on adolescent eating behavior. J Adolesc Health 1996;18:27–34.

62. Neumark-Sztainer D, Story M, Resnick MD, Blum RW. Correlates of inadequate fruit and vegetable consumption among adolescents. Prevent Med 1996;25:497–505.

63. Contento IR, Michela JL, Williams SS. Adolescent food choice criteria: role of weight and dieting status. Appetite 1995;25:51–76.

64. Brook U, Tepper I. High school students' attitudes and knowledge of food consumption and body image: implications for school-based education. Patient Educ Couns 1997;30:283–288.

65. Sobal J, Marquart LF. Vitamin/mineral supplement use among high school students. Adolescence 1994;29:835–843.

66. Krowchuk DP, Anglin TM, Goodfellow DB, et al. High school athletes and the use of erogenic aids. Am J Dis Child 1989;143: 486–489.

67. Massad SJ, Shier NW, Koceja DM, Ellis NT. High school athletes and nutritional supplements: a study of knowledge and use. Int J Sport Nutr 1995;5:232–245.

68. Garner DM, Olmsted MP, Polivy J. The eating disorder inventory: a measure of cognitive-behavioral dimensions of anorexia nervosa and bulimia. In: Anorexia nervosa: recent developments in research. New York: Alan R. Liss 1983: 173–184.

69. Garner DM, Garfinkel PE. The eating attitudes test: an index of the symptoms of anorexia nervosa. Psychol Med 1979;9:273–279.

70. Dummer GM, Rosen LW, Heusner WW, et al. Pathogenic weight-control behaviors of young competitive swimmers. Phys Sportsmed 1987;15:75–86.

71. Rosen LW, McKeag DB, Hough DO, Curley V. Pathogenic weight-control behavior in female athletes. Phys Sportsmed 1986; 14:79–86.

72. Rosen LW, Hough DO. Pathogenic weight-control behaviors of female college gymnasts. Phys Sportsmed 1988;16:140–146.

73. Sundgot-Borgen J. Eating disorders in female athletes. Sports Med 1994;17:176–188.

74. Wilmore JH. Eating and weight disorders in the female athlete. Int J Sport Nutr 1991;1:104–117.

75. Kagan DM, Squires RL. Eating disorders among adolescents: patterns and prevalence. Adolescence 1984;19:15–29.

76. Winkler MCR, Vacc NA. Eating-disordered behavior in girls. Elem

School Guid Counsel 1989;24: 119–127.

77. Killen JD, Hayward C, Litt I, et al. Is puberty a risk factor for eating disorders? Am J Dis Child 1992; 146:323–325.

78. Attie I, Brooks-Gunn J. Development of eating problems in adolescent girls: a longitudinal study. Devel Psychol 1989;25:70–79.

79. Brown C. The continuum: anorexia, bulimia, and weight preoccupation. In: Brown C, Jasper K, eds. Consuming passions. Toronto: Second Story, 1993:53–68.

80. Ciliska D. Why diets fail. In: Brown C, Jasper K, eds. Consuming passions. Toronto: Second Story, 1993 :80–90.

81. Melnyk MG, Weinstein E. Preventing obesity in black women by targeting adolescents: a literature review. J Am Diet Assoc 1994;94: 536–540.

82. Lucas AR, Huse DM. Behavioral disorders affect food intake: anorexia nervosa and bulimia nervosa. In: Shils ME, Olson JA, Shike M, eds. Modern nutrition in health and disease. 8th ed. Philadelphia: Lea and Febiger, 1994:979.

83. Brownell KD, Rodin J. Prevalence of eating disorders in athletes. In: Brownell KD, Rodin J, and Wilmore JH, eds. Eating, body weight, and performance in athletes: disorders of modern society. Philadelphia: Lea & Febiger, 1992:128–145.

84. Brownell KD, Steen SN. Weight cycling in athletes: effects on behavior, physiology, and health. In: Brownell KD, Rodin J, Wilmore JH, eds. Eating, body weight and performance in athletes: disorders of modern society. Philadelphia: Lea & Febiger, 1992:159–171.

85. Leon GR. Eating disorders in female athletes. Sports Med 1991;12;219–227.

86. Nattiv A, Agostini R, Drinkwater B, Yeager KK. The female athlete triad: the interrelatedness of disordered eating, amenorrhea, and osteoporosis. Clin Sports Med 1994;13:405–418.

87. Putukian M. The female triad: eating disorders, amenorrhea, and osteoporosis. Sports Med 1994; 78:345–356.

88. Taub DE, Blinde EM. Eating disorders among adolescent female athletes: influence of athletic participation and sport team membership. Adolescence 1992; 27:833–848.

89. Braisted JR, Mellin L, Gong EJ, Irwin CE Jr. The adolescent ballet dancer: nutritional practices and characteristics associated with anorexia nervosa. J Adol Health Care 1985;6:365–371.

90. Garner DM, Garfinkel PE, Rockert W, Olmsted MP. A prospective study of eating disturbances in the ballet. Psychother Psychosom 1987;48:170–175.

91. Lundholm JK, Littrell JM. Desire for thinness among high school cheerleaders: relationship to disordered eating and weight control behaviors. Adolescence 1986;21: 573–579.

Chapter 13

Optimal Nutrition for the Mature Adult in Health and Disease

Alice H. Lichtenstein

Currently, approximately 12.5% of Americans are over the age of 65. This is expected to increase to approximately 20% by the year 2025. Along with this shift in the demographic makeup of the United States will come demands for nonpharmacologic means of maintaining function with advancing age. A better understanding of the nutrient needs of older Americans is essential.

The 1989 Recommended Dietary Allowances (RDA) distinguish between nutrient needs of adults aged 25 to 50 and those over the age of 51. No further distinction or allowance is made for individuals in their 70s, 80s, and 90s. However, the well-documented changes that occur with advancing age, e.g., decreased lean muscle mass and increased fat mass or reduction in gastric acid secretion, will have an impact on energy and nutrient requirements, respectively. The lack of more specific recommendations for the mature adult is the consequence of limited information on which to base precise recommendations and the tremendous variability in physiologic age within each chronologic age category (21).

In this chapter, current guidelines and recommendations will be reviewed and special considerations regarding the mature adult population will be discussed. Additionally, specific dietary issues aimed at delaying the onset of degenerative diseases will be addressed. The focus of this chapter is on the healthy mature adult segment of the population and what dietary recommendations can be made to prolong this period. On an encouraging note, evidence suggests that within a population, those individuals age 70 and older who score relatively high on diet assessments have better survival rates (10,17,40). A recent assessment of a large cohort of elderly people in Europe suggested that elderly people today are consuming a diet lower in total fat and higher in micronutrient density than they were 20 years ago (44). The micronutrients for which elders still are at risk for low intakes were identified as vitamins B_6 (increased requirement and low intake) and B_{12} (decreased absorption and low intake), vitamin D (low sun exposure, low intake, impaired metabolism), calcium (low intake), zinc (low intake), and iodine (low intake in some areas).

CURRENT RECOMMENDATIONS FOR OPTIMAL NUTRITION IN MATURE ADULTS

As indicated earlier the only distinction made in the RDAs for the mature adult population is for individuals age 51 and over compared with ages 25 to 50. It is anticipated that as the new Daily Recommended Intakes (DRI) become available, nutrient needs for the mature adult will be treated separately (24,37,38).

A survey of the nutrients for which RDAs have been established indicates that no distinction is made between adults below and above age 50 for protein; vitamins A, D, E, K, C, B_6, and B_{12}; folic acid; calcium; phosphorus; magnesium; zinc; iodine; and selenium. The nutrients for which a distinction has been made between the two age categories are thiamine, riboflavin, and niacin for women and men, and iron for women. The lower RDA for iron for women is a reflection of the decreased losses after the cessation of menses. The primary functions of thiamine, riboflavin, and niacin are as co-factors in energy metabolism. Therefore, requirements are related to energy requirements. The lower thiamine, riboflavin, and niacin RDAs for older women and men are a reflection of lower energy needs.

NUTRITION AND THE MATURE ADULT: SPECIAL CONSIDERATIONS

The area of nutrition and the mature adult is broad and can be discussed from a number of different perspectives (13). The approach that will be taken in this chapter is consideration of the changes that both physiologic and psychosocial factors can contribute to the development of compromised nutrient status. Stated in another way, we consider separately the actual aging-related changes in nutrient requirements resulting from declines in organ systems, which impair absorption or utilization of nutrients, changes in the ability of older individuals to acquire and prepare foods of adequate nutrient content, and changes in psychosocial situations that conspire to have a negative impact on the nutrient quality or consumption of meals. Accommodations made for all three areas are critical for maintaining adequate nutrition with increasing age are addressed.

Physiologic Factors

There is strong evidence that nutrient needs change as a result of the aging process (39). These changes are, for the most part, related to changes in the functioning of organ systems, which have an impact on the use of specific nutrients (Table 13-1). As an individual ages, there is a decline in the rate of hydrochloric acid secretion by the stomach and digestive juices by the pancreas and small intestine (4). The resulting hypochlorhydria has a negative impact on vitamin B_{12} absorption. Similarly, declines in hepatic and biliary function raise the potential for nutrient intoxication and alter the availability of bile acids (39). A decline in absorptive capacity of the gastrointestinal system and motility can impair efficient use of ingested foods. High-protein diets superimposed on renal disease can result in membrane damage (39.) A weakening of the muscles of the large intestine can result in constipation and diverticulitis.

Clearly the effect of aging on nutrient balance is multifactorial and nutrient-specific. Older adults have been reported to need less vitamin B_6 in response to increased protein intake relative to younger adults (32). Age-related decline in intestinal vitamin D receptor protein concentration has been estimated to account for 12% to 30% of the age-related change in calcium absorption (22).

Impairments or decreases in the functioning of the heart, blood vessels, and kidneys can result from the normal demands on everyday life. Changes in body composition (decreased lean muscle mass and increased fat mass) result in a decrease in basal metabolic rates, energy needs, and capacity for physical activity (16). Increased use of prescription and nonprescription medications, chronic drug therapy, and decreased capacity of the liver to metabolize drugs can compromise nutrient unitization. All these factors need to be addressed on a regular basis by the health care provider.

Activities of Daily Life

Integral to ensuring optimal nutriture in the older adult is retaining the desire to eat a variety of foods and the capacity to obtain and prepare these foods on a daily basis. Disabilities related to vision, dexterity, and mobility can make food

Table 13-1 Physiologic Changes Contributing to Compromised Nutrient Status in Mature Adults

SYSTEM	CHANGE
Digestive system	↓ hydrochloric acid secretion ↓ digestive juice secretion (pancreas, small intestine) ↓ absorptive capacity ↓ GI motility ↑ malabsorption ↓ muscle tone in large intestine ↑ chronic blood loss from ulcers and hemorrhoids
Liver	↓ hepatic and biliary function ↓ rate of detoxification
Heart	↓ cardiac output ↓ strength and flexibility of blood vessels
Kidneys	↓ blood flow ↓ glomerular filtration
Senses	↓ acuity of vision and hearing ↓ taste (loss of taste buds, mainly salt and sweet) ↓ smell
Skin	↓ synthesis of vitamin D
Body composition	↓ lean muscle mass and ↑ fat mass ↓ physical activity
Immune system	↓ T cell-mediated function ↑ susceptibility to infection and malignancy
Pharmacokinetics	↑ prescription and nonprescription drug use ↑ chronic drug therapy ↓ capacity to metabolize drugs
Mouth	↓ salivary secretion ↑ altered bite pattern from tooth loss

GI, gastrointestinal tract.

acquisition and preparation difficult and have a severe impact on variety and quality in the diet (Table 13-2). Difficulty in opening jars, cans, or bubble-packaged foods because of arthritis or diminished strength can lead to a decrease in variety and ability to consume preferred foods. Decreased taste and smell acuity can lead to poor appetite. These factors can turn mealtime into a negative and frustrating experience. Coupled with decreased energy needs and capacity for consuming large quantities of food, the importance of consuming a nutrient-dense diet takes on an increased level of urgency.

Psychosocial Factors

In addition to dealing with declines in physical capacity associated with aging, there are also changes in the social situation that can have an impact on nutritional status (Table 13-3). Loss of a spouse and other family members with whom meals

Table 13-2 Activities of Daily Life Changes Contributing to Compromised Food Intake in Mature Adults

FACTOR	CHANGE
Oral cavity	↑ periodontal disease
	↑ ill-fitting dentures
	↓ salivary gland function
Mobility	↓ physical activity
	↓ respiratory capacity
	↓ lean muscle mass (strength, physical disability)
	↑ physical isolation
Senses	↓ acuity, which leads to
	↓ appetite (taste, smell, sight)
Dexterity	↑ arthritic involvement in finger and hand joints
	↑ tremor
	↓ manual dexterity
Energy needs	↓ energy requirements
	↓ caloric intake
	↓ volume

Table 13-3 Psychosocial Changes Contributing to Compromised Food Intake in Mature Adults

FACTOR	CHANGE
Companionship	↑ loss of spouse
	↑ social isolation
	↑ loss of companions
	↓ social interaction secondary to
	↓ mobility
Mental state	↑ depression
	↑ mental deterioration (dementia)
	↑ alcoholism
	↑ loneliness
	↑ chronic disease
Economic	↑ fixed income (poverty)
	↓ choice and availability
	↓ quantity needs
	↓ variety
Nutrition knowledge	↑ susceptibility to food fads
Housing	→ change in status (loss of home)

were shared and for whom meals may have been prepared is common. This can lead to increased social isolation, especially during mealtime, and decreased interest or desire to prepare and consume healthful meals.

Because of deterioration in mental or economic status, mature adults are frequently faced with having to adapt to a new living environment. This can result in dramatic changes in meal timing, food preparation, and food choices. The onset of chronic disease states can further limit food choices and

make the older individual susceptible to the lures of food fads that promise the fountain of youth and drain scarce resources for food purchases. Depression frequently accompanies the aging process in individuals unable or without the support to make the necessary adaptations. These individuals are at increased risk of alcoholism. All these factors may lead to diminished interest in food and poor food consumption patterns. Coupled with declines in economic status, which frequently challenge older individuals, the probability of malnutrition increases.

NUTRIENT REQUIREMENTS OF THE MATURE ADULT

This section will summarize the most common concerns about altered nutrient requirements associated with aging. It is not comprehensive, and clearly, many unanswered questions remain, primarily because of lack of data. Detailed reviews of the topic have been published (37,49).

Little data exist that suggest that there is a generalized decline in nutrient absorption or use with increasing age. General views on the subject range from "qualitatively grossly comparable" (43) to "potential small declines." Part of the difficulty in assessing the nutrient needs of mature adults is the difficulty in separating changes in nutrient needs caused by the aging process per se from changes secondary to physiologic changes, which occur with increased prevalence in older individuals. Clearly, the decline in energy needs attributable to changes in body composition and activity levels predisposes elders to compromised nutrient status and increases the importance of choosing nutrient-dense diets (21).

Vitamins

Table 13-4 summarizes some of the major issues concerning vitamin requirements in the elderly. In no case has a clear-cut increase in requirement based on decreased absorption or metabolism been identified as resulting from increased age (37). However, two factors need to be taken into consideration when assessing the potential for vitamin insufficiency in the elderly. One is inadequate intake caused by impairments in activities of daily life (Table 13-2) or psychosocial factors (Table 13-3). The second is changes in nutrient use secondary to the aging process.

One of the best-documented examples of an increased nutrient requirement secondary to changes inherent in the aging process is that of atrophic gastritis and the accompanying hypochlorhydria. This condition effects an estimated 30% of individuals over age 60 (37). A consequence of hypochlorhydria is impaired absorption of food protein–bound vitamin B_{12} and bacterial overgrowth in the stomach and proximal small intestine; bacteria compete with the body for vitamin B_{12}.

Another well-documented example of an increased nutrient requirement secondary to changes inherent in the aging process is that of vitamin D. Skin changes associated with aging result in decreased efficiency of the skin to convert the provitamin 7-dehydrocholesterol to active vitamin D. Additionally, it appears that, with increased age, many target tissues of vitamin D, either sites of activation (hydroxylation) or response (intestine and bone), become resistant.

Table 13-4 Special Considerations in Vitamin Requirements in Mature Adults	
NUTRIENT	**SELECTED CONSIDERATIONS**
Vitamin A	→ or ↑ absorption
	→ selective deficiency in elderly
Vitamin C	→ pharmokinetics
	→ half-life
Vitamin D	→ absorption
	→ hepatic hydrolyzation of vitamin D
	↓ skin synthesis
	↓ sun exposure
	↓ renal response to PTH for hydrolyzation of 25-hydroxyvitamin D
	↑ resistance of bone and intestine to 1,25-dihydroxyvitamin D
Vitamin E	?
	↑ indicators of cell-mediated immunity in elderly
Vitamin K	? significance of bacterial synthesis
Thiamin	→
Niacin	→
	? conversion of tryptophan to niacin
	? impact of altered vitamin B_6 requirement
Riboflavin	→
Vitamin B_6	→ bioavailability
	→ in response to change in protein intake
	→ or ↑ requirement
Vitamin B_{12}	↑ requirement, if atrophic gastritis is present
Folic acid	→
Biotin	?
Pantothenic acids	?

PTH, parathyroid hormone.

Table 13-5 Special Considerations in Mineral Requirements in Mature Adults	
NUTRIENT	**SELECTED CONSIDERATIONS**
Calcium	↓ absorption efficiency
	↓ ability to ↑ absorption efficiency in response to low intake
	2° ↓ status due to ↓ renal production of 1,25-dihydroxyvitamin D
	2° ↓ status due to ↓ response of small intestine to 1,25-dihydroxyvitamin D
	↓ intake due to ↑ lactose intolerance
Zinc	↓ absorption efficiency
	→ adaption to low-zinc diet
Magnesium	→ absorption
	→ renal resorption
Iron	→ due to hypochlorhydria
Selenium	?
Copper	→ absorption efficiency
	↑ adaption to low-copper diet
Chromium	?
Iodine	↓ intake

This problem is further compounded by diminished renal hydroxylation of 25-hydroxyvitamin D and responsiveness of the small intestine to 1,25-hydroxyvitamin D. These issues are particularly important in light of the increasing prevalence of lactose intolerance and the resulting lower calcium intake with advancing age.

Concern regarding zinc nutriture in the elderly has been raised. Some evidence suggested compromised efficiency of intestinal absorption with advancing age. Despite this, evidence also suggests that the ability of older individuals to adapt by increasing efficiency of absorption in response to low zinc intake remains intact (49).

Data concerning magnesium, iron, and copper suggest no independent effect of age on dietary requirements. Data for selenium, chromium, iodine, and other essential minerals on which to base specific requirements for the mature adult are too limited at this time. As for vitamin requirements, there is a tremendous amount of interest in the field at this time, and it is anticipated that the issues related to the effect of aging on mineral status will be clarified in the near future.

PHYSIOLOGIC DISORDERS COMMON IN MATURE ADULTS

Nutrient-related chronic diseases of middle and later years include cardiovascular disease, cancer, diabetes, hypertension, and osteoporosis; disorders of dentition and associated senses; and declines in immune, cognitive, and gastrointestinal function. Other disorders, such as tuberculosis, pneumonia, pressure sores, and alcohol abuse, occur with increased frequency in elderly people. In some cases, the goals of nutrient recommendations for the mature adult are aimed at delaying the onset of chronic disease, while in others they are aimed at

For many other vitamins, as listed in Table 13-4, too little information is available to assess whether nutrient use or metabolism are altered during the aging process and whether those alterations are of sufficient magnitude to have an impact on nutrient requirements. This area is currently of interest and no doubt in the coming years more information will become available.

Minerals

Table 13-5 summarizes some of the major issues concerning vitamin requirements in the elderly. Limited data are available on the topic (49). In some cases, conclusions are drawn on the basis of a single study.

Concern has been raised regarding the adequacy in calcium intakes in mature adults. Evidence suggests that the elderly may have increased calcium requirements on the basis of apparent decreases in the efficiency of calcium intestinal absorption and compromised ability to increase efficiency of absorption in response to a low-calcium diet.

treatment or accommodation to the disorder, or some combination of the two.

Dentition and Associated Senses

With increasing age, there tends to be a decrease in the sense of taste and smell. These changes include loss of taste buds, mainly those involving salt and sweet, resulting in greater sensitivity to acid and bitter (26). Another change often observed in older individuals is diminished sense of smell. It has been observed that older individuals with poor odor perception have a lower nutrient intake than individuals with good odor perception (15). Salivary secretions have been noted to decrease with increased age. Changes in bite pattern from partial or complete extraction or loss of teeth are common in the elderly. Poorly fitted dentures can make eating a painful and distasteful chore. The prevalence of root caries is higher in older than in younger adults (33). The increased incidence of tooth disease in the elderly has been related to high levels of sugar consumption (33).

Any one or a combination of these factors can alter and restrict acceptable foods. Making food and nutrition recommendations for an older individual should include an assessment of dentition and possible limitations regarding food textures and methods of preparation. Counseling to avoid substitution of high-sugar foods of low-nutrient density for foods that are difficult to chew should be encouraged. It is also critical to suggest alternatives that are acceptable both from a cultural and economic perspective. Clearly, older adults are at risk for excluding specific food groups and having inadequate nutrient intake.

Cardiovascular Disease

The rate of cardiovascular disease increases with age, especially after menopause in females (42). Cross-cultural studies have revealed a positive correlation between rates of cardiovascular disease and both blood cholesterol levels and saturated fat intake. The American Heart Association (23) and the National Cholesterol Education Program (11) recommend restricting total fat to 30% or less of calories, saturated fat to less than 10%, monounsaturared fat to 10% to 15%, polyunsaturated fat to up to 10%, and cholesterol to less than 300 mg/day for all individuals over age 2. For individuals with total cholesterol levels of more than 200 mg/dL, saturated fat is further restricted to less than 7% of calories and cholesterol to less than 200 mg/day. No specific recommendations are made for older individuals. It has been clearly shown that older individuals, both men and women, respond to diets meeting these criteria with significant reductions in total and low-density lipoprotein (LDL) cholesterol levels (25,41). There is no evidence that diets meeting such recommendations pose a risk to older individuals, and such diets should therefore be encouraged.

Osteoporosis

Osteoporotic fractures affect 50% of females and 30% of males over age 50 (35). Bone loss, i.e., age-related or type II osteoporosis, is associated with the aging process. This is contributed to by loss of estrogen (in women), decreased calcium absorption from the gut, decreased calcium resportion from the kidney, decreased physical activity, decreased efficiency of

vitamin D metabolism, and decreased calcitriol production secondary to hyperparathyroidism (12,35). In the elderly, calcium balance is favorably affected by vitamin D intake, whereas it is negatively affected by high sodium, protein, alcohol, and caffeine intakes (12).

Recent work has suggested that supplemental calcium (500 mg/day) in postmenopausal women living in latitudes north of 42° north may be enhanced by an additional 100 IU to 700 IU of vitamin D per day, with the goal of minimizing bone loss from the spine and whole body but not the femoral neck (8). Because serum osteocalcin and plasma calcidiol fluctuate seasonally as a result of sun exposure, vitamin D intake is particulary important during the period of winter and spring in these women. Over a 3-year period, both men and women over age 65 who were given a dietary supplement of 500 mg of calcium and 700 IU of vitamin D have been reported to exhibit moderately reduced bone loss as measured in the femoral neck, spine, and total body, and importantly, a reduced incidence of nonvertebral fractures (9). These data strongly support maintenance of intake and perhaps supplementation in the elderly with both calcium and vitamin D.

Diabetes and Glucose Intolerance

The incidence of abnormal glucose homeostasis, specifically non–insulin-dependent diabetes mellitus (NIDDM), increases with age. The hallmarks of the disease are insulin resistance and impaired insulin secretion (36). Changes in lifestyle factors in older individuals have been found to be efficacious in the treatment of the disorder (3). These changes include instituting a daily exercise program (even in frail individuals), weight loss, and dietary modification aimed at decreasing simple carbohydrate intake and increasing fiber intake. A diet with 50% to 60% carbohydrate, predominantly complex, and 30 to 35 grams of fiber would be consistent with these recommendations (19). Since individuals with diabetes or glucose intolerance are at increased risk for the development of cardiovascular disease, these recommendations would be merged with restrictions in total fat (≤30%), saturated fat (<10%), and cholesterol (<300 mg per day). If the individual is hypercholesterolemic (>200 mg/dL) future restrictions as outlined above should be instituted.

Hypertension

The risk of developing elevated blood pressure increases with age. This risk is increased by weight gain during the adult years. A number of clinical trials have demonstrated clear benefits of the treatment of hypertension in the elderly (20). Preventing weight gain or normalizing body weight is an important strategy. From a nutrient perspective, sodium restriction has been found to be a useful treatment in some patients. Older hypertensive individuals appear to be more responsive to sodium restriction that younger hypertensive individuals (19). There is also evidence that coupling decreased sodium intakes with increased potassium intake may lead to improved blood pressure control (7).

Caution has been suggested regarding sodium restriction. Limited data suggest that sodium restriction is accompanied by lower intakes of energy, and accordingly, lower intakes of fat, protein, carbohydrate, calcium, and other nutrients (29). Some of these changes may be favorable, e.g., decreased energy intake in an older overweight individual;

however, some changes, e.g., lower calcium intake, can tax an already low intake. This cautionary note is particularly pertinent in light of the recent results from the Dietary Approaches to Stop Hypertension (DASH) study. Independent of sodium restriction, hypertensive subjects achieved maximum blood pressure reduction after consuming diets high in fruits, vegetables, and low-fat dairy products compared with diets rich in fruits and vegetables alone (1).

Immune Function

The most commonly associated age-related change in the immune response is cell-mediated function (27). It has recently been reported that vitamin E supplementation increases in vivo immune response in healthy elderly subjects (28). This potential increased need of older subjects for vitamin E has been suggested to be secondary to age-associated increased free radical formation and lipid peroxidation. At this time, it appears appropriate to recommend that older subjects consume diets with at least the minimum levels of vitamin E as defined by the RDAs. Further research is needed to determine whether the recommended levels should be increased.

Cancer

The incidence of cancer shows tremendous variability on the bases of worldwide distribution and type and site in the body. However, the incidence of all types of cancer increases with age. Support for a diet-cancer incidence link comes from data suggesting markedly divergent food consumption patterns and incidence rates of cancer among different population groups (45). The topic is too broad and the data too circumstantial to present more than a general overview. It has been suggested that to decrease the risk of certain cancers (listed in parentheses), the following dietary components should be considered: decreased alcohol intake (laryngeal), increased calcium and vitamin D intake (stomach, colon, breast), decreased fat intake (breast, colon, prostate), increased fiber intake (breast, colon), increased antioxidant vitamins, including vitamin A and beta-carotene, vitamin C, vitamin E, and trace elements, or orange and dark-green vegetable intake (wide range of sites) (6,19,45,46,48). It is likely that in the near future, as more data become available, this area will become clearer. Fortunately, general dietary recommendations to reduce cancer risk are consistent with the general dietary guidelines for the United States population.

SUMMARY

There is a progressive decline in organ function and change in body composition with advancing age. Diet, throughout the life-cycle, is related to the onset of many degenerative diseases that have a disproportionally high incidence in the mature adult. The overall aim of dietary recommendations for the older individual should be first to maintain optimal general health and function for as long a period as possible, and second, to forestall the development and progression of chronic disorders. Evidence suggests that there is a direct relationship between the nutrient quality of the diet and survival rates in the elderly. Although recommendations for specific nutrients for older individuals are not as yet available, the nutrient needs of the elderly are at least as great as that of their younger counterparts. Because of decreased metabolic rates and activity levels, which result in deceased energy requirements, special consideration needs to be given to individual food choices. Additionally, potential changes in living environment, economic status, mental health, and ability to acquire and prepare food can have a significant impact on food intake patterns that must be addressed on a regular basis. Emerging evidence suggests that active nutrient intervention with respect to cardiovascular disease, osteoporosis, diabetes, hypertension, immune function, and possibly cancer can help either forestall the development or help halt the progression of these disorders in the elderly. Dangerous is the attitude of either the mature adult or health care provider who believes that an individual is so old that they do not have to worry about nutrition. Our definitions for old age and expectations for the period of time individuals can live an active, productive, and independent life are expanding. Similarly, our concern and efforts toward intervention during this period with regard to encouraging and enabling the maintenance of optimal nutrition patterns should keep up with this trend.

This project has been funded at least in part with federal funds from the U.S. Department of Agriculture, Agricultural Research Service, under contract number 53/3-K06-5-10. The contents of this article do not necessarily reflect the views or policies of the US Department of Agriculture, nor does mention of trade names, commercial products, or organizations imply endorsement by the United States government.

REFERENCES

1. Appel LJ, Moore TJ, Obarzanek E, et al. A clinical trial of the effects of dietary patterns on blood pressure by the DASH Collaborative Research Group. N Engl J Med 1997;336:1117–1124.

2. Bostick RM, Potter JD, Sellers TA, et al. Relation of calcium, vitamin D, and dairy food intake to incidence of colon cancer among older women. The Iowa Women's Health Study. Am J Epidemiol 1993;137:1302–1317.

3. Brown DF, Jackson TW. Diabetes: 'tight control' in a comprehensive treatment plan. Geriatrics 1994;49:24–29.

4. Byrd D, Russell JM. Malabsorption in an elderly patient. Gastroenterologist 1993;1:287–290.

5. Campbell WW, Crim MC, Dallal GE, et al. Increased protein requirement in elderly people: new data and retrospective reassess-ments. Am J Clin Nutr 1994;60:501–509.

6. Cattaruzza MC, Maisonneuve P, Boyle P. Epidemiology of laryngeal cancer. Eur J Cancer 1996;32B:293–305.

7. Cutler JA. Combination of lifestyle modification and drug treatment in management of mild-moderate hypertension: a review of randomized clinical trials. Clin Exper Hypertens 1993;15:1193–1204.

8. Dawson-Hughes B, Harris SS, Krall EA, et al. Rates of bone loss in postmenopausal women randomly assigned to one or two dosages of vitamin D. Am J Clin Nutr 1995; 61:1140–1145.

9. Dawson-Hughes B, Harris SS, Krall EA, Dallal GE. Effect of calcium and vitamin D supplementation on bone density in men and women 65 years of age or older. N Engl J Med 1997;337:670–676.

10. De Groot LC, van Staveren WA, Burema J. Survival beyond age 70 in relation to diet. Nutrition Reviews 1995;54:212–221.

11. Expert Panel. Summary of the second report of the National Cholesterol Education Program Expert Panel on detection, evaluation, and treatment of high blood cholesterol in adults. JAMA 1993; 269:3015–3023.

12. Faine MP. Dietary factors related to preservation of oral and skeletal bone mass in women. J Prosthetic Dent 1995;73:65–72.

13. Feldman EB. Aspects of the interrelations of nutrition and aging: 1993. Am J Clin Nutr 1993;581: 1–3.

14. Fereday A, Gibson NR, Cox M, et al. Protein requirements and ageing: metabolic demand and efficiency of utilization. Brit J Nutr 1997;77:685–702.

15. Griep MI, Verleye G, Franck AH, et al. Variation in nutrient intake with dental status, age, and odor perception. Eur J Clin Nutr 1997; 50:816–825.

16. Hoffman N. Diet in the elderly: needs and risk. Med Clin North Am 1993;77:745–756.

17. Houston DK, Johnson MA, Daniel TD, Poon LW. Health and dietary characteristics of supplement users in an elderly population. Inter J Vit Min Res 1997;67:183–191.

18. James WP, Nelson M, Ralph A, Leather S. Socioeconomic determinants of health: the contribution of nutrition to inequalities in health. Brit J Med 1997;314:1545–1549.

19. Johnson K, Kligman EW. Preventive nutrition: disease-specific dietary interventions for older adults. Geriatrics 1992;47:39–49.

20. Kaplan NM. The promises and perils of treating the elderly hypertensive. Am J Med Sci 1993;305: 183–197.

21. Kerstetter JE, Holthausen BA, Fitz PA. Nutrition and nutritional requirements for the older adult. Dysphagia 1993;8:51–58.

22. Kinyamu HK, Gallagher JC, Prahl JM, et al. Association between intestinal vitamin D receptor, calcium absorption, and serum 1,25 dihydroxyvitamin D in normal young and elderly women. J Bone Min Res 1997;12:922–928.

23. Krauss RM, Deckelbaum RJ, Ernst N, et al. Dietary guidelines for healthy American adults. Circulation 1996;94:1795–1800.

24. La Rue A, Koehler KM, Wayne SJ, et al. Nutritional stauts and cognitive functioning in a normally aging sample: a 6-year reassessment. Am J Clin Nutr 1997;65:20–29.

25. Lichtenstein AH, Ausman L, Carrasco W, et al. Effects of canola, corn, and olive oil on fasting and postprandial plasma lipoproteins in humans as part of a National Cholesterol Education Program Step 2 Diet. Arterio Thromb 1993;13: 1533–1542.

26. Lipson LG, Bray GA. Energy. In: Nutritional aspects of aging. Vol. 1. Linda H. Chen, ed. Boca Raton, FL: CRC Press, 1986.

27. Meydani SN, Wu D, Santos MS, Hayek MG. Antioxidants and immune response in aged person: overview of present evidence. Am J Clin Nutr 1995;62(suppl):1462S –1476S.

28. Meydani SN, Meydani M, Blumberg JB, et al. Vitamin E supplementation and in vivo immune response in healthy elderly subjects: a randomized controlled trial. JAMA 1997;277:1380–1386.

29. Morris CD. Effect of dietary sodium restriction on overall nutrient intake. Am J Clin Nutr 1997; 65(suppl):687S–691S.

30. National Research Council. Recommended dietary allowances. 10th ed. Washington, DC: National Academy Press, 1989.

31. Paterson WG. Dysphagia in the elderly. Can Fam Phys 1996;42: 925–932.

32. Pannemans DLE, Van Den Berg H, Westerterp KR. The influence of protein intake on vitamin B$_6$ metabolism differs in young and elderly humans. J Nutr 1994;124: 1207–1214.

33. Papas AS, Joshi A, Palmer CA, et al. Relationship of diet to root caries. Am J Clin Nutr 1995; 61(suppl):423S–429S.

34. Prince RL, Dick IM, Lemmon J, Randell D. The pathogenesis of age-related osteroporotic fracture: effects of dietary calcium deprivation. J Clin Endocrin Metab 1997;82:260–264.

35. Prince RL, Diet and prevention of osteoporotic fractures. NEJM 1997;337:701–702.

36. Ruoff G. The management of non–insulin-dependent diabetes mellitus in the elderly. J Fam Pract 1993;36:329–335.

37. Russell RM, Suter RP. Vitamin requirements of elderly people: an update. Am J Clin Nutr 1993;58: 4–14.

38. Russell RM. New views on the RDAs for older adults. J Am Diet Assoc 1997;515–518.

39. Russell RM. The impact of disease states as a modifying factor for nutrition toxicity. Nutr Rev 1997; 55:50–53.

40. Sahyoun NR, Jacques RF, Russell RM. Carotenoids, vitamins C and E, and mortality in an elderly population. Am J Epidemiol 1996; 144:501–511.

41. Schaefer EJ, Lichtenstein AH, Lamon-Fava S. Efficacy of National Cholesterol Education Program Step 2 diet in normolipidemic and hypercholesterolemic middle-aged and elderly men and women. Arterio Thromb Vasc Biol 1995;15:1079–1085.

42. Schaefer EJ, Lichtenstein AH, Lamon-Fava S. Lipoproteins, nutri-

tion, aging, and atherosclerosis. Am J Clin Nutr 1995;61(suppl): 726S–740S.

43. Schlienger JL, Pradignac A, Grunenberger F. Nutrition of the elderly: a challenge between facts and needs. Horm Res 1995;43: 46–51.

44. Schroll M, Vellas B. Second European Congress on nutrition and health in the elderly. Age 1996;7: 136–181.

45. Serra-Majem L, Va Vecchia C, Ribas-Barba L. Changes in diet and mortality from selected cancers in southern Mediterranean countries, 1960–1989. Eur J Clin Nutr 1993;47(suppl):S25–S34.

46. Stahelin HB, Gey KF, Eichholzer M. Plasma antioxidant vitamins and subsequent cancer mortality in the 12-year follow-up of the prospective Basel Study. Am J Epidemiol 1991;133:766–775.

47. Suter PM, Russell RM. Vitamin requirements of the elderly. Am J Clin Nur 1987;45:501–512.

48. Watson R, Leonard T. Selenium and vitamins A, E, and C: nutrients with cancer prevention properties. J Amer Diet Assoc 1986; 86:505–510.

49. Wood RJ, Suter PM, Russell RM. Mineral requirements of elderly people. Am J Clin Nutr 1995;62: 493–505.

Chapter 14

Nutrition 101: The Concept of Nutritional Status and Guides for Nutrient Intakes, Eating Patterns, and Nutrition

Johanna T. Dwyer

This chapter provides an overview of the tools that are available for evaluating dietary intakes of individuals. It describes the concepts of dietary status, nutritional status, and some simple tools for measuring them. The dietary reference intakes, which are the standards for nutrient intakes that are used in the United States and Canada, are described and their uses are discussed. The food guide pyramid, which provides food-based recommendations based on the dietary reference intakes, is described. The Dietary Guidelines for Americans (DGA), recommendations to help guide Americans in altering their current intakes in more healthful directions, are summarized. The Nutrient Adequacy Index (NAI), a simple means of evaluating the balance, variety, and adequacy of intakes on the basis of these standards, is described. Finally, national goals for promoting health and preventing disease that involve nutrition are summarized.

THE CONCEPT OF NUTRITIONAL STATUS AND ITS MEASUREMENT

Nutritional status is an aspect of health status that results from the intake, absorption, and utilization of food and from the operation of infection, trauma, and metabolic factors that may be of pathologic significance. Dietary status is one aspect of nutritional status that refers to an individual's consumption of foods, food groups, or nutrients. Dietary status and nutritional status are not necessarily similar, since food consumption is not the only factor that is involved in determining if dietary intakes are sufficient to maintain health. Nutritional status assessment usually includes anthropometric, biochemical, clinical, and dietary examinations; collection of relevant

characteristics; and history of the individual that may be relevant to eating and metabolism. Table 14-1 summarizes the reasons why several indices of malnutrition are necessary. In addition to the many forms of malnutrition, each assessment method measures different stages in the development of malnutrition, and each method has its limitations. Therefore, several different measures that tap many characteristics and different levels of effects are usually employed.

The forms of malnutrition are several. Common terms used to describe them are listed in Table 14-2. The concept of nutritional status and its measurement have been discussed elsewhere in greater detail (1). The clinical signs of malnutrition and their effects on weight or height and on functions, such as the activities of daily living and quality of life, are the end result of a pathologic process, which is often present earlier in biomarkers, organ systems, tissues, and individual cells. Alterations in biochemical and hematologic measurements often reflect this in an earlier preclinical phase. If diet is the cause of the malnutrition, dietary alterations are usually apparent for days, weeks, or months before metabolism is altered and changes in biochemical measurements are present.

This chapter focuses on only one of the factors involved in nutritional status assessment—dietary intake. The rationale for measuring dietary intake is that many dietary factors affect nutritional status. These include the amount and the forms in which the nutrient is present in the diet, which may affect absorption, the presence of other nutrients or food constituents with biologic effects, and the presence of pathogens in the diet.

The usual goal of examining dietary intake is to obtain an estimate of habitual intake, either by measuring diet

Table 14-1 Forms of Malnutrition and Their Descriptive Clinical Terminology

FORM AND CAUSE OF MALNUTRITION	CLINICAL TERMINOLOGY	COMMENTS
Dehydration: inadequate fluid intake to meet bodily needs	Dehydration	Often occurs secondary to fever, exertion, or very warm, dry climate, or because of diets with high solute loads or drugs that have diuretic effects.
Starvation: virtually totally inadequate intakes of all nutrients	Marasmus, emaciation, cachexia	Occurs with prolonged fasting; withholding of fluids worsens its effects.
Protein-calorie malnutrition	Kwashiorkor, protein-calorie malnutrition	Often occurs secondary to disease and infection, probably via cytokine-mediated responses to acute infection or trauma, e.g., HIV infection, sarcopenia caused by inadequate intake of protein or cytokine-mediated responses to insult.
Vitamin, mineral, or other specific nutrient deficiencies	Pellagra (niacin/tryptophan deficiency), scurvy (ascorbic acid deficiency), rickets and osteomalacia (vitamin D deficiency in children and adults, respectively), iron deficiency anemia (iron deficiency), nutritional anemia (iron, vitamin B_6, folic acid, or vitamin B_{12} deficiency), essential fatty acid deficiency	Often occur secondarily to inadequate food intake or inadequate dietary quality. May also occur as conditioned deficiencies secondary to disease.
Increased diet-related chronic disease risk factors resulting from imbalances of nutrients	Excess of saturated fat, cholesterol, and other atherogenic and thrombogenic dietary lipids (hyperlipidemias and perhaps altered clotting factors); excess of salt or sodium (hypertension risk factors)	Imbalances or excesses of energy-yielding nutrients or related substances may give rise to metabolic aberrations and increase risks of ill health, especially in those with certain genetic patterns.
Obesity: excess food energy intake or insufficient energy output	Excess food energy, regardless of source, gives rise to obesity and overweight	Physical inactivity may increase likelihood of excess energy intakes.
Alcohol excess	Alcoholism, problem drinking	At very high levels of alcohol intake, all persons develop physical signs of chronic disease; at lower levels of intake, some individuals are particularly susceptible.
Excess of other specific nutrients (vitamins, minerals, others)	Specific toxicities vary: hypervitaminosis A (vitamin A), hypervitaminosis D (vitamin D), fluorosis (fluoride), etc.	Intakes that exceed the upper level of the DRIs generally increase risk of compromising one or more body functions. The functions involved vary from nutrient to nutrient.
Toxicity: excesses of other constituents in food, drink, or supplements	Names vary depending on substance; lead poisoning, lathyrism, etc.	Many substances other than nutrients in food and supplements may cause illness.
Foodborne disease	Food poisoning or food intoxication: salmonellosis, botulism, staphylococcal food poisoning, and others. Parasites, such as beef tapeworm, may cause problems. Prions or viruses, as in bovine spongiform encephalopathy	Food is the carrier for a microorganism, virus, or parasite, or a toxin produced by bacteria.

directly or by report. Because most health effects depend on usual or habitual intake, the report should span a sufficiently long period of time (e.g., many days or weeks) to be representative of usual intake. Only representative intakes over relatively long periods are meaningful when the goal is to assess the effects of diet on nutritional status. There are many methods of assessing dietary intake. These are reviewed elsewhere (2). Although they all have their limitations, at least they do provide a picture of food and nutrient consumption that may be useful for purposes of planning intakes or assessing what has been eaten.

The major shortcoming of most dietary assessment methods is that while they furnish a general profile of nutrient intakes, they are less accurate in providing information on the absolute amounts of different nutrients that are consumed. Most dietary assessment methods depend heavily on the eater's report, since it is very difficult to observe everything a person eats. As such, they may be biased. People may forget what they

Table 14-2 Why Multiple Indicators of Nutritional Status Are Needed
Multiple forms of malnutrition exist. See Table 14-1 for some examples. *The causes of malnutrition vary.* Some forms of malnutrition are caused by deficient quality or quantity of diet alone (primary malnutrition), but most are secondary to disease or social or psychological problems and may occur even in the face of adequate and appropriate food in the environment. Many different pieces of information are necessary to arrive at an understanding of how these causes interact. *No single indicator for all the forms of malnutrition exists.* The most sensitive, least costly, and most specific indicators of malnutrition vary from nutrient to nutrient. Even for a specific form of malnutrition, indicators vary with respect to how sensitive, specific, valid, and reliable they are. *Severity of malnutrition varies.* Milder forms require different and more sensitive indicators (e.g., measures of tissue or blood stores) than the more severe (which may be evident with anthropometric or clinical measures alone).

eat or report inaccurately because they want to appear to conform to what the questioner wants to hear, or they may unconsciously change what they eat when they are actually writing down what they eat. Therefore, information on dietary intakes is never perfectly accurate. These errors are usually quite large; perhaps 20% or more. Forgetting is a particular problem when people are asked to remember what they have eaten over the past day or weeks. When people are given lists of foods and asked to record the frequency with which they usually eat them, they often overestimate how much they eat. If they are asked to keep food records or diaries, they frequently change what they eat to make the recording task simpler or because they are surprised at how much they eat and decide to eat less to make their intakes appear more "balanced."

Because of the problems involved in obtaining accurate information on food intakes, if very precise estimates of intakes are necessary, as is the case in research studies, often other measures that reflect intakes of some nutrients are used. The problems are that the biochemical and other measures that are used are very specific, usually only reflect intakes of a single nutrient rather than the overall diet, and may require blood or urine samples. Therefore, biochemical and other measures of diet and nutritional status also have their limitations for practical studies.

Dietary intake assessment is used because it is less expensive than a full-fledged nutritional status assessment, and it often provides much useful information. It can identify those who are at high risk of malnutrition because they are eating too little, too much, or imbalanced amounts of foods

and nutrients. Dietary assessment also helps clarify and strengthen assumptions about the presumed causes of changes in nutritional status from anthropometric, biochemical, clinical, and other characteristics of the individual. Related questioning may reveal many environmental factors that influence dietary intakes and nutritional status, such as climate, living conditions, exposure to pathogens, and socioeconomic conditions.

Dietary status assessment only measures what an individual eats, not what is actually metabolized. Therefore, it may miss other causes of poor nutritional status, and thus it is narrower than nutritional status assessment. Although dietary assessment is potentially an extremely sensitive indicator of malnutrition, since it reflects a very early stage in the development of the pathology, in fact, it is often not useful by itself. Dietary data are less precise and reliable than biochemical and anthropometric indices. Because they are usually obtained by report from the patient or respondent, they are usually more subject-dependent and vary more in validity and reliability from one person to the next. It is difficult to determine whether suspected deficits in dietary intake actually result from diet or from errors in reporting. Therefore, dietary information must be combined with other types of data to fully assess nutritional status.

DIETARY REFERENCE INTAKES

The Dietary Reference Intakes (DRI) are standards used for nutrient intakes. They are quantitative estimates of nutrient intakes to be used for planning and assessing diets for healthy people. They are a conjoint effort of Health Canada and the Food and Nutrition Board of the U.S. National Academy of Sciences to develop dietary reference intakes that are used in formulating recommendations of nutrients for their citizens. They are also used as the basis for other materials providing food-based dietary guidance. The rationale and current status of the projects and recommendations to date are discussed. The issue of exportability of such recommendations is examined, and the next steps in going forward with the process are outlined.

Overview of the Dietary Reference Intakes
The DRIs are multiple reference points that serve as dietary standards for various uses (3,4), instead of the single reference values used in our countries in the past. The availability of new data on many nutrients; potential "candidate" nutrients; new concepts that recommendations should also reduce risks for chronic disease and excessive intake, if possible; and new user needs made a revision of existing recommendations imperative. The new DRIs include the estimated average requirement (EAR), the recommended dietary allowance (RDA), or, if it cannot be calculated, the adequate intake (AI), and the upper intake level (UL). The first three of these categories of DRI are defined with specific criteria of nutrient adequacy. The UL, in contrast, is defined by a specific indicator of excess.

Reference weights and heights for adults and children on which the dietary recommendations are based are derived from recent population-based surveys of the United States.

Criteria on Which Recommendations are Based

The criteria of adequacy upon which nutrient needs are formulated are critical. The possibilities vary: These include the best level to determine the risk of an individual becoming deficient in the nutrient, but another possibility may relate to reducing the risk of chronic degenerative diseases. Each EAR, RDA, and AI is described in terms of a selected criterion or criteria of adequacy. For example, the criterion for folic acid among women in the childbearing years is based on a combination of biochemical indicators, such as red cell folate, and secondarily, plasma homocysteine and serum folate levels. A separate recommendation is made for women capable of becoming pregnant to reduce the level of neural tube defects.

Prevention of chronic disease is a focus of some nutrient adequacy determinations. For example, calcium was selected to be a level of intake sufficient to provide retention of calcium during growth and minimize bone loss during adulthood. In the case of fluoride, the amount needed to decrease rates of dental caries was selected. However, the factual basis for preventing chronic disease was judged to be insufficient for other nutrients, including phosphorus, magnesium, vitamin D, the B vitamins, and choline.

Recommended Dietary Allowance

The recommended dietary allowance (RDA) is the average daily dietary intake level that is sufficient to meet the nutrient requirements of nearly all (97% to 98%) healthy persons of a specific gender at a particular stage of life and age or physiologic condition, such as pregnancy or lactation. The only use of the RDA is to serve as a goal for individuals.

To establish an RDA, agreement on the criterion to be used to set the EAR is the first issue that must be addressed. This criterion is used to assess adequacy. Then the appropriate cutoff must be established for each criterion to determine the difference between what is considered an adequate and an inadequate level of nutritional status. To do this, there must be sufficient data on individuals who are consuming levels of intake at which some reach the suggested cutoff for the criterion and at which others do not. It is also necessary to have an understanding of the distribution of requirements among individuals in the group from whom the requirement is estimated. When nutrient requirements are skewed for a population, other approaches are used to find the 97th to 98th percentile to set the RDA.

Current RDAs and AIs are provided in Tables 14-3 and 14-4. These are the values that should be used for planning individual intakes. Note that many of the values have not yet been revised and updated; this is a time-consuming process. A revision of all the RDAs will not be completed for several more years. For nutrients that have not yet been reviewed, values from the 1989 RDAs should be used as the standard.

The RDAs are not appropriate for assessing the diets of either individuals or groups or for planning diets for groups.

Estimated Average Requirement

The estimated average requirement (EAR) is another DRI value that is essential for setting the RDA. The EAR is the amount of a nutrient that is estimated to meet the requirement of half the healthy individuals in a specific life-stage and gender group. The EAR is used to assess adequacy of intakes of population groups and, along with knowledge of the distribution of requirements, to develop RDAs. The EAR is the lowest level of a nutrient eaten chronically that will maintain a defined level of nutriture. Before setting an EAR, a specific criterion of adequacy must be chosen. This selection is based on a careful review of the literature. Among the criteria that may be used, reduction of disease risk may be considered, along with other health parameters. Ideally, the standard deviation (SD), i.e., an estimate of the variability of requirements, is desirable. It is assumed that the distribution of requirements is normal. If the SD is not available, then an assumed coefficient of variation (CV) is used, usually of 10%. Under these circumstances, the RDA is assumed to be $1.2 \cdot EAR$. Conversely, if this CV is 15%, the RDA is $1.3 \cdot EAR$.

Adequate Intake

The adequate intake (AI) is a recommended daily intake level based on observed or experimentally determined approximations of nutrient intake in a group of healthy people. It is used when an RDA cannot be determined. The AI is based on observed or experimentally determined estimates of a group's nutrient intake. The main use of the AI is as a goal for the nutrient intake of individuals. These AIs are usually based on observed levels of intake that appear to maintain an acceptable level of health or growth. The AI, therefore, is an indication that experts believe that sufficient data on requirements are not present and that more research needs to be done. The AI is set at a level that is expected to cover the needs of at least 98% of people, but it might cover the needs of fewer or more since the EAR cannot be estimated. Unfortunately, the degrees to which AIs exceed average requirements probably differ among nutrients and population groups.

In the reports of the DRI to date, AIs rather than RDAs are proposed for all nutrients for infants up to age 1, and for calcium, vitamin D, fluoride, pantothenic acid, biotin, and choline for persons of all ages. RDAs are provided for all the other nutrients.

Recommended individual intake guidelines, such as the RDA and AI, should not be used inappropriately. Both the RDA and AI are appropriately used for setting goals for intakes of individuals. However, greater uncertainty surrounds the AI.

Upper Intake Level

Nutrients within a certain range of intake are essential for human well-being and life. However, at excessive levels nutrients share the possibility of producing adverse effects. Also, at dietary levels, human experience is considerable on intakes at levels found in food. However, it is only in the past few decades that single concentrated sources of nutrients have become available, and the possibility of higher intakes is now more likely. At present, there is no evidence to suggest that nutrients consumed at recommended intake levels of the RDA and AI present a risk of adverse effects to most persons. However, there is a possibility that, given that there are higher amounts of nutrients in fortified food and nonfood sources

Table 14-3 Dietary Reference Intakes

Food and Nutrition Board, Institute of Medicine-National Academy of Sciences Dietary Reference Intakes: Recommended Intakes for Individuals

Life-Stage Group (Age)	Calcium (mg/day)	Phosphorus (mg/day)	Magnesium (mg/day)	Vitamin D (µg/day)a,b	Fluoride (mg/day)	Thiamin (mg/day)	Riboflavin (mg/day)	Niacin (mg/day)c	Vitamin B6 (mg/day)	Folate (µg/day)d	Vitamin B12 (µg/day)	Pantothenic Acid (mg/day)	Biotin (µg/day)	Cholinee (mg/day)
Infants														
0–6 mo	210*	100*	30*	5*	0.01*	0.2*	0.3*	2*	0.1*	65*	0.4*	1.7*	5*	125*
7–12 mo	270*	275*	75*	5*	0.5*	0.3*	0.4*	4*	0.3*	80*	0.5*	1.8*	6*	150*
Children														
1–3 yr	500*	460	80	5*	0.7*	0.5	0.5	6	0.5	150	0.9	2*	8*	200*
4–8 yr	800*	500	130	5*	1*	0.6	0.6	8	0.6	200	1.2	3*	12*	250*
Males														
9–13 yr	1300*	1250	240	5*	2*	0.9	0.9	12	1.0	300	1.8	4*	20*	375*
14–18 yr	1300*	1250	410	5*	3*	1.2	1.3	16	1.3	400	2.4	5*	25*	550*
19–30 yr	1000*	700	400	5*	4*	1.2	1.3	16	1.3	400	2.4	5*	30*	550*
31–50 yr	1000*	700	420	5*	4*	1.2	1.3	16	1.3	400	2.4	5*	30*	550*
51–70 yr	1200*	700	420	10*	4*	1.2	1.3	16	1.7	400	2.4f	5*	30*	550*
>70 yr	1200*	700	420	15*	4*	1.2	1.3	16	1.7	400	2.4f	5*	30*	550*
Females														
9–13 yr	1300*	1250	240	5*	2*	0.9	0.9	12	1.0	300	1.8	4*	20*	375*
14–18 yr	1300*	1250	360	5*	3*	1.0	1.0	14	1.2	400g	2.4	5*	25*	400*
19–30 yr	1000*	700	310	5*	3*	1.1	1.1	14	1.3	400g	2.4	5*	30*	425*
31–50 yr	1000*	700	320	5*	3*	1.1	1.1	14	1.3	400g	2.4	5*	30*	425*
51–70 yr	1200*	700	320	10*	3*	1.1	1.1	14	1.5	400	2.4f	5*	30*	425*
>70 yr	1200*	700	320	15*	3*	1.1	1.1	14	1.5	400	2.4f	5*	30*	425*
Pregnancy														
≤18 yr	1300*	1250	400	5*	3*	1.4	1.4	18	1.9	600h	2.6	6*	30*	450*
19–30 yr	1000*	700	350	5*	3*	1.4	1.4	18	1.9	600h	2.6	6*	30*	450*
31–50 yr	1000*	700	360	5*	3*	1.4	1.4	18	1.9	600h	2.6	6*	30*	450*
Lactation														
≤18 yr	1300*	1250	360	5*	3*	1.5	1.6	17	2.0	500	2.8	7*	35*	550*
19–30 yr	1000*	700	310	5*	3*	1.5	1.6	17	2.0	500	2.8	7*	35*	550*
31–50 yr	1000*	700	320	5*	3*	1.5	1.6	17	2.0	500	2.8	7*	35*	550*

* This table presents Recommended Dietary Allowances (RDAs) in bold type and Adequate Intakes (AIs) in ordinary type followed by an asterisk (*). RDAs and AIs may both be used as goals for individual intake. RDAs are set to meet the needs of almost all (97% to 98%) individuals in a group. For healthy breastfed infants, the AI is the mean intake. The AI for other life-stage and gender groups is believed to cover needs of all individuals in the group, but lack of data or uncertainty in the data prevent being able to specify with confidence the percentage of individuals covered by this intake.

a As cholecalciferol. 1 µg cholecalciferol = 40 IU vitamin D.

b n the absence of adequate exposure to sunlight.

c As niacin equivalents (NE). 1 mg of niacin = 60 mg of tryptophan; 0–6 months = preformed niacin (not NE).

d As dietary folate equivalents (DFE). 1 DFE = 1 µg food folate = 0.6 µg of folic acid (from fortified food or supplement) consumed with food = 0.5 µg of synthetic (supplemental) folic acid taken on an empty stomach.

e Although AIs have been set for choline, there are few data to assess whether a dietary supply of choline is needed at all stages of the life cycle, and it may be that the choline requirement can be met by endogenous synthesis at some of these stages.

f Because 10% to 30% of older people may malabsorb food-bound B12, it is advisable for those older than 50 years to meet their RDA mainly by consuming foods fortified with B12 or a supplement containing B12.

g In view of evidence linking folate intake with neural tube defects in the fetus, it is recommended that all women capable of becoming pregnant consume 400 µg of synthetic folic acid from fortified foods and/or supplements in addition to intake of food folate from a varied diet.

h It is assumed that women will continue consuming 400 µg of folic acid until their pregnancy is confirmed and they enter prenatal care, which ordinarily occurs after the end of the periconceptional period—the critical time for formation of the neural tube.

Reproduced by permission from Institute of Medicine, Food and Nutrition Board. Dietary reference intakes. Washington DC: National Academy Press, 1998, Copyright 1998 by the National Academy of Sciences. Courtesy of the National Academy Press.

Table 14-4 Recommended Dietary Allowances

FOOD AND NUTRITION BOARD, NATIONAL ACADEMY OF SCIENCES—NATIONAL RESEARCH COUNCIL RECOMMENDED DIETARY ALLOWANCES,[a] REVISED 1989 (ABRIDGED) DESIGNED FOR THE MAINTENANCE OF GOOD NUTRITION OF PRACTICALLY ALL HEALTHY PEOPLE IN THE UNITED STATES

Category	Age (yr) or Condition	Weight[b] (kg)	(lb)	Height[b] (cm)	(in)	Protein (g)	Vitamin A (µg RE)[c]	Vitamin E (mg α-TE)[d]	Vitamin K (µg)	Vitamin C (mg)	Iron (mg)	Zinc (mg)	Iodine (µg)	Selenium (µg)
Infants	0.0–0.5	6	13	60	24	13	375	3	5	30	6	5	40	10
	0.5–1.0	9	20	71	28	14	375	4	10	35	10	5	50	15
Children	1–3	13	29	90	35	16	400	6	15	40	10	10	70	20
	4–6	20	44	112	44	24	500	7	20	45	10	10	90	20
	7–10	28	62	132	52	28	700	7	30	45	10	10	120	30
Males	11–14	45	99	157	62	45	1000	10	45	50	12	15	150	40
	15–18	66	145	176	69	59	1000	10	65	60	12	15	150	50
	19–24	72	160	177	70	58	1000	10	70	60	10	15	150	70
	25–50	79	174	176	70	63	1000	10	80	60	10	15	150	70
	51	77	170	173	68	63	1000	10	80	60	10	15	150	70
Females	11–14	46	101	157	62	46	800	8	45	50	15	12	150	45
	15–18	55	120	163	64	44	800	8	55	60	15	12	150	50
	19–24	58	128	164	65	46	800	8	60	60	15	12	150	55
	25–50	63	138	163	64	50	800	8	65	60	15	12	150	55
	51	65	143	160	63	50	800	8	65	60	10	12	150	55
Pregnant						60	800	10	65	70	30	15	175	65
Lactating	1st 6 mo					65	1300	12	65	95	15	19	200	75
	2nd 6 mo					62	1200	11	65	90	15	16	200	75

Note: This table does not include nutrients for which Dietary Reference Intakes have recently been established (see Dietary Reference Intakes for Calcium, Phosphorus, Magnesium, Vitamin D, and Fluoride [1997] and Dietary Reference Intakes for Thiamin, Riboflavin, Niacin, Vitamin B₆, Folate, Vitamin B₁₂, Pantothenic Acid, Biotin, and Choline [1998]).
a The allowances, expressed as average daily intakes over time, are intended to provide for individual variations among most normal persons as they live in the United States under usual environmental stresses. Diets should be based on a variety of common foods to provide other nutrients for which human requirements have been less well defined.
b Weights and heights of Reference Adults are actual medians for the U.S. population of the designated age, as reported by the NHANES II study. The median weights and heights of those under 19 years of age were taken from Hamill et al (1979). The use of these figures does not imply that the height-to-weight ratios are ideal.
c Retinol equivalents. 1 retinol equivalent = 1 µg retinol or 6 µg β-carotene.
d α-Tocopherol equivalents. 1 mg d-α tocopherol = 1 α-TE.
Reproduced by permission from National Research Council, Subcommittee on the Tenth Edition of the RDAs, Food and Nutrition Board. Recommended dietary allowances. 10th ed. Washington DC: National Academy Press, 1989. Copyright 1989 by the National Academy of Sciences. Courtesy of the National Academy Press.

such as supplements, these sources may pose a risk of adverse health effects.

The tolerable upper intake level (UL) is the highest level of chronic and usual daily nutrient intake that is likely to pose no risk of adverse health effects to almost all individuals in the general population (5). The higher the intake increases above the UL, the greater the risk of adverse effects. The UL limits include intake from food, water, and nonfood sources, such as nutrient supplements and pharmacologic preparations. The word *tolerable* is used because the meaning is that individuals should be able to tolerate this level of intake. However, it does not imply that this level is desirable. Many individuals are using large amounts of nutrients for curative or treatment purposes. Those who are being treated by a physician should recognize that the UL is not an intended level of a nutrient. As intake increases above the UL, the risk of adverse effects increases. The UL is not a level at which there is a beneficial effect; it describes the intake level at which there is a high probability that the dose of the nutrient can be tolerated biologically. If certain total intake amounts have been associated with toxicity, this is stated. In a few cases, it may be that toxicities are only associated with supplements or drugs.

Adverse effects are any significant alterations in the structure or function of the human being or any impairment of a physiologically important function. Also, intakes of one nutrient may alter the health benefits conferred by another to create adverse nutrient-nutrient interactions: this is also considered an adverse health effect.

Risk assessments describe the relationships between exposure to an agent, such as a nutrient, and the likelihood that adverse health effects will occur in the exposed populations. Consideration of a constant set of scientific principles involved in the process of risk assessment is used to set ULs. Risk assessment is a systematic method for evaluation of the probability of adverse health events occurring in humans from excess exposure to an environmental agent, such as a nutrient or food component. The vital point is that all evaluations and judgments are explicit, and evidence is provided to document conclusions. Both qualitative and quantitative types of evidence must be considered. ULs are set by reviewing the literature to determine levels at which no observed adverse effects are noted (NOAEL), or the lowest level of intake associated with observed adverse effects. Then an uncertainty factor is applied to reduce the intake level from the lowest adverse effect level to insure that even the most sensitive persons would not be affected by the UL dose chosen. At present, for many nutrients there is not enough evidence to develop a UL. For many nutrients, data are so limited that a UL cannot be determined. The process of identifying hazards, assessing dose-responses, assessing intake, and then characterizing risk and evaluating risk most expand. The risk is expressed as the fraction of the exposed populations, if any, that have nutrient intakes in excess of the estimated ULs. ULs are not always certain values that are fixed in stone. Risk assessment includes both data- and inference-related scientific uncertainties. In addition to risk assessments, it may be necessary to address public health concerns about the significance of the risk, the technical feasibility of achieving various degrees of risk control, and economic and social costs of such control. Safety and lack of it are not absolutes.

For many nutrients, ULs are not available. Often,

although intakes are available, there are no data on adverse effects of taking large amounts of nutrients, or data are often anecdotal in nature. Thus, a UL cannot be established. This does not mean that there is no risk of adverse effects from high intake; in fact, when data about adverse effects are very limited, extra caution may be warranted. The data that exist are often scanty or drawn on studies to address the questions.

Risk-risk assessments may sometimes be more useful than risk-benefit studies; e.g., the risks of taking the nutrient versus the risk of not taking the nutrient or supplement.

Current Status of the DRI Revisions

The first order of business has been to convene panels of experts on nutrients to develop recommendations. A report on calcium and related nutrients was issued in 1997 that included recommendations for calcium (AI), phosphorus, magnesium, fluoride, and vitamin D (6). A report on folic acid and other B vitamins was issued in 1998 (7). The panel on "antioxidant" nutrients (ascorbic acid, vitamin E, and possibly others) and a panel on the uses of the DRIs are now meeting. Reactions to date have been positive, and food-based recommendations will soon be discussed (8).

Not all of the DRIs are yet available, and for the present, the 1989 RDAs are used for nutrients for which DRIs have not yet been set (9).

Uses Outside the U.S.: Are the DRIs Exportable?

DRI recommendations are probably more exportable to other countries than they used to be, but less than they may need to be, in our increasingly global economy during the next millennium.

Some elements of the DRI process are clearly exportable. The evidence-based review of the scientific literature is certainly so; other experts can review the evidence and come to their own conclusions. Clearer distinctions are made between considerations based on fact and judgments. Also, economic realities, usual intakes, and historical precedents are better separated from considerations of requirements than ever before: these aspects of the process are also useful. The EAR and UL, which are determined largely by human biology, should theoretically be useful in other countries. However, the functional criteria used to set requirements are many, and the most appropriate ones for each country may vary with expert judgment and health realities. Other countries may wish to choose other end points or interpret the data differently.

Exportability may be limited in other ways as well. Food and nutrient intakes of populations vary, as do environmental factors. Population profiles, resource constraints, and expert judgment may lead to the choice of different criteria for adequacy, with the result that EAR, RDA, AI, and UL values chosen may change.

So far, the DRI committees have not set recommendations for intakes of nutrients for populations—only for individuals. Population recommendations for nutrient intakes are likely to be much more environment- and culture-bound than estimates of requirements and are likely to vary much more from country to country than are RDA, EAR, or UL. This is because not only do average intakes of nutrients differ greatly from one country to another, but also so do the distributions of intakes. The shape of these distributions of nutrient intakes is probably very wide in some countries and narrow in others.

Recommended levels for population intakes must take into account not only EARs but also these distributions of nutrient intakes within the population. Also, the strategies (e.g., fortification, supplementation, nutrition education, limitation of excessive intakes) that may be adopted for bringing intakes into an optimal range may vary from one country to another and be subject to resource and environmental constraints. The desired percentage of the population having access to or actually achieving intakes that meet whatever criteria are chosen for the DRI will also vary from one country to another, and success involves political will as well as scientific judgment.

The notion of exporting the DRI recommendations is therefore untested, and results would probably vary, depending on the specific DRI and nutrient that are being considered. Indeed, the Canadian-American process still does not cover all of North America; Mexico was unable to participate in the early part of the process but may join in the effort soon. Finally, it goes without saying but goes better said that North America is not the world repository of all nutrition science wisdom and truth. Experts in other countries no doubt have much to add to the process and product and may develop even sounder recommendations as a result of their further deliberations. Finally, since science is constantly changing and growing, there is always a need for revision, as new data become available. The DRIs were conceived as a first attempt and not as the last word, so there is room for change and diversity. Diversity in expert judgments may help to drive science forward to seek firmer evidence.

Next Steps for the DRI

The Canadians and Americans have a great deal to do before their tasks are completed. Reference documents for experts must be developed for each nutrient. This process is time-consuming and expensive. A document on the appropriate uses of each dietary standard and how professionals should interpret them is sorely needed, since these are new concepts for many. The thorny issue of population recommendations must be addressed. Finally, recommendations for the public with respect to healthy diets and providing examples of dietary patterns must be developed. These are likely to be country-specific.

The collaborative effort between Canada and the U.S. has been intellectually satisfying, productive, and personally gratifying. A common standard of DRIs in North America will hopefully thrive and expand in the third millennium. For other countries, the DRI recommendations, which are more evidence-based than ever before, deserve examination. The DRIs may serve as useful compendia to review for other nations' own efforts. Exportability and importability judgments are more difficult to make. Certainly there is still something to be said for diverse efforts strengthening the final product, and since all science is subject to revision as new evidence emerges, constant review is needed in any event. Other expert groups in other countries will no doubt have useful suggestions and improvements from which we can learn. Before the DRIs travel, some of them may need visas! Perhaps, by the end of the next century, these differences can be done away with altogether, but for now, a certain amount of diversity in the requirements may be healthy. To learn more about the Canadian-U.S. DRIs, the World Wide Web will keep you in touch at http://www2.nas.edu/fnb.

USES OF THE RDI

Assessing the Adequacy of Groups

The most appropriate ways to evaluate the intakes of groups are to use the EARs when they are available. The proportion of individuals below the fiftieth percentile can be measured: these individuals are at greater risk of dietary inadequacy. Defining the percent of the population with intakes below the RDAs as being at risk is specifically not appropriate and will overestimate the proportion truly at risk because of the very definition of the RDA. The AI is probably close to the group mean intake. If the mean intake of a group is at or above the AI, we can be confident that there are unlikely to be major shortfalls for intake of the nutrient. The AI is a good target for planning group intakes. It is not possible to quantitatively assess risk of inadequacy with AIs; however, qualitative statements can be made. The difficulties of assessing toxicity with the UL must aslo be considered. With respect to assessing intakes of individuals, the best criterion is to compare intakes to the EAR.

DIETARY GUIDELINES FOR AMERICANS

The Dietary Guidelines for Americans (10) are recommendations to help guide dietary choices that Americans make. They are targeted to people over age 2; such recommendations are not appropriate for small infants and toddlers who are not yet consuming family fare.

The dietary guideline recommendations have changed somewhat over the years, but in general they have stayed quite constant. Table 14-5 compares the 1980 and 1995 versions of the DGA. The guidelines emphasize not only getting enough

Table 14-5 Comparisons of the Dietary Guidelines for Americans (DGA) in 1980 and 1995 (Most Recent Revision)	
DGA 1980	**DGA 1995**
Eat a variety of foods	Eat a variety of foods
Maintain desirable weight	Balance the food you eat with physical activity; maintain or improve your weight
Avoid too much fat, saturated fat, and cholesterol	Choose a diet with plenty of grain products, vegetables, and fruits
Eat foods with adequate starch and fiber	Choose a diet low in fat, saturated fat, and cholesterol
Avoid too much sugar	Choose a diet moderate in sugar
Avoid too much sodium	Choose a diet moderate in salt and sodium
Drink alcohol in moderation, if you drink	If you drink alcoholic beverages, do so in moderation

food but also balance, variety, and moderation in consumption patterns to decrease diet-related risks of chronic degenerative diseases.

Note that the messages have evolved from proscriptive suggestions that centered on foods and dietary constituents to avoid to more prescriptive recommendations about positive dietary behaviors. Also, as scientific evidence has increased, the emphasis and content have changed somewhat. Current DGA recommend that to stay healthy, one should eat a variety of foods, maintain or improve one's weight by balancing food intake with physical activity, and choose a diet that is plentiful in grain products and vegetables and fruits; moderate in salt, sodium, and sugars; and low in fat, saturated fat, and cholesterol. Those who consume alcoholic beverages should do so in moderation.

Note that the guidelines are qualitative for the most part, recommending patterns of food choices and food groups, rather than very specific amounts of foods or nutrients. This qualitative emphasis reflects their educational purpose. Some of the guidelines are more quantitative. For example, the variety goal is defined more precisely in the text that accompanies the dietary guidelines to include specific servings from the food guide pyramid that is discussed below. Also, specific goals are provided for dietary fats, since the basis for evidence on intakes of this nutrient is very well developed.

Many other sets of guidelines are also available. Among the better known alternative guidelines are the recommendations of the National Academy of Sciences (11). In most respects, these guidelines are similar to the DGAs.

Providing guidelines is one thing; incorporating them into our daily lives is quite another. Recommendations for putting DGAs into action are available and deserve careful reading by health professionals and others (12).

FOOD GUIDE PYRAMID

The US Department of Agriculture introduced the food guide pyramid in 1992 (Figure 14-1) (13). The pyramid

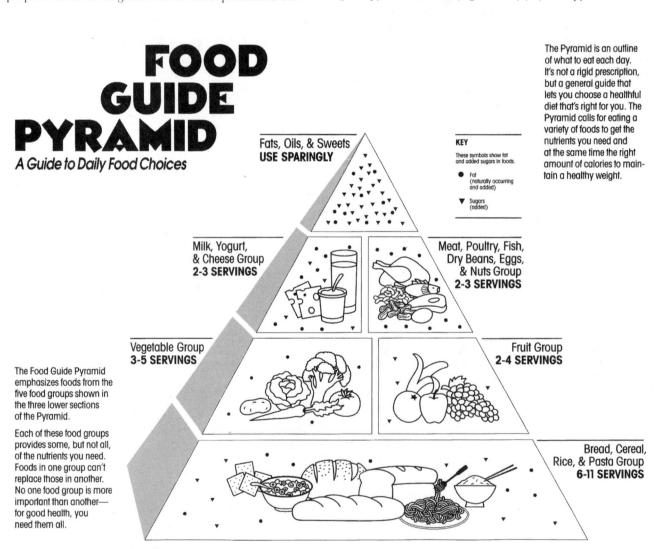

Figure 14-1 The U.S. Department of Agriculture food guide pyramid. (SOURCE: U.S. Department of Agriculture and the U.S. Department of Health and Human Services. Provided by the Education Department of the National Cattleman's Beef Association.)

Table 14-6 Serving Size and Number for Various Food Groups in the USDA Food Pyramid

Food Group	Serving Size	Women and Some Older Adults	Children, Teenage Girls, Active Women, and Most Men	Teenage Boys and Active Men
Calorie Level*		About 1600	About 2200	About 2800
		No. of Servings		
Bread group	1 slice bread; ½ cup cooked rice, pasta, or cooked cereal; 1 oz. ready-to-eat cereal	6	9	22
Vegetable group	½ cup chopped raw or cooked vegetables; 1 cup of leafy raw vegetables	3	4	5
Fruit group	1 piece of fruit or melon wedge; ¾ cup juice; ½ cup canned fruit; ¼ cup dried fruit	2	3	4
Milk group	1 cup milk or yogurt; 1.5 to 2.0 oz. cheese	2–3	2–3[a]	2–3[a]
Meat group	2.5 to 3.0 oz. of cooked lean meat, poultry, or fish; count ½ cup of cooked beans; 1 egg; 2 Tbsp. peanut butter as 1 oz. lean meat (about 1/3 serving)	2 (5 oz.)	2 (6 oz.)	3 (7 oz.)

* Calorie levels assume choices are low-fat, lean foods from the five major food groups, using foods from the fats, oils, and sweets group sparingly.

[a] Women who are pregnant or breastfeeding, teenagers, and young adults to age 24 need 3 servings.

provides a simple graphic tool that assists people in choosing healthy dietary patterns that are varied, balanced, and moderate. The pyramid suggests the number of recommended servings per day from each food group. The reason for dividing foods into groups is that each of the food groups provides some, but not all, of the nutrients people eat every day. It emphasizes the importance of consuming a menu that starts with plenty of breads, cereals, rice and pasta, vegetables, and fruits; of choosing two to three servings from the milk group and two to three servings from the meat group, with an emphasis on foods low in fats, sugars, and alcohol; and of avoiding excessive energy intakes.

The serving sizes suggested are provided in the pyramid. The amount people eat at a sitting may be more than just one serving: for example, a dinner portion of spaghetti would count as two or three servings of pasta. Table 14-6 provides the serving sizes and number of servings that conform to usual calorie intakes of various groups. No serving sizes are given for fats, oils, and sweets. These should be limited, especially if there is a need to lose weight. Fats, oils, sweets, and alcohol provide calories but relatively few vitamins or minerals.

HEALTHY EATING INDEX

The Healthy Eating Index (HEI) is a summary measure of people's overall diet quality. In a sense, it is a "report card" on how well Americans are eating (14,15). It consists of a score that is the sum of ten components, each representing a different aspect of a healthful diet. The first five components measure the degree to which a person's diet conforms to the USDA food guide pyramid's recommendations for servings from the five major food groups: grains (bread cereal, rice, and pasta); vegetables; fruits; milk (milk, yoghurt, and cheese); and the meat group (meat, poultry, fish, dry beans, eggs, and nuts). The sixth component measures total fat consumption as a percentage of total food energy intake (i.e., calories). The seventh component focuses on saturated fat consumption as a percentage of total food energy intake. The eighth component measures total cholesterol intake; the ninth, total sodium intake; and the tenth focuses on the variety in a person's diet. Each of these ten components has a maximum score of 10 and a minimum score of zero. A high score on a component indicates that intakes are close to the recommended ranges or amounts, as stated in the USDA food guide pyramid, the DGAs, or similar authoritative guidance. Low scores indicate less compliance with recommended ranges or amounts of nutrients. Thus, the maximum overall score for the ten components combined is 100.

The latest "report card" on the nation's eating habits was compiled using HEI data from the 1994 to 1996 Continuing Survey of Food Intakes by Individuals, a nationally representative food consumption survey (16). Most people could improve their intakes. Approximately 12% of the population has a good diet, with an HEI score over 80, and 18% has a poor diet, as signified by HEI scores of less than 51. Special areas needing improvement

Table 14-7 Permissible Health Claims for Foods

HEALTH CLAIM	COMMENTS
Calcium and osteoporosis	A calcium-rich diet is linked to a reduced risk of osteoporosis, a condition in which the bones become soft or brittle.
Fat and cancer	A diet low in total fat is linked to a reduced risk of some cancers.
Saturated fat and cholesterol and heart disease	A diet low in saturated fat and cholesterol can help reduce the risk of heart disease.
Fiber-containing grain products, fruits, and vegetables, and cancer	A diet rich in high-fiber grain products, fruits, and vegetables can reduce the risk of some cancers.
Fruits, vegetables, and grain products that contain fiber and heart disease	A diet rich in fruits, vegetables, and grain products that contain fiber can help reduce the risk of heart disease.
Sodium and high blood pressure	A low-sodium diet may help reduce the risk of high blood pressure, which is a risk factor for heart attacks and strokes.
Fruits and vegetables and some cancers	A low-fat diet rich in fruits and vegetables (foods that are low in fat and may contain dietary fiber, vitamin A, or vitamin C) is linked to a reduced risk of some cancers.
Folic acid and neural tube birth defects	Women who consume 0.4 mg of folic acid daily reduce their risk of giving birth to a child affected with a neural tube defect.

are consumption of fruit and milk and milk products. Boys, aged 15 to 18, tended to have lower quality diets. African Americans, people with low incomes, and those with a high school diploma or less education also had lower quality diets (17). More definitive reports on nutritional status are issued periodically by the federal government. These provide detailed discussions of dietary patterns and nutrients (18).

OTHER METHODS FOR DIETARY ASSESSMENT

There are many different methods for assessing dietary intakes. The appropriate method depends on what question is being asked. Also, the choice of method depends on whether food patterns, food groups, individual foods, or nutrients are the units that are of greatest interest. The various dietary assessment methods and their pros and cons are discussed elsewhere in depth (19,20), and the reader should consult these sources to determine what tools are the most appropriate.

NUTRIENT LABELING

One other consumer education and awareness tool deserves special mention: nutrient labeling. Processed food products have had ingredient labeling, with ingredients listed by weight, for many years. These are helpful for persons who want to include or avoid certain food ingredients in their diets for health or cultural reasons. For those who were knowledgeable about the nutrient content of foods, such listings were also helpful in providing information about what products contained.

New tools on labels now make it even easier for consumers. Nutrient labeling of processed foods was first made mandatory in 1993. The nutrition facts panel provides information about fat and other nutrient content in standardized serving sizes. It is a tool to help people select healthy diets by labeling the nutrient content for standard portion sizes of most processed packaged foods. Today, the vast majority of such foods are labeled, and efforts are being made to extend labeling to other foods, such as fresh fruits and vegetables, meats, poultry, and fish. In addition to these steps, over-the-counter vitamin and mineral supplements are labeled using a standard known as the USRDA, which provides a comparison to nutrient standards.

Over the last few years, nutrient content claims and health claims have also been permitted on foods (21). Nutrient content claims on food labels, such as "low in fat" or "good source of dietary fiber" are specified so that the same standard is used on all foods of the same type. Health claims describe the relationship between a nutrient or food and a disease; these provide additional information for consumers. Table 14-7 presents some current allowable health claims for foods.

PROMOTING HEALTH, PREVENTING DISEASE: OBJECTIVES FOR THE NATION

Starting in 1980 and at the beginning of every decade thereafter, the Department of Health and Human Services has convened public, private, and voluntary groups to update the plan and assess progress toward achieving it. It is now customary to issue a "mid-course review" halfway through the decade to make mid-term corrections and to redirect resources, if this should prove to be necessary.

The current prevention plan is entitled "Healthy People 2000" (24). The overall goals are general ones. They are to increase the span of healthy life, reduce health disparities among Americans, and to achieve access to preventive services for all Americans. For each life stage, there are specific objectives stated in terms of reducing mortality in the various areas. Goals are also set for each priority area. Nutrition is considered as one of these areas. In the Healthy People 2000 document, there are 27 nutrition-related objectives (Table 14-8). They deal with health status; risk reduction and service-related issues; and set measurable objectives in each area. The latest review of progress was done in 1995 (25). (See Chapter 11 for details.)

Progress in nutrition has been substantial in some areas, and slower in others (26). For example, substantial

Table 14-8 Year 2000 Goals in Nutrition

HEALTH STATUS

Reduce coronary heart disease death to no more than 100:100,000 people.
Revise the rise in cancer deaths to achieve a rate of no more than 130:100,000.
Reduce overweight to a prevalence of no more than 20% among people aged 20 and older and no more than 15% among adolescents aged 12 to 19.
Reduce growth retardation among low income children aged 5 and younger to less than 10%.

RISK REDUCTION OBJECTIVES

Reduce dietary fat intakes to an average of ≤30% of total calories and average saturated fat intake to <10% of total calories among people over age 2.
Increase complex carbohydrate and fiber-containing foods in the diets of adults to 5 or more daily servings for vegetables (including legumes) and fruits and to 6 or more daily servings for grain products.
Increase to at least 50% the proportion of overweight people aged 12 and older who have adopted sound dietary practices combined with regular physical activity to attain an appropriate body weight.
Increase calcium intake so that at least 50% of youth aged 12 through 24 and 50% of pregnant and lactating women consume 5 or more servings daily of foods rich in calcium and at least 50% of people aged 25 and older consume 2 or more servings daily.
Decrease salt and sodium intake so that at least 65% of home cooks prepare foods without adding salt, at least 80% of people avoiding use of salt at the table, and at least 40% of adults regularly practice modified or lowered sodium use.
Reduce iron deficiency to <30% among children aged 1 through 4 and among women of childbearing age.
Increase to at least 75% the proportion of mothers who breastfeed their babies in the early postpartum period and to at least 50% the proportion who continue breastfeeding until their babies are 5 to 6 months old.
Increase to at least 75% the proportion of parents and caregivers who use feeding practices that prevent baby bottle tooth decay.
Increase to at least 85% the proportion of people aged 18 and older who use food labels to make nutritious food selections.

SERVICES AND PROTECTION OBJECTIVES

Achieve useful and informative nutrition labeling for virtually all processed foods and at least 40% of fresh meat, poultry, fish, fruits, vegetables, baked goods, and ready-to-eat carry-away foods.
Increase to at least 5000 brand items the number of processed food products that are reduced in fat and saturated fat content.
Increase to at least 90% the proportion of restaurants and institutional food service operations that offer identifiable low-fat, low-calorie food choices, consistent with the Dietary Guidelines for Americans.
Increase to at least 80% the receipt of home food services by people aged 65 and older who have difficulty in preparing their own meals or are otherwise in need of home-delivered meals.
Increase to at least 75% the proportion of the nation's schools that provide nutrition education from preschool through twelfth grade, preferably as part of a high-quality school health education curriculum.
Increase to at least 50% the proportion of worksites (with ≥50 employees) that offer nutrition education or weight management programs for employees.
Increase to at least 75% the proportion of primary care providers who provide nutrition assessment and counseling or referral to qualified nutritionists and dietitians.

progress has been made in reducing coronary artery disease deaths; in lessening the prevalence of growth retardation among low income children aged 5 and under; in reducing average dietary fat intakes; in increasing the availability of reduced-fat processed foods and of low-fat, low-calorie restaurant food choices; in worksite nutrition, weight management programs, and weight control programs; and in increasing the prevalence of informative nutrient labeling on processed foods. Progress has been slight but positive for breastfeeding in the early postpartum period; it has been much slower in sustaining breastfeeding after that. Among the greatest disappointments have been the increases instead of decreases in the prevalence of overweight in adults and children, in adopting appropriate weight loss practices, and in increasing consumption of foods rich in calcium.

Where does particular attention need to be paid in setting objectives for the future? Certainly all of these objectives deserve continued attention. In addition, over time, new objectives have emerged. These goals are discussed at greater length in Chapter 11.

SUMMARY

Dietary intake is only one facet of nutritional status, but it is an important one. The DRIs, such as the RDA and UL, provide useful guides for planning and evaluating intakes of nutrients. Other tools, such as the USDA food pyramid, are helpful food-based recommendations that, if followed, ensure that the RDA are met. The DGAs provide recommendations for altering current intakes in more healthful directions. The NAI provides a simple tool for evaluating the balance, variety, and adequacy of intakes based on the food guide and DGAs. Health professionals can use these simple tools to plan and assess their own diets and those of their clients. For many practical purposes, these tools will suffice. For more elaborate planning and assessment, other tools may be necessary.

Finally, the year 2000 nutritional goals for promoting health and preventing disease provide additional useful health targets toward which to aim.

This project has been funded at least in part with federal funds from the U.S. Department of Agriculture, Agricultural Research Service, under contract number 53/3-K06-5-10. The contents of this article do not necessarily reflect the views or policies of the US Department of Agriculture, nor does mention of trade names, commercial products, or organizations imply endorsement by the United States government.

REFERENCES

1. Dwyer JT. Concept of nutritional status and its measurement. In: Himes JH. Anthropometric assessment of nutritional status. New York: Wiley Liss Inc., 1991:5–28.

2. Dwyer JT. Dietary assessment. In: Shils M, Shike M, and Olsen JA. Modern nutrition in health and disease. Philadelphia: Lea and Febiger: 1995.

3. Institute of Medicine, Food and Nutrition Board. How should the recommended dietary allowances be revised? Washington, DC: National Academy Press, 1994.

4. The development and use of the dietary reference intakes. Nutrition Reviews 1997;55:319–352.

5. Food and Nutrition Board, Institute of Medicine, National Academy of Sciences. A risk assessment model for establishing upper intake levels for nutrients. Washington, DC, June 1998.

6. Institute of Medicine, Food and Nutrition Board. Dietary reference intakes: calcium, phosphorus, magnesium, vitamin D and fluoride. Washington, DC: National Academy Press, 1997.

7. Institute of Medicine, Food and Nutrition Board. Dietary reference intakes: folic acid and B vitamins. Washington, DC: National Academy Press, 1998.

8. National Institute of Nutrition. Dietary reference intakes. Rapport (Canada) 1998;13:1–7.

9. National Research Council, Subcommittee on the Tenth Edition of the RDAs, Food and Nutrition Board. Recommended dietary allowances. 10th ed. Washington, DC: National Academy Press, 1989.

10. U.S. Department of Agriculture/ U.S. Department of Health and Human Services. Dietary guidelines for Americans. 4th ed. USDA Home and Garden Bulletin 1995;232 (December).

11. National Research Council, Committee on Diet and Health, Food and Nutrition Board. Diet and health: implications for reducing chronic disease risk. Washington, DC: National Academy Press, 1989.

12. Committee on Implementation of the Diet and Health Report. Improving America's diet and health: from recommendations to action. Washington, DC: National Academy Press, 1991.

13. U.S. Department of Agriculture. The food guide pyramid. Home and Garden Bulletin, 1992; 252.

14. Kennedy ET, Ohls J, Carlson S, and Fleming K. The healthy eating index: design and applications. J Am Diet Assoc 1994;95:1103 –1108.

15. Variyam JN, Blaylock J, Smallwood D, and Basiotis PP. USDA's healthy eating index and nutrition information. U.S. Department of Agriculture. Economic Research Service Technical Bulletin No 1866, Washington, DC, 1998.

16. U.S. Department of Agriculture, Agricultural Research Service. February 1994–95 continuing survey of food intakes by individuals and 1994–96 diet and health knowledge survey and related materials. CD-ROM. U.S. Department of Agriculture, Washington, DC, 1998.

17. Bowman SA, Lino M, Gerrior SA, and Basiotis PP. The healthy eating index 1994–96. U.S. Department of Agriculture, Center for Nutrition Policy and Promotion, CNPP 5, Washington, DC, 1998.

18. Life Sciences Research Office, Federation of American Societies of Experimental Biology. Nutrition monitoring in the United States: an update report on nutrition monitoring. Prepared for the U.S. Department of Agriculture and U.S. Department of Health and Human Services, No. (PHS) 99-122-5. U.S. Public Health Service, Washington, DC, September 1989.

19. Dwyer JT. Dietary assessment. In: Shils ME, Olsen JA, and Shike M, eds. Modern nutrition in health and disease. Philadelphia: Lea and Febiger, 1992.

20. Thompson FE, Byers T, eds. Kohlineier L, guest ed. Dietary assessment resource manual. J Nutr 124; No. 11S 2245–2311S.

21. Wilkening VL. FDA's regulations to implement the NLEA. Nutrition Today 1993;(Sept–Oct):13–20.

22. U.S. Department of Health and Human Services. Healthy people: the Surgeon General's report on health promotion and disease prevention. U.S. Department of Health and Human Services, Washington, DC, 1979.

23. Office of the Assistant Secretary for Health, U.S. Department of Health and Human Services. Promoting health, preventing disease: objectives for the nation. U.S. Department of Health and Human Services, Washington, DC, 1980.

24. U.S. Department of Health and Human Services. Healthy people 2000: full report with commentary. U.S. DHHS. Publication No. (PHS) 91-5028, Washington, DC.

25. U.S. Department of Health, Education, and Welfare, Public Health

Service. Healthy people 2000: midcourse review and 1995 revisions. U.S. Department of Health and Human Services, Washington, DC, 1995.

26. Lewis CJ, Crane NT, Moore BJ, and Hubbard VS. Healthy people 2000: report on the 1994 nutrition progress review. Nutrition Today 1994;29:6–14.

Chapter 15

Nutrition for Elite Athletes

Joan E. Benson
E. Wayne Askew

NUTRITIONAL CONDITIONING FOR ELITE COMPETITION

Although the discipline of sports nutrition has been a visible feature of competitive athletics for almost two decades, there is still some confusion about the impact of nutrition research on actual diets of elite performers. Relatively few diet surveys have been performed on athletes at the highest level since the 1970's, and those surveys that exist reveal a wide variation in dietary intake (1). Although few elite athletes and coaches argue the importance of nutrition preparation to peak athletic performance, recent surveys of young athletes in particular revealed that they failed to recognize nutritional practices critical to the demands of their sport activities and were unable to meet the energy requirements for high performance (2).

The nutritional intake of elite athletes during training periods and surrounding race or performance day is an important determinant of their ability to compete at the level of full potential. But while the athlete's physical training and rest program is well defined and understood by coaching and training staff, nutritional preparation is often less well managed and is more likely to the sacrificed to the demands of training and travel schedules. In addition, elite athletes and their advisors are often victims of the "nutrition elixir syndrome," indulging in drastic or ineffective measures, such as steroid or diuretic abuse or expensive vitamin, herbal, or hormone supplements, which are at the least costly and at worst, unhealthy or banned substances.

In this chapter, we will review the nutritional recommendations for elite performance, address the issue of ergogenic aids, and provide practical suggestions for athletes in training and competition.

THE ROLE OF CARBOHYDRATES IN EXERCISE
Optimizing Glycogen Stores

Of all dietary factors that influence elite performance, carbohydrate is overwhelmingly the most important. A reduction of body stores of carbohydrate and blood glucose is related to the perception of fatigue and the inability to maintain high-quality performance. This has been clearly shown with aerobic, endurance events of moderate intensity and more than 90 minutes duration. At intensities ranging between 60% and 80% of maximum aerobic power, e.g., a moderate intensity distance training run, the major source of fuel (60% to 70%) is muscle carbohydrate, or glycogen. Numerous studies have demonstrated that the capacity to exercise at these intensities for prolonged periods is directly related to the pre-exercise muscle glycogen level. Carbohydrate stores may also have relevance for athletes involved in short, high intensity, repetitive events, especially if body weight control is an issue (e.g., gymnastics or wrestling) (3). In prolonged competition, after 1 to 3 hours of continuous running, cycling, or swimming at 65% to 80% of maximal oxygen uptake or after repeated bouts of intense sprints or routines (at ≥85% of maximal oxygen uptake) muscle stores of carbohydrate, or glycogen, become depleted and fatigue makes further high-level activity impossible.

How much and what type of dietary carbohydrate an athlete should consume to achieve and maintain optimal levels of muscle glycogen depend on the intensity and duration of exercise and the amount of muscle activated. In general, elite athletes are no different from the population at large in benefiting from a diet low in fat and high in nutritious carbohydrate sources, such as grains, fruits, vegetables. Where athletes differ is in the amount of energy they expend and therefore the amount of food they must consume. Endurance athletes often train intensely for 90 continuous minutes or more and expend 1000 to 1400 kcal in the process. These athletes generally must eat approximately 50 kcal of food per kilogram of body weight—for example, 3500 kcal a day for a 70-kg athlete (4). At least half, but more ideally 60% to 70% of those calories for elite endurance trainers should be from carbohydrate—roughly 7 to 9 g of carbohydrate per kilogram of body weight. This amounts to 500 to 600 g of carbohydrate a day, and an enormous volume of food. Table 15-1 contains a list of common high-carbohydrate foods. High-carbohydrate, but less nutritious, foods such as energy bars, sports drinks, candy, and low-fat cookies are often useful to supplement a diet of this type. However, in the week before an important competition, many elite athletes are interested in taking measures that will maximize muscle carbohydrate stores.

Glycogen Loading or Supercompensation

To supercompensate muscle glycogen stores during the week before elite competition, endurance athletes have resorted to a variety of dietary and training strategies. Muscle glycogen supercompensation will only have benefit in sporting activities that involve high intensity exercise lasting longer than 90 minutes. Marathons, long-distance swimming, cross-country ski races, 30-km runs, soccer, cycling time trials, and triathalons are all appropriate activities for supercompensation. Shorter duration activities, such as football games, 10-km runs, downhill ski races, most swimming events, basketball games, and most track and field events, don't benefit from supercompensation and may in fact be hampered by this technique.

Bergstrom et al (5) were the first to describe a method to supercompensate muscle glycogen stores. Six subjects consumed a normal mixed diet for 3 days, exercised to exhaustion, and then consumed a low-carbohydrate diet for three days. As a result, muscle glycogen as measured by muscle biopsy procedure decreased from 106 mmol/kg of muscle to 11 mmol/kg of muscle. The subjects then consumed a diet with 82% of calories from carbohydrate for the next 3 days—increasing muscle carbohydrate to 204 mmol/kg—nearly double the baseline glycogen concentration. In a second study by Ahlborg et al (6), study subjects repeated the protocol of exercise to exhaustion followed by a very low (2% of calories) carbohydrate intake for 1 day, and then a high (95% of calories) carbohydrate intake for 3 days—with similar results. Exhaustive exercise and depletion of muscle carbohydrate with dietary restriction potentiates muscle glycogen synthesis. However, exercising to exhaustion during the week before an important competition increases the risk of injury and the risk that an athlete will not be in peak physical condition for competition. And such drastic dietary measures required in this "classic method" of glycogen loading are difficult to implement, especially if an athlete is on the road. Fortunately, research by Sherman et al (7) indicates that muscle glycogen can be supercompensated using a less drastic approach. He found that progressively reducing training beginning 1 week before competition and ending with a rest day, and at the same time increasing dietary carbohydrate from 50% of calories to 70% (or from 4 g of carbohydrate per kilogram of body weight to 10 g) the last 3 days before the race, would result in virtually the same muscle glycogen content as the more drastic, classic approach.

Carbohydrate Feeding Before Exercise

High-carbohydrate meals eaten within 6 hours of competition can ensure glycogen stores are saturated. A low-fat meal containing 100 to 200 g of carbohydrate consumed 2 to 6 hours before competition will prevent hunger and improve endurance, especially if glycogen stores are not full, but the athlete should not experiment with new foods at this time. Food consumed just before exercise should supply carbohydrate that can elevate or maintain blood glucose levels

Table 15-1 Low-Fat, High-Carbohydrate Foods
SOURCES WITH 30 g OF CARBOHYDRATE PER SERVING
Breads Bagel, 1 small Bun, 1 hamburger or hot dog English muffin, 1 Low-fat crackers, 10 pieces **Pasta and Rice** Macaroni, noodles, spaghetti (cooked, plain or with tomato sauce), 1/2 cup Ravioli (spinach), 1/2 cup Rice, brown or white, cooked, 1/4 cup Rice-a-Roni or other pilaf (prepared without fat), 1/2 cup **Miscellaneous** Burrito (bean), 1 Flour Tortilla, 2 Granola bar, 1
SOURCES WITH 15 g OF CARBOHYDRATE PER SERVING
Breads and Cereals Bread (all kinds), 1 slice Breadstick, 2 Roll, wheat or white, 1 Cooked cereal, 1/2 cup Cold cereal, 3/4 to 1 cup Pancake or waffle, 1 (5″ diameter) **Snacks** Low-fat chips, 1 oz Low-fat cookies, 1 oz Popcorn (low-fat microwave), 3 cups Pretzels (3-1/8″ long), 25 **Beans, Lentils, and Peas** Baked beans, 1/4 cup Other beans (kidney, navy, black, pinto, etc.), 1/2 cup Lentils or peas, 1/2 cup **Soup** Bean (all), 1/2 cup Noodle soup, 1 cup Minestrone, 1 cup **Vegetables and Fruits** Corn, potatoes, winter squash, and yams, 1/2 cup Canned fruit in syrup (all, drained), 1/3 cup Fresh fruit (all types), 1/2 cup

without increasing insulin secretion. Insulinemia could reduce the availability of fatty acids as an energy substrate. It has also been suggested that foods with a high glycemic index, consumed within 2 hours of competition, may lead to hypoglycemia at the onset of exercise and resultant fatigue, again as a result of insulinemia. Theoretically, a low glycemic index (GI) pre-event carbohydrate should optimize the availability of both glucose and fatty acids for use by the muscles and be superior to glucose or other high GI foods. Consuming low GI foods in the 2 hours before competition may also moderate the decline in blood glucose that occurs in the beginning of exercise, reduce reliance on glycogen as a fuel, and increase lipid use by muscles, although there is insufficient evidence to claim that these metabolic changes would translate into improved performance. Table 15-2 lists a number of foods by glycemic index. Fruits, pasta, and rice are examples of low GI foods, and although the GI of sports drinks have not been published, drinks high in

glucose would presumably have the highest GI and those with more fructose or sucrose would be lower. Craig (8) reviewed many exercise studies using fructose feedings before exercise, and the trend was toward no increase in either blood glucose or insulin levels. Although one study (9) noted a glycogen-sparing effect of pre-exercise fructose compared with glucose or water alone, this was not seen in subsequent studies involving high intensity bouts of exercise in which muscle glycogen would be more limiting. In addition, no performance benefit was noted in most experiments for fructose compared with glucose. In general, while blood glucose was maintained at higher levels during the initial period of exercise relative to high GI carbohydrates like glucose, more subjects complained of gastrointestinal distress after fructose ingestion, probably because of its slow rate of absorption and osmotic effects. However, there may be benefit to fructose ingestion before exercise when used in combination with other carbohydrate sources. For example, muscle glycogen sparing

---

Table 15-2 Glycemic Ranking of Common Foods

BREADS, GRAINS, CEREALS

High Glycemic Index (70–95)
Waffle
Doughnut
Bagel, all types
Rice, instant
White bread
Rice Krispies cereal
Grape Nuts Flakes cereal
Corn flakes
Cheerios cereal
Moderate Glycemic Index (55–70)
Whole wheat bread
Cornmeal
Bran muffin
White and brown rice
Shredded Wheat cereal
Grape Nuts cereal
Life cereal
Oatmeal
Low Glycemic Index (15–55)
Bulgur
Spaghetti, white or whole wheat
Wheat kernels
Barley
All Bran cereal

FRUITS, STARCHY VEGETABLES, AND BEANS

High Glycemic Index (70–95)
Watermelon
Baked potato
Instant potatoes
Mashed potatoes
Carrots
Moderate Glycemic Index (55–70)
Raisins
Pineapple
Green peas
Sweet potatoes

Low Glycemic Index (15–55)
Banana
Grapes
Orange
Pear
Apple
Baked beans
Garbanzo beans
Lentils
Kidney beans
Soy beans

BEVERAGES, SWEETS, AND SNACKS

High Glycemic Index (70–95)
Rice cakes
Jelly beans
Graham crackers
Corn chips
Life Savers candy
Honey
Moderate Glycemic Index (55–70)
Sucrose (table sugar)
Soft drinks
Orange juice
Ice cream
Angel food cake
Popcorn
Wheat crackers
Oatmeal cookies
Low Glycemic Index (15–55)
Apple juice
Yoghurt, sweetened
Milk, all types
Chocolate
Banana cake
Peanuts
Potato chips (regular)
Fructose
Lactose

---

and performance enhancement were observed in athletes consuming a mixture of glucose polymers and fructose when compared to glucose polymers alone (8). Therefore, consuming fluids containing small amounts of fructose with other carbohydrate sources before activity may benefit some athletic activities, but again, it is critical that the athlete experiment with pre-event feedings during training sessions to determine tolerance.

Carbohydrate Ingestion During Competition

After 1 to 3 hours of continuous exercise at 70% to 80% of maximum aerobic power, athletes tire as a result of carbohydrate depletion. Carbohydrate feedings during exercise can delay fatigue by as much as 30 to 60 minutes by allowing the exercising muscles to rely mostly on blood glucose for energy late in exercise—not by sparing muscle glycogen utilization. Research by Lamb and Brodowicz (10) and Murray et al (11) has shown that consuming carbohydrate beverages during exercise can improve performance, but the optimal form of carbohydrate to provide (glucose, glucose polymers, sucrose, or fructose) and the concentration of the fluid are often in question. Results of recent research by Jackson et al (12) suggest that a 6% sucrose solution consumed during exercise enters the bloodstream as rapidly as plain water, is associated with improved exercise endurance, and has a favorable influence on cardiovascular and thermoregulatory function in trained cyclists. The consumption of glucose, glucose polymers, or sucrose in a 6% solution during exercise has a similar and beneficial effect on exercise performance. Performance improvements occur when athletes consume at least 30 to 70 g of carbohydrate each hour during activities that are longer than 90 minutes (3). Fructose ingestion, however, is not associated with exercise improvement, possibly because fructose is preferentially removed by the liver, is slow to be metabolized into glucose, and is therefore not readily available to the working muscle.

Combining carbohydrate with electrolytes (CE) appears to have superior ergogenic effects compared with either alone, particularly in activities lasting more than 1 hour, and possibly in other competition scenarios as well. In a study by Below et al (13), eight well-trained cyclists exercised at 80% of maximum oxygen consumption (Vo_2max) for 50 minutes. This was followed by a cycling performance test that required completion of a set amount of work in the shortest time possible, simulating a sprint finish. The men randomly received CE in a 6% solution as an electrolyte solution alone, carbohydrate as glucose polymers, or water alone. Both carbohydrate-containing solutions provided 79 g glucose polymers. The set amount of work was performed more quickly by the CE group (9.93 minutes) compared to electrolyte alone (10.51 minutes), carbohydrate alone (10.55 minutes), or water (11.34 minutes). In summary, consuming carbohydrates or carbohydrate with electrolytes in solution during endurance activities will increase time to exhaustion and improve performance.

Glycogen Resynthesis

Recovery after exercise poses an important challenge to the extreme athlete. Restoring liver and muscle glycogen, as well as fluid and electrolytes lost in sweat, is critical, especially in tournament situations, when competition takes place over a series of days or when training is intense. Rapid resynthesis of muscle glycogen stores is aided by the immediate intake of, in particular, high GI carbohydrates after competition stops, at a rate of 1 gm/kg of body weight every 2 hours (14), leading to a total intake of 7 to 10 g of carbohydrate per kilogram of body weight over 24 hours. Provided adequate carbohydrate is consumed, it appears that the frequency of intake, the form (liquid versus solid), and the presence of other macronutrients do not affect the rate of glycogen storage. Only about 5% of the muscle glycogen used is resynthesized each hour after exercise, so at least 20 hours are required for complete restoration after exhaustive exercise.

In summary, elite endurance athletes benefit from careful attention to adequate carbohydrate intake during training, the week before competition, and immediately before competition, as well as during exercise and postevent. Saturating glycogen stores and maintaining blood glucose levels during and before exercise enhance all aspects of endurance performance. Reestablishing muscle and liver glycogen levels after competition or rigorous workout improves recovery and optimizes subsequent training activities.

THE ROLE OF FAT IN EXERCISE

Fat Oxidation During Exercise

The importance of fat metabolism in providing energy for exercise is well documented (15). Carefully controlled metabolic studies show that fat can provide a major portion of the energy required to support low- to moderate-intensity exercise (16,17). An important adaptive metabolic response to exercise training is an increase in the capacity of skeletal muscle to oxidize fatty acids (16). Despite the fact that fat is a major provider of substrate during exercise and that an increase in the enzymic capability to oxidize fat is part of the overall biochemical adaptation to exercise training, dietary manipulations to increase carbohydrate intake remain the major avenue available to athletes to enhance performance through dietary means. This focus on carbohydrate has shifted somewhat in recent years as the result of studies that have demonstrated that increasing fat utilization during exercise may be an indirect route to sparing or reserving the athlete's limited carbohydrate stores for the final stages of exercise when glycogen is depleted or oxygen is in such short supply that fat cannot be aerobically oxidized (18).

Regulation of Fat Oxidation During Exercise

Randle et al (19) in 1964 proposed that increased fatty acid oxidation concomitantly reduces glucose uptake and oxidation by reducing the activity of certain key enzymes of the glycolytic pathway. This relationship, referred to as the *glucose-fatty acid cycle*, has guided our understanding of the relationship between fat and carbohydrate metabolism during the past 30 years. Recent investigations of the roles of the glucose-fatty acid cycle in sustained exercise, however, indicate that regulatory control described by Randle et al (fat oxidation regulates carbohydrate metabolism) may not hold under the conditions of intense exercise. While the glucose-fatty acid cycle seems to operate in muscle at rest and during low-intensity exercise (20), the same control may not operate in human skeletal muscle during intense exercise (21). The ability of fat to regulate carbohydrate metabolism in humans during exercise may be more limited than previously believed. Coyle et al (22) have provided evidence that suggests that the converse of the Randle hypothesis is actually true under the conditions of intense exercise, e.g., carbohydrate metabolism regulates its own oxidation and, indirectly, the oxidation of fat. Fat oxidation during exercise is inhibited by preexercise feedings that elicit hyperglycemia and hyperinsulinemia and increased glycolytic flux. The net effect of carbohydrate ingestion before exercise minimizes the release of free fatty acids (FFA) and reduces their oxidation by skeletal muscle. Carbohydrate ingestion, however, does not exert the same inhibition of medium-chain fatty acid oxidation (22). The oxidation of medium-chain fatty acids, such as octanoic acid, by skeletal muscle does not seem to be influenced by carbohydrate ingestion. When included with carbohydrate feeding during exercise, medium-chain fatty acids seem to spare carbohydrate from oxidation during exercise (23). This unique characteristic of medium-chain fatty acids to act synergistically with ingested carbohydrate may have dietary implications for elite athletes who wish to access additional energy sources during exercise to spare glycogen stores.

Dietary Enhancement of Fat Oxidation in Elite Athletes

Studies with animal (24,25) and human (26,27) models have demonstrated that artificially raising blood FFA and stimulating their uptake by the injection or infusion of heparin before and during exercise can prolong endurance time, presumably by sparing carbohydrate. Because of unacceptable risk associated with heparin, these manipulations are neither safe nor practical methods of increasing fat utilization. Some investigators have attempted to make fat more quantitatively available by feeding high-fat diets. However, high-fat diets, with some exceptions (28–30), have typically resulted in reduced performance (31,32). With a long enough period (approximately 2 weeks) of dietary adaptation, muscle enzymes can adapt and increase their ability to provide energy through fatty acid and ketone body oxidation (33,34). Moderate-intensity exercise following a period of adaptation to a high-fat diet can be supported as well, if not better, than exercise supported by a normal fat diet (28–30). This research has stimulated interest in the concept of *fat loading*, drawing the inevitable parallel to carbohydrate loading. Fat loading, however, has not led to the same consistent enhancement of performance that has characterized carbohydrate loading (18). The problem seems to lie with the inherent differences in pathways of absorption of carbohydrate and fat, as well as the necessity for enzymic adaptation in the case of high-fat diets, but not high-carbohydrate diets. Dietary glucose can be absorbed directly across the gut into the blood, where it is readily available for metabolism by the liver and muscle. Long-chain fatty acids, on the other hand, must be packaged into chylomicrons in the intestinal mucosa and absorbed into the lymphatic circulation, from which they ultimately become available to muscle after liberation by lipoprotein lipase. Not all fatty acids are restricted to travel through the lymphatic system, however. Medium-chain triglycerides (MCT) provide medium-chain fatty acids (C-8-12) that can be absorbed from the gut similar to glucose by passing directly into the portal blood. These medium-chain fatty acids are then rapidly taken up and oxidized by muscle, independent of enzymic transport systems (such as carnitine acyltransferase), sparing some glucose in the process, thereby prolonging the capacity for exercise. MCT do not seem to be ergogenic by themselves, but when administered in combination with carbohydrate, may exert a beneficial effect upon endurance performance (23).

The focus of energy provision from lipid metabolism during exercise has shifted from adipose tissue and plasma FFA to fatty acids provided by locally stored intramuscular triglycerides (35,36). Although some conflicting data exist regarding the importance of intramuscular triglycerides (IMTG) as fuel for muscular contraction (32,37), recent stable-isotope tracer studies indicate that IMTG may represent a quantitatively important "local store" of energy for contracting muscle, similar to muscle glycogen (17,36,38). This observation has led some investigators to suggest that it may be important for endurance athletes to replenish IMTG after exercise (32). Based on available evidence, elite endurance athletes probably have a rapid turnover of IMTG (16). However, we do not currently have enough information to recommend specific dietary programs for rapid replenishment of muscle triglycerides. As discussed earlier, short-term high-fat diets will increase IMTG concentrations but may not benefit performance (32). Effective dietary manipulations designed to replenish muscle triglyceride stores preferentially over adipose triglyceride stores are currently not established but may be important research areas in the future.

It is premature to recommend high-fat diets, fat loading, or alternative forms of fat, such as MCT, to elite athletes. It is, however, possible that elite athletes may be metabolically better positioned by genetics or training adaptations to take advantage of the potentially larger stores of energy from dietary (MCT) or stored (IMTG) fat. Energy from carbohydrate is limited by the amount that can be stored before exercise and also by the amount that can be absorbed from the gut during exercise. It makes 'metabolic sense" to look to the potentially larger energy stores of dietary medium-chain fatty acids and IMTG as energy sources for elite athletes to capitalize on to support their increased energy expenditure needs.

PROTEIN NUTRITION FOR ELITE ATHLETES

Although it is known that carbohydrate and fat are major fuels used for sport, more recent information shows there is increased protein utilization during exercise and, under certain conditions, protein may contribute significantly to energy metabolism. Therefore, the amount of protein elite athletes need has come under question. The current RDA of 0.8 g/kg of body weight per day has been challenged as being inadequate for athletes. Nitrogen balance studies in endurance and strength athletes have reported that the requirement for protein may be between 1.2 and 1.8 g/kg body weight per day, respectively (39). Differences in experimental approaches and in the type of subjects studied could account in part for the wide range in protein values. Meredith et al (40) examined young and middle-aged endurance-trained men consuming 0.6 g/kg, 0.9 g/kg, or 1.2 g/kg of body weight per day of high-quality protein over three separate 10-day periods, while maintaining training and constant body weight. The minimum protein requirement to maintain positive nitrogen balance was 0.94 g/kg of body weight per day, an amount

17% greater than the RDA. Friedman and Lemon (41) reported protein requirements of 1.14 g/kg to 1.39 g/kg per day, an amount 42% to 74% higher than the current RDA, for five well-trained endurance runners. Why high intensity endurance exercise increases protein need is unknown. Endurance exercise causes an increased utilization of several amino acids, especially the branched-chain amino acids, as fuel. Factors such as high exercise intensity and long-duration endurance training appear to promote a greater amino acid oxidation (42). In addition, muscle damage occurs with endurance exercise, especially if it includes an eccentric component—increasing protein needs for repair. It therefore seems likely that elite endurance athletes could benefit from a protein intake of between 1.0 g/kg and 1.5 g/kg per day, an amount closely reflecting the usual American diet.

The debate regarding optimal protein needs of strength athletes, such as weight lifters, football players, and field athletes, is an old one. Although strength training can be intense, each bout is very brief, making it unlikely that amino acid oxidation plays an important role in providing energy for this type of exercise—carbohydrates are the major fuel. However, recent evidence indicates that actual requirements are higher than those of more sedentary individuals. Some data even suggest that high-protein diets can enhance the development of muscle mass and strength when combined with heavy resistance exercise training (43), but it would appear that substantial individual variability exists. Five of the ten elite weight lifters studied by Clejowa et al (44) were found, by nitrogen balance methods, to be consuming inadequate protein even when their protein intake was 250% of the RDA. One of the five athletes consumed a diet containing inadequate total energy, but four of the 5 were consuming adequate calories. In a review article, Lemon (43) concluded that a diet providing approximately 1.5 g/kg to 2.0 g/kg per day (180% to 250% of the RDA) is required for strength athletes, providing calorie needs are met. In fact, perhaps the most important single factor determining protein/amino acid need is the adequacy of energy intake. Insufficient calorie intake elevates protein needs. Some data indicate that strength athletes who consume 12% to 15% of their total energy intake as protein can maintain positive nitrogen balance. Meredith (45) reported that 0.5 g/kg to 0.6 g/kg per day was sufficient to maintain nitrogen balance in seven men who habitually weight-trained 7 hours a week and consumed approximately 4200 cal/day. This amount of protein, though low, was equivalent to 12% of total kilocalories and in line with recommendations for the general public. However, Torun et al (46) found that five subjects who consumed diets consisting of 100% of the RDA for protein and adequate total energy experienced a decreased cell mass (measured by potassium [40]) over 6 weeks of strength training. With continued training and an increase in protein intake to 200% of RDA, cell mass increased. Finally, impressive gains in strength (5%) and size (6%) were observed over several months of strength training in world-class weight lifters when they increased their dietary protein from 225% to 438% of the RDA (47). The lack of adequate controls, however, makes these data difficult to interpret.

The lack of agreement in the literature makes it difficult to define the influence of diet on strength development. If energy intake is adequate, then athletes can increase muscle strength and size while consuming the protein RDA. However, it is likely that some athletes can experience greater gains in muscle mass and strength with higher intakes of protein.

Amino Acid Supplements

Whether specific amino acids have a role in elite performance is in question. There appears to be little scientific evidence to support the hypothesis that amino acid supplementation may enhance the physiologic responses to strength training when athletes consume dietary protein within the recommended guidelines (48). However, athletes in weight-controlled sports, such as wrestling, may benefit from supplementation of branched-chain amino acids (BCAA) while restricting calories for weight loss purposes. Mourier et al (49) provided a group of wrestlers who were restricting their calories with BCAA and compared them with a hypocaloric group who received no amino acid supplement. Compared to the control group, the BCAA-supplemented group exhibited a significant reduction in visceral adipose tissue after 19 days, with no change in aerobic and anaerobic capacities. Another study investigating the influence of BCAA supplementation on loss of body mass and muscle power in high-altitude trekkers showed positive results (50). Sixteen subjects took either a dietary supplement of BCAA (5.76 g/day, 2.88 g/day, and 2.88 g/day of leucine, isoleucine, and valine, respectively) or placebo in a controlled double-blind manner. While fat mass dropped in both groups during the 21-day trek, the BCAA group showed a significantly increased lean mass of 1.5% as opposed to no change in the placebo group. There was also a significant increase in arm muscle cross-sectional area in the BCAA group compared with the placebo group. It appears that BCAA may prevent muscle loss during chronic hypobaric hypoxia and may be similarly useful to athletes undergoing calorie restriction.

Vegetarianism

A final question then remains, Can an elite athlete be also a vegetarian? And the answer is, conditionally, yes. Although meat, chicken, fish, eggs, and milk provide high-quality proteins for tissue growth and repair, essential amino acids can be derived from plant sources, especially if calories are adequate. However, weight-controlled athletes and performers such as gymnasts and dancers may find it very difficult to meet protein needs from a purely plant-based diet. There is even some evidence that increasing plant fiber may contribute to the problem of menstrual dysfunction in elite female athletes. Of further concern is the problem of obtaining adequate minerals, such as iron and zinc, in a diet lacking animal protein sources. Iron and zinc deficiencies are the most noted drawbacks of vegetarian or modified vegetarian diets and are the most common dietary deficiencies among athletes (51,52). The recommended intake of iron and zinc for women is 18 mg/day and 12 mg/day, respectively, and for men, 10 mg of iron and 15 mg of zinc per day. All types of meat contain heme iron, which is more bioavailable than nonheme, or plant, sources or supplements. Certainly iron deficiency anemia will impair physical performance, and it is likely that iron depletion marked by low plasma ferritin levels (but without anemia) affects performance as well. A lack of meat sources of zinc may contribute to or increase the potential for the development of low blood zinc concentrations in athletes. Among the 25 major sources of zinc in the U.S. diet, meat items comprise the top 10. Zinc absorption from some plant sources is limited by their content of fiber and phytate. Zinc deficiency would certainly impair physical activity because of the critical role of zinc in regulating lactate dehydrogenase activity, AMP-deaminase, and other zinc-dependent enzymes. Zinc deficiency results in decreased muscle strength and endurance, although the effects of low zinc status on performance are unclear. If the vegetarian diet is vegan, i.e., free of dairy products, the problem of consuming adequate calcium, especially for young female elite performers, becomes a concern as well, especially in view of the new recommendations for calcium intake in the range of 1200 to 1500 mg/day. As vegetarian styles of eating become more popular, athletes must understand how to plan so that adequate nutrients are obtained. Adding good plant sources of iron and zinc, such as whole grains and beans, and calcium sources, such as broccoli and tofu, to the diet can improve mineral status, but supplementation of these nutrients is usually warranted for strict vegetarians.

WATER AND ELECTROLYTE REQUIREMENTS DURING COMPETITION AND TRAINING

Most elite athletes are well aware of the need to maintain hydration during competition. The adverse effects of various levels of dehydration range from reduced work capacity at a 2% loss of weight in water to likely collapse at a 7% loss. Although increased thirst is experienced at only 1% loss of body weight, it is difficult to restore water balance during heavy exercise, even with continuous attention to drinking. At 3% loss of body weight, hemoconcentration occurs and urinary output is reduced. A 20% to 30% decrement in physical work capacity occurs at only a 4% loss of weight in water (53). Restoring lost water is essential to peak performance, but there is much debate over the best method for fluid replacement. Gisolfi (54) showed that fluid absorption occurs during exercise and is not reduced until the exercise approaches 60% to 70% of maximum capacity. One can absorb between 1.9 and 2.3 liters of water per hour, and the presence of glucose in solution increases both water and sodium absorption. Consequently, if minerals are added, then glucose or glucose polymers must be added to the sports drink as well. Greater quantities of fluid are absorbed from CE beverages than from plain water under all conditions (10).

The American College of Sports Medicine (ACSM) established recommendations for fluid replacement during sports activity that vary as the duration of exercise increases. These recommendations include pre-exercise, during exercise, and postexercise needs for fluid, carbohydrate, and electrolytes (55).

Events of Less Than 1 Hour

Competitive events that last less than 1 hour (e.g., track events, some cycling events, cross-country skiing) will range in intensity from 75% to 100% of Vo_2max. During such activities, it is difficult to ingest fluid, and most athletes won't sacrifice the time to drink. Also, gastric emptying is reduced at intensities exceeding 75% of Vo_2max, and drinking could

produce distress and bloating. Therefore, achieving proper hydration before competition is the primary concern in short duration events. In addition, since glycogen depletion can occur during high-intensity exercise of less than 1 hour, the addition of a low GI carbohydrate to the pre-event drink may be beneficial. In summary, 300 to 500 mL of a 6% to 10% carbohydrate beverage should be ingested 15 minutes before competition, and 500 to 1000 mL of cool (5°C to 15°C) plain water should be consumed during competition, as tolerated.

Events Lasting 1 to 3 Hours

Competitions of longer duration (e.g., marathon runs, cycling road races) are characterized by intensities of about 65% to 90% of Vo_2max. The primary concern during these events is to replace body water losses and to provide a source of energy. Events lasting 1 to 3 hours can result in hyperthermia and dehydration as well as glycogen depletion. The amount of fluid needed during competition depends on the sweat rate, which can vary greatly with individuals. Although the amount of fluid needed to provide adequate carbohydrate from a 6% solution is 500 mL to 1000 mL per hour, in all likelihood this amount would be inadequate to replace water lost in sweat. The ACSM guideline is to replace with 100 mL to 200 mL every 2 to 3 km of a run or approximately 200 mL every 15 minutes during a bike race. The pre-event fluid for events lasting 1 to 3 hours should be plain water, or a dilute low GI solution, rather than a glucose or glucose polymers solution. Again, fat metabolism should be promoted early in these events, and the inclusion of a high GI carbohydrate in the pre-event solution could increase insulinemia, thus inhibiting the release of free fatty acids into the bloodstream. For events lasting from 1 to 3 hours, 300 to 500 mL of fluid should be ingested before the race, and 800 to 1600 mL per hour of a cool 6% to 8% carbohydrate solution containing 10 to 20 mEq of sodium per liter should be consumed during exercise. The sodium is added to improve intestinal absorption of the fluid and to improve the taste of the solution.

Events Lasting More Than 3 Hours

In events lasting more than 3 hours (e.g., triathalon, ultra-marathon, century and double-century cycling competitions), intensities will range from 30% to 80% of Vo_2max. The hydration concerns encompass meeting fluid needs, replacing lost electrolytes, and providing carbohydrate for energy. This type of competitive activity has resulted in hyponatremia or water intoxication resulting in coma when electrolyte-free solutions were ingested during competition (55,56). Therefore, fluids consumed during ultra-distance events should contain 20 to 30 mEq of sodium per liter. The carbohydrate concentration should be 6% to 8%, and the pre-event fluid should be plain water. The question surrounding the replacement of potassium in competition fluids is not easily answered. Sweat concentrations of potassium are small (57). However, rehydration of the intracellular fluid compartment appears to be enhanced by potassium. Therefore, to replace the small amount of potassium lost in sweat and to stimulate the rehydration of the intracellular spaces, the addition of 3 to 5 mEq per liter of potassium to the sports drink may be beneficial. In summary, for endurance events of more than 3 hours, one should drink 300 to 500 mL of plain water before the competition and 500 to 1000 mL per hour of cool 6% to 8% carbohydrate solution with 20 to 30 mEq of sodium during exercise. Adding 3 to 5 mEq of potassium may be beneficial.

Postexercise Fluid Recovery

Although as much as 65% of body water lost in sweat and respiration during exercise can be replenished during competition by diligent fluid consumption, significant losses are inevitable and need to be replaced over the 24-hour recovery period. The goal should be regaining the athlete's precompetition weight. A liberal intake of water and carbohydrate during the first 2 hours of recovery will greatly improve performance in subsequent athletic events. Fluid replacement is significantly enhanced when 40 mEq of sodium is included in postcompetition beverages (58). This concentration of salt is about the maximum that is palatable.

ERGOGENIC AIDS TO ELITE PERFORMANCE

As long as competitive sports have existed, athletes have attempted to improve their performance by ingesting a variety of vitamins, herbs, and other potentially bioactive substances. Products offering promises of improved ergogenic performance clutter pharmacy, supermarket, and health food store shelves, while clinical trial evidence supporting these claims is only sporadically provided. Sometimes the use of such substances during competition is unethical, and a number are included on the International Olympic Committee's list of banned substances (58a). We will review the most common ergogenic compounds used by elite athletes, and offer evidence supporting or discounting their usefulness as available.

Caffeine

Caffeine has a long history of use in athletic competition. Although it is now a controlled or restricted drug in the athletic world, most athletes that consume caffeine beverages before competition never approach the urinary level of 12 µg/mL, which is the legal limit for caffeine. Numerous studies performed in the 1990s have shown improvements in endurance exercise (59,60) as well as intense, short-duration activities after caffeine ingestion (61). Jackman et al (61) tested 14 subjects after they ingested either caffeine or placebo, with an intense protocol in which they performed a series of maximal interval bouts, followed by a maximal effort to exhaustion. Caffeine ingestion resulted in a significant increase in endurance (4.93 min versus 4.12 min for placebo) demonstrating that caffeine can be an effective ergogenic aid for exercise as brief as 4 to 6 minutes. How much caffeine is required to provide optimal performance, while avoiding gastrointestinal distress and disqualification from competition, and the proper timing of the dose are of concern. Pasman et al (59) experimented with different doses of caffeine (0 mg/kg, 5 mg/kg, 9 mg/kg, and 13 mg/kg) on well-trained cyclists. Caffeine doses were administered in random order in a double-blind trial. One hour after ingestion, subjects cycled until exhausted at 80% of Vo_2max. A significant increase in endurance performance was found for all caffeine levels compared with placebo, and no differences in endurance performance were found between the three dosages of caffeine. However, only the lowest dose of caffeine (5 mg/kg) resulted in postexercise urine caffeine concentrations below the doping limit of the International Olympic Committee. This suggests that a dose-response relation between caffeine and endurance time does not exist; therefore, taking higher doses unnecessarily exposes athletes to risk of disqualification. Other studies have shown ergogenic effects at doses of 3 mg/kg, 5 mg/kg, and 6 mg/kg of caffeine without exceeding the limit of 12 µg/mL allowed in urine (62,63). A 70-kg person could drink about six regular-sized (6 ounce) cups of drip coffee 1 hour before exercise, exercise for 1.0 to 1.5 hours and still not approach the urinary caffeine limit postexercise. French et al (64) tested whether a large dose of caffeine (10 mg/kg) taken immediately before the start of endurance exercise would improve performance. Six males who were not habitual caffeine users and who were experienced marathon runners exercised on a treadmill for 45 minutes at 75% of Vo_2max. Treadmill speed was then increased by 2 miles per hour until exhaustion. During the caffeine trial, the athletes ran further than either the control or placebo conditions ($p < 0.05$). These results suggest that endurance athletes can use caffeine just before exercise. How caffeine increases endurance time is unclear. By increasing free fatty acids in the bloodstream and increasing fat metabolism, it is believed that caffeine may help spare glycogen use early in exercise. Caffeine also appears to stimulate the transport of potassium into inactive tissues, thereby lowering plasma potassium levels. It has been postulated that the lower serum potassium helps maintain the excitability of cell membranes in contracting muscles, thereby prolonging endurance activity. However, more research into the mechanisms of caffeine's ergogenic effects is needed.

Creatine and Creatine Monohydrate

Power lifters and sprinters supplement with creatine to increase energy production and speed recovery after high intensity exercise. Creatine phosphate is rapidly converted into adenosine triphosphate (ATP) for muscle contraction, and research supports that supplementing with 1- to 5-g doses of creatine for 5 days increases muscle concentrations of the compound and stimulates creatine phosphate resynthesis after exercise (65,66). Volek et al (67) found that creatine supplementation resulted in a significant improvement in peak power output during five sets of jump squats and a significant improvement in repetitions during five sets of bench presses compared with placebo in a group of 14 active men. Several studies have shown improved cycling sprint performance after supplementation with creatine monohydrate for 5 days, compared to placebo (68,69), but others have shown no improvement of sprint performance in swimmers (70), runners (71,72), and cyclists (73) provided with similar supplementation regimens. This conflict in study results suggests that more research to determine optimal dosing protocols and specific sport application for creatine supplements is needed.

Ginseng

Ginseng is an herb that has a long history of medicinal use in Asian countries. Elite athletes in the U.S. and other countries ingest ginseng in the belief that it will improve work capacity and physiologic responses during and immediately after exercise; however the data supporting these contentions are conflicting. Several European clinical trials conducted by Forgo et al (74–76) using elite athletes have shown pronounced ergogenic affects after supplementing with

200 mg/day of ginseng. However, a recent placebo-controlled trial failed to duplicate these findings. Engels et al (77) recruited 36 healthy men into randomized double-blind placebo-controlled research, using two dose levels of ginseng—200 mg/day and 400 mg/day for 8 weeks. The three groups were compared at the end of the study period with respect to changes in Vo_2max, respiratory gas exchange, heart rate, and perceived exertion during maximal and submaximal exercise. The mean habitual activity levels among study groups were not significantly different either before or after the test. The researchers found that supplementation with ginseng, at both high and low doses, had no effect on any of the physiologic and psychologic parameters examined compared with placebo. Chronic ginseng intake was not associated with a change in oxygen use nor did it result in an improvement of aerobic work capacity. This research reflects the findings of Morris et al (78) who also failed to note any physiologic and work performance effects of varying doses of ginseng during intense exercise. The discrepancy between these findings and those of Forgo may be the result of differences in study population—elite athletes versus fit healthy adults. However, Pieralisi et al (79) noted that the effects of ginseng may be more pronounced in persons with lesser aerobic capacity than in those with very high Vo_2max levels. In any case, more research is needed to clarify the usefulness of ginseng to elite sports performance.

Carnitine

Carnitine plays a central role in fatty acid (FA) metabolism. The main function of carnitine is to transport FA from the cytosol into the mitochondrial matrix for beta-oxidation. Although carnitine is supplied by both the normal diet and by endogenous biosynthesis, many athletes believe that supplementing with carnitine will improve muscle use of FA as an energy source during endurance exercise. In theory, enhanced FA oxidation would spare glycogen and postpone fatigue. Since supplemental carnitine can increase muscle levels of the compound in those who are deficient, and since the level of carnitine in skeletal muscle and the capacity of FA oxidation are coupled, it is logical that athletes would be interested in dosing with additional carnitine. However, Heinonen (80) reviewed a series of studies which showed that carnitine supplementation under normal conditions and low doses does not necessarily increase muscle carnitine levels in normal, healthy subjects. In addition, studies on the effects of carnitine supplementation on physical performance have generally shown no improvement. While Marconi et al (81) found a 6% increase in Vo_2max in a group of men supplemented with carnitine, subsequent investigations could not replicate these results (82–85). In fact, these later studies concluded that despite carnitine loading, heart rate, pulmonary ventilation, oxygen consumption, and respiratory quotient remained unchanged, as did blood lactate and pyruvate levels during rest and exercise. In summary, carnitine supplementation increased neither exercise tolerance nor FA oxidation during exercise in trained individuals. Cooper et al (86) loaded 10 experienced male marathon runners with 4 g of carnitine for 10 days, but failed to detect an improvement in marathon performance. Oyono-Enguelle et al (87) studied 10 healthy sedentary men who received 2 g/day of carnitine for 4 weeks. During a 1-hour cycling exercise at 50% Vo_2max there were no changes in

physiologic variables or in the levels of circulating metabolites, causing the researchers to conclude that supplemental carnitine does not increase FA oxidation. In short, the evidence supporting the use of carnitine as an ergogenic aid in humans is scarce, and although there are theoretical points favoring the potential ergogenic effects of carnitine supplementation, it cannot be recommended to healthy athletes until more positive evidence is provided.

UNIQUE NUTRIENT REQUIREMENTS: DO ELITE ATHLETES NEED SUPPLEMENTAL ANTIOXIDANTS?

Exercise and Oxidative Stress

Exercise is associated with increased production of free radicals (88–91). Free radical formation leading to oxidative stress is believed to contribute to undesirable changes in cell membranes and, if unchecked, can contribute to the development of chronic disease (90,92). Free radical formation occurs in athletes and nonathletes alike, but the rate of formation of these damaging reactive species may be greater in athletes working at high rates of energy expenditure and using increased amounts of oxygen. Humans have developed defense mechanisms that help control free radical damage (92). A significant portion of these defense mechanisms is comprised of "sacrificial" antioxidants. These antioxidant nutrients are supplied by the diet and consist of vitamins (vitamins A, C, and E) or vitamin precursors, such beta-carotene (provitamin A). Plant phytochemicals, such as flavonoids, polyphenols, and other complex organic molecules, ingested as part of the diet are also potent antioxidants that can neutralize free radicals. A second defense against free radicals resides in tissue antioxidant enzyme systems, such as superoxide dismutase (SOD) and glutathione peroxidase (GPx). These enzyme systems require certain mineral cofactors (SOD: Zn^{++}, Cu^{++}, Mn^{++}; GPx: Se^{++}) for optimum functioning. Studies of exercise and oxidative stress indicate that athletes may generate a larger number of free radicals than sedentary individuals (90,93). Lines of evidence pointing to increased free radical production during exercise include increased levels of indirect indicators of oxidative stress in breath, blood, and urine (93,94). Animal studies showing decreased levels of muscle cell membrane antioxidants, such as vitamin E, and reduced levels of glutathione after exercise have provided further indirect evidence of increased oxidative stress (95,96). Inflammation from muscle overuse or injury, metabolic "pressure" on the electron transport chain with resultant electron leakage, intermittent periods of anoxia and reoxygenation, and increased catecholamine production all could potentially contribute to increased free radical production during exercise (97).

The Elite Athlete and Oxidative Stress

The elite athlete who trains longer and harder than other athletes or who trains in cold, hot, or high-altitude environments may be subject to even greater oxidative stress risk than other less active athletes (98). Increased free radical production associated with exercise seems to argue in favor of supplemental antioxidants in the athlete's diet. However, two offsetting arguments can be offered that indicate that although athletes do indeed generate more free radicals, they may not necessarily

Table 15-3 Estimated Safe Dietary Intakes of Antioxidant Vitamins

VITAMIN	RDA[a]		SAFE DAILY SUPPLEMENT RANGE[b]
	MALES	FEMALES	MALES AND FEMALES
Vitamin E[c]	6.7 IU	5.4 IU	30–800 IU
Vitamin C	60 mg	60 mg	50–1000 mg
Vitamin A[d]	3300 IU	2664 IU	<10,000 IU

[a] Recommended dietary allowances. 10th ed. Washington, DC: National Academy Press, 1989.
[b] Based upon several sources, including the 1989 RDA; Cohen RD, Braunstein NS. Vitasearch reference guide to vitamins and minerals. Newmarket, NH: Vitasearch, 1996:2–6; and McNamara LR. Medical resource manual for nutritional supplementation. 3rd ed. Vinyard, UT: First Image, 1997:59–63.
[c] 0.67 IU = 1 mg TE.
[d] Most supplements utilize beta-carotene as safer precursor for vitamin A, RE = 3.33 IU from retinol = 6 µg, beta-carotene = 10 IU from beta-carotene.

have a greatly increased risk of oxidative stress (94). A vigorous physical training program that incorporates exercise bouts leading to increased free radical production also leads to an increased level or activity of antioxidant enzymes such as SOD and, presumably, greater endogenous free radical protection (90). Additional protection may also result from increased food intake. Elite athletes who train hard have increased caloric needs. If the athlete consumes increased quantities of a mixed diet to meet those increased energy needs, it is likely, but not assured, that an increased dietary intake of antioxidant vitamins and phytochemicals will result. Long-term antioxidant supplement–oxidative stress studies with exercising athletes are lacking; hence, it is not possible to recommend supplemental antioxidants in a quantitative manner (similar to quantities of these vitamins known to be needed to prevent classical deficiency diseases).

Dietary Antioxidants: Supplements Versus Diet

The relative safety of antioxidants, such as vitamin E and vitamin C (99), and the evidence that supplemental vitamin E (and to some extent, vitamin C) improves cell membrane fluidity and oxygen transfer by preventing free radical damage to membranes (95,96,100) argues in favor of prophylactic antioxidant supplementation for elite athletes. Recommendations to increase the polyunsaturated fatty acid (PUFA) content of the diet as a general measure to reduce serum cholesterol, to increase red blood cell membrane fluidity, and to improve oxygen diffusion capacity at lung and muscle tissue capillary sites (101,102) may also require additional dietary antioxidants to protect these PUFA from peroxidation (103,104). A general dietary recommendation can be made for elite athletes, recreational athletes, and nonathletes alike to increase their intake of dietary sources of vitamins A, E, and C and phytochemicals from fruits and vegetables. However, some athletes are not able or willing to select good sources of antioxidant-containing foods for their daily diet. Additionally, some key antioxidant nutrients, such as vitamin E, are difficult, if not impossible, to consume from dietary sources in quantities adequate to meet levels associated with effective antioxidant protection. This argues for a possible role of a dietary antioxidant supplement for elite athletes as prophylaxis for the control of oxidative stress that exceeds normal levels of free radical production. Table 15-3 lists levels of daily antioxidant vitamin intake that are considered to be safe for human consumption. The antioxidant nutrients vitamin C, E, and beta-carotene are generally safe and well tolerated (99). One exception is that vitamin E may exacerbate the tendency toward bleeding in people deficient in vitamin K taking the anticoagulant drug warfarin. Garewal and Diplock (99) have reviewed the safety of antioxidant vitamins and conclude that based on toxicity criteria alone, these nutrients are ideally suited for a putative disease-preventive application. Their use does not require any toxicity monitoring except in unusual circumstances. Excessively high intakes may be associated with unacceptable risk for side effects and are not needed to control the level of oxidative stress associated with chronic exercise. An important unanswered question is whether commercial synthetic antioxidant supplement mixtures are as effective in controlling oxidative stress as food products containing plant-based phytochemical antioxidants. Until this question is resolved, athletes should be advised to consume a diet containing at least five servings of fruits and vegetables per day. Vitamin E is a safe and potentially useful dietary supplement (and probably the most important single antioxidant nutrient) to add to the elite athlete's diet.

REFERENCES

1. Grandjean AC. Diets of elite athletes: has the discipline of sports nutrition made an impact? J Nutr 1997;127(suppl):S874–S877.

2. van Erp-Baart, Saris WH, Binkhorst BA, et al. Nationwide survey on nutritional habits in elite athletes. Int J Sports Med 1989;10(suppl):S3–S10.

3. Walberg-Rankin J. Dietary carbo-hydrate as an ergogenic aid for prolonged and brief competitions in sport. Int J Sport Nutr 1995;5(suppl):S13–S28.

4. Brotherhood JR. Nutrition and sports performance. Sports Med 1984;1:350–389.

5. Bergstrom J, Hermansen L, Saltin B. Diet, muscle glycogen and physical performance. Acta Physiol Scand 1967;71:140–150.

6. Ahlborg B, Bergstrom J, Brohult J, et al. Human muscle glycogen content and capacity for prolonged exercise after different diets. Foersvarsmedicin 1967;3:85–99.

7. Sherman WM, Costill DL, Fink WJ, et al. The effect of exercise and diet manipulation on muscle

glycogen and its subsequent use during performance. Int J Sports Med 1981;2:114–118.

8. Craig BW. The influence of fructose feeding on physical performance. Am J Clin Nutr 1993; 58(suppl):815S–819S.

9. Levine L, Evans WJ, Cadarette BS, et al. Fructose and glucose ingestion and muscle glycogen use during submaximal exercise. J Appl Physiol 1983;55: 1767–1771.

10. Lamb DR, Brodowicz GR. Optimal use of fluids of varying formulation to minimize exercise-induced disturbances in homeostasis. Sports Med 1986;3: 247–274.

11. Murray R, Eddy DE, Murray T, et al. The effect of fluid and carbohydrate feedings during intermittent cycling exercise. Med Sci Sports Exerc 1987;19: 597–604.

12. Jackson DA, Davis JM, Broadwell MS. Effects of carbohydrate feeding on fatigue during intermittent high-intensity exercise in males and females. Med Sci Sports Exer 1995;27(suppl): S223.

13. Below PR, Mora-Rodriquez R, Gontelez-Alonzo J, et al. Fluid and carbohydrate ingestion independently improve performance during 1 hr of intense exercise. Med Sci Sports Exer 1995;27: 200–210.

14. Burke LM. Nutrition for post-exercise recovery. Aust J Sci Med Sport 1997;29:3–10.

15. Turcotte LP, Richter RE, Kiens B. Lipid metabolism during exercise. In: Hargreaves M, ed. Exercise metabolism. Champaign, IL: Human Kinetics, 1995:99–130.

16. Coggan AR, Williams BD. Lipid metabolism during exercise. In: Hargreaves M, ed. Exercise metabolism. Champaign, IL: Human Kinetics, 1995:177–210.

17. Phillips SM, Green HJ, Tarnopolsky MA, et al. Effects of training duration on substrate turnover and oxidation during exercise. J

Appl Physiol 1996;81: 2182–2191.

18. Sherman WM, Leenders N. Fat loading: the next magic bullet? Int J Sport Nutr 1995;5(suppl): S1–S12.

19. Randle PJ, Newsholme EA, Garland PB. Regulation of glucose uptake by muscle: effects of fatty acids, ketone bodies and pyruvate, and of alloxan-diabetes and starvation, on the uptake and metabolic fate of glucose in rat heart and diaphragm muscles. Biochem J 1964;93:652–664.

20. Newsholme EA. An introduction to the roles of the glucose-fatty acid cycle in sustained exercise. In: Biochemistry of exercise. Champaign, IL: Human Kinetics, 1996:119–125.

21. Spriet LL, Dyk DD. The glucose-fatty acid cycle in skeletal muscle at rest and during exercise. In: Biochemistry of exercise. Champaign, IL: Human Kinetics, 1996:127–155.

22. Coyle EF, Jeukendrup AE, Wagenmakers AJM, Saris WHM. Fatty acid oxidation is directly regulated by carbohydrate metabolism during exercise. Am J Physiol 1997;273:E268–E275.

23. Van Zyl CG, Lambert EV, Hawley JA, et al. Effects of medium chain triglyceride ingestion on fuel metabolism and cycling performance. J Appl Physiol 1996; 80:2217–2225.

24. Rennie MJW, Winder WW, Holloszy JO. A sparing effect of increased plasma fatty acids on muscle and liver glycogen contents in the exercising rat. Biochem J 1976;156:647–655.

25. Hickson RC, Rennie MJ, Conlee RK, et al. Effects of increased plasma free fatty acids on muscle glycogen utilization and endurance. J Appl Physiol 1977; 43:829–833.

26. Costill DL, Coyle EF, Dalsky G, et al. Effects of elevated plasma FFA and insulin on muscle glycogen utilization during exercise. J Appl Physiol 1977;43:695–699.

27. Vukovich MD, Costill DL, Hickey MS, et al. Effect of fat emulsion infusion and fat feeding on muscle glycogen utilization during cycle exercise. J Appl Physiol 1993;75:2774–2780.

28. Phinney SD, Bistrian BR, Evans WK, et al. The human metabolic response to chronic ketosis without caloric restriction: preservation of submaximal exercise capacity with reduced carbohydrate oxidation. Metabolism 1983;32:796–776.

29. Muoio DM, Leddy JJ, Horvath PJ, et al. Effect of dietary fat on metabolic adjustments to maximal VO_2 and endurance in runners. Med Sci Sports Exercise 1994;26:81–88.

30. Lambert EV, Speechly DP, Dennis SC, et al. Enhanced endurance in trained cyclists during moderate intensity exercise following 2 weeks adaptation to a high fat diet. Eur J Appl Physiol 1994; 69:287–293.

31. Helge JW, Richter EA, Kiens B. Interaction of training and diet on metabolism and endurance during exercise in man. J Physiol 1996;492:293–306.

32. Starling RD, Trappe TA, Parcell AC, et al. Effects of diet on muscle triglyceride and endurance performance. Metabolism 1997;82:1185–1189.

33. Miller WC, Bryce GR, Conlee RK. Adaptations to a high fat diet that increased exercise endurance in male rats. J Appl Physiol 1984;56:78–83.

34. Conlee RK, Hammer RL, Winder WW, et al. Glycogen repletion and exercise endurance in rats adapted to a high fat diet. Metabolism 1990;39:289–294.

35. Oscai LB, Esser K. Regulation of muscle triglyceride metabolism in exercise. In: Biochemistry of exercise. Champaign, IL: Human Kinetics, 1996:105–125.

36. Martin WH. Effect of endurance training on fatty acid metabolism during whole body exercise. Med Sci Sports Exercise 1997;29: 635–639.

37. Kiens B, Essen-Gustavsson B, Christiensen NJ, et al. Skeletal muscle substrate utilization during submaximal exercise in man: effect of endurance training. J Physiol 1993;469: 459–478.

38. Romijn JA, Coyle EF, Sidossis LS, et al. Regulation of endogenous fat and carbohydrate metabolism in relation to exercise intensity and duration. Am J Physiol 1993;265:E380–E391.

39. Lemon PW. Is increased dietary protein necessary or beneficial for individuals with a physically active lifestyle? Nutr Rev 1996;54(suppl):S169–S175.

40. Meredith CN, Zacklin MJ, Frontera WR. Dietary protein requirements and body protein metabolism in endurance-trained men. J Appl Physiol 1989;66: 2850–2856.

41. Friedman JE, Lemon PWR. Effect of chronic endurance exercise on retention of dietary protein. Int J Sports Med 1989;10:118–123.

42. Lemon PWR. Protein and exercise: update 1987. Med Sci Sports Exerc 1987;19(suppl): S179–S190.

43. Lemon PW. Protein and amino acid needs of the strength athlete. Int J Sport Nutr 1991;1: 127–145.

44. Celejowa I, Homa M. Food intake, nitrogen and energy balance in Polish weightlifters during a training camp. Nutr Metabol 1970;12:259–274.

45. Meredith CN, O'Reilly KP, Evans WJ. Protein and energy requirements of strength-trained men. Med Sci Sports Exerc 1992; 24(suppl):S71.

46. Torun B, Scrimshaw NS, Young VR. Effect of isometric exercises on body potassium and dietary protein requirements of young men. Am J Clin Nutr 1977;30: 1983–1993.

47. Dragan GI, Vasiliu V, Georgescu E. Effect of increased supply of protein on elite weight lifters: milk proteins. TE Galesloot, BJ Tinbergen, eds. Wageningen: The Netherlands, 1985:99–103.

48. Kreider RB, Miriel V, Bertun E. Amino acid supplementation and exercise performance: analysis of the proposed ergogenic value. Sports Med 1993;16:190–209.

49. Mourier A, Bigard AX, de Kerviler E, et al. Combined effects of caloric restriction and branched-chain amino acid supplementation on body composition and exercise performance in elite wrestlers. Int J Sports Med 1997;18:47–55.

50. Schena F, Guerrini F, Tregnaghi P, et al. Branched-chain amino acid supplementation during trekking at high altitude: the effects on loss of body mass, body composition and muscle power. Eur J Appl Physiol 1992; 65:394–398.

51. Lamanca JJ, Haymes EM. Effects of low ferritin concentration on endurance performance. Int J Sport Nutr 1992;2:376–385.

52. Singh A, Deuster PA, Moser PB. Zinc and copper status in women by physical activity and menstrual status. J Sports Med Phys Fit 1990;30:29–36.

53. Greenleaf JE. Problem: thirst drinking behavior, and involuntary dehydration. Med Sci Sports Exerc 1992;24:645–651.

54. Gisolfi CV. Sports science exchange: exercise, intestinal absorption, and rehydration, Sports Physiology/Biochemistry. 1991;4.

55. American College of Sports Medicine. Position stand on exercise and fluid replacement. Med Sci Sports Exerc 1996;28: i–vii.

56. Noakes TD, Goodwin N, Rayner BL, et al. Water intoxication: a possible complication during endurance exercise. Med Sci Sports Exerc 1985;17: 370–274.

57. Frizzell RT, Lang GH, Lawrence DC, et al. Hyponatremia and ultramarathon running. JAMA 1986;255:722–726.

58. Robinson S, Robinson AH. Chemical compounds of sweat. Physiol Rev 1954;34:202–204.

58a. United States Olympic Committee. Guide to banned medications. Sports Mediscope 1988;7:1–5.

59. Gisolfi CV, Duchmann SM. Guidelines for optimal replacement beverages for different athletic events. Med Sci Sports Exerc 1992;24:679–684.

60. Bucci LR. Nutrients as ergogenic aids in exercise and sport. Boca Raton, FL: CRC Press, 1989: 344–361.

61. Pasman WJ, van Baak MA, Jeukendrup AE, et al. The effect of different dosages of caffeine on endurance performance time. Int J Sports Med 1995;16:225–230.

62. Graham TE, Spriet LL. Performance and metabolic responses to a high caffeine dose during prolonged exercise. J Appl Physiol 1991;71:2292–2298.

63. Jackman M, Wendling P, Friars D, et al. Metabolic catecholamine and endurance responses to caffeine during intense exercise. J Appl Physiol 1996;81: 1658–1663.

64. Graham TE, Spriet LL. Metabolic, catecholamine and exercise performance responses to varying doses of caffeine. J Appl Physiol 1995;78:867–874.

65. Trice I, Haymes EM. Effects of caffeine ingestion on exercise-induced changes during high-intensity, intermittent exercise. Int J Sports Nutr 1995;5:37–44.

66. French C, McNaughton L, Davis P, et al. Caffeine ingestion during exercise to exhaustion in elite distance runners. J Sports Med Phys Fitness 1991;31: 425–432.

67. Harris RC, Soderlund K, Hultman E. Elevation of creatine in resting and exercised muscle of normal subjects by creatine supplementation. Clin Sci 1992;83: 367–374.

68. Greenhaff PL. Creatine and its application as an ergogenic aid.

Int J Sport Nutr 1995;5(suppl): S100–S110.

69. Volek JS, Kraemer WJ, Bush JA, et al. Creatine supplementation enhances muscular performance during high-intensity resistance exercise. J Am Diet Assoc 1997;97:765–770.

70. Jacobs I, Bleue S, Goodman J. Creatine ingestion increases anaerobic capacity and maximum accumulated oxygen deficit. Can J Appl Physiol 1997;22: 231–243.

71. Casey A, Constantin-Teodosiu D, Howell S, et al. Creatine ingestion favorably affects performance and muscle metabolism during maximal exercise in humans. Am J Physiol 1996; 271:E32–E37.

72. Mujika I, Chatard JC, Lacoste L, et al. Creatine supplementation does not improve performance in competitive swimmers. Med Sci Sports Exerc 1996;28: 1435–1441.

73. Redondo DR, Dowling EA, Graham BL, et al. The effect of oral creatine monohydrate supplementation on running velocity. Int J Sport Nutr 1996;6: 213–221.

74. Terrillion KA, Kolkhorst FW, Dolgener FA, et al. The effect of creatine supplementation on two 700 m maximal running bouts. Int J Sport Nutr 1997;7: 138–143.

75. Barnett C, Hinds M, Jenkins DG. Effects of oral creatine supplementation on multiple sprint cycle performance. Aust J Sci Med Sport 1996;28:35–39.

76. Forgo I, Kirchdorfer AM. On the question of influencing the performance of top sportsmen by means of biologically active substances. Artzl Prax 1981;33: 1784–1786.

77. Forgo I. Effect of drugs on physical performance and hormone system of sportsmen. Munch Med Wochenshr 1983; 125:822–824.

78. Forgo I, Schimert G. The duration of effect of the standardized

ginseng extract G115 in healthy competitive athletes. Notabene Medici 1985;15:636–640.

79. Engels HJ, Wirth JC. No ergogenic effects of ginseng (Panax ginseng, CA Meyer) during graded maximal aerobic exercise. J Am Diet Assoc 1997;97: 1110–1115.

80. Morris AC, Jacobs I, McLellan TM, et al. No ergogenic effects of ginseng ingestion. Int J Sport Nutr 1996;6:263–271.

81. Pieralisi G, Rpiari P, Vecchiet L. Effects of a standardized ginseng extract combined with dimethylaminoethanol bitartrate, vitamins, minerals, and trace elements on physical performance during exercise. Clin Ther 1991;13:373–382.

82. Heinonen OJ. Carnitine and physical exercise. Sports Med 1996;22:109–132.

83. Marconi C, Sassi G, Carpinelli A, et al. Effects of L-carnitine loading on the aerobic and anaerobic performance of endurance athletes. Eur J Appl Physiol 1985;54:131–135.

84. Soop M, Bjorkman O, Cederbald G, et al. Influence of carnitine supplementation on muscle substrate and carnitine metabolism during exercise. J Appl Physiol 1988;64:2394–2399.

85. Greig C, Finch KM, Jones DA, et al. The effect of oral supplementation with L-carnitine on maximum and submaximal exercise capacity. Eur J Appl Physiol 1987;56:457–460.

86. Trappe SW, Costill DL, Goodpaster B, et al. The effects of L-carnitine supplementation on performance during interval swimming. Int J Sports Med 1994;15:181–185.

87. Vukovich MD, Costill DL, Fink WJ. Carnitine supplementation: effect on muscle carnitine and glycogen content during exercise. Med Sci Sports Exerc 1994;26: 1122–1129.

88. Cooper MB, Jones DA, Edwards RHT, et al. The effect of

marathon running on carnitine metabolism and on some aspects of muscle mitochondrial activates and antioxidant mechanisms. J Sports Sci 1986;4:79–87.

89. Oyono-Enguelle S, Freund H, Ott C, et al. Prolonged submaximal exercise and L-carnitine in humans. Eur J Appl Physiol 1988;58:53–61.

90. Jenkins RR. Exercise, oxidative stress and antioxidants: a review. Int J Sports Nutr 1993;3: 356–375.

91. Alessio H. Exercise-induced oxidative stress. Med Sci Sports Exerc 1993;25:213–217.

92. Kantner MM. Free radicals, exercise and antioxidant supplementation. Int J Sports Nutr 1994;4: 205–220.

93. Sen C. Oxidants and antioxidants in exercise. J Appl Physiol 1995; 79:675–686.

94. Halliwell B, Gutteridge JMC. Free radicals in biology and medicine. 2nd ed. Oxford: Clarendon, 1989:86–179, 416–508.

95. Haramaki N, Packer L. Oxidative stress indices in exercise. In: Sen CK, Packer L, Hanninen O, eds. Exercise and oxygen toxicity. New York: Elsevier, 1994:77–87.

96. Clarkson PM. Antioxidants and physical performance. Critical Rev Food Sci Nutr 1995;35: 131–141.

97. Kagan VE, Spirichev VB, Serbinova EA, et al. The significance of vitamin E and free radicals in physical exercise. In: Wolinsky I, Hickson JF, eds. Nutrition in exercise and sport. 2nd ed. Boca Raton, FL: CRC Press, 1993:185–213.

98. Tidus PM, Houston ME. Vitamin E status and response to exercise training. Sports Med 1995;20: 12–23.

99. Singh VN. A current perspective on nutrition and exercise. J Nutr 1992;122:760–765.

100. Askew EW. Environmental and physical stress and nutrient

requirements. Am J Clin Nutr 1995;61(suppl):631S–637S.

101. Garewal HS, Diplock AT. How safe are antioxidant vitamins? Drug Safety 1995;13:8–14.

102. Alessio HM, Goldfarb AH, Cao G. Exercise-induced oxidative stress before and after vitamin C supplementation. Int J Sports Nutr 1997:1–9.

103. Guezennec CY, Nadaud JF, Sabatin F, et al. Influence of polyunsaturated fatty acid diet on the hemorrheological response to physical exercise in hypoxia. Int J Sports Nutr 1989;10:286–201.

104. Aguilaniu B, Flore P, Perrault H, et al. Exercise-induced hypoxaemia in master athletes: effects of a polyunsaturated fatty acid diet. Eur J Appl Physiol 1995; 72:44–50.

Chapter 16

Communicating the Message About Sound Nutrition and Other Healthy Lifestyle Practices: Challenges and Opportunities

Barbara Moore
Idamarie Laquatra

As educators and communicators we are in the midst of an "evolution." Technology is rapidly changing, altering how, when, and where we see, hear, and experience communication. Health professionals are taking advantage of these new technologies by harnessing the tools of communication to reach the public. Public relations and marketing principles are being used to craft health-promoting, disease-reducing campaigns. Although the specific objectives differ, in general, the campaigns are designed to increase awareness and educate, and ultimately to effect a change in behavior conducive to health (1).

Developing a powerful health promotion campaign requires an understanding of the process of behavior change and familiarity with learning principles. A model of generating and delivering health communications can then be followed so that the campaign can flow in an organized manner for optimal effect.

Knowing how individuals change their behaviors results in program goals that are reasonable and likely to be achieved. A model of change that has been quite helpful in understanding behavior change is the trans-theoretical approach developed by Prochaska and DiClemente (2). Originally designed for the treatment of addictive behaviors, the trans-theoretical approach has been applied to behavior change in general (3). The initial model identified four stages of change people pass through as they alter their behaviors (2). Further study of people involved in the process of self-change resulted in an expansion to a six-stage model. The six stages are: precontemplation, contemplation, preparation, action, maintenance, and termination (4).

During the precontemplation stage, individuals may not be aware or may resist becoming aware of a problem or solution to the problem. Precontemplators process less information about their problems and spend less time and energy becoming more self-aware (2). In this stage would be sedentary individuals who have never thought of incorporating physical activity into their lives. They view the negative aspects of physical activity as far outweighing the positive ones. As individuals progress to contemplation, which may occur as a result of developmental or environmental changes, they begin to think about change and become more conscious about themselves and their problems. An individual in this stage might be someone who recently celebrated a fiftieth birthday and is in the process of reevaluating his or her health.

The preparation stage is one of decision making and commitment to take action. Individuals in the preparation stage have a plan. Purchasing a gym membership and planning the days for attendance in the time frame of the next month would be markers for individuals in this stage.

The action stage is characterized by specific activities, such as goal setting and skill acquisition, which the person undertakes to deal with a problem. During this stage it is critical that individuals believe their own efforts play a role in success. Also, they must accept the responsibility for changing. A previously sedentary person in the midst of an exercise program is an example of someone in the action stage.

During the maintenance stage, the individual deals with the issue of relapse. This involves learning how to sustain motivation and provide self-reinforcement to avoid slipping back into previous behaviors. Termination refers to the stage individuals reach when they have no temptation to return to their old lifestyles even when faced with high-risk situations. They feel confident they will not relapse.

People do not pass through the stages of change in a linear fashion. They more commonly follow a cyclical pattern during the change process. Additionally, some people can become lodged in a particular stage of change and seem unable to progress to later stages. To help someone, health professionals must tailor their approach to address the individual's stage of change. On a broader basis, campaigns should be designed to help individuals move from one stage to another. For example, helping precontemplators progress to the contemplation stage requires informational messages that increase awareness and communicate the advantages for changing behavior. Individuals in the action stage benefit from choices they can make as they alter their behaviors.

Health professionals armed with good intentions can unwittingly cause resistance to change. Three major pitfalls must be recognized and successfully avoided. The first pitfall is a lack of understanding of what is important to the individual. Practitioners are often disappointed and frustrated when people they are trying to help fail to change and continue to engage in behaviors that are contrary to good health. Moving through the stages of change hinges on how important changing is to the individual. The individual must believe the benefits of changing outweigh the disadvantages. Knowing the needs of the person helps practitioners identify what is important. If the change is more important to the health professional than to the individual who is doing the changing, chances are the change will not occur.

The second pitfall has to do with the types of goals for behavior change that are set. Practitioners are trained to set goals for change that are ideal for health. Unfortunately, these may be goals that are unrealistic (5). When the 1995 Dietary Guidelines for Americans (DGA) were released, the most noticeable change in wording was for the weight guideline. Not only did it emphasize both diet and physical activity, but it also stressed both weight maintenance and weight loss. The 1990 guideline, "maintain a healthy weight," was based on the presumption that a healthy weight could be achieved and maintained (6). The Committee recognized that such a goal may be impossible for the large number of overweight people in the United States, given the high rates of relapse after weight loss. The new guideline, "balance the food you eat with physical activity—maintain or improve your weight," emphasizes weight maintenance as a more realistic goal (6)—at least for some people.

Related to unrealistic goals are inflated expectations for what can be accomplished through a health promotion campaign. It takes time for people to pass through the stages of change. A review of the effectiveness of community action as a strategy for health promotion indicated that even methodologically adequate projects have failed to show major gains in reducing health risk behaviors (7). The authors recommended that practitioners accept that gains in public health will appear small and take time and that behaviors that are less threatening be targeted before tackling the more ingrained behaviors (7).

The third major pitfall involves the methods used for encouraging change. Resistance to change is increased when tactics such as advice giving, threatening, warning, and moralizing are used (5). Although such tactics may briefly capture media interest, in the long run, they produce no or, worse still, negative effects on health behaviors. During the developmental stages of any health promotion campaign, therefore, health professionals should understand the needs of the target audience; recognize the importance of setting small, realistic goals; accept that change is a slow process; and focus on positive messages and actions.

A good grasp about how people learn is also required if campaigns are to be effective. Health professionals often rely on giving information to help people change behaviors (8). While a lack of knowledge certainly may contribute to lack of change, it usually is not the only reason people do not acquire health-promoting behaviors. Indeed, a randomized, controlled trial that tested the efficacy of an information booklet to increase the duration of breastfeeding did not have any significant effect on breastfeeding behavior. The authors suggested that use of written materials alone had limited efficacy and that such a single intervention be combined with more individualized support for greater effectiveness (9).

A health promotion campaign must be relevant to the needs of the audience and have a clear purpose and appropriate content at the right level and pace. A variety of teaching and learning methods are needed to engage individuals because the audience expects to enjoy their learning. In addition, individuals value opportunities to try out what they have learned with feedback about progress (10). Understanding the sources of information important to a target population, using appropriate targeting media, and combining them with a hands-on intervention to involve the patient may be important in not only reaching patients but also in influencing their behaviors (11). An example of a campaign with these characteristics was reported by Lee et al (11). The study was designed to examine the impact of a multimedia campaign on patient behavior in eye care. The well-integrated educational effort had an additional component of patient involvement by use of a simple self-administered screening device. Individuals were surveyed one year after they mailed in a contrast sensitivity screening card during a focused multimedia educational campaign. Those who failed the screening test were much more likely to have had an eye examination in the year after the campaign (11).

TOOLS FOR A HEALTH PROMOTION CAMPAIGN

One approach to developing a health promotion campaign is "social marketing," a process in which commercial marketing concepts and techniques are applied to social and health issues (12). There have been controversy and debates swirling around the use of social marketing techniques in the public health sector (13–15). We believe that there are benefits to using marketing strategies in health promotion; social marketing can be viewed as a valuable tool for developing effective campaigns. In the for-profit sector, marketing strategies include research conducted with consumers to learn about their needs and behaviors. Such research is a cost-effective way to better target the message and the type of communications used.

The Centers for Disease Control and Prevention (CDC) developed a 10-step model for the development, pre-testing, refinement, delivery, and evaluation of health messages for targeted audiences (16). Arguments have been made to alter the model slightly to be more in line with those used by health educators and commercial marketers (17). The revised model is shown in Table 16-1.

As Table 16-1 indicates, the needs, preferences, beliefs, and attitudes of the target population are taken into account in designing and implementing interventions. This is critical, because a public health message must be highly personal to be relevant and effective (11). Setting communication objectives should include the action the person should take as a result of the communication (12). Consumers have indicated that they want directions—they want to know how and what to do. Rather then saying, "Increase fruits and vegetables in your diet," a more powerful message would provide helpful ways to achieve the goal (6). Furthermore, providing choices can enhance motivation. Giving three choices has been shown to be more effective for motivating people than giving just one choice, but more than three seems to have no additional effect (4).

When message concepts are identified, they must move beyond the clinical and epidemiologic research basis. Such facts rarely motivate. Consumers look for specific reasons, meaningful in their lives, to change (6).

Knowing the target audience will help to identify the communication vehicles that should be used. Communication vehicles include the Internet, television, newspapers, magazines, direct mail, and public relations (e.g., news releases to the media, press conferences). Media programs for public health campaigns tend to rely on vehicles such as brochures and public service announcements (PSAs) without evaluating their usefulness (12). PSAs may or may not be effective, depending on their design and what they expect people to do. In a review of methods used in Project LEAN (Low-Fat Eating for America Now), a national nutrition campaign in which the aim is to reduce dietary fat consumption, it was found that despite their attractiveness and wide use, PSAs did not greatly enhance the impact of the campaign message on the target audience. The campaign achieved more from well-placed publicity than from unpaid PSAs (8). On the other hand, Shape Up America!, a national initiative to promote healthy weight and physical activity, used PSAs featuring its

founder, former Surgeon General C. Everett Koop. The spots featured a toll-free telephone hotline, which people could call to be connected to the Shape Up America! clearinghouse, an information and referral service that operated on a 24-hour basis during the PSA campaign. During the three-month period that the PSAs were aired, more than 10,600 individuals called the clearinghouse and received materials free of charge.

Knowledge of the target audiences' media habits can be used to select the appropriate channels for communication. For example, a study of smoking prevention interventions found that mass media combined with school intervention resulted in significantly lower smoking prevalence within a higher risk sample (18). Careful analysis of the target groups found that higher risk groups consistently reported frequent use of radio, cable television (MTV), and network television programs. Using purchased media time to optimize exposure proved to be beneficial.

Once the communication channels are chosen, messages and materials appropriate for the channels can be developed. A promotion plan that includes a timeline is the next step. The promotion plan should include partnerships with other organizations. Not only will this provide support, but it will also result in more widespread involvement for the program on the national and local levels (8).

AN EXAMPLE OF A HEALTH PROMOTION CAMPAIGN

Shape Up America! is a public health initiative that was launched in December 1994 to elevate healthy weight as a priority concern. With the ultimate goal of stimulating behavioral change, Shape Up America! is conducting a broad-based educational initiative to encourage a better diet and increased physical activity in all individuals and a modest weight loss in overweight people that can be maintained over time. Shape Up America! is the only privately funded, national program committed solely to education about the importance of healthy weight, an improved diet, and increased activity.

The Shape Up America! initiative is supported by 46 nonprofit organizations that comprise its coalition. The coalition includes food, nutrition, medical, public health, physical fitness, sports, and special constituency groups that provide an important grassroots network for communicating obesity-related messages to the general public, health care professionals, employers, community leaders, policy makers, and the media. With a combined membership of approximately 41 million, the potential range of influence of the Shape Up America! coalition is very significant.

Since the inception of Shape Up America! in 1994, the initiative has concentrated on communicating four messages that are central to the Shape Up America! mission:

1. Add a total of 30 extra minutes of physical activity a day, using such conventional means as walking and climbing the stairs.
2. Eat a sensible, well-balanced diet that is low in fat and includes a variety of foods with plenty of grains, fruits, and vegetables.

Table 16-1 The Revised CDC Framework for Health Communication

STEPS

1. Review background information
2. Analyze and segment target audiences
3. Set communication objectives
4. Identify message concepts and pretest
5. Select communications channels
6. Create messages and materials, and pretest
7. Develop promotion plan
8. Implement communication strategies
9. Assess effects
10. Collect feedback

SOURCE: Donovan R. Steps in planning and developing health communication campaigns: a comment on CDC's framework for health communication. Public Health Reports 1995;110:215–217.

---

3. Achieving or maintaining a healthy weight is possible. You can do it!

4. Help others to achieve a healthy weight.

While these messages are essential to combating obesity in America, getting them before the public in a compelling way has always been a challenge. Therefore, Shape Up America! focused its 1996 educational activities around high-impact media designed to engage Americans on the issue of healthy weight and motivate them to take action.

Recognizing the growing power of the Internet as an information source, in October 1996, Shape Up America! unveiled a new cyberspace clinic (www.shapeup.org) where the public, health professionals, policy makers, and the media can get the latest facts on obesity-related issues. Incorporating state-of-the-art interactive technology, the Internet site is designed to inform individuals on a personal basis about weight management, while also helping physicians and other healthcare professionals to treat obese patients effectively. Within the first month of operation, five Internet information resources had voted the site one of the best information tools on the Internet. These endorsements, plus extensive publicity in the consumer and technology media, have resulted in over 500,000 visits to the cyberspace clinic every week or approximately 2 million hits a month (Figure 16-1). One component of the website is the CYBERkitchen, an interactive feature that translates into real-life terms the meaning of messages about how to balance the food you eat with physical activity. Along with helping the visitor calculate his or her daily calorie and fat levels, the website features breakfast, lunch, and dinner selections; a customized shopping list; and selected recipes.

In support of the Surgeon General's Report on Physical Activity and Health, Shape Up America! teamed up with TOPS (Take Off Pounds Sensibly), an international nonprofit weight-loss support group with 300,000 members worldwide and a coalition member, to unveil its national walking campaign. To celebrate the development of this new community-based initiative, Shape Up America! hosted a special walk for about 2000 TOPS members who joined with their Congressmen from all across the country to promote the health benefits of walking. As the next step, TOPS sent campaign implementation kits to local chapters that will be promoting walking clubs in their localities on an ongoing basis. Further, Shape Up America! is distributing TOPS kits to each member of the Shape Up America! coalition to encourage walking on a national scale.

Besides the potential for elevating the value of walking at the community level, this walking campaign sets out a course of action for creating local walking clubs, recruiting walkers, locating walking routes, and establishing mileage goals as incentives. This effort is further being reinforced through the participation of Shape Up America! in the Partnership for a Walkable America (PWA), whereby Shape Up America! is providing assistance on evaluating communities and in removing barriers to walking and other forms of nonautomotive transportation.

Shape Up America! has also targeted the medical community in its efforts. To encourage physicians to intervene with their adult obese patients and to provide responsible,

state-of-the-art guidance for such interventions, Shape Up America! teamed up with its coalition member, the America Obesity Association (AOA), to develop obesity treatment guidance. Guidance for Treatment of Adult Obesity is the first comprehensive medical guide that takes into account the various complications of obesity and recommends a logical progression of treatment options tied to the patient's degree of health risk. To generate nationwide awareness among the medical community for this guidance document, Dr. Koop held a major news conference in Washington, DC, and gave special interviews on major television networks. In addition, national and local stations aired over 175 television stories coast to coast. At the same time, the release of the obesity treatment guidance was covered by every major wire service and news bureau, resulting in widespread newspaper and radio coverage as well as articles and commentaries in many of the leading medical journals.

Shape Up America! is also building public awareness and interest in combatting obesity by providing the public, educators, community leaders, the media, and policy makers with a steady stream of new and compelling information about healthy weight, physical activity, and sensible eating. Its news bureau generates news stories and, in 1996 alone, the campaign was featured in over 1000 newspaper articles and in more than 75 television features on issues related to healthy weight.

For a program like Shape Up America!, which hopes to go beyond public awareness and actually produce behavior change, the results to date document the potential of this initiative to make an impact on people's lives. To change behavior will require a sustained effort of time and resources and a strong commitment to be patient enough to see change.

A major issue for this and every other public health initiative is funding. There is an ongoing need for staff to locate and consider new funding sources and strategies and, at the same time, to aggressively design and implement educational program initiatives. Yet private sector initiatives have a number of distinct advantages over similar initiatives in the government sector:

1. They can act more quickly because of reduced layers of review.

2. The language used in educational materials is less encumbered by political interference.

3. They have lower overhead because they can staff on an as-needed basis.

The not-for-profit community has sought creative alliances with the commercial sector to communicate key messages. Although controversial, the advantage of such alliances is a dramatically increased reach to the target audience. A major drawback is the need to jointly craft messages so that they do not distort or mislead and serve the purposes of both organizations.

There is a need to craft even wider alliances that include the financial strength and resources of the government sector with the remarkable outreach of the commercial sector. We believe the private not-for-profit sector is the logical midwife of such alliances and is an excellent mechanism for future initiatives.

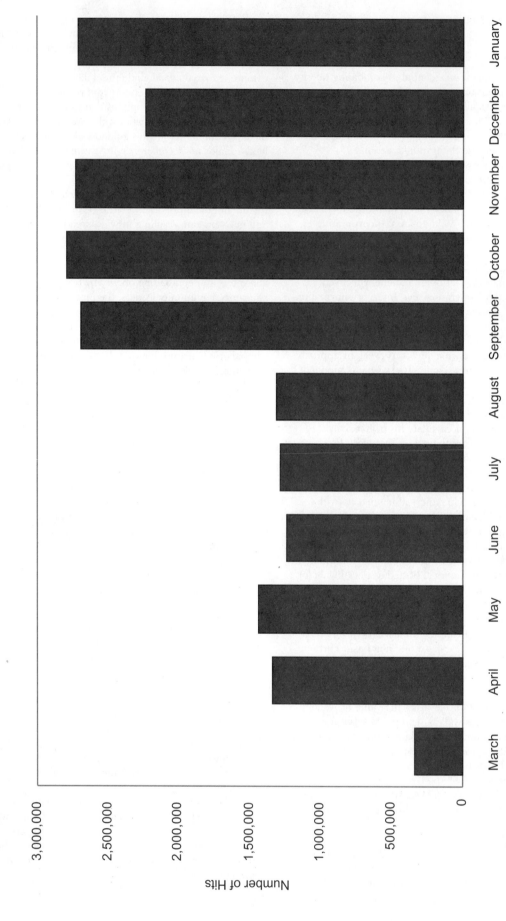

Figure 16-1 Shape Up America! website hits March 1997 through January 1998 (website URL is www.shapeup.org).

REFERENCES

1. Green LW, Kreuter MW. Health promotion as a public health strategy for the 1990s. Ann Rev Public Health 1990;11: 319–334.

2. Prochaska JO, DiClemente CO. Toward a comprehensive model of change. In: Miller WR, Healther N, eds. Treating addictive behaviors: processes of change. New York: Plenum Press, 1986:3–27.

3. Greene GW, Rossi SR, Reed GR, et al. Stages of change for reducing dietary fat to 30% of energy or less. J Am Diet Assoc 1994; 94:1105–1110.

4. Prochaska JO. Why do we behave the way we do? Can J Cardiol 1995;11(suppl):20A–25A.

5. Botelho RJ, Skinner H. Motivating change in health behavior: implications for health promotion and disease prevention. Primary Care 1995;22:565–589.

6. Kennedy E, Meyers L, Layden W. The 1995 dietary guidelines for Americans: an overview. J Am Diet Assoc 1996;96:234–237.

7. Hancock L, Sanson-Fisher RW, Redman S, et al. Community action for health promotion: a review of methods and outcomes 1990–1995. Am J Prev Med 1997;13:229–239.

8. Samuels SE. Project LEAN—lessons learned from a national social marketing campaign. Public Health Rep 1993;108: 45–53.

9. Curro V, Lanni R, Scipione F, et al. Randomised controlled trial assessing the effectiveness of a booklet on the duration of breast-feeding. Arch Dis Child 1997;76: 500–504.

10. Daines J, Daines C, Graham B. Adult learning: adult teaching. Nottingham: University of Nottingham, 1993:15.

11. Lee PP, Linton K, Ober RR, et al. The efficacy of a multimedia educational campaign to increase the use of eye care services. Ophthalmology 1994;101: 1465–1469.

12. Sutton SM, Balch GI, Lefebvre RC. Strategic questions for consumer-based health communications. Public Health Rep 1995;110:725–733.

13. Montazeri A. Social marketing: a tool not a solution. J Roy Soc Health 1997;117:115–118.

14. Vanden Heede FA, Pelican S. Reflections on marketing as an inappropriate model for nutrition education. J Nutr Educ 1995; 27:141–145.

15. Lefebvre RC, Lurie D, Goodman LS, et al. Social marketing and nutrition education: inappropriate or misunderstood? JNE 1995;27: 146–150.

16. Roper WL. Health communication takes on new dimensions at CDC. Public Health Rep 1993;108: 179–183.

17. Donovan RJ. Steps in planning and developing health communication campaigns: a comment on CDC's framework for health communication. Public Health Rep 1995;110:215–217.

18. Flynn BS, Worden JK, Secker-Walker RH, et al. Long-term responses of higher and lower risk youths to smoking prevention interventions. Prev Med 1997; 26:389–394.

Part III.

SPORTS MEDICINE AND ORTHOPEDICS

Edited by
Angela Smith

Introduction to Sports Medicine and Orthopedics

Angela Smith

To many, sports medicine is synonymous with injury treatment. Of course, modern sports medicine includes not only the care of physical and mental disorders of sport and fitness activity participants but also prevention of potential problems. This section focuses on the musculoskeletal system and discusses the role of exercise in preventing bone loss, prevention of injuries during exercise, evaluation of those injuries that do occur, and general principles of treatment and rehabilitation of those injuries.

Approximately 50% of injuries sustained during sport and fitness activities could be avoided. Methods of injury prevention include preparing for new activity in a graduated, progressive manner and careful attention to factors such as equipment and playing conditions. Rehabilitation of previous injuries is critical to avoid recurrent or additional injury.

Victoroff discusses the evaluation and initial treatment of acute sports injuries. He provides clinical tips on evaluation of an injured participant at all the typical venues, from on the field to in the office. He also recommends appropriate indications for expensive or sophisticated tests and for referral to a specialist.

Injured athletes often expect physical therapy as a component of their treatment. Those treating the athlete may be uncertain of the science or the efficacy of different therapeutic treatments. Wickham, Schmidtt, and Snyder-Mackler lend insight into what is and is not known about commonly used modalities.

Krivickas and Sheehan carry rehabilitation treatment to the next step, suggesting therapeutic modalities and therapeutic exercise regimens tailored to both the injury and the individual. Both Krivickas and Victoroff offer guidelines for criteria for return to sport and physical activity.

Jaffe and Drinkwater address the relationship of exercise to bone strength. Jaffe's discussion of the female athlete triad of disordered eating, amenorrhea, and osteoporosis looks at a problem that involves multiple organ systems and requires a multidisciplinary approach for treatment. Drinkwater updates the role of exercise in prevention and treatment of postmenopausal osteoporosis. As new data have become available in the last decade, recommendations have frequently evolved. Drinkwater reminds us that adequate bone-loading exercise represents only one leg of a three-legged stool that includes sufficient estrogen and adequate nutrients—the stool doesn't stand if any of the three are missing.

Although this section is intended to have a clinical focus, future research can be expected to lead to continued improvements in injury prevention strategies and musculoskeletal injury evaluation and treatment. Exercise is clearly required for the development and maintenance of healthy bones and muscles. A gradually progressing training program prevents injuries and rehabilitates injured structures as well. The authors offer clinical insights and "pearls" certain to be useful in counseling those concerned about a healthy lifestyle.

Chapter 17

Female Athlete Triad: Clinical Evaluation and Treatment

Rebecca Jaffe

The female athlete triad was first named in the early 1990s by a group of women who noted the association of disordered eating, amenorrhea, and osteoporosis. In May 1993, a conference was convened to identify what was known and what needed to be better understood about the triad (1). If the potential problems of the triad for athletes were to go unchecked, the consequences to the individual's health could be catastrophic. Therefore, the group set out to educate all who observe, care for, or suffer from symptoms of the triad. This effort was made in order to stave off the potential dangers of not identifying individuals at risk, while emphasizing the strongly positive effects of sport and fitness activites for the vast majority of female athletes (2).

The evaluation of the patient who is suspected of being subject to the triad is not necessarily a simple task. It is a multifactorial problem that has many known and unknown consequences, including the potential for premature death. Patients suffering from the triad often are secretive and lie to health practitioners during traditional history and physical evaluations. Although older women may develop the disorder, adolescents are the group most affected. Adolescents may be more susceptible because they are attempting to balance a number of factors in their lives, including good health, peak performance, and issues related to appearance and self-esteem (3).

Evaluation of the separate parts of the triad may prove more rewarding and helpful in attempting to evaluate each individual. Fitting all pieces of the puzzle together to develop a cautious and thoughtful care plan is imperative. It seems clear that aggressive, early interventions may prevent the otherwise expected poor outcomes.

AMENORRHEA

The first and easiest clinical entity to identify is amenorrhea, or lack of menses. Amenorrhea is an unnatural suppression of menses. In athletes, it may be a result of an energy imbalance resulting from excessive expenditures of energy without the necessary compensatory caloric ingestion. In all females, amenorrhea is identified and defined as follows:

- Primary amenorrhea occurs in a girl who has never had a menstrual cycle at the chronologic age of 16, or 2 years after the development of secondary sex characteristics.

- Secondary amenorrhea occurs in a girl who has had at least one menstrual cycle but has ceased having cycles thereafter.

- Oligomenorrhea has several different definitions. We use the definition of irregular cycles with gaps of 3 months or more between cycles.

There is an overwhelming belief among athletes that menses hinder performance. This is a myth perpetuated by many athletes and coaches. The medical literature shows that despite the fact that athletes believe menses affect their ability to perform, many women have won gold medals at the Olympics and set world records while menstruating. There is a significantly higher prevalence of menstrual disorders among women athletes compared with the general female population (4).

In obtaining a patient's history, one should try to establish whether there is an apparent cause for the lack of cycles. Questions about sexual activity, galactorrhea, late menarche, medications, previous episodes of amenorrhea associated with exercise, body hair, and fatigue should be part of an interview. Certain elite sports activities are related to a higher incidence of these disorders. They include long distance running, gymnastics, and classical ballet. Also at increased risk are cyclists, rowers, and swimmers. The history should also include symptoms related to eating disorders or osteoporosis, discussed later in this chapter.

On physical examination, it is important to examine the patient's body hair distribution, establish her Tanner stage, study her body habitus, and perform a pelvic examination. Body fat assessment may be helpful, although there is no specific critical level at which menses cease. Checks for virilization—hirsutism, acne, and clitoromegaly—are important.

If all appears normal, laboratory evaluation is indicated. A serum human chorionic gonadotropin (hCG) test should exclude pregnancy, the most common reason for an athlete to have amenorrhea. In addition, serum prolactin, thyrotropin (TSH), and follicle-stimulating hormone (FSH) tests should be done to exclude most pituitary, thyroid, or ovarian causes of amenorrhea. If the patient is hirsute, a dehydroepiandrosterone sulfate (DHEAS) determination should also be made (5).

Individuals who have symptoms of the triad or with isolated athletic amenorrhea will have no identifiable laboratory cause for their amenorrhea. There may be multifactorial explanations for their lack of cycles, including pathogenic methods of weight control, excessive training or exertion, "stress," low body mass index (BMI less than 19), and reproductive immaturity. The common pathway seems to be that there is loss of control at the hypothalamic level, with loss of the normal pulsatility of gonadotrophin-releasing hormone (GnRH) (6).

Other tests can include energy imbalance testing in a metabolic chamber and progestin challenge tests, but neither of these tests will help to differentiate patients with the triad from those with nonathletic amenorrhea. The progestin challenge test involves administering 10 mg of progestin a day, for 10 days, then determining whether menstrual bleeding occurs after progestin withdrawl. If bleeding occurs, there is adequate estrogen priming the uterus. Women with these symptoms and findings should have menses induced periodically, because unopposed estrogen puts them at risk for endometrial hyperplasia and uterine adenocarcinoma. If no bleeding occurs, an estrogen-progestin challenge is done. Some physicians use a traditional birth control pill pack to perform this test. Other physicians use up to 1.25 mg of conjugated estrogen for 25 days and supplement the final 14 days with 10 mg of progestin. The end result should be withdrawal bleeding in previously menstruating women with true athletic amenorrhea.

DISORDERED EATING AND EATING DISORDERS

The second facet of the triad—eating disorders or disordered eating—is much more difficult to establish in an uncooperative patient. It impairs both athletic and cognitive functioning, may induce hypoglycemia and electrolyte disturbances, and can cause long-term, complex psychological problems.

Eating disorder is a Diagnostic and Statistical Manual, fourth edition (DSM-IV) diagnosis with established criteria.

Two eating disorders are included in the current edition. Anorexia nervosa is defined by four criteria: the fear of being fat, disordered body image, refusal to maintain a weight more than 85% of that expected for height, and amenorrhea (if appropriate for age). There are two forms of anorexia, a restrictive type and a binge-purge type. An anorexic person may experience one or both forms at various times in life. Bulimia nervosa is defined by recurrent binge eating, binge-purge cycling on average at least two times a week for at least 3 months, an obsessive concern with body shape and weight, and distorted body image. There are two forms of bulimia: the purging form with use of vomiting, laxatives, and diuretics, and the nonpurging form with fasting or excessive exercise.

Disordered eating is a continuum between poorly balanced diets and overt DSM-IV eating disorders. Societal pressure to lose weight and look thinner plays a role, and for athletes, this pressue is amplified. These messages come from advertisements, peers, coaches, family, and even strangers. Two athletic groups are thought to be at higher risk for disordered eating. Athletes who participate in aesthetic sports like gymnastics, figure skating, ballet, dance, and cheerleading have been indoctrinated to appear a certain way. Athletes such as judo competitors, rowers, wrestlers, and jockeys who must meet a certain weight to compete are also at risk. Sometimes the aberrant desire for extremely low weight maintenance may be a symptom of underlying emotional distress. Up to 74% of female athletes engage in some kind of abnormal eating pattern (7), although good studies are few. These pressures to "make weight" are now seen among male athletes as well and have negative health implications.

It frequently becomes apparent when taking a patient's history that the athlete lacks understanding of the role of nutrition in performance. Warning signs of the female athlete triad include a secretive nature of responses to questioning about food intake and excessive exercising. Asking the same or similar questions in different formats and at different times during the patient encounter may help the practitioner discover those women who are being covert about their problem. Severe weight changes and a family history of eating disorders are also possible indicators of this diagnosis.

During the physical examination, examine the patient without clothing. Some of these patients wear baggy and deceptive clothing and may even use weights in their clothing to deceive health care workers about their weight. Hair may be excessively brittle. The skin might be dry, and fine lanugo hair may appear. Russell's sign, an abrasion on the dorsum of the knuckles caused by self-induced vomiting, may be present. Intermittent parotid swelling should be recognized as a warning signal of bulimia. New dental caries in an adult are potential signs of an eating disorder. Arrhythmias and bradycardias are the predominant cardiac finding in patients with eating disorders. These individuals may be hypotensive or have orthostatic hypotension.

Results of laboratory studies are not diagnostic for the triad or eating disorders. These patients may be anemic or have liver and kidney abnormalities because of their aberrant eating habits. Some clinicians recommend tests including complete blood cell (CBC) count, a serum iron level (even if hemoglobin level is normal), total iron-binding capacity (TIBC), erthrocyte sedimentation rate (ESR), a chemistry panel, thyroid functions, and urinalysis (expecting ketonuria, at a minimum, to be present). Alpha-carotene serum concentrations have been reported to be higher in individuals with eating disorders. A serum estradiol (E_2) level is helpful in patients who have the triad; it may influence treatment plans. But results of all studies may be normal.

Additional tests may include eating disorder surveys, which may be helpful in individuals for whom the diagnosis is elusive. Multiple inventories are commercially available. Although there has not been concensus regarding a single best screening test, the Eating Disorders Inventory (EDI) and Eating Attitudes Test (EAT) are widely used. An electrocardiogram (ECG) may be indicated if the physical examination suggests dysrhythmia or severe bradycardia.

Patients with disordered eating may have long-standing problems with self-esteem. These athletes may have difficulty seeking solutions to their problems and an inability to handle stress. The eating problem may first be seen as a coping mechanism and later as a control issue. Individuals with severe eating disorders may require hospitalization to prevent morbidity and mortality. Cognitive-behavioral therapy is the psychological treatment of choice. Treatment is multidisciplinary, typically including the primary physician, dietitian, physical therapist, athletic trainer, coach, and possibly others.

OSTEOPOROSIS

Osteoporosis, or bone weakness to the point of fracture, occurs as a consequence of the nutritional and hormonal aspects of the triad. Individuals who have eating disorders and are amenorrheic are at an extremely high risk for bone fragility (8). Peak bone mass, typically achieved early in a woman's third decade, is an important determinant of osteoporosis and fracture risk (9).

Athletes with osteoporosis may give a history of multiple occult fractures, recurrent fractures, or stress fractures. Nutritional history, including caloric and calcium intake, will be helpful in identifying those at risk. A drug history is important, since steroids, thyroid hormone, anti-seizure medication, antacids, laxatives, furosemide, and heparin can all lead to osteoporosis. At risk are thin, white women whose calcium intake has been poor. Positive family history is a risk factor. The athlete may also give a history of amenorrhea.

The most widely accepted test for osteoporosis at this time is the dual energy x-ray absorptiometry (DEXA) scan; it is reproducible and cost-effective. The World Health Organization (WHO) has defined osteoporosis on the basis of norms and standard deviations (SD) from the normal in healthy young women. WHO defines women as osteopenic if their bone density is between 1.0 and 2.4 SD below the mean; osteoporosis is defined as readings with an SD of 2.5 or more below the mean. If osteoporosis is apparent on plain-film radiographs, the athlete has already lost at least 35% of the bone mineral at that site.

If an athlete has a diagnosis of osteoporosis, one must look for primary and secondary causes of the disease. The history and physical examination direct the workup. Age is also a factor in determining the extent of the workup. In adolescent athletes, the minimum workup should include a CBC count, SMA-18, and thyroid function tests. Serum estradiol levels are also helpful: Levels of less than 35 μg/dL in postmenopausal women lead to bone degradation, and low levels in young women are even more worrisome. Elevated cortisol levels have been identified as a laboratory marker for osteopenia in patients with anorexia nervosa.

Once an athlete has a diagnosis of one component of the triad, she should be carefully checked for the other two. The patient's trust is crucial. The physician must approach the patient in a nonthreatening, nonjudgmental way. The physician should understand the patient's dedication to her sport and related activities. Each patient may benefit from one or both of the generalized recommendations of some decrease in activity and increase in caloric intake on a daily basis (10,11).

There are many case studies of women with the triad and the multiple fractures they endure. Some young female athletes who are amenorrheic, yet physically very active, have been found to have measured bone mineral densities similar to 70-year-old women (12). Heredity has a role, but it appears that external forces play a much larger role for some athletes.

The approach to athletes with an overt eating disorder must be multidisciplinary, including dietitian, psychologist or psychiatrist, and primary physician working together with the patient. The athlete's coach, physical therapist, and additional physicians are also typically involved in her treatment. These health professionals should have experience treating athletes and be knowledgeable about the triad.

Education of young women athletes is critical in prevention of the triad as well as later intervention. The athlete must understand how important fueling her body is to her performance and well-being (11). Athletes should know the caloric makeup of their diet as well as the calcium content of the food they eat. They should be instructed in obtaining their basic calorie needs, usually 1200 calories plus the additional calories for the activities they perform. Calcium intake should preferentially come from food rather than supplements. Intake should be no less than 1000 mg/day, but preferably 1500 mg/day. Energy intake should be optimized for size, age, and exercise intensity. Food diaries, counseling, contracts, and advance meal planning can all be successful strategies to guide athletes to better nutrition (13). Education about body fat measurements is also important. There is no optimal level of body fat with regard to success in a particular sport. There are usual ranges of body fat percentages for elite competitors in a given sport. Typically, many factors other than weight and percentage of body fat alone determine competitive success.

Athletes should be made aware that having regular menses is a sign of good health and is important to their long-term health. The fact that there is a relationship between exercise intensity and energy consumption needs to be clearly defined.

All patients, athletic or not, should be queried about their calcium intake. At puberty, a young woman has gained 70% of her peak bone mass. The final consolidation to maximize the mineral content of her skeleton occurs by age 30. Young athletic women must maintain adequate calcium intake to maximize bone mineral content. Young amenorrheic athletes should have a calcium intake of 1500 to 2000 mg daily to try to prevent bone loss. The stronger the young adult skeleton, the longer it takes to get to a fracture threshold once age-related bone loss begins (14). Weight-bearing activity (especially high-impact activities) and strength training aid in achieving and maintaining optimized peak bone mass (15,16).

Recommendations about the use of estrogen therapy to improve bone mineral content in these patients are mainly based on a postmenopausal model. In postmenopausal women, estrogen helps to maintain bone integrity. Adequate studies of estrogen therapy have not been done in the premenopausal woman with the triad. We do find that the athletes who have low estradiol levels are the ones who have osteoporosis with the triad. The addition of estrogen via oral contraceptive medication has been anecdotally reported to improve healing in women with previously nonhealing stress fractures (17). Currently, there are no long-term, large studies to verify that exogenous estrogen will benefit bone density in these young women. The American Academy of Pediatrics has endorsed the optimization of calcium intake and a decrease in exercise intensity to treat these patients (4).

There are many ways to build self-esteem with physical activity. We must educate coaches, competition judges, parents, and peers on the best way to encourage athletics. Comments about weight can have a lifelong impact on these impressionable athletes. Clearly, negative comments about body habitus can direct a young girl down a dangerous path. Support of the athlete, especially one who is demonstrating signs of underlying emotional distress, is necessary. Teaching these young women realistic, reasonable goals for dieting and weight control is highly desirable. Never encourage any kind of purging, or skipping meals, for weight control. Athletes need to build an identity less reliant on appearance for self-esteem and competence (18).

The health care provider must gain the patient's trust and be nonthreatening and nonjudgmental toward these goal-oriented and competitive young women. More research and clinical collaboration are needed to define how specific interventions may play a positive role in preventing the potential consequences of the female athlete triad.

REFERENCES

1. Yeager KK, Agostini R, Nattiv A, et al. The female athlete triad: disordered eating, amenorrhea, osteoporosis. Med Sci Sports Exerc 1993;25:775–777.

2. Otis CL, Drinkwater B, et al. ACSM position stand: the female athlete triad. Med Sci Sports Exerc 1997; 29:i–ix.

3. Mansfield MJ, Emans SJ. Anorexia nervosa, athletics, and amenorrhea. Pediatr Clin N Amer 1989; 36:533–549.

4. American Academy of Pediatrics, Committee on Sports Medicine. Amenorrhea in adolescent athletes. J Pediatr 1989.

5. Marshall L. Clinical evaluation of amenorrhea in active and athletic women. Clin Sports Med 1994; 13:2.

6. Haberland CA, et al. A physician survey of therapy for exercise-associated amenorrhea: a brief report. Clin J Sports Med 1995;5: 246–250.

7. Benson JE, Engelbert-Fenton KA, Eisenman PA. Nutritional aspects of amenorrhea in the female athlete triad. Int J Sports Nutr 1996;6:134–145.

8. Rencken MC, Chesnut CH, Drinkwater BL. Bone density at multiple skeletal sites in amenorrheic athletes. JAMA 1996;276: 238–240.

9. Micklesfield LK, Lambert EV, Fataar AB, et al. Bone mineral density in mature, premenopausal ultramarathon runners. Med Sci Sports Exerc 1995;27:688–696.

10. Heltand ML, Haarbo J, Christiansen C, et al. Running induces menstrual disturbances but bone mass is unaffected except in amenorrheic women. Am J Med 1993;95:53–60.

11. Dueck CA, Matt KS, Manore MM, et al. A diet and training intervention program for the treatment of athletic amenorrhea. Int J Sport Nutr 1996;6:24–40.

12. Warren MP, Fox RP, DeRogatis AJ, et al. Osteopenia in hypothalamic amenorrhea: a 3-year longitudinal study. J Clin Endocrinol Metab 1996;81:437–442.

13. Franztaher NT, Dhuper S, Warren MP, et al. Nutrition and the incidence of stress fractures in ballet dancers. Am J Clin Nutr 1990;51: 779–783.

14. Kadel NJ, Teitz CC, Kronman RA. Stress fractures in ballet dancers. Am J Sports Med 1992;20: 445–449.

15. Robinson TL, Snow-Harter C, Taaffee DR, et al. Gymnasts exhibit higher bone mass than runners despite similar prevalence of amenorrhea and oligomenorrhea. J Bone Min Res 1995;10: 26–35.

16. Heinonen A, Oja P, Kannus P, et al. Bone mineral density in female athletes representing sports with different loading characteristics of the skeleton. Bone 1995; 17:197–203.

17. Hergenroeder AC. Bone mineralization, hypothalamic amenorrhea, and sex steroid therapy in female adolescents and young adults. J Pediatr 1995;126: 683–689.

18. Nattiv A, Agostini R, Drinkwater B, Yeager K. The female athlete triad: the inter-relatedness of disordered eating, amenorrhea, and osteoporosis. Clin Sports Med 1994;13:2.

Chapter 18

Injury Prevention

Angela Smith

Several studies have suggested that up to 50% of sport injuries among children and adolescents can be prevented (1). These studies have pointed to flexibility, muscle strength, careful and appropriate training methods with gradual progression, and complete rehabilitation of previous injuries as being the most important factors in prevention of new injury. Few published studies address injury prevention among older athletes, although similar principles likely apply.

Both intrinsic and extrinsic factors relate to injuries. Some of an individual's attributes or deficits may be hereditary and fixed, but some intrinsic problems may be correctable. For example, an athlete can perform specific exercises to strengthen and stretch the quadriceps and hamstring muscles. Stronger, more flexible muscles are more likely than weak, inflexible muscles to absorb sudden forces that might tear the muscle or strain a knee ligament. As with intrinsic factors, many extrinsic factors may be under the athlete's control, but others—such as weather—are not.

INTRINSIC FACTORS

Intrinsic factors that might cause injury include weak bones and soft tissues, ligament laxity, muscle and joint inflexibility, and bone and joint architecture. Overuse injuries have particularly been studied in regard to intrinsic factors (2). Lysens et al profiled college physical education students to determine who might be most likely to develop overuse injuries. They found that the profile of the individual who was prone to developing overuse injuries had lax ligaments and weak and inflexible muscles (3).

Several studies have shown that one of the most frequent causes of injury is a previous injury to the same region (4,5). The most likely reason for this finding is incomplete rehabilitation or incomplete healing of the original injury. Inadequate strength, flexibility, and endurance are likely predictors of injury recurrence. Aerobic fitness may also play an important role in predicting injury or reinjury. A study of U.S. Army trainees found that lower performance on a 1-mile run test correlated with training period injuries in both men and women (6).

Strength

Bone

Stronger bones are less likely to break when exposed to either a single macrotraumatic force or repetitive microtraumatic impacts. Bone mineral content may be abnormally low from metabolic bone disease, poor nutrition, or lack of sufficient loading of the bone. Altered hormonal regulation of bone formation and remodeling occurs in postmenopausal or senile osteoporosis and in the female athlete triad of disordered eating, amenorrhea, and osteoporosis (7). Corticosteroids also disrupt the normal coupling of bone formation and resorption. Asthmatics and patients with inflammatory bowel disease who are treated chronically with corticosteroids may be predisposed to the development of stress fractures when they change activity level.

Bone strength is determined by genetic potential, nutrition (8), and weight-bearing and resistance exercise (9). The peak bone mineral content for most young women seems to be determined by the late teen years or early in the third decade (10). The bone mineral content for young men does not maximize until the middle or later years of the third

209

decade. Bone adapts to the stresses placed upon it. Limbs that undergo greater amounts of impact activities tend to have stronger bones (11,12) and stronger muscles. Resistance activities that strengthen the muscles but do not load the bones longitudinally do not appear to strengthen the long bones as much as impact loading activities. For example, young female swimmers have been found to have lower bone mineral content in their spine and lower extremities than do sedentary controls. Conversely, competitive gymnasts and figure skaters have much greater bone mineral content of the lower extremities than competitive swimmers and sedentary women (12,13).

When an athlete stops using a limb temporarily, during illness or injury for example, not only muscle strength but bone strength is lost. The bone loss may take more than a year to rebound to the previous level once activity is resumed. Periods of immobilization and non–weight-bearing should therefore be kept as brief as possible during an injury.

Muscle

Strong muscles aid in injury prevention in several ways. Strong muscles stabilize joints, protect adjacent structures by dissipating forces, and are less likely to sustain strain injury under tension (14).

Muscle configuration is genetically determined to a significant extent. Physical activity, nutrition, and hormones also influence the muscle size and contractile properties. Women and prepubertal boys can normally make significant muscle strength gains with exercise. Women and boys who use exogenous anabolic steroids may develop muscle size similar to that seen in adult men, who have much higher levels of testosterone than typical women and prepubertal boys.

Since there is such a wide range of normal muscular configurations, it is very useful to compare one side of the body against the other when examining for muscle atrophy. Of course, such comparison cannot be used in individuals with significant side-to-side hereditary differences, as found in individuals with hemihypertrophy or other congenital anomalies, for example.

Other Soft Tissues

The strength of other soft tissues, such as ligaments and tendons, also plays a role in injury risk. Although specific collagen deficiencies that predispose apparently normal people to ligament and tendon injuries have not been clearly defined, their presence seems likely. An athlete who has ruptured one Achilles tendon is more likely than other similar athletes to rupture the opposite one. The same is true for anterior cruciate ligaments, although here there may be additional anatomic and mechanical factors involved in ligament rupture.

Flexibility

The relationship of muscle and joint flexibility to injury remains controversial. However, several carefully performed studies have shown that certain specific flexibility deficits are or may be associated with specific injury patterns. Few scientific studies support that injury is caused by the flexibility deficit, but several studies indicate a relationship between the two (15–17). In addition, in clinical practice, resolution of the flexibility deficit—without any other treatment—rapidly leads to resolution of pain for some of these injuries.

Joints

The intrinsic flexibility or range of motion of a joint is determined by both the bony configurations and the surrounding soft tissues. During growth, the articulating bones can be altered to provide an athlete with an increased range of motion. This is seen in the notched neck of the dorsal aspect of the talus in ballet dancers and basketball players.

The soft-tissue constraints of a joint include the joint capsule, its ligaments, meniscal cartilages (in some joints, such as the knee), and the muscles that cross the joint. The viscoelastic behavior of connective tissue (its ability to elongate passively by processes known as creep, with stress relaxation) appears genetically determined. The total range of motion of the ligaments and joint capsules can likely be influenced by repetitive stretching. For example, dancers who work beginning in childhood to increase the range of motion of their hip joints to well beyond that of the average population are often able to maintain that extreme flexibility even into adulthood, as long as they continue to practice the range-of-motion exercises on a regular basis.

Muscles

The flexibility of the musculature, including the musculotendinous junctions and the tendons themselves, is also influenced by the genetic makeup of an individual's collagen. Those with Ehlers-Danlos or Marfan's syndromes, for example, have abnormal extensibility of their connective tissue. Within the normal range of flexibility is a spectrum, which ranges from athletes who must perform stretching exercises many times daily to maintain a level of flexibility that just barely provides minimum range of motion for their activities to athletes who stretch only briefly as part of warm-up, yet have maximum range of motion. Adult men tend to have less soft-tissue flexibility than children and adult women.

The muscle-tendon unit has viscoelastic properties that allow it to lengthen gradually and maintain the increased length for a period of time, probably several hours (18). It can also elongate relatively permanently by adding new sarcomeres. A muscle stretches farther if it is warm than it does if it is cold (19). It elongates best when a slow, passive stretch is applied to a relaxed, warm muscle. The greatest temporary gains in muscle lengthening are made within the first 20- to 30-second application of a stretching force. With each subsequent 20- to 30-second period, less additional elongation is attained. After the third or fourth stretching cycle within a short period of time, minimal additional gains are made (18,20).

Muscle flexibility can readily be improved with appropriate exercise by most people of all ages. The causes of flexibility deficits and the best flexibility exercises to make up the deficit vary with the person's age, however. In adolescence, there is a dynamically changing relationship between the bone length and the muscle length because of growth. As the bone grows longitudinally, the muscle lags behind slightly, only growing as it is stretched fully. Typically, muscles that cross two joints are not stretched through their full range of motion on a regular basis, so that they tend to be the ones with flexibility deficits among growing children and adolescents. Among adults, muscles that cross two joints are also the ones most at risk for strain injury. Adult tissues are also less readily extensible. More thorough warm-up and slower stretching are required to allow more time for muscle relaxation and elongation.

Several studies have noted relationships between flexibility deficits and overuse injuries, but none clearly demonstrates a causal relationship. Smith, Stroud, and McQueen found a relationship between quadriceps inflexibility and all types of anterior knee pain among adolescent elite figure skaters (15). The relationship between hamstring flexibility and patellofemoral pain was also found in young adults studied by Stroud and colleagues (21). Ireland and Micheli found a relationship between inflexibility of the gastrocnemius muscle and calcaneal apophysitis (16). Among patients with unilateral calcaneal apophysitis, they found that the injured side averaged approximately 6° of ankle dorsiflexion with the knee extended, but the uninjured side averaged approximately 10° of ankle dorsiflexion. Patients with bilateral apophysitis had dorsiflexion of approximately 6° bilaterally. Previous unpublished studies by Smith and Stroud have suggested that average ankle dorsiflexion, with the knee extended, among adolescent athletes is approximately 12°. These numbers also correspond to studies of adult hip fractures, where adults who had more than 10° of ankle dorsiflexion were less likely to sustain hip fracture than those who did not have adequate ankle dorsiflexion.

Age-Related Changes
Osteoporosis

The most frequent cause of osteoporosis is aging. As the bone mineral content decreases, less force is required to cause a fracture—either from repetitive microtrauma or from a single traumatic event. Postmenopausal women who start an exercise program to decrease their risk of osteoporotic fractures may sustain a stress fracture if the exercise program is not gradually progressive, so that the bones and surrounding soft tissues adapt. Once age-related bone mineral loss has occurred, little can be regained with exercise and medication. Although only a small percentage of bone mass can be regained, risk factors for falls that lead to fracture in the elderly can be reduced by aerobic and strength training programs (22).

Articular Cartilage

Changes in articular cartilage that occur with aging alter the molecular composition, compressibility, and water content. The specific changes in cartilage during midlife and later and the effects of exercise on articular cartilage of older people are not known. However, no study has linked repetitive pounding exercise, such as jogging, with articular cartilage degeneration (23). Conversely, evidence suggests that better subchondral bone quality, which may develop with repetitive loading of the bone with sufficient but not excessive force, may protect the overlying cartilage.

Soft Tissues

With aging, connective tissue elasticity decreases, leading to decreased flexibility of musculotendinous units as well as liga-
ments and joint capsules (24). Another non-preventable change is slowed nerve conduction velocity. However, although muscle mass and strength decline with age, the amount and quality of physical activity influence the rate of decline. Ligaments and their insertions also undergo change with decreased loading. As an individual ages and performs less strenuous and less frequent activity, ligament collagen synthesis decreases so that collagen synthesis and degradation are no longer balanced (25). In addition, resorption of bone at ligament insertion sites weakens the bone-ligament interface (25). Studies to date have not clarified whether the decreased strength and stiffness of ligaments with aging is related primarily to changes in activity level or changes in the ability of the ligament cells to respond to exercise with appropriate matrix macromolecule formation. However, one study of exercising dogs found no difference between the mechanical properties of the medial collateral ligaments or the flexor digitorum profundus tendons of dogs who ran on a treadmill 5 days a week, wearing a weighted vest, for up to 10 years, and caged controls (25).

Psychological State

Anxiety and tiredness have been associated with injury risk among gymnasts (26). Life stress and poor social support correlate with injury among collegiate athletes (27). A study of athletic young adults found injury more likely in those with stressful life events, a dominant personality, and exhaustion (28). Since many adults use exercise as a means to relieve stress, emotionally stressed exercisers may need to pay greater attention than usual to painful signals that may provide early warning of an injury.

EXTRINSIC FACTORS
Training Program
Gradual Increase

One of the most common causes of repetitive stress injury is rapid increase in one or more parameters of the exercise program, such as distance, speed, or intensity. A rule of thumb that is clinically successful is to increase either distance or speed in a given week and to increase by no more than 10% per week. Similarly, if distance or speed is increased, intensity should not be increased at the same time.

Changes in technique cause muscle groups to contract in new patterns and to different degrees. Bones and soft tissues require adaptation time, so new techniques should initially be practiced for only a limited number of repetitions. Similar limitations should be placed on the practicing of new skills in order to decrease the risk of injury.

Protective Equipment
Event Equipment

Some sports utilize specific equipment, such as (soccer) goals, (baseball) bases, or (gymnastics) parallel bars. To decrease risk of injury, goals and equipment such as bars and rings should be well secured to the ground. Recent innovations designed to further decrease injury risk include breakaway bases in baseball and softball, spring-loaded floors for gymnastics, and padded goalposts.

Player's Personal Equipment

Participants in many sport activities have protective equipment available. Helmets decrease the risk and severity of head injuries from bicycling, in-line skating, white-water kayaking, canoeing, football, hockey, and equestrian sports. Helmets should fit well, be comfortable, and be worn regularly to be effective. Helmet liners should be changed periodically to maintain effective shock absorption.

Other protective headgear includes eye masks or goggles, face masks, mouthguards, and ear protectors. All protective equipment must interfere as little as possible with the athlete's ability to see, hear, and maneuver. Protective pads or semi-rigid guards are standard for sports such as football, hockey, and soccer. The use of some types of protective equipment, such as football helmets, has actually led to other types of injuries, because athletes feel armored and can inflict damage to others or themselves by using the protective equipment offensively.

Since ankle and knee injuries occur so frequently, several studies have investigated protective braces. Knee braces are not recommended prophylactically, because there is not convincing evidence that bracing prevents either medial collateral or anterior cruciate ligament injuries in a normal knee. Available evidence suggests that some players are more aggressive when wearing protective knee braces and may even be more likely to sustain injury (29,30). Ankle-stabilizing braces have been shown to decrease the incidence of ankle sprains (31). Ankle taping is also effective in decreasing ankle injuries, but loses effectiveness after 20 minutes.

Athletic footwear should provide sport-specific stabilization and adequate shock absorption. The amount and location of cushioning is also specific to the sport. For example, shoes for distance running should have sufficient heel cushioning to decrease forces at heel strike. Conversely, excessive heel padding in a basketball or tennis shoe could interfere with lateral stability on side-to-side motion. Unfortunately, some athletes cannot use sole cushioning because of the functional or aesthetic requirements of the sport. Gymnasts must be able to feel the balance beam to perform this difficult discipline. On the other hand, cushioned shoes for gymnasts that could dissipate landing forces on the other apparatus are apparently rejected for only aesthetic reasons. Athletes should be encouraged to use the proper shoe for each type of training. For example, a soccer player does not need to perform distance running in the spiked shoes used for play but can use cushioned running shoes with a firm heel counter for the distance exercise.

Environment
Playing Surface

Playing surfaces should be dry (assuming that is the appropriate state for the sport), without holes, rocks, or ruts. Swimming and diving venues should be clear of unseen objects, and areas for diving must be of appropriate depth.

Rules Safety

Most sports have some rules that relate to safer play. Fouls and technical deductions encourage players to participate in a safe manner. Sports-governing bodies may disallow certain moves, such as back flips and the "head banger" lift in figure skating, because of safety considerations. Little League rules now restrict the number of innings a child can pitch to reduce the incidence of deforming elbow and shoulder injuries (1).

Of course, some sports consist of multiple intentional collisions. In these sports, the rules disallow certain types of contact that are thought to be particularly likely to cause severe injury. For example, football rules against spear tackling have decreased the incidence of severe cervical spine injury and paralysis (32).

Coaching and Supervision

Coaches, officials, and any supervisory assistants in an athletic activity play an extremely important role in injury prevention. They must know and enforce the rules of the game (1). They should understand and use safe training principles. In addition, they must recognize the need for water and nourishment breaks to fuel the mind to avoid injury-prone situations and fuel the muscles for protective maneuvers.

PREPARTICIPATION EVALUATION AND RETURN TO ACTIVITY AFTER INJURY
Preparticipation Evaluation

Examination of the musculoskeletal system, when focusing on injury prevention, should include several particular aspects. First, observation of the extremities includes right-to-left comparison of symmetry of muscle bulk and limb length. Symmetry of muscles (medial versus lateral and anterior versus posterior) can also be checked. The range of motion of each major joint should be tested to ensure that normal range of motion is present and is equal to the opposite side. Decreased pronation or supination of a forearm, for example, may indicate a previously unrecognized synostosis of the radius and ulna, which could predispose to injuries of the remainder of the kinetic chain of that upper extremity. Similarly, full extension of one knee and hyperextension of the opposite knee could indicate a mechanical block in the knee that does not hyperextend.

Joint laxity can be checked. Individuals who have more lax joints than average may be predisposed to injuries, particularly once their muscles fatigue and cannot protect the loose joints. However, there is controversy over this area. Some have suggested that joints with looser ligaments might be able to deform to a greater extent before the ligaments are actually injured, so that they are less likely to suffer injury, rather than more likely.

The flexibility of the major muscle groups should also be examined. Lower extremity muscle flexibility should be examined in any athlete, with the exception of those few athletes who do not use their lower extremities at all. Upper extremity flexibility, particularly of the muscles of the shoulder girdle, is mainly important for those who do weight-bearing on their upper extremities (wrestlers and gymnasts) or who are engaged in throwing (or similar) sports, such as pitching and playing tennis.

Finally, muscle strength of the left and right sides should be compared when appropriate. Recognize that many athletes have dominance of one side because of the particular sport, and the muscles on that side should be expected to be stronger and of greater size. Knowledge of the specific muscle groups needed for a particular activity is helpful when examining for muscle deficit.

If there is a history of any type of injury, a complete examination of the injured area and associated areas should be performed. It is especially important to ascertain full return to normal strength and endurance of the muscles, as well as proprioceptive qualities.

Although prevention of musculoskeletal injuries is the focus of this chapter, the preparticipation examination includes a directed history and physical examination of all the systems. Athletes who are missing a paired organ, such as a kidney or testicle, have potentially more serious consequences if the remaining organ is injured, so greater protection may be required. Athletes with poorly controlled medical conditions, such as severe asthma or diabetes mellitus, may need to consider special precautions, such as more frequent breaks from activity or snacks to maintain mental clarity and to provide the working muscles with sufficient oxygen and energy to protect the athlete. An athlete with a seizure disorder should not swim unsupervised or in murky water (33).

The preparticipation examination also provides an excellent opportunity for counseling regarding sports nutrition, proper warm-up, strength training, stretching, and excessive risk-taking.

At Time of Injury Treatment

Another opportunity for interval evaluation and counseling is immediately before allowing return to unrestricted activity. If the athlete has not already achieved full range of motion, strength, flexibility, muscle endurance, and aerobic capacity, the remainder of the therapeutic exercise program should be covered. Equally important is the plan for a gradual return to full activity so that early reinjury is avoided. Athletes should understand that the longer they have been away from a particular activity, the longer is the period required for tissues and the cardiovascular system to adapt to the demands of the activity.

The return-to-participation visit is another opportunity for counseling. Especially important areas to cover include risk-taking, proper warm-up, and use of any recommended protective equipment. This may be one of the most receptive moments for the athlete. Reminding a participant that the most frequent cause of athletic musculoskeletal injury is a previous injury to the same region may provide additional motivation for completing the recommended exercise program and resuming activity gradually.

Counseling those who would like to participate in sport and fitness exercise occurs regularly in clinical offices. Participants can significantly reduce their risk of injury from the activities by appropriate preparation. If injury does occur, the patient may be particularly interested in learning ways to prevent future recurrent or other injuries, and counseling on injury prevention methods may be especially productive.

REFERENCES

1. Smith AD, Andrish JT, Micheli LJ. The prevention of sport injuries of children and adolescents. Med Sci Sports Exerc 1993;25(suppl): 1–7.

2. Krivickas LS. Anatomical factors associated with overuse sports injuries. Sports Med 1997;24: 132–146.

3. Lysens RJ, Ostyn MS, Auweele YV, et al. The accident-prone and overuse-prone profiles of the young athlete. Am J Sports Med 1989; 17:612–619.

4. Caine D, Cochrane B, Caine C, Zemper E. An epidemiologic investigation of injuries affecting young competitive female gymnasts. Am J Sports Med 1989;17:811–820.

5. Garrick JG, Gillien DM, Whiteside P. The epidemiology of aerobic dance injuries. Am J Sports Med 1986;14:67–72.

6. Jones BH, Bovee MW, Harris JM, et al. Intrinsic risk factors for exercise-related injuries among male and female Army trainees. Am J Sports Med 1993;21:705–710.

7. Nattiv A, Agostini R, Drinkwater B, Yeager KK. The female athlete triad: the inter-relatedness of disordered eating, amenorrhea, and osteoporosis. Clin Sports Med 1994;13:405–418.

8. Frusztajer NT, Dhuper S, Warren MP, et al. Nutrition and the incidence of stress fractures in ballet dancers. Am J Clin Nutr 1990;51: 779–783.

9. Suominen H. Bone mineral density and long term exercise: an overview of cross-sectional athlete studies. Sports Med 1993;16: 316–330.

10. Teegarden D, Proulx WR, Martin BR, et al. Peak bone mass in young women. J Bone Miner Res 1995;10:711–715.

11. Robinson TL, Snow-Harter C, Taaffe DR, et al. Gymnasts exhibit higher bone mass than runners despite similar prevalence of amenorrhea and oligomenorrhea. J Bone Miner Res 1995;10:26–35.

12. Slemenda CW, Johnston CC. High intensity activities in young women: site specific bone mass effects among female figure skaters. Bone Miner 1993;20: 125–132.

13. Cassell C, Benedict M, Specker B. Bone mineral density in elite 7- to 9-yr-old female gymnasts and swimmers. Med Sci Sports Exerc 1996;28:1243–1246.

14. Taylor DC, Dalton JD, Seaber AV, Garrett WE. Experimental muscle strain injury: early functional and structural deficits and the increased risk for reinjury. Am J Sports Med 1993;21:190–194.

15. Smith AD, Stroud L, McQueen C. Flexibility and anterior knee pain in adolescent elite figure skaters. J Pediatr Orthop 1991;11:77–82.

16. Micheli LJ, Ireland ML. Prevention and management of calcaneal apophysitis in children: an overuse

syndrome. J Pediatr Orthop 1987; 7:34–38.

17. Smith AD. Reduction of injuries among elite figure skaters: a 4-year longitudinal study. Med Sci Sports Exerc 1991;23(suppl):151.

18. Hughes HG, Schwellnus MP. The effect of static stretch duration and frequency on hamstring musculotendinous flexibility. Med Sci Sports Exerc 1998;30(suppl): S25.

19. Strickler T, Malone T, Garrett WE. The effects of passive warming on muscle injury. Am J Sports Med 1990;18:141–145.

20. Taylor CC, Seaber AB, Garrett WE Jr. Response of muscle-tendon units to cyclic repetitive stretching. Trans Orthop Res Soc 1985;10:84.

21. Stroud L, Smith AD, Kruse RW. The relationship between increased femoral anteversion in childhood and patellofemoral pain in adult-hood. Orthop Trans 1989;13:554.

22. Hurley BF, Hagberg JM. Optimizing health in older persons: aerobic or strength training? Exerc Sports Sci Rev 1998;26:61–90.

23. Gordon SL, Premen AJ. Structure and function of cartilage: adult and age-related changes. In: Gordon SL, Gonzalez-Mestre X, Garrett WE, eds. Sports and exercise in midlife. Rosemont, IL: American Academy of Orthopedic Surgeons, 1993:155–176.

24. Vuori I. Environmental risk factors of exercise and sport injuries. In: Gordon SL, Gonzalez-Mestre X, Garrett WE, eds. Sports and exercise in midlife. Rosemont, IL: American Academy of Orthopedic Surgeons, 1993:43–60.

25. Buckwalter JA, Woo SL-Y. The response of ligaments to exercise. In: Gordon SL, Gonzalez-Mestre X, Garrett WE, eds. Sports and exercise in midlife. Rosemont, IL: American Academy of Orthopedic Surgeons, 1993:133–154.

26. Kolt GS, Kirkby RJ. Injury, anxiety, and mood in competitive gymnasts. Percept Mot Skills 1994; 78:955–962.

27. Petrie TA. Psychosocial antecedents of athletic injury: the effects of life stress and social support on female collegiate gymnasts. Behav Med 1992;18: 127–138.

28. Mechelen WV, Twisk J, Molendijk A, et al. Subject-related risk factors for sports injuries: a 1-yr prospective study in young adults. Med Sci Sports Exerc 1996;28: 1171–1179.

29. Grace TG, Skipper BJ, Newberry JC, et al. Prophylactic knee braces and injury to the lower extremity. J Bone Joint Surg 1988;70:422–427.

30. Teitz CC, Hermanson BK, Kronmal RA, Diehr PH. Evaluation of the use of braces to prevent injury to the knee in collegiate football players. J Bone Joint Surg 1987; 69:2–9.

31. Sitler M, Ryan J, Wheeler B, et al. The efficacy of a semirigid ankle stabilizer to reduce acute ankle injuries in basketball: a randomized clinical study at West Point. Am J Sports Med 1994;22:454–461.

32. Torg JS, Vegso JJ, Sennet B. The national football head and neck injury registry, 14-year report on cervical quadriplegia, 1970–1984. JAMA 1984;254: 3439–3443.

33. Zupanc ML. Therapeutic drug use and epilepsy in sports. In: DeLee JC, Drez D, eds. Orthopaedic sports medicine: principles and practice. Philadelphia: W.B. Saunders, 1994:341–345.

Chapter 19

Injury Rehabilitation Principles

Lisa S. Krivickas
Daniel J. Sheehan

A GENERAL APPROACH TO INJURY REHABILITATION

Rehabilitation is the process of restoring the greatest possible function and health to the athlete. The ideal result of the rehabilitation process is a return to full sports participation with the physical capacity to meet one's full athletic potential and avoid future injury. A key concept in the rehabilitation of musculoskeletal injuries is SAID, or "specific adaptation to imposed demands." The body's tissues adapt to increased demands placed upon them by various athletic activities, and a failure to adapt to increased demands rapidly enough can result in an overuse injury. The rehabilitation process should ensure that the injured tissue adapts adequately to the demands placed on it.

The rehabilitation of an injured athlete is a team effort with team members including the athlete (and his or her parents, if a child), physicians, physical therapists, occupational therapists, athletic trainers, coaches, and, in some cases, a sports psychologist. The implementation of an injury rehabilitation program begins with goal setting. The following goals should be part of any program, independent of the specific nature of the injury:

1. Eliminate pain.
2. Achieve tissue healing with restoration of normal tissue properties.
3. Reduce deleterious effects of immobilization.
4. Restore full strength to the injured tissue.
5. Restore a range of motion (ROM) comparable to that of the uninjured limb.
6. Restore strength comparable to that of the uninjured limb.
7. Restore muscle endurance.
8. Restore normal proprioception.
9. Correct biomechanical, technique, flexibility, or strength deficits that may have contributed to the injury.
10. Maintain cardiovascular fitness and sports-specific skills during the rehabilitation period.

Other goals may be more specific and are determined based on the particular injury, the performance level of the athlete, and the athlete's age and gender.

Saal has described an 8-phase rehabilitation process designed to restore function to the injured athlete (1). These phases are outlined in Table 19-1. Each phase will be discussed in detail throughout the course of this chapter. The rehabilitation process should follow an orderly progression, with athletes progressing to the next stage only after fulfilling specific criteria in the preceding stage. In addition, the program must be individualized; cookbook algorithms do not produce optimal results. The time at which each phase is initiated and the amount of time required to complete the phase depends on the type of tissue injured, the severity of the injury, and whether or not the injury requires surgical management. The majority of sports musculoskeletal injuries can be managed nonoperatively, but many fractures, meniscal tears, grade 3 ligament sprains, and complete tendon tears require surgical intervention. If surgery is performed, the timing of the rehabilitation phases depends on the integrity of the surgical repair (e.g., in cases of ligament reconstruction,

215

Table 19-1 Eight Phases of the Rehabilitation Process
Phase I: Control inflammation. Phase II: Control pain. Phase III: Restore joint range of motion and soft tissue-extensibility. Phase IV: Improve muscular strength. Phase V: Improve muscular endurance. Phase VI: Develop specific sport-related biomechanical skill patterns (coordination training). Phase VII: Improve general cardiovascular endurance. Phase VIII: Establish maintenance programs.

Table 19-2 Deleterious Effects of Immobilization on Tissue	
Bone	Decreased bone formation Normal bone resorption Osteoporosis or osteopenia Decreased cortical bone mass Decreased ability to withstand tensile and compressive loads Calcium mobilization
Cartilage	Decreased water content Decreased glycosaminoglycan content Decreased resistance to compressive loads Decreased cartilage thickness
Tendon and Ligament	Decreased collagen synthesis Impaired collagen matrix organization Decreased tensile strength Atrophy
Muscle	Decreased muscle mass Type I fiber atrophy Fiber type conversion (I to IIa, IIa to IIb) Decreased oxidative enzyme levels (SDH, CPK) Decreased fuel storage (creatine, glycogen) Decreased intracellular water Increased extracellular water

meniscal repair, internal fracture fixation) and the rate of postoperative tissue healing.

Injury to Bone

The rehabilitation of injuries to bone is influenced by the time required for fracture healing, the degree of immobilization required for adequate healing, and weight-bearing restrictions. Injuries to bone can be broadly divided into two categories: 1) traumatic fractures and 2) stress fractures or reactions. Traumatic fractures usually require immobilization, often with a cast or internal or external fixation, and at least 4 to 6 weeks of non–weight-bearing. During this healing phase, rehabilitation must focus on maintaining flexibility and strength of the uninvolved joints and limbs as well as maintaining cardiovascular fitness. Once mobilization of the injured limb and weight-bearing are allowed, load must be gradually increased to avoid overloading the bone, which has been weakened by immobilization. After 6 weeks of non–weight-bearing, lower extremity cortical bone mass declines by approximately 15% (2).

Stress injuries to bone generally do not require immobilization and can be treated with relative rest rather than non–weight-bearing. Pain is a useful guide in determining how much activity may be tolerated. If pain is present with weight-bearing, the activity level should be reduced. Depending on the location and severity of the stress reaction or fracture, the period of relative rest required for tissue healing may range from a few weeks to several months. A few stress fractures known to have prolonged clinical courses or grave consequences if they progress to complete fracture, require a period of non–weight-bearing, nonloading, or immobilization similar to that for traumatic fractures; these difficult stress fractures include femoral neck stress fractures, stress fractures of the anterior cortex of the midshaft of the tibia, the Jones fracture (base of the fifth metatarsal), navicular stress fractures, and olecranon stress fractures (3–5).

Cartilage Injury

Sports injuries affecting cartilage include osteochondral injuries, osteochondritis dissecans, and meniscal injuries. As is true for bone and most other tissues in the musculoskeletal system, loading and motion are important to maintain the optimal mechanical properties and chemical composition of cartilage. Table 19-2 summarizes the deleterious effects of

immobilization on various tissues, including cartilage. The content of water and glycosaminoglycan in articular cartilage decreases with immobilization (6), diminishing the cartilage's ability to withstand compressive loads. In contrast, a recent study suggested that immobilization actually increases meniscal water content but decreases proteoglycan content, which has an overall adverse effect on the viscoelastic compressive properties of the meniscus (7).

Cartilage is relatively avascular, with poor healing and regeneration properties. Thus, allowing time for tissue healing is not an important consideration in the rehabilitation of all cartilage injuries. Often, the focus of rehabilitation is pain relief, followed by controlled mobilization. Exceptions to this rule are osteochondral lesions, in which the goal is healing of the underlying bone, and meniscal tears treated with surgical repair. Traditionally, patients undergoing meniscal repair have been restricted from full ROM and weight-bearing for at least 4 to 6 weeks after surgery. However, recent studies suggest that allowing unrestricted ROM and weight-bearing, as tolerated, immediately postoperatively does not have long-term adverse impact on healing and allows a more rapid return to athletic activity (8).

Ligament Injury

Ligamentous injuries occur both as a result of microfailure from repetitive loading within the physiologic range and as a result of acute trauma, with loads exceeding those in the physiologic range. In grade 1 sprains, only a few of the collagen fibers are disrupted; in grade 2 injuries, enough collagen fibers are disrupted to produce joint laxity; in grade 3 sprains, total rupture of the ligament occurs. Healing of the ligament following grade 3 sprains does not occur without surgical repair. However, ligamentous healing is not always necessary for return of function. Scar tissue may develop and effectively substitute for ligament function in the case of isolated medial collateral ligament tears and rupture of certain ankle ligaments.

Ligament remodels in response to the loads placed on it, and a prolonged period of time is necessary for ligaments to regain full tensile strength after a period of immobilization or surgery. Following an 8-week period of immobilization, 12 months is required for ligaments to regain their baseline strength and stiffness (9). However, if non–weight-bearing or protected motion is allowed, ligament mechanical properties are better maintained (10). After surgical repair of a ligament, controlled loading promotes healing by improving the matrix organization, accelerating collagen synthesis, and increasing graft weight (11). Most surgeons now advocate accelerated rehabilitation programs, which allow ROM exercises and immediate weight-bearing after ligament repair or reconstruction (12). In contrast to older philosophies of rehabilitation, the pace of the rehabilitation program does not need to be based on the time required for graft maturation. Graft strength is actually greatest at the time of reconstruction; the graft progressively weakens postoperatively as it undergoes avascular necrosis and then strengthens as new collagen forms and the graft becomes ligamentized. This is a very slow process, requiring more than a year for the graft to obtain its maximal strength. If complete ligament ruptures are not repaired surgically, the goal of the rehabilitation program is to strengthen muscles that stabilize the joint and functionally substitute for the torn ligament. Again, ROM exercises and weight-bearing may begin as soon as tolerated without increasing inflammation.

Muscle and Tendon Injury

Muscle and tendon injuries are the most common sports injuries. Injuries to muscle include contusions and strains. Strains most frequently occur at the musculotendinous junction in muscles crossing two joints (13,14). More severe strains also cause disruption of muscle fibers within the muscle belly (15). Tendon injuries include the degenerative tendinoses (without a significant inflammatory component) and tendonitis, which is accompanied by inflammation and is usually caused by overuse. The healing of an acute tendon injury occurs in 3 stages: an inflammatory stage (first 6 days), a fibroblastic or proliferative stage (days 5 to 21), and a remodeling and maturation stage (begins about day 20) (16). The rehabilitation of muscle and tendon injuries does not require immobilization unless surgical repair is performed. As with other tissues, immobilization has several deleterious effects on muscle, including loss of muscle mass and atrophy of type 1 fibers. Loss of muscle mass occurs exponentially, with 50% of the overall decrease in mass occurring during the first 4 to 6 days of immobilization. Interestingly, this process can be delayed by immobilizing a muscle in a lengthened position (17). Applying a tensile force to the tendon during the fibroblastic stage facilitates optimal organization of newly synthesized collagen fibrils. Active ROM and strengthening begin as soon as pain and inflammation are under control. With muscle contusions and tears, minimizing

hemorrhage is critical to prevent the development of myositis ossificans.

CONTROLLING PAIN AND INFLAMMATION

Obtaining rapid control of inflammation, limiting joint effusion and edema, and minimizing hemorrhage after an acute injury decrease pain and accelerate the rehabilitation process. Applying the components of rest, ice, compression, and elevation (RICE) is the most effective means of controlling pain and inflammation. Rest involves a short period of non–weight-bearing or nonloading for the injured extremity. It may also include using splints or braces to protect a damaged structure from further stress, which might exacerbate the inflammatory process. Protective braces of this type include ankle braces, which prevent inversion after a lateral sprain, and knee braces, which prevent the application of valgus stress after a medial collateral ligament sprain. With some muscle contusions, especially those to the quadriceps, it is advisable to rest the muscle in an elongated position. Elevating the injured part above the level of the heart, when feasible, reduces blood flow and can thus assist with limiting effusion, edema, and hemorrhage. Compression of the limb with an elastic sleeve or bandage performs a similar and complementary function. Ice decreases tissue metabolism and blood flow and also has an analgesic effect. Ice should be applied for 10- to 15-minute treatment periods and then removed for an equal period of time before being reapplied. Caution must be exercised in using cryotherapy near superficial nerves; injury to the common peroneal nerve at the fibular head has been reported as a complication of prolonged ice application (18). Contrast baths, which consist of alternating heat with cold therapy, are especially helpful for decreasing edema and inflammation caused by ankle and foot injuries. Galvanic electrical stimulation may also help control inflammation and edema. This modality is discussed, along with other forms of electrical stimulation, in the next section of this chapter. Once the acute inflammation is controlled, heating modalities may also be used for pain relief.

Nonsteroidal anti-inflammatory drugs (NSAIDs) reduce both inflammation and pain. Inflammation is suppressed by inhibiting the synthesis and release of prostaglandins, which act as mediators of inflammation. However, there is some controversy surrounding NSAID use for acute injuries because some degree of inflammation may be beneficial in promoting eventual tissue healing. Animal studies have shown that ibuprofen and indomethacin slow bone healing (19,20). However, indomethacin appears to augment tensile strength of ligaments and tendons when used after injury (21–23). NSAIDs alter tendon fibroblast (24) and chondrocyte synthetic function in vitro, but no deleterious clinical effect has been demonstrated. After muscle strain injuries, NSAIDs did not adversely influence the recovery of contractile and tensile strength in one study (25), but in another study, they delayed the regenerative response in injured muscle (26). The use of NSAIDs for treatment of soft-tissue injuries is generally safe and often provides significant pain relief. In fact, the analgesic effect may be much more important than the anti-inflammatory effect; the inflammatory response may continue even in the presence of NSAIDs, because nonprostaglandin mediators of inflammation, such as histamine, serotonin, and oxygen radicals, are not inhibited (27). In addition, some prostaglandins actually have anti-inflammatory effects (28). Overall, recovery time from a variety of minor soft-tissue injuries is decreased by NSAID use (29).

Occasionally either oral or injected corticosteroids are used to control acute pain and inflammation. These authors do not advocate the use of oral corticosteroids for management of acute musculoskeletal injuries; the potential side effects appear to outweigh any benefit. One exception to this rule is the management of acute cervical or lumbar radiculopathies in which a 1-week rapidly tapering course of prednisone may be helpful. Corticosteroid injections do not have a role in the management of acute sports injuries. If given before participation in sports, they may mask pain and predispose the athlete to further injury. Corticosteroids should never be injected into tendons or ligaments as they produce structural weakening and predispose to rupture; in addition, they inhibit the synthetic function of tendon cells, slowing the healing process (30). Repeated joint injections impair protein synthesis and cause deterioration of articular cartilage (31).

USE OF MODALITIES

Cold

Cryotherapy is used in the management and rehabilitation of acute soft-tissue injuries because of its ability to decrease inflammation, edema, and pain (32,33). The physiologic effects of cold application are summarized in Table 19-3. Inflammation is delayed by sympathetic-mediated vasoconstriction, which decreases blood flow. The work of Lehmann and DeLateur has shown that, following 10 minutes of ice application to the thigh, muscle is cooled a maximum of 2°C in a person with 1 cm of subcutaneous fat and not at all in a person with 2 cm of subcutaneous fat; in the thinner person, the cooling penetrates to a depth of 2 cm within the muscle (34). Whether or not cold can actually reduce edema remains controversial; several animal studies have not found any reduction in edema with cryotherapy (35,36). The mechanism by which cold produces analgesia is also not clearly understood; it may increase the pain threshold via the gate theory of Melzack and Wall (37,38) or increase endogenous production of endorphins (39). Some authors have suggested that cold produces analgesia by slowing sensory nerve conduction velocity; however, this reasoning is faulty because nerve conduction velocity slowing without conduction block does not produce any clinical symptoms. Contraindications to cryotherapy include Raynaud's phenomena, cryoglobulinemia, cold-induced urticaria, and paroxysmal cold hemoglobinemia, all of which are rare in athletes.

Modes of cold application include ice packs, ice cups (for massage), ice slurries (bucket of water and ice in which a foot and ankle may be immersed), chemical ice packs, gel packs, and electrical compression cooling systems. Ice is as good as or superior to all other cooling modalities. Chemical and gel packs are dangerous because they can burn the skin if punctured. Ice massage can usually be tolerated for 5 to 10 minutes, and the ice should not be left stationary over the skin. Ice and cold packs may be applied for up to 20 minutes at a time. During the first 48 to 72 hours following an acute injury, the injured area should be iced frequently (every 2 hours is ideal, while the injured person is awake). Tissue warms up more slowly than it cools, and time must be allowed for warming between icing sessions. Once an exercise program and functional activities are begun, ice application after therapy sessions or workouts helps to control pain and swelling.

Heat

Muscle and joint temperature affect flexibility, and heating modalities can be used to enhance the increase in ROM achieved by stretching. Heating increases the extensibility of collagen, a major component of tendon and joint capsules (40,41). The increased ROM achieved with heating is probably a result of increased elongation of the tendon rather than a further elongation of the muscle. Heat also has a beneficial effect on the major spinal reflexes, decreasing the sensitivity of the muscle spindle reflex and increasing the firing rate of the Golgi tendon organ in response to stretch (42,43); this is the physiologic basis of muscle spasm relaxation with heat application. Animal studies have shown that warming-up muscle and tendon by preconditioning it with electrically stimulated isometric contractions increases extensibility; although muscle temperature was not directly measured in these experiments, it was hypothesized that the warm-up elevated temperature to produce increased collagen extensibility (44).

The beneficial effects of heat are summarized in Table 19-4. In addition to enhancing flexibility, heat can assist with

Table 19-3 Physiologic Effects of Cryotherapy
Decreases muscle spindle activity
Decreases muscle spasm
Decreases pain
Reduces edema
Vasoconstriction
Decreases blood flow
Decreases metabolic rate
Reduces deposition of inflammatory mediators
Decreases collagen extensibility
Increases joint stiffness

Table 19-4 Physiologic Effects of Heat
Decreases muscle spindle sensitivity
Increases Golgi tendon organ firing rate
Decreases muscle spasm
Decreases pain
Acute edema exacerbation
Chronic edema resolution
Vasodilation
Increases blood flow
Increases lymphatic and venous drainage
Increases metabolic rate
Enhances removal of metabolic waste products
Increases capillary permeability
Increases collagen extensibility

the resolution of chronic edema and decrease pain. The mechanism by which heat relieves pain is not clear but may involve the gate theory (37). Absolute contraindications to the use of heating modalities include acute inflammation or bleeding, lack of normal cutaneous sensation, infection, malignancy, and impaired circulation. In the past, concerns were raised about using ultrasound over open epiphyses and metal implants; application is now believed to be safe in both of these situations (45–48), but ultrasound should not be used over bone cement (methyl methacrylate) (39). Likewise, the use of ultrasound over a fluid-filled space, such as over the spinal cord following laminectomy, is contraindicated.

In the rehabilitation of sports injuries, heating modalities usually may be applied 48 hours after injury. The most common modes of heat application are hot packs, whirlpools, contrast baths, and ultrasound. Heat is most useful when applied at the beginning of a therapy session before stretching soft tissues (40). Hot and cold are similar in that both decrease pain and muscle spasm; however, their effects on tissue metabolism, blood flow, joint stiffness, and acute edema are opposite. After the first 48 hours, whether to use hot or cold depends to some extent on athlete preference. In addition to their direct effects on soft tissue, both types of therapy may have positive emotional, motivational, or placebo effects; the interaction with a therapist or trainer administering the treatment may play an important role in these indirect benefits (49).

Moist heat is applied in the physical therapy setting by using hydrocollator packs made of a silica gel with a cotton covering. The packs are stored in a tank of water heated to 70°C to 80°C. To maintain maximum heating, the packs should be replaced with hot ones every 8 to 10 minutes. Maximum heating occurs at the surface of the skin (6°C temperature increase) with an increase in subcutaneous tissue temperature of only 1°C at a depth of 1 to 2 cm; thus, no true muscle heating occurs (50). In the home setting, heating pads specifically designed for use with wet towels (so as not to create an electrical safety hazard) may be used to apply moist heat.

Whirlpool treatment is useful for facilitating ROM exercise after injury to the ankle or knee joint; upper extremity treatments are somewhat more cumbersome. A treatment session usually lasts 15 to 20 minutes and should be followed by stretching. To avoid increasing core body temperature, the lower extremity should not be immersed in water warmer than 40.5°C or the upper extremity in water hotter than 43°C. Contrast baths increase blood flow to the injured extremity and assist with mobilization of chronic edema. The usual protocol consists of soaking for 4 to 5 minutes in hot water or a whirlpool (40.5°C to 43°C) followed by 1 to 2 minutes in cold (10°C to 15°C) water. This sequence is repeated four or five times, ending with cold immersion. Contrast baths are useful after workout sessions for those returning to play after ankle sprains.

Ultrasound and Phonophoresis

Ultrasound is the most effective modality for deep tissue heating. Short-wave and microwave diathermy were used for deep heating in the past but are now primarily of historical interest. Ultrasound is a form of conversion heating in which acoustic energy is converted to heat. Ultrasound generates heat at interfaces where tissue density changes. The greatest temperature increase occurs at the bone and soft-tissue interface, i.e., within the joint itself (51). In experiments using the hip joint of live pigs, standard ultrasound treatment increased temperature at the surface of the bone 3.5°C, with the maximal temperature increase of 4.5°C occurring within the cortical bone (52). Thus, ultrasound is particularly effective for heating deep structures, such as tendons and the joint capsule. Because the density change between subcutaneous fat and muscle is slight, these tissues are not heated significantly. Clinically, ultrasound is useful in the treatment of chronic tendonosis and bursitis, because it decreases pain, improves tissue extensibility and response to stretching, and may assist with mobilization of chronic edema. There is not convincing evidence to support that ultrasound enhances resorption of calcium deposits in calcific tendonosis. Ultrasound also preferentially heats fibrous scar tissue within muscle and may assist with lysis of adhesions. Ultrasound should not be used over areas of myositis ossificans, because it might accelerate calcification by increasing the local metabolic rate. Recent studies have demonstrated that low-intensity pulsed ultrasound treatments accelerate fracture healing (53,54).

Ultrasound treatments must be administered by a therapist familiar with the use of the equipment. The therapist must select the appropriate frequency and intensity settings based on the athlete's body habitus and the joint being treated. Depth of penetration is inversely related to frequency. A conductive gel applied to the skin or immersion of the limb in water prevents sound wave dissipation at the skin-air interface. The ultrasound transducer head should be moved continually in slow circular strokes to prevent overheating of tissue at any one location. Treatments generally last 5 to 10 minutes. Multiple areas (i.e., anterior, posterior, and lateral aspects of the joint) must be treated to adequately heat large joints, such as the shoulder and hip. The athlete should not experience discomfort during the treatment; pain indicates that the periosteum is being overheated, and intensity should be reduced.

Ultrasound has nonthermal effects that are poorly understood from a scientific standpoint. These nonthermal effects are known as cavitation, acoustic streaming, and standing wave production. They are most prominent when high frequencies, which produce minimal heating, are used. Cavitation refers to a vibrational effect of the ultrasound waves, which causes gas bubbles within tissue to expand and then burst, possibly causing tissue damage (55). Acoustic streaming refers to movement of particulate matter away from the ultrasound wave front and is thought to be the driving force behind phonophoresis, but it too may produce cellular damage (56). Standing waves are produced by the superimposition of resonant frequencies of sound waves and may cause abnormalities in blood flow (56). Neither cavitation nor standing wave formation occurs when ultrasound is used at standard clinical intensities (1.0 to 2.5 W/cm^2) with a stroking movement of the applicator. A newer ultrasound technique, which requires further research, is pulsed ultrasound delivered at a frequency designed to produce primarily nonthermal effects. This technique may be found to assist with decreasing inflammation in acute traumatic injuries in which traditional ultrasound treatment is initially contraindicated (57).

Phonophoresis is a technique that uses the nonthermal properties of ultrasound, primarily acoustic streaming, to purportedly drive medication into tissue. It is most commonly used to administer hydrocortisone. However, there is not enough thorough literature documenting the depth of tissue penetration and drug concentration within the tissues being treated. Several studies have failed to show significant intra-articular drug concentration after treatment (58–60). Injection is a much more reliable method of insuring delivery of a specific quantity of drug into a target tissue.

Electrical Stimulation

Three forms of electrical stimulation are used in the management and rehabilitation of sports injuries. Transcutaneous electrical nerve stimulation (TENS) may be used to decrease both acute and chronic pain associated with an injury. High-voltage electrical stimulation may be used to reduce edema in the acute injury phase, to decrease muscle atrophy during postoperative immobilization, and possibly to enhance muscle strengthening. Iontophoresis is a form of electrical therapy, analogous to phonophoresis, which is advocated by some clinicians for delivery of drug into soft tissues.

TENS application is an art rather than a science. Literature on both the mechanism of action and the physiologic effects of TENS is contradictory. The gate theory (37) is frequently used to explain the mechanism by which TENS produces analgesia, but other investigators have suggested that TENS provides generalized analgesia by increasing central nervous system (CNS) endorphin levels (61,62). Conventional TENS consists of electrical stimulation at 60 to 100 Hz at an intensity ranging from one to three times the sensory threshold and probably works via the gate theory. Low-frequency, or "acupuncture-like," TENS is performed at 0.5 to 10.0 Hz and three to five times the sensory threshold for 20 to 30 minutes; it is less comfortable than conventional TENS, which generally can be tolerated for hours. Low-frequency TENS is more likely to stimulate endorphin release. TENS units for home use cost more than $500, and we reserve their use for athletes in whom all other methods of decreasing pain to a level that allows participation in a rehabilitation program have failed. Reported success rates for pain relief vary from 30% (placebo level) to 90% (63). Two populations in which TENS seems to have the greatest benefit are those with postoperative knee (64–66) and back pain (67). The beneficial effects of TENS diminish over time when it is used for extended periods. Factors that appear to influence the TENS success rate are the stimulating parameters, electrode placement, tissue generator and duration of pain, concurrent medications and treatments, and patient expectations.

High-voltage electrical stimulation (HVS) produces involuntary muscle contraction, which can strengthen muscle (68,69) and prevent atrophy. However, numerous studies have shown that the rate and degree of strength increase obtained with HVS in normally innervated muscle are no greater than that obtained with exercise alone (63,70). In addition, tetanic electrical stimulation can be uncomfortable and poorly tolerated. A technique called "Russian stimulation," consisting of stimulation at 2500 Hz, was reported in 1977 by a scientist from the Soviet Union as producing increases in strength much greater than those possible with strength training alone; although some athletes still use this technique, its efficacy has

never been substantiated (71,72). To effectively increase strength, HVS would have to produce a more forceful contraction than the athlete's maximal voluntary contraction, and this does not occur (71).

In the injured athlete, HVS may be useful when voluntary muscle contraction is inhibited by pain, swelling, or immobilization; a common application of HVS is to decrease loss of quadriceps strength and muscle atrophy after knee surgery (73–75). The beneficial effects of HVS in this setting may be caused by a combination of muscle re-education, encouragement of early contraction, and pain relief. Physiologic muscle recruitment does not occur with electrically stimulated contractions. Rather than recruiting type 1 fibers before type 2, the fibers closest to the stimulating electrode are recruited first; this limits the functional transfer of strength gains. In some studies, HVS has helped to maintain isometric strength, thigh girth, and myofibrillar adenosine triphosphatase (ATPase) during immobilization, but it does not preserve speed of muscle contraction or glycogen stores (73,76). Other studies have failed to show any benefit of HVS beyond that which can be achieved with isometric contractions alone (77). HVS also increases local circulation and lymphatic flow (78) and reduces vascular "leakiness," thus diminishing edema formation (79). This application of HVS is especially useful for reducing the swelling associated with acute ankle sprains.

Iontophoresis uses electrical current flow to introduce electrically charged molecules into subcutaneous tissue. Some practitioners recommended iontophoresis as a method of delivering corticosteroids to joints to treat musculoskeletal injuries. However, as with phonophoresis, there is no sound evidence demonstrating that any significant quantity of drug penetrates deeper than the skin (80). Injection is a much more reliable method of delivering a given quantity of drug into a joint or soft tissue. At present, iontophoresis should be considered experimental and therefore, as having a limited role in the rehabilitation of injured athletes.

Massage and Manual Therapy

Massage and manual therapy can be useful adjuncts to a rehabilitation program when performed by knowledgeable practitioners; on the other hand, they can be painful or harmful when performed incorrectly. Soft-tissue massage enhances muscle relaxation, which may be beneficial before a stretching session. Some of the more aggressive forms of compression massage (petrissage), such as friction massage, help break up scar tissue and adhesions within injured muscle. In some instances, massage may also enhance fluid mobilization, reducing edema. Manipulation performed by a chiropractor, a physical therapist, or an osteopathic physician may relieve acute back pain in instances where neurologic deficits and fractures have been excluded. A complete review of these techniques is beyond the scope of this chapter.

FLEXIBILITY TRAINING

Once the acute pain and inflammation associated with an injury have subsided, normal ROM must be restored to the injured joint or muscle. In some cases, a flexibility deficit may have contributed to the development of the acute injury, and one goal of the rehabilitation program is to improve flexibility beyond its pre-injury state. Flexibility training is essential for both rehabilitation and prevention of injury recurrence.

Flexibility has been defined as the ROM of a joint or series of joints that is influenced by muscles, tendons, ligaments, bones, and bony structures (81,82). When comparing the contributions of muscle, tendon, and ligament to joint ROM, muscle is by far the greatest contributor. Gajdosik has challenged this definition of flexibility, suggesting that muscle flexibility is a physiologic phenomenon requiring simultaneous measurement of the length-tension relationship of muscles as they are lengthened passively without muscle activation (83).

Muscle flexibility is muscle- and joint-specific and influenced by the age, gender, and possibly the race of the individual. Static flexibility differs from dynamic flexibility because dynamic flexibility depends on the strength of antagonist muscles to move the limb and on the freedom of the limb to move, i.e., the lack of other constraining factors. For example, a ballet dancer with excellent static hamstring flexibility may be able to perform a split on the floor with ease; however, if she has weak hip flexors or hip pain impairing the ability to move her leg, she may have poor dynamic flexibility and be unable to lift her leg to even 90° when standing. Neuromuscular factors, such as reflex activity, strongly influence both static and dynamic flexibility. Temperature of muscle also influences flexibility because of its effect on collagen extensibility.

The muscle-tendon unit is viscoelastic in its mechanical behavior. When a pure elastic material is stretched, it returns to its initial length when the stretch is released. When a purely viscous material is stretched, its rate of deformation is proportional to the force applied, and it does not return to its original length when the stretch is released. Viscoelastic materials combine these properties such that the phenomena of stress relaxation, creep, hysteresis, and strain-rate dependence occur (see Table 19-5 for definitions).

Taylor and his colleagues (84) have studied the viscoelastic properties of the muscle-tendon unit using a model consisting of rabbit extensor digitorum longus and tibialis anterior with an intact neurovascular supply. This work suggests that muscle length gains achieved by stretching are not rapidly reversible. These studies also help explain why ballistic stretching may be harmful and ineffective. A rapid stretching velocity increases tension and energy storage in muscle, which may increase risk and severity of injury. In addition, ballistic stretching is not held long enough to allow stress relaxation or creep to occur. Summarizing the work of Taylor et al (84), it appears that most muscle lengthening occurs during the first 12 to 18 seconds of a stretch and during the first four stretch cycles.

Several correlation studies have demonstrated significant associations between flexibility deficits and specific types of injuries. A study of adolescent elite figure skaters found an association between anterior knee pain syndromes and hamstring, rectus femoris, and gastrocnemius-soleus muscle tightness (85). Adults with increased femoral anteversion and patellofemoral pain syndrome have tighter hamstring muscles than those with increased femoral anteversion without patellofemoral pain syndrome (86). In a prospective study of collegiate physical education students, Lysens et al (87) found that muscle inflexibility was associated with an increased incidence of overuse injuries. Knapik et al (88) found that colle-

Table 19-5 Behavior of Viscoelastic Materials

BEHAVIOR	DEFINITION
Stress relaxation	Less force is required over time to maintain a given increase in length during a sustained stretch.
Creep	A fixed force is applied to a material, and continued slow deformation occurs.
Strain rate dependence	A slow stretch (strain) produces more elongation than a fast stretch.
Hysteresis	More energy is absorbed during a stretch than is released when the stretch is terminated; the material absorbs energy when stretched.

giate female athletes with asymmetric lower extremity flexibility developed more lower extremity injuries.

We have (89) studied the relationship between lower extremity muscle tightness and lower extremity injuries in college athletes using a 10-point muscle tightness scale. We found that for each additional point on the muscle tightness scale, risk of injury increased by 23%. When the data were analyzed by gender, we found that men had significantly tighter muscles than women, and muscle tightness was not associated with injury incidence in women. It may be that the women in this study had achieved a threshold flexibility level necessary to avoid increased risk of injury.

The three major forms of stretching are ballistic, static, and proprioceptive neuromuscular facilitation (PNF). Ballistic stretching consists of rapid bouncing motions, which tend to have relatively high force and velocity, increasing the risk of muscle injury. Although effective, this form of stretching is not recommended. It activates the spindle reflex, which is counterproductive, and it is more likely than other stretching methods to produce muscle soreness. Static stretching is an effective means of improving flexibility. Advantages are that it minimizes activation of the spindle reflex, activates the Golgi tendon reflex if held long enough, does not require a partner, and is unlikely to cause muscle soreness. A static stretch must be held for at least 6 seconds in order to fully activate the Golgi tendon reflex (90).

PNF stretching was popularized by Knott and Voss (91). There are several different techniques of PNF stretching, but they all involve isometric contraction and relaxation of the muscle being stretched. Two of the most popular PNF techniques are contract-relax (CR) and contract-relax agonist-contract (CRAC). To stretch the hamstrings using the CR technique, the subject lies supine while a partner passively performs a straight leg raise on the subject. The subject then contracts his hamstrings while the partner resists movement of the leg; when the subject relaxes his hamstrings, the partner pushes the straight leg raise further, increasing hip ROM. Using the CRAC technique, the subject would contract his quadriceps while the partner was assisting the straight leg raise. The PNF stretching techniques were devised to take advantage of neurophysiologic principles such as autogenic and reciprocal inhibition, which are believed to alter spinal reflexes. Autogenic inhibition refers to stimulation of the Golgi tendon organ produced by contraction of the muscle that is being stretched. Reflex inhibition is believed to occur when the CRAC technique is used; contraction of the opposite muscle induces relaxation of the muscle being stretched. One drawback of the PNF techniques is that most require a partner, and some training is necessary to perform the exercises properly.

Several investigators have compared the efficacy of ballistic, static, and PNF stretching programs. All three methods result in increased flexibility, but it is not clear which technique is most effective. Lucas and Koslow (92) found that the three techniques all increased hamstring ROM by similar amounts. Other studies have found PNF stretching to be more effective than either ballistic or static stretching (93–95). The work of Godges et al (96) in healthy college males found a single bout of static stretching to increase hamstring ROM more than a single session of combined soft-tissue massage and PNF stretching. Moore and Hutton (97) compared static, CR, and CRAC hamstring stretching protocols in college-aged female gymnasts. The CRAC method produced the greatest hamstring EMG activity while the hamstrings were supposed to be relaxed and was perceived as being the most painful stretching technique; in addition, it was less effective than either the static or CR stretches. Overall, the static stretch was perceived as most effective because it produced the greatest increase in ROM and was least painful.

In summary, it appears that both PNF and static stretching have similar levels of effectiveness in healthy young adults. If a PNF technique is used, the CR method may be preferable to the CRAC method because it is less painful and less likely to produce co-contraction of the muscle being stretched.

Based on the few studies (84,94,98) that have addressed the appropriate frequency, duration, and intensity of stretching programs, we make the following recommendations:

1. Either static, PNF, or a combination of both types of stretches should be prescribed.

2. The CRAC PNF technique should be used with caution, because it may be more painful than other techniques and may encourage co-contraction of the muscle being stretched.

3. Ballistic stretching should not be prescribed.

4. Stretching must be performed at least three times per week to improve flexibility, but daily stretching will probably result in greater, faster gains in flexibility.

5. Each stretch should be performed at least three times and held for 15 to 30 seconds during each stretching session.

STRENGTH TRAINING

Once the injured joint or limb is pain-free, strengthening exercise should be initiated within a ROM comfortable for the athlete. Full joint ROM does not need to be present to begin strengthening; flexibility training should be continued concurrently. For example, isometric quadriceps sets can be performed even while the knee is immobilized in extension. If

pain persists or time must be allowed for tissue healing before strengthening the muscles about an injured joint, strengthening of muscles acting on adjacent joints may be initiated. The entire body acts as a kinetic chain; allowing disuse weakening of muscles surrounding uninjured joints affects biomechanics when the athlete returns to activity and may place additional stress on the injured joint or structure.

Strengthening exercises may be classified as involving *isometric, isotonic,* or *isokinetic* muscle contractions or as *functional exercises.* In addition, both *eccentric* and *concentric* isotonic and isokinetic training can be performed. Another way of classifying strength training exercises is as *closed kinetic chain* or *open kinetic chain* exercises. These terms are defined, along with their advantages and disadvantages and clinical examples, in Table 19-6.

Isometric exercises are performed without any appreciable change in joint position or muscle length and can be performed with or without the use of weights. Quadricep sets and straight leg raises with ankle weights are isometric exercises commonly prescribed early in the course of rehabilitation of patellofemoral pain syndrome. Isometric strengthening exercises are least effective in terms of improving dynamic function and sports-related skills, but they are useful for helping to prevent atrophy in muscles around acutely injured, painful joints. If an injured limb tolerates only isometric exercise, the noninjured contralateral limb can be used to perform isotonic or isokinetic exercise, which may enhance strength gain in the injured limb via the "crossover effect," in which exercising one limb may produce strength gains in the opposite limb (99,100).

Isotonic and isokinetic strengthening exercises are both effective means of restoring strength following injury. Taken literally, the term *isotonic* means that tension or torque remains constant throughout the contraction. In real life, this is not possible because muscle tension changes with joint angle. For this reason, some exercise physiologists have replaced the term *isotonic* with *dynamic* (101). Isotonic exercises can be performed using the body as a weight (without special equipment), using machines, or using free weights. Isotonic exercises using machines are useful early in the rehabilitation process because movement is restricted to a single plane. Use of machines, including those with cams that attempt to vary resistance (such as Universal and Nautilus), allows the athlete to strengthen injured muscles with relatively little risk of further injury. These machines come closer to a true isotonic or constant force contraction than do exercises using body weight or free weights. Use of free weights is often the most advanced step in the strengthening component of a rehabilitation program. With free weights, the athlete must incorporate the ability to isolate specific muscles, as well as balance skills, symmetry, and, to some extent, proprioception.

A form of strength training closely related to isotonic exercises has been termed *isodynamic* and refers to the use of elastic cords or bands with variable resistance. This method of strengthening allows incorporation of sport-specific movement patterns into the exercise program. The equipment is also inexpensive and easily transportable.

Isokinetic strengthening requires specially designed weight-lifting machines. The underlying principle is that by keeping the angular velocity about a joint constant, muscle groups can exert maximal torque throughout the entire

Table 19-6 Types of Muscle Actions

Term	Definition	Clinical Example	Advantage	Disadvantage
Static (Isometric)	Muscle contraction without change in joint position	Straight leg raise with ankle weights for quadriceps strengthening	Possible when joint is immobilized or painful	Effort-dependent; does not follow specificity of training principle
Dynamic (Isotonic)	Contraction with constant tension or torque through ROM	Nautilus (Independence, VA) weight-lifting machines; free weights (theoretically)	Strengthens through entire ROM	Strengthening not equally effective through whole ROM
Dynamic (Isokinetic)	Contraction with constant angular velocity and variable resistance	Cybex (Medway, MA) machines	Allows objective strength (torque) measurement; low risk of injury	Requires expensive equipment; nonphysiologic
Isodynamic	Exercise with elastic cords or bands providing variable resistance	Theraband (Hygienic Corp., Algron, OH) rotator cuff strengthening exercises	Incorporates sport-specific movement patterns; inexpensive, portable equipment; low injury risk	Effort-dependent
Functional	Exercises using sport-specific skills	Cycling, rowing	Physiologic; does not require special equipment; trains timing and proprioception	Not possible if weight-bearing limited
Concentric	Contraction with muscle shortening	Biceps curl	Relatively safe; positive feedback during ROM	Force generation not uniform through ROM
Eccentric	Contraction with muscle lengthening	"Negatives": slowly lowering the weight after a biceps curl	Produces high forces; often simulates functional activities	Increased risk of muscle or tendon injury and delayed-onset muscle soreness
Open Kinetic Chain	Distal limb moves through space; usually single joint movement	Knee extensions with ankle weights	May be sport-specific (kicking, throwing)	Produces unnatural shear forces across joint
Closed Kinetic Chain	Distal limb fixed; multiple proximal joints move	Squats, push-ups	Physiologic joint loading; encourages agonist and antagonist co-contraction; trains balance and proprioception	Not possible if weight-bearing limited

ROM, range of motion.

ROM. Isokinetic dynamometers are often used to measure strength, enabling assessment of rehabilitation progress and side-to-side comparisons. No human movements involved in either normal daily activities or athletics are truly isokinetic. In addition, the speed required for many sports skills cannot be achieved by isokinetic dynamometers. In one study, participants in isokinetic and isotonic strengthening programs made similar gains in strength, but those who trained isokinetically gained strength quicker and experienced less postworkout soreness (102).

Both isotonic and isokinetic contractions may be eccentric or concentric. Eccentric contractions generate greater force, are more efficient, and are more likely to produce injury or delayed onset muscle soreness (103–105). The more rapid the eccentric contraction, the greater the force it is able to generate; the converse is true for concentric contractions

(i.e., slower contractions generate greater force). Figure 19-1 illustrates the relationship between force, speed, and type of contraction. Because of the high force generated by eccentric contractions, it is critical that they be incorporated into the final stages of a sports rehabilitation program. Eccentric contractions are involved in decelerating the humerus after throwing and in landing from jumps. A strengthening program that emphasizes eccentric contractions is especially beneficial for rehabilitation of tendon injuries because the tendon is maximally loaded (16).

An additional form of strengthening exercise has been termed *functional exercise*, because it improves strength through what are considered functional activities (at least for the athlete). Examples of functional exercises used to strengthen the quadriceps and hamstrings after a knee injury include jumping rope, using a pogo stick, stationary cycling, and

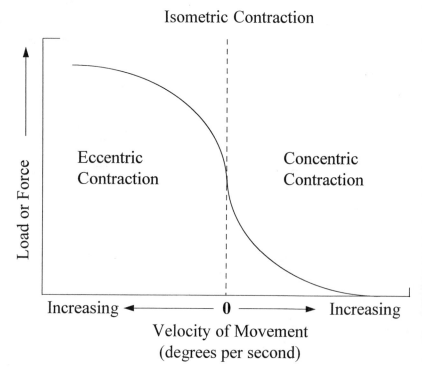

Figure 19-1 Graph demonstrating the relationship between force, velocity, and muscle contraction type.

Isometric Contraction

Eccentric Contraction

Concentric Contraction

Load or Force

Increasing ← 0 → Increasing

Velocity of Movement
(degrees per second)

jumping on a trampoline. These may be used in place of isokinetic exercises when isokinetic dynamometers are not available (106).

Plyometrics are strengthening exercises that involve rebounding and use the viscoelastic properties of muscle in the performance of both concentric and eccentric contractions. The exercises involve high joint loading and impact forces; thus they should not be added to the rehabilitation program until almost complete healing of the injury has taken place. This form of strengthening simulates sports skills such as rebounding on the basketball court or tumbling in gymnastics.

Prescription of *closed kinetic chain exercises* has become increasingly popular over the last 10 years. The distal part of the extremity is fixed while multiple proximal joints move. The lower extremity is used in this manner when weight-bearing. In *open chain exercises*, the distal end of the limb moves through space, and one joint is primarily moved. Kicking is one of the few sport-related open chain lower extremity activities. In contrast to the lower extremity, the upper extremity is used primarily in an open chain fashion. An exception is gymnasts who bear weight on their upper extremities. Closed chain exercises are favored because they reduce unnatural shear force across joints and encourage co-contraction of agonist and antagonist muscles, thus assisting with joint stabilization (107–110).

When a strengthening program is prescribed, three principles must be followed: 1) specificity of training, 2) maximal loading, and 3) progression of loading (16). Strength gains are greatest at the joint angle at which isometric exercises are performed, for the specific type of contraction (concentric versus eccentric), in the ROM and plane in which isotonic exercises are performed, and at the velocity at which isokinetic exercises are performed (111–114). However, strength gained by training at high speeds transfers better to

lower speed activities than vice versa (115,116). The greater the overload to which a muscle is subjected, the more rapid is the gain in strength. However, to avoid injury, one must gradually build up to the maximal load. Many strength programs are based on the gradual addition of progressive resistance. This concept initially was described by DeLorme (117,118). No single algorithm for a progressive resistance exercise (PRE) program has been proven to be superior to the other variants. A simple PRE program can be devised by identifying a weight that can be lifted 8 to 12 times (usually 70% to 80% of the one repetition maximum). The athlete then completes three sets with rest periods in between. A set consists of lifting the weight as many times as possible. If the weight cannot be lifted at least eight times during the last set, it should be reduced. If it can be lifted 12 times during all sets, it should be increased by 10% (101). To increase strength, the workout should be performed at least three times per week. If one wishes to improve power, a lighter weight should be used and lifted rapidly 15 to 20 times per set.

PROPRIOCEPTIVE TRAINING

Currently, proprioception retraining is a very popular component of rehabilitation after athletic injuries. Several studies have demonstrated physiologic changes in muscle firing patterns that seem to support this practice. Anecdotally and conceptually, it seems that proprioception retraining may hasten recovery and decrease risk of re-injury, but randomized clinical trials have not yet been performed to confirm this idea.

Proprioception is a sensory modality that allows the athlete to detect joint movement (kinesthesia) and joint position (119). Motor programming and neuromuscular control needed for athletic performance and prevention of injury require adequate proprioceptive function. Mechanoreceptors, including Ruffini's corpuscles, Pacinian corpuscles, muscle spindles, and Golgi tendon organs, contribute afferent input to the proprioceptive pathways. These mechanoreceptors and other sensory receptors in the skin, retina, and semicircular canals supply information to the CNS. At the level of the spinal cord, spinal reflexes may also contribute to motor control; only a portion of proprioceptive input reaches the cortex. Injury to the skin, muscles, tendons, ligaments, and the joint capsule may damage mechanoreceptors and disrupt proprioceptive function. Age and osteoarthritis also produce proprioceptive deficits (120–123). Sharma et al (123) proposed that impaired proprioception precedes the development of osteoarthritis. Proprioceptive deficits impair the athlete's ability to perform sport-specific motor skills, producing poor athletic performance and increasing the risk of injury or re-injury. Proprioceptive retraining is an important aspect of rehabilitation after ankle, knee, and shoulder injury or surgery. Figure 19-2 depicts the manner in which proprioceptive deficits and injury are interrelated.

Freeman et al (124) proposed that altered proprioception may account for functional instability following ankle sprains and suggested using a wobble board to retrain proprioception. Electromyographic (EMG) studies have documented alterations in the muscle firing patterns in the lower leg in patients with chronic ankle injuries and in patients undergoing proprioceptive retraining. Lofvenberg et al (125) documented a delay in reaction time of the peroneus longus and tibialis anterior muscles in patients with a history of chronic lateral ankle instability. Sheth et al (126) compared ankles receiving proprioceptive training using a wobble board to untrained ankles, both of which were subjected to a simulated ankle sprain. In the untrained ankles, invertor and evertor muscles fired simultaneously. After 8 weeks of ankle disk training, the peroneus longus fired earlier than the tibialis anterior and posterior muscles, helping to protect the ankle from an inversion sprain. Konradsen et al demonstrated the ability of afferent input from the calf muscles to substitute for proprioceptive input from the lateral ankle ligaments (127).

Many of the studies concerning knee proprioception have focused upon the effects of anterior cruciate ligament (ACL) deficiency and ACL reconstruction. The ACL contains proprioceptive mechanoreceptors and probably plays both a mechanical role and a sensory role in knee instability

(128–130). Several studies have demonstrated proprioceptive deficits in the ACL-deficient knee (131–133). Closed chain weight-bearing exercises have been recommended to enhance neuromuscular coordination and proprioceptive retraining in the ACL-deficient knee (133,134).

Theoretically, ACL deficiency produces proprioceptive loss, which in turn causes a delay in hamstring muscle firing, which contributes to and worsens knee instability. Delayed firing patterns of the hamstring muscles have been documented by measuring the reflex hamstring contraction latency (RHCL) in ACL-deficient patients (135,136). Although the utility of the RHCL as a measure of proprioception is controversial (137), Beard et al (138) have shown improvement in the RHCL and function in ACL-deficient patients who underwent a rehabilitation program specifically designed to enhance proprioception. The proprioceptive retraining program included closed kinetic chain exercises and wobble board, stationary bike, and plyometric functional exercises. This program was more effective than a routine hamstring and quadriceps strengthening program.

Patients with a history of recurrent shoulder dislocations have proprioception deficits, and surgery partially restores proprioception in patients undergoing capsulolabral reconstruction (139). Borsa et al (140) suggest that a shoulder rehabilitation program including dynamic stabilization activities with axial loading and coactivation of shoulder muscles may improve shoulder proprioception and stability.

Knee and ankle bracing and taping improve joint proprioception and thus may enhance performance and decrease risk of injury. Feuerbach et al (141) tested proprioception both with and without a stirrup-style ankle orthosis after the lateral ankle ligaments (anterior talofibular and calcaneofibular) were anesthetized. The brace significantly improved ankle proprioception. The mechanism of improvement may be stimulation of cutaneous mechanoreceptors. Other investigators (142–144) have found significant improvements in knee proprioceptive function when either a knee sleeve or an elastic bandage is worn.

MUSCLE ENDURANCE TRAINING

Once adequate strength has been restored, muscles must be endurance-trained to prevent a decline in strength and

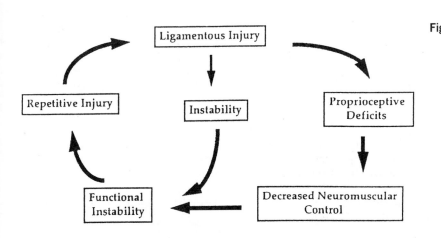

Figure 19-2 Paradigm depicting the interrelationship between joint instability, proprioceptive deficits, and injury. (Reproduced by permission from Lephart SM, Henry TJ. The physiologic basis for open and closed kinetic chain rehabilitation for the upper extremity. J Sport Rehab 1996;5:71–87.)

performance with fatigue. Muscle fatigue contributes to both acute and overuse sports injuries. Muscle fatigue predisposes the athlete to fall or fail to successfully complete a skill, resulting in injury. In team sports, such as football and basketball, the frequency of injury is highest during the last half of a game. A skier whose quadriceps muscles are fatigued is more likely to fall and sustain acute ligamentous injury to the knee. Wojtys et al (145) have demonstrated that anterior tibial translation in healthy knees increases when the hamstrings and quadriceps muscles become fatigued. Fatigue of the scapular stabilizers, particularly the serratus anterior, can predispose swimmers to develop rotator cuff tendonitis (146). Fatigue of the deep plantar flexors is probably an etiologic factor in the development of tibial and metatarsal stress fractures (147,148). An animal model of muscle strain injuries demonstrated that although fatigued muscles are injured at the same length as nonfatigued muscles, they can withstand less force and absorb less energy before injury (149).

Local muscle endurance may be expressed as a ratio. A predetermined number of maximal contractions is performed, and the ratio of the force generated by the first contraction to the force generated by the last contraction quantifies endurance. The endurance ratio may be calculated from measurements made on an isokinetic dynamometer and used to assess the progress of a muscle endurance building program. Muscle endurance is primarily determined by the aerobic capacity of the muscle. Endurance training converts some type 2B (fast, glycolytic) to 2A (fast, oxidative, and glycolytic) fibers. Muscles with the highest proportion of type 1 fibers have the greatest endurance.

Endurance training is accomplished by performing a high number of repetitions with moderate or low resistance. Ideally, one should use an endurance training load close to, or slightly higher than, the load muscle is subjected to during athletic activities. Steadman has devised an endurance training program that incorporates training to enhance both aerobic and anaerobic local muscle endurance (150). Anaerobic endurance is important for skills requiring explosive strength or bursting activity. Steadman's program consists of a series of high-repetition moderate-weight sets followed by rapid low-resistance sets performed until fatigue. Following fatigue, a maximal isometric contraction is held for 1 minute.

CARDIOVASCULAR FITNESS

Maintaining cardiovascular fitness is a crucial component of all sports rehabilitation programs. First, maintaining cardiovascular fitness allows an athlete to return to his or her previous level of competition more rapidly once the musculoskeletal injury has been adequately rehabilitated. With detraining, Vo_2max declines much more rapidly than muscle strength. If a runner with a leg injury did not perform aerobic training for several weeks, his Vo_2max would drop, and muscle capillary number and mitochondrial acitivity would decrease (151,152). Fortunately, the rapid decline in cardiovascular fitness is somewhat attenuated in athletes who have endurance trained for long periods of time (153,154). Nevertheless, if routine low to moderate level physical activity takes the place of athletic training, all training benefits dissi-

pate within 2 to 8 months (155). In addition, if an athlete does not maintain cardiovascular fitness while injured, he or she is more likely to sustain another injury when returning to sport. For example, a gymnast who becomes deconditioned from a cardiovascular standpoint while rehabilitating an ankle injury returns to the gym and attempts to perform a full floor routine. Because she is fatigued and short of breath on her last tumbling pass, she does not use optimal technique and is unable to complete her twisting in the air; she sustains a knee ligament injury when landing.

The mode of cardiovascular training should be as sport-specific as possible, e.g., runners should run, swimmers should swim, cyclists should cycle. However, because of the location of an athlete's injury, this is not always possible. If athletes involved in running sports are unable to bear full weight on their lower extremities, they may use a bicycle ergometer, swimming, or pool running to maintain aerobic fitness. As injury healing progresses, they may switch to a stair climber or cross-country ski machine; lower extremity joint impact forces are less with these forms of exercise than with running. Swimmers with upper extremity injuries may maintain fitness by swimming with a kick board using the legs only. The intensity of cardiovascular training should also be modeled after the demands of an athlete's sport. Distance runners require pure aerobic training and need to train for longer periods of time than do middle distance runners or sprinters. Football players must perform in short bursts of activity; thus, their cardiovascular training program must have an anaerobic as well as an aerobic component.

Exercise intensity should be based on measurements of either heart rate or Vo_2max. Measurement of Vo_2max requires specialized equipment; the heart rate reserve (HRR) method of exercise intensity prescription is more practical in most clinic settings. Using Karvonen's formula, maximum heart rate (HR_{max}) is estimated as 220 minus age. The HRR is HR_{max} minus the resting heart rate (HR_{rest}). To improve aerobic fitness, recreational athletes need to train at 70% to 80% of their HRR (65% to 75% of Vo_2max) and competitive athletes at 80% to 90% of their HRR (75% to 85% of Vo_2max). The training heart rate is HR_{rest} plus the appropriate percentage of HRR (156). The amount of training needed to maintain cardiovascular fitness while recuperating from injury is dictated by the athlete's sport. For a football player, 20 to 30 minutes of conditioning three times per week may be sufficient. A marathoner may require an hour of aerobic training 6 days per week. When initiating a cardiovascular conditioning program, the intensity should be low enough that the athlete can perform the activity for the target time duration. While maintaining this duration, the intensity is gradually increased until it reaches the target level.

Programs have been developed to specifically train anaerobic capacity (157). Those participating in sports with significant anaerobic demands benefit from interval training (158). A typical interval training program consists of 3- to 5-minute periods of intense aerobic activity alternating with rest periods. Initially the rest period should be the same length as the exercise interval. As training progresses, the length of the rest periods may be progressively reduced until they are 50% the length of the exercise interval. During the rest period, the HR should drop to at least 50% of the HRR or less before beginning the next exercise interval.

BRACING, TAPING, AND ORTHOTICS

The use of braces, taping, and orthotics is commonly considered part of a rehabilitation program. Scientific literature supporting the adjunctive use of such devices is scant. Braces can be divided into three major categories: prophylactic (designed to prevent injury), rehabilitation (used during the rehabilitation process), and functional (designed to be worn during play as a substitute for an injured ligament). The efficacy of bracing and taping is discussed in reference to the rehabilitation of acute ankle and knee injuries. The use of shoe inserts or orthotics in the rehabilitation of a variety of lower extremity overuse injuries is reviewed.

The ankle sprain is one of the most common sports injuries, and taping and bracing have long played a role in its management. When tape is initially applied, it restricts motion in inversion. However, after 10 to 20 minutes of exercise, most of the motion control is lost because of stretching of the tape (159). Tape, when used regularly for an entire competitive season, is more expensive than most ankle braces, and its application is labor-intensive. The three types of commonly prescribed ankle braces are the elastic sock variety, cloth lace-on, and semirigid plastic stirrup style. Most studies comparing the efficacy of different styles of braces show the greatest motion limitation with the stirrup brace as well as the least loss of efficacy after exercise. Several studies have examined the effect of bracing on performance and show slight reductions in jumping ability and running speed (159,160); other studies have not shown any adverse effects of bracing on performance (161). The work of Surve et al (162) showed a fivefold reduction in reinjury rate of soccer players wearing a stirrup brace; Sitler et al (163) also showed a significant decrease in injury rate among West Point cadets wearing braces. Concern has been expressed that restricting motion at the ankle shifts force transmission to the knee and may predispose it to more frequent or severe injury, but this has not been substantiated (163). Overall, the best method of preventing ankle injury is to develop strong evertor muscles (164). If a brace is prescribed, its use must be accompanied by an aggressive peroneal muscle strengthening program. Prescribing a brace without an appropriate rehabilitation program to accompany it is worse than no brace at all; it gives athletes a false sense of security while contributing to further weakening of the peroneal muscles.

Knee braces are often prescribed during rehabilitation of ligamentous knee injuries, whether the injury is treated nonsurgically or surgically. Rehabilitation braces are designed to allow early protected and controlled motion while tissue healing occurs, thus avoiding the deleterious effects of immobilization. They are commonly used following collateral and cruciate ligament injuries as well as after ligament reconstruction. These braces generally have unilateral or bilateral metal uprights with hinges that can be set to control flexion and extension. The braces also provide some resistance to varus and valgus movement, but they are not designed to control ligamentous stress. Rehabilitation braces are designed to be worn for a limited period of time and thus should be relatively inexpensive off-the-shelf, rather than custom-made, designs. Extensive biomechanical studies, such as those performed on prophylactic and functional braces, have not been undertaken for rehabilitation braces (165). The few studies

that have been performed show that 15° to 20° of motion occurs beyond that dictated by the setting of the hinge (166). Thus, if one wishes to limit extension to 15° less than full extension, the extension stop should be set at 25° to 30° (167).

Transitional rehabilitation braces are lighter weight and less restrictive than standard rehabilitation braces, allowing low level functional activity such as jogging; they are not designed for full sports participation. Once the rehabilitation process is near completion, a functional knee brace may be prescribed as a "substitution" for a torn ligament. These braces are designed for use during full sports participation, must be individually fitted, and usually are custom-made and considerably more expensive than rehabilitation braces.

Functional knee braces are prescribed primarily for the ACL- or posterior cruciate ligament (PCL)-deficient knee or to protect ligament grafts after surgery. Numerous biomechanical studies have been performed to assess the efficacy of these braces in protecting the knee from abnormal motion or excessive ligamentous loading. None of the currently available functional braces are capable of protecting the knee from abnormal translations and rotations, even at subphysiologic loads (168,169). Likewise, the braces do not have any effect on ACL strain (170). The primary reason for this inability to control motion is the inability to rigidly fix the brace to the limb. Functional braces may have some potentially beneficial neuromuscular effects. They seem to promote the development of a "quadriceps avoidance" gait in ACL-deficient patients (171) and may improve proprioception of the knee joint, but this has not yet been concretely demonstrated (172). Several adverse effects of bracing have also been reported. These include increased heart rate and oxygen consumption (173), decreased knee extension and flexion torque (174), and increased fatigue (175). Subjectively, patients using functional braces have reported fewer symptoms and better performance (176). However, there are not any objective clinical outcome studies documenting a decreased incidence of degenerative osteoarthritis, reinjury, or graft disruption with functional bracing. Based on available information, a good strengthening program and muscle re-education is as effective as any currently available brace for controlling abnormal knee motion and forces.

Bracing and taping are also often employed during the rehabilitation of patellofemoral pain syndrome (PFPS). The primary goal of these braces is to control abnormal patellar tracking and decrease pain. Braces used for this purpose include infrapatellar straps, elastic sleeves with buttresses designed to control patellar motion, and braces with rigid lateral uprights and an extension stop. McConnell taping is a taping technique designed to promote normal firing patterns in the vastus medialis and correct abnormal patellar tracking (177). No studies have clearly shown that either bracing or taping can effectively alter patellar tracking or position (178,179). Improved knee extension torque has been reported in patients with PFPS after both bracing and taping (180), but Kowall et al did not find any beneficial effect of adding patellar taping to a rehabilitation program when patients receiving physical therapy alone were compared with those receiving taping and therapy (181). Multiple studies have shown improvement in symptoms with a combination of physical therapy and bracing or taping (182,183), but none have compared bracing plus therapy to bracing alone. We believe that an aggressive rehabilitation program that includes lower extremity flexibility training and closed chain quadriceps strengthening exercises is as effective or more effective than any form of bracing or taping.

Pronation and foot malalignment are implicated in a variety of lower extremity overuse injuries. Orthotics are often prescribed as part of the rehabilitation process to correct pronation or foot malalignment, but whether they actually achieve this goal is debatable. Foot orthotics can be divided into two categories, functional and accommodative. Functional orthotics attempt to realign the foot by placing the subtalar joint in a neutral position; they are constructed of a rigid or semirigid material that will maintain the foot in the desired position. Accommodative orthotics are prescribed to improve weight distribution by bringing the support surface up to meet the foot; these orthotics are fabricated from a softer material that will mold to the foot and accommodate deformities. Accommodative orthotics are generally prescribed for treatment of cavus feet to distribute pressure over a greater surface area. Some feet are treated best with a hybrid of the functional and the accommodative orthotic.

Kilmartin and Wallace (184) reviewed the literature on functional foot orthotics and concluded that they have little effect on knee motion or alignment but do reduce rear foot movement. Studies of the effect of orthotics on knee alignment have shown that orthotics may reduce the static Q angle but do not alter the dynamic Q angle (182). In addition, orthotics affect the knee differently in walking and running. Orthotics have been shown to decrease both maximum pronation and the velocity of rear foot movement (185), which theoretically decreases the work required by supinating muscles such as the medial soleus. This reduction in work load should benefit those with overuse injuries related to medial soleus overload, such as medial tibial stress syndrome and tibial stress fractures. On the other hand, no research has proven the advantage of placing the foot in a supinated position (184). Orthotic prescription is based on the clinical determination of subtalar joint neutral position, and no objective, repeatable method for determining the neutral point has been devised.

In summary, orthotics may be useful in the treatment and rehabilitation of overuse injuries in which excessive pronation is thought to be an etiologic factor, but firm evidence of benefit is lacking. Subjectively, orthotics appear to be beneficial; 78% of the runners in the study by James et al (186) reported benefit from the use of orthotics. Because orthotics (especially if rigid) may alter the biomechanics and loading of the lower extremity, potentially, their use might contribute to the development of new overuse injuries, including stress fractures. If used, functional orthotics should be one part of a comprehensive treatment program and not the sole treatment.

CORRECTING INJURY RISK FACTORS

An important aspect of the rehabilitation process is identifying and correcting or eliminating factors that may have contributed to injury development. These factors can be broadly categorized as extrinsic, or environmental, factors and intrinsic factors. Extrinsic factors include footwear, braces, sports equipment, playing surface, and training regimen. Intrinsic factors include diet, overall health status and fatigue level, anatomic malalignment, and sport-specific technique and biomechanics.

Improperly designed or poorly fitted running shoes, golf shoes, skating boots, ski boots, or other footwear may contribute to injury. In runners, inadequate footwear is most often associated with stress fractures. The most important considerations in selecting an athletic shoe are cushioning, stability, and flexibility. The shock absorption properties are determined primarily by the construction of the midsole. The age of a shoe is inversely proportional to its shock-absorbing properties. Most running shoes lose a significant portion of their shock absorbing capability after 500 to 1000 miles. The two basic materials used for midsole construction are ethyl vinyl acetate and polyurethane; polyurethane is denser, heavier, and more durable. Recently, shoes have been designed with air encapsulated in the midsole (airsoles); these systems are more resistant to compaction than polyurethane and are therefore more durable. The stability of a shoe enhances the ankle's ability to avoid inversion and eversion forces; stability is increased by using a board or combined last (contains a fiber board between the upper portion of the shoe and the midsole) rather than a slip last, a semi-curved as opposed to a curved last, and a firm heel counter. The importance of shoe stability and cushioning depends on both the shape of the foot and the athlete's sport. Rigid cavus feet have good stability but are poorly cushioned; flexible flat feet are better-cushioned but less stable (187). Excessively flexible forefeet on football shoes are associated with the development of "turf toe" (first metatarsophalangeal joint sprain). Cleats are an important part of many athletic shoes. In general, the longer and more rigid the cleats, the firmer the foot fixation and the greater the incidence of knee and ankle injuries. An excellent review of the literature comparing various styles of cleats and their association with injury has been written by Clanton (188).

The overall health of the athlete may play a role in injury development and thus should be addressed during rehabilitation. If athletes are overly fatigued as a result of poor nutrition, inadequate sleep, or excessive stress, they are more likely to make mental errors, which lead to falls and injury. Health professionals working with athletes must identify general health and lifestyle factors contributing to injury. Of particular concern is the female athlete triad, consisting of disordered eating, amenorrhea, and osteoporosis, which predisposes to the development of stress fractures. The female athlete triad is especially prevalent among athletes involved in "appearance" sports, such as gymnastics, figure skating, and ballet. In addition, distance runners may be pressured to maintain low body weight because coaches believe this will improve their times.

Anatomic malalignment, particularly in the lower extremity, is associated with a number of overuse injuries (189). Although rehabilitation cannot alter bony alignment, the rehabilitation professional must recognize malalignment as a risk factor for overuse injuries so that a flexibility and strengthening program may be designed to minimize its deleterious effects.

Developing the proper biomechanics and technique for sport-specific skills is important not only for producing optimal performance but for preventing injury. When an athlete is ready to return to play, it is often helpful to analyze the biomechanics of the skill during which the athlete was injured to determine whether an alteration in technique and biomechanics might prevent future injury. Swimmers often develop rotator cuff tendonitis and impingement syndrome. Improper stroke mechanics, such as excessive internal rotation of the arm at entry in the freestyle or butterfly strokes and high elbow recovery with the elbow leading the hand, encourage impingement (190). On the other hand, increasing body roll and alternate side breathing may decrease problems with impingement. Pitchers develop overuse injuries of the shoulder and elbow when they lack adequate upper trunk and hip rotation during the cocking phase. Pelvis and trunk rotation transfers energy up the kinetic chain from the feet into the throwing arm; without this energy transfer, the pitch is slower, and the muscles about the shoulder and elbow are overworked in an attempt to compensate for the force deficit. In a properly executed pitch, a large percentage of the ball's velocity comes from the legs, hips, and trunk. Cervical spine injuries in both American football players and English and Welsh rugby players are caused by specific tackling techniques; in both sports, rule changes have significantly decreased the number of serious spine injuries (191,192). Among ballet dancers, forced turnout in those with limited external rotation at the hip, known as "screwing the knees," is an important etiologic factor in the development of patellofemoral stress syndrome and tibialis posterior and flexor hallucis longus tendonitis (193).

RETURN TO PLAY CRITERIA

General guidelines for return to play criteria are proposed in Table 19-7 (194). Obviously, these guidelines must be applied in a flexible manner, and the individual situation of each athlete must be considered. The injured athlete serves as his or her own "control" when determining whether flexibility and strength are adequate for return to full participation. If an extensive preseason examination was performed (before injury), the clinician may use this information to establish the athlete's baseline strength and flexibility levels. If a flexibility or strength deficit is believed to have contributed to the development of the injury, as is the case with many overuse syndromes, this deficit should be corrected before return to full participation, or the injury will recur; in these cases, one may wish to see better-than-baseline strength or flexibility before return to play. When baseline data are unavailable, the contralateral limb may be used as a control. Isokinetic testing is useful for following strength and power gains during the rehabilitation process. Objective strength measurements are important, even though they may not correlate with functional performance, because athletes may have 20% to 30% side-to-side strength differences without being aware of them.

Relative rest or activity modification is the key to rehabilitation of many injuries. While rehabilitating an injury, the athlete can often participate in some sport-specific skills and activities in addition to performing aerobic conditioning to maintain overall fitness. For example, a female gymnast with a wrist injury can perform dance elements on the floor exercise and balance beam as well as aerial elements that do not

Table 19-7 Return to Play Criteria
Full ROM after neck or back injury
90% of full ROM after extremity injury
Normal strength with side-to-side difference of <20%
Normal neurologic examination
No swelling of injured joint
No uncontrolled joint instability
Able to run, jump, and perform sport-specific skills without pain
Not taking pain medication
Able to demonstrate:
Proper warm-up
Performance of prescribed flexibility and strength programs
Recommended use of heat and cold
Use of prescribed taping or bracing
Understands risks and potential consequences of reinjury

ROM, range of motion.

require upper extremity weight-bearing. Male gymnasts may continue to train on the high bar, rings, parallel bars, and pommel horse while rehabilitating knee and ankle injuries.

The performance of sport-specific skills must be built into all rehabilitation programs before the athlete is cleared for full participation. For the tennis player with an upper extremity injury, this might involve beginning with slow-paced ground strokes, both forehand and backhand, advancing to short and then longer volleys, and serving at progressively faster speeds. For throwing athletes, a return to throwing should progress from lobbing the ball with a fluid motion and proper form to throwing progressively greater distances at higher velocities with a decreased arc. Following a lower extremity injury, the redevelopment of running and cutting skills should occur in an orderly fashion. Athletes should progress from fast walking to jogging and then to running. During the early phases of this progression, the athlete must be observed closely to make sure that muscle substitution patterns, which alter biomechanics and may predispose to the development of other injuries, do not occur. When the athlete can run at 75% of preinjury speed without pain or other symptoms, drills emphasizing direction changes, such as running figures-of-eight, can be started (194). Finally, jumping activities, sprinting, and cutting are introduced.

Once an injury has been rehabilitated adequately such that full return to sports is allowed, the training load must be gradually increased to the preinjury level to avoid the development of additional overuse injuries. For endurance sports, such as distance running, cycling, and swimming, a good rule of thumb is to begin workouts at 50% of the preinjury distance and a comfortable pace. Distance may be increased 10% every 3 to 4 days, as long as the athlete remains pain-free, until the target training load is achieved. Once the desired training distance has been reached, speed should be increased gradually. During and after return to full participation, the athlete should continue with a maintenance strength and flexibility program to help prevent injury recurrence.

REFERENCES

1. Saal J. General principles and guidelines for rehabilitation of the injured athlete. Phys Med Rehab: State of the Art Reviews 1987;1:523–536.

2. Uhthoff HK, Jaworski ZFG. Bone loss in response to long-term immobilisation. J Bone Joint Surg Br 1978;60-B:420–429.

3. Eisele SA, Sammarco G. Fatigue fractures of the foot and ankle in the athlete. J Bone Joint Surg Am 1993;75-A:290–298.

4. Rettig AC, Sherbourne KD, McCarroll JR, et al. The natural history and treatment of delayed union stress fractures of the anterior cortex of the tibia. Amer J Sports Med 1988;16:250–255.

5. Torg JS, Pavlov H, Cooley LH, et al. Stess fractures of the tarsal navicular. J Bone Joint Surg Am 1982;64-A:700–712.

6. Akeson WH, Woo SLY, Amiel D, et al. The connective tissue response to immobility: biochemical changes in periarticular connective tissue of the immobilized rabbit knee. Clin Orthop Rel Res 1973;93:356–362.

7. Djurasovic M, Aldridge JW, Grumbles R, et al. Knee joint immobilization decreases aggrecan gene expression in the meniscus. Amer J Sports Med 1998;26:460–466.

8. Shelbourne KD, Patel DV, Adsit WS, et al. Rehabilitation after meniscal repair. Clin Sports Med 1996;15:595–612.

9. Noyes FR. Functional properties of knee ligaments and alterations induced by immobilization. Clin Orthop Rel Res 1977;123:210–242.

10. Klein L, Heiple KG, Torzilli PA, et al. Prevention of ligament and meniscus atrophy by active joint motion in a non-weight bearing model. J Orthop Res 1989;7:80–85.

11. Buckwalter JA, Woo SL. Effects of repetitive loading and motion on the musculoskeletal tissues. In: DeLee JC, Drez D, eds. Orthopaedic sports medicine. Philadelphia: WB Saunders, 1994:60–72.

12. Irrgang JJ. Modern trends in anterior cruciate ligament rehabilitation: nonoperative and postoperative management. Clin Sports Med 1993;12:797–813.

13. Garrett WE. Muscle strain injuries: clinical and basic science aspects. Med Sci Sports Exerc 1990;22:436–443.

14. Garrett WE, Safran MR, Seaber AV, et al. Biomechanical comparison of stimulated and nonstimulated skeletal muscle pulled to failure. Am J Sports Med 1987;15:448–454.

15. Hasselman CT, Best TM, Seaber AV, et al. A threshold and continuum of injury during active stretch of rabbit skeletal muscle. Am J Sports Med 1995;23:65–73.

16. Hawary RE, Stanish WD, Curwin SL. Rehabilitation of tendon injuries in sports. Sports Med 1997;24:347–358.

17. Booth FW. Time course of muscular atrophy during immobilization of hindlimbs in rats. Environ Exerc Physiol 1977;43:656–661.

18. Bassett FH, Kirkpatrick JS, Engelhardt DL, et al. Cryotherapy-induced nerve injury. Am J Sports Med 1992;20:516–518.

19. Tornkvist H, Lindholm TS, Netz P, et al. Effect of ibuprofen and indomethacin on bone metabolism reflected in bone stength. Clin Orthop Rel Res 1984;187:255–259.

20. Ro J, Sudmann E, Martin PF. Effect of indomethacin on fracture healing in rats. Acta Orthop Scand 1976;47:588–599.

21. Carlstedt C, Madsen K, Wredmark T. The influence of indomethacin on tendon healing: a biomechanical and biochemical study. Arch Orthop Trauma Surg 1986;105:332–336.

22. Vogel HG. Mechanical and chemical properties of various connective tissue organs in rats as influenced by non-steroidal antirheumatic drugs. Connec Tissue Res 1977;5:91–95.

23. Dahners LE, Gilbert JA, Lester GE, et al. The effect of a nonsteroidal antiinflammatory drug on the healing of ligaments. Am J Sports Med 1988;16:641–646.

24. Almekinders LC, Baynes AJ, Bracey LW. An in vitro investigation into the effects of repetitive motion and nonsteroidal antiinflammatory medication on human tendon fibroblasts. Am J Sports Med 1995;23:119–123.

25. Obremsky WT, Seaber AV, Ribbeck BM, et al. Biomechanical and histologic assessment of a controlled muscle strain injury treated with piroxicam. Am J Sports Med 1994;22:558–561.

26. Mishra DK, Friden J, Schmitz MC, et al. Anti-inflammatory medication after muscle injury. J Bone Joint Surg (Am) 1995;77A:1510–1519.

27. Almekinders LC. Anti-inflammatory treatment of muscular injuries in sports. Sports Medicine 1993;15:139–145.

28. Belch JJF. Eicosanoids and rheumatology: inflammatory and vascular aspects. Prostaglandins Leukotrienes and Essential Fatty Acids: Reviews 1989;36:219–234.

29. Lereim P, Gabor I. Piroxicam and naproxen in acute sports injuries. Am J Med 1988;84:45–49.

30. Buckwalter JA, Woo SL. Tissue effects of medications in sports injuries. In: DeLee JC, Drez D, eds. Orthopaedic sports medicine. Philadelphia: WB Saunders, 1994:73–79.

31. Mankin HJ, Conger KA. The acute effects of intra-articular hydrocortisone on articular cartilage in rabbits. J Bone Joint Surg Am 1966;48-A:1383–1388.

32. Schaubel HJ. The local use of ice after orthopedic procedures. Am J Surg 1946;72:711–714.

33. Basur RL, Shephard E, Mouzas GL. A cooling method in the

treatment of ankle sprains. Practitioner 1976;216:708–711.

34. Lehmann JF, DeLateur BJ. Therapeutic heat. In: Lehman JF, ed. Therapeutic heat and cold. Baltimore: Williams and Wilkins, 1990:417–581.

35. McMaster WC, Liddle S. Cryotherapy influence on posttraumatic limb edema. Clin Orthop Rel Res 1980;150:283–287.

36. Matsen FA, Questad K, Matsen AL. The effect of local cooling on postfracture swelling: a controlled study. Clin Orthop Rel Res 1975; 109:201–206.

37. Melzack R, Wall PD. Pain mechanisms: a new theory. Science 1965;150:971–979.

38. Bini G, Cruccu G, Hagbarth KE, et al. Analgesic effect of vibration and cooling on pain induced by intraneural electrical stimulation. Pain 1984;18:239–248.

39. Lehmann JF, DeLateur BJ. Diathermy and superficial heat, laser, and cold therapy. In: Kottke FJ, Lehman JF, eds. Krusen's handbook of physical medicine and rehabilitation. Philadelphia: WB Saunders, 1990:283–367.

40. Lehmann J, Massock A, Warren C, et al. Effect of therapeutic temperatures on tendon extensibility. Arch Phys Med Rehabil 1970;51:481–487.

41. Gersten J. Effect of ultrasound on tendon extensibility. Am J Phys Med Rehabil 1955;34:362–369.

42. Ottoson D. The effects of temperature on the isolated muscle spindle. J Physiol 1965;180: 636–648.

43. Mense S. Effect of temperature on the discharges of muscle spindles and tendon organs. Pflugers Archives 1978;374:159–166.

44. Safran MR, Garrett WE, Seaber AV, et al. The role of warmup in muscular injury prevention. Am J Sports Med 1988;16:123–129.

45. Irrgang JJ, Sawhney R. Rehabilitation for childhood and adolescent orthopaedic sports-related injuries. In: Stanitski CL, DeLee JC, and Drez D, eds. Pediatric and adolescent sports medicine. Philadelphia: WB Saunders, 1994:498–519.

46. Vaughen JL, Bender LF. Effects of ultrasound on growing bone. Arch Phys Med Rehabil 1959; 40:158–160.

47. Lehmann JF, Brunner GD, Martinis AJ, et al. Ultrasonic effects as demonstrated in live pigs with surgical metallic implants. Arch Phys Med Rehabil 1959;40:483–488.

48. Lehmann JF, Lane KE, Bell JW, et al. Influence of surgical metal implants on the distribution of the intensity in the ultrasonic field. Arch Phys Med Rehabil 1958;39:756–760.

49. Havorson GA. Therapeutic heat and cold for athletic injuries. Phys Sports Med 1990;18:87–94.

50. Lehmann JF, Silverman DR, Baum BA, et al. Temperature distributions in the human thigh produced by infrared, hot pack, and microwave applications. Arch Phys Med Rehabil 1966;47:291–298.

51. Lehmann JF, McMillon J, Brunner GD, et al. Comparative study of the efficiency of short-wave, microwave, and ultrasound diathermy in heating the hip joint. Arch Phys Med Rehabil 1959;38:510–512.

52. Lehmann JF, DeLateur BJ, Warren CG, et al. Heating produced by ultrasound in bone and soft tissue. Arch Phys Med Rehabil 1967;48:397–401.

53. Heckman JD, Ryaby JP, McCabe J, et al. Acceleration of tibial fracture-healing by non-invasive, low-intensity pulsed ultrasound. J Bone Joint Surg Am 1994;76A: 26–34.

54. Kristiansen TK, Ryaby JP, McCabe J, et al. Accelerated healing of distal radial fractures with the use of specific low-intensity ultrasound. J Bone Joint Surg Am 1997;79A:961–973.

55. Lehmann JF, Herrick JF. Biologic reactions to cavitation, a consideration for ultrasonic therapy. Arch Phys Med Rehabil 1953; 34:86–98.

56. Dyson M. Non-thermal cellular effects of ultrasound. Br J Cancer 1982;45:165–171.

57. Cox JS. Heat modalities. In: DeLee JC, Drez D, eds. Orthopaedic sports medicine principles and practice. Philadelphia: WB Saunders, 1994:208–212.

58. Oziomek RS, Perrin DH, Herold DA, et al. Effect of phonophoresis on serum salicylate levels. Med Sci Sports Exerc 1991;23: 397–401.

59. Muir WS, Magee FP, Longo JA, et al. Comparison of ultrasonically applied vs. intra-articular injected hydrocortisone levels in canine knees. Orthop Rev 1990;19: 351–356.

60. Bare AC, McAnaw MB, Pritchard AE, et al. Phonophoretic delivery of 10% hydrocortisone through the epidermis of humans as determined by serum cortisol concentrations. Phys Ther 1996; 76:738–749.

61. Almay BGL, Johansson F, Knorring LV, et al. Long-term high frequency transcutaneous electrical nerve stimulation (hi-TENS) in chronic pain: clinical response and effects on CSF-endorphins, monoamine metabolites, substance P–like immunoreactivity (SPLI) and pain measures. J Psychosomat Res 1985;29:247–257.

62. Hughes GS, Lichstein PR, Whitlock D, et al. Response of plasma beta-endorphins to transcutaneous electrical nerve stimulation in healthy subjects. Phys Ther 1984;64:1062–1066.

63. Basford JR. Electrical therapy. In: Kottke FJ, Lehmann JF, eds. Krusen's handbook of physical medicine and rehabilitation. Philadelphia: WB Saunders, 1990:375–401.

64. Smith MJ, Hutchins RC, Hehenberger D. Transcutaneous neural stimulation use in postoperative knee rehabilitation. Am J Sports Med 1983;11:75–82.

65. Arvidsson I, Eriksson E. Postoperative TENS pain relief after knee surgery. Orthopedics 1986;9: 1346–1351.

66. Jensen JE, Conn RR, Hazelrigg G, et al. The use of transcutaneous neural stimulation and isokinetic testing in arthroscopic knee surgery. Am J Sports Med 1985;13:27–33.

67. Jensen JE, Etheridge GL, Hazelrigg G. Effectiveness of transcutaneous electrical neural stimulation in the treatment of pain: recommendations for use in the treatment of sports injuries. Sports Med 1986;3:79–88.

68. Laughman RK, Youdas JW, Garrett TR, et al. Strength changes in the normal quadriceps femoris muscle as a result of electrical stimulation. Phys Ther 1983;63:494–499.

69. McMiken DF, Todd-Smith M, Thompson C. Strengthening of human quadriceps muscles by cutaneous electrical stimulation. Scand J Rehab Med 1983;15: 25–28.

70. Currier DP, Mann R. Muscular strength development by electrical stimulation in healthy individuals. Phys Ther 1983;63:915–921.

71. Walmsley RP, Letts G, Vooys J. A comparison of torque generated by knee extension with a maximal voluntary muscle contraction vis-a-vis electrical stimulation. J Orthop Sports Phys Ther 1984;6: 10–17.

72. Owens J, Malone T. Treatment parameters of high frequency electrical stimulation as established on the electro-stim 180. J Orthop Sports Phys Ther 1983; 4:162–168.

73. Wigerstad-Lossing I, Grimby G, Jonsson T, et al. Effects of electrical muscle stimulation combined with voluntary contractions after knee ligament surgery. Med Sci Sports Exerc 1988;20:93–98.

74. Morrissey MC, Brewster CE, Shields CL, et al. The effects of electrical stimulation on the quadriceps during postoperative knee immobilization. Am J Sports Med 1985;13:40–45.

75. Gould N, Donnermeyer D, Gammon GG, et al. Transcutaneous muscle stimulation to retard disuse atrophy after open meniscectomy. Clin Orthop Rel Res 1983;178:190–197.

76. Stanish WD, Valiant GA, Bonen A, et al. The effects of immobilization and of electrical stimulation on muscle glycogen and myofibrillar ATPase. Can J Appl Spt Sci 1982;7:267–271.

77. Singer KM. Electrical stimulation in sports medicine. In: DeLee JC, Drez D, eds. Orthopaedic sports medicine: principles and practice. Philadelphia: WB Saunders, 1994:213–227.

78. Clemente FR, Matulionis DH, Barron KW, et al. Effect of motor neuromuscular electrical stimulation on microvascular perfusion of stimulated rat skeletal muscle. Phys Ther 1991;71: 397–406.

79. Reed BV. Effect of high voltage pulsed electrical stimulation on microvascular permeability to plasma proteins: a possible mechanism in minimizing edema. Phys Ther 1988;68:491–495.

80. Chantraine A, Ludy JP, Berger D. Is cortisone iontophoresis possible? Arch Phys Med Rehabil 1986;67:38–40.

81. Anderson B, Burke ER. Scientific, medical, and practical aspects of stretching. Clin Sports Med 1991;10:63–86.

82. Corbin CB. Flexibility. Clin Sports Med 1984;3:101–117.

83. Gajdosik RL. Flexibility or muscle length? Phys Ther 1995;75:238–239.

84. Taylor D, Dalton J, Seaber A, et al. Viscoelastic properties of muscle-tendon units: the biomechanical effects of stretching. Am J Sports Med 1990;18:300–309.

85. Smith AD, Stroud L, McQueen C. Flexibility and anterior knee pain in adolescent elite figure skaters. J Pediatr Orthoped 1991;11:77–82.

86. Stroud L, Smith AD, Kruse R. The relationship between increased femoral anteversion in childhood and anterior knee pain in adulthood. Orthop Transact 1989;13:554.

87. Lysens RJ, Ostyn MS, Auweele YV, et al. The accident-prone and overuse-prone profiles of the young athlete. Am J Sports Med 1989;17:612–619.

88. Knapik JJ, Bauman CL, Jones BH, et al. Preseason strength and flexibility imbalances associated with athletic injuries in female collegiate athletes. Am J Sports Med 1991;19:76–81.

89. Krivickas LS, Feinberg JH. Lower extremity injuries in college athletes: relation between ligamentous laxity and lower extremity muscle tightness. Arch Phys Med Rehabil 1996;77:1139–1143.

90. Shellock FG, Prentice WE. Warming-up and stretching for improved physical performance and prevention of sports-related injuries. Sports Med 1985;2: 267–278.

91. Voss D. Proprioceptive neuromuscular facilitation: patterns and techniques. 3rd ed. Philadelphia: Harper, 1985.

92. Lucas RC, Koslow R. Comparative study of static, dynamic, and proprioceptive neuromuscular facilitation stretching techniques on flexibility. Percep Motor Skills 1984;58:615–618.

93. Sady SS, Wortman M, Blanke D. Flexibility training: ballistic, static, or proprioceptive neuromuscular facilitation? Arch Phys Med Rehabil 1982;63:261–263.

94. Wallin D, Ekblom B, Grahn R, et al. Improvement of muscle flexibility: a comparison between two techniques. Am J Sports Med 1985;13:263–268.

95. Etnyre BR, Lee EJ. Chronic and acute flexibility of men and women using three different stretching techniques. Res Quar Exerc Sport 1988;59:222–228.

96. Godges JJ, MacRae H, Longdon C, et al. The effects of two stretching procedures on hip

range of motion and gait economy. J Orthop Sports Phys Ther 1989;10:350–357.

97. Moore MA, Hutton RS. Electromyographic investigation of muscle stretching techniques. Med Sci Sports Exerc 1980;12:322–329.

98. Bandy WD, Irion JM. The effect of time of static stretch on the flexibility of hamstring muscles. Phys Ther 1994;74:845–852.

99. Hellebrandt FA, Waterland JC. Indirect learning: the influence of unimanual exercise on related muscle groups of the same and the opposite side. Am J Phys Med Rehabil 1962;41:45–55.

100. Hellebrandt FA, Parrish AM, Houtz SJ. Cross education—the influence of unilateral exercise on the contralateral limb. Arch Phys Med Rehabil 1947;28:76–85.

101. Young JL, Press JM. The physiologic basis of sports rehabilitation. Phys Med Rehab Clin 1994; 5:9–36.

102. Pipes TV, Wilmore JH. Isokinetic vs. isotonic strength training in adult men. Med Sci Sports Exerc 1975;7:262–274.

103. Friden J, Sjostrom M, Ekblom B. Myofibrillar damage following intense ecentric exercise in man. Int J Sports Med 1983;4:170–176.

104. Knuttgen HG, Petersen FB, Klausen K. Oxygen uptake and heart rate responses to exercise performed with concentric and eccentric muscle contractions. Med Sci Sports Exerc 1971;3:1–5.

105. Komi PV, Buskirk ER. Effect of eccentric and concentric muscle conditioning on tension and electrical activity of human muscle. Ergonomics 1972;15:417–434.

106. Paulos LE, Grauer JD. Exercise. In: DeLee JC, Drez D, eds. Orthopaedic sports medicine principles and practice. Philadelphia: WB Saunders, 1994:228–243.

107. Yack HJ, Collins CE, Whieldon TJ. Comparison of closed and open kinetic chain exercise in the anterior cruciate ligament-deficient knee. Am J Sports Med 1993;21:49–54.

108. Lutz GE, Palmitier RA, An KA, et al. Comparison of tibiofemoral joint forces during open-kinetic-chain and closed-kinetic-chain exercises. J Bone Joint Surg Am 1993;75A:732–739.

109. Stuart MJ, Meglan DA, Lutz GE, et al. Comparison of intersegmental tibiofemoral joint forces and muscle activity during various closed kinetic chain exercises. Am J Sports Med 1996;24:792–799.

110. Palmitier RA, An K-N, Scott SG, et al. Kinetic chain exercise in knee rehabilitation. Sports Med 1991;11:402–413.

111. Rosentsweig J, Hinson M, Ridgway M. An electromyographic comparison of an isokinetic bench press performed at three speeds. Res Q 1975;46:471–475.

112. Moffroid MT, Whipple RH. Specificity of speed of exercise. Phys Ther 1970;50:1692–1700.

113. Scudder GN. Torque curves produced at the knee during isometric and isokinetic exercises. Arch Phys Med Rehabil 1980;61:68–73.

114. Rasch PJ, Morehouse LE. Effect of static and dynamic exercises on muscular strength and hypertrophy. J Appl Physiol 1957;11:29–34.

115. Lesmes GR, Costill DL, Coyle EF, et al. Muscle strength and power changes during maximal isokinetic training. Med Sci Sports Exerc 1978;10:266–269.

116. Coyle EF, Feiring DC, Rotkis TC, et al. Specificity of power improvements through slow and fast isokinetic training. J Appl Physiol 1981;51:1437–1442.

117. DeLorme TL. Restoration of muscle power by heavy resistance exercise. J Bone Joint Surg Am 1945;27:645–667.

118. DeLorme TL, Watkins AL. Technics of progressive resistive exercise. Arch Phys Med Rehabil 1948;29:263–273.

119. Lephart SM, Pincivero DM, Giraldo JL, et al. The role of proprioception in the management and rehabilitation of athletic injuries. Am J Sports Med 1997; 25:130–137.

120. Skinner HB, Barrack RL, Cook SD. Age-related decline in proprioception. Clin Orthoped 1984; 184:208–211.

121. Barrett DS, Cobb AG, Bentley G. Joint proprioception in normal, osteoarthritic and replaced knees. J Bone Joint Surg 1991;73B:53–56.

122. Barrack RL, Skinner HB, Cook SD, et al. Effect of articular disease and total knee arthroplasty on knee joint-position sense. J Neurophysiol 1983;50:684–687.

123. Sharma L, Pai Y-C, Holtkamp K, et al. Is knee joint proprioception worse in the arthritic knee versus the unaffected knee in unilateral knee osteoarthritis? Arthritis Rheumatism 1997;40:1518–1525.

124. Freeman MAR, Dean M, Hanham I. The etiology and prevention of functional instability of the foot. J Bone Joint Surg 1965;47B:669–677.

125. Lofvenberg R, Karrholm J, Sundelin G, et al. Prolonged reaction time in patients with chronic lateral instability of the ankle. Am J Sports Med 1995; 23:414–417.

126. Sheth P, Yu B, Laskowski ER, et al. Ankle disk training influences reaction times of selected muscles in a simulated ankle sprain. Am J Sports Med 1997; 25:538–543.

127. Konradsen L, Ravn JB, Sorensen AI. Proprioception at the ankle: the effect of anaesthetic blockade of ligament receptors. J Bone Joint Surg Br 1993;75B:433–436.

128. Schultz RA, Miller DC, Kerr CS, et al. Mechanoreceptors in human cruciate ligaments: a his-

tologic study. J Bone Joint Surg Am 1984;66-A:1072–1076.

129. Haus J, Halata Z. Innervation of the anterior cruciate ligament. Int Orthop 1990;14:293–296.

130. Johansson H, Sjolander P, Sojka P. A sensory role for the cruciate ligaments. Clin Orthop 1991; 268:161–178.

131. Barrack RL, Skinner HB, Buckley SL. Proprioception in the anterior cruciate deficient knee. Am J Sports Med 1989;17:1–6.

132. Corrigan JP, Cashmen WF, Brady MP. Proprioception in the cruciate deficient knee. J Bone Joint Surg 1992;74-B:247–250.

133. Borsa PA, Lephart SM, Irrgang JJ, et al. The effects of joint position and direction of joint motion on proprioception sensibility in anterior cruciate ligament-deficient athletes. Am J Sports Med 1997;25:336–340.

134. Synder-Mackler L. Scientific rationale and physiological basis for the use of closed kinetic chain exercise in the lower extremity. J Sport Rehabil 1996; 5:2–12.

135. Beard DJ, Kyberd PJ, Fergusson CM, et al. Proprioception after rupture of the anterior cruciate ligament: an objective indication of the need for surgery? J Bone Joint Surg Br 1993;75-B:311–315.

136. Wojtys E, Huston LJ. Neuromuscular performance in normal and anterior cruciate ligament-deficient lower extremities. Am J Sports Med 1994;22:89–104.

137. Jennings AG, Seedhom BB. Proprioception in the knee and reflex hamstring contraction latency. J Bone Joint Surg Br 1994;76-B: 491–494.

138. Beard DJ, Dodd CAF, Trundle HR, et al. Proprioception enhancement for anterior cruciate ligament deficiency. J Bone Joint Surg Br 1994;76-B:654–659.

139. Lephart SM, Warner JP, Borsa PA, et al. Proprioception of the shoulder in normal, unstable, and post-

surgical individuals. J Shoulder Elbow Surg 1994;3:371–380.

140. Borsa PA, Lephart SM, Kocher MS, et al. Functional assessment and rehabilitation of shoulder proprioception for glenohumeral instability. J Sports Rehab 1994; 3:84–104.

141. Feuerbach JW. Effect of an ankle orthosis and ankle ligament anesthesia an ankle joint proprioception. Am J Sports Med 1994;22: 223–229.

142. Perlau R, Frank C, Fick G. The effects of elastic bandages on human knee proprioception in the uninjured population. Am J Sports Med 1995;23:251–255.

143. McNair PJ, Stanley SN, Strauss GR. Knee bracing: effects of proprioception. Arch Phys Med Rehabil 1996;77:287–289.

144. Barrett DS. Proprioception and function after anterior cruciate reconstruction. J Bone Joint Surg Br 1991;73-B:833–837.

145. Wojtys EM, Wylie BB, Huston LJ. The effects of muscle fatigue on neuromuscular function and anterior tibial translation in healthy knees. Am J Sports Med 1996; 24:615–621.

146. Scovazzo ML, Browne A, Pink M, et al. The painful shoulder during freestyle swimming: an electromyographic cinematographic analysis of twelve muscles. Am J Sports Med 1991;19:577–582.

147. Sepulchre P, Blaimont P, Pasteels J. Douleurs tibiales internez chez les coureurs a pied. Inter Orthop 1988;12:217–221.

148. Sharkey NA, Ferris L, Smith TS, et al. Strain and loading of the second metatarsal during heel-lift. J Bone Joint Surg Am 1995; 77A:1050–1057.

149. Mair SD, Seaber AV, Glisson RR, et al. The role of fatigue in susceptibility to acute muscle strain injury. Am J Sports Med 1996; 24:137–143.

150. Steadman JR. Rehabilitation after knee ligament surgery. Am J Sports Med 1980;8:294–296.

151. Klausen K, Andersen LB, Pelle I. Adaptive changes in work capacity, skeletal muscle capillarization, and enzyme levels during training and detraining. Acta Physiol Scand 1981;113:9–16.

152. Henrikssson J, Reitman JS. Time course of changes in human skeletal muscle succinate dehydrogenase and cytochrome oxidase activities and maximal oxygen uptake with physical activity and inactivity. Acta Physiol Scand 1977;99:91–97.

153. Madsen K, Pedersen PK, Djurhuus MS, et al. Effects of detraining on endurance capacity and metabolic changes during prolonged exhaustive exercise. J Appl Physiol 1993;75:1444–1451.

154. Coyle EF, Martin WH, Bloomfield SA, et al. Effects of detraining on responses to submaximal exercise. J Appl Physiol 1985;59: 853–859.

155. Responses and long term adaptations to exercise: physical activity and health: a report of the Surgeon General. Atlanta: U.S. Dept. of Health and Human Services, 1996:61–80.

156. Latin RW. Preseason conditioning: aerobic power. In: Mellion MB, Walsh WM, and Shelton GL, eds. The team physician's handbook. Philadelphia: Hanley and Belfus, 1990:27–33.

157. Medbo JI, Burgers S. Effect of training on the anaerobic capacity. Med Sci Sports Exerc 1990; 22:501–507.

158. Tabata I, Nishimura K, Kouzaki M, et al. Effects of moderate-intensity endurance and high-intensity intermittent training on anaerobic capacity and Vo_2max. Med Sci Sports Exerc 1996;28: 1327–1330.

159. Greene TA, Hillman SK. Comparison of support provided by a semirigid orthosis and adhesive ankle taping before, during, and after exercise. Am J Sports Med 1990;18:498–506.

160. Burks RT, Bean BG, Marcus R, et al. Analysis of athletic perfor-

mance with prophylactic ankle devices. Am J Sports Med 1991; 19:104–106.

161. Pienkowski D, McMorrow M, Shapiro R, et al. The effect of ankle stabilizers on athletic performance: a randomized prospective study. Am J Sports Med 1995;23:757–762.

162. Surve I, Schwellnus MP, Noakes T, et al. A fivefold reduction in the incidence of recurrent ankle sprains in soccer players using the sport-stirrup orthosis. Am J Sports Med 1994;22: 601–606.

163. Sitler M, Ryan J, Wheeler B, et al. The efficacy of a semirigid ankle stabilizer to reduce acute ankle injuries in basketball. Am J Sports Med 1994;22:454–461.

164. Ashton-Miller JA, Ottaviani RA, Hutchinson C, et al. What best protects the inverted weightbearing ankle against further inversion? Evertor muscle strength compares favorably with shoe height, athletic tape, and three orthoses. Am J Sports Med 1996;24:800–809.

165. Black KP, Raasch WG. Knee braces in sports. In: Nicholas JA, Hershman EB, eds. The lower extremity and spine in sports medicine. St. Louis: CV Mosby, 1995:987–998.

166. Millet CW, Drez D. Knee braces. In: DeLee JC, Drez D, eds. Orthopaedic sports medicine: principles and practice. Philadelphia: WB Saunders, 1994:1468–1474.

167. Cawley PW, France P, Paulos LE. Comparison of rehabilitative knee braces: a biomechanical investigation. Am J Sports Med 1989; 17:141–146.

168. Cawley PW, France EP, Paulos LE. The current state of functional knee bracing research: a review of the literature. Am J Sports Med 1991;19:226–233.

169. Liu SH, Mirzayan R. Current review: functional knee bracing. Clin Orthop Rel Res 1995;317: 273–281.

170. Beynnon BD, Pope MH, Wertheimer CM, et al. The effect of functional knee braces on strain on the anterior cruciate ligament in vivo. J Bone Joint Surg Am 1992;74A:1298–1312.

171. DeVita P, Hunter PB, Skelly WA. Effects of a functional knee brace on the biomechanics of running. Med Sci Sports Exerc 1992;24:797–806.

172. Branch TP, Hunter R, Donath M. Dynamic EMG analysis of anterior cruciate deficient legs with and without bracing during cutting. Am J Sports Med 1989;17:35–41.

173. Highgenboten CL, Jackson A, Meske N, et al. The effects of knee brace wear on perceptual and metabolic variables during horizontal treadmill running. Am J Sports Med 1991;19:639–643.

174. Wojtys EM, Kothari SU, Huston LJ. Anterior cruciate ligament functional brace use in sports. Am J Sports Med 1996;24:539–546.

175. Styf JR, Lundin O, Gershuni DH. Effects of a functional knee brace on leg muscle function. Am J Sports Med 1994;22:830–834.

176. Mishra DK, Daniel DM, Stone ML. The use of functional knee braces in the control of pathologic anterior knee laxity. Clin Orthop Rel Res 1989;241:213–220.

177. McConnell JS. The management of chondromalacia patella; the long-term solution. Austr J Phys 1986;32:215–223.

178. Larsen B, Andreasen E, Urfer A, et al. Patellar taping: a radiographic examination of the medial glide technique. Am J Sports Med 1995;23:465–471.

179. Bockrath K, Wooden C, Worrell T, et al. Effects of patella taping on patella position and perceived pain. Med Sci Sports Exerc 1993;25:989–992.

180. Lysholm J, Nordin M, Ekstrand J, et al. The effect of a patella

brace on performance in a knee extension strength test in patients with patellar pain. Am J Sports Med 1984;12:110–112.

181. Kowall MG, Kolk G, Nuber GW, et al. Patellar taping in the treatment of patellofemoral pain: a prospective randomized study. Am J Sports Med 1996; 24:61–66.

182. Palumbo PM. Dynamic patellar brace: a new orthosis in the management of patellofemoral disorders. Am J Sports Med 1981;9: 45–49.

183. Greenwald AE, Bagley AM, France EP, et al. A biomechanical and clinical evaluation of a patellofemoral knee brace. Clin Orthop Rel Res 1996;324:187–195.

184. Kilmartin TE, Wallace WA. The scientific basis for the use of biomechanical foot orthoses in the treatment of lower limb sports injuries: a review of the literature. Br J Sports Med 1994;28: 180–184.

185. Smith LS, Clarke TE, Hamill CL. The effects of soft and semirigid orthoses upon rearfoot movement on running. J Am Podiatr Med Assoc 1986;76: 227–233.

186. James SL, Bates BT, Osternig LR. Injuries to runners. Am J Sports Med 1978;6:40–50.

187. Frey C. Footwear and stress fractures. Clin Sports Med 1997;16: 249–257.

188. Clanton TO. Etiology of injury to the foot and ankle. In: DeLee JC, Drez D, eds. Orthopaedic sports medicine: principles and practice. Philadelphia: WB Saunders, 1994:1642–1704.

189. Krivickas LS. Anatomical factors associated with overuse sports injuries. Sports Med 1997;24: 132–146.

190. Taunton JE, McKenzie DC, Clement DB. The role of biomechanics in the epidemiology of injuries. Sports Med 1988;6: 107–120.

191. Cantu RC, Mueller FO. Catastrophic spine injuries in football. J Spinal Disord 1990;3:227–231.

192. Silver JR, Gill S. Injuries of the spine sustained during rugby. Sports Med 1988;5:328–334.

193. Quirk R. Common foot and ankle injuries in dance. Orthop Clin N Amer 1994;25:123–133.

194. Saal JA. Rehabilitation of the injured athlete. In: DeLisa JA, ed. Rehabilitation medicine: principles and practice. Philadelphia: JB Lippincott, 1993: 1131–1164.

Chapter 20

Osteoporosis and Exercise

Barbara L. Drinkwater

A recent Roper poll found that 88% of the women surveyed believed that exercise prevented osteoporosis. When asked about the most effective treatment for osteoporosis, 87% voted again for exercise. While it is true that physical activity has an important role to play in decreasing the risk of osteoporotic fractures later in life, there is no evidence that exercise—or even exercise plus calcium—can completely prevent the accelerated bone loss that occurs in the early postmenopausal years. When studies first appeared describing the beneficial effects of exercise on bone, there was some hope that weight-bearing physical activity could indeed prevent the bone loss that leads to osteoporotic fractures. Over the years, that optimism has waned as study after study has reported minimal improvement in the bone mineral density (BMD) of postmenopausal women following 12 to 24 months of an exercise protocol. Many scientists studying osteoporosis have concluded that the main benefit of exercise for older women relates more to keeping them active, avoiding the bone loss that would occur if they were sedentary, and decreasing the risk of falling by improving muscular strength, balance, coordination, and flexibility, thereby decreasing the risk of a hip fracture (4,14).

Osteoporosis has been thought of as a woman's disease for so long that there is very little useful information available about the role of exercise is preventing or delaying bone loss in men. Yet men also are at risk for osteoporotic fractures. More than 2 million men in the United States may have osteoporosis now and more than 3 million men are at future risk of the disease. Although fewer men than women experience hip fractures, the mortality rate in men in the first 6 months after fracture is almost twice that of women (18). Risk factors for men are the same as those for women with one exception—men do not have an abrupt decrease in testos-terone levels similar to the decrease in estrogen that women experience at menopause. While many women have inadequate knowledge about how to prevent osteoporosis, the majority of men do not recognize that they are at risk, do not understand the consequences of the disease, and do not know how it can be prevented.

OSTEOPENIA AND OSTEOPOROSIS DEFINED

The World Health Organization has established a standard for evaluating the results of bone density tests, i.e., dual energy x-ray absorptiometry (DXA) scans, based on the values for healthy young adults. Women whose BMD falls above 1.0 SD below the young normal mean have a normal bone density. Those who are between −1.0 and −2.5 SD below the young normal mean are defined as osteopenic. When BMD is more than 2.5 SD below the young normal mean, the diagnosis is osteoporosis, or severe osteoporosis if a fracture has already occurred. Rather than use the term *standard deviation*, the distance of the BMD from the mean is expressed as a T score. In most DXA databases, a difference of one SD represents a 10% to 11% change in BMD. Many postmenopausal women have already experienced moderate to severe bone loss and fall within the osteopenic or osteoporotic categories. The average increase in BMD in prospective exercise studies is simply not enough to raise the BMD of most women in these categories to normal, although even a slight increase in BMD is better than continuing to lose bone. What is seldom stated in these studies, however, is that the gain in BMD quickly disappears unless the woman continues to exercise at the same level of intensity.

A number of new devices designed to measure BMD at

peripheral sites, primarily the forearm, finger, and calcaneus, are now on the market. Smaller and less expensive than the table DXA machines, they are used primarily as a screening tool and are especially useful in rural areas, where access to the standard DXA is limited. However, using them with athletes can be problematic. Nattrass et al (21) have found that the site-specific loading of some sports can result in misleading results. Masters runners, for example, on average have a positive T score at the calcaneus and a negative T score at the lumbar vertebrae, radius, finger, and proximal femur. In contrast, masters rowers have a positive T score at the finger and proximal radius and negative T scores at the calcaneus, lumbar vertebrae, and proximal femur. T scores at peripheral sites in women masters athletes may reflect the bone loading characteristics of their sport rather than their risk for osteoporosis.

THE ROLE OF EXERCISE

It is important to understand how physical activity affects bone, the effect of age on the response of bone to exercise, and the interaction of exercise, nutrition, and hormones in ensuring bone health. For 44% of the women in the Roper study, the source of information about osteoporosis was the media, whose expertise to evaluate research in the exercise and bone field is questionable. When exercise is used as an experimental variable, the design and protocol of the studies must be evaluated as carefully as those of clinical trials of pharmaceutical agents. For example, results from exercise studies that did not randomize subjects, allowing them instead to select either the exercise or control group, could have led to biased and erroneous conclusions. Other studies have failed to quantify the exercise protocol, had small sample sizes with inadequate power to detect significant differences, used activities that did not stress the skeletal site where BMD was measured, failed to report compliance, and ignored confounding variables such as age, weight, nutrition, menstrual cycle irregularities, and use of oral contraceptives (6).

All exercise is not equal. Forty-nine percent of the

women in the Roper poll identified walking as the best exercise to build bone, and 75% of those who do exercise named walking as their primary source of activity. While there is no doubt that an aerobic activity such as walking is essential for good health, the activity must produce an internal strain within bone that exceeds its usual range to be an osteogenic stimulus (10,25). Walking is walking. Whether from room to room within the house or outside around the block, there is no difference in the mechanical loading on the skeleton and therefore no stimulus to increase bone mass. A number of physical activities labeled "exercise" do not exceed the threshold level for stimulating bone formation. Swimming, for example, is both an exercise and a sport, but competitive swimmers usually have bone densities similar to or even lower than nonathletes (23), presumably because they exercise in a weightless environment. On the other hand, some forms of manual labor do load specific skeletal sites beyond their customary range, even though the activity is not considered exercise per se. It is the load on the bone, not the specific activity, that provides the osteogenic stimulus. The results of the Roper poll suggest that women do not know what type of activity is most beneficial for their bones (Figure 20-1).

For most older women, remaining physically active does not increase BMD but does prevent the bone loss that occurs inevitably if they become inactive. Women should not be discouraged from walking for exercise. It is an excellent overall activity, particularly for older women. The woman who goes out for a brisk walk three or four times a week may not increase her bone mass, but the overall benefit to a number of physiologic systems will help her remain active as she ages and avoid the bone loss that would occur if she were to become sedentary. However, believing that exercise can prevent osteoporosis may lead many women to avoid therapies that have been proven to prevent postmenopausal bone loss.

Is Osteoporosis a Pediatric Disease?

At the same time that confidence in the ability of exercise to increase bone density in older women is declining, there is increased interest in factors that determine peak bone mass

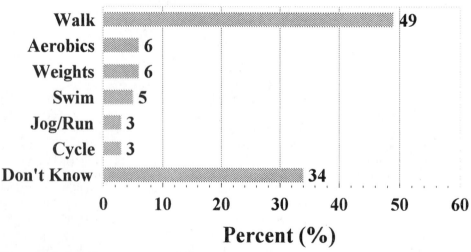

Figure 20-1 Activities women aged 50 and older believe are most effective in building bone.

during childhood and adolescence and, in particular, the role of exercise in enabling children and adolescents to maximize their peak bone mass. Bailey and Martin (2) were among the first to explore how physical activity affects bone within this "window of opportunity." Their results and those of other investigators suggest that the developing skeleton responds more readily to mechanical loading, not only by increasing BMD but by developing a bone structure more resistant to fracture. Physicians are an important conduit for educating parents about the importance of physical activity for their children during these critical years.

Does Exercise Prevent Bone Loss in Adult Women and Men?

For adult women and men, ages 20 to 50, the challenge is to maintain their peak bone mass. While athletes of both sexes usually have significantly higher bone density than nonathletes, it is difficult to find similar differences between active and sedentary women in the third decade. Mazess et al (19) divided college women into quartiles of activity level; measured BMD at the spine, femoral neck, and radius; and found no differences in BMD related to the quartile of activity level at any site. Similar results were reported for young Finnish women by Heinonen et al (13). Results such as these demonstrate once again that activity per se is not sufficient to markedly increase bone density. Even among athletes, a higher BMD is found only at those skeletal sites specifically loaded by the sport (9,11,12). Mechanical or gravitational loading of the skeleton, not cardiovascular fitness, determines bone health.

However, if men and women remain active throughout adult life they can expect to have a higher BMD at any age than those who choose a sedentary lifestyle (1,24). This does not mean they can disregard other factors that influence bone mass. For women, the concept of a three-legged stool—legs representing exercise, calcium, and estrogen—and the question, "Which leg is unnecessary if we want to keep the stool standing?" emphasizes the point that an absence of any one factor can have a detrimental effect on bone.

Does Exercise Prevent Postmenopausal Bone Loss?

Researchers whose studies appear to show an increase in BMD in postmenopausal women have uniformly selected sedentary women not on hormone replacement therapy (HRT) as subjects. Baseline BMD in these women represents not only the effect of decreased estrogen levels but also the result of inactivity. Increasing the stress on the skeleton may have partially reversed the negative effect of inactivity, but the increase in bone mass has been slight, usually less than 3%. More importantly, no one has continued to monitor the bone density of these women in the years following the conclusion of the study. When Dalsky et al (5) re-examined the bone density of their exercise group 1 year after the conclusion of training, they found that bone density had reverted to pre-training levels. Whether it would have continued to decrease in ensuing years is unknown.

Using only sedentary women as subjects in exercise studies, as most investigators have, maximizes any benefit to be gained from increasing activity. What most women do not realize is that BMD gained as a result of exercise remains only as long as that same level of stress is maintained.

"Detraining" affects the skeleton as it does aerobic power, strength, and flexibility; when the activity stops, the benefits of the training program are lost.

Interaction of Exercise and Estrogen

If the experience of young amenorrheic athletes can be generalized to postmenopausal women, one would have to conclude that exercise cannot compensate for the decrease in endogenous estrogen levels after menopause. Several investigators (3,7,17) have reported that female athletes with secondary amenorrhea have a lumbar spine density averaging approximately 84% that of eumenorrheic controls, a value comparable to that seen in 50-year-old women. The bone loss in these athletes is generalized throughout the skeleton and includes the proximal femur, femoral shaft, and tibia (20,22). If the strenuous training programs of the hypoestrogenic female athlete cannot protect her from losing bone, it is unlikely that exercise can provide adequate protection against bone loss after menopause. If a woman does decide to rely on exercise to prevent osteoporosis, a bone density measurement should be done at that time and again 1 or 2 years later to determine how effective the exercise has been. Without monitoring BMD, the first indication that bone has been lost is likely to be an osteoporotic fracture.

On a positive note, when exercise is combined with HRT, the increase in BMD is greater than with either intervention alone at the lumbar spine and for the skeleton as a whole (Figure 20-2) (16). Neither intervention, alone or combined, had any effect at the ultradistal site of the wrist and results at the proximal femur were mixed. Both HRT and exercise had a positive effect on BMD at the femoral neck and trochanter, but the combination of the two had no more effect than each alone.

Exercise Prescription

Exercise is "prescribed" not only in terms of the type of activity, but also the frequency and duration of the training sessions and the intensity of the physical effort. Sedentary women who are worried about their risk for osteoporosis and want to know what type of exercise is best for "building bone" should be encouraged to engage in a variety of activities that use all the major muscle groups in the body. Walking is an excellent activity for these women. They are unlikely to incur an injury, which would deter them from future activity, and they can make it a social activity by walking with a friend. By slowly increasing the distance and pace and choosing a course with some hills, they can reap aerobic benefits while getting in the exercise "habit." To increase bone mass requires going one step further and placing a greater demand on the bones. Weight training appears to satisfy many of the basic principles required for increasing bone density. It can be designed to stress those skeletal areas most at risk for osteoporotic fracture, and the resistance or weight can be slowly increased as the muscles become stronger. Like other physiologic systems, bone will adapt to a given level of stress and will not continue to improve unless the workload is increased.

Compliance is always a major problem when attempting to encourage sedentary women to follow through with their good intentions and continue their exercise program. It is difficult to convince large numbers of women that they should exercise today to prevent a problem 10 or 20 years

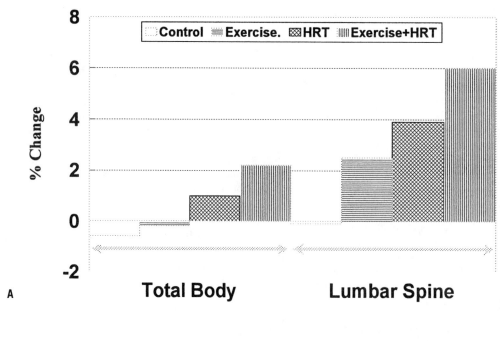

A

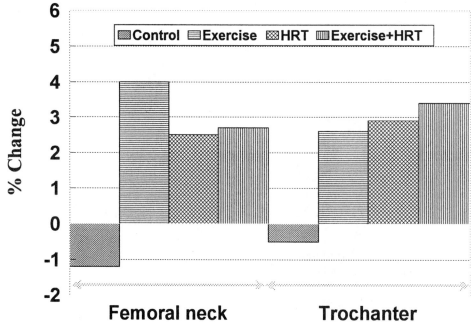

B

Figure 20-2 The percent change in bone density in (a) the total body and lumbar spine and (b) the femoral neck and greater trochanter after 11 months of: 1) a weight-bearing exercise program, 2) hormone replacement therapy (HRT), 3) the combination of exercise and HRT, and 4) a control group. (Figure drawn from data in Kohrt WM, Snead DB, Slatopolsky E, Birge SJ Jr. Additive effects of weight-bearing exercise and estrogen on bone mineral density in older women. J Bone Miner Res 1995;10:1303–1311.)

in the future. It is particularly difficult to be convincing when the evidence suggests that there will be very little return, as judged by increases in bone density, for their effort. Rather than looking at exercise solely as a means of preventing osteoporosis, the emphasis should be on the overall health benefits that accrue from being physically active.

For more active women, backpacking, cross-country skiing, rowing, and other fairly strenuous activities are all good choices. Although these activities may not markedly increase bone mass, they do improve cardiovascular fitness and at the same time provide some beneficial stimulus to the bones. Women in this group may have been led to believe that their active lifestyle will protect them from osteoporosis. They need to know that there is no evidence that exercise is an alternative to hormone replacement or other therapy at menopause but should be considered an adjunct therapy.

REFERENCES

1. Alekel L, Clasey JL, Fehling PC, et al. Contributions of exercise, body composition, and age to bone mineral density in premenopausal women. Med Sci Sports Exerc 1995;27:1477–1485.

2. Bailey DA, Martin AD. Physical activity and skeletal health in adolescents. Pediatr Exerc Sci 1994;6:330–347.

3. Cann CE, Martin MC, Genant HK, Jaffe RB. Decreased spinal mineral content in amenorrheic women. JAMA 1984;251:626–629.

4. Cooper C, Wickham C, Coggan D. Sedentary work in middle life and fracture of the proximal femur. Br J Industrial Med 1990;47:69–70.

5. Dalsky G, Stocke KS, Eshani AA, et al. Weight-bearing exercise training and lumbar bone mineral content in postmenopausal women. Ann Intern Med 1988; 108:824–828.

6. Drinkwater BL. Does physical activity play a role in preventing osteoporosis? Res Q Exerc Sport 1994;65:197–206.

7. Drinkwater BL, Nilson K, Chesnut CH III, et al. Bone mineral content of amenorrheic and eumenorrheic athletes. N Engl J Med 1984;311:277–281.

8. Farmer ME, Harris T, Madans JH, et al. Anthropometric indicators and hip fractures: the NHANES 1 epidemiological follow-up study. J Am Geriatr Soc 1989;37:9–16.

9. Fehling PC, Alekel L, Clasey J, et al. A comparison of bone mineral densities among female athletes in impact loading and active loading sports. Bone 1995;17:205–210.

10. Frost HM. The role of changes in mechanical usage set points on the pathogenesis of osteoporosis. J Bone Miner Res 1992;7: 253–261.

11. Hamdy RC, Anderson J, Whalen KE, Harvill LM. Regional differences in bone density of young men involved in different exercises. Med Sci Sports Exerc 1994;26:884–888.

12. Heinonen A, Oja P, Kannus P, et al. Bone mineral density of female athletes in different sports. Bone Miner 1993;23:1–14.

13. Heinonen A, Oja P, Kannus P, et al. Bone mineral density in female athletes representing sports with different loading characteristics of the skeleton. Bone 1995;17:197–203.

14. Joakimsen RM, Magnus JH, Fonnebo V. Physical activity and predisposition for hip fractures: a review. Osteoporos Int 1997;7: 503–513.

15. Kannus P, Haapasalo H, Sankelo M, et al. Effect of starting-age of physical activity on bone mass in the dominant arm of tennis and squash players. Ann Intern Med 1995;123:27–31.

16. Kohrt WM, Snead DB, Slatopolsky E, Birge SJ Jr. Additive effects of weight-bearing exercise and estrogen on bone mineral density in older women. J Bone Miner Res 1995;10:1303–1311.

17. Marcus R, Cann C, Madvig P, et al. Menstrual function and bone mass in elite women distance runners. Ann Intern Med 1985; 102:158–163.

18. Jacobsen SI, Goldberg J, Miles TP, et al. Race and sex difference in mortality following fracture of the hip. Amer J Public Health 1992; 82:1147–1150.

19. Mazess RB, Barden H. Bone density in premenopausal women: effect of age, dietary intake, physical activity, smoking, and birth-control pills. Am J Clin Nutrition 1991;53:132–142.

20. Myburgh KH, Bachrach LK, Lewis B, et al. Low bone density at axial and appendicular sites in amenorrheic athletes. Med Sci Sports Exerc 1993;25: 1197–1202.

21. Nattrass SM, Drinkwater BL. Does mechanical loading of peripheral skeletal sites affect prediction of axial BMD? J Bone Miner Density 1998;23:S315. Abstract.

22. Rencken ML, Chesnut CH, Drinkwater BL. Bone density at multiple skeletal sites in amenorrheic athletes. JAMA 1996;276:238–240.

23. Risser WL, Lee EJ, LeBlanc A, et al. Bone density in eumenorrheic female college athletes. Med Sci Sports Exerc 1990;22:570–574.

24. Suominen H, Rahkila P. Bone mineral density of the calcaneous in 70- to 81-yr-old male athletes and a population sample. Med Sci Sports Exerc 1991;23:1227–1233.

25. Turner CH. Homeostatis control of bone structure: an application of feedback theory. Bone 1991;12: 203–217.

Chapter 21

Evaluation of Acute Sports Injuries of the Adult

Brian N. Victoroff

ACUTE EVALUATION OF SPORTS INJURIES

Musculoskeletal injuries comprise a major proportion of the problems encountered and treated by primary care physicians in the office setting. The gradual increase in popularity of heavy recreational physical activity and the continued need for manual labor in society ensure that this will continue to be the case. The key to understanding and treating these injuries lies in careful anatomic diagnosis. Once an anatomic diagnosis is made, treatment is based on physiologic principles and common sense. Some noteworthy exceptions do occur and represent special cases of diagnostic dilemma or require alternative treatment. In this chapter, we summarize the diagnostic and therapeutic approach to common musculoskeletal injuries sustained by adults, including contusions, ligamentous sprains, musculotendinous strains, fractures, dislocations, and meniscal injuries.

Health care providers have the opportunity to evaluate and treat their patients' sports injuries in a number of contexts: as on-field physicians or trainers covering sporting events, in sports injury clinics or club settings, or in private offices as either primary providers or referred specialists. Acute, observed injuries afford unique opportunities for immediate evaluation of injury. This can be helpful or difficult. On the one hand, it is useful to be the first person evaluating an acute injury, because the injury is appreciated in context, the initial appearance of the injury is evident, and early interventions can be guided appropriately. On the other hand, acute sports injuries occur in a public setting with many interested observers interjecting helpful and occasionally not-so-helpful suggestions.

Many physicians providing on-field care are accompa-

nied by a certified athletic trainer. Injury triage during sporting events is usually managed by the trainer, who evaluates the patient on the field and determines whether the patient may safely move to the sideline or should be assessed by the physician before moving. Following the on-field assessment, the athlete should be taken to the sideline, training room, or emergency medical facility (as appropriate), where distractions are minimized and a more thorough evaluation can be completed.

Most injuries are to extremities. Evaluation of extremity injuries should proceed in an organized fashion, with a progressive assessment algorithm. The initial assessment should concentrate on the appearance of the whole patient, including the position of the injured extremity, the patient's response to the injury, the ability of the patient to move the extremity, and any potential impediments to the examination, such as equipment, uniforms, or clothing. Physical examination follows a step-wise, systematic pattern. Direct observation is followed by palpation, including assessment of the peripheral pulses and neurologic function. Patients with obvious deformity or inability to move the injured extremity should be splinted appropriately and transported for radiographs and further evaluation. If the integument is intact and the patient can move the involved extremity, the examination should include testing for gross stability. If gross stability is confirmed, the patient is permitted to move the joint progressively as tolerated. If patients are able to bear weight, they are permitted to walk. Once an injured athlete can walk comfortably, careful jogging is permitted along the sidelines. If the injury permits painless jogging, then functional tests, such as windsprints and figure-of-eight running patterns, should be undertaken before permitting the athlete to return to participation. Failure to complete any stage of the progressive functional assessment restricts the athlete from play until further assessment is completed.

The majority of adults sustaining injuries in sports are evaluated by a physician in an office setting—hours to days after the injury—in a controlled environment with minimal distraction. Disadvantages in this situation include possibly inaccurate recall of the mechanism of injury, as well as swelling, pain, and muscle spasm that may adversely affect the assessment of the injury. Pain and spasm may interfere with the clinician's ability to perform a complete examination of the area. When this is the case, appropriate radiographs should be done to rule out fracture or dislocation. The injuries may then be re-evaluated at a second visit, once the swelling, pain and inhibition have resolved. Few musculoskeletal injuries, aside from acute dislocations, require urgent surgical intervention. In most cases, acute musculoskeletal injuries requiring urgent intervention are self-evident, but specialty consultation may be useful when the diagnosis is unclear.

Initial treatment for soft-tissue injuries sustained by adults in the setting of sports often is guided by nonphysicians, including patients, teammates, certified athletic trainers, personal trainers, physical therapists, or well-meaning friends and family. Most physicians play their primary role in the subacute management of sports injuries. The interventions initiated by the care provider at this stage of treatment correlate predictably with the physiologic response to injury. The fundamental concepts guiding treatment at this stage include accurate assessment, pain control, protection from reinjury or worsening of injury, and control of both the inflammatory and the compensatory physiologic responses to injury. These fundamentals serve as guiding principles for the management of the specific types of injury discussed below.

Injuries included under the rubric of acute sport injuries include those sustained during participation in actual sports. However, many industrial injuries are similar to sports injuries and can be evaluated and treated by algorithms identical to those used for sports injuries. In this context, laborers may be considered similar to professional athletes in their goals for rehabilitation and recovery.

CONTUSIONS

Contusions represent by far the most common injuries sustained by adults in athletics or laborers in the course of their work duties. The severity of contusion injury is related to the kinetic energy of the wounding force, including: 1) the velocity and mass of the structures involved; 2) the specific anatomic structure receiving the impact—in particular, the thickness and resilience of soft tissue and the presence of adipose or muscle mass overlying bone; and 3) the phase of muscle contraction. Contracted muscle may provide some protective function, as maximal contraction of the muscle in an animal model lessens the impact response to a muscle contusion (1). The impact response of limbs with relaxed muscles is taken up primarily by underlying bone because the force is transmitted through the muscle, while maximally contracted muscle decreases the force transmission to bone and lessens the impact response.

Most contusion injuries represent superficial

hematomas, with minor bleeding from ruptured subdermal and subcutaneous capillaries. This allows hemorrhage into the interstitium, generally occupying the subcutaneous tissue without significant deep components. Injuries of greater magnitude may cause fascial or muscular injury with intramuscular hematomas. Even more severe trauma in heavily muscled extremities or blows to areas relatively unprotected by muscle (e.g., the anterior tibia) may result in transmission of force to the bone with periosteal or bone contusion.

Superficial contusion injuries are not serious and can generally be expected to recover rapidly regardless of treatment. Notable exceptions occur when substantial hemorrhage creates intramuscular or subfascial liquid hematomas associated with significant disruption of muscle fibers. These injuries must be considered a higher grade injury and require more aggressive treatment and appropriate follow-up.

Evaluation and Treatment

A clinician faced with a contusion injury often encounters the dilemma of deciding when to obtain radiographs. In the case of contusions to extremities, the general guidelines are based on the function of the extremity. If the patient can move the extremity painlessly, radiographs may be unnecessary. If the patient is unable to actively move the affected joint through a range of motion without significant pain, appropriate radiographs may be needed to rule out fracture. Any later failure to recover along the anticipated course would be reasonable indication for obtaining radiographs. While this general guideline may be applied to injuries of the extremities, abdominal and trunk contusions may represent a manifestation of internal injury, and the threshold for obtaining screening radiographs is lower.

Most contusions can be treated appropriately applying the RICE (rest, ice, compression, and elevation) concept. This treatment of musculoskeletal injuries enjoys well-deserved, wide application. For contusions, cryotherapy in the form of application of ice packs or cold packs plus compression is helpful. Patients should be instructed to apply cold with gentle compression to the affected area as soon as possible after the injury. This treatment reduces the capillary hemorrhage and therefore the magnitude and severity of the contusion. Patients should be cautioned to avoid thermal injury to their skin by avoiding application of the ice directly to the skin. The ice or cold pack may be used in conjunction with compressive bandages. Application of compressive cold packs is most important in the initial hemorrhage phase after a contusion injury and becomes less effective over time. It is unlikely that application of cold beyond 48 hours from injury significantly affects the natural history. Elevation of the affected extremity during the initial hours after injury also lessens the severity of the contusion. Moving the extremity out of a dependent position reduces capillary filling pressure and probably decreases the amount of bleeding from injured vascular structures. As with compression, the elevation of the injured extremity is most effective in the first 12 to 24 hours, after which the effect is diminished.

Return to Participation

Once a contusion has reached a steady state wherein the ecchymosis is no longer expanding and the extremity may be moved through range of motion without pain, most patients are able to return to participation. They should be cautioned to use appropriate protective padding and to monitor the injured area for increased ecchymosis or decreased function. Ecchymosis from contusions, in most cases, persists long after the pain and dysfunction from the contusion have resolved and generally is not reason for concern.

Special Cases

Occasionally, contusion injuries may be severe, such as deep muscle contusions, which may be accompanied by fascial or muscle fiber disruption with the formation of a large hematoma. Deep muscle contusion may cause substantial bleeding with development of intramuscular hematoma and, in rare cases, compartmental syndrome.

Intramuscular hematoma is seen occasionally in quadriceps contusions (Figure 21-1). This has been described frequently in contact sports and is the reason for the rigid padding over the anterior thigh used by most football players. Deep muscular hematoma in the anterior quadriceps may cause substantial muscular inhibition and loss of extension strength, which may manifest as buckling of the knee during gait. This could be misinterpreted as a more severe quadriceps rupture or intra-articular knee injury. In addition, deep muscle contusions may manifest some long-term difficulties, such as muscle fibrosis with effective shortening, intrafascial adhesions, and deposition of heterotopic bone within the muscle as the hematoma is replaced by osteoid, which may be converted to bone. Heterotopic ossification within the quadriceps muscle can be substantially disabling to an athlete's performance, with a propensity for reduced range of motion in the affected extremity, persistent tenderness, and a greater likelihood of reinjury. Excision of heterotopic ossification is done with

guarded prognosis and a substantial likelihood of recurrence. Interestingly, the immature woven bone of heterotopic ossification is markedly similar to rapidly forming bone seen in some primary neoplasms of bone, such as osteogenic sarcoma. Appropriate injury history must accompany biopsies of areas of heterotopic bone to prevent this potential misinterpretation.

Rarely, compartment syndrome may occur in the setting of deep muscle contusion. Compartment syndrome occurs when direct soft-tissue trauma results in bleeding, causing increased interstitial pressure within an anatomically confined muscle compartment. The increased pressure may interfere with circulation and function of the muscle and ultimately compromise neurovascular components within the compartment. Untreated compartment syndrome can result in permanent neurovascular injury and tissue necrosis. Most compartment syndromes manifest soon after injury but occasionally may develop gradually after injury. A patient with compartment syndrome typically presents with pain out of proportion to that expected for the degree of injury; palpable or visible swelling of the involved compartment; pain on passive stretch of muscle within the involved compartment; and manifestations of ischemia such as pallor, cyanosis, or reduced pulses. Occasionally, the manifestations of compartment syndrome are subtle and may be missed on clinical examination. A patient with suspected compartment syndrome should be evaluated rapidly by measuring the pressures of the compartments concerned. Elevated compartment pressure is an indication for urgent surgical decompression by release of the tight skin and fascia.

Deep muscle contusions represent a reasonable case for immobilization of the extremity for a limited period. It is probable that this, accompanied by a compressive wrap, can

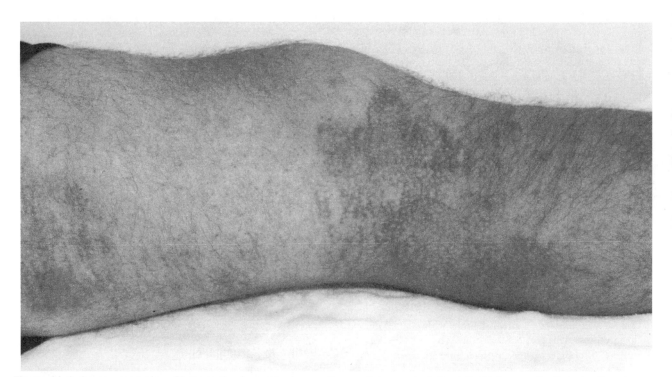

Figure 21-1 Severe contusion. Photograph of a contusion on the medial aspect of the left thigh, manifesting significant subcutaneous ecchymosis.

significantly reduce the amount of hemorrhage occurring within the muscle and affect the rate of recovery. For large quadriceps contusions, some success has been gained with immobilization in the position of knee flexion, maintaining the quadriceps at maximal length for the first 24 hours after the injury until the bleeding subsides (2). It is likely that maintenance of muscle at full excursion length and early restoration of motion reduce the potential for muscle fibrosis and fascial adhesions. In the early phase of treatment, protected weight-bearing may be needed to prevent buckling of the knee. Appropriate rehabilitation includes application of physical therapy modalities and gradual progression of activities. Athletes may return to participation when the hemorrhage is stable, full range of motion has returned to the hip and knee, and full or nearly full quadriceps contraction strength is recovered, as measured by isokinetic muscle testing.

In summary, contusions remain the most common injuries sustained in sports. Most represent minor hematomas and can be treated with early application of gentle compression and cryotherapy. Once the hematoma is stable and full range of motion and protective muscle contraction have returned, athletes may return to participation with appropriate padding. Special cases include deep hematoma affecting muscle and the rare occurrence of compartmental syndrome, both of which require more aggressive intervention.

LIGAMENTOUS INJURIES: SPRAINS

Skeletal ligaments are fibrous bands comprised of bundles of collagen fibrils. They make up the major structural component of joint capsules. Ligaments act as the primary stabilizers of skeletal joints. They originate from bone and insert into bone on the opposite side of a joint. The most severe manifestation of ligament sprain is seen in joint dislocation.

Disruption of a ligament's function may occur from an intrasubstance rupture or may be associated with an avulsion fracture of the bone. The ligament may detach from the bone, or a fragment of bone may be broken off, with the ligament remaining attached to the fragment. A semantic problem is encountered wherein the definition of sprain is subject to interpretation. Most sprains are defined anatomically; however, the exact wording depends on the degree of specificity. For example, a sprain injury to an ankle may be described in reference to the joint, i.e., "ankle sprain"; the location on the joint, i.e., "lateral ankle sprain"; the ligament complex involved, i.e., "lateral collateral ligament sprain"; or the specific fiber bundle, i.e., "anterior talofibular ligament sprain." Any and all of these descriptions of the same injury may be appropriate and which description is applied depends on the circumstance.

Clinicians should be as accurate as possible and as specific as necessary when describing sprains. For example, an anterior talofibular ligament disruption would be appropriately described as such among referring physicians; however, the same injury might be described as a lateral ankle sprain in consultation with a concerned parent.

Grading Ligament Injuries

A general consensus exists among musculoskeletal practitioners that ligament injuries manifesting as sprain be graded on a scale of 1 to 3. Grade 1 sprains may be described in lay terms as a *stretch injury*. These represent disruption of a small proportion of the ligament fibers, with primarily microscopic injury. There is no significant loss of continuity of the ligament, no change in the structural properties of the ligament, and most importantly, no resultant joint pathologic laxity. A grade 2 sprain could be described as a partially torn ligament. In these cases, there is macroscopic injury to the affected ligament with significant alteration in structural properties, manifesting as a compromise of ligament stiffness. In these cases, manual testing for joint stability demonstrates significant laxity when compared to the opposite (intact) side. However, despite significant side-to-side difference in joint excursion, an end point remains on manual testing. One might ask in this circumstance whether the "intact" fibers of the injured ligament are stretched—having sustained grade 1, or microscopic injury, as well. This is highly likely and probably depends on the specific ligament complex involved. Grade 3 injuries might be described simply as a completely torn ligament, wherein enough fibers are torn to result in loss of continuity of the ligament, loss of function of the ligament, and joint instability. Manual testing will reveal a soft or absent end point.

Manifestations of ligament injury depend on the grade of severity of the injury and the specific joint involved.

In general, grade 1 sprains demonstrate minimal or no swelling. Tenderness to palpation and mild pain with stressing the ligament are noted. As disruption of fiber architecture is limited, there tends to be less hemorrhage in the area of injury and minimal ecchymosis. Patients generally are able to place the involved extremity through a range of motion with pain only at the extremes of the range of motion. Mild muscle inhibition and guarding may occur, but usually there is not loss of function.

Grade 2 injuries, despite the relatively poor vascularity of ligaments, often are accompanied by significant joint hemarthrosis. This will manifest as swelling, possibly accompanied by gradual onset of ecchymosis (Figure 21-2). Patients experience pain on active motion of the involved joint and, for weight-bearing joints, pain on ambulation. Usually these injuries are moderately painful. Patients tend to protect the joint, avoiding the extremes of range of motion and, for weight-bearing extremities, exhibit an antalgic gait.

Grade 3 sprains are accompanied by significant pain. Patients may have perceived a tearing sensation or a pop at the time of injury. Hemarthrosis occurs rapidly with accompanying ecchymosis. Patients avoid weight-bearing on lower extremity joints, and significant muscle inhibition and guarding are seen.

The components of the ligament injury, including fiber disruption with instability, hemorrhage, muscle inhibition, and guarding, represent clinical manifestations, which must be addressed in the treatment of sprain injuries.

Clinical Assessment of Sprains

Acute (on-field) assessment of sprain injuries includes all components of a traditional examination, with visual observation, palpation, and manipulative tests accompanied by a progressive functional examination. Injured athletes should be moved to the sideline, where fewer distractions permit better assessment. If gentle mechanical testing confirms stability and the

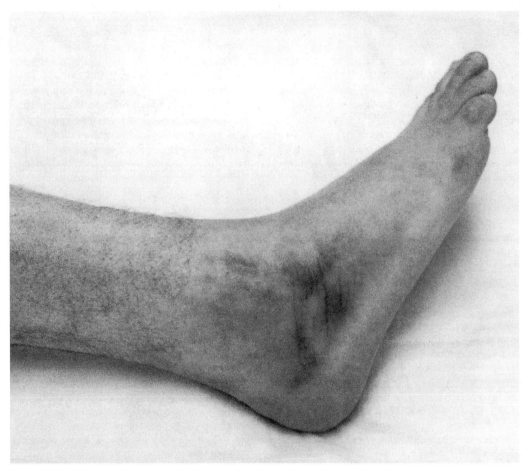

Figure 21-2 Right ankle sprain. Significant ecchymosis may develop soon after a lateral ankle sprain. This usually appears distal to the lateral malleolus and proximal to the lateral edge of the plantar surface.

athlete can place the involved joint through a range of motion with minimal inhibition, functional progressive tests should be employed. When an athlete is able to move the joint with minimal pain, he or she is permitted to attempt to walk. If walking is painless, the athlete may try light jogging or, in the case of upper extremity joints, simple functional testing such as tossing a ball or swinging a bat. If the athlete is able to jog, a final functional test imitating the demands of the sport should be completed before being allowed to return to play. This may consist of sprinting on the sidelines with rapid change of direction or throwing a ball with speed. Athletes able to complete the functional tests generally are permitted to resume play. Any obvious structural instability, clinically significant hemarthrosis, limitation in range of motion, or failure to successfully complete a transition test is reasonable grounds for discontinuance of play and further workup of the injury.

Office examination for sprain injury should concentrate on all of the parameters described above. Frequently, patients seen in the office have developed significant swelling, hemarthrosis, muscle guarding, and inhibition owing to the time interval since injury. Guarding and inhibition may compromise the accuracy of a physical assessment. For example, a patient with a significantly swollen sprained ankle may not allow stability testing to a degree necessary to demonstrate a side-to-side stability difference. In this circumstance, it is prudent to temporarily immobilize an extremity or mobilize it in a protected manner until repeat examination can be performed when the swelling has subsided. Often, the repeat examination is more accurate and may obviate the need for sophisticated and costly imaging modalities such as magnetic resonance imaging (MRI). Radiographs should be obtained for all joint injuries manifesting with significant hemarthrosis, lack of range of motion, or clinically evident instability.

Grading Injuries

As implied above, there is significant subjectiveness in the grading of ligament injury severity. Determination of grades 1 to 3 is in some cases accompanied by a quasi-objective measurement system. For example, Hughston et al (3) grade laxity of the medial collateral ligament of the knee according to the amount of joint opening seen with displacing forces, as follows: grade 0 is normal, grade 1 is a joint opening 1 to 4mm, grade 2 is 5 to 9mm, and grade 3 is 10 to 15mm. Obviously, the accurate measurement of joint opening by millimeters demands significant experience and still may be inconsistent among examiners. A similar grading system is not used routinely for stress testing of the ankle joint, but both joints may be evaluated appropriately using a grading system similar to that described above. According to the general grading system applied to the medial collateral ligament of the knee, Hughston grade 0 injuries would demonstrate no laxity on abduction stress testing when compared to the contralateral side, grades 1 and 2 would manifest with significant laxity but with a definite end point, and grade 3 tears would manifest with an absent or soft end point. Most practitioners are capable of distinguishing between these general grades of injury severity with a cooperative patient. This form of grading represents an attempt to make subjective findings objective enough to be practical. Special tests and more refined measurements of joint laxity, such as the KT 1000 instrument for anterior cruciate ligaments or stress radiographs for ankle instability, generally should be used in the setting of more severe injuries and specialty care.

Ligament Injury and Healing

Effective interventions used in the initial stages after a sprain injury address components of the inflammatory response to injury. Tissue trauma occurring in sprains releases breakdown products of injured tissue, which trigger an inflammatory response, including vasodilation and leakage of fluid (plasma) and cells. These cells, including platelets and leukocytes, release tissue growth factors (TGF) and cytokines into damaged tissue. Growth factors such as tissue growth factor–beta (TGF–β) induce cells to produce extracellular matrix, and other cytokines stimulate cell proliferation, particularly of white blood cells and fibroblasts. These tissue responses are responsible for the swelling, edema, and pain experienced with sprain injuries. They also introduce the initial phase of the ligament repair response.

The treatment of sprain injury by application of elevation, compression, and cold addresses these tissue responses to inhibit the vasodilatation and extravasation of fluid and cells, thus limiting the resultant pain and hopefully hastening the transition to recovery.

A clinician's intervention after sprain injury can significantly affect the outcome of healing. Because of the relatively poor vascularity of ligaments in comparison to other skeletal soft tissues, the initial inflammatory phase after ligament injury takes longer than in general wound healing. Newly formed bundles of collagen fibers initially are disorganized and oriented irregularly. Collagen bundles gradually become oriented along the line of application of force across the ligament, and scar tissue becomes less cellular over time. Mechanical stress applied by functional loading to the joint affects the reorientation of collagen fiber bundles and increases fibril size and density. While gradual healing occurs, scar matrix in the ligament matures and is reorganized to resemble closely the original ligament. However, the scar matrix always remains slightly disorganized and hypercellular microscopically, and injured ligaments tend to compensate for this by hypertrophy. Immobilization of an injured ligament promotes a protracted state of catabolism in the ligament, with degradation of the structural matrix, leading to progressive atrophy and lack of mechanical strength. Controlled motion optimizes organized ligament repair. Therefore, the rehabilitation conditions (immobilization versus mobilization, weight-bearing versus non–weight-bearing, and application of functional stress) influence the appearance and biologic properties of healing ligaments. This basic principle influences a clinician's choices regarding rehabilitation.

Ligament Remodeling

Following the initial inflammatory response, the injured tissue enters a cellular recovery phase. Several days after injury, the hematoma begins to organize with recruitment of inflammatory cells for the phagocytosis of necrotic tissue and fibroblasts to initiate the repair response. Tissue matrix is synthesized by fibroblasts as the necrotic tissue and clot are replaced by disorganized matrix and granulation tissue. In this phase of recovery, the initial pain of the injury is resolved and ligament remodeling starts. During the ensuing weeks, ligament remodeling begins, and it is at this stage that the application of controlled motion assists with the remodeling of ligament tissue along the lines of applied stress. Patients are encouraged to move the affected extremity while protected from excessive nonphysiologic stresses. In an animal model of ligament injury, Woo (4) evaluated the repair tissue in rabbits with injured medial collateral ligaments (MCL). Animals that were permitted cage activity with an isolated MCL injury demonstrated organized healing of the ligament and the strong repair. Animals with combined MCL and anterior cruciate ligament (ACL) injuries were noted to have disorganized and incomplete remodeling of the MCL during healing. This effect was thought to be attributable to the exposure of nonphysiologic stresses to the unstable joint from the accompanying cruciate ligament instability.

It is the application of the principle of controlled motion that explains the utility of protective functional bracing for recovery of sprain injuries. Most ligament injuries complete remodeling within 4 to 6 months of injury with some exceptions. Bracing is appropriately maintained throughout this period. The duration of the bracing regimen depends on the grade of injury and the specific ligament injured. Once ligament remodeling is completed, patients with residual laxity may require long-term bracing for participation in heavy activities or surgical intervention, depending on the context. Few ligaments recover their full tensile strength after injury, but in most cases this does not result in a clinically significant ligament instability.

Treatment of Sprains

Treatment goals for sprain injuries may be separated into early and late phases. In the early postinjury phase, primary treatment goals include: 1) controlling local hemorrhage, edema, and pain; 2) restoring joint motion; and 3) protecting the healing ligament from further injury. In the later phase, once acute manifestations of injury have subsided, goals are advanced to include: 1) establishment of compensatory strength, 2) restoration of joint proprioception, and 3) protection of the joint from reinjury on return to use.

Regardless of the severity of sprain, early treatment within the first 48 to 72 hours is RICE. The concept of rest is relative; a minor (grade 1) ankle sprain is rested by avoidance of heavy physical activity, while a severe (grade 3) sprain with hemarthrosis may require temporary cast application and non–weight-bearing as the most extreme manifestation of rest. Cold and compression are useful modalities in these injuries and should be applied as soon as possible after the injury. Elevation is also important in grade 2 and more serious sprains of the lower extremities. These initial interventions are designed to inhibit acute swelling caused by hemorrhage and soft-tissue edema and secondarily reduce the pain and accompanying joint inhibition.

General treatment methods for the rehabilitation phase of sprains includes joint mobilization (stretching), strengthening of agonist muscles, proprioception enhancement (coordination), and protection of the injured joint from any residual laxity that may remain.

Proprioceptive deficit occurs in conjunction with ligament injury for several reasons (5–10). Proprioceptive organs demonstrated in most ligaments include pacinian corpuscles, Ruffini's end organs, muscle spindles, and free nerve endings, which may be injured along with the fibrous structure of the injured ligament, reducing the afferent input from the injured joint. Joint effusion and hemarthrosis result in compromised neuromuscular feedback and inhibition of muscles crossing the affected joint (11–13). In addition, proprioceptive input from joints is often perceived at the end range when maximal or near-maximal ligament tension is achieved, so this mechanism is compromised when a ligament has sustained enough injury to be functionally lengthened. Retraining for proprioception is possible and may be successful in restoring functional stability and preventing reinjury. This has been demonstrated in a laboratory setting for knee injuries and in the practical setting of elite athletics (14,15).

The application of these general concepts to treatment of sprain injury depends on the severity of sprain. Grade 1 sprains are easily treated with minimal intervention. Application of the RICE regimen should be started early. Most patients do not require immobilization, and recovery from grade 1 sprains may be anticipated to occur within days from the injury. Most patients do not require formal rehabilitation.

Grade 2 sprains are treated initially in the same manner. Control of edema and pain can be enhanced using nonsteroidal anti-inflammatory medications (NSAIDs) prudently. Recalling the importance of functional mobilization, controlled motion is applied effectively in these injuries, followed by sequential rehabilitation. Grade 2 sprains generally heal without need for surgical intervention or cast immobilization. Recovery proceeds over a period of weeks. Athletes or laborers may require some significant period of abstention from play or labor during the rehabilitative process. Return to full participation in athletics or full duty at work is determined on the basis of the patient's performance on controlled functional testing. Occasionally a return to an uncontrolled work environment may require a formal work assessment and simulation program for laborers. The transition back to play or work necessitates cooperation among the patient, clinician, and therapist who collaborate in the process.

Grade 3 sprains are treated initially with the RICE regimen. Gross instability often necessitates temporary immobilization. Again, recalling the concept of ligament remodeling along the lines of applied stress, immobilization should be limited to the acute phase with appropriate bracing and sequential rehabilitation used to permit optimal ligament remodeling. Surgery is indicated in selected cases of grade 3 sprain, depending on the specific joint injury and patient demands.

Residual joint instability after remodeling may be significant, depending on the ligament complex and joint involved. A distinction should be made between the joint *laxity* and clinical *instability*. A patient may manifest significant laxity on manual testing; however, no functional deficit may be perceived. Conversely, patients may experience significant functional deficit and joint instability, which does not correlate precisely with the laxity detected on manual testing. Instability probably occurs as the result of a combination of biomechanical compromise and loss of joint proprioception. The rehabilitative phase of treatment for sprain injury addresses both these concerns. Compensatory muscle strengthening is directed at enhancing the power and reaction time of agonist muscles crossing the unstable joint. Occasionally, specific muscle groups may be emphasized to enhance protective strength; for example, lateral ligament instability of the ankle may be reduced significantly with a guided program for strengthening of the tibialis anterior and peroneal muscle groups. Patients with recurrent ankle sprains have demonstrated a reduced ratio of dorsiflexion to plantar flexion ankle strength, and recovery of the normal strength ratio while simultaneously emphasizing peroneal strength may compensate for lateral ankle ligament laxity (16).

In summary, optimizing compensatory strength and recovery of proprioception in the rehabilitation phase may effectively restore stability even in cases when ligament laxity remains detectable. Patients for whom these measures do not restore functional stability may be considered candidates for long-term bracing or surgical reconstruction.

The following cases illustrate these rehabilitation concepts.

Case 1

A 17-year-old girl sustained an inversion injury of her left ankle while playing basketball. She experienced immediate pain on the lateral aspect of the ankle and could not continue playing. Physical examination the following day demonstrated point tenderness over the lateral ankle ligaments, nearly full range of motion with pain at the extremes of the range of plantar flexion and dorsiflexion, mild discomfort on inversion stress testing with no significant guarding, and no compromise of lateral collateral ligament laxity on side-to-side joint testing. This patient was instructed to apply ice packs to the ankle for 24 to 48 hours. She was permitted full weight-bearing with a gradual progression to activities as tolerated. No formal referral to physical therapy was necessary, and this patient had a high probability of good outcome without long-term compromise of joint function.

Case 2

A 35-year-old man sustained a valgus-twisting injury to his right knee while descending stairs rapidly at his work place. He had a sense of tearing or an audible pop with acute onset of knee pain and mild swelling. Physical examination the following day in the office revealed localized swelling around the medial side of the knee but minimal intra-articular hemarthrosis. Range of motion was painful at the extremes of extension and flexion. Tenderness was elicited at the medial joint line, and on valgus stress testing, the patient experienced pain with significant medial joint opening, compared with the opposite side, but a definite end point. Radiographs were obtained in this circumstance and results were negative, so treatment for a grade 2 sprain initiated. Initial application of ice, compression, and elevation, accompanied by abstention from heavy activity, was recommended. The patient was offered a limited prescription for anti-inflammatory medications. The healing collateral ligament was protected with a functional range of motion brace permitting flexion and extension but protecting against varus and valgus instability. Formal physical therapy was used to guide recovery of full range of motion and strength. A repeat physical examination within 10 days to 2 weeks of injury—when acute swelling and pain had subsided—was justified to confirm the diagnosis and guide rehabilitation. This patient was be able to return to work within 6 weeks of the injury and could expect full or nearly full recovery without functional deficits. A collateral ligament brace would be used for one season of sports participation.

Case 3

A 49-year-old woman sustained an inversion injury to her right ankle at her home. She had immediate pain and rapid onset of swelling and was evaluated in the emergency room, where results of radiographs were noted to be normal. On clinical examination, the patient manifested marked swelling of the lateral aspect of the ankle, reduction in active range of motion, and pain on attempted active motion. The ankle was held in a protective position of slight plantar flexion, and the patient was unable to bear weight comfortably. Manipulative testing at the initial examination failed to disclose instability resulting from inhibition and guarding from pain.

Radiographs should be obtained in this case, and if results were negative, this would be interpreted as grade 3 injury. Repeat examination after the acute hemarthrosis resolves is important. Initial treatment and recommendations include the RICE regimen, along with application of temporary immobilization in the form of a splint or cast. The patient should be protected from weight-bearing and encouraged to elevate the extremity as much as possible over the next several days. Between 10 days and 3 weeks from injury, controlled motion should be allowed and sequential physical therapy started. Controlled weight-bearing in a functional brace is permitted after sequential rehabilitation. The rehabilitation sequence should concentrate initially on recovery of full range of motion and joint proprioception using balance and coordination drills, followed by strengthening of agonist muscles—foot dorsiflexors and evertors, in particular. This patient may experience significant residual laxity and require bracing for participation in heavy activities and athletics. Surgery may be applied in selected cases of grade 3 sprain, although in the ankle, acute surgical repair after grade 3 sprains has not been proven definitively to provide a better outcome than late reconstruction and therefore is recommended infrequently.

In summary, sprains represent injuries to ligaments. They are graded 1 through 3, according to severity. Grade 1 and 2 ligament injuries generally heal well without significant residual laxity. Grade 3 sprains may require an initial period of immobilization, followed by functional bracing and occasionally, surgery. Initial application of rest, ice, compression and elevation (RICE) is a universal concept appropriate for the initial treatment of all of these injuries. Late rehabilitation involves joint mobilization, strengthening of agonist muscles, recovery of proprioception, and protection for joints with residual laxity.

DISLOCATIONS

Joint dislocations present some of the most serious manifestations of capsuloligamentous injury. In the setting of sport, the immediate deformity and pain experienced by the athlete attracts attention and generates marked concern among observers. While the pain response and visible deformity may be intimidating, this appearance may not reflect directly the severity of the injury. The severity of soft tissue and cartilage injury, the treatment regimen, and the prognosis of dislocation injuries vary widely depending on the joint involved and the energy imparted to the affected extremity. Despite the wide variability, some general principles do apply to the initial and long-term treatment of dislocations and the prognosis for recovery or recurrent instability.

Most dislocations occur as a result of passive forces applied indirectly across a joint. For example, most anterior shoulder dislocations result from a combination of external rotation, abduction, and extension applied to the arm, whereas posterior dislocations may occur with a fall onto an outstretched, forward-flexed arm. Rarely does a shoulder dislocation occur as the result of a direct blow to the joint. This principle applies in most cases of dislocation.

The energy imparted to the dislocated joint correlates with the severity of ligament injuries sustained and the probability of articular cartilage damage. In general, the greater the articular congruity of the dislocated joint, the more force is required to result in dislocation. For example, in the shoulder, the glenohumeral articulation provides little articular congruity, and the glenohumeral ligament complex allows maximum mobility. This may be an adaptation to brachiation locomotion. While this provides benefit in the form of a highly mobile joint, it permits the shoulder to be relatively vulnerable to dislocation injury. The force required to dislocate a shoulder, therefore, is relatively small and the likelihood of severe ligament injury and articular cartilage damage also relatively small (Figure 21-3).

At the other end of the spectrum, the human hip joint represents a highly congruous bony articulation with a relatively constrained range of motion and greater inherent stability. Therefore, the energy required to cause a hip dislocation is extreme. Most hip dislocations occur in the context of motor vehicle accidents with enormous energy imparted indirectly across the hip joint, resulting in dislocation. Because of this inherent stability and the large forces required to dislocate, hip dislocation is more likely to be accompanied by serious soft-tissue injury, articular cartilage damage, or fracture of the femoral head or acetabulum (Figure 21-4).

In the middle of the spectrum lies the elbow joint, which is unique in that the bony articular congruity is maximal while the joint is in extension when the olecranon is engaged within the olecranon fossa. This may be an adaptation to knuckle-walking in primates, which are known to maintain the elbow joint in extension while weight-bearing. In flexion, the articular congruity is decreased and soft-tissue restraints play a greater role in maintaining elbow stability. For this reason, most elbow dislocations are thought to occur in a position of slight flexion. The severity of trauma imparted to the articular surfaces and soft tissues stabilizing the elbow joint may, therefore, range widely,

Figure 21-3 Anteroposterior radiograph demonstrating an anterior subcoracoid dislocation of the right shoulder (glenohumeral joint). The relatively unconstrained shoulder joint generally permits dislocation without significant bone injury.

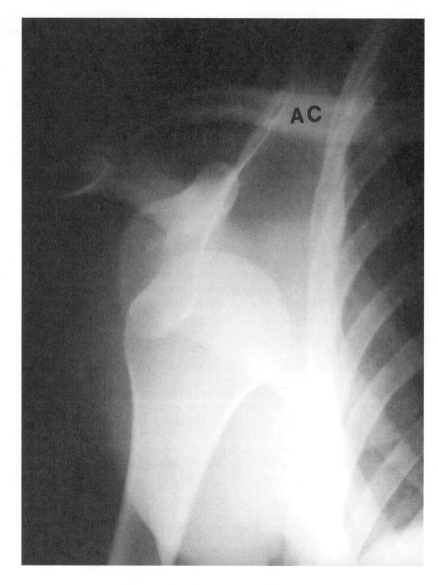

depending on the position of the elbow at injury and severity of the applied force.

Major concerns addressed in the treatment of joint dislocation include: 1) potential vascular or neurologic compromise occurring as a result of the dislocation; 2) reduction of the deformity and restoration of joint congruity; 3) maintenance of the reduction; and 4) rehabilitation. Each is considered in turn.

The significant forces applied to a joint to result in dislocation and the marked anatomic deformity that occurs may cause significant vascular or neurologic injury. Joints such as the knee and hip are particularly vulnerable to neurologic or vascular injury. Knee dislocations usually involve significant force, and associated injury to the popliteal artery is not unusual. Common findings include intimal tears and arterial spasm. While reduction of knee dislocations is generally fairly easy, most authors agree that the high probability of popliteal artery injury justifies vascular imaging by arteriogram or noninvasive duplex scanning to rule out intimal tears, which could cause catastrophic arterial occlusion if undetected.

Vascular injury in hip dislocation is unique because of the particular vulnerability of the blood supply to the femoral head. The retinacular vessels, which run along the femoral neck, may be torn by the initial traumatic event and remain compressed while the hip is dislocated. For the best chance of avoiding avascular necrosis of the femoral head, hip dislocation should be considered an emergency and reduced as soon as possible. Delay in reduction and repeated unsuccessful attempts at closed reduction are thought to contribute significantly to the risk of avascular necrosis.

In the shoulder, neurologic and vascular injury occur relatively infrequently. However, depending on the severity of the trauma, components of the brachial plexus—in particular, the axillary nerve—may sustain significant injury. Considering these examples, it is apparent that careful sensory and motor neurologic testing should be performed and documented both before and after manipulative reduction of any joint.

Most manipulative reductions of dislocated joints occur in the emergency room setting, with appropriate radiographs taken before and after reduction and access to pain medica-

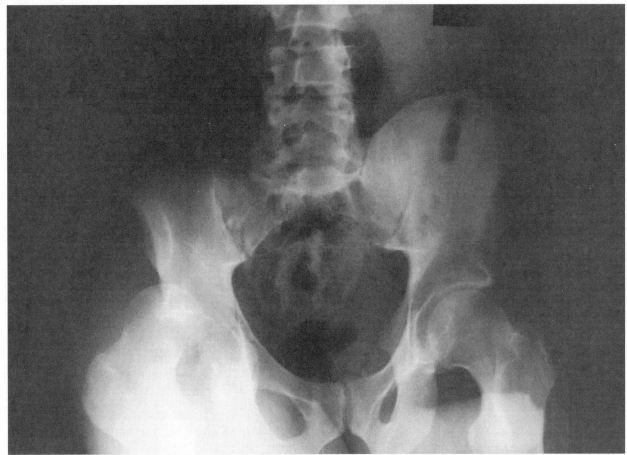

Figure 21-4 Anteroposterior radiograph of the pelvis and hips demonstrating a posterior dislocation of the right hip. The relatively constrained hip joint requires greater energy for dislocation. Hip dislocations may be accompanied by fracture of the posterior wall and weight-bearing dome of the acetabulum, as demonstrated in this radiograph.

tion and intravenous sedation. However, occasionally circumstances may mandate an attempt at manipulative reduction in the field. Significant vascular compromise with cyanosis or absent pulses, a remote setting, or delayed access to an emergency medical facility represents a relative indication for on-field reduction. The caregiver is faced with conflicting arguments in this setting. The well-intentioned goals of alleviating pain and permitting recovery of vascular flow to an extremity argue in favor of acute manipulative reduction. On the other hand, the caregiver is forced to make this decision without the benefit of prereduction radiographs, which could disclose a periarticular fracture that might represent a contraindication to closed manipulation. In general, when access is available, it is prudent to postpone attempts at manipulative reduction and apply temporary splinting until the patient can be transported to an appropriate facility for radiographs.

The physiologic response to acute dislocation usually includes significant muscle spasm as the body attempts to stabilize the injured joint. Muscle spasm increases over the first few hours after injury. For this reason, successful closed reduction may actually be more difficult to treat (without intravenous sedation and pain medication) in patients who have been splinted and transported than in those treated on the field. Proponents of early reduction cite this as a relative argument in favor of on-field manipulation of dislocated joints.

If emergency services are not readily available and circumstances mandate early intervention, it is reasonable to perform manipulative reduction. Gradual longitudinal traction applied to the affect extremity in an attempt to restore anatomic length and alignment often is effective in reducing a dislocated joint and bears relatively little risk of worsening the injury. Unsuccessful reduction attempts should not be repeated. The extremity should be splinted and the patient transported to an appropriate facility for radiographs and further treatment as indicated.

Following successful reduction, the physical examination should be repeated, concentrating on the careful assessment of the neurologic and vascular status of the extremity. Postreduction radiographs should be obtained. The position of immobilization depends on the specific joint and any associated fracture. The initial goal should be to prevent early redislocation or subluxation. Some joints, such as the hip or the proximal interphalangeal joints of the fingers, are inherently stable as long as there is no fracture, so they rarely require lengthy immobilization after reduction. Other joints, such as the shoulder and elbow, may be vulnerable to recurrent instability, depending on position. After reduction of an anterior dislocation, the shoulder should be protected in a position of adduction and internal rotation and kept out of the vulnerable position of abduction and external rotation during the initial recovery period. This is easily maintained with a sling and swathe. After reduction of an elbow dislocation, the joint tends to be stable in a position of flexion and unstable in extension and supination, so a posterior splint is applied in a position of flexion and neutral rotation during the initial recovery period.

Aftercare for dislocations, including the duration of immobilization and the time for beginning rehabilitative exercises, must be considered specifically for each joint. In general, it is best not to immobilize any dislocated joint for a long period, as arthrofibrosis with disorganized scar formation and loss of motion may result. In most cases, strict immobilization is only required for several days after a dislocation before motion therapy is started. Acknowledging that most dislocations represent significant ligament injuries, it is important to recall that ligament remodeling is optimized by protected motion. Functional bracing or careful monitoring by a physical therapist can protect a dislocated extremity from recurrent dislocation while introducing a gradual, progressive functional rehabilitation program.

Necessity for Surgery

The need for surgical reconstruction after joint dislocation is highly variable and dependent on the specific joint involved. Dislocations of the knee represent high-energy injuries with severe damage to ligamentous structures. Most require surgical intervention in the form of ligament reconstruction to restore functional stability. Dislocations of the hip, while usually stable after successful reduction, may include other problems, such as osteochondral fractures of the femoral head or later avascular necrosis. For the shoulder, the risk of recurrent instability is highly dependent on the patient. Active adolescent patients have a high probability of recurrent instability and will be more likely to require surgery (17–20). Patients over age 40 are much less likely to experience recurrent instability after shoulder dislocation but are more likely to sustain injuries to the rotator cuff (21,22). Other joints, such as the ankle and patella, are vulnerable to osteochondral injury at the time of dislocation. While they may recover stability, continued disability attributable to the osteochondral fracture may require surgical intervention.

In summary, articular dislocations generally occur as the result of forceful, indirect trauma. The force required to create a dislocation and the probability of concomitant bone or articular cartilage injury relates to the shape of the injured joint. Unconstrained, mobile joints are more vulnerable to instability but less vulnerable to articular injury, and highly constrained joints are less vulnerable to dislocation but more susceptible to articular cartilage injury or fracture. It is generally recommended that manipulative reductions be performed in the setting of an emergency trauma center where prereduction radiographs and careful evaluation of the neurovascular status can be completed. Occasionally, limited access to emergency facilities or vascular compromise may mandate manipulative reduction on the field. Most safe reductions can be achieved with gradual longitudinal traction. Regardless of the location of the reduction maneuver, postreduction radiographs and careful examination are imperative. The likelihood of recurrent instability and the course of progressive rehabilitation depend on the specific joint injured. Rehabilitation regimens follow the same concepts as those for severe

sprains, emphasizing progressive functional motion applied early with protection of the vulnerable joint until tissue healing or surgical reconstruction restores stability.

ACUTE FRACTURES

Although fractures occur less often than soft-tissue injuries in sports, they often required prolonged periods of immobilization or surgical intervention for treatment. Healing rates range from weeks to months. Associated soft-tissue injuries and muscle atrophy may take additional months, or even years, for full recovery.

Fractures typically occur with one of three mechanisms: 1) direct force, 2) associated with dislocation, 3) or noncontact. Most fractures occur from direct force application. The direction of the load applied may be bending, twisting (torsion), or axial loading. Most fractures probably occur from a combination of these mechanisms. For example, as an athlete falls on an outstretched hand, the forearm may rotate, causing one of the forearm bones to bend over the other, as an axial load is being applied simultaneously. An example of a fracture that occurs from a pure bending mechanism is a direct blow, such as a soccer player's foot directly contacting another player's tibia, with enough force to break it. The severe and potentially catastrophic football tackling injury that consists of the athlete's cervical spine flexing slightly so that the normal lordosis is straightened, and immediately followed by axial loading, can result in marked displacement of one cervical vertebra relative to another, as well as displacement of the compression fracture fragments of the cervical vertebra itself.

Fractures may occur during joint dislocation, but some fractures actually occur as the joint is being relocated. Common examples of fracture-dislocations include the humeral head, the patellofemoral joint, and articulations of the finger joints.

Finally, fractures can occur as noncontact injuries. The tibial eminence may be avulsed by the anterior cruciate ligament in noncontact hyperextension or deceleration injuries. Similarly, a severe ankle sprain may include an avulsion fracture of the distal fibula.

Evaluation of injuries that are potentially fractures includes physical examination of the injured area and of the adjacent joints both proximal and distal to the injury. It also includes careful evaluation for possible compartmental syndrome and examination of the neurovascular status of the limb (or of the entire body, if the injury involves the spinal column). If there is deformity, marked swelling, or bony tenderness, radiographic evaluation is indicated. Further imaging, such as computed tomographic (CT) scanning, may be needed to completely evaluate a possible fracture.

Treatment

Initial treatment is splinting of the injured region. When deformity is noted, the best recommendation is generally to splint the limb in its present position, rather than to attempt correction of deformity in the field. Exceptions to this include significant neurovascular compromise where possible permanent damage to the limb could occur before the patient is transported to an appropriate treatment venue. At times, reduction of a deformed limb may be appropriate in the field when carried out by a trained individual who has first evaluated this situation fully enough to have made a provisional diagnosis before any reduction is attempted. The appropriate splint for someone with a suspected spinal column injury is a spine board, with appropriate lateral and rotational stabilization.

The next phase of treatment, following determination of accurate diagnosis, is stabilization of the fracture. Typically, the fracture should be stabilized in an anatomically reduced position. Stabilization methods include splinting, cast immobilization, internal fixation with metal implants, or external fixation with intraosseus pins and an external frame. Once the fracture is stabilized, the next phase of treatment is protected mobilization. The length of time before mobilization depends on fracture pattern, and type of treatment. For example, rehabilitation of an athlete's tibia fracture treated with intramedullary rodding might include range of motion exercises for the knee and ankle immediately after surgery, followed by early weight-bearing and rapid return to functional strengthening exercises. Conversely, a distal radius fracture treated by closed reduction and an above-elbow cast typically requires 4 to 6 weeks of immobilization in the initial cast, followed by an additional 4 weeks in a below-elbow cast or splint. In this situation, rehabilitation of the biceps and triceps cannot begin until the shorter cast or splint is applied.

Return to Play

Return to participation principles are identical to those for sprains, strains, and dislocations. They include full or nearly full range of motion of the joints of the extremity, strength sufficient for safe participation, and adequate proprioception. The amount of range of motion and strength must be determined by the requirements that particular sports make of the injured limb.

MUSCULOTENDINOUS INJURIES: STRAINS

Strain refers to injury of musculotendinous units. Usually this means an acute disruption of muscle fibers in the region of the musculotendinous junction. The definition may be extended to include tendon rupture, muscle rupture, and avulsion of tendinous insertions from bone. Strain injuries seem to have a predilection for transitional areas of stiffness of the musculotendinous unit, such as the junction between muscle and tendon or between tendon and bone. Force apparently concentrates in these transitional areas—a recurrent theme in musculoskeletal biomechanics.

The clinical appearance of strain injury generally manifests as an acute, painful episode. Patients perceive pain in the injured extremity associated with disability ranging from mild, with pain on resisted contraction, to severe, with functional deficit and inability to move an affected joint. A grading system similar to that used for ligament sprains may be applied to strain injury. Grade 1 injuries represent strains in which a small percentage of muscle fibers is torn, with intact fascia. Muscle disruption is found on a microscopic level, with little macroscopic damage and minimal disability. Grade 2 injuries involve a larger proportion of the muscle fibers, with significant hemorrhage. Fascial disruption may occur and result in functional deficit, but muscle contraction is possible

and the affected extremity may be moved—but with pain. Grade 3 muscle strain injuries are characterized by complete or near-complete rupture of the muscle-tendon unit, affecting the surrounding fascia with hemorrhage. Most strains present with marked weakness or inability to move a joint affected by the muscle, and significant pain.

Risk factors for strain injury relate to the strength, mode of contraction, flexibility, fiber type, anatomy, and contraction phase of the involved muscle. Weak or fatigued muscles are more vulnerable to strain injury. This factor is the reason that strain injuries occur more often to wrestlers participating in practices and tournaments where they are required to compete while fatigued than to those participating in individual matches. In addition to strength, flexibility of muscles correlates with vulnerability to injury. Stiffer muscles are more prone to strain injury than supple, elastic muscles. Factors affecting the stiffness of the musculotendinous unit include preactivation (warm-up) and resting length of the muscle. The vulnerability of a stiffer musculotendinous unit may explain in part the tendency for adolescents to sustain muscle injuries during their rapid growth phase, when musculotendinous units are continually accommodating to increasing bone length and adapting to a new resting tension.

The type of activity and mode of contraction of the muscle-tendon unit also contribute to vulnerability to strain injury. Muscles stretched passively are more prone to acute strain than muscles contracted actively. In addition, muscles are more vulnerable to strain during eccentric contraction (the muscle is lengthened while being contracted) than during concentric contraction (the muscle shortens while contracting). These factors are underscored in rabbit and rat models when the musculotendinous junction is stretched to failure. Contracting muscle is found to absorb more energy than passively stretched muscle (1). These muscles are thought to act as energy absorbers, and stronger, more flexible muscles may absorb more energy before failure than weaker and fatigued muscles.

Finally, anatomy and fiber type also contribute to risk of strain injury. Biarticular muscles—those crossing two joints (such as the biceps brachii and rectus femoris)—are more vulnerable to strain injury than muscles crossing only one joint. The proportion of fiber types 1 (slow twitch) and 2 (fast twitch) also correlates with vulnerability to strain. Muscles with a higher percentage of type 2 fast twitch fibers, which are more often used in ballistic, rapid acceleration-deceleration activities, are more prone to strain injury (23–25).

The histology of muscle strain injury follows a predictable course. Immediately upon injury, disruption occurs at or near the musculotendinous junction. Rupture of muscle tissue and fascia results in bleeding with the possibility of collection of significant hematoma. This hematoma may be constrained within the surrounding fascial compartment or leak through a rent in the fascia into the subcutaneous space. The amount of extravasation correlates with the site of injury, with injuries occurring primarily in the muscle being accompanied by more bleeding, and injuries to tendons—which are relatively avascular—having less bleeding. This is particularly true of injuries of sheathed tendons, such as flexor tendons of the hand, which are accompanied by little or no significant hemorrhage.

Leakage of fluid and cells is followed by release of growth factors and cytokines in damaged tissues. In the first days following muscle injury, necrosis of muscle fibers occurs, accompanied by macrophage infiltration within the disrupted fibers. Proliferation of inflammatory cells is followed by clearing of necrotic muscle fibers and proliferation of granulation tissue, leading to muscle regeneration and fibrosis. Several days after injury, a prominent increase in fibrosis occurs, with an increase in connective tissue between the muscle fibers. Within granulation tissue, high concentrations of fibronectin and chemoattractants lead to the migration of fibroblasts between the necrotic tendon stumps or into the area of muscle injury for healing. Reorganization of the cell-rich fiber network occurs, and while healing proceeds, the area becomes less cellular and musculotendinous fibers become oriented in the direction of mechanical stress.

Strain injuries occurring within muscle, or at the musculotendinous junction, may be considered significantly different from pure tendinous injuries, and healing of tendons—as with ligaments—depends on their environment. As seen with ligament healing, the highly organized, remodeled scar tissue in tendon healing resembles the tendon grossly but never perfectly exhibits its anatomic features. A good approximation is achieved, but residual weakness or increased stiffness at the repair site, attributable to increased collagen, may be responsible for the compromised biomechanical behavior of ruptured tendons after healing. It is probable that, as long as scar exists within a musculotendinous unit, this will remain an area of force concentration and reduced resiliency. Strain injuries occurring within muscle or at musculotendinous junctions are in a favorable environment for healing, with a higher potential for recovery. As the muscle-tendon unit is followed into the sheathed tendon, the potential for recovery is less as tendons are avascular and tendons within sheaths are bathed in synovial fluid. True tendon ruptures are more likely to require surgical repair to restore continuity. Remodeling of musculotendinous injury is, in part, dependent on the applied stress and, as do ligaments, tendons tend to remodel with more anatomic fiber orientation when a controlled, subthreshold stress is applied.

Treatment of Strains

The clinical appearance and treatment of musculotendinous injuries may be considered according to grade. Grade 1 strain injuries manifest with mild swelling and minimal or no ecchymosis. Point tenderness is noted on physical examination and pain occurs, primarily with resistance testing. Generally, range of motion without resistance of the affected extremity will be painless in a grade 1 strain. Most injuries at this level heal with little or no intervention. Treatment should be based on physiologic principles: 1) inhibition of the initial hemorrhage; 2) suppression of the inflammatory reaction responsible for initial pain; and 3) rapid rehabilitation. Patients are counseled to apply cold and compression as soon as possible after the injury. Oral NSAIDs are useful in the first 5 to 7 days. Once the initial pain of injury is gone, heat may be used before stretching. Active stretching, starting as early as possible after injury, is helpful in restoring function and reducing recovery time.

Patients follow a progressive rehabilitation program based on milestones. For example, when contraction of the muscle is pain-free, strengthening may proceed. When full, painless contraction and full strength recover, patients may be permitted gradual progression to activities. Little to no long-term sequelae are expected from a grade 1 strain injury, and patients generally do not perceive any deficit.

In the case of the grade 2 injury, the clinical appearance is more severe. Patients may have perceived a pop or tearing sensation. Acute pain is noted and gradual onset of swelling and ecchymosis seen. On physical examination, weakness is noted on resistance testing, although contraction of the muscle with motion of the affected joint is noted. In these cases, the initial hemorrhage is significant, and the early application of cold and compression is important. As with grade 1 strains, patients sustaining grade 2 strains may benefit significantly from the use of NSAIDs. Gentle muscle stretching is instituted early, and the joint is permitted motion within the tolerable range. Rehabilitation is progressive, following milestones. These patients may benefit from the observation and guidance of a physical therapist. This is particularly relevant when return to heavy labor or sports is a goal. Return to heavy activities is delayed until full strength is regained on manual or instrumented testing.

The appearance of grade 3 musculotendinous strain injury is characteristic. These are often quite painful, accompanied by a perception of a tearing or a pop. Hemorrhage is significant, with probable disruption of fascia or tendon sheath, and ecchymosis is evident within hours of the injury. On physical examination, palpation of the edematous extremity may identify a significant defect, and no effective contractile function is noted. In many cases, more than one musculotendinous unit crosses the involved joint, and patients may be able to generate significant motion in the context of the complete muscle tear. This may be seen in cases of Achilles tendon rupture, where patients can generate active ankle plantar flexion with the tibialis posterior and toe flexors. This also may be seen in quadriceps tendon ruptures in which the lateral and medial retinacula remain intact and active quadriceps contraction and straight-leg raise are achievable. In these circumstances, it is possible to miss a clinically significant tendon rupture.

Treatment of grade 3 strains includes the previously mentioned regimen of application of cold and compression, elevation when possible, and resting of the affected extremity. As the initial hemorrhage stabilizes and the inflammatory phase begins, NSAIDs are helpful. In some cases, immobilization is warranted, particularly when extremity function is lost. Immobilization accompanying compression can also help reduce the initial hemorrhage.

The specific treatment for grade 3 musculotendinous injuries varies widely, depending on the location of the injury and the musculotendinous unit involved. For example, rupture of sheathed flexor tendons in the hand generally requires surgery (depending on the location of the rupture), but a tear of the medial gastrocnemius muscle in the calf rarely requires surgical intervention and is likely to go on to full healing without significant deficit. As a general rule, strain injuries occurring within muscle do not require surgical intervention, whereas tendon ruptures are much more likely to require surgery. The most commonly encountered tendon ruptures seen by musculoskeletal care providers include rupture of the long head of the biceps brachii, rupture of the quadriceps or patellar tendon, Achilles tendon tears, and rotator cuff tears. Most often, rupture of the biceps tendon presents a cosmetic problem, as the biceps sags with gravity to be bundled into the distal arm. This is accompanied by a small strength deficit, because elbow flexion benefits from significant redundancy of muscles. Surgical repair in this circumstance generally is considered optional. Quadriceps and patellar tendon disruption usually preclude active knee extension and have a poor prognosis for spontaneous healing. These are more likely to be treated surgically with acute or subacute repair, followed by protective bracing and rehabilitation. Tears of the Achilles tendon compromise plantar flexion strength significantly and affect walking. The sheathed Achilles tendon can heal without surgery, and these can be treated in a cast with the ankle joint maintained in a position of plantar flexion to appose the torn tendon ends. However, the rerupture rate after nonoperative treatment for Achilles tendon ruptures tends to be higher than after surgery, and this must be weighed against the potential risks of surgical intervention in the decision making for these injuries. Rotator cuff tendon ruptures have a wide spectrum of clinical presentations, from gradual degenerative attrition to acute rupture. Treatment is considered on a case-by-case basis with a variety of options, ranging from conservative rehabilitation to surgical reconstruction.

In summary, strain injuries represent tears of musculotendinous units. They tend to occur in areas of transition of stiffness, such as the myotendinous junction or at the insertion site of a tendon. Biarticular muscles that are stretched passively and fatigued muscles, as well as muscles contracting eccentrically and not preconditioned (warmed up), are more vulnerable to strain injury. Strain injury histology follows a predictable course of hemorrhage, inflammation, repair, and remodeling. Treatment for musculotendinous injuries is based on physiologic principles, with immediate treatment, usually with cold and compression, followed by early institution of rehabilitation. Rehabilitation emphasizes active contraction and controlled passive stretching as soon as possible. A gradual progression of activities is undertaken using objective measurements as guidelines.

Prevention of muscle strain injury is implied by the risk factors for injury. Resilience to injury is optimized with appropriate warm-up. Preparatory warm-up for heavy activity requires both preactivation and stretching, both of which are known to increase the ability of the muscle to absorb energy and prevent injury. Preparatory conditioning in the form of strengthening is also protective. These principles serve as the foundation for athletic conditioning and can also be applied effectively in the setting of work simulation.

MENISCUS TEARS

The menisci serve crucial roles in knee function. They are load-sharing structures, absorbing and dissipating weight-bearing force and protecting articular cartilage. The menisci also function in conjunction with ligaments as secondary stabilizers of the knee. Meniscal injuries in adults may vary widely in regard to the early manifestations and presentation of injury and the potential long-term outcome. Meniscus injuries often occur as secondary injuries in conjunction with significant ligament tears.

Evaluation of meniscal injuries in the adult generally is straightforward. However, it is of paramount importance to interpret meniscal injuries within their context; the recommendations for treatment and prognosis for recovery from meniscus injury depend greatly on whether the injury occurs in the context of a ligament injury or as an isolated tear; and the pre-injury condition of the knee, in particular, the existence of concomitant osteoarthrosis.

Most meniscal injuries that happen in the workplace or during sports occur as a result of indirect trauma. Menisci sustain significant stress when weight-bearing and torque are applied across the knee. This may be seen in circumstances of forceful and ballistic twisting injuries, as seen in football, basketball, and wrestling, which account for the greatest number of meniscal injuries occurring in sports. Meniscal injuries may also be sustained with relatively minor trauma, such as the repetitive hyperflexion position maintained during certain activities in the workplace or at home, e.g., gardening. It is likely that the majority of meniscal injuries are acquired outside of the context of sports participation, and many occur as a component of osteoarthrosis (26).

Acute meniscal injuries sustained during sport or labor often present a characteristic history. Patients have an acute or subacute onset of pain, often localized to one side of the knee. This is followed by persistence of pain, and the gradual development of effusion over several days. Acutely meniscal tears occasionally displace and become dislodged into a nonanatomic position within the knee. This often creates a locking symptom in which full extension or, less frequently, full flexion is blocked mechanically. An acutely locked knee is very painful, and patients tend to guard the knee, avoiding attempts at motion. Muscle spasm accompanies this guarding and makes physical examination difficult. Patients in this condition are often evaluated in an emergency setting and negative results on radiographs are followed by an MRI scan to confirm the presence of a displaced meniscal tear. More often, however, acute locking symptoms do not occur. The patient has either no mechanical obstruction to motion or occasional mild catching symptoms. These manifest as a transient painful click or pop, often followed by a sense of relief. In many cases, patients do not have signs of mechanical catching or locking, and the persistence of pain and effusion motivates them to seek medical care.

Evaluation of patients suspected of sustaining meniscus injury begins with a detailed history, which most often strongly suggests the diagnosis. The patient evaluation must include examination for concomitant ligament injury and instability patterns, along with assessment for any evidence of preexisting osteoarthritis, regardless of how mild. The physical examination for a meniscus tear should concentrate on the following salient features.

Range of Motion

Limitation in range of knee motion when compared with the contralateral extremity is seen in most patients with significant meniscal injury. For patients with locked, displaced meniscal fragments, this limitation is very obvious, most often manifesting as a failure to achieve full extension. Patients resist efforts to manipulate the joint forcefully into extension. Attempts at manipulation with the goal of reducing displaced meniscal fragments should be limited to experienced examiners. More often, the limitation of motion manifests as pain in flexion. This may be attributable to the compression of damaged meniscal tissue in the posterior aspect of the knee or, more simply, attributable to reduction of the potential knee joint capsular volume caused by hyperflexion, so most patients with a significant effusion are uncomfortable in a position of hyperflexion.

Effusion

Most patients with acute or subacute meniscal tears present with significant knee effusion. Tense effusions are less common than those seen with acute ligament injuries. More often, small submaximal effusions are detected, which may be chronic, persisting for months.

Joint Line Tenderness

Tenderness at the medial or lateral joint line is the most sensitive and specific test for meniscus tear (27–29). Excluding patients with concomitant ligament injury or significant osteoarthritis, most patients with a meniscus tear have tenderness located precisely at the joint line, more often posterior-medial or posterior-lateral, depending on the location of tear.

Provocative Tests

Many provocative tests have been described to diagnose meniscus tears. Most of these are a combination of flexion, compression, and rotation, with or without accompanying varus or valgus stress to compress the posterior aspect of the medial or lateral meniscus, respectively (30–32). It is essential to differentiate patients who have pain with these provocative maneuvers from those who have pain simply from being placed into a hyperflexed position, and it is easy to misinterpret pain with hyperflexion as a positive provocative sign for meniscal pathology.

A patient presenting with a history suggestive of meniscus pathology and physical examination consistent with the diagnosis should be evaluated for concomitant osteoarthritis. Plain radiographs offer a helpful diagnostic adjunct. All patients with suspected meniscus injuries should have posterior-to-anterior plain radiographs obtained while weight-bearing with the knees flexed at 45° (33). The 45° flexion posterior-to-anterior weight-bearing radiograph is a highly sensitive method of demonstrating subtle joint space narrowing associated with early osteoarthrosis. It is crucial to determine this; the reason is related to prognosis. An isolated meniscal injury occurring in a younger patient without significant chondral damage bears a very good prognosis for treatment and a likelihood of meniscal repair as a treatment alternative. However, patients with osteoarthritis who have accompanying degenerative meniscus tears have a significantly worse prognosis for treatment. It is for this reason that the flexion weight-bearing radiograph must be obtained *before* considering sophisticated imaging modalities such as MRI. Patients with meniscal symptoms in the context of osteoarthritis generally do not require MRI to confirm the degenerative meniscus tear, as meniscal degeneration is implicit if asymmetric joint space narrowing is demonstrated. In this context, the patient should be treated first for acute exacerbation of osteoarthrosis before considering arthroscopy for meniscectomy.

MRI should be reserved for patients in whom the diagnosis remains uncertain after appropriate physical examination and assessment with plain radiographs. MRI obtained on a high-quality machine with an appropriate magnet of 1.5 tesla or greater, evaluated by an experienced reader, can provide a high degree of sensitivity and specificity for meniscal pathology (34).

As with the assessment for meniscus pathology, the plan for treatment must be made within the context in which the meniscal injury occurs. Patients sustaining locked displaced meniscus injuries are unable to walk until the meniscus is treated. If the knee can be manipulated and extension restored, there remains a high probability of recurrent displacement and locking. Therefore, patients sustaining locking episodes are appropriately counseled to have arthroscopic evaluation and treatment as soon as it is convenient. Patients with locked knees recalcitrant to manipulation require arthroscopy. The majority of patients presenting with meniscus tears, however, suffer from subacute symptoms of long standing. Most are able to ambulate well, but complain of joint line pain accompanied by recurrent effusion. These patients with chronic meniscal tears may require arthroscopic surgery for partial meniscectomy or, in selected cases, meniscus repair. Intervention is not urgent in these circumstances and can be arranged when convenient for the patient. There is some evidence that a significant delay in treatment may reduce the capacity for meniscal healing in the context of an attempted meniscus repair (35). However, this is by no means certain and it is not unreasonable to permit patients a trial of protected weight-bearing with anti-inflammatory medications as long as appropriate follow-up is arranged. These patients should be counseled to avoid repetitive stress on the knee, particularly in positions of hyperflexion.

While a reasonable argument can be made that a patient with recurrent mechanical symptoms of catching may be causing more injury to their knee by continuing to bear weight, patients without significant mechanical symptoms are probably at low risk for accumulating damage in their knee if there is a delay in treatment. A reasonable compromise would be to permit patients a period of protected weight-bearing with a cane or crutches, with the goal of mobilizing rapidly to full weight-bearing, possibly with the assistance of a physical therapist. Patients who can transition successfully to full weight-bearing may gradually increase their activities, if they are vigilant in observing the knee. Recurrent mechanical symptoms, effusion, or persistent pain are appropriate indications for further assessment and consideration for possible surgery.

For patients with meniscus pathology occurring in conjunction with osteoarthritis, the decision to undergo surgery for the meniscus must be undertaken with caution. The prognosis for arthroscopy in the context of osteoarthritis is poorer than that for meniscus tears occurring in an otherwise pristine knee. Patients should be counseled carefully about the guarded prognosis and offered nonoperative treatment alternatives before having arthroscopy.

The load-sharing function of the meniscus and the occurrence of osteoarthritis in knees having undergone meniscectomy are well documented (36). In the setting of arthroscopy and partial meniscectomy, the greater the area of resection of meniscus, the more weight transfer and force transmission sustained to the articular cartilage along with a higher probability of development of osteoarthritis in the involved knee (37). For this reason, surgical treatment of meniscus tears should always include a primary goal of achieving repair if possible. Unfortunately, the majority of meniscal tears occur in the relatively avascular inner portion of the meniscus, with a poor prognosis for healing, and are treated with partial meniscectomy. Short-term outcome from partial meniscectomy in an otherwise normal knee is excellent. Generally, the less meniscus that is removed, the better.

As stated above, meniscectomy occurring in the context of osteoarthritis may have a significant beneficial effect; however, the ultimate long-term prognosis must be based on the natural history of osteoarthritis and not on the diagnosis of meniscus tear. Most patients can expect a return to normal or near-normal knee function after partial meniscectomy or successful repair. Patients undergoing meniscectomy with excision of a large portion of meniscal tissue may be counseled appropriately to alter their activities to avoid repetitive impact loading, if possible, to protect the articular surfaces and prolong the functional lifetime of the involved knee.

REFERENCES

1. Crisco JJ, Hentel KD, Jackson WO, et al. Maximal contraction lessens impact response in a muscle contusion model. J Biomech 1996; 29:1291–1296.

2. Ryan JB, Wheeler JH, Hopkinson WJ, et al. Quadriceps contusions: West Point update. Am J Sports Med 1991;19:299–304.

3. Hughston JC, Andrews JR, Cross MJ, Moschi A. Classification of knee ligament instabilities. Part 1: the medial compartment and cruciate ligaments. J Bone Joint Surg 1976;58A:159–172.

4. Woo SL, Young EP, Ohland KJ, et al. The effects of transection of the anterior cruciate ligament on healing of the medial collateral ligament: a biomechanical study of the knee in dogs. J Bone Joint Surg 1990;72A:382–392.

5. Gross MT. Effects of recurrent lateral ankle sprains on active and passive judgements of joint position. Phys Ther 1987;67:1505–1509.

6. Smith RL, Brunolli J. Shoulder kinesthesia after anterior glenohumeral joint dislocation. Phys Ther 1989;69:106–112.

7. Garn SN, Newton RA. Kinesthetic awareness in subjects with multiple ankle sprains. Phys Ther 1988;68:1667–1671.

8. Barrack RL, Skinner HB, Buckley SL. Proprioception in the anterior cruciate deficient knee. Am J Sports Med 1989;17:1–6.

9. Lephart SM, Fu FH, Borsa PA, et al. Proprioception of the knee and shoulder joint in normal, athletic, capsuloligamentous pathological, and post-reconstruction individuals. Orthop Trans 1995;18:1157.

10. Victoroff BN, Greenwald AE, Rosenberg TD, Newhouse K. Knee proprioception in ACL intact, deficient and reconstructed knees: effects of starting position and angular velocity. Poster presentation at the American Academy of Orthopaedic Surgeons 64th Annual Meeting, San Francisco, February 1997.

11. Spencer JD, Hayes KC, Alexander IJ. Knee joint effusion and quadriceps reflex inhibition in man. Arch Phys Med Rehabil 1984;65:171–177.

12. Fahrer H, Rentsch HU, Gerber NJ, et al. Knee effusion and reflex inhibition of the quadriceps: a bar to effective retraining. J Bone Joint Surg 1988;70B:635–638.

13. Jensen K, Graf BK. The effects of knee effusion on quadriceps strength and knee intraarticular pressure. Arthroscopy 1993;9: 52–56.

14. Tropp H, Askling C, Gillquist J. Prevention of ankle sprains. Am J Sports Med 1985;13:259–262.

15. Ihara H, Nakayama A. Dynamic joint control training for knee ligament injuries. Am J Sports Med 1986;14:309–315.

16. Baumhauer JF, Alosa DM, Renstrom AF, et al. A prospective study of ankle injury risk factors. Am J Sports Med 1995;23:564–570.

17. Rowe CR, Sakellaides HT. Factors related to recurrences of anterior dislocations of the shoulder. Clin Orthop 1961;20:40–48.

18. McLaughlin HL, MacLellan DI. Recurrent anterior dislocation of the shoulder. Part 2: a comparative study. J Trauma 1967;7:191–201.

19. Henry JH, Genung JA. Natural history of glenohumeral dislocation—revisited. Am J Sports Med 1982;10:135–137.

20. Hovelius L, Eriksson K, Fredin H, et al. Recurrences after initial dislocation of the shoulder: results of a prospective study of treatment. J Bone Joint Surg 1983;65A:343–349.

21. Neviaser RJ, Neviaser TJ, Neviaser JS. Concurrent rupture of the rotator cuff and anterior dislocation of the shoulder in the older patient. J Bone Joint Surg 1988; 70A:1308–1311.

22. Sonnabend DH. Treatment of primary anterior shoulder dislocation in patients older than 40 years of age: conservative versus operative. Clin Orthop 1994;304: 74–77.

23. Garrett WE Jr. Injuries to the muscle-tendon unit. Instr Course Lect 1988;37:275–282.

24. Garrett WE Jr, Almekinders L, Seaber AV. Biomechanics of muscle tears in stretching injuries. Trans Orthop Res Soc 1984;9:384.

25. Garrett WE Jr, Califf JC, Bassett FH III. Histochemical correlates of hamstring injuries. Am J Sports Med 1984;12:98–103.

26. Baker BE, Peckham AC, Pupparo F, Sanborn JC. Review of meniscal

injury and associated sports. Am J Sports Med 1985;13:1–4.

27. Anderson AF, Lipscomb AB. Clinical diagnosis of meniscal tears: description of a new manipulative test. Am J Sports Med 1986;14:291–293.

28. Fowler PJ, Lubliner JA. The predictive value of five clinical signs in the evaluation of meniscal pathology. Arthroscopy 1989;5:184–186.

29. Terry GC, Tagert BE, Young MJ. Reliability of the clinical assessment in predicting the cause of internal derangements of the knee. Arthroscopy 1995;11:568–576.

30. Apley AG. The diagnosis of meniscus injuries. J Bone Joint Surg 1947;29:78–84.

31. Henning CE, Lynch MA, Glick KR. Physical examination of the knee. In: Nicholas JA, Herschman EB, eds. The lower extremity and spine in sports medicine. St. Louis: CV Mosby, 1985:685–689.

32. McMurray PP. The semilunar cartilages. Br J Surg 1942;29:407–414.

33. Rosenberg TD, Paulos LE, Parker RD, et al. The forty-five-degree posteroanterior flexion weight-bearing radiograph of the knee. J Bone Joint Surg 1988;70A:1479–1483.

34. Polly DW Jr, Callaghan JJ, Sikes RA, et al. The accuracy of selective magnetic resonance imaging compared with the findings of arthroscopy of the knee. J Bone Joint Surg 1988;70A:192–198.

35. Henning CE, Lynch MA, Yearout KM, et al. Arthroscopic meniscal repair using an exogenous fibrin clot. Clin Orthop 1990;252:64–72.

36. Fairbanks TJ. Knee joint changes after meniscectomy. J Bone Joint Surg 1948;30B:664–670.

37. Baratz ME, Fu FH, Mengato R. Meniscal tears: the effect of meniscectomy and of repair on intraarticular contact areas and stress in the human knee: a preliminary report. Am J Sports Med 1986;14:270–275.

Chapter 22

Scientific Basis for the Use of Modalities in Sports Medicine

Robbin Wickham
Laura Schmitt
Lynn Snyder-Mackler

When an athlete is injured, therapeutic modalities can be used to create a better environment for healing. Thermal and electrotherapeutic agents do not accelerate biologic healing, but they can be manipulated to maximize the effectiveness of treatment. This chapter provides the health care professional who treats athletes with an overview of the scientific basis for the use of therapeutic modalities. Superficial application of heat and cold, ultrasound, phonophoresis, iontophoresis, and basic electrotherapy application are discussed.

CRYOTHERAPY

Cryotherapy is the most commonly used physical agent in sports medicine. Cold can diminish the inflammatory response and help to control inflammation after it occurs. Pain and swelling are the hallmarks of an inflammatory response, and cold has a direct effect on both. Many agents can be used to apply cold to the body, including ice packs, ice massage, chemical cold packs, cold or ice water, and commercial compressive cold devices. Cold has been well studied, and evidence for its effectiveness in treatment of acute inflammatory conditions and muscle soreness is strong. Physiologic effects of cold include decreasing tissue temperature with simultaneous effects on inflammation, blood flow, pain, muscle spasm, metabolism, and muscle strength and function.

The ability of superficial cold application to decrease tissue temperatures is a result of temperature gradient, conduction of temperature, and duration of application. The best conductor of heat is water and therefore, crushed ice, ice water baths, and ice massage (where ice is placed directly on the skin and melts as it moves, leaving a film of water between the skin and the ice cup) provide a large temperature gradient with excellent conduction. Superficial tissues cool rapidly and therefore skin temperature may not be a good indication of cooling at deeper tissue depths. Superficial cooling modalities do not appear to be able to cool deep structures. Levy et al (1) found no temperature difference between a control group and a group who received 90 minutes of cold therapy via a Cryo/Cuff (AirCast, Summit, NJ) in either the glenohumeral joint or subacromial space. Superficial application of ice does significantly cool superficial structures, even when the part is not directly exposed. Metzman et al (2) found that the presence of a synthetic or a plaster cast does not prevent the lowering of skin temperature by crushed ice packs applied to the surface of the casts. The skin temperature of legs in synthetic casts decreased an average of 10.4°C while the temperature of legs in plaster casts decreased an average of 11.0°C after approximately 60 minutes of application (2).

Zemke et al (3) found ice massage promoted maximal tissue cooling more quickly than other cryotherapy methods. Ice massage is an aggressive cryotherapeutic agent and is most beneficial for treatment of a localized area. For larger areas, cold whirlpools or ice baths can provide similar cooling effects, as long as a dependent position is not a concern. If a localized treatment area or a dependent position is undesirable, a cold compression unit can be used in combination with elevation.

Studies of healthy subjects generally show increase in threshold to experimentally induced pain with cold application (4). In studies of patients' responses to cryotherapy, however, the literature is conflicting regarding pain relief from cold (5–8). As Zemke pointed out, cold application produces superficial analgesia in 2 to 5 minutes; however, most of the time, the target tissue is much deeper (e.g., muscle) (3,9,10). Pain perception is not just nociception. Experiential and behavioral components of pain perception add complexity to the assessment of the effectiveness of any physical agent for pain management. Ernst and Fialka (11) speculate that increased pain threshold results from the anti-nociceptive effect on the gate control system, decreased nerve conduction, reduction in muscle spasm, and prevention of edema after injury. Cold can decrease pain by decreasing nerve conduction and slowing the transmission of pain impulses. Pain can also be indirectly influenced. Michlovitz infers pain reduction is also caused by a counter-irritant effect of ice application, leading to decreased pain perception via the gate theory (12).

Cold causes vasoconstriction and when applied to an acute injury can help delay local hemorrhage and inflammation. Vasoconstriction contributes to decreased blood flow to the injured area; consequently, the precursors of inflammation can be controlled. Weston et al (13) observed a decrease in blood volume in the injured area after a 20-minute application of cold gel pack to acute ankle sprains. For the first 24 to 48 hours after injury, ice application is the treatment modality of choice. When cold is applied in a timely manner, cellular metabolism can be decreased reducing the hypoxic effects of injury (14).

Edwards et al (15) investigated cold therapy after arthroscopic anterior cruciate ligament (ACL) reconstruction in a prospective, randomized study. They found no difference among three groups (i.e., Cryo-Cuff with ice; Cryo-Cuff with room temperature water; no Cryo-Cuff) in blood loss, analgesic use, range of motion (ROM), and visual-analog pain (15). Speer et al (16) prospectively studied 50 patients after shoulder surgery. Twenty-five patients used a cryotherapy device and 25 did not. In this study, however, the cryotherapy group had less pain, less swelling, and needed fewer analgesic agents, both immediately after surgery and after 10 days. Shroeder et al (17) also found applying ice and compression after ACL reconstruction significantly reduced swelling, pain, and consumption of analgesic medications. A recent critical review of the literature on treatment of soft-tissue injuries of the ankle found evidence to support judicious early use of cryotherapy in the treatment of these injuries (18).

The influence of cold on muscular strength and function is a concern when treating athletes. Reports of strength changes after application of ice show conflicting results. Much of the discrepancy appears to be related to the duration of application. When ice is applied for shorter periods of time (5 to 10 minutes), enhanced muscle performance has been demonstrated (19). Studies measuring strength after longer applications of cold (20 min/hr for 5 hours, 20 minutes, and 25 minutes, respectively) have shown decreases in muscle performance (20–22). However, Evans et al (23) found no significant changes in agility following ice immersion for 20 minutes. They attributed this finding to decreasing the joint temperature without affecting large muscles and concluded strength deficits are observed when large muscles are cooled. When the joint is cooled, power and strength are not affected as greatly and, therefore, no change in agility was seen. The current recommendation is to avoid vigorous work immediately after cryotherapy to avoid potential tissue damage.

Although few, contraindications include hypersensitivity to cold (e.g., Raynaud's disease, cold urticaria), diminished or absent sensation, and compromised circulation. There have been several reported cases of injuries to peripheral nerves induced by exposure to ice (5,24,25). Nerves lying close to the skin surface (e.g., peroneal, ulnar, lateral femoral cutaneous, and supraclavicular) are particularly susceptible to cold-induced injury (25). Duration of exposure to ice as well as intensity of cooling should be considered to avoid injury to these structures. Padding over the nerve minimizes injury.

Cryotherapy is effective and safe. There are few contraindications. Application is simple and inexpensive. The only danger occurs with long duration applications at low temperatures. The evidence for effectiveness of cryotherapy in the treatment of acute musculoskeletal injuries is strong in theory and practice.

SUPERFICIAL HEAT

Superficial heat, in the form of moist heat packs or warm whirlpools, is most frequently used in sports medicine as an adjunct to the rehabilitation program or training and conditioning. The therapeutic effects of increased circulation and muscle relaxation are beneficial before exercise to accelerate warm-up of the muscles. Tissue temperature must be elevated to 40°C to 45°C to achieve these effects (26–29). Alleviation of pain following heat treatment is largely attributable to relaxation of the muscles.

The depth of the target tissue and the thermal agent choice (superficial or deep) need to be considered when the goal is to increase tissue extensibility. When studying the application of superficial heating and cooling followed by static stretching in 24 subjects, Taylor et al and Henricson et al (30,31) found that the greatest increases in ROM occurred after application of heat in conjunction with stretching; however, the effect was not statistically greater than stretching alone. Wessling et al (32) demonstrated deep-heat modalities improved the efficacy of static stretching over superficial heat modalities. The evidence is largely theoretical, but clinically, superficial heat is often used before stretching superficial muscles. Because heating increases blood flow, the increased tissue temperature rapidly dissipates after removal of the heat source. If superficial heating is used in combination with or in preparation for stretching, the stretch should immediately follow or be performed concurrently with the application of heat, avoiding dissipation of the heat and increasing the effectiveness of the stretch.

Superficial heat should not be used in acutely inflamed areas. Likewise, heat should not be used over an area of active infection. If sensation or circulation is impaired, only gentle heating should be used and skin should be monitored for signs of distress.

HYDROTHERAPY

Whirlpool baths are commonly used to treat athletic injuries and as an adjunct to training and conditioning. Typically, the warm whirlpool temperature is between 102°F and 105°F and the cold whirlpool temperature is 55°F to 60°F. The physiologic effects of superficial heat and cold application are evoked using water as a medium. Hydrotherapy provides an environment for the entire limb to be immersed in water, increasing surface area coverage. Exercises can be performed simultaneously. The main disadvantage of whirlpools is that the limb is positioned in a dependent position. When swelling is a concern, therefore, the whirlpool may not be a good therapeutic option.

ULTRASOUND

Therapeutic ultrasound is a physical agent that can increase tissue temperature at a depth of 3 to 5 cm. Ultrasound is a unique thermal modality. Both thermal and nonthermal effects (cavitation, acoustical streaming, and micromassage) are produced. Cavitation refers to the vibration of cellular gas bubbles found in body fluids. When cavitation is stable, gas bubbles expand and contract; however, when unstable, the gas bubbles may implode and release energy, causing tissue damage (33,34). Unstable cavitation has not been demonstrated with application of therapeutic ultrasound. Acoustical streaming is the movement of fluids along the boundaries of cell membranes as a result of the mechanical pressure wave and may affect cell membrane and vascular wall permeability. Micromassage is oscillation at the cellular level resulting from ultrasonographic mechanical energy.

Ultrasound is delivered by moving the ultrasound head over the affected area with a hydrophilic coupling agent between the ultrasound head and the body part. Uniform contact with the skin surface is maintained throughout the treatment. Kimura et al (35) found temperature increases to be greatest when ultrasound was applied at angles of 80° and 90° to the skin surface. Careful consideration of size of the treatment area, depth of target tissue, desired temperature increase, and output intensity over time can make treatment application more reproducible as well as more effective (36).

Ultrasound can be delivered in continuous or pulsed modes. Continuous mode ultrasound produces thermal and nonthermal effects; pulsed ultrasound produces only nonthermal effects. Pulsed ultrasound has been shown to aid the healing of chronic decubitus ulcers but has not been shown to be helpful in the treatment of musculoskeletal conditions (37,38). When vigorous heating is desired, the dose is determined by turning the intensity up until the patient perceives warmth. Recommended treatment times vary from 5 to 10 minutes but are largely dependent on the size of the area to be treated. Rimington et al (39) and Draper et al (40) determined ultrasound should not be administered after ice therapy if thermal effects are desired.

Clinical indications for ultrasound include joint contracture, scar tissue, muscle spasm, and inflammation. Since ultrasound can deliver thermal effects to depths of 5 cm, significant heating of joint structures and consequent increases in tissue extensibility can occur. Decreased viscoelastic properties of collagen and inhibition of neural activity can result from vigorous heating (35). Reed et al (41) studied joint displacement after application of ultrasound and reported that the concept of clinical heating to increase tissue extensi-

bility is supported, but the magnitude of the temperature change was not significant. Draper et al (27) found a 5°C temperature increase following a 3 MHz ultrasound treatment decayed by 3°C within the first 5 minutes. Clinically, this finding underscores the importance of stretching during or immediately after application of ultrasound.

Ultrasound is produced by an electrical "ringing" of a synthetic crystal. The resonant frequency of the ultrasound head is inversely proportional to the depth of penetration. Until recently, most ultrasound devices sold in the United State were 1.0 MHz, which penetrates up to 5 cm. Recently, 3.0 MHz devices have become available for use in superficial applications of vigorous heat and in areas where bone lies close to the skin surface.

Precautions include performing ultrasound over superficial bone (e.g., lateral epicondyle) because the mechanical energy generated can cause vibration of the periosteum, eliciting pain. In this instance, to avoid periosteal pain caused by sound beam reflection off the bone, a 3.0 MHz sound head is used. The ultrasound head should be kept moving at all times to prevent burning or the deleterious nonthermal effects.

PHONOPHORESIS

Phonophoresis is the introduction of a medication through the skin using the mechanical force of ultrasound. The drug is transmitted in its molecular form to the tissue, where it can have a local or a systemic effect. The medications are typically compounded with a coupling medium. Cameron and Monroe (42) examined some of the base formulations commonly used in compounding the medication. They found that corticosteroid gel, methyl salicylate cream, and unmedicated ultrasound gel and lotion transmitted more than 80% of the ultrasound energy, but hydrocortisone creams, mixtures of hydrocortisone in ultrasound gel, and petrolatum-based ointments transmitted less than 40% of the sound waves. Generally, lipid-based coupling media do not transmit ultrasound and are poor choices for phonophoresis. Likewise, if the medication itself does not transmit ultrasound, compounding it in a medium with good transmission does not necessarily result in increased transmission.

When using phonophoresis, one must know the depth of penetration of the ultrasound energy. Tissues lying deeper than 5 cm from the skin are not good candidates for treatment with phonophoresis, unless a systemic response is desired. The area treated should be pre-heated and ultrasound should be applied at a level to cause thermal elevation in the skin and subsequently increase blood flow to maximize the systemic effects of phonophoresis. When local effects are desired, ultrasound parameters that minimize heating can be used to decrease drug transportation away from the treatment area (43).

Medications used in phonophoresis include anesthetics, such as lidocaine, to numb surrounding tissues; analgesics to locally reduce pain; anti-inflammatory medications, such as adrenal corticosteroids, to inhibit inflammation; and counter-irritants to induce pain relief by over-stimulating the large afferent nerves (44). The only contraindication to phonophoresis distinct from those for ultrasound is allergy to the medication.

The basic research demonstrates mixed results regarding the effectiveness of ultrasonic delivery of medication to subdermal tissue. Bare et al (45) examined serum cortisol levels after phonophoresis of a 10% hydrocortisone acetate gel (1.0 MHz frequency, 1.0 W/cm^2 intensity, 5 minutes duration). They found no increase in serum cortisol levels within 15 minutes of treatment. Griffen et al found a 100% increase in cortisol concentration in muscle and a 146% increase in neural tissue after cortisone was introduced with ultrasound at intensities of 0.1 to 3.0 W/cm^2, frequencies of 0.09 to 3.60 MHz, over 5 to 51 minutes (46,47). The highest level of cortisol concentration was seen in treatments involving low-intensity and long-duration phonophoresis. Oziomek et al found no increase in serum salicylate levels after a 5-minute phonophoresis treatment with a salicylate-containing formula at doses of 1.5 W/cm^2 pulsed at 50%, 1.5 W/cm^2 continuous, or "sham" ultrasound (48). The studies involving animal models often used doses that caused tissue destruction, limiting the applicability to human subjects.

Clinicians have also performed studies to evaluate the ability of phonophoresis to decrease pain and inflammation in a variety of clinical conditions. Smith et al (49) found no difference in pain reduction in patients with shin splints when dexamethasone-lidocaine phonophresis was added to the treatment regimen. Ciccone et al (50) found no change in soreness associated with induced delayed-onset muscle soreness after trolamine salicylate phonophoresis, but ultrasound alone increased pain. The results can be interpreted in several ways. First, the anti-inflammatory properties of the medication may have decreased the thermal effect of the ultrasound on the tissue. Another explanation may be that the medication decreased the penetration of the soundwaves so that tissue heating did not occur. Patient perception of trigger-point pain was decreased after six phonophoresis treatments with a dexamethasone and lidocaine mixture (51). Griffen et al (52) found patients with osteoarthritis or joint and muscle pathology reported less pain and had more ROM after three treatments of hydrocortisone phonophoresis. Finally, Shin and Choi (53) found an increase in pressure pain threshold and decrease in pain on a visual analog scale in patients who received indomethacin phonophoresis for temporomandibular joint pain. Ultrasound can be used to deliver anti-inflammatory medications to local subcutaneous tissues at therapeutic concentrations to provide pain relief and increase function. It would appear that careful selection of medication formulation can improve the efficacy of phonophoresis.

IONTOPHORESIS

Iontophoresis transports a charged particle (ion) across the skin when direct current is applied to an aqueous solution containing the ion. The medication in use must therefore form an ionic solution in water. The stratum corneum is the primary barrier to movement of ions across the skin (54); therefore, ions tend to move preferentially through the sweat glands, where permeability is greater (55,56).

Direct current causes a predictable acidic chemical reaction under the anode (positive electrode) and a basic chemical reaction at the cathode (negative electrode). The medication is then driven across the skin by electrostatic repulsion (like charges repel each other). Negative ions are delivered at the cathode and positive ions are delivered at the anode. The skin carries a negative charge at physiologic pH and when positively charged ions are driven into the subdermal tissue from the anode, the resulting concentration gradient forces water into the subdermal tissue. Ionic materials dissolved in the water are carried along via iontohydrokinesis (57). This helps explain the reported use of the positive electrode to transport dexamethasone, a negative ion.

The ideal solution for iontophoresis has several important characteristics. The medication should ionize in water and have high conductivity. The solution should contain few to no other ions to decrease competition for current. Finally, the drug should be soluble at high concentration and over the range of pH changes that occur at the active electrode (58).

Dexamethasone sodium phosphate is the most widely used medication in iontophoresis and many researchers and clinicians have examined its effectiveness in reducing pain and dysfunction associated with musculoskeletal inflammation (59–64). Bertolucci (59) demonstrated a decrease in pain after dexamethasone iontophoresis in tendinitis conditions but no change in pain or ROM in patients with adhesive capsulitis. Plantar fasciitis symptoms decreased sooner in patients treated with dexamethasone iontophoresis than in those who did not receive iontophoresis, although no significant difference was found at 1-month follow-up between the group receiving traditional physical therapy and the group receiving traditional physical therapy with iontophoresis (60). Hasson and colleagues (62) found a decrease in pain associated with delayed-onset muscle soreness after dexamethasone iontophoresis but saw no difference in quadriceps maximum isometric contraction, peak torque, or work. Glass and associates (65) used radiolabeled dexamethasone to determine the depth of drug penetration with iontophoresis. They were able to isolate the drug from the skin, muscle, synovium, joint capsule, tendon, and cartilage, demonstrating that iontophoresis can effectively introduce medications into the subcutaneous tissues.

Other medications used in iontophoresis treatments include hydrocortisone, lidocaine, acetic acid, magnesium sulfate, sodium salicylate, and iodine. In a study by DeLacerda (66), 12 college athletes had complete relief of pain from shin splints after one to six treatments of hydrocortisone iontophoresis. Tissue and serum levels of hydrocortisone were not obtained after treatment, but the relief of inflammatory symptoms indicates tissue level penetration at a minimum. Local anesthesia has been induced before injection (67) and during office-based dermatologic procedures using lidocaine (68). Lidocaine is also frequently added to the active electrode when dexamethasone is administered to provide pain relief as well as anti-inflammatory properties. Results of acetic acid iontophoresis to decrease calcification in an abnormal location have been mixed. Perron et al (69) found acetic acid iontophoreses to be ineffective in reducing the size of the calcium deposit in patients with calcific tendinitis of the shoulder when compared with the control group. In a single case study of quadriceps femoris myositis ossificans, however, Wieder (70) reported a 98% decrease in ossified mass after nine treatments of acetic acid iontophoresis with restoration of full ROM and function. The results of Wieder's study should be interpreted cautiously because it is uncertain whether the treatment caused the decrease in the calcific mass or if the resorption was part of the natural resolution of myositis ossificans. Weinstein and Gordon (71) found magnesium iontophoresis to be effective in reducing pain and improving function in patients with subdeltoid bursitis. Iontophoresis of salicylates was effective in eliminating plantar warts with only two or three treatments (72). Iodine iontophoresis has been used to reduce postsurgical scar tissue between tendon and bone (73).

Iontophoresis should not be used in patients intolerant of electical stimulation or allergic to the medication or preservatives or on overdamaged skin or new scar tissue. Caution must be exercised during treatment over insensate areas.

Iontophoresis has been shown to be effective in the treatment of a variety of musculoskeletal disorders. Iontophoresis is noninvasive and may be better tolerated by patients than injection. In general, if there is no improvement in the patient's symptoms within four treatments, iontophoresis should be discontinued.

ELECTRICAL STIMULATION

Electrical stimulation is often used in rehabilitation of athletic injuries to reduce pain, minimize the effects of disuse on the muscular system, assist with strengthening, decrease muscle spasm, and promote tissue healing. That we intuitively believe electricity can have a positive effect on biologic tissues is certainly indicated by the plethora of scientific studies attempting to elucidate the exact effect of electrical stimulation on the neuromuscular system.

Pain Control

Pain is the No. 1 reason patients seek medical care. In the United States, the yearly medical costs associated with pain management are in the billions of dollars. Consequently, the management of pain symptoms is a goal of all medical professionals. The earliest documented accounts of pain control through electrical stimulation date back to A.D. 48 when Scribonis Largus described the use of electrical shocks from the torpedo fish to reduce the pain of headache and gout (74). In more recent times, electrical stimulation has been used to control or alleviate pain from numerous musculoskeletal conditions. Three modes of stimulation are commonly used to manage pain. Sensory level stimulation is used to stimulate the large-diameter myelinated sensory neurons. The amplitude or intensity is set at sensory level with a high frequency (10 to 100 pulses per second [pps]) and a phase duration of 50 to 100 microseconds. Motor level stimulation produces muscle contraction at frequencies of less than 10 pps (usually in the range of 1 to 4 pps) with a pulse duration of 100 to 300 microseconds. Noxious level stimulation is applied at frequencies of 50 to 100 pps at high current intensities.

Over the past 25 years, electrical stimulation (ES) has been used to treat pain associated with many musculoskeletal disorders. Ersek (75), Marchand et al (76), and Cheng et al (77) reported greater pain reduction and improved function for patients with low back pain who were treated with ES. Not all studies showed positive results with ES treatment. Deyo et al (78) and Herman et al (79) failed to show a greater decrease in pain when ES was included in the plan of care for patients with low back pain versus treatment without ES. Zizic et al (80) reported improvement in pain, function, and global assessment in patients with knee osteoarthritis after ES treatment. Sensory level ES was found to be as effective as acetaminophen with codeine in controlling pain associated with acute traumatic conditions such as sprains, contusions, fractures, and lacerations (81). Denegar et al (82) found that ES significantly reduced the pain associated with induced delayed-onset muscle soreness compared with sham ES and no treatment. Pain relief was also enhanced when ES was applied to acupuncture points compared to application of ES over sham acupuncture points (83). Overall, the literature supports the use of ES to manage pain, but the clinician is cautioned that pain is a symptom of an underlying pathology so treatment must also be directed at correcting the source of the pain.

Another method for decreasing pain using electrical stimulation is high-intensity electrical stimulation. Manal et al (84) advocate the use of high-intensity electrical stimulation to control pain in a noncontractile tissue. The area to be treated must be localized and cannot be referred from another structure. Parameters for stimulation include 2500 Hz AC modulated at 50 bursts/sec, 50% duty cycle, 12 seconds on and 8 seconds off (a.k.a. Russian current). The current is increased to the maximum level that the patient can tolerate (not the patient's comfort level). Interelectrode analgesia is usually seen within the first 5 minutes of treatment and can last hours or even days. Early control of pain allows the patient to engage in a more progressive rehabilitation program, leading to a faster return to previous activity levels. This is important not only for the elite athlete but also for the weekend warrior who must carry on with daily activities.

Strengthening

The desire to enhance athletic performance beyond that level attainable through an intensive volitional training program led athletes, coaches, and medical professionals to explore the use of electrical stimulation in increasing strength. Studies have examined the most effective electrode size (85), electrode placement patterns (86), stimulators (87), wave form (88), and frequency (89) in an attempt to generate an electrical stimulation–enhanced training program that gives the athlete a competitive edge.

Electrical stimulation has been used to strengthen the abdominal muscles (90), trunk muscles (91–93), latissimus dorsi (94), and the quadriceps (95–98). Stimulation of the abdominal musculature combined with exercise induced greater strength gains than stimulation alone or exercise alone (90). Subjects receiving low-frequency electrical stimulation showed increased isokinetic back muscle strength similar to that observed in a group performing exercise alone. Low frequency and medium-to-high frequency electrical stimulation promoted increased endurance of the trunk muscles (91). McQuain (92) found that subjects receiving electrical stimulation to the lumbar paraspinal muscles had increased isometric back extension strength compared with the exercise only control group. In a patient with segmental hypermobility at L5-S1, electrical stimulation and exercise increased stability at that level and allowed the patient to return to usual activities of daily living (ADLs) and recreational activities (93). Electrical stimulation of the latissimus dorsi muscle of swimmers resulted in an increase in isometric, concentric, and eccentric peak torque and decreased times on swimming tasks (94). Delitto et al (95) demonstrated that simultaneous stimulation of the quadriceps and hamstrings after ACL reconstruction led to increased strength gains in both muscles compared with voluntary muscle contraction. He also used high-intensity electrical stimulation to the quadriceps femoris muscle of an elite weight lifter for a total of 6 weeks over a 4-month period (no stimulation for 4 weeks, stimulation for 4 weeks, no stimulation for 4 weeks, and stimulation for 2 weeks) in conjunction with weight training to increase weight-lifting capacity on three competitive lifts. This training program led to an increase in type 1 muscle fiber area with a decrease in 2a and 2b area on muscle biopsy (96). Selkowitz (97) and Snyder-Mackler et al (98) found high-intensity electrical stimulation improved quadriceps strength over exercise alone in healthy subjects (97) and in those who had undergone ACL reconstruction (98). Electrical stimulation has been shown to improve strength in healthy muscle as well as in muscle impaired by injury or disuse. Whether strength gains result from retraining the nervous system to recruit more motor units or to changes in recruitment pattern or fiber type, the outcome is ultimately the same—namely, improved function.

Tissue Healing

Recently, researchers have focused on manipulating the electrical potential through an externally applied electrical stimulus to promote tissue healing (99). Bettany et al (100) demonstrated a reduction in injury-induced edema formation in frog limbs after treatment with high-voltage pulsed current (HVPC). Griffen et al (101) found an increased healing rate of pressure ulcers after 5, 10, 15, and 20 treatments with HVPC compared with ulcer healing under traditional wound care techniques. Kloth and Feeder (102) likewise found improved healing in decubitus ulcers after treatment with HVPC (105 Hz, 100 to 175 V, 50 microsecond intraphase interval). Electrical stimulation is also used to promote bone healing in fractures with delayed bony healing, including the tibia and scaphoid. Three methods of stimulation have been applied to fracture sites: a percutaneous direct current bone stimulator (103), an implanted direct current stimulator (104,105), and an external pulsed electromagnetic field (PEMF) stimulator (106,107). While there have been no studies to evaluate the effectiveness of electrical stimulation on the healing rate of human tendons or ligaments, scientists have conducted animal studies to provide preliminary guidelines and efficacy data. Daily treatment for 2 weeks with anodal current via an implanted electrode led to increased tensile strength in the Achilles tendon of rats after surgical tenotomy (108). Akai et al (109) found that electrical stimulation at the defect restored tensile stiffness more rapidly to the patellar ligament in rabbits compared with the nonstimulated ligaments.

In an attempt to elucidate a mechanism to increase soft-tissue healing, Bourguignon et al (110) examined the effect of electrical stimulation HVPC on the synthesis of protein and DNA by fibroblasts. Results demonstrated the greatest protein and DNA synthesis with 50 V and 75 V, respectively, using a cathodal current, and a pulse rate of 100 pps. Use of these parameters in the clinical setting is likely to provide the best environment for wound healing.

Electrical stimulation should not be used over demand-type pacemakers, over the pregnant uterus, over the eyes, or transcutaneously. Careful monitoring is recommended when electrical stimulation is used in an area with decreased sensation.

EMG BIOFEEDBACK

Electromyographic (EMG) biofeedback involves the use of a voltmeter to make electromyographic measurements. EMG biofeedback is used to improve motor unit recruitment to generate stronger voluntary muscular contraction and to inhibit muscular contraction to promote relaxation of overactive muscles. Biofeedback is not as useful for eliciting muscle contraction in patients with spastic neuromuscular diseases as it is in those with an intact central nervous system (CNS).

EMG biofeedback can be used over any superficial muscle. The purpose is to give the patient or athlete immediate feedback regarding performance regardless of whether the desired outcome is to increase or reduce muscle contraction. Studies have demonstrated increased strength gains (111,112) improved motor learning, and neuromuscular re-education (113–116). Draper et al (111) compared exercise with biofeedback, exercise with electrical stimulation, and exercise alone and found biofeedback with exercise enhanced quadriceps muscle contraction to a greater extent than electrical stimulation with exercise or exercise alone after ACL reconstruction. Levitt et al (112) concluded that biofeedback with exercise improved extensor torque and quadriceps muscle recruitment after knee arthroscopy. Norris (113) used biofeedback during lumbar stabilization exercises to retrain the patient to contract the abdominal muscles without flexing the lumbar spine. Reid et al (114) and Young (115) demonstrated effective muscle re-education using biofeedback in patients with shoulder instability. The patients had improved function and reduced occurrence of instability. A significant improvement was found in the patellofemoral congruence angle after a 3-week training period with biofeedback to emphasize vastus medialis oblique (VMO) muscle contraction (116).

Because voluntary muscle contraction is a necessity during sports and other daily activities, it seems obvious that providing feedback during the performance of the desired movement pattern would lead to improved motor learning by reinforcing the correct movement. The use of EMG biofeedback provides information about the strength of contraction and can help eliminate substitution of stronger muscles.

Sometimes the desired action is not stronger contraction of a muscle but rather decreased activity to promote muscle relaxation. Rokicki and associates (117) found biofeedback during relaxation training exercises led to decreased incidence of headaches in patients with tension headaches. Biofeedback is also used clinically to assist with muscle relaxation of the hamstrings during stretching at end-range extension following ACL reconstruction and during shoulder elevation strengthening exercises to decrease substitution of the upper trapezius muscle.

SUMMARY

We have reviewed the scientific basis and evidence for the use of thermal agents and electrotherapy in rehabilitation of sports injuries. The evidence ranges from theoretical to strong with the best support for the use of cryotherapy, continuous ultrasound, iontophoresis, EMG biofeedback for enhancing muscle activity, and neuromuscular electrical stimulation for strengthening muscle. Other agents that are commonly used in sports settings (e.g., pulsed ultrasound, phonophoresis, superficial heating for increasing flexibility) are supported by weak evidence. A better understanding of the support in the literature for the use of these therapeutic agents should allow for more effective treatments of athletes with musculoskeletal injuries.

REFERENCES

1. Levy AS, Kelly B, Lintner S, et al. Penetration of cryotherapy in treatment after shoulder arthroscopy. Arthroscopy 1997; 13:461–464.

2. Metzman L, Gamble JG, Rinsky LA. Effectiveness of ice packs in reducing skin temperature under casts. Clin Orthop 1996;330: 217–221.

3. Zemke J, Andersen J, Guion W, et al. Intramuscular temperature responses in the human leg to two forms of cryotherapy: ice massage and ice bag. J Orthop Sports Phys Ther 1998;27:301–307.

4. Carman K, Knight K. Habituation to cold-pain during repeated cryokinetic sessions. J Athl Train 1992;27:223–230.

5. Lessard L, Scudds R, Amendola A, et al. The efficacy of cryotherapy following arthroscopic knee surgery. J Orthop Sports Phys Ther 1997;26:14–22.

6. Basur RL, Shepard E, Mouzas GL. A cooling method in the treatment of ankle sprains. Practitioner 1976;216:708–711.

7. Kirk JA, Kersley GD. Heat and cold in the physical treatment of rheumatoid arthritis of the knee. Ann Phys Med 1968;9: 270–274.

8. Williams J, Harvey J, Tannenbaum H. Use of superficial heat versus ice for the rheumatoid arthritic shoulder: a pilot study. Physiother Can 1986;38:8–13.

9. Bugaj R. The cooling, analgesic, and rewarming effects of ice massage on localized skin. Phys Ther 1975;55:11–19.

10. Waylonis GW. The physiologic effects of ice massage. Arch Phys Med Rehabil 1967;47:37–42.

11. Ernst E, Fialka V. Ice freezes pain? a review of the clinical effectiveness of analgesic cold therapy. J Pain Symptom Manage 1994;9:56–59.

12. Rennie GA, Michlovitz S. Biophysical principles of heating and superficial heating agents. In: Thermal agents in rehabilitation. Philadelphia: FA Davis, 1996:107–138.

13. Weston M, Taber C, Casagranda L, et al. Changes in local blood volume during cold gel pack application to traumatized ankles. J Orthop Sports Phys Ther 1994;19:197–199.

14. Knight KL. Temperature changes resulting from cold. In: Knight KL, ed. Cryotherapy in sport injury management. Champaign, IL: Human Kinetics, 1995:59–76.

15. Edwards DJ, Rimmer M, Keene GC. The use of cold therapy in the postoperative management of patients undergoing arthroscopic anterior cruciate ligament reconstruction. Am J Sports Med 1996;24:193–195.

16. Speer KP, Warren RF, Horowitz L. The efficacy of cryotherapy in the postoperative shoulder. J Shoulder Elbow Surg 1996;5:62–68.

17. Schroeder D, Passler HH. Combination of cold and compression after knee surgery: a prospective randomized study. Knee Surg Sports Traumatol Arthrosc 1994; 2:158–165.

18. Oglivie-Harris DJ, Gilbart M. Treatment modalities for soft tissue injuries of the ankle: a critical review. Clin J Sports Med 1995;5:175–186.

19. McGown HL. Effects of cold application on maximal isometric contraction. Phys Ther 1967;47: 185.

20. Paddon-Jones DJ, Quigley BM. Effect of cryotherapy on muscle soreness and strength following eccentric exercise. Int J Sports Med 1997;18:588–593.

21. Cross KM, Wilson RW, Perrin DH. Functional performance following an ice immersion to the lower extremity. J Athletic Train 1996; 31:113–116.

22. Ruiz DH, Myrer JW, Durrant E, et al. Cryotherapy and sequential exercise bouts following cryotherapy on concentric and eccentric strength in the quadriceps. J Athl Train 1993;28:320–323, 360–361.

23. Evans T, Ingersoll C, Knight K, et al. Agility following the application of cold therapy. J Athl Train 1995;30:231–234.

24. Moeller JL, Monroe J, McKeag DB. Cryotherapy-induced common peroneal nerve palsy. Clin J Sports Med 1997;7:212–216.

25. Malone TR, Englehardt DL, Kirkpatrick JS, et al. Nerve injury in athletes caused by cryotherapy. J Athl Train 1992;27:235–237.

26. Castel JC. Therapeutic ultrasound. Rehabil Ther Prod Rev 1993;Jan/Feb:22–32.

27. Draper DO, Richard MD. Rate of temperature decay in human muscle following 3 MHz ultrasound: the stretching window revealed. J Athl Train 1995;30: 304–307.

28. Gertsen J. Effect of ultrasound on tendon extensiblity. Am J Phys Med 1955;34:362–369.

29. Lehman JF, Delateur BJ. Therapeutic heat. In: Lehman JF, ed. Therapeutic heat and cold. Baltimore: Williams & Wilkins, 1990: 417–581.

30. Taylor B, Waring C, Brashear T. The effects of therapeutic application of heat or cold followed by static stretch on hamstring muscle length. J Orthop Sports Phys Ther 1995;21:283–286.

31. Henricson AS, Fredriksson K, Persson I, et al. The effect of heat and stretching on the range of hip motion. J Orthop Sports Phys Ther 1984;13:110–115.

32. Wessling D, DeVane D, Hylton C. Effects of static stretch versus static stretch and ultrasound combined on triceps surae muscle extensibility in healthy women. Phys Ther 1987;67:674–679.

33. Lehman JF, Guy AW. Ultrasound therapy. In: Reid J, Sikov MR, eds. Interaction of ultrasound and biological tissues. DHEW Pub (FDA) 73-8008, Session 3:8, pp. 141–152, 1971.

34. Lehman J, Herrick J. Biologic reactions to cavitation, a consideration for ultrasonic therapy. Arch Phys Med Rehabil 1955;36:282.

35. Kimura I, Gulick D, Shelly J, et al. Effects of two ultrasound devices and angles of application on the temperature of tissue phantom. J Orthop Sports Phys Ther 1998;27:27–31.

36. Draper DO, Castel JC, Castel D. Rate of temperature increase in human muscle during 1 MHz and 3 MHz continuous ultrasound. J Orthop Sports Phys Ther 1995;22:142–150.

37. Green S, Buchbinder R, Glazier R, et al. Systematic review of randomized controlled trials of interventions for painful shoulder: selection criteria, outcome assessment, and efficacy. BMJ 1998;316:354–360.

38. Nykanen M. Pulsed ultrasound treatment of the painful shoulder a randomized double-blind, placebo-controlled study. Scand J Rehabil Med 1995;27:105–108.

39. Rimington SJ, Draper DO, Durrant E, et al. Temperature changes during therapeutic ultrasound in the precooled human gastrocnemius muscle. J Athl Train 1994;29:325–327.

40. Draper DO, Schulthies S, Sorvisto P, et al. Temperature changes in deep muscles of humans during ice and ultrasound therapies: an in vivo study. J Orthop Sports Phys Ther 1995;21:153–157.

41. Reed B, Ashikaga T. The effects of heating with ultrasound on knee joint displacement. J Orthop Sports Phys Ther 1997;26:131–137.

42. Cameron MH, Monroe LG. Relative transmission of ultrasound by media customarily used for phonophoresis. Phys Ther 1992;72:142–148.

43. Byl NN. The use of ultrasound as an enhancer for transcutaneous drug delivery: phonophoresis. Phys Ther 1995;75:539–553.

44. Byl NN, McKenzie A, Halliday B, et al. The effects of phonophoresis with corticosteroids: a controlled pilot study. J Orthop Sports Phys Ther 1993;18:590–600.

45. Bare AC, McAnaw MB, Pritchard AE, et al. Phonophoretic delivery of 10% hydrocortisone through the epidermis of humans as determined by serum cortisol concentrations. Phys Ther 1996;76:738–749.

46. Griffen JE, Touchstone JC. Ultrasonic movement of cortisol into pig tissues: Part 1: movement into skeletal muscle. Am J Phys Med 1963;42:77–85.

47. Griffen JE, Touchstone JC, Liu AC-Y. Ultrasonic movement of cortisol into pig tissues: Part 2: movement into paravertebral nerve. Am J Phys Med 1965;44:20–25.

48. Oziomek RS, Perrin DH, Herold DA, et al. Effect of phonophoresis on serum salicylate levels. Med Sci Sports Exerc 1991;23:397–401.

49. Smith W, Winn F, Parette R. Comparitive study using four modalities in shin splints treatments. J Orthop Sports Phys Ther 1986;8:77–80.

50. Ciccone CD, Leggin BG, Callamaro JJ. Effects of ultrasound and trolamine salicylate phonophoresis on delayed-onset muscle soreness. Phys Ther 1991;71:666–678.

51. Moll MJ. A new approach to pain: lidocaine and decadron with ultrasound. USAF Med Serv Digest 1979;30:8–11.

52. Griffen JE, Echternach JL, Price RE, et al. Patients treated with ultrasonic driven hydrocortisone and with ultrasound alone. Phys Ther 1967;47:594–601.

53. Shin SM, Choi JK. Effect of indomethacin phonophoresis on the relief of temporomandibular joint pain. Cranio 1997;15:345–348.

54. Banga A, Panus PC. Clinical applications of iontophoretic devises in rehabiltation medicine. 1999 (in press).

55. Grimnes S. Pathways of ionic flow through human skin in vivo. Acta Derm Venereol 1984;64:93–98.

56. Burnette RR, Ongpipattanakul B. Characterization of pore transport properties of excised human skin during iontophoresis. J Pharm Sci 1988;77:132–137.

57. Gangarosa LP, Park NH, Wiggins CA, et al. Increased penetration of nonelectrolytes into mouse skin during iontophoretic water transport (iontohydrokinesis). J Pharmacol Exp Ther 1980;212:377–381.

58. Banga AK, Chien YW. Iontophoretic delivery of drugs: fundamentals, developments and biomedical applications. J Control Release 1988;7:1–24.

59. Bertolucci LE. Introduction of antiinflammatory drugs by iontophoresis: double blind study. J Orthop Sports Phys Ther 1982;4:103–108.

60. Gudeman SD, Eisele SA, Heidt RS, et al. Treatment of plantar fasciitis by iontophoresis of 0.4% dexamethasone: a randomized, double-blind, placebo-controlled study. Am J Sports Med 1997;25:312–316.

61. Harris PR. Iontophoresis: clinical research in musculoskeletal inflammatory conditions. J Orthop Sports Phys Ther 1982;4:109–112.

62. Hasson SM, Wible CL, Barnes WS, Williams JH. Dexamethasone iontophoresis: effect on delayed muscle soreness and muscle function. Can J Sport Sci 1992; 17:8–13.

63. Li LC, Scudds RA, Heck CS, Harth M. The efficacy of dexamethasone iontophoresis for the treatment of rheumatoid arthritic knees: a pilot study. Arthritis Care Res 1996;9:126–132.

64. Schiffman EL, Braun BL, Lindgren BR. Temporomandibular joint iontophoresis: a double-blind randomized clinical trial. J Orofacial Pain 1996;10:157–165.

65. Glass JM, Stephen RL, Jacobson SC. The quantity and distribution of radiolabeled dexamethasone delivered to tissue by iontophoresis. Int J Derm 1980;19:519–525.

66. DeLacerda FG. Iontophoresis for treatment of shinsplints. J Orthop Sports Phys Ther 1982;3:183–185.

67. Petelenz T, Anenti I, Petelenz RJ, et al. Mini set for iontophoresis for topical analgesia before injection. Int J Clin Pharmacol Ther Toxicol 1984;22:152–155.

68. Maloney JM, Bezzant JL, Stephen RL, et al. Iontophoresis administration of lidocaine anesthesia in office practice: an appraisal. J Dermatol Surg Oncol 1992;18:937–940.

69. Perron M, Malouin F. Acetic acid iontophoresis and ultrasound for the treatment of calcifying tendinitis of the shoulder: a randomized control trial. Arch Phys Med Rehabil 1997;78:379–384.

70. Wieder DL. Treatment of traumatic myositis ossificans with acetic acid iontophoresis. Phys Ther 1992;72:133–137.

71. Weinstein MV, Gordon A. The use of magnesium sulfate iontophoresis in the treatment of subdeltoid bursitis. Phys Ther Rev 1958; 38:96–98.

72. Gordon AH, Weinstein MV. Sodium salicylate iontophoresis in the treatment of plantar warts. Phys Ther 1969;49:869–870.

73. Tannenbaum M. Iodine iontophoresis in reducing scar tissue. Phys Ther 1980;60:792.

74. Kellaway P. The William Osler medal essay: the part played by electrical fish in the early history of bioelectricity and electrotherapy. Bull Hist Med 1946;20:112–137.

75. Ersek RA. Low back pain: prompt relief with transcutaneous neuro-stimulation: a report of 35 consecutive patients. Orthop Rev 1976;5:27–31.

76. Marchand S, Charest J, Li J, et al. Is TENS purely a placebo effect? A controlled study on chronic low back pain. Pain 1993;54:99–106.

77. Cheng RSS, Pomeranz B. Electrotherapy for chronic musculoskeletal pain: comparison of electroacupuncture and acupuncture-like transcutaneous electrical nerve stimulation. Clin J Pain 1987;2:143–149.

78. Deyo RA, Walsh NE, Martin DC, et al. A controlled trial of transcutaneous electrical nerve stimulation (TENS) and exercise for chronic low back pain. N Engl J Med 1990;322:1627–1634.

79. Herman E, Williams R, Stratford P, et al. A randomized controlled trial of transcutaneous electrical nerve stimulation (Codetron) to determine its benefits in a rehabilitation program for acute occupational low back pain. Spine 1994;19:561–568.

80. Zizic TM, Hoffman KC, Holt PA, et al. The treatment of osteoarthritis of the knee with pulsed electrical stimulation. J Rheumatol 1995;22:1757–1761.

81. Ordog GJ. Transcutaneous electrical nerve stimulation versus oral analgesic: a randomized double blind controlled study in acute traumatic pain. Am J Emerg Med 1987;5:6–10.

82. Denegar CR, Perrin DH. Effect of transcutaneous electrical nerve stimulation, cold, and a combination treatment on pain, decreased range of motion, and strength loss associated with delayed onset muscle soreness. J Athl Train 1992;27:200–206.

83. Hidderley M, Weinel E. Clinical practice: effects of TNES applied to acupuncture points distal to a pain site. Int J Palliat Nurs 1997;3:185–188.

84. Manal TJ, Snyder-Mackler L. Electrotherapy for pain management: high intensity electrical stimulation shows promising results. Rehab Manage 1997; June/July:56–57.

85. Alon G. High voltage stimulation: effects of electrode size on basic excitatory responses. Phys Ther 1985;65:890–895.

86. Barnett S, Cooney K, Johnston R. Electrically elicited quadriceps femoris muscle torque as a function of various electrode placements. J Clin Electrophysiol 1991;3:5–8.

87. DeDomenico G. Maximum torque production in the quadriceps femoris muscle group using a variety of electrical stimulators. Aust J Physiother 1986;32:51–55.

88. Sander TC, Schrank EC, Kelln BM, et al. Differences in torque generation by trial and three different waveforms. J Clin Electrophys 1994;6:10–13.

89. Balogun JA, Onilari OO, Akeju OA, et al. High voltage electrical stimulation in the augmentation of muscle strength: effects of pulse frequency. Arch Phys Med Rehabil 1993;74:910–916.

90. Alon G, McCombe SA, Koutsantonis S, et al. Comparison of the effects of electrical stimulation and exercise on abdominal musculature. J Orthop Sports Phys Ther 1987;8:567–573.

91. Kahanovitz N, Nordin M, Verderame R, et al. Normal trunk muscle strength and endurance

in women and the effect of exercises and electrical stimulation. Part 2: comparative analysis of electrical stimulation and exercises to increase trunk muscle strength and endurance. Spine 1987;12:112–118.

92. McQuain MT, Sinaki M, Shibley LD, et al. Effect of electrical stimulation on lumbar paraspinal muscles. Spine 1993;18:1787–1792.

93. Starring DT. The use of electrical stimulation and exercise for strengthening lumbar musculature: a case study. J Orthop Sports Phys Ther 1991;14:61–64.

94. Pichon F, Chatard JC, Martin A, et al. Electrical stimulation and swimming performance. Med Sci Sport Exerc 1995;27:1671–1676.

95. Delitto A, Rose SJ, McKowen JM, et al. Electrical stimulation versus voluntary exercise in strengthening thigh musculature after anterior cruciate ligament surgery. Phys Ther 1988;68:660–663.

96. Delitto A, Brown M, Strube MJ, et al. Electrical stimulation of quadriceps femoris in an elite weight lifter: a single subject experiment. Int J Sport Med 1989;10:187–191.

97. Selkowitz DM. Improvement in isometric strength of the quadriceps femoris muscle after training with electrical stimulation. Phys Ther 1985;65:186–195.

98. Snyder-Mackler L, Delitto A, Bailey SL, et al. Strength of the quadriceps femoris muscle and functional recovery after reconstruction of the anterior cruciate ligament. J Bone Joint Surg 1995;77A:1166–1173.

99. Wojtys EM, Carpenter JE, Ott GA. Electrical stimulation of soft tissues. Instr Course Lect 1993;42:443–452.

100. Bettany JA, Fish DR, Mendel FC. Influence of high voltage pulsed direct current on edema formation following impact injury. Phys Ther 1990;70:219–224.

101. Griffen JW, Tooms RE, Mendius RA, et al. Efficacy of high voltage pulsed current for healing of pressure ulcers in patients with spinal cord injury. Phys Ther 1991;71:433–442.

102. Kloth LC, Feedar JA. Acceleration of wound healing with high voltage, monophasic, pulsed current. Phys Ther 1988;68:503–508.

103. Brighton CT. Treatment of nonunion of the tibia with constant direct current (1980 Fitts Lecture, AAST). J Trauma 1981;21:189–195.

104. Paterson D. Treatment of nonunion with a constant direct current: a totally implantable system. Orthop Clin North Am 1984;15:47–59.

105. Cundy PJ, Paterson DC. A ten-year review of treatment of delayed union and nonunion with an implanted bone growth stimulator. Clin Orthop 1990;259:216–222.

106. Fontanesi G, Traina GC, Giancecchi F, et al. Slow healing fractures: can they be prevented? (Results of electrical stimulation in fibular osteotomies in rats and in diaphyseal fractures of the tibia in humans.) Ital J Orthop Traumatol 1986;12:371–385.

107. Borsalino G, Bagnacani M, Bettati E, et al. Electrical stimulation of human femoral intertrochanteric osteotomies: double-blind study. Clin Orthop 1988;237:256–263.

108. Owoeye I, Spielholz N, Fretto J, et al. Low-intensity pulsed galvanic current and the healing of tenotomized rat Achilles tendon: preliminary report using load-to-breaking measurements. Arch Phys Med Rehabil 1987;68:415–418.

109. Akai M, Oda H, Shirasaki Y, et al. Electrical stimulation of ligament healing: an experimental study of the patellar ligament of rabbits. Clin Orthop 1988;235:296–301.

110. Bourguignon GJ, Bourguignon LYW. Electric stimulation of protein and DNA synthesis in human fibroblasts. FASEB J 1987;1:398–402.

111. Draper V, Lyle L, Seymour T. EMG biofeedback versus electrical stimulation in the recovery of quadriceps surface EMG. Clin Kinesiol 1997;51:28–32.

112. Levitt R, Deisinger JA, Wall JR, et al. EMG feedback-assisted postoperative rehabilitation of minor arthroscopic knee surgeries. J Sports Med Phys Fitness 1995;35:218–223.

113. Norris CM. Spinal stabilization: 5. An exercise programme to enhance lumbar stabilisation. Physiotherapy 1995;81:138–146.

114. Reid DC, Saboe LA, Chepeha JC. Anterior shoulder instability in athletes: comparison of isokinetic resistance exercises and an electromyographic biofeedback re-education program—a pilot program. Physiother (Can) 1996;48:251–256.

115. Young MS. Electromyographic biofeedback use in the treatment of voluntary posterior dislocation of the shoulder: a case study. J Orthop Sports Phys Ther 1994;20:171–175.

116. Ingersoll CD, Knight KL. Patellar location changes following EMG biofeedback or progressive resistive exercises. Med Sci Sports Exerc 1991;23:1122–1127.

117. Rokicki LA, Holroyd KA, France CR, et al. Change mechanisms associated with combined relaxation/EMG biofeedback training for chronic tension headache. Appl Psychophysiol Biofeedback 1997;22:21–41.

Part IV.

PREVENTIVE MEDICINE

Edited by
Bill Hettler

Introduction to Preventive Medicine

Bill Hettler

When one considers that there are entire textbooks devoted to the subject of preventive medicine, it is obvious that this section is limited to a subset of the important topics surrounding prevention. A particular focus of the section is some of the more interesting applications afforded to the field of prevention by the advent of computer technology. At no time in human history have computers played such an important role in assisting individuals in making positive lifestyle changes.

Medical economics has also emerged as an important player in promoting greater emphasis on preventive medicine. As more and more of our citizens are being enrolled in managed care organizations, there are increased incentives to implement preventive medicine within the health care delivery systems.

Other forces that have also changed the landscape permanently include direct advertising to the public by drug companies, the fitness industry, and regular health features on television and in the popular press. Every major news program has regular features that focus on a wide variety of health topics.

The number of websites devoted to prevention and health has been increasing exponentially. The challenge to those of us who are in health care delivery is to assist the consumer in finding the quality and avoiding the nonsense.

The opening of communication systems to consumers has enabled individuals with specific health concerns to find others who have similar interests or, better yet, have been successfully managing the particular problem or issue. The willingness of individuals to assist strangers has been reported in a number of instances.

Just as when new pharmaceuticals are introduced, there is always the downside possibility that undesirable side effects might follow the introduction of new technology. One such negative side effect may be Internet addiction. There have been numerous anecdotal reports highlighting the negative consequences of Internet overuse.

As we enter the twenty-first century, there is no question that the field of medicine is being influenced by the information age. In this section, you will find information on a wide variety of topics. The chapter by Molly Mettler of Healthwise in Boise, Idaho, describes some preliminary results of an exciting new program that assists patients with decision making support regarding their personal health concerns. In this program, the use of the Healthwise Handbook along with

"dial help" systems that use a computer-based knowledge base has demonstrated efficacy in decreasing the cost of care, while increasing self-advocacy for personal health management. It is likely that this type of system will become a mainstream resource as we progress further into the information age.

In Chapter 25, this author has been joined by his daughter, Joeli Hettler, a chief resident in pediatrics, to discuss the use of the World Wide Web and the Internet for preventive medicine activities. The observations and conclusions of an emerging physician may provide a useful perspective for the reader. This chapter has focused on a wide range of topics. There is no question that, by the time this book actually is in print, there will have been significant advances in the resources available to both practicing professionals and consumers.

At the same time, while the World Wide Web and Internet resources are rapidly expanding, CD-ROM resources are also increasing in absolute numbers and breadth of topic. Linda Chapin, Executive Director of the National Wellness Institute, brings her experience and training as a dentist and as the chief executive officer of a national organization serving health promotion professionals to the issue of CD-ROM and other technology resources in this field. Linda has been an active participant in the expanded use of technology as an adjunct to serving the professional needs of National Wellness Association members.

There is an accelerated rate of conversion of scientific journals from print to electronic format. An entirely new system of publishing and compensation for authors is in the works. We are living in an exciting era.

This author encourages all readers to become part of the information age. My recommendations are simple:

- If you do not own a computer, buy one.
- If you do not have access to the Internet, sign up.
- If you do not have email, get an email account.
- If you do not know how to use any of the above, hire a bright junior high school student to teach you.

There you have it; it may seem simple-minded, but it worked for me. I encourage you to enjoy the rapidly increasing availability of useful, readily accessible, high-quality information.

Chapter 23

Physician-Directed Medical Self-Care

Bill Hettler

This chapter focuses on the natural evolution that is occurring within modern medicine. More and more physicians are encouraging individual patients to take appropriate actions based on the best science and outcomes research available. The transformation of patient education from the clinical office setting to the home, work site, church, school, public library, and other community buildings is a reality.

Probably one of the best early examples of physician-directed medical self-care is the progress that has been made in the care of people with diabetes. If you think about the early days of diabetes care, you will recall that physicians were actively involved in the daily decision making concerning diet, insulin doses, exercise, and other medications. After a short period of time, it became obvious to the patients as well as the physicians that much of this management could be assumed by the patients themselves.

In addition, improvements in technology have made this physician-directed medical self-care safe, less expensive, and less intrusive. Initially, home testing was limited to urine testing. Later, finger-stick blood chemistry analysis was brought to the home. Today, there are computerized decision support machines that provide high-tech support for the patient who is learning to manage their diabetes at home. Naturally, in this era of managed care, there are enormous cost savings associated with this activity.

This one example is instructive, but is just one example of a major shift that is occurring as we enter the twenty-first century. The bigger picture is that our nation and the world are in transition as we leave the industrial age economic base and move rapidly, sometimes frighteningly fast, into the information age. The explosion of technology-based resources and public access to these resources has created a totally unantici-

pated opportunity to improve useful life expectancy through the delivery of health information, decision support software, self-help support groups, and multimedia resources. If you have the right equipment, these resources are now available 24 hours per day, in virtually any location on the planet.

Digital delivery via satellite transmission, cellular phone, microwave wide area networks, and direct phone connection is now a reality. Individual patients are, more and more, becoming providers of medical information as well as recipients of medical care. The medical self-care movement has been learning to use the massive computerized system that enables people with similar concerns to find each other and share their successes and failures in real time.

The best online self-help projects are managed in such a way that the professionals are included, as valuable resources to the mix of participants. This inclusion is helpful to the professionals as well as to the lay participants. This author has gained insights by viewing the messages in a self-help online chat room. By reading the comments of hundreds of participants that all are organized around specific issues, I was able to understand (from the patient's perspective) issues that, without this online resource, would have taken years of time in an office practice setting. Listening to (reading) the comments provided online accelerated my learning about the real issues that influence patient decision making and their compliance with recommendations that might be made via physician. Appendix 23-1 will give some glimpses in one such group.

This author has had 10 years of experience delivering physician-directed self-care for patients who have asthma. My first exposure to the phrase *physician-directed self-care* was from listening and viewing a videotape designed for continuing medical education. The resource person in this videotape was Dr. Roger Bone, a national expert in respiratory disease. Dr. Bone was highly motivated to encourage his patients to get actively involved in the management of their asthma, because he had witnessed tragic, unnecessary loss of life because of delays in care or inappropriate care provided to asthma patients.

For the last 10 years, I have been teaching a class at the university level, entitled Asthma Self-Care. This course is conducted in an independent study format, with heavy reliance on Internet delivery of content, multimedia resources, and links to resources on a worldwide basis. The course encourages participants to view professionals as resources who can be used to assist in the management of their asthma. Over the years, I have been amazed at the level of misinformation that has existed, sometimes for years, in the minds of these asthma patients.

It is amazing to me, and frustrating as well, to realize that in spite of the explosion of knowledge about the care of asthma, the death rate from asthma in the United States continues to rise. We must identify the barriers that exist between the knowledge that has been accumulated and the use of that knowledge by people who actually have the problem. This is true for most of the common conditions that interfere with useful life expectancy and quality of life.

Physician-directed medical self-care can be delivered through a variety of systems. Some of the systems include:

- The Internet and the World Wide Web
- Interactive CD-ROM
- Videotape resources
- Audiotape systems
- Automated fax back systems
- Computerized decision support software
- Dedicated medical self-care television networks
- Topic-specific online chat rooms and forums
- Newsletters and journals
- Talk radio

It is this author's opinion that the most dramatic and least expensive delivery system will involve the Internet and the World Wide Web. Almost all of the other resources listed above can be delivered most efficiently through the use of the Internet and World Wide Web. Michael McDonald, MPH, a health and human ecology director for the Environmental Science and Policy Institute, has predicted that communication speed will grow by a factor of 10 million and computing power will increase by a factor of 10,000 by the year 2003. He suggests that when these two predictions are combined, the combination will produce machines a billion times more powerful than those that exist today.

As the medical profession becomes more comfortable with computer technology and other audiovisual delivery systems, this massive increase in processing power and storage capacity can assist us in our goals to improve the quality of life and lower the cost of care for the patients we serve. For the time being, the Internet and World Wide Web seem to be the most efficient delivery system.

This chapter, in fact, is being written using voice recognition software. At this point in the article, I have been using regular conversation that is recognized efficiently by the software, which then places the words directly on the screen. While I am creating this document, I can switch back and forth to resources on the World Wide Web or physically present in the form of books and journals on my desk.

INTERACTIVE CD-ROM RESOURCES

The dramatic reduction in the cost of CD-ROM recorders, video capture technology, and multimedia editing software has made it possible for individual physicians, nurses, and patient educators to create their own multimedia self-care resources. A CD-ROM recorder can be purchased for less than $500. For about the same amount of money, a video capture device can be installed in a home computer. This device enables the user to capture video clips that have been developed privately by the user or purchased from professional sources. Using multimedia editing software, which often is included with the video capture device, one can create customized patient education materials.

The cost of blank media for CD-ROM production is less than $2 per disk. Capturing images electronically by using scanners, digital cameras, and video cameras is commonplace in many American grade schools. This author has personally observed third graders capturing and editing videotape information. They were successful in creating educational materials that could be used by other students anywhere in the world. This is an enormous step forward.

Just 10 years ago, the cost of creating videodisc interactive technology was more than $100,000 per topic. When it comes to educational technology, there are hundreds of companies actively working to create user-friendly software that physicians can use to create practice-specific, physician-directed self-care materials. The emphasis today on chronic disease care management and demand management will drive greater use of these resources in the larger managed care arena.

The use of microcomputers to create customized videotape resources is also a reality. This also is a grade-school skill in many locations. As the students in our schools today begin to graduate and seek jobs, it will be realistic for the larger clinics to include customized videotape production as one of the expectations in the job description of health educators or medical self-care leaders.

LOST POTENTIAL

Each day in America, there are hundreds of high-quality video productions created by news programs in local television stations. Many of these programs could be captured, cataloged, and stored for later use by medical self-care production facilities. Obviously, a system must be created to give proper credit and compensation to the original producers of such materials. The ability of current technology to manage a database of these resources makes this a feasible concept.

Audiotape production has also enjoyed significant technologic advances. Microcomputers, high-quality microphones, and editing software make it possible for any health care provider to create customized decision support audiotapes that can be given to the patient to reinforce the instructions or procedures recommended for the care of their problems. The cost of such production and duplication of the audiotapes is minimal.

Another innovation that can work in many locations is automated fax back systems. There are turnkey systems available that enable a medical office or clinic to provide automated patient information at very low cost. The systems are easily customized and can be managed by clerical staff. The health professionals must create the content, but once this content is created, patients can easily access instructions or materials of their choice through fax technology.

There are similar automated systems that involve voice messaging. Many of the systems enable the user, by the use of touch-tone input, to select specific information of their choice. This technology is also cost-effective and is being used particularly in the technical support area of computer companies. Logic tree structures are created that enable the user to be quickly moved to the resources that will assist them in solving their problems. This same procedure can be used to assist patients in finding the answers they need to make decisions in a self-care mode.

Computerized decision support systems are also evolving as we approach the end of the twentieth century. There is an excellent description of one of the systems in Chapter 24.

There are numerous dedicated television networks evolving that are topic-specific. For example, the American Health Network offers 16 hours per day of dedicated health information materials. It is likely that in the future, partnerships will evolve between providers of medical care and the industries that provide the products necessary for optimal care to jointly sponsor continuous fee television channels of interest to the public.

There are hundreds of online chat rooms and public forums already in existence. There have been numerous anecdotal reports of the value and, in some cases, dramatic lifesaving outcomes from some of these activities. There have also been some interesting negative outcomes.

One situation was reported at a national medical self-care meeting. This case involved a nationally funded double-blind study involving experimental treatments for a rare disorder. The report stated that many of the participants in the study were communicating in a rare disease forum sponsored by one of the national online services. As the patients who were participating in this study began to discuss their experiences, it became clear that the patients taking the active ingredient noticed an increased frequency of urination. One participant made the observation that if you did not have to get up and go to the bathroom in the middle of the night, it was likely you were taking the placebo. At this point, many of the participants who presumed they were taking the placebo went back to their investigators and asked to be put on the active drug. This was true, even though the active drug had not yet been proven to be effective for their condition. The multi-site trial had to be canceled. In spite of this occurrence, this author is convinced that open communication between and among people who have rare disorders is a highly desirable activity.

There are hundreds of examples of self-help groups providing not only assistance to the patients who participate but also to the professionals who view or participate in these forums.

TELECOMMUNICATION AND PHYSICIAN-DIRECTED MEDICAL SELF-CARE

TelePractice and Cleveland State University have developed telecommunication systems that facilitate the integration of patient self-care with clinical care. The systems empower patients to do self-care while having the guidance of their private physician. These TelePractice systems provide patients with:

- Health education
- Access to physicians
- Health reminders
- Social support
- Automated monitoring
- Triage

The initial use of the TelePractice system was for the management of pregnant patients, drug abuse in patients, and newborns.

The TelePractice system is a proprietary turnkey system that is integrated into the existing phone system. Through a computer interface and proprietary software, patients are able to record questions and receive recorded answers at a later date. Recorded questions and answers are organized in a talk-show format and shared with other callers. This type of system is called a voice information service (VIS). The VIS market is growing rapidly. There are a number of companies that provide recorded health and other education messages, which can be obtained through touch-tone telephones. Instead of recording public notice messages about general concerns, one TelePractice product, Community Rap, has managed to allow experts to record answers to specific callers' questions. Furthermore, the system is educational for people who may not have any question and may just wish to listen to questions left by others.

Imagine a system in which the physician can leave prerecorded answers to the most commonly requested issues. These systems are totally automated. Through a simple voice tree, the patient can select the topic of their concern 24 hours a day without the use of a microcomputer or Internet connection.

In one evaluation of such systems, conducted in the inner city of Cleveland, Ohio, it was found that all clinic patients, regardless of their socioeconomic level, were able to gain access to the phone system. Everyone lived within range of at least a pay phone or a phone of a neighbor that could be used.

Many professionals work in environments that provide voice mail. The competition for voice mail systems is fierce. The top five companies that provide voice mail control more than 50% of the market. While it is true that none of these companies have products that focus on unique aspects of health care delivery, the systems can easily be adapted to provide a logic tree–structured delivery system for frequently asked questions. TelePractice has developed a system that is called care mail. The price of this system initially was under $2000 per year. The system included features that would permit the physician to remind patients about their appointments, follow up with patients who failed to return at a designated appointment, send current reminders for those with chronic conditions, and send reminder notices about the preparation required for various diagnostic procedures.

Preliminary studies on these systems have indicated a high level of satisfaction among patient users, regardless of socioeconomic level. Arthur D. Little Inc., in a publication entitled "Can Telecommunications Help Solve America's Health-Care Problems?," has projected that telecommunications systems could reduce health care costs by $30 billion annually.

INFORMED MEDICAL DECISION MAKING USING INTERACTIVE VIDEO

One of the most thoroughly studied uses of interactive video was the shared decision making programs created by the Foundation for Informed Medical Decision-Making in Hanover, New Hampshire. The president and CEO of the foundation, Joseph F. Kasper, has stated, "There is no substitute for the compassionate and knowledgeable care of a well-meaning clinician. But where quality of life issues are involved, the best medical decision fully involves the patients. For such involvement, the patient needs accurate, balanced, complete information."

Dr. Kasper and his colleagues have demonstrated that the use of interactive video can dramatically improve the quality of patient education when it comes to serious medical issues, such as benign prostatic hyperplasia, low back pain, mild hypertension, breast cancer surgery, and breast cancer adjuvant therapy.

What exactly is interactive video? Interactive video is the merging of video disk technology with PC-based microcomputers. The advantage of video disk or CD-ROM–based video material is that the user can almost instantly have access to a specific segment of material. In the old days—10 years ago—videotape was the standard delivery system. When using videotape, one must wait until the tape has been forwarded or reversed to the proper location. The access time for a video disk or CD-ROM–based video resource is less than a second. This is clearly an advantage for the viewer.

This technology allows the physician to provide, in his or her own words and gestures, the desired information, in a consistent, reliable, and painless format. In addition, the microcomputer can document that the patient reviewed the material. This is particularly useful when it comes to issues of informed consent.

When information is presented to a patient using balanced, interactive video, the choices made by the patient are more likely to be "true choices." The research conducted by Kasper et al demonstrated that patients with benign prostatic hyperplasia were much less likely to choose a surgical course of treatment if they had participated in the interactive video presentation on that topic. As one might guess, this caused some amount of consternation among the urologists in that area.

COMPREHENSIVE HEALTH ENHANCEMENT SUPPORT SYSTEM

Another important example of physician-directed medical self-care is a program developed at the University of Wisconsin–Madison. The program is entitled Comprehensive Health Enhancement Support System or as it is commonly known, CHESS. CHESS is a PC-based system designed to provide health care consumers with the information, referrals, decision support, and social support necessary for them to become empowered partners in the management of their own disease and health care. Individual CHESS workstations are installed either in patients' homes or community sites like clinics, community centers, and public libraries and are linked together through modems to a central host computer, which supports communication with other workstations.

Initial topic areas developed under the CHESS program are AIDS/HIV infection, breast cancer, adult children of alcoholics, sexual assault, stress, and substance abuse. The CHESS system providers users with a wide range of integrated services.

Questions and Answers is a compilation of answers to hundreds of common questions about each topic. The answers are brief overviews with references to where more detailed information can be found both in other CHESS services and outside of CHESS. CHESS offers a collection of several hundred articles, brochures, and templates. The articles cover a broad range of topics and are presented at different levels of complexity. The articles are drawn from scientific journals, newsletters, and the popular press.

Getting Help/Support This section help users understand what health and social services are available, how they work, how to find a good provider, and how to be an effective and active consumer.

The Personal Stories This section of CHESS provides real-life accounts of living with and coping with health crises. The stories were collected and written by trained journalists. CHESS users can read 300- to 500-word overviews and more detailed expansions on specific topics.

Ask an Expert This section of CHESS permits the users to ask health care experts anonymous questions. Most of the questions received a confidential response within 24 hours of submission.

Discussion Group This component of CHESS is very popular. It permits anonymous, nonthreatening communication among people affected by the specific health crisis. Message centers are identified by code name. Users share information, experiences, hopes and fears, and give and receive support. This system facilitates discussion and creates a safe environment for the sharing of different perspectives on common issues.

Decision Aid This component of CHESS helps people through the hard decisions that often are necessary. Users are encouraged to consider their various options and the implications of each possible choice. Two different types of decision support are available. Tailored programs help users with specific decisions, such as how to tell a friend about being HIV-positive or what type of breast cancer treatment to choose. The second model can be used for any decision. Both programs use multi-attribute utility models for the analysis.

Action Plan The action plan component of CHESS helps users implement a new decision. Once the new decision is made, specific steps must be outlined to assure a positive outcome. This component of the program asks the user how they propose to implement a decision; helps them analyze their strengths and weaknesses, support, and barriers; and predicts a likelihood of success.

Health Charts The health charts system enables a user to automatically keep a diary of important health-related information, including symptoms, medications, weight, and other important variables.

The CHESS program also provides a dictionary that includes easy-to-understand definitions of over 850 medical and health-related terms.

PHYSICIAN-DIRECTED SELF-CARE SOFTWARE

There are an increasing number of computerized decision support systems created by physicians. One such system has been created by Roger L. Gould. Dr. Gould has named his system Interactive Health System, Inc., which produces problem-solving methods and software to assist individuals with personal growth.

Dr. Gould believes that individuals can maintain ownership of problems and accelerate decision making and taking action toward resolution of problems, if proper tools are at their disposal. Gold believes that interactive software is the optimum tool to facilitate this process. The software 1) leads the user through pathways of revelatory thinking; 2) evokes sensitive personal data in specific, concrete, bite-sized pieces; 3) is nonjudgmental and nonthreatening; 4) produces results with gratifying speed; and 5) generates hard copy printouts for durable learning and reinforcement.

Dr. Gold has produced programs for use in professional clinics, work sites, and schools. The programs have addressed such issues as stress management, moods, foods and will power, reality problem solving, therapeutic learning, and stress.

Dr. John Greist, a psychiatrist in Madison, Wisconsin, has developed a number of physician-directed software packages that assist patients in managing their blood levels of various psychotherapeutic agents. Dr. Greist has found that the majority of patients can learn quickly to use software to maintain their medications in a therapeutic range.

APPENDIX 23-1

Taken from: http://www.aboutwomen.com/addiction/messages/69.html
Posted by M on October 09, 1997 at 18:37:45:
In reply to: zyban [bupropion] posted by C on October 05, 1997:

I started taking zyban on a Friday night. Each pill is 150 mg and you take 2 a day while you are still smoking. Smoke as much as you want because on day 8 you put a patch on and stop smoking. I had a dry mouth and the jitters for about a week and a half. I didn't really notice the insomnia part because I took my pills at 6am and 6pm. The zyban did cut my urge to want to smoke the first week, but I forced myself to continue smoking because this was my last week of doing it.

I put a 14 mg patch on for a week and then the following week I put on a 7 mg patch for 5 days. I took myself off of the patch because I am sick and tired of being addicted to nicotine. After being on zyban for a month I had to go back to the Dr. to get another prescription. He didn't want to give it to me because he doesn't believe in mind altering drugs. But he gave me some free samples of wellbutrin, enough for a month. He told me to start cutting back on them, so now I only take 1 pill a day, in the morning, with my coffee. I'm still on the 150 mg dose.

The package you get with zyban tells you to be on it for 7–12 weeks. If you have health insurance have your Dr. prescribe wellbutrin because insurance doesn't cover zyban and it's about $81.00.

For the most part I'm doing OK. I have had a couple of smokes, but it's been nothing that I've enjoyed. I haven't gained any weight. As a matter of fact, I've lost a couple

of pounds. I was surprised at that. Overall I do feel a lot better and I'm breathing easier.

Posted by JD on October 29, 1997:
In reply to: Zyban (Wellburin, bupropion), Smoking, Melatonin, and DHEA posted by JH on June 15, 1997:

My start-day on Zyban is Oct. 1st with a first no-smoke day of Oct. 9th (my 51st birthday) . . . During the months leading up to this planned date I have grown more and more apprehensive about the potential suffering, but now as it draws very near, I have actually noticed myself looking forward to it . . . I sort of feel as if I am psychologically prepared (and spiritually, I hope) . . . A recovering alcoholic with one year of sobriety (also Oct. 9th), I am viewing tobacco similarly to alcohol . . . I have been destroying my lungs and they NEED a rest . . . which I'm about to give them . . . Overwhelmed by the idea of not smoking for the REST OF MY LIFE, I plan to take it one day at a time . . . "I'll just rest my lungs TODAY" . . . I believe the addage that, in this life, pain is inevitable, but suffering is optional . . . So, I'll report how Zyban is helping with the pain as long as it lasts . . . and try to enjoy my recovery without succumbing to the temptation of "partying in my suffering". . . .

Posted by MR on October 20, 1997:
In Reply to: Zyban (Wellburin, bupropion), Smoking, Melatonin, and DHEA posted by JH on June 15, 1997:

My husband had a heart attack 2 weeks ago. He is 46 years old and has smoked since he was 8 to 10 years old. The doctor has put him on zyban to help him stop

(Continued)

smoking. We read the info that came with the medication. The really scary part was when they kept taking about seizures. I am going to call our family doctor on monday and ask him about melatonin and see if he will prescribe that instead. The zyban is about $1.40 per pill. He is supposed to take 2 per day and has enough prescription for 60 days. This is expensive but not as expensive as smoking both money and health wise. Thank you for providing this information so that I could check this out and get new insight into exactly what zyban was supposed to accomplish in this whole process. I will try to keep you updated on his progress and what the doctor says. Thanks again for caring.

Posted by DH on October 23, 1997:
In Reply to: Zyban (Wellburin, bupropion), Smoking, Melatonin, and DHEA posted by JH on June 15, 1997:

Contrary to JB's response, some insurance companies DO pay for Zyban. Within 5 days of our doctor telling us that Prudential Prucare HMO wouldn't pay for it, we found out that they do indeed include that as part of their approved Rx drugs which yields only a $5 copay to the client. This obviously transpired within the past 2 or 3 weeks.

"We" includes myself and my wife . . . I have found more successful results in smoking susession by using the "patch" and simply telling myself that I'm better off without the cigs. I tried the Zyban and found no assistance. My wife, on the other hand, is using the Zyban to squelch her nicotine appetite and is having respectable success with it.

Best of luck to all interested,
DH

Posted by C on October 25, 1997:
In Reply to: Re: Zyban (Wellburin, bupropion), Smoking, Melatonin, and DHEA posted by JD on October 23, 1997:

Today I Quit smoking! I have been on Zyban for a week, and feel great. I am using the patch (14 mg) with the zyban so my actual withdrawl symptoms would not be so bad even without the zyban. The last few days I found myself smoking out of habit, rather than craving. This was nice and encouraging as my quit date approached. Today I really feel great and think I can beat this thing. In the past when I've tried to quit, I became nasty, snapish, verbally abusive and felt like a tight spring that wanted to hit someone! (not like myself at all)

I also in past attempts felt very tired and wanted to sleep all the time. With Zyban I have a lot more energy today than I did when smoking!

I wouldn't say that Zyban relaxes me, more the opposite . . . but with a good energy.

The side effects of jitters, and insomnia did not bother me past the first days, but the dry mouth has stayed with me. The dangerous side effects I understand are seizures, but occur in people with existing medical conditions. (anyone please feel free to correct me on this) Good Luck . . . I hope I've helped . . . C

Posted by SW on October 27, 1997:

I've been on Zyban since Oct. 6. My quit date was Oct. 15 and I have not had a cigarette since! No patches, no gum, nothing. I feel great mentally and physically. Only side effects were dry mouth for the first week, since then I am side-effect free. I rarely have an urge to smoke, I really don't even think about it. Zyban is my miracle drug! I've been smoking for 28 years. If anyone has been on Zyban for more than 30 days I would love to hear from you. Good luck to everyone!

Posted by L on October 26, 1997:

Had been a smoker for over 30 years and always wanted to quit, but did not want to gain weight. Changed my eating habits this summer to lose a few pounds and gear up for my quitting day. After four weeks of not smoking, am pleased to see no weight gain. I did have to cut back on the 150 mg dose by splitting my pill in half. I also found that by taking my first dose at 5am and my second dose at 1pm, am not having trouble sleeping. Good luck to all of you! If I can change my ways, you can too!

Posted by KW on November 06, 1997:

I am a 61 year old woman who has been smoking since age 15. I am very lucky; I am in perfect health and have taken very few medications throughout my life; am very happy and upbeat; am owner of a travel agency and work full time in the office and escorting tours. I am a heavy smoker and am intent on quiting for several reasons. I spend so much of my time smoking, I am embarrased about the habit and I want to continue to feel good.

I am concerned about the chance of having seizures but in reading through the messages this seems to be of little concern.

My husband smokes and this concerns me but I know that I cannot make him quit . . . it is a decision that needs to be made by each individual. I hope I am successful in stopping smoking while living in a smoke filled house. But I am determined.

Thanks for listening to a frightened lady. Any suggestions will be greatly appreciated!

Chapter 24

The Patient and Self-Care: Implications for Medical Practice

Molly Mettler
Donald W. Kemper

Whatever people do to recognize, prevent, treat and manage their own symptoms and health problems can be called medical self-care. The woman who takes aspirin for her headache, the man who monitors his own blood pressure, and the teenager who treats her own acne all practice self-care. Self-care is practiced by all people, in all cultures, virtually every day. When encouraged and supported by physicians and other health care providers, patient self-care can contribute greatly to the quality and positive outcomes of medical care.

Health plans, businesses, and clinics are turning to a very old idea—people taking care of themselves—to engage consumers in their own care management. By offering programs and resources to teach patients how to manage common or chronic illnesses at home, payers and providers are expecting to see informed and knowledgeable consumers making a positive difference in both the quality and cost of health care.

Self-care programs are on the rise across the country, reaching millions of people with books, pamphlets, classes, and telephone hot lines. This chapter explores the history of self-care, the benefits of active self-care for both patient and physician, some case studies of self-care working within different populations, and five simple steps to help your patients become your partners in care.

INCIDENCE OF SELF-CARE

Vickery defines medical self-care as "actions taken by an individual with respect to a medical problem," which places the emphasis on individual decision making (1). When confronted with a symptom or health problem, the practice of self-care encompasses a variety of possible activities by either the patient or by caregivers. "Preventing, treating, and managing" health problems can comprise a host of activities, including taking no action; watchful waiting; self-diagnosis; seeking advice from friends and family; self-medication with over-the-counter drugs and home remedies; restricting activity; consulting books, magazines, and online electronic databases; and asking advice of pharmacists and others with professional training (2–4).

The pervasiveness of what has been humorously described as "people practicing medicine without a license" is well illustrated by a study that Demers et al conducted (5). They analyzed all the health problems recorded by 107 subjects over a 3-week period. They found that less than 6% of the problems received professional medical care. Of the 348 recorded illness episodes or health problems, 24.7% were not treated, 67.6% were treated with self-initiated self-care measures, and 2.3% were treated with self-care measures after getting telephone advice from a health professional (Figure 24-1).

Most of the health care in this country consists of what people do for themselves. Other studies done in North America, Europe, and Scandinavia confirm what Demers and his colleagues found: that 80% to 90% of symptoms are first treated at home, either by watching and waiting, by using over-the-counter medicine or a cultural remedy that has been passed down, or by employing information gathered from friends and loved ones, the communications media, or books (6,7).

When we consider that 8 out of 10 health problems are handled at home by laypersons without any intervention from a medical professional, we must recognize patients as the

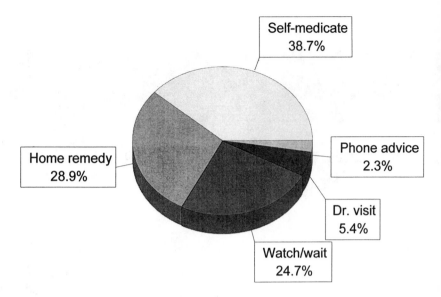

Figure 24-1 What people do when they have a health problem. (Based on data from Demers R, et al. An exploration of the dimensions of illness behavior. J Fam Pract 1980;11:1085–1092. Used by permission.)

Self-medicate 38.7%

Phone advice 2.3%

Dr. visit 5.4%

Watch/wait 24.7%

Home remedy 28.9%

primary providers of their own care. However, self-care has been the most overlooked part of the health care system. Lay consumers are the "hidden providers" of health care.

THE HISTORY OF SELF-CARE

History itself supports the layperson's role in health care. Since the beginning of civilization, the majority of health care has been provided by the individual and the family. Ancient Greek and Babylonian texts record the importance of daily living patterns in maintaining health (8). Nor are books on self-care a twentieth century phenomenon. In 1747, the Reverend John Wesley, founder of the Methodist Church, published a popular self-care book, *Primitive Remedies* (9). The modern interest in self-care had a resurgence in the 1970s with such books as *Our Bodies, Our Selves*, published by the Boston Women's Health Collective, and *How to be Your Own Doctor Sometimes* (10,11).

These days self-care has become big business. Dozens of texts detailing common illnesses and injuries and what to do about them are available through bookstores, managed care organizations, employers' benefits departments, Medicare, Medicaid, and other health insurance programs. Employers and insurers are distributing self-care manuals in part to assist their employees and subscribers in providing good, sensible family care and also to ensure the appropriate use of medical services (12). (See the consumer resources information in the box on this page.)

The question arises: "Is all this self-care good for the patient?" The dangers of self-care were addressed by Wilkinson, who studied the self-care actions of 340 subjects over a 2-week period. In only 2% of cases were the actions assessed as "inappropriate and potentially harmful" (13). Simply put, most people provide sound and appropriate self-care for their health problems most of the time.

CONSUMER RESOURCES

Johnson RV. The Mayo Clinic Complete Book of Pregnancy & Baby's First Year. New York: William Morrow & Co., 1994.

Kemper DW, et al. Healthwise Handbook. 13th ed. Boise, ID: Healthwise, Inc., 1997.

Kemper DW. It's About Time: Better Health Care in a Minute (or Two). Boise, ID: Healthwise, Inc., 1993.

Kemper DW, et al. La salud en casa: Guia practica de Healthwise. 11th ed. Boise, ID: Healthwise, Inc., 1994.

Larson DE, ed. Mayo Clinic Family Health Book. 2nd ed. New York: William Morrow, 1996.

Lorig K, Holman H, Sobel D, et al. Living a Healthy Life with Chronic Conditions: Self-Management of Heart Disease, Arthritis, Stroke, Diabetes, Asthma, Bronchitis, Emphysema, and Others. Palo Alto, CA: Bull Publishing, 1994.

Mayo Clinic and Mayo Medical School. Everything You Need to Know About Medical Tests. Springhouse, PA: Springhouse, 1996.

Mettler M, Kemper DW. Healthwise for Life: Medical Self-Care for Healthy Aging. 2nd ed. Boise, ID: Healthwise, Inc., 1996.

Pantell R, Fries JF, Vicker D, et al. Taking Care of Your Child. 4th ed. Reading, MA: Addison Wesley, 1993.

Vickery D, Fries JF. Take Care of Yourself. 6th ed. Reading, MA: Addison Wesley, 1996.

BENEFITS OF PATIENT SELF-CARE FOR THE PHYSICIAN

Is your role as a *medically-trained* health care provider to remind patients "just who is the doctor here" and discourage patient self-activation? Or, do you better serve these hidden providers of care by entering into a partnership with your patients that helps them provide the very best care to themselves and their families and to get the very best care from their interactions with you?

Although self-care is practiced by the patient, it is also complementary to the physician's practice of medicine. At its best, building self-care skills raises patient confidence and competence and reinforces a positive doctor-patient relationship. Physicians, nurses, and other health care providers play a vital role in encouraging patients to become involved in their own care.

How might your practice be affected by working with informed patients who consider you to be a partner, rather than the sole supplier, of their health care? Training in self-care skills and access to self-care information for your patients can make a significant contribution to them in quality, cost, and appropriateness of health care.

Quality

Improving the quality of care given at home helps prevent complications and improves health outcomes. With accurate information, people can provide appropriate home treatment to manage symptoms and often prevent an illness from getting worse. Consider the patient who successfully self-treats and manages an upper respiratory infection, thus lessening the chance that he or she may develop a secondary bacterial infection. In chronic illnesses as well, self-care is the mainstay of effective treatment. The successful management of chronic problems like hypertension, heart disease, arthritis, and diabetes is based as much on the quality of home treatment and self-management as it is on the quality of professional care.

Good self-care includes knowing when to seek professional help. Getting to the right doctor at the right time has a tremendous impact on the quality of care received. With accurate information and support from their doctors and other health care providers people make more knowledgeable and appropriate decisions about the need for and the urgency of seeking professional care. Recently, a middle-aged man with a history of hypertension called into a community-based nurse advice line complaining of headache, dizziness, visual disturbance, and arm numbness. The nurse convinced him to seek a medical evaluation. He called back later to say, "Thank you for giving me another chance at life," and to report that he was now managing his illness with medication and lifestyle changes (14).

The role of self-care does not end when your patient walks through your clinic doors. Even after the physician is involved, self-care and disease self-management play a big role in the quality of care. When patients present an accurate history of symptoms, your diagnoses are more apt to be accurate. When your patients prepare properly for diagnostic tests, there are fewer false findings. Overall, active patient involvement results in better outcomes and a greater level of patient satisfaction (15).

Cost for Value

Medical self-care reduces health care costs primarily by reducing use of services. In a review of studies focusing on medical self-care interventions, six of the seven studies reviewed demonstrated a reduction in visits to physicians. The magnitude of the reductions is relatively consistent, with five of the seven studies reporting a 7% to 15% drop in visit rates (16).

In one study conducted by a managed care company, health claims for people who had received a self-care guide and attended a self-care workshop were 15% to 90% lower for participants in five of six categories: sore throats, knee sprains, upper respiratory infections, allergies, and stomachaches. The sixth category, ear infections, actually showed a 50% increase in claims. But as program organizers pointed out, the self-care information directed consumers to see a doctor for ear infections (17).

One large U.S. health maintenance organization (HMO) implemented a comprehensive self-care program for its members and staff. The goals were to improve members' self-care skills and appropriate use of services (visits and calls) while reducing unnecessary use of services, to enhance visit and telephone accessibility, and to integrate self-care into medical care delivery (18).

Two years later, 90% of the people who had received the medical self-care guide had used it at least once, resulting in a decrease in overall use of services. The HMO recorded a drop of more than 15% in emergency room visits (19).

Appropriate use of and reductions in office visits and emergency room visits makes great economic sense in the ever-widening world of capitated care. *The Wall Street Journal* has reported that of 90 million emergency room visits made in this country every year, more than 50% of them were for minor problems, such as sore throats, resulting in unnecessary bills totaling more than $5 billion a year (20).

Appropriateness

For physicians who are practicing in a fee-for-service environment and are somewhat economically dependent on visits by patients for acute, self-limiting illness, perhaps the promise of reduced utilization does not hold strong appeal. However, when viewed in the context that your patients and their families are already practicing self-care and that active involvement brings better outcomes and greater satisfaction, doesn't it make sense to help them do the very best job possible?

Appropriateness and relevance are added to health care through consumer involvement in medical decision making. Considering patient preferences and values in medical decision making is steadily gaining ground as a viable component of patient care. Patients report being more satisfied with both the care they receive and the physician providing that care if they are included in the decision making process (21).

Patient-centered medical care helps avoid medical treatments that are not in the consumer's best interest. When major medical decisions need to be made, such as when to opt for an angioplasty, patients often assume a passive role, thus removing their own values from the decision making process. By encouraging shared medical decision making, the patient's values are included as a part of the decision process and help increase both the appropriateness and relevance of the care.

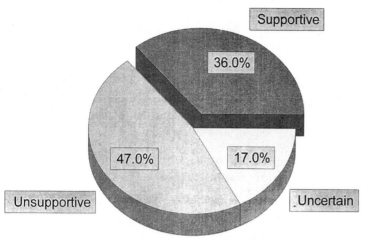

Figure 24-2 Physician attitudes: 1979. (Source: Linn LS, Lewis CE. Attitudes toward self-care among practicing physicians. Medical Care 1979;18:183–190.)

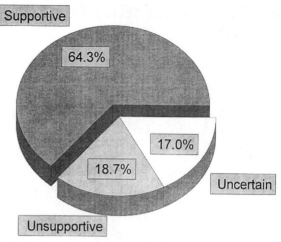

Figure 24-3 Physician attitudes: 1995. (Unpublished data, from Healthwise, Incorporated, 1996.)

TRADE-OFF OR PAYOFF? A SHIFT IN PHYSICIAN ATTITUDES

Physician attitudes toward a more informed and self-activated patient are changing. In 1979, Linn and Lewis measured attitudes held by physicians toward patient self-care and patient involvement in care. Then, close to half of physicians surveyed were not supportive of patients becoming actively involved in their own care (22). Using the same questionnaire, researchers found that attitudes had changed substantially by the mid-1990s; almost two-thirds of physicians surveyed were now supportive of patient self-care (Figures 24-2 and 24-3).

Still, not all providers welcome the "informed patient" with open arms. Physicians have expressed real concerns that the informed patient isn't always *well-informed* and that questioning patients tend to be more work than passive patients (24). Perhaps this perspective needs to be reframed. Physicians who cultivate an open partnership with their patients agree that passive patients tend to assign their physicians all the responsibility for their health and opt out of any personal control or input into their well-being. On the other hand, patients who share in decision making power also share some of the responsibility for the outcome and are more likely to concur with the diagnosis and comply with the treatment regimen.

How do these concepts play out in populations who are either medically underserved or economically disadvantaged? Health Service, Empowerment, and Transformation (SET) of Denver and Albuquerque is a medical self-care program targeted at uninsured working families, Medicaid families, and single and teen mothers. Each family attends a 2-hour workshop and is given a self-care kit that includes a self-care handbook. In addition, each family is given three stamped, self-addressed postcards that are to be returned as the manual and kit are used. The returned postcards indicated that families who had self-care education took care of health problems at home 77% of the time. Further evaluation studies indicate a 46% reduction in inappropriate use of the emergency room and a 17% reduction rate in office visits (25).

An experimental program for 280,000 people living in Idaho is seeking to make a difference in the quality and cost of health care by engaging everyone in a four-county area to play an active role in their health care. (See "The Healthwise Communities Project" in the box below.) The project is for everyone in four counties, whether they are insured or not, educated or not, and with access to care or not. Approximately 13% of the population is uninsured, and 9% are below the poverty level.

Research on the program's impact on quality outcomes, cost, and satisfaction is being undertaken by Oregon Health Sciences University. They are using randomized population surveys, in-depth analysis of insurers, employers, the Health Care Financing Administration (HCFA) and Medicaid claims data, direct analysis of hospital data for selected procedures, and trend analysis in the target area and two control communities in the Northwest. Preliminary findings indicate that 69% of those people in the target area who indicated that they had received the self-care handbook at their homes have used the book to identify or manage a common illness or injury (26).

Blue Cross of Idaho, one of the program sponsors, analyzed customer claims filed 1 year before and 1 year after everyone in the four counties received their free medical self-care guide. The preliminary findings are that emergency room visits declined an average of 18% in the target area (27).

SHARED MEDICAL DECISION MAKING

Projects like Healthwise Communities demonstrate the significant advances to medical self-care now possible as a result of recent improvements in information technology. In the past, in-depth medical information was restricted to those few patients who had access to medical libraries and were willing to pore over relevant articles in the medical literature. Today, new technology has lifted those restrictions. Now, patients can get high-quality, in-depth information on almost any health problem easily and inexpensively over the Internet and other

THE HEALTHWISE COMMUNITIES PROJECT

The Healthwise Communities Project is a community-wide health initiative designed to help 280,000 Idahoans become the best-informed medical consumers in the world. The goals of the project are to improve health care quality and reduce health care costs by making fundamental changes in the way doctors and patients work together.

Thanks to a $2.1 million grant from The Robert Wood Johnson Foundation and contributions from insurers, hospitals, and local corporations, the Healthwise Communities Project seeks to help residents become more active participants in their own health care. The underlying philosophy of the project is that, with sound medical information, patients and their doctors can work together to improve the health care system and lower costs. Project services are free for everyone in the four-county area. Services include:

- A free 335-page self-care guide, *The Healthwise Handbook*, which has been mailed to every home in the area

- A telephone advice line staffed by specially trained registered nurses

- Information "stations" in over 40 locations, providing access to medical reference books and the Healthwise Knowledgebase, a comprehensive health information database written for consumers

- Access to the Knowledgebase from home on the World Wide Web at http://www.hcp.org

- Consumer self-care workshops

- Seminars for health providers to learn better ways of supporting the "empowered" health consumer

Two studies on the impact of Healthwise Communities both show a drop in emergency room visits and suggest that widespread, consumer-focused health care management efforts can lower health care utilization and costs.

In a study conducted by Blue Cross of Idaho, one of the sponsors of the project, the number of emergency room visits for enrollees dropped by 18% in the first year of the program. Patient claims data 12 months before distribution of the handbook were compared with utilization patterns 12 months after distribution. As a comparison, Blue Cross of Idaho researchers also looked at ER visits for enrollees in two adjacent counties that did not receive the self-care materials. Blue Cross researchers estimate that the handbook distribution saved the health plan over $365,000.

An earlier study was done by Oregon Health Sciences University (OHSU) measuring the extent to which people were actually using the health information distributed by Healthwise. When asked whether they had used the Healthwise Handbook or health information within the last few months, 71% of Idaho respondents said "yes." In two control communities with access to health information but no concerted community-wide initiative, 44% of Montana respondents and 48% of Oregon respondents reported using a self-care guide or other health information. OHSU also asked whether using a reference book saved a visit to the doctor. In Idaho, 62% said it had saved a visit; in Montana, 61%, and in Oregon, 53%.

As for saving a trip to the emergency room, the OHSU study showed that 33% of Idaho respondents said the book saved a visit to the ER; in Montana, 32%, and in Oregon, 28%.

Preliminary studies such as these seem to seem to indicate that involving consumers and patients in their care can improve quality and lower health care costs.

---

electronic information sources installed at public libraries, medical centers, and worksites.

More and more, in response to patient interest and demand, managed care organizations, health insurers, and hospital systems are providing free access to such information sources.

"INFORMATION THERAPY": THE ROLE OF THE PHYSICIAN IN SHARED DECISION MAKING

In addition to writing prescriptions for drugs or ordering further diagnostic tests, doctors may also want to add "information therapy" to their repertoire of treatment options. Using new technologies, physicians can play a direct role in ensuring that their patients have access to medically reliable and unbiased consumer health information. With information therapy, once a diagnosis is established and before major treatment decisions are made, physicians can direct patients to review specific sections of the information before the office visit to set the treatment plan. "Prescription information," getting the right information to the right patient to help him or her get to the right decision, then becomes a powerful tool in the doctor-patient partnership. When the patient comes to the visit informed, physician and patient can work collaboratively in deciding which treatment options best meet the needs and preferences of the patient.

FROM PATIENT TO PARTNER: FIVE SIMPLE STEPS

In a world of troubled patients and 10-minute physician visits, mutually satisfying doctor-patient communication is a challenge. To get the best health care, patients must be willing and encouraged to become more involved as active partners with their doctors. The doctor's language, attitude, and influence can go a long way toward inspiring this partnership for better health. To encourage your patients to become your partner in their care:

1. Support their practice of self-care. Let your patients know that you expect them to provide care to them-

selves and their families. Many patients are worried that their physicians disapprove of self-care (or alternative care) measures and simply don't report them. Let your patients know that you are willing to work in partnership with them.

2. Ask them to watch and record symptoms at the first sign of a health problem. Encouraging your patients to keep a record of symptoms helps you make an accurate diagnosis and involve them in the decision making process.

3. Help them to prepare for office visits. Recognize that patients often feel hurried through an appointment. Show them how to get more value from their time with you by preparing a simple Doctor Visit Prep List (see Table 24-1), which includes guidelines on presenting the chief complaint first, sharing their hunches and fears about what is wrong, and listing the three top questions they want answered. By giving patients clear instructions on how to prepare their remarks and questions, you can hopefully bypass the dreaded "laundry list" of complaints and get right to the heart of the matter.

4. Select and recommend self-care information your patients can trust. Take the time to review a variety of self-care handbooks and other information sources. Then, recommend the sources that you trust to all of your patients. Your confidence in the information will add value to it for your patients. And your encouragement to seek information will greatly reinforce the patient's willingness to become involved in their own health care.

5. Invite and listen to your patients' preferences and values regarding their own care. True shared decision making goes beyond simply outlining the patient's options for treatment. It means eliciting their input and perspectives on what they hope the outcomes will be for them *as individuals*. Each patient you work with brings his or her own personality and spirit into the encounter. Some are risk-adverse, some are risk-takers. Some seek aggressive treatment, others are more conservative in their approach. However, most patients won't add or share their points of view unless they are invited to do so.

For some of your patients, these simple steps toward improved communication and better quality care represent a large, if

---

Table 24-1 Components of a Doctor Visit Prep List for Patients

Before your visit to the doctor:
- Prepare a symptom list.

- Highlight your chief complaint (your main concern).

- Write down 2–3 questions you want answered most.

- Write down your hunches about what is wrong.

- Make a list of your medications.

Used by permission from: It's about time: better health care in a minute (or two). ©Copyright 1993 by HEALTHWISE Incorporated, PO Box 1989, Boise ID 83701. Copying of any part of this material is not permitted without express written permission of HEALTHWISE, Incorporated.

---

not frightening, leap. Many patients have been taught that doctors are not to be questioned, much less "partnered with." You can help your patients become better medical consumers by believing in and supporting the important role they play, and by making available resources that enhance and improve their medical consumer skills.

The culture of health care is changing. In the emerging culture, the patient is accepted as a primary provider of care, and the physician is recognized as a partner, rather than a strict purveyor of care. What brings the patient and providers together as partners is accurate and helpful information, a willingness to work together for good health, and a belief that both patient and provider input is necessary for the practice of good medicine. In essence, we need to "reinvent" the patient's role in health care, and by doing so, improve health care quality and reduce health care cost.

REFERENCES

1. Vickery D. Medical self-care: a review of the concept and program models. Amer J Health Promo 1986;(Summer):23–28.

2. Verbrugee L, Ascione F. Exploring the iceberg: common symptoms and how people take care of them. Medical Care 1987;25:539–569.

3. Elliott-Bins C. An analysis of lay medicine: fifteen years later. J R Coll Gen Pract 1986;36:542–544.

4. Levin L, Idler E. Self-care in health. Ann Rev Pub Health 1983; 4:181–201.

5. Demers R, Altamore R, Mustin H, et al. An exploration of the dimensions of illness behavior. J Fam Pract 1980;11:1085–1092.

6. Williamson J, Danaher K. Self care in health. London: Croom Helm, 1978:39.

7. Dean K, Holst E, Wagner MG, et al. Self-care of common illnesses in Denmark. Medical Care 1983; 21:1012–1032.

8. Sigerist H. History of medicine. vol. 1. Oxford: Oxford University Press, 1951.

9. Wesley J. Valuable primitive remedies. 1747.

10. Boston Women's Health Book Collective. Our Bodies, Ourselves.

New York: Simon and Schuster, 1971.

11. Sehnert K. How to be your own doctor sometimes. New York: Grosset and Dunlap, 1975.

12. Stevens L. Emphasizing active partnerships. Healthplan 1996;July/August:77–80.

13. Wilkinson I, Darby DN, Mant A. et al. Self-care and self medication: an evaluation of individuals' health care decisions, Medical Care 1987;25:965–978.

14. Case history from the Healthwise Line, Healthwise Communities Project, Boise, Idaho, December 6, 1996.

15. Greenfield S, Kaplan S, Ware JE Jr, et al. Expanding patient involvement in care: effects on patient outcome. Ann Intern Med 1985;3:448–457.

16. Kemper D, Lorig K, Mettler M, et al. The effectiveness of medical self-care interventions: a focus on self-initiated responses to symptoms. Patient Edu Counsel 1993; 21:29–39.

17. Sandberg M. Self-care programs produce immediate results. Managed Healthcare 1994:July.

18. Larson P. The Kaiser Permanente self-care program: enhancing quality, satisfaction, accessibility and cost-effectiveness with member education. Paper presented at the International Federation of Health Funds meeting, Capetown, South Africa, March 1998.

19. Davis S. Idaho group hopes to reengineer the patient. Reengineering the Hospital 1998;4:1–4.

20. The Wall Street Journal, February 4, 1997.

21. Kaplan SH, Greenfield S, Gandek B, et al. Characteristics of physi-cians with participatory decision-making styles. Ann Intern Med 1996;124:497–504.

22. Linn LS, Lewis CE. Attitudes toward self-care among practicing physicians. Medical Care, 1979; 17:183–190.

23. Healthwise Incorporated, Physician Attitude Survey, 1995.

24. Dudley TE, Falvo DR, Podell RN, et al. The informed patient poses a different challenge. Patient Care 1996;October15:128–132, 134, 136–138.

25. Health SET report, June 25, 1995.

26. Hibbard J, et al. Idaho community health survey follow-up. Oregon Health Sciences University, 1997.

27. LeMay C. People learning E.R. means emergency. The Idaho Statesman, January 22, 1998.

Chapter 25

The Internet and Preventive Medicine

Joeli Hettler
Bill Hettler

WHAT IS PREVENTIVE MEDICINE?

One of the best ways to explore the modern view of preventive medicine is to use the Internet. It is possible, from the comfort of one's home or office, to visit the Web sites of major preventive medicine training sites. In addition, one can also visit the Web sites of the three most prominent professional organizations related to preventive medicine: the American Board of Preventive Medicine (http://www.abprevmed.org), the American College of Preventive Medicine (http://www.acpm.org), and the Association of Teachers of Preventive Medicine (ATPM) (http://www.atpm.org). Table 25-1 contains a more extensive list of Web sites on preventive medicine.

Who Actually Practices Preventive Medicine?

Prevention, in its broadest sense, it practiced by all physicians and other health professionals who help their patients stay healthy. Preventive medicine, however, also is a distinct medical specialty, one of the 25 recognized by the American Board of Medical Specialties.

The specialty of preventive medicine is based on our knowledge that promoting health and preventing disease require work with both individuals and communities. The distinctive aspects of preventive medicine include knowledge and competence in:

- Biostatistics
- Epidemiology
- Environmental and occupational health

The Contributions of Preventive Medicine

Today we take for granted the many contributions of preventive medicine. It is easy to forget that 100 years ago, 1 out of every 10 babies born in the United States died before its first birthday. Today fewer than 1 in 100 suffer this fate.

The nineteenth century advances in sanitary sciences and food hygiene were followed by major achievements: immunization against deadly diseases such as diphtheria, smallpox, and polio and the control of rheumatic fever, typhoid and other infections.

Recent contributions of preventive medicine include: the discovery of the role of tampons in toxic shock syndrome, research on the prevention of cancer through dietary change, the establishment of programs to prevent and limit the spread of AIDS and tuberculosis, and the development of methodologically sound recommendations for clinical preventive services. Preventive medicine has contributed substantially to a better understanding of occupational diseases, such as black lung, and to a more complete knowledge of human physiology in hazardous environments, such as outer space. Preventive medicine has improved the lives of untold millions (1).

- The social planning, administration, and evaluation of health services and behavioral aspects of health and disease
- The practice of prevention in clinical medicine

Table 25-1 Preventive Medicine and Related Sites on the World Wide Web
The American College of Preventive Medicine Home Page http://www.acpm.org/
Health-Promotion Conferences Directory http://wkweb2.cableinet.co.uk/healthpro/conf/conflist.htm
Welcome to The National Center For Health Promotion http://www.welltech.com/nchp/welcome.htm
Fourth International Conference on Health Promotion http://www.ki.se/phs/wcc seh/events/ichp4.html
World Health Organization's Jakarta Conference, 1997 Menu http://who.ultralab.anglia.ac.uk/
Health Promotion Outcomes http://rubble.ultralab.anglia.ac.uk/WHO Approach to HPR/Outcomes.html
Preventive Medicine Links http://weber.u.washington.edu/~sphcm/academic/pmrlink.html
The Preventive Medicine Center of Hartford, CT http://www.prevmedctr.org/
American College of Preventive Medicine http://www.social.com/health/nhic/data/hr2000/hr2043.html
PREVENTION'98 http://www.prevention-meeting.org
Internet Journal of Health Promotion: Health Promotion on the Internet http://www.monash.edu.au/health/IJHP/1995/1/
Health Promotion http://www.uky.edu/Education/KHP/khpheal.html
World Health Day 1996 Home Page http://www.who.ch/whday/1996/HealthyCity.html

The American Board of Preventive Medicine grants certificates to physicians who have demonstrated special knowledge and competence in the specialty and successfully passed a written examination. Postgraduate training in preventive medicine consists of 3 years of supervised training in any one of three areas: general preventive medicine or public health; occupational medicine; or aerospace medicine. Specialists in general preventive medicine or public health focus their skills on population groups, such as the residents of a particular community or state or the patient population of a health center, hospital, or health maintenance organization (HMO). Occupational physicians focus on health and safety in the workplace. The community associated with aviation, including passengers, is the domain of the aerospace physician.

Preventive medicine specialists work in a wide variety of settings, including public health and community agencies, outpatient and primary care settings, managed care organizations, industry, and academia. These physicians usually engage in multiple activities, including planning, administration, and evaluation of disease prevention and health promotion programs and research, teaching, and direct patient care.

There are more than 5000 physicians nationally who are board-certified in preventive medicine. Postgraduate training takes place in 85 residency programs accredited by the Accreditation Council for Graduate Medical Education in

which about 435 residents are annually enrolled. For more information, see the Careers in Preventive Medicine Section Web site (http://www.acpm.org/careers.htm) or contact the College by e-mail at info@acpm.org.

HOW WELL ARE PHYSICIANS DOING AT PRACTICING PREVENTIVE MEDICINE?

How well are physicians doing at practicing preventive medicine? A recent *Journal of the American Medical Association* article suggests not so well:

> Physician counseling of patients regarding health risk behaviors should be greatly improved if the U.S. Preventive Services Task Force recommendations are to be fulfilled. Improvement is especially needed in regard to alcohol consumption, safe sex, and seat belt use. Physicians also need to be more vigilant in properly identifying and counseling low-income patients at risk in regard to diet and exercise and high-income patients who smoke.
>
> JAMA EDITOR'S NOTE—The U.S. Preventive Services Task Force recommends that physicians assess health behaviors of all patients and discuss changing behavior with those at risk. This survey of Massachusetts employees asked about their health behaviors and whether their physician had ever addressed their health risks. Patients were not receiving the recommended advice: at best, 73% of those with inadequate exercise had the issue discussed by a physician; at worst, only 16% of those who inconsistently used seat belts had the issue discussed by a physician. Low-income patients, who were more likely to smoke than high-income patients, were more likely to have smoking discussed by a physician. Ironically, although low-income patients were more likely to be obese and need exercise, high-income patients were more likely to have diet and exercise discussed by a physician. This survey, the first to examine the relationship to patient income and discussion of health risk behaviors, emphasizes the importance of assessing health behaviors among all patients (2).

INFORMATION AGE ACCELERATES MAJOR PARADIGM SHIFTS

As the information age continues to influence all sectors of our society, there is no doubt that the field of preventive medicine will be fundamentally changed by the citizen empowerment that is occurring. This empowerment comes from the substantial increases in available health information systems readily available. In addition, medical care providers and consumers alike are beginning to recognize that the medical model, based primarily on industrial age values and attitudes, once taught us that physicians were in charge of "their" patients' lives. In reality, research is showing us that positive health status is more likely to be a result of positive lifestyle choices than use of medical care. Positive lifestyle choices are more likely to be the result of community and cultural norms than a result of purchasing medical care.

One health policy authority provides the following perspective in his recent book, *Purchasing Population Health*:

> Despite the massive resources it consumes, the U.S. health care system remains under stress. While we are global leaders in technical accomplishments in medicine, the amount of health we achieve per dollar invested is far from optimal. So far, both market and regulatory reforms have failed to address or even acknowledge this reality. The fundamental argument of this book, drawing from many disciplines such as medicine, economics, sociology, ethics, and management, is that we will not maximize the amount of health we achieve until a measure of health outcome becomes the purchasing standard for both the private and the public sectors (3).

THE MAJOR PARADIGM SHIFT

Shifting Attention from Preventive Medicine to Health Promotion and Wellness

Health promotion consists of the development of lifestyle habits that healthy individuals and communities can adopt to maintain and enhance the state of well-being. The ultimate goal is the optimization of health. Health promotion addresses individual responsibility, while preventive services can be fulfilled by health providers (4).

Ilona Kickbusch, Director of the Division of Health Promotion, Education, and Communication of the World Health Organization, has provided valuable insights via the Internet. Director Kickbusch reminded an audience about the World Health Organization definition of health: "Health is a state of complete physical, mental, and social well-being and not merely the absence of disease or infirmity" (5).

One journal editor defines health promotion as the following: "It is any combination of health education, and related organizational, political, and economic intervention designed to facilitate behavioral and environmental changes conducive to health" (6). This definition stresses the interdisciplinary nature of health promotion.

Definition of Wellness

Wellness is an active process of becoming aware of and making choices toward a more successful existence. The key words in this first sentence are process, aware, choices, and success.

Process means that we never arrive at a point were there is no possibility of improving.

Aware means that we are by our nature continuously seeking more information about how we can improve.

Choices mean that we have considered a variety of options and select those that seem to be in our best interest.

Success is determined by each individual to be their personal collection of accomplishments for their life.

Wellness is multidimensional. A popular model adopted by many university, corporate, and public health programs encompasses six dimensions: social, occupational, spiritual, physical, intellectual, and emotional.

Using a definition that is this broad-based can be a strength as well as a weakness. The definition is useful in that it emphasizes the influences of many dimensions on the well-being of individuals. Using a definition that is so broad-based, especially to describe a program or position, can easily be seen as more casual and less professional. In spite of that concern, there is a growing list of *Fortune* 500 corporations, major medical centers, and hospitals that are have created "wellness" departments or programs.

An excellent glossary of terms related to health promotion can be obtained from the World Health Organization Web site. WHO has created one of the most up to date and complete compilations of definitions of terms related to the promotion of population health. It can be found at http://www.who.ch/hpr/hep/documents/glossary.pdf.

Preventive medicine is no longer the only term used in most health professional settings. People who have a "wellness" or "health promotion" orientation are more likely to be perceived as doing something relevant to the populations being served. Preventive medicine is a medical specialty. The specialty origins are founded firmly in the "medical model."

Health promotion and wellness are much more modern terms, which include population-based activities. Practitioners of preventive medicine represent a wide range of professionals, with wide-ranging beliefs and practices.

For the purposes of this chapter, we use all three terms, *preventive medicine*, *health promotion*, and *wellness*, to relate to health-promoting activities conducted by or for individuals and groups.

Rapid Expansion of Web-Based Resources

A preliminary Internet search using the phrases preventive medicine, health promotion, and wellness was done in November 1997. This activity was repeated in mid-June of 1998 using exactly the same search program and phrases. Table 25-2 demonstrates the rapid increase in resources being added to the Internet.

The term *wellness* is obviously more commonly used than the others. The increase of 60% in documents over a 7-month period indicates that there are significantly more Web pages being developed that contain the term *wellness* than *preventive medicine* and *health promotion* combined. While these data are certainly anecdotal, and clearly not all the sites have

Table 25-2 Increase in Number of Websites for Specific Subjects			
Search Phrase	**No. of Documents Matching Query**		**Increase (%)**
	November 5, 1997	**June 20, 1998**	
Preventive Medicine	18,823	23,474	25
Health Promotion	28,640	43,773	52
Wellness	222,381	355,810	60

credible resources, there is clearly a more rapid increase in the topics health promotion and wellness than in preventive medicine.

USE OF THE INTERNET FOR WELLNESS AND HEALTH PROMOTION ACTIVITIES

E-Mail and Listserves

Many leaders agree that e-mail is the most valued element of the Internet. Most professionals, once involved, have found the use of e-mail to be a major leap forward in accomplishing their goals and objectives in wellness and health promotion. Many professionals regularly subscribe to a number of listserves. Health promotion and wellness listserves are essentially e-mail connections among professionals who are willing to share information on a regular basis about their efforts in promoting health and wellness. It is common for a member to post a question or dilemma to the listserve and to find that within 30 minutes, there are helpful responses. Many professionals are involved in health policy decisions. A listserve focused on the issues of health policy enhances their productivity.

Members of a professional organization are usually able to locate a listserve that focuses on the needs and interests of their organization. Some listserves can easily generate more than 12,000 messages a year. Trying to keep up with the volume of material available is like trying to get the proper amount of water needed for hydration by sipping from a fully charged firehouse. It can be done, but there is some risk involved.

Fortunately, many authors have an e-mail client software package that automatically deposits those messages in a separate folder, so that they do not clog up day-to-day computer activities.

The use of e-mail, which provides the opportunity to attach graphic files or text files, for regular communication has increased the efficiency of sharing information with colleagues around the world. We realize that some readers may not enjoy such a collaborative relationship in their work setting. As a matter of fact, some of their plans and activities could be labeled as trade secrets, and therefore, for some, the advantages of this electronic sharing may not exist.

The health professionals of the twenty-first century will be more efficient if they develop skills in using the major elements and services available on the Internet. The ability of people with similar interests to locate each other and share information is facilitating collaboration.

Online Chat Rooms and Real-Time Communication

Many of us have read or heard news accounts of events in which a person, participating in an online chat room, separated from another person by as much as 5000 miles, was able to take action that resulted in saving the life of one of the participants. In one such documented case, the participant noticed that one individual was becoming incoherent. Using the Internet, they were able to locate the nearest emergency services and get help for the person in jeopardy. In these cases, because of online real-time communication, it was noticed that someone was having difficulties. In these cases,

the observer of the difficulties was able through another form of communication, a phone, to contact the authorities in the location where the individual was in a crisis.

While these are certainly exciting events that do attract news coverage, they are not the regular day-to-day business activities for those of us who work in wellness and health promotion. In this chapter, we outline some of the main uses of the Internet that apply to wellness and health promotion.

One significant breakthrough related to the Internet and real-time communication is the refinement of face-to-face video communication. Using inexpensive (<$150), lightweight (<1 lb) videocameras and an Internet connection, people anywhere in the world can meet face-to-face. There are no additional costs for the connection. Once you buy the camera and the Internet connection, you can experience true distance videoconferencing.

Decision Support and Problem-Focused Support Services

Another remarkable advantage of the Internet is the ability for people involved in personal prevention activities to have 24-hour-a-day decision support and group support when they are encountering difficulties. For people attempting some major life change, the availability of other people who have experienced that same situation and their willingness to share their successes and failures electronically, 24 hours a day, has been a godsend. Dr. John Grohol has provided links to a number of support groups that are available on the World Wide Web, most in the Usenet format. Most people are familiar with the two main functions of the Internet, i.e., e-mail and Web sites, but there are a number of other services available over the World Wide Web that do not involve e-mail or Web site browsing. Usenet News Groups is one such service. These services are usually focused on a specific topic or concern. An example might be "survivors of sexual assault." There are similar services available in the form of Web-based chat rooms. One link to these services is can be found at Dr. Grohol's Web site (http://www.grohol.com).

News That You Can Use: Web-Based Information, News, and E-Journals

Every major news site on the World Wide Web has new health and wellness information posted each day. *Time* magazine, *USA Today*, *The New York Times*, CNN, *The Washington Post*, *The Chronicle of Higher Education*, and *Journal of the American Medical Association* are all examples of sites with free Web-based content that is updated daily. In addition to these traditional news sources going online, there are hundreds of corporate Web sites that are offering high-quality health-promoting content just to generate traffic to their Web pages. More than a year ago, the Mayo Clinic hired three full-time writers to provide daily new content for their consumer-oriented Web pages.

The Internet also provides users with the ability to view presentations and major conference addresses in real time or delayed, asynchronous format. We can get a more complete picture of this changing scene by reviewing this portion of an address by Director Kickbusch:

> The most crucial defining factor of any health promotion strategy is that it starts out from health creation:

"Health is created where people live, love, work, and play."

Health is created and lived by people within the settings of their everyday life; where they learn, work, play, and love.

This could seem like a trivial statement—actually it is a revolution in health thinking. It was pioneered by Aaron Antonovsky and is best reflected in his seminal work, *Unraveling The Mystery of Health; How People Manage Stress and Stay Well*. Antonovsky argues convincingly that the key question health research must ask is: "What creates health?" It is the interaction between environments and people in the process of everyday life that creates a pattern of health—of the individual, the family, the community, the nation, and the globe. Antonovsky went on to develop a scale called "the sense of coherence" (SOC), which links a person's sense of comprehensibility, manageability, and meaningfulness to health status. His research indicates that a high SOC tends to correlate with good health.

While Antonovsky restricted his research to the SOC of individuals, others such as R. Evans and P. Stoddart have indicated that it might apply to communities, even nations. For example they put forward the hypothesis of a relationship between collective self-esteem and health using the very high Japanese life expectancy as an example—a factor that could prove very important as Asia continues to grow and develop.

A key challenge for health promotion based on a salutogenic model therefore is to develop strategies that strengthen the sense of coherence (and self-esteem) of individuals and social groups. Health promotion has transformed this not only into a vision of environments that are supportive to health, but also into practical networks and projects concerned with creating a healthy school, a health-promoting hospital, a healthy workplace, a healthy city, to name just a few (7).

Further searches for the work of Ilona Kickbusch reveal not only the full text of other recent presentations and articles, but also the actual Powerpoint slide presentations, which can be viewed on the World Wide Web. An example can be found at: http://odphp.osophs.dhhs.gov/pubs/HP2000/kickbusch.htm.

The ability to review her major address in full-text format and then save the entire document for later review is an example of the power of the Internet in increasing communication, ease of access, filing for future use, and the ability to forward an idea to colleagues. The Internet also provides a much more efficient system for contacting an author. If you have ever tried to contact the author of a book or publication in the pre–Internet days, you may have experienced the difficulties in tracking down an author or researcher. Today there are several search programs that will enable people to locate an individual by name, location, Internet domain, or country.

Web-Based Support for Behavior Change

Another recent development that has been made more generally available because of Internet access is the transtheoretical model for behavior change developed by James Prochaska and his colleagues at the University of

Rhode Island. Web site address for his main page is http://www.uri.edu/research/cprc/ttm.htm.

From the Cancer Prevention Research Center (CPRC) Web site:

Stages of Change

Five stages of change have been conceptualized for a variety of problem behaviors. The five stages of change are precontemplation, contemplation, preparation, action, and maintenance. Precontemplation is the stage at which there is no intention to change behavior in the foreseeable future. Many individuals in this stage are unaware or underaware of their problems. Contemplation is the stage in which people are aware that a problem exists and are seriously thinking about overcoming it but have not yet made a commitment to take action. Preparation is a stage that combines intention and behavioral criteria. Individuals in this stage are intending to take action in the next month and have unsuccessfully taken action in the past year. Action is the stage in which individuals modify their behavior, experiences, or environment in order to overcome their problems. Action involves the most overt behavioral changes and requires considerable commitment of time and energy. Maintenance is the stage in which people work to prevent relapse and consolidate the gains attained during action. For addictive behaviors this stage extends from six months to an indeterminate period past the initial action (8).

Dr. Prochaska and colleagues have provided Web-based access to a number of assessment tools that they use in their behavior change work. It is possible to refer your clients to these Web sites so that they might determine their readiness for change for a variety of health-promoting lifestyle issues.

Another valuable resource that is available to our field is the Web-based patient-client handouts that are available. There are hundreds of sites at which very useful, up-to-date information has been made available on the World Wide Web. Frequently, some clinicians give their "connected" patients a set of Web sites instead of a handout. Patients can then seek out this information and choose which, if any, they want to print. In some cases, patients may just want to provide a bookmark to their own browser system so that they can refer back to this information whenever there is interest.

Many health professionals are in the process of creating behavior change guides and educational programs using the World Wide Web as the delivery system. One such system we have been creating is a set of pages to assist health professionals in learning more about smoking cessation. The title of the program is "The History and Future of Smoking Cessation." We now have a number of tools available to assist us in helping people change that behavior. Some samples of these Web pages can be viewed in the near future. Further notices will be made available through the National Wellness Institute Web site, which is http://www.wellnessnwi.org.

Web-Based Assessment Tools

Another major resource that has become available for clients of wellness and health promotion professionals is assessment materials. There are literally hundreds of personal health assessment services that are now available on the World Wide Web. Some of these services are free; others have some user fee attached. It is not unusual for a university level course to rely heavily on the World Wide Web for assessment, quizzes, and projects. Listed in Table 25-3 are the links to a number of assessment tools that were used in one such course.

E-Mail Addresses for Examples of Listserves

Health Policy   HEALTHPOL@HOME.EASE.LSOFT.COM

Health
Promotion
(College
Health)   hlthprom@relay.doit.wisc.edu

TAGFAM   TAGFAM@MAELSTROM.STJOHNS.EDU
(Gifted and
Talented)

Search Programs and Search Robots: Search While You Sleep

There are 50 or more programs on the World Wide Web that can be used to find specific information desired. You can find information by subject, language, date, topic, author, country, domain, or file size. Some of these programs are specifically designed to locate individuals. A well done summary of intelligent agents, multi-search engines, and individual search engines can be found on the Web at: http://www.philb.com. One of the most important skills for the professional of the twenty-first century is to be able to wade through the enormous volume of documents made available to find the best quality information.

There are intelligent robot software systems that search the Internet 24 hours a day. The software is instructed to search for topics of interest; the software tracks and delivers the information to your computer desktop on a continuous basis.

An example of this type of service can be downloaded free from the Pointcast Network home page: http://www.pointcast.com/.

Clinical Practice Guidelines for Providers and Consumers

Another important effect that the Internet has had on the field of preventive medicine is the immediate availability of clinical practice guidelines; two of the full statements from the American College of Preventive Medicine Web site are provided in Appendix 25-1 and Appendix 25-2. The two topics selected for demonstration purposes are cervical cancer screening and screening mammography for breast cancer. These guidelines, complete with references, are available with the click of a mouse to any clinician as well as the public at large. It is very possible today that a patient may be better informed than their clinician. The empowerment that occurs when patients have full access to the original information can be revolutionary. The next generation of patients will have even greater comfort with finding the answers to their questions online, and the role of health professionals will likely change into a new form of assisting.

We will close this chapter with one last example of the information infrastructure supporting the empowerment of citizens. The federal government has made the National Library of Medicine and the Medline search services available to the public at large. Any citizen, with the help of a librarian, can find the information most relevant to topics of interest. Since the cost of computers continues to drop each month, we can expect even broader availability of the resources necessary to take advantage of the Internet and other online resources.

Table 25-3 An Example of Assessment Tools on the World Wide Web	
TOOL	**WEBSITE ADDRESS**
Keirsey Temperament Test	http://sunsite.unc.edu/jembin/mb.pl
Life Expectancy	http://www.northwesternmutual.com/games/longevity/longevitymain.html
Center For Financial Well-Being	http://www.healthycash.com/center/
World's Smallest Political Quiz	http://www.self-gov.org/quiz.html
Men: Test Your Knowledge Of Women's Health	http://www.coolware.com/health/medical_reporter/quiz.html
Basal Metabolism Rate	http://www.room42.com.nutrition/basal.shtml
A Quick Ready "Reckoner" to Calculate Your Daily Energy and Fat Intake	http://www.st-ivel.co.uk/2146.htm
How Well Am I Eating Calculator	http://homearts.com/helpers/calculators/ddiary.htm
STD Risk Profiler	http://www.unspeakable.com/profiler/profiler.html
STD Quiz	http://www.unspeakable.com/nph-survey.cgi?tag=std
The "What You Can Say" Guide for Safer Sex	http://www.unspeakable.com/unspeakable/unspeak.html
Target Heart Rate Calculator	http://www.stevenscreek.com/goodies/hr.shtml
Calorie Calculator	http://www.stevenscreek.com/goodies/jcalories.shtml
LifeScan	http://wellness.uwsp.edu/Health_Service/services/lifeScan.shtml
Stress Assess	http://wellness.uwsp.edu/Health_Service/Services/stress.shtml
LiveWell	http://wellness.uwsp.edu/Health_Service/services/livewell/index.shtml

REFERENCES

1. The contributions of preventive medicine. American College Preventive Medicine Web site. Available at: http://www.acpm.org/whatis.htm.

2. Olson CM. The relationship between patient income and physician discussion of health risk behaviors. JAMA 1997;278:1412–1417.

3. David A. Kindig. *Purchasing Population Health.* Ann Arbor, MI: University of Michigan Press, 1997.

4. U.S. Dept. of Health, Education and Welfare. Healthy people 2000. Washington, DC: U.S. Dept. of Health, Education, and Welfare, 1979.

5. WHO glossary web site: http://www.who.ch/hpr/hep/documents/glossary.pdf.

6. Michael O'Donnell, editor of the American Journal of Health Promotion.

7. Kickbusch I. Building the prevention agenda for 2010: lessons learned. Keynote address at the Health People 2000 Consortium Meeting, New York, November 15, 1996.

8. Cancer Research Prevention Web site: http://www.uri.edu/research/cprc.

APPENDIX 25-1
PRACTICE POLICIES AND GUIDELINES: CERVICAL CANCER SCREENING

Burden of Suffering

It is estimated that approximately 15,000 women will be diagnosed with invasive carcinoma of the cervix and 4800 women will die from this disease in 1995 (1). Rates for carcinoma in situ peak between the ages of 20 and 30, and the incidence of invasive cervical cancer increases with age (2). Twenty-five percent of all invasive cervical cancers occur in women over age 65. Any woman who has been sexually active is at risk for cervical cancer (3). Additional risk factors include early onset of sexual intercourse (4,5); history of multiple sexual partners (5); history of sexually transmitted disease, especially human papillomavirus (HPV) (6) and HIV infection (7); smoking (8); and never having been screened (9).

Description of Preventive Measures

The Papanicolaou (Pap) smear is used to screen for cervical cancer to detect lesions when they are still highly curable (10). The lead time from the development of precancerous lesions to invasive cancer is estimated at 8 to 9 years (2). The American College of Obstetricians and Gynecologists (ACOG) recommends obtaining cellular samples from both the endocervical canal (using an endocervical brush) and from the portio, which includes the entire transformation zone (11). Use of both an endocervical brush and a spatula has been shown to collect a better sample of cells than either a spatula alone or a spatula used in combination with a cotton-tipped swab (12).

Evidence of Effectiveness

A recent meta-analysis reports that the ranges for sensitivity and specificity of a single screening Pap test for detecting cervical intraepithelial neoplasia (CIN) grades I and II are from 14% to 99% and from 24% to 96%, respectively (13). The wide range of reported sensitivity can be attributed to differences in screening technique, i.e., insufficient sampling of cells, inadequate slide preparation, laboratory accuracy and reporting (14), and differences in the manner in which the investigators define sensitivity (13). False-negative test results may allow a lesion to progress to more advanced disease before it is detected, whereas false-positive test results can lead to anxiety and unnecessary tests (3,14). No randomized controlled trials to test the effectiveness of Pap smears for prevention of cervical cancer have been conducted; it is unlikely that such trials will ever be conducted because of ethical considerations (3,15). However, case-control studies have clearly demonstrated that women with invasive cervical cancer were less likely to have been screened compared to controls (3,14), and decreased mortality and incidence of invasive cervical cancer have been described in populations following implementation of Pap screening (16).

Public Policy Considerations

Two major issues with important public policy considerations are cost and patient compliance. Estimates from mathematical models indicate that regular triennial screening would achieve 91% to 96% of the benefit of annual screening, while greatly reducing the cost, potential harms, and inconvenience (14). Increasing the screening interval from 1 to 3 years would reduce the total number of smears obtained (on the more than 77 million American women at risk) by two-thirds (3). The recommendation of many current guidelines that three initial annual screens be performed has been shown by mathematical modeling to have substantial cost with little benefit (14). Advocates of annual testing, however, have concerns about patient compliance; women may receive Pap tests at a frequency lower than guidelines, and a 3-year interval is more difficult to track than a 1-year interval. Results from a mathematical model, however, show that even if women are not screened precisely every 3 years, screening at 4 years retains 99% of the effectiveness of the 3-year interval (14).

For women over age 65 with a history of regular screening and negative results, continued screening produces diminishing yields and increasing costs (17). Screening is more cost-effective, however, for women over age 65 with a history of inadequate screening (3,17). Similarly, efforts to expand screening to women who have not undergone regular Pap testing (and who are often at increased risk for cervical cancer) may offer a more dramatic public health benefit than adjusting screening protocols for women who are already undergoing regular testing.

Recommendations of Other Groups

The American Academy of Family Physicians (AAFP) (2) and the U.S. Preventive Services Task Force (USPSTF) (3) recommend that Pap screening be instituted with the onset of sexual activity or at age 18, if the sexual history is unreliable. The ACOG, American Cancer Society (ACS), and National Cancer Institute (NCI) suggest that screening begin with the onset of sexual activity or at 18 years of age, whichever occurs first (2,18). Most major authorities recommend that after three normal annual smears, screening frequency may be decreased at the discretion of the physician and patient. The Canadian Task Force on the Periodic Health Examination (CanTF) requires only two normal smears before decreasing the frequency (19). The American College of Physicians (ACP) (20) and CanTF recommend screening every 3 years for most women; in women at increased risk for cervical cancer, they recommend screening more frequently (19).

The USPSTF recommends ending screening at age 65, provided there is documentation of regular screening with consistently normal smears within the previous 9 years. The CanTF states that screening may be stopped at age 69 (19). The ACP recommends cessation of screening at age 65, or at age 75 if not screened in the 10 years before age 66 (20).

The USPSTF also specifies in its recommendations that specimens should be submitted to laboratories with adequate quality control measures and that thorough follow-up of test results be ensured.

Rationale Statement

The key controversies surrounding cervical cancer screening include the number of initial annual screens, the screening interval, and when screening may be discontinued. The International Agency for Research on Cancer Working Group reported in its evaluation of cervical cancer screening programs that women who had two or more initial negative smears had a greater relative protection against invasive cervical cancer than women who had one initial smear (21). Retrospective studies (15,21,22) have found that obtaining Pap smears 3 years apart is as effective as annual screening for detecting cervical cancer in its early stages (noninvasive, or stage I). Mathematical modeling estimates suggest that screening past age 65 is inefficient and may be discontinued in women who have a history of regular negative results (17).

Recommendations of the American College of Preventive Medicine

Screening for cervical cancer by regular Pap tests should be performed in all women who are or have been sexually active and should be instituted after a woman first engages in sexual intercourse. If the sexual history is unknown or considered unreliable, screening should begin at age 18. At least two initial screening tests should be performed 1 year apart. For women who have had at least two normal annual smears, the screening interval may then be lengthened at the discretion of the patient and physician after considering the presence of risk factors, but should not exceed 3 years. Screening may be discontinued at age 65 if the following criteria are met: the woman has been regularly screened, has had two satisfactory smears, and has had no abnormal test results within the previous 9 years. For all women over age 65 who have not been previously screened, three normal annual smears should be documented prior to discontinuation of screening. Clinicians should use proper techniques in collecting specimens, should submit them to qualified cytopathologic laboratories for analysis, and should provide appropriate follow-up on test results.

References for Appendix 25-1

1. Wingo PA, Tong T, Bolden S. Cancer statistics, 1995. CA 1995;45:8–30.

2. U.S. Department of Health and Human Services/Public Health Service. Adults/Older adults screening: Papanicolaou smear. In: Clinician's handbook of preventive services. Washington, DC: U.S. Government Printing Office, 1994.

3. U.S. Preventive Services Task Force. Screening for cervical cancer. In: Guide to clinical preventive services: an assessment of the effectiveness of 169 interventions. Baltimore: Williams and Wilkins, 1989.

4. Terris M, Wilson F, Smith H, et al. Epidemiology of cancer of the cervix. V. The relationship of coitus to carcinoma of the cervix. Am J Public Health 1967;57:840–847.

5. Brinton LA, Hamman RF, Huggins GR, et al. Sexual and reproductive risk factors for invasive squamous cell cervical cancer. J Natl Cancer Inst 1987;79:23–30.

6. Schiffman MH. Recent progress in defining the epidemiology of human papillomavirus infection and cervical neoplasia. J Natl Canc Inst 1992;84:394–398.

7. Maiman M, Fruchter RG, Serur E, et al. Human immunodeficiency virus infection and cervical neoplasia. Gynecol Oncol 1990;38: 377–382.

8. Winklestein W. Smoking and cervical cancer—current status: a review. Am J Epidemiol 1990;131:945–957.

9. Stenkvist B, Bergstrom R, Eklund G, Fox CH. Papanicolaou smear screening and cervical cancer: what can you expect? JAMA 1984;252:1423–1426.

10. Van Nagell JR, Higgins RV, Powell DR. Invasive cervical cancer. In: Knapp RC, Berkowitz RS, eds. Gynecologic oncology. 2nd ed. New York: McGraw-Hill, 1993.

11. Cervical cytology: evaluation and management of abnormalities. Washington, DC: American College of Obstetricians and Gynecologists, 1993. ACOG Technical Bulletin, no. 183.

12. Chalvardjian A, DeMarchi WG, Bell V, Nishikawa R. Improved endocervical sampling with the cytobrush. Can Med Assoc J 1991;144: 313–317.

13. Fahey MT, Irwig L, Macaskill P. Meta-analysis of Pap test accuracy.

Am J Epidemiol 1995;141:680–689.

14. Eddy DM. Screening for cervical cancer. Ann Intern Med 1990; 113:214–226.

15. Bearman DM, MacMillan JP, Creasman WT. Papanicolaou smear history of patients developing cervical cancer: an assessment of screening protocols. Obstet Gynecol 1987;69:151–155. (Erratum in Obstet Gynecol 1987; 69:660.)

16. Dickinson L, Mussey ME, Kurland LT. Evaluation of the effectiveness of cytologic screening for cervical cancer. II. Survival parameters before and after inception of

screening. Mayo Clin Proc 1972;47:545–549.

17. Fahs MC, Mandelblatt J, Schechter C, Muller C. Cost-effectiveness of cervical cancer screening for the elderly. Ann Intern Med 1992; 117:520–527.

18. American Cancer Society. Summary of American Cancer Society recommendations for the early detection of cancer in asymptomatic people. CA 1993;43: 42–46.

19. Canadian Task Force on the Periodic Health Examination. The Canadian guide to clinical preventive health care. Ottawa: Canada Communication Group, 1994.

20. Common screening tests. Philadelphia: American College of Physicians, 1991.

21. International Agency for Research on Cancer, Working Group on Evaluation of Cervical Cancer Screening Programs. Screening for squamous cervical cancer: duration of low-risk after negative results of cervical cytology and its implications for screening policies. Br Med J 1986;293:659–664.

22. MacGregor JE, Moss SM, Parkin DM, Day NE. A case-control study of cervical cancer screening in northeast Scotland. Br Med J 1985;290:1543–1546.

SOURCE: Hawkes AP, Kronenberger CB, Mackenzie, TD. Cervical cancer screening: American College of Preventive Medicine Practice Policy Statement. Am J Prev Med 1996;12:342–344.

APPENDIX 25-2
AMERICAN COLLEGE OF PREVENTIVE MEDICINE RECOMMENDATION FOR SCREENING MAMMOGRAPHY FOR BREAST CANCER

Burden of Suffering

Breast cancer is the most frequently diagnosed cancer and is the second leading cause of cancer death among women in the United States. Projected for 1996 are 184,300 new cases of breast cancer and 44,300 breast-cancer deaths. The 5-year survival rate is 84% for Caucasian, non–Hispanic women and 69% for African-American women (1). Risk factors for breast cancer include age, family history (FH), and familial cancer syndrome (FCS), as well as hormonal factors such as early menarche, late menopause, late parity, and nulliparity; however, the majority of women with breast cancer have no known risk factors. Risk factors, pathogenesis, prognosis, and course differ significantly in premenopausal and postmenopausal breast cancer (2).

Description of Preventive Measures

Mammography is one of several screening tools for detecting early breast cancer. Other measures, such as clinical and self-examinations, will be addressed in future practice policy statements. During mammography, the breast should be compressed and two views taken. Plain film or xeromammography are appropriate (3). Sensitivity is dependent on the quality of the equipment, competence of the radiology staff, and the density of the breast tissue.

    Since implementation of the Mammography Quality Standards Act in 1994, all U.S. mammography centers must be certified by the Food and Drug Administration.

Evidence of Effectiveness

Estimates of mammography sensitivity range from 75% to 90% with specificity from 90% to 95%. The positive predictive value of mammography for breast cancer ranges from 20% in women under age 50 to 60% to 80% in women aged 50 to 69. Randomized clinical trials (RCTs) have demonstrated a 30% reduction in breast cancer mortality in women 50 to 69 years who are screened annually or biennially with mammograms (4). The data on women under age 50 are less clear. Conclusions regarding the value of mammography in these women are hampered by inadequately designed studies, including failure of randomization and inadequate sample size, low compliance in the intervention group, and high screening rates (cross-over) in the control groups (5,6). A few studies have suggested adverse effects on mortality in the early years after screening implementation, but both the occurrence and potential etiology of these effects are poorly understood (6,7). Even with meta-analysis, the combined sample sizes are too small to reach conclusions regarding the efficacy of screening women under age 50 (8). Likewise, data are sparse regarding efficacy of screening mammograms in women older than age 69. Constantly updated analyses of research on the effectiveness of mammograms for particular groups are available through the National Cancer Institute by calling 1-800-4-CANCER.

Public Policy Considerations

Currently, compliance with mammography guidelines is low, especially among women over age 60, those with low socioeconomic status, and ethnic minority women. Estimates vary widely; 10% to 60% of women report having had mammograms in the preceding year, depending on the population and geographic area under consideration (9). Low utilization of mammography has been blamed on financial and insurance barriers, lack of education, and most importantly, lack of encouragement by a physician (10). Both primary care physicians and specialist physicians should encourage their patients to have routine mammography: a recommendation from a physician is the most important motivator for patients. Medical offices can improve patient compliance by using reminder systems, ancillary health personnel for health education, and a comprehensive approach to preventive services. Cost-effectiveness estimates of mammography screening—based on methodology, population, and interval—vary widely; it is estimated that breast cancer screening costs $3400 to over $83,000 per life-year saved (11). The potential cost-effectiveness of screening is higher when screening older populations, partly because the incidence of breast cancer increases with age.

Recommendations of Other Groups

The ACS, American College of Radiology, and ACOG recommend screening mammography for women aged 40 to 49 every 1 to 2 years and annually after age 50. The American College of Physicians recommends biennial screening for women aged 50 to 74 years. The American Academy of Family Physicians, which recommends mammography screening for women over age 50, is currently updating its guidelines. The CanTF recommends annual mammography for women aged 50 to 69 and recommends against mammography screening for women aged 40 to 49. Similarly, the USPSTF recommends mammography screening every 1 to 2 years for women aged 50 to 69.

Rationale

Population-based mammography screening aims to reduce morbidity and mortality from breast cancer by early detection and treatment of occult malignancies. There is ample evidence from a variety of well-conducted RCTs that annual or biennial mammography is effective in reducing breast cancer mortality in women aged 50 to 69 years. The college provides no recommendations for women under age 50 because of lack of evidence of the efficacy of screening in this group and differences between premenopausal and postmenopausal women in breast density, breast cancer incidence, sensitivity and specificity of mammography, incidence of false-positive results, tumor growth, mortality rates, and the

suggestion of increased mortality with mammography screening. Although data are sparse regarding the efficacy of mammography screening in women over age 69, similarities between women aged 50 to 69 and older women in terms of breast density, sensitivity and specificity of mammography, tumor growth, mortality rates, and response to treatment, coupled with the higher incidence of breast cancer in this age group, point to a need to screen older women whose health would permit breast cancer treatment (12). Lack of outcome evidence makes it difficult to develop specific recommendations for high-risk women.

Low-Risk Women

Low-risk women are those with no family history, familial cancer syndrome, or prior cancer. There is inadequate evidence for or against mammography screening of women under age 50. Women between ages 50 and 69 should have annual or biennial, high-quality, two-view mammography. Women aged 70 or older should continue undergoing mammography screening provided their health status permits breast cancer treatment.

Higher-Risk Women

Women with a family history of premenopausal breast cancer in a first-degree relative or those with a history of breast or gynecologic cancer may warrant more aggressive screening. Women with these histories often begin screening at an earlier age, although there is no direct evidence of effectiveness to support this practice. The future availability of genetic screening may define new recommendations for screening high-risk women (13,14).

The college recommends further research to clarify the risk-benefit ratio of mammography screening for breast cancer in women under age 50, particularly to identify women in this age group who benefit most from screening. To compensate for inadequate sample size, another well-designed RCT, a meta-analysis using individual (rather than summary) data, or a well-designed population-based cohort or case-control study is needed. Further studies should address whether menopausal status rather than age is a better predictor of the utility of mammography screening and whether recommendations should be modified for women taking hormone replacement therapy.

References for Appendix 25-2

1. Parker S, Tong L, Bolden S, Wingo P. Cancer statistics, 1996. CA 1996;46:8–9.

2. Colditz G. Epidemiology of breast cancer: findings from the nurses health study. CA 1993;71(suppl): 1480–1489.

3. Hendrick RE. Mammography quality assurance: current issues. Cancer 1993;72(suppl):1466–1474.

4. Elwood JM, Cox B, Richardson AK. The effectiveness of breast cancer screening by mammography in younger women. Online J Clin Trials 1993;2:Doc. no. 32.

5. Miller AB, Baines CJ, To T, et al. Canadian national breast screening study 1: breast cancer detection and death rates among women ages 40–49 years. Can Med Assoc J 1992;147:1459–1498.

6. Nystrom L, Rutqvist I, Wall S, et al. Breast cancer screening with mammography: overview of Swedish randomized trials. Lancet 1993;341:973-978.

7. Vogel V. Screening younger women for breast cancer. J Natl Cancer Inst 1994;16:55–60.

8. Kopans D. Screening for breast cancer and mortality reduction among women 40–49 years of age. CA 1994;74(suppl):311–322.

9. Caplan LS, Wells BL, Haynes S. Breast cancer screening among older racial-ethnic minorities and whites: barriers to early detection. J Gerontol 1992;47:101–110.

10. Fox SA, Stein JA. The effect of physician-patient communication on mammography utilization by different ethnic groups. Med Care 1991;29:1065–1082.

11. Brown ML, Fintor L. Cost-effectiveness of breast cancer screening: preliminary results of a systematic review of the literature. Breast Cancer Res Treat 1993;25: 113–118.

12. Moskowitz M. Guidelines for screening for breast cancer: is a revision in order? Radiol Clin North Am 1992;30:221–233.

13. Bondy M, Lustbader E, Halabi S, et al. Validation of a breast cancer risk assessment model in women with a positive family history. J Natl Cancer Inst 1994;86:620–624.

14. Thompson W. Genetic epidemiology of breast cancer. CA 1994; 74(suppl):279–287.

SOURCE: Ferrini R, Mannino E, Ramsdell E, et al. Screening mammography for breast cancer: American College of Preventive Medicine Practice Policy Statement. Am J Prev Med 1996;12:340–341.

Chapter 26

The Internet, CD-ROMs, and Other Electronic Resources in Medicine, Health Education, and Health Promotion

Linda Chapin

This chapter is intended to provide a brief review of electronic products and services that have been developed to assist people in learning more about medicine, health education, health promotion, and wellness. As the cost of multimedia computers continues to drop, more and more families, companies, and professionals are gaining an appreciation for the advantages of multimedia formats. This article will focus on:

- Products and services to assist health professionals
- Products intended specifically for families
- Products designed for children
- The major connective services

BACKGROUND INFORMATION

The American public is rapidly gaining an appreciation for and an interest in the power of access to health information. The emerging technologies that facilitate the dissemination of health information will accelerate the growth of this interest. There are numerous competing and complementing approaches being evaluated. The evolution of sharing health information among the humans of our planet has included oral traditions, pictographs, scrolls, carvings, pottery, leather works, beads, jewelry, books, handouts, support groups, counseling, radio, television, newspapers, magazines, film strips, posters, audio tapes, recordings, videotapes, videodisks, interactive fax systems, computer bulletin boards, computer conferencing, special interest groups, CD ROMs, interactive computer programs, simulation systems, virtual reality systems, decision support software, and artificial intelligence.

Almost all of these methods are still in use today. The advent of technologic breakthroughs has dramatically expanded the possibilities of applying the best information to the decision making process of the average citizen.

The reality of the merging technologies of video, audio, telephones, and computers has been the result of the following breakthroughs (some expensive, and some not perfected):

- The conversion of audio and video communication into a digital format that can be read by a laser system: this permits almost instantaneous access to any section of a collection. This also permits the imbedding of audio or video forms of information within interactive computer systems.

- Digital data compression techniques now allow the transmission of audio and video information through existing phone and cable lines. Additional breakthroughs are needed to increase the speed of the process.

- The use of fiber-optic wiring systems has dramatically increased the capacity to transmit information. The speed and volume of data that can be sent over fiber optics are almost limitless.

- There are hundreds of companies working on equipment that will facilitate the seamless access of desired information through phones and smart television systems. Interactive television and phone conferencing have been a reality for years.

How can we maximize the availability of all this progress to assist people in gaining the highest level of functioning that they desire? The information highway can aid patients in assessing their health and lifestyle with assessment tools online and aid patients in gaining information with consultative support and interactive programs.

Lifestyle Assessment and Medical Triage

- The ability to examine one's lifestyle in the privacy of one's home is a theoretical advantage.
- Obtaining information on the most current recommendations for health screenings would be more convenient at home.
- Availability of information on self-care could decrease the need for some visits to clinics.
- Interactive computer-assisted mental health assessments, monitoring, and guidance have been demonstrated to be cost-effective for certain problems.

Telemedicine, Consultation, and Decision Support

- Exploring the problem an individual has can be facilitated by human-assisted computer systems or totally automated decision support systems.
- Seeking availability of clinical expertise that matches the variable personal needs and beliefs of the consumer can only be efficiently done by computers.
- Searching the gigantic array of relevant data to assist people with rare or common disorders can only be done in a timely way by the use of computers.
- Computer-assisted decisions can avoid missing the rare etiology or the complicating coexisting condition.

Treatment and Outcomes

- Support groups can add to the understanding of the process of recovery and therefore improve healing times and decrease unnecessary clinic visits.

CD-ROM TECHNOLOGY

Just a few years ago the costs of creating CD-ROMs were prohibitively expensive for most purposes. However, in the last few years, the cost of the equipment required to produce CD-ROMs has dropped dramatically. This has led to an explosion of products being created to assist health professionals in finding the information they need to help their patients or clients. In the field of medicine and nursing, many of the products are not yet taking full advantage of the multimedia potential. In some cases, they have merely converted a text from its book format to a CD-ROM format. The programmers and developers, however, are quickly gaining an insight into the expansion of audio, video, and advanced searching capabilities.

One of the exciting uses of CD-ROM technology is in the ability to provide continuing education credits for health professionals using the multimedia format. It is possible to interview test subjects and have real voices providing the information to the professional. Most of the products that I have seen so far have been designed for the medical profession. However, I expect that very quickly this approach will be used for all of the health professions. There are now catalogues available that limit their offerings strictly to medical

CD-ROM applications. As evidence for how fast this field is developing, one of the *oldest* medical CD-ROM catalogs brags on its cover that it has been "your medical CD-ROM source since 1991." This particular catalogue is one of the most comprehensive medical sources identified to date.*

One of the most powerful features of the resources being created for professionals on CD-ROM is the search ability. One example is *MAXX: The Electronic Library of Medicine. MAXX* includes 24 textbooks on a single CD. Included with this library of books is a search engine that can find a single term or phrase across all textbooks in a split second. There is a history window that lets the user record each step that they make as they flip through multiple books. The ability to find information quickly will assist professionals in providing better care in a more timely fashion. The product is updated quarterly.

The next major step that I see is the development of translations of all medical knowledge into language that the average citizen can understand. My vision is that libraries and other centers in the community will become resource centers to help people find out more about the things that are of concern to them.

Consider that there are two gigantic health-focused collections of knowledge being created. Health professionals are assembling one (see Table 26-1). The growing self-help movement is assembling the other. The self-help knowledge base is being created on CompuServe, Prodigy, America Online, and the Internet. As these two major efforts begin to share information, there is dramatic potential for improving the quality of care and the understanding of the needs of our citizens. It is not uncommon for health professionals to participate in the growing number of online self-help discussion groups, chat rooms, listserves, Usenet groups, and other groups.

Why Would Health Professionals Join Online Self-Help Groups?

The professionals who participate in online self-help groups are able to gain insights from the views of the large numbers of people on the Web. The same experience might take years to accumulate by seeing people who might have that problem or interest as they appear, much more rarely, as a part of their clinical caseload. This is particularly true when we consider rare disorders.

Medical Self-Care on CD-ROM

There are a growing number of CD-ROM products that can be described as decision support software. These products help people explore their symptoms and learn about possible causes. In most cases, these products avoid sophisticated jargon and terminology not familiar to the average family. These products are not intended to replace medical care but are intended to assist people in deciding how they might choose to use medical care and to learn more about the problems they might encounter. There is a growing diversity of programs available, ranging from *Dr. Schuller's Home Medical Advisor Pro* to the *Better Homes and Gardens Healthy Cooking CD Cookbook*.

---

*If you would like your own copy of their catalog, they have a toll-free number: 1-800-227-CMEA.

Two of the best decision support CDs that I reviewed are the *Mayo Clinic Family Health Book* and *Dr. Schuller's Home Medical Advisor Pro*. Both of these programs provide a useful format that allows the individual to search on the basis of symptoms or diseases. Most consumers easily understand most of the terminology used. While both products use graphic images and sounds along with an occasional video clip, much of the material is straight text format. It appears in *Dr. Schuller's Home Medical Advisor* that one of the producers had a fascination with scuba diving. There are numerous video clips that are weakly connected to the rest of the product. It appears as if the authors were trying to fill up the disk with some underwater footage they happened to have available. *The Mayo Clinic Family Health Book* has been created by IVI Publishing with much of the material being adapted from the Mayo Clinic's well-known series of books designed for patient education. The disk has an excellent section covering anatomy and has plenty of connections that permit the user to follow an interest from one topic to another. The format is easy to use and has an excellent help system. There is animation and audio narration that assist the user in learning more about the product.

Another large group of CD-ROMs in the medical self-care field center around assisting people with understanding medications. Here again, the Mayo Clinic has come forward with an excellent product entitled *The Mayo Clinic Family Pharmacist*. This product allows the user to search on the basis of the knowledge of the name of a product or the disease entity that is of concern. Synonyms are frequently included, so that an individual looking for hypertension might also find their interests met by looking under high blood pressure. Another real advantage of *The Mayo Clinic Family Pharmacist* is that it can help people identify medications based on drug ID number, color, shape, and size. The product also includes a useful section on first aid.

Another product that helps people understand their medications is the *Health Soft Complete Guide to Prescription and Non-Prescription Drugs*. While the only multimedia feature of this product is that it has the ability to pronounce any pharmaceutical name included on the disk, the product is easy to use. These are pictures available for many of the products listed. As with other pharmacy programs, this program allows you to search by generic name or trade name. Even though physicians try to provide detailed information about the medications they prescribe for patients, and pharmacists are obligated to provide counseling in most states, I believe there is a great need for these types of products. Even if the physician, nurse, or pharmacist had taken the time to try to explain the possible side effects and hazards associated with various medications, the amount of information the patient will remember is small. Many of the undesirable outcomes in medicine are the result of interactions of medications or conflicts with over-the-counter medications that are taken along with prescriptions.

Additional medical self-care products that I have reviewed include *The Total Heart*, produced by the Mayo Clinic. This is an excellent product that provides detailed information about the anatomy and physiology of the heart, the prevention of avoidable heart disease, and the treatment of heart disease if it should occur. The interface is slick and easy to use. There are true 3-D animations and plenty of

information that might help individuals who themselves are suffering from heart disease. There are detailed discussions concerning the causes, symptoms, and risks of heart disease and what to do in cardiac emergencies. Another nice feature of this product is that if there are words that you do not understand, there is a definition included in the medical dictionary portion of the program. Another contribution made by Mayo Clinic to the CD-ROM library is the *Mayo Clinic Sports, Health, and Fitness CD*. This excellent product includes use of full animation and multimedia capabilities. The product helps the individual to assess their fitness level, analyze their preferences, explore nutritional issues, and create their own personal fitness program. The program includes a personal journal and tracking capabilities.

ANATOMY PROGRAMS

The next grouping of products for the home is related to helping people understand their anatomy and physiology. The three best products that I have reviewed are *A.D.A.M. The Inside Story*, *BodyWorks*, and *The Ultimate Human Body*. *A.D.A.M. The Inside Story* provides entertainment and animation and can be used by adults and children. Adults have the ability to censor some of the genital anatomy through use of a fig leaf option. *A.D.A.M.* also provides interviews with a physician who can explain how to detect, treat, and avoid common illnesses. The product includes puzzles that provide the user with an opportunity to learn how various sections of human anatomy can be properly aligned.

The *BodyWorks* product does not provide as slick an interface as *A.D.A.M. The Inside Story*, but it does provide the user with plenty of animation as well as 3-D models. One of the criticisms of *BodyWorks* is that most of the figures are men. Interestingly enough, even one of the figures that includes ovaries appears to be a man. The pronunciation of medical terms is done in a computer synthesized voice, whereas *A.D.A.M. The Inside Story* uses human voices that have been recorded.

The Ultimate Human Body is another slick interface product to help people understand the anatomy. There are plenty of animations and illustrations to show how different parts of our anatomy and physiology function. One of the interesting features of the product is that you can slowly move through the anatomy by simply clicking on an organ that might hide something behind it. This highly detailed product is one that would be of interest for children as well as adults.

Programs Designed for Children

Although some components of the products that I have reviewed earlier might be appropriate for children, the Mayo Clinic has released two products that are designed specifically for young people. The first one is entitled *AnaTomy* which is subtitled *An Adventure Into The Human Body*. This product is entertaining and informative. The participants enter a small spaceship and travel through the human body exploring and interacting with different components of anatomy and physiology. My children enjoy the games and can't help but learn while they are playing the games at different sites in the body.

The interface for this product is not as sophisticated as some of the other Mayo Clinic products, but the children did not seem to mind. As most children do, they quickly figured out what it took to make this product work and were satisfied with the use of arrow keys and other keyboard controls. The product appears to be best designed for a game pad, which unfortunately, we did not have.

The other product that we have reviewed from Mayo is entitled *Safety Monkey*. These products are designed to be fun and educational. As *Safety Monkey* travels around through the house and yard, the children help him identify safety hazards and take corrective action where appropriate. Another product that has been created specifically for kids is entitled *Body Park: Anatomy, Nutrition, Health, and Safety For Kids*. This product teaches children how their bodies work, the impor-

tance of good nutrition, general health and safety tips, memory skills, problem solving, and how the five senses work. This is a virtual entertainment product that is aimed at grade school and younger children. Two other products that have been released by Digital Theater are entitled *What Would You Do? At Home* and *What Would You Do? First Aid*. Each of these products covers situations that might occur and provides children with solutions for common situations or problems.

THE INFORMATION SUPER HIGHWAY

The major services that include health promotion and wellness resources are America Online CompuServe, The Microsoft Network, Prodigy, and of course, the universal

---

Table 26-1 Partial List of Current CD-ROM Offerings

Journals
The Journal of Hand Surgery: American Edition, British and European Edition
Pediatrics Review and Education Program/Red Book
Pediatrics On Disc
Pediatric Infectious Disease Journal
Annals of Internal Medicine
New England Journal Of Medicine
American Family Physician
Internal Medicine Compact Libraries
Internal Medicine
Single-Journal Full-Text Archive
AIDS Compact Library

General Reference
BiblioMed Essential Medical Reference
Quick Medical Reference
Physicians GenRx
AskRx Plus
A.D.A.M. Obstetrics and Gynecology
A.D.A.M. Orthopaedics of the Lower Limb
A.D.A.M. Scholar Series
A.D.A.M. Comprehensive
A.D.A.M. Standard
A.D.A.M. Essentials
A.D.A.M. Studio

Practice Management
Flash Code
Ophthalmic Practice Management
CodeManager '97

Medical Graphics
MediClip Medical Clip Art
LifeART Collections

Books on CD-ROM
MAXX: The Electronic Library of Medicine
CMEA's STAT!-Ref Plus Library with Quarterly Updates
STAT!-Ref Starter Edition
STAT!-Ref Student Edition
Stein's Internal Medicine, 4th Edition, on CD-ROM
Textbook of Dermatology
The Complete Year Book Collection on SilverPlatter
Year Books on Disc

Continuing Medical Education (CME) on CD-ROM
Family Practice Recertification
Clinical Dermatology Illustrated: A Regional Approach
Mayo Clinic Proceedings on CD-ROM
Scientific American SAM-CD
PrimePractice
PrimePratice Single Issues
SilverPlatter Multimedia Accelerated Learning Series
American College of Allergy and Immunology 1993 Annual Meeting
Pediatric Airway Obstruction
Pigmented Lesions of the Skin
The Etiology of Cancer
Diagnosis of Pulmonary Embolus: A Clinician's Approach
Atlas of Clinical Rheumatology

Patient Education
Mayo Clinic Family Health Book
Mayo Clinic Family Pharmacist
Mayo Clinic: The Total Heart
Breast Self-Examination

Medline on CD-ROM
BiblioMed Urology Series on CD-ROM
BiblioMed Citation Series
BiblioMed Gastroenterology Series
Knowledge Finder Medline Series
Unabridged Journals
Unabridged Journals (continued)
CANCERLIT
Health Planning and Administration
Core Journals
Core Journals (continued)
Specialty Series
Physicians' Silver Platter Medline
Cardiology
Dermatology
Family Practice
Gastroenterology
Occupational and Environmental Medicine
Orthopedics
Pediatrics
Surgery
Comprehensive Medline

Table 26-2 Audiovisual Materials

Procedural Videotapes
The Web-based catalog of these videos offers online
  compressed sample viewing.
Dermatology Procedures for the Primary Care Physician
Cardiac Stress Testing For the Primary Care Physician
Clinical Ophthalmology: Symptoms, Signs, and
  Management
Office Orthopedics: Essentials I
Office Orthopedics: Essentials II
Airway Cam Intubation Video
The Video Atlas of Human Anatomy
Primary Care Psychiatry Video Series
3-D Pelvic Anatomy
Suburethral Fascia Lata Sling

CMEA Audio Cassette Series
Office Gynecology and Women's Health
Pediatrics Review Course
Internal Medicine: A Comprehensive Review
Office Orthopedics and Bone Radiology
Primary Care Essentials
Wilderness Medicine Review Course
Primary Care Review Course
Cardiology in Primary Care
Practical Dermatology for the Primary Care Physician

Table 26-3 Leading Organizations in Health Promotion and Wellness

American Journal of Health Promotion
1660 Cass Lake Road, Suite 104
Keego Harbor, MI 48320
Phone: (248) 682-0707
Fax: (248) 682-1212
Web: www.healthpromotionjournal.com
E-mail: ajhealthp@aol.com

Association for Worksite Health Promotion
60 Revere Drive, Suite 500
Northbrook, IL 60062
Phone: (847) 480-9574
Fax: (847) 480-9282
Web: www.awhp.com
E-mail: awhp@awhp.org

Health Media, Inc.
130 S. First Street
Ann Arbor, MI 48104
Phone: (734) 623-0000
Fax: 734-623-0003

Healthwise
2601 N. Bogus Basin Rd
PO Box 1989
Boise, ID 83701
Phone: (208) 345-1161
Fax: (208) 345-1897
Wed: www.healthwise.org
E-mail: moreinfo@healthwise.org

National Wellness Institute, Inc.
1300 College Court
PO Box 827
Stevens Point, WI 54481
Phone: (715) 342-2969
Fax: (715) 342-2979
Web: www.wellnessnwi.org
E-mail: nwi@wellnessnwi.org

Wellness Councils of America
Community Health Plaza, Suite 311
7101 Newport Avenue
Omaha, NE 68152
Phone: (402) 572-3590
Fax: (402) 572-3594
Web: www.welcoa.org
E-mail: welcoa@neonramp.org

Internet. There is a continued explosion in the number of people using these services. There are self-help groups, forums, special interest groups, news groups, bulletin board services, and hundreds of other subsets of connection available to the interested user. As more and more people become connected and share more and more information about how to get things done, there will be greater problem solving potential.

As the knowledge being created, by users, is edited and combined with the packaging and search capabilities of CD-ROM products, it is likely that people will be better able to solve their problems and find the resources that they need. With Microsoft making a major entry into the interface market for the information superhighway, it is likely that there will be a second explosion of use of all the services, particularly Internet. I am not suggesting that we will replace human interaction, but I am suggesting that people will be learning more and more about the things that they need to know to get the best that professionals have to offer. The use of the information superhighway for scientific publishing activity is increasing at such an accelerated pace that if you read it in print, it's out of date. There are clear benefits for professionals to getting connected and taking advantage of the information that is available.

Part V.

WOMEN'S HEALTH

Edited by
Kathryn M. Rexrode
JoAnn E. Manson

Introduction to Women's Health

Kathryn M. Rexrode
JoAnn E. Manson

Women's health in many respects is similar to men's health; however, certain issues are of particular concern to women, either by virtue of the overwhelming burden of certain diseases (such as breast cancer, osteoporosis, and domestic violence), the unique incidence of a disease in women (e.g., menopause), or in the way that treatment options (coronary heart disease) or risks and benefits (physical activity) may differ for women. These chapters are meant to help clinicians understand issues that are of particular interest for women, so that they may offer better counsel on disease prevention and treatment for their female patients.

Estrogen replacement therapy in the management of menopausal symptoms as well as for potential long-term health protection is one of the most controversial areas in women's health. Kathryn Martin outlines the areas of consensus as well as controversy, emphasizing the need to separate the goals, risks, and benefits of short-term versus long-term therapy. Since definitive evidence about the balance of absolute risks and benefits is lacking, the decision about hormone replacement therapy must be made by each woman with her care provider, weighing personal risks and benefits. This chapter should help clinicians in that important discussion.

Nanette Wenger details the high burden of coronary heart disease in women. Many women and some clinicians are still unaware of the facts. While many risk factors are similar for men and women, diabetes appears to be a stronger risk factor in women than men and estrogen status is clearly a coronary risk factor that is unique to women. Hypertension and hypercholesterolemia are more prevalent in older women than older men. Although on average they develop coronary disease later in life than men, once women develop clinical manifestations of coronary heart disease, they tend to have less favorable outcomes. Whether this is a true gender difference, a reflection of greater comorbidity in women, or a gender bias in treatment requires further research.

Ursula Matulonis reviews modifiable risk factors for breast cancer. While many women list breast cancer as their number one health fear, few know how diet and lifestyle factors, including alcohol intake, physical activity, weight, and hormonal therapy, may affect their breast cancer risk. This chapter should serve as a valuable resource in counseling women about how to modify their risk. Further research in this area of prevention is clearly warranted and ongoing.

Osteoporosis is a major cause of disability and mortality in older women and has received inadequate attention in the past. With an improved understanding of the important role of lifestyle factors, especially physical activity and nutrition, in preventing osteoporosis and the recent availability of numerous treatment options, the toll exacted on women by this condition could be significantly reduced. Meryl LeBoff reviews state-of-the-art knowledge on primary prevention and treatment of osteoporosis, indications for screening, and the role of the clinician in managing this complex condition that disproportionately afflicts women.

Regular physical activity is central to optimal health in both women and men. Bensenor, Rexrode, and Manson review the clinical and epidemiologic evidence that exercise reduces risk of cardiovascular disease, type 2 diabetes mellitus, osteoporosis, and certain forms of cancer, as well as relieves stress and improves emotional well-being. Issues unique to women, such as the complex balance of benefits and risks of prolonged vigorous exercise in women, menstrual and reproductive effects of exercise, the "female athlete triad," the role of resistance training, and exercise during pregnancy, are addressed. Clinician counseling regarding the health benefits of physical activity and the prescription of appropriate exercise programs can substantially improve the health of women.

The overwhelming burden of domestic violence falls upon women, although both men and women can be perpetrators. Deborah Prothrow-Stith and Jacqueline Kral detail the scope of the problem as well as the health consequences of domestic violence. Health providers should screen all women for a history of domestic violence and provide referrals to mental health providers, shelters, violence prevention services, and victim support groups for those that need them. This chapter should help clinicians approach this difficult and important issue in women's health.

Chapter 27

Estrogen Therapy for the Menopause

The medical management of menopause continues to be a topic of controversy. While many of the benefits of estrogen therapy have been well established (treatment of estrogen deficiency symptoms, prevention of osteoporosis, and improvement in lipid profiles), the potential risks, in particular those related to breast cancer, are of great concern. Many postmenopausal women are candidates for hormone replacement therapy (HRT), but many choose not to take it due to fear of breast cancer or concerns about potential side effects and continued menstrual bleeding. Therefore, making choices about potential therapies after menopause can be a difficult one for both women and their health care providers.

An important principle of HRT is the notion of short-term vs. long-term use, as both the goals of therapy and risk-benefit profiles are quite different. While most perimenopausal and postmenopausal women are candidates for short-term HRT (with the exception of those with a history of breast cancer), there is no general consensus yet as to who should or should not receive long-term HRT. Other new areas of clinical investigation in the field of menopause and HRT include the possible impact of estrogen on cognitive function, the role of exogenous androgen replacement for libido, and the role of a new class of drugs known as selective estrogen receptor modulators (SERMs). Given this rapidly changing field, it is likely that the medical management of menopause will continue to evolve in the coming years.

EPIDEMIOLOGY

The average age of menopause in recent epidemiologic studies is approximately 51, although the range considered to be normal is quite wide, as menopause can occur in normal women anytime between the ages of 42 and 58 (1). Life expectancy for women has gradually increased and is now estimated to be approximately 78 years. Therefore, for most women, up to one-third of their total lifespan occurs after the menopause. This aging of the population has raised many important questions about the public health impact of menopause. While estrogen replacement was historically used short term to treat only the symptoms of the menopause, more recently the emphasis has been on long-term use of estrogen to prevent both osteoporosis and coronary heart disease (CHD). Unopposed estrogen use is known to be associated with an increased risk of endometrial hyperplasia and cancer (2), a risk that can be prevented with the routine addition of a progestin (3). However, there are concerns that long-term use of estrogen might also be associated with an increased risk of breast cancer (4).

PHYSIOLOGY AND ENDOCRINOLOGY

Although menopause is defined clinically as permanent cessation of menses, the neuroendocrine and ovarian changes leading up to the menopause occur over a 5- to 10-year period referred to as the perimenopausal transition. The groundwork for menopause begins in utero, and by the sixth month of fetal life the human ovary contains approximately 6 to 7 million oocytes (5). However, after this peak, a degenerative process known as follicular atresia begins until there are no remaining oocytes at the time of menopause. Fewer than 1% of oocytes are lost via ovulation, the remainder are lost via atresia, a process which is poorly understood.

Endocrine changes seen during menopause include changes in ovarian sex steroid biosynthesis and pituitary gonadotropin secretion. The premenopausal ovary contains three functioning compartments: the stroma, follicle, and corpus luteum. After menopause, however, the only remaining functional compartment is the stroma, the site of androgen production. Testosterone and androstenedione production rates decrease after menopause, but whether this decline in androgens is associated with a decline in libido or sexual function has not been established. The postmenopausal ovary appears to make little or no estrogen, and circulating estrogen in postmenopausal women is derived primarily from peripheral conversion of androstenedione to estrone (6).

The earliest endocrine finding during the peri-menopausal transition is a selective rise in serum FSH, which is often seen in women over age 40 with ovulatory cycles (7,8). This is thought to be due primarily to a decrease in serum estradiol secretion across the cycle, although a decrease in other ovarian hormones such as inhibin might also be playing a role (8).

CLINICAL FINDINGS

The earliest clinical finding during the perimenopausal transition is a decrease in cycle length. It has been demonstrated that ovulatory women over age 40 have a mean cycle length of 25 days compared to 30 days in 18- to 30-year-old controls, while 45-year-old women have a mean cycle length of only 23 days (7). Although most women initially will experience these short cycles, many then develop long, anovulatory cycles that may be interspersed with the shorter, ovulatory ones. The reasons for this waxing and waning of ovarian activity are unclear, but might reflect a difference in the responsiveness of the remaining oocytes, or a difference in the types of FSH the pituitary secretes during the perimenopausal transition.

Genitourinary atrophy is another common problem because the vagina and the outer third of the urethra are estrogen-responsive tissues. Therefore, patients often experience vaginal dryness, dyspareunia, and urinary symptoms that mimic urinary tract infection. All of these symptoms are responsive to estrogen.

The vasomotor flush is the most common clinical finding of the menopause. Approximately 75% of women having a natural menopause will experience flushes, as will as many as 90% of women who have surgical menopause (9). There are two components to a flush. The hot flash describes the subjective feeling of warmth prior to any physiologically measurable change. The hot flush is the physiologically measurable change and is characterized by visible redness in the chest, neck, and face, usually followed by sweating in the same distribution. Nocturnal hot flushes are more common than daytime hot flushes, and sleep deprivation is a common result. Studies have demonstrated nocturnal flushes with corresponding waking episodes, using skin temperature and EEG recordings (10). This is clinically relevant as many of these women experience insomnia-related symptoms such as fatigue, irritability, and depression. It has been demonstrated that treatment of these symptomatic women with estrogen results in

improved sleep latency, and an increased percentage of REM sleep (11).

Another clinical finding is osteoporosis, defined as a decrease in bone mass per unit volume, its major consequence being fractures. It is estimated that 15 to 20 million persons in the United States have osteoporosis and that there are over 1 million fractures annually with total medical costs in the range of $6 billion to $10 billion. There is abundant evidence that exogenous estrogen treatment prevents bone loss in this population (12,13).

The most important clinical finding is coronary heart disease. It has been demonstrated that the relative risk of coronary disease in premenopausal women from the ages of 45 to 54 compared to men of the same age is approximately 1:15 (14). By age 65, the risk in women approximates that seen in men. Estrogen deficiency appears to play a role, and there is experimental evidence in animals, as well as epidemiologic evidence in humans, that suggests that estrogen is cardioprotective (see below).

RISKS OF HORMONE REPLACEMENT THERAPY

The incidence of gallbladder disease and the need for cholecystectomy appear to be increased in estrogen users vs nonusers (15). The increased risk of endometrial hyperplasia and carcinoma with unopposed estrogen use has been well documented. For example, in one study, short-term users of estrogen (less than one year of use) appeared to have no increased risk of cancer, while the long-term users had a five-fold increased risk (2). The risk of thromboembolic disease appears to be higher among current HRT users (36).

It is known that addition of a progestin to HRT dramatically reduces the risk of endometrial cancer. While the dose and type of progestin are obviously important, there are data suggesting that the duration of progestin exposure is equally important. The incidence of hyperplasia with unopposed estrogen in one study was 18% to 32%, with a decrease to 3% to 4% if a progestin is added for 7 days, with a further reduction to 0% for 12 to 13 days of progestin (3). The current trend clinically is to give a low dose of medroxyprogesterone acetate (5 mg) for 12 to 13 days (the low dose to minimize metabolic complications and the 12 to 13 days to maximize endometrial protection).

The degree of risk of breast cancer secondary to estrogen replacement has not been conclusively established. Individual observational studies and meta-analyses have reported conflicting results, with many reporting no increase in breast cancer risk, while some report an increased breast cancer risk after many years of use (16–19). A recent report from the Nurses' Health Study saw an age-dependent increase in breast cancer risk after only 5 years of use (4). More recently, the Collaborative Group on Hormonal Factors in Breast Cancer re-analyzed approximately 90% of the available epidemiologic evidence and concluded that the relative risk of developing breast cancer increased by a factor of 1.023 for each year of HRT use after menopause (20). This increase is the same as that seen for the effect of delaying menopause by 1 year. Five or more years of HRT use was associated with a relative risk of breast cancer of 1.35 (95% CI, 1.21–1.49) (20).

Several conclusions can be drawn from the current breast cancer literature: 1) there is no evidence that short-term use of replacement estrogen (up to 3 years) is associated with an increase in breast cancer risk. The recent 3-year PEPI (Postmenopausal Estrogen/Progestin Intervention Trial) would support this notion (21). 2) An increase in breast cancer risk is likely with long-term use (longer than 5 to 10 years), although the magnitude of such an increase is still debated. 3) The impact of progestins on breast cancer remains controversial. Unlike the endometrium, where progestins have an antimitotic and therefore protective effect, this does not appear to be the case for breast tissue. Current studies that have attempted to examine the impact of progestins on breast cancer have shown an increase, a decrease, and no effect on breast cancer risk (19). Table 27-1 summarizes some of these results.

BENEFITS OF HORMONE REPLACEMENT THERAPY

Estrogen is effective for relieving vasomotor flushes and genitourinary atrophy. Prevention of osteoporosis with estrogen is also well established, and there is abundant epidemiologic evidence that estrogen is cardioprotective (19). Many studies have demonstrated that estrogen prevents bone loss, while a steady rate of bone loss is seen in untreated women (12). If estrogen is discontinued at any point, bone loss resumes (12). The dose required to prevent bone loss is conjugated estrogen 0.625 mg or its equivalent. Progestins appear to have a synergistic effect with estrogen on bone in preliminary studies, although the dose required to see this effect is quite high (22). There is also evidence that estrogen might be associated with a decreased risk of colon cancer, although this effect is diminished after discontinuing therapy (23).

Table 27-1 Effect of Combined HRT on the Relative Risk of Disease

	Duration of HRT (years)	RR	95% CI[a]
Coronary heart disease	Any	0.60[b]	0.20–0.60
Breast cancer	<2	1.14	0.91–1.45
	2–4.9	1.20	0.99–1.44
	5–9.9	1.46	1.22–1.74
	>=10	1.46	1.20–1.76
Hip fracture	>=10	0.46	0.30–0.69
Endometrial cancer	Any	1.0	0.6–1.2

[a] CI indicates confidence interal.
[b] Represents the estimate derived from unopposed estrogens.
Reproduced by permission from Col NF, Eckman MH, Karas RH, et al. Patient-specific decisions about hormone replacement therapy in postmenopausal women. JAMA 1997;277:1140–1147. Copyright 1997, American Medical Association.

GONADAL STEROIDS AND THE CARDIOVASCULAR SYSTEM

There are many ways that sex steroids can affect the cardiovascular system, via changes in blood pressure, carbohydrate metabolism, the coagulation system, lipoprotein metabolism, and direct effects on the vasculature. While it had initially been calculated that all of estrogen's beneficial effect was mediated through lipids, it is now thought that lipid changes account for only 30% of the apparent reduction in CHD risk, with the rest being related to the direct vascular effects (24).

Many of the effects of estrogen are dose-dependent. Short-term use of conjugated estrogen (0.625 mg) has not been associated with increases in blood pressure (25). This is in contrast to oral contraceptive use, for example, where blood pressure elevations are seen in some women (26). Carbohydrate metabolism is affected only by very high doses of estrogen in postmenopausal women. For example 50–100 μg of ethinyl estradiol causes an abnormal glucose tolerance test, while replacement doses of estrogen do not (27).

While it had previously been thought that there was no increase in the risk of thromboembolic events with hormone replacement therapy (28,29) and that replacement doses of estrogen do not increase clotting factors (30), recent reports from three observational studies (31–33) suggest that there might indeed be an increase in the relative risk of deep venous thrombosis and pulmonary embolism in estrogen users vs. nonusers (although the absolute risk remains very small).

Estrogen improves lipid profiles (increased HDL, decreased LDL), while progestins cause a worsening (34). In addition, estrogen appears to be an antioxidant as LDL is less oxidized in its presence (35). Unopposed estrogen has been shown to increase HDL concentrations by approximately 10% and HDL_2 levels by as much as 25% (36). The PEPI Trial has demonstrated that medroxyprogesterone acetate, a synthetic progestin used commonly as part of hormone replacement therapy, appears to negate some of the increases in HDL seen with unopposed estrogen, although a modest HDL increase is still seen in the presence of medroxyprogesterone (21). It was also observed that oral micronized progesterone (200 mg/day for 14 days) had no negative impact on HDL (21), leading many to argue that micronized progesterone should be the progestin of choice for postmenopausal women. Micronized progesterone has limitations, however, that have limited its widespread use for HRT. First, it has not been FDA approved, and therefore, has not been commercially available (although it may be approved and available soon). While there are pharmacies who prepare micronized progesterone capsules, quality control is always an issue. In addition, the endometrial protective effects of 200 mg micronized progesterone as used in the PEPI trial have not been as well established as those for medroxyprogesterone acetate. However, for those patients who cannot tolerate medroxyprogesterone acetate, micronized progesterone is a reasonable alternative.

There are a number of observations that suggest that estrogen has direct vascular effects. Platelet aggregation studies before and after estrogen suggest that estrogen suppresses platelet function (37). In a primate model, estradiol blocks the abnormal vasomotor (vasoconstrictive) response to acetylcholine in atherosclerotic arteries (38). Finally, angiography studies in women have demonstrated that estrogen is a potent vasodilator (39), which is not surprising as gonadal steroid receptors are known to be present in vessel walls (40).

The epidemiologic data to date overwhelmingly support the notion that estrogen reduces the risk of CHD (24). A cardiac catheterization study of postmenopausal women with coronary artery stenoses at baseline demonstrated that 10-year survival was significantly better in those women who took estrogen when compared to those who did not (41). In this same study, women with normal coronary arteries at baseline who then took estrogen also had somewhat better survival than nonusers of estrogen, although the differences were not statistically significant. Therefore, while the observational studies suggest that estrogen replacement is important for the primary prevention of CAD, estrogen also appears to be important for secondary prevention as well.

More recently, data has been published from a clinical trial known as the HERS study (Heart and Estrogen/Progestin Replacement Study) suggesting that estrogen might actually be harmful for women with established CHD (41a). In this prospective trial of 2763 women on placebo or combined continuous HRT, no overall reduction in risk of CHD events was seen (nonfatal myocardial infarction or sudden coronary death). In a timetable analysis, the risk of CHD events in year 1 was higher in women taking HRT vs. placebo. However, there was then a trend towards a protective effect by year 4. A possible explanation for these observations is that the pro-thrombotic effect of estrogen dominates during early therapy, but that later lipid effects result in a reduction of CHD risk. This time lag would be consistent with many of the lipid-lowering agent studies, in which a reduction in CHD risk is not seen for the first 1 or 2 years. Based on the findings of the HERS study, it seems reasonable to continue HRT in those women who are already receiving therapy. However, initiating HRT in women with newly established CHD might increase risk in the first year of therapy.

While short term lipid studies suggest that progestins would negate some of the beneficial effects on CHD, recent epidemiologic data suggests that HDL levels are similar in combined HRT users compared to unopposed estrogen users (42), suggesting that progestins might not have the negative impact that was initially feared. The best evidence to date that progestins do not affect the risk of myocardial infarction comes from the Nurses' Health Study, where the protective effect against CHD was the same in women on unopposed estrogen vs. those on combined HRT (43).

ESTROGEN AND COGNITIVE FUNCTION

Dementia is an important concern for postmenopausal women as the prevalence of dementia (including Alzheimer's disease) doubles every 5 years after age 65 (44). However, despite its severity and prevalence, there are few effective treatment or prevention strategies. There have been a number of observations that suggest estrogen might be important for cognitive function in women. For example, estrogen promotes the growth of cholinergic neurons in animal models as well as in humans (45). In addition, estrogen has a possible impact on adrenergic and serotonergic pathways (via suppression of monoamine oxidase) that are important for learning and memory (46). Finally, in the rat, estrogen maintains neuronal

circuitry in several brain regions important for cognition (47).

In women, studies of the impact of estrogen on cognitive function have been variable. Most observational studies have failed to control for depression and education, variables that have an important impact on cognitive test results. One carefully designed prospective cohort study reported on results of 12 cognitive function tests in 800 postmenopausal women (48). These tests were administered 15 years after women initially entered the cohort. The authors observed an age-related decline in test performance, but no difference between estrogen users and nonusers (adjusted for age and education).

There are a number of small, short-term clinical trials designed to look at the impact of estrogen on cognitive function. While estrogen improves performance on cognitive testing in women who are symptomatic with vasomotor flushes and insomnia, a beneficial effect of estrogen in asymptomatic women has not yet been established (49).

A lower risk of Alzheimer's disease in postmenopausal estrogen users vs. nonusers has been seen in some epidemiologic studies (50). In a recent meta-analysis, eight case-control studies and two prospective cohort studies looking at the impact of estrogen on dementia risk were reviewed (49). When the outcome evaluated was any type of dementia (including Alzheimer's disease), the summary odds ratio was 0.71 (95% CI, 0.53–0.96). This issue will be further addressed in the context of the Women's Health Initiative Memory Study, where cognitive function and the risk of dementia (including Alzheimer' disease) will be followed in 8000 postmenopausal women treated with HRT vs. placebo for 10 years.

ISSUES OF ANDROGEN REPLACEMENT

The known decrease in ovarian androgen production rates and circulating androgen levels has given rise to concern that menopause might be associated with a decline in libido in postmenopausal women. In fact, an age-associated decline in sexual desire has been observed in both men and women. However, it is unclear whether this decline in libido seen in postmenopausal women is age or menopause related, as studies to date in women have not shown a significant correlation between libido and serum estradiol or testosterone levels (51). Studies designed to look at the effect of androgen replacement on libido and sexual function in postmenopausal women have had significant methodological problems. In particular, variables such as previous sexual difficulties, marital problems, sexual dysfunction in the partner, and subject mood are often not taken into account. Therefore, it is difficult to draw meaningful conclusions from this literature.

The symptoms of vaginal dryness and dyspareunia are common in postmenopausal women and are related to estrogen deficiency. Both symptoms respond to standard replacement doses of estrogen. How to treat a decline in libido is far more difficult, and data on the effectiveness of exogenous testosterone replacement in women have been inconsistent. However, in one small but carefully designed study, estrogen plus testosterone implants were observed to be better for sexual desire and function than estrogen implants alone (52). Other studies have shown improved libido only when serum testosterone levels are maintained at 200 ng/dL or higher (53). Oral testosterone preparations have been associated with a decrease in serum HDL concentrations (54), while this has been less of a problem with parenteral preparations. Other side effects of exogenous androgen administration include hirsutism and acne, of particular concern when serum testosterone levels are maintained in a supraphysiologic range. Newer studies using novel delivery systems for testosterone administration are currently in progress.

NEW THERAPEUTIC AGENTS

A new class of drugs, known as SERMs (selective estrogen receptor modulators), have unusual pharmacology in that they act as estrogens or anti-estrogens at different tissues. Both the estrogen agonist and antagonist effects are mediated through the estrogen receptor, but through different estrogen response elements (one termed the raloxifene response element) (55). This modulation of multiple DNA response elements could explain the tissue selectivity of these agents.

Tamoxifen and clomiphene citrate are examples of drugs in this category, but have limited utility for hormone replacement in postmenopausal women. The newest available agent, raloxifene, has been shown to be a useful agent for the treatment of osteoporosis in 600 postmenopausal women with low or normal bone density (an estrogen agonist effect) (56). In this same study, raloxifene also appeared to have an estrogen agonist effect on lipids, and an estrogen antagonist effect on the endometrium and breast. Potential limitations of the drug include vasomotor flushes and a lack of demonstrated protective effect against CHD. While data in postmenopausal women might predict a lowered risk of CHD due to a favorable impact on lipids (decrease in total cholesterol and LDL) (56), primate data have demonstrated that raloxifene is similar to placebo with regards to development of atherosclerosis (57).

HORMONE REPLACEMENT REGIMENS

There are three main categories of hormone replacement therapy for postmenopausal women: unopposed estrogen, cyclic combined estrogen plus progestin, and continuous combined estrogen plus progestin. The choice of regimen is based on patient preference, the number of years since the patient's last episode of menses, and the presence or absence of a uterus.

Unopposed Estrogen

Unopposed estrogen is used primarily for those women who have undergone hysterectomy, as there is no rationale for adding a progestin except to reduce the risk of estrogen-associated endometrial hyperplasia and cancer. However, some women are unable to tolerate progestins (in particular, the depressive effects of medroxyprogesterone acetate). In this instance, unopposed estrogen is sometimes prescribed, although yearly endometrial biopsies are mandatory. The dose of estrogen used for HRT is conjugated estrogen 0.625 mg or its equivalent given daily. Endometrial cancer risk has been shown to be identical whether the estrogen is given daily or in a cyclic fashion (58).

Bleeding Patterns on Continuous Unopposed Estrogen

In a large prospective, randomized, 1-year multicenter study of 1724 postmenopausal women, amenorrhea was seen in approximately 75% of cycles in those on unopposed estrogen, with irregular spotting or bleeding occurring in the remaining 25% (59).

Cyclic Combined Hormone Regimens

The most popular cyclic regimen until recently had been conjugated equine estrogen (CEE) 0.625 mg on days 1 to 25 of the calendar month, with medroxyprogesterone acetate (MPA) 10 mg added on days 16 to 25. More recently, lower doses of MPA have been used to minimize the negative impact on lipids. In addition, the progestin is now usually given for 12 to 14 days as this has been shown to maximize the endometrial protective effect (60). Therefore, a typically prescribed regimen is CEE 0.625 mg on days 1 to 25, with MPA 5 mg on days 13 to 25. However, there is no proven reason for stopping the estrogen at the end of the month, and in fact, many women become symptomatic with vasomotor flushes during this interval. Therefore, CEE 0.625 mg daily, with MPA 5 mg on days 1 to 13, is a reasonable cyclic regimen for the patient with a uterus. Moving the progestin to the beginning of the calendar month helps with patient compliance.

Bleeding Patterns on Cyclic Combined Hormone Regimens

From 80% to 90% of women on cyclic combined hormone regimens have a monthly withdrawal bleed (59,60). Although bleeding is often light, any menstrual bleeding becomes a significant lifestyle concern for the older postmenopausal patient. In general, bleeding occurs after the last dose of progestin has been administered. However, up to 25% of women bleed before the completion of the progestin (60). There are conflicting data about bleeding patterns and the need for endometrial biopsy. The American College of Obstetrics and Gynecology has recently issued guidelines for endometrial biopsy based on the currently available literature, with endometrial sampling recommended if menstrual bleeding occurs before day 6 of the progestin (in a patient taking a cyclic regimen) (61).

Continuous Combined Hormone Regimens

Because the cyclic combined hormone regimens result in withdrawal bleeding in the majority of patients, there has been increasing emphasis on the use of continuous, combined regimens as a way of inducing amenorrhea (daily progestin exposure eventually results in an atrophic endometrium). The most commonly used continuous regimen in the U.S. is daily CEE 0.625 mg with MPA 2.5 mg. There are now many studies demonstrating that this regimen is protective against endometrial hyperplasia and cancer, including the PEPI Trial and the Menopause Study Group (21,62).

Bleeding Patterns on Continuous Combined Hormone Regimens

While the goal of the continuous, combined regimens is to induce amenorrhea, the main drawback has been irregular bleeding, which often persists for many months. While it had initially been claimed that most women eventually develop amenorrhea, most early clinical studies were difficult to interpret as they were relatively small and the dropout rate was as high as 62% (largely due to bleeding) (63). Data from the Menopause Study Group, the large prospective study referred to above, has demonstrated that the prevalence of bleeding is related to the number of years since menopause. Those women who were more than 3 years past clinical menopause were less likely to experience the bleeding and were more likely to develop amenorrhea by the end of 1 year (when compared to women who were less than 3 years since menopause). This is likely due to the fact that those who are further from menopause already have an atrophic endometrium, and are less likely to bleed. The American College of Obstetrics and Gynecology recommends endometrial biopsy in those taking a continuous combined regimen if the bleeding is unusually heavy, lasts longer than 10 days, or persists beyond the sixth month of therapy (61).

Other Estrogen Preparations

Equivalent doses (to 0.625 mg of CEE) of other estrogen preparations include: micronized estradiol 1–2 mg; estropipate 1.25 mg; and ethinyl estradiol 5–10 µg. Ethinyl estradiol is an extremely potent estrogen that is used for oral contraceptive preparations rather than hormone replacement regimens. The equivalent dose of transdermal estradiol would be 0.05 mg delivered daily in a 3- or 7-day patch respectively. Intramuscular injections of estrogen are also available but have no particular advantage given their variable absorption. Vaginal estrogen creams (conjugated estrogen and estradiol) are also available and in general are used for treatment of atrophic vaginitis. Systemic absorption of vaginal estrogen is extremely efficient, and therefore risk and benefit considerations are the same as those for the transdermal estrogens (both avoid first pass hepatic metabolism).

Low Dose Oral Contraceptives

Low dose oral contraceptives are often prescribed for the perimenopausal patient who has become symptomatic and seeks treatment. These are often women aged 40–50 who are technically still candidates for oral contraception (per FDA guidelines). In this instance, a pill containing 20 µg of ethinyl estradiol can be given, a dose which provides symptomatic relief and contraception, while sometimes providing better bleeding control than conventional HRT.

WHO SHOULD RECEIVE HRT?

There is still no general consensus in the field on who should receive HRT, although guidelines such as those provided by the American College of Physicians have attempted to aid the clinician in this decision-making process (19). A recent decision-analysis by Col and colleagues provides the clinician with an algorithm for who should and who should not receive HRT (based on using 6 months of prolonged life as the definition of clinically significant benefit) (64). This particular analysis supports more widespread use of HRT. However, these types of decision analyses will need to be modified as more epidemiologic data becomes available, particularly with regards to breast cancer risk.

Short-term versus long-term HRT is an important distinction for both clinicians and patients as the goals of therapy and risk-benefit profiles of short-vs. long-term use are quite different. Short-term HRT refers to 3 years or less of treatment, the goal of therapy being management of estrogen deficiency symptoms. Nearly all peri- or postmenopausal women (with the exception of those with a personal history of breast cancer) are candidates for short-term treatment, given the lack of evidence for an increase in breast cancer risk with 3 years of use. However, short-term use does not confer any long-term benefits for the cardiovascular system or bone. Long-term HRT refers to 3 years or more of treatment, its goal being prevention of disease: osteoporosis, CHD, and possibly Alzheimer's disease. However, when using HRT long term, the increased risk of breast cancer becomes relevant. Decision analyses such as that described above are based on long-term use of HRT. Therefore, when counseling patients about HRT, the distinction between short and long-term HRT is an important one, given the different risk-benefit profile.

SUMMARY

Short-term HRT is a reasonable therapeutic option for most postmenopausal women who seek relief of estrogen deficiency symptoms. On the other hand, the decision to continue HRT long term is a more difficult one, for both the clinician and patient. While long-term estrogen has been demonstrated to prevent osteoporosis and its associated fractures, and may reduce the risk of CHD by approximately 50%, there also appears to be an increased risk of breast cancer with long-term estrogen use. Therefore, the risks and benefits must be carefully weighed for each individual.

It is possible that estrogen has other benefits as well, including a reduction in the risk of Alzheimer's disease and colon cancer. However, these benefits are not well established. Like the cardiovascular benefit of estrogen, results of randomized clinical trials from the Women's Health Initiative are awaited to resolve many of these issues. In the meantime, the development of the SERMs raises the possibility that one of these newer agents will have all of the properties needed to replace exogenous estrogen-progestin therapy, i.e., one that acts as an estrogen agonist on the cardiovascular system, bone, and central nervous system, while having an estrogen antagonist effect on the endometrium and breast. Other alternative therapies that are now receiving attention for the management of menopause include acupuncture, dietary modifications (phytoestrogens), and herbal therapies. It is likely that postmenopausal women will have many more therapeutic options from which to choose in the future.

REFERENCES

1. Hammar M, et al. Climacteric symptoms in an unselected sample of Swedish women. Maturitas 1984;6:345.

2. Shapiro S, et al. Risk of localized and widespread endometrial cancer in relation to recent and discontinued use of conjugated estrogens. N Engl J Med 1985;313:969.

3. Whitehead M, Hilliard T, Crook D. The role and use of progestogens. Obstet Gynecol 1990;75(suppl):59.

4. Colditz GA, Hankinson SE, Hunter DJ, et al. The use of estrogens and progestins and the risk of breast cancer in postmenopausal women. N Engl J Med 1995;332:1589–1593.

5. Richardson S, et al. Follicular depletion during the menopausal transition: evidence for accelerated loss and ultimate exhaustion. J Clin Endocrinol Metab 1987;65:231.

6. Grodin J, et al. Source of estrogen production in postmenopausal women. J Clin Endocrinol Metab 1973;36:207.

7. Sherman B, et al. The menopausal transition: analysis of LH, FSH, estradiol, and progesterone concentrations during menstrual cycles of older women. J Clin Endocrinol Metab 1976;42:629.

8. MacNaughton J, Banah M, McCloud P, et al. Age related changes in follicle stimulating hormone, luteinizing hormone, oestradiol and immunoreactive inhibin in women of reproductive age. Clin Endocrinol 1992;36:339–345.

9. McKinlay SM, Jeffreys M. The menopausal syndrome. Br J Prev Soc Med 1974;28:108.

10. Erlik Y, Tatargn IV, Meldum DR, et al. Association of waking episodes with menopausal hot flashes. JAMA 1981;245:1741.

11. Schiff I, Regestein Q, Tulchinsky D, et al. Effects of estrogens on sleep and psychological state of hypogonadal women. JAMA 1979;242:2405.

12. Christiansen C, Christiansen MS, Transbol I. Bone mass in postmenopausal women after withdrawal of estrogen/gestagen replacement therapy. Lancet 1981;1:459–461.

13. Lufkin EG, Wahner HW, O'Fallon WM. Treatment of postmenopausal osteoporosis with transdermal estrogen. Ann Intern Med 1992;117:1–9.

14. Gordon T, Kanne WB, Hjortland M, et al. Menopause and coronary heart disease: the Framingham study. Ann Intern Med 1976;89:157–161.

15. Grodstein F, Colditz GA, Stampfer MJ. Postmenopausal hormone use and cholecystectomy in a large prospective study. Obstet Gynecol 1994;83:5–11.

16. Bergkvist L, Adam HO, Persson I, et al. The risk of breast cancer after estrogen and estrogen-progestin replacement. N Engl J Med 1989;321:293–297.

17. Dupont WD, Page DL. Menopausal estrogen replacement therapy and breast cancer. Arch Int Med 1991;151:67–72.

18. Steinberg KK, Thacker SB, Smith J, et al. A meta-analysis of the effect of estrogen replacement therapy on the risk of breast cancer. JAMA 1991;265:1985–1990.

19. Grady D, Rubin SM, Petitti DB, et al. Hormone therapy to prevent disease and prolong life in postmenopausal women. Ann Intern Med 1992;117:1016–1037.

20. Collaborative Group on Hormonal Factors in Breast Cancer. Breast cancer and hormone replacement therapy: collaborative reanalysis of data from 51 epidemiologic studies of 52,705 women with breast cancer and 108,411 women without breast cancer. Lancet 1997;350:1047–1059.

21. The Writing Group for the PEPI Trial. Effects of estrogen or estrogen/progestin regimens on heart disease risk factors in postmenopausal women. JAMA 1995;273:199–208.

22. Gallagher J, Kable W, Goldgar D. Effect of progestin therapy on Cortical and Trabecular Bone: Comparison with Estrogen. Am J Med 1991;90:171–178.

23. Grodstein F, Martinez E, Platz E, et al. Postmenopausal hormone use and risk for colorectal cancer and adenoma. Ann Int Med 1998;128:705–712.

24. Stampfer MJ, Colditz GA. Estrogen replacement therapy and coronary heart disease: a quantitative assessment of the epidemiologic evidence. Prev Med 1991;20:47–63.

25. Wren BG, Routledge AD. The effect of type and dose of oestrogen on the blood pressure of postmenopausal women. Maturitas 1983;5:135.

26. Chasan-Taber L, Willett WC, Manson JE, et al. Prospective study of oral contraceptives and hypertension among women in the United States. Circulation 1996;94:483.

27. Thom M. Effect of hormone replacement therapy on glucose tolerance in postmenopausal women. Br J Obstet Gynaecol 1997;84:776.

28. Devor M, et al. Estrogen replacement therapy and the risk of venous thrombosis. Am J Med 1992;92:275–282.

29. Boston Collab Drug Surveillance Program. Surgically confirmed gallbladder disease, venous thromboembolism, and breast tumors in relation to postmenopausal estrogen therapy. N Engl J Med 1974;290:15.

30. Notelovitz M, et al. Combination estrogen and progestogen replacement therapy does not adversely affect coagulation. Obstet Gynecol 1993;62:596.

31. Jick H, Derby LE, Myers MW, et al. Risk of hospital admission for idiopathic venous thromboembolism among users of postmenopausal oestrogens. Lancet 1996;348:981–983.

32. Grodstein F, Stampfer M, et al. Prospective study of exogenous hormones and risk of pulmonary embolism in women. Lancet 1996;348:983–987.

33. Daly E, Vessey MP, Hawkins MM, et al. Risk of venous thromboembolism in users of hormone replacement therapy. Lancet 1996;348:977–980.

34. Ottoson UB. Subfractions of high-density lipoprotein cholesterol during estrogen replacement therapy: a comparison between progesterone and natural progesterone. Am J Obstet Gynecol 1985;151:746.

35. Subbiah MTR, Kessel B, Agrawal M, et al. Antioxidant potential of specific estrogens on lipid peroxidation. J Clin Endocrinol Metab 1993;77:1095–1097.

36. Lobo RA. Effects of hormonal replacement on lipids and lipoproteins in postmenopausal women. J Clin Endocrinol Metab 1991;73:925–930.

37. Bar J, Tepper R, Fuchs J, et al. The effect of estrogen replacement therapy on platelet aggregation and adenosine triphosphate release in postmenopausal women. Obstet Gynecol 1993; 81:261–264.

38. Williams JK, Adams MR, Klopfenstein HS. Estrogen modulates responses of atherosclerotic coronary arteries. Circulation 1990; 81:1680–1687.

39. Lieberman EH, Gerhard MD, Uehata A, et al. Estrogen improves endothelium-dependent, flow-mediated vasodilation in postmenopausal women. Ann Intern Med 1994;121:936–941.

40. Ingegno MD, Money SR, Thelmo T, et al. Progesterone receptors in the human heart and great vessels. Lab Invest 1998;59:353–356.

41. Sullivan JM, VanderZwaag R, Hughes JP, et al. Estrogen replacement and coronary artery disease: effect on survival in postmenopausal women. Arch Intern Med 1990;150:2557–2562.

41a. Hulley S, Grady D, Bush T, et al. for the Heart and Estrogen/progestin Replacement Study (HERS) Research Group. Randomized trial of estrogen plus progestin for secondary prevention of coronary heart disease in postmenopausal women. JAMA 1998;280:605–613.

42. Nabulsi AA, Folsom AR, White A, et al. Association of hormone-replacement therapy with various cardiovascular risk factors in postmenopausal women. N Engl J Med 1993;328:1069–1075.

43. Grodstein F, Stampfer M, Manson J, et al. Postmenopausal estrogen and progestin use and the risk of cardiovascular disease. N Engl J Med 1996;335:453.

44. Evans DA. Estimated prevalence of Alzheimer's disease in the United States. Milbank Q 1990;68:267–289.

45. Toran-Allerand CD, Miranda RC, Bentham WD, et al. Estrogen receptors colocalize with low affinity nerve growth factor receptors in cholinergic neurons of the basal forebrain. Proc Natl Acad Sci USA 1992;89:4668–4672.

46. Aylward M. Plasma tryptophan levels and mental depression in postmenopausal subjects: effects of oral piperazine-oestrone sulfate. IRCS Med Sci 1973;1:30–34.

47. Matsumoto A. Synaptogenic action of sex steroids in developing and adult neuroendocrine brain. Psychoneuroendocrinology 1991;16:25–40.

48. Barrett Connor E, Kritz-Silverstein D. Estrogen replacement therapy and cognitive function in older women. JAMA 1993;269:2637–2641.

49. Yaffe K, Sawaya G, Lieberburg I, et al. Estrogen therapy in postmenopausal women: effects on cognitive function and dementia. JAMA 1998;279:688–695.

50. Pagannini-Hill A, Henderson VW. Estrogen deficiency and the risk of Alzheimer's disease in women. Am J Epidemiol 1994;140:256.

51. Myers LS, Dixen J, Morrissette D. Effects of estrogen, androgen, and progestin on sexual psychophysiology and behavior in postmenopausal women. J Clin Endocrinol Metab 1990;70:1124–1131.

52. Davis SR, McCloud P, Strauss BJ. Testosterone enhances estradiol's effects on postmenopausal bone density and sexuality. Maturitas 1995;21:227–236.

53. Sherwin BB, Gelfand MM, Schuber R. Postmenopausal estrogen and androgen replacement and lipoprotein lipid concentrations. Am J Obstet Gynecol 1987;156:414–419.

54. Youngs DD, Hoogwerf BJ, Schover LR. Circulating lipid and lipoprotein concentrations with oral estrogen-androgen hormone replacement therapy. Cleve Clin J Med 1992;59:357–358.

55. Yang NN, Venugopalan M, Hardikar H, et al. Identification of an estrogen response element activated by metabolites of 17B-estradiol and raloxifene. Science 1996;273:1222–1224.

56. Delmas PD, Bjarnason NH, Mitlak BH. Effects of raloxifene on bone mineral density, serum cholesterol concentrations, and uterine endometrium in postmenopausal women. N Engl J Med 1997;337:1641–1647.

57. Clarkson TB, Anthony MS, Jerome CP. Lack of effect of raloxifene on coronary artery atherosclerosis of postmenopausal monkeys. J Clin Endocrinol Metab 1998;83:721–726.

58. Schiff I, Sela HK, Cramer D, et al. Endometrial hyperplasia in women on cyclic or continuous estrogen regimens. Fertil Steril 1982;37:79–82.

59. Archer DF, Pickar JH, Bottiglioni F. Bleeding patterns in post-

menopausal women taking continuous combined or sequential regimens of conjugated estrogens with medroxyprogesterone acetate. Obstet Gynecol 1994;83: 686–692.

60. Whitehead M, Townsen P, Pryse-Davies J, et al. Effects of various types and dosages of progestogens on the postmenopausal endometrium. J Reprod Med 1982;27:539–548.

61. ACOG Technical Bulletin 1992; 166:1–8.

62. Woodruff JD, Pickar JH. Incidence of endometrial hyperplasia in postmenopausal women taking conjugated estrogens (Premarin) with medroxyprogesterone acetate or conjugated estrogens alone. Am J Obstet Gynecol 1994; 170:1213–1216.

63. Hillard T, Siddle N, Whitehead M, et al. Continuous combined conjugated equine estrogen-progestogen therapy: effects of medroxyprogesterone acetate and norethindrone acetate on bleeding patterns and endometrial histologic diagnosis. Am J Obstet Gynecol 1992;167:1–7.

64. Col NF, Eckman MH, Karas RH, et al. Patient-specific decisions about hormone replacement therapy in postmenopausal women. JAMA 1997;277:1140–1147.

Chapter 28

Coronary Heart Disease in Women: Prevention, Diagnosis, and Treatment

Nanette K. Wenger

Although traditionally considered a disease predominantly of men, coronary heart disease is the major cause of mortality for adult women in the United States, accounting for more than 250,000 deaths annually (1). Coronary heart disease among women has a greater age dependency than that seen for men; 1 in 9 U.S. women aged 45 to 64 years has clinical evidence of coronary heart disease as compared with 1 in 3 women over age 65. Women are consistently about a decade older than men at any initial manifestation of coronary heart disease and as much as 20 years older at the occurrence of myocardial infarction (2). Nonetheless, almost 20,000 U.S. women younger than age 65 die from myocardial infarction each year, and more than one third of these women are younger than age 55. With progressive aging of the population, the prevalence of coronary heart disease is likely to escalate among older women unless successful preventive interventions are undertaken across the life span (3). Although the ratio of male-female deaths is elevated in all age groups, as the U.S. population has aged and with greater numbers of women in this aged population, more women than men currently die from coronary heart disease each year. Moreover, coronary heart disease is a substantial contributor to hospitalizations and to physician visits for women.

It is important to recognize that coronary heart disease is a highly lethal disease for women. Women have less favorable outcomes following both myocardial infarction (4) and myocardial revascularization procedures than do their male counterparts. The age-adjusted coronary death rate is 25% to 30% higher for U.S. black women than for white women, and the myocardial infarction death rate for black women is double that for white women. The age-adjusted risk for coronary heart disease is also greater in black women aged 25 to

54 years than in their white counterparts (5). A major contemporary public health challenge, documented in recent surveys, is that U.S. women do not understand their vulnerability to coronary heart disease, not even listing heart disease among their major perceived health problems (6,7).

PREVENTION OF CORONARY HEART DISEASE IN WOMEN

Coronary risk factors are highly prevalent in U.S. women of all racial and ethnic groups (8,9). Seventy percent of all women in the U.S. have at least one major coronary risk factor. This already high percentage increases in older women, because of the increased prevalence of a number of coronary risk factors with aging. There is a prominent female to male crossover in several risk factors associated with aging. Although hypertension and hypercholesterolemia are more prevalent at younger ages in men than in women, their prevalence is greater in older women than in older men.

Based on information from the National Center for Health Statistics (1991), of women between the ages of 20 and 74, more than one third had hypertension; more than one quarter each had hypercholesterolemia, were cigarette smokers, or were overweight; and 6 of 10 U.S. women have a sedentary lifestyle, making this the most prevalent coronary risk attribute for women.

Coronary risk factors are more prevalent and tend to cluster among women with less favorable socioeconomic and educational status, mandating intensive attention to coronary risk reduction in these underserved populations. Attention to socioeconomic circumstances is particularly relevant for

312

elderly women, in that almost twice as many U.S. women as men aged 65 years and older are likely to be at the poverty level; poverty rates are particularly high among black, Hispanic, and native American women. Additionally, the report of a Commonwealth Fund survey (10) shows that U.S. women older than age 65 are less likely to undertake preventive measures, including diet and exercise.

Although women share with men the traditional coronary risk factors, some risk attributes are unique to women, prominent among which is estrogen status and the use of postmenopausal hormone therapy.

Cigarette Smoking

Twenty-three percent of U.S. women older than age 18 currently smoke cigarettes. Cigarette smoking triples the risk for myocardial infarction, even among premenopausal women, with the greatest risk present among women already at high risk due to both older age and the prevalence of other coronary risk factors. Cigarette smoking increases coronary risk in women in a dose-dependent fashion, although even smoking fewer than five cigarettes daily doubles the coronary risk.

Cigarette smoking lowers the age at initial myocardial infarction more for women than for men (11). Smoking also lowers the age at menopause, on average 1.5 to 2 years, with the longer period in menopausal status potentially augmenting coronary risk.

Smoking cessation measures have been far more effective among men than women, with the result that currently equal numbers of women and men in the United States smoke cigarettes. Within two years of smoking cessation, former smokers decrease their cardiovascular mortality risk by 24% (12); within 3 to 5 years of cessation, the coronary risk approaches that of women who had never smoked. The benefit of smoking cessation is evident in women with coronary heart disease as well, both increasing survival and decreasing reinfarction (13). The benefit does not lessen at older ages (13), reinforcing the recommendation that smoking cessation be encouraged for women even at advanced ages.

Diabetes Mellitus

Diabetes is a far more important risk factor for coronary heart disease in women than in men, essentially negating the gender protective effect (14). Data from the Nurses' Health Study show that maturity-onset diabetes was associated with a three- to sevenfold increase in the risk of a cardiovascular event (15). After age 45, women are twice as likely as men to develop diabetes, with the result that diabetes is an important contributor to the multifaceted increased coronary risk factor prevalence in older women, compared with the status at younger ages.

In the Nurses' Health Study, the incidence of diabetes was reduced among women who exercised regularly (16). Thus a regular exercise regimen should be part of the preventive strategy for women at high risk for diabetes, such as those who have had gestational diabetes or those with a strong family history of diabetes mellitus.

Diabetes adversely affects both the in-hospital and the long-term prognosis once myocardial infarction occurs, with the prognosis substantially worse for diabetic women than for diabetic men (17). Diabetic women have a doubled risk of reinfarction and a fourfold increase in the risk of development of heart failure. Additionally, among women who undergo both coronary artery bypass graft surgery and percutaneous transluminal coronary angioplasty, more women than men are diabetic; diabetes likely contributes to their less favorable procedural outcomes.

Hypertension

More than half of the white women and almost 80% of the black women older than age 45 have hypertension, with the racial discrepancy more pronounced for women than for men. Seventy-one percent of U.S. women older than age 65 have hypertension; hypertension is more prevalent in women than men after age 65. At young to middle age, hypertension is more prevalent in men than in women, but levels of systolic blood pressure continue to rise among women with increasing age, at least to age 80. Thus the prevalence of hypertension in women increases dramatically with older age, particularly the prevalence of isolated systolic hypertension (9). Based on data from the U.S. National Health Examination Follow-up Survey (NHEFS), obesity, and in particular central obesity with its associated hyperinsulinemia and insulin resistance, appear more important contributors to hypertension for women than for men.

Because of the increase in hypertension with aging, blood pressure should be measured annually, even among older women; the woman who was normotensive in early menopause may well develop hypertension at an older age. In the Systolic Hypertension in the Elderly Program (SHEP), control of isolated systolic hypertension in persons age 55 or older reduced the occurrence of stroke, fatal cardiovascular events, and nonfatal cardiovascular events in both genders; women comprised 57% of the study cohort (18). Because of the limited numbers of women included in most other clinical trials of antihypertensive therapies, information remains conflicting regarding gender-specific outcome, particularly questions of whether women respond differently to specific antihypertensive therapies than do men. Subgroup meta-analysis suggested comparable treatment benefit for women and men in terms of relative risk; absolute risk reduction by treatment seemed dependent on untreated risk (19).

Lipid Abnormalities

Women have higher levels of HDL cholesterol than men across the lifespan, with HDL cholesterol levels decreasing only minimally at menopause and later. Low levels of HDL cholesterol appear to place women at particularly high risk, typically when associated with high triglyceride levels. An increase of 10 mg/dL in HDL cholesterol in the Framingham Heart Study was associated with a 40% to 50% decrease in the risk of coronary events for women.

LDL cholesterol levels are lower in women in their premenopausal years than for comparably aged men; however, LDL cholesterol levels in women rise progressively with aging, particularly following menopause, such that LDL cholesterol levels in elderly women are higher than those in elderly men (20). In a large number of population studies, total cholesterol levels (predominantly reflecting LDL cholesterol levels) continue to predict coronary risk in older women (21). Although the cholesterol-coronary heart disease relationship is less prominent for black than for white women (22,23), once clinical coronary heart disease becomes evident, black women have less favorable outcomes than do white women.

The benefit of cholesterol lowering for women with coronary heart disease has been well-documented in several recent randomized controlled clinical trials. In the Scandinavian Simvastatin Survival Study (4S) (24), lowering cholesterol by the use of simvastatin in patients who had myocardial infarction decreased major coronary events comparably in women and men, 35% and 34% respectively. Women constituted 19% of the study cohort, and benefit was maintained at older age for both women and men. Among postinfarction patients with average cholesterol levels in the CARE (Cholesterol and Recurrent Events) trial (25), lowering cholesterol with pravastatin reduced death or recurrent infarction by 40% in women in contrast to 26% in men, with women representing 14% of the study population. More recently, benefit was evident for women in the Australian LIPID (Long-term Intervention with Pravastatin and Ischemic Disease) and the AFCAPS-TexCAPS (Air Force/Texas Coronary Atherosclerosis Prevention Study) trial.

Optimal lipid lowering in women thus has the potential to provide substantial benefit. Nonetheless, among women with defined coronary heart disease enrolled in the Heart and Estrogen/Progestin Replacement Study (HERS) between 1993 and 1994, most had LDL cholesterol levels that exceeded NCEP treatment goals even though 47% were taking a lipid-lowering drug (26).

Obesity

Obesity has increased in prevalence in the U.S. in both genders (9), but is particularly prominent in populations with lower educational and income levels. The 1991 U.S. National Center for Health Statistics report states that 50% of black women and more than 35% of white women are at 20% or greater than desirable weight. Obesity imparts a two- to fourfold increase in coronary risk for women, at least in part related to the unfavorable effect of obesity on blood lipid levels, glucose tolerance, and blood pressure.

The distribution of body fat appears important in that central obesity, characterized by a waist-to-hip ratio of more than 0.8, substantially increases the coronary risk for women (27). Central obesity is characteristically associated with lower levels of HDL cholesterol, high triglyceride levels, insulin resistance, and hypertension.

Weight control can substantially improve the cardiovascular risk profile. Fourteen-year follow-up data from the Nurses' Health Study (28) confirm a direct relationship between increased body weight and mortality from all causes without excess mortality in lean women when smokers were excluded. However, substantial fluctuations in weight are also associated with increased coronary risk.

Sedentary Lifestyle

Physical inactivity, the most prevalent coronary risk factor in women, is an independent risk factor for coronary heart disease; physical inactivity predominates in populations with lower education and income levels (29). Those studies of physical activity where gender-specific data are available show a 50% lower coronary risk for physically active than physically

inactive women. In these studies, coronary risk was decreased by habitual exercise even at older age, with modest habitual leisure time activity, equivalent to 30 to 45 minutes of walking three times weekly, reducing myocardial infarction risk by 50% (30). Questionnaire data confirmed a graded inverse association between physical activity and mortality from all causes in postmenopausal women as well (31).

Because of these documented benefits, there is concern about the lower rate at which physicians refer women compared to men to exercise rehabilitation following a coronary event, with this discrepancy being particularly prominent for elderly women (32). This under-referral raises concern because of the documented benefits of physical activity in improving exercise tolerance for older women, as well as the potential for coronary risk reduction in the cardiac rehabilitation setting. Nonetheless, because musculoskeletal injuries are more prominent among elderly women than elderly men when high-impact exercise is undertaken, an exercise regimen for women of older age should be characterized by low-impact aerobic activity of low-to-moderate intensity (33).

Aspirin and Antioxidants

Although men older than age 40 appear to derive a preventive benefit against myocardial infarction from the routine use of aspirin, the observational data available for women are conflicting. Because of the less frequent occurrence of myocardial infarction in women, the risk of hemorrhagic stroke associated with aspirin use in women may be potentially disproportionate to the benefit attributable to the reduction in myocardial infarction (34). Data from randomized clinical trials are required for firm recommendations.

Data for both women and men are also limited and conflicting regarding the role of antioxidant therapies (35), and for interventions designed to alter homocysteine levels.

Postmenopausal Hormone Therapy

Postmenopausal hormone therapy is discussed in detail in Chapter 27.

Despite ample documentation of several plausible biologic mechanisms for estrogen benefit (36–39), and a large number of observational studies of postmenopausal hormone use suggesting a substantial reduction in coronary risk (40), particularly among current users, no randomized clinical trial data of postmenopausal hormone therapy are available that provide clinical outcome results. Although data from the randomized Postmenopausal Estrogen/Progestin Intervention (PEPI) trial (41) document an intermediate outcome, an improvement in the cardiovascular risk factor profile among women randomized to unopposed estrogen and several estrogen/progestin combinations, the clinical risk-benefit ratio of hormone use must be precisely ascertained. The HERS trial failed to find a benefit for secondary prevention of heart disease (26). Potential risks, particularly for breast cancer (29,42,43), as well as for venous thromboembolism (44–46), must be compared with the benefits in a randomized clinical trial setting, such as the ongoing large-scale trial in the Women's Health Initiative. The same scientific rigor must be applied to the evaluation of postmenopausal hormone use as is the case for other pharmacologic preventive therapies.

Diagnosis of Coronary Heart Disease in Women

Evaluation of chest pain in women poses a challenge. Although the characteristics of the history of chest pain are important in selecting the appropriate test procedures, the clinical history alone, even if compatible with angina pectoris, is inadequate to make a diagnosis of coronary heart disease. In the Coronary Artery Surgery Study (CASS) Registry, among patients referred to coronary arteriography by their treating physician to evaluate chest pain syndromes of sufficient severity to warrant consideration for coronary artery by-pass graft surgery, 50% of the women, as compared with 17% of the men, had minimal or no coronary atherosclerotic obstruction.

Because the initial presentation of coronary heart disease in women is more likely to be chest pain than myocardial infarction, the reverse of the pattern for men, the clinical descriptors of the chest pain are valuable to define the appropriate diagnostic procedures (47,48). Men with chest pain typical for angina pectoris have a 93% likelihood of having significant coronary disease; in a number of series only 60% to 75% of women with chest pain typical for angina had significant coronary disease, with one quarter to one half of these having multivessel coronary disease. For this group of women with a high likelihood of coronary disease, either exercise-based or other stress testing or coronary arteriography is a reasonable initial diagnostic approach (48). For women considered to have probable angina pectoris, i.e., those whose chest pain had some features characteristic yet some atypical for angina, there was a 30% to 40% prevalence of significant coronary disease and a 4% to 22% occurrence of multivessel disease. In this intermediate likelihood group, exercise-based or other stress testing is particularly of value. When the chest pain symptoms were nonspecific, only about 5% of the women had evidence of coronary disease, and virtually none had multivessel disease, such that exercise-based testing is unlikely to be of diagnostic value in this subset (48). In patients older than age 65, it is important to note that exertional chest pain is associated with a gender-neutral risk of coronary death (49).

Although the optimal timing and selection of noninvasive diagnostic procedures remains controversial, substantial advances have occurred in the selection and utilization of noninvasive test procedures for women with chest pain. Until this decade, women with chest pain syndromes compatible with or suggestive of angina pectoris had far less aggressive investigation and management than did their male counterparts. With the delineation of the high prevalence and substantial lethality of coronary heart disease in women, there have been major changes in the pattern of clinical care. In a number of studies reported through the early 1990s, women suspected or defined to have coronary heart disease were less often referred for diagnostic and therapeutic interventions and, in particular, were less likely to undergo invasive tests. Given the evolving and expanding database regarding women's cardiovascular health, physicians are currently less likely to attribute a woman's chest pain symptoms to noncoronary causes or psychologic etiologies. Objective testing is now undertaken earlier in women with chest pain syndromes to ascertain those for whom coronary heart disease is the underlying etiology.

Exercise Testing

Exercise testing remains the cornerstone of the noninvasive evaluation of chest pain syndromes in women. However, the predictive accuracy of any noninvasive diagnostic test to evaluate chest pain syndromes in women is limited by their lower prevalence of coronary disease, and particularly of multivessel disease, except at older age; this results in a lower pretest likelihood of disease for young and middle-aged women. Given the low pretest likelihood of coronary heart disease in young and middle-aged women, a normal exercise test result with a test of adequate intensity has powerful predictive value for excluding coronary heart disease; this negative predictive value is comparable to that for men (50,51). At older ages, when the pretest likelihood of coronary disease increases, the frequent inadequate intensity of the exercise accomplished (due either to deconditioning or to comorbid problems limiting the ability of older women to exercise) reduces the diagnostic value of exercise electrocardiography. The results of exercise-based testing are dependent on the intensity of the exercise performed and the severity of the abnormalities induced; thus the abnormal test data reflect both the severity and the extent of the underlying coronary arterial obstruction and the adequacy of the intensity of exercise (52).

An additional factor contributing to the lower sensitivity and specificity of the exercise electrocardiogram for women is their higher prevalence of baseline ECG repolarization abnormalities, particularly those associated with hypertension, left ventricular hypertrophy, mitral valve prolapse, and possibly related to hormonal effects. Data from the Coronary Artery Surgery Study (CASS) confirm that, in the presence of a normal resting electrocardiogram and a reasonable exercise tolerance enabling an adequate test, there is comparable diagnostic value of the exercise electrocardiogram for women and for men. In the CASS Registry, exercise electrocardiography provided valuable prognostic information as well; it significantly predicted subsequent 16-year survival for both women and men. In the CASS Registry, women classified as at low-to-intermediate risk had a 30% to 79% survival rate compared with the women classified as at high risk, who had a 44% survival rate (53).

Radionuclide Studies

Radionuclide-based exercise testing increases the sensitivity and specificity of the exercise test for both women and men. The sensitivity and specificity of thallium 201 imaging is significantly better than that of the exercise electrocardiogram, 75% and 97% versus 34% and 41% respectively (54,55). Exercise radionuclide myocardial perfusion imaging, both with thallium 201 and with technetium 99 sestamibi, either exercise-based or using a pharmacologic challenge, provides better predictive accuracy than does the exercise ECG. Although earlier studies highlighted a large proportion of false-positive tests for women resulting from breast attenuation artifact, the contemporary interpretation using a gender-specific algorithm shows good predictive accuracy of exercise thallium scintigraphy for women (56). Technetium 99 sestamibi perfusion imaging may have advantage over thallium 201 in that there appears to be less attenuation, there is the ability to measure a first pass ejection fraction, and gated imaging acquisition can be performed (57). Pharmacologic radionuclide perfusion studies or pharmacologic echocardiography are advised for women who cannot exercise adequately. Pharmacologic studies, both pharmacologic radionuclide myocardial perfusion imaging and pharmacologic echocardiography, have better predictive accuracy than does the exercise ECG, although the pharmacologic studies in women unable to exercise seem associated with more side effects than are encountered in men.

Exercise radionuclide ventriculography is not recommended for women, as the exercise ejection fraction in both normal women and in elderly patients of both genders does not reliably increase in the absence of coronary disease as it does in younger men; this invalidates the criterion of an exercise-based decrease in ejection fraction as suggestive of coronary disease in these populations.

High sensitivity and specificity, about 86% each even with single vessel coronary disease, is described with either exercise or pharmacologic echocardiography. Limitations of this technique include the inability to obtain an adequate echocardiographic image owing to the chest configuration. Adequate echocardiographic images may be difficult to obtain in obese women and in very elderly patients of both genders. A recent study suggested that in women with abnormal exercise electrocardiograms or exercise thallium tests, dobutamine transesophageal echocardiography was an accurate test to identify those with coronary disease (58).

The roles of positron emission tomography, magnetic resonance imaging and angiography, and ultrafast CT imaging for coronary calcium remain to be ascertained. The advantages of these procedures are the lack of ionizing radiation.

Coronary Arteriography

Coronary arteriography is a major determinant of the access to myocardial revascularization procedures. Whereas a decade ago there was a tenfold greater likelihood of men than women with abnormal noninvasive exercise-based tests being referred for coronary arteriography, there is currently almost comparable referral by gender. Currently there are comparable rates for the performance of revascularization following coronary arteriography, based on the severity of the arterial obstruction. In a Cleveland Clinic cohort, the gender-related differences in referral to coronary angiography after exercise thallium testing were related only to a higher rate of abnormal tests in men. Further, at angiography, women were less likely to have severe coronary disease; the lesser referral of women for myocardial revascularization following coronary arteriography reflects the typically lesser severity of the documented coronary disease. Examination of the outcomes of patients with abnormal noninvasive testing not referred for invasive test procedures or myocardial revascularization show that the long-term outcomes are less favorable for non-revascularized women than for non-revascularized men (59).

In a recent cost-effectiveness analysis, the most expensive diagnostic strategy was initial coronary arteriography, at a cost of about $1500 per patient. Exercise electrocardiography, with subsequent coronary angiography as needed, averaged $1000 per patient. However, exercise echocardiography, although initially expensive, entailed an average cost of about $800 per patient because fewer coronary arteriograms were

performed, with these selected only for patients with exercise-induced new or worsening wall motion abnormalities (60).

TREATMENT OF CORONARY HEART DISEASE IN WOMEN

Myocardial Infarction

The hospital mortality rate for myocardial infarction is higher for women than for men (61), with older women twice as likely as men to die within the initial week following infarction. In the Myocardial Infarction Triage and Intervention Registry (62,63), the hospital mortality was 16% for women as compared with 14% for men. Additionally, 44% of women died within the subsequent year, in contrast to 27% of men. As well as an increased 1-year mortality for women, there is an earlier and more frequent recurrence of nonfatal myocardial infarction among female survivors. Although these gender differences lessen when controlling for older age and comorbidity (64), they do not disappear.

Women who present with myocardial infarction tend to be sicker than men, having a higher Killip class, more tachycardia, atrioventricular block, and pulmonary rales. Among patients presenting to emergency departments with chest pain, men are twice as likely as women to have acute myocardial infarction; when evidence of heart failure accompanies the chest pain in women, their likelihood of myocardial infarction equals that of men (65). Women are more likely to have complications of myocardial infarction that include shock, heart failure, recurrent chest pain and cardiac rupture, and stroke (66–69), although those gender differences also lessen when corrected for older age and comorbidity. Data from the Myocardial Infarction Triage and Intervention Registry define that women were half as likely as men to receive acute coronary catheterization, coronary angioplasty, coronary thrombolysis, or coronary artery bypass graft surgery (70); the contribution of the difference in the application of diagnostic and therapeutic procedures versus the gender issue cannot be ascertained. Additionally, recent data highlight that pharmacotherapeutic interventions for suspected acute myocardial infarction continue to differ by gender (71). In women there was a consistently lower use not only of thrombolytic agents, but also of beta blocking drugs and aspirin.

In the TIMI III Registry Study (72), women with unstable angina or non-Q-wave myocardial infarction had less severe coronary disease than did men. Additionally, although they were less likely to receive intensive anti-ischemic medical therapies, women had less frequent coronary arteriography, and fewer myocardial revascularization procedures. Despite their less severe disease, women had similar outcomes to men; this raises concern that similar outcomes with less severe disease likely constitutes a less favorable result for women compared with men. Women in the TIMI III Registry also were less likely to be treated with beta blocking drugs, aspirin, heparin, and nitroglycerin.

Gender comparisons of the early outcome of acute myocardial infarction in the Third International Study of Infarct Survival (ISIS-3) trial among patients with a clear indication for fibrinolytic therapy showed an unadjusted odds ratio for 35-day mortality of 1.73 (95% CI, 1.61–1.86) for women. Adjustment for age decreased this odds ratio to 1.20

(95% CI, 1.11–1.29) and adjustment for presenting prognostic characteristics to 1.14 (95% CI, 1.05–1.23). A limitation of these data is that more women than men are ineligible for fibrinolytic therapy owing to older age, co-existing conditions, and late presentation after symptom onset (73), all characteristics associated with a less favorable outcome (74).

As regards thrombolytic therapy for acute myocardial infarction, comparable survival benefit for women and men was defined in the GUSTO I trial. This survival benefit was evident despite the excess occurrence of bleeding complications, and particularly intracerebral bleeding with resultant stroke, among women. Despite the decrease in absolute mortality with coronary thrombolysis, gender differences in mortality persisted in the GUSTO I trial, with 30-day mortality rates of 11.3% for women, more than twice that for men (5.5%). In this study women were also more likely to have nonfatal complications of shock, heart hailure, and reinfarction (75,76). Primary angioplasty may be an appropriate alternative for women, owing to their increased risk of intracranial bleeding with coronary thrombolysis. The hospital outcomes of primary percutaneous transluminal coronary angioplasty were equally favorable for women and men in the Primary Angioplasty and Myocardial Infarction (PAMI) trial (77); women who received primary angioplasty had a lesser risk of intracranial bleeding and an improved survival compared with women who received coronary thrombolysis.

Data from the Multicenter Myocardial Ischemia Research Group require attention (78). In stable patients 1 to 6 months following a coronary event, subsequent cardiac event rates were comparable for women and men, although noninvasive testing less frequently identified myocardial ischemia in women.

Of concern is that fewer women than men are referred for cardiac rehabilitation services following myocardial infarction, interventions that can improve their exercise tolerance and functional capacity and offer opportunities for coronary risk reduction as well (32).

Myocardial Revascularization Procedures

During the past decade there has been an almost threefold increase in the rates of coronary artery bypass graft (CABG) surgery and of percutaneous transluminal coronary angioplasty (PCTA) and other transcatheter revascularization procedures in women. Nonetheless, in all reported series, the mortality from CABG surgery is double for women as compared with men. As an example, the hospital mortality rate following CABG surgery was 13% for women as compared with 6% for men in the Myocardial Infarction Triage and Intervention Registry (79). It remains uncertain whether this is a gender issue or whether it represents the confounding factors that women who undergo CABG surgery are generally older, have greater functional impairment, and are more likely to present with severe and unstable angina, such that they have a greater likelihood of urgent or emergency CABG surgery (80,81). Despite the high hospital mortality rate, women in the Coronary Artery Surgery Study who survived the operative hospitalization had a comparable 15-year survival to that for men (82). In addition to the increased surgical mortality rate, lower rates of graft patency, less postoperative symptomatic relief, more frequent perioperative infarction and heart failure, and a greater likelihood of reoperation within

the initial 5 years following CABG surgery are described for women in most published series.

Contemporary data document that the procedural success and safety of PTCA are comparable for women and for men (83,84). Of interest is that comparable results are obtained despite the fact that women tend to be older, and are more likely to have had antecedent heart failure and unstable angina, as well as complicating hypertension, hypercholesterolemia, and diabetes (83,85). In the 1985 NHLBI PTCA Registry (86), twice as many women as men referred for PTCA were considered either inoperable or at high surgical risk, and more women than men had unstable angina. Not surprisingly, at 4-year follow-up more women had died, but myocardial infarction and the need for CABG surgery were comparable. However, women in this PTCA Registry were more likely not only to have residual angina but severe angina and, as a result, were receiving more maintenance antianginal medication. Despite the initial favorable results, women tend to have less favorable long-term survival following PTCA, predominantly related to their older age; they also have less late symptomatic relief. For the newer transcatheter revascularization procedures, higher complication rates and lower success rates occur in women, likely as a result of the large size of these devices compared with the small coronary artery size of women. Although similar rates of restenosis in both genders were described in the CAVEAT trial (87), there is little information as to whether gender differences exist in the rates of restenosis following coronary intravascular procedures.

As was the case with myocardial infarction, fewer women than men are referred to cardiac rehabilitation for exercise training and coronary risk reduction following myocardial revascularization procedures (32). This is particularly true for older women.

It remains uncertain whether the more frequent severe and unstable angina in women referred for myocardial revascularization procedures reflects gender-related differences in clinical presentation; delayed recognition of the disease and referral of women, and in particular older women, by their physicians; or a delayed presentation of women to medical care following symptom onset. Also unknown is whether more women than men refuse myocardial revascularization procedures when these are recommended.

SUMMARY

As we approach the next millennium, there is increased appreciation of the magnitude and ominous prognosis of coronary heart disease in women. As well, the high prevalence of remediable coronary risk factors is also evident.

Once women develop clinical manifestations of coronary heart disease, either myocardial infarction or the requirement for myocardial revascularization procedures, their outcomes are less favorable than seen for their male counterparts. Whether these are true gender differences; or reflect that women are of older age and have greater comorbidity, particularly diabetes and hypertension; or whether these reflect the differences in therapies by gender—a substantially remediable component—remains to be ascertained.

REFERENCES

1. Wenger NK. Coronary heart disease in women: evolving knowledge is dramatically changing clinical care. In: Julian DG, Wenger NK, eds. Women and heart disease. London: Martin Dunitz, 1997:21–38.

2. Lerner DJ, Kannel WB. Patterns of coronary heart disease morbidity and mortality in the sexes: a 26-year follow-up of the Framingham population. Am Heart J 1986;111:383–390.

3. Rich-Edwards JW, Manson JE, Hennekens CH, et al. The primary prevention of coronary heart disease in women. N Engl J Med 1995;332:1758–1766.

4. Wenger NK, Speroff L, Packard B. Cardiovascular health and disease in women. N Engl J Med 1993;329:247–256.

5. Gillum RF, Mussolino ME, Madans JH. Coronary heart disease incidence and survival in African-American women and men: the NHANES I Epidemiologic Follow-up Study. Ann Ietern Med 1997;127:111–118.

6. Legato MJ, Padus E, Slaughter E. Women's perceptions of their general health, with special reference to their risk of coronary artery disease: results of a national telephone survey. J Women's Health 1997;6:189–198.

7. Pilote L, Hlatky MA. Attitudes of women toward hormone therapy and prevention of heart disease. Am Heart J 1995;129:1237–1238.

8. Eaker ED, Chesebro JH, Sacks FM, et al. Cardiovascular disease in women. Circulation 1993;88:1999–2009.

9. National Center for Health Statistics. Health: United States, 1990. Hyattsville, MD: U.S. Public Health Services, Centers for Disease Control; 1991.

10. Commonwealth Fund: Survey of women's health. Lewis Harris, 1993.

11. Hansen EF, Andersen LT, Von Eyben FE. Cigarette smoking and age at first acute myocardial infarction and influence of gender and extent of smoking. Am J Cardiol 1993;71:1439–1442.

12. Kawachi I, Colditz GA, Stampfer MJ, et al. Smoking cessation in relation to total mortality rates in women; a prospective cohort study. Ann Intern Med 1993;119:992–1000.

13. Hermanson B, Omenn GS, Kronmal RA, et al, and Participants in the Coronary Artery Surgery Study. Beneficial six-year outcome of smoking cessation in older men and women with coronary artery disease: results from the CASS Registry. N Engl J Med 1998;319:1365–1369.

14. Barrett-Connor EL, Cohn BA, Wingard DL, et al. Why is diabetes mellitus a stronger risk factor for fatal ischemic heart disease in women than in men? The Rancho Bernardo Study. JAMA 1991;265:627–631.

15. Manson JE, Colditz GA, Stampfer MJ, et al. A prospective study of maturity-onset diabetes mellitus and risk of coronary heart disease and stroke in women. Arch Intern Med 1991;151:1141–1147.

16. Manson JE, Rimm EB, Stampfer MJ, et al. Physical activity and incidence of non-insulin-dependent diabetes mellitus in women Lancet 1991;338:774–778.

17. Liao Y, Cooper RS, Ghali JK, et al. Sex differences in the impact of coexistent diabetes on survival in patients with coronary heart disease. Diabetes Care 1993;16:708–713.

18. SHEP Cooperative Research Group. Prevention of stroke by antihypertensive drug treatment in older persons with isolated systolic hypertension: final results of the Systolic Hypertension in the Elderly Program (SHEP). JAMA 1991;265:3255–3264.

19. Gueyffier F, Boutitie F, Boissel J-P, et al. Effect of antihypertensive drug treatment on cardiovascular outcomes in women and men: a meta-analysis of individual patient data from randomized, controlled trials. Ann Intern Med 1997;126:761–767.

20. Kannel WB. Nutrition and the occurrence and prevention of cardiovascular disease in the elderly. Nutr Rev 1988;46:68–78.

21. Manolio TA, Pearson TA, Wenger NK, et al. Cholesterol and heart disease in older persons and women: review of an NHLBL Workshop. Ann Epidemiol 1992;2:161–176.

22. Demirovic J, Sprafka JM, Folsom AR, et al. Menopause and serum cholesterol: differences between blacks and whites. The Minnesota Heart Survey. Am J Epidemiol 1992;136;155–164.

23. Knapp RG, Sutherland SE, Keil JE, et al. A comparison of the effects of cholesterol on CHD mortality in black and white women: twenty-eight years of follow-up in the Charleston Heart Study. J Clin Epidemiol 1992;45:1119–1129.

24. Scandinavian Simvastatin Survival Study Group. Randomised trial of cholesterol lowering in 4444 patients with coronary heart disease: the Scandinavian Simvastatin Survival Study (4S). Lancet 1994;344:1383–1389.

25. Sacks FM, Pfeffer MA, Moye LA, et al, for the Cholesterol and Recurrent Events Trial Investigators. The effect of pravastatin on coronary events after myocardial infarction in patients with average cholesterol levels. N Engl J Med 1996;335:1001–1009.

26. Schrott HG, Bittner V, Vittinghoff E, et al, for the HERS Research Group. Adherence to National Cholesterol Education Program treatment goals in postmenopausal women with heart disease: the Heart and Estrogen/Progestin Replacement Study (HERS). JAMA 1997;277:1281–1286.

27. Kaplan NM. The deadly quartet: upper-body obesity, glucose intolerance, hypertriglyceridemia, and hypertension. Arch Intern Med 1989;149:1514–1520.

28. Willett WC, Manson JE, Stampfer MJ, et al. Weight, weight change,

and coronary heart disease in women: risk within the "normal" weight range. JAMA 1995;273: 461–465.

29. Anda RF, Waller MN, Wooten KG, et al. Behavioral risk factor surveillance, 1988. MMWR CDC Surveill Summ 1990;39:1–21.

30. Lemaitre RN, Heckbert SR, Psaty BM, et al Leisure-time physical activity and the risk of nonfatal myocardial infarction in postmenopausal women. Arch Intern Med 1995;155:2302–2308.

31. Kushi LH, Fee RM, Folsom AR, et al. Physical activity and mortality in postmenopausal women. JAMA 1997;277:1287–1292.

32. Wenger NK, Froelicher ES, Smith LK, et al. Clinical practice guideline number 17: Cardiac rehabilitation. Rockville, MD: Agency for Health Care Policy and Research and the National Heart, Lung, and Blood Institute, U.S. Department of Health and Human Services, Public Health Service, 1995. AHCPR Publication No. 96-0672.

33. Pollock ML, Carroll JF, Graves JE, et al. Injuries and adherence to walk/jog and resistance training programs in the elderly. Med Sci Sports Exerc 1991;23:1194–1200.

34. Manson JE, Stampfer MJ, Colditz GA, et al. A prospective study of aspirin use and primary prevention of cardiovascular disease in women. JAMA 1991;266:521–527.

35. Kushi LH, Folsom AR, Prineas RJ, et al. Dietary antioxidant vitamins and death from coronary heart disease in postmenopausal women. N Engl J Med 1996;334:1156–1162.

36. Samaan SA, Grawford MH. Estrogen and cardiovascular function after menopause. J Am Coll Cardiol 1995;26:1403–1410.

37. Wenger NK: Postmenopausal hormone therapy: is it useful for coronary prevention? (plausible mechanisms and available data). Cardiol Clin North Am 1998;16: 17–25.

38. Grodstein F, Stampfer M. The epidemiology of coronary heart disease and estrogen replacement in postmenopausal women. Prog Cardiovasc Dis 1995;38:199–210.

39. Guetta V, Cannon RO III. Cardiovascular effects of estrogen and lipid-lowering therapies in postmenopausal women. Circulation 1996;93:1928–1937.

40. Heckbert SR, Weiss NS, Koepsell TD, et al. Duration of estrogen replacement therapy in relation to the risk of incident of myocardial infarction in postmenopausal women. Arch Intern Med 1997; 157:1330–1336.

41. The Writing Group for the PEPI Trial. Effects of estrogen or estrogen/progestin regimens on heart disease risk factors in postmenopausal women: the Postmenopausal Estrogen/Progestin Interventions (PEPI) trial. JAMA 1991;273:199–208.

42. Grodstein F, Stampfer MJ, Colditz GA, et al. Postmenopausal hormone therapy and mortality. N Engl J Med 1997;336:1769–1775.

43. Collaborative Group on Hormonal Factors in Breast Cancer. Breast cancer and hormone replacement therapy: collaborative reanalysis of data from 51 epidemiological studies of 52,705 women with breast cancer and 108,411 women without breast cancer. Lancet 1997;350:1047–1059.

44. Daly E, Vessey MP, Hawkins MM, et al. Risk of venous thromboembolism in users of hormone replacement therapy. Lancet 1996;348:977–980.

45. Jick H, Derby LE, Myers MW, et al. Risk of hospital admission for idiopathic venous thromboembolism among users of postmenopausal oestrogens. Lancet 1996;348: 981–983.

46. Grodstein F, Stampfer MJ, Goldhaber SZ, et al. Prospective study of exogenous hormones and risk of pulmonary embolism in women. Lancet 1996;348:983–987.

47. Guiteras Val P, Chaitman BR, Waters DD, et al. Diagnostic accu-

racy of exercise ECG lead systems in clinical subsets of women. Circulaton 1982;65:1465–1474.

48. Chaitman BR, Bourassa MG, Lam J, et al. Noninvasive diagnosis of coronary heart disease in women. In: Eaker ED, Packard B, Wenger NK, et al, eds. Coronary heart disease in women. New York: Haymarket Doyma, 1987:222–228.

49. LaCroix AZ, Guralnik JM, Curb JD, et al. Chest pain and coronary heart disease mortality among older men and women in three communities. Circulation 1990; 81:437–446.

50. Weiner DA, Ryan TJ, McCabe CH, et al. Exercise stress testing: correlations among history of angina, ST-segment response and prevalence of coronary-artery disease in the Coronary Artery Surgery Study (CASS). N Engl J Med 1979;301: 230–235.

51. Hlatky MA, Pryor DB, Harrell FE Jr, et al. Factors affecting sensitivity and specificity of exercise electrocardiography: multivariable analysis. Am J Med 1984;77:64–71.

52. Hung J, Chaitman BR, Lam J, et al. Noninvasive diagnostic test choices for the evaluation of coronary artery disease in women: a multivariate comparison of cardiac fluoroscopy, exercise electrocardiography and exercise thallium myocardial perfusion scintigraphy. J Am Coll Cardiol 1984;4:8–16.

53. Weiner DA, Ryan TJ, Parsons L, et al. Long-term prognostic value of exercise testing in men and women from the Coronary Artery Surgery Study (CASS) Registry. Am J Cardiol 1995;75:865–870.

54. Melin JA, Wijns W, Vanbutsele RJ, et al. Alternative diagnostic strategies for coronary artery disease in women: demonstration of the usefulness and efficiency of probability analysis. Circulation 1985;71: 535:542.

55. Friedman TD, Greene AC, Iskandrian AS, et al. Exercise thallium-201 myocardial scintigraphy in women: correlation with coronary arteriography. Am J Cardiol 1982;49:1632–1637.

56. Goodgold HM, Rehder JG, Samuels LD, et al. Improved interpretation of exercise T1-201 myocardial perfusion scintigraphy in women: characterization of breast attenuation artifacts. Radiology 1985; 165:361–366.

57. Cerqueira MD. Diagnostic testing strategies for coronary artery disease: special issues related to gender. Am J Cardiol 1995;75: 52D–600.

58. Laurienzo JM, Cannon RO III, Ouyyumi AA, et al. Transesophageal dobutamine stress echocardiography for detection of coronary artery disease in women presenting with chest pain: comparison with other standard tests. J Am Coll Cardiol 1995;25:62A-63A. Abstract.

59. Shaw LJ, Miller DD, Romeis JC, et al. Gender differences in the noninvasive evaluation and management of patients with suspected coronary artery disease. Ann Intern Med 1994;120:559–566.

60. Anderson T, Marwick T, Williams MJ, et al. Exercise echocardiography is more cost efficient than exercise ECG as an initial test for evaluation of cardiac symptoms in women. J Am Coll Cardiol 1995; 25:17A–18A. Abstract.

61. Kostis JB, Wilson AC, O'Dowd K, et al, for the MIDAS Study Group. Sex differences in the management and long-term outcome of acute myocardial infarction: a statewide study. Circulation 1994; 90:1715–1730.

62. Maynard C, Litwin PE, Martin JS, et al. Gender differences in the treatment and outcome of acute myocardial infarction: results from the Myocardial Infarction Triage and Intervention Registry. Arch Intern Med 1992;152:972–976.

63. Kudenchuk PJ, Maynard C, Martin JS, et al, for the MITI Project Investigators. Comparison of presentation, treatment, and outcome of acute myocardial infarction in men versus women (The Myocardial Infarction Triage and Intervention Registry). Am J Cardiol 1996; 78:9–14.

64. Coronado BE, Griffith JL, Beshansky JR, et al. Hospital mortality in women and men with acute cardiac ischemia: a prospective multicenter study. J Am Coll Cardiol 1997;29:1490–1496.

65. Zucker DR, Griffith JL, Beshansky JR, et al. Presentations of acute myocardial infarction in men and women. J Gen Intern Med 1997; 12:79–87.

66. Jenkins JS, Flaker GC, Nolte B, et al. Causes of higher in-hospital mortality in women than in men after acute myocardial infarction. Am J Cardiol 1994;73:319–322.

67. Clarke KW, Gray D, Keating NA, et al. Do women with acute myocardial infarction receive the same treatment as men? BMJ 1994; 309:563–566.

68. Adams JN, Jamieson M, Rawles JM, et al. Women and myocardial infarction: agism rather than sexism? Br Heart J 1995;73:87–91.

69. Radford MJ, Johnson RA, Daggett WM Jr, et al. Ventricular septal rupture: a review of clinical and physiological features and an analysis of survival. Circulation 1981;64:545–553.

70. Maynard C, Every NR, Martin JS, et al. Association of gender and survival in patients with acute myocardial infarction. Arch Intern Med 1997;157:1379–1384.

71. McLaughlin TJ, Soumerai SB, Willison DJ, et al. Adherence to national guidelines for drug treatment of suspected acute myocardial infarction: evidence for undertreatment in women and the elderly. Arch Intern Med 1996; 156:799–805.

72. Stone PH, Thompson B, Anderson HV, et al., for the TIMI III Registry Study Group. Influence of race, sex, and age on management of unstable angina and non-Q-wave myocardial infarction: the TIMI III Registry. JAMA 1996;275:1104–1112.

73. Gurwitz JH, McLaughlin TJ, Willison DJ, et al. Delayed hospital presentation in patients who have had acute myocardial infarction. Ann Intern Med 1997;126: 593–599.

74. Malacrida R, Genoni M, Maggioni AP, et al, for the Third International Study of Infarct Survival Collaborative Group. A comparison of the early outcome of acute myocardial infarction in women and men. N Engl J Med 1998; 338:8–14.

75. Weaver WD, White HD, Wilcox RG, et al, for the GUSTO-I Investigators. Comparisons of characteristics and outcomes among women and men with acute myocardial infarction treated with thrombolytic therapy. JAMA 1996;275:777–782.

76. Woodfield SL, Lundergan CF, Reiner JS, et al. Gender and acute myocardial infarction: Is there a different response to thrombolysis? J Am Coll Cardiol 1997;29:35–42.

77. Stone GW, Grines CL, Browne KF, et al. Comparison of in-hospital outcome in men versus women treated by either thrombolytic therapy or primary coronary angioplasty for acute myocardial infarction. Am J Cardiol 1995;75:987–992.

78. Moriel M, Benhorin J, Brown MW, et al, and the Multicenter Myocardial Ischemia Research Group. Detection and significance of myocardial ischemia in women versus men within six months of acute myocardial infarction or unstable angina. Am J Cardiol 1996;77:798–804.

79. Maynard C, Weaver WD. Treatment of women with acute MI: new findings from the MITI registry. J Myocard Ischemia 1992;4:27–37.

80. O'Connor GT, Morton JR, Diehl MJ, et al, for the Northern New England Cardiovascular Disease Study Group. Differences between men and women in hospital mortality associated with coronary artery bypass graft surgery. Circulation 1993;88(part 1):2104–2110.

81. Weintraub WS, Wenger NK, Jones EL, et al. Changing clinical characteristics of coronary surgery patients: differences between men and women. Circulation 1993; 88(part 2):79–86.

82. Davis KB, Chaitman B, Ryan T, et al. Comparison of 15-year survival for men and women after

initial medical or surgical treatment for coronary artery disease: a CASS registry study. J Am Coll Cardiol 1995;24:1000–1009.

83. Welty FK, Mittleman MA, Healy RW, et al. Similar results of percutaneous transluminal coronary angioplasty for women and men with postmyocardial infarction ischemia. J Am Coll Cardiol 1994;23:35–39.

84. Bell MR, Grill DE, Garratt KN, et al. Long-term outcome of women compared with men after successful coronary angioplasty. Circulation 1995;91:2876–2881.

85. Weintraub WS, Wenger NK, Kosinski AS, et al. Percutaneous transluminal coronary angioplasty in women compared with men. J Am Coll Cardiol 1994;24:81–90.

86. Kelsey SF, James M, Holubkov AL, et al, and investigators from the National Heart, Lung, and Blood Institute Percutaneous Transluminal Coronary Angioplasty Registry. Results of percutaneous transluminal coronary angioplasty in women: 1985–1986 National Heart, Lung, and Blood Institute's Coronary Angioplasty Registry. Circulation 1993;87:720–727.

87. Jacobs AK, Faxon DP, Pinkerton CA, et al. Impact of gender on outcome following percutaneous coronary revascularization: the CAVEAT experience. Circulation 1993;88(part 2):1–448. Abstract.

Chapter 29

Breast Cancer: Modifiable Lifestyle Risk Factors

Ursula A. Matulonis

Breast cancer in the United States has a cumulative lifetime incidence of one in eight women. It is second only to lung cancer as the most frequent cause of cancer death among American women (1). Breast cancer represents 30% of new cancer cases per year, and is the leading cancer diagnosed in women. In 1998, 178,700 women in the United States were diagnosed with breast cancer, and 43,500 women died of their disease (1). Research has focused on establishing the etiologies of breast cancer in order to allow modification of risk factors to reduce risk. Established risk factors for breast cancer include older age, having a first degree relative (mother or sister) with breast cancer, nulliparity or late age (over 30) at first birth, early menarche (before age 12, compared to age 15 or greater), late menopause (after age 55), postmenopausal obesity, biopsy-confirmed proliferative breast disease, residency in North America or Europe versus Asia, and higher levels of educational status or income (2–5) (Table 29-1). Rates of breast cancer are lowest in China, India, and Japan, intermediate in South America and Eastern Europe, with the highest rates in North America and Western Europe (2). Many studies have focused on the discrepancy between the incidence of breast cancer in the United States and Western Europe and the comparatively lower incidence in Asia and more underdeveloped countries (2). Cultural variations in lifestyles including diet, exercise, body weight, and menstrual and reproductive patterns have been examined. These variations may ultimately affect breast cancer risk and better explain the high incidence of breast cancer in the United States.

Ultimately, when clear risk factors relating to diet and lifestyle are identified, and several already have been, then modifications can be made in order to impact and reduce risk. Certain risk factors such as diet, exercise, ingestion of hormones, age at first pregnancy and number of pregnancies can be modified. But, at this time, others such as age at menarche and menopause and genetic predisposition to breast cancer are less easily modified. In the United States and in many Western countries, age at menarche has decreased from 16 to less than 13 over the past century (6). This has occurred because of improved childhood nutrition, fewer childhood infections and illnesses, and decreased physical activity during childhood. In addition, the age at first pregnancy has increased and the average number of children per woman has decreased concomitantly with the decrease in age of menarche; this may help to explain the high breast cancer rates in the United States. Some researchers have suggested that decreasing the incidence of breast cancer may be accomplished by delaying menarche, decreasing the time period between menarche to first birth, or by decreasing breast cell division with hormonal therapies (6). Other factors that might be able to modified in order to reduce risk are discussed in this chapter.

DIET

The observed differing breast cancer rates around the world (7) and the acquisition of increased breast cancer risk when migrants' offspring move from low-risk countries to higher risk countries (8,9) suggest that diet is a leading environmental risk for breast cancer. Diets high in fat have been implicated because of the much higher fat content of Western diets compared to diets in underdeveloped or Asian countries (7). Other dietary constituents such as micronutrients, caffeine, alcohol,

Table 29-1 Known Breast Cancer Risk Factors in Women

Increasing age
Family history of breast cancer
Late menopause/early menarche
Postmenopausal obesity
Late first pregnancy
Proliferative breast disease
Significant alcohol consumption (>1 drink/day)
Higher socioeconomic status

soy, isoflavones, and phytochemicals have been examined. Multiple cohort and case-control studies have examined the impact and effect of diet and breast cancer in regards to fat, protein, fiber, and micronutrient intake, with some evidence to support specific recommendations to lessen breast cancer risk. However, these studies have not yet provided information needed for broad dietary changes for the nutritional prevention of breast cancer or attenuation of risk. This section will deal with specific diet constituents and known data for breast cancer risk.

Fat

Fat has been implicated as a risk factor for breast cancer because of its prevalence in Western diets. Animal data have demonstrated an association between fat intake and subsequent increased risk of breast cancer (10,11), but the overall relevance of mice and rat studies to humans has been questioned (12). Animal data have shown that high fat intake promotes mammary tumorigenesis and also significantly increases the size and number of metastatic sites in animals already with cancer (11).

Three types of studies have been used to study diet and breast cancer risk in humans: case-control, cohort, and intervention studies. In case-control studies, the prediagnosis diet in women with breast cancer is compared to the diet of women from the same population who do not have a diagnosis of breast cancer. Case-control studies can be biased by selection bias and recall bias. In selection bias, women who volunteer as controls in a research study may have different dietary habits than women who choose not to be in a study. Recall bias can affect memory about prediagnosis diet. In a review of breast cancer and diet (13), 25 case-control studies were reviewed. In 3, there was an increased risk of breast cancer with fat intake, 12 reported a statistically nonsignificant increase risk, 8 found no association, and 2 found a significant decreased risk. Howe (14) et al reviewed 12 case-control studies, and a statistical summary of all these studies indicated a modest, yet statistically significant result.

In cohort studies or prospective studies, the diet of a large group of women is examined; the diets of women who eventually develop breast cancer are compared to women who do not develop breast cancer. Cohort studies minimize selection bias since the population that develops breast cancer is part of the original group. Recall bias is also minimized since dietary information is collected before breast cancer is diagnosed. Hunter et al reviewed data from 11 prospective studies

(15), and none of these studies demonstrated any significant association between fat intake and incidence of breast cancer when women who consumed the highest amount of fat were compared to those with the lowest fat intake. A pooled analysis of seven prospective studies by Hunter et al (16) revealed no evidence of a positive association between total fat intake and breast cancer risk. This pooled analysis concluded that lowering the amount of total fat intake was unlikely to substantially reduce breast cancer risk.

Most studies have focused on adult premenopausal and postmenopausal women. However, events and exposures occurring during the period between menarche and first full-term pregnancy are thought to be critical for subsequent breast cancer risk, and diet habits during this time period may be important. One recently published study suggests that diet make-up during childhood and adolescence has minimal impact on risk (17). More studies will need to be performed to corroborate these findings before definitive statements may be made about the impact of diet during adolescence.

One other possible explanation for the lack of association is that extremely low fat intake which is below Western standards (reduction of fat intake to less than 20% of food intake) may lessen risk (12,18). In the largest cohort study, the Nurses' Health Study (19), the relative risk for the lowest decile (less than 25% of calories from fat) compared with the highest decile (more than 40% of calories from fat) was 1.2, suggesting no protection even with a lower fat intake and thus casting doubt on the possibility that extremely low fat intakes results in decreased risk.

Specific types of fats may have different cancer-promoting impacts. Animals fed safflower and corn oil, which have high amounts of linoleic acid, demonstrated increased tumor incidence compared with diets high in olive oil (rich in oleic acid) and coconut oil (11). These animal studies have corroborated several studies conducted in Mediterranean countries where there has been an observed decreased risk of breast cancer with a higher intake of monounsaturated fat (in olive oil) (20,21). In the Nurses' Health Study, higher consumption of monounsaturated fat was associated with a lower rate of breast cancer (12). This apparent protective effect of monounsaturated effects merits further study.

An intervention trial is currently underway. The Women's Health Initiative, sponsored by the National Institutes of Health, will compare rates of breast cancer among women randomized to either a usual diet or a diet of 20% or fewer calories derived from fat.

Total fat intake does not appear to be associated with an increased risk of breast cancer in middle-aged and older women. Further studies will be needed to better examine the consequences of fat intake during childhood and both young and later adulthood as well as the impact of certain types of fat on breast cancer risk.

Caffeine

Because of the observation that elimination of caffeine from the diet can provide relief from pain associated with benign breast disease, caffeine was thought to perhaps serve as a risk factor for breast cancer. However, caffeine has not been demonstrated to increase the risk for breast cancer in several case-control and cohort studies (18,22,23).

Fiber

Diets high in fiber have been hypothesized to possibly protect against breast cancer by inhibiting intestinal reabsorption of estrogens that are excreted in the bile. Results of case-control and cohort studies have been difficult to interpret because of variations in measuring fiber amounts as well differences in the types of fiber used in the studies. In a meta-analysis of 10 case-control studies, there was a statistically significant relative risk of 0.85 for an increase of 20 grams per day in dietary fiber (14). In the Nurses' Health Study, there was no protective effect of fiber against breast cancer (19). Rohan et al (24), in a prospective study using high-fiber diets, did demonstrate a statistically significant protective effect, but when the effects of vitamin A were controlled, the significance disappeared. Thus, results are heterogeneous, and no definitive statement of the effects of fiber intake and breast cancer risk can be made at this time.

Vitamins C and E

Three prospective studies have examined the impact of vitamin C intake and the risk of breast cancer, with no significant effect on risk (13,18,25). Ten case-control studies have been performed and were heterogeneous, and no firm conclusions can be made for any benefit for vitamin C intake and protection against breast cancer.

Studies of vitamin E intake and breast cancer risk do not suggest any protective effect (13,18). Case-control study results have been mixed (15). The Nurses' Health Study found no correlation between vitamin E intake and protection against breast cancer (25).

Vitamin A and Beta-carotene

Vitamin A is derived from animal sources, which contain preformed vitamin A (retinol, retinyl esters), and from certain carotenoids that are found in fruits and vegetables. Carotenoids are partially converted to retinol in the intestinal epithelium, and many are potent antioxidants providing possible protection against DNA damage (25,28), thereby producing anti-cancer effects. Vitamin A may exert its protective effects through the regulation of cell differentiation.

The data that are available for vitamin A and breast cancer risk do suggest a modest protective effect for vitamin A. Most studies have been case-control studies, and in a meta-analysis of nine of these studies, total vitamin A, including both preformed vitamin A and carotenoids, had a significant association with breast cancer development (14). But when this meta-analysis examined the individual associations with preformed vitamin A and carotenoids, there was a significant inverse relationship with beta-carotene, but not with preformed vitamin A.

In the prospective Nurses' Health Study (25), there was a modest but significant inverse association between vitamin A and breast cancer. Compared to carotenoids, preformed vitamin A was more strongly associated with a lower risk of breast cancer. In the Nurses' Health Study (25), the effects of both dietary intake of vitamin A and dietary supplements were examined. For nurses who had adequate dietary intake of vitamin A, there was no added benefit to dietary supplements of vitamin A. However, in the nurses who had the lowest quintile of dietary intake, the use of vitamin A supplements (at least 10,000 IU) demonstrated a 50% decrease in the risk of breast cancer compared to women not taking supplements. These findings suggest benefits from vitamin A, rather than some other food constituent that also contains vitamin A. The relationship between total vitamin A intake and breast cancer risk was not exactly linear; women in the highest quintile of vitamin A intake had a 20% lower breast cancer risk compared to women in the lowest quintile. This suggests that only women with a low vitamin A intake are at increased risk.

Therefore, based on case-control studies and cohort studies, both forms of vitamin A, preformed and carotenoids, may be protective against breast cancer, especially in women with low intakes.

Selenium

Five prospective studies have been performed to detect the effect of selenium levels on breast cancer risk (13,18). The Nurses' Health Study, which has provided the longest follow-up data for selenium and risk of breast cancer, found there was no association (26). Of the remaining four cohort studies, Knekt et al (27) did show an increase in breast cancer risk with low selenium levels. This study was performed in Finland, a country with extremely low selenium levels, suggesting a threshold below which low selenium intake will increase breast cancer risk.

Phytoestrogens

Phytochemicals are biologically active non-nutrients, among which phytoestrogens (comprised of lignans and isoflavonoids) are consumed as part of high soyfood diets in countries with known low breast cancer rates (29,30). Soy products have also been shown to increase menstrual cycle length and decrease serum follicular stimulating hormone (FSH) and luteinizing hormone (LH) levels in premenopausal women. In vitro and in vivo studies have demonstrated the anti-angiogenic, estrogenic, anti-estrogenic, and anti-tumor effects of phytoestrogens (30).

Ingram et al's (30) case-control study of phytoestrogens revealed a reduction in breast cancer risk among women with a high intake of phytoestrogens, especially equol and enterolactone, compared to low intake. Since 1991, five other case-control studies have been performed, and three found a reduced risk of breast cancer for premenopausal women, but only one for postmenopausal women (29).

Since another purported antitumor mechanism for phytoestrogens is to bind to the estrogen receptor because of their structural similarity to estrogens, one concern is that phytoestrogens might actually be tumor-promoting. Other concerns are the safety of phytoestrogens in women with estrogen receptor positive breast cancers; more scientific data will be necessary before formal recommendations can be made.

HEIGHT AND BODY MASS INDEX

Several studies examining the relationship between body mass index (BMI) (weight [kg]/height [m^2]) and breast cancer risk have found that BMI and breast cancer risk varies with menstrual status (31). Most studies support an increased risk of breast cancer with postmenopausal obesity and a moderate inverse association with premenopausal women. Examination of the Nurses' Health Study cohort demonstrated that a higher current BMI was associated with lower breast cancer risk before menopause, and after menopause there was a minimally higher risk of breast cancer (32).

Obesity in the postmenopausal woman has also been shown to be associated with a larger tumor size at diagnosis and more extensive nodal involvement as well as a poorer overall survival compared with leaner women (33–35). Obesity may result in delayed detection, higher stage at diagnosis, and more rapid growth of metastases.

The protective effect from obesity in premenopausal women may relate to demonstrated lowered serum estradiol and progesterone levels because of a higher frequency of anovulation (36). In postmenopausal women, serum estrogen is derived mostly from adipose tissue, so estrogen production is directly correlated with body weight and thus BMI (37). Obese women also have lower plasma sex hormone-binding globulin concentration with a resultant increased biologically active estrogen level (38).

Weight gain from age 18 until middle age was unrelated to premenopausal breast cancer but associated with significantly increased risk of postmenopausal breast cancer among women in the Nurses' Health Study. The association was limited to women who had never used postmenopausal hormone replacement therapy. Among these women who never used hormones, a weight gain of 20 kg or more from age 18 to middle age was associated with a relative risk of 1.99 (95% CI, 1.43–2.76) (32).

ALCOHOL

Alcohol consumption is one of the most well-established dietary risk factors for the development of breast cancer (39). Alcohol is an important risk factor since use of alcohol by women in the United States is not uncommon and its use can be modified (40). Popular press coverage of alcohol as a significant risk factor has been limited (41).

Consumption of alcohol and breast cancer risk appear to be dose related (39,42,43). In a recent meta-analysis published in 1994 (43), which incorporated 10 cohort studies and 28 case-control studies, the relative risk for women consuming three drinks per day compared with abstinence was 1.4; these results have also been corroborated by Smith-Warner et al (39) in a pooled analysis of five prospective studies demonstrating a relative risk of 1.41 for intakes of two to five drinks per day, when compared to nondrinkers.

The increased risk of breast cancer and alcohol consumption has been observed in both premenopausal and postmenopausal women. Some studies report larger risks in premenopausal women (44,45), some in postmenopausal women (46) or an equal risk in both (47–49). Some studies have supported a higher risk during earlier ages (7,12), but other studies refute this (47). The type of alcoholic beverage does not appear to impact risk, and most studies indicate that breast cancer risk is increased with consumption of any type of alcohol, including beer, wine, and other spirits (43).

Several possible etiologies exist to explain the increased risk of breast cancer risk from alcohol consumption, including increase in circulating estrogen levels, increased transport of carcinogens into breast tissue, impairment of the immune system, and DNA repair disruption (51). The most well studied has been the resultant augmentation of blood estrogen levels following alcohol consumption. In premenopausal women, plasma estradiol levels increase 20 to 115 minutes following acute alcohol ingestion during the follicular phase of the menstrual cycle (52). However, chronic alcohol consumption in premenopausal women has been shown to increase preovulatory levels of dehydroepiandrosterone sulfate, estrone, and estradiol and luteal phase increases in urinary estrone, estradiol, and estriol (53).

An increase in breast cancer risk has been noted in postmenopausal women taking estrogen replacement therapy (ERT) who have significant alcohol intake. Two (54,55) of three (54–56) cohort studies have demonstrated this interaction between ERT and alcohol use. In postmenopausal women, Ginsburg et al (51) demonstrated a threefold increase in circulating estradiol after acute alcohol ingestion in postmenopausal women taking estrogen. In women taking ERT, estradiol levels increased to 327% of baseline after alcohol administration, and levels rose before peak alcohol levels had been reached. In women not taking ERT, plasma estradiol levels did not change following alcohol consumption. Reasons for the alcohol-related increase in serum estrogen levels are unclear, but possible explanations include increased absorption of estrogen from the gastrointestinal tract or alteration of estradiol metabolism with a decreased conversion of estradiol to estrone.

Alcohol may also act as a carcinogenic promoter by acting as a cocarcinogen, activating procarcinogens, improving cell membrane permeability to carcinogens, and inhibiting the detoxification of carcinogens by direct hepatic impairment (57).

Therefore, based on data demonstrating a relationship between alcohol consumption and risk of breast cancer, those women who are at a higher risk of developing breast cancer should be educated that significant alcohol intake is associated with a higher risk of breast cancer. This is especially true for women who are taking postmenopausal ERT, since the risk of breast cancer is increased threefold with significant concomitant alcohol use. The risks of alcohol intake must be balanced with the demonstrated benefits of moderate alcohol consumption (one to two drinks per day) on reduction of cardiovascular disease, which is the leading cause of death for American women of all ages (58). The mechanism for alcohol's reduction in cardiovascular disease is most likely the result of an increase in high-density lipoprotein cholesterol levels (59) and decreases in platelet aggregability (60).

Because of the benefits of moderate alcohol use and the breast cancer risks of significant alcohol use, which is magnified with concomitant ERT use, the risks and benefits of ERT and alcohol consumption need to be discussed individually with each patient depending on her own breast cancer and cardiovascular disease risk profiles. Other additional complicating medical issues such as osteoporosis or menopausal symptoms must also be factored into the decision-making process.

EXERCISE AND PHYSICAL ACTIVITY

Most epidemiologic studies of physical exercise have demonstrated a reduction in the risk of breast cancer among physically active women. Over 15 case-control and cohort studies have been performed, and most have linked regular exercise with a decreased risk of breast cancer (61,62). However, a definite cause and effect relationship has not been established, nor has the optimal duration, type of exercise, or frequency for optimal impact on a woman's protection against breast cancer (61). Possible explanations for the observed reduction of risk of breast cancer with exercise may include a change in ovulatory characteristics, reduction in obesity, and perhaps immune-based mechanisms (61).

Animal data exists to support a relationship between exercise and breast cancer risk using chemically-induced mammary carcinogenesis in rats. These studies have been performed using various ranges of fat intakes, different carcinogenic agents to induce tumors, and either voluntary or forced exercise (62). In animals induced to have tumor formation, mammary tumor incidence is reduced by exercise when performed at the time of tumor initiation (defined to be complete within 7 days following administration of the carcinogen) (62,63). Some studies, but not all, have shown benefit of exercise during tumor progression (or promotion) (64,65), while some data suggests that exercise enhances tumor promotion (62). These differing results may be a result of forced versus voluntary exercise, differences in the amount and intensity of exercise, and differences in body weight and diet; these factors are also important for the interpretation of human studies.

Thune et al (66) identified 351 women with breast cancer in Norway and compared their level of physical activity to a group of women without breast cancer. Physical activity was scored from 1 (least active, sedentary) to 4 (most active). In this population-based cohort study, physical activity was demonstrated to reduce breast cancer risk, particularly in premenopausal and younger postmenopausal women. For premenopausal women, there was an inverse relationship between activity and risk of breast cancer. For moderate exercise (rating of 2), the adjusted relative risk was 0.77, which dropped to 0.53 for regular exercise. Other case-controlled and cohort studies have supported the concept that exercise reduces the risk of breast cancer, with up to a 60% reduction in risk (61,67–70). However, other studies have refuted this, and in fact have shown an increase in risk with exercise (61,71,72) of from 23% to 60%. As observed in the animal data, interpretation of these studies has been made difficult because of the differences in type, amount, and intensity of exercise, memory recall bias and selection bias observed in case-control studies, and consideration of other breast cancer risks such as alcohol use, family history, and hormonal issues (age at menarche, length of menstrual cycles, age at first pregnancy, and age at menopause).

Several purported mechanisms exist for the observation that exercise decreases breast cancer risk, but so far none have been definitively proven. In humans, much evidence exists linking endogenous hormones to development of breast cancer. Important hormonal events which impart breast cancer risk include age at menarche, age at first pregnancy, and age at menopause (73). Early menarche, and thus early onset of ovulation (74), does have a modest effect on breast

cancer risk, with menarche starting at age 11 or earlier imparting a relative risk of 1.5. Late menopause also increases breast cancer risk, and both early menarche and late menopause effectively allow a longer duration of estrogen production by the ovary. Some researchers have postulated that a woman's lifetime risk of breast cancer is determined by reproductive patterns up to menopause, with the length of time between menarche and first full-term pregnancy to be the most critical period. Thus, the factors which influence a woman's cumulative exposure to estrogen will likely influence breast cancer risk.

In order to decrease breast cancer risk, exercise may change menstrual characteristics, resulting in later age at menarche, fewer ovulatory cycles, and longer length between menstrual periods. Onset of menstruation is delayed in girls who participate in strenuous athletic training such as swimming, running, and ballet (75,76). This delay in menarche may be mediated by an effect on body weight or fat, which are determinants for menarche (61). Other alterations in menstrual characteristics observed in young athletes include secondary amenorrhea, anovulation, and irregular menstrual cycles (77). Delayed menarche has also been associated with lower serum estrogen levels (61).

Exercise can affect body size and decrease obesity, well known risk factors for postmenopausal breast cancer (78). However, heavier premenopausal women may have a decreased risk of breast cancer (79,80). Thus, for postmenopausal women, physical exercise could reduce breast cancer risk by preventing weight gain or enhancing weight loss. Postmenopausal obesity may increase breast cancer risk by increasing circulating free estradiol, free testosterone, and estrone levels (81), as discussed in an earlier section of this chapter.

The immune system has an unknown role in the development of breast cancer. Immune function is generally compromised by extreme high-intensity levels of physical activity (61) and functions at an optimal level during moderate exercise (82). At the cellular level, moderate exercise appears to increase the number and possibly the activity of macrophages, natural killer cells, and lymphokine-activated killer cells (83).

In conclusion, both animal experiments and human epidemiology studies have demonstrated that physical exercise may decrease the risk of breast cancer. Exercise can modify certain characteristics of the menstrual cycle that may be related to breast cancer risk, thereby accounting for the decreased risk of breast cancer. Exercise can further lessen breast cancer risk in postmenopausal women by decreasing body size and reducing obesity, known risk factors for postmenopausal breast cancer. However, before medical care providers can provide specific recommendations on exercise in the prevention of breast cancer, more epidemiologic evidence is needed regarding optimal type, extent, frequency, and duration of physical activity and which time periods within a woman's life can be affected through exercise.

CIGARETTE SMOKING

Cigarettes are undoubtedly the most prevalent known carcinogen in the industrialized world, increasing cancer risk in the respiratory and digestive tracts due to direct exposure to cigarette smoke. Cigarettes have also resulted in increased cancer rates in the bladder, ureters, and pancreas (84). Cigarettes do not appear to significantly increase or decrease the overall risk of breast cancer development (85,86). Women who smoke cigarettes do have estrogen deficiency characteristics, such as increased risk of osteoporosis and early menopause, and decreased risks of endometrial cancer, uterine fibroids, and endometriosis (85,87). This suggests that cigarette smoking has anti-estrogenic effects. Decreased urinary estrogen levels have been found in smokers during the luteal phase of menstruation (88). The anti-estrogenic effect of cigarettes may also be explained by increased hepatic metabolism of estrogens (89). Cigarette smoke may also have carcinogenic effects on the breast because of mutagenic effects; high levels of cigarette mutagens were discovered in breast fluid of non-lactating women (90). It is possible that in breast tissue the direct carcinogenic effects of smoking are counterbalanced by the protective anti-estrogenic effects of cigarette smoking (91). Whether smoking has an effect on breast cancer risk will likely depend on a woman's individual breast cancer risk profile. Women with mutations in either the *BRCA1* or *BRCA2* gene have an approximately 80% chance of developing breast cancer by age 70 (92,93). However, some women with a genetic mutation will not develop breast cancer, and modulation of risk factors may alter their chance of breast cancer development. Cigarette smoking may be a modifiable risk, since there has been a suggestion of a protective effect of cigarette smoking on breast cancer risk in women with *BRCA1* or *BRCA2* gene mutations (94), but this requires further corroborative epidemiologic evidence for confirmation.

USE OF EXOGENOUS ESTROGENS

The benefits of estrogen replacement therapy (ERT) have been well established and documented and include reduced risk of osteoporosis and amelioration of menopausal symptoms such as hot flashes and vaginal dryness. Other possible benefits include reduced risk of cardiovascular disease and attenuation of risk for Alzheimer's disease (95,96).

Estrogen has been implicated, however, in the causation of breast cancer. Direct evidence pointing to estrogen's importance for breast cancer risk is through animal models demonstrating that exogenous estrogen increases mammary tumor development and through in vitro assays showing the growth-promoting effects of estrogen in cultured human breast cancer cells (97).

Human data has also confirmed the importance of estrogen in breast cancer risk (98–100). Excessive estrogenic stimulation of normal breast tissue can increase the number of cell divisions and random genetic errors occurring during breast cell division, which may possibly lead to development of the neoplastic phenotype (97,101). In addition, according to Pike's model (101), a woman's total exposure and timing of exposure to estrogen is critical for breast cancer risk. Age at menarche, first pregnancy, and time of menopause are all critical time points dictating and directing risk. Following a woman's first pregnancy, regardless of age, a short-term increased risk of breast cancer occurs because of hormonal stimulation of breast tissue (97,101). This is followed by a longer-term reduction in risk. An early pregnancy results in

ductal, alveolar, and lobular breast tissue proliferation as a result of high estrogen and progesterone levels as well as breast stem cell differentiation in the terminal ducts and lobules (97,101). This reduction of the stem cell population to more differentiated forms may be the reason for the protection against breast cancer incurred by early pregnancy and may decrease the susceptibility of breast tissue to genetic and exogenous insults.

Cohort studies have supported the concept that long-term ERT (longer than 5 to 10 years) is associated with an increased risk of breast cancer (102). The Nurses' Health Study (99,100) has reported that for women currently taking ERT, there was a significant increase in breast cancer risk. Women taking ERT for 5 to 9 years had a relative increased risk of 1.46, as did women taking ERT for more than 10 years. However, past users of hormonal therapy did not have any increased risk of breast cancer, implying that there are no long-term effects on risk once ERT use has stopped.

The Nurses' Health Study also has examined overall mortality, and current ERT users had a lower mortality compared to non-users (95). However, most of the benefit was observed for women at highest risk for coronary heart disease. Long-term use (more than 10 years) resulted in attenuation of benefit because of a 43% increase in breast cancer mortality. The benefit on overall mortality rate was lost 5 years after stopping use. The Nurses' Health Study also found that addition of a progestin to estrogens does not appear to attenuate the increased risk associated with estrogens, but will reduce the risk of uterine cancer (100,103).

Use of ERT and increased breast cancer risk has been confirmed by a meta-analysis through the Collaborative Group on Hormonal Factors in Breast Cancer (98). Among women currently using ERT, the relative risk of having breast cancer diagnosed increased by 1.023 for each year of use. For women who had used ERT for more than 5 years the relative risk was 1.35. The risk of breast cancer ceased after 5 or more years after cessation of ERT use.

The relationship between breast cancer and oral contraceptives (OC) was also examined by the Collaborative Group on Hormonal Factors in Breast Cancer (104). There was a small increased risk of breast cancer while women were taking combined OC and in the 10 years after stopping use. Relative risk among current users was 1.24; 1 to 4 years after stopping, the risk was 1.16; 5 to 9 years after stopping, it was 1.07. Increased risk of breast cancer ceased 10 years after stopping OC. For both ERT and OC users, the cancers diagnosed were less clinically advanced than those women who had never used ERT or OC.

ERT may increase breast cancer risk in conjunction with other risk factors for breast cancer, and certain populations of women may be at increased risk. The concomitant use of ERT and significant alcohol intake appears to increase substantially the risk of breast cancer. This is discussed earlier in the section on alcohol. Oral contraceptive use in patients with *BRCA1* mutations may increase their risk for breast cancer (105).

Selective estrogen receptor modifiers (SERM's) such as raloxifene, can act as estrogen agonists and result in bone density improvement in postmenopausal women (106) and lower low-density lipoprotein levels (107). Delmas et al (106) studied 601 women who were randomized to placebo, 30 mg,

60 mg, or 150 mg of raloxifene for 2 years. Each dose of raloxifene improved bone density in the lumbar spine and hip, while placebo use resulted in decreased bone density over the 2-year period. In preliminary studies, SERM's may also lower breast cancer and endometrial cancer risk in postmenopausal women (108). Breast cancer risk was lowered by approximately 50% in women who took raloxifene compared to women taking a placebo; endometrial cancer was also lower. Longer follow-up of these studies is needed before definitive recommendations can be made.

Therefore, ERT and OC appear to increase breast cancer risk among current and long-term users. Documented benefits of ERT include decreased risk of osteoporosis and

hip fractures, reduction in menopausal symptoms, and possible decreased risk of cardiovascular disease and Alzheimer's disease. Women should be carefully counseled about the known risks and benefits of ERT and need to understand their own risk factors regarding cardiovascular disease, osteoporosis, and certain cancers, especially breast and uterine. Treatment decisions should be made on an individual basis, weighing the risks and benefits of interventions such as ERT. More research needs to be performed in order to better delineate which groups of women may be more significantly affected by the use of ERT. In addition, SERM's will undoubtedly be used in the future as ERT substitutes and may modify cancer risk.

REFERENCES

1. Landis SH, Murray T, Bolden S, et al. Cancer statistics, 1998. CA Cancer J Clin 1998;48:6–29.

2. Brinton LA, Devesa SS. Epidemiologic factors: incidence, demographics, and environmental factors. In: Harris JR, Lippman ME, Morrow M, and Hellman S, eds. Diseases of the breast. Philadelphia: Lippincott-Raven, 1996:159–168.

3. Brinton LA, Hoover R, Fraumeni JF. Reproductive factors in the aetiology of breast cancer. Br J Cancer 1982;47:757.

4. Brinton LA, Schairer CS, Hoover RN, et al. Menstrual factors and risk of breast cancer. Cancer Invest 1988;6:245.

5. Dupont WD, Page DL. Risk factors for breast cancer in women with proliferative breast disease. N Engl J Med 1985; 312:146.

6. Colditz GA. Fat, estrogens, and the time frame for prevention of breast cancer. Epidemiology 1995;6:209–211.

7. Armstrong B, Doll R. Environmental factors and cancer incidence and mortality in different countries with special reference to dietary practices. Int J Cancer 1975;15:617–631.

8. McMichael AJ, Giles GG. Cancer in migrants to Australia: extending descriptive epidemiologic data. Cancer Res 1988;48:751.

9. Buell P. Changing incidence of breast cancer in Japanese-American women. J Natl Cancer Inst 1973;51:1479–1483.

10. Albanes D. Total calories, body weight, and tumor incidence in mice. Cancer Res 1987;47: 1987.

11. Wynder EL, Cohen LA, Muscat JE, et al. Breast cancer: weighing the evidence for promoting role of dietary fat. J Natl Cancer Inst 1997;89:766–775.

12. Willett WC. Diet and cancer: what do we know? Adv Oncol 1995;11:3–8.

13. Clavel-Chapelon F, Niravong M, Joseph RR. Diet and breast cancer: review of the epidemiologic literature. Cancer Detect Prev 1997;21:426–440.

14. Howe GR, Hirohata T, Hislop TG, et al. Dietary factors and risk of breast cancer: combined analysis of 12 case-control studies. J Natl Cancer Inst 1990;82: 561–569.

15. Hunter DJ, Willet WC. Diet, body build, and breast cancer. Ann Rev Nutr 1994;14:393–418.

16. Hunter DJ, Spiegelman D, Adami H-O, et al. Cohort studies of fat intake and the risk of breast cancer—a pooled analysis. N Engl J Med 1996;334:356–361.

17. Potischman N, Weiss HA, Swanson CA, et al. Diet during adolescence and risk of breast cancer among young women. J Natl Cancer Inst 1998;90:226–333.

18. Hunter DJ, Willett WC. Nutrition and breast cancer. Cancer Causes Control 1996;7:56–68.

19. Willett WC, Hunter DJ, Stampfer MJ, et al. Dietary fat and fiber in relation to risk of breast cancer. JAMA 1992;268:2037.

20. Martin-Moreno JM, Willett WC, Gorgojo L, et al. Dietary fat, olive oil intake and breast cancer risk. Int J Cancer 1994;54:774–780.

21. Trichopoulou A, Katsouyanni K, Stuver S, et al. Consumption of olive oil and specific food groups in relation to breast cancer risk in Greece. J Natl Cancer Inst 1995;87:110–116.

22. Rosenberg L, Miller DR, Helmrich SP, et al. Breast cancer and the consumption of coffee. Am J Epidemiol 1985;122:391–399.

23. Snowden DA, Phillips RL. Coffee consumption and risk of fatal cancers. Am J Public Health 1984;74:820–823.

24. Rohan TE, Howe GR, Friedenreich CM, et al. Dietary fiber, vitamins A, C, and E, and the risk of breast cancer: a cohort study. Cancer Causes Control 1993;4:29–37.

25. Hunter DJ, Manson JE, Colditz GA, et al. A prospective study of the intake of vitamins C, E, and A and the risk of breast cancer. N Engl J Med 1993;329:234–240.

26. Hunter DJ, Morris JS, Stampfer MJ, et al. A prospective study of

selenium status and breast cancer risk. JAMA 1990;264:1128–1131.

27. Knekt P, Aromaa A, Maatela J, et al. Serum selenium and subsequent risk of cancer among Finnish men and women. J Natl Cancer Inst 1990;82:864–868.

28. Peto R, Doll R, Buckley JD, et al. Can dietary beta-carotene materially reduce human cancer rates? Nature 1981;290:201–208.

29. Messina M, Barnes S, Setchell KD. Phytoestrogens and breast cancer. Lancet 1997;350:971–972.

30. Ingram D, Sanders K, Kolybaba M, et al. Case-control study of phyto-estrogens and breast cancer. Lancet 1997;350:990–994.

31. Hunter DJ, Willett WC. Diet, body size, and breast cancer. Epidemiol Rev 1993;15:110–132.

32. Huang Z, Hankinson SE, Colditz GA, et al. Dual effects of weight and weight gain on breast cancer risk. JAMA 1997;278:1407–1411.

33. Tretli S, Haldorsen T, Ottestad L. The effect of pre-morbid height and weight on the survival of breast cancer patients. Br J Cancer 1990;62:299–303.

34. Senie RT, Rosen PP, Rhodes P, et al. Obesity at diagnosis of breast cancer influences duration of disease-free survival. Ann Intern Med 1992;116:26–32.

35. Daniell HW, Tam E, Filice A. Larger axillary metastases in obese women and smokers with breast cancer: an influence by host factors on early tumor behavior. Breast Cancer Res Treat 1993;25:193–201.

36. Potischman N, Swanson CA, Siiteri P, et al. Reversal of relation between body mass and endogenous estrogen concentrations with menopausal status. J Natl Cancer Inst 1996;88:756–758.

37. Hankinson SE, Willett WC, Manson JE, et al. Alcohol, height, and adiposity in relation to estrogen and prolactin levels in postmenopausal women. J Natl Cancer Inst 1995;87:1297–1302.

38. Newcomb PA, Klein R, Klein BE, et al. Association of dietary and life-style factors with sex hormones in postmenopausal women. Epidemiology 1995;6:318–321.

39. Smith-Warner SA, Spiegelman D, Yaun S-S, et al. Alcohol and breast cancer in women: a pooled analysis of cohort studies. JAMA 1998;279:535–540.

40. Schatzkin A, Longnecker MP. Alcohol and breast cancer. Cancer 1994;74(suppl):1101–1110.

41. Houn F, Bober MA, Huerta EE, et al. The association between alcohol and breast cancer: popular press coverage of research. Am J Public Health 1995;85:1082–1086.

42. Willet WC, Stampfer MJ, Colditz GA, et al. Moderate alcohol comsumption and the risk of breast cancer. N Engl J Med 1987;316:1174–1180.

43. Longnecker M. Alcoholic beverage consumption in relation to risk of breast cancer: meta-analysis and review. Cancer Causes Control 1994;5:73–82.

44. Schatzkin A, Jones Y, Hoover RN, et al. Alcohol consumption and breast cancer in the epidemiologic follow-up study of the first National Health and Nutrition Examination Survey. N Engl J Med 1987;316:1169–1173.

45. Van't Veer P, Kok FJ, Hermus RJ, et al. Alcohol dose, frequency, and age at first exposure in relation to the risk of breast cancer. Int J Epidemiol 1989;18:511–517.

46. Ferraroni M, Decarli A, Willett WC, et al. Alcohol and breast cancer risk: a case-control study from Northern Italy. Int J Epidemiol 1991;20:859–864.

47. La Vecchia C, Negri E, Parazzini F, et al. Alcohol and breast cancer: update from an Italian case-control study. Eur J Cancer Clin Oncol 1989;25:1711–1717.

48. Sneyd MJ, Paul C, Spears GF, et al. Alcohol consumption and risk of breast cancer. Int J Cancer 1991;48:812–815.

49. Longnecker MP, Newcomb PA, Mittendorf R, et al. Risk of breast cancer in relation to lifetime alcohol consumption. J Natl Cancer Inst 1995;87:923–929.

50. Harvey EB, Schairer C, Brinton LA, et al. Alcohol consumption and breast cancer. J Natl Cancer Inst 1987;78:657–661.

51. Ginsburg EL, Mello NK, Mendelson JH, et al. Effects of alcohol ingestion on estrogens in postmenopausal women. JAMA 1996;276:1747–1751.

52. Mendelson JH, Lukas SE, Mello NK, et al. Acute alcohol effects on plasma estradiol levels in women. Psychopharmacology 1988;94:464–467.

53. Reichman ME, Judd JE, Longcope C, et al. Effects of alcohol consumption on plasma and urinary hormone concentrations in premenopausal women. J Natl Cancer Inst 1993;85:722–727.

54. Colditz GA, Stampfer MJ, Willett WC, et al. Prospective study of estrogen replacement therapy and risk of breast cancer in postmenopausal women. JAMA 1990;264:2648–2653.

55. Gapstur SM, Potter JD, Sellers TA, et al. Increased risk of breast cancer with alcohol consumption in postmenopausal women. Am J Epidemiol 1992;136:1221–1231.

56. Freidenreich CM. Letter to the editor. Am J Epidemiol 1994;5:541–542.

57. Garro AJ, Lieber CS. Alcohol and cancer. Annu Rev Pharmacol Toxicol 1982;1:267–271.

58. Stampfer MJ, Rimm EB, Chapman Walsh D. Commentary: alcohol, the heart, and public policy. Am J Public Health 1993;83:801.

59. Stampfer MJ, Sacks FM, Salvini S, et al. A prospective study of cholesterol, apolipoproteins, and

the risk of myocardial infarction. N Engl J Med 1991;325:373.

60. Kluft C, Hie AFH, Kooistra PK, et al. Alcohol and fibrinolysis. In: Veenstra J, van der Heij DG, eds. Alcohol and cardiovascular disease. Wageningen, The Netherlands: Pudoc, 1992:45.

61. Gammon MD, John EM, Britton JA. Recreational and occupational physical activities and risk of breast cancer. J Natl Cancer Inst 1998;90:100–117.

62. Friedenreich CM, Rohan TE. A review of physical activity and breast cancer. Epidemiology 1995;6:311–317.

63. Yedniak RA, Layman DK, Milner JA. Influences of dietary fat and exercise on DMBA-induced mammary tumors. Fed Proc 1987;45:1087.

64. Cohen LA, Boylan E, Epstein M, et al. Voluntary exercise and experimental mammary cancer. Adv Exp Med Biol 1992;322: 41–59.

65. Bennink MR, Palmer HJ, Messina MJ. Exercise and caloric restriction modify rat mammary carcinogenesis. Fed Proc 1986;45: 1087.

66. Thune I, Brenn T, Lund E, et al. Physical activity and the risk of breast cancer. N Engl J Med 1997;336:1269–1275.

67. Albanes D, Blair AA, Taylor PR. Physical activity and risk of cancer in the NHANES I population. Am J Public Health 1989; 79:744–750.

68. Bernstein L, Henderson BE, Hanisch R, et al. Physical exercise and reduced risk of breast cancer in young women. J Natl Cancer Inst 1994;86:1403–1408.

69. Mittendorf R, Longnecker MP, Newcomb PA, et al. Strenuous physical activity in young adulthood and risk of breast cancer (United States). Cancer Causes Control 1995;6:347–353.

70. D'Avanzo B, Nanni O, La Vecchia C, et al. Physical activity and breast cancer risk. Cancer Epidemiol Biomarkers Prev 1996;5:155–160.

71. Dorgan JF, Brown C, Barrett M, et al. Physical activity and risk of breast cancer in the Framingham heart study. Am J Epidemiol 1994;139:662–669.

72. Paffenbarger RS, Hyde RT, Wing AL. Physical activity and incidence of cancer in diverse populations: a preliminary report. Am J Clin Nutr 1987;45(1 Suppl): 312–317.

73. Colditz GA, Frazier AL. Models of breast cancer show that risk is set by events of early life: prevention efforts must shift focus. Cancer Epidemiol Biomarkers Prev 1995;4:567–571.

74. Bernstein L, Ross RK. Endogenous hormones and breast cancer risk. Epidemiol Rev 1993;15;48–65.

75. Malina RM, Spirduso WW, Tate C, et al. Age at menarche and selected menstrual characteristics in athletes at different competitive levels and in different sports. Med Sci Sports Exerc 1978;10:218–222.

76. Frisch RE, Wyshak G, Vincent L. Delayed menarche and amenorrhea in ballet dancers. N Engl J Med 1990;303:17–19.

77. Harlow SD, Matanoski GM. The association between weight, physical activity, and stress and variation in the length of the menstrual cycle. Am J Epidemiol 1991;133:38–49.

78. Kelsey JL, Bernstein L. Epidemiology and prevention of breast cancer. Annu Rev Public Health 1996;17:47–67.

79. Ballard-Barbash R, Swanson CA. Body weight: estimation of risk for breast and endometrial cancers. Am J Clin Nutr 1996; 63(3 suppl):437S–441S.

80. Hunter DJ, Willett WC. Nutrition and breast cancer. Cancer Causes Control 1996;7:56–68.

81. Enriori CL, Reforzo-Membrive J. Peripheral aromatization as a risk factor for breast and endometrial cancer in postmenopausal women: a review. Gynecol Oncol 1984;17:1–21.

82. Nieman DC. Exercise, upper respiratory tract infection, and the immune system. Med Sci Sports Exerc 1994;26:128–139.

83. Shephard RJ, Shek PN. Cancer, immune function, and physical activity. Can J Appl Physiol 1995;20:1–25.

84. Schottenfeld D, Fraumeni JF, eds. Cancer epidemiology and prevention. 2nd ed. New York: Oxford University Press, 1996.

85. Baron JA, La Vecchia C, Levi F. The antiestrogenic effect of cigarette smoking in women. Am J Obstet Gynecol 1990;162:502–514.

86. Palmer JR, Rosenberg L. Cigarette smoking and the risk of breast cancer. Epidemiol Rev 1993;15:145–156.

87. Hiatt RA, Fireman BH. Smoking, menopause, and breast cancer. J Natl Cancer Inst 1986;76:833–838.

88. MacMahon B, Trichopoulos D, Cole P, et al. Cigarette smoking and urinary estrogens. N Engl J Med 1982;307:1062–1065.

89. Michnovicz JJ, Hershcoph RJ, Naganuma H, et al. Increased 2-hydroxylation of estradiol as a possible mechanism for the antiestrogenic effect of cigarette smoking. N Engl J Med 1986; 315:1305–1309.

90. Petrachis NL, Maack CA, Lee RE, et al. Mutagenic activity in nipple aspirates of human breast fluid. Cancer Res 1980;40:188–189. Letter.

91. Baron JA, Haile RW. Protective effect of cigarette smoking on breast cancer risk in women with BRCA1 or BRCA2 mutations? J Natl Cancer Inst 1998;90:726–727. Editorial.

92. Easton DF, Ford D, Bishop DT. Breast and ovarian cancer incidence in BRCA1-mutation carriers: Breast Cancer Linkage Consortium. Am J Hum Genet 1995;56:256–271.

93. Tonin P, Ghadirian P, Phelan C, et al. A large multisite cancer family is linked to BRCA2. J Med Genet 1995;32:982–984.

94. Brunet JS, Ghadirian P, Rebbeck TR, et al. Effect of smoking on breast cancer in carriers of mutant BRCA1 or BRCA2 genes. J Natl Cancer Inst 1998;90:761–766.

95. Grodstein F, Stampfer MJ, Colditz GA, et al. Postmenopausal hormone therapy and mortality. N Engl J Med 1997;336:1769–1775.

96. Grodstein F, Stampfer MJ. The epidemiology of coronary heart disease and estrogen replacement in postmenopausal women. Prog Cardiovasc Dis 1995;38:199–210.

97. Hulka BS, Liu ET, Lininger RA. Steroid hormones and risk of breast cancer. Cancer 1994;74:1111–1124.

98. Collaborative Group on Hormonal Factors in Breast Cancer. Breast cancer and hormone replacement therapy: collaborative reanalysis of data from 51 epidemiological studies of 52,705 women with breast cancer and 108,411 women without breast cancer. Lancet 1997;350:1047–1059.

99. Colditz GA, Stampfer MJ, Willett WC, et al. Prospective study of estrogen replacement therapy and risk of breast cancer in postmenopausal women. JAMA 1990;264:2648–2653.

100. Colditz GA, Hankinson SE, Hunter DJ, et al. The use of estrogens and progestins and the risk of breast cancer in postmenopausal women. N Engl J Med 1995;332:1589–1593.

101. Pike MC, Krailo MD, Henderson BE, et al. "Hormonal" risk factors, "breast tissue age" and the incidence of breast cancer. Nature 1983;303:767–770.

102. Steinberg KK, Smith SJ, Thacker SB, et al. Breast cancer risk and duration of estrogen use: the role of study design in meta-analysis. Epidemiology 1994;5:415–421.

103. Antures CMF, Stolley PD, Rosenshein NB, et al. Endometrial cancer and estrogen use: a report of a large case-control study. N Engl J Med 1970;300:9–13.

104. Collaborative Group on Hormonal Factors in Breast Cancer. Breast cancer and hormonal contraceptives: collaborative reanalysis of individual data on 53,297 women with breast cancer and 100,239 women without breast cancer from 54 epidemiological studies. Lancet 1996;347:1713–1727.

105. Ursin G, Henderson BE, Haile RW, et al. Does oral contraceptive use increase the risk of breast cancer in women with BRCA1/BRCA2 mutations more than in other women? Cancer Res 1997;57:3678–3681.

106. Delmas PD, Bjarnason NH, Mirlak N, et al. N Engl J Med 1997;337:1641.

107. Walsh BW, Kuller LH, Wild RA, et al. JAMA 1998;279:1445–1451.

108. Cummings SR, Norton L, Eckert S, et al. Raloxifene reduced the risk of breast cancer and may decrease the risk of endometrial cancer in post-menopausal women: two-year findings from the multiple outcomes of raloxifene evaluation (MORE) trial. Proc Am Soc Clin Oncol 1998;17:2a.

Chapter 30

Osteoporosis

Meryl S. LeBoff

Osteoporosis, a low bone mass that leads to skeletal fragility and fractures, is a major public health problem. More than 75 million Europeans, Americans, and Japanese have osteoporosis or are at risk for osteoporosis (1), and only about 25% are diagnosed. Osteoporosis was thought to be a part of the normal aging process, a silent disease until a patient presented with a forearm, spine, or hip fracture. With advancing age there is an exponential rise in spine and hip fractures in women and men. A 50-year-old woman has a 40% lifetime risk of an osteoporotic fracture (2–4) and a man has up to a 29% risk (5). While spine and forearm fractures may cause pain and disability, hip fractures are the most serious fractures because they may lead to loss of independence and death in up to 20% of patients in the first year (2,6). A woman's risk of a hip fracture is equal to her combined risk of breast, ovarian, and uterine cancer.

Health care expenditures for osteoporosis in the United States are $13.8 billion annually or $38 million a day: 62.4% for inpatient care, 28.2% for nursing home services, and 9.4% for outpatient care (7). With the aging of America, and the increased life expectancy of women and men beyond age 65, these health care costs could rise two- to threefold in the early 21st century. The personal and health care costs of osteoporosis could be reduced by prevention and treatment programs. Osteoporosis has been in the dawn of a new era that will make it possible to prevent the rise in osteoporotic fractures with age. This chapter will review the diagnosis of osteoporosis and the prevention and treatment of this disease.

SKELETAL LIFE CYCLE

Bone is built during adolescence, after which peak bone mass is achieved. About 50% of bone mass is gained during puberty, a critical time to maximize peak bone mass. Women and men lose bone with age at a rate of approximately 0.7% to 1% per year and recent data show that bone loss increases in the eighth and ninth decades (8–12). Women show an early menopausal acceleration of bone loss of approximately 1% to 3% each year (13–15). From young adulthood to old age, women lose 42% of their spinal and 58% of femoral neck bone mass; in the spine and hip, men lose one-fourth and two-thirds that of women, respectively (16). Bone density in a given patient depends on the peak bone mass at maturity and bone loss with menopause and/or age.

RISK FACTORS

Risk factors for osteoporosis include: Caucasian or Asian race, family history of a hip fracture, body weight less than 127 pounds (below the 25th percentile), history of fracture (over age 40), or cigarette smoking. Table 30-1 lists some secondary causes of low bone mass or osteoporosis (17–19). Glucocorticoid therapy is the most common secondary cause of osteoporosis. Osteoporosis develops in an estimated 30% to 50% of glucocorticoid-treated subjects through multiple mechanisms including negative calcium balance, deficient bone formation, and increased bone resorption (20). Anorexia and eating dis-

Table 30-1 Conditions and Medications Associated with Reduced Bone Mass or Osteoporosis

CATEGORY	SPECIFIC CONDITION/MEDICATION
Primary osteoporosis	Juvenile osteoporosis, postmenopausal osteoporosis (Type I), involutional osteoporosis (Type II)
Endocrine abnormalities	Glucocorticoid excess, thyroid excess (supraphysiological), hypogonadism, prolactinomas or anorexia nervosa (hypogonadism), hyperparathyroidism, hypercalciuria
Nutritional deficiency	Vitamin D deficiency
Processes affecting the marrow	Multiple myeloma, leukemia, Gaucher's disease
Immobilization	Spaceflight
Gastrointestinal diseases	Gastrectomy, primary biliary cirrhosis, liver disease, inflammatory bowel disease
Connective tissue disorders	Osteogenesis imperfecta, homocystinuria, Ehlers-Danlos syndrome
Rheumatological disorders	Ankylosing spondylitis, rheumatoid arthritis
Medications	Anticonvulsants, heparin, methotrexate, GnRH agonists and cytoxan (hypogonadism), lithium, Cyclosporine-A

Modified from LeBoff MS. Calcium and metabolic bone disease. In: Medical knowledge self assessment program (MKSAP X), Part C Book 4. Philadelphia: American College of Physicians, 1995:1079–1087.

orders affect 3% of young adults; in addition to nutritional deficiencies, anorexia nervosa is associated with hypogonadism, hypercortisolism, and low adrenal androgen (21) and IGF-1 levels (22). A low bone mass may result from other secondary causes such as hyperthyroidism or supraphysiological doses of thyroid hormone, malabsorption, inflammatory bowel disease (23), hypogonadism, malignancies (e.g., multiple myeloma), and osteomalacia. Hyperparathyroidism results in hypercalcemia, hypercalciuria, nephrolithiasis, and preferential loss of cortical bone (e.g., in the one-third radius of a bone density measurement) (24). The reduced bone mass in alcoholics may result from malnutrition and suppressive effects of ethanol on osteoblasts. Use of a gonadotropin-releasing hormone agonist for the therapy of fibroids or endometriosis induces estrogen deficiency and rapid loss of bone that can be prevented with low-dose estrogen and progesterone therapy (25). Cyclosporine A produces a high-turnover osteoporosis, and cyclosporine and prednisone therapy in organ transplant recipients is associated with low bone mass and fractures (26,27). Other medications, including anticonvulsant therapy, can lead to low bone mass and increased risk of fractures (17).

BONE DENSITY

Bone mineral density (BMD) of the spine, hip, or forearm can be measured rapidly and reproducibly with little radiation exposure using a technique called dual x-ray absorptiometry (DXA) [Figure 30-1]. There is an inverse relationship between BMD and the risk of fracture; a low BMD provides a gradient of risk for fracture. According to prospective studies, a decrease in bone mineral density of more than one standard deviation compared with age-adjusted controls (age 65 or older) is associated with a 1.3- to 2.7-fold increase in relative fracture risk (28). In a woman over age 65, hip bone density is most predictive of the risk of a hip fracture. Body composition (fat and lean tissue) may also be measured sensitively and accurately with DXA (29). The BMD in a patient is compared with that of: 1) young-

normal controls to determine whether there is reduction in BMD from peak bone mass (e.g., t score), and 2) age-matched controls to assess whether the BMD is diminished relative to an age-matched controls (e.g., z score). The World Health Organization (WHO) has developed the following bone density definitions to describe different gradations of low bone mass (6): *Normal* (BMD not more than 1 SD below the young adult mean); *osteopenia (low bone mass)* (BMD between −1 SD and −2.5 SD); *osteoporosis* (BMD below −2.5 SD); *established osteoporosis* (BMD below −2.5 SD, with superimposed fracture(s)).

Who Should Be Tested?

Routine use of bone densitometry to screen all healthy, premenopausal women is not recommended. It is, however, indicated for: 1) estrogen-deficient women at risk for osteoporosis*, to identify those women who might benefit from therapy to protect the skeleton from osteoporosis; 2) patients with evidence of vertebral abnormalities, nontraumatic fractures, or reduced bone mass on x-ray films; 3) patients receiving long-term glucocorticoid therapy; 4) patients with primary or secondary hyperparathyroidism to identify those who would benefit from treatment; and 5) monitoring the clinical response to a treatment intervention—to determine whether the prescribed treatment is effective or whether an alternative therapy should be used.

In addition to bone densitometry, the evaluation of a patient with osteoporosis or a bone mass in the very low range of age-matched controls (for example, z score below −1.5 or −2.0) is directed toward the exclusion of secondary causes of low bone mass or osteoporosis. An evaluation for

---

*According to a National Osteoporosis Foundation cost-effectiveness analysis presented at the American Society for Bone and Mineral Research in 1997, risk factors for osteoporosis include: a family history (first-degree relative) of a hip fracture, personal history of a fracture, low body weight, or smoking (18,19).

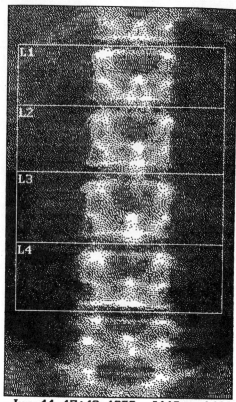

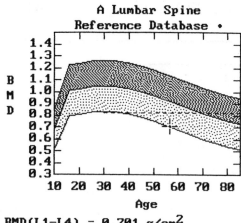

$$BMD(L1\text{-}L4) = 0.701 \text{ g/cm}^2$$

Region	BMD	T(30.0)		Z	
L1	0.635	-2.63	69%	-1.60	78%
L2	0.678	-3.18	66%	-2.04	75%
L3	0.690	-3.58	64%	-2.37	73%
L4	0.779	-3.07	70%	-1.83	79%
L1-L4	0.701	-3.15	67%	-1.97	76%

◆ Age and sex matched
T = peak BMD matched
Z = age matched   TK   11/04/91

·Jun 11 17:42 1998 [113 x 141]
Hologic QDR-2000 (S/N 2413)
Array Spine Medium V4.66A:1

Figure 30-1 Dual x-ray absorptiometry (DXA) of the spine. The patient's bone density is compared with: 1) peak bone mass as the number of standard deviations (SD) relative to the young adult mean (T-score) and 2) age-matched controls as the number of SD relative to and an age-matched cohort (z-score).

secondary causes of osteoporosis includes the measurement of levels of calcium, 25-hydroxy-vitamin D, sensitive thyroid stimulating hormone (TSH), and, in some instances, parathyroid hormone (PTH), liver tests, complete blood count, serum and possibly urinary protein electrophoresis, and urinary calcium and creatinine levels. Additional tests to identify neoplastic or endocrinologic processes and a possible bone biopsy (following a double tetracycline label) should be considered in patients with severe bone loss and in whom primary osteoporosis is uncommon, such as children, African-Americans, premenopausal women, or men under age 60. Correction of the underlying etiology of the osteoporosis may result in marked improvements in BMD.

PREVENTION AND TREATMENT

Treatment of osteoporosis is initiated if the *t* score is below −2.5. Therapy for prevention of osteoporosis is considered for patients with osteopenia and a *t* score between −1 and −2.5. On the basis of a recent National Osteoporosis Foundation cost-effectiveness analysis (which does not apply to the secondary causes of osteoporosis listed in Table 30-1), in a patient without risk factors, therapy to prevent osteoporosis should be started at a *t* score below −2.0 (18,19). In the presence of risk factors (a family history of a fracture, personal history of a fracture after age 40, low body weight, or smoking), therapy should be initiated earlier at a *t* score of −1.5 and with multiple risk factors at a *t* score of −1.0. According to an earlier evaluation of clinical indications for bone densitometry, a *z* score below −1 warranted possible therapy (30).

The therapeutic objectives in patients with osteoporosis are to 1) ameliorate acute or chronic pain associated with a fracture and increase functional capacity, 2) inhibit bone resorption and 3) increase bone formation, a more daunting task, and 4) reduce fractures. A brief period of immobilization, analgesics (e.g., non-steroidal analgesics and non-sedating medications), ice or heat, back braces, and physical therapy are effective for pain control. Physical or occupational therapy, progressive joint mobilization, and exercise are part of the rehabilitation from a fracture.

Healthy Lifestyles

Lifestyle modifications such as eliminating smoking and excessive alcohol intake and insuring participation in regular weight-bearing exercises should be routinely recommended to every patient. Before introducing a therapeutic intervention, it is also important to review a patient's calcium and vitamin D intake, and try to reduce risk factors associated with osteoporosis.

Calcium

If total calcium intake and absorption are inadequate to balance the daily calcium losses, bone loss ensues. Prospective studies show that supplemental calcium is effective in stabilizing cortical bone, particularly in late postmenopausal women and those with a low calcium intake (10,19). Calcium may also contribute to a reduction in fractures (31). According to the Institutes of Medicine in 1997, to prevent negative calcium balance, children and young adults aged 9 to 18 and pregnant women require 1300 mg of elemental calcium daily (Tables 30-2 and 30-3). In pre-pubertal children calcium supplementation raises BMD that may ultimately improve peak bone mass (32). As shown in Table 30-2, women and men aged 50 and younger require 1000 mg and those over age 50 require 1200 mg of elemental calcium daily.

National surveys show that the average calcium intake is about 600 mg/day, one half the current recommended intake. Calcium is optimally consumed in the diet in the form of dairy products and other food sources replete with calcium because of the presence of many other nutrients. Good sources of dietary calcium are shown in Table 30-4. Calcium-fortified orange juice, which contains the same amount of calcium as a glass of milk, provides a practical option for some children and adults. In women and men with insufficient dietary calcium intakes, supplemental calcium such as calcium carbonate or calcium citrate to provide the total calcium intakes listed in Table 30-2 are generally safe, unless there is an underlying disorder of calcium homeostasis. Recent data from a large observational study, however, showed a lower risk of kidney stones when calcium is consumed from dietary rather than supplemental sources (33).

Calcium carbonate is the most widely used supplement, containing 40% of elemental calcium by weight; it should be taken with meals because of poor absorption in achlorhydric patients (34). Calcium citrate contains 24% elemental

Table 30-2 Adults and Required Calcium

Age	How much (mg)
• 9 to >19 years, pregnant or lactating	1000
• 19–50 years	1000
• 51->70 years	1200
Upper limit	2500

SOURCE: Dietary Reference Intake (DRI) Committee, 1997.

Table 30-3 Children and Required Calcium

Age	How much (mg)
• 6 months–1 year	400
• 1–3 years	270
• 4–8 years	500–800
• 9–18 years	1300

SOURCE: Dietary Reference Intake (DRI) Committee, 1997.

Table 30-4 Good Dietary Sources of Calcium

Food	Portion Size	Calcium (mg)
• Skim milk	1 cup	302
• Yogurt, plain		
non-fat	1 cup	452
fruit + low fat	1 cup	314
• Swiss cheese	1.5 oz.	408
• Orange juice		
(with Ca⁺⁺)	1 cup	300
• Frozen yogurt	1/2 cup	103
• Broccoli	1 cup	72

SOURCE: New England Dairy & Food Council.

calcium, has enhanced bioavailability, and is associated with fewer gastrointestinal side effects than calcium carbonate. Normally there is an inverse relationship between calcium intake and absorption. As a result of this homeostatic process, the intake of 1000 mg elemental calcium instead of 500 mg results in 27% lower absorption (35). Thus, to optimize absorption, the calcium content of a supplement should not exceed 500 mg per dose.

Vitamin D

Vitamin D is important for the absorption of calcium and normal mineralization of bone. Advancing age leads to decreased intake of vitamin D, less activation of vitamin D in the skin, less sun exposure, and lower rates of calcium absorption that may adversely affect the skeleton (36–38). It is striking that studies done 30 years ago from Europe and Scandinavia showed an increased incidence of osteomalacia in up to one third of patients with hip fractures (39–41). Vitamin D deficiency may be uncommon in healthy individuals (42). Despite the rising incidence of hip fractures in the elderly in the United States, vitamin D deficiency, although preventable, is often unrecognized (38).

Several lines of evidence indicate that subclinical vitamin D deficiency may lead to fractures. First, vitamin D levels show a seasonal variation with a decrease in winter and spring that parallels the seasonal increase in hip fractures according to some studies (43–45). Second, low vitamin D levels and reduced calcium absorption lead to a compensatory rise in parathyroid hormone (PTH) levels, increased bone turnover, and bone loss; patients with hip fractures show elevated PTH levels, according to some studies (46,47). In a study of patients with acute hip fractures in Boston with no known secondary causes of bone loss, 57% of patients had deficient vitamin D levels (<5 ng/mL) and 37% had secondary hyperparathyroidism with elevated PTH levels (48). Recent data show that vitamin D and calcium therapy lead to suppression of PTH and a rapid reduction in markers of bone turnover (49). In addition, in a prospective study of 3600 elderly women living in residential communities, supplementation with 1200 mg of calcium and 800 units of vitamin D was associated with a 42% reduction of hip fractures in 18 months (50). Dawson-Hughes et al recently showed a 50% reduction in nonverbetral fractures in community-dwelling men and women treated with 500 mg of calcium and 700 units of vitamin D (51).

Shown in Table 30-5 are the recent recommendations for vitamin D according to the Institutes of Medicine in 1997. Replacement doses of vitamin D (400–800 units/day) are often achieved with a multivitamin that contains 400 units of vitamin D and a calcium and vitamin D supplement(s). Treatment of patients with vitamin D deficiency requires higher doses of vitamin D such as Drisdol (200 units/drop or 8000 units/cc), vitamin D (50,000 units), or rarely vitamin D injections. Very large doses of vitamin D may be necessary in patients with malabsorption until the underlying gastrointestinal disorder is treated. While osteomalacia will heal with 1000 units of vitamin D each day, higher doses (e.g., 1000–7000 units/day) will facilitate a more rapid resolution of the bone disease. With pharmacologic doses of vitamin D, careful monitoring of levels of vitamin D and serum and urine calcium is necessary to prevent hypercalcemia and hypercalciuria.

Use of 1,25-dihydroxyvitamin D may stimulate calcium absorption and bone formation (at pharmacologic doses) but has a narrow therapeutic window with risks of hypercalcemia and hypercalciuria. While some studies showed that 1,25-dihydroxyvitamin D administration is ineffective in preserving bone mass in osteoporosis, high doses of 1,25-dihydroxyvitamin D produced some increase in BMD (52).

Exercise

Weight-bearing and strength-training exercises maintain or modestly increase bone mass (53,54). Exercise increases muscle mass and strength, which may lead to improved balance, coordination, and reduced risk of falls. Examples of weight-bearing exercises include walking, jogging, skating, racquet sports, and aerobic exercises. Regular exercises in a mixed exercise program 30 to 45 minutes three times or more a week are advisable as detraining results in a loss of bone mass. (See also Chapter 20.)

Hormone Replacement Therapy

In the absence of contraindications, estrogen therapy is the first choice for the prevention and treatment of osteoporosis because of the potential combined benefit of a reduction in cardiovascular risk (55,56) and bone loss. The apparent cardioprotective effect of estrogens is mediated in part by changes in lipoprotein profiles and by other mechanisms such as vasodilatory and antioxidant effects. Estrogen reduces concentrations of total and LDL cholesterol and raises levels of HDL by increasing the clearance of LDL and the production

of HDL. The use of combined estrogen and progesterone does not appear to attenuate the cardiovascular benefit (56). In addition, estrogen decreases hot flushes and atrophic urogenital changes.

There are several regimens for prescribing hormone replacement therapy. (See also Chapter 27.) To minimize the risk of endometrial hyperplasia or carcinoma, estrogen is administered in sequential regimen with progestin as follows: 1) daily conjugated estrogen (Premarin) 0.625 mg with medroxyprogesterone 5–10 mg the first 12 to 14 days each month (another choice is Premphase, a combination pill with progesterone for 14 days), or 2) estrogen for 25 days each month with a progesterone added on days 12 or 13 to 25 each month. Because sequential estrogen and progestin regimens usually induce cyclical withdrawal bleeding, daily continuous estrogen and progestin regimens that produce atrophy of the endometrium are now used. Continuous regimens include: daily conjugated estrogen 0.625 mg with 2.5 or 5.0 mg medroxyprogesterone (such as Prempro, a combination pill with two progesterone doses). With use of continuous estrogen and progestin regimens, some women develop irregular bleeding in the first 6 months or more and 80% to 85% are amenorrheic at 1 year. Estrogen is administered alone in women who have had a hysterectomy. Transdermal estrogens can prevent bone loss, although not all preparations have been tested for their effects on bone. Transdermal estrogen may be administered as a biweekly estrogen patch using Estraderm or Virelle or a once-a-week Climara patch. Transdermal estrogens do not raise HDL levels so they do confer the full beneficial effects of oral estrogens on lipoproteins. Combination patches that incorporate both estrogen and progesterone in a patch are under evaluation.

Prospective studies show that estrogen replacement decreases indices of bone resorption and increases bone mass (12,57–60). The Postmenopausal Estrogen and Progesterone Intervention (PEPI) Trial evaluated the effects of progesterone and/or estrogen on bone density in a large prospective, randomized, placebo-controlled study of 875 women over 3 years (Figure 30-2) (12). A placebo group was treated with calcium alone (this group lost bone). The following were the other treatment groups: 1) conjugated estrogen (0.625 mg daily), 2) conjugated estrogen in the same dose plus medroxyprogesterone (10 mg daily) for days 1 to 12 each month, and 3) a daily continuous estrogen and progesterone dose (0.625 mg of conjugated estrogen plus 2.5 mg of medroxyprogesterone). In addition, conjugated estrogen was administered in a sequential fashion with 200 μg of micronized progesterone. In all the estrogen and progesterone groups, there was a significant increase of 5.1% in spinal bone density and of 2.2% in hip BMD. Among the adherent participants, there were no significant differences in the bone density response in the different active treatment groups. Older women between the ages of 55 and 64 had a 5.9% increase in their bone density. Previous studies have also shown that late postmenopausal women show a large increase in bone mass (57,61). Those women who had the lowest bone density at baseline had a 6.2% increase in bone mass (Figure 30-2). Thus, hormone replacement therapy has beneficial effects on the skeleton many years after menopause.

A concern in the use of hormone replacement therapy is whether or not this treatment will preserve or increase bone

Table 30-5 Vitamin D by Life-Stage: Adequate Intake[a]	
Age	**How much (units)**
• 1–50 years	200 units
• 51–71 years	400 units
• >70 years	600 units
Upper limit: 2000 units	

[a] Adequate intake: sustain nutritional status and growth.

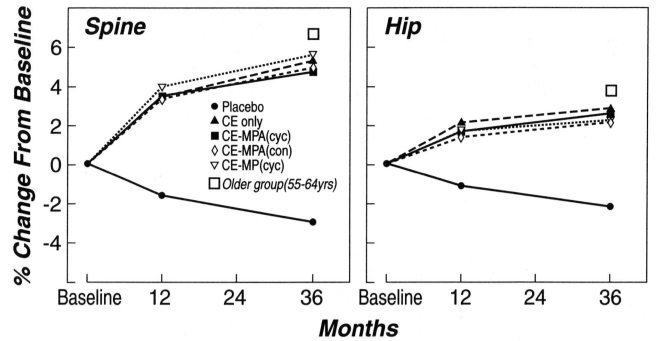

Figure 30-2 The effects of progesterone and/or conjugated estrogen on bone density. Percent change in bone density in adherent participants in the PEPI trial. The following are the descriptors shown herein: CE, conjugated estrogen; MPA, medroxyprogesterone acetate; cyc, cyclical (e.g., sequential therapy); con, continuous; MP, micronized progesterone.

mass. According to the PEPI trial, where pill counts were monitored for compliance, most women on estrogen replacement therapy maintained or increased their bone mass (12). However, in a recent prospective study Rosen et al found that 20% of women lost bone on estrogen replacement therapy, although pill counts were not made (58). Some woman may, therefore, lose bone on estrogen replacement therapy. Adherence to hormone replacement therapy is critically important and physician follow-up and reinforcement is important to ensure this. Estrogen replacement therapy decreases markers of bone breakdown. Chesnut et al recently showed that a large decrement in a marker of bone resorption, the N-telopeptide level, after 6 months of estrogen replacement was associated with an increase in bone mass at 1 year (59). Therefore, a physician might obtain a urine test of bone resorption at 6 months to assess whether certain woman might have the expected increase in bone density at 1 year. The large variability (20%) of this marker of bone breakdown within an individual may confound results if more than one test is not obtained. Bone markers have not, however, consistently predicted the response to therapy using other antiresorptive agents.

A critical question is when to start hormone therapy. Hormone replacement therapy may be instituted at the time of menopause when there is accelerated bone loss, or later in life to prevent the increase in fractures that occurs with age. A recent study by Schneider et al evaluated the efficacy of continuous use of estrogen in women who started therapy at menopause versus late users who commenced estrogen therapy after age 60 (62). These data showed that current users of estrogen who started estrogen at menopause and used it for 20 years had a high bone density of the total hip,

lumbar spine, and forearm that was comparable to the bone density of women over age 60 who had 9 years of estrogen use. Women with the highest bone density at all sites were those who had current and continuous estrogen therapy; previous users of estrogen had the lowest bone densities.

Several studies indicate that estrogen therapy diminishes the risk of fractures. There is little data concerning the effects of estrogen on spine fractures (61,63–65). In a longitudinal cohort study of osteoporotic fractures, Cauley et al showed that women who used hormone replacement therapy for more than 10 years had a marked 73% reduction in the relative risk of hip fractures (65). Similarly, there were marked reductions in the relative risk of wrist fractures (75%) and in all non-spine fractures (40%). Many of the studies of the effects of estrogen on fractures are observational studies and not prospective randomized control studies. The balance of data, however, at present indicate that long-term estrogen therapy (7 to 10 years) is necessary to maximally protect the skeleton and decrease the risk of fractures. Estrogen replacement therapy is approved by the Food and Drug Administration (FDA) for both the prevention and treatment of osteoporosis.

Plant estrogens or phytoestrogens are substances in soy products. These phytoestrogens contain isoflavones that may have estrogen agonist or antagonistic properties. Asian women consume large amounts of soy in their diet. It has been hypothesized that high dietary intake of isoflavones might contribute to the reduced incidence of hip fractures, heart disease, and breast cancer in Asian women compared with women from western societies. In a short-term study in rodents, ipriflavone (an isoflavone derivative) increased bone mass and bone strength (66). In a multicentered, placebo-controlled study of 126 postmenopausal women, ipriflavone increased bone density of the forearm at 1 year (67). Large prospective studies are necessary to demonstrate the effects of soy and its constituents or derivatives on bone and a variety of other clinical endpoints.

Studies show that estrogen replacement therapy may produce a small increase in breast cancer risk (68,69). New data from observational studies indicate that estrogen replacement therapy may delay the onset of and reduce the risk of Alzheimer's disease (70,71). Because of the inherent limitations of observational studies (e.g., healthier, more educated women may take estrogen and this might affect the outcomes), randomized and controlled studies will be necessary to demonstrate a protective effect of estrogen on Alzheimer's disease. Contraindications to estrogen therapy are: breast or endometrial cancer, active liver disease, and active thrombolytic disease (68). Migraine headaches, uterine fibroids, and gallbladder disease are not absolute contraindications to estrogen therapy. Col et al analyzed the risks and benefits of hormone replacement therapy on projected survival and found that estrogen therapy led to increased survival in most women except those with the highest breast cancer risk (for example, two first-degree relatives with breast cancer) (71).

Clinical data from the Nurses' Health Study (72) show that hormone replacement therapy reduces mortality overall by 37%. With long-term use (5 to 10 years), estrogen therapy was associated with a decreased mortality of 20%, as a result of a rise in the number of fatal breast cancers among that group (72). Thus, according to observational studies, or nonrandomized or short-term prospective studies, hormone replacement therapy appears to have beneficial effects on three debilitating diseases that affect postmenopausal women: osteoporosis, cardiovascular disease, and possibly Alzheimer's disease. The Women's Health Initiative, a large prospective randomized trial, should provide conclusive data on the effects of estrogen replacement on osteoporosis, cardiovascular disease, Alzheimer's disease, colon cancer, breast cancer, and other endpoints. Alternative FDA-approved regimens for the treatment and/or prevention of osteoporosis are selective estrogen receptor modulators (SERMs, e.g., raloxifene), the bisphosphonates (e.g., alendronate) or calcitonin (including nasal spray calcitonin).

Selective Estrogen Receptor Modulators

The ideal estrogen will confer the beneficial effects of estrogen on the bone and lipids, and not lead to any increased risk of breast cancer. New drugs named selective estrogen receptor modulators (SERMs) are thought to exert estrogen agonist properties on the bone and lipids and antagonist effects on breast and uterine tissue (73). Tamoxifen, one of the first SERMs, maintains bone mass and lowers total and LDL cholesterol in postmenopausal women with breast cancer (74), but produces a small increase in the risk of endometrial hyperplasia and uterine cancer (75).

Raloxifene (Evista) is the first SERM to be tested in large clinical trials for the effects on bone, lipids, breast and uterus in healthy postmenopausal women. Raloxifene increased spine, total hip, and total body bone density by 2% to 2.5% in women that were randomized to active therapy, compared with women in the placebo group that lost bone (76). The increment in bone density from baseline at these

sites was 1.3% to 1.6%, which is less than that associated with estrogen replacement (76). Raloxifene also decreased markers of bone turnover. In addition, raloxifene reduced LDL cholesterol by 12%, similar to estrogen; however, unlike estrogen, raloxifene had no effect on HDL or triglycerides (77). New data indicate that after 29 months of therapy, raloxifene-treated women showed a 74% reduction in the relative risk of new breast cancers (32 total cases of breast cancer) (78).

Adverse effects of raloxifene therapy include possible hot flashes and a risk of blood clots similar to estrogen replacement therapy. In contrast to estrogen, raloxifene does not stimulate the endometrium, nor does it ameliorate urogenital symptoms associated with menopause. Long-term data will be necessary to determine the effects of raloxifene on fractures, cardiovascular disease, and Alzheimer's disease. Raloxifene (60 mg/day) is approved by the FDA for the prevention but not treatment of osteoporosis. There are many selective receptor modulators including idoxifene, droloxifene, and several other new compounds that are undergoing evaluation for their relative potencies and agonist or antagonist properties on bone, cardiovascular markers, cognitive function, and breast and uterine tissues.

Calcitonin

Calcitonin is a potent inhibitor of osteoclastic-mediated bone resorption. In 1984, injectable calcitonin was approved by the FDA for the treatment of osteoporosis and in 1995 calcitonin nasal spray was approved for the treatment of postmenopausal women (more than 5 years since menopause) with osteoporosis. Nasal calcitonin (Miacalcin) (200 IU/day) increases spinal bone density 2% to 3% compared with placebo, with no apparent effect on hip bone density. Nasal calcitonin reduced spine fractures by 37% (79). Side effects of injectable calcitonin include nausea and flushing. The nasal spray calcitonin is well tolerated, with rhinorrhea as the most common side effect. Both injectable and nasal calcitonin produce a beneficial analgesic response for compression fractures.

Bisphosphonates

Bisphosphonates are analogs of pyrophosphate that are adsorbed onto the hydroxyapatite of bone and inhibit bone resorption. Bisphosphonates have a long half-life and prolonged skeletal retention. Alendronate (Fosamax) (10 mg/day), is FDA approved for the treatment of postmenopausal osteoporosis. Compared with placebo, alendronate increased spinal bone mass 5% to 10% and femoral neck and trochanteric bone density (80,81). Alendronate also produced about a 50% reduction in new spine, hip, and forearm fractures in osteoporotic women (81). Alendronate (5 mg/day) is also FDA approved for prevention of bone loss; this dose was slightly less effective than estrogen on increasing spinal bone density in women under 60 years of age (82). To maximize absorption, alendronate must be taken on an empty stomach with water, and patients should not lie down or take other foods, liquids, or medications for one-half hour. Adverse effects of bisphosphonates include gastrointestinal symptoms, musculoskeletal pain, and impaired mineralization at high doses. Alendronate should be used with caution in patients with active upper gastrointestinal problems (dysphagia, esophageal diseases, gastritis, duodenitis), and is contraindicated in patients with abnormalities of the esophagus (stricture or achalasia). Clinical trials of the efficacy of other bisphosphonates that are potent inhibitors of bone resorption (Table 30-6), are underway.

Combined Use of Estrogen and Other Anti-resorptive Therapy

One question that frequently arises is what is the utility of using a combination of estrogen with another agent if a patient is not responding to monotherapy. Data from Meschia (83) evaluated the effect of calcitonin alone and given twice weekly, compared with calcitonin plus estrogen. In the 1- and 2-year data that compared calcitonin alone or estrogen alone to calcitonin and estrogen together, there was a 10.9% increase in the bone density in the combination therapy group that exceeded either estrogen or calcitonin alone. Etidronate, a bisphosphonate that was not approved for the treatment of osteoporosis in the United States, has an added effect on increasing bone mass in combination with hormone replacement therapy (84). Data of the effects of combination therapy of alendronate with hormone replacement therapy on bone are in progress, although there is no data to support combined use of estrogen and alendronate at this time.

Parathyroid Hormone

Parathyroid hormone (PTH) stimulates bone formation and has anabolic effects on trabecular bone (e.g., spine). In a study in men, injectable PTH (1-34) and 1,25-dihydroxyvitamin D led to a large rise in spinal bone mass, but there was evidence of cortical bone loss (85). In women rendered estrogen deficient from therapy with gonadotropin-releasing hormone, injectable PTH produced a small increase in lateral spine bone mass at 6 months with no effect on hip bone density (86). PTH is administered as intact hormone or fragments [(e.g., hPTH (1-34)]. In women on estrogen therapy, injectable PTH produced large increments in spinal and hip bone density with a slight decrease in vertebral deformities (87). Potential adverse effects of PTH include possible loss of cortical bone when used in conjunction with 1,25-dihydroxvitamin D. There is limited information on the effects of PTH on fracture. Alternative modes of delivery of PTH are under development.

Sodium Fluoride

Sodium fluoride is incorporated into hydroxyapatite, and stimulates bone formation. At high doses (75 mg/day), sodium fluoride produced large incremental gains in bone mineral density but nonvertebral fractures increased. In a 2-year study of 354 osteoporotic women, 50 mg of sodium fluoride and monofluorophosphate increased bone density but did not decrease the incidence of vertebral fractures (88). A slow-release sodium fluoride preparation increased spinal and hip bone density by 4% to 5% and 2.38% per year, respectively, for 4 years and reduced fractures (89). Although recommended for approval by the FDA, slow-release fluoride has not yet been approved. Adverse effects of fluoride include: lower extremity pain, gastrointestinal irritation, and impaired mineralization at high doses. The use of fluoride should be limited to clinical studies.

SUMMARY

Because bone loss is not completely reversible with existing therapies, prevention is essential for optimizing skeletal health. Strategies directed at increasing peak bone mass, including reducing risk factors for bone loss (e.g., inadequate calcium intake, gonadal abnormalities, decreased body fat, cigarette smoking, inactivity, or excessive alcohol intake), and reversing the secondary causes of osteoporosis, may prevent bone loss. Patients should be advised, therefore, to consume adequate vitamin D and calcium, and participate in a regular exercise program.

As we leave the 20th century there is extensive research on the use of hormone replacement therapy, SERMs, new potent bisphosphonates, and growth factors for the treatment and/or prevention of osteoporosis. On the basis of data showing that increased calcium intake can add to bone accretion during adolescence and that interventions such as vitamin D and calcium, estrogen, bisphosphonates, and calcitonin can reduce fractures in older patients, it is never too early or too late to institute preventive strategies or treatments to diminish those fractures that rise exponentially with age.

Table 30-6 Relative Potency of Various Bisphosphonates to Inhibit Metaphyseal Bone Resorption in vivo

AGENT	RELATIVE POTENCY
Etidronate	1
Clodronate	10
Tiludronate	10
Pamidronate	100
Dimethyl pamidronate (mildronate)	500–1000
Alendronate	500–1000
EB 1053[a]	500–1000
Risedronate	1000–5000
BM 21.0955[b] (ibandronate)	1000

[a] Disodium 1-hydroxy-3-(1pyrrolidinyl)-propylidene-1, 1-bisphosphonate.
[b] Nmethyl-N-pentylaminopropane hydroxybisphosphonate.
SOURCE: Kanis JA, Gertz BJ, Singer F, Ortolani S. Rationale for the use of alendronate in osteoporosis. Osteoporos Int 1995;5:1–13.

REFERENCES

1. Consensus Development Statement. Who are candidates for prevention and treatment for osteoporosis? Osteoporos Int 1997;7:1–6.

2. Geelhoed EA, Prince RL. The epidemiology of osteoporotic fracture and its causative factors. Clin Biochem Rev 1994;15:173–178.

3. Melton LJI, Chrischilles EA, Cooper C, et al. Perspective: how many women have osteoporosis? J Bone Miner Res 1992;7:1005–1010.

4. Prince RL, Knuiman MW, Gulland L. Fracture prevalence in an Australian population. Aust J Publ Health 1993;17:124–128.

5. Jones G, Nguyen T, Sambrook PN, et al. Symptomatic fracture incidence in elderly men and women: the Dubbo Osteoporosis Epidemiology Study (DOES). Osteoporos Int 1994;4:277–282.

6. Kanis JA, WHO Study Group. Assessment of fracture risk and its application to screening for postmenopausal osteoporosis: synopsis of a WHO report. Osteoporos Int 1994;4:368–381.

7. Ray NF, Chan JK, Thamer M, Melton LJ III. Medical expenditures for the treatment of osteoporotic fractures in the United States in 1995: report from the National Osteoporosis Foundation. J Bone Miner Res 1997;12:24–35.

8. Ensrud KE, Palermo L, Black DM, et al. Hip and calcaneal bone loss increase with advancing age: longitudinal results from the study of osteoporotic fractures. J Bone Miner Res 1995;10:1778–1787.

9. Riggs BL, Wahner HW, Dunn WL, et al. Differential changes in bone mineral density of the appendicular and axial skeleton with aging. J Clin Invest 1981;67:328–335.

10. Dawson-Hughes B, Dallal GE, Krall EA, et al. A controlled trial of the effect of calcium supplementation on bone density in postmenopausal women. N Engl J Med 1990;323:878–883.

11. Greenspan SL, Maitland LA, Myers ER, et al. Femoral bone loss progresses with age: a longitudinal study in women over age 65. J Bone Miner Res 1994;9:1959–1965.

12. The Writing Group for the PEPI Trial. Effects of estrogen or estrogen/progestin regimens on heart disease risk factors in postmenopausal women: the Postmenopausal Estrogen/progestin Interventions (PEPI) trial. JAMA 1995;273:199–208.

13. Mazess RB, Barden HS, Ettinger M, et al. Spine and femur density using dual-photon absorptiometry in US white women. Bone Miner 1987;2:211–219.

14. Mazess RB. On aging bone loss. Clin Orthop 1982;165:239–252.

15. Ravn P, Hetland ML, Overgaard K, Christiansen C. Premenopausal and postmenopausal changes in bone mineral density of the proximal femur measured by dual-energy x-ray absorptiometry. J Bone Miner Res 1994;9:1975.

16. Riggs BL, Wahner W, Seeman E, et al. Changes in bone mineral density of the proximal femur and spine with aging: differences between the postmenopausal and senile osteoporosis syndromes. J Clin Invest 1982;70:716–723.

17. Cummings SR, Nevitt MC, Browner WS, et al. Risk factors for hip fracture in white women. N Engl J Med 1995;332:767–773.

18. Eddy DM, Johnston CC, Cummings SR, et al. Osteoporosis: cost effectiveness analysis and review of the evidence for prevention, diagnosis and treatment: the basis for a guideline for the medical management of osteoporosis. Osteoporos Int 1998;8(suppl 4):S1–S88.

19. Eastell R. Treatment of postmenopausal osteoporosis. N Engl J Med 1998;338:736–746.

20. Lukert BP, Raisz LG. Glucocorticoid-induced osteoporosis: pathogenesis and management. Ann Int Med 1990;112:352–364.

21. Zumoff B, Walsh BT, Katz JL, et al. Subnormal plasma dehydroepiandrosterone to cortisol ratio in anorexia nervosa: a second hormonal parameter of ontogenic regression. J Clin Endocrinol Metab 1983;56:668–671.

22. Rigotti N, Neer R, Skates S, et al. The clinical course of osteoporosis in anorexia nervosa. JAMA 1991;265:1133–1138.

23. LeBoff MS. Is prolonged use of corticosteroids safe in patients with Crohn's disease? Inflammatory Bowel Dis 1997;3:169–173.

24. Potts JJT. Management of asymptomatic hyperparathyroidism. J Clin Endocrinol Metab 1990;70:1489–1493.

25. Friedman AJ, Daly M, Juneau-Norcross M, et al. A prospective, randomized trial of gonadotropin-releasing hormone agonist plus estrogen-progestin add-back regimens for women with leiomyomata uteri. J Clin Endocrinol Metab 1993;76:1439–1445.

26. Rich GM, Mudge GH, Laffel GL, LeBoff MS. Cyclosporine A and prednisone-associated osteoporosis in heart transplant recipients. J Heart Lung Transplant 1992;11:950–958.

27. Rodino MA, Shane E. Osteoporosis after organ transplantation. Am J Med 1998;104:459–469.

28. Cummings SR, Black DM, Nevitt MC, et al. Bone density at various sites for prediction of hip fractures: the Study of Osteoporotic Fractures Research Group. Lancet 1993;341:72–75.

29. Byrne TA, Morrissey TB, Gatzen C, et al. Anabolic therapy with growth hormone accelerates gain in lean tissue in surgical patients requiring nutritional rehabilitation. Ann Surg 1993;218:400–418.

30. Johnston CCJ, Melton LJI, Lindsay R, Eddy DM. Clinical indications for bone mass measurements. J Bone Miner Res 1989;4:1–28.

31. Recker RR, Hinders S, Davies KM, et al. Correcting calcium nutri-

tional deficiency prevents spine fractures in elderly women. J Bone Miner Res 1996;11:1961–1966.

32. Johnston CC, Jr., Miller JZ, Selmenda CW, et al. Calcium supplementation and increases in bone mineral density in children. N Engl J Med 1992;327:82–87.

33. Curhan GC, Willett WC, Spcizer FE, et al. Comparison of dietary calcium with supplemental calcium and other nutrients as factors affecting the risk for kidney stones in women. Ann Intern Med 1997;126:497–504.

34. Recker RR. Calcium absorption and achlorhydria. N Engl J Med 1985;313:70–73.

35. Heaney RP, Recker RR, Stegman MR, Moy AJ. Calcium absorption in women: relationships to calcium intake, estrogen status, and age. J Bone Miner Res 1989;4:469–474.

36. Dawson-Hughes B. Calcium and vitamin D nutritional needs of elderly women. J Nutr 1996;126: 1165S–1167S.

37. Lips P, Graafmans WC, Ooms ME, et al. Vitamin D supplementation and fracture incidence in elderly persons. Ann Intern Med 1996; 124:400–406.

38. Parfitt AM, Chir B, Gallagher JC, et al. Vitamin D and bone health in the elderly. Am J Clin Nutr 1982;36:1014–1031.

39. Aaron JE, Gallagher JC, Anderson J, et al. Frequency of osteomalacia and osteoporotic fractures of the proximal femur. Lancet 1974;1: 229–233.

40. Chalmers J, Barclay A, Davison AM, et al. Quantitative measurements of osteoid in health and disease. Clin Orthop 1969;63: 196–209.

41. Hordon LD, Peacock M. Osteomalacia and osteoporosis in femoral neck fracture. Bone Miner 1990;11:247–259.

42. Gallagher JC, Kinyamu HK, Fowler SE, et al. Calciotropic hormones and bone markers in the elderly. J Bone Miner Res 1998;13:475–482.

43. Dawson-Hughes B, Harris SS, Krall EA, et al. Rates of bone loss in postmenopausal women randomly assigned to one of two dosages of Vitamin D. Am J Clin Nutr 1995;61:1140–1145.

44. Lips P, Hackeng WHL, Jongen MJM, et al. Seasonal variation in serum concentrations of parathyroid hormone in elderly people. J Clin Endocrinol Metab 1983;57: 204–206.

45. Jacobsen SJ, Goldberg J, Miles TP, et al. Seasonal variation in the incidence of hip fracture among white persons aged 65 years and older in the United States, 1984–1987. Am J Epidemiol 1991;133: 996–1004.

46. Boonen S, Aerssens J, Dequeker J. Age-related endocrine deficiencies and fractures of the proximal femur: implications of vitamin D deficiency in the elderly. J Endocrinol 1996;149:13–17.

47. Chapuy MC, Schott AM, Garnero P, et al. Healthy elderly French women living at home have secondary hyperparathyroidism and high bone turnover in winter. J Clin Endocrinol Metab 1996;81: 1129–1133.

48. LeBoff MS, Kohlmeier L, Franklin J, et al. Compared with osteoporotic controls acute hip fracture patients show high PTH and low vitamin D levels. Paper presented at the Annual Meeting of the Endocrine Society, Minneapolis, June 1997.

49. Prestwood KM, Pannullo AM, Kenny AM, et al. The effect of a short course of calcium and Vitamin D on bone turnover in older women. Osteoporos Int 1996;6:314–319.

50. Chapuy MC, Arlot ME, DuBoeuf F, et al. Vitamin D_3 and calcium to prevent hip fractures in elderly women. N Engl J Med 1992;327: 1637–1642.

51. Dawson-Hughes B, Harris SS, Krall EA, Dallal GE. Effect of calcium and vitamin D supplementation on bone density in men and women 65 years of age or older. N Engl J Med 1997;337:670–676.

52. Gallagher JC, Goldgar D. Treatment of postmenopausal osteoporosis with high doses of synthetic calcitrol: a randomized controlled study. Ann Intern Med 1990;113: 649–655.

53. Dalsky GP, Stocke KS, Ehsani AA, et al. Weight-bearing exercise training and lumbar bone mineral content in postmenopausal women. Ann Int Med 1988;108:824–828.

54. Nelson ME, Fiatarone MA, Morganti CM, et al. Effects of high-intensity strength training on multiple risk factors for osteoporotic fractures: a randomized controlled trial. JAMA 1994; 272:1909–1914.

55. Stampfer MJ, Colditz GA, Willett WC, et al. Postmenopausal estrogen therapy and cardiovascular disease: ten year follow-up from the Nurses' Health Study. N Engl J Med 1991;325:756–762.

56. Grodstein F, Stampfer MJ, Manson JE, et al. Postmenopausal estrogen and progestin use and the risk of cardiovascular disease. N Engl J Med 1996;335:453–461.

57. Lindsay R, Tohme JF. Estrogen treatment of patients with established postmenopausal osteoporosis. Obstet Gynecol 1990;76: 290–295.

58. Rosen CJ, Chesnut CHI, Mallinak NJ. The predictive value of biochemical markers of bone turnover for bone mineral density in early postmenopausal women treated with hormone replacement or calcium supplementation. J Clin Endocrinol Metab 1997;82: 1904–1910.

59. Chesnut CH3, Bell NH, Clark GS, et al. Hormone replacement therapy in postmenopausal women: urinary N-telopeptide of type I collagen monitors therapeutic effect and predicts response of bone mineral density. Am J Med 1997; 102:29–37.

60. El-Hajj Fuleihan G, Brown EM, Curtis K, et al. Effect of cyclical and daily continuous hormone replacement therapy on indices of mineral metabolism. Arch Int Med 1992;152:1904–1909.

61. Lindsay R, Bush TL, Grady DG, et al. Therapeutic controversy: estrogen replacement in menopause. J Clin Endocrinol Metab 1996;81: 3829–3838.

62. Schneider DL, Barrett-Connor E, Morton DJ. Timing of postmenopausal estrogen for optimal bone density: the Rancho Bernardo study. JAMA 1997;277:543–547.

63. Kiel DP, Felson DT, Anderson JJ, et al. Hip fracture and the use of estrogens in postmenopausal women: the Framingham study. N Engl J Med 1987;317:1169–1174.

64. Paganini-Hill A, Ross RK, Gerkins VB, et al. Menopausal estrogen therapy and hip fractures. Ann Int Med 1981;95:28–31.

65. Cauley JA, Seeley DG, Ensrud K, et al. Estrogen replacement therapy and fractures in older women. Ann Intern Med 1995; 122:9–16.

66. Civitelli R, Abbasi-Jarhomi SH, Halstead LR, Dimarogonas A. Ipriflavone improves bone density and biomechanical properties of adult male rat bones. Calcif Tissue Int 1995;56:215–219.

67. Agnusdei D, Adami S, Cervetti R, et al. Effects of ipriflavone on bone mass and calcium metabolism in postmenopausal osteoporosis. Bone Miner 1992;19(suppl): S43–S48.

68. American College of OB-GYN. Hormone replacement therapy: a review of the recent guidelines of the American College of Obstetrics and Gynecology regarding hormone replacement therapy. ACOG Technical Bulletin 1992;166:1–8.

69. Colditz GA, Hankinson SE, Hunter DJ, et al. The use of estrogens and progestins and the risk of breast cancer in postmenopausal women. N Engl J Med 1995;332:1589–1593.

70. Paganini-Hill A, Henderson VW. Estrogen deficiency and risk of Alzheimer's disease in women. Am J Epidemiol 1994;140:256–261.

71. Col NF, Eckman MH, Karas RH, et al. Patient-specific decisions about hormone replacement therapy in postmenopausal women. JAMA 1997;277:1140–1147.

72. Grodstein F, Stampfer MJ, Colditz GA, et al. Postmenopausal hormone therapy and mortality. N Engl J Med 1997;336:1769–1775.

73. Kauffman RF, Bryant HU. Selective estrogen receptive modulators. DN&P 1995;8:531–539.

74. Love RR, Mazess RB, Barden HS, et al. Effects of tamoxifen on bone mineral density in postmenopausal women with breast cancer. N Eng J Med 1992;326:852–856.

75. Fisher B, Costantino JP, Redmond CK, et al. Endometrial cancer in tamoxifen-treated breast cancer patients: findings from the National Surgical Adjuvant Breast and Bowel Project (NSABP). J Natl Cancer Inst 1994;86:527–537.

76. Delmas PD, Bjarnason NH, Mitlak BH, et al. Effects of raloxifene on bone mineral density, serum cholesterol concentrations, and uterine endometrium in postmenopausal women. N Engl J Med 1997;337: 1641–1647.

77. Walsh BW, Kuller LH, Wild RA, et al. Effects of Raloxifene on serum lipids and coagulation factors in healthy postmenopausal women. JAMA 1998;279:1445–1451.

78. Cummings SR, Norton L, Eckert S, et al. Raloxifene reduces the risk of breast cancer and may decrease the risk of endometrial cancer in post-menopausal women: two-year findings from the multiple outcomes of Raloxifene evaluation (MORE) trial. Presented at the American Society of Clinical Oncology, Los Angeles, May 1998.

79. Stock JL, Avioli LV, Baylink DJ, et al. Calcitonin-salmon nasal spray reduces the incidence of new vertebral fractures in postmenopausal women: three-year interim results of the PROOF study. J Bone Min Res 1997;12:S149. Abstract.

80. Liberman UA, Weiss SR, Broll J, et al for the Alendronate Phase III Osteoporosis Treatment Study Group. Effect of oral alendronate on bone mineral density and the incidence of fractures in postmenopausal osteoporosis. N Engl J Med 1995;333:1437–1443.

81. Black DM, Cummings SR, Karpf DB, et al. Randomised trial of effect of alendronate on risk of fracture in women with existing vertebral fractures. Lancet 1996; 348:1535–1541.

82. Hosking D, Chilvers CED, Christiansen C, et al. Prevention of bone loss with alendronate in postmenopausal women under 60 years of age. N Engl J Med 1998; 338:485–492.

83. Meschia M, Brincat M, Barbacini P, et al. A clinical trial on the effects of a combination of elcatonin (carbocalcitonin) and conjugated estrogens on vertebral bone mass in early postmenopausal women. Calcif Tissue Int 1993;53:17–20.

84. Wimalawansa SJ. A four-year randomized controlled trial of hormone replacement and bisphosphonate, alone or in combination, in women with postmenopausal osteoporosis. Am J Med 1998;3: 219–226.

85. Slovik DM, Rosenthal DI, Doppelt SH, et al. Restoration of spinal bone in osteoporotic men by treatment with human parathyroid hormone (1–34) and 1,25-dihydroxyvitamin D. J Bone Min Res 1986;4:377–381.

86. Finkelstein JS, Klibanski A, Schaeffer EH, et al. Parathyroid hormone for the prevention of bone loss induced by estrogen deficiency. N Engl J Med 1994; 331:1618–1623.

87. Lindsay R, Nieves J, Formica C, et al. Randomised controlled study of effect of parathyroid hormone on vertebral-bone mass and fracture incidence among postmenopausal women on oestrogen with osteoporosis. Lancet 1997;350:550–555.

88. Meunier PJ, Sebert JL, Reginster JY, et al. Fluoride salts are no better at preventing new vertebral fractures than calcium-vitamin D in postmenopausal osteoporosis: the FAVO study. Osteoporos Int 1998;8:4–12.

89. Pak CYC, Sakhaee K, Adams-Huet B, et al. Treatment of postmenopausal osteoporosis with slow-release sodium fluoride. Ann Intern Med 1995;123:401–408.

Chapter 31

Physical Activity in Women

Isabela Bensenor
Kathryn M. Rexrode
JoAnn E. Manson

The health benefits of regular physical activity have been documented in numerous large-scale epidemiologic investigations (1–4). There remains considerable uncertainty, however, concerning the optimal frequency, duration, and intensity of physical activity for health benefits. Nonetheless, several leading health organizations, including the US Department of Health and Human Services, the Centers for Disease Control and Prevention (CDC), the American College of Sports Medicine (ACSM), the National Center for Chronic Disease Prevention and Health Promotion, and the President's Council on Physical Fitness and Sports, have agreed on a population-wide goal for physical activity that is judged to be both sufficient to confer health benefits and feasible for most people. The consensus of these organizations, published in *Physical Activity and Health/A Report of the Surgeon General* (5), is that children and adults should set a goal of accumulating at least 30 minutes of moderate-intensity physical activity on most, and preferably all, days of the week. It is important to note that this goal can be reached with moderate degrees of activity divided in several parts during the day.

The most recent data on physical activity patterns in the United States derive from three large-scale population surveys, the National Health Interview Survey (NHIS), the Behavioral Risk Factor Surveillance Study (BRFSS), and the Third National Health and Nutrition Examination Survey (NHANES III). These data demonstrate that approximately one fourth of U.S. adults engage in no regular leisure-time physical activity, and more than 60% fall short of the current exercise guidelines. There is an important gender differential, with the prevalence of physical inactivity in women approximately 1.2 to 1.7 times higher than that in men. There are also racial differences, with more than one third of black and Hispanic women engaging in no leisure-time physical activity as compared with about one quarter of white women. Finally, there is a marked gradient in physical activity in relation to income, with a two- to three fold greater prevalence of physical inactivity among lower income groups.

A broad range of benefits of physical activity have been proposed, including salutary effects on weight control, blood pressure, cholesterol levels, glucose tolerance, coronary heart disease, stroke, cancer, total mortality, osteoporosis, and psychological well-being (Table 31-1). The benefits of physical activity generally far outweigh any risks. In women, there are unique concerns that relate to exercise-induced menstrual dysfunction as well as appropriate physical activity during pregnancy. However, potential hazards can be minimized by specific recommendations that address these issues, as well as recommendations for older persons or those with comorbidity or other special circumstances.

The vast majority of studies of physical activity and health have been conducted in men. Thus, there is a paucity of direct information on the role of exercise in women. In addition, of those studies that have examined this relationship in women, many have been of inadequate sample size to yield conclusive findings. Nonetheless, those studies that have been conducted in women have generally had results comparable to those in men and have supported the conclusion that exercise in women results in a wide range of health benefits.

A central methodologic issue in all studies of physical activity concerns how to measure levels of activity (6,7). The intensity of physical activity is typically measured in METs (work metabolic rate/resting metabolic rate), which are multiples of the resting rate of oxygen consumption during physical activity. One MET represents the approximate rate of

Table 31-1 Effects of Physical Activity

RISK FACTORS

↓	Body weight	↓	Systolic blood pressure
		↓	Diastolic blood pressure
↓	LDL cholesterol		
↑	HDL cholesterol	↓	Type 2 diabetes
↓	Triglycerides	↑	Glycemic control in Type 1 diabetics

CLINICAL OUTCOMES

↓	Coronary heart disease	↓	Total mortality
↓	Stroke		
		↓	Osteoporosis
↓	Endometrial cancer		
↔	Ovarian cancer	↑	Emotional well-being
↓	Breast cancer		
↓	Colon cancer		
↓	Colorectal adenomas		

oxygen consumption of a seated adult at rest, or about 3.5 mL/min per kg. The equivalent energy cost of 1 MET is about 1.2 kilocalories for a 70 kg person or approximately 1 kcal/kg per hr. Moderate physical activity expends 3 to 6 METs and vigorous activity expends more than 6 METs. See Chapter 4 (Table 4-3) for a list of several types of exercise of different intensities and the quantity of METs expended.

Another methodologic concern is the potential for misclassification of physical activity levels. Most studies have used questionnaires or direct interviews that inquired about specific types of physical activity. Many studies have focused on sports participation and other leisure-time physical activity. This raises particular concerns regarding misclassification of activity levels in women, who have only recently begun participating in many of these activities in large numbers, yet who may be quite active in ways not measured by these studies.

Most adults do not need to see a physician before starting a moderate-intensity activity program, but the American College of Sports Medicine recommends that men older than age 40 and women older than age 50 who plan a vigorous program (more than 6 METs) or who have any chronic disease consult a physician before beginning (8). Appropriate moderate-intensity exercise for most adults includes brisk walking, bicycling, running, and swimming, each of which used a range of muscles. Calculating the "target heart rate" is very important for getting the maximum benefit of the exercise. The formula [220 − age (in years)] × 0.7 can be used with any form of exercise to determine maximum target heart rate (9).

Previous recommendations of the American College of Sports Medicine (ACSM) endorsed vigorous endurance exercise for at least 20 minutes, three times a week (10). The more recent recommendation of the CDC and ACSM of 30 minutes of moderately intense physical activity on most, if not all, days of the week has been erroneously interpreted by some as superseding the previous guidelines (8). In fact, the two guidelines are complementary, with the newer recommendation simply more feasible for many people (11). The newer guideline may be particularly important for women, who engage in less leisure-time physical activity than men and for whom there may be unique considerations, including potential reproductive dysfunction with intense physical activity levels.

The following sections review the evidence on physical activity and chronic diseases by specific topics, including unique considerations in women and any gender-specific recommendations.

WEIGHT CONTROL

There is a linear association between body weight and mortality from all causes among middle-aged women (12). Exercise is the only nonpharmacologic method of increasing energy expenditure and is therefore an important tool in maintaining body weight (13), particularly in conjunction with a prudent diet (14). Exercise also acts as an appetite suppressant (15) and enhances dietary compliance during moderate caloric restriction in obese women (16).

The relation between physical activity and presence of cardiovascular disease (CVD) risk factors was assessed cross-sectionally in the European Prospective Investigation into Cancer and Nutrition (EPIC). Body mass index (BMI), waist-hip ratio, and waist circumference were all inversely related to amount of time engaged in leisure-time activities (17). In a study of exercise training among 93 men and women, aged 60 to 70, a 9- to 12-month program of walking and jogging was associated with weight loss in both men and women, with fat lost preferentially from the abdomen and the largest absolute and relative reductions seen at the waist (18).

Repeated weight loss followed by weight gain (weight cycling) may have detrimental metabolic and psychological consequences (19). Regaining weight is also more common among those who do not exercise regularly. In one study of women in California, obese women who regained weight after successful weight reduction were much less likely to exercise regularly than formerly obese women who were successful in maintaining weight loss, with only 34% of relapsers exercising regularly, compared with 90% of those who maintained weight loss (20). The higher prevalence of obesity in minority women and those of lower socioeconomic status may be explained partially by a lower level of recreational physical activity in these groups (21).

Smoking cessation is often followed by weight gain (22), but this effect can be minimized if smoking cessation is accompanied by a moderate increase in the level of physical activity (23).

LIPIDS

Regular exercise has been associated with more favorable lipid plasma profiles in both women and men (24,25). The lipid profile associated with regular exercise includes a lower serum triglyceride level, an elevated high-density lipoprotein (HDL) cholesterol level, and a decreased level of low-density lipoprotein (LDL) cholesterol. These beneficial changes may begin to occur at low to moderate levels of exercise intensity, including intensities lower than those required for physical fitness. Duncan et al (26) compared HDL cholesterol levels in premenopausal women classified into four groups: aerobic walkers (8.0 km/hr), brisk walkers (6.4 km/hr), strollers (4.8 km/hr), and sedentary women. Women in all three exercise groups had HDL cholesterol levels approximately 0.08 mmol/L higher than sedentary women. In contrast, physical fitness, as measured by maximal oxygen uptake, increased with higher intensity of activity in a dose-response manner across the four groups ($p < 0.001$).

In a second cross-sectional study, conducted among 1837 U.S. female runners, HDL cholesterol levels were, on average, 0.133 ± 0.020 mg/dL higher for every additional kilometer run per week, and women who ran more than 64 km/wk had significantly higher mean levels of HDL cholesterol than those who ran less than 48 km/wk (27). In the Postmenopausal Estrogen/Progestin Interventions Trial (PEPI), women who engaged in high-intensity leisure-time physical activity had higher HDL levels than those who engaged in moderate or light physical activity (28).

As regards randomized trial data, in a 2-year trial of randomized exercise among 204 postmenopausal women, there were no significant differences in total HDL cholesterol, HDL_2, or HDL_3 between women who had been assigned to a regular walking regimen and those assigned to a control group (29). In a trial of 88 women randomly assigned to 5 months of resistance-training exercise or control, those allocated to the exercise group experienced significant decreases of 0.33 ± 0.03 mmol/L in total cholesterol and 0.36 ± 0.001 mmol/L in LDL cholesterol levels compared with women in the control group. No significant changes in HDL and triglycerides were seen (30).

Finally, a trial of 116 initially sedentary men and 119 sedentary women allocated participants at random to a traditional, structured exercise program or to physical activity counseling. Both groups achieved high levels of compliance with the CDC/American College of Sports Medicine recommendation of 30 minutes or more of moderate-intensity activity on most, preferably, all days of the week (85% in the structured exercise group and 78% of the physical activity counseling group). Both groups also recorded significant reductions in total cholesterol and total cholesterol/HDL cholesterol ratio. Lack of a non-exercise control group, however, limits the interpretation of these findings (31).

Thus, although the data are not entirely consistent, there is evidence that physical activity may have beneficial effects on several lipid parameters, including triglycerides, total cholesterol, HDL cholesterol, and LDL cholesterol values.

HYPERTENSION

There is a strong relationship between regular physical activity and lower levels of blood pressure (32–34). The efficacy of aerobic exercise for lowering arterial blood pressure was evaluated in a series of nine postmenopausal women with high-normal resting blood pressure or stage I hypertension. Following a 12-week period of regular, moderate-intensity aerobic exercise, mean resting systolic and diastolic blood pressure was significantly lowered by 10/7 mm Hg and 12/5 mm Hg, respectively, in the sitting and standing positions ($p < 0.001$). This reduction was observed in the absence of

changes in maximal aerobic capacity, body weight, or dietary intake (35).

In the EPIC cohort described earlier, there was an inverse association between time spent participating in sports and mean systolic and diastolic blood pressure, with the highest tertile of physical activity correlated with the lowest blood pressure values (17). In a cross-sectional study of women aged 50 to 89, systolic and diastolic blood pressures were lower in women who engaged in regular physical activity compared with those who did not (36).

The Trials of Hypertension Prevention (TOHP), a large-scale, multicenter, randomized clinical trial, tested the efficacy of weight loss induced by a combination of reduced caloric intake and increased exercise on primary prevention of hypertension in men and women. After 18 months, women assigned to a low-calorie diet and regular physical activity had a significant reduction in blood pressure compared with controls, a change accompanied by an average weight loss of 1.8 kg (37).

Thus, physical activity appears to be an effective non-pharmacologic means of lowering blood pressure and should be considered as a first-line treatment strategy, particularly for those with mildly elevated blood pressure (38). Although several studies in women support benefits of physical activity in reducing blood pressure, most data are in men and additional studies in women are needed to ascertain whether there are any important gender differences in this relationship.

GLUCOSE INTOLERANCE AND DIABETES MELLITUS

Glucose Intolerance

Physical training, even in the absence of weight loss, can increase insulin sensitivity and improve glucose tolerance (39–41). Exercise training may affect insulin resistance directly, as well as prevent the accumulation of intra-abdominal fat, which has an important role in insulin resistance (5).

In a study of 25 postmenopausal women who entered an exercise program of either aerobic exercise (treadmill, at 70% to 85% of maximum heart rate) or muscle training with Nautilus equipment for 20 minutes three times weekly, insulin levels at 30 minutes after glucose loading (the first phase of insulin release) were significantly reduced in the treadmill group. Glucose tolerance and insulin response, as measured by area under the curve, were improved in both exercise groups compared with the non-exercising controls (42).

Type 2 Diabetes Mellitus

In the Nurses' Health Study, a large-scale cohort of US female nurses, women who engaged in vigorous activity at least once a week had an age-adjusted relative risk (RR) of 0.67 for type 2 diabetes compared with those who did not exercise weekly. The reduction in risk was present among both obese and non-obese women as well as among those with and without a family history of diabetes (43).

The association between physical activity and the risk of diabetes was recently evaluated in a cohort of men and women aged 35 to 63. In women, after 10 years of follow-up, both a higher total amount of activity and weekly vigorous activity were inversely associated with the risk of diabetes. An age-adjusted relative risk of 2.6 (95% CI, 1.3–5.4) for diabetes was reported for the lowest tertile activity group compared with the highest (44).

While physical activity appears to have an important role in the prevention of type 2 diabetes in women, more data are needed to determine the amounts and types of physical activity that are optimal in preventing this condition.

Type 1 Diabetes Mellitus

Although physical activity has not been shown to play a role in the prevention of insulin-dependent diabetes mellitus (type 1 diabetes mellitus), it can improve the cardiovascular disease risk profile of patients with type 1 diabetes and is associated with improved glycemic control. A 3-month intervention trial evaluated the impact of physical activity on cardiovascular risk factors in persons with type 1 diabetes. There was a linear, dose-response pattern between increased physical activity and loss of abdominal fat and a decrease in blood pressure and lipid-related cardiovascular risk factors, with a marked increase in the HDL_3 cholesterol subfraction. The overall frequency of severe hypoglycemic episodes was reduced from 0.14 to 0.10 per patient-year during the study period (45).

CARDIOVASCULAR DISEASE

Coronary Heart Disease

A large number of epidemiologic studies support a role of physical activity in the prevention of coronary heart disease (CHD) (46). Numerous biologic mechanisms may account for such an effect, including benefits on atherosclerosis, lipids, blood pressure, body weight, glucose tolerance, availability of oxygenated blood, blood clotting, and arrhythmias (5).

In a meta-analysis of studies of physical activity in the prevention of CHD, conducted predominantly in men, a sedentary occupation category was associated with a relative risk of coronary death of 1.9 (95% CI, 1.6–2.2) when compared with an active occupation category. Similar results were seen for non-occupational activity, with a relative risk of coronary death of 1.7 (95% CI, 1.2–2.3) for sedentary compared with high-activity groups (7).

One of the largest studies to assess the relationship of physical activity and cardiovascular disease (CVD) in women is the Iowa Women's Health Study. In this cohort of 40,417 postmenopausal women, after adjustment for potential confounding factors and exclusion of events occurring in the first 3 years of follow-up, those who engaged in moderate physical activity more than four times per week had a significantly lower risk of CVD mortality in comparison to the most sedentary women (RR = 0.53, p-trend = 0.003) (47). There was also an apparent reduction in CVD mortality among those engaging in regular vigorous exercise (RR = 0.20, p-trend = 0.09).

In the Nurses' Health Study (NHS), women in progressively higher walking quintiles, derived from both time spent walking and usual walking pace, had reduced risks of coronary heart disease (12). Vigorous exercise was also associated with reduced risk of CVD events. In the Framingham offspring study, which includes both men and women, there was

an inverse relation between leisure-time physical activity levels and cardiovascular risk (48). The association between physical activity and risk of CVD mortality was evaluated in an analysis utilizing data from three national representative samples in Germany. The analyses included 7749 women and 7689 men. A relative risk of CVD mortality of 0.26 (95% CI, 0.08–0.83) was observed for men spending more than two hours per week in organized sports activities compared with the most sedentary subjects, while the association in women was not reported because there were insufficient numbers of events to permit reliable assessment (49).

As regards case-control data, in the Boston Area Health Study, total physical activity did not differ significantly among female cases with myocardial infarction (MI) and controls, although women who were in the highest quartile of moderate to vigorous activity had nonsignificant risk reductions similar to those seen in men (odds ratio = 0.43) (50). Finally, in a case-control study of leisure-time physical activity and nonfatal MI in postmenopausal women, women in the highest quartile of total energy expenditure had an odds ratio (OR) of 0.40 for MI compared with those in the lowest quartile. Women in the second and third quartiles also had significantly reduced risks. Nonstrenuous physical activity and walking for exercise were also associated with reduced MI risk (51).

Stroke

There is a paucity of data on physical activity and stroke overall and, in particular, in women. Nonetheless, the results of available studies are fairly consistent. In the First National Health and Nutrition Survey I (NHANES I) Epidemiologic Follow-up Study, low levels of nonrecreational activity were associated with an increased risk of stroke in white women aged 65 to 74 years (RR = 1.82; 95% CI, 1.10–3.02) (52). In the Nurses' Health Study, the relationship between total physical activity, as measured by a validated questionnaire from which METs were calculated, and incidence of ischemic and total stroke was examined. Compared with women in the lowest METs quintile, those in the highest quintile had an age- and smoking-adjusted RR of 0.55 (95% CI, 0.38–0.79) for total stroke and 0.48 (95% CI, 0.29–0.81) for ischemic stroke (53). Regular walking was also associated with a reduced risk of stroke (53).

Thus, with respect to cardiovascular disease, regular physical activity is associated with reduced risks of coronary heart disease and stroke in women, although far more data are available for the former. The mechanisms for these benefits appear to include salutary effects on a range of risk factors, including body weight, lipoprotein profile, glucose tolerance, and blood pressure.

CANCER

Cancer is a disease of multifactorial etiology, and different constellations of risk factors appear to be associated with increased risks of different malignancies. For this reason, a number of studies have examined the relationship of physical activity levels with risks of specific cancers, including some unique to women, for which a potential antineoplastic effect of physical activity has been postulated.

Endometrial Cancer

Physical activity may decrease BMI as well as the occurrence of regular ovulatory cycles, both of which have been postulated to reduce the risk of endometrial cancer. Physical activity was inversely related to endometrial cancer risk in two case-control studies. In a study involving 405 endometrial cancer cases and 297 population controls, after adjustment for age, region, parity, smoking, and use of oral contraceptives and postmenopausal estrogens, recent recreational inactivity was associated with increased risks of endometrial cancer (RR for women in the lowest activity tertile = 1.9) (54). The results were similar for recent nonrecreational inactivity (RR in the lowest activity tertile = 2.2). Further adjustment for BMI and nonrecreational activity attenuated the association with recent recreational inactivity (RR = 1.2; 95% CI, 0.7–2.0), while adjustment for BMI and recreational activity did not materially alter the association with nonrecreational inactivity. Analyses of long-term activity patterns also suggested elevated risks among women who were recreationally and nonrecreationally inactive.

In a second study, exercise, occupational activity, and risk of endometrial cancer were evaluated among 232 cases and 631 controls in western New York state. Information was collected on physical activity at four time periods: at age 16 and at 20, 10, and 2 years before the interview. Women who engaged in a moderate amount of vigorous exercise at age 16 and at 20 years before the interview were at reduced risk compared with those who reported no activity, with odds ratios of 0.51 (95% CI, 0.31–0.83) and 0.50 (95% CI, 0.29–0.89), respectively (55). Activity levels 10 and 2 years prior to the interview were more modestly, and not significantly, associated with reduced risks (OR = 0.72 and 0.67, respectively). Occupational physical activity was not related to risk of endometrial cancer.

Ovarian Cancer

Few studies have examined the relationship of physical activity with ovarian cancer. Anovulation induced by physical activity might be expected to reduce risk of ovarian cancer. The association between physical activity and ovarian cancer was assessed among 31,396 postmenopausal women in the Iowa Women's Health Study. Compared with sedentary women, those engaging in regular physical activity had an increased risk of ovarian cancer (RR = 1.5; 95% CI, 1.0–2.2) (56). There was a dose-response pattern with increasing risks associated with increasing frequency of both moderate and vigorous activity, and the associations were unchanged after adjustment for waist-hip ratio and other potential confounding variables. These findings were unexpected and further studies of physical activity and ovarian cancer are needed.

Cancer of the Reproductive System

The occurrence of cancers of the reproductive system (uterus, ovary, cervix, and vagina) was tracked for 5398 living college alumnae, approximately half of whom were former college athletes and half of whom were not. Following adjustment for age, family history, age at menarche, number of pregnancies, use of oral contraceptives and estrogens, smoking, and BMI, the relative risk for reproductive cancer was 2.53 (95% CI,

1.17–5.47) among women who had not participated in college-era athletic programs compared to their athletic peers (57).

Breast Cancer

High levels of physical activity can delay menarche and interrupt regular menstrual cycles, thereby lowering a woman's exposure to estrogen and progesterone. These observations have formed the basis for the hypothesis that regular physical activity may reduce risk of breast cancer.

Three studies of physical activity and breast cancer have reported lower risks of breast cancer among more active women. In the college alumnae study described above, women who had not participated in college athletic programs were at increased risk of breast cancer (RR = 1.86; 95% CI, 1.00–3.47) compared with those who took part in college athletics (57).

In a cohort study in Norway among 25,624 women, aged 25 to 54 at entry, there was a reduction in the risk of breast cancer among women who exercised at least 4 hours per week compared with sedentary women (RR = 0.63; 95% CI, 0.42–0.95) after a median follow-up of 13.7 years. Risk reductions were greater among lean women (BMI < 22.8), premenopausal women, and those who continued to exercise regularly for 3 to 5 years (58). For occupational activity, there was a reduction in risk among those engaged in heavy manual labor compared to women with sedentary occupations (RR = 0.48; 95% CI, 0.25–0.92).

Finally, occupational physical activity and risk of breast cancer was analyzed in a large population-based case-control study in the U.S. that identified cases of breast cancer from four state cancer registries (59). Based on data from 4863 cases and 6783 controls, there was a significant trend toward lower risk of breast cancer with increasing levels of occupational physical activity (p-trend = 0.007). In relation to those with sedentary jobs, women in heavy-activity occupations had an odds ratio for breast cancer of 0.82 (95% CI, 0.63–1.08). For women with jobs requiring medium and light levels of physical activity the odds ratios were 0.86 (95% CI, 0.77–0.97) and 0.92 (95% CI, 0.84–1.01), respectively.

Colorectal Cancer and Adenomas

Regular physical activity can increase intestinal motility and shorten the transit time for elimination of potential carcinogens, providing a basis for a hypothesized benefit of physical activity on risks of colorectal cancer and adenomas.

Numerous studies have suggested an inverse relation of physical activity to risk of colon cancer (60–65). In one, a population-based case-control study in the Seattle area, for men and women combined, moderate- or high-intensity recreational activity was associated with a decreased risk of colon cancer (RR for activity two or more times per week versus none = 0.70; 95% CI, 0.40–1.00) (66). This finding was not materially altered by control for BMI or dietary intake variables. In a population-based cohort in Norway, which included 28,274 women and 53,242 men, physical activity at a level equivalent to walking or bicycling for at least 4 hours a week during leisure time was associated with decreased risk of colon cancer among females when compared with the sedentary groups (RR = 0.62; 95% CI, 0.40–0.97). No such association was observed for occupational activity in women, although this analysis may have been limited by the narrow range of work-related activity in women. Among males, an inverse dose-response effect was observed between total physical activity and colon cancer risk (p-trend = 0.04). No association between physical activity and rectal cancer was observed in males or females (67).

The relationship between physical activity and colorectal adenomas (precursors of cancer) has also been evaluated. In a cohort of US women, there was an inverse association between physical activity and occurrence or progression of adenomas in the distal colon (68), while a second study reported an inverse association in women with leisure-time, but not work-related, physical activity and risk of colorectal adenomas (69). A third study evaluated leisure and occupational physical activity and the risk of colorectal adenomatous polyps in women and men undergoing colonoscopy. After adjusting for potential confounding variables, no association was apparent for leisure-time or occupational activity and risk of polyps in women. In men, statistically significant protective effects were observed for occupational activity, and an association of borderline significance was observed for leisure-time activity (70).

Summary

The available epidemiologic evidence provides support for a protective association between physical activity and risks of endometrial cancer and total reproductive system malignancies. A single study has reported elevated risks of ovarian among more active women. This finding was unexpected, and further studies of this possible association are needed. There is also evidence of a possible protective role of physical activity on risk of breast cancer as well as on risk of colorectal cancers and adenomas.

ALL-CAUSE MORTALITY

A number of studies have demonstrated an inverse association between physical activity and all-cause mortality in women. In the Iowa Women's Health Study, the relationship was examined among 40,417 postmenopausal women, after adjusting for potential confounding variables and excluding women who died or reported cancer or heart disease diagnoses in the first 3 years of follow-up (to minimize confounding by underlying disease). Those who reported regular physical activity had a significantly lower mortality risk than those who did not (RR = 0.77; 95% CI, 0.66–0.90). Both moderate and vigorous activities provided benefit, with a strong monotonic trend of increasing benefit with increasing frequency of activity. For moderate activity, the relative risks for increasing levels of activity, from rarely or never engaging in physical activity to at least four times per week, were 1.0 (referent), 0.76, 0.70, and 0.62 (p-trend < 0.001). For vigorous activity, the corresponding relative risks were 1.0, 0.89, 0.74 and 0.57 (p-trend = 0.06) (47). Among women in the Framingham study, those in the upper two quartiles of physical activity had an overall 16-year mortality rate about 30% lower than women in the two lower quartiles (RR for highest quartile = 0.68; CI, 0.49–0.94) (71).

Physical activity, physical fitness, and all-cause mortality were studied in a cohort of 7080 women and 25,341 men who were examined at a Texas clinic and followed for an average of eight years. There was a strong inverse association between all-cause mortality and level of physical fitness in both men and women (p-trend < 0.001). With regard to physical activity levels, which were based on running habits and involvement in vigorous sports, the most active men were also at lower risk of total mortality than were sedentary men (p-trend = 0.01), but physical activity was not significantly associated with mortality risk in women. The authors suggest that this lack of association in women may be the result of greater misclassification of physical activity in women, who may have engaged in less sports activity but been more physically active in housework, child care, and other energy-expending activities for which women still assume disproportionate responsibility (72).

Physical fitness measured by a maximal treadmill exercise test and risk of all-cause mortality was assessed in a cohort of 10,224 men and 3120 women who were given a preventive medical examination and followed for an average of 8 years. Age-adjusted all-cause mortality rates declined across physical fitness quintiles, from 39.5 per 10,000 person-years in the least fit women to 8.5 per 10,000 person-years in the most fit. Corresponding values for men were 64.0 per 10,000 person-years and 18.6 per 10,000 person-years. Attributable risk estimates for all-cause mortality indicated that a low level of physical fitness was an important risk factor in both men and women (73).

Finally, the Framingham Heart Study analyzed 285 men and women, aged 75 or older, who were grouped in quartiles of physical activity. After adjustments for cardiac risk factors, chronic obstructive pulmonary disease, and cancer, those in the first, second, and third most active quartiles had reduced mortality risks compared with the least active quartile (p-trend = 0.001). The relative risks for successively higher quartiles of activity level were 0.70 (95% CI, 0.38–1.29), 0.26 (95% CI, 0.12–0.55), and 0.39 (95% CI, 0.20–0.77). This trend persisted when deaths in the first 3 years of follow-up were excluded. There was a trend toward reduced mortality among more active men, but this did not attain statistical significance (74).

In summary, data on regular physical activity and overall mortality in women provide strong support for the conclusion that higher levels of regular physical activity are associated with lower all-cause mortality rates.

OSTEOPOROSIS

Osteoporosis is a significant public health problem among older women in developed countries. It is characterized by rapid loss of bone density after menopause—which appears to be directly related to a decrease in estrogen levels—and is associated with increased risks of hip, spine, and wrist fracture. The peak of bone density occurs in adolescence and is determined by many factors, including genetic influences, hormonal factors, and environmental variables, including dietary intake of certain foods (e.g., calcium, which increases bone density, and protein, caffeine, and alcohol, all of which decrease bone density), vitamin D intake, and physical activity.

Others factors associated with osteoporosis include increasing age, early menopause, amenorrhea, cigarette smoking, high parity, and race, with white and Asian women at highest risk. The development of osteoporosis is a function of both peak bone mineral density in adolescence and degree of bone loss after menopause, suggesting that the risk of this condition can be altered by enhancing peak bone density in young women or preventing postmenopausal bone loss. With respect to the influence of physical activity on osteoporosis, the hypothesized benefits relate specifically to weight-bearing exercise, which can increase bone density by stimulating bone growth and trabeculation (75).

In a cross-sectional study of 352 perimenopausal women, after controlling for potential confounding factors, those with higher activity levels had higher bone density at the spine and radius (76). A Canadian case-control study examined the effects of past and recent physical activity on the risk of hip fracture (77). After controlling for recent activity, there were reduced risks of hip fracture among women with moderate (odds ratio = 0.66, 95% CI, 0.45–0.96) and high (odds ratio = 0.54; 95% CI, 0.33–0.88) levels of past physical activity. For recent activity, after adjusting for past activity levels, a similar protective association was observed for women who reported recent moderate activity (odds ratio = 0.61; 95% CI, 0.41–0.90), but not for those in the highest activity group. Possible explanations for the latter finding include chance, increased risk of falls that could offset the benefits of high activity levels, and the potential risks of recent vigorous activity among women who had been inactive in the past and had not accrued the benefits on bone density of regular physical activity at younger ages.

The association between sports participation in adolescence and peri- and postmenopausal bone mineral density (BMD) was studied in 2025 women aged 48 to 58. Women who participated in sports during adolescence had an unadjusted spinal BMD 2.4% higher ($p = 0.001$) than those who had not engaged in athletics. The difference was attenuated, but still significant, after adjusting for age, weight, time since menopause, and duration of estrogen replacement therapy (BMD among athletes 1.4% higher, $p = 0.015$) (78).

Thus, weight-bearing physical activity, particularly at younger ages, appears to be associated with decreased subsequent risks of osteoporosis and fracture. The Surgeon General's report on physical activity and health (5) concludes that weight-bearing physical activity, such as walking, jogging, tennis, rowing, aerobic and strength training, is essential for normal skeletal development during childhood and adolescence and for achieving and maintaining peak bone mass in young adults.

RISKS OF PHYSICAL ACTIVITY

Along with its wide range of benefits, physical activity is also associated with some risks, including possible cardiac events, musculoskeletal injuries, metabolic abnormalities, and menstrual dysfunction (particularly in athletes).

Cardiac Events

The association between vigorous exercise and cardiac events and sudden death has been widely evaluated (79–81). Mittle-man studied 1228 post-MI patients (836 women and 392 men). The estimated relative risk of MI in the hour after heavy physical exertion as compared with less strenuous exercise was 5.9 (95% CI, 4.6–7.7). Among those who usually exercised less than one, one or two, three to four, or five or more times per week, the respective relative risks were 107 (95% CI, 67–171), 19.4 (95% CI, 9.9–38.1), 8.6 (95% CI, 3.6–20.5), and 2.4 (95% CI, 1.5–3.7). The authors concluded that heavy physical exertion can trigger the onset of acute myocardial infarction, particularly in people who are habitually sedentary (82). Nonetheless, it is important to bear in mind that regular physical activity is clearly associated with an overall decrease in cardiovascular disease events that far outweighs the transient risks associated with physical exertion.

In a recent review of the cardiovascular complications of vigorous physical activity, congenital abnormalities in young subjects and atherosclerotic coronary disease in adults were cited as the most frequent causes of exercise-related CVD deaths. The absolute incidence of exercise-related death is low, particularly at younger ages. For high school and college athletes it is approximately 0.75 and 0.13 per 100,000 for males and females, respectively. Routine cardiovascular testing (echocardiography in the young and exercise testing in adults) has limited usefulness because of the rarity of such events, the cost of screening, and poor predictive accuracy of testing for exercise-related events. Physicians should, however, perform routine screening via cardiac auscultation in young athletes, carefully evaluate exercise-related symptoms, and ensure that adults know the symptoms of cardiac ischemia (83).

The Report of the Surgeon General (5) concludes that regular physical activity improves cardiorespiratory fitness and reduces the risk of CVD mortality over the long term, although it can acutely increase risk of untoward cardiac events. The most common causes of death during exercise are myocardial infarction and arrhythmias, with the risk of sudden death greater in typically sedentary people who sporadically engage in a vigorous exercise than it is in those who follow a program of regular physical activity.

Musculoskeletal Injuries and Other Non-Cardiac Events

Musculoskeletal injuries are common in people who engage in regular physical activity. For example, shoulder problems (rotator cuff tendinitis and subtle subluxation and impingement syndrome) are common in women who participate in overhead sports, such as swimming, tennis, and throwing sports (e.g., baseball, softball, javelin) (84). Stress fractures are most common in the lower extremities and are mainly associated with running. Stress fractures occur more commonly in female athletes than male athletes, likely as a consequence of the high prevalence of eating disorders combined with exercise-induced amenorrhea and osteoporosis in young female athletes (85). Table 31-2 shows the specific sites of stress fractures and the activities with which they are most frequently associated. Finally, severe exertion in difficult conditions (e.g., severe heat and humidity) can lead to hyperthermia, electrolyte imbalance, and dehydration, and exercise-provoked asthma can occur in susceptible individuals.

Table 31-2 Specific Sites of Stress Fractures in Women* and Related Sports

TYPE OF STRESS FRACTURE	RELATED SPORTS
Sesamoids (foot)	Distance running, ballet, jumping sports
Metatarsals	Distance running, marching, ballet, jumping sports
Tarsal bones	Distance running, ballet, sprinting, marching, jumping sports
Medial malleolus	Jumping sports, distance running
Tibia	Distance running, jumping sports, ballet
Fibula	Distance running, aerobics, ballet
Patella	Hurdling, jumping sports, running
Femur	Running, ballet, jumping sports
Sacrum	Distance running
Pars interarticularis	Gymnastics, diving, ballet
Ribs	Throwing sports, rowing
Ulna	Racquet sports, fast-pitch softball
Humerus/olecranon	Throwing sports, racquet sports
Acromion	Weight lifting

* All these fractures are more common in women than in men and may be attributed to training surface, training techniques, biochemical abnormalities, and poor conditioning.
SOURCE: Adapted from Reader MT, Dick BH, Atkins JK, et al. Stress fractures. Sports Medicine 1996;22:182–212.

Menstrual Irregularities

A significant issue concerning physical activity in women is the effect exercise can have on menstrual function. The prevalence of menstrual dysfunction is greater in athletes than in the general population (86). Menstrual alterations occur above a specific level of physical activity, although this level differs for each woman. Many factors have been hypothesized to be involved with exercise-induced menstrual irregularities, including loss of fat, elevated ovarian core temperature, increased stress hormone levels, change in the level of endorphins and other neuropeptides, nutrient balance, change in energy levels, and modification of the gonadotropin output. Table 31-3 shows factors associated with menstrual changes in athletes (87).

The effect of strenuous exercise on menstrual function was demonstrated in a study of 28 college-age women who were assigned to a strenuous exercise regimen spanning two menstrual cycles and also randomly allocated to programs of weight loss and weight maintenance (88). All of the women had documented ovulation and luteal adequacy prior to the study. Only 4 of the 28 women had a normal menstrual cycle during the study, with 3 of these being in the weight maintenance group and 1 being in the weight loss group. All women resumed normal cycles within 6 months of training termination.

With the exception of oligomenorrhea and anovulation,

Table 31-3 Primary Factors Associated with Menstrual Changes in Female Athletes

MENSTRUAL REGULARITY	MENSTRUAL IRREGULARITY
Maturity of reproductive axis; established ovulatory cycles	Immaturity of reproductive axis
	Absence of regular ovulatory cycles
Advanced gynecological age	Youth
Parity	Nulliparity
Increased body weight/fat	Decreased body weight/fat
Regular energy diet	Low-energy diet
Gradual increase in activity	Rapid increase in exercise workload
Low-intensity exercise	High-volume, high-intensity exercese
Absence of psychological stress	Presence of psychological stress

SOURCE: Adapted from Carbon R. Female athletes. BMJ 1994;309:254–258.

Table 31-4 Tests to Consider in the Clinical Evaluation of Athletes with Amenorrhea*

- Test for pregnancy
- Serum concentrations of:
  estradiol
  progesterone
  follicle stimulating hormone
  luteinizing hormone
  prolactin
  testosterone, dehydroepiandrosterone
- Thyroid function tests
- Pelvic ultrasonography (preferable to full pelvic examination in young athlete; note that cystic ovaries may be nonspecific)
- Cranial computed tomography or magnetic resonance imaging scan for pituitary tumor (if prolactin concentration is raised)
- Bone density—e.g., dual energy x ray absorptiometry (DEXA)

* All blood tests must be taken after at least 24 hours rest from activity.
SOURCE: Adapted from Carbon R. Female athletes. BMJ 1994;309:254–258.

physical activity is not usually a cause of infertility. Because other conditions, including pituitary tumors, thyroid dysfunction, polycystic ovary syndrome, and premature ovarian failure, may cause amenorrhea in athletes, it is necessary to investigate the cause in all oligomenorrheic and amenorrheic athletes. Table 31-4 describes tests to consider in the clinical evaluation of athletes with amenorrhea (87).

Women with exercise-induced amenorrhea have lower levels of circulating estrogens and may have increased risk of osteoporosis. At particular risk for exercise-related osteoporosis are vigorously active women with low body weight. With respect to the onset of menstruation, some young gymnasts, runners, cyclists, and ballet dancers, especially those with strenuous and demanding exercise regimens, may experience delayed menarche, which has been associated with alterations in skeletal maturation as well as epiphyseal damage. Thus, although regular weight-bearing exercise, particularly at younger ages, is associated with increased bone density in women, amenorrheic athletes have reduced bone density (89), and this may be irreversible or normalize only partially after restoration of menses (90).

Female Athlete Triad

In 1992, the American College of Sports Medicine introduced the term "female athlete triad" to describe a constellation of three disorders whose prevalence in women has increased markedly: disordered eating, amenorrhea, and osteoporosis (91). Disordered eating may include a variety of disturbances, including binging, purging, food restriction, prolonged fasting, and the use of diet pills, diuretics, laxatives, and excessive exercise (84,92). Although many athletes do not meet the strict criteria for anorexia or bulimia, many exhibit symptoms that place them at risk for these conditions (92).

Thus the occurrence of exercise-induced amenorrhea, particularly in women of low body weight who are at increased risk of osteoporosis, underscores the fact that health practices such as regular physical activity, which at a wide range of levels can confer a wide range of benefits, may nonetheless have deleterious consequences at excessive levels.

EMOTIONAL WELL-BEING AND DEPRESSION

Exercise increases levels of endorphins, providing a biologic mechanism to support the increased feeling of well-being often described following physical activity. Exercise can alter norepinephrine release, decrease depression, and may be associated with improved body image and self-esteem, as well as with stress reduction (93–95).

The impact of physical activity on psychological well-being was assessed in a sample of 401 adult men and women in Illinois. More frequent participation in exercise, sports, and physical activities was associated with improved psychological well-being in men and women, after control for potentially confounding factors, including sociodemographic characteristics and weight (96). Farmer et al studied the relationship between physical activity and depressive symptoms in 1900 healthy subjects, aged 25 to 77, in the Epidemiologic Follow-up Study (1982–1984) to the First National Health and Nutrition Examination Survey (NHANES I) (97). Depressive symptomatology, as measured by the Center for Epidemiologic Studies Depression Scale, was examined by sex and race in relation to recreational and nonrecreational physical activity, controlling for age, education, income, employment status, and chronic conditions. Engaging in little or no recreational or nonrecreational physical activity was cross-sectionally associated with depressive symptoms in whites and blacks. After exclusion of those with depressive symptoms at baseline, lack of recreational physical

activity was an independent predictor of depressive symptoms an average of 8 years later in white women. The adjusted odds ratio of depressive symptoms at follow-up was approximately 2 for women with little or no recreational activity compared with women with moderate or high levels of recreational physical activity (95% CI, 1.1–3.2) (97). The Healthy Women Study has also evaluated the relationship between change in physical activity and change in psychological well-being and concluded that women who increased their physical activity also had the smallest increase in depressive and stress symptoms (14). Thus, it appears that regular physical activity can serve as an effective component of efforts by women to maintain emotional well-being and reduce symptoms of depression.

PREGNANCY

Ensuring optimal health of mother and fetus must be the paramount concern during pregnancy. Several issues must be considered in relation to exercise during pregnancy, including potential effects on uterine blood flow, hyperthermia, substrate availability, and uterine contractions. At present, however, there is no clear evidence that exercise-related alterations in these parameters represent a threat to the fetus. Some studies have demonstrated an association between exercise and low birthweight and shortened gestation, but others have not confirmed this observation (98).

Exercise enhances a woman's sensation of well-being in pregnancy, and many studies have reported that women who maintain regular physical activity during pregnancy report fewer typical adverse pregnancy-related symptoms, such as nausea, fatigue, and leg cramps (98,99).

A recent review concluded that volitional exercise during pregnancy was safe for healthy, well-nourished women. There is some evidence of favorable effects of exercise on the course of pregnancy, but there remains substantial uncertainty whether exercise during pregnancy should be actively promoted. At present, therefore, the public health message is not that women should exercise during pregnancy, but that they may (100). According to the American College of Obstetricians and Gynecologists, there are no data in humans to indicate that pregnant women should limit exercise intensity and target heart rates because of potential adverse effects (101). See chapter 35, Exercise and Pregnancy, for a more detailed discussion.

Contraindications to Exercise in Pregnancy

There are a number of medical and obstetric conditions that constitute contraindications to physical activity during pregnancy. These include pregnancy-induced hypertension, preterm rupture of membranes, preterm labor during the prior or current pregnancy, incompetent cervix/cerclage, persistent second- or third-trimester bleeding, and intrauterine growth retardation. Thus, in the absence of either obstetric or medical complications, pregnant women can continue to exercise and derive related benefits. While maternal fitness and sense of well-being may be enhanced by exercise, no level of exercise during pregnancy has been conclusively demonstrated to be beneficial in improving perinatal outcome (102).

CONCLUSION

Physical activity appears to be associated with a wide range of health benefits in women of all ages. One concern in all epidemiologic studies of physical activity is that there may be unmeasured correlates of physical activity that account for the healthier profile of those classified as more active. Most studies, however, have controlled for the effects of known confounding variables. There is also likely to be imprecision in the measurement and classification of physical activity, perhaps particularly in women. Nonetheless, while the precise magnitude of the benefits may be somewhat smaller or larger than those reported in the available studies, it appears reasonable to conclude that there are salutary effects of physical activity on cardiovascular disease risk factors and clinical events, certain cancers, and total mortality. Physical activity at a wide range of levels is also associated with decreased risk of osteoporosis and is associated with improved emotional well-being and reduced symptoms of depression. Regular physical activity poses some risks, but these are generally far outweighed by its benefits. In women, menstrual dysfunction is a concern among those engaging in regular, strenuous activity, and health care providers should be particularly attuned to signs of extreme levels of physical activity that may be a signal of excessive efforts to control weight, requiring intervention and counseling.

The optimal frequency, duration, and intensity of physical activity for overall health remains unclear. However, as more than one quarter of all U.S. women engage in no regular physical activity and nearly two thirds do not meet the current activity guidelines, it is clear that efforts must be redoubled to encourage increased physical activity in women.

REFERENCES

1. Morris JN, Chave SPW, Adam C, et al. Vigorous exercise in leisure-time and the incidence of coronary heart disease. Lancet 1973; 1:333–339.

2. Paffenbarger RS Jr, Wing AL, Hyde RT. Physical activity as an index of heart attack risk in college alumni. Am J Epidemiol 1978;108:161–175.

3. Paffenbarger RS Jr, Hyde RT, Wing AL, Hsieh C-c. Physical activity, all-cause mortality, and longevity of college alumni. N Engl J Med 1986a;314:605–613.

4. Leon AS, Connett J, Jacobs DR Jr, Rauramaa R. Leisure-time physical activity levels and risk of coronary heart disease and death: the Multiple Risk Factor Intervention Trial. JAMA 1987;258: 2388–2395.

5. Physical activity and health: a report of the Surgeon General. Rockville, MD: U.S. Department of Health and Human Services, 1996. DHHS publication no. CDC (S/N 017-023-00196-5).

6. Powell KE, Caspersen CJ, Koplan JP, Ford ES. Physical activity and chronic diseases. Am J Clin Nutr 1989;49:999–1006.

7. Berlin JA, Colditz GA. A meta-analysis of physical activity in the prevention of coronary heart disease. Am J Epidemiol 1990; 132:612–628.

8. Pate RR, Pratt M, Blair SN, et al. Physical activity and public health: a recommendation from the Centers for Disease Control and Prevention and the American College of Sports Medicine. JAMA 1995;273:402–407.

9. Journal Watch: Women's Health/Exercise and your health 1997;2(9).

10. American College of Sports Medicine. Guidelines for graded exercise testing and exercise prescription. 3rd ed. Philadelphia: Lea & Febiger, 1985.

11. Manson JE, Lee IM. Exercise for women: how much pain for optimal gain? N Engl J Med 1996;334:1325–1327.

12. Manson JE, Willet WC, Stampfer MJ, et al. Body weight and mortality among women. N Engl J Med 1995;33: 677–685.

13. Daly PA, Solomon CG, Manson JE. Risk modification in the obese patient. In: Manson JE, Ridker PM, Gaziano JM, Hennekens CH, eds. Prevention of myocardial infarction. New York: Oxford University Press; 1996: 203–273.

14. Owens JF, Matthews KA, Wing RR, Kuller LH. Can physical activity mitigate the effects of aging in middle-aged women? Circulation 1992;85: 1265–1270.

15. Segall KR, Pi-Suniyer FX. Exercise and obesity. Med Clin North Am 1989;73:217–236.

16. Racette SB, Schoeller DA, Kushner RF, Neil KM. Am J Clin Nutr 1995;62:345–349.

17. Pols AA, Peeters PHM, Twisk JWR, et al. Physical activity and cardiovascular disease risk profile in women. Am J Epidemiol 1997;146:322–328.

18. Kohrt WM, Obert KA, Hollosny JO. J Gerontol 1992;47:M99–M105.

19. Ashley FW, Kannel WB. Relation of weight change to changes in atherogenic traits: the Framingham study. J Chronic Dis 1974;27:103–114.

20. Kayman S, Bruvold W, Stern JS. Maintenance and relapse after weight loss in women: behavioral aspects. Am J Clin Nutr 1990; 52:800–807.

21. Jeffery RW, French SA. Socioeconomic status and weight control practices among 20 to 45-year-old women. Am J Public Health 1996;86:1005–1011.

22. The health benefits of smoking cessation: a report of the Surgeon General. Rockville, MD: Office on Smoking and Health, 1990. DHHS publication CDC 90-8416.

23. Kawachi I, Troisis RJ, Rotnitzky AG, et al. Can physical activity minimize weight gain in women after smoking cessation? Am J Public Health 1996;86:999–1004.

24. Taylor PA, Ward A. Women, high-density lipoprotein cholesterol, and exercise. Arch Intern Med 1993;153:1178–1184.

25. Berg A, Frey I, Baumstark MW, et al. Physical activity and lipoprotein lipid disorders. Sports Med 1994;17:6–21.

26. Duncan JJ, Gordon NF, Scott CB. Women walking for health and fitness: How much is enough? JAMA 1991;266:3295–3299.

27. Williams PT. High-density lipoprotein cholesterol and other risk factors for coronary heart disease in female runners. N Engl J Med 1996;334:1298–1303.

28. Greendale GA, Bodin-Dunn L, Ingles S, et al. Leisure, home, and occupational physical activity and cardiovascular risk factors in postmenopausal women. Arch Intern Med 1996;156:418–424.

29. Cauley JA, Kriska AM, LaPorte RE, et al. A two year randomized exercise trial in older women: effects on HDL-cholesterol. Atherosclerosis 1987;66:247–258.

30. Boyden TW, Pamenter RW, Going SB, et al. Resistance exercise training is associated with decreases in serum low-density lipoprotein cholesterol levels in premenopausal women. Arch Inter Med 1993;153:97–100.

31. Dunn AL, Marcus BH, Kampert JB, et al. Reduction in cardiovascular disease risk factors: 6-month results from Project Active. Prev Med 1997;26:883–892.

32. Paffenbarger R, Wing A, Hyde R, Jung D. Physical fitness and incidence of hypertension in college alumni. Ann Epidemiol 1983;117:245–257.

33. Blair SN, Goodyear NN, Gibbons LW, Cooper KH. Physical fitness and incidence of hypertension in healthy normotensive men and women. JAMA 1984;252:487–490.

34. Fagard RH, Follmann D, Elliot P, Suh I. An overview of randomized trials of sodium reduction and blood pressure. J Hypertension 1993;11(suppl):S47–S52.

35. Seals DR, Silverman HG, Reiling MJ, Davy KP. Effect of regular aerobic exercise on elevated blood pressure in post-menopausal women. Am J Cardiol 1997;80:49–55.

36. Reaven PD, Barret-Connor E, Sharon E. Relation between leisure-time physical activity and blood pressure in older women. Circulation 1991;83:559–565.

37. Borhani NO. Significance of physical activity for prevention and control of hypertension. J Human Hypert 1996;10(suppl):S2–S11.

38. Joint National Committee on the Detection, Evaluation, and Treatment of High Blood Pressure. The Sixth Report of the Joint National Committee on the Detection, Evaluation, and Treatment of High Blood Pressure. Arch Intern Med 1997;157:2413–2444.

39. Schneider SH, Amorosa LF, Khachadurian AK, Ruderman NB. Studies on the mechanism of improved glucose control during regular exercise in type 2 (non-insulin dependent) diabetes. Diabetologia 1984;26:355–360.

40. Koivisto VA, Yki-Jarvinen H, de Fronzo RA. Physical training and insulin sensitivity. Diabetes Metab Rev 1988;1:445–481.

41. Ruderman N, Apelian AZ, Schneider SH. Exercise in therapy and prevention of type-II diabetes: implications for blacks. Diabetes Care 1990;13(suppl):1163–1168.

42. van Dam S, Gillespy M, Notelovitz M, Martin D. Effect of exercise on glucose metabolism in postmenopausal women. Am J Obstet Gynecol 1988;159:82–86.

43. Manson JE, Rimm EB, Stampfer MJ, et al. Physical activity and incidence of non-insulin-dependent diabetes mellitus in women. Lancet 1991;338:774–778.

44. Haapanen N, Milunpalo S, Vuori I, et al. Association of leisure time physical activity with the risk of coronary heart disease, hypertension and diabetes in middle-aged men and women. Int J Epidemiol 1997;26:739–747.

45. Lehmann R, Kaplan V, Bingisser R, et al. Impact of physical activity on cardiovascular risk factors in IDDM. Diabetes Care 1997;20:1603–1611.

46. Morris CK, Froelicher VF. Cardiovascular benefits of improved exercise capacity. Sports Med 1993;16(4):225–236.

47. Kushi LH, Fee RM, Folsom AR, et al. Physical activity and mortality in postmenopausal women. JAMA 1997;277:1287–1292.

48. Dannenberg AL, Keller JB, Wilson PWF, Castelli WP. Leisure time physical activity in the Framingham offspring study. Am J Epidemiol 1989;129:76–87.

49. Mensink GBH, Deketh M, Mul M, et al. Physical activity and its association with cardiovascular risk factors and mortality. Epidemiology 1996;7:391–397.

50. O'Connor GT, Hennekens CH, Willet WC, et al. Am J Epidemiol 1995;142:1147–1156.

51. Lemaitre RN, Heckbeert SR, Psaty BM, Siscovick DS. Leisure-time physical activity and the risk of nonfatal myocardial infarction in postmenopausal women. Arch Intern Med 1995;155:2302–2308.

52. Gillum RF, Mussolino ME, Ingram DD. Physical activity and stroke incidence in women and men: the NHANES I Epidemiologic Follow-up Study. Am J Epidemiol 1996;143:860–869.

53. Manson JE, Stampfer MJ, Willet WC, et al. Physical activity and incidence of coronary heart disease and stroke in women. Circulation 1995;91:927.

54. Sturgeon SR, Brinton LA, Berman ML, et al. Past and

present physical activity and endometrial cancer risk. Br J Cancer 1993;68:584–589.

55. Olson SH, Vena JE, Dorn JP, et al. Exercise, occupational activity, and risk of endometrial cancer. Ann Epidemiol 1997;7:46–53.

56. Mink PJ, Folsom AR, Sellers TA, Kushi LH. Physical activity, waist-to-hip ratio, and other risk factors for ovarian cancer: a follow-up study of older women. Epidemiology 1996;7:38–45.

57. Frisch RE, Wyshak G, Albright NL, et al. Lower prevalence of breast cancer and cancer of the reproductive system among former athletes compared to non-athletes. Br J Cancer 1985;52:885–891.

58. Thune I, Brenn T, Lund E, Gaard M. Physical activity and the risk of breast cancer. N Engl J Med 1997;336:1269–1275.

59. Coogan PF, Newcomb PA, Clapp RW, et al. Physical activity in usual occupation and risk of breast cancer (United States). Cancer Causes Control 1997;8:626–631.

60. Wu AH, Paganini-Hill A, Ross RK, Henderson BE. Alcohol, physical activity and other risk factors for colorectal cancer: a prospective study. Br J Cancer 1987;55:687–694.

61. Gerhardsson M, Floderus B, Norell SE. Physical activity and colon cancer risk. Int J Epidemiol 1988;17:743–746.

62. Severson RK, Nomura AMY, Grove JS, Stemmermann GN. A prospective analysis of physical activity and cancer. Am J Epidemiol 1989;130:522–529.

63. Lee I-M, Paffenbarger RS, Hsieh CC. Physical activity and risk of developing colorectal cancer among college alumni. J Natl Cancer Inst 1991;83:1324–1329.

64. Markowitz S, Morabia A, Garibaldi K, Wynder E. Effect of occupational and recreational activity on the risk of colorectal cancer among males: a case-control study. Int J Epidemiol 1992;21:1057–1062.

65. Giovanucci E, Ascherio A, Rimm EB, et al. Physical activity, obesity, and risk of colon cancer and adenoma in men. Ann Int Med 1995;122:327–334.

66. White E, Jacobs EJ, Dailing JR. Physical activity in relation to colon cancer im middle-aged men and women. J Epidemiol 1996;144:42–50.

67. Thune I, Lund E. Physical activity and risk of colorectal cancer in men and women. Br J Cancer 1996;73:1134–1140.

68. Giovanucci E, Colditz GA, Stampfer MJ, Willet WC. Physical activity, obesity, and risk of colorectal adenoma in women (United States). Cancer Causes Control 1996;7:253–263.

69. Sandler RS, Pritchard ML, Bangdiwala SI. Physical activity and the risk of colorectal adenomas. Epidemiology 1995;6:602–606.

70. Neugut AI, Terry MB, Hocking G, et al. Leisure and occupational physical activity and risk of colorectal adenomatous polyps. Int J Cancer 1996;68:744–748.

71. Sherman SE, D'Agostino RF, Cobb JL, Kannel WB. Physical activity and mortality in women in the Framingham Heart Study. Am Heart J 1994;128:879–884.

72. Kampert JB, Blair SN, Barlow CE, Kohl HW. Physical activity, physical fitness, and all-cause and cancer mortality: a prospective study of men and women. Ann Epidemiol 1996;6:452–457.

73. Blair SN, Kohl III HW, Paffenbarger RS, et al. Physical fitness and all-cause mortality. JAMA 1989;262:2395–2401.

74. Sherman SE, D'Agostino RB, Cobb JL, Kannel WB. Does exercise reduce mortality rates in the elderly? experience from Framingham Heart Study. Am Heart J 1994;128:965–972.

75. Lanyon LE. Osteocytes, strain detection, bone modeling and remodeling. Calcif Tissue Int 1993;18(suppl):37S–43S.

76. Zhang J, Feldblum PJ, Fortney JA. Moderate physical activity and bone density among peri-menopausal women. Am J Public Health 1992;82:736–738.

77. Jaglal SB, Kreiger N, Darlington G. Past and recent physical activity and the risk of hip fracture. Am J Epidemiol 1993;138:107–118.

78. Puntilla E, Kröger H, Lakka T, et al. Physical activity in adolescence and bone density in peri- and postmenopausal women: a population-based study. Bone 1997;21:363–367.

79. Vuori I, Makarainen M, Jaasheiainer J. Sudden death and physical activity. Cardiology 1981;68(suppl):1–8.

80. Thompson PD, Funk EJ, Carleton RA, Sturner WQ. Incidence of death during jogging in Rhode Island from 1975 through 1980. JAMA 1982;247:2535–2538.

81. Siscovich DS, Weiss NS, Fletcher RH, Lasky T. The incidence of primary cardiac arrest during vigorous exercise. N Engl J Med 1984;311:874–877.

82. Mittleman MA, MacLure M, Tofler GH, et al. Triggering of acute myocardial infarction by heavy physical exertion: protection against triggering by regular exertion. N Engl J Med 1993;329:1677–1683.

83. Thompson PD. The cardiovascular complications of vigorous physical activity. Arch Intern Med 1996;156:2297–2302.

84. Wiggins DL, Wiggins ME. The female athlete. Clin Sports Med 1997;16:593–562.

85. Reeder MT, Dick BH, Atkins JK, et al. Stress fractures. Sports Med 1996;22:198–212.

86. Shangold M, Rebar RW, Wentz AC, Schiff I. Evaluation and management of menstrual dysfunction on athletes. JAMA 1990;263:1665–1669.

87. Carbon R. ABC of sports medicine: female athletes. BMJ 1994; 309:254–258.

88. Bullen BA, Skrinar GS, Beitins IZ, et al. Induction of menstrual disorders by strenuous exercise in untrained women. N Engl J Med 1985;312:1349–1353.

89. Rencken M, Chestnut CH, Drinkwater BL. Bone density at multiple skeletal sites in amenorrheic athletes. JAMA 1996;276: 238–240.

90. Drinkwater BL, Nilson K, Ott S, et al. Bone mineral density after resumption of menses in amenorrheic athletes. JAMA 1986;256: 380–382.

91. American College of Sports Medicine: The female athlete triad: disordered eating, amenorrhea, osteoporosis: call to action. Sports Med Bull 1992;27:4.

92. Nattiv A, Agostini R, Drinkwater B, Yeager K. The female athlete triad. Clin Sports Med 1994;13: 405–418.

93. Cronan TL, Howley ET. The effect of training on epinephrine and norepinephrine excretion. Med Sci Sports Exerc 1984;5:122–125.

94. Siever LJ, Davis KL. Overview: toward a dysregulation hypothesis of depression. Am J Psychiatry 1985;142:1017–1031.

95. Klein MH, Greist JH, Gurmas AS, et al. A comparative outcome study of group psychotherapy vs. exercise treatments for depression. Int J Mental Health 1985; 13:148–177.

96. Ross CE, Hayes D. Exercise and psychologic well-being in the community. Am J Epidemiol 1988;127:762–771.

97. Farmer ME, Locke BZ, Moscicki EK, et al. Physical activity and depressive symptoms: the NHANES I epidemiologic follow-up study. Am J Epidemiol 1988;128:1340–1351.

98. Sternfeld B. Physical activity and pregnancy outcome. Sports Med 1997;23:33–47.

99. Hall DC, Kauffman DA. Effects of aerobic and strength conditioning in pregnancy outcomes. Am J Obstet Gynecol 1987;157:1199–1203.

100. Sternfeld B, Quesenberry CPJ, Eskenazy B, et al. Exercise during pregnancy and pregnancy outcome. Med Sci Sports Exerc 1995;27:634-640.

101. American College of Obstetricians and Gynecologists. Women and exercise. Washington, DC: ACOG, 1992. ACOG technical bulletin 173.

102. American College of Obstetricians and Gynecologists. Exercise during pregnancy and the postpartum period. Washington, DC: ACOG, 1994. ACOG technical bulletin 189.

Chapter 32

Preventing Violence Against Women: A Health Mandate

Deborah Prothrow-Stith
Jacqueline Kral

Domestic violence is often defined as a pattern of assaultive and coercive behaviors, including physical, sexual, and psychological attacks, that adults or adolescents use against their intimate partners. It may occur in a variety of relationships—married, separated, divorced, dating, heterosexual, gay, and lesbian (1).

Physical abuse can include pinching, slapping, shoving, punching, kicking, or any combination of these. It may also include the use of a weapon. Verbal abuse, done to maintain domination and control over the victim, includes name calling, threats made against the victim and against the victim's family, as well as threats made by the abuser to harm him/herself. Psychological or emotional abuse occurs when the victim's self-worth, self-esteem, and sense of control or safety are questioned. This type of abuse can include threatening gestures and looks. It can also be inflicted verbally, and many times such comments are designed to degrade the victim so that (s)he feels that no other options but this relationship exist. This can lead to feelings of isolation, worthlessness, and depression. These feelings can serve to increase the very serious problem of not reporting abuse, especially for adolescents already struggling with issues of identity and independence (2).

Some definitions of domestic violence omit sexual abuse. Sexual abuse itself ranges from repetitious, unwanted sexual advances and coercion by an abuser to acts such as rape. Sexual abuse also includes "date rape," defined as nonconsensual sex between people who are on a date and/or considered to be in a dating relationship (3). (See Fig. 32-1.)

While both men and women can be perpetrators, men represent the overwhelming majority of reported perpetrators and inflict the most severe injuries on women. As the recipients of the majority of abuse perpetrated by men, a woman's most significant risk factor for abuse is her age. Younger women are disproportionately the victims of violence at the hands of a husband, an ex-husband, a boyfriend, or an ex-boyfriend. Most studies reveal few other factors that distinguish victims from those who are not victims of domestic violence (4,5).

Two large population-based studies in the United States revealed that 3.4% of adult women reported being severely abused by an intimate male partner in the past year, and 11.6% reported less severe acts such as pushing, shoving, and slapping. The National Crime Victimization Survey estimates that 2.5 million women experience violence in a year, 67% at the hands of someone they know. And a 1992 study, using explicit language and a clear definition, estimates 683,000 adult women are raped each year (6).

Though the numbers are shocking, violence against women is more than men physically, verbally, and sexually assaulting women. Women are the grandmothers, mothers, sisters, aunts, nieces, cousins, and friends of every victim and perpetrator of violence. Though girls and women are less often perpetrators of violence, juvenile arrests rates for girls committing violent crimes have dramatically increased. A broader definition of violence against women and a comprehensive family and community approach to prevention and intervention is indicated.

A comprehensive approach to violence is also indicated by the consistent findings showing that children who witness violence or are victims of violence in their early childhood development are at risk for subsequent episodes of violence either as victims or perpetrators. Pynoos et al (7) examined the appearance of posttraumatic stress disorder (PTSD) symp-

Figure 32-1 Power and control wheel. (Reproduced with permission from Cambridge Documentary Films (Cambridge, MA). Study & Resource Guide for the film "Defending Our Lives," p. 12. Adapted from the Domestic Abuse Intervention Project by Elba Crespo-Gonzales.)

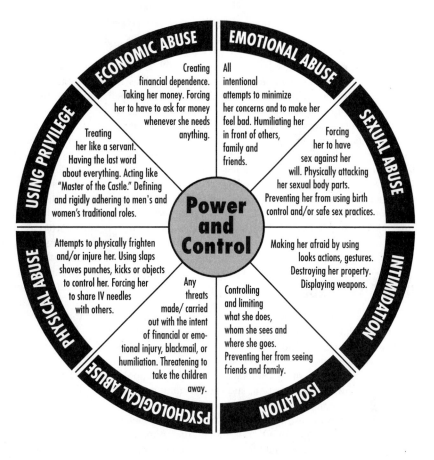

toms in children who experienced a fatal sniper attack on their elementary school and reported a correlation between the type and number of PTSD symptoms and proximity to the violent incident as well as more severe symptoms in children who knew the deceased child.

In addition to acute incidents, other studies report correlations between exposure to chronic violence and distress symptoms (8–12). Lorion et al also described anecdotal reports from their research participants, including reports from teachers and administrators about children who lived in violent settings arriving at school in distress, unable to concentrate or maintain appropriate behavior in class, and who hid in the classroom, afraid to return home or take the bus (13). Clearly, there is a need to address not only the physical threat of violence, but also the potential for psychopathological and/or emotional disturbances in both victims and bystanders, especially in girls and young women (14,15).

Violence against children perpetrated by parents and other family members has been related to those children committing violent acts, and though this is true for both boys and girls, research also shows that girls are more likely than boys to experience physical abuse and sexual abuse at the hands of a family member (16,17). This cycle of violence presents a particular challenge to health care and human service providers.

DATA SOURCES AND STATISTICS

Domestic and family violence is likely to go unreported and police reports are often biased, with families from low socio-economic status being more likely reported. There are not reliable, valid, and consistently used data sets for collection of national population-based incidence data on violence against women. The collection of data on violence against women is complicated by the "hidden" nature of many of these crimes—women may choose not to report abuse due to shame, stigma, previous bad experiences with the criminal justice sector, fear of reprisal from perpetrators, and language and/or cultural barriers. Unfortunately, the United State still lacks a valid and reliable set of methods for the collection of national population-based incidence data on violence against women. The two most widely used data sources, the National Crime Victimization Survey (NCVS) and the Uniform Crime Reports, are likely comprised of severe underestimates.

The NCVS is an ongoing survey of US households regarding their experiences with crime victimization conducted by the Department of Justice. A given household is enrolled in the study for 3 years, during which time the experiences of all household members ages 12 and older are assessed every 6 months, usually in a structured telephone interview. There are several weaknesses in this survey with respect to its ability to count accurately women's experiences with violence. First, the focus of the survey is on "crime." Yet many women who have been or are being victimized by people known to them may not understand that these events constitute crimes. Despite its limitations, improvements have been made in the NVCS. Revisions made in 1993 include questions specifically about events involving neighbors, relatives, coworkers, and friends, as well as questions specifically regarding rape. Whether these amendments adequately address the problem may become clearer in future reports on data collected using this revised strategy.

The Uniform Crime Reports (UCR) are another source of official information on violence against women, but these data are even more limited than those in the NCVS. The UCR are police report data that most police departments in the country voluntarily submit to the Federal Bureau of Investigation for aggregation into a national dataset. These data can tell us how many incidents of violence against women were *reported to the police*, a figure that is obviously biased by factors that inhibit women's willingness to report.

Despite their limitations, the NCVS and the UCR are important because they are routinely collected datasets. They have some potential, therefore, to address trends over time. But they also highlight the relative state of ignorance from which we must form policy on this important topic.

DATING VIOLENCE

Studies have suggested that 28% to 41% of all individuals (teens and adults) will be involved in intimate violence at some point while dating (18) and that 1 out of 10 dating teens has experienced some form of violence in a relationship (19). Another recent survey of 738 students in three high schools, representing inner city, suburban, and rural communities, found that of the 631 students who responded, on average, 17.7% reported some form of physical and/or sexual violence in a dating relationship (20). Overall, though the estimates vary, dating violence is a reality facing many young people and the consequences are severe.

According to the Los Angeles Commission on Assaults Against Women dating violence curriculum, *In Touch with Teens*, dealing with the knowledge or experience of an assault can present unique problems for adolescents because:

*   They have limited access to resources targeted for them.
*   They have feelings of isolation.
*   They may lack support from family and valued peers.
*   They are inexperienced with sex or relationships.
*   They have a desire for independence, while still needing guidance from adults.
*   They experience other stresses that have to do with being an adolescent, such as school and identity issues (21).

These factors can lead to the lack of recognition of abuse. Not recognizing the presence of abuse or having the ability to define abuse is, in part, responsible for the prevalence and lack of reporting of dating violence. Teens, because of their lack of experience in relationships, are at particular risk of nonrecognition, so efforts to design and implement initiatives to prevent dating violence must consider how teens think about violence in the context of a relationship. In addition, gender, race, and previous experience with violence itself have all been associated with how the individual perceives violence in a relationship, either as the victim or the perpetrator (22).

Both females and males can engage in dating violence as the "abuser." Recent studies have shown that physical violence is being equally used by both females and males in dating relationships, however, these findings are highly debated (23). For example, consideration must be given to whether these findings mean that females are more violent and aggressive or if they are in fact more likely to accept responsibility for their actions, possibly being less inhibited to report using physical aggression, as they are traditionally not looked at as "abusers" (24,25).

In addition to reports of use of violence, information has been collected on reasons why teens may choose to use violence against a dating partner. One study found that young women reported that their acts of physical violence resulted from uncontrolled anger, jealousy, self-defense, or retaliation while young men reported that their motivation results from wanting to intimidate, scare, or force their female partner to give them something (26).

Psychological or emotional abuse is consistently reported as the hardest form of abuse to identify (27). However, it is the form of abuse that has the greatest impact on self-perception and confidence. In a recent study looking specifically at the prevalence of psychological abuse within dating relationships, it was found that females reported being the subject of psychological abuse more frequently than males, overall. However, when the researchers categorized their findings between "committed" and "less committed" relationships, meaning married, engaged, or living together versus dating one or more persons, respectively, males reported being the subject of more psychological abuse than females (28).

Again, as with physical violence, these results may be interpreted a number of ways. For example, perhaps women in the "less committed" group do not recognize psychological abuse and therefore underreport it, or men in this group believe they are psychologically abused by their female partner, as such behavior is more consistent with a female stereotype, causing males to overestimate its actual occurrence (29). As teens would seldom fall into the "committed" category, these findings are of interest for dating violence prevention strategy development.

Sexual abuse and rape continue to be one of the most underreported crimes and one of the most difficult crimes to define. The word rape has brutal connotations in our society. Dating, on the other hand, usually conjures up images of excitement, intimacy, expected love, and possible sexual expression. Therefore, "date rape" itself is a contradiction in terms and a confusing phenomenon. Perhaps this explains why sexual abuse within a dating relationship is often not taken seriously, is difficult to label, and often goes unrecognized by victims and assailants. Many victims of date rape are often not aware that a rape has occurred.

The dating relationship is one that has the possibility of culminating in consensual sex, and because of this common expectation, young women are often considered partially at fault if a rape occurs (30). In an anonymous questionnaire administered to college age men and women, 27.5% of the men and 17.5% of the women felt that forcible sex is justifiable when a woman asks a man out on a date, when a women allows the man to pay for the date, and when a woman goes to a man's apartment on or at the end of the date (31). In addition, a similar study also found that forced sex is considered acceptable when a young woman is dressed seductively, or when a dating relationship has been going on for more than 6 months (32). Clearly the cultural norms and expectations of dating relationships in our society have contributed to the occurrence of all abuse within a dating relationship, but especially sexual abuse in youth.

CONTRIBUTING FACTORS

Much of the early research on both sexual assault and domestic violence sought to determine the traits of victims that put them at risk for attack. However, most reviews and larger studies have found few factors that discriminate victims from nonvictims (33,34). The trait of women that has the most significant effect on their risk for violence is one that is entirely beyond their control, namely age. Younger women are at much greater risk for both sexual assault and domestic violence. The previous focus on women's appearance, behavior, and attitudes, much of which smacked of victim blaming, has shifted largely to an approach that emphasizes predisposing traits in perpetrators and the socioenvironmental context of events.

In one of the largest studies of nonincarcerated, undetected perpetrators of sexual assault, Koss et al reported on a sample of approximately 3000 male college students from a nationwide survey of 32 institutions of higher learning (35). Traits they found to be associated with sexual aggression included childhood sexual experiences (both forced and unforced), greater hostility toward women, and acceptance of the use of force in intimate relationships. They also report that "the more serious the self-reported sexual aggression, the more likely that current behavior was characterized by frequent use of alcohol, violent and degrading pornography, and involvement in peer groups that reinforce highly sexualized views of women." These findings have some interesting implications for preventive approaches that address social norms that objectify and denigrate women.

Hotaling et al performed what remains the largest summary analysis of risk markers for domestic violence. Consistent risk markers among men included witnessing violence as a child or adolescent, alcohol abuse, lower educational level, and lower income (36).

Violence in the family of origin, usually measured as violence between the spouses or violent forms of child discipline, is a consistent correlate of both adult domestic violence and dating violence (37–41). This finding is consistent with several theories of the causation of violence against women, particularly a social learning model, which holds that individuals learn what is acceptable and normative behavior from the environment around them—from family, peers, media, and broad social norms. Observing violence in the home of origin appears to increase the risk for men to become perpetrators and for women to become victims.

A factor that appears to be present in many instances of violence against women is substance use—most commonly, alcohol abuse. The National Family Violence Survey of 1985 found a clear trend of increasing prevalence of husband-to-wife violence as the level of drinking by the male partner increased (42). The highest prevalence of violence (19%) was among binge drinkers, a pattern found in other studies as well. It is important to note, however, that the prevalence among abstainers was not zero (it was 6%), and that the majority of binge drinking men did *not* commit violence. In other words, there is not a one-to-one correlation of violence

with drinking. The study found that drinking immediately preceded violence in only about one fourth of cases overall, but in half of cases where the male partner was a high- or binge-level drinker.

There continues to be debate as to whether or not alcohol use "causes" violence against women, or is largely an exacerbating factor. Men who are violent toward women frequently use intoxication as an excuse for their behavior, recognizing (consciously or not) that in American culture we tend to hold individuals less responsible for violence that occurs while under the influence of alcohol.

The causes of dating violence, like domestic violence, are heavily debated, and research has not given any conclusive formula for predicting who is more likely to be an abuser or victim. Theories around issues of societal influence range from the notion that society reinforces the need for hierarchy in relationships, to the negative effect of male peer support, to gender roles and stereotypes (43,44). Though inconclusive, these theories do give a framework in which all, some, or none of these influences can be considered relevant. Other researchers have looked to personal experience with violence as a witness, victim, or perpetrator prior to the dating relationship as a predictor (45,46). Overall, more research is needed.

VIOLENCE AND GIRLS: FROM VICTIMS TO PERPETRATORS

Girls are three times as likely as boys to be the victims of sexual assault (47). In addition, in 1993, at least 603 girls under age 19 were murdered by their partners (48). Research has suggested that one in four women in the United States will be raped, or a victim of attempted rape, by the time they are in their mid-twenties, and three fourths of those rapes or attempted rapes will be committed by someone the victim knows (49). It has also been found that adolescent women who commit homicide rarely kill strangers. While only 13.8% of juvenile male offenders arrested for murder or non-negligent manslaughter killed a parent, stepparent, or other family member, 44% of the juvenile females arrested for these crimes had killed a parent, stepparent, or other family member (50). Despite these horrifying statistics, little is known about the link between victimization and perpetration of violence in adolescent women. It is quite evident from the data, however, that adolescent women are committing more acts of violence than ever before.

In response to this growing crisis, it is imperative that we expand our understanding of the unique risk factors contributing to the rise in the perpetration of violence by adolescent women and challenge the youth violence prevention movement to create programming reflective of the increasingly active participation of young women as violent offenders.

The list of risk factors for violence typically applied to the adolescent population includes: prior victimization, witnessing violence, poverty, family disorganization, and death of or separation from a parent or older sibling (51). This list, however, does not take into consideration the broader experience of being female in this society. It fails to examine the context of the contemporary "culture of violence" in which women of all ages live, as well as the persistent images of violent victimization of women in the media.

It is clear that the link between being a victim of violence and a perpetrator must be explored further if we are to develop effective strategies and programs that assist adolescent women in preventing violence. One study of women incarcerated in juvenile facilities indicated that 62% had been physically abused and 30% said this abuse began between the ages of 5 and 9 (52). This link between victimization and perpetration of violence continues to emerge in the small amount of research being conducted on adolescent women and violence. This link manifests itself at several levels, including victimization as a child, current victimization, witnessing victimization, and perceived victimization, all contributing to the use or perceived need for the use of violence.

The link between victimization and perpetration of violence by adolescent women also relates to beliefs about the use of violence. The Center for Women Policy Studies found that 54% of adolescent women surveyed reported that they believed "girls act violently because they have been victims of violence," and that girls who had been physically abused were twice as likely as girls who had not been abused to view violence as "always okay when someone threatens you." In addition, the same survey found that 82% of girls said they felt justified in being violent if someone tries to force them to have sex, while 23% said that violence is justified if someone starts a "bad rumor" about them (53).

The effect of the media on the use of violence is no longer hypothetical, and several studies have shown an association between viewing violence on television and violent behavior (54,55). By the age of 18, it is estimated that a child has watched 22,000 hours of television and has been exposed to as many as 18,000 televised murders and 800 televised suicides (56). The glamorization of violence, in general, by our culture and the constant portrayal of women as victims of violence by the media contributes simultaneously to the sense of a need for violence and to the vulnerability to violence young women feel. The defensive posture taken by many young women, this idea of choosing either to be a "victim or violator," is reinforced by the reality of the nightly news, which reports the murder of a woman by her spouse, as well as by the lyrics of popular music. The message repeatedly conveyed to young women, and to women in general, is that not only are you a target but that violent retaliation is the only way to not be a victim.

Despite the increasing number of adolescent women who are committing acts of violence, there is a serious dearth of violence prevention programs for adolescent women. According to the Center for the Study of Youth Policy, "there are few, if any, meaningful community-based programs for troubled and delinquent girls." The Office of Juvenile Justice and Delinquency Prevention reports that 50% of all juvenile crime occurs in the 3 hours after school, yet girls are often discouraged from participating in after-school programs because of concern for their safety. There are also fewer resources allocated to programs that specifically focus on girls (57). In addition, a 1991 national survey of state of the art violence prevention programs for adolescents revealed that only 3 programs out of the 51 that responded served a primarily female population, and of the 3, only 1 served potential perpetrators of violence, while 2 served survivors of violence (58).

HEALTH CONSEQUENCES OF VIOLENCE AGAINST WOMEN

Numerous studies have examined the short- and long-term health consequences of violence against women. Immediate physical trauma resulting from both domestic abuse and sexual assault most often affects the head, face, neck, and torso, primarily in the form of contusions, abrasions, and lacerations (59,60). More severe episodes may result in fractures, brain injury, damage to internal organs, or even death. Sexual assault may lead to trauma to the vagina and/or rectum (61), and health risks associated with sexually transmitted diseases (including HIV) and pregnancy (62,63). Both physical and sexual assault may have serious traumatic consequences for pregnant women and their fetuses (64–66).

According to the 1985 National Family Violence Survey, 3% of battered women received medical attention for abuse-related injuries in the past year (67). Among women who experienced severe abuse, this figure was 7.3%. Though shocking, these figures likely underrepresent the number of women with injuries serious enough to "require" medical attention, since batterers may prevent women from seeking help. In fact, nonfatal episodes of violence are often not reported to emergency rooms or anywhere else. The Northeast Ohio Trauma Study showed a 5 : 1 ratio of assaults reported by emergency room personnel to those reported to police. In the absence of a national trauma registry that would include emergency room data there is much less known about nonfatal episodes of violence.

The National Women's Study reported that 24% of rape victims sustained minor injury and 4% sustained serious injury (68). However, a full 49% of victims reported that they feared serious injury or death during their rape, and 40% of women raped within the past 5 years were fearful of contracting HIV/AIDS.

Longer-term somatic consequences of both domestic and sexual abuse that have been cited include chronic pelvic pain, gastrointestinal syndromes, back pain, and headache (69). The incidence of such outcomes, and their relationship to violent victimization, is more difficult to assess than the immediate effects. Temporal associations may become cloudy over time and lack of information in medical records may lead to a dependence on (potentially biased) subjective recall of violence and subsequent symptomatology.

Acute trauma such as rape and assault may also confer an elevated risk for disease, mediated by stress-induced changes in immune functioning (70,71). Investigation with respect to such long-term outcomes specifically following violence has been very limited, however.

Psychological or behavioral sequelae of violent victimization that have been described in the research literature include posttraumatic stress disorder (PTSD), major depression, anxiety disorders, substance abuse, and eating disorders (72–77).

In a national sample of 4008 women, those who had experienced criminal victimization (physical or sexual assault) were much more likely to receive a lifetime (25.8%) or current (9.7%) diagnosis of PTSD than were nonvictims of crime (9.4% and 3.4%, respectively) (78). The same study estimated that approximately 1.3 million women currently suffer from rape-related PTSD (79). A high prevalence of prior violent

Table 32-1 Clinical Presentations Associated with Victimization

- Self neglect, malnutrition, dehydration, failure to thrive
- Depression, anxiety, panic attacks, sleep disorders
- Alcohol, drug abuse
- Aggression towards self and others
- Dissociative states, repeated self-injury
- Somatizing disorders, eating disorders, chronic pain
- Suicide attempts
- Compulsive sexual behaviors, sexual dysfunction
- Lying, stealing, truancy, running away
- Poor adherence to medical recommendations

victimization (50% to 80%) also has been found among psychiatric patients with a range of presenting complaints (80,81).

Major depression is another common outcome of violent victimization. Stets et al (82) reported that 58% of severely abused women had high depression scores, compared to 21% of women not abused. In the National Women's Study, 21% of all rape victims were experiencing a major depressive episode at the time they were interviewed, compared to 6% of women who were not victims of crime (83). This study also found that 13% of rape victims had attempted suicide, compared to 1% of other women. Table 32-1 lists the clinical presentations associated with victimization.

Several studies have found high rates of prior and/or ongoing violence among alcoholic women (84,85). For instance, in a study that compared alcoholic women with a random household sample of women, both moderate and severe husband-to-wife violence were more common in the alcoholic sample (86). One fourth of alcoholic women had been kicked, hit, or hit with a fist, compared to only 5% of those in the random sample. Spousal violence remained a strong predictor of group type even after the data were controlled for alcohol problems in the spouse, income, parental violence, and parental alcohol problems.

Kilpatrick et al (87) found that among rape victims who developed PTSD, 20% had two or more major alcohol-related problems, compared to 1.5% of women who had never been crime victims.

Violence also has the potential to affect women's social health. This can include difficulty functioning at work and reduced ability to enjoy sexual relations (88,89). Even more seriously, some studies indicate that violence may be a risk factor for homelessness (90,91).

The costs associated with violent victimization have been estimated in several studies. Koss et al (92) found that women crime victims, as compared to nonvictims, made twice as many physician visits in the past year (6.9 versus 3.5).

Severity of victimization was the best predictor of yearly physician visits and total outpatient costs in an analysis that controlled for age, income, ethnicity, education, health status, and other life stressors. Most recently, Miller et al (93) estimated the total costs (monetary, mental health, and quality of life) associated with rape, robbery, assault and arson. Total victim costs per crime were $47,424 for rape and $14,738 for assault. Among survivors with physical injury, total costs were $60,376 for rape and $49,603 for assault. For both rape and assault, mental health costs were substantially larger than medical costs and accounted for a major portion of total costs.

RESPONSE OF HEALTH CARE PRACTITIONERS AND THE HEALTH CARE SYSTEM

Although response to rape in most medical settings has been formalized for some time through protocols and wide use of forensic rape kits, there is evidence that women often do not seek medical attention and proper procedures are not always followed. Kilpatrick et al (87) found that only 17% of women had a medical examination following their attack. Among those women who had received rape examinations within the past 5 years, 55% of victims were not counseled about pregnancy testing or pregnancy prevention; 50% were not given information about testing for HIV; and 33% were not provided with information about testing for exposure to sexually transmitted diseases.

Structured response in health care settings to forms of violence against women other than rape, particularly domestic violence, is more recent. The notion that health professionals should be trained to identify and refer patients affected by domestic abuse began to gain real momentum in 1991 when the American Medical Association established its National Coalition of Physicians Against Family Violence. Since that time, training programs and treatment protocols have proliferated.

Violence against women has begun to obtain a small foothold in formal health policy statements. For instance, the Joint Commission on the Accreditation of Healthcare Organizations (JCAHO) passed regulations effective in January of 1992 calling for all hospital emergency departments and hospital-affiliated outpatient care facilities to have protocols and training plans for response to all forms of family violence (94). Similarly, the Council on Ethical and Judicial Affairs of the American Medical Association (AMA) has outlined the ethical duty of physicians to diagnose and treat family violence (95).

The American Medical Association's Diagnostic and Treatment Guidelines on Mental Health Effects of Family Violence (96) offer guidance to physicians around issues of assessing a patient's exposure to violence and abuse. The following is a brief overview of some of the recommended AMA strategies.

How to ask about abuse
- Create a supportive and safe environment and always see patients without their partners.

- Assure confidentiality of any and all disclosures the patient makes and make sure they understand any mandatory reporting requirements you may have.

Table 32-2 Taking the Abuse History

Current History of Abuse
Is the patient currently being hurt or harmed? In the past? Is s/he still at risk? Who is the perpetrator? What kind of access does the perpetrator have to the patient/victim?

Impact of Abuse:
How has the abuse affected her/his psychological health? What is the relationship of abuse to her present symptoms? How does s/he feel about the abuse? How has the abuse affected her/his life—children, work, school, personal relationships?

Options/Resources:
What has s/he tried already? What has worked? What has not? How has this affected hope for change? What other options are seen as available? What does s/he want immediately? In the long run? Where is s/he at in the process of being able to change her/his situation? Who else knows? Who else can help? Who else actually will?

Needs Assessment:
What does s/he need—information, support, shelter, counseling, support group, legal advocacy, mental health/substance abuse services, access to other resources? Can s/he manage this herself, or does s/he need more help with the initial steps? What resources are available in the community: shelter, safe homes, counseling, support groups, legal advocacy? Are there special service needs—cultural, religious, sexual orientation, language, disability, communication? If not, what alternatives exist or could be developed? Are there needs for children or others requiring attention too?

Maintaining a Supportive Relationship:
How is s/he feeling about the fact that you are asking?

- If the patient is willing to discuss or volunteers information about abuse, let them know you appreciate their willingness to tell you, offer services and resources, and make sure they feel safe before leaving.

- Let victims know they are not alone, not responsible, and that you are concerned for their safety.

When to ask about abuse
- All new patients should be asked questions about current or past abuse as part of the initial health screen.

- Health care providers should also periodically revisit the issue of abuse, especially if:

  1) The patient presents a complaint suggesting that abuse should be part of the differential diagnosis.

  2) A woman is contemplating pregnancy or is being seen for the first and subsequent pre-natal visits of each pregnancy.

  3) The patient reports a change in intimate partners.

  4) There are frequent unexplained appointment changes or cancellations.

  5) Physical symptoms do not make sense, do not suggest clear etiology, or fail to respond to treatment.

- See Table 32-2 for suggested questions.

Avoid retraumatization
- Carefully explain all procedures in advance, especially pelvic, rectal, oropharyngeal, and breast examinations, when it is known that sexual abuse was a part of the abuse.

- If hospitalization is necessary, be sensitive to the number of caregivers, introduce new members of the caregiving team, and explain all procedures in advance.

Assess safety
- It is imperative that the patient's safety be evaluated before leaving the medical setting, including physical safety as well as ability to take care of herself.

- Does the patient need immediate shelter or are there friends or family with whom she can stay.

- Evaluate the risk of perpetration of violence against the abuser, such as homicide, or against self, such as suicide.

Unfortunately, significant barriers exist in accomplishing change among health practitioners with regard to addressing violence against women. Violence has received scant attention in the training of most clinicians (97). Lack of knowledge not only of physical outcomes but also of the interpersonal dynamics and sociology of violence hinders the ability to motivate health professionals to improve standards of practice. So long as physicians view topics such as domestic violence as a "Pandora's box" (98), attempts at policy revision may be thwarted by resistance among the rank-and-file.

POLITICAL AND SOCIETAL RESPONSE

The most important new legislative response to the problem of violence against women was the passage of the Violence Against Women Act (VAWA) in 1994. Among the initiatives included in the VAWA are: increased funding for shelters, training of law enforcement officials and judges, education and rape prevention programs, piloting and assessment of youth education on domestic violence, and a national domestic violence hotline.

Most legislation related to violence against women continues to be enacted at the state level, where topics of recent interest have included antistalking measures, restriction of gun access and licenses for individuals convicted of domestic violence crimes, and reclassification of certain crimes involving violence against women as federal offenses. It will require careful evaluation to determine the effectiveness of these formal social controls. Unfortunately, the continued deficit of thorough and accurate information on this problem described at the opening of this chapter tends to hinder attempts to evaluate programs or policies.

It also remains to be seen what effect such legislative changes and other prevention and intervention strategies (e.g., increasing shelter spaces, disseminating media awareness campaigns) will have on social norms or informal social control, which may well remain the key to long-term reductions in the level of violence against women.

PREVENTION AND INTERVENTION

Within the discipline of public health, prevention is viewed as consisting of three separate forms or stages: primary prevention, which is intended to prevent an adverse outcome ever from happening; secondary prevention, which focuses on reducing the occurrence of future adverse events in at-risk populations; and tertiary prevention, which aims to reduce the consequences of adverse events that have already occurred. Secondary and tertiary "prevention" are usually accomplished through a variety of intervention strategies.

Prevention of lung cancer provides a useful and easily understood model of these forms of prevention. Primary prevention of lung cancer can be largely accomplished by reducing the number of individuals who begin smoking, which is by far the leading cause of this cancer. In this way, the cancer is prevented from ever occurring. Secondary prevention targets current smokers to persuade them to reduce or give up smoking, which is putting them at increased risk for lung cancer even if the cancer has yet to develop. Tertiary prevention involves improved medical treatments for cancers that have already emerged, such as early diagnosis and more successful chemotherapy.

The hallmark of a public health approach to violence is a focus on primary prevention. Since the authors of this chapter take a predominantly feminist view of the causes of violence against women, believing that the control and subjugation of women is a root motivating factor in the majority of cases, we believe that the primary prevention of this violence lies in improving the status of women in society. A thorough discussion of the many strategies needed to accomplish such a social transformation is beyond the scope of this chapter. Sparks et al (99) discuss the primary prevention of sexual assault through community programs that might serve to increase women's equality, and Swift (100) provides a description of educational and media-based strategies that address sex-role socialization. However, items that need to be on the agenda include addressing gender stereotypes embedded in our social norms early and often, providing job opportunities for women at compensation equal to that of men, and increasing the number of women in legislative office.

Secondary and Tertiary Prevention

The most important source of both secondary and tertiary prevention of family violence is the shelter system. Shelters and safe houses provide the most crucial need of women and children in crisis: safety. In addition, shelters usually provide group counseling for women and referrals for legal, job training, and housing assistance. They may also provide specialized programs for children of abused women, and often do educational outreach in the local community.

Shelters cannot take on the entire burden of keeping women safe from their abusers, however. There are a variety of legal remedies that are available to women, though the specifics of these interventions tend to vary from state to state.

The police are frequently the first professionals to respond to domestic violence, although the 1985 National Family Violence Survey found that only 7% of all incidents, and 14% of serious incidents, are reported to police (101). In many states, the police are now mandated to arrest the primary aggressor if they have reason to believe that abuse has occurred. The research on mandatory arrest provides a complex picture of this strategy's effects (102). It appears that arrest may have a beneficial effect when the perpetrator is employed and otherwise has a "stake" in society. For perpetrators who are unemployed, it appears that arrest may have the ability to exacerbate the violence.

One of the most frequently used legal remedies for domestic violence is the civil restraining or protective order. These orders are available in all states, though their coverage and provisions may vary. Generally speaking, restraining orders include provisions that require the defendant to stop the abuse, vacate the home (if there is a common domicile), stay a certain distance from the plaintiff, and have no contact whatsoever with the plaintiff except as specified (e.g., for child visitation). Restraining orders can also include orders to surrender custody of minor children, provide child and other financial support, and surrender weapons (particularly guns). Although a restraining order is clearly no guarantee of physical safety, it can provide women with breathing space to assess their situation and plan future actions. Seeking a restraining order may also empower women, particularly in the context of a judge who sends a clear message that the defendant's behavior is illegal and inappropriate, and not deserved by the plaintiff.

Many women who have been abused are entitled to file criminal charges, which could include assault, aggravated assault, kidnapping, property damage, and/or stalking, depending upon the specifics of the case. Unfortunately, it is still relatively rare for men to receive jail sentences in the context of criminal convictions related to nonfatal domestic violence, so women must weigh carefully the pros and cons of this strategy. One other intervention that can be applied in cases of domestic violence is batterer treatment. Most often, men enter batterer treatment as a requirement under probation.

Rape crisis centers operate on the front lines of response to women who are sexually assaulted, dealing not only with the immediate physical and psychological trauma, but also assisting women with long-term recovery. According to Kilpatrick et al (103), there are over 2000 organizations that assist rape victims. Given what is known about the potential for negative physical and mental health outcomes following assault, these centers and their adjunct services play a crucial role in reducing the toll of future morbidity among victimized women.

Although rape continues to be the most underreported violent crime, and arrest rates are extremely low (104), there has been some attempt in the criminal justice sector to address these cases more sensitively. Sex crime units and victim-witness programs may at least reduce the extent to which victims are revictimized by the legal process. Rape shield laws and other legislative reforms may also prove of some benefit to victims, but the evidence that legislative initiatives have accomplished any general deterrent effect is lacking (105).

There are some "personal safety" and resistance strategies that may also have some utility in preventing sexual assault (106). Since women of college age have been found to be at high risk for sexual assault, many institutions of higher learning have instituted prevention programs. Orientation seminars may suggest to women (in a manner that is not victim blaming) that drinking excessively in the presence of male acquaintances or strangers who are also drinking may place women in a situation in which they are more vulnerable to assault. Using escort services across campus late at night is another example of personal safety strategies that may be recommended. However, there are those who criticize these forms of prevention as "victim control," unduly constraining the freedoms of women in society (107). These strategies do not address primary prevention, and may only displace an instance of sexual assault from a less vulnerable target to a more vulnerable one.

Dating Violence Prevention and Intervention

Acknowledging this risk and recognizing that adult women are not the only victims of abuse at the hands of their partners, battered women's service organizations and others have responded by developing prevention and intervention initiatives that target schools. More recently, male batterer programs have taken notice and responded to the increasing numbers of dating violence victims by designing and implementing interventions that target young men who threaten or who have used violence against their partners.

Dating violence prevention initiatives can vary in type and in length, and most are curriculum-based, ranging from 3 to 10 sessions. These curricula help young people to 1) identify the precursors to violence; 2) learn to identify what constitutes abusive behavior; 3) define an appropriate dating behavior; 4) identify socioenvironmental issues that lead to abusive behavior (sex role stereotyping, sexism, homophobia); and 5) find resources for help. In order to provide a dual perspective on the issue, some program operators advocate that classroom curricula be jointly taught by a male and a female facilitator.

Anger management, communication skills, nonviolent conflict resolution, personal empowerment, and relationship-building skills are incorporated into dating violence prevention initiatives. Students are taught the cyclical nature of dating violence, and how the severity of the violence tends to increase with each violent episode (108). Since students, especially teens, seem to be open to accepting how culture and media are influencing their behavior, education around topics like dating violence encourages teens to resist the stereotypes placed upon them by their families, society, and the media.

In addition to curricula, some dating violence prevention initiatives include training peer leaders to help conduct outreach and to increase school awareness around the prevention and recognition of dating violence. It is important to realize that peer-led discussion and peer leaders trained to recognize and to offer assistance to dating violence victims and perpetrators may often be the most effective way of helping both victims and perpetrators find the help they need. Peer leaders may also be useful for collecting information regarding changes in behavior and attitude.

Some initiatives conduct parent education and outreach in conjunction with other programming, as parents are many times unaware of the signs of abuse. Still others have included a component that reaches out to both the victim of abuse and the perpetrator who exhibits the violent and abusive behavior. These interventions may include establishing peer support groups or referring individuals to counseling. Leaders of these groups work closely with schools, parents, and the young victims to help ensure safety.

Creating a Hybrid: Violence Prevention for Young Women

Efforts to educate adolescents about the issues of violence and its prevention typically take the form of school-based curricula. However, in order to prevent violence against women, there is a need for these efforts to go beyond the current standard and for prevention experts to create and evaluate curricula that specifically address the needs of young women.

For example, typical violence prevention curricula are gender-neutral, treating young women and men as existing in the same societal context and typically assuming that they need the same knowledge and skills in order to handle their anger and to resolve conflict nonviolently. These curricula do not usually address the difference between young women's and men's self-awareness of their risk for being a victim, the differences between young women's and men's motivations to commit violent acts, or of the relationship between being a victim and being a perpetrator. As primary prevention tools, these curricula tend to focus on the individual, and expect that the individual will not only be able to change their own behavior but the behavior of others sharing their environment.

At the other end of the spectrum, dating violence curricula tend to define the roles of abuser and victim, and typically assign these roles to males and females, respectively. These curricula also emphasize the effect that society has on expectations in relationships and of the roles women and men have in them. In addition, gender roles, stereotyping, cultural norms, and the influence of the media are integral parts of most dating violence curricula. Defining a healthy relationship and developing nonviolent conflict resolution skills are also a usual part of dating violence prevention curricula. However, since the focus is on dating relationships, these curricula fail to address the larger context of violence in society and other relationships in which nonviolent communication skills are necessary. These curricula also do not usually address prior or current victimization in a relationship or in general.

The integration of a violence prevention curriculum with a dating violence prevention curriculum could, for young women, create a curriculum base in which both their experiences in society as a victim, whether prior, current, witnessed, or perceived, and their potential of being a perpetrator could be examined and discussed, providing a foundation for skill development and awareness not currently addressed by either type of curriculum.

SUMMARY

Though we know that even our best estimates are inaccurately low, violence against women, whether as children, adolescents, or adults, will continue to have an irrevocable effect on millions of families and communities. As health care and human service providers, it is imperative that we expand our understanding of violence against women, and that we approach this issue comprehensively, demanding the resources and policy modifications we need in order to prevent and intervene.

No longer is the victimization of women an issue only for the shelters and crisis centers. Schools are and should continue to be involved with educational efforts focused on preventing violence against women, starting in elementary school with sexual harassment and bullying prevention initiatives, followed by dating and other violence prevention programs in middle and high school. These efforts should make every attempt to include strong parent education and community awareness building components.

Health and human service providers do and should continue to screen children and adolescents for risk factors like a history of family violence, and provide referrals for clients of all ages to appropriate mental health providers, or specific violence prevention services, such as victim support groups, anger management groups, or batterer programs. Health care providers must shed their resistance to assuming a preventive and intervening role, and start treating the entire woman in addition to assisting victims with their physical injuries. Health care and human service providers can also be advocates for better data collection systems, in order to improve the state of knowledge of the victimization of women, and for improvement in the training of future providers.

Finally, the victimization of women in society, whether prior, current, witnessed, or perceived, has not been adequately addressed as a major contributing factor to the increase in the perpetration of violence by adolescent women. The small amount of research that has been done indicates this is an area in need of further research. The need for programs to assist young women in preventing violence is great, and the need for all levels of society to adequately address the link between being a victim and perpetrator of violence as an adolescent woman is urgent.

REFERENCES

1. Domestic violence toolkit and resource manual. The Third Annual Healthier Communities Conference, Austin, TX, October 26–29, 1997.

2. Gamace D. Domination and control: the social context of dating violence. In: Levy B, ed. Dating violence: young women in danger. Seattle: Seal Press, 1991.

3. Parrot A, Bechofer L, eds. Acquaintance rape: the hidden crime. New York: Wiley, 1991.

4. Hotaling GT, Sugarman DB. An analysis of risk markers in husband to wife violence: the current state of knowledge. Violence and Victims 1986;1:101–124.

5. Koss MP, Dinero TE. Discriminant analysis of risk factors for sexual victimization among a national sample of college women. J Consult Clin Psychol 1989;57:242–250.

6. National Center for Victims of Crime, Crime Victims Research and Treatment Center. Rape in America: a report to the nation. Arlington, VA: National Center for Victims of Crime, 1992.

7. Pynoos RS, Frederick C, Nader K, et al. Life threat and posttraumatic stress in school-age children. Arch Gen Psychiatry 1987; 44:1057–1063.

8. Freeman L, Mokros H, Poznanski E. Violent events reported by normal urban school-aged children: characteristics and depression correlates. J Am Acad Child Adolesc Psychiatry 1993;2:419–423.

9. Osofsky J, Wewers S, Hann D, et al. Chronic community violence: what is happening to our children? Psychiatry 1993;56:36–45.

10. Martinez P, Richters J. The NIMH community violence project II: children's distress symptoms associated with violence exposure. Psychiatry 1993;56:22–35.

11. Lorion RP, Saltzman W. Children's exposure to community violence: following a path from concern to research to action. Psychiatry 1993;1:55–65.

12. Fitzpatrick KM, Boldizar JP. The prevalence and consequences of exposure to violence among African-American youth. J Am Acad Child Adolesc Psychiatry 1993;2:424–430.

13. Lorion RP, Saltzman W. Children's exposure to community violence: following a path from concern to research to action. Psychiatry 1993;1:55–65.

14. Emde RN. The horror! The horror! reflection on our culture of violence and its implications for early development and morality. Psychiatry 1993;1:119–123.

15. Durant R, Pendergast R, Cadenhead C. Exposure to violence and victimization and fighting behavior by urban black adolescents. J Adolesc Health 1994;4:311–318.

16. Hechinger F. Fateful choices: healthy youth for the 21st

century. New York: Carnegie Corporation of New York, 1992.

17. RespecTeen. The troubled journey: a profile of American youth. Minneapolis: RespecTeen, 1990.

18. Sirles EA. A consumer's perspective on domestic violence. J Fam Violence 1993;6:267–276.

19. Sugarman DB, Hotaling GT. Dating violence: prevalence, context, and risk markers. In: Pirog-Good M, Stets JE, eds. Violence in dating relationships: emerging social issues. New York: Praeger, 1989.

20. Department of Justice, Federal Bureau of Investigation. Crime in the United States—1993, uniform crime reports. Washington, DC: US Government Printing Office, 1994.

21. Los Angeles Council on Assaults Against Women. In Touch with Teens curriculum, 1994.

22. Carlson BE. Dating violence: student beliefs about consequences. J Interpersonal Violence 1996;11:3–18.

23. LeJeune C, Follette V. Taking responsibility: sex differences in reporting dating violence. J Interpersonal Violence 1994;9:133–140.

24. LeJeune C, Follette V. Taking responsibility: sex differences in reporting dating violence. J Interpersonal Violence 1994;9:133–140.

25. Stets JE, Henderson DA. Contextual factors surrounding conflict resolution while dating: results from a national study. Family Relations 1991;40:29–36.

26. Sugarman DB, Hotaling GT. Dating violence: a review of contextual and risk factors. In: Levy B, ed. Dating violence: young women in danger. Seattle: Seal Press, 1991.

27. Worcester N. A more hidden crime: adolescent battered women. The National Women's Health Network News 1993; July/August.

28. Kasian M, Painter S. Frequency and severity of psychological abuse in a dating population. J Interpersonal Violence 1992;7:350–364.

29. Kasian M, Painter S. Frequency and severity of psychological abuse in a dating population. J Interpersonal Violence 1992;7:350–364.

30. Parrot A, Bechofer L, eds. Acquaintance rape: the hidden crime. New York: Wiley, 1991.

31. Parrot A, Bechofer L, eds. Acquaintance rape: the hidden crime. New York: Wiley, 1991.

32. Parrot A, Bechofer L, eds. Acquaintance rape: the hidden crime. New York: Wiley, 1991.

33. Hotaling GT, Sugarman DB. An analysis of risk markers in husband to wife violence: the current state of knowledge. Violence and Victims 1986;1:101–124.

34. Koss MP, Dinero TE. Discriminant analysis of risk factors for sexual victimization among a national sample of college women. J Consult Clin Psychol 1989;57:242–250.

35. Koss MP, Dinero TE. Predictors of sexual aggression among a national sample of male college students. Ann NY Acad Sci 1988;528:133–147.

36. Hotaling GT, Sugarman DB. An analysis of risk markers in husband to wife violence: the current state of knowledge. Violence and Victims 1986;1:101–124.

37. Hotaling GT, Sugarman DB. An analysis of risk markers in husband to wife violence: the current state of knowledge. Violence and Victims 1986;1:101–124.

38. Henton J, Cate R, Koval J, et al. Romance and violence in dating relationships. J Family Issues 1983;4:467–482.

39. Roscoe B, Callahan JE. Adolescents' self-report of violence in families and dating relations. Adolescence 1985;20:545–553.

40. O'Keefe NK, Brockopp K, Chew E. Teen dating violence. Social Work 1986;Nov/Dec:465–468.

41. Reuterman NA, Burcky WD. Dating violence in high school: a profile of the victims. Psychology 1989;26:1–9.

42. Kaufman Kantor G, Straus MA. The "drunken bum" theory of wife beating. Social Problems 1987;34:213–230.

43. Gamache D. Domination and control: the social context of dating violence. In: Levy B, ed. Dating violence: young women in danger. Seattle: Seal Press, 1991.

44. DeKeseredy W. Woman abuse in dating relationships: the contribution of male peer support. Sociological Inquiry 1990;60:236–243.

45. Sugarman DB, Hotaling GT. Dating violence: a review of contextual and risk factors. In: Levy B, ed. Dating violence: young women in danger. Seattle: Seal Press, 1991.

46. MacEwen K. Refining the intergenerational transmission hypothesis. J Interpersonal Violence 1994;9:350–365.

47. National Center on Child Abuse and Neglect. Child maltreatment 1995: reports from the states of the National Child Abuse and Neglect Data System. Washington, DC: U.S. Dept of Health and Human Services, 1997.

48. Bergman L. Dating violence among high school students. Social Work 1991;37:21–27.

49. Makepeace J. Courtship violence among college students. Family Relations 1981;30.

50. Ewing CP. When children kill: the dynamics of juvenile homicide. Lexington, MA: Lexington Books, 1990.

51. Murphy DE. The causes of youth violence: an overview. In: Youth violence. San Diego: Greenhaven Press, 1992.

51a. Freed D. The number of victims of teenage violence is increasing.

In: Biskup M, Cozic C, eds. Youth violence. San Diego: Greenhaven Press, 1992.

52. Bergman L. The forgotten few: juvenile female offenders. Federal Probation 1989;March: 73–78.

53. Tucker J, Wolfe LR. Victims no more: girls fight back against male violence. Washington, DC: Center for Women Policy Studies, 1997.

54. Slaby R. Combating televison violence. Chronicle of Higher Education 1994;15.

55. Donnerstein E, et al. The mass media and youth aggression. In: Eron L, Gentry J, Schlegel J, eds. Reason to hope. Washington, DC: Gentry and Schlegal, 1994.

56. Hechinger F. Fateful choices: healthy youth for the 21st century. New York: Carnegie Corporation of New York, 1992.

57. Hechinger F. Fateful choices: healthy youth for the 21st century. New York: Carnegie Corporation of New York, 1992.

58. Wilson-Brewer R, et al. Violence prevention for young adolescents: the state of the art of program evaluation. Washington, DC: Carnegie Council on Adolescent Development, 1991.

59. Stark E, Flitcraft A, Zuckerman D, et al. Wife abuse in the medical setting: an introduction for health personnel. Monograph series, no. 7. Rockville, MD: National Clearinghouse on Domestic Violence, 1981.

60. Koss MP, Heslet L. Somatic consequences of violence against women. Arch Fam Med 1992;1: 53–59.

61. Geist RF. Sexually related trauma. Emer Med Clin North Am 1988;6:439–466.

62. Lacey HB. Sexually transmitted diseases and rape: the experience of a sexual assault centre. Int J STD AIDS 1990;1:405–409.

63. Murphy SM. Rape, sexually transmitted diseases and human immunodeficiency virus infection. Int J STD AIDS 1990;1:79–82.

64. Bullock L, McFarlane J. The birth-weight/battering connection. Am J Nurs 1989;89:1153–1155.

65. Satin AJ, Hemsell DL, Stone IC Jr, et al. Sexual assault in pregnancy. Obstet Gynecol 1991;77: 710–714.

66. McFarlane J, Parker B, Soeken E, et al. Assessing for abuse during pregnancy: severity and frequency of injuries and associated entry into prenatal care. JAMA 1992;267:3176–3178.

67. Stets JE, Straus MA. Gender differences in reporting marital violence and its medical and psychological consequences. In: Straus MA, Gelles RJ, eds. Physical violence in American families: risk factors and adaptations to violence in 8145 families. New Brunswick, NJ: Transaction, 1990.

68. National Center for Victims of Crime, Crime Victims Research and Treatment Center. Rape in America: a report to the nation. Arlington, VA: National Center for Victims of Crime, 1992.

69. Koss MP, Heslet L. Somatic consequences of violence against women. Arch Fam Med 1992;1: 53–59.

70. Cohen S, Williamson GM. Stress and infectious disease in humans. Psychol Bull 1991;109: 5–24.

71. Cohen S, Tyrell DA, Smith AP. Psychological stress and susceptibility to the common cold. N Engl J Med 1991;325:606–612.

72. Stark E, Flitcraft A, Zuckerman D, et al. Wife abuse in the medical setting: an introduction for health personnel. Monograph series, no. 7. Rockville, MD: National Clearinghouse on Domestic Violence, 1981.

73. Resnick HS, Kilpatrick DG, Dansky BS, et al. Prevalence of civilian trauma and posttraumatic stress disorder in a national sample of women. J Consult Clin Psychol 1993;61:984–991.

74. Kilpatrick DG, Saunders BE, Amick-McMullan A, et al. Victim

and crime factors associated with the development of crime-related posttraumatic stress disorder. Behavior Therapy 1989;20:199–214.

75. Siegal JM, Golding JM, et al. Reactions to sexual assault: a community study. J Interpersonal Violence 1990;5:229–246.

76. Winfield I, George LK, Swartz M, et al. Sexual assault and psychiatric disorders among a community sample of women. Am J Psychiatry 1990;147:335–341.

77. Steiger H, Zanko M. Sexual traumata among eating-disordered, psychiatric, and normal female groups. J Interpersonal Violence 1990;5:74–86.

78. Resnick HS, Kilpatrick DG, Dansky BS, et al. Prevalence of civilian trauma and posttraumatic stress disorder in a national sample of women. J Consult Clin Psychol 1993;61:984–991.

79. National Center for Victims of Crime, Crime Victims Research and Treatment Center. Rape in America: a report to the nation. Arlington, VA: National Center for Victims of Crime, 1992.

80. Jacobson A, Richardson B. Assault experiences of 100 psychiatric inpatients: evidence of the need for routine inquiry. Am J Psychiatry 1987;144:908–913.

81. Carmen E, Rieker PP, Mills T. Victims of violence and psychiatric illness. Am J Psychiatry 1984;141:378–383.

82. Stets JE, Straus MA. Gender differences in reporting marital violence and its medical and psychological consequences. In: Straus MA, Gelles RJ, eds. Physical violence in American families: risk factors and adaptations to violence in 8145 families. New Brunswick, NJ: Transaction, 1990.

83. National Center for Victims of Crime, Crime Victims Research and Treatment Center. Rape in America: a report to the nation. Arlington, VA: National Center for Victims of Crime, 1992.

84. Swett C, Cohen C, Surrey J, et al. High rates of alcohol use and history of physical and sexual abuse among women outpatients. J Drug Alcohol Abuse 1991;17: 49–60.

85. Miller BA, Downs WR, Gondoli DM, et al. Spousal violence among alcoholic women as compared to a random household sample of women. J Studies on Alcohol 1989;50:533–540.

86. Miller BA, Downs WR, Gondoli DM, et al. Spousal violence among alcoholic women as compared to a random household sample of women. J Studies on Alcohol 1989;50:533–540.

87. National Center for Victims of Crime, Crime Victims Research and Treatment Center. Rape in America: a report to the nation. Arlington, VA: National Center for Victims of Crime, 1992.

88. Resick PA, Calhoun KS, et al. Social adjustment in victims of sexual assault. J Consult Clin Psychol 1981;49:705–712.

89. Feldman-Summer S, Gordon PE, Meagher JR. The impact of rape on sexual satisfaction. J Abnormal Psychol 1979;88:101–105.

90. Bassuk EL, Rosenberg L. Why does family homelessness occur? A case-control study. Am J Public Health 1988;78:783–788.

91. Wood D, Valdez RB, Hayashi T, et al. Homeless and housed families in Los Angeles: a study comparing demographic, economic, and family function characteristics. Am J Public Health 1990;80: 1049–1052.

92. Wood MP, Koss PG, Woodruff WJ. Deleterious effects of criminal victimization on women's health and medical utilization. Arch Int Med 1991;151:343–347.

93. Miller TR, Choen MA, Rossman SB. Victim costs of violent crime and resulting injuries. Health Affairs 1993;12:186–197.

94. Joint Commission on the Accreditation of Healthcare Organizations. Revised standards address possible victims of abuse. Joint Commission Perspectives 1991; March/April.

95. American Medical Association, Council on Ethical and Judicial Affairs. Physicians and domestic violence: ethical considerations. JAMA 1992;267:3190–3193.

96. American Medical Association. Diagnostic and treatment guidelines on mental health effects of family violence. Chicago: American Medical Association, 1995.

97. Tilden VP, Schmidt TA, Limandri BJ, et al. Factors that influence clinicans' assessment and management of family violence. Am J Public Health 1994;84:628–633.

98. Sugg NK, Innui T. Primary care physicans' response to domestic violence: opening Pandora's box. JAMA 1992;267:3157–3160.

99. Sparks CH, Bar On BA. A social change approach to the prevention of sexual violence against women. (Work in Progress Series no. 83-08.) Wellesley, MA: Wellesley College, Stone Center for Developmental Services and Studies, 1985.

100. Swift CF. The prevention of rape. In: Burgess AW, ed. Rape and sexual assault: a research handbook. New York: Garland, 1985.

101. Kaufman Kantor G, Straus MA. Response of victims and the police to assaults on wives. In: Straus MA, Gelles RJ, eds. Physical violence in American families: risk factors and adaptations to violence in 8145 families. New Brunswick, NJ: Transaction, 1990.

102. Schmidt JD, Sherman LW. Does arrest deter domestic violence? Am Behavioral Scientist 1993; 36:601–609.

103. National Center for Victims of Crime, Crime Victims Research and Treatment Center. Rape in America: a report to the nation. Arlington, VA: National Center for Victims of Crime, 1992.

104. McCall GJ. Risk factors and sexual assault prevention. J Interpersonal Violence 1993;8: 227–295.

105. Marsh JC, Geist A, Caplan N. Rape and the limits of law reform. Boston: Auburn House, 1982.

106. Furby L, Fischhoff B. Rape self-defense strategies: a review of their effectiveness. Eugene, OR: Eugene Research Institute, 1986.

107. Sparks CH, Bar On BA. A social change approach to the prevention of sexual violence against women. (Work in Progress Series no. 83-08.) Wellesley, MA: Wellesley College, Stone Center for Developmental Services and Studies, 1985.

108. Bergman L. Dating violence among high school students. Social Work 1992;37:21–27.

RESOURCES

Victim Support

National Domestic Violence Hotline
1-800-799-SAFE

Programs and Information Centers on Domestic Violence and Sexual Assault

Duluth Domestic Intervention Project
206 West Fourth Street
Duluth, MN 55806
212-722-2781

The Family Violence Project
Resource Center on Domestic Violence, Child Protection and
    Custody
National Council of Juvenile and Family Court Judges
P.O. Box 8970
Reno, NV 89507
(800)527-3223 or (702)784-4829

National Battered Women's Law Project
275 7th Avenue, Suite 1206
New York, NY 10001
212-741-9480

National Clearinghouse for the Defense of Battered Women
125 S. 9th Street. Suite 302
Philadelphia, PA 19107
800-903-0111

National Coalition Against Domestic Violence
National Office
P.O. Box 18749
Denver, CO 80218-0749
303-839-1852

National Maternal and Child Health Clearinghouse
8201 Greensboro Drive, Suite 600
McLean, VA 22120
(703)821-8955, exts. 254/265

National Network to End Domestic Violence
701 Pennsylvania Avenue, NW, Suite 900
Washington, DC 20004
800-903-0111

National Resource Center on Domestic Violence
Pennsylvania Coalition Against Domestic Violence
6400 Flank Drive, Suite 1300
Harrisburg, PA 17112
800-537-2238

Center for the Prevention of Sexual and Domestic Violence
1914 North 34th, Suite 105
Seattle, WA 98103
(206)634-1903

Teen Dating Violence Prevention and Intervention Programs

The Family Violence Prevention Fund
383 Rhode Island Street, Suite 304
San Francisco, CA 94103-5133
(415)252-8900

Los Angeles Commission on Assaults Against Women/
    Teen Abuse Prevention Program
6043 Hollywood Blvd., Suite 200
Los Angeles, CA 90028
213-462-1281

Project H.A.R.T.
Progressive Youth Center
311 North Lindbergh Blvd.
St. Louis, MO 63141
314-993-3566

SafePlace
P.O. Box 19454
Austin, TX 78760
512-445-5776

Programs and Information Centers on Domestic Violence and Sexual Assault for Gays and Lesbians

Community United Against Violence
973 Market Street, Suite 500
San Francisco, CA 94103
415-333-HELP

Fenway Community Health Center's Victim Recovery
    Program
7 Haviland Street
Boston, MA 02115
617-267-0900

Gay and Lesbian Anti-Violence Project
647 Hudson Street
New York, NY 10014
212-807-0197

Part VI.

OBSTETRICS AND GYNECOLOGY

Edited by
Hope A. Ricciotti

Introduction to Obstetrics and Gynecology

Hope A. Ricciotti

The field of obstetrics and gynecology has evolved over the years into a combination of specialty care and preventive care for women. The focus of the chapters in this section are those aspects of preventive care related to obstetrics and gynecology. There is a large overlap between what is considered the realm of women's health and that of obstetrics and gynecology. One such aspect, hormone replacement therapy in menopause, is found in Section V, Women's Health.

The author of the first chapter in this section, Mimi Yum, reviews important aspects of preconceptional care. Preconceptional planning is important to incorporate in all preventive care for any woman of childbearing age, since the vast majority of pregnancies are unplanned. Dr. Yum highlights folic acid in the prevention of neural tube defects and reviews the relationship of some common medical problems and their effect on pregnancy. She discusses some simple preventive measures to enhance pregnancy outcomes.

Hope Ricciotti discusses the nutritional aspects of maintaining a healthy pregnancy. She reviews the basic components of a healthy diet in pregnancy, as well as some precautions. She considers pregnancy an excellent "teaching time," a period in a woman's life when she is interested in learning preventive habits that may then continue for a lifetime.

Susan Hellerstein reviews the literature on exercise in pregnancy. She reviews the basic physiology of exercise in pregnancy. She then discusses a series of studies on exercise and pregnancy, and concludes that there appear to be no adverse sequelae in the offspring of pregnant women who exercised. Mothers who exercise during pregnancy have been shown to have a decrease in some of the discomforts of pregnancy.

Certified lactation consultant Lisa Litchfield McSherry reviews the physiology of breastfeeding and some basic techniques. She summarizes the results of many studies confirming the health benefits seen in breastfed babies. She reviews problems related to breastfeeding, including mastitis, poor weight gain in newborns, engorgement, and poor latch-on. She details the latest issues regarding pumping and storing breastmilk.

Sexually transmitted diseases and vaginitis are common gynecologic problems seen by a multitude of primary care providers. Devora Lieberman and Toni Huebscher review the literature regarding the currently available contraceptive methods and their efficacy. Finally, a chapter by Carol London details the latest CDC guidelines and treatments for these commonly encountered problems.

Chapter 33

Preconceptional Care

Mimi R. Yum

Prenatal care is a fundamental component of preventive medicine. It is commonly recognized that good prenatal care is associated with improved pregnancy outcomes. This concept today has been broadened to include preconceptional care. Preconceptional care has taken on greater importance in our current health care environment for a number of reasons. Our knowledge of how various environmental exposures and medical illnesses affect fertility and fetal development has grown. Our ability to detect and in some instances treat maternal and fetal disease has improved. Our understanding of how pregnancy affects underlying maternal medical conditions has been enhanced. And the number of potentially affected pregnancies has grown as more older women are electing to have children. The purpose of providing preconceptional care is to identify risk, whether based on medical history, family history, or social factors; to educate the patient and her partner in order to assist them in optimizing conditions for a healthy conception and pregnancy as well as to prepare them for possible complications; and to intervene when appropriate to improve the outcome of a pregnancy.

In our present health care environment, many women are receiving their gynecologic as well as general medical care from primary care providers. It is the rare patient who will see her gynecologist for the express purpose of obtaining preconceptional guidance. In fact, approximately 40% of pregnancies in the United States are unintended. But even in the case of a planned pregnancy, the newly pregnant patient will seldom see her obstetrician before 7 or 8 weeks of gestation. At this point, the crucial phases of organogenesis have already taken place. Thus, the primary care physician is uniquely positioned to have a positive effect on early pregnancy and fetal development by incorporating preconceptional care into the routine history and physical of any woman of reproductive age. With an eye to this objective, the physician can assess risk and then provide appropriate counseling and management for the patient for whom future childbearing is a real possibility.

AGE

Extremes of age are associated with complications in pregnancy. Adolescent patients are probably at higher risk because of social factors and lack of prenatal care rather than physiologic immaturity. Higher rates of adolescent pregnancy have been associated with poorer socioeconomic conditions as well as current substance use.

In older patients, however, there is an increased medical risk that can be attributed to a higher prevalence of chronic medical conditions such as hypertension and diabetes. In addition, as women age, their risk of having a child with a chromosomal abnormality increases (1). Patients can be educated of this biologic fact and, when appropriate, can be counseled regarding options for prenatal diagnosis, namely chorionic villi sampling (CVS) and amniocentesis.

Despite the different reasons for their higher risk, both teenagers and older women will more commonly experience complications such as preeclampsia and intrauterine growth retardation in their pregnancies. Women at both ends of the age spectrum can successfully carry pregnancies to term and deliver healthy infants; however, the clinician should caution these patients and provide age-appropriate counseling, be it contraceptive education or preconceptional guidance.

GYNECOLOGIC HISTORY

A careful gynecologic history is of obvious importance in helping the clinician identify potential factors that may affect future fertility and pregnancies. By reviewing a patient's menstrual history, notably frequency and duration of menses, the physician and the patient can gain a sense of ovulatory status. For instance, irregular or infrequent menses may predict future difficulty in conceiving as they are often symptoms of oligoovulation or anovulation. The patient should be made aware of the need for greater latitude in timing a pregnancy. Such a patient, particularly if she is of advanced age, may wish to seek fertility counseling and treatment sooner in the process.

A preconceptional visit affords the physician an opportunity to screen for and treat sexually transmitted diseases before they can affect a future pregnancy. Sexually transmitted infections and their sequelae have been associated with spontaneous abortions, preterm labor and delivery, preterm rupture of membranes, chorioamnionitis, congenital infections, and even fetal demise. Additionally, untreated gonorrhea and chlamydial infections may lead to pelvic inflammatory disease, both symptomatic and silent, that can increase the risk of ectopic pregnancies as well as infertility. All patients who are sexually active should be offered testing for gonorrhea, chlamydia, syphilis, HIV, and hepatitis B. Since HIV and hepatitis B are both chronic infections that can be transmitted to the unborn fetus, knowledge of a positive status may influence a patient's reproductive choices. Such patients should not be pressured to avoid future pregnancy; rather they should be informed of the treatments available to them during pregnancy and to their infants postpartum that can significantly reduce the risk of infection in the offspring.

A history of herpes simplex virus in the patient or her partner is also important to elicit. Patients with a positive history or with a partner with a positive history should be counseled of the significance of this condition in pregnancy and delivery. If the patient has prodromal symptoms or a lesion when she goes into labor, the standard of care is delivery by cesarean section in order to prevent neonatal infection. The risk of neonatal infection is greatest in the event of a primary lesion.

The performance of Pap smears is already a routine component of a general examination by most primary care providers. Patients should be questioned about a history of abnormal Pap smears. The evaluation and treatment of cervical dysplasia, particularly in the case of a high-grade intraepithelial lesion (CIN II or CIN III), is much simpler and more straightforward in the nonpregnant patient. Patients with a history of treatment for cervical dysplasia with a cone biopsy, in a small percentage of cases, should be made aware of the possibility of cervical incompetence that could result in a second trimester loss of the fetus. Since suspected cervical incompetence can be treated successfully with a cervical cerclage, it is important for such a patient to seek early obstetric care.

Other gynecologic procedures have potential consequences for future childbearing. For instance, a history of tubal surgery may predispose a patient toward ectopic pregnancy. A patient with this history should be given appropriate warnings. Prior uterine surgery such as a myomectomy may necessitate cesarean delivery. The patient should be asked to obtain operative notes of prior gynecologic procedures for review.

Patients should be questioned regarding in utero exposure to diethylstilbestrol (DES). Exposure to this hormone, which was prescribed to pregnant women between the late 1940s and 1971, can cause malformations of the reproductive tracts of unborn female infants. In addition to performing a careful examination of affected women, the clinician should alert them of their increased risk of spontaneous abortion, cervical incompetence, and preterm delivery. They should be offered referral to a maternal-fetal medicine specialist early in pregnancy.

REPRODUCTIVE HISTORY

A woman's previous reproductive history is of great value in helping the clinician identify risk factors that may complicate future conception or pregnancy. Appropriate preconceptional counseling can best be provided after a thorough reproductive history is obtained, including past spontaneous abortions, therapeutic abortions, ectopic pregnancies, and deliveries.

It is estimated that 25% to 30% of pregnancies result in first-trimester spontaneous abortions (2). One or two such losses need not necessarily mandate a systematic workup. Recurrent pregnancy loss, generally defined as three or more spontaneous abortions, is considered pathologic, and should therefore prompt an investigation. If the patient is of advanced age, the clinician and the patient may wish to initiate a workup after one or two losses. This type of evaluation is best performed when the patient is not pregnant. The primary care physician can start by screening for an underlying medical condition such as diabetes mellitus, thyroid disease, and autoimmune disease, each of which can contribute to recurrent miscarriages. If no such condition is diagnosed, the patient should then be referred to a gynecologist to rule out a structural or hormonal abnormality. Referral of the patient and her partner to a geneticist should also be strongly considered in order to investigate the possibility of cytogenetic causes. Approximately 5% of recurrent abortions can be attributed to a parental chromosomal rearrangement such as a translocation (3).

A history of a single second-trimester miscarriage, however, is considered abnormal and should prompt an investigation prior to a subsequent pregnancy. The same etiologies of recurrent first-trimester abortions can be responsible for a second-trimester loss. Another important diagnosis to consider is cervical incompetence. This condition is characterized by painless dilatation of the cervix due to a structural or functional cervical defect. Patients at risk include those with a history of cervical trauma, which may have resulted from a dilatation and curettage procedure, a previous delivery, or cervical surgery, as mentioned above, such as a cone biopsy. Although an unequivocal history of cervical incompetence is often difficult to elucidate, any patient with a suspicious history should be strongly counseled to seek early obstetric care in a future pregnancy.

The patient should be questioned regarding all previous deliveries, including mode of delivery, complications during pregnancy or labor and delivery, infant outcome and health, and birthweights. Previous complications may alert the physician to the possiblity of future risk and the need for close surveilance or intervention. For instance, the physician can help a couple with a previous infant with a neural tube defect to reduce their risk of having another affected child (there is a recurrence rate of approximately 2%) by prescibing folate preconceptionally at a dose of 4 mg/day (4). This dose may be started 1 month prior to pregnancy and continued for the first 3 months of gestation. The birth of a child with a genetic disorder or mental retardation should prompt a referral to a geneticist prior to future pregnancy.

While couples who have been actively trying to conceive without success may have already sought the care of a specialist, the primary care physician may occasionally encounter a patient with an unrecognized infertility problem. Infertility is generally defined as the failure to conceive after 1 year of unprotected intercourse, although the criteria are looser in the case of an older patient. While such a patient may not be actively seeking to become pregnant at the time of her visit, she should be cautioned that a planned conception may require time and possible intervention.

MEDICAL HISTORY

By reviewing the medical history, the clinician can preliminarily assess the effect that a patient's existing medical conditions may have on a future pregnancy and a developing fetus and, conversely, the effect the pregnancy may have on the mother's health. This gives the primary care provider the opportunity to modify medical care or medication if appropriate, to consult specialists as necessary, and to educate the patient and her partner.

While many medical conditions if recognized and appropriately managed can be compatible with a healthy mother and infant, pregnancy may seriously compromise maternal health in the case of certain diseases. For example, patients with New York Heart Association class III or IV cardiac disease have a 7% mortality rate with pregnancy (5). Similarly, pulmonary hypertension, aortic coarctation, severe renal disease, valvular heart disease, and history of congestive heart disease are associated with poor pregnancy outcomes. These conditions are relatively strong contraindications to pregnancy.

Hypertension

As more women of advanced age are electing to have children, hypertension is an increasingly common condition of women who are contemplating pregnancy or who are pregnant. Prior to pregnancy, primary causes of hypertension should be ruled out. Essential hypertension can be managed successfully throughout pregnancy, although these patients should be counseled about their increased risk of complications such as preeclampsia, pregnancy-induced hypertension, intrauterine growth retardation, and placental abruption. Blood pressure should be well controlled prior to conception, with diet and exercise as a first-line treatment. If medication is necessary, patients can be managed on an antihypertensive that is not contraindicated in pregnancy. These include beta-blockers, alpha-methyldopa, and calcium-channel blockers. Angiotensin-converting enzyme inhibitors are strictly con-

traindicated, as they have been associated with serious fetal renal dysfunction (6).

Diabetes Mellitus

While the existence of diabetes does not necessarily preclude a healthy pregnancy or infant, it is a disease that should be carefully managed before conception and throughout pregnancy. Poor glycemic control at the time of conception and during organogenesis is associated with an increased rate of spontaneous abortions and congenital anomalies. Most studies concur that diabetics with poor glycemic control are two to three times more likely to have a child with an anomaly compared to a nondiabetic mother. These anomalies may be quite serious and even fatal, including cardiovascular malformations, neural tube defects, and anomalies of the genitourinary and gastrointestinal systems. Patients and their physicians should aim for a glycosylated hemoglobin level of less than 7% to 8% before attempting pregnancy. The range of acceptable blood glucose values is much tighter throughout pregnancy, with fasting glucose between 60 mg/dL and 90 mg/dL and 2-hour postprandial glucose of less than 120 mg/dL. Non-insulin-dependent diabetics must switch from oral hypoglycemics to insulin therapy before pregnancy, while insulin-dependent patients will often see an increase in their insulin requirement. Multiple complications have been associated with diabetes in pregnancy, including preeclampsia, intrauterine fetal demise, intrauterine growth retardation or macrosomia, neonatal respiratory distress syndrome, and acceleration of maternal end organ disease. A diabetic woman should be fully aware that a pregnancy requires considerable commitment by her in order to maintain her own and her infant's health.

Seizure Disorder

Women with seizure disorders face an increased risk of giving birth to infants with congenital anomalies, notably cleft palate or lip, cardiac defects, and neural tube defects. Whether this risk is due to the seizure disorder itself or to antiseizure medications has not been clearly elucidated. If a patient has been free of seizures for at least 2 to 3 years, a trial off medication can be attempted before she becomes pregnant. While ideally a patient would be off medication and free of seizures at the time of conception and during pregnancy, this is not possible for many epileptic patients. It may be unsafe and unwise for affected women to discontinue their medication. Therefore it is the responsibility of the physician to emphasize the importance of continuing medication throughout the pregnancy. The physician may be able to reduce the risk of fetal malformations by altering the patient's medication regimen, however. The anticonvulsant with the lowest teratogenic profile is phenobarbital, which is not apparently associated with specific congenital malformations. Valproic acid, phenytoin, and carbamazepine, on the other hand, all have significant teratogenic potential. Both valproic acid and carbamazepine are associated with a 1% risk of neural tube defects. Phenytoin is associated with a constellation of anomalies known as fetal hydantoin syndrome, including mental retardation, cleft palate, microcephaly, and abnormal facies. Again, a trial on phenobarbital would be best attempted in the nonpregnant state.

Phenylketonuria

Women with phenylketonuria (PKU), a disease characterized by the inability to metabolize phenylalanine, require strict nutritional counsel prior to conception. Many affected women discontinue a phenylalanine-restricted diet once they reach their teen years as elevated levels of the amino acid have not been considered dangerous to the mature nervous system. During pregnancy, however, these elevated levels are quite devastating to the fetus, causing cardiac defects, microcephaly, severe mental retardation, and intrauterine growth retardation. This occurs whether or not the fetus itself is affected with PKU. Women with PKU who are considering pregnancy should therefore resume a phenylalanine-restricted diet.

Asthma

Asthma is another condition frequently seen in women of childbearing age. The effects of pregnancy on this condition vary tremendously from individual to individual. It is commonly stated that one third of pregnant patients experience improvement of their disease, one third experience deterioration, while one third see no change. Patients should be strongly counseled to continue necessary maintenance medication such as beta-agonist and steroid inhalers before and during pregnancies. The effects of such medication on a developing fetus are minimal or none while the possible consequences of inadequate treatment can be serious.

Thyroid Disease

Thyroid disorders commonly affect women of reproductive age. Overt thyroid disease often results in infertility or early fetal wastage. A euthyroid state should be achieved prior to pregnancy, either medically or surgically, if indicated in the case of refractory thyrotoxicosis. Poorly controlled hypothyroidism in pregnancy has been associated with a slightly increased risk of complications such as preeclampsia, low birthweight, and fetal demise (7). Inadequately treated hyperthyroidism may result in fetal complications of preterm delivery and preeclampsia and maternal complications such as cardiac arrhythmias and congestive heart failure (8). It should be strongly emphasized to women with hypothyroid and hyperthyroid conditions that medication should be continued before conception and throughout pregnancy. Thyroid function should then be periodically evaluated during the course of pregnancy. The infants of hyperthyroid mothers may require closer surveillance in utero and postnatally as they are also at risk for developing thyroid dysfunction as a result of maternal transmission of antithyroid medication or thyroid-stimulating antibodies.

Mental Health

It is crucial that the clinician not overlook mental health and well-being in evaluating preconceptional patients. As in the case of other chronic medical conditions, psychiatric disorders should be well controlled prior to attempting conception. Patients with a history of psychiatric conditions should recognize that pregnancy and the puerperium can induce a maelstrom of physical and psychologic changes that may exacerbate preexisting disease. Current use of psychoactive medications should be reviewed. While many women may wish to stop their medication at the time of conception and

during pregnancy, it may be not be medically expedient to discontinue medication despite unknown teratogenicity. The risks of uncontrolled maternal disease in many cases will outweigh potential fetal risk from drug exposure. These patients may be referred to a genetics specialist for in-depth counseling. The primary care provider and obstetrician should work in conjunction with a patient's mental health care provider to promote the optimal treatment plan.

MEDICATIONS

An important aspect of preconceptional counseling is reviewing with the patient her list of medications and discussing possible effects on a developing fetus. As stated above, patients with underlying medical conditions need to have their disease well controlled to optimize their own health as well as that of the fetus while pregnant; thus they must continue the medications essential to controlling their disease. There are, however, certain drugs with such great teratogenic potential that, if the drug cannot be discontinued, the patient should be counseled to avoid pregnancy. These include isotretinoin, warfarin, some chemotherapeutic agents, tetracycline, and androgenic medications. In some cases, an alternative with lower teratogenicity can be safely prescribed.

In general, most over-the-counter medications, such as acetaminophen and other nonsteroidals, antacids, and cold medicines pose minimal or no risk with casual use before a pregnancy is recognized. Once pregnancy is confirmed, of course, patients should be cautioned to avoid any medication not specifically approved by their providers.

FAMILY HISTORY

A preconceptional visit is the optimal time to perform risk assessment based upon the family history of the patient and her partner. Careful questioning may reveal a positive family history of a genetic disease that should prompt a referral to genetics counseling (Table 33-1). With current advancements in molecular genetics, both genetic testing and prenatal diagnosis have an expanded role in preconceptional and obstetric care. Even with an unremarkable family history, certain ethnic groups are at increased risk for having children affected with a genetic disease; thus carrier status for a number of conditions should also be determined prior to conception (Table 33-2). For example, an individual of Ashkenazic Jewish or French Canadian background has a 1 : 30 chance of being a carrier

Table 33-1 Genetic Diseases
Hemoglobinopathies
Sickle cell disease
B-thalassemia
Alpha-thalassemia
Hemophilia
Muscular dystrophy
Mental retardation, known fragile X or unexplained
Cystic fibrosis

Table 33-2 Carrier Screening

Disease	Ethnic Group	Screening Test
Sickle cell anemia	African, Caribbean, Latin American, Mediterranean, West Indian	Hemoglobin electrophoresis
Beta-thalassemia	African, Indian, Mediterranean, Southeast and East Asian	Complete blood count with indices
Alpha-thalassemia	African, Chinese, Filipino, Southeast Asian	Complete blood count with indices
Tay-Sachs disease	Eastern European, French Canadian, Ashkenazi Jews	Assay for enzyme hexosaminidase A
Cystic fibrosis	Northern European, positive family history	DNA analysis

for Tay-Sachs disease, an autosomal recessive disease that is characterized by fatal degeneration of the nervous system.

By providing these services before pregnancy to couples at risk, the clinician is giving them greater power over their reproductive future. While many of these couples will accept the risks and still elect to have children, others may choose options that would have been closed to them once a pregnancy occurred, including remaining childless, adoption, preimplantation diagnosis, and chorionic villi sampling.

SOCIAL HISTORY

The preconceptional period is the optimal time to educate patients of the risks posed by their behaviors and environmental exposures. This early counseling gives the patient and her partner an opportunity to modify parameters under their control before exposing their unborn child.

Smoking

Although cigarette smoking is universally recognized to be unhealthy to mother and fetus, 20% to 30% of women of reproductive age continue to smoke (9). While many women assert that they will quit smoking once pregnant, it is of greater benefit to the patient to begin the process prior to pregnancy. Smoking is associated with an increased risk of spontaneous abortions, preterm labor, and low-birthweight infants. There is evidence that it is also associated with placental abruption. Nicotine medication may be useful for heavier smokers and may, if necessary, be continued in pregnancy if the patient is unable to decrease smoking to fewer than 10 to 15 cigarettes a day.

Alcohol

Ethanol alcohol is one of the most common potentially teratogenic substances to which pregnant women expose their unborn infants. Fetal alcohol exposure is the leading cause of mental retardation and is associated with a variety of other congenital defects and developmental deficiencies, including intrauterine growth retardation, facial dysmorphism, microcephaly, and behavioral problems. In one study, fetal alcohol syndrome was seen in the children of 11% of women who drank 1 to 2 ounces of alcohol a day during the first trimester (10). No threshold amount of alcohol has been proven to be safe to the fetus; therefore women considering pregnancy should be advised to avoid any alcohol consumption. On the other hand, patients that have had a drink or two before a pregnancy was recognized should be reassured that there is no evidence that minimal exposure causes a significant risk. Another compelling reason to avoid alcohol is its strong association with trauma and abuse.

Substance Abuse

Cocaine, heroine, and marijuana are among the more common illicit substances used by young women. Cocaine causes vasoconstriction that decreases uterine blood flow. This can result in spontaneous abortions, placental abruption, preterm labor and delivery, and intrauterine growth restriction. The habitual use of heroin and other opiates, though not associated with malformations, can result in a neonatal withdrawal syndrome that can be quite severe. Marijuana, though not definitely linked to congenital anomalies in human studies, has been associated with teratogenicity in animal studies. Marijuana, however, does affect judgment and lucidity that can clearly impair the safety of a user. Patients should be questioned regarding drug use in a nonjudgmental manner, educated of the effects of such usage on a pregnancy, and offered treatment if appropriate.

Environmental Exposures

Patients should be questioned regarding environmental and occupational exposures. In particular, women should try to avoid exposure to organic chemicals in the periconceptional period as they have been associated with spontaneous abortions. Some additional substances that may have abortifacient effects include anesthetic gases, benzene, ethylene oxide, arsenic, and lead (11).

Domestic Violence

Domestic violence is an important issue to address in the evaluation of women of all ages, although it is of particular significance preconceptionally. Pregnant women are too frequently victims of sexual and physical abuse. As with medical problems, assessment and intervention can be less complicated when the patient is not pregnant. Every clinician's office should have the names and numbers of local resources and social services available for any patient for whom this is a potential issue.

PHYSICAL EXAMINATION

A general physical examination should be performed with special attention to blood pressure, weight, and pelvic examination. The general examination may uncover underlying medical conditions that are best managed prior to pregnancy. If the pelvic examination reveals abnormal findings that may complicate conception or childbearing, the patient can be referred for further evaluation and possible treatment.

COUNSELING

In addition to the identification of specific risk factors, a preconceptional visit allows the primary care provider to provide general counsel that will benefit the low-risk patient as well.

Folate

By taking folate in the periconceptional period, women can significantly reduce their risk of having a child with a neural tube defect. With an incidence of 1–2 per 1000 live births, neural tube defects are the second most common major birth defect in the United States, following congenital heart anomalies. There is a wide range in the severity of the defect, from malformations that are incompatible with life to mild disease that results in functional deficits. While there is a genetic component, the etiology of neural tube defects is multifactorial, with 95% occurring in infants of women with no identifiable risk factor. Multiple studies have confirmed a decrease in the incidence of neural tube defects in women who took folate in the periconceptional period. One large, multicentered case-control study demonstrated a relative risk of 0.4 with folate therapy (12).

For this reason, the Centers for Disease Control and Prevention (CDC) (4) have recommended a daily dose of 400 μg for all women of reproductive age. Patients at higher risk of having a child with a neural tube defect, including diabetics, patients on anticonvulsants or patients with a positive family history or a previously affected infant, should consume 4 mg a day. This dose has been associated with a 75% decrease in recurrence in families with a previous history (13). Both high- and low-risk women should initiate folate therapy one month before pregnancy and continue through the first 3 months of gestation. No reduction of risk is seen when folate is started after 6 weeks of gestation. Most prenatal vitamin formulations contain 400 μg of folate. This can be prescribed for patients planning for a pregnancy. Other dietary sources of folate include dark green leafy vegetables, organ meats such as liver and kidney, and fortified cereals. As of January 1998, grain, flour and cereal products are fortified with folate as per the Food and Drug Administration's recommendations (14).

Nutrition

Women trying to conceive should eat a healthy well-balanced diet. The nutritional needs of the pregnant woman are very similar to what any healthy adult should eat. During pregnancy, an additional 300 to 500 calories per day are needed, depending upon the level of physical activity. The majority (more than 50%) of calories should come from carbohydrates. Approximately 60 g of protein per day are needed, which is just 10 g more than nonpregnant women need. Approximately 30% of calories should come from fat. Meals should be based upon such foods as pasta, potatoes, grains, and fresh vegetables, with meat or other protein sources serving as accompaniments. This style of eating is what any healthy adult female should consume, and the preconceptional period is an ideal time to reinforce this.

Exercise

Pregnant and nonpregnant women alike reap benefits from mild to moderate exercise. Ideally, women should be fit and exercising before pregnancy. Once pregnant, patients should not initiate a new and more strenuous exercise regimen. Preconceptional counseling, therefore, is an ideal time to encourage women to begin a regular exercise routine, as many are motivated at this time. Staying active can reduce some of the discomforts of pregnancy such as backache, constipation, fatigue, and swelling. Exercise can also improve energy level, mood, and self-image. It is thought that physically fit women may have an easier labor as well. Patients trying to become pregnant should avoid elevating body temperature above 38°C (100.4°F). Most forms of exercise are safe in pregnancy, including walking, swimming, jogging, and bicycling. Exercises that may result in abdominal trauma should be carefully considered and possibly avoided, particularly for the less skilled; these include skiing, surfing, and rollerblading.

Vaccinations

The preconceptional period is the optimal time to make sure that a patient's immunization record is up to date. Table 33-3 shows the recommended schedule of immunizations. Patients can be tested for rubella immunity as well as varicella immunity if they are uncertain of previous exposure or illness. Although congenital rubella and varicella are rare, both infections are potentially devastating to the unborn infant. Nonimmune women should be vaccinated, then should defer pregnancy for three months.

Table 33-3 Recommended Immunizations

IMMUNIZATION	FREQUENCY	PATIENTS	SAFE IN PREGNANCY?
Diptheria/tetanus	Every 10 years	All	Yes
Influenza	Annually	Susceptible individuals	Yes
Pneumococcal	Once	Susceptible individuals	Yes
Hepatitis B	Once (3 shots)	At risk individuals	Yes
MMR	Once	All	No
Varicella	Once	Susceptible individuals	No

Additional Precautions

Preconceptional patients should be cautioned about some mundane, seemingly harmless activities.

Some *cats*, particularly outdoor cats, are carriers of a protozoan called Toxoplasma gondii. Congenital toxoplasmosis, though rare, is a potentially devastating infection that may result in intrauterine growth retardation, nonimmune hypdrops, hydrocephalus, and microcephaly. Manifestations of infection may not be apparent until well after birth. Vertical transmission to fetuses occurs in 60% of acutely infected pregnant women (15). Women can minimize their risk of acute infection in the periconceptional period by avoiding fecal matter of cats (including that in litter boxes) and by not consuming raw meat, both of which can house sporulated cysts that can be transmitted transplacentally. Many women may be serologically immune without previous known infection. This is best determined prior to pregnancy by measuring IgG and IgM titres, ideally in a reference laboratory.

Heat exposure in very early gestation has been linked to an increased risk of neural tube defects (16). Heat sources may be external, in the form of hot tubs or saunas, or internal, the result of high fevers or strenuous exercise. Patients should be alerted to these dangers. Most situations are easily avoided. In the event of high fevers, acetaminophen can be taken.

The effect of *caffeine* on a developing fetus is controversial. Studies have produced conflicting results. One prospective study demonstrated no increased risk of spontaneous abortions or intrauterine growth retardation with moderate caffeine consumption, defined as less than 300 mg/day (the equivalent of two to three cups of coffee) (17). Another study revealed an approximately twofold increase in risk of spontaneous abortion with moderate caffeine consumption in early pregnancy and heavy consumption in the preconceptional period. Patients can be apprised of the two schools of thought. Similarly, there is no clear evidence on the effects of *aspartame*. Long-term effects of this artificial sweetener are not known. Many patients attempting to become pregnant will wish to avoid these substances.

CONCLUSION

In the spirit of preventive health care and improved patient education, the importance and demand for preconceptional counseling has grown. The primary care provider can play a key role in determining the health of a mother and child even before a pregnancy begins. Preconceptional evaluation and counseling should become a standard component of the primary care of any woman of childbearing age.

REFERENCES

1. Hook EB. Rates of chromosome abnormalities at different maternal ages. Obstet Gynecol 1981;58: 282–285.

2. Wilcox AJ, Weinberg CR, O'Connor JF, et al. Incidence of early pregnancy loss. N Engl J Med 1988; 319:189.

3. Portnoi MF, Joye N, van den Akker J, et al. Karyotype of 1142 couples with recurrent abortion. Obstet Gynecol 1988;72:31–34.

4. Centers for Disease Control and Prevention. Recommendations for the use of folic acid to reduce the number of cases of spina bifida and other neural tube defects. MMWR 1992;41:1–7.

5. Sullivan JM, Ramanathan KB. Management of medical problems in pregnancy: severe cardiac disease. N Engl J Med 1985; 313:304.

6. Hanssens M, Keirse MJNC, Vankelecom F, et al. Fetal and neonatal effects of treatment with angiotensin-converting enzyme

inhibitors in pregnancy. Obstet Gynecol 1991;78:128–135.

7. Davis LE, Leveno KL, Cunningham FG. Hypothyroidism complicating pregnancy. Obstet Gynecol 1988; 72:108.

8. Davis LE, Lucas MJ, Hankins GDV, et al. Thyrotoxicosis complicating pregnancy. Am J Obstet Gynecol 1989;160:63.

9. Centers for Disease Control. Cigarette smoking among reproductive-aged women: behavioral risk factor surveillance system—1989. MMWR 1991;40:719–723.

10. Leuzz RA, Scoles KS. Preconception counseling for the primary care physician. Med Clin North Am 1996;80:337–374.

11. Barlow S, Sullivan FM. Reproductive hazards of industrial chemicals: an evaluation of animal and human data. New York: Academic Press, 1982.

12. Werler MM, Shapiro S, Mitchell AA. Periconceptional folic acid

exposure and risk of reccurrent neural tube defects. JAMA 1993;269:1257–1261.

13. MRC Vitamin Study Research Group. Prevention of neural tube defects: results of the Medical Research Council Vitamin Study. Lancet 1991;338:131–137.

14. American College of Obstetricians and Gynecologists. FDA orders food fortification with folic acid. ACOG Newsletter 1996;40:1–2.

15. Desmonts G, Couvreur J. Congenital toxoplasmosis: a prospective study of 378 pregnancies. N Engl J Med 1974;290:1110.

16. Milunsky A, Ulcickas M, Rothman KJ, et al. Maternal heat exposure and neural tube defects. JAMA 1992;268:882–885.

17. Mill JL, Homes LB, Aarons JH, et al. Moderate caffeine use and the risk of spontaneous abortion and intrauterine growth retardation. JAMA 1993;269:593–597.

Chapter 34

Nutrition in Pregnancy

Hope A. Ricciotti

There is nothing mysterious about getting the proper nutrition during pregnancy. A well-balanced diet containing a variety of foods will almost automatically have the proper mix of nutrients. Eating foods in their natural, unprocessed form will ensure their wholesomeness. This style of eating is good not only for pregnancy, but is a pattern that may be continued for a lifetime.

Pregnancy is an excellent "teaching time"—many women quit smoking, exercise more regularly, and begin eating well. These are habits that may be continued for a lifetime. Since women are often the ones who determine what the family eats and how they exercise, the whole family may benefit from their healthier lifestyles.

FOOD PYRAMID

Pregnant women should eat a well-balanced diet by selecting foods from the food pyramid. The food pyramid was created to replace the basic four food groups, and teaches about nutrient adequacy while guarding against nutrient excesses. Pregnant women should eat 6 to 11 servings from the bread, cereal, rice and pasta group; 3 to 5 servings from the vegetable group; 2 to 4 servings from the fruit group; 2 to 3 servings from the milk, yogurt, and cheese group; 2 to 3 servings from the meat, poultry fish, beans, eggs, and nuts group. Fats, oils, and sweets should be used sparingly. The pyramid illustrates the dietary guidelines both for pregnancy and general health: eat a variety of foods; choose a diet low in fat, saturated fat, and cholesterol; emphasize vegetables, fruits, and grain products; use sugar only in moderation (Fig. 34-1).

DIETARY REQUIREMENTS

The dietary requirements during pregnancy are very similar to what any healthy adult female should eat. At least half of the calories in the diet should come from carbohydrates, and 30% of calories should come from fat. Sixty grams of protein per day are needed. This means that meals should be based upon foods such as pasta, potatoes, grains, and fresh vegetables, with meat or other protein sources serving more as a garnish.

Carbohydrates

More than 50% of calories should come from carbohydrates, including such foods as pasta, potatoes, rice, bread, and bagels. No specific number of grams of carbohydrate are recommended because the amount of carbohydrate in the diet depends on caloric needs, which are highly variable. This often comes as a surprise to patients, many of whom believe they should be protein loading during pregnancy. But it is carbohydrates that should make up the majority of the diet, both in pregnancy and throughout life.

Protein

Only a moderate amount of protein, just 60 g per day, is required during pregnancy. This is an increase of 10 g over the nonpregnant state. This is not a large increase: 10 g of protein are found in 1 oz of chicken or 1/3 cup of yogurt. The average pregnant female in the United States eats much more protein than is needed—on average, from 75 to 110 g per day (1). Vegetarians will need more than 10 g of additional protein since extra protein is needed if it all comes

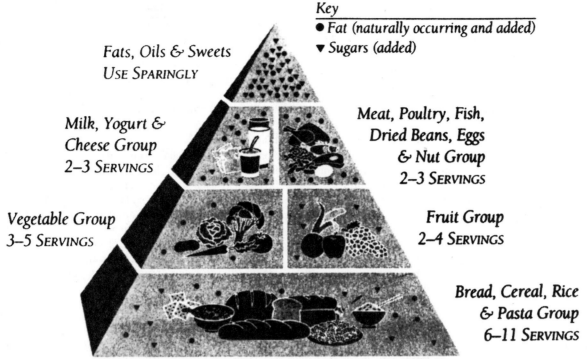

Figure 34-1 The food pyramid. (SOURCE: The Food Guide Pyramid. Washington DC: U.S. Department of Agriculture, Human Nutrition Information Service, 1992. Home and Garden Bulletin No. 252.)

from vegetable sources. Most vegetable proteins do not supply all eight essential amino acids, but different plant foods may be consumed in combination in order to become complete proteins. Combining vegetable proteins in this manner is biologically the same as eating protein from meat but requires that slightly more protein be consumed. A vegetarian diet is safe in pregnancy, as long as dairy products are included. A strict vegan diet is not recommended, since it tends to be deficient in vitamin B_{12} and zinc.

Fat

During pregnancy, 30% of calories should come from fat. The body stores fat in order to support the fetus as it grows and to enable women to breastfeed postpartum. In addition, a certain amount of fat is needed in the diet to help produce steroid hormones and utilize the fat-soluble vitamins A, D, E, and K. Thus, pregnancy is not a time when a diet very low in fat should be eaten. Eating enough fat, though, is generally not a problem for Americans, who often obtain more than 50% of their daily calories from fat.

The concentrations of cholesterol and lipoproteins found in the blood increase appreciably during pregnancy. These increases are thought to be from the stimulating effect of estrogen and progesterone on the liver, and synthesis of these substances is independent of diet. Thus, levels of cholesterol, HDL, and LDL are all elevated during pregnancy. Therefore, pregnancy is not a time to screen for lipid abnormalities. After delivery, however, the concentrations of these substances decrease to their prepregnancy levels, and there is no known association of these elevated levels during pregnancy with any disease states.

RECOMMENDED DIETARY ALLOWANCES

The Food and Nutrition Board of the National Academy of Sciences has published the Recommended Dietary Allowances (RDAs) periodically since 1943. RDAs are based on a combination of estimates and clinical research data. The values, which are neither means nor averages, are adjusted near the top of the normal range in order to encompass the needs of most people. Therefore, many individuals eat a diet that is nutritionally adequate for them but that may not meet the RDAs.

Dietary allowances for most substances increase during pregnancy. According to the 1989 recommendations (2), during gestation:

- the RDAs for iron, folic aid, and vitamin D double
- the RDAs for calcium and phorphorus increase by one half
- the RDAs for pyridoxine and thiamine increase by one third
- the RDAs for protein, zinc, and riboflavin increase by one fourth
- the RDAs for all nutrients except vitamin A increase by less than one fifth
- there is no increase in the RDA for vitamin A since it is adequately stored in the body

Many nutrients are required in larger amounts during pregnancy, with the major ones being iron, folic acid, and calcium. All can be found in a well-balanced diet, with the exception of iron. For this reason, a prenatal vitamin or iron supplement may be prescribed.

Iron

The iron requirements of pregnancy are about 1000 mg/day. This includes 500 mg used to increase the maternal red blood cell mass, 300 mg transported to the fetus, and 200 mg to compensate for normal daily iron losses by the mother (mainly by cells sloughed into the bowel).

During pregnancy the blood volume increases by 50%. The plasma increase is more than the red blood cell increase, creating a "physiologic anemia." This increase prepares women for the 500 cc average blood loss that occurs during vaginal deliveries, and the 1000 cc average blood loss during cesarean sections. The iron requirements of pregnancy are not constant, but increase remarkably during the third trimester. The fetus receives almost all the iron transported to it during the last 12 weeks of pregnancy.

The National Academy of Sciences currently recommends that 30 mg of ferrous-iron supplements be prescribed for pregnant women daily because the iron content of the typical American diet and the iron stores of many women are not sufficient to provide the iron required during pregnancy. In the past it was controversial as to whether non-anemic pregnant women should receive routine iron supplementation. Most American obstetricians favored the practice, while those in Britain and Europe generally considered it unnecessary. Studies of iron stores (serum ferritin levels) have shown that the average pregnant women who does not take supplements, although not anemic, is significantly iron deficient at term (3).

The purpose of iron supplementation during pregnancy is not to raise or even to maintain the maternal hemoglobin concentration, and it is not to prevent iron deficiency in the fetus. Rather, the purpose of maternal supplementation is to prevent iron deficiency in the mother. Iron is actively transported to the fetus by the placenta against a high concentration gradient, and fetal hemoglobin levels do not correlate with maternal levels (4). Maternal iron deficiency does not appear to lead to reduced fetal iron stores.

It has been estimated that women who are iron sufficient at the beginning of pregnancy and who do not take iron supplements during pregnancy need about 2 years after delivery to replenish their iron stores from dietary sources. Because many women have a shorter interval than this between pregnancies and because many do not have an ideal diet, iron supplementation is recommended on a routine basis. To ingest more iron from dietary sources alone would simultaneously provide an undesirable excess of calories. Because calcium, magnesium, and other minerals can inhibit absorption (such as when taken with antacids or in multivitamins), it is most effective to prescribe simple iron supplements alone. Iron needs are slight during the first 4 months of pregnancy, and therefore it is not always necessary to provide supplemental iron during this time. Withholding iron supplementation during the first trimester of pregnancy avoids the risk of aggravating nausea and vomiting, which is very common in early pregnancy.

The necessary 30 mg of iron can be found in dosage forms of 150 mg of ferrous sulfate, 300 mg of ferrous gluonate, or 100 mg of ferrous fumarate. Some preparations come combined with a stool softener to counteract the constipating effect that iron (and pregnancy) has on the digestive system.

Iron-rich foods (Table 34-1) include beef, chicken, collard greens, kale, spinach, Swiss chard, turkey, and wheat germ. The body's absorption of iron from the diet and from supplements may be enhanced by combining iron-containing foods or supplements with foods containing vitamin C. Conversely, caffeine and phytic acid (found in tea) inhibit the absorption of iron in the body. Cooking meals in cast-iron cookware will provide additional iron.

Folic Acid

Preconceptionally, folic acid deficiency has been linked with neural tube defects. In the United States, approximately 4000 pregnancies each year are affected by the two most common neural tube defects: spina bifida and anencephaly. An estimated 2500 infants per year are born with neural tube defects. At least half of these neural tube defects could be prevented if all women capable of becoming pregnant consumed 0.4 mg of folic acid daily during the periconceptional period (28 days before through 28 days after the last menstrual period) (5).

Neural tube closure is complete by 4 weeks after conception, which is 6 weeks after the last menstrual period. Most women do not know they are pregnant prior to missing their period, which is 2 to 3 weeks after conception. Thus preventing neural tube defects with folic acid requires advance planning. It is important to remind women of childbearing age to take folic acid when trying to conceive.

Presently the U.S. Public Health service recommends that 0.4 mg of folic acid be given to women daily when trying to conceive. Prenatal vitamins contain at least 0.4 mg of folic acid, as do many multivitamins. However, some multivitamins contain only 0.3 mg of folic acid, so it is important for patients to check the label. In addition, folic acid supplements alone may be taken, many of which are in 0.8-mg formulations, which are safe and have few side effects.

Folic acid in this amount can easily be obtained in the diet, although this has not been studied in the prevention of neural tube defects in controlled trials. Good dietary sources of folic acid are dark green leafy vegetables, legumes, nuts, and fruits (Table 34-2). Note that more folic acid is destroyed by microwave cooking than by any other cooking method. Also, this vitamin is lost whenever high temperatures or large amounts of water are used in cooking.

Table 34-1 Sources of Iron

Apricots	Kidney beans
Beef	Navy beans
Black beans	Pinto beans
Blackstrap molasses	Prunes
Broccoli	Pumpkinseeds
Chicken	Shrimp
Chickpeas	Spinach
Clams	Swiss chard
Collard greens	Tofu
Egg yolks	Tuna
Enriched breads and cereals	Turkey
Kale	Wheat germ

Calcium

The fetus requires approximately 30 g of elemental calcium be deposited in its skeleton by the time of full-term delivery (6). The fetus is efficient at obtaining this calcium. If maternal nutritional intake is not adequate, fetal mineralization may occur at the expense of the maternal skeleton. This may increase the risk for osteoporosis later in life, although there is insufficient evidence at this point to determine this with certainty.

Approximately 75% of women between the ages of 18 and 30 do not receive the RDA for calcium in their diet. The current RDA for calcium for adult women is 800 mg of elemental calcium per day, 1200 mg in pregnancy, and 1600 mg in lactation. Pregnancy is characterized by increased absorption efficiency of calcium. The absorption of calcium by the intestine is influenced by various factors. Calcium intake, vitamin D, parathyroid hormone, calcitonin, and estrogen all contribute to the efficiency with which calcium is absorbed from the gastrointestinal tract. It is also important to keep in mind that competitive inhibition of absorption of calcium can occur between certain nutrients. Many pregnant women are not only adjusting their diet but also are taking prenatal vitamins and iron supplements, all of which may result in competitive inhibition of absorption of calcium.

Bones are in a very active phase of growth from birth until approximately 20 years, and although growth may stop at age 20, bone density may increase until age 35. Therefore, it is important to maintain calcium intake during pregnancy, because most pregnant women are of the age at which their own skeleton depends upon adequate nutrition for proper growth and development.

Calcium probably has an important role in hypertensive cardiovascular disorders in pregnant and nonpregnant women. In clinical intervention trials involving young nonpregnant healthy women and women with mild hypertension, calcium supplementation was associated with an overall reduction in blood pressure (7).

Several studies have also examined the effects of calcium supplementation on blood pressure during pregnancy and its effect on the development of preeclampsia. There has been near unanimity in the observed phenomenon that calcium supplementation of approximately 2 g of elemental calcium (5 g of calcium carbonate) per day results in an overall lowering of blood pressure and an overall reduction in the incidence of hypertensive disorders of pregnancy (8). A multicenter trial under the auspices of the National Institute of Health is being conducted at this time to test this hypothesis. It is currently not recommended to supplement calcium routinely in pregnancy. However, patients should be encouraged to ensure adequate calcium intake in their diet. Dairy products are a rich source of calcium, as are dark green leafy vegetables such as kale, collards, broccoli, and bok choy. Also available are calcium-fortified fruit juices, which contain an amount of calcium equivalent to that in milk (Table 34-3). It is difficult to meet calcium requirements without consuming dairy products. Individuals who do not consume milk or milk products may require calcium supplementation. Some substances can hinder the absorption of calcium, including oxalic acid (found in spinach and Swiss chard) and phytic acid (found in tea and in the outer layers of whole grains). Both of these form insoluble compounds with calcium, binding it in such a way that it cannot be absorbed from the intestine.

Vitamins

There is no need to take any vitamin supplement other than folic acid in the preconceptional period and iron during the remainder of pregnancy. The Subcommittee on Dietary Intake and Nutrient Supplements during Pregnancy of the National Academy of Sciences maintains that healthy American women should be encouraged to get the vitamins they need from their diet rather than from supplements. The subcommittee points out that there is a much greater risk of overdose from supplements than from foods (9). For example, exposure to levels of 5000 IU of vitamin A has been associated with birth defects. Beta carotene and other carotenoids are plant-synthesized precursors of vitamin A that are partially converted to vitamin A in the body, but are not associated with teratogenesis.

Retinoids affect the development of neural-crest cells and may interfere with the closure of the neural tube. A specific group of malformations, the "retinoic acid embryopathy," has been described, with abnormalities of craniofacial, cardiac, thymic, and central nervous system structures. Recent data has indicated a teratogenic effect of vitamin A at levels not far above those currently recommended (10). Preformed vitamin A (but not carotenoids), in excess of 10,000 IU, was associated with defects of cranial neural-crest tissue, compared to the babies whose mothers consumed 5000 IU or less per day. It is therefore recommended to limit preformed vitamin A in supplements to 5000 IU or less.

Although in the United States prenatal vitamins are routinely given, they generally are needed only by high-risk

Table 34-2 Sources of Folic Acid	
Asparagus	Lean beef
Broccoli	Legumes
Chicken	Nuts
Collard greens	Potatoes
Corn	Spinach
Egg yolks	Squash
Fish	Swiss chard
Fruits	Tomatoes
Kale	Turnip greens

Table 34-3 Sources of Calcium	
Blackstrap molasses	Kale
Bok choy	Legumes
Broccoli	Milk or skim milk
Buttermilk	Mangoes
Cheese	Sesame seeds
Collard greens	Tofu
Fortified juices	Turnip greens
Frozen yogurt	Whole grains
Ice cream	Yogurt

groups such as adolescents and smokers, who frequently have inadequate diets. This is important information with which one can reassure nauseated women in early pregnancy. Many women in the first trimester are too nauseated to tolerate prenatal vitamins, but feel that they may be harming their babies by not taking them. They can be counseled to take folic acid alone until 6 weeks after the last menstrual period, and then can resume prenatal vitamins or iron when they are feeling better.

Salt

More sodium is needed during pregnancy than at any other time of life, but virtually all women meet this need with their normal intake of salt. There is a net accumulation of about 1000 mEq of sodium during pregnancy (11). In the past, pregnant women were told to restrict salt to prevent edema and preeclampsia, but this has not been found to be helpful. Dependent edema in the lower extremities is caused by venous compression by the weight of the uterus and is a normal part of pregnancy, particularly in the third trimester. Restricting sodium or fluid intake will not decrease edema or affect the development of preeclampsia. Taking diuretics is not advised and may be dangerous. There is, therefore, no need to restrict salt or fluid intake during pregnancy. Healthy pregnant women may salt food to taste.

WEIGHT GAIN

Many women think of pregnancy as a time when they can eat as much as they wish and anything they want without worrying about weight gain or fat content. Nothing could be further from the truth. In fact, the calories that pregnant women generally require is only 15% more than the needs of nonpregnant women. This translates to 300 to 500 calories per day, depending on the mother's weight and activity.

The total weight gain recommended during pregnancy is 25 to 35 lb for women of normal weight. Underweight women may gain up to 40 lb, and overweight women can safely limit weight gain to 15 lb (Table 34-4). During pregnancy, "eating to appetite" results in an average weight gain of 28 lb (12).

There is a positive correlation between weight gain in pregnancy and birthweight of the newborn. Independent of weight gain during pregnancy, there is also a positive relationship between prepregnancy weight and birthweight (13). Women who begin pregnancy underweight or gain less than the recommended amount are more likely to have a small-for-gestational-age infant. Women who begin pregnancy overweight or gain more than the recommended weight are more likely to have a large-for-gestational-age infant. However, fetal weight is not related to maternal weight gain among women who are obese (>135% ideal body weight) (14,15). Finally, woman who gain above the recommended amounts have an increased risk for cesarean section, even when factored independently of birthweight (16).

During the first trimester, the required weight gain is small (3 to 6 lb). During the second and third trimester, 6 to 12 lb should be gained each trimester (1/2 to 1 lb per week). These gains are only rough guides; many women's weight

gain patterns deviate considerably from these. It is best to focus on the overall pattern of gain rather than the week-to-week or even the monthly weight gain.

It is important to emphasize to women who may have difficulties with such rapid changes in their bodies that very little of this weight gain is fat. About 2 to 3 lb are from increased fluid retention, 3 to 4 lb are from increased blood volume, 1 to 2 lb from breast enlargment, 2 to 3 lb from enlargment of the uterus, and 2 to 3 lb from amniotic fluid. At term, the baby may weigh approximately 6 to 8 lb and the placenta 1 to 2 lb. A 4 to 6 lb increase in maternal stores of fat are important to protect the fetus against nutritional deprivation in the third trimester and support lactation after birth (Table 34-5).

Postpartum Weight Retention

An almost universal anxiety among new mothers is whether they will lose the weight they gained during pregnancy. The strongest factor contributing to postpartum weight retention is excessive prenatal weight gain. Data from the 1988 National Maternal and Infant Health Survey showed that women who gain more than the Institute of Medicine weight guidelines gained a median of 5.6 lb postpartum, compared to 2.2 lb for those who gained within the recommended weight range (17).

Loss of excess weight from pregnancy is unlikely to occur after the first year postpartum, so an increase of even a few pounds is likely to be permanent for many women, and perhaps compounded with each subsequent pregnancy. Long-term obesity can pose serious health threats to women. Heart disease, diabetes, hypertension, some forms of cancer, and overall mortality all have been linked to higher body weights in women (18). Obesity has been increasing in the US population in the past few decades, and currently 27% of white

Table 34-4 Recommended Total Weight Gain During Pregnancy	
For normal-weight women	25–35 pounds
For underweight women	40 pounds
For overweight women	15 pounds

Table 34-5 Components of Weight Gain in Term Pregnancy	
Fluid retention	2–3 lb
Increased blood volume	3–4 lb
Breast enlargement	1–2 lb
Uterus enlargement	2–3 lb
Amniotic fluid	2–3 lb
Baby	6–8 lb
Placenta	1–2 lb
Fat stores	4–6 lb

women and 44% of black women between 20 and 74 years of age are overweight (19).

Assisting all new mothers to return to an appropriate weight postpartum is an important component of perinatal care and can have long-term effects.

OTHER NUTRITION-RELATED ISSUES

Nausea and Vomiting

Nausea and vomiting, or "morning sickness," is present in up to 70% of all pregnancies. Although distressing, morning sickness rarely poses health problems for the mother. In a few individuals, it can cause serious dehydration and electrolyte imbalances, a condition known as hyperemesis gravidarum. In severe cases, hyperemesis may require intravenous fluid and electrolyte restoration. In most women, the nausea and vomiting ceases by the end of the first trimester, and in almost all women by around week 16. There are, however, a few women who have persistent nausea and vomiting until delivery.

The cause of this most troublesome problem has remained elusive. Relaxation of the smooth muscle of the gastrointestinal tract because of high levels of the hormone progesterone likely plays a role. There is some evidence that elevated levels of human chorionic gonadotropin (HCG) may be involved. However, the correlation between high levels of this hormone and the degree of nausea and vomiting is not linear, so some other factor must be involved. There may also be an anxiety or psychological component (20).

Treatment for the nausea and vomiting of pregnancy involves changing the diet to one that is better tolerated. Taking many small meals helps some women since, paradoxically, it seems to relieve the nausea to have the stomach partially filled. Carbohydrates, such as potatoes, bread, rice, crackers, and pasta, served as bland as possible with a minimum of fat and protein, seem to be best tolerated. Patients who are very nauseated in the first trimester should be reassured that eating a well-balanced diet at this point in pregnancy is not critical, and should simply focus on eating and drinking to maintain some caloric intake and hydration. Later in pregnancy, during the second and third trimester, complete nutrition becomes more important. Avoiding prenatal vitamins in the first trimester, other than folic acid until 6 weeks past the last menstrual period, will minimize nausea.

Women may be reassured that the obstetric outcomes of babies of mothers with even severe hyperemesis are no different than babies of mothers without this problem (21).

Heartburn

Heartburn in pregnancy is caused by relaxation of the lower esophageal sphincter. The prevalence of heartburn increases with advancing gestational age: 22% of women in the first trimester, 39% in the second, and 72% in the third trimester experience heartburn. The growing uterus pushes up on the stomach, compounding the problem as pregnancy progresses (22).

Dietary changes may diminish heartburn. Eating many small meals instead of three large ones will help stop food and stomach acid from refluxing into the esophagus. Pillows at bedtime may help. If necessary, antacids may be prescribed.

Constipation

Due to a combination of factors, constipation is a very common problem in pregnancy. Progesterone is a smooth muscle relaxant, which slows the motility of the gastrointestinal tract. Iron supplements can compound constipation. Finally, the uterus mechanically obstructs the colon as it grows larger in the second and third trimester. Patients should be advised to maintain adequate fluid intake, increase the fiber content of the diet, and maintain exercise. When necessary, mild laxatives, such as prune juice, milk of magnesia, bulk-producing substances, or stool-softening agents, may be used.

Toxoplasmosis

Toxoplasma gondii is a protozoan parasite that can infect any warm-blooded animal. When pregnant women are infected with *T. gondii*, the developing fetus may be harmed. Maternal immunity appears to protect against intrauterine parasite transmission. Therefore, for congenital toxoplasmosis to develop, the mother must have acquired the infection during pregnancy. About one-third of North American women acquire protective antibody before pregnancy, and this is higher in those keeping cats as pets. Maternal infection is often subclinical. Common symptoms include fatigue, muscle pains, and lymphadenopathy. The virulence of fetal infection is greater the earlier that infection is acquired. Fetal infection is characterized by low birthweight, hepatosplenomegaly, icterus, anemia, intracranial calcifications, hydrocephaly, microcephaly, and chorioretinitis (23).

The organism is found in cat litter, raw or undercooked meat, and the soil. Pregnant women should be advised not to change cat litter, cook meat well (170° F, which is medium-well to well-done), and to wear gloves when gardening.

Caffeine

Caffeine in large amounts (more than 300 mg per day) has been associated with increased risk for spontaneous abortion and intrauterine growth retardation (24,25). There are approximately 100 mg of caffeine in a cup of coffee, 50 mg in tea, 30 mg soda, and 30 mg in a chocolate bar. Caffeine intake does not increase the risk of premature delivery (26,27) or cause congenital anomalies (28,29).

It is therefore prudent to advise pregnant women to limit their caffeine intake to one cup of coffee or tea daily.

Aspartame

The low-calorie sweetening agent aspartame (Nutrasweet) appears to be safe in pregnancy. Aspartame is broken down in the small intestine into three moieties: aspartic acid, methanol, and phenylalanine. Aspartame, even in abuse doses, does not raise phenylalanine levels in the fetus near the range generally accepted to be associated with mental retardation in the offspring of phenylketonuric heterozygotes. No evidence of risk to the fetus has been demonstrated even with intake of huge amounts of this substance (30,31).

Alcohol

Wine or other alcohol is safe to use in cooking during pregnancy as long as it is simmered for at least five minutes. The cooking process will evaporate the alcohol, leaving the flavor behind.

However, consumption of alcohol in other forms during pregnancy is not advised. Alcohol is a known teratogen, and is responsible for fetal alcohol sydrome. This disorder is characterized by mental retardation, facial anomalies, low birthweight, and behavioral problems, including attention deficit disorder and hyperactivity. Heavy drinking is a major risk to the health of the fetus, and reduction in alcohol intake, even in midpregnancy, can be of benefit. An occasional drink during pregnancy carries no known risk, but no level of drinking is known to be safe (32).

REFERENCES

1,2. Subcommittee on the Tenth Edition of the RDAs, Food and Nutrition Board, Commission of Life Sciences, and National Research Council. Recommended Dietary Allowances, 10th ed. Washington, DC: National Academy Press, 1989.

3. Taylor DJ, Mallen C, McDougall N, et al. Effect of iron supplementation on serum ferritin levels during and after pregnancy. Br J Obstet Gynecol 1982;89:1011–1017.

4. McFee JG. Iron metabolism and iron deficiency during pregnancy. Clin Obstet Gynecol 1979;22:799–808.

5. Werler MM, Shaprio S, Mitchell AA. Periconceptional folic acid exposure and risk of occurrent neural tube defects. JAMA 1993;269:1257–1261.

6. Pitkin RM. Calcium metabolism in pregnancy: a review. Am J Obstet Gynecol 1975;121:724–737.

7. Belizan JM, Villar J, Pineda O, et al. Reduction of blood pressure with calcium supplementation in young adults. JAMA 1983;249:1161–1165.

8. Belizan JM, Villar J, Gonzalez L, et al. Calcium supplementation to prevent hypertensive disorders of pregnancy. N Engl J Med 1991;325:1399–1405.

9. Subcommittee on Nutritional Status and Weight Gain during Pregnancy. Nutrition during Pregnancy. Washington DC: National Academy Press, 1990.

10. Rothman KJ, Moore LL, Singer MR, et al. Teratogenicity of high vitamin A intake. N Engl J Med 1995;333:1369–1373.

11. Fuchs AR, Fuchs F. Physiology and endocrinology of parturition. In: Gabbe SG, Niebyl JR, Simpson JL, eds. Obstetrics: normal and problem pregnancies. 2nd ed. New York: Churchill Livingstone, 1991:132.

12. Hytten FE. Weight gain in pregnancy. In: Hytten FE, Chamberlain F, eds. Clinical physiology in obstetrics. London: Blackwell, 1980.

13. Eastman NJ, Jackson E. Weight relationships in pregnancy: the bearing of maternal weight gain and pre-pregnancy weight on birth weight in full term pregnancies. Obstet Gynecol Surv 1968;23:1003–1025.

14. Abrams B, Laros RK. Prepregnancy weight, weight gain and birth weight. Am J Obstet Gynecol 1986;154:504–509.

15. Parker JD, Abrams B. Prenatal weight gain advice: an examination of the recent prenatal weight gain recommendations of the Institute of Medicine. Obstet Gynecol 1992;79:664.

16. Johnson J, Longmate J, Frentzen B. Excessive maternal weight and pregnancy outcome. Am J Obstet Gynecol 1992;167:353–370.

17. Keppel K, Taffel S. Pregnancy-related weight gain and retention: implications of the 1990 Institute of Medicine Guidelines. Am J Public Health 1993;83:1100–1103.

18. Abrams B, Berman C. Women, nutrition, and health. Curr Prob Obstet Gynecol Fertil 1993;16:30–35.

19. Nutrition monitoring in the United States. 1998. National Center for Health Statistics, Hyattsville, MD: DHHS publication no. (PHS) 99–1255.

20. Depue RH, Bernstein L, Ross RK, et al. Hyperemesis gravidarum in relation to estradiol levels, pregnancy outcome, and other maternal factors: a seroepidemiologic study. Am J Obstet Gynecol 1987;156:1137–1141.

21. Tierson FD, Olsen CL, Hook EB. Nausea and vomiting of pregnancy and association with pregnancy outcome. Am J Obstet Gynecol 1986;155:1017–1022.

22. Marrero JM, Goggin PM, de Caestecker JS, et al. Determinants of pregnancy heartburn. Br J Obstet Gynecol 1992;99:731–734.

23. Cunningham FG, MacDonald PC, Gant NF, et al, eds. Williams Obstetrics. 19th ed. Norwalk CT: Appleton & Lange, 1993.

24. Mills JL, Holmes LB, Aarons JH, et al. Moderate caffeine use and the risk of spontaneous abortion and intrauterine growth retardation. JAMA 1993;269:593–597.

25. Infante-Rivard C, Fernandez A, Gauthier R, et al. Fetal loss associated with caffeine intake before and during pregnancy. JAMA 1993;270:2940–2943.

26. Cook DG, Peacock JL, Feyerabend C, et al. Relation of caffeine intake and blood caffeine concentrations during pregnancy to fetal growth: prospective population based study. BMJ 1996;313:1358–1362.

27. Peacock JL, Bland JM, Anderson HR. Preterm delivery: effects of socioeconomic factors, psychological stress, smoking, alcohol, and caffeine. BMJ 1995;311:531–535.

28. Hinds TS, West WL, Knight EM, et al. The effect of caffeine on pregnancy outcome variables. Nutr Rev 1996;54:203–207.

29. Kurppa K, Holmberg PC, Kuosma E, et al. Coffee consumption during pregnancy and selected congenital malformations: a nationwide case-control study. Am J Public Health 1983;73:1397–1399.

30. Sturtevant FM. Use of aspartame in pregnancy. Int J Fertil 1985;30:85–87.

31. Position of the American Dietetic Association: use of nutritive and nonnutritive sweeteners. J Am Diet Assoc 1993;93:816–821.

32. Bratton RL. Fetal alcohol syndrome: how you can help prevent it. Postgrad Med 1995;98:197–200.

Chapter 35

Exercise and Pregnancy

Susan Hellerstein

A large percentage of women of reproductive age in the United States exercise regularly. With a heightened concern about taking care of oneself during pregnancy, many of these women or those who have previously been sedentary will approach their care providers about beginning or continuing physical fitness programs during pregnancy. Pregnancy can also be viewed as a time when women may be able to establish healthy habits that will endure beyond the pregnancy period. Given the physiologic changes that occur in pregnancy and the stress of acute aerobic exercise, the practitioner must consider what type and level of exercise to recommend to the woman with a normal or a medically complicated pregnancy. This chapter will review the unique physiologic changes occurring in pregnancy that influence exercise tolerance, and review exercise recommendations for pregnancy.

Observations about pregnancy outcomes and physical activity have been published since ancient times. There are biblical references to the easier labor and delivery experience of Hebrew slaves when compared to the more sedentary Egyptian women. Aristotle attributed difficult childbirth to inactive lifestyles of pregnant women (1).

Over time and throughout most of the twentieth century, the common sense concept of exercise in "moderation" had been accepted based on moral and social outlooks rather than on scientific knowledge. A series of manuals for expectant women published in the 1940s through 1960s encouraged exercise through housework and daily walks while discouraging sports and heavy lifting (1). In response to the fitness craze of the 1970s and 1980s, the American College of Obstetrics and Gynecology (ACOG) published a technical bulletin in 1985 that endorsed the safety of and recom-

mended most low-impact aerobic exercise to be performed at maximum maternal heart rate of 140 beats per minute for 15 minutes duration (2). In 1994, ACOG published a less conservative recommendation based on a more recent review of the literature on exercise and pregnancy (3). The bulletin stated that women with normal pregnancies can do most aerobic exercise with no heart rate or time restrictions without compromising fetal growth and development or causing complications of pregnancy, labor, and delivery.

Research on exercise and pregnancy outcomes has been subject to many methodologic challenges. Many of the studies have small sample sizes that limit the power to detect effects. These studies often have conflicting results. Due to the varying definitions of physical activity and outcomes, generalization of results and meta-analysis is difficult. Nonetheless, the practitioner is expected to compile the best available data and make recommendations. The types of studies that can be reviewed include animal models, physiologic studies of response to acute aerobic exercise in pregnancy, and studies of pregnancy outcomes.

PHYSIOLOGY OF EXERCISE IN PREGNANCY

Cardiorespiratory Changes

Hemodynamic changes in pregnancy include an increase in blood volume, heart rate, and cardiac output and a decrease in systemic vascular resistance (4). The supine position can obstruct the inferior vena cava and decrease venous return, thus decreasing cardiac output. Some women are very sensitive to this decrease in cardiac output and will experience supine hypotension.

In pregnancy, an increase in tidal volume and an unchanged respiratory rate result in increased minute ventilation by approximately 50% (5). This results in an increase in arterial oxygen tension. In addition, pregnant women have an increased oxygen uptake and increased baseline oxygen consumption due to an increase in the number of red blood cells, an increase in tissue mass, and an increase in metabolic rate. Maternal-fetal oxygen consumption at rest near the end of pregnancy is 16% to 30% above nonpregnant levels.

Invasive and noninvasive studies of non–weight-bearing submaximal exercise in pregnancy generally show an increase in maternal cardiac output (6). Resting maternal heart rate is elevated up to 15 beats per minute. Studies of maximal exercise and cardiac output during weight-bearing exercise are limited. There may be a reduction of maximal maternal heart rate response to aerobic exercise near the end of pregnancy. However, there is some controversy in the exercise research community on pregnancy's effect on maximal exercise heart rate. Maximal heart rate is higher with weight-bearing exercise than non–weight-bearing exercise. For most women, exercise tests show that maximal exercise performance is decreased, although there may be no change in maximal aerobic capacity in the elite athlete.

There is concern that for some women there is a decrease in tissue oxygen availability during aerobic exercise because of the increase in resting oxygen requirements and the increased work of breathing in pregnancy. However, compared to nonpregnant women, pregnant women have a greater hemoconcentration during exercise due to increased plasma filtration out from the capillary bed and an increased release of red blood cells from the spleen with the increase in catecholamines associated with exercise. These combine to increase the oxygen-carrying capacity of blood with exercise in pregnancy (5).

Uterine Blood Flow

Uterine blood flow during exercise has been assessed by using animal models, noninvasive Doppler studies of uterine and umbilical perfusion, and studies of fetal heart rate responses to exercise. The concern that exercise may result in fetal hypoxia or compromised fetal growth stems from the physiologic hemodyamic respiratory maternal response. During short-term exercise, cardiac output is shifted away from the splanchnic organs to exercising muscles. Splanchnic blood flow may decrease by 50% (7). Animal and human studies have shown a decrease in uterine blood flow during exercise. However, mechanisms that maintain a stable fetal oxygen consumption include an increase in maternal hematocrit with exercise, which increases the oxygen-carrying capacity of blood; an increase in oxygen extraction as blood flow decreases; and blood flow redistribution that favors the placenta over the myometrium (8).

A review of noninvasive Doppler studies of exercise and uteroplacental circulation in humans show conflicting results (4). Some studies show an increase in the vascular resistance of the uterine artery during exercise while others do not. The majority of studies show no change or a decrease in the umbilical artery resistance during and after exercise, and thus no significant change in fetal hemodynamic response to maternal exercise.

Studies of fetal heart rate changes during exercise have shown an increase of 5 to 15 beats per minute in the baseline fetal heart rate (3). There is debate in the literature as to whether reported episodes of fetal bradycardia were truly observed or secondary to motion artifacts. One study (9) showed the incidence of fetal bradycardia during exercise was 1% with submaximal exercise and 10% with maximal exercise. There were no cases of adverse neonatal outcome secondary to fetal heart rate changes associated with exercise. Other studies have documented no increase in fetal heart rate abnormalities, meconium in labor, or low Apgar scores in well-conditioned women who continue to perform aerobic exercise (10).

Hyperthermia

Most of the energy expended in exercise is converted into heat. In nonpregnant women, aerobic exercise increases core body temperature. In pregnancy, base metabolic rate is increased. Most of the heat produced by exercise is dissipated with increased blood flow to the skin, but some may result in an increase in body temperature. Maternal temperature is the primary determinant of fetal temperature, which generally runs 0.5°C higher than maternal temperature.

Animal studies have demonstrated that hyperthermia has a teratogenic effect, resulting in limb and central nervous system defects (5). In a review of hyperthermia in human pregnancy, neural tube defects have been reported in association with hyperthermia in the first trimester. Some studies of hot tub use have suggested a possible first-trimester threshold for teratogenesis of 39.2°C (3).

There have not been direct studies of fetal temperature during human exercise. However, studies of core (vaginal or rectal) temperature in aerobically conditioned pregnant women during exercise show an actual decrease in temperature by 0.3°C in the first trimester and a further decrease with advancing gestation (11). In contrast, maternal skin temperature increases with exercise. There has been no increase in observed rates of neural tube defects or other birth defects in pregnant women who exercise in early pregnancy. This suggests that the observed maternal physiologic adaptation of thermoregulation in pregnancy is protective against hyperthermic teratogenesis.

Metabolic Changes

To meet the metabolic needs of pregnancy an average woman needs to increase her caloric intake by approximately 300 kcal/day. Fasting glucose levels in pregnancy are lower than in the nonpregnant state. When a pregnant woman exercises she uses carbohydrates at a greater rate than when not pregnant. Some studies have shown that exercise has a hypoglycemic effect for the mother (8). The fetus relies on a continuous supply of glucose for fat and protein synthesis. Further studies need to be done to clarify if this metabolic challenge has a detrimental effect on pregnancy outcome.

Musculoskeletal System

The incidence of musculoskeletal injury in pregnancy is not well documented. Theoretically, there is an increased risk of injury due to a shift in the center of gravity, which results in changes in balance. An increase in the hormone relaxin may increase the laxity of the pelvis and other ligaments and joints. Combined with an increase in body weight, this puts stress on weight-bearing joints. The effect of exercise on musculoskeletal injuries in pregnancy needs further study.

EXERCISE AND PREGNANCY OUTCOMES

Thus far we have reviewed the maternal physiologic response to exercise. How do these observed physiologic changes translate into differences in pregnancy outcome? There have been many studies of physical activity associated with work and pregnancy outcomes that may be applicable to recreational activity, but one must acknowledge the potential confounders in applying these results to outcomes associated with aerobic exercise. A review of exercise and its relation to preterm labor, birthweight, length of labor, operative delivery rates, management of gestational diabetes, and maternal well-being follows.

Prematurity and Birthweight

A large number of studies have been published looking at exercise in pregnancy and infant birthweight and gestational age at delivery. With exercise, both epinephrine and norepinephrine levels increase. While epinephrine inhibits uterine contractions, norepinephrine can increase the frequency and strength of uterine contractions (3). A number of studies have shown a significant increase in uterine activity during exercise, with up to a fivefold increase in contraction frequency, but with rapid recovery after exercise (12). However, a transient increase in contraction frequency does not mean an increase in preterm labor or delivery rates.

There are some major limitations in many of the studies of preterm delivery and exercise, including small sample size, varying definitions of physical activity, and retrospective design. Larger prospective randomized studies are needed to definitively sort out this issue.

A meta-analysis of 18 published studies (13) shows no difference in preterm delivery rate and birthweights between exercising and sedentary pregnant women. In another recent review of eight studies of gestational length and exercise done since 1990 (14), only one study showed a significant increase in preterm labor rate. This was in US Army workers whose jobs involved lifting greater that 50 pounds during 80% of work hours, and was not a study of recreational exercise. Two studies (15,16) showed a significant reduction in birthweight with high-intensity exercise or heavy work in the standing position. The average weight difference was 300 to 350 g. There was no difference in head circumferences or crown rump length, with the weight difference due to a decrease in subcutaneous fat (16). No increase in intrauterine growth retardation or in short- or long-term sequelae were observed in the offspring of pregnant women who exercised.

Labor and Delivery

The effects of aerobic exercise on the outcome of labor have been examined. A number of recent studies (17–19) have demonstrated a significantly shortened second stage of labor in women who exercise regularly. Clapp also showed a lower incidence of operative delivery rates (6% versus 20%) and cesarean section rates (6% versus 30%) in women who exer-

cised regularly compared to sedentary women (17). Other studies have not confirmed these findings (9). Randomized prospective studies could better sort out this result and eliminate the selection bias that may account for the differences in labor outcomes.

Maternal Well-Being

With regular exercise in pregnancy women can maintain or improve their aerobic capacity. Some studies show that women who exercise regularly have a decrease in a number of common symptoms, such as fatigue, nausea, leg cramps, and back pain. A trimester-specific study of the temporal relationship between exercise and perceived symptoms showed women were feeling better because they were exercising, not the opposite (8). Other studies show evidence of improved self-esteem, body image, and sleep associated with exercise.

EXERCISE RECOMMENDATIONS
High-Risk Pregnancy

The effect of exercise on the outcomes of many high-risk pregnancies have not been well studied. Exercise is contraindicated for women with hypertension, multiple gestations, premature rupture of membranes, incompetent cervix, persistent second-or third-trimester bleeding, and risk for preterm delivery and intrauterine growth retardation.

Diabetes Mellitus

In contrast, there are an increasing number of studies on exercise and diabetes mellitus in pregnancy. Extensive research on nonpregnant subjects shows that muscle contraction stimulates glucose transport in insulin-sensitive cells (20). Many other factors such as hormones and catecholamines can influence this transport, but these have not been specifically studied in pregnancy. There are limited studies on gestational diabetes mellitus (GDM) and exercise. Due to the increased risk of hypoglycemia in women who have GDM and require insulin, it is prudent to advise these women to exercise only in a medically-supervised environment. Two studies of exercise (21,22) using leisurely walking versus sedentary lifestyles in insulin-dependent pregnant diabetic women showed a modest but insignificant improvement in glucose control with no change in neonatal outcomes. These studies were unable to monitor patient compliance with the exercise program, and perhaps the lack of motivation and compliance with exercise recommendations explains the weak associations found.

In three studies of non–insulin-dependent gestational diabetes and non–weight-bearing exercise (20,23), including one prospective randomized study, there was normalization of blood glucose levels as measured by hemoglobin A_{1C} fasting glucose levels or repeat glucose challenge testing. There was no increase in complication rates, poor neonatal outcomes, uterine activity, or fetal heart rate abnormalities in the women who exercised. Non–weight-bearing exercise was chosen because it seems to favor carbohydrate as a fuel source (24). Exercise for the woman with gestational diabetes may offer a chance to avoid insulin therapy.

The studied exercise protocols for women with non–insulin-dependent gestational diabetes demonstrated the safety of home exercise doing 20 to 30 minutes of exercise at 50% of maximal oxygen consumption (which is perceived as fairly light to moderate) daily after each meal or a hospital-based exercise program with 45 minutes of exercise performed three times a week (20). This was in addition to usual careful fetal-maternal monitoring of women with gestation diabetes mellitus.

Low-Risk Pregnancies

In recommending exercise programs for low-risk pregnant women it is essential to individualize the prescription based on a woman's motivation, previous level of exercise, and an overall health assessment. For healthy women who previously performed regular weight-bearing exercise prior to pregnancy, it is realistic for them to expect a decline in exercise performance of approximately 50% by the third trimester (25,26). A combination of aerobic capacity, fatigue, and morphologic changes account for this decline. Women who wish to begin exercising or to change the type of exercising are better able to maintain high-intensity exercise throughout pregnancy if they choose non–weight-bearing exercise regimens (25,26).

The 1994 ACOG recommendations, which are well founded in the current literature, suggest that there is no reason that low-risk pregnant women need to limit exercise intensity or duration. A summary of the recommendations during pregnancy and postpartum is as follows (3):

1. Maintain regular (3 or more times a week) mild to moderate exercise routines.

2. Avoid the supine position after the first trimester.

3. Modify the intensity of aerobic exercise according to maternal symptoms, stopping when fatigued and before exhaustion.

4. Non–weight-bearing exercises (cycling or swimming) minimize the risk of injury and facilitate continuation during pregnancy, but weight-bearing exercise may be continued.

5. Avoid exercise requiring balance, especially during the third trimester.

6. Maintain adequate caloric intake.

7. Augment heat dissipation in the first trimester with adequate hydration, appropriate clothing, and an optimal environment.

The use of target heart rates to determine optimal exercise intensity is limited in pregnancy. The goals of exercise in pregnancy should include increasing muscular strength, endurance, improving posture and the sense of well-being as well as establishing exercise habits that may endure beyond pregnancy.

REFERENCES

1. Artal R, Wiswell R. Exercise in pregnancy. Baltimore: Williams and Wilkins, 1986.

2. American College of Obstetricians and Gynecologists. Exercise and pregnancy. Washington, DC: ACOG, 1985. ACOG technical bulletin 87.

3. American College of Obstetricians and Gynecologists. Exercise during pregnancy and the postpartum period. Washington, DC: ACOG, 1994. ACOG technical bulletin 189.

4. Veille JC. Maternal and fetal cardiovascular response to exercise during pregnancy. Semin Perinatol 1996;20:250–262.

5. Schick-Boscheto B, Rose N. Exercise in pregnancy. Obstet Gynecol Surv 1991;47:10–13.

6. Wiswell R. Applications of methods and techniques in the study of aerobic fitness during pregnancy. Semin Perinatol 1996;20:213–221.

7. Rowell LB. Human cardiovascular adjustments to exercise and thermal stress. Physiol Rev 1974; 154:75–159.

8. Sternfeld B. Physical activity and pregnancy outcome. Sports Med 1997;23:33–47.

9. Carpenter MW, Sady SP, Hoegsberg B, et al. Fetal heart rate response to maternal exertion. JAMA 1988;259:3006–3009.

10. Clapp J. Exercise in pregnancy: a brief clinical review. Fetal Med Rev 1990;89–101.

11. Clapp JF. The changing thermal response to endurance exercise during pregnancy. Am J Obstet Gynecol 1991;165:1684–1689.

12. Spinnewyn W, Lotgerny F, Strviyk P, Wallenburg H. Fetal heart rate and uterine contractibility during maternal exercise at term. Am J Obstet Gynecol 1996;174:43–48.

13. Lokey EA, Tran ZV, Wells CL, et al. Effects of physical exercise on pregnancy outcomes: a metaanalytical review. Med Sci Sports Exerc 1991;23:1234–1239.

14. Dye T, Oldenaettel D. Physical activity and the risk of preterm labor: an epidemiological review and synthesis of recent literature. Semin Perinatol 1996;20:334–339.

15. Naeye RL, Peters LL. Working during pregnancy: effects on the fetus. Pediatrics 1982;69:724–727.

16. Clapp J, Capeless E. Neonatal morphometrics after endurance exercise during pregnancy. Am J Obstet Gynecol 1990;163:1805–1811.

17. Clapp J. The course of labor after endurance exercise during pregnancy. Am J Obstet Gynecol 1990; 163:1799–1804.

18. Botkin C, Driscoll CE. Maternal aerobic exercise: newborn effect. Fam Pract Res J 1991;11:387–393.

19. Beckman RRB, Beckman CA. Effect of a structured antepartum exercise program on pregnancy and labor outcome primiparas. J Reprod Med 1990;35:704–709.

20. Bung P, Artal R. Gestational diabetes and exercise: a survey.

Semin Perinatol 1996;20:328–333.

21. Hollingsworth DP, Moore TR. Postprandial walking exercise in pregnant insulin dependent diabetic women. Am J Obstet Gynecol 1987;157:1359–1363.

22. Javanovic-Peterson L, Durak EP, Peterson CN. Randomized trial of diet versus diet plus cardiovascular conditioning on glucose levels in gestational diabetics. Am J Obstet Gynecol 1989;161:415–419.

23. Artal R, Masaki D, Khodiguian N, et al. Exercise prescription in pregnancy, weight-bearing versus non–weight-bearing exercise. Am J Obstet Gynecol 1989;161: 1464–1469.

24. Collings CA, Curet LB, Mullin JP. Maternal and fetal responses to maternal exercise program. Am J Obstet Gynecol 1983;145:702–707.

25. Sibley L, Ruhling RO, Caneran-Forth J, et al. Swimming and physical fitness during pregnancy. J Nurse Midwifery 1981;26:3–12.

26. Clapp J. The effect of continuing regular endurance exercise on the physiological adaptations to pregnancy and pregnancy outcome. Am J Sports Med 1996;24:528–529.

Chapter 36

Breastfeeding

Lisa Litchfield McSherry

The impact of the practitioner's counseling upon the pregnant woman's choice of infant feeding method cannot be underestimated. Despite the uniform support of the pediatric world for human milk as the best feeding choice for a newborn, in the United States the majority of women still choose to formula feed. The breastfeeding initiation rate in 1993 was 55.9%. At 6 months, only 19% of these mothers continued to breastfeed their babies (1).

The history of breastfeeding practices show that almost all infants were breastfed either by their mother or by a wet nurse prior to the 1930s. Artificial feeding had a high mortality rate at that point in time. With the development of pasteurized cow's milk in the 1850s, consideration began for the use of cow's milk for infant feeding. However, pasteurized cow's milk spoiled easily because of unavailability of refrigeration. The development of condensed milk that could be canned and transported without spoiling marked the beginning of the lucrative business of selling cow's milk for infant feeding. Initially, this milk was used in addition to breast milk to boost weight gain in infants. Milk laboratories designed for preparing milk exclusively for infants were developed. Unfortunately, many of the ingredients were chosen because of their low cost rather than their nutritional value. Today, formula is the most common infant feeding "choice" of mothers. Formula sales have tripled in the past 10 years, with these companies generating $22 million in revenues daily (2).

Examining one's personal feelings concerning infant feeding methods is important before counseling patients whether to breastfeed. Much of our initial reaction to the breastfeeding dyad of infant and mother is derived from our own heritage, past experiences, and body image. These issues, combined with cultural differences, greatly affect the information that is relayed to our patients. Clinicians continually admit that they have withheld important facts on infant feeding to avoid eliciting feelings of guilt from the pregnant mother-to-be (3).

Breastfeeding remains the first choice of feeding of the American Academy of Pediatrics (AAP) for newborn infants. The AAP recommends exclusive breastfeeding for infants for the first 4 to 6 months and continued breastfeeding for the first year of life (4). The goals for our nation, by the year 2000, are to "increase to at least 75% the proportion of mothers who exclusively or partially breastfeed their babies in the early postpartum period and to at least 50% the proportion who continue breastfeeding until their babies are 5 to 6 months old (5,6).

HEALTH BENEFITS

In third world countries the benefits of human breastmilk are clear: infants who are not breastfed are five times more likely to die of diarrheal illnesses (7). The benefits of human breastmilk in the United States were, until recently, considered to be questionable because of the advanced quality of drinking water and infant formulas. Equivocal beneficial results of research on breastfed infants are now being questioned. We are now discovering that there are greater benefits for newborns who are largely breastfed. Much of the older research on the benefits of breastfeeding described a breastfeeding infant as one who was receiving as little as one to two feedings of breastmilk per day. Stricter criteria in defining a breastfeeding infant has shed new light on the benefits.

Secretory IgA immunoglobulins from human breastmilk

line the mucous membranes of the gastrointestinal tract of the breastfed infant. Secretory IgA is not produced by the infant until 4 months of age, and is not fully produced until 12 months (8). Lactobacillus bifus and lysozyme, enzymes that are found in the intestine of breastfed infants but not in formula-fed infants, discourage the overgrowth of bacteria. Lactoferrin, a protein with strong bacteriostatic properties, is increased in the intestine of the breastfed infant. It binds with iron and competes with other bacteria, such as staphylococci and E. coli, which need iron for growth, keeping them in check (9). Through these exclusive properties, breastfed infants are protected from diarrheal illnesses caused by many viruses and bacteria. There is strong evidence that breastfeeding protects against other infectious diseases, including respiratory syncytial virus, otitis media, and bacteria and meningitis caused by *Haemophilus influenzae* (10).

Variations in the definition of breastfeeding have accounted for many discrepancies in the data on the benefits of breastfeeding. The greatest benefits are derived from exclusive breastfeeding. Newer studies show that exclusive breastfeeding for 4 months can greatly reduce the frequency of gastrointestinal, respiratory tract, and skin infections. One study showed that exclusively breastfed infants at 4 months of age had a lower incidence of gastrointestinal and respiratory illnesses and a higher score on the Denver developmental screening test (11). Even infants who have breastfed and have had an occasional bottle of infant formula (<120 ml/day) were shown to have a much lower incidence of diarrhea and otitis media compared to formula-fed infants (12).

Recent research has shown that the long term benefits of breastfeeding are even more extensive than previously thought. Long term follow-up studies have shown some association between formula feeding and immune system disorders, increased incidence of diabetes mellitis, some lymphomas, and food allergic diseases. As adults, formula-fed infants have an increased risk of Crohn's disease and ulcerative colitis. Formula feeding accelerates the development of celiac disease. Bottle feeding with infant formula appears to be a risk factor for sudden infant death syndrome (SIDS). Possible explanations for the lower association of breastfeeding with SIDS include the facts that breastfeeding infants have shorter periods of sleep, they frequently sleep with their mothers, and they obtain increased immunity from the human milk (13).

ANATOMY AND PHYSIOLOGY

From the embryonic state of the fetus to the adult mother, the human breast develops and prepares itself for breastfeeding. During puberty, estrogens help to form ducts within the breast, a process which continues until age 35. During pregnancy, lobular development begins and 15 to 25 milk ducts develop, ending at the nipple (14). Lobular and alveolar development begin during a woman's first pregnancy (15). Each lobule has several structures connected to one other. At the posterior section of the mammary gland are the alveoli, which comprise the glandular tissue of the breast responsible for milk production. Each individual alveolus is surrounded by myoepithelial cells that contract and push milk into adjoining ductules (16). The small ductules converge into one of the 15

to 25 lactiferous sinuses. These sinuses end as an opening at the tip of the nipple.

The areola around the nipple is the most sensitive part of the breast. It is the stimulation of the areola that starts the sequence of events that are responsible for the milk ejection reflex. The nipple itself is the least sensitive part of the breast.

High levels of progesterone during pregnancy inhibit lactation. When the placenta is expelled during delivery, the drop in progesterone and estrogen triggers the anterior pituitary to release prolactin (17). When the areola is stimulated during suckling, the hypothalamus inhibits the release of dopamine and in turn stimulates the release of prolactin. Prolactin, which is responsible for milk production, increases with pregnancy, peaks at full-term gestation, and increases and decreases with each nursing session.

Nipple/alveola stimulation triggers the posterior pituitary to release oxytocin, which in turn contracts the myoepithelial cells. These contractions push milk through the ductules and sinuses, and the process is commonly referred to as "let down" (18). It is milk removal that dictates milk volume. This intricate system of supply and demand is important to remember when assisting women in the management of breastfeeding.

MANAGEMENT OF LACTATION

Breastfed infants feed more frequently than formula-fed infants. Breastmilk is completely compatible with the human infant's gastrointestinal system and is readily digested. This, combined with the small size of the infant's stomach, results in frequent feeding. In contrast, formula curds in the infant's stomach and tends to delay feedings. It is normal for the breastfed infant to feed 8 to 12 times in a 24-hour period, averaging every 2 to 3 hours (19). This is compared to feedings every 3 to 4 hours in the formula-fed newborn. Breastfed infants are also prone to periods of cluster feeding, where they feed every hour to every hour and a half, most commonly in the evening.

The breastfed infant feeds more frequently than a formula-fed baby during the night. These nighttime feedings are normal and should be encouraged. Practitioners should be alerted if the mother reports long periods of sleep by the infant initially after discharge, as these infants may not be getting adequate nutrition. The old myth of not waking a sleeping baby should not necessarily be followed during the first few weeks of life of the breastfed infant. This is particularly important for lower-weight babies whose serum blood sugar tends to drop, causing them to become more passive when frequent feeding is not maintained (20). Mothers should generally be counseled to avoid letting a breastfed baby sleep more than 4 hours until the infant's weight has been checked in the first 1 to 2 weeks of life, confirming that the infant has gained adequate weight.

Infant feeding times vary greatly from 10 to 45 minutes per feed, with an average of 20 to 30 minutes per feed (21). A typical feeding should start on one breast and continue until the infant shows a loss of interest, either by falling asleep, releasing the nipple, or slowing down of suckling. The initial feeding on the first breast will take from several minutes to half an hour. After the feeding on the first breast, the baby may need to be awakened by such stimulation as undressing the baby, changing the diaper, or repeatedly bringing the baby from a lying position to a sitting position. It is typical for the baby to take the second breast for only a short time (22). Failure of the practitioner to instruct the mother on the frequency and duration of nursing sessions can result in early weaning of the mother-infant dyad. The management of feeding schedules of breastfeeding infants often is a confusing area for both practitioners and family members alike.

The infant should be encouraged to nurse on one breast for a longer period of time than on the other, so that the infant receives an adequate ratio of foremilk to hindmilk. Foremilk is the breastmilk that is expressed during the beginning of the feeding and is high in water content. Hindmilk is higher in cream content and lower in volume, and is largely responsible for good weight gain (23). After a feeding from both breasts, the mother should initiate the next feeding on the breast on which she ended (24).

It is prudent to counsel mothers on strategies to manage their sleeping time, rather than helping the mother to find ways to get her baby to sleep longer periods. Caution should be heeded in advising mothers who complain about lack of sleep and fatigue postpartum regarding supplemental formula. Supplemental formula interferes with the supply-demand component of breastfeeding. The absence of breast stimulation created by the use of supplemental formula feedings will cause a decreased milk supply by eliminating the cue to produce milk. It may be more helpful for the breastfeeding mother to receive advice on ways to increase her sleep while continuing with frequent feedings. It may be helpful for the mother to keep her baby close to her during night feedings or to keep surrounding areas quiet and to try falling asleep during feedings using prone positions (25). A severely fatigued mother may be advised to pump some breastmilk during the day, before noon, and to save it for her support person for a night feeding, allowing the mother a longer stretch of sleep during one portion of the night. This should not be advised until the milk supply is well established, usually 3 to 4 weeks postpartum. Care must be taken for the mother to keep a consistent schedule of pumpings and dropped feedings to avoid overfilling the breasts, which can result in a blocked duct or mastitis (26).

The mother should be instructed on proper positioning and latch-on during the first few days postpartum. It is important for the mother to receive consistent information from physicians, nurses, and family members. The mother should be advised to rotate positions initially to minimize nipple soreness. Once any soreness has passed, the mother may nurse in a position that is the most comfortable for both her and her baby. Three commonly used positions are usually taught to the breastfeeding mother: the cradle position, the football hold (clutch position), and the side lying position (Figure 36-1). The mother is encouraged to use ample pillows in order to support the infant at breast level and to keep the infant turned towards the mother, belly to belly. This positioning keeps the infant latched on properly and helps the mother to avoid neck, shoulder, and back strains (27).

Proper latch-on is achieved by rubbing the infants lips with the mothers nipple and waiting to elicit the infant's rooting reflex. The mother holds her breast with her hand, with her thumb on the top of the breast and her fingers placed under her breast. With this hand positioning, her hand is forming the letter "C" (Figure 36-2). The mother supports the infant's head with her hand or forearm. When the infant opens its mouth widely, the mother quickly moves the infant's head to her breast, allowing the infant to latch on.

When proper latch-on is achieved, the infant's nose, cheeks, and chin should be close to the mother's breast and sometimes touching the breast (Figure 36-2). The mother can use her thumb or forefinger to gently depress the breast to keep the infant's nose from being blocked (28). The presence of cheek dimpling is a sign of improper latch-on. During the assessment of the infant-mother dyad during a feeding, audible swallowing should occur. It is important for the mother to learn proper positioning and latch-on during the first few days postpartum, so that she might avoid some of the common problems associated with breastfeeding her infant.

Sore Nipples

Sore nipples during the first few days of breastfeeding is a common problem for the breastfeeding mother. Many mothers are taught (incorrectly) that nipple soreness is abnormal. However, mild soreness that peaks on days 3 to 6 postpartum and gradually disappears can be normal (29). Skin breakdown, as manifested by cracks, blistered and bruised nipples and areola, is caused by a variety of factors including incorrect positioning and poor latch-on. Therefore, it is important to assess these factors in the infant-mother dyad. It is also important to rule out candidiasis of the nipple and infant thrush as an etiology for sore nipples.

Occasionally sore nipples are caused by ankyloglossia ("tongue tie") of the infant. In this situation, the tongue cannot cover the lower gum line because of a tight frenulum (30). Evidence of ankyloglossia may be observed as a heart-shaped tongue when the infant is crying. Some pediatricians may clip the frenulum once the diagnosis is made.

Encouragement to continue nursing is critical during this period of nipple soreness. This time period is often a difficult one: fatigue, episiotomy pain, cesarean section pain, as well as a major role change for the mother may all be aggravating factors during this stressful time. Reminding new mothers that the soreness is temporary can help. Suggesting that the mother keep a daily pain log can also be helpful. In this way, the patient is taught to score the pain from 1 to 10 during latch-on followed by a secondary assessment at 5 minutes into the nursing session. This daily reminder, through documentation, of diminishing nipple soreness is especially effective even for those mothers with more prolonged periods of soreness, sometimes lasting 6 to 8 weeks.

Treatment of nipple soreness should include a variety of measures. Instructing the mother to air dry her nipples after each nursing session can facilitate the timely healing of damaged nipples. She should express a few drops of colostrum or breast milk from her nipple and spread it around her nipple and areola. The fat content of the breastmilk can help to keep the skin lubricated (31). The mother should be instructed to wear only cotton nursing bras and nursing pads. The new mother must also be sure to avoid washing the breasts with soap. Soap removes many of the skin's natural lubricating oils. Washing with warm water is adequate.

New research shows that the use of a modified lanolin creme applied to the cracked, blistered and/or broken down

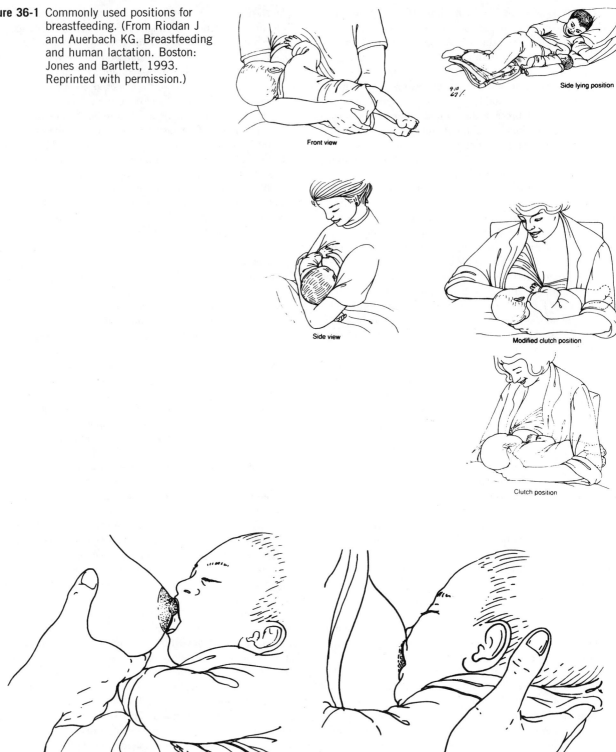

Figure 36-1 Commonly used positions for breastfeeding. (From Riodan J and Auerbach KG. Breastfeeding and human lactation. Boston: Jones and Bartlett, 1993. Reprinted with permission.)

Front view

Side lying position

Side view

Modified clutch position

Clutch position

Latch—on

Figure 36-2 Latch-on process. Left, mother holds breast with baby's mouth gaped open. Right, baby grasping breast in proper latch-on. (From Riodan J and Auerbach KG. Breastfeeding and human lactation. Boston: Jones and Bartlett, 1993. Reprinted with permission.)

nipples can speed up the rate of the healing process. Modified lanolin limits the pesticide residue to 3 parts per million and limits the free lanolin alcohols to 6%, therefore allowing the preparation to be safely used on the nipple without harm to the infant and without wiping the nipple before each nursing session (32).

Occasionally, especially after the use of antibiotics prescribed for the mother or baby, the dyad can develop a candida infection. This presents as a nipple infection in the mother and a thrush infection in the infant's mouth. The mother presents with a new onset of red, burning, and sometimes scaling nipples. The infant presents with white, cheesy patches in the inside of the cheek, tongue, and lips. Both mother and infant need to be treated even if the infection only appears to be active in one of them. The mother's skin may be treated with nystatin or clotrimazole cream for 14 days. The mother should consult her pediatrician for treatment of the infant.

It is helpful to teach new mothers with nipple soreness the techniques of heat application to the breast, breast massage, and manual breastmilk expression. These techniques can usually elicit the let-down response and start a significant amount of dripping breast milk. These steps performed before the infant latches on can help in preventing trauma to the nipple when the infant initially suckles (33). Prenatal nipple preparation and the use of nipple shields are outdated practices that have not been shown to prevent or relieve nipple soreness.

Engorgement

Engorgement is the common phrase for the period of time from 2 to 4 days postpartum when a woman's milk comes in. Until this time, the baby is receiving small amounts of colostrum. Under normal conditions, this period of milk buildup is technically characterized as breast fullness. With breast fullness, the breast is indentable, and the infant can still latch on to the areola. There is some generalized swelling and usually the mother is afebrile (34).

Breast engorgement is characterized by a vascular appearance, with the breast no longer indentable. The breasts are very tender and the mother may develop a low-grade fever (35). Breast engorgement is usually the result of poor breastfeeding management. Without frequent and adequate suckling the breast tissue becomes congested with the accumulation of milk, making it difficult or impossible for the infant to latch on to the breast. Difficult or poor latch-on compounds the situation.

Treatment of engorgement is focused upon decreasing milk stasis in the breast. This is achieved by applying heat, either in the shower or by the direct application of warm compresses to the breasts. Gentle massage can be initiated after heat application to move milk forward. Finally, to remove milk around the areola and soften the breast, the mother may use manual breast expression or an intermittent low-suction breast pump just prior to nursing, so that the infant can resume suckling. Frequent feedings (more than 8 times in 24 hours) should be initiated for approximately 15 minutes per feed, to control breast fullness and in turn prevent engorgement. In some circumstances the mother can be instructed to take acetaminophen, ibuprofen, or a codeine preparation for comfort (36).

Poor Latch-On

One of the greatest challenges in breastfeeding support is the infant who refuses to latch on to the breast. There are many causes, both maternal and infant related. The origin of the problem can be difficult to assess and treatment should include a collaboration between the lactation consultant and the infant's pediatrician. Infant-originated difficulties can result from the use of bottles or pacifiers, a disorganized or ineffective suck, and prematurity and/or low birthweight. Maternal causes may include flat or inverted nipples, improper positioning at the breast, or breast engorgement.

Treatment of the infant who has not learned to latch on effectively to the breast includes step-by-step retraining, and providing the infant with positive reinforcement for proper latch-on. During this process the mother is instructed to continue to put the infant to the breast at least eight times per day. The mother should use heat, massage, and manual expression to elicit dripping milk before the nursing session in order to allow the infant to taste and receive mouthfuls of milk with each proper latch-on. After an unsuccessful nursing session, the mother is instructed to pump her breasts with a hospital grade breast pump and to feed her baby the pumped milk using an alternative feeding method such as syringe, finger, or cup feeding, to avoid nipple confusion from standard bottles (37). It is very important that all pumped milk be fed to the infant to prevent dehydration. It is helpful for the mother to spend time between feedings with the infant on her chest in order to create a positive, calm association with the smell of human milk, and the warmth of her skin. In the case of ineffective sucking or disorganized suckling that does not resolve, the mother should be referred to her pediatrician and a lactation consultant.

In the past, mothers with flat or inverted nipples were encouraged to wear breast shells during the third trimester to help pull the nipple out. The usefulness of breast shells for this purpose is controversial, with newer data not supporting their effectiveness. A better method is the use of the electric breast pump before each feeding, to help pull the nipple out to make it easier to grasp by the infant. During a period of poor latch-on, it is helpful to instruct the mother to compress the breast behind the areola so that the infant is able to quickly latch on. Usually a day or two of this consistent positioning and offering of the breast will retrain a healthy full-term infant with a good suck back to the breast (38). In the event of breast engorgement the treatment is focused on softening the breast to make the nipple easier to grasp. (See the earlier section on engorgement.)

Poor Weight Gain

The two most common reasons given by mothers for abandoning breastfeeding include poor weight gain of the infant and concerns about a low milk supply. Low weight gain caused by low milk supply is actually a diagnosis that is very uncommon. In the first few days postpartum, adequate milk supply may be monitored by the number of urine and stools produced by the infant, as well as overall satiation. Further evidence of a sufficient supply is the observation of breast fullness before feeding and breast softening after feedings.

During the first 3 to 4 days postpartum, the mother produces colostrum at an average volume of 37 mL per day

(39). This high-protein, lower-fat milk, rich in immunoglobulins, is enough nutrition to result in one or two wet diapers and usually one stool per day. When the milk comes in, approximately 3 to 4 days after delivery, the urinary output will increase to four to five wet diapers a day, and one to several stools per day (40). The day after the milk comes in, the urinary output will increase to five to six wet diapers per day, and one to several stools per day (41). At this stage, the infant usually seems satisfied with feedings, and will initiate cluster feedings during a particular time of the day. In the presence of adequate urine and stools, care must be taken not to confuse cluster feeding with low milk supply. In the absence of adequate urine and stools, practitioners should assess the hydration of the infant by both mucous membrane and skin assessment. Because of the low volume of milk produced in the first 3 to 4 days postpartum, babies will usually lose weight, up to 10% of their birthweight. After this time, babies should gain between one half to one ounce per day, and should be back to their birthweight by 2 to 3 weeks after birth (42).

Many pediatricians evaluate babies at 2 weeks postpartum, and if the birthweight has not been regained by this time, will begin to observe babies closely to ensure adequate weight gain. Practitioners may help nursing mothers to ensure adequate weight gain by beginning with a review of the frequency and duration of feedings. In addition, observing a nursing session will allow assurance of proper latch-on and milk swallowing by the baby. Once let down has occurred the suck/swallow ratio is usually one to one, and there should be no dimpling of the infants cheeks (43). Finally, mothers can be assessed for adequate breast glandular tissue by a series of carefully presented questions requarding breast changes during pregnancy. Woman who have not noted breast enlargement during pregnancy can be at risk for low milk supply (44). Problems in these areas, with the accompaniment of low weight gain, may originate from a low milk supply. In addition, consideration should always be given for an organic cause in the newborn with poor weight gain (45).

When babies are found to have poor weight gain, it is advisable for the mother and infant to meet with a lactation consultant to review feeding patterns and techniques in order to increase her milk supply. Emphasis should be given to the frequency of feedings rather that the duration of the infant on the breast. Nursing on both breasts at each feeding should be encouraged to ensure a better milk supply (46). The frequent stimulation of the breast by nursing triggers the let down response, which allows for the removal of a greater volume of milk and in turn cues the body to increase milk production. Occasionally, a consultant will suggest a mother pump her breasts after a predetermined number of feedings, and supplement the infant with this high-fat hindmilk. In addition, practitioners should stress that mothers need to eat and drink well and to sleep as much as possible (47). In very difficult situations, supplemental nursing systems or hormonal stimulation with metoclopramide may be utilized under the supervision of a skilled lactation consultant and pediatrician (48).

Mastitis

Mastitis is a localized breast infection that may develop any time during lactation. It is usually caused by staphylococci, *E.*

coli, and occasionally streptococci. Symptoms may include a reddened, warm area of the breast, temperature of 101°F or greater, general malaise, and muscle aches. Symptoms will often arise suddenly. Woman at risk for infection include those who have a broken area of skin on the nipple area, those who have not properly emptied their breast or have missed a feeding, and those who have a constriction of the breast from clothing or a bra, resulting in a blocked duct. Fatigue can contribute to susceptibility to this infection (49). Mastitis most commonly occurs in the first weeks postpartum, although approximately one-third of cases occur after this period (50).

Treatment for the mother with mastitis includes oral antibiotic therapy (usually dicloxacillin), continuation of frequent breastfeeding, heat and massage before nursing sessions of the affected area, rest, and increased oral fluids (51). For mothers who are experiencing chronic mastitis, low-dose erythromycin can be given for the duration of lactation (52). Culturing the mother's breast milk can often be helpful in identifying the organism.

A blocked duct is often misdiagnosed as mastitis. A blocked duct is characterized by a temperature of less than 101°F, no flu-like symptoms, and a gradual appearance of a mildly painful lump on one area of the breast with little or no warmth. The treatment is the same, but without the administration of antibiotics. It can sometimes be helpful to vary the nursing positions in order to help release the blockage in the duct (53).

NUTRITION AND WEIGHT LOSS DURING LACTATION

The healthy lactating mother will nourish her infant well by selecting foods from the food pyramid: breads and cereals, fruits, vegetables, milk and milk products, and meats and proteins (54). Mothers should be more concerned about consuming enough calories rather than consuming a perfect diet. When eating a well-balanced diet, it is not necessary to take additional vitamins while breastfeeding. It is important to encourage calcium intake in the diet, as the RDA for calcium during lactation is 1500 mg daily. Although certain foods will flavor the breastmilk, mothers can eat whatever foods they wish without worrying that it will negatively affect their breastmilk (55).

When babies are colicky and fully breastfed, there is some research that suggests that the mother's dairy product consumption may be the cause. The mother should eliminate all dairy products from her diet for 1 week. If the baby is then comfortable after feeding, the baby may be sensitive to bovine milk protein. The mother may then add dairy back into the diet slowly, thereby discovering how much or which dairy products are offensive (56).

When mothers are interested in losing weight, they should avoid crash dieting. Eating a balanced diet often will be sufficient for weight loss. Breastfeeding burns approximately 500 calories daily. Lactation mothers can lose up to 2 lb per week without affecting their milk composition. Breastfeeding mothers tend to lose weight during the first 6 months of lactation (57).

Vegetarian breastfeeding women need to pay attention to selecting foods from complementary plant groups in order to receive complete amino acid composition. Vegetarians who consume no dairy products can be deficient in zinc and B$_{12}$ (58).

DRUGS AND LACTATION

When considering the risks and benefits of administering drugs to the breastfeeding mother, the practitioner must review the drug's properties and how the medication will affect the infant through the mother's milk supply. The infant's age should be a consideration when evaluating its ability to metabolize a particular drug. The length of time a drug is administered is also a factor. If the drug has some potential side effects on the infant, but the treatment is short, the mother may be instructed to pump and discard her milk during the time she is taking the drug until it clears her system. If the medication is short acting, the drug may be given after the mother nurses her baby. The route of administration also affects systemic absorption and length of time in the mother's bloodstream (59).

The Committee on Drugs of the American Academy of Pediatrics publishes a list of drugs that are transferred into the mother's breast milk. They give recommendations for drugs that are contraindicated during lactation, drugs that require interruption of breastfeeding, and drugs that are safe to use during lactation. The publication by Briggs et al (59a) is a reliable source when evaluating the safety of medication used by a nursing mother.

PUMPING AND STORAGE

Many women will desire to offer their baby a bottle at some point before their child takes liquids from a cup. The practitioner should encourage the mother to pump breastmilk for use at another time, especially when the mother is exclusively breastfeeding. Because of the risk of nipple confusion, feedings by bottle should not take place before 4 to 6 weeks, until breastfeeding has been well established (60). Waiting this time period allows the mother's milk supply to be tailored for her child's needs. Breastfed babies tend to favor orthodontic-shaped nipples. At 4 to 6 weeks of age, most babies will still accept bottles. Waiting longer than this time period may result in an infant's refusal to bottlefeed. Mothers need to continue offering occasional bottles as little as two to three times per week or as much as once a day so that the infant can remember how to latch on to the bottle tip in order to continue accepting bottlefed milk.

Pumping for this "practice bottle" is best done between feedings in the morning when the mother's milk is most abundant. Keeping in mind the theory of supply and demand, a mother who pumps at the same time every day will begin to produce more milk at this particular time, allowing her body to think that her child was requiring more milk at this time of the day.

There are many different commercial breast pumps available to breastfeeding mothers. When advising a mother which pump to purchase or rent it is important to know for what purpose the mother will be pumping. For occasional use for short and infrequent outings, manual expression, manual pump or battery-operated hand-held pumps work just fine.

These pumps vary in efficiency according to the mother's ability to elicit the let-down reflex. These pumps usually require some breast preparation such as breast massage and relaxation in order to remove a fair amount of milk. Some of these pumps can be time consuming because they only pump one breast at a time.

Mothers returning to employment either part time or full time will require an electric piston-driven hospital-grade pump. These pumps are not only very efficient, but they cycle quickly (an average of 40 times per minute), which closely simulates the suckling rhythm of the infant (about 50 times per minute). The combination of quick cycling and a strong but gentle vacuum quickly elicits the let-down reflex and removes a good amount of milk. These pumps allow mothers the best chance of keeping up their milk supply when away from their babies for prolonged periods of time. Many of these pumps come with a double-breasted pumping option, which allows for a better milk supply by increasing prolactin levels. Most mothers find double pumping desirable since it cuts the pumping time in half.

Auerbach describes three phases of breastfeeding for working mothers. Phase 1, within the first 4 months postpartum, requires the mother to stimulate her breasts with nursing or pump frequently at regular intervals to maintain her milk supply. In Phase 2, when the infant is 4 to 9 months old, mothers can usually reduce pumping to once during her workday and still have an adequate supply when she is home with her baby. Phase 3, when the infant is 9 months or older, is a time period when the mother may not need to pump at all at work and still enjoy a good breastfeeding relationship (61).

The storage guidelines for freshly expressed breast milk are as follows: 6 to 10 hours at room temperature; 72 hours in the refrigerator; and 6 months in a home freezer. The storage guidelines for thawed breast milk are as follows: it should not be stored at room temperature; 24 hours in the refrigerator; and it should not be refrozen (62). Breast milk, because of bacteriostatic properties, lasts longer at room temperature than ever before thought possible (63).

BREAST SURGERY

Most breast reduction surgery involves some sort of "keyhole" technique. This removes a wedge of breast tissue under the breast and preserves the nipple by raising it, while keeping it attached by a flap of tissue. In many instances nerves are severed. Only about 50% of woman who have had breast reduction surgery are able to breastfeed (64). For women attempting to breastfeed after breast reduction surgery, care must be taken to carefully monitor the infant's hydration and weight gain by a lactation consultant and the infant's pediatrician.

For the woman who has undergone breast augmentation, the success of breastfeeding is dependent on where the implant was inserted. If there was an incision near or around the areola, this may interfere with breastfeeding (65). If the incision was made under the axilla, there should be no interference with breastfeeding (66). Another type surgery used to reduce breast sagging, mastopexy, removes excess skin and lifts the breast up. This usually does not interfere with breastfeeding (67).

WEANING

At various points during lactation a mother may decide to wean her baby from breastmilk to either artificial milk (formula) or cow's milk. The American Academy of Pediatrics recommends that babies receive either formula or breastmilk for the first year of life. The reasons mothers may desire to wean vary: returning to employment and not wanting to pump, no longer desiring to breastfeed, or pressure from family, friends, or society to wean a child that might be nursing "too long." Mothers wishing to wean should be informed of their options. For example, mothers who wish to wean because they cannot pump breastmilk at work should still be offered the possibility of breastfeeding in the morning and evening. Keeping in mind the theory of supply and demand when counseling patients, mothers must be reminded that they will likely not have an adequate supply to nurse during the day, even on days when she is home with her baby.

Occasionally a mother needs to wean quickly because of a medical problem or because of an unanticipated separation from her baby. She should try to allow at least 2 to 3 days for her body to adjust to each dropped feeding (68). If time allows, this can be accomplished with her baby, or if time is of the essence, it can be accomplished with an electric breast pump.

Especially after the introduction of solid food, mothers who choose to practice baby-led weaning will notice a decrease in feeding during the course of the first year. After the first year, babies vary in the frequency of breastfeeding. Some babies choose to comfort nurse upon waking, before naps, and before bedtime. Others still continue to nurse frequently. Most babies, if given a choice, will choose to breastfeed for an average of two years. Many women try to lead a baby to more natural weaning by distracting them with other activities during the usual time of nursing. This type of gradual weaning is usually more comfortable for mother and baby. Mothers who nurse beyond the first year in the United States receive much criticism and tend to only breastfeed behind closed doors. It is helpful for practitioners to be accepting of the mother who chooses to continue.

REFERENCES

1. Slusser W, Powers N. Breastfeeding update 1: immunology, nutrition, advocacy. Pediatr Rev 1997;18:111–119.

2,3. Baumslag N, Michels DL. Milk, money, and madness, Westport CT: Bergin & Garvey, 1995.

4. Slusser W, Powers N. Breastfeeding update 1: immunology, nutrition, advocacy. Pediatr Rev 1997;18:111–119.

5. Healthy people 2000. Washington, DC: National Health and Human Services, US Department of Health and Human Services, Public Health Services, 1994. Publication No. (PHS) 91-50213.

6. Lawrence R. Breastfeeding: a guide to the medical profession. St. Louis: Mosby, 1994:1.

7. Lawrence R. Breastfeeding: a guide to the medical profession. St. Louis: Mosby, 1994:149–152.

8,9. Slusser W, Powers N. Breastfeeding update 1: immunology, nutrition, advocacy. Pediatr Rev 1997;18:111–119.

10. Riodan J, Auerbach K. Breastfeeding and human lactation, Boston: Jones and Bartlett, 1993:116–118.

11. Wang Y, Wu S. The effect of exclusive breastfeeding on development and incidence of infection in infants. J Hum Lactation 1996;12:27–30.

12. Dewey K, Heinif J, Nommsen-rivers L. Differences in morbidity between breast-fed and formula-fed infants. J Pediatr 1995;126:696–701.

13. Riodan J, Auerbach K. Breastfeeding and human lactation. Boston: Jones and Bartlett, 1993:505.

14. Riodan J, Auerbach K. Breastfeeding and human lactation. Boston: Jones and Bartlett, 1993:81–92.

15–18. Lawrence R. Breastfeeding: a guide for the medical profession. St. Louis: Mosby, 1994:37–87.

19. Neifert M. Early assessment of the breastfeeding infant. Contemp Pediatr 1996;13:142–166.

20. Riodan J, Auerbach K. Breastfeeding and human lactation. Boston: Jones and Bartlett, 1993:223.

21. Huggins K. The nursing mother's companion. Boston: The Harvard Common Press, 1995:38.

22. Neifert M. Early assessment of the breastfeeding infant. Contemp Pediatr 1996;13:143.

23. Riodan J, Auerbach K. Breastfeeding and human lactation. Boston: Jones and Bartlett, 1993:670.

24. Lawrence R. Breastfeeding: a guide for the medical profession. St. Louis: Mosby, 1994:235.

25. Slusser W, Powers N. Breastfeeding update 2: clinical lactation management. Pediatr Rev 1997;18:147–161.

26. Mohrbacher N, Stock J. The breastfeeding answer book. Schaumburg, IL: La Leche League International, 1991:137–139.

27. Mohrbacher N, Stock J. The breastfeeding answer book. Schaumburg IL: La Leche League International, 1991:47–48.

28. Riodan J, Auerbach K. Breastfeeding and human lactation, Boston: Jones and Bartlett, 1993:220.

29. Riodan J. A practical guide to breastfeeding. Boston: Jones and Bartlett, 1990:229–234.

30. Lawrence R. Breastfeeding: a guide for the medical profession, St. Louis: Mosby, 1994: 242–247.

31. Mohrbacher N, Stock J. The breastfeeding answer book. Schaumburg IL: La Leche League International, 1991.

32. Spangler A, Hildebrant E. The effect of modified lanolin on nipple pain/damage during the first ten days of breastfeeding. Int J Childbirth Educ 1993; 8:15–19.

33. Walker M, Driscoll J. Sore nipples: the new mother's nemesis. Matern Child Nurs J 1989;14:260–265.

34. Riodan J, Auerbach K. Breastfeeding and human lactation. Boston: Jones and Bartlett, 1993:227–228.

35,36. Lawrence R. Breastfeeding: a guide for the medical profession. St. Louis: Mosby, 1994:238–242.

37. Riodan J, Auerbach K. Breastfeeding and human lactation. Boston: Jones and Bartlett, 1993:221.

38. Lawrence R. Breastfeeding: a guide to the medical profession. St. Louis: Mosby, 1994: 249.

39. Riodan J, Auerbach K. Breastfeeding and human lactation. Boston: Jones and Bartlett, 1993:108.

40. Lawrence R. Breastfeeding: a guide for the medical profession. St. Louis: Mosby 1994: 95.

41. Mohrbacher N, Stock J. The breastfeeding answer book.

Schaumburg, IL: La Leche League International, 1991:21.

42–46. Frantz K. The slow-gaining breastfeeding infant, NAACOG's Clin Issues 1992; 3:647–655.

47,48. Desmarais L, Browne S. Inadequate weight gain in breastfeeding infants: assessments and resolutions, La Leche League International. New York: Avery Publishing Group, 1990: Unit 8.

49. Lawrence R. Breastfeeding: a guide for the medical profession. St. Louis: Mosby, 1994: 261–264.

50,51. Riodan J, Auerbach K. Breastfeeding and human lactation. Boston: Jones and Bartlett, 1993:382–384.

52. Lawrence R. Breastfeeding: a guide for the medical profession, St. Louis: Mosby, 1994:264.

53. Mohrbacher N, Stock J. The breastfeeding answer book. Schaumburg, IL: La Leche League International, 1991:137–139.

54. Bertelsen C, Auerbach K. Nutrition & breastfeeding: the cultural connection. In: Lactation Consultant Series, Unit 11. Schaumburg IL: La Leche League International, 1987.

55. Riodan J, Auerbach K. Breastfeeding and human lactation. Boston: Jones and Bartlett, 1993: 352.

56. Riodan J, Auerbach K. Breastfeeding and human lactation. Boston: Jones and Bartlett, 1993:239–240.

57. Riodan J, Auerbach K. Breastfeeding and human lactation. Boston: Jones and Bartlett, 1993:350–352.

58. Bertelsen C, Auerbach K. Nutrition & breastfeeding: the cultural connection. In: Lactation Consultant Series, Unit 11. Schaumburg IL: La Leche League International, 1987.

59. Huggins K. The nursing mother's companion. Boston: The Harvard Common Press, 1995:203–205.

59a. Briggs G, Freeman R. Drugs in pregnancy and lactation. Baltimore: Williams and Wilkins, 1997.

60. Slusser W, Poers N. Breastfeeding update 1: immunology, nutrition, advocacy. Pediatr Rev 1997;18:111–119.

61. Auerbach K. Maternal employment and breastfeeding. In: Lactation Consultant Series, Unit 6. Schaumberg IL: La Leche League International, 1987.

62. Breast milk collection and storage tearsheets. McHenry, IL: Medela, 1994.

63. Auerbach K. Maternal employment and breastfeeding. In: Lactation Consultant Series, Unit 6. Schaumberg IL: La Leche League International, 1987.

64,65. Love S. Dr. Susan Love's breast book. Reading MA: Addison-Wesley, 1995:59–65.

66. Riodan J, Auerbach K. Breastfeeding and human lactation. Boston: Jones and Bartlett, 1993:389.

67. Love S. Dr. Susan Love's breast book. Reading MA: Addison-Wesley, 1995:59–65.

68. Mohrbacher N, Stock J. The breastfeeding answer book. Schaumburg IL: La Leche League International, 1991:115–126.

Chapter 37

Contraception

Devora Lieberman
Toni Huebscher

The purpose of this chapter is to help clinicians assist their patients in making informed, educated choices about the contraceptive method most appropriate for them.

Unintended pregnancy is one of the most critical public health problems in the United States. In 1987, nearly 57% of pregnancies were unintended, and over half of those ended in induced abortion. Unfortunately, a decade later the percentage of pregnancies that are unintended has remained constant. Choosing a method of contraception is an important decision. The information provided by health care practitioners is critical in helping patients to use contraception carefully and consistently. Every study that has followed women after their acceptance of a method of contraception has shown that some users still become pregnant unintentionally. From 3% to 20% of women receiving care from family planning clinics become pregnant within 6 months to 2 years after their visit (1–3). If women who are "using" a method still become pregnant, clinicians have a wide window of opportunity to help women become more effective users of their chosen method.

Who makes the choice? Ideally, users themselves should make the decisions about which method they will choose. The consequences of that choice are great. A method that is not effective for a user will have the consequence of unintended pregnancy. A method that is not safe for an individual user can have serious medical consequences. And a method that does not suit an individual's personal or sexual lifestyle is unlikely to be used correctly or consistently.

Counseling can make a statistically significant difference in outcomes (4,5). Through counseling, patients can chose the most suitable contraceptives. Health care providers can also influence the user's motivation and ability to use a given method correctly.

One approach to effective counseling includes several suggestions. 1) Establish a rapport and mutual respect by providing an atmosphere of privacy and equality. 2) Ascertain what goal the patient has in mind by using a particular method. 3) Interact with the patient by asking questions rather than "explaining" or "educating." 4) Listen to her responses and build on that information. 5) Be a catalyst and facilitator, rather than an "educator" who tends to tell the patient what needs to be done (6). It is important to remember that more than half of all information transmitted in a clinical encounter is forgotten immediately after the visit.

In general, the most important questions about contraceptive methods have to do with their effectiveness and safety. The first factor to consider is the inherent efficacy of the method. Second is the potential for misuse or nonuse by the individual. Methods such as sterilization, implants, and injectables have inherently high efficacy, and by their nature ensure proper and consistent use. Other methods, such as the contraceptive pill and intrauterine device (IUD), have a high theoretical efficacy, but allow for potential misuse, such as forgetting to take pills, or failing to check for IUD strings to ensure continued presence of the IUD. Studies of coitally-related methods such as barrier methods, condoms, and spermicides consistently display a wide range of effectiveness because the potential for misuse or nonuse is high. These methods are also less inherently effective than their noncoitally-related counterparts.

As for safety, contraception itself poses few serious risks to users. In addition, using any contraceptive method is usually safer than pregnancy. The method itself may have inherent safety issues such as risk of hospitalization, surgery, medical side effects, infection, loss of fertility, or even death.

Accidental pregnancy is also associated with similar risks. Each woman must assess her particular risks associated with the chosen method and compare those to the dangers of an unintended pregnancy.

ORAL CONTRACEPTIVES

When used properly, combination oral contraceptives (OCPs) provide highly effective, reversible contraception. With perfect use, OCPs are more than 99% effective in the first year of use. Over the past 30 years, many myths about the risks of OCPs have developed that have caused concern for patients and for their health care providers. Many of the earlier studies, which indicated increased cardiovascular risks including myocardial infarction, cerebral infarction, and markedly elevated risk of venous thromboembolism, were based on formulations containing 50 micrograms (μg) or greater of ethinyl estradiol (7). Studies of the newer, sub-50 μg formulations have not shown the same risks. Use of OCPs by healthy, non-smoking women no longer appears to be associated with an increased risk of either myocardial infarction or stroke (8–11). In fact, given their many noncontraceptive benefits, oral contraceptives should be considered a first choice among women seeking a highly effective, reversible method of contraception.

As listed in patient package labeling, contraindications to OCP use are: active thromboembolism or thromboembolic disorders; history of deep-vein thrombophlebitis or embolic disorders; cerebral vascular or coronary artery disease; presence or personal history of breast cancer; endometrial cancer; undiagnosed abnormal genital bleeding; hepatic adenomas or carcinomas; cholestatic jaundice of pregnancy or jaundice with prior OCP use; and pregnancy (12). Cigarette smoking increases the risk of serious cardiovascular side effects from OCP use, a risk that increases markedly in women over the age of 35. All women who use OCPs should be encouraged to quit smoking. For women over age 35 who continue to smoke, another method should be selected.

OCPs and Breast Cancer

Oral contraceptives were first introduced in 1960. In the past 30 years, an estimated 200 million women worldwide have used them (13). Soon after the use of oral contraceptives was approved, concern was raised that use of exogenous female hormones may result in an increased risk of breast cancer (14). Since then, over 50 epidemiologic studies have been performed to address this association. The results have been inconsistent, an outcome frustrating both to providers and consumers of oral contraceptives.

The possible link between OCPs and breast cancer is important for several reasons. First, breast cancer is the most common cancer among women in the United States (15). Breast cancer is second only to lung cancer as a cause of cancer death among women. Second, oral contraceptives are widely used (16), so even a small effect of OCPs on breast cancer risk will have a large public health impact. Finally, intense media attention and growing public awareness has made breast cancer a primary concern among women and their health care providers.

Although the use of OCPs appears generally not to be associated with breast cancer risk, several studies have reported an increased risk in certain subgroups of women. Some studies have suggested that long-term use of OCPs is related to increased breast cancer risk (17). Other studies have suggested that the timing of OCP use in a woman's life is critical to increasing a woman's risk of breast cancer, particularly as related to her first pregnancy (18–20). The hypothesis that long-term use of OCPs may increase the risk of developing breast cancer at an early age was supported by results from the UK National Case-Control Study (21), reanalyses of two older studies (22,23) and several meta-analyses (24–26).

The largest study investigating the association between breast cancer and OCPs was the Cancer and Steroid Hormone (CASH) Study (27,28). In the 1980s, the Centers for Disease Control and the National Institute of Child Health and Human Development conducted this study, which included 4711 cases of breast cancer and 4676 community-based controls. The CASH study found no overall association between breast cancer and OCP use (OR = 1.0, 95% CI 0.9–1.1). Several other reviews of the health effects of oral contraceptives performed in the same period also found no association between ever having used oral contraceptives and risk of breast cancer (29–31).

Recently, the Collaborative Group on Hormonal Factors in Breast Cancer conducted the largest ever meta-analysis of the worldwide data on the relationship of OCPs to breast cancer (32,33). The group pooled results from 54 epidemiologic studies and comprises data on 53,297 women with breast cancer and 100,239 women without disease. The collaborators conducted numerous statistical analyses to estimate the relative risk of breast cancer by different variables, including those that had raised suspicion in the earlier studies. They studied such variables as age, time since first and last use of OCPs, the type of formulation used, and the extent of spread of disease.

The investigators found that there was no increase in risk with dose or with increasing duration of use. They did note a small increased risk for current users (RR = 1.24) and in the first 10 years after stopping use (RR = 1.16 for 1 to 4 years; RR = 1.07 for 5 to 10 years). There was no excess risk, however, 10 or more years after stopping use. Among young users, the absolute number of breast cancer cases associated with OCP use would be very small, since the incidence of breast cancer among young users is low. This increased risk is subject to detection bias, because users of OCPs have more regular and frequent examinations than nonusers.

As for a woman's background risk factors for breast cancer, OCP use did not increase risk among women with different reproductive histories and those with or without a family history of breast cancer. Another critical finding of the study was that breast cancers in current and former users of OCPs were less advanced than those tumors found in those who never used OCPs. The relative risk of tumor spread compared with local disease was 0.88 for ever-users as compared with never-users. So while young women may be at slightly greater risk of developing breast cancer if they use OCPs, they are more likely to have local disease that is more easily curable.

Ovarian Cancer and OCPs

Ovarian cancer is of major public health concern for women. In 1996, there were almost 27,000 new cases of ovarian cancer in the United States (34). Because early detection of ovarian cancer is difficult due to lack of early warning signs and symptoms and effective screening modalities, ovarian cancer has already metastasized by the time of detection in 75% of women. As a result, ovarian cancer has a dismal 5-year survival rate of 40–45%. Age, race, and family history are important risk factors for the disease. In addition, nulliparous women and women with low parity are also at increased risk.

The increased risk of ovarian cancer among these women appears to be caused by incessant ovulation with continual disruption of the ovarian capsule. Users of oral contraceptives are less likely to develop ovarian cancer than those who never used OCPs (35). The biologic mechanism of this protection is thought to be avoidance of incessant ovulation or suppression or reduction of pituitary gonadotropin levels.

The largest investigation of this issue to date, the Cancer and Steroid Hormone study (CASH), found an average 40% decrease in the future likelihood of ovarian cancer in women who had ever used OCPs (36). This was true for all subtypes of ovarian cancer, and for all doses of OCPs. There is a direct correlation with duration of use and level of protection afforded by OCPs. A protective effect has been found after as little as 3 to 6 months of use. Use for 7 years or more confers a 60% to 80% reduction in risk. The reduction in risk related to duration persists for 15 years or more after cessation of use. This point is particularly important for older users of OCPs, as women who use OCPs in their late thirties and forties will have increased protection during the decade of peak incidence of ovarian cancer.

For women who are at increased risk of ovarian cancer because of a family history of the disease, studies have shown that OCPs can provide primary prevention (37). Gross et al assessed data from the CASH and other studies to estimate the effect of the use of OCPs on the risk of developing ovarian cancer. They found that 10 years of OCP use by women with a positive family history of ovarian cancer can reduce their risk to a level below that for women with a negative family history who never use OCPs.

Endometrial Cancer and OCPs

While ovarian cancer is the most common cause of death among women with gynecologic cancers, endometrial cancer is the most common gynecologic cancer among American women (38). Using OCPs for a year or longer reduces the risk of all subtypes of endometrial cancer. Overall, the risk of endometrial cancer is reduced by approximately 50% in users (39). As with the reduction in risk for ovarian cancer, the amount of reduction is related to duration of use. One year of use reduces the risk by 20%; 2 years reduces the risk by 40%. The risk is reduced by 60% with 4 or more years of use. Again, the CASH study found that the protective effect of OCPs persisted for 15 years or more after cessation of use.

Venus Thromboembolism and OCPs

Prior to 1995, the risk of venous thromboembolism (VTE) was felt to be related to the estrogen component of OCPs. Many studies found that as the dose of estrogen in OCPs decreased, there was a concomitant decrease in the incidence of VTE (40,41). It appeared that the role of progestin, if any,

was minor, and studies on the relationship of VTE to progestin dose in early OCPs did not find an association (42,43).

In 1995, however, several studies were published that called this into serious question. These studies found that the risk of VTE was greater in women taking the newer "third-generation" pills containing desogestrel and gestodene than for women taking the "second-generation" pills containing norethindrone and levonorgestrel (44–47). The publication of these studies led to regulatory action in several European countries, with gestodene and desogestrel-containing formulations being removed from the market. Since that time, even the authors of these studies have come forth to say that the response to their studies was premature. The studies were subject to many biases, particularly diagnosis and prescribing biases (48–51).

While it now appears that third-generation OCPs are no more dangerous than second-generation OCPs with respect to venous thromboembolism, combination OCPs do increase a woman's risk of VTE compared with nonusers. Studies have consistently shown a relative risk of around 3 to 4 for OCP users (52,53). It is important to remember, however, that even this elevated relative risk is significantly below that associated with pregnancy, which carries a relative risk of VTE of 6. In the absence of an acceptable contraceptive option, OCPs will be safer than no method with regard to VTE.

Protein C and protein S are the two most important anticoagulant proteins in the complex clotting cascade. The active form of protein C regulates clot formation by inhibiting clotting activity at the levels of factors V and VIII. Protein S is a necessary cofactor in this inhibition. Protein C requires the presence of protein S in order to exert its anticoagulant effect (54). The effects of OCPs on these clotting factors are minor. In users of OCPs, there is a 10% to 20% increase in fibrinogen, a 10% to 20% decrease in protein S, and no change in protein C (55). There are no data that suggest that these changes have any clinical significance in women with normal protein S and protein C activity (56).

These changes in clotting factors occur to an even greater degree in pregnancy. Protein S levels decrease by about 70% (57). It is believed that these changes occur to protect against hemorrhage at time of delivery. This protective mechanism may be why pregnancy carries with it an increased disposition to the development of venous thrombi.

Protein C and protein S deficiencies together account for about 9% of thrombosis patients (58). In the past few years, a newly discovered entity, activated protein C (APC) resistance and a gene mutation affecting factor V (factor V Leiden), has been found to account for 40% of thrombosis patients. The factor V Leiden mutation, named for the city in the Netherlands where it was discovered, involves a single amino acid substitution in factor V. The variant is resistant to the anticoagulant effect of protein C, leading to continuous clot formation. Factor V Leiden is found in 5% of the general population, and 40% of thrombosis patients (59). APC resistance also occurs in pregnancy, demonstrated in 42% of women at 14 to 20 weeks gestation, and 55% of women at 28 weeks (60).

Women with factor V Leiden who use OCPs are at greatly increased risk of VTE. A recent Dutch study compared nonusers with normal factor V and those with factor V

Leiden to users with and without factor V Leiden (61). They found that normal women who used OCPs had a fourfold increase in the risk of VTE, and women with factor V Leiden who did not use OCPs had an eightfold increase in risk. Factor V Leiden and OCPs appear to act synergistically on the risk of VTE: women who had factor V Leiden and used OCPs had a thirtyfold increase in risk. This risk translated into 28.5 VTE events per 10,000 women years. The risk, therefore, does not represent a substantial increase in practice. Routine screening for factor V Leiden is not recommended. One cost-effectiveness study that addressed the question of routine screening for OCP users found that the cost of preventing one thrombotic death was $44,180,000 (62).

Noncontraceptive Benefits of OCPs

There are many noncontraceptive benefits of OCPs, and OCPs may be used to treat a variety of medical conditions.

Menstrual Cycle Benefits

Most women taking OCPs experience decreased menstrual flow and a reduction in dysmenorrhea (63). This effect has led to the use of OCPs as therapy for some women with dysfunctional uterine bleeding (64), primary dysmenorrhea, or both (65,66). The frequency of dysfunctional bleeding is most common in adolescents and perimenopausal women. For both groups, taking OCPs will reduce the abnormal bleeding and provide effective contraception. Studies have found that up to 60% of adolescents complain of dysmenorrhea. Of those, 14% have missed school as a result (67).

Relief from dysmenorrhea appears to be mediated by reduction in menstrual fluid prostaglandin (68). For older women, effective medical treatment decreases the need for surgical intervention. Both groups may also experience a reduction in iron deficiency anemia (69).

The flip side of the menstrual benefit coin is that among OCP users, about 20% will experience intermenstrual bleeding (70). The incidence of breakthrough bleeding (BTB) tends to decrease and stabilize after 6 months of use. In one randomized controlled clinical trial (71) comparing levonorgestrel and norethindrone triphasic preparations, the incidence for all types of intermenstrual bleeding for all preparations combined was 25.2% in cycle one and dropped to 8.4% by cycle six. Another randomized controlled clinical trial (72) evaluating bleeding patterns and steroid levels in women using OCPs containing varying doses of ethinyl estradiol and norethindrone showed similar findings. The study also suggested that increasing the dose of either the estrogen or progestin is associated with a decreased frequency of intermenstrual bleeding.

For practitioners, the practical implication of this finding is that increasing either the progestin or the estrogen dose when a patient has intermenstrual bleeding that persists after several months may be beneficial. It is also important to note that about 1% to 2% of OCP users will experience amenorrhea for at least one cycle.

Benign Breast Disease

Numerous studies over the past several decades have consistently demonstrated a decreased incidence of benign breast disease among OCP users. The relative risk in these studies

has ranged from 0.3 to 0.7 for users as opposed to nonusers (73–77). The reduction in the risk of fibrocystic breast disease appears to be especially true for those who use OCPs prior to their first full-term pregnancy. The mechanism of this effect seems to be inhibition of breast cell proliferation that normally occurs in the first half of an ovulatory menstrual cycle. The effect is most likely due to the progestin component, as two British studies have found the greatest reduction in risk with higher progestin formulations (78,79). As has been seen with other beneficial effects of the pill, the effect is related to duration of use. The Oxford Family Planning Study found decreasing incidence of both fibroadenomas and chronic cysts with increasing years of use. The protective effect appears to persist for at least 1 year after discontinuation of use.

Functional Ovarian Cysts

The finding that use of combination OCPs could be used to suppress functional ovarian cyst formation is based on older epidemiologic studies (80,81). These data are based on use of older pills containing 50 μg or more of ethinyl estradiol. Newer data using lower estrogen doses, however, find that this effect is severely attenuated. A population-based case control study (82) looked at the effect of current use of both mono- and triphasic pills on the development of functional ovarian cysts. The users of monophasic pills had a relative risk of 0.8 as compared with nonusers. The confidence interval, however, crossed 1 (95% CI, 0.4–1.8), making the difference not statistically significant. The users of triphasic pills actually had a slightly higher relative risk of 1.3 when compared with nonusers. This finding was also not statistically significant (95% CI, 0.5–3.3). Another large cohort study of 7500 women found that, compared to nonusers of OCPs, users had a nonsignificant lower incidence of functional cysts. For low-dose monophasic pills, the relative risk was 0.5 (95% CI, 0.01–1.3); for multiphasic pills, the relative risk was 0.9 (95% CI, 0.3–2.3). The greatest effect was found with higher-dose estrogen pills, with a relative risk of 0.2. Again, the effect was not statistically significant (95% CI, 0.01–1.3). If a patient requires treatment for functional ovarian cysts, therefore, practitioners should consider using an OCP containing 50 μg of ethinyl estradiol. In this case, it is important to weigh the increased risk of cardiovascular events associated with higher-dose pills.

Pelvic Inflammatory Disease

The effect of OCPs on the acquisition of sexually transmitted infections needs to be divided into upper and lower tract infection. From several studies, it is clear that OCPs do not reduce the risk of gonococcal or chlamydial cervicitis, and in fact the use of OCPs is associated with higher rates of detection of chlamydial infection (83,84). The proposed mechanism of increased susceptibility to chlamydia is the cervical ectropion that develops in OCP users, which may make the cervix easier to infect. Even with increased rates of lower tract disease and presence of chlamydia, OCPs appear to protect the upper genital tract from infection. The debate persists, however, about the nature of this protection.

One case-control study evaluated women with symptoms of acute salpingitis who underwent laparoscopy (85). Women who were using OCPs had a significantly lower risk of salpingitis than those using no method or a barrier method (RR = 0.2, 95% CI, 0.1–0.4). Furthermore, of the women who had gonorrhea and/or chlamydia infection of the cervix, those using OCPs were less likely to have the disease spread to the upper tract than women who were not using OCPs. This study found that the protection was greater for gonorrhea than for chlamydia. A follow-up study by the same author, however, found that the protection was greater for chlamydia (86). In this study, women who used OCPs were 50% less likely to develop salpingitis than women who did not use OCPs (RR = 0.5; 95% CI, 0.3–1.0). Women infected only with chlamydia were 80% less likely to develop acute salpingitis than women not using OCPs (RR = 0.2; 95% CI, 0.1–0.6). This study found no protection against PID for OCP users with gonorrhea (RR = 0.9%; 95% CI, 0.3–2.6). When salpingitis occurs in OCP users, however, there is evidence that the tubal disease is milder than in women who do not use OCPs (87).

There are several proposed mechanisms for the protective effect of OCPs on salpingitis. The progestin component of OCPs makes cervical mucus thick, viscous, and less penetrable to both sperm and infectious organisms. OCPs decrease menstrual flow, which results in a less favorable environment for bacterial growth. Less retrograde menstruation will lead to a decrease in the bacterial load deposited in the fallopian tubes. OCPs may also lead to changes in myometrial activity, which results in decreased ascent of bacteria into the tubes.

It is clear from the data that OCPs do not offer any protection from HIV. In fact, a Kenyan study actually found that OCP use is an independent risk factor for seroconversion (RR = 4.5; 95% CI, 1.4–13.8) (88). Possible mechanisms for the increased rate of seroconversion may be a cervical ectropion that makes infection more likely, and the increased risk of infection with chlamydia, which in turn increases the risk of acquiring HIV. Other studies, however, have not supported this finding of an association with HIV and OCP use (89).

Bone Density

It is well understood that postmenopausal loss of bone mass occurs because of gradually declining levels of estrogen (90). A decline in bone density begins for women in their 30s. Up to 10% of bone mass may be lost in the 5 years surrounding menopause (91). As more women over age 35 begin to use OCPs with increasing regularity, interest in the effect of OCPs on bone density has grown. Although the evidence is sometimes contradictory, the majority of studies favor a positive effect of OCPs on bone mineral density. Many of the studies are marred by methodologic flaws, and varying approaches to measuring bone density precludes comparison among them. In a review of the literature on bone-sparing properties of OCPs, DeCherney (92) found 9 studies that support the theory that premenopausal use of OCPs increases bone mineral density.

The fact that 4 studies failed to show a benefit has been attributed to differences in study design or inadequate sample size to detect differences. Furthermore, in young, healthy, premenopausal women, bone density is usually normal, so unless OCPs increase bone density, it is unlikely that an effect will be detected. The duration of some of the studies was only a few years. Those studies that found a positive effect found it only after longer duration of use (93,94). Because of these difficulties in study design, the best way to evaluate the effect of OCPs on bone mass is to assess peri- or postmenopausal women who have a history of OCP use. Studies using this design have found that women who use OCPs for 10 or more years can be expected to have increased bone mineral density (95).

Managing Side Effects
Breakthrough Bleeding

Breakthrough bleeding (BTB) is related to the dose and potency of the estrogen and progestin in a particular formulation, as well as a woman's individual response. If bleeding occurs in a new OCP user, it usually does so only in the first few months of use and will subside without any intervention. There are few randomized prospective studies comparing BTB rates among different formulations, and the reasons for the differing rates of BTB are unclear.

If BTB occurs and persists beyond the first 3 months of use, the clinician must first investigate use patterns. Women on low-dose, sub-50 μg OCPs (as almost all women should be) should take their pills at about the same time every day. A delay of even a few hours can lead to a drop in serum steroid levels with resultant BTB. Chlamydia infection appears to be high among OCP users reporting BTB (96), so it is important to rule out infection in these women.

If cultures are negative and a patient appears to be taking her pills consistently, it may help to switch a patient to a pill with a different category of progestin (e.g. switching from norethindrone to desogestrel, or to norgestrel from norgestimate). If BTB persists, one might consider a 3-month course of a 50 μg pill, or adding 20 μg of ethinyl estradiol. At this point, however, an anatomic cause of bleeding such as an endometrial polyp or submucous myoma may be investigated. Such structural abnormalities may cause bleeding without regard to time in the OCP cycle.

Weight Gain

The perception of an increase in weight is a major reason that women, especially adolescents, cite for discontinuing OCPs. In most instances, weight gain is minimal and unrelated to pill use. Approximately as many women will lose weight as will gain weight on OCPs. In some women, however, weight gain is definitely related to pill use, and rarely can be as much as 10 to 20 lb or more. There are several possible explanations. The weight may be due to fluid retention from either the progestin or the estrogen component. This pattern occurs in the first month or so of use. The estrogen component may cause an increase in subcutaneous fat, which will become apparent after several months of use. The androgenicity of some progestins may have an anabolic effect leading to increased appetite and food intake. The most common reason for weight gain is either an increase in caloric intake, a decrease in caloric output with decreased exercise, or both. Should a patient complain of weight gain on the pill, consider switching to a low-androgen, low-estrogen pill, after appropriate counseling regarding diet and exercise.

There are few well done studies of weight gain with second-generation progestins. Studies of OCPs containing either norgestimate or desogestrel, however, found a maximum mean weight gain of 1 pound after 1 year of use (97,98).

Headache

Common migraines are highly prevalent in the population, affecting about 20% of premenopausal women. Women with common migraine may be allowed a trial of OCPs. If the patient, however, complains of focal neurologic symptoms, such as scotomata, she should select another method due to the increased risk of thrombotic stroke (99). For the rest, there are few data on headaches in OCP users. Selection of the appropriate formulation may be by trial and error with adjustments in the type and potency of progestin. If the headaches cannot be controlled, another method should be selected.

If the headaches occur consistently in the pill-free week, it is possible that the patient is suffering estrogen withdrawal headaches. In this situation, a monophasic pill may be taken continuously, or the placebos may be supplemented with estradiol.

Mood Changes

Changes in mood are highly subjective, and their relation to OCP use is difficult to assess. There are few data that directly compare different formulations, but there is evidence to suggest that the low-dose OCPs have minimal impact on mood. If a patient complains of mood changes or depression, switching to a formulation with a different progestin may help. If there is no relief, another method should be considered.

Nausea

Nausea most often occurs in the first month or two of pill use, or during the first few pills of each cycle. Emesis is rare. If vomiting occurs within one hour of taking the pill, patients should be advised to take a second dose to replace that pill. Many women can control nausea by taking their pills just after a meal or with a snack, or at bedtime. If nausea occurs for the first time after months or years of pill use, it is important to rule out pregnancy. Nausea is primarily related to the estrogen dose, and switching to a 20 μg pill may alleviate the problem.

THE INTRAUTERINE DEVICE

American women differ significantly from their international counterparts in their choice of contraceptive method. In the rest of the world, the intrauterine device (IUD) is the most widely-used reversible method of contraception, chosen by more than 85 million users (100). In the United States, the IUD is used by less than 1% of women using contraception (101). The reluctance of American women to use IUDs can be traced back to the debacle of the Dalkon Shield, which was removed from the market in 1974. Although it has now been more than 20 years since the reports of septic abortions and severe pelvic infections, the perception that IUDs are not safe has persisted among women (102) and their providers (103).

Some women are not considered good candidates for the IUD: women with active, recent, or recurrent infection;

women at high risk for sexually transmitted diseases (candidates should be in mutually monogamous relationships); those with risk factors for HIV infection and/or HIV disease; those with undiagnosed genital bleeding, valvular heart disease, or anatomical abnormalities of the endometrium (such as distortion by myomas); and, in the case of the copper-containing IUD, those with Wilson's disease.

Mechanism of Action

The IUD's main mechanism of contraceptive action in the human is spermicidal, produced by a local sterile inflammatory reaction caused by the presence of the foreign body in the uterus. Tissue breakdown product of these leukocytes are toxic to all cells, including sperm and the blastocyst. The addition of copper increases the inflammatory reaction. Because of the spermicidal action of IUDs, very few, if any, sperm reach the oviducts, and the ovum usually does not become fertilized.

On removal of both copper-bearing and non-copper-bearing IUDs, the inflammatory reaction rapidly disappears. Resumption of fertility after IUD removal is not delayed and occurs at the same rate as resumption of fertility after discontinuation of mechanical methods of contraception, such as the condom and diaphragm.

Types of IUDs

There are currently two types of IUDs available in the United States. The Copper T 380A (Paragard) became available in 1988, and is effective for up to 10 years. The constant dissolution of copper, which amounts daily to less than that ingested in the normal diet, requires it be replaced in this time period. The other is the progesterone-releasing device (Progestasert), which became available in 1976. It is effective for 1 year, and therefore must be replaced annually. The progesterone IUD releases 65 mg of progesterone daily. This amount of hormone release does not cause a measurable increase in peripheral serum progesterone levels. The reservoir of progesterone becomes depleted after about 18 months of use, requiring its replacement by 1 year after insertion. The safety of both devices has been well demonstrated. For many women, particularly those for whom oral contraceptives are contraindicated, the IUD may be the safest and most effective reversible contraceptive option. With its high efficacy and long duration of action, the Copper T 380A may be a viable, non-surgical alternative to sterilization.

Pelvic Infection

The Dalkon Shield left a legacy of fear of an increased risk of pelvic infection associated with IUDs. New research, and reevaluation of earlier studies, have now shown that the increased risk of infection is unique to the Dalkon Shield. The relative risk of developing PID as 15.6 with the Dalkon Shield. Other types of IUDs have a relative risk of PID of 1.5, an epidemiologically trivial number (104). The problem with the Dalkon Shield was its multifilament tail, which facilitated the ascension of bacteria to the upper genital tract. This does not occur with IUDs that have monofilament tails; these types of IUDs have PID rates no different from IUDs without tails (105).

The increased risk of infection with the IUD appears to

be related to insertion. The World Health Organization conducted an international, multicenter study of 23,000 IUD insertions. They found only 81 cases of PID (106). The risk of developing PID was highest in the first 20 days following insertion with an incidence of 10 per 1000 woman-years. After 20 days, PID becomes very rare, with an incidence of 1 per 1000 woman-years. This rate is similar to that of women using no method of contraception (107).

Given that the risk of infection is related to insertion, it would seem intuitive that the use of prophylactic antibiotics would be preventative. Most studies of the use of peri-insertion antibiotics have shown that there is no effect on infection rates or the need for medical removal. A large study of 447 women in Los Angeles prospectively randomized patients to receive either a single dose of 200 mg of doxycycline or placebo 1 hour prior to insertion (108). Only 2 subjects, one from each group, met the diagnostic criteria for acute PID. The overall retention rate was 91% for the antibiotic group, and 89.7% for the placebo group. This difference was not statistically significant. If sexually transmitted infections are common in the population being served, some clinicians choose to provide women with prophylactic antibiotics at the time of IUD insertion. If concern about infection is that high, however, perhaps another contraceptive method should be selected.

Expulsion

The incidence of expulsion is approximately 5% in the first year. Most of these expulsions will occur in the first 3 months of use. Many clinicians, therefore, will ask patients to return 3 months after insertion to check string placement. This also provides an opportunity to discuss management of side effects such as increased menstrual bleeding and cramping. Patients should be encouraged to check for strings following each menstrual period. Factors that have been associated with increased rates of expulsion are nulliparity, young age, immediate postpartum insertion, and the skill and experience of the clinician performing the insertion (109).

Uterine Bleeding and Pain

The most commonly reported side effect of IUDs is increased menstrual bleeding and cramping. In the first year of use, between 5% and 15% of women will discontinue the IUD because of this side effect (110). Very often, these symptoms can be relieved by the use of nonsteroidal anti-inflammatory agents.

While the progesterone-releasing device has been associated with a decrease in the amount of menstrual flow (111), the copper-containing IUD causes a 55% increase in menstrual blood loss. Despite the increase in menstrual flow, this IUD is not associated with iron deficiency anemia.

Spontaneous Abortion and Preterm Delivery

While the IUD is a highly effective method of contraception, it is important to remember that no method is perfect, and unintended pregnancies can occur. Should a pregnancy occur with an IUD in place, there is a risk of spontaneous abortion of 40% to 50% (112). Unlike with the Dalkon Shield, however, there is no increased risk of septic abortion. The risk of spontaneous abortion is even greater if the IUD is left in

place (113). Therefore, the IUD should always be removed if the string is visible. If the woman decides to continue the pregnancy and the IUD is not removed, the risk of preterm labor and delivery is increased nearly fourfold (114). There is no increased risk, however, of birth defects if the IUD is left in place (115).

Ectopic Pregnancy

As stated earlier, the IUD's main mechanism of contraceptive action is the production of a sterile inflammatory reaction in the uterine cavity. If the egg is fertilized, the foreign body reaction acts to prevent implantation of the embryo into the endometrium. Because more inflammatory reaction is present in the endometrial cavity than the oviducts, the IUD prevents intrauterine pregnancy more effectively than it prevents ectopic pregnancy. Overall however, because of the IUD's highly effective contraceptive action, the IUD reduces the incidence of ectopic pregnancy compared to the rate seen in women not using contraception. If a women does conceive with an IUD in place, her chances of having an ectopic pregnancy range from 3% to 9%. Because of this, if a woman conceives with an IUD in place, ectopic pregnancy should first be ruled out.

Return to Fertility

Another concern that many women have is fear of infertility as result of the IUD. Many studies have shown a rapid return to fertility following removal of the device (116,117). The median time to return to fertility following removal of either currently available device is 3 months (118,119).

LEVONORGESTEREL IMPLANTS

Although the availability of levonorgestrel implants (Norplant) in the United States is relatively recent, the development of this method began 30 years ago as a project sponsored by the Population Council. Since then, more than 60,000 women have participated in clinical trials of the system. Since the drug is delivered via a subdermal implant, there is no room for user error. Its high efficacy, combined with its 5 years of potential use, make levonorgestrel implants an excellent contraceptive choice for many women.

The list of contraindications to levonorgesterel use is similar to that of oral contraceptives. The absolute contraindications are genital bleeding of uncertain etiology, known or suspected pregnancy, acute liver disease, active thrombophlebitis or thromboembolic disease, breast cancer, and liver tumors.

Mechanism of Action

The delivery system consists of six Silastic rods, each containing 36 mg of levonorgestrel. In a simple office procedure, the rods are placed subdermally through a small incision, usually in the inner aspect of the upper arm. Following insertion, levonorgestrel can be detected in the bloodstream within 2 hours. Contraceptive concentrations are found within the first day (120). The implants will continue to release adequate amounts of levonorgestrel for 5 years. After the implants are removed, levonorgestrel is undetectable in the circulation after 1 week.

There are several proposed mechanisms by which this system provides its contraceptive effect. The continuous release of levonorgestrel exerts a negative feedback on the cyclicity of gonadotropins that are necessary to produce ovulation. Measurements of luteal phase progesterone indicate that ovulation occurs in 18% of users in the first year of use, and in 60% of users by the fifth year of use. It appears, however, that hormonal patterns are interrupted enough to prevent normal conception, possibly by impairing oocyte maturation (121).

The second proposed mechanism of levonorgestrel action is the maintenance of a thick cervical mucous that is impenetrable to sperm. Studies of beta HCG levels in levonorgesterel users have shown that they do not have a significant fertilization rate, so it does not act as an abortifacient (122).

Should the first two proposed mechanisms fail, levonorgestrel has a third backup method in its effect on the endometrium. Levonorgestrel leads to a mixed proliferative-secretory endometrium. This iatrogenic luteal phase defect makes implantation of those few fertilized eggs rare.

Effectiveness

The overall risk of pregnancy for women who use levonorgestrel is less than 1%. An international, multicenter study of 12,133 woman years of use found that of the 20 pregnancies that occurred, 19 had luteal phase insertions (123). The importance of timing of insertion was further confirmed by another study that found that the majority of pregnancies with levonorgestrel use are present at the time of insertion (124). It is critical, therefore, to ensure that that women are not pregnant at the time of insertion. Levonorgestrel implant insertion is best performed postpartum, immediately after an abortion, or within the first 5 days following the start of a menstrual period.

Managing Side Effects

Almost all users of levonorgestrel will experience side effects at some time during the 5 years of use, most commonly in the first few months. Side effects include irregular menses, headaches, acne, weight change, mastalgia, hyperpigmentation over the implants, hirsutism, hair loss, depression, mood changes, anxiety, nervousness, and galactorrhea. The only side effect for which treatment has been proven effective is irregular bleeding. Should the user find that the side effects interfere with her quality of life, the only option is to remove the implants.

First-year continuation rates for levonorgestrel range between 76% and 90%. First-year continuation rates compare favorably with those for OCPs and IUDs, which average 50% and 75%, respectively. Continuation rates with levonorgestrel decline in a linear fashion, and by the fifth year of use range between 25% and 55% (125).

Menstrual irregularity is by far the most common reason given for requests for removal of the implants (126). In one study, 82% of women complained of irregular bleeding (127). Advising patients of the likelihood of bleeding irregularities prior to insertion may be helpful in avoiding premature removal. After the first 3 months of use, the average number of "bleeding starts" averaged over 1 year is the same as for women with regular 28-day cycles. Over time, the incidence of bleeding episodes declines. Bleeding patterns for individual patients are unpredictable, but have not been shown to lead to anemia.

Several regimens for controlling irregular bleeding in levonorgestrel users have been used with success. One study prospectively randomized women to use either ethinyl estradiol (0.05 mg/day for 20 days), ibuprofen (800 mg three times a day for 5 days), levonorgestrel (30 µg twice a day for 20 days), or placebo (one/day for 30 days) (128). Patients taking placebo averaged 129 days of bleeding in the first year of use. In all of the treatment arms the number of bleeding days was reduced. Ethinyl estradiol reduced the number of days to 77, ibuprofen to 94, and levonorgestrel to 101.

Another study prospectively randomized patients to three treatment arms: ethinyl estradiol (50 µg/day for 20 days), an oral contraceptive (50 µg ethinyl estradiol and 250 µg levonorgestrel for 20 days) or placebo. Women treated with the combination birth control pill bled an average of 2.6 days during treatment compared with 5.4 and 12.3 days in the ethinyl estradiol and placebo groups, respectively (129). Other options include conjugated estrogens (1.25 mg/day) or estradiol (2 mg/day for 7 days). The goal of these regimens is intended to be a temporary aid. They are not intended to provide long-term resolution of irregular bleeding, but rather to stop prolonged bleeding periods of greater than 8 days.

Return to Fertility

Normal ovulatory cycles usually resume during the first month after implant removal. Sivin found that by 1 year following removal, 84% of those attempting pregnancy had conceived.

DEPO-MEDROXYPROGESTERONE ACETATE

Depo-medroxyprogesterone acetate (Depo Provera; DMPA) is the only injectable contraceptive available in the United States. After it had been used for more than 20 years by 30 million women in more than 90 countries, the Food and Drug Administration approved its use for contraception in the United States in 1992. The only absolute contraindications to its use are current coagulation disorders, previous hepatic adenoma, undiagnosed genital bleeding, and pregnancy. Contraception with DMPA may be an ideal choice for women who are seeking highly effective birth control but experience problems with other reversible methods. Some women may choose DMPA because they have difficulty remembering to take oral contraceptive pills daily, experience compliance problems with coitally-related barrier methods, prefer the convenience of one injection every 3 months, develop estrogen-related side effects when taking oral contraceptives, or require the privacy associated with DMPA. Because there is no visible evidence of DMPA use, no one other than the health care provider needs to know that the drug is being used.

Dosage, Administration, and Contraceptive Action

DMPA is a microcrystalline suspension of low solubility that provides a sustained release of progestogen when administered intramuscularly. After deep gluteal or deltoid injection of 150 mg of DMPA, contraceptive plasma levels are reached within 24 hours, and peak plasma concentrations are achieved within 20 days (130). The low solubility of the microcrystals results in delayed absorption from the injection site and prolonged circulating concentrations of the active progestagen. Contraceptive levels of plasma DMPA concentrations are sustained for at least 14 weeks after injection. This allows for a short grace period for those women who are late for their 3-month reinjection visit. Repeated injections of DMPA every 3 months have not been associated with progressive elevation of plasma drug concentrations (131).

As with oral contraceptives, DMPA's contraceptive effect results mainly from its inhibition of ovulation. After administration, DMPA leads to a decline in plasma levels of follicle-stimulating hormone and luteinizing hormone, and LH surges do not occur (132). Further contraceptive effect is achieved by causing the endometrium to become atrophic and unfavorable for implantation of an embryo. DMPA also suppresses estrogen receptors throughout the genital tract, leading to an increased tenacity of cervical mucus that resists sperm penetration, as well as a decrease in tubal motility.

When 150 mg of DMPA is administered every 3 months, its contraceptive efficacy exceeds 99%. Both the expected failure rate and the typical user failure rate are less than 1% per year. A 1986 WHO study found no pregnancies in 607 women (452 woman-years) (133). Failure rates in other studies ranged from 0.1 to 0.7 per 100 woman-years (134).

Timing of the first injection is critical. The optimal time to initiate contraception with DMPA is immediately postpartum, after an abortion, or within the first 5 days of the menstrual cycle. DMPA injection at this point in the menstrual cycle ensures that the recipient is not already pregnant and prevents ovulation during the first month of use (135). After a single injection of 150 mg of DMPA, ovulation does not return for at least 14 weeks (136). Should a woman return for a repeat injection more than 14 weeks after the previous injection, pregnancy must be ruled out.

Noncontraceptive Benefits

There are several noncontraceptive benefits to DMPA.

Reduction of Menstrual Blood Loss

Because the long-term use of DMPA reduces menstrual blood, hemoglobin levels often increase slightly in women using DMPA (137). In women with sickle cell anemia, users of DMPA have increased hemoglobin levels and erythrocyte survival and decreased frequency of painful crises (138).

Gynecologic Benefits

Women who use progestational agents for contraception have a decreased incidence of candidal vulvovaginitis and pelvic inflammatory disease (139,140). Because DMPA is so highly effective in preventing pregnancy, its use reduces the risk of ectopic pregnancy. DMPA also significantly reduces the risk of endometrial cancer (141).

Seizure Disorders

DMPA appears to be a particularly appropriate choice for women with seizure disorders for two reasons. First, use of DMPA results in a decrease in seizure frequency (142). Second, the contraceptive efficacy of DMPA does not appear

to be reduced by concurrent use of anticonvulsants such as phenytoin or carbamazepine.

Problems with DMPA
Menstrual Disturbances

Most women who use DMPA will experience menstrual irregularities, and very few will have regular cycles (143). Episodes of unpredictable irregular spotting and bleeding lasting 7 days or more occur commonly in the first few months of use. In up to 20%, the bleeding may be frequent or prolonged. Heavy bleeding is uncommon, however, reported by less than 5% of women in large studies. Over time, the frequency and duration of spotting and bleeding episodes decreases, and amenorrhea becomes more common. After 1 year of use, approximately 50% of women will develop amenorrhea.

Menstrual disturbance is the most common medical reason for discontinuation of DMPA (144). The mechanism of the irregular bleeding is not well understood, but appears to be related to the progestogen effect on the blood vessels of the endometrium, making them more fragile. In order to reduce dissatisfaction with and discontinuation of DMPA, women should be carefully counseled about expectations. Many women find that amenorrhea is a significant benefit of the method.

Medical intervention is rarely necessary for irregular bleeding as it rarely leads to anemia. Short-term management of the problem is unsatisfactory, although many regimens have been studied (145). Oral estrogen (conjugated estrogen 1.25 mg, or 2 mg of estradiol) for 10 to 21 days will minimize or eliminate bleeding. After the estrogen is discontinued, however, bleeding will frequently recur. Support and counseling by health care providers is critical to help women continue to use the method. Women who remain dissatisfied with the menstrual changes should be advised to select another method.

Return to Fertility

There has been concern about the prolonged delay in return to fertility following use of DMPA. The effects on fertility are short-term only. There is no evidence to suggest that long-term fertility is compromised in either parous or nulliparous women (146). In a large study that evaluated conception rates among 1258 women who discontinued various methods of contraception, pregnancy was delayed in former DMPA users during the first 9 months after discontinuation compared with a mean 3-month delay among women discontinuing oral contraceptives and a mean 5-month delay after intrauterine device removal (147). Within the first 12 months after discontinuation, nearly 70% of former DMPA users had conceived, and more than 90% had conceived by 24 months. Before DMPA contraception is initiated, future childbearing plans should be discussed and patients should be counseled about the possibility of prolonged suppression of ovulation after discontinuation.

Bone Density Changes

Recent controversy surrounding the issue of bone demineralization during treatment with DMPA was sparked by a small study from New Zealand (148). In this cross-sectional study, bone mineral density of 30 women using DMPA for at least 5 years was compared with 30 premenopausal controls. The authors found that the women using DMPA had significantly lower bone mineral density in the lumbar spine and femoral neck in comparison to the premenopausal controls. No clinical evidence of osteoporosis, such as fractures, was noted in the DMPA users, and the reduction in bone density was reversible after the method was discontinued. The decrease in bone mineral density may be related to suppression of ovarian estradiol production. The FDA has recommended that prospective postmarketing studies be performed to further evaluate the effects of DMPA on bone mineral density.

Weight Gain

A mean weight gain of 2 kg in the first year of use has been reported (149). However, 20% to 60% of women lose weight while on DMPA. Weight gain appears to be less in obese women, but can be a significant problem for some women.

Other Clinical Effects

A variety of minor adverse effects have been reported with DMPA use, such as mild headache, abdominal bloating, mood changes, depression, breast swelling, and hair loss. It is important to advise patients about the possibility of side effects with any method of contraception. Because many of these effects may be irreversible for the 14-week life of the injection, pre-injection counseling is particularly important for women considering DMPA.

BARRIER METHODS OF CONTRACEPTION

Diaphragm

The diaphragm was initially developed in the late 1800s in Germany, and reached the United States in the 1920s. Many decades later, it is still one of the more commonly used barrier methods in the United States. The device functions to physically obstruct the flow of sperm through the cervix.

A diaphragm must be carefully fitted by a trained professional who is familiar with female anatomy. The size with the widest diameter that feels comfortable should be used. Following proper fitting, the patient should practice removal and insertion herself, and she should be able to digitally locate her own cervix and pubic symphysis. The patient should feel confident about doing this properly before returning home.

The diaphragm, in order to maximize effectiveness, should be used in conjunction with contraceptive jelly and be left in the vagina for at least 8 hours following coitus. If repeated intercourse occurs during these 8 hours, another dose of contraceptive jelly should be inserted into the vagina without removing the diaphragm. Although it has not been demonstrated conclusively that pregnancy rates are lower when a spermicide is used, it is generally advised that the use of spermicide is prudent. When using the diaphragm, patients should also be cautioned not to leave the device in place for more than 24 hours, as this may result in abrasions or ulcerations of the vaginal mucosa. It has been reported that recurrent urinary tract infections may be one of the most common side effects of the diaphragm (150).

The published failure rates that determine efficacy are extremely sensitive to the consistency of use of the diaphragm. This may be related to the level of comfort the patient has regarding insertion, which may in turn be dependent on certain social or cultural issues. For this reason, researchers frequently divide the data into perfect-use and imperfect-use distinctions (151). Failure of the diaphragm to protect against pregnancy during the first year of use reportedly occurs at a rate of 18% with typical use, and at a rate of 6% with perfect use. Approximately 60% of women continue use of the diaphragm for more than 1 year following initiation (152).

There is limited but consistent data indicating that the diaphragm may offer some protection against transmission of sexually transmitted infection. The device appears to have a protective effect against gonorrhea and chlamydia similar to that of condoms. The relative risk of such infections is reportedly 0.3 to 0.5 in nonrandomized studies (153–155).

Cervical Cap

The cervical cap was first available over 100 years ago. Throughout this time, the popularity of this method has waxed and waned, likely in relation to the availability of alternative methods of contraception.

Issues pertaining to the patient's level of comfort with her own anatomy, as well as education regarding proper insertion and removal of the device, apply equally to the diaphragm as well as to the cervical cap. The cap, while smaller in diameter than the diaphragm, is designed to similarly block the passage of sperm through the cervical os. The cervical cap has the advantage of being able to stay in place for an extended period of time, and may be somewhat more comfortable than the diaphragm for some women. The cap should not be left in the vagina for greater than 48 hours. Some unpleasant features have been reported to be associated with the cervical cap, including increase in vaginal odor, significant time necessary for proper initial fitting of the device, difficulty with removal and reinsertion, dislodgement during coitus, and theoretical increased risk of toxic shock syndrome (156).

Failure rates of the cervical cap are difficult to ascertain because data is limited. In addition, dropout rates are quite high. Such dropout rates have been reported to range from 32.6% (157) to 49.5% (158). Failure rates, if all reported studies of more than 100 woman-users are considered, range from 3.5 to 16 per 100 woman-years of use (159–161).

Condom

Use of the condom protects both partners from acquiring gonorrhea and chlamydia infections. Condoms may also prevent the transmission of viruses, including the herpes virus and HIV. Additionally, condoms have been reported to decrease the incidence of cervical neoplasia, presumably by decreasing to some extent the transmission of the human papilloma virus (162,163).

The incidence of sexually transmitted infections is greatest in the under-25 age group. Because use-failure rates for mechanical barrier methods are highest in this group, it is generally advised that women use an oral contraceptive or other more effective hormonal method of contraception in addition to use of the condom. In so doing, the couple achieves highly effective contraception while preventing sexually transmitted infections. Particularly in the young, this is an important point for contraceptive education (164).

One-year failure rates of condom usage range between 1% and 4% when the women are over 30. In contrast, the failure rates range between 10% and 33% when the female is under 25 (165).

Female Condom

The female condom is a device designed to be used by women to loosely line the vaginal vault during intercourse. It is the first female-controlled barrier method officially recognized as a means for preventing sexually transmitted infection (166). This condom is made of a tubular sheath and two flexible rings. The smaller ring fits into the vagina at the closed end of the condom, and the larger ring is attached to the open end of the sheath, which lies on the vulva. Some studies have indicated that there is a high rate of discontinuation with the female condom. Additionally, patients have reported that it is aesthetically unacceptable, and that the whole device has been pushed into or pulled out of the vagina during intercourse. It likely has similar failure rates to that of the male condom (167–169).

Spermicides (Foams, Creams, Suppositories)

Spermicidal agents usually contain an agent called nonoxynol-9. This substance is a surfactant that immobilizes sperm. It also provides a physical barrier and must be placed into the vagina prior to each act of intercourse. The effectiveness of this method is similar to that of the diaphragm, and increases with increasing age of the user. While surfactants cause irreversible loss of sperm motility, they also affect membranes of bacteria or any parasite that might be present in the vagina. Because of this, a lower incidence of sexually transmitted infections is associated with the use of spermicidal products containing surfactants. However, the surfactants also affect the cells of the vaginal mucosa, and vaginal irritation is occasionally reported by women using these products (170).

EMERGENCY CONTRACEPTION

In the United States every year, 3.5 million women experience unintended pregnancies. While about half of these pregnancies occur because the couple did not use any method of contraception, 47% occur despite the use of contraception (171). Experts estimate that use of emergency contraception could potentially reduce the number of unintended pregnancies in the United States each year by at least 1.7 million (172). With wider use of emergency contraception, nearly 1 million abortions may be averted annually (173). Despite many years of research that support the safety and efficacy of emergency contraception, many clinicians lack information about the appropriate use of the method, and many women remain unaware that such an option exists (174).

The unfortunate use of the term "morning after" further confuses the issue, because some women and health care providers may assume that, in order to be effective, the regimen must be instituted within 24 hours of unprotected intercourse. Actually, treatment with combined oral contraceptives can be effective when begun up to 72 hours following intercourse, and insertion of a copper-containing IUD can be effective up to 7 days later (175). The most well-understood option for emergency contraception is the Yuzpe method, named for the Canadian physician, Albert Yuzpe, who first developed the method. The original regimen consisted of 0.1 mg of ethinyl estradiol and 1.0 mg of dl-norgestrel (2 Ovral) taken within 72 hours of unprotected sex. A second dose is repeated 12 hours later.

Candidates for Emergency Contraception

A woman who has had unprotected intercourse within 72 hours, regardless of the time in the menstrual cycle, is a candidate for emergency contraception (176). In circumstances such as rape or failure of a mechanical barrier method, emergency contraception is the only option for reducing the potential of an unintended pregnancy. The most common reasons women give for seeking emergency contraception are failure to use any method, and failure of a barrier method.

Formulations

In early 1997, the Food and Drug Administration issued a statement supporting the use of certain standard oral contraceptive pills for emergency contraception. Although the FDA decided against mandating that manufacturers apply for this indication or include such information in package labeling, physicians in the United States can legally prescribe hormones for the purpose of emergency contraception. The formulation options are listed in Table 37-1.

Treatment consists of two doses of oral contraceptive pills taken 12 hours apart. Use of an antiemetic before taking the medication may reduce the risk of nausea and vomiting.

Table 37-1 Oral Contraceptive Formulations Used for Emergency Contraception		
TYPE OF PREPARATION	FORMULATION	NUMBER OF PILLS TAKEN WITH EACH DOSE
High-dose monophasic	0.05 mg ethinyl estradiol 0.50 mg norgestrel	2
Low-dose monophasic	0.03 mg ethinyl estradiol 0.30 mg norgestrel	4
Low-dose monophasic	0.03 mg ethinyl estradiol 0.15 mg levonorgestrel	4
Low-dose triphasic	0.30 mg ethinyl estradiol 0.125 mg levonorgestrel (yellow pills only)	4

Mechanism of Action

Although not completely understood, researchers believe that emergency contraceptive pills (ECPs) prevent pregnancy through several mechanisms (177). When estrogens and progestins are taken in high doses, they disrupt the natural hormonal patterns necessary for pregnancy. By altering the endometrium, they prevent implantation. They may also interfere with ovulation, fertilization, or with the luteal phase of the menstrual cycle. ECPS exert their effect before implantation occurs. After that, ECPs have no effect on the pregnancy (178). Other researchers believe that ECPs interfere by inhibiting or delaying ovulation, as well as interfere with the proper functioning of the corpus luteum (179).

Efficacy

Emergency contraception is not a substitute for consistent use of a prophylactic method of contraception, primarily because it is not as effective. When oral contraceptives are used for emergency contraception, they are about 75% effective in preventing pregnancy (180). A simple way to explain this point is to inform women that if 8 out of 100 women would get pregnant from a single act of unprotected intercourse, use of ECPs will reduce that number to 2.

Side Effects

As with any high dose estrogen, the most common side effects are nausea and vomiting. Nausea occurs in up to 50% of women, while vomiting occurs in 25% (181). No studies have found that there is a higher failure rate if vomiting occurs within 3 hours of taking the dose. Nausea and vomiting can be reduced if an antiemetic is taken 1 hour prior to the dose.

Trussell et al found no serious or long-term complications among over 6,300 women who received ECPs. In the United Kingdom, where over 4 million prescriptions were written between 1984 and 1996, only six serious adverse reactions were reported. Of those, only one occurred close enough to the time of administration to suggest that the drug may have been related (182).

Contraindications

While there does not appear to be an increased risk of fetal malformations, the most obvious contraindication to the use of ECPs is an existing pregnancy. A meta-analysis of teratogenicity after exposure to oral contraceptives (including the high doses used with ECPs) found no increased risk of fetal malformations (183).

There have been no studies evaluating the effect of ECPs on women with preexisting contraindications to oral contraceptives. The American College of Obstetricians and Gynecologists does not specify any contraindications to ECPs. It is as yet unknown whether women who take ECPs are at increased risk for breast cancer, blood clots, or migraines. Clinicians must weigh the risks and benefits of ECPs against an unintended pregnancy. For women with severe contraindications to estrogen, alternative methods of emergency contraception may be considered.

Other Hormonal Methods

Other options for emergency contraception include synthetic or conjugated estrogens and danazol. Progestin-only pills may also be considered. Of these, levonorgestrel is the only formulation that has been studied for potential use as an emergency contraceptive. A study that compared the Yuzpe method to levonorgestrel found similar efficacy rates and a decreased incidence of side effects with the levonorgestrel regimen (184). The dosage of the levonorgestrel formulation available in the United States is 20 tablets of progestin-only norgestrel repeated once 12 hours later. As with the Yuzpe method, treatment should be initiated within 72 hours of unprotected intercourse.

Danazol is an androgenic progestin typically used in the treatment of endometriosis. It has also been used in doses of 800–1200 mg as an emergency contraceptive option. Danazol works by interfering with implantation. It has fewer side effects than the Yuzpe method, but its efficacy in randomized controlled trials is poor (185).

IUDs for Postcoital Contraception

The insertion of a copper-containing IUD within 5 days after ovulation or 5 to 7 days after unprotected intercourse is another available option (186). The IUD triggers a sterile inflammation in the endometrium making it hostile for implantation. It also interferes with fertilization by inhibiting sperm transport. Postcoital IUD insertion is highly effective. A meta-analysis that included 20 studies and over 8400 women found a failure rate of 0.1% or lower (187). Insertion of an IUD is an option for women with severe contraindications to oral contraceptives, and is ideal for the woman who plans to continue to use the IUD as her method of contraception.

FEMALE STERILIZATION

Female sterilization by tubal ligation is one of the most popular methods of contraception in the United States. A survey performed in 1995 found that 24% of women aged 15 to 50 years used either female or male sterilization as their method of contraception (188). Every year, approximately 1 million sterilization procedures by tubal ligation are performed.

The risk of sterilization is primarily related to the type of anesthesia used. Women considering sterilization must be advised that the procedure is permanent. Many women are under the misconception that tubes may be easily "untied." Tubal reversal has a variable success rate. In states that mandate insurance coverage for in vitro fertilization, tubal sterilization voids the benefit. Many studies have shown that regret is highest among women who undergo the procedure when they are under age 30.

Effectiveness

Female sterilization was long thought to be the most effective method available for women. Recent data from the U.S. Collaborative Review of Sterilization (CREST), however, demonstrated that sterilization is not as effective in preventing pregnancy as was previously thought (189). This landmark study followed over 10,000 women for 10 years following sterilization. The study found that the risk of pregnancy varies by sterilization method, and persists for years after the procedure. The risk of pregnancy, therefore, is greater for women who opt for the procedure at younger ages. The CREST study found an overall pregnancy rate of nearly 2%: 19.5 pregnancies for every 1000 procedures.

Methods

The only methods of sterilization currently available in the United States are surgical procedures that are performed either by laparoscopy or minilaparotomy. Bipolar coagulation had, in the CREST study, a 10-year cumulative failure rate of .025%, unipolar coagulation a failure rate of 0.75%, silicone rubber band application (Fallope or Yoon rings) a failure rate of 1.8%, and spring clip application (Hulka clips) had a failure rate of 3.6%. Partial salpingectomy when performed following delivery had a low 10-year failure rate of 0.75%, equal to the failure rate of unipolar coagulation. If the partial salpingectomy is performed at a time unrelated to pregnancy, the 10-year failure rate was significantly higher at 2%.

MALE STERILIZATION

Effectiveness

Vasectomy is the most effective method of contraception currently available, with a first year failure rate of 0.15% (190).

As with female sterilization, the procedure must be considered permanent.

Methods

There are two methods of vasectomy that are most commonly performed. The vas can be occluded either via one or two small incisions or with the "no-scalpel" technique. In the latter procedure, the vas is palpated through the scrotal skin, held in place with a ring forceps, and the skin is punctured with dissecting forceps. The vasa are then elevated through the small wounds and occluded. The punctures are small enough that they heal without sutures.

Once they have been isolated, the vasa may be occluded by one of several methods, not unrelated to those methods used for tubal ligation. Options include electro- or thermal cautery, ligation of the cut ends, or removal of a segment of the vas. In the "open-ended" vasectomy, the testicular end of the vas is left open. This procedure allows sperm to drain into surrounding tissues which prevents pressure from building up in the epidydimis.

REFERENCES

1. Harlap S, Kost K, Forrest JD. Preventing pregnancy, protecting health: a new look at birth control choices. New York: The Alan Guttmacher Instititute, 1991.

1a. Furstenberg FF JR, Shea J, Allison P, et al. Contraceptive continuation among adolescents attending family planning clinics. Fam Plann Perspect 1983;15:211–214.

2. Emans SJ, Grace E, Woods ER, et al. Adolescents' compliance with the use of oral contraceptives. JAMA 1987;257:3377–3381.

3. Oakley D, Sereika S, Bogue EL. Oral contraceptive pill use after an initial visit to a family planning clinic. Fam Plann Perspect 1991;23:150–154.

4. Namerow PB, Weatherby M, Williams-Kaye J. The effectiveness of contingency-planning counseling. Fam Plann Perspect 1989;21:115–119.

5. Galen M, Lettenmaier C, Green CP. Counseling makes a difference. Pop Rep [J] No. 35.

6. Oakley D. Rethinking patient counseling techniques for changing contraceptive use behavior. Am J Ob Gyn 1994;176:1585–1590.

7. Prentice RL, Thomas DB. On the epidemiology of oral contraceptives and disease. Adv Cancer Res 1987;49:285.

8. Vessey MP, Villard-Mackintosh L, McPherson K, Yeares D. Mortality among oral contraceptive users: 20 year follow up of women in a cohort study. BMJ 1989;299:1487.

9. Petitti DB, Sidney S, Bernstein A, et al. Stroke in users of low-dose oral contraceptives. N Engl J Med 1996;335:8.

10. Buring JD. Low-dose oral contraceptives and stroke. N Engl J Med 1996;335:53.

11. Lewis MA, Spitzer WO, Heinemann LAJ, et al. Third generation oral contraceptives and risk of myocardial infarction: an international case-control study. BMJ 1996;312:88.

12. Physician's Desk Reference. 49th ed. Montvale, NJ: Medical Economics Data, 1995.

13. Kleinman EL, ed. Hormonal contraception. London: IPPF Medical Publication, 1990.

14. Kalache A, McPherson K, Barltrop K, Vessey MP. Oral contraceptives and breast cancer. Br J Hosp Med 1983;30:278.

15. Kaunitz Am, Benrubi GI, Fryldberg ER, et al. Hormonal contraception and gynecologic cancer: a clinicians guide to the epidemiologic literature. Clinician 1996;14:1.

16. Ory HW, Rosenfeld A, Landman LC. The pill at 20: An assessment. Fam Plann Perspect 1980;12:278.

17. Meirik O, Lund, E, Adami H-O, et al. Oral contraceptive use and breast cancer in young women. Lancet 1986;ii:650.

18. McPherson K, Vessey MO, Neil A, et al. Early contraceptive use and breast cancer: results of another case-control study. Br J Cancer 1987;56:653.

19. Pike MC, Henderson BE, Krailo MD, et al. Breast cancer in young women and use of oral contraceptives: possible modifying effect of formulation and age at first use. Lancet 1983;ii:926.

20. Romieu I, Willett WC, Colditz GA, et al. Prospective study of oral contraceptive use and risk of breast cancer in women. J Nat Cancer Inst 1989;81:1313.

21. UK National Case-Control Study Group. Oral contraceptive use and risk of breast cancer in young women. Lancet 1989;I:973.

22. Wingo PA, Lee NC, Ory HW, et al. Age-specific differences between oral contraceptive use and breast cancer. Obstet Gynecol 1991;78:161.

23. Paul C, Skegg DCG, Spears GFS. Oral contraceptive use and risk of breast cancer. Int J Cancer 1990;46:366.

24. Romieu I, Berlin JA, Colditz GA. Oral contraceptives and breast cancer: review and meta-analysis. Cancer 1990;66:2253.

25. Delgado-Rodriguez M, Sillero-Arenas M, Rodriguez-Contreras R, et al. Oral contraceptives and breast cancer: a meta-analysis. Rev Epidemiol Sante Publ 1991; 39:165.

26. Rushton L, Jones DR. Oral contraceptive use and breast cancer risk: a meta-analysis of variations with age at diagnosis, parity and total duration of oral contraceptive use. Br J Obstet Gynaecol 1992;99:239.

27. The Cancer and Steroid Hormone Study of the Centers for Disease Control and the National Institute of Child Health and Human Development. Oral contraceptive use and the risk of breast cancer. N Eng J Med 1986;315:405.

28. The Centers for Disease Control and Steroid Hormone Study. Long-term oral contraceptive use and the risk of breast cancer. JAMA 1983;249:1591.

29. Prentice RL, Thomas DB. On the epidemiology of oral contraceptives and disease. Adv Cancer Res 1987;49:285.

30. Johnson JH. Weighing the evidence on the pill and breast cancer. Fam Plann Perspect 1989;21:89.

31. Drife JO. The contraceptive pill and breast cancer in young women. BMJ 1989;289:1269.

32. Collaborative Group on Hormonal Factors in Breast Cancer. Breast cancer and hormonal contraceptives: collaborative reanalysis of individual data on 53,297 women with breast cancer and 100,239 women without breast cancer from 54 epidemiologic studies. Lancet 1996;347:1713.

33. Collaborative Group on Hormonal Factors in Breast Cancer. Further results. Contraception 1996; 54(suppl):1S.

34. American Cancer Society. Cancer Facts and Figures-1996. Atlanta: American Cancer Society, 1996.

35. Schlesselman JJ. Cancer of the breast and reproductive tract in relation to use of oral contraceptives. Contraception 1989;40:1.

36. The Cancer and Steroid Hormone Study of the Centers for Disease Control and the National Institute of Child Health and Human Development. The reduction in risk of ovarian cancer associated with oral contraceptive use. N Engl J Med 1987;316:650.

37. Groos TP, Schlesselman JJ. The estimated effect of oral contraceptive use on the cumulative risk of ovarian cancer. Obstet Gynecol 1994;83:419.

38. American Cancer Society. Cancer Facts and Figures-1996. Atlanta: American Cancer Society, 1996.

39. Prentice RL, Thomas DB. On the epidemiology of oral contraceptives and disease. Adv Cancer Res 1987;49:285.

40. Stergachis A. Epidemiology of the noncontraceptive effects of oral contraceptives. Am J Obstet Gynecol 1992;167:1165.

41. Mishell D. Oral contraceptives: past, present, and future perspectives. Int J Fertil 1991; 36(suppl):7.

42. Stadel BV. Oral contraceptives and cardiovascular disease. N Engl J Med 1981;305:672.

43. Gerstman BB et al. Oral contraceptive oestrogen and progestin potencies and the incidence of deep venous thromboembolism. Int J Epidemiol 1990;19:931.

44. World Health Organization Collaborative Study of Cardiovascular disease and Steroid Hormone Contraception. Venous thromboembolic disease and combined oral contraceptives: results of international multicentre case-control study. lancet 1995; 346:1575.

45. World Health Organization Collaborative Study of Cardiovascular disease and Steroid Hormone Contraception. Effect of different progestagens in low oestrogen oral contraceptives on venous thromboembolic disease. Lancet 1995;346:1582.

46. Jick H, Jick SS, Gurewich V, et al. Risk of idiopathic cardiovascular death and nonfatal venous thromboembolism in women using oral contraceptives with differing progestins. Lancet 1995;346:1589.

47. Spitzer WO, Lewis MA, Heinemann LAJ, et al. Third generation oral contraceptives and risk of venous thromboembolic disorders: an international case-control study. BMJ 1996;312:83.

48. Lidegaard O, Milsom I. Oral contraceptives and thrombotic diseases: impact of new epidemiologic studies. Contraception 1996;53:135.

49. Jamin C, de Mouzon J. Selective prescribing of third generation oral contraceptives (Ocs). Contraception 1996;54:55.

50. Spitzer WO. Data from transnational study of oral contraceptives have been misused. BMJ 1995;311:1162. Letter.

51. MacRae K, Kaye C. Third generation oral contraceptive pills: is the scare over the increased risk of thrombosis justified? BMJ 1995;311:1112. Editorial.

52. Farmer RDT, Preston TD. The risk of venous thromboembolism associated with low oestrogen oral contraceptives. J Obstet Gynecol 1995;15:195.

53. Bloemenkamp KWM, Rosendaal FR, Helmerhorst FM, et al. Enhancement by factor V Leiden mutation of risk of deep vein thrombosis associated with oral contraceptives. Lancet 1995; 346:1593.

54. Alving B, Comp P. Recent advances in understanding clotting and evaluating patients with recurrent thrombosis. Am J Obstet Gynecol 1992;167:1184.

55. Speroff L, DeCherney A, Burkman RT Jr, et al. Evaluation of a new

generation of oral contraceptives. Obstet Gynecol 1993;81:1034.

56. Comp PC, Thurnau GR, Welsh J, et al. Functional and immunologic protein S levels are decreased during pregnancy. Blood 1986;69:692.

57. Alving B, Comp P. Recent advances in understanding clotting and evaluating patients with recurrent thrombosis. Am J Obstet Gynecol 1992;167:1184.

58. Kolodziej M, Comp PC. Hypercoaguable states due to natural anticoagulant deficiencies. In: Anderson JW, ed. Current Opinion in Hematology. Philadelphia: Current Science, 1993:301.

59. Koster T, Rosendaal FR, de Ronde H, et al. Venous thrombosis due to poor anticoagulant response to activated protein C.: Leiden Thrombophilia Study. Lancet 1993;342:1503.

60. Cumming AM, Tait RC, Fildes S, et al. Development of resistance to activated protein C during pregnancy. Br J Haematol 1995; 90:725.

61. Vandenbrouke JP, Koster T, Briet E, et al. Increased risk of venous thrombosis in oral-contraceptive users who are carriers of factor V Leiden mutation. Lancet 1994; 344:1453.

62. Altes A, Souto JC, Mateo J, Borrell M, Fontcuberta J. Activated protein C resistance assay when applied in the general population. Am J Obstet Gynecol 1996;176:358.

63. Burkman RT. Modern trends in contraception. Obstet Gynecol Clin North Am 1990;17:759.

64. Larsson G, Milsom I, Linstedt G, Rybo G. The influence of a low-dose combined oral contraceptive on menstrual blood loss and iron status. Contraception 1992;46: 327.

65. Milsom I, Sundell G, Andersch B. The influence of different combined oral contraceptives on the prevalence and severity of dysmenorrhea. Contraception 1990; 42:497.

66. Dawood MY. Dysmenorrhea. Clin Obstet Gynecol 1983;26:719.

67. Klein JR, Litt IF. Epidemiology of adolescent dysmenorrhea. Pediatrics 1981;68:661.

68. Chan WY, Dawood MY. Prostaglandin levels in menstrual fluid of nondysmenorrheic and of dysmenorrheic subjects with or without oral contraceptive or ibuprofen therapy. Adv Prostaglandin Res 1980;8:1443.

69. Peterson HB, Lee NC. The health effects of oral contraceptives: misperceptions, controversies, and continuing good news. Clin Obstet Gynecol 1989;32:339.

70. Burkman RT. Modern trends in contraception. Obstet Gynecol Clin North Am 1990;17:759.

71. Droegemueller W, Katta LR, Bright TG, et al. Triphasic Randomized Clinical Trial: comparative frequency of intermenstrual bleeding. Am J Obstet Gynecol 1989;161:1407.

72. Saleh WA, Burkman RT, Zacur HA, et al. A randomized trial of three oral contraceptives: comparison of bleeding patterns by oral contraceptive type and steroid level. Am J Obstet Gynecol 1993;168:1740.

73. Vessey MP, Doll R, Peto R, et al. A long-term follow-up study of women using different methods of contraception: an interim report. J Biosoc Sci 1976;8:375.

74. Ory H, Cole P, MacMahon B, et al. Oral contraceptives and reduced risk of benign breast diseases. N Engl J Med 1976;294:419.

75. Hislop TG, Threlfall WJ. Oral contraceptives and benign breast disease. Am J Epidemiol 1984; 120:273.

76. Pastides H, Kelsey JL, LiVolsi, et al. Oral contraceptives and fibrocystic breast disease with special reference to its histopathology. J Natl Cancer Inst 1983;71:5.

77. Charreau I, Plu-Bureau G, Bachelot A, et al. Oral contraceptive use and risk of benign breast disease in a French case-control

study. Eur J Cancer Prev 1993; 2:147.

78. Royal College of General Practitioners' Oral Contraception Study. Effect of hypertension and benign breast disease of progestagen component in combined oral contraceptives. Lancet 1977;1:624.

79. Brinton LA, Vessey MP, Flavel R, et al. Risk factors for benign breast disease. Am J Epidemiol 1981;113:203.

80. Peterson HB, Lee NC. The health effects of oral contraceptives: misperceptions, controversies, and continuing good news. Clin Obstet Gynecol 1989;32:339.

81. Prentice RL, Thomas DB. On the epidemiology of oral contraceptives and disease. Adv Cancer Res 1987;49:285.

82. Holt VL, Daling JR, McKnight B, et al. Functional ovarian cysts in relation to the use of monophasic and triphasic oral contraceptives. Obstet Gynecol 1992;79:529.

83. Washington AE, Gove S, Scgacter J, et al. Oral contraceptives, Chlamydia trachomatis infection and pelvic inflammatory disease: a word of caution about protection. JAMA 1985;252:2246.

84. Handsfield HH, Jansen LL, Robert PL, et al. Criteria for selective screening for Chlamydia trachomatis infection in women attending family planning clinics. JAMA 1986;255:1730.

85. Wolner-Hanssen P, Svensson L, Mardh P, et al. Laparoscopic findings and contraceptive use in women with signs and symptoms suggestive of acute salpingitis. Obstet Gynecol 1985;66:233.

86. Wolner-Hanssen P, Eschenbach DA, Paavonen J, et al. Decreased risk of symptomatic chlamydial pelvic inflammatory disease associated with oral contraceptive use. JAMA 1990;263:54.

87. Svensson L, Westrom L, Mardh PA. Contraceptives and acute salpingitis. JAMA 1984;215: 2553.

88. Plummer FA, Simonsen JN, Cameron DW, et al. Co-factors in

male-female sexual transmission of human immunodeficiency virus type 1. J Infect Dis 1991;163: 233.

89. European Study Group. Risk factors for male to female transmission of HIV. BMJ 1989;298: 411.

90. Compston JE. HRT and osteoporosis. In: Khaw KT, ed. Hormone replacement therapy. Edinburgh: Churchill Livingstone, 1992:309.

91. Reproductive health in the perimenopause. Contracept Rep 1993;4:1.

92. DeCherney A. Bone-sparing properties of oral contraceptives. Am J Obstet Gynecol 1996;174:15.

93. Kritz-Silverstrin D, Barrett-Connor E. Bone mineral density in postmenopausal women as determined by oral contraceptive use. Am J Public Health 1993;34: 333.

94. Kleerekoper M, Brienza RS, Schultz LR, et al. Oral contraceptives use may protect against low bone mass: Henry Ford Hospital Osteoporosis Cooperative Research Group. Arch Intern Med 1991;151:1971.

95. Lindsay R, Tohme J, Kanders B. The effect of oral contraceptive use on vertebral bone mass in pre- and postmenopausal women. Contraception 1986;34:333.

96. Krettek SE, Arkin SI, Chaisilwattana P, et al. Chlamydia trachomatis in patients who used oral contraceptives and had intermenstrual spotting. Obstet Gynecol 1993;81:728.

97. Anderson FD. Selectivity and minimal androgenicity of norgestimate in monophasic and triphasic oral contraceptives. Acta Obstet Gynecol Scand 1992; 71(suppl 156):15.

98. Corson SL. Efficacy and clinical profile of a new oral contraceptive containing norgestimate: US clinical trials. Acta Obstet Gynecol Scand 1990;(suppl 152):25.

99. Mattson RH, Rebar RW. Contraceptive methods for women with neurologic disorders. Am J Obstet Gynecol 1993;168:2027.

100. Reinprayoon D. Intrauterine contraception. Curr Opin Obstet Gynecol 1992;4:527.

101. Ortho 1995 Annual Birth Control Study. Raritan, NJ: Ortho Pharmaceutical Corporation, 1995.

102. Forrest JD. Acceptability of IUDs in the United States. In: Bardin CW, Mishell DR Jr, eds. Proceedings from the Fourth International Conference on IUDs. Boston, MA, Butterworth-Heinemann, 1994.

103. Kookier CH, Scutchfield FD. Barriers to prescribing the copper T 380A intrauterine device by physicians. West J Med 1990; 153:279.

104. Tatum HJ. Milestones in intrauterine device development. Fertil Steril 1983;39:141.

105. Potts DM, Champiion CB, Kozuh-Novak M, et al. IUDs and PID. A comparative trial of strings versus stringless devices. Adv Contracept 1991;7:251.

106. Farley TMM, Rosenberg MJ, Rowe PJ, et al. Intrauterine devices and pelvic inflammatory disease: an international perspective. Lancet 1992;339:785.

107. Lee NC, Rubin GL, Borucki R. The intrauterine device and pelvic inflammatory disease revisited: new results from the Women's Health Study. Obstet Gynecol 1988;72:1.

108. Walsh TL, Bernstein GS, Grimes DA, et al. Effect of prophylactic antibiotics on morbidity associated with IUD insertion: results of a pilot randomized controlled trial. IUD Study Group. Contraception 1994;50:319.

109. World Health Organization. Mechanism of action, safety and efficacy of intrauterine devices. Geneva, Switzerland, World Health Organization, 1987. Technical Report Series, 753.

110. Speroff L, Darney PD. A Clinical Guide for Contraception. 2nd ed. Baltimore, MD: Williams & Wilkins, 1996.

111. Milsom I, Andersson K, Jonasson K, et al. The influence of the Gyne-T 390s IUD on menstrual blood loss and iron status. Contraception 1995;52:175.

112. Lewit S. Outcome of pregnancy with intrauterine devices. Contraception 1970;2:47.

113. Foreman H, Stadel BV, Schlesselman S. Intrauterine device usage and fetal loss. Obstet Gynecol 1981;58:669.

114. Chaim W, Mazor M. Pregnancy with an intrauterine device in situ and preterm delivery. Arch Gynecol Obstet 1992;252:21.

115. Layde PM, Goldberg MF, Safra MJ, et al. Failed intrauterine device contraception and limb reduction deformities: a case-control study. Fertil Steril 1979;31:18.

116. Vessey MP, Lawless M, McPherson K, et al. Fertility after stopping use of the intrauterine contraceptive device. BMJ 1983; 286:106.

117. Wilson JC. A prospective New Zealand study of fertility after removal of copper intrauterine contraceptive devices for conception and because of complications: a four-year study. Am J Obstet Gynecol 1992;166: 1208.

118. Cramer DW, Schiff I, Schoenbaum S, et al. Tubal infertility and the intrauterine device. N Engl J Med 1985;312: 941.

119. Belhadj H, Sivin I, Diaz S, et al. Recovery of fertility after use of the levonorgestrel 20mcg/d or copper T 380Ag intrauterine device. Contraception 1986;34:261.

120. Brache V, Alvarez-Sanchez F, Faundes A, et al. Ovarian endocrine function through five years of continuous treatment with Norplant subdermal contraceptive implants. Contraception 1990;41:169.

121. Hatasaka H. Implantable levonorgestrel contraception: 4 years of experience with Norplant. Clin Obstet Gynecol 1995;38:859.

122. Sivin I. Contraception with NOR-PLANT implants. Hum Reprod 1994;9:1818.

123. Sivin I. International experience with Norplant and Norplant-2 contraceptives. Stud Fam Plann 1988;19:81.

124. Frank ML, Poindexter AN III, Corin LM, et al. One-year experience with subdermal implants in the United States. Contraception 1993;48:229.

125. Darney PD, Klaisle CM, Tanner ST, et al. Sustained release contraceptives. In: Ryan KJ, Barbiere RB, Berek JB, eds. Current problems in obstetrics, gynecology and fertility. Chicago: Mosby-Year Book, 1990:87.

126. Walsman S, ed. NORPLANT Levonorgestrel implants: a summary of scientific data. New York: The Population Council, 1990.

127. Darney PD, Atkinson E, Tanner ST, et al. Acceptance and perceptions of Norplant among users in San Francisco, USA. Stud Fam Plann 1990;21:152.

128. Diaz S, Croxatto HB, Pavez M, et al. Clinical assessment of treatments for prolonged bleeding in users of Norplant implants. Contraception 1990;42:97.

129. Alvarez-Sanchez F, Brache V, Thevenin F, et al. Hormonal treatment for bleeding irregularities in Norplant implant users. Am J Obstet Gynecol 1996;174:919.

130. Ortiz A, Hiroi M, Stanczyk FZ, et al. Serum MPA (MPA) concentrations and ovarian function following intramuscular injection of Depo-MPA. J Clin Endocrinol Metab 1977;44:32.

131. Koetsawang S, Shrimanker K, Fotherby K. Blood levels of medroxyprogesterone acetate after multiple injections of depoprovera or cycloprovera. Contraception 1979;20:1.

132. Mishell DR, Kletzky OA, Brenner PF, et al. The effect of contraceptive steroids on hypothalamic-pituitary function. Am J Obstet Gynecol 1977;128:60.

133. WHO Task Force on Long-Acting Systemic Agents for Fertility Regulation. Special programme of research, development and research training in human reproduction: a multicentred phase III comparative clinical trial of depot medroxyprogesterone acetate given three-monthly at doses of 100 mg or 150 mg. I: contraceptive efficacy and side effects. Contraception 1986;34:223.

134. Trussel J, Kost K. Contraceptive failure in the United States: a critical review of the literature. Stud Fam Plann 1987;18:237.

135. Siriwingse T, Snidvongs W, Tantayaporn P, et al. Effect of Depo-medroxyprogesterone acetate on variuos cycle days. Contraception 1982;26:487.

136. Fotherby K, Koetsawang S, Marthrubutham M. Pharmacokinetic study of different doses of Depo provera. Contraception 1980;22:527.

137. Schwallie PC, Assenzo JR. Contraceptive use efficacy study utilizing medroxyprogesterone acetate administered as an intramuscular injection once every 90 days. Fertil Steril 1973;24:331.

138. Ceulaer K, Gruber C, Hayes R, et al. Medroxyprogesterone acetate and homozygous sickle-cell disease. Lancet 1982;2:229.

139. Topppzada M, Onsy FA, Fares E, et al. The protective effect of progestogen-only contraception against vaginal moniliasis. Contraception 1979;20:99.

140. Gray RH. Reduced risk of pelvic inflammatory disease with injectable contraceptives. Lancet 1985;1:1046. Letter.

141. WHO Collaborative Study of Neoplasia and Steroid Contraceptives. Depot-medroxyprogesterone acetate (DMPA) and risk of endometrial cancer. Int J Cancer 1991;49:191.

142. Mattson RH, Cramer JA, Caldwell BV, et al. Treatment of seizures with medroxyprogesterone acetate: preliminary report. Neurology 1984;34:1255.

143. Fraser IS, Weisberg E. A comprehensive review of injectable contraceptives, with special emphasis on depot medroxyprogesterone. Med J Aust 1981;1:1.

144. Belsey EM. Taskforce on Long-Acting Systemic Agents for Fertility Regulation, WHO Special Programme of Research in Human Reproduction. The association between vaginal bleeding patterns and reasons for the discontinuation of contraceptive use. Contraception 1988;38:207.

145. Fraser IS. A survey of different attitudes to the management of menstrual disturbance in women using injectable contraceptives. Contraception 1983;28:385.

146. Pardthiassong T, Gray RH, McDaniel EB. Return of fertility after discontinuation of depot medroxyprogesterone acetate and intrauterine devices in Northern Thailand. Lancet 1980;1:509.

147. Pardthiassong T. Return of fertility after use of the injectable contraceptive Depo Provera: an updated analysis. J Biosoc Sci 1984;16:23.

148. Cundy T, Evans M, Roberts H, et al. Bone density in women receiving depot medroxyprogesterone acetate for contraception. BMJ 1994;308:247.

149. Fraser IS, Holck S. Depot Medroxyprogesterone acetate. In: Mishell DR Jr, ed. Long acting steroid contraception. New York: Raven Press, 1983:1.

150. Mishell DR Jr. Contraception, sterilization, and pregnancy termination. In: Herbst A, Mishell DR Jr, Stenchever M, et al, eds. Comprehensive gynecology. 2nd ed. St Louis: Mosby-Year Book, Inc., 1992:300–301.

151. Tagg PI. The diaphragm: barrier contraception has a new social role. Nurse Pract 1995;20:36–42.

152. Hatcher R, Trussell J, Stewart F, et al. Contraceptive technology. 16th rev. ed. New York: Irvington, 1995:191–211.

153. d'Oro LC, Parazzini F, Naldi L, LaVecchia C. Barrier methods of

contraception, spermicides, and sexually transmitted diseases: a review. Genitourin Med 1994;70: 410–417.

154. Austin H, Louv WC, Alexander J. A case-control study of spermicides and gonorrhea. JAMA 1984;251:2822–2824.

155. Bradbeer CS, Thin RN, Thirumorrthy T. Prophylaxis against infection in Singaporean prostitutes. Genitourin Med 1988;64:52–53.

156. Corson SL, et al. eds. Fertility control. Boston: Little, Brown, 1985:223–239.

157. Koch J. The experience of 372 women using the Prentif contraceptive cervical cap. Distributed to the International Cervical Cap Symposium, Atlanta, May 1983.

158. Boehm D. The cervical cap: effectiveness as a contraceptive. J Nurse Midwife 1983;28:3.

159. Yarros RS. Report of the Illinois Birth Control League, Chicago, 1927.

160. Denniston GC. Presented to meeting of Planned Parenthood Physicians. Denver, October 1980.

161. High rates of pregnancy and dissatisfaction mark first cervical cap trial. Fam Plann Perspect 1981;13:48.

162. Coker AL, Hulka BS, McCann MF, Walton LA. Barrier methods of contraception and cervical intraepithelia neoplasia. Contraception 1992;45:1–10.

163. Parazzini F. Negri E, La Vecchia, et al. Barrier methods of contraception and the risk of cervical neoplasia. Contraception 1989; 40:519–530.

164. Radius SM, Joffe A, Gall MJ. Barrier versus oral contraceptive use: a study of female college students. J Am Col Health 1991; 40:83–85.

165. Scott JR, DiSaia P, Hammond C, et al, eds. Obstetrics and gynecology. 6th ed. Philadelphia: JB Lippincott, 1990:709–713.

166. Gollub EL, Stein ZA. Commentary: the new female condom

item 1 on a women's AIDS prevention agenda. Am J Public Health 1993;83:498–500.

167. Update: barrier protection against HIV infection and other sexually transmitted diseases. MMWR 1993;42:589–597.

168. The female condom. Med Let Drugs Ther 1993;35:123–124.

169. Femidom: a condom for women. Drug Ther Bull 1993;31:15–16.

170. Faundes A, Elias C, Coggins C, et al. Spermicides and barrier contraception. Curr Opin Obstet Gynecol 1994;6:552–558.

171. Harlap S, Kost K, Forrest JD. Preventing pregnancy, protecting health: a new look at birth control choices in the United States. New York: The Alan Guttmacher Institute, 1991.

172. South-to-South Cooperation in Reproductive Health. Consensus statement on emergency contraception. Contraception 1995;52: 211.

173. Trussell J, Stewart F, Guest F, et al. Emergency contraceptive pills: a simple proposal to reduce unintended pregnancies. Fam Plann Perspect 1992;24:269.

174. Derman SG, Peralta LM. Postcoital contraception: present and future options. J Adolesc Health 1995;16:6.

175. Ellertson C. History and efficacy of emergency contraception: beyond Coca-Cola. Fam Plann Perspect 1996;28:44.

176. The American College of Obstetricians and Gynecologists. Emergency contraception. In: ACOG Practice Patterns Washington, DC: ACOG, December 1996.

177. Grou F, Rodrigues I. The morning-after-pill—how long after? Am J Obstet Gynecol 1994;171:1529.

178. Haspels AA. Emergency contraception: a review. Contraception 1994;50:101.

179. Swahn ML, Westlund P, Johannison E, et al. Effect of postcoital contraceptive methods

on the endometrium and the menstrual cycle. Acta Obstet Gynecol Scand 1996;75:738.

180. Trussell J, Stewart F. The effectiveness of postcoital hormonal contraception. Fam Plann Perspect 1992;24:262.

181. Glasier A, Thong KJ, Dewar M, et al. Mifepristone (RU 486) compared with high-dose estrogen and progestogen for emergency postcoital contraception. N Engl J Med 1992;327:1041.

182. Food and Drug Administration. Prescription drug products: certain combined oral contraceptives for use as postcoital emergency contraception. Federal Register 1997;62:8610.

183. Bracken MB. Oral contraception and congenital malformations in offspring: a review and meta-analysis of the prospective studies. Obstet Gynecol 1990; 76:552.

184. Ho PC, Kwan MSW. A prospective randomized comparison of levonorgestrel with the Yuzpe regimen in postcoital contraception. Human Reprod 1993;8: 389.

185. Barnhart KT, Sondheimer SJ. Emergency contraception. Curr Opin Obstet Gynecol 1994;6: 559.

186. Fasoli M, Parazzini F, Cecchetti G, et al. Postcoital contraception: an overview of published studies. Contraception 1989;39:459.

187. Trussell J, Ellerston C. The efficacy of emergency contraception. Fertil Control Rev 1995;4:8.

188. Ortho 1995 Annual Birth Control Study. Raritan, NJ: Ortho Pharmaceutical Corporation, 1995.

189. Peterson HB, Xia Z, Hughes JM, et al. The risk of pregnancy after tubal sterilization: findings from the US Collaborative Review of Sterilization. Am J Obstet Gynecol 1996;174:1161.

190. Trussell J, Hatcher RA, Cates W Jr, et al. A guide to interpreting contraceptive efficacy studies. Obstet Gynecol 1990;76:558.

Chapter 38

Prevention and Treatment of Sexually Transmitted Diseases and Vaginitis

Carol London

Sexually transmitted diseases (STDs) are a group of infections whose major mode of transmission is sexual contact. In this chapter, we will discuss the prevention, diagnosis, and treatment of the most common STDs: gonorrhea, syphilis, chlamydia, herpes, and condyloma. HIV and hepatitis B are also sexually transmitted, and preventive strategies are similar for these infections. However, it is beyond the scope of this chapter to cover the diagnosis and treatment of HIV and hepatitis B. The two most common causes of vaginitis, yeast and bacterial vaginosis, although not sexually transmitted, will also be covered.

In addition, there are minor and less common STDs: lymphogranuloma venereum, granuloma inguinale, chancroid, pediculosis pubis, scabies, molluscum contagiosum, and trichomoniasis. The symptoms, diagnosis, and treatment of these less common diseases are covered in Table 38-1.

Diagnostic and treatment regimens are based on current recommendations at the time of this publication. Since this is a rapidly changing field, the clinician may keep current by utilizing the latest Center for Disease Control (CDC) treatment guidelines.

EPIDEMIOLOGY

In the early 1990s, there was a decline in the incidence of syphilis, gonorrhea, and chlamydia (1). Unfortunately, the increase in the viral STDs, herpes and condyloma, has far surpassed the incidence of all the others combined (2). Traditional public health preventive measures—screening, treatment, contact tracing, and safer sex guidelines—have worked well in combating the bacterial diseases. These methods have

not worked as well for the viral STDs, because of their chronic nature and the lack of curative treatments. Until cures for these diseases are found, it is unlikely we will see much slowing in the epidemic of herpes and condyloma. While the mortality from these diseases will never approach that of AIDS or hepatitis B, the impact on individuals and society in terms of financial and social loss is considerable. It is critical for practitioners in primary care, pediatrics, and obstetrics/gynecology to be skilled in the prevention, screening, and management of STDs.

SEXUAL HISTORY

The cornerstone of screening for STDs is taking an adequate sexual history. While clinicians agree that this is an important part of history taking, most studies show that clinician performance in this area is poor (3). Many reasons have been cited: time limitations, lack of comfort by the clinician, perceived discomfort of the patient, and lack of understanding of risk factors (4). However, studies also show that patients wish to discuss their concerns about STDs and are relieved when clinicians raise the issue (5).

The initial step in any clinician-patient relationship is establishing a rapport and an atmosphere of trust and shared responsibility for the patient's health. Sexuality in our society is a value-laden area. Understanding our own values and beliefs may help us provide nonjudgmental and appropriate care to patients whose values or beliefs may differ from our own.

A sexual history can be obtained in many ways. Basic information is most easily and efficiently obtained by incorpo-

Table 38-1 Symptoms, Diagnosis, and Treatment of Less Common Sexually Transmitted Diseases

Disease (Organism)	Symptoms	Diagnosis	Treatment Choices
Chancroid (*H. ducreyi*)	multiple painful genital ulcers	culture; rule out other causes of genital ulcers	• azithromycin 1 gm PO, single dose • ceftriaxone 250 mg IM, single dose • ciprofloxacin 500 mg b.i.d × 3 days • erythromycin base 500 mg PO q.i.d. × 7 days
Lymphogranuloma venereum (*C. trachomatis*)	transient genital ulcer, inguinal lymphadenopathy	clinical	• doxycycline 100 mg PO b.i.d. × 21 days • erythromycin 500 mg PO q.i.d. × 21 days
Granuloma inguinale (*Calymmatobacterium granulomatis*)	beefy red painless ulcers	biopsy, stain for Donovan bodies	• trimethoprim-sulfa methoxazole DS 1 PO b.i.d × 21 days • doxycycline 100 mg PO × 21 days • ciprofloxacin 750 mg PO b.i.d. × 21 days • erythromycin 500 mg PO q.i.d × 21 days
Trichomoniasis (*T. vaginalis*)	irritating, frothy yellow/green discharge	saline wet mount for motile organisms	• metronidazole 2 g PO, single dose • metronidazole 500 mg b.i.d. × 7 days
Molluscum contagiosum (pox virus)	waxy papules with central cores	clinical stain for inclusion bodies	• curretage • cryotherapy
Pediculosis pubis (*Phthicus pubis*)	pruritis, presense of nits, lice	observation of nits, lice	• permethrin 1% cream, apply and rinse after 10 min • lindane 1% shampoo, apply and rinse after 4 min • pyrethrins with piperonyl butoxide, apply from the neck down and rinse after 8 to 14 hr
Scabies (*Sarcoptes scabiei*)	pruritis, burrows	skin scraping for mites	• lindane 1%, 10 g lotion or 30 g cream, applied from the neck down and rinse after 8 hr

rating it into a patient history questionnaire, which may be filled out prior to the visit. This information can then be reviewed during the visit and any issues can be addressed. A sample sexual history questionnaire is shown in Table 38-2.

A screening history for sexually transmitted diseases should include sexual preference. The incidence of gonorrhea and chlamydia are low in lesbian women, but herpes and condyloma are seen in this population. It is important to ask about any sexual contact with men in the past, to avoid missing possible risk factors.

Contraceptive Method and Risk of STDs

The method of contraception utilized can affect the risk of aquiring STDs. Barrier methods of contraception (condoms and diaphragm) have been shown to decrease transmission of some STDs (6). Oral contraceptives and intrauterine devices may increase risk in some instances (7). If a patient is using a barrier method, any problems or lapses in use should be discussed in order to fully assess risk.

Sexual Relationships

Clinicians should discuss the number and timing of sexual relationships, as this can affect treatment strategies. For example, a woman exposed to a partner with syphilis within the past 3 months would require preventive treatment as well as screening. Exposure more than 3 months prior would

Table 38-2 Sample Sexual History Questionnaire

Sexual preference
Male partners(s) ____past____present
Female partners(s) ____past____present
Sexual relationships
Length of current relationships(s) ____
Monogamous____non-monogamous____
Last sexual contact ____
Last prior sexual contact ____
Number of lifetime sexual partners ____
Past history of sexually transmitted diseases
gonorrhea ____   genital warts ____
chlamydia ____   genital herpes ____
syphilis ____   other ____
Sexual practices
anal intercourse ____
oral sex ____
other ____

require screening and treatment only if infected. The number of partners will clearly affect treatment and teaching strategies. Timing of the last sexual encounter is also significant in its risk for possible pregnancy.

Past History of STDs

Past history may affect screening, teaching focus, and long-term follow-up. It is important when taking a history of previous STDs that clinicians be familiar with lay terms for these infections in order to obtain a full history (8).

Sexual Practices

Some sexual practices increase the risk of contracting an STD if exposed. Because mucous membranes are fragile, anal intercourse increases the risk of contracting most STDs. The practice of having anal followed by vaginal or oral intercourse increases the likelihood of spreading enteric infections.

PRIMARY PREVENTION OF STDS

The goal of primary prevention is avoidance of disease. Strategies for preventing STDs include condom and spermicide use, limiting sexual partners, and safer sexual practices. Hepatitis B is the only sexually transmitted infection for which a vaccine, a traditional primary prevention strategy, is available. All sexually active women should be offered vaccination. Advances in vaccine research continue to offer the hope of an effective primary preventive strategy for other STDs. Currently, research is underway for a vaccine for the herpes and human papilloma viruses (9,10).

SECONDARY PREVENTION OF STDS

Secondary prevention of STDs is aimed at rapid diagnosis and treatment of infected individuals. Patients who present with symptoms, or who are sexual contacts of someone with a known or suspected case of an STD should be screened. Women with suspected STDs should have a thorough physical examination including careful inspection for genital herpes and condyloma, both of which may be relatively asymptomatic and for which no screening tests are available. As part of the examination, screening for gonorrhea, chlamydia, and syphilis should be performed, and HIV counselling and testing offered. Prompt treatment should be initiated. Patients should be instructed to avoid sexual contact until treatment is complete and any follow-up testing is accomplished.

Sexually transmitted diseases should be reported to public health departments. The current reportable STDs are: gonorrhea, chlamydia, syphilis, chancroid, lymphogranuloma venereum, and granuloma inguinale. Many states offer free and easily accessible treatment for women with STDs and their partners. Notification of partners is an important part of prevention for the individual (to avoid reinfection) and the greater community (to reduce the number of new cases). Clinicians can work with patients by identifying possible infected partners and assisting patients in informing their sexual contacts. Discussing ways to inform partners, providing written information, and role playing are all possible strategies. For reportable STDs, contact tracing by public health workers is done in some areas.

BACTERIAL STDS

Gonorrhea

Infection with *Neisseria gonorrhoeae*, although decreasing in recent years, still accounts for a million cases of STDs each year in the United States (11). Symptoms of gonorrhea are often subtle or absent in women. Because of this, many women do not seek treatment until complications such as pelvic inflammatory disease have developed.

Screening

All sexually active adolescents, women with multiple sexual partners, and those who do not use condoms should routinely be screened. Patients at high risk (multiple sexual partners, unsafe sexual practices) should be offered screening every 3 to 6 months. All pregnant women should be screened in the first trimester. If infected or at high risk, screening should be performed at least once again in the third trimester. Women with a sexual partner with gonorrhea should be tested and treated.

Diagnosis

Women with uncomplicated gonorrhea may occasionally present with complaints of yellow vaginal discharge. Upon examination, mucopurulent cervicitis may be present. Symptoms usually develop within 2 weeks of exposure. Cervical culture for gonorrhea is diagnostic. Because of the varied flora of the vagina, Gram's stain is not an accurate tool for diagnosis.

Treatment

Recommended treatment regimens are aimed at curing disease and preventing transmission of disease or the development of complications. Over the years, the emergence of gonorrhea strains resistant to penicillin, spectinomycin, and tetracycline has eliminated the use of these antibiotics as routine therapy. The newer cephalosporins and fluoroquinolones allow for single-dose cost-effective treatments with improved compliance and few side effects. The 1997 CDC treatment regimen for uncomplicated gonorrhea (12) is a choice of a single dose of one of the following: cefixime 400 mg PO; ceftriaxone 125 mg IM; ciprofloxacin 500 mg PO; ofloxacin 400 mg PO.

The selected treatment should be combined with an effective regimen for presumptive coinfection with chlamydia.

Pregnant women should be treated with a recommended cephalosporin. If a pregnant woman is unable to tolerate a cephalosporin, 2 g of spectinomycin IM should be given. Azithromycin or amoxicillin should be given for presumptive coinfection with chlamydia.

Follow-up

All sexual partners within 60 days should be tested and treated. Patients should be seen 1 week after treatment for re-culture and re-interview to assure adequate treatment of sexual partners. One month follow-up visits are also encouraged since this is the time period in which women run the highest risk of reinfection from untreated sexual partners. At each visit, guidelines for safer sex should be reviewed and the patient's own plan for implementing safer sex practices should be reinforced.

Chlamydia

With the advent of simpler more accurate screening for chlamydia infections, a more accurate picture of the incidence of chlamydia has been determined (13). The high incidence of chlamydia coupled with the frequency of silent pelvic infection and its sequelae of infertility and chronic pelvic pain point to the need for adequate screening, diagnosis, and treatment.

Screening

As with gonorrhea, all sexually active adolescents and women with multiple sexual partners who are not using condoms should be routinely screened. All pregnant women should be screened in the first trimester. Infected or at-risk pregnant women should be retested in the third trimester. Women with a sexual partner with chlamydia should be tested and treated.

Diagnosis

Occasionally women will present with a complaint of increased vaginal discharge with or without accompanying itching or irritation. If any symptoms develop, they will be present within 2 weeks of the exposure. Mucopurulent cervicitis may or may not be present. The gold standard for diagnosis remains the culture. Because of the fastidious nature of the organism, in some settings the use of culture is not practical. Culture continues to be recommended in cases with legal ramifications such as rape or child abuse.

The ELISA, immunofluorescent, and polymerase chain reaction (PCR) technology for testing all compare favorably with culture in detecting chlamydia (14). The use of these tests has greatly improved the ability of clinicians to provide routine testing.

Treatment

Treatment regimens selected should provide cure and protect against development of sequelae. Doxycycline has been the standard treatment and is effective and low cost. A newer antibiotic, azithromycin, provides convenient single-dose therapy.

The 1997 CDC treatment guidelines (15) are a choice of: azithromycin 1 g PO, single dose, or doxycycline 100 mg, twice a day for 7 days.

Alternative choices are erythromycin base 500 mg PO, four times a day for 7 days; erythromycin ethyl succinate 800 mg PO, four times a day for 7 days; or ofloxacin 300 mg PO, twice a day for 7 days.

Recommended regimens for pregnant women are a choice of:

- erythromycin base 500 mg PO, four times a day for 7 days, or amoxicillin 500 mg PO, three times a day for 7 days. Alternative choices are erythromycin base 250 mg PO, four times a day for 14 days;

- erythromycin ethylsuccinate 800 mg PO, four times a day for 7 days; or

- azithromycin 1 gm PO, single dose.

Initial data on the safety of azithromycin in pregnancy is reassuring. However, because of the limited follow-up data, the CDC does not currently recommend it for first-line therapy.

Follow-up

Sexual contacts within 60 days should be tested and treated. Test of cure for chlamydia is not considered necessary because treatment failure with these regimens is so low. In addition, false positives in repeat tests done in less than 3 weeks is possible. However, follow-up at 4 weeks is advisable to detect reinfection.

Pelvic Inflammatory Disease

Pelvic inflammatory disease (PID) is a broad term for several upper genital tract disorders including endometritis, salpingitis, tubo-ovarian abscess, and pelvic peritonitis. PID is a serious complication of gonorrhea or chlamydia. These two conditions account for the majority of cases of PID. Other anaerobes such as *Gardnerella vaginalis, Haemophilus influenzae*, enteric gram-negative rods and *Streptococcus agalactiae* have been implicated as coinfective agents (16). The use of an intrauterine device and therapeutic abortion have also been identified as risk factors in the development of PID (17).

Diagnosis

PID is a difficult diagnosis to make because of the spectrum of symptoms that may be present. Unfortunately, the symptoms of PID may be mild and can mimic other disorders. Delay in treatment can lead to more serious sequelae. Because of the impact of PID on long-term health, clinicians should have a low threshold for considering PID and initiating treatment in women with lower abdominal pain (18).

The following CDC guidelines are helpful in making a diagnosis of PID. The minimum criteria are lower abdominal tenderness, adnexal tenderness, and cervical motion tenderness. Treatment for PID should be instituted if these criteria are present and no other cause has been found.

Additional criteria that may support the diagnosis include: oral temperature above 38.0°C, abnormal cervical or vaginal discharge, elevated erythrocyte sedimentation rate, elevated C reactive protein, and positive test for chlamydia or gonorrhea.

The definitive criteria for PID are:

- histopathologic evidence or endometritis on endometrial biopsy

- transvaginal sonography or other imaging techniques showing thickened fluid-filled tubes with or without free pelvic fluid or tubo-ovarian complex

- laparoscopic abnormalities consistent with PID

Treatment

Treatment regimens selected must be broad spectrum in order to cover the most common pathogens. Even when chlamydia and gonorrhea cultures from the cervix are negative, the organisms may still be present elsewhere in the reproductive tract, and therefore need to be covered by the antibiotic chosen. Opinions of experts differ as to whether hospitalizing patients improves outcomes.

The CDC guidelines suggest two oral regimens that have been shown to provide broad-spectrum coverage for the common pathogens in PID (19). Regimen A consists of ofloxacin 400 mg PO twice a day for 14 days, plus metronidazole 500 mg PO twice a day for 14 days. Regimen B consists of doxycyline 100 mg PO every 12 hours for 14 days, plus one of the following: a single dose of ceftriaxone 250 mg IM; or a single dose of cefoxitin 2 g IM plus probenecid 1 g PO; or another third-generation cephalosporin.

Women treated as outpatients for PID should be re-examined 72 hours after initiating therapy. Patients who do not respond within 72 hours after instituting treatment should be re-evaluated and parenteral therapy considered.

The CDC gives the following criteria for considering hospitalization (20):

- surgical emergencies such as appendicitis are in the differential diagnosis

- the patient is pregnant

- failure to respond clinically to oral antimicrobial therapy

- inability to follow or tolerate an outpatient regimen

- severe illness, nausea and vomiting, or high fever

- current immunodeficiency (HIV infection with low CD-4 counts, immunosuppressive therapy, or other disease affecting the immune system)

The 1997 CDC guidelines (21) for parenteral therapy are cefotetan 2 gm IV every 12 hours or cefoxitin 2 gm IV every 6 hours. Both should be combined with doxycycline 100 mg IV or orally every 12 hours. Another parenteral regimen recommended by the CDC is clindamycin 900 mg IV every 8 hours plus gentamycin loading dose IV or IM (2 mg/kg of body weight) followed by a maintenance dose (1.5 mg/kg of body weight) every 8 hours.

A single daily dose of gentamycin may be substituted. Parenteral therapy may be stopped 24 hours after the patient is clinically improved. Continued oral therapy should consist of doxycycline 100 mg PO twice a day or clindamycin 450 mg PO four times a day for a total of 14 days. If a tubo-ovarian abscess is present, doxycycline and clindamycin or metronidazole may be combined to better cover anaerobes.

Follow-up

Women should be re-examined 72 hours after initiating therapy. Substantial clinical improvement should be confirmed (decreased fever, diminished abdominal or cervical motion tenderness). If not improved, patients should have further diagnostic evaluation and perhaps surgical intervention. Examining and rescreening for gonorrhea and chlamydia at 4 to 6 weeks is also recommended to discover reinfection and relapse before the infection progresses.

Syphilis

Syphilis is caused by the spirochete *Treponema pallidum*. Despite dramatic decreases in the number of cases in homosexual males, the incidence of syphilis has been increasing overall during the last decade. The rise of cases in youth, newborn, black, and drug-using groups is probably responsi-

ble for the increased number of outbreaks. Approximately 130,000 cases of syphilis are diagnosed each year in the United States (22).

Screening

Sexually active young women should be offered screening for syphilis. Drug-using women or partners of drug users, particularly users of cocaine and intravenous drugs, should be screened (23). All HIV-positive women should be tested because of the high incidence of coinfection and the possibility of rapid progression of disease. Pregnant women should be screened in the first trimester and high-risk women should be tested at least once again in the third trimester. Women whose sexual contacts have syphilis should be tested and prophylactically treated if re-exposed within 3 months.

Symptoms

Patients can present for diagnosis in any stage of syphilis and with a broad spectrum of symptoms.

The first, or *primary*, stage of syphilis, consists of the incubation period and the genital lesion (chancre) stage. Incubation is from 9 to 90 days, with the majority of patients developing a primary lesion at approximately 21 days. The primary lesion is a nonpainful beefy-colored ulcer with a well-defined, indurated border. The exudate is usually clear or gray. Inguinal lymphadenopathy is usually present on the side of the body that the lesion appeared. The chancre usually appears at the site of moist friction during sexual contact, which allows the spirochetes to enter the skin. These lesions commonly appear on the vulva, vaginal walls, cervix, mouth, or rectum. Because these lesions are generally nonpainful and can be in areas difficult to visualize, many women do not notice the lesions or seek treatment. Even without treatment, the lesions disappear in 1 to 2 weeks.

In the *secondary* stage, the spirochetes multiply and the disease develops systemic manifestations. Lymphadenopathy, flulike symptoms, and a variety of lesions and rashes can occur. Symptoms of secondary syphilis can develop up to 3 months after the primary lesion, but generally the symptoms occur 6 weeks after the chancre.

The classic palmar and plantar rash can be macular or papular-squamous. Rashes on the trunk and extremities can also occur. Lesions in the moist creases, including the mouth, genital area, and skin folds, can occur. Flat lesions with gray membranes are called mucous patches and can sometimes be confused with oral thrush. Papular lesions, condyloma lata, can also occur. Their wartlike appearance may be confused with condyloma acuminata, or genital warts. The lesions of syphilis are soft, moist, and friable, while genital warts are dry and not as soft or friable. Alopecia, or patch hair loss, can occur on the scalp, eyebrows and eyelashes. Without treatment, symptoms resolve on their own in 2 to 10 weeks. Symptoms can recur for several years.

In *latent syphilis*, no symptoms are present. For epidemiologic purposes, latency is divided into early latent and late latent syphlis. Early latent syphilis is generally defined as the first year of infection, a time when transmission is more likely. Late latent syphilis is defined as the period from the first year of infection until tertiary symptoms appear.

Symptoms of *tertiary syphilis* can occur from 1 to 2 years

after infection or as late as 30 or 40 years later. In tertiary syphilis, the skin, bones, heart, blood vessels, and nervous system can be affected. The damage can be serious, leading to crippling, blindness, heart disease, and death. With the discovery of penicillin, the occurence of tertiary syphilis is rare. However, in recent years the increasing number of immunocompromised people with AIDS has caused some more unusual and serious complications of tertiary and neurosyphilis to appear (24).

Diagnosis

Primary lesions and most lesions of secondary syphilis can be examined using darkfield microscopy. The presence of spirochetes is diagnostic except in oral lesions, where the oral flora can have nonpathogenic spirochetes present. The intracacies of handling and special equipment necessary for darkfield microscopy can make it difficult to use this technique for diagnosis.

Serological testing for nontreponemal antibodies can also be performed. The VDRL and rapid plasma reagin (RPR) are the most commonly performed tests. Nontreponemal tests become positive at approximately that time a primary lesion appears but can also take up to a month after the appearance of the lesion to turn positive. If a primary lesion is suspected and the blood test is negative, serial weekly serologies can be performed. The antibody titers rise in secondary syphilis, usually begin to decline in latency, and can become negative in late syphilis. The nontreponemal tests can be falsely positive when other conditions are present, such as acute bacterial or viral illnesses, arthritis, lupus, drug addiction, hepatitis, alcoholism, and pregnancy. Therefore the treponemal tests FTA-ABS or MHA-TP should be used as confirmatory tests when the nontreponemal tests are positive, in order to rule out false positives.

Treatment

The 1997 CDC treatment guideline (25) for primary and secondary syphilis is a single dose of benzathine penicillin G, 2.4 million units IM. For early latent syphilis, the CDC recommends a single dose of benzathine penicillin G, 2.4 million units IM. Late latent syphilis and tertiatary syphilis without neurosyphilis should be treated with benzathine pencillin G, 7.2 million units IM, administered in 3 doses of 2.4 million units at weekly intervals. The regimen for neurosyphilis is crystalline penicillin G, 18–24 million units, administered as 3–4 million units IV every 4 hours for 10 to 14 days.

Pregnant women who are allergic to penicillin can be skin tested and should be desensitized and treated with penicillin in order to avoid congenital syphilis.

Nonpregnant women with primary, secondary, and early latent syphilis who are allergic to penicillin should be treated with doxycycline 100 mg PO twice a day for 14 days, or tetracycline 500 mg PO four times a day for 14 days. Late latent syphilis in patients allergic to penicillin should be treated with doxycycline 100 mg PO twice a day for 28 days, or tetracycycline 500 mg PO four times a day for 28 days. Because there are no adequate studies on the efficacy of non-penicillin therapy, patients should be followed up carefully. If treatment failure is suspected, the patient should be desensitized and treated with penicillin.

Follow-up

Patients with syphilis should have follow-up serologies at 3 to 6 month intervals to determine cure and detect reinfection. A failure to see a fourfold decline in early syphilis after 6 months should be considered treatment failure. Increasing titers should be considered reinfection. Patients with treatment failure should be re-evaluated for HIV, and some experts recommend cerebrospinal fluid (CSF) evaluation. The response to treatment in latent syphilis is less clear. However, patients whose titers do not decrease or who have increasing titers should be re-evaluated and retreated. Patient with neurosyphilis should have follow-up CSF examination every 6 months until there is a normal cell count. Children born to women with syphilis should be fully evaluated at birth and treated as indicated.

Casefinding in syphilis is an important aspect of primary prevention. Because of the length of incubation, casefinding can prevent disease and limit transmission. Syphilis is a reportable disease and in many states public health staff are available for casefinding. Sexual contacts within 3 months of diagnosis of patients with primary and secondary syphilis should be tested and treated prophylactically with a treatment regimen adequate for early latent syphilis. Sexual contacts within six months of diagnosis of a patient with secondary syphilis or within a year of early latent syphilis should be tested and treated if infected.

VIRAL STDS
Genital Herpes

Genital herpes is a viral illness caused by the herpes simplex virus (HSV). HSV II is the cause of genital disease approximately 80% of the time. HSV I, which is primarily found in oral lesions ("cold sores"), can also be a cause of genital disease. Although not a reportable disease, the incidence is estimated at 500,000 cases in the United States annually, with over 50 million people infected (26).

Screening

Women who present with genital ulcers, or who are sexual contacts of partners with a genital ulcer, should be examined for genital herpes. No routine screening tests are available. Current antibody testing is not specific enough to be used for screening. Because congenitally acquired herpes can cause devastating effects on the central nervous system of the neonate, pregnant women with genital lesions during pregnancy should be examined. Patients with herpes acquired in the latter part of pregnancy or with primary lesions at the time of delivery can potentially transmit the virus to the newborn. These patients and their newborns should be cared for in consultation with a neonatologist.

Surveillance cultures of pregnant women with a previous history of herpes simplex virus infection, but without active lesions, are not necessary, and vaginal delivery is acceptable. Cesarean delivery is performed if primary or recurrent lesions are present at the time of labor. If lesions are noted at the time of labor or immediately subsequent to delivery, the neonate should be monitored carefully and treatment instituted if necessary.

Diagnosis

Patients initially infected with the herpes virus can progress to a primary outbreak in 2 to 20 days. The virus can also be asymptomatic and become dormant in the basal ganglia. Herpes is recurrent in about 50% of patients. The number of recurrences and severity is impossible to predict. They vary from one to two times a year with just a few pinhead-size ulcers to eight or more outbreaks with multiple painful lesions. The amount of initial innoculation of virus, host resistance, and the strain of the virus are all theories of why the disease varies from one person to another. Frequently, the symptoms can be difficult for the patient to identify. Some patients will experience a distinct prodrome lasting from a few hours to days. Patients describe the prodrome as burning, itching, or a "pins and needle" sensation at the site of outbreak. Recent research indicates that subclinical disease and shedding, the presence of virus without symptoms, is very common and may be a source of transmission (27).

Treatment

No cure is available for herpes. Treatment is aimed at limiting symptoms and controlling transmission. Treatment usually consists of a combination of antiviral therapies, comfort or complementary treatments, and patient education.

In first outbreaks, antiviral therapy can decrease symptoms, length of outbreak, and viral shedding. Antivirals do not affect the recurrent viral course of the disease.

Recommended treatment choices for primary outbreaks are acyclovir 400 mg PO three times a day or 200 mg five times a day for 7 to 10 days; famcyclovir 250 mg PO three times a day for 7 to 10 days; or valcyclovir 1 g PO twice a day for 7 to 10 days (28).

Patients diagnosed with herpes need education and support to deal with this chronic, contagious, sexually transmitted infection. Knowledge enpowers the patient and allows them some control over the disease. Patients should be counselled regarding the natural course of the disease, how to identify symptoms or prodromes, and how to decrease transmission to sexual partners. Dealing with sexual partners can be particularly difficult for patients. Role playing and meeting with the patient and her partner is often helpful. Some patients do not cope well with the diagnosis and it seriously affects their self-image and self-esteem. These patients can be helped by individual counselling and support groups. The American Social Health Association (P.O. Box 100, Palo Alto, CA 94302) provides education and sponsors support groups.

Patients can sometimes identify "trigger factors" for recurrences. Trigger factors can be either exogenous, such as friction, sex, heat, or tight clothing, or endogenous such as stress, fluctuation in hormones, change in circadian rhythms, or other illnesses. Patients who can identify trigger factors can sometimes eliminate the factors or, if not, allow time to institute therapy or avoid sexual transmission. Comfort measures that some patients have found helpful are aluminum acetate (Burow's solution) soaks, and applications of topical anesthetic agents. Some women will have severe pain upon urination, particularly in primary outbreaks. Making a "funnel" (such as with a toilet paper roll) that covers the urethra and avoids

urine splashing on ulcers, pouring a pitcher of tepid water over the genital area while urinating, or urinating in a bath of warm water are all helpful.

Antiviral therapy can be useful in recurrent disease. It can be used episodically to shorten the length of outbreaks and decrease discomfort. It can also be used as suppressive therapy to decrease or eliminate outbreaks. It appears that suppressive therapy decreases viral shedding and thus decreases transmission. The CDC recommendations for episodic treatment (29) are acyclovir 400 mg three times a day or 800 mg twice a day for 5 days; or acyclovir 200 mg five times a day for 5 days; or famcyclovir 125 mg twice a day for 5 days; or valacyclovir 500 mg twice a day for 5 days.

The CDC recommendations for daily suppressive therapy (30) are acyclovir 400 mg twice a day; famcyclovir 250 mg twice a day; valacyclovir 500 mg twice a day or 1000 mg once a day.

Antiviral drugs during pregnancy for recurrent herpes are not currently recommended routinely. Antivirals can be used for primary infections during pregnancy or for life-threatening disease (31).

Follow-up

Patients with a primary outbreak should be encouraged to return for a follow-up visit for counseling. Patients on suppressive therapy for recurrent genital herpes should have their therapy reviewed on a yearly basis. Because the natural course of the disease is to lessen over time, patients should consider a trial of stopping treatment every 1 to 2 years to see how they respond without therapy.

Genital Warts

Genital warts, or condyloma acuminata, are caused by the human papilloma virus (HPV). Most genital warts are caused by types 6, 11, 16, 18, 31, and 33, with a total of 24 different human papilloma viruses identified. Types 16, 18, 31, and 33 are strongly associated with cervical dysplasia and may be a contributing factor in cervical and other genital cancers (32).

In young adults aged 15 to 49, approximately 15% are infected with HPV, for a total of 20 million people (33). Subclinical disease is thought to be common. The role of viral shedding is unknown.

Screening

All women presenting with genital lesions or whose sexual partners have genital lesions should be examined for genital warts. Because genital warts are common in young sexually active adults and are generally painless, women should be examined for warts during all routine pelvic examinations. DNA hybridization and PCR can identify the virus, but are too expensive for routine screening and are generally used in research only.

Diagnosis

The incubation period for genital warts appears to be 3 months or longer. Genital warts can present in a variety of ways. They can have the classic verrucous or "cauliflower" appearance, or can be dome-shaped or almost flat. While generally flesh colored, they may also be pigmented or have a thick keratitic layer.

Lesions can appear anywhere on the genitals. They occur at sites of friction where the virus enters the body, most commonly in the introitus, labial folds, perineum, anus, and around the clitoris. They can also be found on the vaginal walls and cervix, where they are usually flat and hypopigmented. Subclinical disease, especially on the cervix, can occur. Occasionally, patients note itching or discomfort, particularly if warts are large or become irritated with intercourse.

Most warts are diagnosed by inspection alone. Use of 10% acetic acid topically on lesions will make them appear white, and can be helpful in diagnosis. Biopsy is not routinely recommended, but is often performed for lesions that do not respond to treatment or have an unusual appearance. Pap smears should be done on all patients with genital lesions. Women with abnormal Pap smears and HPV should have colposcopy performed, with directed biopsies of any areas that appear abnormal.

Treatment

Treatment modalities fall into two classes, cytodestructive and immunity enhancing. These can be further divided into clinician- and patient-applied. No single treatment has been identified as superior, and treatment decisions are based upon type and location of lesions, cost, and clinician or patient preference.

Clinician-applied treatments include cryotherapy, podophyllin, trichloroacetic acid or bichloroacetic acid, interferon, and surgery. Cryotherapy involves applying liquid nitrogen to freeze and destroy the warts. It is applied every 1 to 2 weeks. It is quick and relatively painless, and it can be accurately applied even to small warts. A disadvantage is the difficulty in storage of liquid nitrogen, which may not be practical for low-volume practices.

Podophyllin resin 10% or 25% is applied to warts every 1 to 2 weeks. It is relatively inexpensive and easy to use. However, it is caustic, and because it is liquid it can irritate surrounding tissues.

TCA or BCA is applied every week to 2 weeks. It is inexpensive and relatively easy to use. TCA and BCA are watery liquids and can easily get on tissues surrounding warts. Applying petroleum jelly to surrounding areas prior to using TCA or BCA is helpful.

Interferon is thought to have antiviral and immunostimulating properties. It is injected into the base of the wart three times per week. It is generally not recommended for first-line therapy because of expense, difficulty of administration, and systemic side effects including fever and flulike reactions.

Generally, all of the clinician-applied therapies take three to six treatments. A switch to another therapy is recommended if there is no response after three treatments or if lesions are not completely cleared after six treatments. Laser therapy of lesions may also be considered in these cases.

Patient-applied therapies, podofilox and imiquimod, are convenient for patients but generally take time to effect a cure. For many women, visualizing the warts can be difficult. Clinicians may apply the first treatment in order to demonstrate the application technique to the patient. Podofilox 5% solution or gel can then be applied twice a day for 3 days, followed by no treatment for 4 days, for up to four cycles. Imiquimod 5% cream, an immunomodulator, is the newest treatment in the therapy arsenal. It is applied in the evening three times per week for up to 16 weeks. It should be washed off after 6 to 8 hours.

Pregnant women should not use podophyllin, podofilox, or imiquimod. Because warts can grow faster during pregnancy, most clinicians recommend treatment with one of the other modalities. HPV 6 and 11 can cause laryngeal papillomatosis in infants. The mode of transmission is unknown and preventive cesarean section is not recommended (34).

Follow-up

Most recurrences occur within the first 3 months after treatment. Patients should be encouraged to inspect for recurrences and return for treatment if they occur. Because visualizing the genital area is difficult for patients, some clinicians offer patients follow-up visits.

Since the course of disease is varied and the mechanism of transmission is unknown, patients need a great deal of support and counselling. They should be encouraged to have their sex partners examined even if the partners have no apparent symptoms. Condoms are helpful in avoiding transmission, but exactly where and how the virus is transmitted is unknown. Women should be counselled to have yearly Pap smears.

VAGINITIS
Yeast Vaginitis

Yeast vaginitis, or vulvovaginal candidiasis, is one of the most common causes of vaginitis, with 75% of women reporting at least one episode (35). In addition, at least one recurrence is reported by 40% to 50% of women. Several strains of yeast have been identified as causes, with the most common being *Candida albicans*. Other strains identified include *C. lubrata*, *C. tropicalis*, *C. krusei*, *C. paraprilosis*, *C. lasitaniae*, and *S. cervisiae*. Many cofactors are thought to increase the likelihood of developing yeast vaginitis, including pregnancy, the use of oral contraceptives, and antibiotics. These factors affect the pH and normal flora in the vagina, which allows the yeast to multiply and cause disease. Underlying diseases that affect the immune system, such as diabetes and HIV, have also been identified as factors in recurrent disease. Finally, factors such as sex, tight or occlusive clothing, high carbohydrate diets, and personal hygiene practices are all thought to be possible contributing factors, but very little scientific research has been done.

Diagnosis

Women with classic symptoms present with burning, pruritis, erythema, and occasionally superficial fissures on the vulva, perineum, and introitus. The vaginal discharge is white, "cottage cheese" in appearance, and often clings to the walls of the vagina. Occasionally, the symptoms are milder or less apparent. Other disorders, including contact dermatitis, skin diseases that cause lichenification, and carcinoma can be confused with yeast infections. It is important to differentiate yeast from these conditions, particularly in patients who appear to have recurrent symptoms or who do not respond to treatment.

Microscopic examination of vaginal secretions using 10% potassium hydoxide (KOH) which reveals hyphae and budding is diagnostic. The pH is usually less than 4.5. Some strains of yeast are difficult to identify under the microscope. A culture is also diagnostic. It is important to note that yeast can be found normally in the vagina and patients who are asymptmatic do not require treatment.

The availability of over-the-counter antifungal medications has made proper diagnosis of yeast more difficult. Patients should be counselled to seek medical care for a first episode, if symptoms do not resolve with treatment, or if symptoms are recurrent.

Treatment

The CDC 1997 treatment guidelines recommend all of the intravaginal azoles as potential treaments for yeast vaginitis. Also recommended is an oral regimen consisting of one dose of 150 mg of oral fluconazole. Pregnant women may use any of the topical treaments, but at least a 7-day treatment course is recommended (36).

Some experts have classified yeast infections into noncomplicated and complicated disease, to further assist in making treatment decisions. Uncomplicated disease is defined as mild, sporadic, nonrecurrent yeast vaginitis, in a woman with normal immunity and probable infection with C. albicans. These cases can usually be treated with any of the therapies, including treatment courses of 7 days or less. Patients with complicated disease, severe symptoms, recurrent disease, decreased immunity, or infection with strains other than C. albicans may require longer treatment courses of 10 to 14 days.

Treatment for patients with chronically recurring disease, generally defined as four or more times in a year, has not been well studied. The 1997 CDC recommendations are for a 10 to 14 day regimen followed by a maintenance dose of ketoconazole 100 mg daily.

Complementary treatments, such as acidophilus pills and increased consumption of yogurt, have been tried in order to increase lactobaccilli and improve local immunity. Loose clothing and improved personal hygiene have also been recommended, but there is little scientific data on this.

Bacterial Vaginosis

Bacterial vaginosis (BV) is the reason for 10 million office visits per year, with prevalence ranges from 5% to 25% of women (37). BV is believed to be a polymicrobial infection characterized by a replacement of the normal vaginal flora lactobaccilli species with high concentrations of anaerobic bacteria. Prevotella, porphymonas, bacteroides, *Peptococcus*, mycoplasma, *Ureaplasma*, and mobiluncus species have all been found in women with this syndrome. A link between these anaerobes in pregnancy and premature rupture of membranes, preterm labor, and preterm birth has been described (38). BV has also been implicated as a cofactor in postpartum and postsurgical endometritis, and in pelvic inflammatory disease (39,40).

Although most commonly found in sexually active women, BV does not appear to be a sexually transmitted disease. Treament of sexual partners does not seem to decrease the incidence of disease.

Screening

Women presenting with vaginal discharge should be evaluated for BV. However, no simple screening test has been determined. Since BV has been associated with serious sequelae, researchers are currently evaluating the need for screening tests and routine treatment of asymptomatic pregnant and presurgical patients.

Diagnosis

Women with BV will often present with a thin creamy white or grey vaginal discharge with a fishy (amine) odor. Pruritis, erythema, or pain are generally absent. Approximately 50% of women are asymptomatic. The following guidelines (41) are helpful in making a diagnosis:

- Discharge is homogeneous, white, noninflammatory, and smoothly coats the vaginal walls
- Clue cells (epithelial cells whose borders are obscured and covered with bacteria) are present on saline wet-prep microscopic examination of vaginal discharge
- The pH of vaginal fluid is greater than 4.5
- There is a fishy (amine) odor before or after addition of 10% KOH (whiff test) to vaginal discharge

Gram's stain to evaluate the relative number of bacterial morphologies is considered diagnostic. However, culture for *Gardnerella vaginalis* is not considered specific for infection, since about one half of all normal woman will have cultures positive for *Gardnerella*.

Treatment

Treatment of BV is aimed at alleviating symptoms. Some authorities are suggesting that women who are symptomatic or who are at high risk for preterm labor be treated. Many clinicians are considering treatment of asymptomatic BV prior to therapeutic abortion or other surgical procedures performed through the vagina.

CDC guidelines (42) for first-line therapy of nonpregnant women are metronidazole 500 mg PO twice a day for 7 days; clindamycin cream 2%, one full applicator (5 g) intravaginally at bedtime for 7 days; or metronidazole gel 0.75%, one full applicator (5 g) intravaginally twice daily for 5 days. Alternative regimens include metronidazole 2 g PO in a single dose, or clindamycin 300 mg PO twice a day for 7 days.

The 2-g single dose of oral metronidazole is convenient but is considered less efficacious than the 7-day oral or intravaginal treatment. Patients taking metronidazole should avoid consuming alcohol during treatment and for 24 hours after completion. Clindamycin cream is oil-based and may weaken the integrity of condoms and diaphragms. Patients should consult the package insert of these products.

The CDC recommended (43) first-line therapy for pregnant women is metronidazole 250 mg PO three times a day for 7 days. Alternate regimens are metronidazole 2 gm PO in a single dose; clindamycin 300 mg PO twice a day for 7 days; or metronidazole gel 0.75%, one full applicator twice a day for 5 days.

Pregnant women with a previous history of preterm labor with symptomatic or asymptomatic disease can be treated with these regimens. Low-risk women can also be treated in order to alleviate symptoms.

Follow-up

Routine follow-up when symptoms have resolved is not necessary. However, recurrence is common and patients should be encouraged to seek treatment if symptoms return. Alternative treatments can be used for recurrent disease. Partner treatment and evaluation are not recommended, although some clinicians will treat partners of women with recurrent disease.

REFERENCES

1,2. Kassler WJ, Caters W Jr. The epidemiology and prevention of sexually transmitted diseases. Urol Clin North Am 1992;19: 1–12.

3. Boekeloo BO, Marx ES, Kral AH, et al. Frequency and thoroughness of STD/HIV risk assessment by physicians in a high risk metropolitan area. Am J Public Health 1991;81: 1645–1648.

4. Maheux B, Haley N, Rivard M, et al. STD risk assessment and risk reduction counseling by recently trained family physicians. Acad Med 1995;70: 726–728.

5. Wiens A, Brazman R. A rationale and method for the sexual history in family practice. J Fam Prac 1997;5:213–215.

6. O'Connell ML. The effect of birth control methods on sexually transmitted disease/HIV risk. J Obstet Gyn Neonat Nurs 1996;225:476–480.

7. Harrison HR, Costin M, Meder JB, et al. Cervical clamydia trachomatis infection in university women: relationship to history, contraception, ectopic, and cervicitis. Am J Obstet Gynecol 1985;153:244–251.

8. Andrist LC. Taking a sexual history and educating clients about safe sex. Nurs Clin North Am 1988;23:959–973.

9. Bourne N, Stanberry LR, Bernstein DI, et al. DNA immunization against experimental genital herpes simplex virus infection. J Infect Dis 1996; 173:800–807.

10. Frazer IH. The role of vaccines in the context of STDs: HPV vaccine. Genitourin Med 1996;12:1398–1403.

11. Rice RJ, Roberts PL, Handsfield HH. Sociodemographic distribution of gonorrhea incidence: implications for prevention and behavioral research. Am J Public Health 1991;81:125–128.

12. Centers for Disease Control and Prevention. 1997 sexually transmitted disease treatment guidelines. Atlanta: U.S. Dept. of Health and Human Services, Public Health Services, Centers for Disease Control, Center for Prevention Services, Division of STD/HIV Prevention, 1997:1–116.

13,14. Blanding J, Hirsch L, Stranton N, et al. Comparison of the Clearview Clamydia, the PACE assay, and culture for detection of chlamydia trachomatis from cervical specimens in a low prevalence population. J Clin Microbiol 1993;31: 1622–1625.

15. Centers for Disease Control and Prevention. 1997 sexually transmitted disease treatment guidelines. Atlanta: U.S. Dept. of Health and Human Services, Public Health Services, Centers for Disease Control, Center for Prevention Services, Division of STD/HIV Prevention, 1997:1–116.

16. Centers for Disease Control at Preoenta. Sexually transmitted disease treatment guidelines. MMWR 1993;42:RR-14.

17. Task Force On Intrauterine Devices, Special Programme of Research, Development and Research Training in Human Reproduction, WHO. PID associated with fertility regulating agents. Contraception 1984;30:1–21.

18–21. Centers for Disease Control and Prevention. 1997 sexually transmitted disease treatment guidelines. Atlanta: U.S. Dept. of Health and Human Services, Public Health Services, Centers for Disease Control, Center for Prevention Services, Division of STD/HIV Prevention, 1997:1–116.

22. Kassler WJ, Cates WJ. The epidemiology and prevention of sexually transmitted diseases. Urol Clin North Am 1992;10: 1–12.

23. Garnett GP, Aral SO, Hoyle DV, et al. The natural history of syphilis: implications for the transmission dynamics and control of infection. Sex Transm Dis 1997;24:185–200.

24–25. Centers for Disease Control and Prevention. 1997 sexually transmitted disease treatment guidelines. Atlanta: U.S. Dept. of Health and Human Services, Public Health Services, Centers for Disease Control, Center for Prevention Services, Division of STD/HIV Prevention, 1997:1–116.

26. Corey L. The current trends in genital herpes: progress in prevention. Sex Transm Dis 1994;21:538–544.

27. Wald A, Zeh J, Barnum G, et al. Suppression of subclinical shedding of herpes simplex virus type II with acyclovir. Ann Intern Med 1996;12:8–15.

28–31. Centers for Disease Control and Prevention. 1997 sexually transmitted disease treatment guidelines. Atlanta: U.S. Dept. of Health and Human Services, Public Health Services, Centers for Disease Control, Center for Prevention Services, Division of STD/HIV Prevention, 1997:1–116.

32. Walboumers JM, Van den Brat AJ, Snyders PJ, et al. The diagnosis of human papilloma virus (HPV) by polymerase chain reaction in cervical scrape. Paper presented at: International Cervical Cancer Symposium, 1991; Saint Lucia, W Indies. Abstract 25.

33. Schneider A, Loutsky LA. Natural history and epidemiological features of genital HSV infection. IARC Sci Pub 1992;119:25–52.

34. Centers for Disease Control and Prevention. 1997 sexually transmitted disease treatment guidelines. Atlanta: U.S. Dept.

of Health and Human Services, Public Health Services, Centers for Disease Control, Center for Prevention Services, Division of STD/HIV Prevention, 1997:1–116.

35. Mead PB. Epidemiology of bacterial vaginosis. Am J Obstet Gynecol 1993;169:446–449.

36. Centers for Disease Control and Prevention. 1997 sexually transmitted disease treatment guidelines. Atlanta: U.S. Dept. of Health and Human Services, Public Health Services, Centers for Disease Control, Center for Prevention Services, Division of STD/HIV Prevention, 1997:1–116.

37. Hill GB. The microbiology of bacterial vaginosis. Am J Obstet Gynecol 1993;169:450–455.

38. McGregor JA, French JI, Seo K. Premature rupture of membranes and bacterial vaginosis. Am J Obstet Gynecol 1993; 169:463–466.

39. Soper DE. Bacterial vaginosis and post-operative infection. Am J Obstet Gynecol 1993; 169:467–469.

40. Hillier SL, Kiviat NB, Howes SE, et al. Role of bacterial vaginosis-associated microorganisms in endometritis. Am J Obstet Gynecol 1996;177S: 435–441.

41–43. Centers for Disease Control and Prevention. 1997 sexually transmitted disease treatment guidelines. Atlanta: U.S. Dept of Health and Human Services, Public Health Services, Centers for Disease Control, Center for Prevention Services, Division of STD/HIV Prevention, 1997:1–116.

Part VII.

PULMONARY MEDICINE

Edited by
Donald A. Mahler

Introduction to Pulmonary Medicine

James M. Rippe

The area of pulmonary medicine has experienced significant advances in how daily lifestyle actions and practices such as physical activity and minimizing exposure to environmental toxins (e.g., cigarette smoking) can result in a dramatic impact on pulmonary function. This section reviews current knowledge and the linkages between lifestyle and respiratory function.

The section opens with a chapter by Schwartzstein showing how elements of history obtained from the patient may relate to the physiology and clinical significance of respiratory symptoms. The chapter by Casaburi takes this knowledge into the laboratory to describe how currently available assays of pulmonary function may help elucidate pulmonary disease.

Asthma represents a common, distressing, and potentially dangerous condition for over 14 million individuals. As D'Alonzo and Ciccolella point out, prevention and treatment of this disease rest on the use of both nonpharmacologic and pharmacologic interventions. In particular, the daily habits and activities of patients with asthma play a significant role in disease management and prevention. The authors discuss in detail the lifestyle practices that can result in substantial differences in both short- and long-term health and quality of life in individuals with asthma.

The chapter by Orenstein and Cerny on cystic fibrosis reminds us that this is one of the most common life-shortening diseases in Caucasian populations. The authors present a comprehensive description of cystic fibrosis and emphasize how lifestyle practices such as regular physical activity can make an important therapeutic difference in this common, inherited condition.

The chapter by Mahler and Mejia on chronic obstructive pulmonary disease provides a state-of-the-art summary of modern knowledge of this condition as well as a structured clinical approach, including lifestyle measures, to decrease both morbidity and mortality. The section concludes with a chapter by Ries on pulmonary rehabilitation. The author reminds us that COPD is now the fourth leading cause of death in the United States. However, modern pulmonary rehabilitation programs can play a very significant role in reducing both morbidity and mortality in this common, frequently lifestyle-related condition.

Chapter 39

Respiratory Symptoms

Richard M. Schwartzstein

Shortness of breath, cough, and wheezing are among the most common complaints expressed by patients seeking medical care. As in most areas of medicine, the evaluation of patients with respiratory symptoms rests in large part upon a comprehensive and insightful history obtained by the physician. Although the information offered spontaneously by the patient is the starting point in the evaluation of any problem, knowledge of the pathophysiology and the differential diagnoses underlying the symptoms allows the physician the opportunity to probe further, to determine which areas of the physical examination require special attention, and ultimately to narrow if not eliminate the radiographic and laboratory testing required to confirm the diagnosis.

Often there is a confusion between respiratory symptoms and signs. For example, a patient is described as being "short of breath" as part of the physical examination. In fact, symptoms can only be described by the patient. We may speculate that a patient is experiencing respiratory discomfort based on the observations that accessory muscles of ventilation are being recruited, that the respiratory rate is elevated, or that the patient is unable to speak in full sentences. Nevertheless, we must rely on what the patient tells us to accurately describe the symptoms themselves.

In obtaining a history from patients with respiratory symptoms, however, physicians are often hampered by the lack of personal experience they and their patients may have had with these sensations previously. Unlike sensations of "pain," which are common to even healthy individuals over the course of months and years and the experience of which can be drawn upon when describing new events, breathing discomfort may only have been experienced with exercise, and wheezing not at all. Thus, it is important to consider the

findings of new research that have led to the development of a language of dyspnea, and factors such as the timing of the symptoms and conditions that precipitate them or help to relieve the discomfort.

This chapter focuses on the elements of the history obtained from the patient that help us to understand the physiologic and clinical significance of respiratory symptoms. The utility of pulmonary function tests and discussions of specific disease states such as asthma and chronic obstructive pulmonary disease (COPD) will be addressed in other chapters. When pertinent, the chapter covers how specific elements of the physical examination, in concert with the symptoms reported, can greatly narrow the differential diagnosis.

DYSPNEA

Definition

The word *dyspnea* derives from the Greek term for difficult breathing, but has come to represent a more global set of sensations that can be grouped as "respiratory discomfort." Dyspnea, or breathlessness, may be experienced by healthy individuals when exercising to the limits of their aerobic capacity, may represent primary pulmonary or cardiac disease, or may be a manifestation of a severe metabolic acidosis. Although there are no data on the prevalence of dyspnea in the general population, the conditions most commonly associated with this symptom lead to large expenditures of healthcare dollars. Coronary artery disease (CAD), for example, is the leading cause of mortality in the United States and myocardial ischemia is often associated with dyspnea (1). Congestive heart failure (CHF) is the primary reason for hos-

433

pital admission in the medicare population, and breathlessness is the most common complaint of patients suffering from heart failure. Furthermore, there are approximately 25 million people in the United States who suffer from asthma and COPD and for whom the cost of managing their disease is in excess of $10 billion annually (2). When one adds to these groups patients with interstitial lung disease, pulmonary emboli, respiratory infections, and lung cancer, it is readily apparent that this symptom is one with which a physician may be confronted on a daily basis. Consequently, it is critical that doctors have a clear understanding of the best methods to elicit the nuances of this symptom in order to garner clues about the underlying diagnosis.

Physiology of Dyspnea

Although a detailed review of the physiology of dyspnea is beyond the scope of this chapter, it is important to understand the basic principles that underlie the sensations of respiratory discomfort (3). Dyspnea associated with respiratory disorders appears to arise as a result of a variety of physiologic mechanisms that involve stimulation of receptors in the upper airways, lungs, and chest wall as well as peripheral and central chemoreceptors (Figure 39-1). In addition, there are believed to be neural discharges, termed *corollary discharges*, between the motor and sensory cortex that are activated when

ventilation is consciously increased. The physiology of cardiac dyspnea is less well understood, but likely involves many of these same mechanisms as well as others unique to low cardiac output states. A summary of common cardiopulmonary conditions and the associated pathophysiologic bases for dyspnea is outlined in Table 39-1.

In the presence of increased mechanical loads on the respiratory system (e.g., airway obstruction or decreased pulmonary compliance associated with interstitial lung disease), the motor cortex must increase the neural signals sent to the ventilatory muscles to overcome the load and maintain appropriate levels of arterial carbon dioxide ($Paco_2$). These outgoing messages, or efferent signals, are associated with a simultaneous corollary discharge to the sensory cortex that is hypothesized to provide the individual with a sense of how much "effort" or "work" is being expended in the act of breathing (4). Dyspnea associated with muscle weakness (e.g., myasthenia gravis, Guillain-Barré syndrome) is also attributable to this mechanism. The intensity of dyspnea under conditions of mechanical loading may be affected by the relative motion of the lungs and chest wall in response to the neural signals being transmitted to the ventilatory muscles (i.e., when the system does not respond as expected for a given level of neural drive to breathe, dyspnea results). This discrepancy between the output of the respiratory centers and the

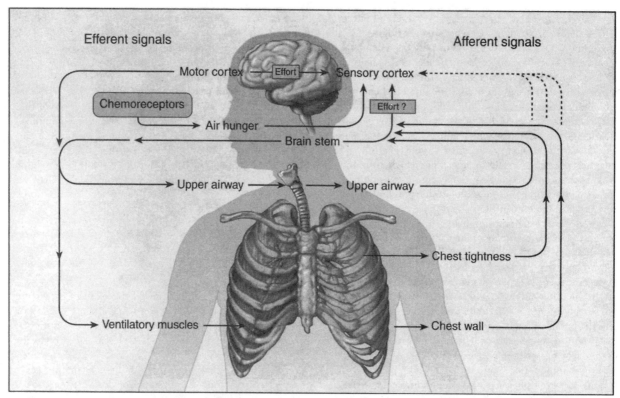

Figure 39-1 Physiologic mechanisms producing dyspnea. The sensations of breathing discomfort that are grouped under the term *dyspnea* result from stimulation of a range of receptors throughout the respiratory system as well as from a corollary discharge that is hypothesized to arise from the motor cortex when efferent neural discharges are sent to the ventilatory muscles. Qualitative phrases used to describe the sensations are noted based on existing experimental evidence (see text for discussion). (Reproduced by permission from Manning HL, Schwartzstein RM. Pathophysiology of dyspnea. N Engl J Med 1995;333:1547–1553. Copyright 1995 Massachusetts Medical Society. All rights reserved.)

Table 39-1 Relationship of Possible Mechanisms of Dyspnea in Selected Conditions	
CONDITION	MECHANISM
Asthma	Increased sense of effort
	Stimulation of irritant receptors in airways
Neuromuscular disease	Increased sense of effort
COPD	Increased sense of effort
	Hypoxia
	Hypercapnia
	Dynamic airway compression
Pulmonary embolism	Stimulation of receptors in pulmonary vasculature or right atrium (?)
Congestive heart failure	Stimulation of J-receptors in lung
	Stimulation of receptors in pulmonary vasculature (?)
	Hypoxia
	Stimulation of ergoreceptors (?)
Deconditioning	Stimulation of ergoreceptors (?)

Modified from Manning HL and Schwartzstein RM. Pathophysiology of dyspnea. N Engl J Med 1995;333: 1547–1553.

mechanical response of the system has been termed *efferent-afferent* or *neuromechanical dissociation* (5,6).

Conditions that result in an increase in a reflex or automatic increase in the neural output from the respiratory control centers in the brainstem are also associated with breathing discomfort, generally described as a sense of "air hunger," or an increased "urge to breathe." Stimulation of the peripheral chemoreceptors by hypoxia and hypercapnia and central chemoreceptors by hypercapnia and metabolic acidosis is presumed to produce dyspnea by this mechanism. Stimulation of receptors in the lungs may also result in an increase in ventilation and be responsible for part of the breathlessness in these conditions (e.g., asthma and pulmonary embolism).

Further evidence for the role of pulmonary receptors in the generation of breathing discomfort is provided by studies of bronchoconstriction. This condition is associated with a sensation of chest tightness (7–9). Inhalation of lidocaine to block airway receptors has been shown to reduce the discomfort resulting from methacholine-induced bronchospasm but not that associated with external resistive loads (10).

Cardiac dyspnea may occur in settings in which systolic or diastolic function is impaired and the heart must operate at high levels of left ventricular diastolic pressure in order to generate an appropriate cardiac output. This leads to increases in pulmonary capillary wedge pressure and, in some instances, to the transudation of fluid into the pulmonary interstitium and alveoli. Consequently, the lung becomes stiffer or less compliant, which increases the mechanical load on the respiratory system, and hypoxia may ensue. Further-

more, the increase in pulmonary vascular pressures may directly lead to respiratory discomfort.

In states associated with low cardiac output, there may be reduced blood flow to the ventilatory muscles, resulting in muscle weakness and fatigue (11). CHF also appears to alter respiratory control mechanisms, leading to increased levels of ventilation compared to control subjects for any given level of exercise (12). As noted previously, factors that stimulate the neural drive to breathe may lead to dyspnea. Finally, there appear to be receptors (ergoreceptors) in the peripheral muscles that are sensitive to increases in the byproducts of anaerobic metabolism and may contribute to the increased ventilation and breathing discomfort associated with low cardiac outputs (13).

Qualities of Dyspnea

Is all dyspnea the same? Do patients with CHF, COPD, pulmonary embolism, and asthma all experience the same sensation when they complain of respiratory discomfort? Can we discern different types of dyspnea by the questions we ask patients? In recent years, a number of studies have demonstrated that dyspnea, like pain, is comprised of multiple, qualitatively distinct sensations and that attention to the "language of dyspnea" can provide insights into a patient's disease.

Physicians have long recognized that the term *pain* subsumes many different sensations and that qualitative distinctions among the different types of pain can yield important information about the pathologic etiology of the discomfort. Questionnaires were developed to assist in the categorization of painful sensations (14) and these were applied to patients with a variety of syndromes. Patient responses permitted distinctions to be made among disease states (15,16).

This approach has been applied recently to patients with breathing discomfort. Utilizing a questionnaire (Table 39-2) derived from interviews with patients and studies in

Table 39-2 Descriptors of Dyspnea
1. My breath does not go in all the way.
2. My breathing requires effort.
3. I feel that I am smothering.
4. I feel a hunger for more air.
5. My breathing is heavy.
6. I cannot take a deep breath.
7. I feel out of breath.
8. My chest feels tight.
9. My breathing requires more work.
10. I feel that I am suffocating.
11. I feel that my breath stops.
12. I am gasping for breath.
13. My chest is constricted.
14. I feel that my breathing is rapid.
15. My breathing is shallow.
16. I feel that I am breathing more.
17. I cannot get enough air.
18. My breath does not go out all the way.
19. My breathing requires more concentration.

Reprinted with permission from Simon PM, Schwartzstein RM, Weiss JW, et al. Distinguishable sensations of breathlessness induced in normal volunteers. Am J Resp Crit Care 1989;140: 1021–1027. © American Lung Association.

which normal subjects were made breathless while performing a range of ventilatory tasks (17), Simon et al demonstrated that various cardiopulmonary conditions associated with dyspnea could be characterized by a unique set of verbal phrases (7). These findings were confirmed by Elliott et al in an investigation using a similar approach, but with an expanded questionnaire (8). The responses offered by patients when asked to describe their breathing discomfort have been shown to be reproducible over time (9).

From these and related studies, a language of dyspnea is beginning to emerge (Table 39-3). Patients with bronchoconstriction, primarily in association with asthma but occasionally with CHF, frequently describe a sensation of "chest tightness." The presence of increased mechanical loads, which is typical of airway obstruction, interstitial disease, and chest wall abnormalities, usually results in a sensation of increased "effort or work" of breathing. Neuromuscular weakness also produces a sensation of increased effort to breathe. Significant hyperinflation, as is seen in patients with severe emphysema, may lead to a sensation of an "inability to get a deep breath" (18). In experimental conditions, acute hypercapnia has been shown to produce a discomfort characterized as "air hunger," or an increased urge to breathe (19). This sensation is also present with other conditions associated with an increased stimulus to breathe (e.g., severe asthma, pulmonary embolism, acute hypoxia). One must remember that many conditions are characterized by multiple pathophysiologic derangements and patients may express several of these sensations simultaneously (e.g., an asthma patient with chest tightness related to bronchoconstriction and an increased effort of breathing associated with hyperinflation and airway resistance).

Deconditioning, the inability to achieve maximal work loads with physical activity because of reduced aerobic capacity of the heart and muscles, afflicts normal individuals as well as patients with cardiopulmonary disease. It deserves special attention because too often patients with underlying pathologic problems and reduced functional capabilities are assumed to be limited by their disease when, in fact, they are restricted by deconditioning, a state that can be corrected with an exercise program (20,21). For example, patients with asthma, when asked why they had reduced exercise capacity, stated that it was because of their asthma; yet when subjected to formal exercise testing, these individuals were limited by cardiovascular deconditioning rather than airway reactivity (20). Similarly, patients with COPD, even those with severe airway obstruction ($FEV_1 < 40\%$ of predicted), are often limited by leg fatigue rather than by poor ventilatory reserve (22). Dyspnea associated with deconditioning has been characterized as "heavy breathing" or "breathing more" (9) or as "huffing and puffing." Patients relate that their lungs and chest seem to expand normally, and that air moves in and out freely. It is important that the physician be alert to the presence of deconditioning since it, unlike many chronic lung problems, is treatable. Although the patient may assume the lung disease is responsible for the limited exercise capability, careful questioning may elicit the information needed to diagnose deconditioning.

When questioning a patient who complains of shortness of breath, it is best to inquire about the nature of the "breathing discomfort." This phrase is a generic term that can be used to address the problem and then allows you to elicit specific qualities of the patient's distress without biasing the individual toward a particular sensation. At times it may be helpful to show the patient a dyspnea questionnaire and ask him or her to select up to three phrases that best describe the breathing discomfort. Be alert to the possibility that a patient may have different sensations (and different kinds of dyspnea due to different problems) under varying conditions (e.g., a patient with interstitial lung disease and superimposed airway reactivity, or a patient with asthma who also is deconditioned). It is also important to distinguish between dyspnea that is secondary to chest wall pain and breathing discomfort that is a primary sensation. For example, patients with a fractured rib may have severe pain with inspiration and express a sensation of "inability to get a deep breath" or "air hunger" despite the absence of pulmonary or cardiovascular pathology.

ESSENTIALS OF THE HISTORY

Timing: Acute Versus Chronic Dyspnea

There are a relatively small number of conditions that result in an abrupt onset of breathing discomfort (Table 39-4). These tend to be associated with sudden changes in airway resistance (bronchospasm), hypoxemia (obstruction of the airways by secretions with acute ventilation/perfusion mismatch), or sudden increases in pulmonary vascular pressures (cardiac ischemia or pulmonary embolism). Often, with treatment (e.g., administration of a bronchodilator or nitroglycerin), these conditions improve as rapidly as they begin. On occasion, dyspnea may develop acutely in a patient with a chronic pulmonary disease and limited pulmonary reserve whose system is then subjected to a sudden metabolic stress

	Table 39-3 The Language of Dyspnea: Association of Qualitative Descriptors and Physiologic Mechanisms of Shortness of Breath	
QUALITATIVE DESCRIPTORS	**PATHOPHYSIOLOGY**
Chest tightness or constriction	Bronchoconstriction, interstitial edema (asthma, myocardial ischemia)
Increased work or effort of breathing	Airway obstruction, neuromuscular disease, chest wall disease (COPD, moderate to severe asthma, myopathy, kyphoscoliosis)
Inability to get a deep breath	Hyperinflation (COPD, asthma)
Air hunger, need to breathe, urge to breathe	Increased drive to breathe (CHF, pulmonary embolism, moderate to severe airway obstruction)
Heavy breathing, rapid breathing, breathing more	Deconditioning

Table 39-4 Acute Causes of Dyspnea

Bronchospasm
   Acute asthma
   Acute interstitial edema
Hypoxemia
   Acute mucous plugging of airways
   Pulmonary embolism
   Pneumothorax
Increases in Pulmonary Vascular Pressures
   Myocardial ischemia
   Pulmonary embolism
Sudden Increased Demand for Ventilation
   Acute metabolic acidosis

(e.g., a patient with severe COPD who develops an infection with a high fever and metabolic acidosis). The need to increase ventilation under these conditions to meet the increased demands for oxygen consumption and/or carbon dioxide elimination may result in a combination of an increased sense of effort or work of breathing as well as a sense of an increased urge to breathe.

Chronic dyspnea tends to develop slowly over the course of weeks or months. Often the patient has difficulty pinpointing the exact onset of the symptom or attributes it to a respiratory infection that, despite resolution of all the systemic aspects of the illness, left him or her with chronic breathing discomfort. Not infrequently, the date that a patient gives up cigarette smoking is, in retrospect, related consciously or unconsciously to the onset of dyspnea. Causes of chronic dyspnea include COPD, progressive interstitial lung disease, pleural effusions, worsening chest wall deformities, chronic CHF, and recurrent pulmonary emboli. The chronicity of these conditions may be masked by changes in lifestyle. Faced with the increasingly difficult task of walking up a flight of stairs to his or her apartment, the patient with COPD may decide to move to a home in a building served by elevators or live on the ground floor. Children are called upon to do the shopping. Deconditioning becomes superimposed on the underlying cardiopulmonary disorder. Now, even routine tasks become uncomfortable, and the patient may present to the physician complaining of seemingly new symptoms over the course of a few weeks. The reality is that the patient has a chronic condition and is only able to avoid recurring dyspnea because of avoidance of physical activity.

Timing: Night Versus Day

Nocturnal dyspnea, awakening in the middle of the night with acute respiratory distress, can be an extremely frightening experience for a patient. The majority of cases are due to one or more of three problems: 1) bronchospasm, 2) aspiration, and 3) CHF.

Patients with asthma may have worsening symptoms at night because of a trough in the level of their bronchodilator medications, triggering of bronchospasm by gastroesophageal reflux through a reflex mediated by the vagus nerve when acid enters the esophagus, or as a result of exposure to allergens localized to the bedroom. The sensations experienced are usually similar to asthma attacks that occur during the day

(e.g., chest tightness and increased effort to breathe) although the precipitating factors are generally different. At times, the patient may have cough without discernible wheezing (see the discussion below). The association of the symptoms with changes in the home environment (e.g., new carpeting or a new pet) may give clues to the diagnosis.

Recurrent aspiration as a cause of nocturnal dyspnea can be a very elusive diagnosis. Reports of witnessed aspiration or gagging are relatively rare. The presence of partially digested food on the patient's pillow is infrequently reported but is very suggestive of regurgitation and aspiration if present. The diagnosis is usually entertained in a patient with a history consistent with gastroesophageal reflux, infiltrates on chest radiograph in dependent portions of the lung, and an absence of a history of asthma.

The onset of nocturnal dyspnea characterized as a sense of air hunger or a suffocating feeling is most typical of CHF and is generally termed *paroxysmal nocturnal dyspnea* (PND). Clues to the diagnosis of PND include the presence of peripheral edema and the relief of the respiratory discomfort shortly after the patient assumes an upright position. Redistribution of edema fluid to the central circulation during the night with consequent increases in pulmonary vascular pressures in a patient with compromised left ventricular function is believed to be the pathophysiologic basis for this condition. Acute myocardial ischemia at night may mimic PND, but is unlikely to have a recurring pattern, may be associated with chest pain, and is less likely to be relieved by sitting upright.

Rest dyspnea that occurs during the day; is associated with tachypnea and normal gas exchange, pulmonary function, and chest radiograph; and never occurs at night is suggestive of the hyperventilation syndrome. These patients often complain of a sense of air hunger or urge to breathe, but appear quite comfortable at night while asleep.

Position

Dyspnea that occurs with or is relieved by changes in position should prompt a consideration of abnormalities in the ventilatory pump (i.e., the muscles of ventilation and the configuration of the chest wall, focal abnormalities in the lung that lead to hypoxemia when blood flow is increased to that area, or redistribution of fluid into the central circulation in patients with a history of CHF).

Orthopnea, dyspnea that occurs when the patient is in the recumbent position, can result from several abnormalities. The most common explanation is a redistribution of fluid from the legs into the central circulation, leading to an increase in pulmonary vascular pressures in a patient with CHF and compromised cardiac function. Given the very rapid onset and resolution of this symptom with change in position, dyspnea in this situation probably is secondary to stimulation of intracardiac (possibly the right atrium) or pulmonary vascular receptors, rather than the development of interstitial edema. In patients who are very obese or who have a distended abdomen due to ascites, the large abdomen reduces the compliance of the chest wall and increases the work of breathing. This phenomenon is exacerbated by the recumbent position since gravity is no longer pulling the abdomen away from the diaphragm. Patients with cervical spinal cord injury who lack active intercostal inspiratory muscles may also suffer from orthopnea.

Arteriovenous malformations (AVMs) in the pulmonary circulation lead to shunting of blood from the right to the left side of the heart (i.e., the blood never passes through the pulmonary capillaries and is sent to the systemic circulation with a low oxygen saturation). Any position that increases the gravity-dependent flow of blood through the AVM will lead to worsening hypoxemia and dyspnea. Focal areas of atelectasis or pneumonia will lead to similar gas exchange derangements when the body position is such that blood flow to that region of lung is enhanced. Consequently, the guiding principle in these circumstances is "good lung down" when positioning a patient to maximize gas exchange and minimize dyspnea.

Platypnea is a term that refers to the development of tachypnea and hyperventilation when the patient is in the upright position. It is physical finding rather than a symptom, although the patient may also complain of breathing discomfort. The exact mechanism for this finding is unclear, but it probably relates to the presence of pathology at the lung bases with stimulation of pulmonary receptors or worsening gas exchange when blood flow is increased to these areas with the patient upright.

COUGH
Definition and Physiology
A cough is a sudden expiratory maneuver, associated with high intrathoracic pressures, to clear secretions and foreign material from the airways. An effective cough requires the ability to take a large inspiratory volume that allows one to utilize the elastic recoil of the lungs and chest wall in the production of high intrathoracic pressures. Full attainment of these pressures also requires the ability to seal the glottis and to recruit expiratory muscles. The sound of the cough is associated with the sudden opening of the glottis and the subsequent explosive release of pressurized intrathoracic gas with vibration of the vocal cords. This vibration may help to loosen secretions from the larynx.

Conditions which impair inspiratory or expiratory muscle function lead to weakened cough. In addition, patients with vocal cord paralysis or tracheostomy are unable to seal the glottis and cannot generate the high intrathoracic pressure needed to clear secretions most effectively. These patients are at increased risk for lower respiratory infection and may complain of an increased sense of chest congestion.

Although we think of cough primarily as a mechanism to clear airway secretions, the triggers for cough are complex. Stimulation of irritant receptors in the larynx, trachea, and large airways can lead to cough. In addition, stretch receptors and C fibers in the interstitium of the lung may also produce a cough when activated (e.g., in interstitial pneumonitis or fibrosis). Cough may also be a manifestation of pleural irritation, and can be produced by a reflex mechanism triggered by the reflux of acid from the stomach to the esophagus. Finally, a rare cause of cough is stimulation of the tympanic membrane; we have seen one case of a patient with a chronic cough who had a small insect trapped in the external auditory canal.

Clinical Causes of Cough
The most common etiologies of cough are outlined in Table 39-5. In considering the differential diagnosis for this

symptom, it is useful to consider acute versus chronic coughs and to further subdivide patients with chronic cough into those with a normal versus abnormal chest radiograph.

Acute Cough

The most common cause of acute cough is a respiratory infection. These coughs tend to be associated with the production of sputum and are often accompanied by a "raw" sensation in the substernal area. A feeling of chest congestion may also be present. Fever, malaise, and other systemic symptoms of a viral or bacterial infection are likely to coexist.

Subclinical bronchospasm is another cause of acute (as well as chronic) cough. In patients with mild asthma, wheezing may not be present. Sudden exposures to allergens, cold air, or exercise may result in transient cough. A high index of suspicion, along with appropriate pulmonary function tests, is needed to make this diagnosis.

Inhalation of toxic fumes (e.g., cleaning agents, smoke) can produce a cough as a result of damage to the airway epithelium. Airway hyperreactivity may also result. As with acute infections, a raw sensation is often present in the substernal area. Dyspnea commonly accompanies these exposures. Aspiration of a foreign body (e.g., food particle or, in the case of a child, a small toy) may not be recalled by the patient. A cough may ensue immediately but, in some cases, can be delayed for hours or days. A focal wheeze is appreciated on examination of the chest in some cases, and a postobstructive penumonia can follow if the foreign material occludes the greater portion of an airway.

Chronic Cough with Clear Chest Radiograph

The scenario of chronic cough without significant dyspnea and with a normal chest radiograph is commonly seen both by physicians in primary care and by pulmonary specialists. This entity has been well studied (23,24), and the vast majority of patients will have one or a combination of three findings: postnasal drip, airway reactivity, and gastroesophageal reflux.

Table 39-5 Common Clinical Causes of Cough
Acute Cough
Respiratory infection, airway inflammation
Bronchospasm
Aspiration
Chronic Cough With Clear Chest Radiograph
Postnasal drip
Bronchospasm
Gastroesophageal reflux
Chronic bronchitis
Bronchiectasis
Endobronchial neoplasms
Chronic Cough With Abnormal Chest Radiograph
Interstitial lung disease
Recurrent aspiration
Endobronchial neoplasm
Indolent infections (e.g. *Pneumocystis carinii* pneumonia, tuberculosis)

Postnasal drip is a common complication of perennial rhinitis as well as a sequela of upper respiratory infections. Secretions from the posterior nasopharynx descend to the larynx and result in an irritating feeling or a "tickle" in the throat. The cough may be nonproductive or the patient may note small amounts of white sputum. If there is a history of chronic sinus infections, purulent sputum can be present. Typically, the cough will worsen when the patient assumes a supine position to go to sleep, both because of a worsening of the nasal drainage in that position and a greater awareness of the "irritation" in the absence of the usual distractions one has during the day. Not uncommonly, patients will not be aware of a "drip," per se, but, when questioned about the source of the cough (i.e., where the cough seems to be originating), they will localize it to the throat rather than the chest. It is important in these situations to inquire about frequent "throat clearing" during the day. If the patient is not aware of this, a family member should be questioned as well. Often one will note the frequent throat clearing during the interview session. A history of allergies should be sought, particularly if the frequency or severity of the cough varies with the seasons. However, in most cases, the patient will be unaware of specific allergens and skin testing may be necessary if symptoms persist despite treatment.

Hyperactive airways without wheezing can present as chronic cough and have been termed *cough variant asthma* (25). In a patient without a prior history of asthma, the symptoms will often follow a respiratory infection. The systemic symptoms associated with the infection will clear over several weeks, but the cough will persist. In many cases, the cough will resolve spontaneously in 8 to 12 weeks, but it can continue indefinitely. Typically, the cough will be nonproductive or lead to small amounts of clear to white sputum. In contrast to cough associated with postnasal drip, patients with subclinical bronchospasm will localize the origin of the cough to the chest. It is important to inquire about factors that exacerbate the cough. Exposure to cold air, exercise, smoke, and toxic fumes characteristically worsens cough arising from airway reactivity. Spirometry is often normal when patients are seen by their physician, and the diagnosis may be made based on response to a therapeutic trial of bronchodilators or by bronchial provocation tests.

Gastroesophageal reflux completes the triad of common causes of chronic cough. It may produce cough on its own or exacerbate the symptom in a patient with airway reactivity. Patients with this problem typically have a nonproductive cough and localize the origin of the symptom to the chest. A history of heartburn or reflux symptoms is helpful but is frequently absent. In addition to asking about heartburn, one should inquire about "waterbrash," the sudden sensation of a sour taste in the mouth, which is typical of reflux of gastric contents.

Other less common causes of chronic cough with a normal chest radiograph include bronchiectasis, chronic bronchitis, and bronchial carcinoid. Patients with bronchiectasis typically have a cough productive of purulent sputum, although upper lobe disease, which tends to drain well throughout the day, may be associated with a dry cough or scant secretions. Sputum is often purulent and occasionally streaked with blood. A history of one or more pneumonias in the past is helpful in making the diagnosis, but is neither sensitive nor specific. Patients with bronchiectasis are susceptible to recurring respiratory infections that tend to be associated with low-grade fever and worsening cough and sputum production. The presence of *Pseudomonas aeruginosa* on repeated sputum cultures is very suggestive of this condition. Although the chest radiograph is often normal, focal areas of fibrosis or fibrocystic disease may be present, and CT scans of the chest are quite sensitive in defining the extent of disease.

Chronic bronchitis is defined as cough present for 3 or more months of the year for at least 2 years and is the result of chronic inflammation of the airways induced by cigarette smoking. The cough is typically most pronounced early in the morning and tends to diminish as the day progresses. Patients localize the cough to the chest. Sputum is gray to green in color and occasionally mixed with blood. Due to associated airway obstruction, these patients can have dyspnea on exertion.

Endobronchial neoplasms in central airways can produce cough and, in the absence of a significant airway obstruction leading to focal atelectasis, will usually have a normal chest radiograph. Although bronchogenic carcinoma can present with this picture, especially if the patient is more than 40 years old and has a significant smoking history, we typically think of bronchial adenomas, or carcinoid tumors, in this setting. These tumors, which usually behave as very low-grade malignancies with a small potential for distant metastases, may have a polypoid appearance that, in some cases, leads to a positional cough (i.e., a cough that is present primarily when the patient assumes a particular position). This quality is assumed to be secondary to intermittent airway obstruction from the adenoma that correlates with that particular position.

Chronic Cough with an Abnormal Chest Radiograph

Interstitial lung disease typically presents with the gradual onset of dyspnea on exertion, but may have cough as a prominent associated symptom or as the only manifestation of the disease in its early stages. The cough is localized to the chest by the patient and is nonproductive. In severe cases, the symptom can be quite debilitating and refractory to cough suppressants. In approximately 90% of cases, the chest radiograph will demonstrate an increase in interstitial markings on presentation (26). For those patients with normal chest radiographs but suspected interstitial disease, high-resolution computerized tomography (CT) scans are a very sensitive tool for confirming the diagnosis (27). Additional clues that can be gleaned from the interview with the patient include an occupational history (e.g., exposure to inorganic or organic dusts), the presence of joint symptoms or peripheral skin nodules to suggest collagen-vascular disease (e.g., rheumatoid arthritis, systemic lupus erythematosus), and eye symptoms or lower extremity joint pain that would be indicative of sarcoidosis.

As noted above, endobronchial neoplasms can present as a chronic cough. Bronchogenic carcinomas in the central airways are often associated with partial or complete obstruction of a segmental or lobar bronchus leading to focal atelectasis or volume loss on the chest radiograph. Mediastinal lymphadenopathy may also be seen. The cough is typically nonproductive but may give rise to intermittent hemoptysis.

Although we typically think of cough associated with lower respiratory infections as having an acute presentation, there are many indolent infections that can present with a chronic cough and a paucity of systemic symptoms. *Pneumocystis carinii* pneumonia in patients with human immunodeficiency virus (HIV) disease, for example, can develop over several weeks to months as a nonproductive cough with gradually progressive dyspnea on exertion. Similarly, reactivation of mycobacterium tuberculosis can present with cough, fatigue, and mild weight loss in its early stages. Chest radiographs usually provide evidence of the underlying infection.

Essentials of the History

After determining whether the cough is acute or chronic, the next useful distinction to make in patients presenting with cough is to determine if dyspnea and/or systemic symptoms are part of the symptom complex. The presence or absence of purulent sputum is helpful in diagnosing many infectious problems. Localizing the cough to the throat versus the chest is extremely useful in patients with chronic cough and no dyspnea since cough originating from an irritation in the throat is likely due to postnasal drip.

Timing of the cough, particularly for chronic cough, is quite useful. Morning cough tends to be associated with chronic bronchitis and bronchiectasis. Evening and nocturnal cough is more typical of postnasal drip, gastroesophageal reflux, and airway reactivity. Exercise-induced cough should make one consider bronchospasm and interstitial lung disease.

Finally, positionally related cough may provide essential clues to the diagnosis. Cough that worsens in the supine position may reflect postnasal drip or gastroesophageal reflux, whereas symptoms that are reproducible when lying on one side or the other or when leaning forward may be indicative of a transient airway obstruction from a bronchial adenoma.

HEMOPTYSIS

Definition and Physiology

Hemoptysis refers to the coughing or expectoration of blood or blood-tinged sputum. As a general principle, the term is reserved for blood that originates in the lower respiratory tract (i.e., below the larynx). In some cases, however, it may be difficult to determine whether the blood is coming from the posterior nasopharynx or the gastrointestinal tract, especially if vomiting is associated with a paroxysm of cough. It is worth noting that the normal tracheobronchial tree should not bleed even in the presence of a coagulopathy. Thus, hemoptysis in the setting of anticoagulation should be considered as a potentially pathologic finding.

There are four major sources of blood in the lower respiratory tract: airways, pulmonary parenchyma, pulmonary circulation, and bronchial circulation. Inflammation or irritation of the airways, as is seen with acute pulmonary infections, chronic bronchitis, or foreign body aspiration, can result in what are usually small amounts of hemoptysis, often mixed in with sputum. Bleeding from the pulmonary parenchyma occurs with pulmonary infarction or contusion. With pulmonary AVMs or greatly elevated pressures in the pulmonary circulation from mitral stenosis, bleeding may occur as well.

Finally, the bronchial circulation may give rise to hemoptysis in patients with bronchiectasis or large intrapulmonary cavities.

Massive hemoptysis is typically defined as greater than 600 mL of blood in 24 hours. Patients commonly overestimate the amount of blood they have expectorated because of the anxiety that results from this symptom. Therefore, it is very important to compel the patient to be as explicit as possible when quantifying the amount of blood. One should show the patient, and others who witnessed the episode, various-sized containers to assist them in making an estimate of the quantity expectorated. While massive hemoptysis can occur from an endobronchial carcinoma, it is more commonly associated with erosions of bronchial vessels in large intrapulmonary cavities or with bronchiectasis (28).

Etiology

There are six etiologic categories to be considered when evaluating a patient with hemoptysis (Table 39-6). Determining which category is applicable for your patient will be based to a great extent on the nature of symptoms other than the hemoptysis itself.

Infections of the lower respiratory tract lead to inflammation of airways and can cause bleeding. This is most common with bacterial tracheobronchitis, but can occur as well with bacterial pneumonias. Atypical infections (e.g., viruses and *Mycoplasma pneumoniae*) are less common explanations. Typically, hemoptysis in the setting of an acute infection will be small in quantity (<50 mL) and will last less than 1 week with resolution coincident with improvement in the other associated symptoms (e.g., cough, fever, malaise). Bronchiectasis and chronic bronchitis are chronic inflammatory conditions of the lung that often lead to acute infections. Each is associated with occasional episodes of blood-streaked sputum on occasion, most typically in the presence of an acute infection that leads to increased sputum production. As noted above, bronchiectasis infrequently leads to massive hemoptysis.

Pulmonary neoplasms, most commonly bronchogenic carcinoma, are a common cause of hemoptysis. This diagnosis should be considered particularly in patients who are over age 40 and have a significant smoking history, and in whom the hemoptysis extends over more than a 10-day period (29). Patients with a history of an extrathoracic malignancy that can metastasize to the lungs (e.g., breast carcinoma or sarcoma) are also at increased risk of pulmonary neoplasm as a cause for hemoptysis. Bleeding in the setting of neoplasm usually occurs in the absence of other symptoms and presents as frank blood without sputum.

Table 39-6 Etiologic Categories for Hemoptysis
Pulmonary infections
Neoplasms
Collagen-vascular and immunologic lung diseases
Cardiovascular diseases
Aspiration of foreign bodies
Chest trauma with pulmonary contusion

Hemoptysis in association with joint symptoms, rashes, dyspnea, or renal dysfunction raises the specter of collagen-vascular diseases. In particular, the pulmonary-renal syndromes, (e.g., systemic lupus erythematosis, Wegener's granulomatosis, and Goodpasture's syndrome) may present with hemoptysis as part of their symptom complex. In most cases, bleeding is not an isolated finding.

Cardiovascular causes of bleeding include AVMs, pulmonary emboli, pulmonary edema, and mitral stenosis. Pulmonary edema classically produces pink sputum and there is evidence on lung biopsy of hemosiderin-laden macrophages consistent with pulmonary hemorrhage. Gross blood, however, is uncommon in CHF unless the patient also has a coagulopathy. Bleeding may be the first symptom of an AVM and massive hemoptysis has been reported (30). Hemoptysis from pulmonary emboli or mitral stenosis usually occurs in the presence of other symptoms such as dyspnea and chest discomfort.

Aspiration of foreign bodies can lead to hemoptysis either by causing direct trauma to the airways or by leading to local inflammation. Pulmonary contusions result most commonly from blunt trauma to the chest (e.g., automobile accidents) and are associated with other evidence of trauma such as rib fractures, pneumothorax, and cardiac contusion. Hemoptysis in these settings is usually small in quantity.

Essentials of the History

As noted above, may of the clues about the etiology of hemoptysis derive from evaluation of other symptoms. Thus, attention must be paid to a focused history designed to eluicidate information that will permit you to place the patient into one of the categories outlined in Table 39-6. With respect to the bleeding itself, careful quantification of the hemoptysis is important along with details on the duration of the symptom. The presence of a history of cigarette smoking clearly raises the risk of a bronchogenic carcinoma. Finally, the presence of blood with sputum raises the probability that one is dealing with an infectious or inflammatory cause for the hemoptysis.

WHEEZING

Definition and Physiology

Wheezing is a sound that emanates from lower airways (i.e., below the larynx) and results from turbulent flow. It is a "continuous" sound, as compared to the intermittent or staccato sounds that accompany chest congestion with mucus in the airways, and may be described as occurring during expiration, inspiration, or throughout the respiratory cycle. It is both a symptom, a sound that the patient reports he or she has heard in association with breathing, as well as a physical finding if the physician appreciates the sound during examination of the patient.

The sound is produced by turbulent flow through narrowed airways and in some cases may reflect the rapid oscillation of the airway walls (31). Airway narrowing can result from a variety of problems including bronchospasm, airway inflammation and mucous hypersecretion, mucosal edema, airway collapse, and endobronchial obstructions (Table 39-7). As a general principle, physicians distinguish wheezing, a sound originating in the lower airways, from stridor, which is

Table 39-7 Common Causes of Wheezing
Primary airway reactivity (e.g., asthma)
Interstitial edema
Airway inflammation and mucous hypersecretion
Endobronchial obstruction (e.g., neoplasm or foreign body)
Vocal cord dysfunction

primarily an inspiratory sound, qualitatively similar to wheeze, but arising from the larynx and upper airways. Because the transmural pressure across the intrathoracic airways favors expansion of the airways during inspiration (due to negative pleural pressures), inspiratory wheezing is relatively uncommon. In contrast, the extrathoracic airways tend to collapse during inspiration (atmospheric pressure surrounding the airway is greater than the negative pressure inside it), making any narrowing more prominent. Thus, wheezing that worsens during inspiration is likely to be secondary to an obstruction in the extrathoracic airways, whereas wheezing that is more pronounced on expiration is probably coming from the intrathoracic airways. When the intensity of wheezing seems quite constant throughout the respiratory cycle, one should consider a fixed obstruction.

Etiology

The most common cause of wheezing is asthma although, as noted above in the discussion of cough, asthma may occur in the absence of wheeze. Historical information key to the diagnosis of asthma includes factors that precipitate wheezing that are suggestive of airway reactivity, such as allergens, cold air, and exercise, and a favorable response to inhaled bronchodilators. Physician examination and pulmonary function testing are usually sufficient to confirm the diagnosis. Mucous hypersecretion associated with infections and airway inflammation may also lead to wheezing. Since these lower tract infections can also produce transient airway hyperreactivity, it may be difficult to distinguish this from asthma. A rapid disappearance of the wheeze in association with cough or bronchopulmonary hygiene, however, is suggestive of mucous hypersecretion as the underlying etiology.

Cardiac asthma, wheezing in association with increased pulmonary capillary pressures and interstitial edema, is another major cause of wheezing. Generally, there will be other evidence of CHF in the history (orthopnea, paroxysmal nocturnal dyspnea) and physical examination (distended jugular veins, S_3 gallop, peripheral edema). However, acute CHF secondary to myocardial ischemia may be difficult to distinguish from asthma in a patient with a history of airway reactivity.

Partial endobronchial obstructions can lead to focal or localized wheezing although the patient may not recognize the focal origins of the sound nor be able to localize any internal sensations in association with the wheeze. Bronchogenic neoplasms, either carcinomas or adenomas, as well as aspirated foreign bodies can lead to focal wheezing.

Wheezing may originate from the upper airways when laryngospasm is present. This symptom may be extremely difficult to distinguish from asthma by history alone.

Frequently, this condition occurs in young women, often with a history of emotional difficulties, and commonly is treated as asthma for months or years before the definitive diagnosis is recognized (32). Some clues to the diagnosis are a very rapid onset of symptoms and the association of psychological stress with wheezing episodes. Direct visualization of the vocal cords during an attack can confirm the diagnosis.

Swelling of the vocal cords secondary to infection, allergic reactions, or chemical or smoke inhalation narrows the upper airway, increases turbulent flow, and may lead to wheezing that is typically termed *stridor*. The sound is high-pitched and most prominent during inspiration because of the propensity for the narrowing to worsen with negative pressure in the upper airway relative to the atmospheric pressure in the surrounding tissues. The insult that causes the laryngeal edema may also lead to spasm of the lower airways and classical wheezing. Urticaria and angioedema commonly accompany allergic reactions that produce laryngeal edema.

Essentials of the History

Confronted with a patient complaining of wheezing, the physician's questions focus largely on associated symptoms that may provide clues to underlying cause. Is there evidence of respiratory infection and increased secretions (increased mucus in airways)? Is the wheezing episodic and precipitated by exposure to allergens, fumes, or cold air (asthma)? Does the wheezing occur in association with chest pain or the development of peripheral edema (CHF)? Are there pruritis and swelling of the lips and tongue to suggest an allergic reaction and possible laryngeal edema?

The presence of chest tightness is suggestive of either asthma or CHF with myocardial ischemia as the cause of the wheezing. Onset of symptoms at night is consistent with either diagnosis, asthma or CHF, but the wheezing is more likely to subside with assumption of the upright posture in CHF than when the symptom is due to asthma.

Worsening of the symptom during inspiration is suggestive of an upper airway etiology. Localization of the sound on physical examination raises the possibility of a focal endobronchial obstruction or narrowing.

HOARSENESS

Definition and Physiology

Hoarseness is a coarse, somewhat muffled quality to the voice. Since vocalization depends upon modulation of the movement of air out of the lungs and the associated vibration of the vocal cords, conditions that interfere with normal vibration tend to result in distortion of and diminution in the intensity of the sound. Causes of hoarseness can be grouped physiologically into two categories: those that arise from thickening, inflammation, or ulceration of the vocal cords, and those that are due to weakness or paralysis of the muscles that control movement of the cords (Table 39-8). In the former situation, the pathology of the vocal cords themselves prevents normal vibration. In the case of weakness or paralysis of the muscles controlling the cords, the cords either become fixed in position or lose the capability to resist the movement of air.

Table 39-8 Common Causes of Hoarseness
Thickening, inflammation, or ulceration of the vocal cords
Viral infections
Inhalation of irritant gases
Use of inhaled steroids
Granulomatous disease
Trauma
Vocal cord neoplasms
Weakness of muscles controlling vocal cord motion
Neurologic diseases involving the bulbar muscles
Myasthenia gravis
Botulism
Polio
Damage to the recurrent layrngeal nerve
Trauma
Mediastinal tumors
Thoracic aortic aneurysm

Etiology

Edema of the vocal cords can result from a number of infectious and noninfectious causes. Viral infections of the upper respiratory tract are commonly associated with laryngeal edema and hoarseness. Inhalation of irritant gases including smoke can also produce this finding as can prolonged shouting or overuse of the voice. Use of inhaled steroids in high doses for asthma has led, in some cases, to thickening of the cords and hoarseness as well.

Ulcerations and neoplasms of the vocal cords interfere with normal motion and vibration. Ulceration most typically results from prolonged placement of an endotracheal tube. Infections such as tuberculosis and typhoid fever as well as collagen-vascular diseases, such as systemic lupus erythematosus, have also been associated with vocal cord ulceration. Granulomas (which can follow chronic irritation of the cords), polyps, and carcinomas similarly interfere with normal vibration and present with hoarseness as the primary symptom.

Weakness or paralysis of the muscles controlling movement of the vocal cords is due either to general neurologic conditions that affect the bulbar muscles, or to local factors that interfere with the function of the laryngeal nerves that supply these muscles. Myasthenia gravis, botulism, and polio are examples of the former. The most common causes of damage to the laryngeal nerves are trauma, including blunt or penetrating injuries of the neck or thorax as well as surgical damage, and neoplasms. The path of the recurrent laryngeal nerve takes it into the apical thorax on the right side, where it passes under the subclavian artery, and under the aorta on the left. Invasion of the mediastinum by carcinomas or extension of tumor into mediastinal lymph nodes can lead to damage of the nerve and hoarseness. Thoracic aortic aneurysms with an expanding aortic arch may also cause damage to the recurrent laryngeal nerve on the left.

Essentials of the History

The quality of hoarseness does not vary in a consistent and specific way based on the etiology of the symptom. In contrast, the rapidity with which the hoarseness develops is an important clue to the underlying problem. Infectious causes of hoarseness tend to develop over hours or a day or two. Similarly, hoarseness developing secondary to trauma to the recurrent laryngeal nerve will be acute in onset. In contrast, neurologic conditions that lead to weakness of the bulbar muscles, damage to the recurrent laryngeal nerve from mediastinal or thoracic neoplasms, and growths on the vocal cords typically develop over the course of weeks or months.

Associated symptoms also provide important information about the etiology of the hoarseness. The presence of fever, cough, and head congestion suggests an upper respiratory infection. Hemoptysis in the absence of infectious symptoms raises the specter of bronchogenic carcinoma. Muscle weakness involving the extremities signals a diffuse neurologic disorder.

SNORING

Definition and Physiology

Snoring is defined as noisy breathing during sleep and may be a "normal" finding in approximately 10% of the population (33). However, snoring with the mouth open does imply an element of upper airway obstruction. Oral snoring results from vibration of the soft palate and faucial pillars. The likelihood that snoring will occur is dependent upon the size of the airway, the tone of the soft tissue structures in the airway, and the individual's body position. As discussed above (see the discussion of upper airway wheezing), the intraluminal pressure in the hypopharynx becomes negative during inspiration, which favors collapse of the airway because of the relatively greater pressure (atmospheric) surrounding it. If the airway is already narrowed because of increased fat in the soft tissues, as can be seen in obese patients or those treated with systemic corticosteroids, or edema, the propensity for airway obstruction and snoring is increased. Conditions that reduce the muscle tone of the surrounding tissue (e.g., alcohol, sedative agents) further increase the risk of airway obstruction. Rapid eye movement (REM) sleep is associated with decreased muscle tone, and snoring occurs most commonly during this phase of sleep.

The tongue is a major component of the anterior wall of the hypopharynx, and movement of the tongue can contribute to upper airway obstruction. When the tongue falls posteriorly, obstruction is worsened. Patients who sleep in the supine position are more likely to have snoring or more severe obstruction because of the propensity of the tongue to be pulled posteriorly by gravity.

Etiology

While snoring can be a normal finding in individuals, particularly when the muscles of the upper airway become flaccid as the result of the ingestion of alchohol or benzodiazepines, it may be the first sign of obstructive sleep apnea. In this condition, snoring may give way to apneas with cessation of airflow during complete obstruction of the airway. Intermittent hypoxia occurs and, in patients with underlying lung disease, chronic hypercapnia may follow. Patients typically will complain of daytime hypersomnolence and may have morning headaches, difficulty concentrating, and enuresis. Associated findings include hypertension and evidence of right ventricular overload.

Children with large tonsils or adenoids may be brought to the physician by a parent concerned about the child's snoring. Significant airway obstruction, however, is unusual in this clinical setting.

Essentials of the History

Snoring, unlike many symptoms, is less likely to be reported by the patient than by the patient's spouse or roommate. Thus, it is important to include anyone who has witnessed the patient's sleep when obtaining the history about snoring. First, one must clearly distinguish whether the snoring is occurring during mouth or nasal breathing. Nasal snoring is generally not considered indicative of a pathologic process. Second, the physician should try to ascertain whether there have been episodes of apnea, either central (when there is no evidence of airflow or chest wall movement) or obstructive (no airflow but intact chest wall motion). Additional questions are focused on the features of the obstructive sleep apnea syndrome as outlined above.

The chronicity of the snoring and associated changes in weight or drug and alcohol use are also important pieces of information. A middle-aged individual, for example, whose snoring dates back to adolescence and who has otherwise been well is likely to have a benign condition. On the other hand, an individual whose snoring is only 6 months old and began in association with a 50-lb weight gain should be considered for possible obstructive sleep apnea, especially if there is evidence of hypersomnolence or right ventricular failure.

SUMMARY

With an understanding of the physiology underlying respiratory symptoms, physicians can gain valuable insights into the disease processes afflicting their patients. The lungs and upper airways have fairly limited ways to respond to pathologic changes. Thus, the number of types of symptoms experienced by patients with respiratory diseases is small. The challenge is to understand the nuances of the descriptions of the sensations and the sounds that patients report, and to ask probing questions that elicit these subtle distinctions. With this knowledge, and the information gleaned from physical examination, diagnoses can often be made with little if any corroborative laboratory testing, the patient is spared unnecessary risks and discomfort, and healthcare resource utilization is optimized.

Acknowledgment: This work was supported in part by a grant from the Merck Company Foundation.

REFERENCES

1. Cook DG, Shaper AG. Breathlessness, lung function, and risk of heart attack. Eur Heart J 1988;9:1215–1222.

2. Higgins M. Epidemiology of obstructive pulmonary disease. In: Cassaburi R, Petty TL, eds. Principles and practice of pulmonary rehabilitation. Philadelphia: WB Saunders, 1993:10–17.

3. Manning HL, Schwartzstein RM. Pathophysiology of dyspnea. N Eng J Med 1995;333:1547–1553.

4. McCloskey DI. Corollary discharges: motor commands and perception. In: Brookhart JM, Mountcastle VB, eds. Handbook of physiology, sect. 1. The nervous system, vol II. Bethesda, MD: American Physiological Society, 1981:1415–1447.

5. Schwartzstein RM, Manning HL, Weiss JW, Weinberger SE. Dyspnea: a sensory experience. Lung 1990;168:185–199.

6. O'Donnell DE, Webb KA. Exertional breathlessness in patients with chronic airflow limitation. Am Rev Respir Dis 1993;148:1351–1357.

7. Simon PM, Schwartzstein RM, Weiss JW, et al. Distinguishable types of dyspnea in patients with shortness of breath. Am Rev Respir Dis 1990;142:1009–1014.

8. Elliott MW, Adam L, Cockroft A, et al. The Language of breathlessness: use of verbal descriptors. Am Rev Respir Dis 1991;144:826–832.

9. Mahler DA, Harver A, Lentine T, et al. Descriptors of breathlessness in cardiorespiratory diseases. Am J Respir Crit Care Med 1996;154:1357–1363.

10. Taguchi O, Kikuchi Y, Hida W, et al. Effects of bronchoconstriction and external resistive loading on the sensation of dyspnea. J Appl Physiol 1991;71:2183–2190.

11. McParland C, Krishnan B, Wang Y, Gallagher C. Inspiratory muscle weakness and dyspnea in chronic heart failure. Am Rev Respir Dis 1992;146:467–472.

12. Rubin SA, Brown HV. Ventilation and gas exchange during exercise in severe chronic heart failure. Am Rev Respir Dis 1984;129:S63.

13. Clark A, Poole-Wilson P. Breathlessness in heart disease. In: Adams L, Guz A, eds. Respiratory sensation. New York: Marcel Dekker, 1996:263–283.

14. Melzack R. The McGill Pain Questionnaire: major properties and scoring methods. Pain 1975;27:277–299.

15. Dubuisson D, Melzack R. Classification of clinical pain descriptions by mulitple group discriminate analysis. Exp Neurol 1976;51:480–487.

16. Hunter M, Philips C. The experience of headache—an assessment of the qualities of tension headache pain. Pain 1981;10:209–219.

17. Simon PM, Schwartzstein RM, Weiss JW, et al. Distinguishable sensations of breathlessness induced in normal volunteers. Am Rev Respir Dis 1989;140:1021–1027.

18. O'Donnell DE, Bertley JC, Chau LK, Webb KA. Qualitative aspects of exertional breathlessness in chronic airflow limitation: pathophysiologic mechanisms. Am J Respir Crit Care Med 1997;155:109–115.

19. Banzett RB, Lansing RW, Brown R, et al. "Air hunger" arising from increased P_{CO_2} persists after complete neuromuscular block in humans. Respir Physiol 1990;81:1–17.

20. Garfinkel SK, Kesten S, Chapman KR, Rebuck AS. Physiologic and nonphysiologic determinants of aerobic fitness in mild to moderate asthma. Am Rev Respir Dis 1992;145:741–745.

21. Sue DY, Wasserman K, Moricca RB, Casaburi R. Metabolic acidosis during exercise in patients with chronic obstructive pulmonary disease. Chest 1988;94:931–938.

22. Killian KJ, Summer E, Jones NL, Campbell EJM. Dyspnea and leg effort during incremental cycle ergometry. Am Rev Respir Dis 1992;145:1339–1345.

23. Irwin RS, Curley FJ, French CL. Chronic cough: the spectrum and frequency of causes, key components of the diagnostic evaluation, and outcome of specific therapy. Am Rev Respir Dis 1990;141:640–647.

24. Poe RH, Harder RV, Isreael RH, Kallay MC. Chronic persistent cough: experience in diagnosis and outcome using an anatomic diagnostic protocol. Chest 1989;95:723–728.

25. Corrao WM, Braman SS, Irwin RS. Chronic cough as the sole presenting manifestation of bronchial asthma. N Engl J Med 1979;300:633–637.

26. Epler GR, McLoud TC, Gaensler EA, et al. Normal chest roentgenograms in chronic diffuse infiltrative lung disease. N Engl J Med 1978;298:934–939.

27. Wells AU, Hansell DM, Rubens MB, et al. The predictive value of appearances on thin-section computed tomography in fibrosing alveolitis. Am Rev Respir Dis 1991;148:1076–1082.

28. Knott-Craig CH, Oostuizen JG, Rossouw G, et al. Management and prognosis of massive hemoptysis. J Thorac Cardiovasc Surg 1993;105:394–397.

29. Jackson CV, Savage PJ, Quinn DL. Role of fiberoptic bronchoscopy in patients with hemoptysis and a normal chest roentgenogram. Chest 1985;87:142–144.

30. Ference BA, Shannon TM, White

RI, et al. Life-threatening pulmonary hemorrhage with pulmonary arteriovenous malformations and hereditary hemorrhagic telangiectasia. Chest 1994;106:1387–1390.

31. Hollingsworth HM. Wheezing and stridor. Clin Chest Med 1987;8:231–240.

32. Christopher KL, Wood RP, Eckert RC, et al. Vocal-cord dysfunction presenting as asthma. N Engl J Med 1983;308:1566–1570.

33. Cooper KR. Hoarseness and snoring. In: Glauser FL, ed. Signs and symptoms in pulmonary medicine. Philadelphia: J.B. Lippincott, 1983:86–96.

Chapter 40

Use of Pulmonary Function and Cardiopulmonary Exercise Laboratories for Diagnostic Testing

Richard Casaburi

Laboratory science is an integral component of the practice of pulmonary medicine. Over the years, testing modalities designed by pulmonologists have been found to be useful for patients with nonpulmonary disease, as well. The largest pulmonary-based laboratories offer a wide range of tests. However, two tests are the mainstays of many of these laboratories: pulmonary function testing and cardiopulmonary exercise testing. This chapter is intended as a primer in the principles and utility of these two tests. References are given to more comprehensive treatments of these topics. For the interested reader, references to other tests commonly offered in comprehensive pulmonary laboratories are offered below:

- Bronchial provocation (1,2)
- Lung elastic recoil and lung compliance (3,4)
- Airway resistance (3,5)
- CO_2 and O_2 chemosensitivity (3,6,7)
- Infant pulmonary function (8)
- Sleep disturbances (9)
- Respiratory muscle strength and endurance (10,11)
- Arterial blood gas analysis (12)

PULMONARY FUNCTION TESTING

Pulmonary function testing consists of a set of physiologic measurements that serves to detect lung dysfunction, assists in the differential diagnosis of lung disorder, and yields an assessment of the severity of lung disease. In pulmonary function testing, we wish to know: 1) if the lung is stiff (i.e., if lung compliance is low), 2) if the resistance to airflow is high, 3) if

airflow and pulmonary blood flow go evenly to all areas of the lung, and 4) if alveolar gases exchange freely with the pulmonary capillary blood. Although pulmonary function testing does not provide direct measurement of these qualities (e.g., lung compliance is not measured), a series of tests indirectly evaluate all these aspects of function. These tests are designed to be quick, efficient, and essentially noninvasive. Further, pattern analysis of pulmonary function test abnormalities can distinguish among the major classes of pulmonary diseases:

1. It is possible to distinguish between obstructive lung disease with a substantial reversible component (i.e., asthma) and chronic obstructive pulmonary disease (COPD). It is often possible to determine whether COPD is predominantly of the bronchitic (prominent airway inflammation) or emphysemic (prominent alveolar destruction) varieties.

2. The presence of restrictive lung disease can be detected. In these conditions the air volume of the lung during a maximum inspiratory effort is decreased. These conditions include disorders of the lung parenchyma (e.g., fibrosis, lung masses, pneumonia, pneumonectomy) or limitations to chest wall expansion (rib cage deformities, severe obesity, pleural effusion).

3. Pulmonary vascular disease can be inferred from deficits in gas transfer from alveoli to blood. Further, it is possible to distinguish between disorders in which pulmonary capillaries are dysfunctional but alveoli are intact (e.g., pulmonary emboli, pulmonary vasculitis) and disorders in which both alveoli and pulmonary vasculature are destroyed or nonfunctional (e.g., pulmonary fibrosis, pneumonia, pneumonectomy).

Pulmonary function testing is a mature science; a similar set of tests is offered by most laboratories. Further, normal values are available, so that abnormalities can be defined by statistical contrast with a normal population (13,14). After examination of large groups of normal subjects, regression equations have been derived based on a subject's height, age, and gender. A small correction for race is often employed.

Lung Volumes

Figure 40-1 illustrates the static lung volumes. The tidal volume (V_T) is the volume inspired and expired during unforced breathing. Inspiratory capacity (IC) is the volume inspired with a maximal effort after a normal exhalation. The expiratory reserve volume (ERV) is the volume exhaled with a maximal effort after a normal exhalation. The inspiratory reserve volume (IRV) is the volume inhaled with a maximal effort after a normal inhalation. The vital capacity (VC) is the volume exhaled when going from a maximal inhalation to a maximal exhalation. These volumes can be measured fairly simply when the patient respires into a volume displacement spirometer or an airflow measuring device (in which volume is calculated by integration of airflow rate). Of these volumes, the most useful in disease diagnosis is vital capacity. In fact, the earliest use of pulmonary function testing occurred when Hutchinson measured vital capacity in a large population of Londoners in the 1840s (15). *Vital capacity is reduced in restrictive disease. It is also usually reduced in obstructive lung disease, because air trapping limits the ability to empty the lungs.*

Other lung volumes pictured in Figure 40-1 cannot be measured by spirometry. The residual volume (RV) is the volume of air remaining in the lungs after a maximal exhalation. The functional residual capacity (FRC) is the volume of air in the lung after a normal exhalation. The total lung capacity (TLC) is the volume of air in the lungs at the end of a maximal inhalation. As can be seen in the figure, some of these volumes are interrelated (for example, TLC = FRC + IC; RV = FRC − ERV). Generally, FRC is measured and RV and TLC are calculated using spirometrically measured volumes. There are three commonly used methods to measure FRC.

Nitrogen washout measures the volume of nitrogen in the lung at the end of an exhalation (16,17). Since the lung gas contains 79% N_2, the FRC can be easily calculated if the volume of nitrogen in the lung at end exhalation is known. Conceptually, the nitrogen washout test involves transferring this volume of nitrogen out of the lung where it can be measured. To do this, the patient respires through a breathing valve. At end exhalation, the gas supplied through the inspiratory port is changed from air to 100% oxygen (i.e., 0% nitrogen). Thereafter, the nitrogen contained in the gas exhaled through the expiratory port is derived solely from the nitrogen originally residing in the lung gas. Over the next few minutes the nitrogen concentration in the lung progressively declines as it is diluted by the inspired 100% O_2. After about 7 minutes, virtually no nitrogen remains in the lung gas; it all has been exhaled. The volume of nitrogen exhaled can be measured if the exhalate is collected in a gas bag; it is calculated as the product of the final volume of the bag and the nitrogen concentration in the gas. In modern measurement systems, however, a gas collection bag is not utilized. The exhaled nitrogen concentration and gas flow rate are continuously measured; the product of these two signals is summed over the entire washout period to yield the total nitrogen volume exhaled.

The second commonly used measure of FRC is helium dilution (18,19). In this test, at the end of a normal exhalation the patient begins to rebreathe from a gas bag of known volume and known concentration of helium. At the end of several minutes of rebreathing, the helium is evenly distributed between the bag gas and the lung gas. The following equation describes the process:

$$V_B F_{He}^B = (V_L + V_B) F_{He}^E$$

Since no helium resides in the lung before the test begins, the volume of helium in the gas bag before equilibration begins (left side of the equation) equals the volume of helium in the lung-bag system after equilibration (right side of the equation), where V_B is the bag volume, F_{He}^B and F_{He}^E are the helium fractional concentrations initially in the gas and at equilibrium, and V_L is the volume of the lung at FRC. Since V_B, F_{He}^B, and F_{He}^E are measured, V_L can be calculated.

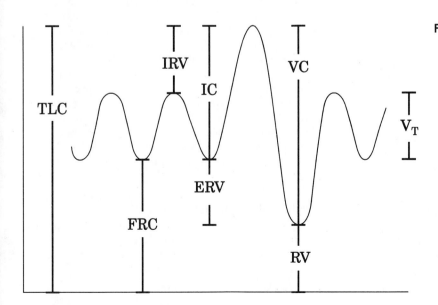

Figure 40-1 Subdivisions of pulmonary lung volumes. V_T, tidal volume; IC, inspiratory capacity; ERV, expiratory reserve volume; IRV, inspiratory reserve volume; VC, vital capacity; RV, residual volume; TLC, total lung capacity; FRC, functional residual capacity.

Body plethysmography is the third commonly utilized method of FRC measurement (5,20). The patient sits within an airtight phone booth–sized box and breathes through a mouthpiece connected to the outside of the box. The mouthpiece is briefly occluded and the patient pants against the closed orifice. The pressure fluctuation in the lung gas is measured at the mouth during the panting maneuver. The volume change of the thorax produced by this pressure fluctuation in the lung gas is measured indirectly from the pressure fluctuation within the body plethysmograph. The larger the volume of gas within the lung, the larger is the volume change of the thorax for a given pressure fluctuation. To a good approximation, this yields:

$$V_L = \frac{\Delta V}{\Delta P} P$$

where V_L is lung volume (that is, FRC), P is barometric pressure minus water vapor pressure, and ΔV and ΔP are the pressure and volume fluctuations produced by panting.

Measured by any one of these three techniques FRC, when added to the spirometrically measured inspiratory capacity, allows calculation of TLC. *TLC is often greater than predicted in obstructive lung disease. However TLC is always low in restrictive lung disease. In fact, a lower than predicted TLC is the* sine qua non *of restrictive lung disease.*

Lung Flow Rates

Most inferences regarding lung flow rates are derived from the forced expiratory vital capacity maneuver (21,22). After a full inspiration, air is forcefully exhaled, with the maneuver prolonged (for at least 6 seconds) until no more gas can be exhaled. Figure 40-2 shows the time course of lung volume change, which can be measured directly by a volume displacement spirometer, or indirectly by an airflow transducer (in which volume is measured by integrating flow rate). In the lung with high airway resistance, it will take longer to complete the expiration. Forced expiration (rather than forced inspiration) is studied, since the airway compression from the positive intrathoracic pressures during expiration will increase airway resistance, especially in the patient with obstructive airway disease. Although there are several ways of expressing the "slowness" with which the forced expired volume is exhaled (23), the most common are based on FEV_1, the forced expiratory volume exhaled in the first second of the expiration. Figure 40-2 shows typical curves from a healthy subject and from patients with obstructive and restrictive lung disease. Clearly, FEV_1 is reduced in both obstructive and restrictive lung disease. However, when expressed as a fraction of the exhaled vital capacity (VC), FEV_1/VC is low in obstructive lung disease and is normal (and may be high) in restrictive lung disease. In fact, *a low FEV_1/VC is the* sine qua non *of obstructive lung disease*. In a healthy subject FEV_1/VC is roughly 0.8; in an obstructed patient, the value can be much lower.

An indication of whether a substantial reversible component exists in airway obstruction is obtained by repeating the forced expiratory vital capacity maneuver after a bronchodilator is inhaled. Typically, a beta agonist drug with a short onset of action is used (e.g., albuterol) (24). An increase in FEV_1 of 12% or greater (coupled with an increase in FEV_1 of at least 200 mL) is generally taken as an appreciable bronchodilator response, although other criteria have been proposed (25,26). It is important to note that the failure to elicit an appreciable FEV_1 increase from an acute administration of bronchodilator does not imply that bronchodilators will not be clinically useful when given for a prolonged period of time.

Maldistribution of Ventilation

In an ideal lung, inhaled gas will go evenly to all alveoli. In normal lungs, ventilation is not distributed evenly because of a modest gravity-based tendency for more inspired gas to go to basilar alveoli because their distending pressure is greater (27). In lung disease, particularly in obstructive lung disease, maldistribution of ventilation can be much worse. Regional differences in segmental airway resistance and airspace compliance will markedly affect the rate of filling and emptying of regional airspaces, yielding dramatic maldistribution of ventilation.

Assessing maldistribution of ventilation assumes greater importance based on contentions that abnormalities in this aspect of lung function may be an earlier manifestation of obstructive lung disease than changes in spirometry (28).

The most commonly used measure of maldistribution of ventilation in pulmonary function testing is the single breath oxygen (SBO_2) test (3,29,30). In this test, the patient, while breathing through a mouthpiece, first exhales fully and then inhales fully a breath of 100% O_2. At this point, the O_2 concentration differs in different parts of the lung. Areas with low airway resistance will tend to receive more of the breath and will have a relatively low N_2 concentration (high O_2 concentration). Areas with high airway resistance will tend to receive less of the 100% O_2 breath and will have a relatively high N_2 concentration. The trachea and large airways will contain no N_2 (100% O_2). The patient is then asked to exhale slowly, while the exhaled volume and nitrogen concentration in the exhalate are continuously measured. Figure 40-3 shows a typical plot of N_2 concentration versus exhaled volume in a patient with appreciable maldistribution of ventilation. The first gas exhaled originates in the trachea and large airways; it has no nitrogen. Thereafter, there is a rapid rise in N_2 concentration as alveolar gas begins to appear. The first alveolar gas originates from alveoli served by lower-resistance airways; as the exhalation proceeds, lung units with higher-resistance airways have a greater contribution. Therefore, there is a gradual increase in the nitrogen concentration; the slope of this phase serves as an index of maldistribution of ventilation. By convention, the increase in percentage of N_2 over the half liter of exhalation between 0.75 and 1.25 liters is measured and this value is multiplied by 2 (to yield the percentage of N_2 increase per liter exhaled). Values greater than 2% to 3% N_2 increase per liter signify abnormal maldistribution of ventilation (28,31).

Pulmonary Gas Transport

It is important to assess the effectiveness of alveolar-capillary gas transport since gas transport is the lung's primary mission (32). The amount of gas flowing through a membrane in a given period of time is influenced by:

1. Thickness of the membrane

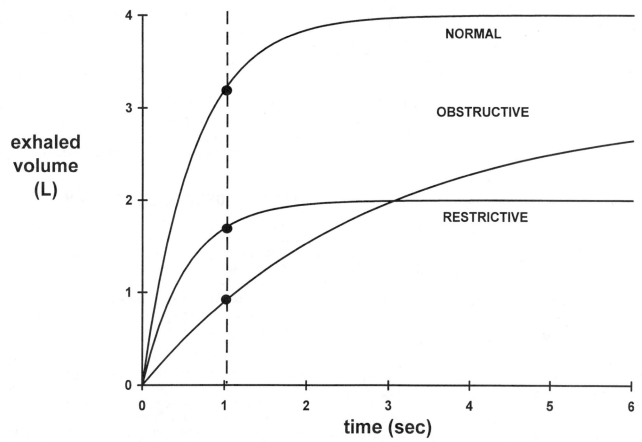

Figure 40-2 Forced vital capacity maneuver. The time course of expired volume is plotted. Typical curves for a normal subject, a patient with obstructive lung disease, and a patient with restrictive lung disease are illustrated.

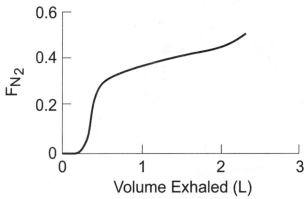

Figure 40-3 The single breath oxygen test. The patient inhales a full breath of 100% oxygen; the percentage of nitrogen in the exhalate is plotted as a function of the volume exhaled. The high slope of this relation between 0.75 and 1.25 liters of exhaled volume indicates substantial maldistribution of ventilation (see text).

2. Composition of the membrane
3. Area of the membrane
4. Gas species traversing the membrane
5. Partial pressure gradient for a given gas species across the membrane

The first three factors are the properties of the alveolar-capillary barrier that we wish to assess. The two gas species of interest (factor 4) are oxygen and carbon dioxide. Since carbon dioxide diffuses through biologic membranes much more readily than does oxygen, it is the diffusion characteristics for oxygen in which we are most interested. However, the partial pressure gradient across the alveolar capillary barrier (factor 5) for oxygen is difficult to assess; alveolar Po_2 varies regionally, and the mean capillary Po_2 is difficult to compute (5). Over 80 years ago, a solution to this problem was described (33). Instead of oxygen, carbon monoxide (CO) (which has diffusion characteristics somewhat similar to oxygen) is used as the test gas. CO has the substantial advantage that the capillary partial pressure is approximately zero, irrespective of the alveolar partial pressure. CO is avidly bound by hemoglobin (210 times more avidly than oxygen); any CO that enters the pulmonary capillary blood is immediately removed from the plasma by red cell hemoglobin. The capacity for CO removal is so high that pulmonary blood flow does not influence CO uptake during the maneuver. [However, the red cell membrane does offer some impedance to CO diffusion; as a result, hematocrit is a determinant of carbon monoxide diffusion (34)]. Thus, the pressure gradient for CO can be assessed solely by measuring alveolar CO concentration.

The test that has evolved, with refinements introduced

in the 1950s (35), is known as the diffusing capacity for carbon monoxide of the lung (D_LCO) (36–38). In this test, a maximal exhalation is followed by a maximal inhalation of the test gas. The breath is held for 10 seconds, after which the patient exhales fully. Figure 40-4 depicts the time course of alveolar CO following the inhalation of the test gas containing 0.3% CO. The initial alveolar concentration is determined by the dilution of the inspired bolus in the alveolar gas. Thereafter, the alveolar CO concentration declines exponentially, as CO diffuses into the blood. The better the diffusion characteristics of the alveolar capillary interface, the lower will be the alveolar concentration of CO at the end of the 10-second breath hold. The calculated D_LCO is proportional to the difference between the initial and final CO concentrations.

Measuring alveolar CO concentration is, of course, not possible; in practice, what is measured is the concentration of CO in a sample of the gas exhaled after the 10-second breath hold. The initial alveolar CO concentration is calculated ingeniously! A second gas species is included in the test gas. It is an inert (or nearly inert) gas that only minimally diffuses from alveolar gas to blood; helium, neon, or methane is the common choice. Figure 40-4 shows the alveolar time course of the inert gas if the test gas contains 0.3% of both CO and the inert gas. Since the inert gas concentration stays constant throughout the breath hold, the inert gas concentration at the end of the breath hold is equal to the CO concentration at the beginning of the breath hold.

Common causes of reduced D_LCO (39) include loss of alveolar surface area (e.g., pulmonary resection, pulmonary fibrosis, pneumonia) and reduced lung capillarity (e.g., pulmonary vascular disease, pulmonary embolism) or a mixture of the two (e.g., emphysema). Uncommonly, reduced D_LCO can be ascribed to an increased alveolar-capillary diffusion distance (e.g., pulmonary alveolar proteinosis, *Pneumocystis carinii* pneumonia). D_LCO is increased above predicted levels when recruitment of the pulmonary vascular bed increases (e.g., exercise, mild congestive heart failure, left-to-right shunt).

Indications for Pulmonary Function Testing

These rapid, noninvasive tests find use in several circumstances (40,41):

1. Differential diagnosis of lung disease
2. Assessing severity of lung disease
3. Evaluation of operative risk
4. Evaluation of response to therapy
5. Screening at-risk populations (e.g., cigarette smokers) for early manifestations of lung disease (42,43).

CARDIOPULMONARY EXERCISE TESTING

Exercise intolerance is one of the cardinal manifestations of disease. Since mobility is such an important part of life, exercise intolerance invariable depresses the quality of life. Understanding the source of the patient's complaints is a necessary prerequisite for formulating effective therapy. Cardiopulmonary exercise testing studies the human machine under operating conditions. Composing a physiologically based differential diagnosis of exercise intolerance is the major application of this testing modality.

There are other indications for cardiopulmonary exercise testing, however. These include: disability evaluation, assessment of the results of therapy, preoperative evaluation, and defining the need for oxygen supplementation. This introduction to the techniques and utility of cardiopulmonary exercise testing first discusses the physiologic requirements for performing exercise. Next, methods and instrumentation for exercise testing are reviewed. The patterns of abnormality that can be used to diagnose specific disease states are presented. Finally, the specific indications for exercise testing are evaluated.

Physiologic Requirements for Exercise

Because a central feature of this testing method is analyzing the respired gases, and because the majority of testing is performed in the pulmonary laboratory, the misunderstanding

Figure 40-4 Conceptual underpinning of the single breath diffusing capacity (D_LCO) maneuver. Typical time course of alveolar gas concentrations during a 10-second breath hold following a full inhalation of a gas containing 0.3% carbon monoxide (CO) and 0.3% methane. Carbon monoxide diffuses across the alveolar-capillary interface during the breath hold; its alveolar concentration decreases exponentially. Methane is relatively inert; its concentration remains nearly constant (see text).

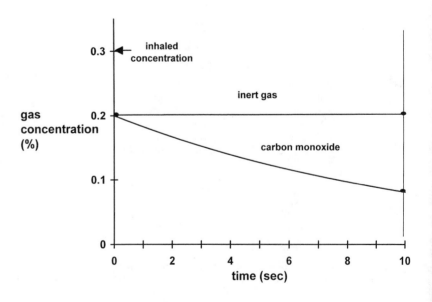

sometimes arises that this is a "pulmonary exercise test." However, the key concepts underlying cardiopulmonary exercise testing are that 1) exercise requires an integrated response of a number of organ systems and failure of any of these organ systems results in exercise intolerance, and 2) distinct patterns of response of CO_2 and O_2 exchange measured at the mouth can be assigned to dysfunction of specific organ systems.

Figure 40-5 is a schematic representation of the systems that are required to interact in order to perform exercise; this schematic was first formulated by Wasserman et al (45) 30 years ago. On the left are the exercising muscles. In order to produce the high-energy phosphate compounds necessary for muscle contraction and relaxation, food substrates (predominantly fats and carbohydrates) must be metabolized. This takes place in the muscle cell cytosol and mitochondria. The supply of fat or carbohydrate is not usually a limiting factor, but their processing requires an adequate supply of oxygen and requires that carbon dioxide be eliminated. In fact, just a moderate rate of exercise requires about a twentyfold increase in O_2 consumption and CO_2 production by the exercising muscle. The whole body has to gear up to supply the oxygen and eliminate the carbon dioxide. A reasonable case can be made for the statement that the most important function of the cardiovascular system is to provide oxygen and eliminate CO_2. The heart has to pump blood at an appropriate rate. The blood it pumps must have a high capacity for transporting O_2 and CO_2. Further, the blood must be directed to the exercising muscle by appropriate vasodilation of the vascular bed of the exercising muscle and vasoconstriction of nonexercising beds. The final link in the chain is the pulmonary system, whose function is to take oxygen from (and excrete CO_2 to) the atmosphere. To do this, blood has to be directed to ventilated alveoli; this requires control of the pulmonary vasculature to ensure a balance between ventilation and perfusion. Pulmonary ventilation is adjusted, mainly keyed on CO_2 (46,47), to respond to the increased requirements of exercise. Thus, it can be appreciated that although the rate of uptake of oxygen and output of CO_2 can be measured in the respired gas, these measurements have relevance to the function of all these interlinked subsystems.

It is worth considering the consequences of an inadequate response to exercise. A simplified schematic of the biochemical processes underlying energy production in the muscle is shown in Figure 40-6. The muscle cell burns glucose (the preferred fuel of the muscle for exercise of short duration) and turns it into CO_2 and water plus energy. But the cell needs an adequate supply of oxygen to complete this process. This is referred to as *aerobic* energy production. If the supply of oxygen is not adequate for a given level of exercise, this pathway cannot suffice. However, there is a backup pathway although this pathway is a much less efficient method of energy production. A side product of this *anaerobic* pathway is lactic acid. Lactic acid builds up in the muscle and is one reason why exercise tolerance is reached (48). Thus the acceleration of lactate production (and a consequent increase of lactic acid level in the blood) is a sign that oxygen supply is starting to be inadequate (49). This is illustrated by showing the responses of three groups of subjects to exercise (Figure 40-7). On the abscissa is the oxygen requirement for a given level of exercise and on the ordinate is the blood lactate the exercise engenders. In normal subjects blood lactate doesn't rise until a work rate is reached which requires 1 liter/min or so of oxygen uptake—the equivalent of a quick walk. Athletes can do much more exercise without producing lactate. In contrast, patients with heart disease produce lactate at work rates involved in a slow walk on level ground. It can be appreciated that the work rate at which lactate starts to be produced is an important index of exercise tolerance. It is known as the *anaerobic threshold* (also known as the lactic acidosis threshold) and is an important measurement to make during exercise testing (50).

Fortunately, there are ways to detect the anaerobic threshold without sampling blood. Lactic acid is a strong acid. When it is produced, it must be buffered by the bicarbonate system. As blood lactate increases, blood bicarbonate is consumed (51,52). However, bicarbonate buffering generates CO_2, which adds to the CO_2 generated by aerobic metabolism. The consequences of this are seen in Figure 40-8. As work rate is steadily increased, both O_2 uptake and CO_2 output steadily increase. Note that at about 130 W (watts), CO_2 output increases out of proportion to O_2 uptake. This

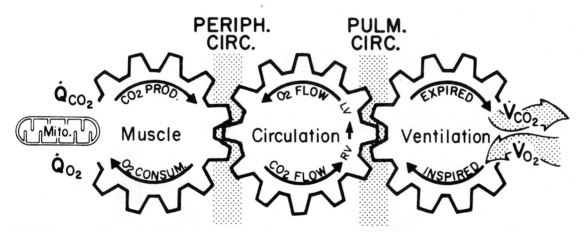

Figure 40-5 Schematic diagram indicating the interlinked processes required for oxygen and carbon dioxide exchange between the muscle cell and the environment. (Reproduced by permission from Wasserman K, Hansen JE, Sue DY, et al. Principles of exercise testing and interpretation. 2nd ed. Philadelphia: Lea & Febiger, 1994.)

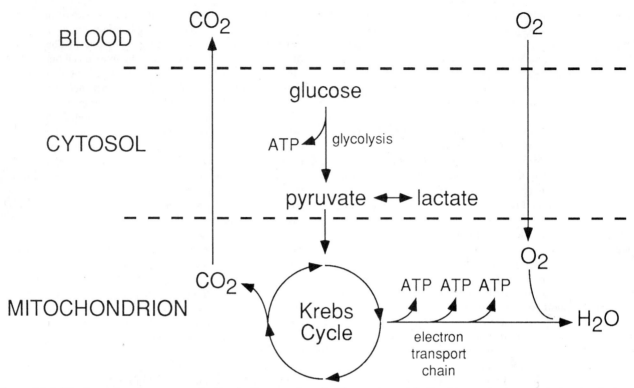

Figure 40-6 Biochemistry of energy production in the muscle cell. Glucose is metabolized to produce pyruvate by glycolysis. Pyruvate enters the tricarboxylic acid (TCA) cycle, which yields substrate for oxidative phosphorylation. This mechanism yields a large number of high-energy phosphate (ATP) molecules per molecule of glucose metabolized. However, an adequate supply of oxygen is required for this mechanism. If oxygen is inadequate, glycolysis can continue (with a small rate of ATP generation), but lactic acid is an obligatory product.

extra CO_2 output is from bicarbonate buffering of lactate; therefore, the anaerobic threshold of this subject is approximately 130 W.

An effective method to detect the anaerobic threshold during an exercise test in which work rate is progressively increased is shown in the top panel of Figure 40-9. By plotting CO_2 output versus oxygen uptake, we can see that they increase in parallel until CO_2 output accelerates. The acceleration in CO_2 output represents CO_2 produced by lactic acid buffering and defines the anaerobic threshold (53–55).

In cardiopulmonary exercise testing there are two variables that are used to gauge whether exercise tolerance is normal or abnormal. The anaerobic threshold defines the range of work rates that can be sustained for a long period of time. The maximum oxygen uptake defines the peak exercise capacity, but one that can be sustained for only a short period of time.

Methods and Instrumentation for Exercise Testing

Cardiopulmonary exercise testing, as it is generally performed, consists of a very specific examination with a standardized exercise stimulus and a well-defined group of response variables. There has been a debate as to the most desirable mode of exercise to use, with most proponents preferring either the treadmill or the cycle ergometer. Each has advantages. Treadmill exercise, because it involves a somewhat greater muscle mass, generally engenders roughly 10% higher maximum oxygen uptake. The cycle ergometer is cheaper, more compact, and somewhat safer. However, the important advantage of the cycle ergometer is that the rate at which work is performed can be precisely measured. With the treadmill, speed and grade are set, but pacing strategy and (especially) gripping the handrails appreciably influence the work rate (56). The ability to precisely quantitate work rate is important in establishing patterns of abnormality (see below).

The exercise test is designed to take no more than 20 minutes. After 3 minutes of recording resting responses and 3 minutes of unloaded pedaling, work rate is steadily increased (either in 1-minute steps, or continuously, in a "ramp" pattern). The rate at which work rate is incremented is selected [based on an *a priori* estimate of the patient's exercise tolerance (44)] to produce exhaustion within 8 to 12 minutes (57). The key variables monitored during cardiopulmonary exercise testing include the composition and flow rate of the respired air, but electrocardiographic and blood gas variables are usually measured as well. Instrumentation has been developed to automate the process (58). The key capability of these devices is to measure ventilation and gas exchange (oxygen uptake and CO_2 output) on a breath-by-breath basis (59,60). This requires simultaneous measurement of the time course of CO_2 partial pressure (P_{CO_2}) and O_2 partial pressure (P_{O_2}) in the respired air as well as airflow. Conceptually, this involves

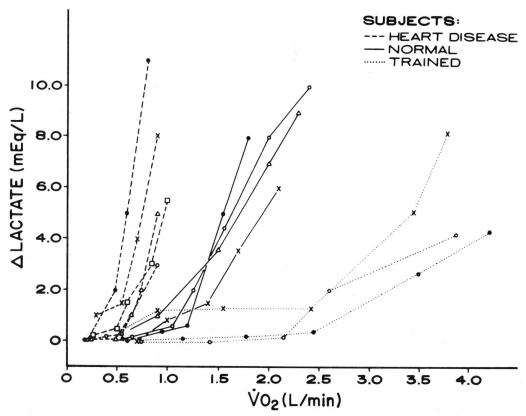

Figure 40-7 Responses to progressive increases in work rate in three groups of subjects: patients with cardiovascular disease, healthy sedentary subjects, and athletes. In each group, arterial blood lactate increases once a certain metabolic rate ($\dot{V}_{O_2}$) is exceeded (the anaerobic threshold), although the anaerobic threshold differs substantially among groups. (Reproduced by permission from Wasserman K, Hansen JE, Sue DY, et al. Principles of exercise testing and interpretation. 2nd ed. Philadelphia: Lea & Febiger, 1994.)

Figure 40-8 Gas exchange responses to incremental cycle ergometer exercise of a typical subject. After 3 minutes of rest and 3 minutes of unloaded cycling, work rate is increased 20 W each minute. $\dot{V}_{CO_2}$ increase parallels $\dot{V}_{O_2}$ increase until about 130 W. At this point $\dot{V}_{CO_2}$ accelerates out of proportion to $\dot{V}_{O_2}$. This excess CO_2 is the result of bicarbonate buffering of lactic acid. (Reproduced by permission from Wasserman K, Hansen JE, Sue DY, et al. Principles of exercise testing and interpretation. 2nd ed. Philadelphia: Lea & Febiger, 1994.)

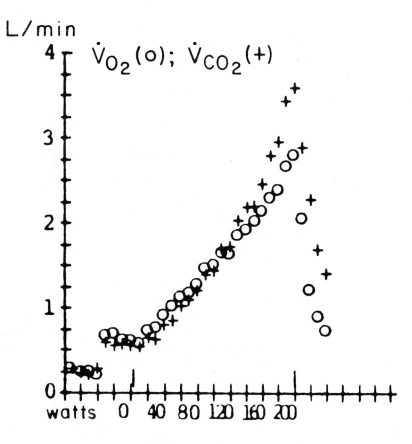

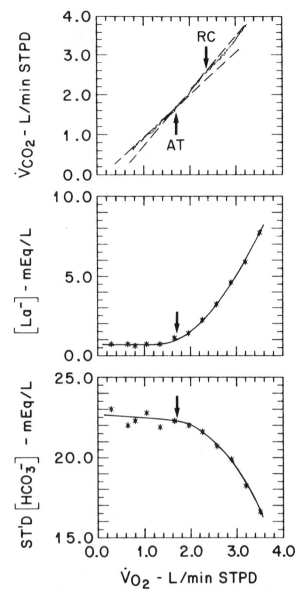

Figure 40-9 Determination of the anaerobic threshold (AT). This determination from gas exchange data is most reliably discerned by plotting CO_2 output ($\dot{V}_{CO_2}$) as a function of oxygen uptake ($\dot{V}_{O_2}$) (top panel). The upward deflection of $\dot{V}_{CO_2}$ marks the anaerobic threshold. As shown in the middle and bottom panels, blood lactate rises and blood bicarbonate falls at approximately the same $\dot{V}_{O_2}$. RC, point of respiratory compensation for the metabolic acidosis. (Reproduced by permission from Wasserman K, Hansen JE, Sue DY, et al. Principles of exercise testing and interpretation. 2nd ed. Philadelphia: Lea & Febiger, 1994.)

dividing the breath into a large number of time intervals and assuming that over each one both airflow and gas concentration are constant (a time interval of a 1/50 or 1/100 of a second is appropriate). This is simplest to consider for CO_2. For each time interval, the quantity of CO_2 that leaves the body is calculated as the product of the volume of air that leaves the lips and the fraction of that gas that is CO_2. This product is summed over the whole breath to give the total volume of CO_2 exhaled within the breath.

The heart of the cardiopulmonary exercise testing system is a digital computer. Software development has made calibration procedures, data collection, data display, and final report generation straightforward. During these tests, the patient breathes through a mouthpiece with a nose clip in place. For many years the pneumotachograph was the standard device for measuring airflow. It measures the pressure drop across a low-resistance screen, but it has to be placed an appreciable distance from the mouth to get a smooth airflow profile and to keep the screen from getting clogged up with saliva. This requires that a breathing valve be interposed. New devices have been introduced—one is based on the hot wire principle. Airflow cools a heated wire, changing its resistance and creating an electrical signal. Another new transducer utilizes the pitot tube principle; it measures the pressure difference created by air flowing past a series of holes in a plastic tube. These newer devices can measure airflow without requiring a breathing valve.

Modern gas analyzers for CO_2 and O_2 are small, stable, and rapidly responding. The CO_2 analyzers are based on the infrared absorption of CO_2; the O_2 analyzers are based on paramagnetic or fuel cell principles. Because breath-by-breath gas exchange analysis requires simultaneous measurement of airflow and gas concentrations, it is necessary to precisely compensate for the transport delay for gas to flow from the mouthpiece to the gas analyzers (usually approximately 0.5 second). Further, newer sampling line tubing selectively allows water vapor to escape as the sampled gas passes through the tubing; the gas is dry when it arrives at the analyzers and this simplifies metabolic rate calculations.

Other variables need to be measured as well. Heart rate is usually detected from the R-R interval of a three-lead ECG configuration. In most tests, 12-lead ECG recordings are made every 2 minutes during exercise. These monitors must be especially designed for rejection of motion artifact. Blood pressure is measured either manually by auscultation or by automated cuff (61). Pulse oximeters allow estimation of arterial oxygen saturation, although some investigators have defined problems with accuracy associated with exercise (62,63).

In some cardiopulmonary exercise tests it is necessary to sample arterial blood (in order to accurately assess the gas exchange properties of the lung). This is usually accomplished by inserting an arterial cannula, although obtaining single blood samples by radial artery puncture is sometimes adequate. For arterial blood analysis, blood gas and co-oximeter measurements establish oxygenation and acid-base status during exercise. Blood lactate levels are sometimes measured as well.

Defining Patterns of Abnormality

Once the test has been performed, computerized analysis is performed and both tubular and graphic summaries are prepared. The graphic summary is of greatest help. Standardized multipanel graphic montages have been perfected that allow a range of insights to be obtained (44,64). Table 40-1 is an outline of some of the key derived variables. The first ques-

Table 40-1 Derived Variables Contributing to Exercise Testing Interpretation

Exercise Tolerance	$\dot{V}o_2$max
	Anaerobic threshold
Gas Exchange Limitation	V_D/V_T
	$P(_A - a)o_2$
	$\dot{V}_E/\dot{V}co_2$
	O_2 saturation
Cardiovascular Limitation	$\Delta\dot{V}o_2/\Delta WR$
	$\dot{V}o_2$/HR
	Heart rate reserve
	Blood pressure
	Electrocardiogram
Ventilatory Limitation	Breathing reserve

tion to ask is whether exercise tolerance is reduced. There are well-defined normal values for maximal oxygen uptake ($\dot{V}o_2$max) based on age, height, and gender (44,65) and any value less than 80% of predicted can be defined as abnormal. A low $\dot{V}o_2$max indicates that, working at maximum effort, some component of the system is not adequate. Similarly, abnormality of the anaerobic threshold can be defined (44,65). The anaerobic threshold has the special virtue that it is *not* effort-dependent. $\dot{V}o_2$max can be low because of inadequate effort, but a low anaerobic threshold cannot be the result of poor effort.

Exercise testing diagnosis can be divided into three areas of inference: gas exchange limitation, cardiovascular limitation, and ventilatory limitation. Gas exchange limitation means that the lungs do not adequately transport CO_2 and O_2. The first two measures listed in Table 40-1 are the preferable variables to assess, but both require arterial blood sampling. The ratio of dead space to tidal volume (V_D/V_T) defines the fraction of the exhaled tidal volume that is ineffective in clearing CO_2 from the lungs. This can be calculated from the mass balance equation:

$$\frac{V_D}{V_T} = 1 - \frac{k}{Paco_2(\dot{V}_E/\dot{V}co_2)} \qquad (40\text{-}1)$$

where ventilation ($\dot{V}_E$) and CO_2 output ($\dot{V}co_2$) are measured from the respired air and arterial Pco_2 ($Paco_2$) is measured from arterial blood analysis. V_D/V_T normally is lower during exercise than at rest; values above 0.3 during exercise are abnormal and indicate that there are alveoli that are being ventilated but not perfused. The efficiency of oxygen exchange is assessed by calculating the difference between the calculated ideal alveolar Po_2 (Pao_2) and measured arterial Po_2 (Pao_2). For room air breathing at sea level, this is approximated by the equation:

$$P(_A - a)o_2 = 150 - Paco_2/R - Pao_2 \qquad (40\text{-}2)$$

where R is the gas exchange ratio ($\dot{V}co_2/\dot{V}o_2$). During exercise, $P(_A - a)o_2$ is normally approximately 15 mm Hg (although higher values are seen in the healthy elderly); an

elevated value is usually an indicator of poor matching of ventilation to perfusion. The other two measures of gas exchange abnormalities listed in Table 40-1 are noninvasive, but less reliable. Pulse oximetry is sometimes inaccurate during exercise and, because it estimates oxygen saturation rather than partial pressure, moderate degrees of hypoxemia may not be reliably detected (66). $\dot{V}_E/\dot{V}co_2$ is the number of liters of gas that must be exhaled to exhale 1 liter of CO_2; during exercise values are normally 30 or less. However, as can discerned from Equation (40-1), elevated values can be seen either with abnormal pulmonary gas exchange (i.e., high V_D/V_T), or with primary hyperventilation (i.e., low $Paco_2$).

The key to diagnosis of cardiovascular abnormalities from cardiopulmonary exercise testing is the realization that oxygen uptake is primarily a cardiovascular, not a pulmonary variable (67). The Fick equation dicates that:

$$\dot{V}o_2 = \dot{Q}(Cao_2 - CVo_2) \qquad (40\text{-}3)$$

where $\dot{Q}$ is cardiac output and Cao_2 and CVo_2 are arterial and mixed venous O_2 content, respectively. Thus, oxygen uptake is closely linked to cardiac output. Further, the rate of increase of $\dot{V}o_2$ with work rate is dictated by biochemical efficiency (68). This translates into approximately 10 mL/min of $\dot{V}o_2$ for every watt increase in work rate during the incremental phase of the exercise test (69). This will occur unless oxygen is not being transported to the muscle and the muscle is forced to do work without adequate oxygen (70). A low slope of the $\dot{V}o_2$-work rate curve means that the cardiovascular system is failing to deliver oxygen adequately to the site of metabolism in the muscles. By dividing both sides of Equation (40-3) by heart rate, the following is derived:

$$\dot{V}o_2/HR = SV(Cao_2 - CVo_2) \qquad (40\text{-}4)$$

where $\dot{V}o_2$/HR is known as *oxygen pulse*, the volume of oxygen extracted from the blood by the lung with each heart beat, and SV is stroke volume. Therefore, if oxygen pulse fails to increase normally with work rate, it is usually a sign that stroke volume is not increasing normally. Cardiovascular abnormalities are also often accompanied by a low anaerobic threshold. The heart rate reserve is the difference between the predicted maximal heart rate (usually calculated as $220 - age$) and the observed peak heart rate. In healthy subjects the heart rate reserve is usually low; a high heart rate reserve may indicate poor effort or that exercise is limited by noncardiac factors. The electrocardiogram and blood pressure responses are, of course, also important indicators of the cardiovascular response.

Composing a differential diagnosis when a cardiovascular limitation to exercise is detected is an important part of exercise test interpretation. Table 40-2 presents the basic strategy. A cardiovascular limitation accompanied by electrocardiographic abnormalities or by certain patterns of blood pressure response suggests cardiac disease. When accompanied by disproportionate leg pain, peripheral vascular disease is likely. In the setting of substantial pulmonary gas exchange abnormalities, pulmonary vascular disease is probably the mechanism of cardiovascular abnormalities in the exercise response. Since poor cardiovascular oxygen transport from any cause will be detected, anemia, hypoxemia, or carboxyhemoglobinemia will yield a

Table 40-2 Differential Diagnosis of Cardiovascular Limitation to Exercise
• Cardiac disease: accompanied by ECG or blood pressure abnormalities
• Peripheral vascular disease: accompanied by disproportionate leg pain
• Pulmonary vascular disease: accompanied by abnormal pulmonary gas exchange
• Poor blood oxygen transport: accompanied by anemia, hypoxemia, or carboxyhemoglobinemia
• Muscular deconditioning: accompanied by a history of a sedentary life style

cardiovascular limitation to exercise. Finally, failure to transfer oxygen from the muscle capillaries to the site of metabolism because of deconditioning (or, less commonly, to a specific myopathy) will yield a cardiovascular limitation (usually of mild degree), and is usually accompanied by a history of a sedentary lifestyle.

Ventilatory limitation is seen when the demands of exercise exceed the ability to ventilate the lungs (71). This limitation is usually due to a combination of an elevated level of ventilation for a given level of exercise caused by poor gas exchange function (and/or ventilatory stimulation from lactic acidosis) and impaired lung mechanics. A measure of this limitation is the breathing reserve, defined as the difference between the maximal voluntary ventilation and the peak ventilation observed during exercise. The maximal voluntary ventilation is determined from resting spirometric measures (44).

Indications for Cardiopulmonary Exercise Testing
Determining the Cause of Exercise Intolerance

Exercise testing is capable of narrowing the differential diagnosis of exercise intolerance (72,73). Unlike other testing modalities that primarily examine one organ system's function (e.g., pulmonary function test, ECG stress test), the cardiopulmonary exercise test yields diagnoses in several organ systems. In many situations, it is more efficient to order exercise testing early in a patient's evaluation for unexplained exercise intolerance.

Evaluating Disability

In evaluating the lack of ability for a certain level of a specific type of performance, exercise testing is often useful (74). Measurement of the anaerobic threshold and maximum oxygen uptake indicates the levels of exercise subjects are able to tolerate in sustained tasks and in short bursts, respectively. Moreover, a substantial literature documents exercise testing's utility in evaluating impairment from occupational exposure (75). Malingering is usually easily detected: The patient will have a low peak oxygen uptake but a normal anaerobic threshold, and high ventilatory and heart rate reserves.

Cardiopulmonary exercise testing has specifically been found of value in assessing impairment in chronic lung disease. In interstitial lung disease, exercise testing assists in early diagnosis and assessing dysfunction and, possibly, determining prognosis (76,77). In cystic fibrosis, exercise testing has been shown to be useful in defining prognosis and assisting with management (78). In COPD patients preparing to undergo a program of rehabilitative exercise, exercise testing helps to rule out cardiac contraindications.

Preoperative Evaluation

It may be argued that an operative procedure and heavy exercise are similar in that they are both severe stressors of multiple organ systems. In patients with cardiac disease, exercise testing can help to predict mortality following major surgery (79,80). For the patient requiring lung cancer resectional surgery, exercise testing helps to determine the amount of lung that can safely be resected and can help predict the likelihood of postsurgical complications (81–84). Exercise testing is commonly used in assessing risk of lung transplantation (85), volume reduction surgery (86,87), and cardiac transplantation (88).

Assessing the Results of Therapy

If testing is performed before and after a therapeutic intervention, objective evidence of improvement in exercise tolerance can be obtained. Exercise training results in increased maximum $\dot{V}O_2$ and anaerobic threshold (89). Changes in the physiologic responses to submaximal work rates are also seen [e.g., for heavy exercise levels, ventilatory response is substantially reduced (90)]. These measurements have proven useful in evaluating the effectiveness of exercise training in several patient groups (91). The benefits of heart and lung transplantation have been quantified (92,93). The results of a wide range of pharmacologic interventions can be evaluated [e.g., bronchodilators, corticosteroids, cardiac inotropic agents (94), pulmonary vasodilators].

REFERENCES

1. Sterk PJ, Fabbri LM, Quanjer PH, et al. Official statement of the European Respiratory Society: airway responsiveness: standardized challenge testing with pharmacological, physical and sensitizing stimuli in adults. Eur Respir J 1993;6(suppl 16):53–83.

2. Anderson SD. Diagnosis and management of exercise-induced asthma. In: Gershwin ME, Halpern GM, eds. Bronchial asthma. Principles of diagnosis and treatment. 3rd ed. Totowa, NJ: Humana Press, 1994:513–547.

3. Murray JF, Nadel JA. Textbook of respiratory medicine. 2nd ed. Philadelphia: WB Saunders, 1994.

4. Dawson A. Elastic recoil and compliance. In: Clausen JL, ed. Pulmonary function testing: guidelines and controversies. New York: Academic Press, 1982:193–204.

5. Comroe JH, Forster RE, DuBois AB, et al. The lung: clinical physiology and pulmonary function tests. 2nd ed. Chicago: Year Book, 1962.

6. Read DJC. A clinical method for assessing the ventilatory response to carbon dioxide. Australas Ann Med 1967;16:20–32.

7. Rebuck AS, Campbell EJM. A clinical method for assessing the ventilatory response to hypoxemia. Am Rev Respir Dis 1974;109:345–350.

8. Pfaff JK, Morgan WJ. Pulmonary function in infants and children. Pediatric Clin North Am 1994; 41:401–423.

9. Kryger MH, Roth T, Dement WC. Principles and practice of sleep medicine. 2nd ed. Philadelphia: WB Saunders, 1994.

10. Black LF, Hyatt HRE. Maximal respiratory pressures: normal values and relationship to age and sex. Am Rev Respir Dis 1969;99:696–702.

11. Nickerson BG, Keens TG. Measuring ventilatory muscle endurance in humans as sustainable inspiratory pressure. J Appl Physiol 1982;52:768–772.

12. Hansen JE. Arterial blood gases. Clin Chest Med 1989;10:227–237.

13. Official Statement of the American Lung Society. Lung function testing: selection of reference values and interpretative strategies. Am Rev Respir Dis 1991; 144:1202–1214.

14. Ghio AJ, Crapo RO, Elliott CG. Reference equations used to predict pulmonary function. Chest 1990;97:400–403.

15. Hutchinson J. On the capacity of the lungs and on the respiratory functions, with a view of establishing a precise and easy method of detecting diseases by the spirometer. Trans Med Soc Lond 1846;29:137–252.

16. Jalowayski AA, Dawson A. Measurement of lung volume: the multiple breath nitrogen method. In: Clausen JL, ed. Pulmonary function testing: guidelines and controversies. New York: Academic Press, 1982:115–140.

17. Darling RC, Cournand A, Richard DW Jr. Studies on the intrapulmonary mixture of gases: III: an open circuit method for measuring residual air. J Clin Invest 1940;19:609–618.

18. Meneely GR, Ball CO, Kory RC, et al. A simplified closed circuit helium dilution method for the determination of the residual volume of the lungs. Am J Med 1960;28:824–831.

19. Holmgren A. Determination of the functional residual volume by means of the helium dilution method. Scand J Clin Lab Invest 1954;6:131–136.

20. Zarins LP, Clausen JL. Body plethysmography. In: Clausen JL, ed. Pulmonary function testing: guidelines and controversies. New York: Academic Press, 1982:141–153.

21. Official Statement of the American Thoracic Society. Standardization of spirometry. 1994 update. Am J Respir Crit Care Med 1995;152:1107–1136.

22. Sobel BJ. Spirometry and forced flow studies. In: Chisud EL, ed. The selective and comprehensive testing of adult pulmonary function. Mount Kisco, NY: Futura 1983:29–75.

23. Morris JF. Spirometry in the evaluation of pulmonary function. West J Med 1976;125:110–118.

24. Casaburi R, Adame D, Hong CK. Comparison of albuterol to isoproterenol as a bronchodilator for use in pulmonary function testing. Chest 1991;100:1597–1600.

25. Hansen JE, Casaburi R, Goldberg AS. A statistical approach for assessment of bronchodilator responsiveness in pulmonary function testing. Chest 1993;104:1119–1126.

26. Shim C. Response to bronchodilators. Clin Chest Med 1989;10:155–164.

27. West JB. Respiratory physiology— the essentials. 5th ed. Baltimore: Williams and Wilkins, 1994.

28. Buist AS, Ross BB. Quantitative analysis of the alveolar plateau in the diagnosis of early airway obstruction. Am Rev Respir Dis 1973;108:1078–1098.

29. Ruppel G. Gas distribution tests. In: Manual of pulmonary function testing. St. Louis: C.V. Mosby, 1979:52–64.

30. Comroe JH, Fowler WS. Lung function studies VI: detection of uneven alveolar ventilation during a single breath of oxygen. Am J Med 1951;10:408–413.

31. Buist AS. Closing volumes and flow-volume studies. In: Chusid EL, ed. The selective and comprehensive testing of adult pulmonary function. New York: Futura, 1983: 55–65.

32. Weibel ER. The pathway for oxygen. Cambridge, MA: Harvard University Press, 1984.

33. Krogh M. The diffusion of gases through the lungs of man. J Physiol (Lond) 1915;49:271–296.

34. Roughton FJW, Forster RE. Relative importance of diffusion and chemical reaction rates in determining rate of exchange of gases in the human lung, with special reference to true diffusing capacity of pulmonary membrane and volume of blood in the lung capillaries. J Appl Physiol 1957; 11:290–302.

35. Ogilvie CM, Forster RE, Blakemore WS, et al. A standardized breath holding technique for the clinical measurement of the diffusing capacity of the lung for carbon monoxide. J Clin Invest 1957; 36:1–17.

36. Official Statement of the American Thoracic Society. Single breath carbon monoxide diffusing capacity (transfer factor): recommendations for a standard technique. Am Rev Respir Dis 1987;136:1299–1307.

37. Official Statement of the American Thoracic Society. Single-breath carbon monoxide diffusing capacity (transfer factor)—1995 update. Am J Respir Crit Care Med 1995; 152:2185–2198.

38. Huang YCT, Macintyre NR. Real-time gas analysis improves the measurement of single-breath diffusing capacity. Am Rev Respir Dis 1992;146:946–950.

39. Ayers LN, Ginsberg ML, Fin J, et al. Diffusing capacity, specific diffusing capacity and interpretation of diffusion defect. West J Med 1975;123:255–264.

40. Crapo RO. Pulmonary function testing. N Engl J Med 1994;331:25–30.

41. AARC Clinical Practice Guideline. Spirometry. Respir Care 1991;36:1414–1717.

42. Law M, Tang JL. An analysis of the effectiveness of interventions intended to help people stop smoking. Arch Intern Med 1995;155:1933–1941.

43. Siafakes NM, Vermeire P, Pride NB, et al. Optimal assessment and management of chronic obstructive pulmonary disease (COPD). Eur Respir J 1995;8:1398–1420.

44. Wasserman K, Hansen JE, Sue DY, et al. Principles of exercise testing and interpretation. 2nd ed. Philadelphia: Lea and Febiger, 1994.

45. Wasserman K, Van Kessel AL, Burton GG. Interaction of physiologic mechanisms during exercise. J Appl Physiol 1967;22:71–85.

46. Wasserman K, Whipp BJ, Casaburi R. Respiratory control during exercise. In: Handbook of physiology—the respiratory system II. Bethesda, MD: American Physiological Society, 1986:595–619.

47. Casaburi R, Whipp BJ, Wasserman K, et al. Ventilatory and gas exchange dynamics in response to sinusoidal work. J Appl Physiol 1977;42:300–311.

48. Westerblad H, Lee JA, Lännergren J, et al. Cellular mechanisms of fatigue in skeletal muscle. Am J Physiol 1991;261:C195–C209.

49. Koike A, Hiroe M, Adachi H, et al. Cardiac output-O_2 uptake relation during incremental exercise in patients with previous myocardial infarction. Circulation 1992;85:1713.

50. Wasserman K, Whipp BJ. Exercise physiology in health and disease. Am Rev Respir Dis 1975;112:219–249.

51. Beaver WL, Wasserman K, Whipp BJ. Bicarbonate buffering of lactic acid generated during exercise. J Appl Physiol 1986;60:472–478.

52. Stringer W, Casaburi R, Wasserman K. Acid-base regulation during exercise and recovery in humans. J Appl Physiol 1992;72:954–961.

53. Wasserman K, Beaver WL, Whipp BJ. Gas exchange theory and the lactic acidosis (anaerobic) threshold. Circulation 1990;81(suppl II):II-14–II-30.

54. Beaver WL, Wasserman K, Whipp BJ. A new method for detecting anaerobic threshold by gas exchange. J Appl Physiol 1986;60:2020–2027.

55. Sue DY, Wasserman K, Moricca RB, et al. Metabolic acidosis during exercise in patients with chronic obstructive pulmonary disease. Chest 1988;94:931–938.

56. Chester EH, Belman MJ, Bahler RC, et al. Multidisciplinary treatment of chronic pulmonary insufficiency: 3: the effect of physical training on cardiopulmonary performance in patients with chronic pulmonary disease. Chest 1977;72:695–702.

57. Buchfuhrer MJ, Hansen JE, Robinson TE, et al. Optimizing the exercise protocol for cardiopulmonary assessments. J Appl Physiol 1983;55:1558–1564.

58. Casaburi R, Cotes JE, Prefaut C. Equipment, measurements and quality control in clinical exercise testing. In: Clinical exercise testing with reference to lung diseases. Eur Respir Mon 1997;6:72–87.

59. Beaver WL, Wasserman K, Whipp BJ. On-line computer analysis and breath-by-breath graphical display of exercise function tests. J Appl Physiol 1973;34:128–132.

60. Lamarra N, Whipp BJ. Measurement of pulmonary gas exchange. In: Maud PJ, Foster C, eds. The physiological assessment of human

fitness. Champaign, IL: Human Kinetics, 1995:19–35.

61. Ramsey M. Blood pressure monitoring: automated oscillometric devices. J Clin Monit 1991;7:56–67.

62. Hansen JE, Casaburi R. Validity of ear oximetry in clinical exercise testing. Chest 1987;91:333-337.

63. Clark JS, Votteri B, Ariagno RL, et al. Noninvasive assessment of blood gases. Am Rev Respir Dis 1992;145:220–232.

64. Wasserman K. Diagnosing cardiovascular and lung pathophysiology from exercise gas exchange. Chest 1997;112:1091–1101.

65. Hansen JE, Sue DY, Wasserman K. Predicted values for clinical exercise testing. Am Rev Respir Dis 1984;129(suppl):549–555.

66. Carlin BW, Clausen JS, Ries AL. The use of continuous oximetry in the prescription of long-term oxygen therapy. Chest 1988;94:239–241.

67. Wasserman K. New concepts in assessing cardiovascular function. Circulation 1988;78:1060–1071.

68. Whipp BJ, Wasserman K. Efficiency of muscular work. J Appl Physiol 1969;26:644–648.

69. Hansen JE, Casaburi R, Cooper DM, et al. Oxygen uptake as related to work rate increment during cycle ergometer exercise. Eur J Appl Physiol 1988;57:140–145.

70. Hansen JE, Sue DY, Oren A, et al. Relation of oxygen uptake to work rate in normal men and men with circulatory disorders. Am J Cardiol 1987;59:669–674.

71. Casaburi R. Exercise training in COPD. In: Casaburi R, Petty TL, eds. Principles and practice of pulmonary rehabilitation. Philadelphia: WB Saunders, 1993:204–224.

72. Sue DY, Wasserman K. Impact of integrative cardiopulmonary exercise testing on clinical decision making. Chest 1991;99:981–992.

73. Martinez FJ, Stanopoulos I, Acero

R, et al. Graded comprehensive cardiopulmonary exercise testing in the evaluation of dyspnea unexplained by routine evaluation. Chest 1994;105:168–174.

74. Oren A, Sue DY, Hansen JE, et al. The role of exercise testing in impairment evaluation. Am Rev Respir Dis 1987;135:230–235.

75. Sue DY. Exercise testing in the evaluation of impairment and disability. Clin Chest Med 1994;15:369–387.

76. Kelley MA, Daniele RP. Exercise testing in interstitial lung disease. Clin Chest Med 1984;5:145–156.

77. Augstí C, Xaubet A, Roca J, et al. Interstitial pulmonary fibrosis with and without associated collagen vascular disease: results of a 2 years follow up. Thorax 1992;47:1035–1040.

78. Nixon PA, Orenstein DM, Kelsey SF, et al. The prognostic value of exercise testing in patients with cystic fibrosis. N Engl J Med 1992;327:1785–1788.

79. Older P, Hall A. The role of cardiopulmonary exercise testing for preoperative evaluation of the elderly. In: Wasserman K, ed. Exercise gas exchange in heart disease. Armonk, NY: Futura, 1996:287–297.

80. Older P, Smith R, Courtner P, et al. Preoperative evaluation of cardiac failure and ischemia in elderly patients by cardiopulmonary exercise testing. Chest 1993;104:701–704.

81. Colman NC, Schraufnagel DE, Rivington RN, et al. Exercise testing in evaluation of patients for lung resection. Am Rev Respir Dis 1982;125:604–606.

82. Gilbreath EM, Weisman IM. Role of exercise stress testing in preoperative evaluation of patients for lung resection. Clin Chest Med 1994;15:389–403.

83. Olsen GN. The evolving role of exercise testing prior to lung resection. Chest 1989;95:218–225.

84. Bolliger CT, Wyser C, Roser H, et al. Lung scanning and exercise testing for the prediction of postoperative performance in lung resection candidates at increased risk for complications. Chest 1995;108:341–348.

85. Howard DK, Iademarco EJ, Trulock EP. The role of cardiopulmonary exercise testing in lung and heart-lung transplantation. Clin Chest Med 1994;15:405–420.

86. Cooper JD, Trulock EP, Triantafillou AN, et al. Bilateral pneumectomy (volume reduction) for chronic obstructive pulmonary disease. J Thorac Cardiovasc Surg 1995;109:106–119.

87. Sciurba FC, Rogers RM, Keenan RJ, et al. Improvement in pulmonary function and elastic recoil after lung-reduction surgery for diffuse emphysema. N Engl J Med 1996;334:1095–1099.

88. Stevenson LW, Sietsema K, Tillisch JH, et al. Exercise capacity for survivors of cardiac transplantation or sustained medical therapy for stable heart failure. Circulation 1990;81:78–85.

89. Casaburi R. Physiologic responses to training. Clin Chest Med 1994;15:215–227.

90. Casaburi R, Storer TW, Wasserman K. Mediation of reduced ventilatory response to exercise after endurance training. J Appl Physiol 1987;63:1533.

91. Casaburi R, Patessio A, Ioli F, et al. Reduction in exercise lactic acidosis and ventilation as a result of exercise training in obstructive lung disease. Am Rev Respir Dis 1991;143:9–18.

92. Casaburi R. Deconditioning. In: Fishman AP, ed. Pulmonary rehabilitation. New York: Marcel Dekker, 1996:213–230.

93. Levy RD, Ernst P, Levine SM, et al. Exercise performance after lung transplantation. J Heart Lung Transplant 1993;12:27–33.

94. Hansen JE, Sue DY, Oren A, et al. Relation of oxygen uptake to work rate in normal men and men with circulatory disorder. Am J Cardiol 1987;59:669–674.

Chapter 41

Asthma

Gilbert E. D'Alonzo
David E. Ciccolella

Asthma is an inflammatory disease of the airways characterized by intermittent symptoms, including chest congestion, cough, and wheezing. These symptoms are associated with airway hyperresponsiveness and variable airflow obstruction.

Approximately 14.5 million individuals in the United States have asthma (1,2). Therefore, the prevalence of asthma is approximately 5% to 7%. Despite the constant development of new medications to treat asthma over the last decade, there has been a rising hospitalization rate, and it remains a frequent cause of absenteeism from both school and work. Most concerning is that approximately 6000 deaths from asthma occur in the United States each year (2).

The prevention and treatment of this disease are highly dependent upon a variety of interventions, both nonpharmacologic and pharmacologic. The daily habits and activities of patients with asthma play an important role in disease management and prevention. Minor alterations in lifestyle practices can make substantial differences in the long-term health of the asthmatic patient.

This chapter focuses on the traditional asthma topics of pathogenesis, diagnosis, and treatment. More importantly, the environmental issues important to asthma are discussed. Asthma symptom prevention and enhanced control of this disease are stressed and the effect of exercise, occupation, stress, and pregnancy on asthma is discussed.

CLINICAL FEATURES

Clinical symptoms of asthma are dyspnea, cough, chest congestion and tightness, and noticeable wheezing. Milder cases of asthma may only be recognized by a cough, which is worse at night, or dyspnea during or following exertion. In more severe attacks, some or all of the symptoms have been occurring over several days before the patient seeks medical help; however, a minority of patients have a rapid onset of severe symptoms over just a few minutes or hours. In very severe attacks, respiratory failure may occur, requiring tracheal intubation and mechanical ventilation in order to avoid death.

An asthma patient may be able to identify a certain trigger that destabilizes his or her asthma. Often, symptoms occur during exercise, viral infection, exposure to furry or feathered animals, or exposure to environments laden with dust, mold, smoke, or other noxious fumes or chemicals. Even changes in weather, emotions such as laughing and crying, and menses may destabilize the asthmatic patient. There are certain patients who have attacks following the ingestion of aspirin or other medications. Eczema, hay fever, rose fever, or a family history of asthma is often associated with asthma, but their presence is not required for its diagnosis.

The asthmatic, when not having asthma, will often have a normal physical examination. However, in patients who are having asthma the physical examination commonly reveals an increase in respiratory rate with a prolonged expiratory time and wheezing. On forced expiration the wheezing becomes accentuated and coughing generally occurs. With more severe asthma the use of the accessory muscles of ventilation occurs, the chest appears to be hyperinflated, and the patient may be diaphoretic and not able to speak in full sentences. A clinical classification for the severity of asthma is found in Table 41-1 (3).

Table 41-1 Classification of Asthma by Disease Severity (Prior to Treatment)				
	MILD INTERMITTENT	MILD	MODERATE PERSISTENT	SEVERE
Symptom Frequency	≤Twice a week	>Twice a week <one a day	Daily	Continuous
Severity of Attacks	Less severe and brief	Can affect activity	Can last days and limit activity	Frequent and severe
Nocturnal Frequency	≤Twice a month	>Twice a month	>one a week	Frequent
Lung Function FEV$_1$ or PEFR % Predicted	≥80%	≥80%	60% to 80%	<60%
PEFR Variability	<20%	20% to 30%	30%	>30%

PATHOGENESIS

Airway narrowing leading to increased airway resistance and airflow obstruction in asthma occurs through three major mechanisms:

1. Airway smooth muscle contraction
2. Increased airway lumen debris
3. Airway wall thickening from inflammation, edema, and over time, fibrosis (3)

In asthma, damaged epithelial cells detach from the mucosal surface of the airways. Airway wall thickening occurs in patients with persistent asthma as a result of the unimpeded inflammatory process. The effects of inflammation accumulate over time, leading to smooth muscle hypertrophy, epithelial basement membrane thickening, connective tissue deposition, and proliferation and hypertrophy of mucus-secreting glands (Figure 41-1). All of these factors contribute to progressive airflow obstruction, which is further compromised by the presence of thick tenacious mucus, ineffective mucociliary clearance, and edema in the walls of the bronchi, especially during an acute asthmatic exacerbation. Finally, episodic smooth muscle contraction further leads to the variability of symptoms in asthma.

Multiple mechanisms produce airway inflammation, and they involve a variety of interactions between inflammatory cells and numerous proinflammatory and inflammatory mediators. The asthmatic inflammatory cell matrix is made up of mast cells, macrophages, eosinophils, and activated lymphocytes. Both immune and nonimmune factors can activate the asthma disease process. When an asthmatic is exposed to a specific activating antigen, the release of a variety of mediators occurs via high-infinity immunoglobulin (IgE) receptors, which are found on bronchial mast cells, and low-infinity IgE receptors on macrophages and eosinophils. Lymphocytes control these processes. Both antibody-mediated and cell-mediated immune system processes are involved. The chemical mediators from these activated cells can directly contract airway smooth muscle, stimulate mucous secretion, enhance vascular permeability, and result in airway edema, all of which contribute to airflow obstruction. Furthermore, some mediators actually attract other inflammatory cells and activate them, and these activated cells further damage the airway. The cellular inflammatory reaction involves the release of preformed mediators from granules and rapidly generated mediators, including cytokines, histamines, a variety of

leukotrienes, and prostaglandins. Part of the inflammatory reaction causes a disruption of airway epithelial cell wall integrity. A loss of epithelial integrity allows increased permeability to inhaled allergens and other triggering substances and decreases mucociliary clearance of airway debris. The loss of epithelial integrity exposes nerve endings, which partially explains the enhanced cholinergic-mediated airway hyperreactivity found in asthma. Furthermore, the loss of epithelial integrity predisposes asthma patients to bacterial and viral infections.

Inflammation can be acute or chronic. The acute inflammatory response involves early recruitment of cells to the airway. This is followed by an evolving inflammatory reaction, as recruited and resident cells are activated and produce a complex pattern of inflammation. Chronic inflammation is characterized by a persistent level of cell damage and an ongoing level of repair that is unable to keep up with the ongoing damaging process. Chronic inflammation can lead to permanent airway damage.

Airway inflammation induces airway hyperresponsiveness (Figure 41-2). This hyperresponsiveness, along with the inflammatory changes of the airways, contributes further to airflow obstruction. In a susceptible individual, exposure to a variety of environmental risk factors leads to airway inflammation. Certain triggers may not only activate but also propagate inflammation and drive airway responsiveness to a more hyperresponsive state. The magnitude of airway hyperresponsiveness seems to correlate with the activity of airway inflammation. Furthermore, airway hyperresponsiveness seems to correlate with the clinical symptoms and signs of asthma.

Airway hyperresponsiveness, which is measured as the ease with which airways narrow in response to various nonsensitizing physical or chemical stimuli, is a hallmark of asthma. Hyperresponsiveness is assessed by measuring airflow before and after the inhalation of increasing doses of inhaled methacholine or histamine (Figure 41-3). Hyperresponsive airways will develop obstruction at lower cumulative doses of these chemicals than normal airways. This increased "twitchiness" of the airways is thought to protect the lungs from the detrimental effects of irritating inhalants. Airway hyperresponsiveness is not unique to the diagnosis of asthma. Hyperresponsive airways are found in other airway inflammatory diseases, like chronic bronchitis and sarcoidosis. It is important to note that the treatment of asthma, by improving airway inflammation, does diminish airway responsiveness. But airway hyperreactivity may not always be eradicated by the

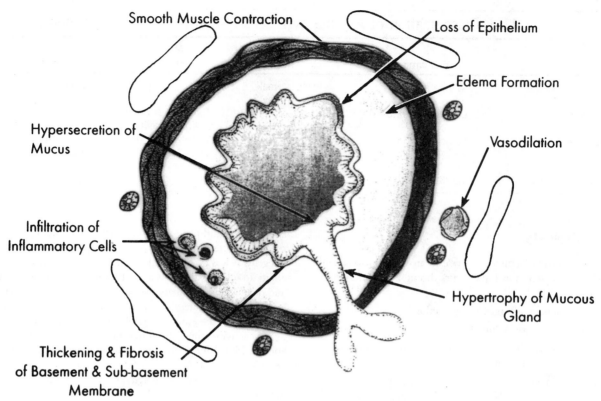

Figure 41-1 Changes in airway morphology in asthma.

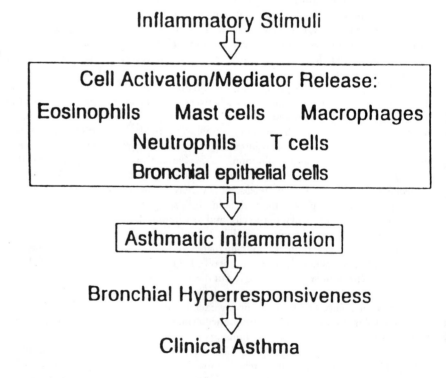

Figure 41-2 Steps involved in the asthmatic inflammatory cascade. These include the introduction of inflammatory stimuli to cell activation and mediator release, to asthmatic inflammation and bronchial hyper-responsiveness, and finally clinical asthma.

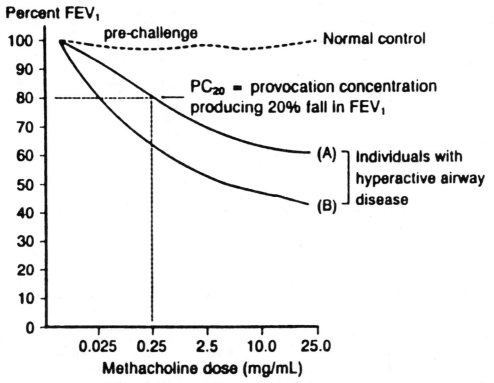

Dose-response curves of methacholine challenge

Figure 41-3 People with asthma have hyperresponsive ("twitchy") airways that are overly sensitive to immunologic or nonimmunologic stimuli (asthma "triggers"). Bronchial provocation testing can serve as a useful tool in measuring this bronchial hyperresponsiveness. Although helpful in confirming asthma diagnoses, such testing tends to be used mainly in clinical research.

use of antiinflammatory therapy, thus suggesting additional factors contributing to airway responsiveness.

MONITORING DISEASE ACTIVITY

The goals of asthma therapy are to prevent symptoms and help the patient achieve normal lung function and activity, especially during exercise; prevent exacerbations of asthma, no matter how mild, and certainly minimize the need for emergency department visits or hospitalizations; meet patient and family expectations and satisfaction with asthma care; and lastly, provide optimal pharmacotherapy with minimal adversity (3).

In order to ensure that these goals are met, periodic assessments and ongoing monitoring of asthma are recommended (3). If the patient has minimal signs and symptoms, with optimal airflow during exertion and sleep, then overall patient-perceived quality of life improves.

Physician assessment and patient self-assessment are part of the asthma monitoring process. Spirometry is recommended at the time of initial assessment, during treatment, and when changes in symptoms or home monitoring of peak expiratory flow rate (PEFR) have occurred (3,4).

A spirometer is a simple device used to measure certain lung volumes and airflows (5,6). The patient takes a deep breath and forces air from the lungs until all flow has ceased (Figure 41-4). With a cooperative and motivated effort, spirometric values are very reproducible. The forced expiratory volume in 1 second (FEV_1) is the most important airflow measurement. The asthmatic patient often has a reduction in the FEV_1 (see Figure 41-4). In fact, in the asthmatic, airflow obstruction is shown by a decrease in the forced expiratory volumes, the forced vital capacity (FVC), the FEV_1, and a decreased FEV_1/FVC ratio. These measurements are generally taken in the doctor's office or in a pulmonary function laboratory. On the other hand, the asthmatic subject can measure airflow on a daily basis, or at multiple times if necessary. Using a small hand-held device, which is generally made of durable plastic, peak expiratory flow rates can be measured in a reproducible fashion.

The inflammation in asthma, which causes the pathologic abnormalities in the airways, results in airway narrowing, increased airflow resistance, and airflow obstruction. Airway smooth muscle contraction, which is a reversible abnormality, further contributes to the airflow obstruction. Asthma, being a reversible obstructive airflow disease, waxes and wanes. With these changes, there are alterations in FEV_1 and PEFR (Figure 41-4). There are also variable needs for the use of medication to relieve symptoms. As the asthmatic becomes better controlled with therapeutic interventions, overall airflow improves, variability in airflow over each 24-

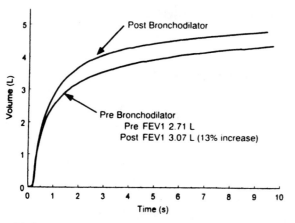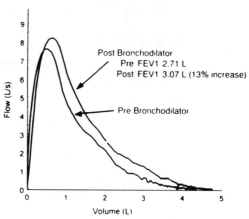

Figure 41-4 Administration of an inhaled bronchodilator improves airflow significantly. The panel on the left shows the FEV$_1$ spirographic improvement; the panel on the right shows the improvements in PEFR and subsequent flows by using flow volume curves.

hour time period decreases, and the need for "rescue" medication to relieve symptoms substantially decreases. As all of these factors change, overall quality of life improves. This translates into better sleep at night and resistance to asthma exacerbation during exposure to certain environmental challenges, like exercise or cigarette smoke.

It is very important to train patients to recognize symptom patterns that indicate improper asthma control. For certain patients, a written action plan based on signs and symptoms, and when necessary, changes in PEFR, can be helpful in the management process. The more chronic and severe the asthma, the greater is the importance of a written action plan.

THERAPY OF ASTHMA
Environmental Control
Environmental control measures, such as allergen avoidance, should always be included in asthma management strategies (3). Additionally, the patient should make a valid attempt to try to avoid potential airway irritants on a daily basis. Exposure of asthma patients to certain irritants or allergens increases asthma symptoms and often precipitates exacerbations. As a team, the physician and patient should do everything possible to identify those exacerbating allergens and irritants. The patient's history of likely sensitivity to seasonal allergens and employing skin testing or in vitro blood testing to assess the sensitivity to perennial allergens can be helpful. After identifying these allergens, it is important to use these positive tests in the context of the patient's medical history.

Certain environmental exposure rules should be followed. If an asthmatic knows what irritants or allergens destabilize his or her disease, everything should be done to avoid these exposures. Exposure to tobacco smoke should be avoided (7,8). Asthmatic patients should not receive beta blocker therapies (9,10) or foods that contain sulfites (11), preservatives that often exacerbate the asthmatic condition. Aspirin and other nonsteroidal antiinflammatory agents should be avoided (12,13), especially in patients who have

nasal polyps. Finally, rhinosinusitis (14) and gastroesophageal reflux (15), which are two additional conditions that have been implicated as asthma destabilizers, should be controlled.

Perhaps the most important step in controlling allergen-induced asthma is to reduce exposure to relevant indoor and outdoor allergens. All warm-blooded pets can cause allergic reactions. If there are pets in the patient's home and the patient is sensitive to that animal, then the animal should be removed from the house (3). At a minimum, the animal should be kept out of the patient's bedroom, it should be kept clean (16), and all airducts that lead into the bedroom should be covered with a filter.

House dust mite allergen is a major environmental factor in asthma (3). House dust mites are universal in areas of high humidity, which includes most of the United States. In addition to high humidity, mites depend upon human dander for survival. Mites thrive in mattresses, pillows, carpets, upholstered furniture, and soft toys. Since we generally spend most of our home time in the bedroom, it is the most important location to control. In patients who are house dust mite sensitive and demonstrate a clinical picture consistent with allergy to the mite allergens, there are a variety of desirable control measures that should be considered (17). Mattresses should be encased in an allergen-impermeable cover, as should the pillow. The sheets and blankets on the patient's bed should be rinsed in hot water on a weekly basis. If possible, indoor humidity should be maintained at less than 50%, and carpets, upholstered furniture, and stuffed animals should be removed from the area. There are a variety of chemical agents available for killing mites and denaturing the antigens, but these agents are not as effective as the environmental control measures mentioned.

If cockroach infestation is present in the home, it is very important to institute chemical control measures to reduce this antigen load (3). Asthma severity seems to increase with increasing levels of cockroach antigen. When chemical agents are used to control infestation, the home should be well ventilated and the patient should not return to the home until the odor has substantially dissipated.

Molds are fungi, which proliferate in humid environments, especially homes that have dampness problems. Creating a drier environment by fixing old water leaks and eliminating water sources reduces mold growth. Reducing indoor humidity to less than 50% substantially limits mold growth. A variety of tree, grass, and weed pollens and seasonal mold spores contribute to the outdoor allergen loads that affect many asthmatic patients. By staying indoors with the windows closed, generally in an air-conditioned environment, patients with outdoor allergen problems can be relatively protected. Pollen and spore counts are highest during the midday and afternoon, at periods of brightest sunlight. For the asthmatic who has a significant outdoor allergen problem, conducting outdoor activity shortly after sunrise or before sunset can result in a reduced pollen exposure.

A variety of measures can be taken to reduce allergen load in the home by modifying indoor air. Vacuuming carpets twice a week, preferably with a cleaner loaded with a high-efficiency particulate air filter, can reduce house dust accumulation, but the patient should not be in the room when the vacuuming is occurring. Air conditioning and the use of a dehumidifier are helpful. Humidifiers and evaporative coolers are not recommended for use around dust mite–sensitive patients with asthma. Indoor air cleaning devices should not substitute for the measures previously described. High-efficiency particulate air filters and electrostatic precipitating filters have been shown to reduce certain animal dander, mold spores, and the particulate from tobacco smoke. However, these devices do not have an impact on house dust mite and cockroach allergens, which are heavy particulates and do not remain airborne, and thus are not effected by air filtering.

Allergen immunotherapy can be helpful in certain asthmatic patients (3,18,19). However, it is preferable to have clear evidence of a relationship between asthma symptoms and exposure to the allergen in question. Finally, symptoms should be nearly perennial and difficult to control with pharmacotherapy alone. The whole concept of allergen immunotherapy is under constant debate, in terms of long-term benefit. If allergen immunotherapy is started, it should be given under the careful guidance of a well-trained physician immunotherapist who is capable of treating any life-threatening reaction that may occur (20). The immunotherapy should be directed at a single or only a very few allergens. Multiple-allergen mixes should be avoided. Finally, the course of allergen therapy is typically 3 to 5 years in duration, but a recognizable favorable improvement in asthma should occur early in treatment.

Pharmacologic Therapy

The pharmacologic treatment of asthma includes two broad categories of drugs: bronchodilators that relax airway smooth muscle and antiinflammatory drugs that reduce the influx of inflammatory cells and the release and/or effects of a large variety of chemical mediators from these cells.

Bronchodilators include short- and long-acting beta-adrenergic receptor agonists (beta-agonists), methylxanthines, and anticholinergics. Antiinflammatory agents include glucocorticoids, chromones (cromolyn and nedocromil), and leukotriene blockers.

In the chronic management of asthma, pharmacologic therapy is given by the oral or inhalation route, but inhalation therapy seems to be the preferred because of the higher concentration of medication directly delivered to the lungs, often with greater efficacy and lower risk of adverse effects (21). The inhalation of medication can be performed through a small-volume nebulizer or a metered-dose inhaler. An inhaler is sometimes attached to a tube spacer device, in order to reduce certain oropharyngeal adverse effects and, for some patients, enhance aerosol drug delivery into the lungs (3,22).

Medications are now characterized into two general treatment classes: long-term controller medications, which are used to achieve and maintain control of chronic asthma, and quick-relief medications, or relievers, which treat acute symptoms during an asthma exacerbation (Table 41-2) (3). However, even though there are a variety of controllers, the most effective medications for long-term therapy are those that have clearly demonstrated antiinflammatory effects.

Chronic Controllers

Corticosteroids are the most potent and effective antiinflammatory medications available for the management of asthma. The inhaled form of medication from a metered-dose inhaler, often attached to a spacer device, is used for the long-term control of asthma. Systemic corticosteroids, administered orally, are used to gain control of asthma following a period of destabilization and are avoided for long-term control by optimizing inhaled corticosteroid therapy and using additional controller therapies. However, some patients with severe chronic disease may require systemic corticosteroid therapy on a regular basis. Corticosteroids reduce airway inflammation and airway hyperresponsiveness. Furthermore, glucocorticoids prevent asthmatic exacerbations and bronchial wall remodeling, known to occur with chronic inflammation and responsible for the development of fixed airflow obstruction later in life (23–26).

There are many different products and delivery devices for the administration of inhaled corticosteroids, and their per-inhalation doses vary (3). For the most part, these therapies should not be used more than twice a day and no more than four inhalations each time, for compliance purposes. Most importantly, the lowest daily dose of an inhaled corticosteroid should be used in order to control disease.

Cromolyn and nedocromil sodium are nonsteroidal, antiinflammatory inhalative medications used in the chronic management of mild and moderate asthma. The mechanisms of action of these medications are not fully understood (3). However, they prevent bronchospasm caused by an inhaled

Table 41-2 Controller and Quick-Relief Therapies for Asthma

CONTROLLERS	QUICK RELIEVERS
Inhaled corticosteroids	Short-acting beta$_2$ agonists
Cromolyn	Ipratropium
Nedocromil	Systemic corticosteroids
Leukotriene modifiers	
Long-acting bronchodilators	
Systemic corticosteroids	

allergen and have been shown, with long-term use, to decrease nonspecific bronchial hyperreactivity, decrease asthma symptoms, and improve airflow obstruction (27,28). These therapies are used as initial long-term controller medication for children and adolescents, but their response seems to be less predictable than that of inhaled steroid therapy.

Another group of drugs that are best classified as antiinflammatory agents, which have recently been released for the treatment of asthma, are the leukotriene blockers. These are oral therapies that block certain chemicals called leukotrienes, which are by-products of the arachidonic acid–metabolic pathway, and they are potent bronchoconstrictors and inflammatory stimulants in humans. These leukotrienes are released from a variety of inflammatory cells, such as eosinophils and mast cells, and not only induce bronchoconstriction but increase vascular permeability, mucous secretion, and other inflammatory cells, which when they come to the airway site, are activated and release other powerful chemicals that propagate the inflammatory state even further (29). Leukotriene blockers improve lung function, diminish asthma symptoms, and reduce the need for the rescue use of short-acting inhaled beta agonists. Their efficacy has been shown in patients with mild to moderate asthma, and generally the improvements that are seen are modest in nature when compared to inhaled corticosteroid therapy. Furthermore, these agents have been shown to reduce bronchoconstriction caused by exercise, aspirin, and inhaled allergen exposure (30).

Theophylline, a methylxanthine compound, seems to control asthma for unclear reasons, but it does act as a modest bronchodilator and may have certain antiinflammatory effects as well (31,32). When theophylline is administered in a sustained-release oral theapy form, it has a long duration of action and can further control asthma when used in combination with inhaled corticosteroid therapy (33). Theophylline should be considered as an alternative controller therapy to that of inhaled corticosteroids (3). Theophylline's narrow therapeutic margin of safety, multiple medication interactions, and weak bronchodilating effect have placed it as a third-line controller therapy for chronic asthma. It is often used in patients with moderate to severe asthma after inhaled corticosteroid therapy has been optimized and a second-line controller therapy, such as a leukotriene blocker or a long-acting beta agonist, has been employed. For each patient using theophylline, there must be dose individualization to optimize efficacy, but more importantly, to minimize the potential for drug toxicity.

Short-acting, rapid-onset beta$_2$-agonist inhalative therapy is used as first-line therapy during asthma exacerbation (3). However, there are certain sustained-release oral beta-agonist tablets and a long-acting inhaled beta-agonist that should be used as controller therapy, in addition with antiinflammatory therapy, in the management of chronic asthma. Patients with moderate and severe asthma generally require at least two, if not three, controller medications to optimize their pharmacologic therapy (3). Beta agonists, which are more selective for the beta$_2$ receptor, are preferred. Long-acting tablets and inhaler beta$_2$-agonist therapies can have a duration of action at least of 12 hours, far longer than that of the beta agonists that are used by inhalation for the acute control of symptoms (34). These agents relax airway smooth muscle by stimulating adenylyl cyclase, an enzyme located on airway smooth muscle cells, increasing intracellular cyclic adenosine monophosphate (AMP), which relaxes airway smooth muscle.

Quick-Relief Medications

In order to achieve immediate relief of bronchoconstriction and the discomforting symptoms associated with asthma, quick-relief medications, such as nearly immediate onset short-acting beta$_2$ agonists and anticholinergics are employed. Short-acting beta$_2$ agonists relax airway smooth muscle within minutes and improve airflow. These agents are the drugs of choice for treating acute asthma symptoms and exacerbations (3). They are also used for preventing exercise-induced bronchospasm (3). Inhaled anticholinergic therapy, such as ipratropium bromide, can also be used as a bronchodilator in this setting, but a beta agonist should be used first. Ipratropium may provide some additional benefit during a severe asthmatic exacerbation (3).

Systemic corticosteroid therapy can speed the resolution of airflow obstruction and reduce the rate of replapse of treated severe asthma (1). Therefore, systemic corticosteroid therapy is used in more serious asthma exacerbations, as part of the quick-relief medical plan.

Short-acting beta$_2$-agonist therapy, like albuterol, should only be used for the symptomatic relief of asthma. Therefore, the use of this medication can serve as a marker of asthma stability or instability. The more albuterol necessary to control symptoms, the greater is the influence of airway inflammation that is present, and the stronger is the need for initiation or optimization of inhaled antiinflammatory therapy. Using a short-acting beta$_2$-agonist inhaler at the rate of one or more canisters per month has been associated with an increase in asthma morbidity and mortality (35). In fact, the majority of chronic asthma patients in this country should be able to be controlled to a level of mild episodic asthma. Mild episodic asthmatics have two or less mild asthmatic attacks a week. Therefore, if more than four puffs of a short-acting beta agonist are used weekly, then enhanced asthma control is necessary. A well-controlled asthmatic should only need one or two canisters of a short-acting beta$_2$ agonist per year, not counting the therapy that would be used to prevent exercise-induced bronchospasm. This may be the case for nearly 70% to 80% of asthmatics, excluding only the relatively small percentage of patients who have severe asthma and, despite aggressive controller therapy, continue to require their albuterol inhaler on a frequent basis.

MANAGEMENT OF ASTHMA ACCORDING TO SEVERITY CLASSIFICATION

A stepwise approach has been proposed for the pharmacologic therapy of chronic asthma (3) (Figure 41-5). The amount and frequency of medication is dictated by asthma severity. Therapy is directed toward treating airway inflammation. Therefore, controller therapies are emphasized, with antiinflammatory therapy considered to be mainstay. Controller therapies are often initiated at a higher level than the patient's step of severity at the onset in order to gain immediate control of disease. After control has been achieved, then

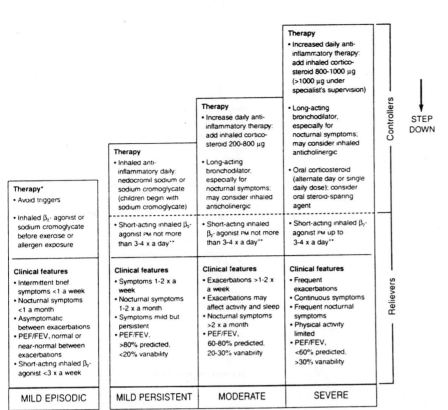

Figure 41-5 Stepwise approach to asthma management.

STEP DOWN

Therapy
- Increased daily anti-inflammatory therapy: add inhaled cortico-steroid 800-1000 µg (>1000 µg under specialist's supervision)
- Long-acting bronchodilator, especially for nocturnal symptoms; may consider inhaled anticholinergic
- Oral corticosteroid (alternate day or single daily dose); consider oral steroid-sparing agent

- Short-acting inhaled β_2- agonist PM up to 3-4 x a day**

Clinical features
- Frequent exacerbations
- Continuous symptoms
- Frequent nocturnal symptoms
- Physical activity limited
- PEF/FEV, <60% predicted, >30% variability

Therapy
- Increase daily anti-inflammatory therapy: add inhaled cortico-steroid 200-800 µg
- Long-acting bronchodilator, especially for nocturnal symptoms; may consider inhaled anticholinergic

- Short-acting inhaled β_2- agonist PM not more than 3-4 x a day**

Clinical features
- Exacerbations >1-2 x a week
- Exacerbations may affect activity and sleep
- Nocturnal symptoms >2 x a month
- PEF/FEV, 60-80% predicted, 20-30% variability

Therapy
- Inhaled anti-inflammatory daily: nedocromil sodium or sodium cromoglycate (children begin with sodium cromoglycate)

- Short-acting inhaled β_2- agonist PM not more than 3-4 x a day**

Clinical features
- Symptoms 1-2 x a week
- Nocturnal symptoms 1-2 x a month
- Symptoms mild but persistent
- PEF/FEV, >80% predicted, <20% variability

Therapy*
- Avoid triggers
- Inhaled β_2- agonist or sodium cromoglycate before exercise or allergen exposure

Clinical features
- Intermittent brief symptoms <1 a week
- Nocturnal symptoms <1 a month
- Asymptomatic between exacerbations
- PEF/FEV, normal or near-normal between exacerbations
- Short-acting inhaled β_2- agonist <3 x a week

Controllers / Relievers

| MILD EPISODIC | MILD PERSISTENT | MODERATE | SEVERE |

*Anti-inflammatory therapy may be used during exacerbations

**Increasing PM β_2- agonist use is an indication to increase anti-inflammatory therapy

therapy is reduced or stepped down. Step-down therapy (see Figure 41-5) is essential if one is to identify the minimum medication necessary to maintain disease control. During this process, it is helpful that airflow is monitored and correlated with asthma symptoms and signs and the supplemental use of the inhaled short-acting beta$_2$ agonist. Patients may relapse if inhaled corticosteroids are completely discontinued (36).

Patients with intermittent symptoms are treated with an inhaled beta$_2$ agonist, which has a quick onset and short duration of action. Albuterol by metered-dose inhaler or nebulizer, used on an as-needed basis, is the quick-relief therapy of choice, but other medications can be used (3). However, when any one of these medications is being used on more than two occasions each week for the relief of asthma, then the patient no longer has episodic asthma and must be classified as having a more persistent form of asthma. Persistent asthma is most effectively controlled with the daily long-term use of a controller medication, specifically, an antiinflammatory therapy. Inhaled glucocorticoid therapy is most often used and should be added to the beta-agonist therapy, which still should be used on an as-needed basis (33,37,38).

The clinician must treat each individual patient, paying attention to the needs and circumstances of the patient in his or her step-wise treatment process. In order to initially gain disease control, it is often necessary to initiate antiinflammatory therapy at a more aggressive level than that required in the long run by the patient's actual clinical disease severity. This often helps establish quicker disease control, and then therapy can be reduced. Many times a short course of sys-temic corticosteroid therapy is used to gain control, along with a reasonable, perhaps more intermediate, daily dose of inhaled corticosteroids. Once asthma is controlled, oral therapy is quickly reduced and stopped. Within a brief period of time, inhaled corticosteroid may even be reduced to a lower daily dose. Control is monitored during this treatment process. With reduced inflammation, asthma symptoms and signs should improve, PEFR should increase, and the variability in airflow over each 24-hour time period should decrease, and finally, the dependency on the rescue use of inhaled albuterol should decrease. Enhanced control should eliminate nocturnal awakenings and activity limitation. Overall, the patient should start to feel "normal."

With regular follow-up visits, the clinician should be able to reduce inhaled corticosteroid therapy by 10% to 25% every 2 to 3 months, until a low daily dose is achieved and disease control is maintained. A chronic asthmatic who is completely withdrawn from inhaled corticosteroid therapy often relapses (36). Therefore, there should be an excellent reason why inhaled corticosteroid therapy or other antiinflammatory controller therapy is completely discontinued. If there is difficulty in gaining control or maintaining control with reasonable doses of controller therapy, then an asthma specialist should be consulted.

This discussion has focused on inhaled corticosteroid therapy as the antiinflammatory medication of first choice. However, other antiinflammatory therapies can be used in the first-line management of persistent asthma. These medications include inhaled cromolyn and nedocromil sodium and oral leukotriene blocker therapy (3). This point is particularly important for children and other patients who are unable to use inhaled corticosteroid therapy on a regular basis, perhaps because of the occurrence of bothersome local adverse effects such as dysphonia and thrush.

If optimal control of asthma is difficult to achieve or be maintained, then the following factors must be considered:

1. Patient medication adherence and administration technique.

2. The need for a transient increase in antiinflammatory therapies in order to reestablish control.

3. A careful review of certain self-management behaviors or even psychosocial problems. Environmental control issues must be carefully reviewed for adherence and technique.

4. It is often necessary to step up therapy to a higher level, often instituting a second- or third-line controller therapy.

Most patients with moderate and severe chronic asthma require not only a higher daily dose of inhaled corticosteroid therapy but a second- or third-line controller medication. These medications include a sustained-release theophylline (39), a long-acting inhalative like salmeterol (40,41), and perhaps leukotriene blocker therapy (42). However, before going to higher daily doses of an inhaled corticosteroid it is better to institute second- and even third-line controller therapy in order to enhance disease control, thereby improving the asthma patient's overall quality of life. Salmeterol and theophylline may be especially helpful in controlling nocturnal breakthrough symptoms.

The most severe persistent asthmatic population requires high daily doses of an inhaled corticosteroid in addition to other controller therapies in an effort to reduce the need for daily, every-other-day, or frequent bolus-taper courses of systemic corticosteroid therapy. This group of patients should see an asthma specialist on a regular basis.

Asthma Complications

Complications from asthma can occur acutely or chronically. An acute asthmatic attack is associated with a variety of complications, including pneumothorax, pneumomediastinum, a variety of cardiac arrhythmias, lung atelectasis, and respiratory failure. Rarely, death can occur. The young and the elderly are at particular risk for death because the severity of their disease is either not appreciated or is ignored. Asthma death can be sudden in onset, possibly associated with laryngospasm. However, most asthmatic deaths are slow in evolution to the point at which respiratory failure occurs as a multitude of metabolic problems develop (43). Table 41-3 shows the numerous factors that have been implicated in asthma mortality.

With poorly controlled asthma over a long period of time irreversible airflow obstruction develops (44,45). Recurrent airway infection is associated with fixed airflow obstruction (46). In a few patients, allergic bronchopulmonary aspergillosis occurs, often with mucoid airway impaction and secondary bacterial infection. Allergic bronchopulmonary aspergillosis associated with asthma is characterized by episodes of severe recurrent asthmatic exacerbations (47).

Table 41-3 Factors Associated with Asthma Mortality
Disease-Related
• Nocturnal asthma
• Laryngospasm
• Large diurnal PEFR variations
• Recent hospitalization (within 2 months)
• Chronic instability
Physician-Related
• Inadequate assessment
• Failure to monitor therapy
• Treatment delay
• Corticosteroids and rescue bronchodilators underprescribed
• Inappropriate sedative therapy
• Inadequate disease education
Patient-Related
• Failure to recognize deterioration
• Failure to seek help
• Ignoring nocturnal symptoms
• Noncompliance
Medication under- and overuse
Failure to avoid environmental stimuli
Therapy-Related
• Medication toxicity
• Inadequate corticosteroid therapy

Fever can be associated with this condition, as can chest pain. Mucous impaction causes transient infiltrates to develop on the chest x-ray, usually in the upper lung fields. Associated blood eosinophilia and an increased serum IgE level are associated with allergic bronchopulmonary aspergillosis, but a positive skin prick test and serum precipitating antibodies to the fungus *Aspergillus fumigatus* are confirmatory for this particular form of chronic asthma. This condition generally requires high doses of inhaled corticosteroids each day, often with oral corticosteroid therapy.

Immunotherapy

Skin testing is widely used to diagnose clinical allergies (48). The procedure involves intracutaneous delivery of a small amount of an aqueous antigen solution. The dose is regulated. The antigen for each skin test combines with IgE antibody affixed to mast cells and certain mediator substances, usually histamine, with a release from the mast cells causing a reaction. The reaction is local vasodilatation and edema. The so-called wheal and flare reactions appear within 20 minutes. There is a standardized scoring system for determining the reactivity of each antigen that is injected. Often, an immediate wheal and flare reaction is followed by a late-phase reaction that involves more erythema and edema.

There are two types of skin tests. The epicutaneous test is often referred to as the *scratch* or *prick technique*. Also, there is an *intracutaneous* or *intradermal test*. These skin tests are generally easy to perform and cause little patient discomfort. Also, there are certain advantages and disadvantages to either the epicutaneous or the intracutaneous skin test (48). Finally, a variety of medications can inhibit a skin test reaction (antihistamines and tricyclic antidepressants).

The discovery of IgE as the antibody responsible for allergic reactions has lead to the development of certain blood tests which can measure the amount of IgE in response to certain allergens. This form of in vitro testing is called *radioimmunoabsorbent testing* (RAST) (48). Skin testing is less expensive than in vitro tests, often providing results within 1 hour. Skin tests are more sensitive than in vitro tests. When the skin test is positive, the patient can see the positive skin test, which often encourages the patient to enhance their compliance with environmental control measures. RAST does not require expertise in technique, no allergen extracts are necessary, there is no risk of an allergic systemic reaction, and it can be performed on patients who are taking medications that often suppress the skin test reaction.

When a positive result is found with skin testing or RAST, the clinician is obliged to look for clinical significance of the positive allergy test in the context of the patient's medical history. If this relationship is clear and the allergen cannot be avoided and it is difficult to control symptoms with pharmacologic therapy, then immunotherapy should be considered. Allergen immunotherapy should be administered by a physician in the office or the hospital where facilities are available to treat the serious adverse reactions that can occur as a result of this form of therapy (20). It is better to use immunotherapy for a single allergen; the more allergens that are being treated for, the higher is the incidence of failure (3). Although multiple-allergen mixes are used for immunotherapy, there are only a few studies that clearly support this practice (18,19). Finally, allergy immunotherapy is typically administered for 3 to 5 years. Immunotherapy should not be used until environmental control has been maximized.

There is a paucity of information that supports the use of immunotherapy in the treatment of asthma, but this therapy is definitively helpful in the management of allergic rhinitis, especially in children (49). Despite the paucity of supportive data for immunotherapy and asthma, there are many allergy specialists who believe that this form of therapy is helpful. Immunotherapy is felt to reduce not only the frequency of symptoms but the extent of symptoms and to minimize the need for bronchodilator medications in the control of asthma. Immunotherapy is most effective for seasonal pollens and house dust, with some success in pet allergy, particularly cat. Immunotherapy is not a cure, but as said previously, it does, at times, reduce asthma and allergic rhinitis symptoms and signs. The success of immunotherapy is dependent upon the blending of the allergic history with the results of either skin testing or serologic testing to identify potential allergens. In other words, the patient's clinical setting should blend with the objective information obtained from skin testing and RAST serology, before the likelihood for immunotherapy as a helpful treatment intervention can be predicted.

There are certain risks associated with immunotherapy. The most common reaction to an allergy shot is swelling, erythema, and pruritus at the site of the injection. This type of a reaction is usually short-lived and can be minimized by using topical antiinflammatory therapy in the form of a cream or an oral antihistamine. The most serious reaction from an allergy shot is called anaphylaxis. Anaphylaxis can occur rather quickly after the administration of the allergy shot. Therefore, immunotherapy should be performed in the presence of a physician experienced in treating anaphylaxis.

Sufficient time should be allowed for the reaction to occur, if it will develop, so most patients have to stay in a physician's office for a period of 15 to 30 minutes after each injection. Anaphylaxis can be treated. Less serious reactions include nasal congestion and sneezing, asthma itself, difficulty swallowing and talking because of a swollen tongue or larynx, and a sensation of lightheadedness. With these reactions, there are often an increase in heart rate and perhaps even a slight change in blood pressure. An anaphylactic reaction includes all of the above but also more profound changes in heart rate and blood pressure, even vascular collapse and death.

Exercise and Asthma

Exercise-induced asthma (EIA) is defined as a reversible decrease in airflow obstruction that occurs during or after exercise (50,51). In asthmatics, EIA is prevalent. Nearly 90% of asthmatics have EIA and patients with allergic rhinitis and even normal relatives of asthmatics can demonstrate this phenomenon. As with asthma, the common symptoms are wheezing, shortness of breath, cough, and what the patient describes as an inability to take in a full breath of air during or following exercise. Typically, the symptoms start several minutes after exercise has stopped and usually improve within 1 to 2 hours, even without medication. The typical fall in airflow is seen between 5 and 20 minutes after exercise (Figure 41-6).

Exercise-induced asthma is thought to be associated with the exchange of heat and water that occurs in the airways during exercise in which minute ventilation is increased. Because of the high minute ventilation there is a cooling and drying effect on the airway that somehow influences airway inflammation in a way that expresses itself more intensely (51,52). During exercise, the airways cool down as minute ventilation increases. This cooling and drying effect of the airways sets the stage for the rapid rewarming of the airways that occurs with resting, which likely triggers bronchoconstriction.

Well-controlled chronic asthma should include the control of asthma during and following exercise. It is realistic to believe that if chronic asthma is controlled, patients can participate in exertional, even athletic, activities at a reasonable level to maintain body conditioning and enjoy themselves. However, there are certain interventions that should be followed to control exercise-induced asthma.

Exercise-induced asthma can be diagnosed simply for the majority of patients. We have had the experience of measuring PEFRs prior to exercise. After an exercise challenge, perhaps running 1 mile at a moderate pace, airflow is remeasured sequentially at 5, 15, and 30 minutes. The exercise-induced asthmatic often drops airflow within this time period. When airflow falls, especially when associated with symptoms consistent with asthma, the diagnosis can be made. This evaluation process can be done by a physician or under the guidance of a physician by instructed individuals such as trainers or coaches. Patients that are known to have asthma should be screened for EIA breakthrough. Also, individuals that may be at high risk for EIA should be screened. We have found that as many as 14% of high-performance athletes will have bronchial hyperresponsiveness, including bronchoconstriction associated with exertion. Often, EIA or perhaps better labeled

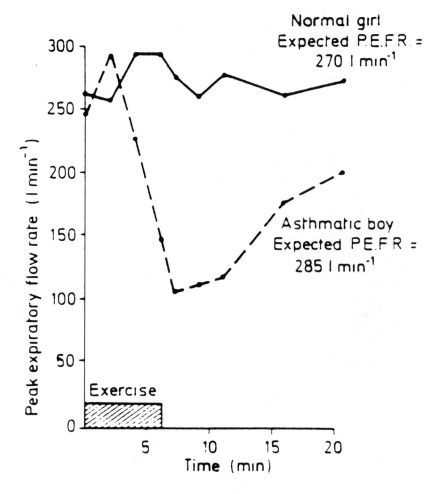

Figure 41-6 Response to exercise of an asthmatic boy and a healthy girl of similar size whose resting PEFRs were within the normal range. The asthmatic boy developed a typical attack of EIA.

for some patients, EIB, can seriously and adversely affect athletic performance.

The prevention and control of EIA or EIB can be accomplished by both nonpharmacologic and pharmacologic approaches. Before an athletic workout or competition, certain nonpharmacologic interventions can be helpful in preventing or minimizing EIB. The use of an extended warm-up session and certain special breathing techniques that help minimize oral hyperventilation and also promote relaxation can be helpful in the treatment process. Even hypnosis has been used to minimize, if not control, EIA.

Sometimes it is important to choose a sport that does not require sustained exercise, perhaps baseball, golf, or even weight lifting, rather than continuous long-duration activities such as long-distance running, basketball, or aerobic dancing. When the exercise is performed, it is good to avoid cold, dry environments. A warm (but not too warm) and moist environment can often be helpful in minimizing EIA. As mentioned above, the use of a warm-up period to try to avoid asthma symptoms can be very helpful. In the preexercise phase the patient should begin warming up slowly to loosen the muscles and elevate the heart rate. With the beginning of a light sweat the patient can perform the exercise at or close to his or her maximum exertion for up to 5 minutes and then take a rest. More accomplished athletes can continue this warm-up process recurrently for 30 to 40 minutes. Eventually, the athlete is ready to perform at full capacity for a longer period

of time. Another strategy is to do brief bouts of exercise for 2 to 3 minutes followed by 3 to 5 minutes of rest. These repetitive exertional challenges should occur over a 30- or 40-minute period. Again, when the athlete is ready to pursue maximum performance for an extended period of time he or she will be less likely to have a more clinically significant asthmatic attack. It is important for the individual athlete to find out which warm-up protocol works best for him or her. In fact, some athletes must warm up for a period as long as an hour.

Just as important as warming up appropriately is concentrating on certain breathing maneuvers during and following exercise. Symptoms can be reduced by breathing warm, humid air rather than cold, dry air. Therefore, swimmers are likely to tolerate their disease better than football players. Certain athletes, during exertion, have learned to breathe through their nose instead of their mouth. This is a hard technique to master. However, when athletes learn how to breathe through their nose, especially during periods where heavy breathing is unnecessary, the air that is brought into their lungs is humidified and heated and thus stimulus to the airways is minimized. Furthermore, with exertion, hyperventilation occurs. By breathing deeper and more slowly, the cooling and drying effect of the hyperventilation phenomena can be minimized. Finally, it is not only the type of sport that one plays but the position selected. For example, a lineman in football is at less risk than a running back.

The postexercise period is also very important. The cool-down phase after a workout or competition should involve taking deep slow breaths. Cooling down in a warmer environment, but not too warm, can be helpful.

Often, drug therapy is necessary to prevent EIA or EIB. There are numerous inhaled beta-agonist medications that can be used shortly before exercise and even during and after exercise to prevent or relieve asthma symptoms (3). Beta agonists, when administered by inhalation, will prevent EIA in more than 80% of EIA patients. Administering a short-acting inhaled beta agonist approximately 15 to 30 minutes before exercise provides protection for 2 to 3 hours. When asthma breaks through, these medications can be safely administered by a metered-dose inhaler. Salmeterol has been shown to prevent EIA for 10 to 20 hours (53), so it is helpful for prolonged prevention when the athlete will reexpose himself or herself to the exercise challenge over this time period. Other therapies can be used in addition to the beta agonist. Inhaled cromolyn or nedocromil can be taken approximately 30 minutes to 1 hour prior to exercise, often in addition to the preexercise use of the short-acting inhaled beta agonist for further control in those patients who fail single preventative therapy (54,55). Remember, most EIA occurs in chronic asthmatics. It is crucial to control chronic asthma with the regular use of controller therapies. When chronic asthma is controlled, the frequency and severity of EIA are reduced (56).

Occupational Asthma

A variety of substances in the workplace have been implicated in the development of asthma, including a large variety of animal proteins, grain and wood dust, cotton dust, chemical compounds such as isocyanates and hydrides, metal salts, and even pharmaceuticals (57) (Table 41-4). It is extremely important to recognize occupational asthma as soon as possible, because the likelihood of complete resolution of symptoms decreases over time (58,59). Occupational asthma is suspected when either the patient or the clinician realizes that there is a relationship between asthma symptoms and work exposure. Many times, the patient will improve on the days that he or she is away from the workplace, particularly during vacations, providing an important clue. Sometimes, coworkers have similar symptoms, and sometimes asthma can occur during the night. Serial peak flow measurements at work and away from work can help diagnose occupational asthma. Occasionally, a bronchial challenge, done in a specialized laboratory with a suspected allergen or irritant from the workplace, can be helpful diagnostically (60,61). Unfortunately, some patients will have persistent asthma despite removal of the inciting substance. A variety of chemicals, dust, and other particulates can sensitize the airways and actually induce chronic asthma. This is different than allergen- or irritant-induced asthma, in which these substances aggravate preexisting asthma but don't actually initiate the disease process. This condition is known as *reactive airways dysfunction syndrome* (RADS), and the respiratory symptoms may last for years.

The management of occupational asthma can be difficult. Often, the employee must avoid the triggering substance. The use of respiratory protection by wearing a ventilator mask can be helpful. Many times, the patient must completely avoid exposure to the initiating agent; therefore, a new job position may be necessary.

Table 41-4 Select Causes of Allergic and Nonallergic Occupational Asthma

	SUBSTANCE	OCCUPATIONS
	Allergic	
High Molecular Weight	Animal protein	Laboratory workers
	Papain	Brewers, lens workers
	Wheat flour	Bakers, millers
	Trypsin	Plastic workers, pharmaceutical workers
	Soybean dust	Farmers, food workers
	Vegetable gums	Printers, food workers
Low Molecular Weight	Platinum	Jewelers, refiners
	Trimellitic anhydride	Plastic and epoxy resin workers
	Phthalic anhydride	Plastic and epoxy resin workers
	Nonallergic	
	Isocyanates	Spray painters, foundry workers
	Polyvinylchloride	Meat wrappers
	Western red cedar	Carpenters

Stress

Asthma is not a psychosomatic illness. However, there is emerging evidence that stress plays an important role in precipitating asthma exacerbation and may act as a risk factor for the increased prevalence of this disease (62). Since emotional upset does contribute to the asthma symptom picture, a variety of psychological interventions may be necessary to enhance overall asthma care. Stress exacerbation of asthma may involve enhanced generation of proinflammatory cytokines (63), but more importantly, psychosocial factors associated with stress influence the asthmatic's personal sphere and often lead to a poor outcome (64,65). Conflict that develops between the patient, the family, and the medical staff often interferes with appropriate asthma care. It is true that the poorly controlled chronic asthmatic can despair and his or her disease can have a significant negative effect on personal relationships and family life, as well as self-image. Uncontrolled asthma can reduce overall quality of life. Enhanced asthma control, and careful discussion of these issues with the patient and family, can help the overall asthmatic care process. The asthmatic who needs psychosocial assistance should take the advantage of appropriate professional counseling. There are a variety of psychologically oriented approaches to asthma care that can be helpful, including family counseling, educational seminars, and even psychotherapy, to name a few. Ignoring one's asthma symptoms and neglecting to use medication can seriously affect overall asthma control, and these issues should be brought to the table for discussion. Asthma education has been associated with enhanced confidence in the patient's management of chronic asthma (3).

Food Hypersensitivity

Food allergens are not a common precipitant of asthma (3). Foods can be an important cause of anaphylaxis in both adults and children (66,67). Lower respiratory tract symptoms are uncommon, even with positive double-blind food challenges (68). Certain foods contain sulfites, and sulfite sensitivity has been described in patients. Wheezing, cough, and shortness of breath after eating shrimp, certain dried fruits, or processed potatoes, or after drinking beer or wine, may be related to sulfite sensitivity. When a food hypersensitivity reaction is suspected, the foods associated with this reaction should be avoided. In general, food products that contain sulfites should be avoided by asthmatics.

The term *food allergy* is often used too loosely. Certain foods cause adverse reactions that should be characterized as *food intolerances*. The mechanisms for these reactions do not involve an allergy-mediated mechanism. For example, lactose intolerance, in which there is a deficiency of the enzyme necessary to digest milk, induces abdominal discomfort and diarrhea when one consumes milk or other dairy products. This is not due to allergy; the reaction is a food intolerance. In fact, many adverse reactions associated with sulfite-containing foods should be classified as a food intolerance rather than a food allergy.

The approach to the diagnosis of food hypersensitivity is controversial. Through a thorough history, the clinician develops a suspicion for the problem. The intolerance is confirmed through a blind food challenge. It is best to employ a double-blind food challenge. Another way of diagnosing the problem would be to employ food elimination from the diet (69). If a specific food is suspected, it is eliminated from the diet; if symptoms improve, then a presumptive diagnosis is made. On the other hand, if symptoms persist, then the food is replaced in the diet and other causes for the symptoms are explored. If on the other hand, the symptoms do disappear during the period in which the food is eliminated and recur when the food is replaced in the diet, then a double-blind, placebo-controlled food challenge should be arranged. A more complicated situation is when the patient does not have a specific suspicion about which food or foods are causing an adverse body reaction. This presents for a more complex elimination process. Symptoms which persist after 2 weeks on a carefully designed strict elimination diet are not likely related to the ingested substances. Symptoms which vanish on an elimination diet may then be explored in an algorithmic fashion (Figure 41-7). Elimination diets are not helpful for patients whose symptoms are sporadic.

A food challenge may be helpful in uncovering either an allergy or an intolerance. A double-blind, placebo-controlled food challenge is most helpful (69). A variety of vehicles are used to disguise the food that is being used, and some food challenges employ opaque capsules using dehydrated or dried food substances. A reasonable protocol that can be used for a simple food challenge has been described by Bock (69). For those patients who present with a history of an immediate reaction, the food challenge can be performed in the physician's office. On the other hand, many patients describe delayed reactions, and the patient has to be instructed to contact the office when symptoms begin. For food allergy and adverse reactions that are delayed, it is rare to have a severe or life-threatening reaction, so the risk involved in such a challenge is small. However, if the history of the patient suggests a more severe reaction, then hospitalization may be necessary to perform the food challenge. Multiple food challenges are more complex to perform. The placebo challenge should be entwined with the multiple food challenges, which are usually performed in a singular or individual fashion at home. Careful diary keeping is necessary, and the physician must be available for the patient if a more significant adverse reaction occurs. It is best to refer a patient who needs a multiple food challenge test to a regional center that has expertise in these diagnosistic techniques.

There is no completely acceptable and highly reliable laboratory hypersensitivity test that can be used for the diagnosis of food allergy or intolerance (69). Immune mechanisms are best documented by skin testing or food challenging, as described. Gastroenteropathies, perhaps due to milk, soy, and gluten proteins, are examples of food intolerances that are not associated with the detection of an IgE immune-mediated reaction.

Foods that contain monosodium glutamate (MSG) or other sulfating agents and yellow food dye No. 5 can sometimes be associated with asthma symptoms. In fact, it is advisable for asthmatics to avoid these food additives altogether. Old-container foods may be another category which should be avoided by asthmatics. These foods include beer, wine, a variety of baked goods, buttermilk, sour cream, cheeses, cider, dried fruits, mushrooms, smoked meats and fish, and especially, leftovers. The third food group that I have been impressed with as an asthmatic trigger and that is associated with anaphylaxis is peanuts and other nuts, including the products derived from these nuts. As the asthmatic avoids foods that have been identified as being potential triggers, longitudinal challenges of these foods may be necessary over time to verify whether the food problem is either ongoing or the patient has "outgrown" the problem (69).

Monosodium glutamate (MSG), a flavor enhancer, is often found in a variety of specialty food preparations. Sulfites, used as preservatives for some foods, may also be found in certain medications. Sulfites act as antioxidants and prevent fruit and vegetable discoloration. Sulfites can be added to lettuce to prevent leaves from going limp and browning. When a sulfite is added to potatoes, whiteness is preserved. Sulfites can be placed on seafood and meats to prevent discoloration. For a while, sulfites were added to bronchodilating solutions, used in nebulizer treatments for asthma. It is important to read the food product label or inquire of the chef as to whether or not a sulfite has been used to preserve the food that the asthmatic is about to eat. Obviously, these foods and medications should be avoided.

Medication-Induced Asthma

The ingestion of aspirin in sensitive individuals may result in nasal congestion, eye irritation, and asthma exacerbation and usually occurs rapidly after ingestion, often within 30 minutes (70). Four to twenty percent of asthmatics are sensitive to aspirin and related compounds, especially a variety of nonsteroidal antiinflammatory agents. Severe and even fatal asthma exacerbations have been associated with aspirin ingestion. Adult patients with severe persistent asthma who have nasal polyps should be carefully instructed not to use any aspirin or aspirin-like medication. Safe alternatives to aspirin

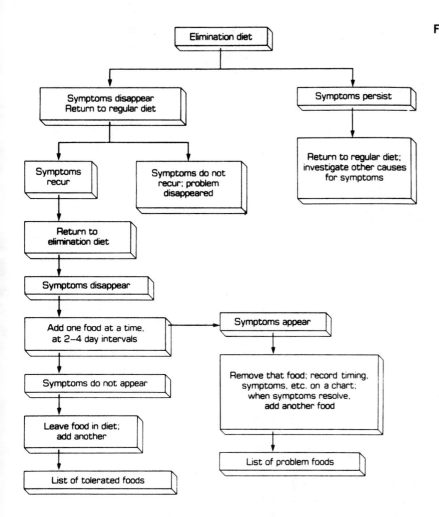

Figure 41-7 Algorithm for evaluation of possible food hypersensitivity in cases in which no specific food is suspected. These situations are more complicated, and they require the use of an elimination diet. Symptoms persisting beyond 14 days of an elimination diet are not likely due to ingested food. (Adapted with permission from Bock SA. Food allergy: a primer for people. New York: Vantage, 1988.)

include acetaminophen and salsalate (71,72). Nasal polyposis and chronic rhinosinusitis occur in nearly 90% of the patients with aspirin sensitivity (Samter's syndrome). The prevalence of aspirin sensitivity increases with age and the severity of asthma. There is no known familial predilection to aspirin sensitivity. It is not known to be associated with atopy. The mechanism appears to be related to inhibition of the enzyme cyclooxygenase, in which arachidonic acid metabolites are passed through the leukotriene pathway resulting in increased production of the leukotrienes C4, D4, and E4 (the slow-reacting substance of anaphylaxis) (73). Therefore, medications that interfere with leukotriene synthesis are helpful in the management of aspirin-induced asthma.

Tartrazine or yellow food dye No. 5 can induce asthma symptoms in some individuals. As mentioned previously, this food coloring is found in a number of foods, but it is been found in some medications. Soft drinks, pastries, and candies can have yellow food dye No. 5, and the asthmatic should read labels carefully to avoid such foods and medications.

Beta-blockers, including a variety of eyedrop preparations, can induce asthma symptoms and should be avoided in asthmatic patients (74,75). The more cardioselective beta-blockers may be better tolerated by the asthmatic (76), but in order to be safe, a patient with asthma should avoid beta-blocker therapy, unless this form of medication is unavoidable for the cardiac or eye condition. Fortunately, there are satisfactory alternatives to beta-blockers for most of these patients.

Gastroesophageal Reflux

Gastroesophageal reflux means that some of the acidic liquid contents of the stomach regurgitate into the esophagus. This fluidy substance is irritating to the esophagus. The gastroesophageal reflux material does not have to be aspirated into the lungs to induce asthma. Reflux of the acidic fluid into the esophagus likely destabilizes asthma by enhancing the cholinergic autonomic nervous system influence. Gastroesophageal reflux should be suspected in patients with poorly controlled asthma, particularly those who have nocturnal symptomatic breakthrough (3). Reflux symptoms do not have to be present, which makes the diagnosis difficult. However, when gastroesophageal reflux is symptomatic, patients usually describe the sensation of "heartburn." A patient who has a hiatal hernia is at particular risk for gastroesophageal reflux.

If gastroesophageal reflux is suspected, medical management (77,78) includes: 1) avoiding eating food and drinking liquids within 3 hours prior to bedtime ; 2) elevating the head of the bed at night by using 6 to 8-in. blocks; 3) eating smaller, and if necessary, move frequent meals; 4) using appropriate pharmacologic therapy, often antacid therapy or a histamine receptor blocker; and 5) cessation of alcohol, cigarettes, and caffeinated foods. Also, theophylline can reduce lower esophageal sphincter tone and predispose the asthmatic to gastroesophageal reflux.

If the medical management, as described above, fails, then further evaluation and other treatment options should be considered. Some patients may have to have further diagnostic interventions like an upper gastrointestinal x-ray series or esophagogastroduodenoscopy, and others may have to be referred to a surgeon for evaluation.

Pregnancy and Asthma

The risk of asthma exacerbation during pregnancy is higher for woman who had asthma before becoming pregnant. For the patient who has had asthma and is now pregnant, there is a chance that the asthma will remain the same or actually get better, or it may intensify (79). Whatever way the asthma changes during the first pregnancy, it is likely that similar symptoms will occur with subsequent pregnancies. Patients with more severe and difficult to control asthma, generally have worse symptoms during pregnancy. As a general rule, one third of all pregnant asthma patients improve during pregnancy, one third remain the same, and one third have a worsening of their disease. It is important for every asthma patient who becomes pregnant to be carefully managed medically during obstetrical care.

Asthma may also have an effect on pregnancy. It is important to point out that uncontrolled asthma is a risk for the fetus. A mother whose asthma is well controlled and free of complications imposes no additional risk to the fetus.

If asthma medications are necessary during pregnancy, one must keep in mind the benefit of keeping asthma under control against the small potential risk for adverse effects from the asthma medications during pregnancy. The majority of asthma medications that are used in practice present little to no risk during pregnancy, although prospective well-designed and well-controlled clinical trials do not exist for most medications that are used during pregnancy. Both systemic and inhaled corticosteroids can be used during pregnancy. Beta-agonist inhalative therapy should be used to treat asthma symptom breakthrough. Allergy immunotherapy can be continued during pregnancy but should not be altered. Furthermore, allergy immunotherapy should not be instituted during pregnancy.

Topical inhalative therapy should be selected over systemic therapies during pregnancy. Over-the-counter medications should be avoided. The obstetrician and the patient's primary care provider should work together to create the safest treatment scenario for the asthmatic patient who is pregnant. When questions arise, the local asthma expert, generally an allergist or pulmonary specialist, should be consulted.

REFERENCES

1. Adams PF, Marano MA. Current estimates from the National Health Interview Survey. Vital Health Stat 1995 1994;10:94.

2. Centers for Disease Control and Prevention. Asthma mortality and hospitalization among children and young adults—United States, 1990–93. MMWR 1996;45: 350–353.

3. National Heart, Lung, and Blood Institute. Guidelines for the diagnoses and management of asthma. Expert panel report II. Publication #97-4051. Washington, D.C.: National Institutes of Health, 1997.

4. Li JP, O'Connell EJ. Clinical evaluation of asthma. Ann Allergy Asthma Immunol 1996;76:1–13.

5. American Thoracic Society. Lung function testing: selection of reference values and interpretive strategies. Am Rev Respir Dis 1991;144:1202–1218.

6. American Thoracic Society. Standardization of spirometry: 1994 update. Am J Resp Crit Care Med 1995;152:1107–1136.

7. Jindal SK, Gupta D, Singh A. Indices of morbidity and control of asthma in adult patients exposed to environmental tobacco smoke. Chest 1994;106:746–749.

8. Marquette CH, Saulnire F, Leroy O, et al. Long-term prognosis of near-fatal asthma: a six year follow-up study of 145 asthmatic patients who underwent mechanical ventilation for a near-fatal attack of asthma. Am Rev Respir Dis 1992; 146:76–81.

9. Schoene RB, Abuan T, Ward RL, Beasley CH. Effects of topical betaxolol, timolol, and placebo on pulmonary function in asthmatic bronchitis. Am J Ophthalmol 1984;96:86–92.

10. Odeh M, Oliven A, Bassan H. Timolol eye drop-induced fatal bronchospasm in an asthmatic patient. J Fam Pract 1991;32: 97–98.

11. Taylor SL, Bush RK, Selner JC, et al. Sensitivity to sulfited foods among sulfite-sensitive subjects with asthma. J Allerg Clin Immunol 1988;81:1159–1167.

12. Szczeklik A, Gryglewski RJ, Czerniawska-Mysik G. Clinical patterns of hypersensitivity to nonsteroidal anti-inflammatory drugs and their pathogenesis. J Allerg Clin Immunol 1997;60: 276–284.

13. Spector SL, Wangaard CH, Farr RS. Aspirin and concomitant idiosyncrasies in adult asthmatic patients. J Allerg Clin Immunol 1979;64:500–506.

14. Watson WT, Becker AB, Simmons FE. Treatment of allergic rhinitis with intranasal corticosteroid in patients with mild asthma: effect on lower airway responsiveness. J Allerg Clin Immunol 1993;91: 97–101.

15. Nelson HS. Gastroesophageal reflux and pulmonary disease. J Allerg Clin Immunol 1984;73: 547–556.

16. Klucka CV, Ownby DR, Green J, Zoratti E. Cat shutting of Fel d I is not reduced by washing, Allerpet C spray or acepromazine. J Allerg Clin Immunol 1995;95:1164–1171.

17. Platts-Mills TAE, Tovey ER, Mitchell EB, et al. Reduction of bronchial hyperreactivity during prolonged allergen avoidance. Lancet 1982;2:675–678.

18. Abramson MJ, Puy RM, Weiner JM. Is allergen immunotherapy effective in asthma? A meta-analysis of randomized controls. Amer J Respir Crit Care Med 1995;151:967–974.

19. Creticos PS, Reed CE, Norman PS, et al. Ragweed immunotherapy in adult asthma patients. N Engl J Med 1996;334:501–506.

20. American Academy of Allergy and Immunology Board of Directors. Guidelines to minimize the risk from systemic reactions caused by immunotherapy with allergenic extracts. J Allerg Clin Immunol 1994;93:811–812.

21. Newhouse MT, Dolovich MB. Control of asthma by aerosols. N Eng J Med 1986;315:870–874.

22. Lipworth BJ. New prospectives on inhaled drug delivery and systemic bioavailability. Thorax 1995;50:105–110.

23. Barnes PJ, Pedersen S. Efficacy and safety of inhaled corticosteroids in asthma. Am Rev Respir Dis 1993;148:S1–S26.

24. Jeffrey PK, Godfrey RW, Adelroth E, et al. Effects of treatment on airway inflammation and thickening of basement membrane reticular collegen in asthma. Am Rev Respir Dis 1992;145:890–899.

25. Kamada AK, Szefler SJ, Martin RJ, et al, and the Asthma Clinical Research Network. Issues in the use of inhaled corticosteroids. Am J Respir Crit Care Med 1996;153:1739–1748.

26. Barnes PJ. Inhaled glucocorticoids for asthma. N Engl J Med 1995;332:868–875.

27. Lal S, Darow PD, Venho KK, Chatterjee SS. Nedocromil sodium is more effective than cromolyn sodium for the treatment of chronic reversible obstruction. Chest 1993;104: 438–447.

28. Schwartz HJ, Blumenthal M, Brady R, et al. A comparison study of the clinical efficacy of nedocromil sodium placebo. Chest 1996;109: 945–952.

29. Henderson WR Jr. The role of leukotrienes in inflammation. Ann Intern Med 1994;121:686–697.

30. Holgate ST, Brandding P, Sampson AP. Leukotriene antagonist and synthesis inhibitors: new directions in asthma therapy. J Allerg Clin Immunol 1996;98:1–13.

31. D'Alonzo GE. The effect of theophylline on the chronobiology of inflammation in asthma. In: Kummer L, ed. Monograph: Asthma. Structural basis—theophylline today. New York: Springer-Verlag, 1995:163–185.

32. Vassallo R, Lipsky JJ. Theophylline: Recent advances of its mode of action and uses in clinical practices. Mayo Clinic Proc 1998;73:346–354.

33. Weinberger M, Hendeles L. Theophylline in asthma. N Engl J Med 1996;334:1380–1388.

34. D'Alonzo GE, Nathan RA, Henochowicz S, et al. Salmeterol xinafoate as maintenance therapy compared with albuterol in patients with asthma. JAMA 1994;271:1412–1416.

35. Spitzer WO, Suissa S, Ernst P, et al. The use of beta-agonist and the risk of death and near death from asthma. N Engl J Med 1992;226:506.

36. Waalkens HJ, VanEssen-Zandvliet EE, Hughes MD, et al. Cessation of long-term treatment with inhaled corticosteroid (budesonide) in children with asthma results in deterioration. Am Rev Respir Dis 1993;148:1252–1257.

37. VanEssen-Zandvliet EE, Hughes MD, Waalkens HJ, et al. Effects of 22 months of treatment of inhaled corticosteroids and/or beta-2-agonists on lung function, airway responsiveness, and symptoms in children with asthma. Am Rev Respir Dis 1992;146: 547–554.

38. Kerstjens HAM, Brand PLP, Hughes MD, et al. A comparison of bronchodilator therapy with or without inhaled corticosteroid therapy for obstructive airways disease. N Engl J Med 1992;327: 1413–1419.

39. Nassif EG, Weinberger M, Thompson R, Huntley W. The value of maintenance theophylline in steroid-dependent asthma. N Engl J Med 1981;304:71–75.

40. Greening AP, Ind P, Northfield N, Schall G. Added salmeterol versus higher-dose corticosteroid in asthma patients with symptoms on existing inhaled corticosteroid. Lancet 1994;344:219–224.

41. Woolcock A, Lundbach B, Ringdal N, Jacques LA. Comparison of addition of salmeterol to inhaled steroids with doubling of the dose of inhaled steroid. Am J Respir Crit Care Med 1996;153:1481–1488.

42. Israel E, Cohn J, Dube L, Drazen JM. Effective treatment with zileuton, a five-lipoxygenase inhibitor in patients with asthma: a randomized control trial. JAMA 1996; 275–931–936.

43. Benatar SR. Fatal asthma. N Engl J Med 1986;314:423–429.

44. Djukanovic R, Roche WR, Wilson JW, et al. Mucosal inflammation in asthma. Am Rev Respir Dis 1990; 142:434–457.

45. Laitinen A, Laitinen LA. Airway morphology: endothelium/basement membrane. Am J Respir Crit Care Med 1994;150:S14–S17.

46. Busse WW, Lemanske RF, Stark JM, Calhoun WJ. The role of respiratory infections in asthma. In: Holgate ST, Austen KJ, Lichtenstein LM, Kay AB, eds. Asthma: physiology, immunopharmacology and treatment. London: Academic Press, 1993:345–353.

47. Roy B, D'Alonzo GE. Allergic bronchopulmonary aspergillosis: diagnosis and management. JAOA 1996;96:S17–S20.

48. Riott IM, Brostoff J, Male DK. Immunology. London: Gower Medical Publishing, 1985: Chapters 19, 25.

49. Slater JE, Kaliner MA. Allergic

rhinitis. Am J Asthma Allergy 1989;2:101–106.

50. Wilkerson LA. Exercise-induced asthma. JAOA 1998;98: 211–215.

51. McFadden ER Jr., Gilbert IA. Exercise-induced asthma. N Engl J Med 1994;330:1362–1367.

52. Anderson SD. Issues and exercise-induced asthma. J Allergy Clin Immunol 1985; 76: 763–772.

53. Kemp JP, Dockhorn RJ, Busse WW, et al. Prolonged effect of inhaled salmeterol against exercise-induced bronchospasm. Am J Respir Crit Care Med 1994;151:1612–1615.

54. Woolley M, Anderson SD, Quigley BM. Duration of turbutaline sulfate cromolyn sodium alone and in combination on exercise-induced asthma. Chest 1990;97: 39–45.

55. Alpazzaz NK, Neale NG, Patel KR. Dose-response study of nebulized nedocromil sodium in exercise-induced asthma. Thorax 1989; 44: 816–819.

56. Vathenen AS, Knox AJ, Wisniewski A, Tattersfield AE. Effect of inhaled budesonide on bronchialre-activity to histamine, exercise, and eucapnic dry air hyperventilation in patients with asthma. Thorax 1991;46:811–816.

57. Chan-Yeung M, Lam S. Occupational asthma. Am Rev Respir Dis 1986;133:686.

58. Pisati G, Baruffini A, Zedda S. Toluene diisocyanate induced asthma: outcome according persistance or cessation of exposure. Br J Intern Med 1993;50: 60–64.

59. Chan-Yeung M, MacLean L, Paggiaro PL. Follow-up study of 232 patients with occupational asthma caused by Western Red

Cedar (THUJA plicata). J Allergy Clin Immunol 1987;79: 792–796.

60. Lopez M, Salvaggio JE. Diagnostic methods and occupational allergic lung disease. Clin Rev Allergy 1986;4:289.

61. Paterson BF, Patterson R, Grammar LC. Pathogenesis of occupational lung disease. Clin Rev Allergy 1986;4:303.

62. Busse WW, Kiecolt-Glaser JK, Coe C, et al. NHLBI Workshop summary. Stress and asthma. Am J Respir Crit Care Med 1995; 151:249–252.

63. Friedman EM, Coe CL, Ershler WP. Bidirectional effects of interleukin-1 on immune responses in Rhesus monkeys. Brain Behav Immun 1994;8:87–99.

64. Brush J, Mathe A. Psychiatric aspects. In: Weiss EB, Stein M, eds. Bronchial asthma. Boston: Little, Brown, 1993:1121–1131.

65. Strunk RC, Mrazek DA, Woolfson-Fehrman GS, et al. Physiological and psychological characteristics associated with death due to asthma in childhood: a case-controlled study. JAMA 1985;254: 1193–1198.

66. Goldbert TM, Patterson R, Pruzansky JJ. Systemic allergen reactions to ingested antigens. J Allergy 1969;44:96–107.

67. Sampson HA, Mendelson L, Rosen JP. Fatal and near-death fatal anaphylatic reactions to food in children and adolescents. N Engl J Med 1992;227:380–384.

68. James JM, Bernhisel-Broadent J, Sampson HA. Respiratory reactions provoked by double-blind food challenges in children. Am J Respir Crit Med 1994;149:59–64.

69. Bock SA. Food allergy: A primer for people. New York: Vantage, 1988.

70. Pleskow WW, Stevenson DD, Mathison DA, et al. Aspirin-sensitive rhinosinusitis/asthma: spectrum of adverse reactions to aspirin. J Allergy Clin Immunol 1983;71: 574–579.

71. Szczeklik A, Gryglewski RJ, Czerniawska-Mysik G. Clinical patterns of hypersensitivity to non-steroidal anti-inflammatory drugs and their pathogenesis. J Allergy Clin Immunol 1977;60:276–284.

72. Settipane RA, Schrank PJ, Simmon RA, et al. Prevalence of cross-sensitivity with acetaminophen in aspirin-sensitive asthmatic patients. J Allergy Clin Immunol 1995; 96:480–485.

73. Szeklic A. The cyclooxygenase theory of aspirin-induced asthma. Eur Respir J 1990;3:588–593.

74. Odeh N, Oliven A, Bassan H. Timolol eyedrop-induced fatal bronchospasm in an asthmatic patient. J Fam Pract 1991;32: 97–98.

75. Schoene RB, Abuan T, Ward RL, et al. Effects of topical betaxolol, timolol and placebo on pulmonary function in asthmatic bronchitis. Am J Ophthalmol 1984;97: 86–92.

76. Dunn TL, Gerber MJ, Shen AS, et al. The effect of topical ophthalmologic instillation of timolol and betaxolol on lung function in asthmatic subjects. Am Rev Respir Dis 1986;133:264–268.

77. Nelson HS. Gastroesophageal reflux in pulmonary disease. J Allergy Clin Immunol 1984;73: 547–556.

78. Hixson IJ, Kelley CL, Jones WN, et al. Current trends in pharmacotherapy of gastroesophageal reflux disease. Arch Intern Med 1992;152:717–723.

79. D'Alonzo GE. The pregnant asthmatic patient. Semin Perinatol 1990;14:119–129.

Chapter 42

Cystic Fibrosis

David M. Orenstein
Frank J. Cerny

Cystic fibrosis (CF) has been known for decades as one of the most common inherited life-shortening diseases in white populations. Although at an incidence of 1 per 3300 live births (1), it is not as common as the familial hyperlipidemias (1 to 2 per 100 for the combined hyperlipidemias; 1 per 500 for familial hypercholesterolemia), it is considerably more life-shortening, with median survival having just reached past 30 years in 1996. (1) CF is a multisystem disorder, affecting epithelial cells throughout the body. It is inherited as an autosomal recessive trait. The gene for CF is located on the long arm of chromosome 7. It encodes a protein dubbed CFTR (the cystic fibrosis transmembrane conductance regulator) because it serves as a cyclic (adenosine monophosphate AMP)–dependent chloride channel and is also important in regulating other aspects of ion transport. In CF epithelial cells, there is relative impermeability to chloride and an overactive sodium channel.

The ion transport defect clearly explains one hallmark of CF, namely, the abnormally high concentration of sodium and chloride in sweat, which serves as the basis for the gold standard diagnostic test for CF. In the sweat test, sweating is stimulated by iontophoresis of pilocarpine into the skin of the forearm, and sweat is collected and analyzed quantitatively. The concentration of sodium and chloride is so much higher in people with CF than in normal controls that there is virtually no overlap between populations.

Despite the clarity of the connection between the epithelial cellular defect and the sweat abnormality, the individual pathophysiologic steps between epithelial ion transport abnormalities and the other clinical manifestations of cystic fibrosis are not yet completely worked out.

The principal manifestations of CF are in the lungs and digestive system. It is the lungs that account for the huge majority of CF morbidity and mortality. Patients suffer from bronchial obstruction and infection, beginning in the smallest peripheral airways and progressing proximally. Typically, patients are well, but have episodic worsening of bronchial infection and inflammation, often in association with viral illnesses. Increased cough, wheeze, shortness of breath, or a combination of these symptoms characterizes these episodes of pulmonary exacerbation. These episodes may be self-limited, or may respond to treatment with antibiotics, bronchodilators, and airway mucus-clearing techniques such as chest percussion, vibration, and postural drainage. With repeated bouts of infection and inflammation, there is a gradual decline in the patients' baseline health, reflecting progressive destruction of lung tissue. This progression leads eventually to respiratory failure and death. Aggressive treatment—both maintenance and in response to increased symptoms—almost certainly is responsible for the amazing improvement in prognosis seen in cystic fibrosis in the past few decades. When the disorder was first described in 1938, life expectancy was uniformly dismal, with death occurring within the first year or two of life. With the institution of comprehensive treatment programs in the 1950s, length and quality of patients' lives began to improve. Median survival for CF patients in the United States reached 31.3 years in 1996 (1).

The digestive manifestations of CF are largely a result of the cellular defect in the pancreas, apparently leading to ductular obstruction, which prevents digestive enzymes from reaching the intestine, and results in malabsorption of nutrients, principally fat and protein. The "textbook picture" of undiagnosed CF is a poorly nourished young child with large malodorous stools and a (compensatory) voracious appetite.

Supplying adequate calories for patients with CF is a continual challenge, despite the availability of effective pancreatic enzyme supplements. High-calorie oral supplements or even enteral nighttime feeds via gastrostomy or jejunostomy tubes may be used.

RESPONSES TO EXERCISE IN CF

Cardiopulmonary

The increased demand for oxygen delivery and carbon dioxide removal during exercise is met through augmentation of pulmonary gas exchange and cardiac output. The normal pulmonary response is characterized by an increase in total minute ventilation $\dot{V}_E$ and its components, tidal volume (V_t) and breathing frequency (Fb) (Figure 42-1). These ventilatory adjustments are made in such a way as to optimize alveolar ventilation and minimize ventilation of non-gas-exchanging areas of the lung (i.e., conducting airways and areas of the lung with little or no blood perfusion), called *dead space*. The lung pathology associated with CF results in progressively greater mismatching of pulmonary ventilation and perfusion, resulting in increases in dead space. In order to compensate for the increased dead space, patients increase $\dot{V}_E$. This increase in $\dot{V}_E$ is adequate to ensure maintenance of alveolar ventilation and therefore adequate gas exchange for patients with mild to moderate lung dysfunction. As lung dysfunction worsens, with further increases in dead space, the elevated $\dot{V}_E$ is insufficient to maintain alveolar ventilation, resulting in decreases in arterial oxygen levels (measured noninvasively by oximetry as a desaturation of arterial hemoglobin) and increases in carbon dioxide levels (see Figure 42-1). Although is difficult to predict precisely which patients will be unable to maintain normal arterial blood gases on the basis of changes in lung function, there is no doubt that the exercise limitation is related to pulmonary dysfunction. Improving pulmonary function with aggressive inpatient treatment results in increased exercise tolerance (2).

Pulmonary hyperinflation associated with CF alters respiratory mechanics during exercise. The hyperinflation makes it difficult to increase tidal volume during exercise (Figure 42-1). Therefore, the exercise-induced increase in $\dot{V}_E$ is accomplished primarily by increases in breathing frequency. This breathing strategy exacerbates the disease-related increases in dead space because with relatively shallow breathing, more of each breath remains in the dead space of the conducting airways. In addition, increased breathing frequency in the face of airway obstruction elevates the energy requirements for breathing. The pulmonary response to exercise in CF, then, is characterized by an increased requirement for ventilation in the face of a decreased ability to meet this requirement. As a consequence, progression of the disease is characterized by an inability to maintain blood gases during exercise and a pulmonary-related reduction in work capacity. In those patients who experience oxyhemoglobin desaturation during exercise in room air, supplemental oxygen can block that desaturation, and lower both heart rate and minute ventilation for submaximal workloads, but does not increase maximal work capacity (3).

Exercise induces cough in many CF patients (4) and also increases mucus clearance over rest, although perhaps not to the extent that chest physiotherapy with percussion and postural drainage does (5).

The cardiac response to exercise is normal. Exercise heart rate and cardiac output are within normal limits during submaximal exercise in CF patients (6). Further, increasing cardiac contractility with digoxin has no effect on the exercise response, indicating that the cardiac system does not limit exercise capacity in these patients (7).

Exercise in the Heat

The sweat defect in patients with cystic fibrosis was discovered as diSant' Agnese et al pursued the dramatic occurrence of heat prostration in a large and disproportionate number of children with CF in New York during a heat wave in 1948 (8). Since that early description, many infants with CF have been recognized as presenting with hyponatremic, hypochloremic alkalosis (9), presumably as a result of excess sweat losses of these ions. Yet, once past infancy, CF patients can exercise safely in the heat, with normal core body temperature, heart rate, and hormonal (aldosterone, renin) responses (10). They produce sweat at a normal rate, but continue to have abnormally high sodium and chloride concentrations in that sweat (10). Further, perhaps because their sweat is close to isotonic and their intravascular contents do not become hypertonic, they underestimate their fluid losses, and when guided by thirst alone, drink less than they have lost, and less than their non-CF peers (11).

EXERCISE PROGRAMS

Exercise as Therapy

As noted above, exercise has been noted to induce cough in many CF patients (4) and, since cough is part of the mucus clearance mechanism, has been promoted as part of the treatment of the pulmonary disease (4). Some form of exercise can be performed safely by most patients, with CF making this an attractive treatment possibility. The actual effectiveness of exercise in promoting mucus clearance is unclear. It is clearly better than rest (12), but one study suggests that it is not as effective as traditional chest physical therapy with percussion and postural drainage (5). Equivocal results are related to the difficulty in measuring mucus clearance through sputum collection or movement of a radiolabeled substance in the airways.

Despite common limitations in exercise tolerance, CF patients are able to undertake, and benefit from, prolonged exercise programs. A few patients have been able to complete 42-km marathon runs (13). There is near unanimity among studies that exercise tolerance (14) and cardiopulmonary fitness, as defined by peak oxygen consumption $\dot{V}o_2$ (5,15), is increased in patients participating in exercise programs. The effects of exercise programs on pulmonary function have been less consistent. Some studies have shown no changes in pulmonary function (15), whereas others, most notably Zach et al's (12,16), have shown an improvement in pulmonary function (Figure 42-2). CF patients participating in upper body weight training showed decreased residual volume, suggesting lessened pulmonary overinflation and air trapping (17). There are indications that, even if regular exercise does not improve pulmonary function, it may slow the normal deterio-

478   Part VII   Pulmonary Medicine

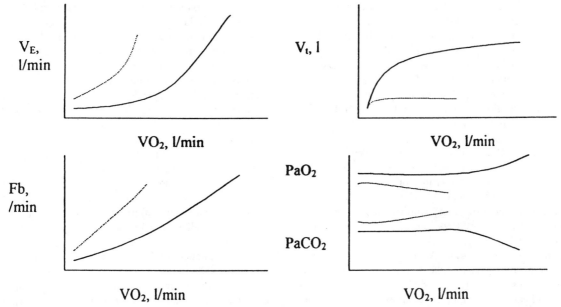

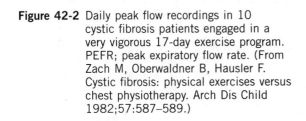

Figure 42-1 The relationship between increasing levels of energy expenditure, as measured by oxygen consumption (V_{O_2}) minute ventilation (V_E), tidal volume (V_t), breathing frequency (Fb), and arterial O_2 and CO_2 (Pa_{O_2} and Pa_{CO_2}). The solid line indicates the response in healthy individuals, the dashed line the response in patients with severe lung dysfunction.

Figure 42-2 Daily peak flow recordings in 10 cystic fibrosis patients engaged in a very vigorous 17-day exercise program. PEFR; peak expiratory flow rate. (From Zach M, Oberwaldner B, Hausler F. Cystic fibrosis: physical exercises versus chest physiotherapy. Arch Dis Child 1982;57:587–589.)

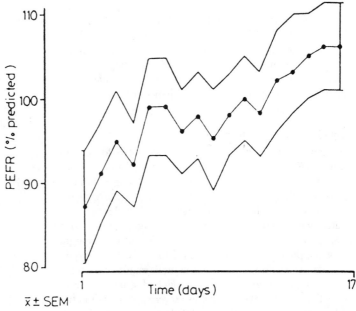

ration of pulmonary function (18). In no study has exercise training been associated with worsened pulmonary function.

Several studies have examined the effects of specific ventilatory muscle endurance training (19–21). Keens et al employed specific ventilatory muscle exercise (sessions of hyperpnea) and nonspecific upper body exercise (swimming and canoeing) in a CF summer camp setting. He found that these exercises increased ventilatory muscle endurance in these CF patients (20). Since general exercise tolerance in people with CF is limited by ventilatory mechanics, Asher et al (19)

wondered if increasing ventilatory muscle endurance could increase overall exercise tolerance. They found that they were able to increase ventilatory muscle endurance in their CF patients, but this improved ventilatory muscle endurance did not result in overall improved exercise tolerance. Similar to Asher's studies, Sawyer et al (21) found improved ventilatory muscle endurance after a specific ventilatory muscle training program, but in contrast to Asher, did find this resulted in an increase in general exercise tolerance. At this point it's hard to explain the different results from these similar studies.

Importantly, exercise programs have also been shown to bring about a decrease in dyspnea (22). The mechanism of this lessened dyspnea has not been explained, but in adults with non-CF chronic obstructive lung disease, it has been suggested that repeated bouts of exercise dull the dyspnea sensation, or increase patients' tolerance of that sensation (22). In other words, nothing changes except one's ability to tolerate the unpleasant sensation of difficult breathing. Even if this is the case, lessened unpleasant sensation can hardly be considered anything but good.

In subjects without CF, repeated bouts of exercise in the heat bring about the physiologic changes (termed *heat acclimation*) that convey improved tolerance of exercise and heat stress (e.g., performing the same task with lower core body temperature, lower heart rate, and with the production and loss of a more dilute sweat). Repeated bouts of exercise in the heat are nearly as successful in patients with cystic fibrosis in bringing about heat acclimation: After 8 days in a row of 90-minute sessions on an exercise bike in a heat chamber at 38°C, CF patients have a significantly lower core body temperature and heart rate in response to an exercise bout than they had on day 1 (23). However, CF patients do not decrease the concentration of sodium and chloride in their sweat as their normal peers are able to do (23). Between the sessions of exercise and heat stress, they are able to regulate their fluid and salt intake based on thirst and taste alone, such that they maintain body weight and serum electrolyte concentrations fairly precisely (23).

For subjects without CF, aerobic fitness is associated with better prognosis (lower death rates from all causes) (24). In CF, aerobic fitness has higher correlation with 8-year survival than any other parameter studied, including pulmonary function and nutritional state (25); the most fit tertile of patients had nearly three times the chances of surviving 8 years than the least fit tertile.

Exercise Programming

Structured exercise programs such as camps (16,20) or gymnasium (15) classes improve exercise tolerance and, in cases where the activity is of higher intensity and longer duration, pulmonary function (12,16). Unstructured programs, such as those promoted at home or through self-selected sports-related activity, are less successful in eliciting positive changes in fitness or pulmonary function (26). It is not surprising that, as for the population at large, most patients with CF require constant external motivation to maintain regular exercise.

Exercise programs can be designed for any patient with cystic fibrosis, regardless of disease severity. Although patients with severe pulmonary disease have lower exercise tolerance than those with mild disease (27), these patients too can profit from exercise training (15). Most experts recommend exercise testing for patients with severe disease (for example, FEV_1 < 50% predicted) in order to identify the workloads at which patients develop severe dyspnea, oxyhemoglobin desaturation, or both. In this way, exercise prescriptions can be given for intensities below those that induce intolerable dyspnea or desaturation. In most cases, patients can regulate the exercise intensity themselves, seeking a "pleasantly tired" feeling (28, p 193), pushing harder if they are just pleasant, easing off if they are just tired. This informal intensity grading system has correlated closely with heart rates in the range of 70% to

85% of each patient's own maximum heart rate as measured with a maximal exercise test (18).

For patients who experience oxyhemoglobin desaturation during exercise, supplemental oxygen can diminish the degree of desaturation, as well as decrease heart rate and minute ventilation for submaximal workloads (3). Oxygen supplementation during exercise can make an exercise program feasible for those patients who would otherwise have had desaturation during exercise (29,30). Most patients undergoing such oxygen-assisted exercise are able to increase their maximum workload on a progressive exercise test, as well as their maximum oxygen consumption (29).

Regular exercise can be performed safely by CF patients during hospital admission (2). Patients admitted to the hospital who are nonambulatory can perform bedside exercises using small weights or elastic tubing. Oxygen saturation should be monitored during exercise in these patients and oxygen supplementation used as needed to maintain saturation above 90%.

Exercise programs for CF patients should include the basic elements of any good program (i.e., flexibility, strength, and endurance). Although one study has shown small improvements in pulmonary function with strength training, most successful programs have been primarily aerobic, including jogging (15), swimming (12,31), cycling (5), or a combination of exercise modalities (16,20). Programs that have included specific upper body exercises such as canoeing (20), as well as those that have emphasized jogging (15) have stimulated improvements in ventilatory muscle endurance. There is no evidence that patients with CF adapt to regular exercise any differently than a healthy population. CF patients should therefore be encouraged to exercise regularly. Patients may have to stop periodically through their exercise sessions to cough, but this is to be encouraged, and non-CF observers need to know that the hard-coughing CF patients pose no contagious hazard to anyone else, nor does the sometimes frightening coughing pose a hazard to the patients themselves.

NUTRITIONAL CONSIDERATIONS

Nutritional Requirements

Patients with CF have increased nutritional requirements. The disease-related inability to digest lipids, if not treated properly, can result in malnutrition. The pulmonary disease of CF, with its associated increased work of breathing, also increases energy requirements (32). Increased energy requirements, with decreased ability to meet these requirements, results in an energy deficit, which becomes worse as the disease progresses. Chronic energy deficit leads to weight loss and increasing difficulty meeting the energy demands of even simple tasks of daily living. Hubbard (33) recommends that patients be counseled to increase caloric intake to 150% of the recommended RDA. Nutritional counseling should be individualized and take into account the increased caloric demands of regular exercise.

Exercise and Nutrition in CF

The increased energy demands for exercise must be considered in conjunction with the nutritional and energy demands of CF. Once patients become malnourished, body fat and, eventually, lean body mass can decrease. The primary energy fuels for exercise lasting more than 15 minutes are lipids. A disease-related deficit of lipid fuels, if complicated by pulmonary limitations, will reduce the capacity to perform long-lasting activities. Likewise, a chronic energy deficit will limit the availability of carbohydrate as a fuel, further limiting exercise tolerance. In order to prescribe exercise for these patients, pancreatic enzyme replacement must approach optimal and energy deficits must be avoided. Muscle function appears to be maintained such that only small decreases in strength are noted until the disease becomes severe, when the strength reduction is related to malnutrition-related decreases in muscle mass (6). Likewise, anaerobic performance is maintained at near-normal levels until the malnutrition of severe disease is present (34).

SUMMARY

Cystic fibrosis affects exercise tolerance through the pulmonary disease, increased energy expenditure, nutritional deficits, and excessive sweat salt losses. Yet, virtually every CF patient can engage in some form of exercise, deriving such benefits as increased exercise tolerance, improved cardiopulmonary fitness, decreased sensation of shortness of breath, perhaps improved airway mucus clearance, improved tolerance to exercise in the heat, and even improved survival. These patients should be encouraged to exercise, and professionals knowledgeable in the effects of exercise in CF should help design their exercise programs.

REFERENCES

1. FitzSimmons S. Cystic fibrosis data registry report for 1996. Bethesda, MD: Cystic Fibrosis Foundation, 1997.

2. Cerny FJ, Cropp GJ, Bye MR. Hospital therapy improves exercise tolerance and lung function in cystic fibrosis. Am J Dis Children 1984;138(3):261–265.

3. Nixon PA, Orenstein DM, Curtis SE, Ross EA. Oxygen supplementation during exercise in cystic fibrosis. Am Rev Respir Dis 1990;142(4):807–811.

4. Mellins R. Pulmonary physiotherapy in the pediatric age group. Amer Rev Respir Dis 1974;110(suppl 2):137–142.

5. Salh W, Bilton D, Dodd M, Webb AK. Effect of exercise and physiotherapy in aiding sputum expectoration in adults with cystic fibrosis. Thorax 1989;44(12):1006–1008.

6. Lands L, Heigenhauser G, Jones N. Cardiac output determination during progressive exercise in cystic fibrosis. Chest 1992;102:1118–1123.

7. Coates AL, Desmond K, Asher MI, et al. The effect of digoxin on exercise capacity and exercising cardiac function in cystic fibrosis. Chest 1982;82(5):543–547.

8. diSant' Agnese P, Darling R, Perera G, Shea E. Abnormal electrolyte composition of sweat in cystic fibrosis of the pancreas. Pediatrics 1953;12:549–563.

9. Beckerman R, Taussig L. Hypoelectrolytemia and metabolic alkalosis in infants with cystic fibrosis. Pediatrics 1979;63:580–583.

10. Orenstein DM, Henke KG, Costill DL, et al. Exercise and heat stress in cystic fibrosis patients. Pediatr Res 1983;17(4):267–269.

11. Bar-Or O, Blimkie C, Hay J, et al. Voluntary dehydration and heat intolerance in cystic fibrosis. Lancet 1992;339(March 21):696–699.

12. Zach M, Purrer B, Oberwaldner B. Effect of swimming on forced expiration and sputum clearance in cystic fibrosis. Lancet 1981;ii:1201–1203

13. Stanghelle JK, Skyberg D. Cystic fibrosis patients running a marathon race. Int J Sports Med 1988;1(37):37–40.

14. Andreasson B, Jonson B, Kornfalt R, et al. Long-term effects of physical exercise on working capacity and pulmonary function in cystic fibrosis. Acta Paediatr Scand 1987;76(1):70–75.

15. Orenstein DM, Franklin BA, Doershuk CF, et al. Exercise conditioning and cardiopulmonary fitness in cystic fibrosis: the effects of a three-month supervised running program. Chest 1981;80(4):392–398.

16. Zach M, Oberwaldner B, Hausler F. Cystic fibrosis: physical exercise versus chest physiotherapy. Arch Dis Child 1982;57(8):587–589.

17. Strauss G, Osher A, Wang C-I, et al. Variable weight training in cystic fibrosis. Chest 1987;92:273–276.

18. Orenstein D. Exercise tolerance and exercise conditioning in children with chronic lung disease. J Pediatr 1988;112(6):1043–1047.

19. Asher MI, Pardy RL, Coates AL, et al. The effects of inspiratory muscle training in patients with cystic fibrosis. Am Rev Respir Dis 1982;126(5):855–859.

20. Keens TG, Krastins IR, Wannamaker EM, et al. Ventilatory muscle endurance training in normal subjects and patients with cystic fibrosis. Am Rev Respir Dis 1977;116(5):853–860.

21. Sawyer EH, Clanton TL. Improved pulmonary function and exercise tolerance with inspiratory muscle conditioning in children with cystic fibrosis. Chest 1993;104:1490–1497.

22. O'Neill P, Dodds M, Phillips B, et al. Regular exercise and reduction of breathlessness in patients with cystic fibrosis. Br J Dis Chest 1987;81:62–69.

23. Orenstein D, Henke K, Green C. Heat acclimation in cystic fibrosis. J Appl Physiol 1984;57:408–412.

24. Blair S, Kohl HI, Paffenbarger RJ, et al. Physical fitness and all-cause mortality. JAMA 1989;262:2395–2401.

25. Nixon P, Orenstein D, Kelsey S, Doershuk C. The prognostic value

of exercise testing in patients with cystic fibrosis. N Engl J Med 1992;327:1785–1788.

26. Blomquist M, Freyschuss U, Wiman LG, Strandvik B. Physical activity and self treatment in cystic fibrosis. Arch Dis Child 1986;61(4):362–367.

27. Cropp GJ, Pullano TP, Cerny FJ, Nathanson IT. Exercise tolerance and cardiorespiratory adjustments at peak work capacity in cystic fibrosis. Am Rev Respir Dis 1982;126(2):211–216.

28. Orenstein D. Cystic fibrosis: a guide for patient and family. 2nd ed. Philadelphia: Lipincott-Raven, 1997.

29. Heijerman H, Bakker W, Sterk P, Dijkman J. Oxygen-assisted exercise training in adult cystic fibrosis patients with pulmonary limitation to exercise. Int J Rehabil Res 1991;14:101–115.

30. Darbee J, Cerny F. Exercise testing and exercise conditioning for children with lung dysfunction. In: Irwin S, Tecklin J, eds. Cardiopulmonary physical therapy. St. Louis: Mosby, 1995:563–578.

31. Edlund LD, French RW, Herbst JJ, et al. Effects of a swimming program on children with cystic fibrosis. Am J Dis Children 1986;140(1):80–83.

32. Hirsch JA, Zhang SP, Rudnick MP, et al. Resting oxygen consumption and ventilation in cystic fibrosis. Pediatr Pulmonol 1989;6(1):19–26.

33. Hubbard V. Nutritional considerations in cystic fibrosis. Sem Respir Med 1985;6:308–313.

34. Cabrera M, Lough M, Doershuk C, DeRivera G. Anaerobic performance—assessed by the Wingate test—in patients with cystic fibrosis. Pediatr Exerc Sci 1993; 5:78–87.

Chapter 43

Chronic Obstructive Pulmonary Disease

Donald A. Mahler
Roberto Mejia

EPIDEMIOLOGY

Chronic obstructive pulmonary disease (COPD) includes both chronic bronchitis and emphysema. Chronic bronchitis is defined as cough productive of daily sputum for 3 months in each of 2 successive years; emphysema is defined as abnormal permanent enlargement of the airspaces distal to the terminal bronchioles accompanied by destruction of their walls and without fibrosis (1). The 1993 National Health Interview Survey estimated that 14 million American adults had chronic bronchitis and 2 million had emphysema (2). In persons over the age of 55 years COPD is recognized in approximately 10% to 15% of the population. The prevalence of the disease appears to be stable or even decreasing in men, but increasing in women (3). Over the past 5 years COPD has become the fourth leading cause of death in the United States (1).

The impact of COPD on morbidity is even greater than on mortality. For example, patients with moderate to severe disease are often limited in their ability to perform activities of daily living and to work. Frustration, anxiety, and/or depression are frequent sequelae of these functional limitations. COPD accounts for 5% of physicians' office visits and more than 13% of hospitalizations (4). Thus, COPD is an enormous cause of disability among affected individuals. Even though there has been a reduction in cigarette smoking in the United States, morbidity and mortality due to COPD will continue to be a problem because of the long latency period before clinical disease is evident and the increased overall life expectancy in our aging population.

RISK FACTORS AND NATURAL HISTORY

The three established risk factors for COPD are cigarette smoking, hereditary alpha$_1$-antitrypsin (AAT) deficiency, and exposure to occupational and environmental dusts and gases (5). Cigarette smokers have a higher prevalence of lung function abnormalities and experience a greater annual rate of decline in expiratory flow rates. Only about 15% to 20% of those who smoke cigarettes actually develop COPD; presumably, this is due to genetic predisposition.

Alpha$_1$-antitrypsin is a serum protein produced in the liver and normally found in the lung, where its main role is the inhibition of neutrophil elastase. There are numerous variants of AAT, but more than 95% of persons in the severely deficient category are homozygous for the Z allele, designated Pi (protease inhibitor) ZZ. Most of these individuals are Caucasians of northern European descent. Severe AAT deficiency leads to premature emphysema with the median onset of dyspnea by 40 years of age in smokers. The diagnosis is made by measuring the serum AAT level followed by Pi typing for confirmation. The indications for testing include the onset of COPD by or before the age of 50 years, a predominance of basilar emphysema, and a family history of AAT deficiency or of COPD onset before age 50 (1).

Occupational exposure to cadmium, silica, and dusts has been linked with reasonable causal evidence to the development of COPD. The particular jobs with increased risk include mining, furnace/metal works, working with wood, paper, and cement, construction workers, grain workers, farmers, and cotton workers. Air pollution is considered as a possible risk factor for COPD.

In healthy nonsmokers the forced expiratory volume in one second (FEV_1) declines by approximately 30 mL per year in men starting about the age of 35 to 40 years. Those individuals who have COPD and continue to smoke have a two- to threefold greater decline in FEV_1 than observed in normals. After smoking cessation the rate of lung function decline slows to about that seen in nonsmokers of the same age. Respiratory infections in individuals with COPD usually cause airway inflammation and lead to decreases in lung function that may last for up to 90 days.

PATHOPHYSIOLOGY AND SYMPTOMS

COPD is charaterized by expiratory airflow obstruction as demonstrated by a decreased FEV_1/forced vital capacity (FVC) ratio (usually < 70%). The causes of airflow obstruction are increased airway secretions, inflammation and edema of the walls of the airways, bronchoconstriction, and/or loss of the alveolar attachments to bronchioles caused by the destructive changes in emphysema.

In chronic bronchitis there is enlargement of mucous glands, and respiratory bronchioles display a mononuclear inflammatory process. Membranous bronchioles less than 2 mm in diameter show varying degrees of mucous plugging, goblet cell metaplasia, inflammation, increased smooth muscle, and distortion caused by fibrosis.

There are different types of emphysema based on the anatomic location. Centriacinar emphysema begins in the respiratory bronchioles and spreads peripherally; it occurs typically with long-standing cigarette smoking and involves the upper lung zones. Panacinar emphysema involves the entire alveolus uniformly; it is seen generally with homozygous AAT deficiency and predominates in the lung bases.

In the vast majority of patients with COPD there is an overlap of both chronic bronchitis and emphysema such that features of both conditions may be present. The major symptom of patients with chronic bronchitis is a productive cough, whereas dyspnea on exertion is the primary complaint of those with emphysema. Although many patients experience one or both of these symptoms for some time, the individual patient does not usually seek medical attention until symptoms interfere with his or her ability to perform daily tasks. Patients with COPD usually select descriptors of dyspnea that relate to the work or effort associated with breathing (6). For breathlessness the person frequently and mistakenly attributes the difficulty breathing to "getting old" or "being out of shape." Wheezing may also occur, but it is a far more common symptom in asthma than in COPD. For most patients with COPD there is a gradual progression of dyspnea over months to years (7). Although many patients and physicians assume that increased breathlessness is due to a worsening of the airflow obstruction, it is imperative to measure lung function because weight gain and/or deconditioning may also cause an increase in dyspnea.

LABORATORY FINDINGS

Pulmonary function tests should be obtained in order to establish the diagnosis of obstructive airway disease (FEV_1/FVC < 70%) and to determine the severity (based on FEV_1 percentage of predicted). Measurement of the single breath diffusing capacity (D_Lco) is helpful to evaluate for emphysema (a reduced D_Lco due to destructive changes).

A current chest radiograph is important to evaluate for any parenchymal abnormalities, heart size, pulmonary vasculature, and possible pleural disease. Hyperinflation of the lung fields may or may not be evident depending on the severity of disease.

Oximetry should be performed as an estimate of oxygen saturation in all patients with COPD. Arterial blood gases are recommended for patients with a FEV_1 < 50% predicted (1).

A baseline 12-lead electrocardiogram is useful. If pulmonary hypertension or right ventricular hypertrophy is suspected, then an echocardiogram is indicated.

STAGING

At the present time there is no established staging system that provides quantitative information regarding morbidity and mortality in patients with COPD. However, the American Thoracic Society has proposed that patients with COPD can be classified into three stages based on severity of disease (Table 43-1).

Table 43-1 Proposed Staging System for Patients with COPD

Stage 1
- $FEV_1 \geq 50\%$ predicted
- Compromises the majority of patients
- COPD has *minimal* impact on health-related quality of life
- Will usually be cared for by a generalist
- The presence of severe dyspnea warrants additional studies and evaluation by a respiratory specialist

Stage 2
- FEV_1 35% to 49% predicted
- Includes a minority of patients
- COPD has *significant* impact on health-related quality of life and results in large per capita healthcare expenditure
- Usually merits evaluation by a respiratory specialist and may receive continuing care by a specialist

Stage 3
- $FEV_1 < 35\%$ predicted
- Includes a minority of patients
- COPD has *profound* impact on health-related quality of life and results in large per capita healthcare expenditure
- Usually will be under the care of a respiratory specialist

Adapted from American Thoracic Society. ATS statement: Standards for the diagnosis and care of patients with chronic obstructive pulmonary disease. Am J Respir Crit Care Med 1995;152(suppl):S82–S83.

OUTCOME MEASURES

The traditional approach has been to measure lung function, particularly FEV_1, as an objective parameter to follow the course of the disease and to assess response to therapy. However, patients are most interested in relief of dyspnea and in improvement in their ability to function along with health-related quality of life (HRQOL). Therefore, it is appropriate to use valid, reliable, and responsive instruments to measure dyspnea and HRQOL in patients with COPD (8). These instruments may be classified as discriminative (How severe is the dyspnea or HRQOL?) or evaluative (Has dyspnea or HRQOL changed?).

Various multidimensional instruments are available to quantify dyspnea based on activities of daily living (Table 43-2). The Baseline (BDI) and Transition (TDI) Dyspnea Indexes include functional impairment, magnitude of task, and magnitude of effort as three components that provoke breathlessness (9). The BDI is a discriminative instrument that includes specific criteria at a single point in time. The TDI is an evaluative instrument that measures changes in the three components compared with the baseline state. The Chronic Respiratory Disease Questionnaire (CRQ) was developed as an evaluative instrument to measure HRQOL in patients with lung disease (10). Dyspnea is one of four dimensions included in the CRQ. The patient rates the severity of dyspnea based on the five most common activities that caused dyspnea over the past 2 weeks. Serial applications are performed to measure changes in the CRQ dyspnea score.

Dyspnea can also be measured during a cardiopulmonary exercise test using either the visual analog scale (VAS) (11) or the 0–10 category-ratio (CR-10) scale developed by Borg (12). The most useful approach to measure dyspnea during exercise is to examine a range or continuum of responses (13). For example, the slope and intercept of the relationship between power production on the cycle ergometer and the dyspnea response obtained at each minute of exercise can be calculated.

Studies using either clincial dyspnea ratings or measures of dyspnea during exercise have demonstrated improvements with various interventions such as bronchodilator medications, pulmonary rehabilitation, and lung volume reduction surgery (14).

Both generic and disease-specific instruments are used to measure HRQOL in patients with COPD (8). The Medical Outcomes Study short-form 36-item questionnaire (15) and the Nottingham Health Profile (16) are two commonly used generic instruments, whereas the CRQ (10) and the St. George's Respiratory Questionnaire (17) are widely used as disease-specific instruments. For individual or group clinical trials evaluating a new therapy or procedure disease-specific instruments are more appropriate because patients and physicians find the items more relevant. However, if the clinical outcome of a treatment currently exists, then a generic HRQOL instrument may be used to provide complementary information. Such data may expand the impact or scope of the therapy, and previously unrecognized adverse effects may be detected.

TREATMENT

Once the diagnosis of COPD has been established, the patient should be educated about the disease and encouraged to be an active participant in preventive care, in maintaining an active lifestyle, and in the various forms of therapy. A general approach to the management of COPD is shown in Figure 43-1.

Smoking Cessation

The physician should express strong and continued interest in smoking cessation for the patient with COPD. Encouragement and counseling from the physician can frequently make the difference for successful smoking cessation. The clinician should help the patient move through the five stages from smoking to nonsmoking status (precontemplation, contemplation, preparation, action, and maintenance). It is important for the patient to set a "quit date." Nicotine replacement therapy (chewing gum or transdermal patches) may be prescribed to control withdrawl symptoms (18). Other pharmacologic therapy such as bupropion hydrochloride may be prescribed (19). Group smoking cessation programs may be beneficial for some individuals. Behavioral modification and/or psychotherapy can also make a difference for individuals' efforts to stop smoking cigarettes. Initial failure is common, and it is the responsibility of the physician to continue to enquire, encourage, and enable the person in smoking cessation.

Preventive Care

Avoidance of second-hand smoke and other airborne irritants should be emphasized. An annual influenza immunization should be routine maintenance of all patients with COPD. The pneumococcal polysaccharide vaccine contains 23 types of the *Streptococcus pneumoniae* bacteria, and immunization is recommended for patients with chronic respiratory disease; revaccination should be considered after 6 years. Maintenance of an appropriate body weight, particularly reduction of excess body fat, is an important part of preventive care and health maintenance.

Bronchodilator Therapy

The major purpose for prescribing bronchodilator medications is for relief of symptoms since there is no current

Table 43-2 Multidimensional Instruments Used to Measure Dyspnea Based on Activities of Daily Living	
YEAR PUBLISHED	**NAME OF INSTRUMENT**
1984	Baseline (BDI) and transition (TDI) dyspnea indexes (8)
1987	Chronic respiratory disease questionnaire (dyspnea is one of four components of quality of life) (9)
1987	University of San Diego shortness of breath questionnaire (41)
1994	Dyspnea questionnaire (42)

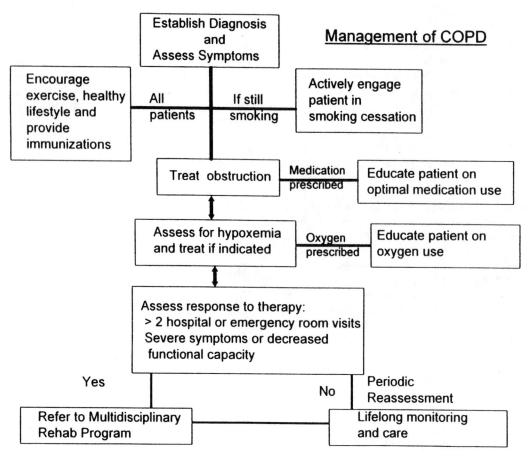

Management of COPD

Figure 43-1 General approach to the management of COPD as recommended by the ATS Statement on the Standards for the Diagnosis and Care of Patients with Chronic Obstructive Pulmonary Disease. (Reproduced with permission from American Thoracic Society. ATS statement: standards for the diagnosis and care of patients with chronic obstructive pulmonary disease. Am J Respir Crit Care Med 1995;152(suppl):S84. © American Lung Association.)

evidence that regular use of pharmacotherapy can alter the course of disease or prolong survival (1). The following approach has been adapted from the American Thoracic Society statement on the diagnosis and care of patients with COPD (1): *All patients should be instructed in the appropiate technique of using a metered-dose inhaler (MDI)* (Table 43-3):

1. *For mild, variable symptoms,* particularly breathlessness, one to two puffs of a short-acting beta$_2$-agonist MDI can be used every 2 to 6 hours as needed. These include albuterol, pirbuterol, and terbutaline as the most commonly used short-acting beta$_2$-agonists. Belman et al (20) reported that albuterol improved exertional breathlessness by reducing dynamic hyperinflation and by enhancing neuroventilatory coupling (the relationship between diaphragmatic function and the corresponding tidal volume during breathing).

2. *For mild to moderate continuing symptoms,* two to six puffs of ipratropium bromide MDI are recommended every 6 to 8 hours *plus* the use of a short-acting beta$_2$-agonist MDI either as needed or four times a day. The combination of ipratropium and albuterol in a single MDI may be more effective than either of the two agents alone and should improve patient compliance (21).

Table 43-3 Instructions for Patients for Appropriate Use of a Metered-Dose Inhaler

1. Shake the inhaler.
2. With the mouthpiece down place it about 2 in. away from your mouth; open your mouth widely, and tilt your head back slightly. (Alternatively, the mouthpiece can be placed in your mouth.)
3. After a normal breath out, breathe in very slowly. At the same time press or actuate the aerosol inhaler so that the aerosol is caught into the air being inspired.
4. Continue to breathe in very slowly (5 to 10 seconds).
5. After you have breathed in fully, hold your breath for 10 seconds or as long as possible. This allows the aerosol to settle deep into the lungs.
6. Wait 1 to 2 minutes, and then take a second puff of the aerosol medication.

Salmeterol xinafoate, an inhaled long-acting beta$_2$ agonist that lasts 12 hours, may be considered as twice-a-day therapy for daily and continuous symptoms due to COPD (22).

3. *If the response to step 2 is unsatisfactory*, (i.e., the patient continues to have daily symptoms), add sustained-release theophylline either once or twice a day. Initial treatment should be with a low dose and adjusted after several days with a target theophylline of 8 to 12 mg/L. Karpel et al (23) showed that combination therapy with albuterol (two puffs), ipratropium (two puffs), and theophylline was superior to ipratropium alone or to the combination of albuterol and theophylline over a 6-hour time period. The physician must be aware that several medications and conditions may affect the metabolism of theophylline (1).

4. *If control of symptoms remains suboptimal*, it is essential to make sure that the patient is using the MDI correctly. Direct observation of the inhalation technique is "key." If the individual has difficulty, a spacer device should be tried. An alternative consideration is to use an ultrasonic nebulizer to deliver the bronchodilator aerosol. A brief (10 to 14 days) course of oral prednisone (20–40 mg) may be tried, although a published meta-analysis suggests that patients with COPD who receive oral corticosteroid therapy will have a 20% or greater improvement in baseline FEV$_1$ approximately 10% more often than similar patients receiving placebo (24). Clearly, if there is no "clinically important" improvement, then the corticosteroid should be stopped. If improvement occurs, it is common practice to prescribe an inhaled corticosteroid with the intent to reduce airway inflammation although the exact role of inhaled corticosteroids in the long-term treatment of COPD is unclear. Several studies are currently evaluating the effect of inhaled corticosteroids on the course of COPD.

For all four classes of bronchodilators used in the treatment of COPD the benefits of the medication must be considered relative to the risks and possible side effects.

Antibiotics

Acute bronchitis is common in patients with COPD and can contribute to bronchoconstriction and increased symptoms. Although it is estimated that about 50% of these episodes are due to viral infections, it is reasonable to prescribe an antibiotic if two of three changes develop (purulent sputum, increased volume of sputum, and increased dyspnea) (25). The major bacteria to be considered are *Streptococcus pneumoniae*, *Haemophilus influenzae*, and *Moraxella catarrhalis*. The choice of the antibiotic is usually made clinically because a sputum culture is not cost-effective and may delay treatment. In patients with severe COPD recurrent or persistent episodes of acute bronchitis may be due to gram-negative bacteria. In such cases a cephalosporin or fluoroquinolone antibiotic should be prescribed.

Oxygen

The present indications for long-term oxygen therapy are (1):

- Arterial oxygen tension (Pao2) $\leq$ 55 mm Hg or arterial oxygen saturation (Sao$_2$) $\leq$ 88%.

- In the presence of cor pulmonale or polycythemia, oxygen should be prescribed if the Pao$_2$ is 55 to 59 mm Hg or if the Sao$_2$ $\geq$ 89%.

If the patient meets one of these criteria at rest, then oxygen should be prescribed during exercise and sleep as well, but titrated to the appropriate flow rate to achieve an Sao$_2$ $\geq$ 90%. If the individual is normoxemic at rest but desaturates during exercise or sleep (Pao$_2$ $\leq$ 55 mm Hg), oxygen should be prescribed for these indications. The purpose of oxygen therapy is to prevent tissue hypoxia. Furthermore, long-term oxygen therapy will reduce pulmonary hypertension, improve exercise tolerance, enhance neuropsychological function, and reverse secondary polycythemia.

Pulmonary Rehabilitation

The major goals of pulmonary rehabilitation are to reduce symptoms, particularly dyspnea, and to improve functional status. Evidence-based guidelines for pulmonary rehabilitation have recently been published by a joint committee of the American College of Chest Physicians and the American Association of Cardiovascular and Pulmonary Rehabilitation (26). Detailed informaion is provided in Chapter 44 of this section.

Nutrition

Patients with COPD often lose weight during the course of their disease; this condition has been termed the *pulmonary cachexia syndrome* (27). It is estimated that between 19% and 60% of patients are malnourished (28,29). In COPD malnutrition is clearly associated with a decline in clinical status and predicts accelerated mortality (30). Although the reasons for the weight loss are not fully understood, an increase in resting energy expenditure and an elevated level of serum tumor necrosis factor alpha are important factors for the observed weight loss (31,32).

Clinical trials of nutritional intervention in patients with COPD have included variable study designs, but a few general conclusions can be made. Studies conducted in inpatients have involved small numbers of subjects (6 to 12 patients) and are of short duration (1 to 3 weeks). Although oral nutrient supplementation has been associated with an increase in body weight and respiratory muscle strength, none of these investigations reported improvements in dyspnea or health-related quality of life. Outpatient studies typically lasting 2 to 3 months show modest increases in body weight (<5 kg) with protein-calorie supplementation, but improvements in muscle strength, walking distance, dyspnea ratings, and quality of life have been inconsistent (27). Using enteral feedings in malnourished patients with COPD over a 16-day period, Whittaker et al (33) reported that refed patients demonstrated significant increases in weight gain and in respiratory mouth pressures. In another study Donahue et al (34) gave patients with COPD who had a severe reduction in body weight nocturnal enteral supplementation to maintain a total daily caloric intake greater than two times the measured resting energy expenditure over a 4-month period. Despite this aggressive approach there was only a mean weight gain of 3.3 kg, and the majority of the increase in body weight occurred in body fat. These collective results suggest that nutritional support programs are limited in patients with COPD, especially in the absence of a comprehensive rehabilitative program designed to enhance muscle strength and/or endurance (27).

Strategies to Reduce Dyspnea

The experience of dyspnea is the most bothersome complaint of patients with COPD and impacts substantially on their general health status (35). Additional treatment options should be considered for the patient who remains symptomatic and frustrated by breathlessness despite smoking cessation, use of preventive measures, optimal medical therapy, oxygen therapy if indicated, and pulmonary rehabilitation.

1. *Coping.* Various coping strategies may be be presented and practiced with the individual in an attempt to relieve the intensity and/or distress of difficult breathing (36). These include positioning, pursed-lips breathing, activity modification, and energy conservation, as well as social support. Furthermore, distraction strategies such as relaxation, biofeedback, music, hypnosis, and visualization techniques may be considered. Attention strategies focus on monitoring breathlessness, increasing knowledge about illness management, and using self-care to reduce dyspnea.

2. *Pharmacology.* Although many patients with progressive COPD experience anxiety and depression, the role of anxiolytic medications remains uncertain. A practical approach is to consider anxiolytic therapy in selected individuals in whom anxiety appears to have a major impact on their sense of breathlessness. Opiates should be considered for individual patients who are extremely limited by disabling dyspnea unresponsive to other treatments; potential side effects should be described (37). In patients with "end-stage" COPD opiates should be used for relief of severe breathing distress similar to the use of these medications for severe pain.

3. *Surgery.* Bullectomy is one of the surgical options. Patients with COPD may develop large bullae that can expand over time and compress normal lung parenchyma. In many of these individuals dyspnea appears to be the consequence of anatomical changes in chest wall and of abnormal mechanics of breathing. In general, bullectomy (resection of the lung bulla) should be considered if the bulla occupies at least one third of the hemithorax and it compresses adjacent lung tissue (38). A computerized tomograph of the chest is indicated to evaluate the preoperative anatomy. Improvement in dyspnea may be due to a decrease in airway resistance, improvements in diaphragm function, and/or reduced hyperinflation of the lung.

Lung volume reduction surgery is another surgical option for the treatment of severe emphysema. Dynamic hyperinflation of the lung develops in response to physical exertion in many patients with moderate to severe COPD. The consequences of the hyperinflation are an increase in the elastic recoil of the lung (intrinsic positive end-expiratory pressure) and shortening of the vertical muscle fibers of the diaphragm; collectively, these alterations contribute to the experience of exertional breathlessness in COPD. Resection of approximately 20% of upper lobe can reduce the hyperinflation and improve the mechanics of breathing as well as dyspnea in patients with severe emphysema. (39,40). The procedure has been performed with either a median sternotomy or by thorascopy. At the present time a multicenter prospective study cosponsored by the National Heart, Lung and Blood Institute and by the Health Care Finance Agency is evaluating the efficacy of this procedure compared with standard treatment of pulmonary rehabilitation.

REFERENCES

1. American Thoracic Society. ATS statement: Standards for the diagnosis and care of patients with chronic obstructive pulmonary disease. Am J Respir Crit Care Med 1995;152(suppl):S77–S120.

2. National Center for Health Statistics. Current estimates from the National Health Interview Survey. Vital and health statistics, Series 10. No. 190. Washington, D.C.: U.S. Department of Health and Human Services (PHS), 1993:95–1518.

3. Mannino DM, Brown C, Giovino GA. Obstructive lung disease deaths in the United States from 1979 through 1993. Am J Respir Crit Care Med 1997;156:814–818.

4. Cydulka RK, McFadden ER, Emerman CL, et al. Patterns of hospitalization in elderly patients with asthma and chronic obstructive pulmonary disease. Am J Respir Crit Care Med 1997;156:1807–1812.

5. Buist AS. Risk factors for COPD. Eur Respir J 1996;6(review 39):253–258.

6. Mahler DA, Harver A, Lentine T, et al. Descriptors of breathlessness in cardiorespiratory diseases. Am J Respir Crit Care Med 1996;154:1357–1363.

7. Mahler DA, Tomlinson D, Olmstead EM, et al. Changes in dyspnea, health status, and lung function in chronic airway disease. Am J Respir Crit Care Med 1995;151:61–65.

8. Mahler DA, Jones PW. Measurement of dyspnea and quality of life in advanced lung disease. Clin Chest Med 1997;18:457–469.

9. Mahler DA, Weinberg DH, Wells CK, et al. The measurement of dyspnea: contents, interobserver agreement, and physiologic correlates of two new clinical indexes. Chest 1984;85:751–758.

10. Guyatt GH, Berman LB, Townsend M, et al. A measure of quality of life for clinical trials in chronic lung disease. Thoraax 1987;42:773–778.

11. Gift AG. Validation of a vertical visual analogue scale as a measure of clinical dyspnea. Rehabilitation Nurs 1989;14:323–325.

12. Borg GAV. Psychophysical bases of perceived exertion. Med Sci Sports Exerc 1982;14:377–381.

13. Mahler DA, Horowitz MB. Perception of breathlessness during exercise in patients with respiratory disease. Med Sci Sports Exerc 1994;26:1078–1081.

14. Mahler DA, Guyatt GH, Jones PW. Clinical measurement of dyspnea. In: Mahler DA, ed. Dyspnea. New York, Marcel Dekker, 1998:149–198.

15. Ware JE Jr, Sherbourne CD. The MOS short-form health survey (SF-36). 1. Conceptual framework and item selection. Med Care 1992;30:473–481.

16. Hunt SM, McEwen J, McKenna SP. Measuring health status. London, Croom Helm, 1986.

17. Jones PW, Quirk FH, Baveystock CM. The St. George's respiratory questionnaire. Respir Med 1991; 85(suppl):25–31.

18. Henningfield JE. Nicotine medications for smoking cessation. New Engl J Med 1995;333:1196–1203.

19. Hurt RD, Sachs DPL, Glover ED, et al. A comparison of sustained-release bupropion and placebo for smoking cessation. New Engl J Med 1997;337:1195–1202.

20. Belman MJ, Botnick WC, Shin JW. Inhaled bronchodilators reduce dynamic hyperinflation during exercise in patients with chronic obstructive pulmonary disease. Am J Respir Crit Care Med 1996;153:967–975.

21. Combivent Inhalation Aerosol Study Group. In chronic obstructive pulmonary disease, a combination of ipratropium and albuterol is more effective than either agent alone. Chest 1994;105:1411–1419.

22. Ramirez-Venegas A, Ward J, Lentine T, Mahler DA. Salmeterol reduces dyspnea and improves lung function in patients with COPD. Chest 1997;112:336–340.

23. Karpel JP, Kotch A, Zinny M, et al. A comparison of inhaled ipratropium, oral theophylline plus inhaled β-agonist, and the combination of all three in patients with COPD. Chest 1994;105:1089–1094.

24. Callahan CM, Dittus RS, Kataz BP. Oral corticosteroid therapy for patients with stable chronic obstructive pulmonary disease. Ann Intern Med 1991;114:216–223.

25. Anthonisen NR, Manfreda J, Warren CPW, et al. Antibiotic therapy in exacerbations of chronic obstructive pulmonary disease. Ann Intern Med 1987;106:196–204.

26. ACCP/AACVPR Pulmonary Rehabilitation Guidelines Panel. Pulmonary rehabilitation. Chest 1997; 112:1363–1396.

27. Donahue M. Nutritional support in advanced lung disease: the pulmonary cachexia syndrome. Clin Chest Med 1997;18:547–561.

28. Laaban JP, Kouchakji B, Dore MF, et al. Nutritional status of patients with chronic obstructive pulmonary disease and acute respiratory failure. Chest 1993;103:1362–1368.

29. Saudny-Unterberger H, Martin JG, Gray-Donald K. Impact of nutritional support on functional status during an acute exacerbation of chronic obstructive pulmonary disease. Am J Respir Crit Care Med 1997;156:794–799.

30. Gray-Donald K, Gibbons L, Shapiro SH, et al. Nutritional status and mortality in chronic obstructive pulmonary disease. Am J Respir Crit Care Med 1996;153:961–966.

31. Schols AMWJ, Fredrix EWHM, Soeters PB, et al. Resting energy expenditure in patients with chronic obstructive pulmonary disease. Am J Clin Nutr 1991; 54:983–987.

32. DiFrancia M, Barbier D, Mege JL, et al. Tumor necrosis factor—alpha levels and weight loss in chronic obstructive pulmonary disease. Am J Respir Crit Care Med 1994;150: 1453–1455.

33. Whittaker J, Ryan C, Buckley P, et al. The effects of refeeding on peripheral and respiratory muscle function in malnourished chronic obstructive pulmonary disease patients. Am Rev Respir Dis 1990;142:283–288.

34. Donahue M, Mancino J, Constantino J, et al. The effect of an aggressive nutritional support regimen on body composition in patients with severe COPD and weight loss. Am J Respir Crit Care Med 1994;147:A313.

35. Mahler DA, Faryniarz K, Tomlinson D, et al. The impact of dyspnea and physiologic function on general health status in patients with chronic obstructive pulmonary disease. Chest 1992;102:395–401.

36. Carrieri-Kohlman V, Gormley JM. Coping strategies for dyspnea. In: Mahler DA, ed. Dyspnea. New York, Marcel Dekker, 1998: 287–320.

37. Stulbarg MS, Belman MJ, Ries AL. Treatment of dyspnea: physical modalities, oxygen, and pharmacology. In: Mahler DA, ed. Dyspnea. New York, Marcel Dekker, 1998:321–361.

38. O'Donnell DE, Webb KA, Bertley JC, et al. Mechanisms of relief of exertional breathlessness following unilateral bullectomy and lung volume reduction surgery in emphysema. Chest 1996;110:18–27.

39. Cooper JD, Patterson GA, Sundaresan RS, et al. Results of 150 consecutive bilateral lung volume reduction procedures in patients with severe emphysema. J Thorac Cardiovasc Surg 1996;112: 1319–1330.

40. Martinez FJ, Montes de Oca M, Whyte RI, et al. Lung-volume reduction improves dyspnea, dynamic hyperinflation, and respiratory muscle function. Am J Respir Crit Care Med 1997;155:1984–1990.

41. Archibald CJ, Guidotti TL. Degree of objectively measured impairment and perceived shortness of breath with activities of daily living in patients with chronic obstructive lung disease. Can J Rehabilitation 1987;1:45–54.

42. Lareau SC, Carrieri-Kohlman V, Janson-Bjerklie S, et al. Development and testing of the pulmonary functional status and dyspnea questionnaire. Heart Lung 1994;23:242–250.

Chapter 44

Pulmonary Rehabilitation

Andrew L. Ries

ORIGINS OF PULMONARY REHABILITATION: EPIDEMIC AND NATURAL HISTORY OF COPD

The origins of comprehensive pulmonary rehabilitation programs parallel the epidemic rise in morbidity and mortality due to chronic obstructive pulmonary disease (COPD) over the past 50 years. Chronic lung diseases, such as COPD, are major causes of death and disability in the modern world. In the United States, COPD is now the fourth leading cause of death. The overall prevalence is approximately 4% to 6% in men and 1% to 3% in women; in adults over age 55, COPD is recognized in approximately 10% to 15%. In spite of the decrease in cigarette smoking in recent years, morbidity and mortality caused by COPD continue to rise because of the cumulative effects of smoking over many years (1–5).

Patients with COPD typically present late in the course of a chronic, progressive, largely irreversible disease process. Because of the large reserve in normal lung function, there is a long asymptomatic or preclinical period in which the person who has smoked for years "without problem" begins to note breathlessness with physical activities previously accomplished without difficulty. This may be attributed to age or "being out of shape." Reduced expiratory flow rates may be detected at this stage. Later, the individual often comes to medical attention after a critical event, such as a respiratory infection from which he or she "just never recovered." The person will often attribute the onset of illness to this time. In truth, this event just pushed the already diseased lungs over the clinical edge of recognition—much like a rope weakened by progressive fraying will break when "only" a small weight is attached.

ROLE OF PULMONARY REHABILITATION IN THE TREATMENT OF COPD

Because COPD is a chronic disease, the primary goals of management should be directed toward preventive health strategies of slowing progression and reducing complications. Secondary goals are to improve symptoms and function and treat reversible components of disease. Important preventive treatment strategies include control of cigarette smoking, chronic bronchodilator treatment, influenza and pneumococcal vaccination, oxygen therapy for hypoxemic patients, and, in appropriate patients, pulmonary rehabilitation (6).

Rehabilitation programs for patients with chronic lung diseases are well established as a preventive healthcare strategy that can enhance standard therapy in order to control and alleviate symptoms and optimize functional capacity (1,7–11). The primary goal of any rehabilitation program is to restore the patient to the highest possible level of independent function, to improve functioning and quality of life. This goal is accomplished by helping patients and significant others to learn more about lung disease, treatment, and coping strategies and to become actively involved in providing their own health care and becoming more independent in daily activities and less dependent on health professionals and expensive medical resources. Rather than focusing solely on reversing the disease process, rehabilitation attempts to improve the disability from disease.

Many pulmonary rehabilitation strategies have been developed for patients with disabling COPD. However, rehabilitation has been applied successfully to patients with other chronic lung conditions such as interstitial diseases, cystic

491

fibrosis, bronchiectasis, thoracic cage abnormalities, and, most recently, before and after surgical procedures such as lung transplantation and lung volume reduction surgery and after treatment for lung cancer (12–15). Pulmonary rehabilitation is appropriate for any patient with stable chronic lung disease who is disabled by symptoms of the underlying disease or by related treatment or complications.

DEFINITIONS OF PULMONARY REHABILITATION

In 1974, the American College of Chest Physicians' Committee on Pulmonary Rehabilitation adopted the following definition (16):

> Pulmonary rehabilitation may be defined as an art of medical practice wherein an individually tailored, multidisciplinary program is formulated which through accurate diagnosis, therapy, emotional support, and education, stabilizes or reverses both the physio- and psychopathology of pulmonary diseases and attempts to return the patient to the highest possible functional capacity allowed by his pulmonary handicap and overall life situation.

This definition focuses on three important features of successful rehabilitation:

1. *Individual.* Patients with disabling lung disease require individual assessment of their needs, individual attention, and a program designed to meet realistic individual goals.

2. *Multidisciplinary.* Pulmonary rehabilitation programs provide information and expertise from several healthcare disciplines that are integrated by experienced staff into a comprehensive, cohesive program tailored to the needs of each patient.

3. *Attention to physiopathology and psychopathology.* To be successful, pulmonary rehabilitation pays attention to psychological and emotional problems as well as helping to optimize medical therapy to improve lung function.

A newer definition was developed by an NIH workshop on pulmonary rehabilitation research that reviewed the scientific evidence and future research opportunities (17). It emphasizes key aspects as the multidimensional services, interdisciplinary team, involvement of patients and families, and individual goals for independence and function in the community.

Pulmonary rehabilitation is a multidimensional continuum of services directed to persons with pulmonary disease and their families, usually by an interdisciplinary team of specialists, with the goal of achieving and maintaining the individual's maximum level of independence and functioning in the community.

Pulmonary rehabilitation is typically provided by a multidisciplinary team of healthcare professionals that may include nurses, respiratory and physical therapists, psychologists, exercise physiologists, or others with appropriate expertise (18). Specific team makeup depends upon the resources and expertise available, but usually includes at least one full-time staff member. The team serves in a support function for the patient

and his or her primary care physician or healthcare provider. The role of the physician in the pulmonary rehabilitation team is primarily to assist in patient evaluation and with setting individual patient and team goals, as well as in providing administrative and general support. Within this general framework, successful pulmonary rehabilitation programs have been established in both outpatient and inpatient settings and with different formats. The keys to success are dedicated, enthusiastic staff, familiar with the problems of pulmonary patients, who can relate well to and motivate them.

PATIENT SELECTION

Any patient with symptomatic chronic lung disease is a candidate for pulmonary rehabilitation (Table 44-1). Appropriate patients are aware of disability from their disease and are motivated to be active participants in their own care in order to improve their health status.

Criteria based on arbitrary lung function parameters or age alone should not be used in selection for pulmonary rehabilitation (8,11). Pulmonary function is not a good predictor of symptoms, function, or improvement after rehabilitation in individuals (19). In general, selection should be based upon an individual's disability and functional limitation from respiratory symptoms, potential for improvement, and motivation to participate actively in a comprehensive self-care program.

Other factors are also important in evaluating candidates. Pulmonary rehabilitation is not generally a primary mode of therapy. Patients should generally be evaluated and stabilized on standard therapy before beginning a program. They should not have other disabling or unstable conditions that might limit their ability to participate fully and to concentrate.

The ideal patient for pulmonary rehabilitation, then, is one with functional limitation from moderate to severe lung disease who is stable on standard therapy, not distracted or limited by other serious or unstable medical conditions, willing and able to learn about his or her disease, and motivated to devote the time and effort necessary to benefit from a comprehensive care program.

PATIENT EVALUATION

The initial step in pulmonary rehabilitation is screening patients to ensure appropriate selection and to set realistic individual and program goals. The evaluation process includes

---

Table 44-1 Patient Selection Criteria for Pulmonary Rehabilitation

Symptomatic chronic lung disease
Stable on standard therapy
Functional limitation from disease
Relationship with primary care provider
Motivated to be actively involved in and take
   responsibility for own health care
No other interfering or unstable medical conditions
No arbitrary lung function or age criteria

the following components: interview, medical evaluation, psychosocial assessment, diagnostic testing, and goal setting (Table 44-2).

The screening interview is an important first step. It serves to introduce the patient to the program as well as to review the patient's medical history and identify psychosocial problems and needs. Significant others should be included. Communication with the primary care physician is important, establishing the vital link for the rehabilitation staff in clarifying questions prior to the program and facilitating recommendations during and after treatment. Care and attention in this initial evaluation help in setting goals compatible with everyone's expectations as well appropriate to program objectives.

Reviewing the medical history helps identify the patient's lung disease and assess its severity. Other problems that might preclude or delay participation may be identified. Available laboratory data should be reviewed including pulmonary function and exercise tests, rest and exercise arterial blood gas measurements, chest radiographs, electrocardiogram, and pertinent blood tests. Program staff can then determine the need for additional information or action before the program.

Planning an appropriate rehabilitation program requires accurate, current information. The complexity of testing procedures performed depends upon individual patient and program goals, as well as the facilities and expertise available.

Pulmonary function testing is used to characterize lung disease and quantify impairment. Spirometry and lung volume measurements are most useful; other tests such as diffusing capacity, airway resistance, and maximal respiratory pressures to assess muscle strength can be added as needed.

Exercise testing helps to assess the patient's exercise tolerance and to evaluate blood gas changes (hypoxemia or hypercapnia) with exercise. This may also uncover comorbid conditions (e.g., heart disease). The exercise test is also used to establish a safe and appropriate prescription for subsequent training. This is most easily performed with the type of activity planned for training (e.g., treadmill for a walking training program) [20].

Table 44-2 Components of a Comprehensive Pulmonary Rehabilitation Program

Patient Evaluation
  Interview
  Medical evaluation
  Diagnostic testing
    Pulmonary function
    Exercise
    Arterial blood gases/oximetry
  Psychosocial assessment
  Goal Setting
Program Content
  Education
  Respiratory and chest physiotherapy instruction
  Exercise
  Psychosocial support

Measurement of arterial blood gases at rest and during exercise is important because of the frequent but unpredictable occurrence of exercise-induced hypoxemia [21]. Blood gas sampling during exercise makes testing more complex. Noninvasive estimation of arterial oxygen saturation by cutaneous oximetry is useful for continuous monitoring, but has limited accuracy (e.g., 95% confidence limits for cutaneous oximetry = ±4% to 5% saturation) [20,22].

Successful rehabilitation requires attention not only to physical problems but also to psychological, emotional, and social ones [23]. Patients with chronic illnesses experience psychosocial difficulties as they struggle to deal with symptoms they may not fully understand. Neuropsychological and cognitive impairment is common in patients with chronic lung disease [24]. This cannot be accounted for solely on the basis of age, depression, or physical disease and is possibly related to or exacerbated by the effects of hypoxemia on the brain. Commonly, patients become depressed, frightened, anxious, sedentary, and dependent upon family members, friends, and medical services to provide for their needs. In one study, Jensen reported that high stress and low social support were better predictors of subsequent hospitalizations than severity of illness in patients with obstructive lung disease [25].

Progressive dyspnea is a frightening symptom, and may lead to a vicious "fear-dyspnea" cycle: With progressive disease, less exertion results in more dyspnea, which produces more fear and anxiety, which, in turn, leads to more dyspnea. Ultimately, the patient avoids any physical activity associated with both of these unpleasant symptoms. Patients also become overly concerned with other physical problems and psychosomatic complaints. Sexual dysfunction and fear are common, often unspoken consequences of chronic lung disease.

In order to address these problems, the initial evaluation should include an assessment of the patient's psychological state and close attention to psychosocial factors during screening interviews, such as family and social support, living arrangement, activities of daily living, hobbies, and employment potential. Cognitive impairment that may limit ability to participate fully can be identified. Family members or friends may provide valuable insight and should be included in the screening process and program whenever possible.

After evaluating a patient's medical, physiologic, and psychosocial state, it is important to set specific goals that are compatible with each individual's disease, needs, and expectations. Goals should be realistic given the objectives of the program. Significant others should be included in this process so that everyone understands what can and cannot be expected.

PROGRAM CONTENT

Comprehensive pulmonary rehabilitation programs typically include several key components: education, respiratory and chest physiotherapy instruction, psychosocial support, and exercise training (see Table 44-2).

Education

Successful pulmonary rehabilitation depends upon the understanding and active involvement of patients and those important for their support. Education is an integral component;

even patients with severe disease can gain a better understanding of their disease and learn specific means to deal with problems (26). Instruction can be provided individually or in small groups, but should be adapted to different learning abilities. Typical topics covered include: how normal lungs work, what chronic lung disease is, medications, nutrition, travel, stress reduction and relaxation, when to call your doctor, and planning a daily schedule. Individual instruction and coaching may be provided on the use of respiratory therapy equipment and oxygen, breathing techniques, bronchial drainage, chest percussion, energy saving techniques, and self-care tips. The general philosophy is to encourage patients to assume responsibility for and become partners with their physician in providing their own care (27).

Despite the importance of education, it is unlikely that knowledge alone will lead to improved health status. It is more difficult to change attitudes and behaviors. Patients require specific, individualized strategies with instruction and reinforcement. Thus, education is a necessary, but not sufficient component of pulmonary rehabilitation.

Respiratory and Chest Physiotherapy Techniques

Patients with chronic lung disease use, abuse, and are confused about respiratory and chest physiotherapy techniques. In pulmonary rehabilitation, each patient's needs for respiratory care techniques can be assessed and instruction provided in proper use. These may include: chest physiotherapy techniques to control secretions: breathing retraining techniques to relieve and control dyspnea and improve ventilatory function; and proper use of respiratory care equipment including nebulizers, metered-dose inhalers, and oxygen.

Patients with chronic lung diseases have abnormal lung clearance mechanisms that make them more susceptible to problems with retained secretions and infection. Therefore, rehabilitation programs teach chest physiotherapy techniques for secretion control, such as controlled coughing, postural drainage, and chest vibration and/or percussion (28). These are important for patients with excess mucous production during exacerbations and as routine preventive measures for patients with chronic sputum production.

Breathing Retraining Techniques

Instruction in breathing techniques such as diaphragmatic and pursed lips breathing is aimed at helping patients relieve and control breathlessness, improve ventilatory pattern (i.e., slow respiratory rate and increase tidal volume), prevent dynamic airway compression, improve respiratory synchrony of abdominal and thoracic musculature, and improve gas exchange. A review of studies evaluating these techniques indicates that improvement in symptoms (e.g., dyspnea) is more consistent than measurable changes in physiologic parameters (1,28–30).

The diaphragmatic breathing technique was described by Barach and Miller as a maneuver in which the patient coordinates abdominal wall expansion with inspiration and slows expiration through pursed lips. The primary effect is to slow respiratory rate and increase tidal volume (29,30).

Pursed lips breathing is the other technique often taught to pulmonary patients, particularly those with COPD. Pursed lips breathing was observed by Laennec as early as 1830 and advocated as a physical exercise for pulmonary patients in the early part of the twentieth century. It is a maneuver assumed naturally by many patients in which the lips are used to narrow the airway during expiration. The aims are to slow the expiratory phase and maintain positive airway pressure in order to "keep the airways open" and improve ventilatory efficiency (28–30).

Oxygen Therapy

For patients who require chronic oxygen therapy, available methods of oxygen delivery can be reviewed to help select the best system for their needs. Supplemental oxygen is beneficial for patients with severe resting hypoxemia. Long-term, continuous oxygen therapy has been shown to improve survival and reduce morbidity in hypoxemic patients with COPD (1,31,32). Benefits of supplemental oxygen for nonhypoxemic patients or for patients with hypoxemia only under certain conditions (e.g., exercise, sleep) are less clearly defined.

Although continuous oxygen therapy is feasible and safe, maintaining patients on oxygen presents several challenges. Handling equipment is particularly difficult for physically disabled and frail patients. Therefore, it is important to assess each patient's oxygen needs and provide instruction in appropriate techniques.

Several new developments have improved the efficiency of gas delivery and patient compliance with continuous therapy. Liquid oxygen provides more gas with less weight than tanks of compressed gas, particularly in portable systems. Also, transtracheal delivery may increase efficiency, reducing flow rates and prolonging duration of portable sources, as well as improving compliance and avoiding problems with nasal catheters. However, patients need careful instruction in caring for and maintaining the catheter (33).

Exercise

Exercise is important in pulmonary rehabilitation. There is considerable evidence of favorable responses to exercise training in patients with chronic lung diseases. Benefits are both physiologic and psychological. Patients may increase their maximum capacity and/or endurance for physical activity, even though lung function does not usually change. Patients may also benefit from learning to perform physical tasks more efficiently. Exercise training provides an ideal opportunity for patients to learn their capacity for physical work and to use and practice methods for controlling dyspnea (e.g., breathing and relaxation techniques) (7,9,34).

Principles of exercise testing and training for patients with lung disease differ from those derived in normals or other patient populations because of differences in the limitations to exercise and the problems encountered in training (34). Many approaches have been used in pulmonary rehabilitation. To be successful, the program should be tailored to the individual patient's physical abilities, interests, resources, and environment. For general application, techniques should be simple and inexpensive. As in normals and other patients. benefits are largely specific to the muscles and tasks involved in training. Patients tend to do best on activities and exercises for which they are trained. Walking programs are particularly useful. They have the added benefit of encouraging patients to expand social horizons. In inclement weather, many patients can walk indoors (e.g., shopping malls). Other types of exercise (e.g., cycling, swimming) are also effective. Patients should be encouraged to incorporate regular exercise into daily activities they enjoy (e.g., golf, gardening).

Since many patients with chronic lung disease have limited exercise tolerance, emphasis during training should be placed on increasing endurance. Changes in endurance are often greater than changes in maximal exercise tolerance (19,35). This allows patients to become more functional within their physical limits. An increase in maximum exercise is also possible as patients gain experience and confidence with their exercise program.

Exercise Prescription

Selecting training targets based on percentages of maximum heart rate or Vo_2 are well established in normals or other patients. In patients with chronic lung diseases, however, the best method of choosing an appropriate training prescription is less clearly defined. Exercise tolerance in pulmonary patients is typically limited by maximum ventilation and breathlessness. Such patients frequently do not reach limits of cardiac or peripheral muscle performance (34).

Many patients with lung disease can be trained at high percentages of maximum that approach or even exceed the maximum level reached on the initial exercise test. In one study, 52 patients with moderate to severe COPD were able to perform endurance exercise testing at an average workload of 95% of baseline maximum exercise tolerance (36). After 8 weeks, these patients were training at 86% of the baseline maximum workload. In fact, many patients with severe COPD were exercising at levels exceeding baseline maximum. In another study in 59 patients with moderate to severe COPD, Carter et al trained patients at levels near their ventilatory limits (37). At baseline, after training, and 3 months later, they reported mean peak exercise ventilation of 94% to 100% of measured maximum voluntary ventilation. These findings suggest that even patients with advanced disease can be trained successfully at or near maximal levels.

Therefore, some pulmonary rehabilitation programs define exercise targets and progression during training more by symptom tolerance than by targets based on heart rate, work level, or other physiologic measurement. Ratings of perceived symptoms (e.g., breathlessness) help teach patients to exercise to "target" levels of breathing discomfort (34).

A typical approach would be to begin training at a level that the patient can sustain with reasonable comfort for several minutes. Increases in time or level are then made according to the patient's symptom tolerance. Patients are encouraged to exercise daily and increase endurance up to 15 to 30 minutes of continuous activity. This helps them achieve a goal of improving their tolerance for tasks of daily living that often require a period of sustained activity.

Blood Gas Changes

A major problem in planning a safe exercise program for patients with lung disease is the potential worsening of hypoxemia with exercise. Patients who may not be hypoxemic at rest can develop changes in arterial oxygenation that cannot be predicted reliably from resting measurements of pulmonary function or gas exchange. Normal individuals do not become hypoxemic with exercise. In patients with obstructive lung disease, Pao_2 changes unpredictably during exercise (21). In patients with mild COPD, Pao_2 typically does not change or may even improve with exercise. However, in patients with moderate to severe COPD, Pao_2 may increase, decrease, or not change. On the other hand, patients with interstitial lung disease commonly develop worsening oxygenation with exercise. Therefore, it is important to evaluate rest and exercise oxygenation. Such testing is also used to prescribe oxygen therapy at rest and with physical activity. With the availability of convenient, portable systems for ambulatory oxygen delivery, hypoxemia is not a contraindication to safe exercise training.

Upper Extremity Training

Exercise programs for pulmonary patients typically emphasize lower extremity training (e.g., walking). However, many patients with chronic lung disease report disabling dyspnea for daily activities involving the upper extremities (e.g., lifting, grooming) at work levels much lower than for the lower extremities. Upper extremity exercise is accompanied by a higher ventilatory demand for a given level of work than for lower extremity exercise. Since training is generally specific to the muscles and tasks used in training, upper extremity exercises may be important in helping pulmonary patients cope better with common daily activities. This type of training may be particularly important in patients recovering from thoracic surgery (7).

Ventilatory Muscle Training

The potential role of ventilatory muscle fatigue as a cause of respiratory failure and ventilatory limitation in patients with chronic lung disease has stimulated attempts to train the ventilatory muscles. Techniques of isocapnic hyperventilation, inspiratory resistive loading, and inspiratory threshold loading have been shown to improve function of these muscles in both normals and in patients. In normals, respiratory muscles do not limit exercise tolerance; therefore, specific respiratory muscle training is unlikely to be of clinical benefit. In patients with COPD, who have been studied most extensively, improvement in general exercise performance from ventilatory muscle training alone has not been demonstrated consistently. Thus, the role of such training incorporated routinely in pulmonary rehabilitation has not been clearly established (7,38).

Psychosocial Support

An essential component of pulmonary rehabilitation is psychosocial support provided to help patients combat symptoms reflecting progressive feelings of hopelessness and inability to cope with their progressive chronic lung disease (39). Psychosocial support is provided best by a warm and enthusiastic staff who can communicate effectively with patients and devote the time and effort necessary to understand and motivate them. Significant others should be included in activities so that they can understand and cope better with the patient's disease. Support groups are also effective. Patients with severe psychological disorders may benefit from individual counseling and therapy. Psychotropic drugs should generally be reserved for patients with more severe psychological dysfunction.

RESULTS OF PULMONARY REHABILITATION

Several comprehensive reviews substantiate the practices and expected results of pulmonary rehabilitation (Table 44-3) (7,9–11). A recent evidence-based document developed by an expert panel provided a succinct review of the published literature, made recommendations from this review, and rated the strength of evidence supporting these recommendations (Table 44-4) (7).

Three recently published randomized clinical trials demonstrate important and significant benefits of pulmonary rehabilitation for patients with COPD, including improvements in exercise performance, symptoms, and key elements of quality of life. In a randomized clinical trial of rehabilitation versus an education program in 119 patients with COPD, Ries et al reported a highly significant improvement in exercise endurance after rehabilitation that was maintained up to 18 months later (35). This was associated with a significant decrease in perceived symptoms of breathlessness and muscle fatigue during exercise as well as improvement in maximum exercise tolerance, reported breathlessness with daily activities, and self-efficacy for walking. Two other recently published randomized trials reported shorter-term benefits favoring pulmonary rehabilitation over conventional treatment. Goldstein et al in Canada reported significant improvement in exercise tolerance, dyspnea, and quality of life after 6 months in 45 patients receiving 8 weeks of inpatient pulmonary rehabilitation followed by 16 weeks of supervised outpatient care compared to 44 patients who received conventional care from their own physicians (40). Finally, Wijkstra et al in The Netherlands reported significant improvement in exercise tolerance and quality of life in 28 patients who were randomly allocated to a home pulmonary rehabilitation program for 12 weeks compared to 15 patients who received no rehabilitation (41).

Improvements in exercise performance and physical activity have been reported consistently as a result of pulmonary rehabilitation. Casaburi et al reviewed 37 published studies of exercise training in more than 900 patients with COPD (9). Nearly unanimously, these studies demonstrated improvement in exercise endurance and/or maximum exercise tolerance.

Pulmonary rehabilitation emphasizes educating patients and significant others to be actively involved in their own care, improve their understanding of disease, and learn practical ways of coping with disabling symptoms. Studies that have examined the effects of education have shown that even patients with severe disease can learn to understand their disease better. However, education alone does not typically

---

Table 44-3 Results of Pulmonary Rehabilitation

Decrease In:
  Medical resources utilization (e.g., hospitalizations, emergency rooms)
  Respiratory symptoms (e.g., breathlessness)
  Psychological symptoms (e.g., depression, fear)
Increase In:
  Quality of life
  Physical activity
    Exercise tolerance (endurance and/or maximum level)
    Activities of daily living
  Knowledge
  Independence
Return to Work Possible
No Change in Lung Function
? Prolonged Survival

Table 44-4 Summary of Recommendations of the Pulmonary Rehabilitation Guidelines Panel Convened by the American College of Chest Physicians and American Association of Cardiovascular and Pulmonary Rehabilitation

COMPONENT/OUTCOME	RECOMMENDATION	GRADE*
Lower Extremity Training	Lower extremity training improves exercise tolerance and is recommended as part of pulmonary rehabilitation	A
Upper Extremity Training	Strength and endurance training improves arm function; arm exercises should be included in pulmonary rehabilitation	B
Ventilatory Muscle Training	Scientific evidence does not support the routine use of ventilatory muscle training in pulmonary rehabilitation; it may be considered in selected patients with decreased respiratory muscle strength and breathlessness	B
Psychosocial, Behavioral, and Educational Components and Outcomes	Evidence does not support the benefits of short-term psychosocial interventions as single therapeutic modalities; longer-term interventions may be beneficial; expert opinion supports inclusion of educational and psychosocial intervention components in pulmonary rehabilitation	C
Dyspnea	Pulmonary rehabilitation improves the symptom of dyspnea	A
Quality of Life	Pulmonary rehabilitation improves health-related quality of life	B
Healthcare Utilization	Pulmonary rehabilitation has reduced the number of hospitalizations and days of hospitalizations	B
Survival	Pulmonary rehabilitation may improve survival	C

* Rating of quality of scientific evidence (A, B, or C).
Reproduced with permission from Ries AL, Carlin BW, Carrieri-Kohlman V. Pulmonary rehabilitation: Joint ACCP/AACVPR evidence based guidelines. Chest 1997;112:1363–1396.

lead to improved health status. Patients also require specific, individual strategies for changing behavior along with encouragement, practice, and positive feedback.

Pulmonary rehabilitation has been shown to produce cost-effective benefits for patients with chronic lung disease. Several studies have analyzed hospital and medical resource utilization before and after rehabilitation (7). Given the high costs of acute care hospitalizations for these often sick patients, the potential savings from a reduction in hospital days alone are significant.

SUMMARY

Pulmonary rehabilitation is an established, effective preventive healthcare strategy that can enhance standard therapy in order to control and alleviate symptoms and optimize functional capacity for patients with chronic lung diseases. A comprehensive program includes a careful initial evaluation and components of education, instruction in respiratory and chest physiotherapy techniques, exercise conditioning, and psychosocial support. Proven benefits include improvement in exercise tolerance, respiratory symptoms, psychological symptoms, quality of life, knowledge, and independence and a reduction in use of healthcare resources. After pulmonary rehabilitation, pulmonary patients become more knowledgeable about their disease, more actively involved in their own appropriate health care, and easier for their primary care physicians to manage.

REFERENCES

1. American Thoracic Society. Standards for the diagnosis and care of patients with chronic obstructive pulmonary disease (COPD) and asthma. Am Rev Respir Dis 1995; 152:S78–S121.

2. Centers for Disease Control and Prevention. Mortality patterns—United States, 1993. MMWR 1996;45:161–164.

3. Feinleib M, Rosenberg HM, Collins JG, et al. Trends in COPD morbidity and mortality in the United States. Am Rev Respir Dis 1989; 140:S9–S18.

4. Mannino DM, Brown C, Giovino GA. Obstructive lung disease deaths in the United States from 1979 through 1993. Am J Respir Crit Care Med 1997;165:814–818.

5. Sherrill DL, Lebowitz MD, Burrows B. Epidemiology of chronic obstructive pulmonary disease. Clin Chest Med 1990;11:375–387.

6. Ries AL. Preventing COPD: You can make a difference. J Respir Dis 1993;14(6):739–749.

7. Ries AL, Carlin BW, Carrieri-Kohlman V. Pulmonary rehabilitation: joint ACCP/AACVPR evidence based guidelines. Chest 1997;112:1363–1396.

8. American Association of Cardiovascular and Pulmonary Rehabilitation, Connors G, Hilling L, eds. Guidelines for pulmonary rehabilitation programs. Champaign IL: Human Kinetics, 1993.

9. Casaburi R, Petty TL, eds. Principles and practice of pulmonary rehabilitation. Philadelphia: WB Saunders, 1993.

10. Hodgkin JE, Connors GL, Bell CW, eds. Pulmonary rehabilitation: guidelines to success. 2nd ed. Philadelphia: JB Lippincott, 1993.

11. Ries AL. Position paper of the American Association of Cardiovascular and Pulmonary Rehabilitation: scientific basis of pulmonary rehabilitation. J Cardiopulm Rehabil 1990;10:418–441.

12. Foster S, Thomas HM. Pulmonary rehabilitation in lung disease other than chronic obstructive pulmonary disease. Am Rev Respir Dis 1990; 141:601–604.

13. Biggar DG, Malen JF, Trulock EP, et al. Pulmonary rehabilitation before and after lung transplantation. In: Casaburi R, Petty TL, eds. Principles and practice of pulmonary rehabilitation. Philadelphia: WB Saunders, 1993.

14. Craven JL, Bright J, Dear CL. Psychiatric, psychosocial, and rehabilitative aspects of lung transplantation. Clin Chest Med 1990;11:247–257.

15. Ries AL. Pulmonary rehabilitation in patients with thoracic neoplasm. In: Aisner J, Arriagada R, Green MR, et al, eds. Comprehensive textbook of thoracic oncology. Baltimore: Williams & Wilkins, 1996.

16. American Thoracic Society. Pulmonary rehabilitation. Am Rev Respir Dis 1981;124:663–666.

17. Fishman AP. Pulmonary rehabilitation research: NIH workshop summary. Am J Respir Crit Care Med 1994;149:825–833.

18. Ries AL, Squier HC. The team concept in pulmonary rehabilitation. In: Fishman AP, ed. Pulmonary rehabilitation. New York: Marcel Dekker, 1996.

19. Niederman MS, Clemente PH, Fein AM, et al. Benefits of a multidisciplinary pulmonary rehabilitation program: improvements are independent of lung function. Chest 1991;99:798–804.

20. Ries A. The role of exercise testing in pulmonary diagnosis. Clin Chest Med 1987;8:81–89.

21. Ries AL, Farrow JT, Clausen JL. Pulmonary function tests cannot predict exercise-induced hypoxemia in chronic obstructive pulmonary disease. Chest 1988;93:454–459.

22. Ries AL, Farrow JT, Clausen JL. Accuracy of two ear oximeters at rest and during exercise in pulmonary patients. Am Rev Respir Dis 1985;132:685–689.

23. Dudley DL, Glaser EM, Jorgenson BN, et al. Psychosocial concomitants to rehabilitation in chronic obstructive pulmonary disease: part 1: psychosocial and psychological considerations; part 2: psychosocial treatment; part 3: dealing with pyschiatric disease (as distinguished from pyschosocial or psychophysiologic problems). Chest 1980;77:413–420, 544–551, 677–684.

24. Prigatano GP, Grant I. Chronic obstructive pulmonary disease: a behavioral perspective. In: McSweeny AJ, Grant I, eds. Neuropsychological correlates of COPD. New York: Marcel Dekker, 1988.

25. Jensen PS. Risk, protective factors, and supportive interventions in chronic airway obstruction. Arch Gen Psychiatry 1983;40: 1203–1207.

26. Neish CM, Hopp JW. The role of education in pulmonary rehabilitation, J Cardiopulmonary Rehabil 1988;11:439–441.

27. Ries AL, Moser KM, Bullock PJ, et al. Shortness of breath: a guide to better living and breathing. 5th ed. St. Louis: Mosby–Year Book, 1996.

28. Rochester DF, Goldberg SK. Techniques of respiratory physical therapy. Am Rev Respir Dis 1980;122(suppl):133–146.

29. Barach AL. Breathing exercises in pulmonary emphysema and allied chronic respiratory disease. Arch Phys Med Rehabil 1955;36:379–390.

30. Miller WF. Physical therapeutic measures in the treatment of chronic bronchopulmonary disorders: methods for breathing training. Am J Med 1958;24:929–940.

31. Medical Research Council Working Party. Long-term domiciliary oxygen therapy in chronic hypoxic cor pulmonale complicating chronic bronchitis and emphysema. Lancet 1981;1:681–686.

32. Nocturnal Oxygen Therapy Trial Group. Continuous or nocturnal oxygen therapy in hypoxemic chronic obstructive lung disease: a clinical trial. Ann Intern Med 1980;93:391–398.

33. Tiep BL, Lewis MI. Oxygen conservation and oxygen-conserving devices in chronic lung disease: a review. Chest 1987;92:263–272.

34. Ries AL. The importance of exercise in pulmonary rehabilitation. Clin Chest Med 1994;15(2): 327–337.

35. Ries AL, Kaplan RM, Limberg TM, et al. Effects of pulmonary rehabilitation on physiologic and psychosocial outcomes in patients with chronic obstructive pulmonary disease. Ann Intern Med 1995; 122:823–832.

36. Punzal PA, Ries AL, Kaplan RM. Maximum intensity exercise training in patients with chronic obstructive pulmonary disease. Chest 1991;100:618–623.

37. Carter R, Nicotra B, Clark L, et al. Exercise conditioning in the rehabilitation of patients with chronic obstructive pulmonary disease. Arch Phys Med Rehabil 1988; 69:118–122.

38. Belman MJ. Ventilatory muscle training and unloading. In: Casaburi R, Petty TL, eds. Principles and practice of pulmonary rehabilitation. Philadelphia: WB Saunders, 1993.

39. Glaser EM, Dudley DL. Psychosocial rehabilitation and psychopharmacology. In: Hodgkin JE, Petty TL, eds. Chronic obstructive pulmonary disease: current concepts. Philadelphia: WB Saunders, 1987.

40. Goldstein RS, Gort EH, Avendano MA, et al. Randomised controlled trial of respiratory rehabilitation. Lancet 1994;344:1394–1397.

41. Wijkstra PJ, Van Altena R, Kraan J, et al. Quality of life in patients with chronic obstructive pulmonary disease improves after rehabilitation at home. Eur Respir J 1994; 7:269–273.

Part VIII.

BEHAVIORAL PSYCHOLOGY

Edited by
Bess H. Marcus

Introduction to Behavioral Psychology

Bess H. Marcus

Behavior therapy is a set of techniques derived from the principles of learning theory. Learning theory describes how unhealthy behaviors are learned through classical conditioning, instrumental conditioning, and modeling. These unhealthy behaviors and their healthy counterparts can be understood in terms of stimulus, response, and reinforcement. Although multiple intervention approaches have been utilized to enhance physical activity behavior and weight management and to decrease smoking behavior, few have been critically evaluated to determine their efficacy. Behavioral approaches have been the most carefully evaluated, and review articles in the areas of smoking cessation, weight management, and exercise promotion all reveal the effectiveness of these strategies. In this section authors delineate the health problems of sedentary lifestyle, smoking, and obesity and describe how applying psychological theory, particularly behavior therapy, to interventions has furthered the field of health promotion. This esteemed group of authors also delineate critical next steps for moving forward both clinical and public health research, practice, and policy.

In their chapter on applying psychological theories to promote healthy lifestyles, Michael Fotheringham and Neville Owen describe how psychological theories and models have been used by practitioners and policy makers to justify, shape, and focus many small- and large-scale efforts, from the consulting room to the whole population. They then review a selection of theories and models that illustrate the content and style of psychological thought being applied to health behavior. Fotheringham and Owen's focus is on theories or models that are either well established now or emerging as potentially useful in the field.

Pat Dubbert and Barbara Stetson describe the prevalence of sedentary lifestyle, the nature of behavioral and cognitive interventions, and a review of the application of these theoretically grounded interventions to promote active lifestyles in their chapter on cognitive and behavioral approaches to enhancing exercise participation. They illustrate the efficacy of different interventions in both clinical and public health settings. Dubbert and Stetson's review covers details of interventions, including the use of contracting, reinforcement, modeling, providing cues and prompts, methods to enhance motivation for behavior change, and monitoring and altering what people say to themselves.

In their chapter on behavioral approaches to enhancing smoking cessation, Karen Emmons and Stefania Maggi describe the nature of the public health problem that cigarette smoking creates, the areas of research that have shown promise, and the areas where future work is needed. They provide information on the health and social consequences of smoking, the reasons why people smoke, and their motivations for quitting, and they review important behavioral approaches to enhancing smoking cessation. Emmons and Maggi point out that even effective intervention approaches will only work for a subset of smokers, and there is not one treatment approach that will work with all smokers. A stepped-care model is described wherein individuals are matched to cessation strategies based on their motivational level and previous experience with cessation.

In their chapter on behavioral approaches to enhancing weight loss and maintenance, Teresa King, Elizabeth Lloyd, and Matt Clark detail the prevalence of obesity, why it is a public health problem, and the effective behavioral strategies for impacting weight loss and maintenance. They discuss societal factors contributing to overweight and detail the nature of behavior therapy and why it has become the most widely used formal treatment for losing weight. For each of the behavioral approaches reviewed, information is provided on how the intervention was developed, which behavioral principles guided its conceptualization, how the strategy is utilized, and the efficacy of the approach.

Chapter 45

Applying Psychological Theories to Promote Healthy Lifestyles

Michael J. Fotheringham
Neville Owen

Applying psychological theories to promoting healthy lifestyles has become a major area of research in health psychology and is having a significant impact on program development and broader public health policy initiatives (1,2). Here, we review a selection of theories and models that illustrate the content and style of psychological thought being applied to health behavior. We draw on material from clinical settings and on research that has focused on community-wide health promotion. The broader range of theories and models that have arisen from research on promoting healthy lifestyles has been reviewed thoroughly elsewhere (3–5). Formal theories and broader theoretical or conceptual models have been very influential in the development and evaluation of practical health promotion programs for several decades (4). Theories and models of the determinants and dynamics of health-related behaviors have been used by practitioners and policy makers to justify, shape, and focus many small- and large-scale efforts, from the consulting room to the whole population.

The comprehensiveness of these theories and their applications to a wide range of health behaviors and to different settings have become part of an extensive research enterprise. In the late 1970s, the general characteristics of health behavior research were described as being oriented toward either psychological or sociologic paradigms (6,7). Today, a more multidisciplinary approach is appropriate as other disciplines, subdisciplines, and interdisciplinary fields such as behavioral epidemiology, behavioral medicine, health psychology, and health promotion contribute to a wider understanding of the personal, social, organizational, and environmental determinants of health. There is less of a focus on intraindividual variables and more explicit efforts to systematically address the broader contextual determinants of health behaviors. The

need for broader multidisciplinary approaches to research and practice in health psychology and health promotion has being recognized by a number of commentators (1,2,8,9).

Here, we describe a subset of the many theories in the field. A number of other influential theories and models could have been included in this review—for example, Bandura's social learning and self-efficacy theories and other social behavior and self-regulation theories (10–13). Social learning theory has been highly influential, and constructs derived from it (particularly self-efficacy) have been incorporated into a number of other theories and models (1–4), including the theories and models we describe in this chapter. Numerous accounts of the applications of social learning theory and its derivations can be found in the literature (2,4).

In this chapter, we have chosen to focus on a selection of theories and models that we believe give a sense of the scope and style of theoretically driven health behavior research—theories that are either well established now or are emerging as potentially useful in the field. Those we describe in this chapter are the Health Belief Model, the Theory of Reasoned Action, Protection Motivation Theory, the Health Promotion Model, and the Transtheoretical Model. The main components and structure of each theory or model are described, along with examples drawn from its use in research.

HEALTH BELIEF MODEL

One of the most influential models of health behavior has been the Health Belief Model (HBM) (14–16). The HBM takes a value-expectancy approach, which holds that behavior is determined by beliefs, including an expectation of the value of the behavior (17). The HBM posits that beliefs about health consist of "perceived susceptibility," "perceived severity," "perceived benefits," and "perceived barriers' (Figure 45-1).

The predictive utility of the HBM was examined in a study of 111 mothers of children being treated for acute asthma episodes. Significant associations were found between the majority of HBM components and measures of adherence to prescribed treatments; mothers' perceptions of the threat of illness were particularly strongly related to adherence (19). Other studies have produced mixed results when using the HBM to predict health behaviors, including treatment adherence and preventive health behaviors (20–22). Rosenstock et al attempted to increase the explanatory power of the HBM by expanding the model to include self-efficacy (confidence in ability to perform a required action) (11,23,24). This construct was not included in the original HBM, because the main focus of the model had been on explaining short-term and often single actions (for example, immunization or specific screening programs), in which self-efficacy was not considered to be a significant influence (25).

Criticisms of the HBM have identified several concerns (26,27): 1) Some of the relationships between the model's variables have not been clearly defined; 2) some determinants have not received sufficient empirical testing, such as "cue to action" or "intention to comply"; and 3) there has been little standardization of the measurement of psychosocial variables described in the model. There may be too many variables involved in the HBM for it to be tested in a single study, and the relationships between some of the variables are imprecisely specified. Thus, the theory can be difficult to falsify (28). Further, the HBM is a multiplicative model, but many studies testing the model have been conducted in an additive fashion (27).

The HBM has been subject to much testing and criticism because of its long history and standing in the health behavior field. It now has a useful place in accounting mainly for shorter-term, single-action behaviors. Other more recent theoretical frameworks now give more tailored accounts of other health behavior domains. This is particularly the case for long-term and habitual behavior patterns, as we will show later in this chapter, particularly in relation to the Transtheoretical Model.

PENDER'S HEALTH PROMOTION MODEL

Pender's Health Promotion Model (29) was developed to describe and explain adherence and other health-enhancing behaviors as a complement to models of health protection.

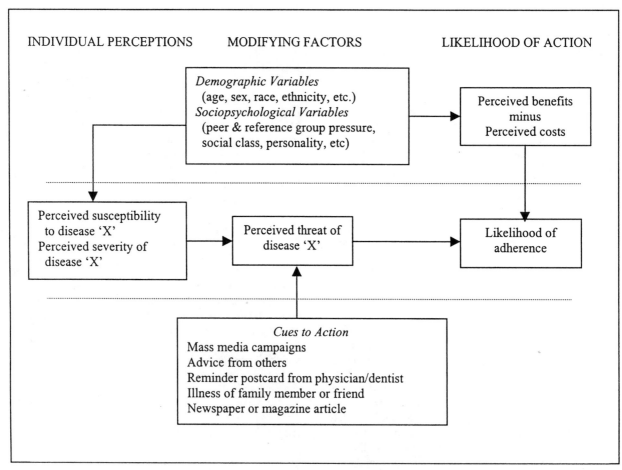

Figure 45-1 The health belief model and adherence with a medical regimen. (Adapted from Dunbar J, Stunkard AJ. Adherence to diet and drug regimen. In: Levy RI, Rifkind BM, Dennis BH, Ernst N, eds. Nutrition, lipids, and coronary heart disease: A global view. New York: Raven Press, 1979:391–423.)

This model is similar to the Health Belief Model, but it refines that model by introducing more order among the HBM component variables. This theoretical innovation answers one of the main criticisms of the HBM—that the relationships between some variables are imprecisely defined (28).

The Health Promotion Model emphasizes cognitive influences on behavior. The primary mechanisms are cognitive-perceptual factors, which are said to influence the likelihood of a health-promoting behavior being performed (Figure 45-2). Foremost among these factors are "importance of health" and the "perceived control of health" (i.e., health value and health locus of control) (30). This model incorporates these factors as direct influences on health behavior. Another factor considered in this model is the definition of health held by the individual, which has been found to be an important determinant of health-related behavior in a number of investigations (31–33).

The Health Promotion Model suggests that the effect of cognitive-perceptual factors on health-promoting behavior is mediated by factors such as biological characteristics and situational variables. The Health Promotion Model recognizes the impact of interpersonal influences, including the expectations of others, the health-related behavior of family members, and relationships with health professionals.

The final component of the Health Promotion Model is "cues to action," which may be either intrinsic or extrinsic. Pender (29) suggests as an example that "feeling good" as a result of exercise may act as an intrinsic cue for continuing exercise, whereas health promotion programs may act as extrinsic cues for initiatives to be more active.

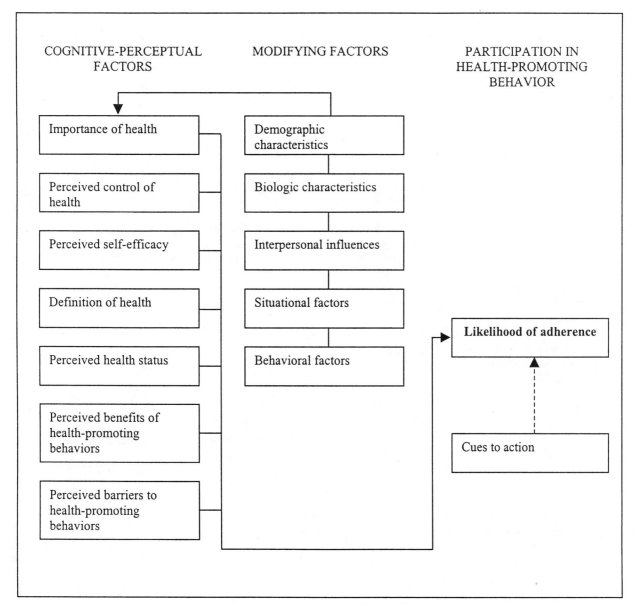

Figure 45-2 Pender's health promotion model. (Adapted from Pender NJ. Health promotion in nursing practice. 2nd ed. Norwalk, CT: Appleton & Lange, 1987.)

The foundations of this model within the constructs of the Health Belief Model, and the improvements made on that model, make the Health Promotion Model potentially valuable.

THEORY OF REASONED ACTION

Fishbein et al's Theory of Reasoned Action (TRA) is a theory of behavior developed from traditions of cognitive and social psychology (34–36). According to the TRA, the performance of a volitional health behavior may be predicted from an intention to perform that behavior (37). An intention to perform a health behavior is a function of attitudes toward that behavior, and of the relevant social norms. Attitudes toward the health behavior are formed from beliefs in the consequence of that behavior, weighed by the value of that consequence. Social norms are conceived as the expectations of significant others, modified by desire to comply with those expectations (Figure 45-3).

An investigation testing the explanatory power of the TRA in relation to adherence behavior of hypertensive patients used path analysis to demonstrate the goodness of fit of the model (38). Dietary, smoking, and exercise behaviors were directly influenced by behavioral intentions, which in turn were directly influenced by motivation to comply and attitudes and indirectly influenced by perceptions of the beliefs of others. That is, the main structure of the TRA was consistent with the findings of this investigation. Other studies have found the TRA to be predictive of health behaviors, including preventive health behaviors (24,39,40), exercise (41), weight control (42), and use of medication (26) and healthcare facilities (43).

In contrast to the lack of specification of structural relationships between HBM variables, the formulation of the TRA is highly specific, both in the relationship between the elements of the model, and in the measurement of these elements (26,44,45). Although such specificity can facilitate cross-study comparisons, it also means that new belief items must be generated when investigating new behaviors (45). The TRA describes health behavior in "rational" or cognitive terms; there is no emotional component in this model. Personality and other psychosocial variables are seen to influence behaviors and behavioral intentions indirectly by their impact on the weighting of the model's components (27,34,44). Further, the TRA does not take into account the barriers and supports for carrying out behavioral intentions (27). A more recent evolution of the TRA that has not been so extensively tested is the Theory of Planned Behavior (TPB). The TPB is an extension of the TRA, with the addition of the construct of perceived behavioral control (46,47), a construct similar to Bandura's self-efficacy (11,24). In the TPB, perceived behavioral control is defined in terms of control beliefs (concerning the absence or presence of supports or barriers to the performance of an activity) and perceived power (the facilitating or inhibiting impact of each of these supports and barriers). Although the TPB and this operationalization of perceived behavioral control have not received extensive testing to date, some evidence suggests that this theory is potentially useful for predicting health behavior (47). Although broadly related to the self-efficacy construct, perceived behavior control can be seen as having elements that could distinguish it as a unique and independent construct.

PROTECTION MOTIVATION THEORY

Protection Motivation Theory (PMT) (48–50) was originally developed to explain the use of fear appeals used in health promotion messages, and was later expanded to encompass other health-related behaviors. According to this model, fear

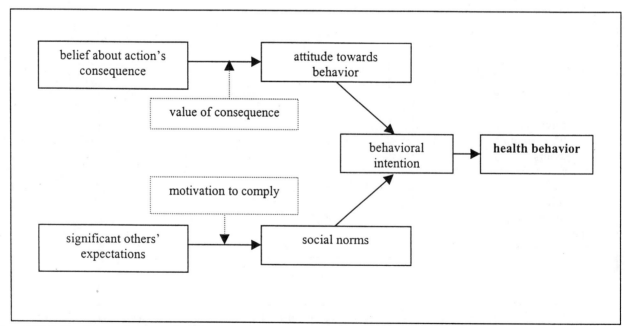

Figure 45-3 The theory of reasoned action.

appeals consist of three components: 1) the degree of noxiousness of a threatened event, 2) the probability of the event, and 3) the efficacy of a protective response (49).

PMT posits that information from various sources (environmental, social, and intrapersonal) initiates two cognitive processes: threat appraisal and coping appraisal. These relate to maladaptive and adaptive responses, respectively. Threat appraisal consists of intrinsic and extrinsic rewards to the maladaptive response, minus the severity of the threat and the probability of being exposed to it. Coping appraisal consists of an appraisal of one's ability to cope with or avert a health threat, mediated by the costs of the adaptive response. The amount of protection motivation elicited by an information source is described as a function of the threat and coping appraisals. It is argued that protection motivation is best measured in terms of behavioral intentions, as described in the TRA (50).

A recent revision of PMT includes the sequential ordering of the appraisal components and the social context of the health threat (51) (Figure 45-4). The introduction of sequential ordering is consistent with the finding that the processing of appraisal information and the appraisal outcome occur consecutively rather than simultaneously (52).

The utility of PMT was assessed using path analysis in relation to the AIDS-related behavior of 84 heterosexual and 147 homosexual adults (53). Results indicated that PMT did fit

the data, accounting for 73% of the variance in behavior of heterosexual subjects and 44% of the variance in homosexual subjects. Other studies have successfully utilized PMT in relation to other health behaviors, such as exercise (54), preventive self-examinations, and cancer-preventive behavior (55).

Unlike the TRA, PMT does not assume that the individual acts in a purely rational manner. This model adds an emotional component to the constructs of the TRA. A limitation of PMT is its focus on fear appeals and other health promotion messages. As such, the application of this model is most useful for intervention studies in which patients' health behavior is examined before and after a health education campaign. PMT may be less applicable to long-term maintenance of health behavior in the absence of intervention.

TRANSTHEORETICAL MODEL

Stage-based theories and models of behavioral change have generated considerable interest among health behavior researchers since the early 1980s (56). Such frameworks also have had considerable appeal to practitioners and policy makers (4). Although a number of stage-based frameworks have been applied to health behavior (56,57), it is arguable that the most influential of these has been the Transtheoretical Model (TTM).

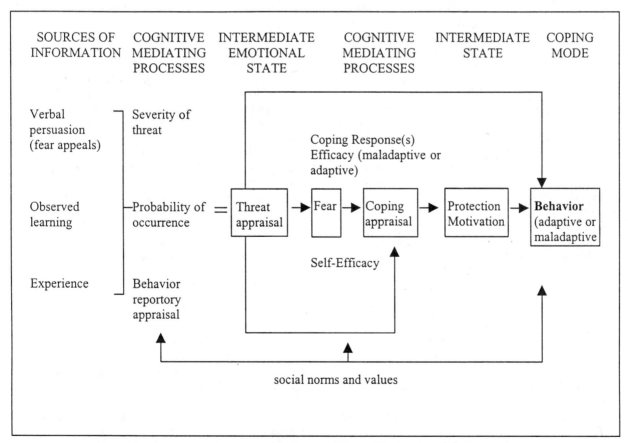

Figure 45-4 Protection motivation theory. (Adapted from Tanner JF, Hunt JB, Eppright DR. The protection motivation model: A normative model of fear appeals. J Mark 1991;55:36–45.)

Table 45-1 Pros (Advantages) and Cons (Disadvantages) of a Health-Related Behavior: The Example of Exercise
Pros • I would be healthier if I exercised more regularly. • I would feel better about myself if I exercised more regularly. • Other people would respect me more if I exercised more regularly. Cons • I would probably be sore and uncomfortable if I exercised more regularly. • If I exercised more regularly, my family and friends would get to spend less time with me. • I would feel that I was wasting my time if I exercised more regularly.

SOURCE: Marcus BH, Owen N. Motivational readiness, self-efficacy and decision making for exercise. J Appl Soc Psychol 1992;22:3–16.

The TTM proposes, as its core construct, a set of stages (58,59). It focuses on both current behavior and future behavioral intentions, and provides a framework that classifies motivational readiness for behavior change (60,61). Thus, behavior change is not seen as an all-or-nothing phenomenon, or a state of action versus inaction (60).

The five stages (58) that form the core of the TTM are:

- Precontemplation, in which change is not being considered

- Contemplation, in which change is considered

- Preparation, in which an individual takes small steps towards change

- Action, involving the initial modification of the habit

- Maintenance, when the change is sustained over 6 months or more.

Although discrete, identifiable stages of change, reflecting varying degrees of readiness to modify behavior, have been proposed by others (56,57), a virtue of the TTM is its recognition of the importance of a broad set of stages, including the early stages of change (62). In the TTM, change is viewed as a continuum, with individuals leaving and reentering at different points. Relapse is a key element of any stage-based model of behavioral change (57,63). In relapse, individuals may lose resolve and abandon new behavior patterns, feel guilty, and lose confidence and revert to their previous habits, with probable recycling through the earlier stages of precontemplation or contemplation.

The TTM has been employed to examine a range of health behaviors as diverse as smoking cessation, exercising, quitting cocaine use, safe sex, sun-screen use, mammography screening, and delinquent behavior (64–66). As well as identifying those who are ready to modify behavior, a key feature of the TTM is its emphasis on examining transitions between the various stages by integrating components of other theories.

Self-efficacy is a key theoretical construct within the TTM, as well as in other models of health behavior. According to self-efficacy theory, confidence in the ability to perform a particular behavior is strongly associated with the actual ability to perform that behavior (24). Self-efficacy beliefs have been shown to be associated with the performance of a diverse range of health-related behaviors (67,68). Studies of health-related behaviors have shown that, compared to those in the later stages, individuals in the early stages of change have little confidence in their ability to change (69,70). The relationships between self-efficacy and the stage of change tend to be consistent for a range of behaviors (66).

The other main constructs within the TTM are decisional balance (69,71) and processes of change (72). Decisional balance is the relative weighting of perceptions of the personal benefits associated with a behavior or behavior change, and the perceived costs or disbenefits of such activities (71). Table 45-1 lists examples of perceived benefits (the "pros") and perceived costs (the "cons") of physical activity. A standardized "decisional balance" score may be derived by subtracting total standardized cons scores from total standardized pros scores (69).

Processes of change are those cognitive and behavioral activities that relate to a range of affective, information-seeking, problem-solving, and other initiatives that may act to encourage or discourage change in behavior, or may influence the precursors of such change. Table 45-2 gives definitions of the 10 processes of change described in the TTM.

The decisional balance and processes of change constructs have been shown to be systematically associated with stages of change. Decisional balance varies as a function of stage (66,69,72). Early stages (precontemplation and contemplation) are associated with higher ratings of the disadvantages (cons) of change and lower ratings of the advantages (pros) of change. In the later stages in the model (action and maintenance), ratings of the cons of change are lower and ratings of the pros of change are higher. The cognitive and behavioral processes of change in the TTM have complex relationships with the stages, and further research will begin to identify those processes that are most significant (72).

Other stage-based models of health behavior change focus on dimensions different to those postulated by the TTM. Weinstein et al (56) described the attributes of a number of stage-based models and consider how these may or may not be helpful in different health behavior domains. For example, the TTM may give a strong account of stages that are highly relevant to smoking cessation (58–60), to exercise adoption (61,64,65,69), and to a number of other health behaviors (66). However, stage-based models that more strongly incorporate perceptions of risk may provide more powerful explanations of the decisions and behaviors associ-

Table 45-2 Processes of Change Within the Transtheoretical Model	
PROCESS	**DEFINITION**
Consciousness Raising	Increasing information about self and problem
Self-Reevaluation	Assessing how one feels and thinks about oneself with respect to a problem
Self-Liberation	Choosing and commitment to act or belief in ability to change
Counterconditioning	Substituting alternatives for problem behaviors
Stimulus Control	Avoiding or countering stimuli that elicit problem behaviors
Reinforcement Management	Rewarding oneself or being rewarded by others for making changes
Helping Relationships	Being open and trusting about problems with someone who cares
Dramatic Relief	Experiencing and expressing feelings about one's problems and solutions
Environmental Reevaluation	Assessing how one's problem affects physical environment
Social Liberation	Increasing alternatives for nonproblem behaviors available in society

SOURCE: Prochaska JO, DiClemente CE, Norcross JC. In search of how people change: Applications to addictive behaviors. Am Psychol 1992;47:1102–1114.

ated with the adoption of health-related precautions such as domestic radon gas testing and implementing specific protective measures (56). Of the stage-based theories, the TTM appears at present to be capturing the imagination of many in the field of health behavior research (4,66). The TTM has so far been a highly influential and productive theoretical framework with many broad applications (60,64,66).

There has been a strong intuitive appeal to practitioners and policy makers of a discrete set of stage categories that may be applied to major health behaviors such as smoking and physical activity (4,64). By organizing and adapting well-established constructs such as stages, decisional balance, and self-efficacy, the TTM has arguably increased the potential influence and policy relevance of health behavior theories more generally. At present, there is a large body of evidence that demonstrates that the TTM has a number of useful organizing constructs that can be shown to be meaningfully related in empirical data and psychometric studies (4).

The TTM has nevertheless been criticized on the basis of what are argued to be broader limitations of stage-based theories (11). The TTM is one of a number of stage-based models of health behavior (56,57), and it is unlikely that a single model can account for all of the specific relevant mechanisms likely to influence the wide diversity of health behaviors—behaviors which take place in a broad range of environmental, social, and organizational contexts.

SUMMARY

Of the models presented in this paper, the Health Belief Model has arguably been highly influential. However, refinement of the HBM has been minimal and some aspects of the model have rarely been applied in empirical evaluations. Pender's Health Promotion Model has been developed from the HBM, with the addition of an ordering of the HBM's main elements, thus answering one of the main criticisms of the HBM, although this new model has yet to be empirically validated. The Theory of Reasoned Action, in contrast, has been tested in a more specific manner, a process made easier by the more detailed formulation of this model.

Protection Motivation Theory has developed from a perspective similar to that of the HBM, but has focused on the use of fear arousal in health-promoting messages. The Transtheoretical Model has built on earlier stage-based frameworks and provides a comprehensive account of behavioral change.

Many other theories not described here also provide accounts of key issues, such as the importance of observational learning, or the role of risk perceptions, health beliefs, and attitudes in health behavior (1–4). Table 45-3 provides a summary of the key variables used in the major theories and models applied to promoting healthy lifestyles.

The focus of the theories and models we have described has been to a large extent on intraindividual and the more proximal social determinants of healthy lifestyles. These models (particularly Pender's Health Promotion Model) do attempt, at least through assessing perceived social norms, to incorporate broader social and environmental variables. However, by their very nature, psychological models tend to deal largely with intraindividual characteristics, an emphasis upon which may limit their explanatory power, insofar as these characteristics explain health behavior (21,25). Externally verifiable social factors, such as the expectations of others, can also influence health behavior (30). To the extent that these factors are predictive of health behavior, models that exclude them limit their ability to account for health behavior. By focusing mainly on aspects of the individual, these models may facilitate victim blaming (25). That is, the role of uncontrollable social, economic, and environmental influences is not properly considered in the explanation of individuals' health-compromising behaviors—the assumption being that it is up to the individual to take personal responsibility for change, or for not "choosing" to change.

There are some major challenges in developing theories that focus less on the individual and account more comprehensively for how the physical environment and social and organizational contexts impact on healthy lifestyles. Such "ecological" models tend to be somewhat generic in their focus (4,73). Addressing, in a more specific, theoretically grounded fashion, the influence of contexts and setting on health-related behavior is a challenging new area of research (74). Such research may help to extend the

Table 45-3 Descriptions of the Key Variables Used in the Major Theories of Health-Promoting Behavior

- Perceived probability that a particular outcome will occur
- Perceived severity of a health outcome
- Perceived effectiveness of the precaution
- Perceived internal rewards from current behavior
- Perceived external rewards from current behavior
- Self-efficacy
- Normative beliefs (strength of the desire of another person that the individual perform a particular behavior)
- Motivation to comply with the other person's desire
- Perceived costs and barriers to action
- Perceived value of a nonhealth outcome
- Health consequences under alternative behavior
- Consequences of alternative behavior other than health effects
- Health consequences under current behavior
- Consequences of current behavior other than health effects

SOURCE: Weinstein N. Testing four competing theories of health-protective behaviour. Health Psychol 1993;12:324–333.

applications of psychological theories to understanding and influencing a wider range of determinants of healthy lifestyles (75,76). The major challenges for the range of disciplines involved in health behavior research are to relate partic-ular psychological theories and models to particular behaviors and contexts, and to account more systematically and specifically for the influences of environmental factors on health behaviors.

REFERENCES

1. Green LW, Kreuter MW. Health promotion planning: an educational and environmental approach. Mountain View, CA: Mayfield, 1991.

2. Winett RA, King AC, Altman DG. Health psychology and public health: an integrative approach. New York: Pergamon, 1989.

3. Glanz K, Lewis FM, Rimer BK, eds. Health behavior and health education: theory, research and practice. San Francisco: Jossey-Bass, 1990.

4. Glanz K, Lewis FM, Rimer BK, eds. Health behavior and health education: theory, research, and practice. 2nd ed. San Francisco: Jossey-Bass, 1996.

5. Weinstein N. Testing four competing theories of health-protective behaviour. Health Psychol 1993; 12:324–333.

6. Stone GC. Psychology and the health system. In: Stone GC, Cohen F, Adler NE, eds. Health psychology: a handbook. San Francisco: Jossey-Bass, 1979:47–75.

7. Kirscht JP, Rosenstock IM. Patients' problems in following recommendations of health experts. In: Stone GC, Cohen F, Adler NE, eds. Health psychology: a handbook. San Francisco: Jossey-Bass, 1979: 189–216.

8. Hinde RA. Developmental psychology in the context of other behavioral sciences. Dev Psychol 1992; 28:1018–1029.

9. Suedfeld P. Environmental factors influencing maintenance of lifestyle change. In: Stuart RB, ed. Adherence, compliance and generalization in behavioral medicine. New York: Brunner/Mazel, 1982: 125–144.

10. Bandura A. Social foundations of thought and action: a social cognitive theory. Englewood Cliffs, NJ: Prentice-Hall, 1986.

11. Bandura A. Self-efficacy: the exercise of control. New York: W.H. Freeman, 1997.

12. Triandis HC. Interpersonal behavior. Monterey, CA: Brooks/Cole, 1977.

13. Leventhal H, Zimmerman R, Gutmann M. Compliance: a self-regulation perspective. In: Gentry D, ed. Handbook of behavioral medicine. New York: Guilford, 1984:369–436.

14. Rimer BK. Perspectives on intra-personal theories in health education and health behavior. In: Glanz K, Lewis FM, Rimer BK, eds. Health behavior and health education: theory, research, and practice. San Francisco: Jossey-Bass, 1990:140–157.

15. Rosenstock IM. Historical origins of the health belief model. Health Educ Monogr 1974;2:328–335.

16. Rosenstock IM, Kirscht JP. The health belief model and personal health behavior. Health Educ Monogr 1974;2:470–473.

17. Feather NT. Subjective probability and decision under uncertainty. Psychol Rev 1959;66:150–164.

18. Dunbar J, Stunkard AJ. Adherence to diet and drug regimen. In: Levy RI, Rifkind BM, Dennis BH, Ernst N, eds. Nutrition, lipids, and coro-

nary heart disease: a global view. New York: Raven Press, 1979: 391–423.

19. Becker MH, Radius SM, Rosenstock IM, et al. Compliance with a medical regimen for asthma: a test of the health belief model. Public Health Rep 1978; 93:268–277.

20. Bond GG, Aiken LS, Somerville SC. The health belief model and adolescents with insulin-dependent diabetes mellitus. Health Psychol 1992;11:190–198.

21. Janz NK, Becker MH. The health belief model: a decade later. Health Educ Q 1984;11:1–47.

22. Kasl SV. The health belief model and behavior related to chronic illness. Health Educ Monogr 1974;2:433–454.

23. Rosenstock IM, Strecher VJ, Becker MH. Social learning theory and the health belief model. Health Educ Q 1988;15:175–183.

24. Bandura A. Selt-efficacy: Toward a unifying theory of behavioral change. Psychol Rev 1977;84: 191–215.

25. Rosenstock IM. The health belief model: explaining health behavior through expectancies. In: Glanz K, Lewis FM, Rimer BK, eds. Health behavior and health education: theory, research, and practice. San Francisco: Jossey-Bass, 1990:39–62.

26. Ried LD, Christensen DB. A psychosocial perspective in the explanation of patients' drug taking behavior. Soc Sci Med 1988;27: 277–285.

27. Wallston BS, Wallston KA. Social psychological models of health behavior: an examination and integration. In: Baum A, Taylor SE, Singer JE, eds. Handbook of psychology and health, vol. 4. Social psychological aspects of health. Hillsdale, NJ: Lawrence Erlbaum, 1984:23–53.

28. de Groot A. Methodology. Foundations of inference and research in the behavioral sciences. Trans. JAA Spiekerman. The Hague: Mouton, 1969.

29. Pender NJ. Health promotion in nursing practice. 2nd ed. Norwalk, CT: Appleton & Lange, 1987.

30. Fotheringham MJ, Sawyer MG. Adherence to medical recommendations in childhood and adolescence. J Paediatr Child Health 1995;31:72–78.

31. Bishop GD, Converse SA. Illness representations: a prototype approach. Health Psychol 1986;5: 95–114.

32. Lau RR, Hartman KA. Common sense representations of common illnesses. Health Psychol 1983;2: 167–185.

33. Skelton JA, Croyle RT. Mental representations in health and illness. New York: Springer-Verlag, 1991.

34. Fishbein M. Toward an understanding of family planning behavior. J Applied Soc Psychol 1972;2: 214–227.

35. Fishbein M. A theory of reasoned action: some applications and implications. In: Page MM, ed. 1979 Nebaska Symposium on motivation. Lincoln: University of Nebraska Press, 1980.

36. Fishbein M, Ajzen I. Beliefs, attitudes, intention and behavior: an introduction to theory and research. Reading, MA: Addison-Wesley, 1975.

37. Egger G, Spark R, Lawson J. Health promotion strategies and methods. Sydney: McGraw-Hill, 1991.

38. Miller P, Wikoff R, Hiatt A. Fishbein's model of reasoned action and compliance behavior of hypertensive patients. Nurs Res 1992; 41:104–109.

39. Brubaker RG, Wickersham D. Encouraging the practice of testicular self-examination: a field application of the theory of reasoned action. Health Psychol 1990;9: 154–163.

40. Terry DJ, Gallois C, McCamish M, eds. The theory of reasoned action: its application to AIDS-preventive behavior. Oxford, UK: Pergamon, 1993.

41. Valois P, Desharnais R, Godin G. A comparison of the Fishbein and

Ajzen and the Triandis attitudinal models for prediction of exercise intention and behavior. J Behav Med 1988;11:459–472.

42. Saltzer EB. Locus of control and intention to lose weight. Health Educ Monogr 1978;6:118–128.

43. Hendricks SJ, Freeman R, Sheilham A. Why inner city mothers take their children for routine medical and dental examination. Community Dent Health 1990;7:33–41.

44. Kippax S, Crawford J. Flaws in the theory of reasoned action. In: Terry DJ, Gallois C, McCamish M, eds. The theory of reasoned action: its application to AIDS-preventive behavior. Oxford: Pergamon, 1993: 253–269.

45. Mullen PD, Hersey JC, Iverson DC. Health behavior models compared. Soc Sci Med 1987;24:973–981.

46. Ajzen I. The theory of planned behavior. Organ Behav Hum Decis Process 1991;50:179–211.

47. Montaño DE, Kasprzyk D, Taplin SH. The theory of reasoned action and the theory of planned behavior. In: Glanz K, Lewis FM, Rimer BK, eds. Health behavior and health education: theory, research, and practice. 2nd ed. San Francisco: Jossey-Bass, 1996: 85–112.

48. Prentice-Dunn S, Rogers RW. Protection motivation theory and preventive health: beyond the health belief model. Health Educ Res 1986;1:153–161.

49. Rogers RW. A protection motivation theory of fear appeals and attitude change. J Psychol 1975; 91:93–114.

50. Rogers RW. Cognitive and physiological processes in fear appeals and attitude change: a revised theory of protection motivation. In: Cacioppo JT, Petty RE, eds. Social psychophysiology: A sourcebook. New York: Guilford, 1983:153–176.

51. Tanner JF, Hunt JB, Eppright DR. The protection motivation model: a normative model of fear appeals. J Mark 1991;55:36–45.

52. Scherer KR. Emotions as a multi-component process: a model and some cross-cultural data. In: Scherer P, ed. Review of personality and social psychology, vol. 5. Beverly Hills, CA: Sage, 1984:37–63.

53. Van der Velde FW, Van der Pligt J. AIDS-related health behavior: coping, protection motivation, and previous behavior. J Behav Med 1991;14:429–451.

54. Fruin DJ, Pratt C, Owen N. Protection motivation theory and adolescents' perceptions of exercise. J Appl Soc Psychol 1992;22:55–69.

55. Rippetoe PA, Rogers RW. Effects of components of protection-motivation theory on adaptive and maladaptive coping with a health threat. J Pers Soc Psychol 1987; 52:596–604.

56. Weinstein ND, Rothman AJ, Sutton R. Stage theories of health behaviour: conceptual and methodological issues. Health Psychol 1998; 17:1–10.

57. Brownell KD, Marlatt GA, Lichtenstein E, et al. Understanding and preventing relapse. Am Psychol 1986;41:765–782.

58. DiClemente CC, Prochaska JO, Fairhurst SK, et al. The process of smoking cessation: an analysis of the precontemplation, contemplation and preparation stages of change. J Consult Clin Psychol 1991;59(2):295–304.

59. Prochaska JO, DiClemente CC. Stages and processes of self-change of smoking: toward an integrative model of change. J Consult Clin Psychol 1983;51: 390–395.

60. Abrams DB. Treatment issues: towards a stepped-care model. Tob Control 1993;2(suppl):S17–S37.

61. Marcus BH, Eaton CA, Rossi JS, et al. Self-efficacy, decision making, and stages of change: an integrative model of physical exercise. J Appl Soc Psychol 1994;24: 489–508.

62. Rossi JS, Rossi SR, Velicer WF, et al. Motivational readiness to control weight. In: Allison DB, ed. Handbook of assessment methods for eating behaviors and weight-related problems: measures, theory, and research. Thousand Oaks, CA: Sage, 1995:387–430.

63. Marlatt GA, Gordon JR, eds. Relapse prevention. New York: Guilford, 1985.

64. Donovan RJ, Owen N. Social marketing and population interventions. In: Dishman RK, ed. Advances in exercise adherence. Champaign, IL: Human Kinetics, 1994:249–290.

65. Owen N, Crawford D. Health promotion: perspectives on physical activity and weight control. In: Johnston M, Johnston D, eds. Health psychology. London: Pergamon, 1998.

66. Prochaska JO, Velicer WF, Rossi JS, et al. Stages of change and decisional balance for 12 problem behaviors. Health Psychol 1994; 13(1):39–46.

67. O'Leary A. Self-efficacy and health. Behav Res Ther 1985;23: 437–451.

68. Strecher VJ, McEvoy-DeVellis B, Becker MH, et al. The role of self-efficacy in achieving health behavior change. Health Educ Q 1986; 13(1):73–91.

69. Marcus BH, Owen N. Motivational readiness, self-efficacy and decision making for exercise. J Appl Soc Psychol 1992;22:3–16.

70. Marcus BH, Selby VC, Niaura RS, et al. Self-efficacy and the stages of exercise behavior change. Res Q Exerc Sport 1992;63:60–66.

71. Janis IL, Mann L. Decision making: a psychological analysis of conflict, choice, and commitment. New York: Collier Macmillan, 1977.

72. Prochaska JO, DiClemente CE, Norcross JC. In search of how people change: applications to addictive behaviors. Am Psychol 1992;47:1102–1114.

73. Stokols D. Establishing and maintaining healthy environments: toward a social ecology of health promotion. Am Psychol 1992;47: 6–22.

74. McLeroy KR, Bibeau D, Steckler A, et al. An ecological perspective on health promotion programs. Health Educ Q 1988;15:351–377.

75. Sallis JF, Owen N. Ecological models. In: Glanz K, Lewis FM, Rimer BK, eds. Health behavior and health education: theory, research, and practice. 2nd ed. San Francisco: Jossey-Bass 1996: 403–424.

76. Sallis JF, Owen N. Physical activity and behavioral medicine. Beverly Hills, CA: Sage, 1998.

Chapter 46

Cognitive and Behavioral Approaches to Enhancing Exercise Participation

Patricia M. Dubbert
Barbara A. Stetson

Recent research has produced exciting new information about the health benefits of an active lifestyle (1,2). Lack of adequate physical activity is now acknowledged as an independent risk factor for important causes of premature death and disability in modern cultures. Unfortunately, knowledge of the importance of healthful physical activity is not sufficient. Surveys repeatedly show that the majority of adults in developed countries fail to meet even the most recent moderate activity guidelines. Discovering the most effective methods of changing physical activity habits remains an important challenge for behavioral and public health scientists (2).

Interventions for changing exercise and physical activity that are derived from experimental psychology and theories of behavior change are now included in many health promotion programs. Behavioral intervention methods are characterized by a focus on specific behavior and factors that can be manipulated to influence the behavior that is the target of change. However, cognitive-behavioral theorists and interventionists also acknowledge the influence of biological variables on behavior and the importance of internal events, including thoughts and emotions. Cognitive interventions focus on changing the cognitions that are thought to facilitate or hinder behavior, and rely on verbal or written reports to assess the otherwise unobservable events that are the focus of change. Cognitive interventions have been studied and applied in the same systematic manner as those that focus on observable behaviors. The two types of interventions are often used in combinations of cognitive-behavioral interventions.

In this chapter, we illustrate a variety of cognitive and behavioral interventions for promoting exercise and physical activity with examples of applications from clinical and public health promotion settings. These theory-based interventions include the use of contracting, reinforcement, modeling, providing cues and prompts, methods to enhance motivation for behavior change, and monitoring and altering what people say to themselves. Our purpose is to show how these intervention strategies can be applied in real-world community and clinical settings for the promotion of exercise and physical activity. We do not attempt to provide a critical review of the physical activity and exercise intervention literature. Comprehensive narrative and meta-analytic reviews are available for the interested reader (2–4). Notably, a quantitative meta-analysis of 127 intervention studies found that interventions with the largest effects used principles of behavior modification (4).

BEHAVIORAL CONTRACTING AND REINFORCEMENT

Reinforcement interventions can be very effective when a behavior reliably changes in response to consequences that can be manipulated by the interventionist. The intrinsic (internally generated) motivation for physical activity seems to be insufficient to maintain an active lifestyle for many teens and adults. Arranging for some kind of extrinsic motivation, such as a reward or recognition for increases in physical activity or compliance with an exercise prescription, is a very common type of reinforcement intervention. Behavioral contracts typically involve a written agreement that specifies the behavior-consequence arrangements and often includes tangible rewards for compliance or forfeiting something of value for noncompliance. Although reinforcement interventions are appealing, they are not always feasible because, in real life, it is often difficult to control the consequences of exercise behavior. For example, we know very little about how to make exercise enjoyable for people who say they don't like it, and we also don't have a good understanding of why some people continue exercising even when it becomes harmful to them. The following are some examples of reinforcement interventions that have successfully changed physical activity and exercise.

Contracting and Lottery Intervention in a Physical Activity Class

Epstein et al (5) conducted a demonstration of the effects of contract and lottery interventions on attendance at aerobics classes with 41 women college students. Over two academic quarters, students were assigned to five groups. Three of the groups had contracts for attendance, one group had a lottery for attendance, and the final group was a no-treatment control. Participants in the attendance contracting groups were required to deposit $5 prior to the beginning of the experiment; they received $1 back for each week that they attended four of the five exercise sessions. The amount of exercise required (running distances from 1 to 2 miles) within the five classes varied. Participants in the lottery group were required to deposit $3 prior to the beginning of the experiment to purchase the lottery prize. They earned chances in the lottery each week that they attended at least four of five sessions. At the end of the quarter, the winner received a gift certificate. Participants in the control group did not deposit any money, and there were no additional contingencies for attendance and exercise. Analyses of attendance data showed that the mean number of classes attended by participants in the contracting groups were similar (15 to 16 sessions) and better than attendance for the control group (11.5 sessions). Performance on a 12-minute walk-run test also indicated that participants in several of the contract groups improved in fitness more than control group participants, providing indirect validation of the differences in adherence.

Contracting and Incentives in a Worksite Health Promotion Program

Incentives for exercise participation have also been used in worksite health promotion programs. Robison et al (6) studied the effects of behavioral contracting with a group of 137 university faculty and staff involved in a worksite program. Participants included young to middle-aged men and women in several academic buildings and departments; those in five of the buildings received the experimental behavioral interventions whereas those in the sixth received the exercise program alone. Participants were recruited at a health fair and all received individual assessment and counseling including a prescription for vigorous exercise. The program utilized several behavioral intervention components, but we emphasize the contracting and incentive components here.

Experimental intervention participants completed a contract specifying types of exercise to be performed and names of people who would serve as witnesses for each completed session for a 6-month period. All contracts specified a minimum of four sessions per week and a duration of 30 minutes per session; intensity varied according to the baseline fitness testing and individual prescriptions. Participants were asked to explain their goals to potential verifiers and ask for their support. They received special forms each week that had to be signed by the witnesses in order to get credit for completing the exercise sessions. The incentives for the program came from a deposit of $40 requested from each participant as a "bet" on himself or herself. Each week, participants who completed four verified sessions received a return of their money for that week; if they failed to complete four sessions, they lost their money. The money forfeited by those who failed to meet their weekly requirements was distributed to members of teams in which all participants had met their goals. Verified sickness or injury was a valid excuse for nonattendance and did not result in loss of money. The money was distributed at the end of the 6-month period. Additional incentives were also utilized; the team with the most money at the end of the 6 months received $150, and individuals in each site earned chances for a $50 cash lottery depending on the number of weeks they fulfilled their contracts. The program for the control participants did not include any of the incentives.

At the end of the 6 months, the contracting and incentive groups averaged 97% adherence, compared with only 19% for the control group. Treadmill performance also improved significantly for the experimental participants whereas there was no change for controls. The authors noted that the control site had a much greater proportion of female participants, but the effect of this difference on the study outcome was not known. Specific costs of each program component were not described, but the total costs were described by the authors as involving a "minimal resource investment" including 15 hours away from the worksite during the 6-month period.

Reinforcement of Increases in Physical Activity or Decreases in Sedentary Behavior in Obese Children

The American population is growing more obese as better laborsaving devices are invented, which give people more free time to spend in sedentary activities such as watching television and playing electronic games. Epstein et al have studied a variety of ways to increase physical activity in obese children. Most recently they have been attempting to find ways to reduce the amount of time the children spend in sedentary leisure activities that compete with healthful physical activity. In a recent study, Epstein compared interventions that were designed to specifically reinforce increases in exercise or decreases in competing sedentary behavior (7). Obese children 8 to 12 years of age were randomly assigned to different physical activity promotion interventions within the context of a comprehensive obesity treatment program that employed many behavioral interventions. Children attended weekly treatment meetings for 4 months, and then less frequent meetings and measurements for a year. All children received information about the benefits of increased physical activity and the negative effects of sedentary activity, but the groups differed in the kinds of activities that were targeted for change. All children recorded time spent in physical activity and sedentary activity in a habit book. Parents and children were requested to review the book each evening and parents were trained to praise the children for performing the desired behaviors.

The program also involved contracting, in which parents provided agreed-upon reinforcers (not food) to their children for meeting their goals. Participants in the increased physical activity group were reinforced for accumulating a specified number of points representing a certain amount of energy expenditure each week. Participants in the decreased sedentary behavior group were reinforced for decreasing the amount of time spent in these activities on a weekly schedule. Participants in a third group were reinforced both for a combination of increased activity and decreased sedentary activity.

Children in all three groups lost weight and improved their fitness, but the participants in the group that targeted decreased sedentary behavior showed the greatest improvement in weight. The combined group results were between the other two groups. Another important outcome measure for this study involved the children's preferences for different types of activities; children in the decreased sedentary behavior group showed a greater increase in preference for high-intensity physical activities than the children in the group reinforced for increasing activity. The authors contend that the results support the importance of designing interventions not only for directly increasing physical activity but also to decrease access to sedentary behaviors that compete with being active. Reinforcing decreases in sedentary behavior without specifying how that time would be used may have been effective in part because it created an opportunity for the children to exercise more control over how they spent their more physically active time. This perceived control could have enhanced the reinforcing value of the alternative activities, allowing for better maintenance over time.

PROVIDING CUES OR PROMPTS FOR PHYSICAL ACTIVITY

People respond, sometimes with little or no awareness, to a myriad of external and internal stimuli every day, and some of these exert powerful control over choices to engage in physical activity and exercise. Behavioral interventionists often recommend that people try to add cues or prompts for exercise behavior to their environment. External cues are easier to work with than internal cues. For example, workout gear left in a prominent place or writing in exercise "dates" on a weekly schedule can serve as effective reminders to engage in regular physical activity. Interpreting feelings of fatigue and dysphoria as signals of a need for physical activity instead of a sedentary distraction may often be appropriate but also more difficult to achieve. Physical activity intervention researchers have demonstrated that at least two types of prompts can reliably promote increased physical activity: signs encouraging physical activity and telephone call reminders.

Posting a Sign Encouraging Physical Activity
Brownell et al (8) studied the effects of a very simple and cost-effective intervention designed to increase physical activity in the natural environment by placing a sign in public places where people had a choice between using stairs or an escalator. The sign showed a bloated, tired-looking heart with the message "Your heart needs exercise . . ." taking the escalator and a fit, cheerful heart climbing the stairs with the message "Here's your chance." In the first study, observations were

made in a shopping center, a bus terminal, and a train station, where an escalator and stairs were located in close proximity. In the second experiment, observations were made at a commuter train station over several months. In both experiments, the researchers found that the sign stimulated more people to use the stairs. Posting the sign during the intervention phases of the experiments doubled or tripled the percentage of people using the stairs, but the majority still chose the escalator. The design of the second experiment allowed the researchers to evaluate the effects of the sign over time. They observed that stair use remained at the higher level during the 15 days while the sign was posted and dropped after the sign was removed, but remained higher than baseline for at least a month. Stair use was back to the preintervention level at a 3-month follow-up.

Telephone Calls from Exercise Staff to Support Home-Based Exercise
Telephone contacts between interventionists and people exercising at distant locations can serve as cues for adhering to an exercise plan. A series of studies has demonstrated the efficacy of home-based exercise for promoting fitness in healthy middle-aged populations (9–11). In a 6-month exercise adoption study, King et al evaluated the effects of brief telephone contacts for prompting exercise compliance in healthy sedentary adults given a prescription for a home-based program. All participants were given an individualized instruction including a 15-minute face-to-face meeting with staff and a 15-minute videotape. Exercise intensity was individually determined from treadmill testing, and participants were given heart rate monitors to enable them to keep track of their home exercise intensity. All were instructed to exercise four times per week for 30 minutes per session. Participants were also told about behavioral principles for promoting exercise. Following the instruction, participants randomly assigned to a control condition had contacts with the exercise program staff only if they did not return exercise logs for 2 or more weeks. Those assigned to the experimental group received an average of 10 five-minute telephone calls from staff. The telephone contacts were used to discuss progress and to provide support and guidance. In anticipation of the calls, participants may have tried harder to meet their goals. The additional counseling and support most likely were also important ingredients. At the end of the 6 months, participants in the telephone prompt condition showed significant increases in fitness, whereas the no-prompt group did not show improvements.

MODELING

The saying "Do as I say, not as I do" conveys an appreciation for the importance of observational learning. Children and adults learn a great deal about the importance of physical activity and how to exercise in a safe and enjoyable way by watching others. Modeling is likely to be most effective when the model is perceived as similar to the observer, when the observer has an opportunity to attend to the behavior without distractions, when the modeled skills are not too complex (or build on one another over time), and when the modeled behavior achieves a positive outcome (12). There are few studies in which modeling has been evaluated as a component in physical activity promotion programs. We present two examples of the application of modeling interventions, both illustrating the successful use of this type of intervention with individuals with special physical activity challenges.

Peer Modeling to Assist Independent Ambulation Skills

Gouvier et al (13) presented a case report of a 2½-year-old child with complete L4 spina bifida who was enrolled in a program to help her learn to ambulate independently. After 3 months, she never used her walker spontaneously and cried whenever she wore her braces. She had no behavioral problems other than resisting the walking training program. After observational data were collected for a 2-week period, the researchers implemented a simple intervention consisting of transferring the patient into a class with a 4-year-old girl who had been walking with fixed braces and a walker for several years. This would allow the child who had successfully mastered walking to serve as a model for the younger child. After the two children had attended school together for 8 days, the researchers again observed the younger child and found that she no longer cried or needed assistance using her walker. A final observation 1 month later confirmed that the improvements were being maintained.

Videotape Modeling to Improve Gait and Balance in Elderly Residents of a Care Facility

Five women with IQ scores in the mental retardation range who were at risk for falls because of poor balance participated in a study of videotape modeling of gait and balance exercises. Neef et al (14) videotaped the women performing a 25-minute sequence of therapeutic exercises including side steps, cross-over steps forward and backward, high steps, static bipedal toe raises, and side glide and hops. The tape was then used for minimally supervised training sessions over a period of several months. Observations showed the women were able to match performance on the tape with minimal staff prompting. In a second study, the researchers found that using videotapes of peers who were friends of the participants was also effective. The videotapes were a very cost-effective intervention. The training produced improvements in gait and balance, although changes were different across subjects. In addition, two subjects who had a history of frequent falls had no falls during the exercise intervention phases.

SELF-MONITORING, SELF-MANAGEMENT, AND COGNITIVE INTERVENTIONS

Many behavioral change programs recommend that participants keep a diary or log to record the behavior they are trying to change. Self-monitoring is very helpful when people perform the health behavior on their own in home and community settings where observation by the interventionist is not feasible. Self-monitoring is also important when the target of change is what people are thinking or saying to themselves. Self-monitoring can increase awareness of these influences on behavior and can give the individual more control over his or her own behavior change process. Detailed self-monitoring can help participants or interventionists working with them identify external and internal factors that seem to be associated with success or failure in meeting behavioral goals. Participants are often encouraged to set up self-management programs in which they reward themselves when they meet specified goals. They can also use self-monitoring of thoughts about the behavior to challenge unrealistic or negative thoughts that get in the way of making progress.

Self-Monitoring of Home-Based Exercise

The importance of self-monitoring in promoting physical activity and fitness was evaluated in a study by Noland (15) that compared a self-monitoring intervention with an intervention in which someone else recorded and rewarded the participants' exercise. Men and women who had not been exercising on a regular basis were assigned to one of three groups: self-monitoring, reinforcement, or control. All participants received a free fitness assessment and exercise prescription. Participants had different exercise prescriptions depending on whether their goals were fat reduction or cardiovascular fitness. They were encouraged to exercise with someone if possible and could join an exercise class if they wished. At the end of the 18-week period, they were reassessed.

The self-monitoring participants received standardized forms to record all exercise performed during leisure time, whether they achieved their recommended heart rate, the duration, date, and type of exercise, and whether they exercised alone or with a group. They were to mail these in to the researcher every 2 weeks (telephone calls were used to prompt those who were late mailing in their forms, but this was only needed in a few cases). In the reinforcement group, the participants reported their exercise to a significant other they had selected. The significant other recorded the same information as in the self-monitoring group and mailed the forms in to the researcher on the same schedule. In addition, each time the participant reported exercise, the recorder was to give him or her a token. After collecting nine tokens, the participant could exchange them for a reward. Most of the participants chose their spouse, a parent, or a child as their recorder. The control group participants were told not to keep written records of their exercise and not to use a reward system.

At the end of the 18-week period, the self-monitoring and reward groups showed improvement on their fitness tests, while the control group did not. Both the self-monitoring and reward groups reported significantly more frequent exercise than the control group. Questionnaire and log data for both intervention groups indicated these participants exercised about two times a week for 30 minutes each session throughout the summer (which was less than the goal of three times per week).

Daily or Weekly Self-Monitoring for Home-Based Exercise

In an exercise maintenance phase for adults who had already completed 6 months of home-based exercise training, King et al (11) randomly assigned participants to daily exercise self-monitoring or to weekly self-monitoring conditions. Exercise instructions and self-monitoring information were the same for both groups. The daily self-monitoring group mailed their completed diaries to the staff each month and also received mailings of exercise adherence tips. The weekly monitoring group mailed in their completed diaries every 3 months and did not receive the mailings. Postintervention measurements for this phase of the study revealed that participants assigned to daily self-monitoring reported significantly more exercise sessions than those who self-monitored weekly. Both groups maintained improved fitness compared with baseline. This was consistent with previous research showing that people are more successful in changing behavior when self-monitoring is close in time to the target behavior (12).

Self-Monitoring and Self-Management for Patients with Lung Disease

Atkins et al (16) evaluated several different types of interventions to help patients with chronic obstructive pulmonary disease increase their walking behavior. Patients received exercise prescriptions and then were randomly assigned to one of five experimental groups. Two of the groups were instructed in behavioral strategies based on self-management and the notion that a high-frequency behavior can often be used as a reinforcer for a low-frequency behavior (17). Patients were asked to identify behaviors that were very likely to occur in their daily lives (such as drinking a morning cup of coffee). Then patients were asked to sign a contract stating that this activity would be contingent upon completing their walking assignments. Patients kept a daily log of walking and other exercise, recording information on the time of day, distance covered, total minutes spent walking, heart rate, and any reasons for not walking (such as illness, travel). They were given a runner's watch, which they could earn by keeping their self-monitoring records, but it was up to the patient to implement the self-management program for reinforcing walking. After 3 months, participants in these groups showed significant improvements in exercise tolerance compared with the control patients.

Monitoring and Changing What People Say to Themselves

Self-monitoring also has an important role in another kind of intervention, which is designed to help people recognize and change the negative thoughts that may discourage them from accomplishing their behavioral goals. In the study with chronic obstructive lung disease patients described in the preceding paragraph, Atkins et al tested a cognitive modification strategy designed to change negative thoughts. As in the previously described intervention, interventionists took a 5-minute sample walk with patients. They worked with patients to help them recognize and self-monitor negative self-statements that might interfere with walking, such as "I can't walk without getting short of breath so what is the use?" Negative self-statements such as these may actually lead to patients talking themselves out of trying to exercise. After recognizing such maladaptive thoughts, however, the individual can actively work on replacing them with more positive thoughts that will encourage continued effort. In Atkins' study, interventionists took short walks with the patients and modeled for them how to make positive, goal-oriented self-statements, such as "I am already halfway to my goal; if I keep going, I can make it."

At the end of the intervention phase, cognitive modification patients had similar gains in fitness to the self-monitoring and self-management patients described in the

previous section. However, another group of patients, which received a combination of all of the self-management and cognitive modification strategies (including a relaxation training component) improved most of all. The combined group was the only one with scores that were consistently better than an attention control group across a variety of measures, including general quality of life. This study demonstrated that a combination of cognitive and behavioral strategies for increasing physical activity could be implemented by patients with chronic disease at home, with the help of an interventionist, and that the increased walking was enough to produce significant improvements in fitness.

MOTIVATIONAL INTERVENTIONS

Recent health promotion intervention studies have shown increasing recognition of the importance of interventions that enhance participants' commitment to behavior change as well as how to actually make the changes required. Too often, interventionists eagerly launch into prescribing goals and strategies for change without establishing the participant's readiness for action and are then disappointed by the participant's "resistance" (18). Lifestyle change, such as finding time for at least 30 minutes of moderate exercise each day, can be fairly difficult for many people. Adding more physical activity means giving up something else that seems important to them. Effective interventionists recognize that people usually have some ambivalence about any change and structure their interventions to help tip the balance in favor of the desired change. In this section, we present some methods that can be used with people who are not yet fully committed to a lifestyle change such as increasing their physical activity.

Decision Balance Sheet for Attending an Exercise Class

Hoyt et al (18a) conducted an experiment that tested the effects of motivational balance sheets on attendance at an early morning exercise class. The early morning class was a voluntary activity for university women, mostly faculty wives, and the experiment included women who had signed a class roster with their phone numbers. The intervention was delivered during a telephone call by one of the experimenters. After asking for background information, that experimenter asked the woman if she could give 10 to 15 minutes to answer some questions concerning people's decisions to engage in health improvement programs. Participants were then asked to get some writing materials. They were told that research indicated that writing down advantages and disadvantages of a decision could help them think of factors they did not originally consider. The women were then asked to take a minute to write down each of the following: 1) what they would gain for themselves from regularly attending the class, 2) what they would lose for themselves by attending the class, 3) what others would gain, and 4) what others would lose. Another group of women were asked to go through the decisional balance procedure, but with respect to smoking (if they did not smoke, they wrote down gains and losses for continuing not to smoke). All the women then heard a 2-minute audiotape recording that strongly recommended regular and frequent attendance at the class and were given an opportunity to ask any questions. They were also asked not to discuss the telephone call with other class members. A third group was not contacted at all. The women's exercise class attendance was monitored for 7 weeks following the telephone calls. Women who had completed the exercise class decisional balance sheet attended almost twice as many class sessions (about twice per week) as women in the smoking decisional balance and in the no-contact control group.

Motivational Interviewing to Promote Exercise in a Diabetes Management Program

Cognitive-behavioral interventions targeting exercise have frequently been used in the context of weight control and cardiovascular risk management programs. In an innovative pilot study conducted with older obese women with non-insulin-dependent diabetes, exercise was targeted for change along with diet and blood glucose (19). Participants were 22 women over age 50, 41% of whom were African-American. All participated in a group-based behavioral weight control intervention that consisted of 16 weekly sessions stressing adherence to moderate calorie restriction, low-fat diet, regular activity, and blood glucose monitoring. Group sessions followed a structured written protocol, and participants self-monitored all target behaviors and were provided with weekly reviews and feedback of diary-generated information. The primary mode of physical activity was walking.

Participants were randomly assigned to the standard cognitive-behavioral weight control program or the same program with three individualized sessions that utilized motivational interviewing techniques derived from interventions that have been shown to improve other problem behaviors such as alcohol abuse (18). Motivational interviewing sessions were conducted at the beginning and midway through treatment. These sessions addressed ambivalence about making changes, formulated individuals' goals in behavioral terms, elicited motivational self-statements, and engaged each participant in problem solving regarding obstacles to behavior change. Participants generated a list of costs and benefits of making changes, and the behavioral steps involved in making changes were addressed. The interviewers also used self-monitoring records to identify discrepancies between each participant's current status and his or her goals; this was done in a manner aimed at promoting participants' self-efficacy for behavior change. Interviewers refrained from confrontation, asked open-ended questions, and used reflective listening to elicit each participant's own personal concerns about his or her health status, benefits of behavior change, and reasons not to change. Participants' own words were used to summarize the information generated, and personal goals were developed in a collaborative fashion. Outcome data were available for 16 of the participants; overall, the motivational interviewing group demonstrated better program adherence than the standard behavioral intervention group, including higher attendance, completion of more diaries, more frequent blood glucose monitoring, and a tendency toward more days of exercise.

Motivationally Tailored Interventions in a Worksite Wellness Program

Marcus et al have conducted studies of interventions to increase motivation and increase physical activity in commu-

nity (20) and worksite settings (21). For a recent multiple-worksite study, a series of five self-help manuals were developed, each designed to match one of the five stages of motivational readiness for change (20). For example, the manual for participants at the lowest stage of motivation (precontemplators) was entitled, "Do I Need This?" Its content emphasized increasing awareness of the benefits of activity and encouraging participants to think about what barriers prevented them from becoming more active. The manual for participants at the next level of motivation was entitled, "Try It You'll Like It". Its content emphasized decision making, including reasons to become active and reasons for staying inactive. It also included information on setting realistic goals, rewarding oneself, and eliciting support from others. The other three manuals were entitled, "I'm On My Way," "Keep It Going," and "I Won't Stop Now" for participants who were beginning to increase activity, those who had been active for only a few months, and for those who had been active for a long time, respectively. About 2 to 3 weeks after completing a set of assessment questionnaires (on company time), participants received the manual best matched to their current activity and motivation for exercise. They also received a letter explaining the program. One month later, they received the next manual in the series, another copy of the original manual, and a second personalized letter. Finally, after the 3-month assessment, they received the entire set of five manuals and another individually tailored letter. The researchers compared the effects of providing the motivationally tailored manuals to the effects of providing a standardized intervention consisting of five manuals on physical activity that had been developed by a well-known association that produces high-quality health education materials for the public.

The interventions were offered to employees in 11 companies, and 903 people completed all the study assessments. The employees who had received the motivational intervention were not different in demographic, health, or exercise characteristics at the beginning of the study. However, postintervention assessment showed that those who received the motivational manuals were more likely to report progression in their exercise stage and associated changes in time spent in physical activity.

APPLICATIONS OF COGNITIVE-BEHAVIORAL INTERVENTION PACKAGES FOR PHYSICAL ACTIVITY IN REHABILITATION AND PRIMARY CARE SETTINGS

The success of behavioral interventions in promoting change in different kinds of health behaviors has led to their integration with standard procedures in clinical treatment programs. In high-risk populations, changes in physical activity are often targeted along with diet, smoking, and medication regimens as part of a program package. Studies of such programs demonstrate that cognitive and behavioral interventions can be successfully implemented not only by behavioral experts such as psychologists but also by other healthcare professionals who have received training in these approaches to behavior change. Outcomes often reflect the interactions between the behavioral intervention strategies and other dimensions of exercise such as program structure and intensity and the physical setting.

Cognitive and Behavioral Interventions in Cardiac Rehabilitation

DeBusk et al (22) conducted a well-controlled evaluation of a home-based case management approach to coronary risk factor modification with several hundred post–myocardial infarction patients at five hospitals affiliated with a health maintenance organization. The program was physician-directed, with specially trained nurses conducting the smoking cessation, exercise training, and diet-drug therapy for hyperlipidemia. Patients were recruited on the third day of their hospitalization or as soon as their medical condition stabilized and were randomly assigned to a usual care condition or the special behavioral intervention in addition to usual care.

The special intervention condition included teaching participants to self-monitor behavior change targets, set realistic subgoals, use feedback of progress to motivate and promote health, and use incentives and seek social support to sustain behavior change efforts. Nurses started the intervention with a videotape and had patients begin self-monitoring exercise and other behaviors while still in the hospital. Exercise rehabilitation was not generally provided by the health maintenance organization during the study but was available at various community facilities for a fee. The exercise training component of the special intervention was initiated in the period between hospital discharge and the postdischarge treadmill exercise test. Patients received an activity prescription of walking briskly for at least 20 minutes per day at an intensity that did not cause cardiac symptoms. Following testing, patients received individualized prescriptions. The nurse case managers instructed patients on duration, frequency, intensity, warm-up, regulation of exercise intensity, and recognition of and response to cardiac symptoms.

Case managers contacted patients by telephone 2 weeks after the start of exercise training. Telephone prompts were then conducted at monthly intervals until the sixth month to evaluate any exercise-related problems. At 6 and 12 months post–myocardial infarction, patients were instructed on maintenance strategies. The total intervention time per patient was approximately 9 hours, with 1 hour devoted specifically to exercise. At 6 months, patients receiving the special intervention had significantly higher functional capacity compared with patients receiving usual care and had significantly increased their capacity since beginning the program. This study highlights the benefits of cognitive-behavioral strategies by providers not traditionally trained in behavioral interventions. The positive outcomes are particularly notable in light of the high-risk population and the minimal healthcare professional time required.

Promotion of Physical Activity by Providers in Primary Healthcare Clinics

Primary care interventions could have widespread public health impact because of the numbers of patients seen on a regular basis. Although physician-based interventions could be especially effective, their implementation may not be perceived as feasible in many settings given the considerable barriers of limited time, lack of reimbursement for health promotion counseling, lack of training in behavioral counseling methods, and lack of perceived effectiveness as a counselor (23). Project PACE (Physician-based Assessment and Counseling for Exercise) was developed to overcome these barriers and allow for cost-effective counseling of healthy sedentary adults.

An efficacy trial of PACE was conducted using a quasi-experimental design, matching control physicians to intervention physicians on patient demographics and medical specialty (23). Seventeen physician offices participated in the study, with specialties including family medicine, obstetrics/gynecology, and internal medicine. Participants were 225 sedentary adults who were scheduled for a check-up visit and who had no history of coronary heart disease or other conditions that could limit mobility. In order to control for training time, physicians in the intervention condition were trained to deliver the PACE intervention and those in the control condition received training in current procedures for diagnosing and treating hepatitis. Patients' baseline activity information and demographic information were obtained by telephone prior to the doctor's office visit.

The PACE intervention involved use of motivational stage-based interventions for patients classified according to their responses to brief questionnaires completed while they waited for their appointments. During the visit, the physician reviewed the questionnaire with the patient and counseled the patient regarding benefits of exercise, goals, and behavioral strategies according to stage-matched protocols. Each counseling session required 3 to 5 minutes. Intervention patients were also contacted by telephone for a 10-minute booster session with research staff to answer questions and discuss progress. If requested, exercise tip sheets on relevant topics were mailed. Control patients did not receive counseling or phone calls.

Follow-up information on patient activity patterns was obtained by telephone interview 4 to 6 weeks following the scheduled office visit. A subsample of patients participated in physical activity monitoring with an electronic accelerometer. Significant changes in activity levels were observed for patients receiving the PACE counseling. Fifty-two percent of the intervention patients moved from being a sedentary "contemplator" to "active" exercising, compared with only 12% of the control patients. Intervention patients reported a significantly greater number of minutes per week spent walking and also had greater activity counts on accelerometer measures.

SUMMARY

There is much important information about the effects of cognitive and behavioral interventions for exercise promotion across time, settings, and populations that will only be known through additional research. Although they have been incorporated into large-scale community prevention studies, cognitive and behavioral interventions for promoting physical activity and exercise have primarily been developed and tested in settings in which trained providers worked directly with individuals or small groups of individuals. We do not yet know what is the best way to apply the kinds of cognitive and behavioral techniques described in this chapter in attempts to change the behaviors of very large groups of people, such as the population of an entire city or state. Until recently, most studies of cognitive-behavioral interventions for physical activity and exercise have also been of brief duration. Results from studies with longer follow-up suggest that people who successfully increase their physical activity tend to relapse to lower levels of activity within 6 months, or—at most—a year or two, unless there is some kind of follow-up. Most exercise promotion programs combine the use of several types of cognitive and behavioral interventions, and there are very few studies that have examined the efficacy of the individual program components. Because of this, we often still do not know which components are most important, how big a "dose" of the intervention is required, or under what circumstances they are needed to make up a successful package. With a few notable exceptions (24,25), there is as yet very little research on interventions that promote adherence to briefer bouts of moderate activity and the new "lifestyle physical activity" recommendations (1). Nevertheless, the examples we have discussed show that there are many situations in which cognitive and behavioral approaches can help people increase physical activity or adhere to exercise prescriptions. We believe that new, creative applications of cognitive and behavioral strategies and further developments in the theories that guide these interventions will continue to extend the effectiveness of current approaches.

REFERENCES

1. Pate RR, Pratt M, Blair SN, et al. Physical activity and public health: a recommendation from the Centers for Disease Control and Prevention and the American College of Sports Medicine. JAMA 1995;273:402–407.

2. U.S. Department of Health and Human Services. Physical activity and health: a report of the Surgeon General. Atlanta, GA: U.S. Department of Health and Human Services, Centers for Disease Control and Prevention, National Center for Chronic Disease Prevention and Health Promotion, 1996.

3. Dishman RK, Sallis JF. Determinants and interventions for physical activity and exercise. In: Bouchard C, Shephard RJ, Stephens T, eds. Physical activity, fitness, and health. Champaign, IL: Human Kinetics 1994:214–238.

4. Dishman RK, Buckworth J. Increasing physical activity: a quantitative synthesis. Med Sci Sports Exerc 1996;28(6):706–719.

5. Epstein LH, Wing RR, Thompson JK, Griffin W. Attendance and fitness in aerobics exercise. Behav Modif 1980;4(4):465–479.

6. Robison JI, Rogers MA, Carlson JJ, et al. Effects of a 6-month incentive-based exercise program on adherence and work capacity. Med Sci Sports Exerc 1992;24(1):85–93.

7. Epstein LH, Valoski AM, Vara LS, et al. Effects of decreasing sedentary behavior and increasing activity on weight change in obese children. Health Psychol 1995; 14(2):109–115.

8. Brownell KD, Stunkard AJ, Albaum JM. Evaluation and modification of exercise patterns in the natural environment. Am J Psychiatry 1980;137(12):1540–1545.

9. Gossard D, Haskell WI, Taylor CB, et al. Effects of low and high intensity home-based exercise training on functional capacity in healthy middle aged men. Am J Cardiol 1986;57:446–449.

10. Juneau M, Rogers F, DeSantos V, et al. Effectiveness of self-monitored, home-based moderate-intensity exercise training in middle-aged men and women. Am J Cardiol 1987;60:66–70.

11. King AC, Taylor CB, Haskell WL, DeBusk RF. Strategies for increasing early adherence to and long-term maintenance of home-based exercise training in healthy middle-aged men and women. Am J Cardiol 1988;61:628–632.

12. Bandura A. Social foundations of thought and action: a social cognitive theory. Englewood Cliffs, NJ: Prentice-Hall, 1986.

13. Gouvier WD, Richards JS, Blanton PD, et al. Behavior modification in physical therapy. Arch Phys Med Rehabil 1985;66:113–116.

14. Neef NA, Bill-Harvey D, Shad D, et al. Exercise participation with videotaped modeling: effects on balance and gait in elderly residents of care facilities. Behav Ther 1995;26:135–151.

15. Noland MP. The effects of self-monitoring and reinforcement on exercise adherence. Res Q Exerc Sport 1989;60(3):216–224.

16. Atkins CJ, Kaplan RM, Timms RM, et al. Behavioral exercise programs in the management of chronic obstructive pulmonary disease. J Consult Clin Psychol 1984;52: 591–603.

17. Premack D. Reinforcement theory. In: Levine D, ed. Nebraska symposium on motivation. Lincoln: University of Nebraska Press, 1965:123–180.

18. Miller WR, Rollnick S. Motivational interviewing. New York: Guilford, 1991.

18a. Hoyt MF, Janis IL. Increasing adherence to a stressful decision via a motivational balance-sheet procedure: a field experiment. J Pers Soc Psychol 1975;31:833–839.

19. Smith DE, Heckemeyer CM, Kratt PP, Mason DA. Motivational interviewing to improve adherence to a behavioral weight control program for older obese women with NIDDM. Diabetes Care 1997;20: 52–54.

20. Marcus BH, Banspach SW, Lefebvre RC, et al. Increasing the adoption of physical activity among community participants. Am J Health Promotion 1992;6:424–429.

21. Marcus BH, Emmons KM, Simkin-Silverman L, et al. Evaluation of motivationally-tailored versus standard self-help physical activity interventions in the workplace. Am J Health Promotion 1998;12: 246–253.

22. DeBusk RF, Houston N, Superko R, et al. A case-management

system for coronary risk factor modification after acute myocardial infarction. Ann Intern Med 1994;120:721–729.

23. Calfas KJ, Long BJ, Sallis JF, et al. A controlled trial of physician counseling to promote the adoption of physical activity. Prev Med 1996;25:225–233.

24. Dunn AL, Garcia ME, Marcus BH, et al. Six-month physical activity and fitness change in Project Active, a randomized trial. Med Sci Sports Exerc 1998;30:1076–1083.

25. Dunn AL, Marcus BH, Kampert JB, et al. Comparison of lifestyle and structured interventions to increase physical activity and cardiorespiratory fitness. JAMA 1999;281:327–334.

Chapter 47

Behavioral Approaches to Enhancing Smoking Cessation

Karen M. Emmons
Stefania Maggi

Cigarette smoking is an intractable public health problem that poses a great threat to the health of the entire population. Although significant strides have been made to reduce smoking prevalence among certain segments of the population, there are important areas in which gains have been minimal. The purpose of this chapter is to provide a brief overview of the health and social consequences of smoking, to review reasons for smoking and motivations for quitting, and to review key behavioral approaches to enhancing smoking cessation. This is not a comprehensive review, but rather a summary of the most effective approaches to date, and of the most promising strategies that are currently being studied.

HEALTH CONSEQUENCES OF SMOKING

Cigarette smoking continues to be the leading preventable cause of chronic disease, especially for coronary heart disease (CHD) and cancer (1–4). Cigarette smoking accounts for 18% of all newly diagnosed (5), and is associated with, cancer of the lung, oral cavity, larynx, esophagus, bladder, kidney, pancreas, stomach, cervix, and colon. Smoking accounts for 20% of all heart disease (6). In addition, prospective studies from several different countries have found that smokers have a two- to fourfold increased incidence of CHD, and a two- to fourfold greater risk of sudden death than nonsmokers. Smoking also increases risk of stroke in both men and women, with smokers having a twofold greater risk of stroke compared to nonsmokers; this risk is dose-dependent, and appears to be strongest in younger groups (7). Although cigarette smoking is an independent risk factor for both CHD and cancer, it also interacts synergistically with other risk factors (e.g., hypertension, diabetes, occupational exposures to carcinogens) to further increase risk. Further, smoking plays a primary role in the development of several respiratory diseases, including chronic obstructive pulmonary disease and emphysema. Maternal smoking during pregnancy is associated with low birth weight, spontaneous abortions, and other serious pregnancy complications and birth defects (8). In utero exposure to maternal smoking has also been associated with deficits in the child's lung function, increased risk of respiratory illness in early infancy, and growth retardation groups (7), and exposure to parental smoking postpartum is associated with sudden infant death syndrome (SIDS).

Smoking is also a major contributor to preventable mortality. Worldwide, about 3 million people die each year from smoking-related diseases (9); it is estimated that by the year 2025 this figure will rise to over 10 million deaths per year. In 1990, over 430,000 smokers in the United States alone died from smoking-related diseases, accounting for 26% of all deaths among men and 17% of deaths among women (10). Forty percent of the smoking-related deaths are from heart disease, 19% from lung cancer, 33% from other cancers, 6% from stroke, and 2% from other diseases (9). Estimates from a prospective evaluation of 1.2 million individuals in the American Cancer Society's Cancer Prevention Study II found that from 1982 to 1986, the overall mortality ratio was 2.22 for men and 1.60 for women who smoked 1 to 20 cigarettes per day, and 2.43 for men and 2.10 for women who smoked more than 20 cigarettes per day. In 1993, the estimated smoking-attributed costs for medical care, lost work, and productivity exceeded $97 billion. If these costs were to be borne by smokers in the form of cigarette taxes, the price of each pack of cigarettes would have to rise to $4 (7). Unaccounted for in these estimates is the cost of illness among nonsmokers who become ill as a result of exposure to second-hand smoke, which is related to the development of both lung cancer (11) and heart disease (12).

SMOKING PREVALENCE AND EPIDEMIOLOGY

Although the prevalence of cigarette smoking has decreased in the United States and much of the developed world over the past 2 decades, it is increasing in many developing countries. It is estimated that there are 1.1 billion smokers worldwide. In 1996, 23.6% of the U.S. population were smokers (13). Educational level is the most important predictor of smoking status; 35.6% of individuals with 9 to 11 years of education smoke, compared to 16.5% of those with a college degree (14). The socioeconomic disparity in smoking status found in the United States is also observed worldwide, with estimates suggesting that by the year 2025 only 15% of the world's smokers will live in rich countries. Although the gender gap in smoking prevalence has narrowed considerably, men still smoke at a slightly but significantly higher rate than women (27% versus 22.6%, respectively) (15). Differences among racial/ethnic groups also exist; smoking prevalence is highest among individuals categorized as American Indian or Alaskan Native (41.9%); smoking prevalence is virtually equivalent among whites and African-Americans (27.3%). Gender by race interactions have also been found (with smoking prevalence being higher among African-American than white men, and lower among African-American than white women), and other subgroup differences in smoking among minority groups have been noted (16).

Cigarette smoking among younger individuals remains a major public health concern. Nearly all smoking initiation occurs before high school graduation, and each day 3000 teenagers start to smoke. Among high school seniors, the prevalence of daily cigarette smoking decreased from 29% to 19.5% from 1976 to 1984. Since 1984, however, there has been little reduction in smoking prevalence among adolescents, with the current prevalence at 19%. Of note however, smoking prevalence among African-American youth decreased dramatically, from 27% in 1976 to just 4% in 1990; smoking prevalence among African-American youth has been under 10% since 1986 (14).

PREVALENCE OF SMOKING CESSATION

Despite the fact that about one quarter of the U.S. population still smokes, it has been estimated that 50% of all adults in the United States who ever smoked regularly have quit (17). This represents a remarkable shift in the health behaviors of the U.S. population. Approximately 5% to 10% of smokers quit smoking on their own and remain abstinent for 12 months. Cessation rates are initially much higher among those who participate in smoking cessation programs, but abstinence rates decline significantly over time. An examination of trends in smoking cessation outcomes, for example, revealed that the average 6- and 12-month abstinence rates are roughly 30% to

35% (18); programs that focus specifically on relapse prevention tend to have slightly better outcomes. Although some may consider these outcomes to be disappointing, they are significant from a public health perspective, especially in light of the enormous economic and health costs of smoking. It is also important to recognize that relapse may be an important part of the cessation process. Smokers who have been successful in achieving long-term abstinence report having stopped and relapsed multiple times prior to ultimate long-term cessation. Therefore, relapse should not be considered failure, but rather a step toward the ultimate goal of long-term cessation.

The availability of pharmacologic aids (e.g., nicotine gum, transdermal nicotine patch) for smoking cessation has helped to increase cessation rates. Nicotine replacement therapies (NRTs) have been developed in order to provide nicotine without the adverse health consequences associated with the constituents of cigarettes, and therefore give the smoker a means to reduce nicotine withdrawal symptoms while simultaneously dealing with the behavioral and psychological components of smoking cessation. Studies of NRT have yielded a doubling of smoking cessation rates over that found with placebo, particularly for smokers who are heavily dependent on nicotine (19). In addition, combining NRT with behavioral intervention strategies, such as those described later in this chapter, has been found to further increase smoking cessation rates.

REASONS FOR SMOKING

It is clear that smoking is the result of multiple determinants that range from social, psychological, economic, and physiologic (20–23). *Social factors* have typically been considered to be of most importance in the *initiation* of smoking. However, recent evidence focusing on smoking among lower income populations, where smoking prevalence remains the highest, suggests that social factors are also very important in the *maintenance* of smoking behavior. For example, having a partner who smokes is one of the most important predictors of postpartum relapse among women who quit smoking during pregnancy (24). In addition, an evaluation of smoking among the social networks of employees in manufacturing workplaces suggests that social norms, particularly related to social pressure, social support, and social rewards, are important predictors of readiness to change and self-efficacy, which are two key predictors of smoking cessation (25). Further, many former smokers cite social pressure as an important impetus for quitting smoking.

Research in the past decade has also examined the relationship between smoking and *psychological factors*, most notably depression (26,27). Individuals with a history of mood disorder are more likely to smoke, and the incidence of current depression and severity of depression have been found to have a linear relationship with smoking status. Among all smokers, dysphoric mood is a common antecedent of relapse (26,28). Further, depressed smokers are 40% less likely to quit, compared to their nondepressed counterparts (26). Smokers with a history of depression also experience more severe withdrawal symptoms when they quit smoking (29). There have also been some reports in the literature of increased risk of developing depressive symptomatology following smoking cessation, especially among those with *a priori* mood disturbance, which may in turn affect long-term maintenance (30). The few studies that have investigated the efficacy of antidepressant medications in smoking cessation have been equivocal; the recent Agency for Health Care Policy Research (AHCPR) Smoking Guideline concluded that, because of the paucity of data in this area, no recommendations about the use of antidepressant medication for smoking cessation can be made. This is an area in which a tremendous amount of research is under way, and it is anticipated that more outcome data regarding existing and new products will be available in the near future.

There is also a need to investigate nonpharmacologic strategies for addressing the relationship between smoking and depression. One innovative study for which preliminary data are available compared a smoking cessation program to smoking cessation plus a cognitive-behavioral treatment for depression (31). This study was conducted among 179 smokers who had a history of major depression, but were not currently depressed. Although there were no main effects, there was a treatment by craving interaction, such that smokers who reported high craving for cigarettes had significantly higher quit rates in the combined smoking/depression intervention. Of note, only one third of the sample reported an increase in depressive symptomatology after quitting smoking. Further research is needed to elucidate the role of depression in smoking cessation outcomes, and to identify the most effective intervention strategies for targeting smokers with a history of depression.

Economic factors also play an important role in smoking behavior. Smoking, like many other risk factors for chronic disease, is more prevalent among lower socioeconomic groups (32,33). A large quantity of research has documented the impact of social conditions on both health and health behaviors (34–39). It is not surprising that health behaviors as well as health outcomes are strongly related to social conditions. Distal social structural forces clearly shape people's day-to-day experiences (40), such that even when individuals are interested in changing their health habits, it may be difficult to control the target health behaviors (41). For example, Hillary Graham has conducted an excellent analysis of the impact of social and economic factors on smoking among women in England (23). Graham concluded that different dynamics drive the smoking habits of low-income women, compared to middle- and upper-income women. She identified four categories of influence, including: 1) everyday responsibilities (e.g., child care, caring for other family members) and patterns of paid work; 2) material circumstances (e.g., housing situation, partner's employment, income and benefit status, access to transportation and telephone); 3) social support and social networks (e.g., relationships with partner, family, and friendship networks, feelings of belonging); and 4) personal and health resources (e.g., physical and psychosocial health, health beliefs, health behaviors, alternative coping strategies). Following an extensive qualitative study and analysis, she concluded that low-income women use smoking as a means of coping with their economic pressures and the resulting demands placed on them to care for others. Having to care for more, while simultaneously living on less, provided the context in which relatively few of the low-income women who were

studied attempted or succeeded at smoking cessation. Compared to women who had never smoked or who had successfully quit smoking, the continuing smokers tended to be caring for others in circumstances that constrained, rather than supported lifestyle change. Graham concluded that the overall pattern of difficulties and disadvantage faced by low-income women who smoke suggests that their adaptive capacity may already be taxed to the limit. This work emphasizes the importance of addressing social contextual factors in intervention strategies for smoking cessation whenever possible.

The *physically addictive properties* of nicotine are also well known. Like other psychoactive drugs (e.g., cocaine, heroin, alcohol), nicotine serves as a reinforcer of its use, and meets criteria for abuse liability in humans. The nicotine withdrawal syndrome, which is now well characterized (42), includes craving to use nicotine, irritability, anxiety, difficulty concentrating, restlessness, and increased appetite. Nicotine addiction is pervasive among smokers and can be a key barrier to long-term abstinence. This is an area in which there have been considerable treatment advances in the past several years, with the advent of NRTs and other products designed to help the nicotine dependent smoker (see Chapter 5). However, in addition to biologic processes, addictions are also affected by behavioral and psychological processes. The fact that smoking has an addictive component does not obviate the use of behavioral, educational, social, and policy strategies to promote cessation. The focus of this chapter is on behavioral intervention strategies for smoking cessation. It should be noted that the efficacy of many of these strategies can be improved by combining them with NRT, particularly for the more physically dependent smoker.

MOTIVATION TO QUIT SMOKING: IMPLICATIONS FOR BEHAVIORAL INTERVENTIONS

Historically, most smoking cessation interventions have been skill-based, and thus have been designed to exclusively target smoking *cessation*, with very little emphasis placed on helping individuals who were not planning to quit. However, a large body of work conducted in the past decade has clearly demonstrated that motivation is an important component of the behavioral change process (43–46). Rather than using a "one size fits all" approach, smoking intervention efforts should be matched to smokers' readiness, or level of motivation for cessation. For example, a smoker who is only beginning to contemplate cessation would not benefit from a smoking cessation program focused on *how* to quit. Instead, efforts to raise this smoker's awareness about the negative aspects of smoking might be more likely to increase his or her readiness to quit. For smokers who are very interested in smoking cessation and ready to take the next steps toward quitting, action-oriented intervention strategies such as those outlined in this chapter are most appropriate.

BEHAVIORAL SMOKING CESSATION STRATEGIES

Substantial scientific and community resources have been dedicated to efforts to increase rates of smoking cessation (7,47).

Strategies that have been used range from extensive media-based campaigns addressing prevention and cessation for the general public, to interventions tailored toward the individual. The purpose of this section is to present the variety of *components* that are most commonly included in behavioral smoking cessation interventions, beginning with assessment strategies and concluding with strategies that can be effective adjuncts to behavioral intervention components (e.g., pharmacologic treatments, physical activity). The subsequent section is a review of the various *types of cessation programs* that contain these intervention components, including minimal contact (e.g., self-help interventions, mass media interventions) and intensive interventions (e.g., individual and group counseling). Regardless of the mode of delivery, most smoking cessation programs focus on providing the behavioral skills thought to be necessary for achieving initial cessation and for maintaining abstinence.

Based upon the principles of classic behaviorism, most of the treatment programs for smoking cessation aim to modify and extinguish the smoking habit (48). The earliest behavioral approaches viewed cigarette smoking merely as a measurable behavior that was guided by principles of respondent and operant conditioning. Newer behavioral approaches, however, recognize the complexity of the interactions between psychological and physiologic factors that contribute to the smoker's career (31). Moreover, the evidence that nicotine is a highly addictive drug led to the inclusion of NRT in smoking cessation interventions. Although medications such as transdermal nicotine patches and nicotine gum are not behavioral strategies, they are often used to help the client cope with nicotine withdrawal symptoms so to maximize the effects of behavioral intervention strategies. The remainder of this section reviews the key components of behavioral smoking interventions.

Assessment

The AHCPR Smoking Cessation Guideline summarizes recommendations for smoking cessation specialists, highlighting key components of quality smoking cessation programs. One key concept is the importance of a thorough assessment before treatment initiation, which allows the provider to assess the smokers' need for motivational, behavioral, and pharmacologic strategies. It is recommended that healthcare providers screen *all patients* regarding their smoking status at every contact; if a patient is interested in cessation, his or her appropriateness for NRT should be determined. A more detailed or specialized assessment to gauge potential for successful quitting can also be very informative. Some factors have been found to be particularly relevant to smoking cessation, and should be included in an assessment. These include an indication of how much the person wants to quit smoking (motivational level), the level of confidence in one's ability to quit smoking (self-efficacy), how much support for quitting is provided by friends and relatives (social support), the presence of other psychiatric conditions (e.g., depression, anxiety), and the level of stress the person is experiencing. A thorough assessment phase also includes an opportunity for the smoker to consider his or her future plans regarding smoking, and to set some goals about cessation. Some people may feel that they will eventually want to quit, but are not ready yet. In that case they may decide they want to reduce the number of cig-arettes smoked for a certain amount of time before they actually quit. Other smokers may be ready to change, and they may set cessation as their short-term goal. Whichever is the case, the role of the counselor is to make sure that the client is prepared for the target behavior change and sets goals that are realistic (49).

Behavioral Intervention Components

Several behavioral strategies are typically combined into cessation programs. These typically include self-monitoring, stimulus control, social support, nicotine fading, cold turkey, goal setting, and behavioral and cognitive coping strategies. Newer strategies that can be used as adjuncts to behavioral approaches include pharmacologic interventions and physical activity.

Self-Monitoring

Smoking is a complex behavior that can be greatly affected by mood and other social factors. Self-monitoring requires smokers to keep track and record the number of cigarettes smoked, and the circumstances surrounding each cigarette smoked. The goal is to identify key patterns that influence each individual's smoking behavior. Self-monitoring produces a written record, or "baseline," of the individual's smoking, and also provides a way to keep track of the progress made throughout the quitting process. A preprinted card or piece of paper that can be inserted in or attached to the cigarette pack is commonly used since it is thought to facilitate the client's self-monitoring; computerized devices are also available. Self-monitoring records typically include the time, place, and circumstances surrounding each cigarette smoked, but can also be customized to include categories that an individual feels are most relevant to his or her situation. The primary purpose of self-monitoring is usually to establish smoking patterns and to document progress in reducing the number of cigarettes smoked. However, the information collected via self-monitoring can also be used to identify and understand key events that may have influenced relapse among quitters who later experience a slip.

Stimulus Control

Smoking is thought to be a learned behavior that is strengthened through repeated associations with the immediate positive consequences of smoking, as well as with interpersonal and environmental factors. In other words, over years of smoking, an individual builds repeated associations with cigarette smoking and key physiologic and psychological cues (e.g., stress, relaxation, key environmental stimuli). Studies have demonstrated that recent quitters have physiologic responses to smoking-related cues, suggesting that these associations are strong and lasting (50,51). If multiple environmental cues trigger urges to smoke across a large variety of situations, then quitting can be a much more difficult process. Stimulus control strategies for smoking cessation are often utilized to break and extinguish the positive associations smokers have between environmental variables and smoking. Accordingly, stimulus control techniques include the rearrangement of the external cues that trigger smoking as well as the alteration of the consequences of smoking. For example, a smoker can minimize the number of cues to smoke by watching TV in a different room than he or she is used to smoking in, by going for coffee in a smoke-free restaurant rather than one where smoking is allowed, or by temporarily eliminating foods and/or activities that are associated with smoking (e.g., having a drink with friends after work, drinking coffee).

As a first step, smokers use self-monitoring to establish the circumstances that typically govern their smoking. Based on this data, they develop active strategies for breaking the relationship between cues that trigger their smoking and their smoking behavior. Smokers can either alter these triggers, or totally avoid the triggers to the extent possible. For example, many smokers tend to smoke in specific and predictable locations (e.g., in the car, on the telephone, while drinking coffee). Once these situations or triggers are identified, smokers can begin to reduce the number of cigarettes they smoke in these circumstances. Over time, the number of situations that trigger the urge to smoke will be greatly reduced. Another stimulus control strategy is to allow smoking only in "deprived" or unpleasant circumstances, such as a garage or basement, in which there are no other secondary gains provided (e.g., watching TV, socializing). Not only does this reduce the number of smoking-related cues, but it may also create new associations between smoking and environmental cues that are not pleasant. As the smoker begins to perceive smoking as a negative event (e.g., having to leave a favorite TV show or an engaging conversation in order to go to the basement and smoke), he or she may start to perceive smoking as an unpleasant experience that is less reinforcing.

Nicotine Fading

Nicotine fading is a procedure that is intended to address both psychological and pharmacologic factors (52–55). The rationale behind this strategy is that cigarettes are physically addicting for many smokers, and gradually reducing their nicotine intake will reduce the intensity of their withdrawal symptoms when they quit. In this approach, smokers first identify the nicotine content of their cigarettes; after they set a quit date, they approach it by switching brands to progressively lower nicotine content cigarettes over a period of a few weeks. Nicotine fading is often combined with self-monitoring of the progress toward lower nicotine intake, providing smokers with immediate feedback about their efforts. Nicotine fading seems to be effective at increasing self-efficacy and assisting more addicted smokers in the cessation process (40). However, this strategy is of limited usefulness with smokers whose usual brand of cigarettes is low in nicotine. Further, many smokers may compensate for the reduced nicotine content of the lower-nicotine brands by changing their smoking pattern (e.g., inhaling more deeply, smoking more of each cigarette), which will maximize the amount of nicotine they receive even from low-nicotine cigarettes. One way to reduce this compensatory smoking may be to increase smokers' awareness of this tendency, and to highlight the importance of not changing their smoking typology. Another alternative for reducing the amount of nicotine consumed prior to quitting is to reduce the number of cigarettes smoked per day. This strategy has the added benefit of reducing the number of situations in which the individual smokes, and thus helps him or her adjust gradually to dealing with more and more situations without smoking.

Cold Turkey

In contrast to the nicotine fading procedure, "cold turkey" is a strategy in which smokers give up cigarettes on a specific day, with no intermediate reductions in smoking rate. The smoker typically selects a quit date on which he or she will stop smoking completely. This strategy is most effective if the individual prepares for the quit date by developing coping strategies. A strong emphasis on relapse prevention is also recommended as part of the quitting preparation process. Regardless of whether the individual decides to quit cold turkey or gradually, using nicotine fading, setting a target quit day in advance is an important strategy for maximizing the changes of successful quitting.

Coping Strategies

Smoking cessation programs may include training in either behavioral coping skills, cognitive coping skills; or both. *Behavioral coping strategies* are thought to help the individual identify and substitute smoking related behaviors with effective non-smoking behaviors. Examples may be eliminating ashtrays from home or work or substituting other behaviors for smoking, such as eating or exercising. Relaxation is another type of behavioral coping strategy that may work particularly well for the large percentage of smokers who report smoking because of stress, or who are extremely anxious about the prospect of quitting (26). The rationale for using relaxation training is that people tend to relapse more often when they are experiencing negative emotional states (28,56). It is believed that training a person to self-induce a relaxation state will increase his or her ability to cope with negative emotions and with stressful situations. Examples of relaxation techniques may include taking deep breaths and practicing deep muscle relaxation. As smokers learn to identify parts of their bodies that are tense, they can also learn to utilize relaxation strategies to produce a state of calmness across a variety of situations.

Cognitive coping skills are those that aim to change the way the individual thinks about smoking and its consequences. That is, most smokers associate smoking with pleasurable sensations, such as relaxation and socializing. Many smokers also feel that they will be unable to cope with negative mood situations without smoking. Cognitive strategies focus on helping smokers learn to reframe the way they think about smoking, and view it as a negative behavior (e.g., smoking gets in the way of doing things that are important to me). Cognitive strategies also focus on breaking cessation down into smaller steps, and shifting the focus from "I can't ever smoke again," to "I'm not going to smoke today." Smokers are typically taught to avoid self-defeating attributions and the resulting negative emotional reactions that promote continued smoking.

Use of coping strategies is particularly important in high-risk situations, not only to avoid relapse but also to increase self-efficacy about ability to cope with urges to smoke (8). In contrast, failure to cope initiates a chain of events in which diminished self-efficacy may lead to a slip, and perhaps to a full-blown relapse (57,58).

Pharmacological Interventions

Between 46% and 90% of smokers experience at least some withdrawal symptoms when abstinent (59,60). For these smokers, withdrawal symptoms can be a significant barrier to quitting and remaining abstinent. The administration of pharmacologic adjuncts such as transdermal nicotine patches, nicotine gum, and nicotine nasal sprays is intended to alleviate the symptoms that smokers experience in the first phase of the quitting process. The levels of nicotine delivered by these products allow smokers to gradually reduce their nicotine levels, rather than to experience the abrupt elimination of this addictive substance. Transdermal nicotine patches have been found to double 6- and 12-month quit rates, compared to placebo; the nicotine patch is considered to be an effective aid to smoking cessation (19,61). A variety of other nicotine replacement products and nicotine-free drugs are currently being evaluated as smoking cessation aids; among the nicotine-free drugs that are currently being evaluated is the antidepressant bupropion, better know as Zyban, which has been recently approved by the Food and Drug Administration as a prescription drug for the indication of smoking cessation. Although large-scale evaluations are needed to determine Zyban's ultimate utility as smoking cessation strategy, there seems to be some evidence of its efficacy (96,97).

Physical Activity

Recent evidence suggests that physical activity may provide a healthful alternative to smoking that enhances the achievement of smoking cessation and decreases the likelihood of relapse following smoking cessation (62–64). Physical activity has several benefits to offer individuals who are trying to quit smoking. First, participation in vigorous activity in particular may reduce the weight gain associated with smoking cessation. Second, exercise may moderate mood changes, and thus be helpful as a coping mechanism for managing negative affect as well as nicotine withdrawal (65–69). Although additional large-scale randomized trials are needed to determine the overall efficacy of exercise as an adjunctive smoking cessation strategy, there is sufficient evidence in the literature to suggest that exercise may be helpful to a large number of smokers as they enter the smoking cessation process.

TYPES OF SMOKING CESSATION MATERIALS AND PROGRAMS

Smoking cessation programs typically combine several of the components discussed in the previous section. There are a variety of smoking cessation programs, which vary in format and intensity. Orleans et al (70) make a distinction between minimal-contact strategies and more intensive counseling-based interventions, which represent two ends of a continuum. Minimal-contact interventions range from the use of self-help material to the addition of adjunctive pharmacotherapy and/or follow-up telephone counseling. In a medical setting, minimal-contact interventions may consist of a brief assessment of smoking history, personalized medical advice to quit smoking, and self-quitting guides. More intensive treatment, on the other hand, typically includes structured and intensive contact, either on an individual basis or in a group setting.

This section presents a brief review of minimal-contact intervention strategies (self-help interventions, media-based interventions, and Web site interventions), as well as more intensive smoking cessation programs (counseling, group, and community-based treatment programs).

Minimal-Contact Interventions

Minimal-contact interventions are considered most appropriate for population-based efforts, in which the goal is to disseminate cessation-related information to broad segments of the population. These types of intervention strategies are likely to be most effective with individuals who have had previous success with minimal-contact strategies, and are recommended as the first course of action for individuals who haven't previously tried to quit (71).

Self-Help Interventions

Self-help materials are an important starting point for many smokers who are considering cessation (44). In fact, about 90% of U.S. smokers report having quit without the help of a smoking cessation program (72). Self-help materials may play an important role in the success of many smokers in that these written materials, videotapes, or audiotapes provide a wide range of information on "do-it-yourself" quitting strategies. The purposes of self-help materials are typically to: 1) increase smokers' motivation to change their smoking habit; 2) target all stages of the cessation process; 3) address health and social consequences of smoking; and 4) address strategies for quitting, maintenance of nonsmoking behavior, and relapse prevention (73). Self-help manuals may stress the importance of identifying a quitting date, training in relaxation techniques, or other coping strategies. They can also be tailored to specific populations, including pregnant women or cultural minorities (74). Self-help interventions have been found to be cost-effective, although the quit rates produced are lower than those found for more intensive strategies (44). For a comprehensive list of self-help materials available for healthcare providers, see Orleans et al (70).

The addition of NRT to self-help materials has not been found to increase quit rates (44); to the contrary, some studies have found that this treatment combination yielded poorer outcomes compared to self-help alone (75). There is some evidence from a study of volunteers that suggests that computer-generated personalized feedback, designed to enhance smokers' self-efficacy about quitting, significantly increases initial and long-term cessation rates (76); however, these results were not replicated in a study with nonvolunteer smokers (77,78).

Telephone counseling, as an adjunct to self-help materials, has recently received considerable research attention (79,80). Telephone contacts may be a practical alternative to follow-up visits and may be effective in boosting adherence to self-quitting protocols, promoting initial cessation, and aiding long-term abstinence (81). Telephone counseling may follow a face-to-face visit at which the client received smoking cessation self-help material, or may be conducted only over the telephone. Studies that have incorporated telephone counseling follow-up with self-help materials have found some intervention effects, although these effects have not typically been long-lasting (77,82,83). Efforts to improve the effectiveness of telephone-based intervention strategies are underway.

Smoker Quitlines

Smoker hotlines or "quitlines" are another minimal-contact intervention that use the telephone as a channel for delivery. Telephone quitlines are different from telephone counseling in that they are reactive (the smoker initiates the call); in contrast, telephone counseling involves proactive outreach to the smoker. Quitlines range from prerecorded nonsmoking messages (84) to hotline counselors who do crisis intervention with callers who have recently relapsed (28). The 1-800-4-CANCER help line is an NCI hotline in which all counselors are trained to provide behavioral smoking cessation counseling for smokers at different stages of change, as well as to provide self-help resources that apply to the callers' specific needs (85). Quitlines have been found to increase smoking cessation rates (86), although it has been found that only about 1% to 2% of the population are likely to use these hotlines (44,87).

Internet Web Sites

Since computers and the Internet have become more and more accessible, several home pages addressed to smokers have recently appeared. Although the efficacy and popularity of smoking cessation materials on the Internet have not yet been assessed, it is possible that they will be preferred to other intervention approaches by some smokers. Advantages of the Internet include that it can be easily accessed through a home computer, and also that it provides immediate access to the information requested. Some home pages provide menus of choices on a variety of issues related to smoking, as well as complete smoking cessation packages at no direct cost. In 1996, Wellness Web presented the "Patient's Network," a Web site that touches on numerous health topics, including a smoker's clinic. Similarly, the Centers for Disease Control and Prevention recently opened a Web site called "Tobacco Information & Prevention Sourcepage," and the Cancer Society of New Zealand recently opened the site "Lifestyle Smoke-Free." No outcome data are yet available by which to evaluate the effectiveness of these Web-based interventions.

Media-based programs

Network television has been another channel for delivery of minimal smoking cessation interventions. Televised programs for smoking cessation may be included in the context of the local news programs (88), or broadcast independently for consecutive days (89). One advantage of media-based programs is that they greatly increase the penetration of smoking cessation materials into the general population of smokers (44). They may include motivational messages, training in coping strategies and relapse prevention, and a focus on social influences and social norms.

Intensive Smoking Cessation Programs

Healthcare providers have been found to play a very important role in the smoking cessation process. Brief, physician-delivered interventions have been found to increase smoking cessation rates, and as a result the AHCPR guideline recommends that healthcare providers counsel all smokers about their smoking behavior. However, despite the importance of incorporating healthcare providers into smoking cessation efforts, there is consistent evidence of a strong dose-response relationship between treatment intensity and smoking cessation outcome. Therefore, more intensive programs are often recommended in terms of effectiveness, particularly for individuals who have been unsuccessful in previous attempts to quit using minimal intervention strategies, those who have particular difficulties in maintaining abstinence, and those who are nicotine-dependent (90). Smokers who have little social support for quitting in their personal network or who have low self-efficacy about quitting may also benefit from more intensive interventions. Smokers may chose among a variety of intensive treatment programs, according to their personal preferences for individual versus group counseling.

In the context of individual counseling, the smoker typically meets with the therapist and discusses a variety of issues that relate to smoking and that may be relevant to quitting. The therapist's role may be that of enhancing motivation and self-efficacy, as well as providing training in coping skills and quitting strategies, and focusing on relapse prevention. Also, the use of pharmacologic adjuncts may be included for those smokers who are nicotine-dependent. Group counseling may touch on similar issues, in a context where clients share their quitting experience with other smokers. Group counseling may be particularly effective for people who have poor social support. Based on an extensive review of the literature, the AHCPR Guideline (19) recommends that smoking intervention programs should include at least four to seven sessions of 20 to 30 minutes in length, and should extend over at least 2 weeks. The guideline also recommends that cessation programs include coping skills training and problem-solving strategies, along with a strong emphasis on support for quitting efforts.

There are several agencies that promote smoking cessation and offer formal treatment programs (e.g., American Lung Association, American Cancer Society, local departments of health). In addition, community-based organizations can provide important smoking cessation resources. For example, in many minority communities the church takes on an important role in promoting smoking cessation (91–93). Smoking cessation programs promoted by the church may include some of the cognitive-behavioral strategies discussed in this chapter, in conjunction with lifestyle and religious messages. These programs may be particularly helpful for people for whom spirituality and religion play a significant role (94).

SUMMARY

This chapter has presented a variety of smoking cessation strategies that have been found to be important components of effective interventions. However, it should be noted that each of these strategies may be effective for only a subset of smokers; that is, it is not likely that all smokers will benefit from each of the strategies outlined, but rather from specific strategies that build upon their skills and needs. Although individual smokers are often the best judge of what smoking cessation approach will suit them best, a stepped-care model has been advocated, wherein individuals would be matched to cessation strategies based on their motivational level and previous experience with cessation (95). Strategies recommended for use range from least intensive (e.g., self-help) to most intensive (e.g., medication plus psychological intervention). Stepped-care approaches hold promise and deserve full-scale testing. Given the clear role that socioeconomic factors play in smoking status, it is likely that the most effective interventions in the future will also focus attention on social contextual issues that operate to maintain smoking behavior. Incorporating smoking cessation interventions into the mission of existing community-based organizations will also increase the likelihood that these strategies are disseminated to the target populations that have the highest smoking prevalence.

This research was supported in part by Grants 1RO1CA77780, 1RO1CA73242, and 1RO1HL50017 from the National Institutes of Health, and grants from Liberty Mutual Insurance Group, Aetna, the Boston Foundation, and NYNEX.

REFERENCES

1. U.S. Department of Health and Human Services. The health consequences of smoking: cancer: a report of the Surgeon General. Rockville, MD: Public Health Service, Office on Smoking and Health, 1982.

2. U.S. Department of Health and Human Services. The health consequences of smoking: cardiovascular disease: a report of the Surgeon General. Rockville, MD: Public Health Service, Office on Smoking and Health, 1983.

3. U.S. Department of Health and Human Services. The health consequences of smoking: chronic obstructive lung disease: a report of the Surgeon General. Rockville, MD: Public Health Service, Office on Smoking and Health, 1984.

4. U.S. Department of Health and Human Services. The health consequences of smoking: cancer and chronic lung disease in the workplace: a report of the Surgeon General. Rockville, MD: Public Health Service, Office on Smoking and Health, 1985.

5. U.S. Department of Health and Human Services. The health consequences of smoking for women: a report of the Surgeon General. Bethesda, MD: U.S. Department of Health and Human Services, Public Health Services, Office of the Assistant Secretary for Health, Office on Smoking and Health, 1980.

6. American Heart Association. Heart and stroke statistical update. Dallas, TX: American Heart Association, 1997.

7. U.S. Department of Health and Human Services. Reducing and health smoking: 25 years of progress: a report of the Surgeon General. Rockville, MD: Public Health Service, Office on Smoking and Health, 1989.

8. U.S. Department of Health and Human Services. The health benefits of smoking cessation. Rockville, MD: Centers for Disease Control, Center for Chronic Disease Prevention and Health Promotion, Office on Smoking and Health, 1990.

9. Glanz K, Brekke M, Harper D, et al. Evaluation of implementation of a cholesterol management program in physicians' offices. Health Educ Res 1992;7:151–163.

10. Peto R, Lopez AD, Boreham J, et al. Mortality from smoking in developed countries 1950–2000. New York: Oxford University Press, 1994.

11. USEP Agency. Respiratory health effects of passive smoking: lung cancer and other disorders. Washington, DC: Office of Health and Environmental Assessment, Office of Research and Development, 1992.

12. Kawachi I, Colditz GA, Speizer FE, et al. A prospective study of passive smoking and coronary heart disease in women. Circulation 1997;95:2374–2379.

13. Centers for Disease Control and Prevention. CDC surveillance summaries. Atlanta: U.S. Department of Health and Human Services, Public Health Service, 1996.

14. Centers for Disease Control and Prevention. Cigarette smoking among adults—United States, 1994. MMWR 1994;45:588–590.

15. MMWR. Total 24.7%, men 27%, women 22.6%. MMWR 1997;46:51.

16. King TK, Borrelli B, Black C, et al. Minority women and tobacco: implications for smoking cessation interventions. Ann Behav Med 1997;19(3):301–313.

17. American Cancer Society. Cancer facts and figures. New York: American Cancer Society, 1986.

18. Shiffman S. Smoking cessation treatment: any progress? J Consult Clin Psychol 1993;61:718–722.

19. U.S. Department of Health and Human Services. Smoking cessation guidelines: agency for Health Care Policy and Research. Atlanta, GA: Centers for Disease Control and Prevention, 1996.

20. Orleans CT, Slade J. Nicotine addiction: Principles and management. New York: Oxford University Press, 1993.

21. Abrams DB, Emmons KM, Niaura R, et al. Tobacco dependence: an integration of individual and public health perspectives. In: Nathan P, McCrady B, Langenbucher J, Frankenstein W, eds. Annual review of addictions treatment and research. New York: Pergamon Press, 1991.

22. Emmons KM. Health behaviors in a social context. In: Berkman IF, Kawachi I, eds. Social

epidemiology. Oxford: Oxford University Press 1999 (in press).

23. Graham H. When life's a drag: women, smoking and disadvantage. London: HMSO, 1993.

24. McBride CM, Pirie PL, Curry SJ. Postpartum relapse to smoking: a prospective study. Health Educ Res 1992;7.

25. Sorensen G, Emmons KM, Stoddard A, et al. Social norms of smoking among blue collar workers (under review).

26. Anda RF, Williamson DF, Escobedo LG, et al. Depression and the dynamics of smoking. JAMA 1990;264:1541–1545.

27. Glassman AH, Helzer JE, Covey LS. Smoking, smoking cessation and major depression. JAMA 1990;264:1546–1549.

28. Shiffman S. A relapse prevention hotline. Bull Soc Psychologists Substance Abuse 1982;1:50–54.

29. Covey LS, Glassman AH, Stetner F. First lapses to smoking: within-subjects analysis of real-time reports. J Consul Clin Psychol 1996;62(2):366–379.

30. Borrelli B, Niaura R, Keuthen NJ, et al. Development of major depressive disorder during smoking-cessation treatment. J Clin Psychol 1996;57(11):534–538.

31. Brown RA, Emmons KM. Behavioral treatment of cigarette dependence. In Cocores JA, ed. The clinical management of nicotine dependence. New York: Springer-Verlag, 1991.

32. Pierce JP, Fiore MC, Novotny TE, et al. Trends in cigarette smoking in the United States: educational differences are increasing. JAMA 1989;56–60.

33. Novotny TE, Warner, KE, Kendrick JS, Remington PL, Smoking by blacks and whites: socioeconomic and demographic differences. Am J Psychiatry 1988;78.

34. Adler NE, Boyce T, Chesney MA, et al. Socioeconomic status and health: the challenge of the gra-

dient. Am Psychologist 1994;49:15–24.

35. Marmot MG, Bobak M, Davey Smith G. Explanations for social inequalities and health. In: Amick BC, Levine S, Tarlov A, Walsh DC, eds. Society and health. London: Oxford University Press, 1996.

36. Wilkinson RG. Income distribution and life expectancy. BMJ 1992;304.

37. Marmot MG, Adelstein AM, Robinson N, Rose G. The changing social class distribution of heart disease. BMJ 1978;2:1109–1112.

38. Kennedy BP, Kawashi I, Prothow-Stith D. Income distribution and mortality: cross-sectional ecological study of the Robin Hood index in the United States. BMJ 1996;312:1004–1007.

39. Krieger N, Rowley D, Hermann AA, et al. Racism, sexism, and social class: implications for studies of health, disease, and well-being. Am J Prev Med 1993;9:82–122.

40. Amick BC, Levine S, Tarlov AR, Walsh DC. Society and health. In: Patrick DL, Wickizer TM, eds. Community and health. Oxford: Oxford University Press, 1995.

41. Lacey LP, Manfredi C, Balch G, et al. Social support in smoking cessation among black women in Chicago public housing. Public Health Rep 1993;108(3):387–394.

42. American Psychiatric Association. Diagnostic and statistical manual of mental disorders. Washington, D.C.: American Psychiatric Association, 1980.

43. Abrams DB, Biener L. Motivational characteristics of smokers at the worksite: a public health challenge. Int J Prev Med 1992;21:679–687.

44. Curry SJ. Self-help interventions for smoking cessation. J Consult Clin Psychol 1993;61:790–803.

45. Miller WR, Rollnick S. Motivational interviewing: preparing people to change addictive

behavior. New York: Guilford Press, 1991.

46. Prochaska J, DiClemente C. Self change processes, self efficacy and decisional balance across five stages of smoking cessation. New York: Alan R. Liss, 1983.

47. Schwartz JL. Review and evaluation of smoking cessation methods: the United States and Canada, 1978–1985. Washington, D.C.: Division of Cancer prevention and Control, National Cancer Institute, U.S. Department of Health and Human Services, Public Health Service, National Institutes of Health, 1987.

48. Bernstein DA. Modification of smoking behavior: an evaluative review. Psychol Bull 1969;71:418–440.

49. Strecher UJ, Seijts GH, Latham GP, et al. Goal setting as a strategy for health behavior change. Health Educ Q 1995;22:190–200.

50. Niaura R, Abrams D, DeMuth B, Pinto R. Responses to smoking related stimuli and early relapse to smoking. Addict Behav 1989;14:419–428.

51. Abrams D, Monti P, Carey K, et al. Reactivity to smoking cues and relapse: two studies of discrimination validity. Behav Res Ther 1988;26:225–233.

52. Foxx RM, Brown RA. Nicotine fading and self-monitoring for cigarette abstinence or controlled smoking. J Appl Behav Anal 1979;12:111–125.

53. Beaver C, Brown RA, Lichtenstein E. Effects of monitored nicotine fading and anxiety management training on smoking reduction. Addict Behav 1981;6:301–305.

54. Brown RA, Lichtenstein E, McIntyre KO, Harrington-Kostur J. Effects of nicotine fading and relapse prevention on smoking cessation. J Consult Clin Psychol 1984;52.

55. Lando HA, McGovern PG. Nicotine fading as a nonaversive

alternative in a broad-spectrum treatment for eliminating smoking. Addict Behav 1985;10.

56. Brandon SL, Tiffany ST, Baker TB. The process of smoking relapse. In: Tims F, Leukfeld C, eds. Relapse and recovery in drug abuse. Rockville, M.D.: National Institute on Drug Abuse, 1986.

57. Marlatt GA, Gordon JR. Determinants of relapse: implications for the maintenance of behavior change. In: Davidson PO, Davidson SM, eds. Behavioral medicine: Changing health lifestyles. New York: Bruner/Mazel, 1980.

58. Marlatt GA, Gordon JR. Relapse prevention. New York: Guilford Press, 1985.

59. Hughes JR, Gust SW, Pechacek TF. Prevalence of tobacco dependence and withdrawal, Am J Psychiatry 1987;144: 205–208.

60. Jarvik ME, Hatsukami DK. Tobacco dependence. In Ney T, Gale A, eds. Smoking and human behavior. New York: John Wiley & Sons, 1989.

61. Richmond RL, Kehoe L, de Almeida Neto AC. Three years continuous abstinence in a smoking cessation study using the nicotine transdermal patch. Heart 1997;78:6:617–618.

62. Marcus BH, Albrecht AE, Niaura RS, Thompson PD. Usefulness of physical exercise for maintaining smoking cessation in women. Am J Cardiol 1991;68:406–407.

63. Marcus BH, Albrecht, AE, King TK, et al. The efficacy of exercise as an aid for smoking cessation in women: a randomized control trial. Arch Int Med 1999 (in press).

64. Marcus BH, Emmons KM, Simkin LE, et al. Smoking and smoking cessation in women: a review. Med Exerc Nutr Health 1994;3: 17–31.

65. Folkins CH, Sime WE. Physical fitness training and mental

health. Am Psychol 1981;36: 373–389.

66. Abrams DB, Monti PM, Pinto RP, et al. Psychological stress and coping in smokers who relapse or quit. Health Psychol 1987;6: 289–303.

67. Carmody TP. Affect regulation, nicotine addiction, and smoking cessation. J Psychoactive Drugs 1989;21:331–342.

68. Shiffman S. Relapse following smoking cessation: a situational analysis. J Consult Clin Psychol 1986;50:71–86.

69. Shiffman S. Coping with temptations to smoke. J Consult Clin Psychol 1984;52:261–267.

70. Orleans CT, Slade J. Nicotine addiction: principles and management. New York: Oxford University Press, 1993.

71. Abrams DB, Emmons KM, Niaura RD, et al. Tobacco dependence: an integration of individual and public health perspectives. In: Nathan PE, Langenbucher JW, McCrady BS, Frankenstein W, eds. The annual review of addictions treatment and research. Elmsford, NY: Pergamon Press, 1991.

72. Fiore MC, Novotny TE, Pierce JP. Methods used to quit smoking in the United States: do cessation programs help? JAMA 1990; 263.

73. Glynn TJ, Boyd GM, Gruman JC. Essential elements of self-help/minimal intervention strategies for smoking cessation. Health Educ Qu 1990;17:329–345.

74. Lando HA, Gritz ER. Smoking cessation techniques, JAMA 1996;51:31–34.

75. Harackiewicz JM, Blair LW, Sansone C, et al. Nicotine gum and self-help manuals in smoking cessation: an evaluation in a medical context. Addict Behav 1998;13:319–330.

76. Curry SJ, Wagner EH, Grothaus LC. Evaluation of intrinsic and extrinsic motivation interventions with a self-help smoking cessa-

tion program. J Consult Clin Psychol 1991;59:318–324.

77. Curry SJ, McBride CM, Louie D, et al. Randomized trial of self-help smoking cessation interventions with non-volunteer smokers. Hamburg, Germany: Paper presented at the Second International Congress of Behavioral Medicine, 1992.

78. Louie D, McBride CM, Curry SJ. Comparison of volunteers and nonvolunteers receiving a self-help smoking cessation booklet and personalized feedback. New York: Paper presented at the 13th annual meeting of the Society of Behavioral Medicine, 1992.

79. Curry S, McBride C, Grothaus L, et al. A randomized trial of self-help materials, personalized feedback, and telephone counseling with nonvolunteer smokers. J Consult Clin Psychol 1995;63: 1005–1014.

80. Zhu SH, Tedeschi GJ, Anderson CM, Pierce JP. Telephone counseling for smoking cessation: what's in a call? J Counseling Development 1996;75:93–102.

81. Orleans CT, Schoenbach VJ, Wagner EH, et al. Self-help quit smoking interventions. Effects of self-help materials, social support instructions, and telephone counseling. J Consult Clin Psychol 1991;59:439–448.

82. Lando HA, Hellerstedt WL, Pirie PL, McGovern PG. Brief supportive telephone outreach as a recruitment and intervention strategy for smoking cessation. Am J Public Health 1992;82: 41–46.

83. Orleans, CT, Rimer BR. Enhancing adherence to cancer control regimens: clear horizons. 1992; unpublished research report.

84. Dubren R. Self-management by recorded telephone messages to maintain non-smoking behaviors. J Consult Clin Psychol 1977; 45:358–360.

85. Anderson DM, Duffy K, Hallett CD, Marcus AC. Proactive health education and patient counseling through telephone help lines.

Public Health Rep 1992;107: 278–283.

86. Ossip-Klein DJ, Giovino GA, Megahed N, et al. Effects of a smoker's hotline: results of a 10-county self-help trial. J Consult Clin Psychol 1991;59:325–332.

87. Lichtenstein E, Glasgow RE, Lando HA, et al. Telephone counseling for smoking cessation: rationales and meta-analytic review of evidence. Health Educ Res 1996;11:243–257.

88. Kviz FJ, Crittenden KS, Belzer LJ, Warnecke RB. Psychosocial factors and enrollment in a televised smoking cessation program. Health Educ Q 1991;18:445–461.

89. Thompson B, Curry SJ. Characteristics and predictors of participation and success in a televised smoking cessation activity. Am J

Health Promotion 1994;8:175–177.

90. Lando HA. Formal quit smoking treatments. In: Orleans CT, Slade J, eds. Nicotine addiction: principles and management. Oxford: Oxford University Press, 1993.

91. Lasater TM, Becker DM, Hill MN, Gans KM. Synthesis of findings and issues from religious-based cardiovascular disease prevention trials. ALP 1997;7:S46–S53.

92. Voorhees CC, Stillman FA, Swank RT, et al. Heart, body, and soul: impact of church-based smoking cessation interventions on readiness to quit. Prev Med 1996;25: 277–285.

93. McFarland MI. When five become twenty-five: a silver anniversary of the five-day plan to stop smoking. Adventist Heritage 1986;11:557–564.

94. Stillman FA, Bone LR, Rand C, et al. Heart, body, and soul: a church-based smoking cessation program for urban African Americans. Prev Med 1993;22: 335–349.

95. Abrams D, Orleans T, Niaura R, et al. Integrating individual and public health perspectives for treatment of tobacco dependence under managed health care: a combined stepped-care and matching model. Ann Behav Med 1996;18:290–304.

96. Goldstein M. Buproprion sustained release and smoking cessation. J Clin Psychiatry 1997;59(4):66–72.

97. Hurt RD, Sachs DP, Glover ED, Offord KP, Johnston JA. A comparison of sustained-release bupropion and placebo for smoking cessation. N Engl J Med 1997;337:1195–1202.

Chapter 48

Behavioral Approaches to Enhancing Weight Loss and Maintenance

Teresa K. King
Elizabeth E. Lloyd
Matthew M. Clark

The prevalence of obesity in this country is increasing at an alarming rate, creating a major public health concern. In 1960, approximately one quarter of American adults were estimated to be overweight. At present, one third of American adults are estimated to be overweight (1). The factors that contribute to the prevalence of obesity in our society (a bountiful supply of inexpensive and highly appealing food, less reliance on manual labor at home and work, and sedentary leisure activities) seem to have established firm roots. Thus, the pattern of an increasing prevalence of obesity is expected to continue. This is extremely troubling given that excess body weight is a risk factor for coronary heart disease, the leading cause of death in the United States. Excess body weight is also associated with a host of other adverse health outcomes, resulting in tremendous costs to our health care system (2).

BEHAVIORAL STRATEGIES FOR WEIGHT LOSS

Given that the societal factors contributing to overweight are not likely to change any time in the near future, strategies are needed that allow individuals to modify behaviors in a permanent fashion. Behavior therapy is the most widely used formal treatment for losing weight (3). Behavior therapy is a set of techniques derived from the principles of learning theory. Learning theory posits that maladaptive behaviors are learned through classical conditioning, instrumental conditioning, or modeling. Behavior can be understood in terms of stimulus, response, and reinforcement. Although multiple treatments for obesity exist, few of these have been critically evaluated to determine their efficacy. Studies generally support the use of behavioral approaches, whether alone or in combination with

a very-low-calorie diet or pharmacotherapy, as more effective than traditional approaches for weight loss (3,4). The purpose of this chapter is to review several key behavioral approaches to weight loss and maintenance. For each approach, we describe how the intervention was developed; that is, we present the behavioral principles that guided its conceptualization, describe how the strategy is utilized, and review research on its effectiveness.

Stimulus Control

Stimulus control is a term used to describe a set of procedures that seek to alter the antecedent stimuli that control behavior (5). Stimulus control applied to weight management is directed toward modifying factors that serve as cues for inappropriate eating (6). Initially, obese individuals were presumed to be particularly responsive to various internal and external triggers to eating, such as mood, time of day, activity, and sight of particular foods (7). Although more recent work suggests that this increased responsivity to these cues is not specific to the obese, targeting and altering an individual's triggers for eating remain integral components of most behavioral weight loss programs for adults, as well as for children (6,8,9).

Stimulus control strategies may be divided into several categories: limiting the times and places associated with eating, reducing exposure to food by storing it out of sight, limiting activities associated with eating, and reducing the purchase of problematic foods, thereby breaking "automatic" eating responses (8,10,11). In one study (12) participants were randomly assigned to one of the following intervention conditions: control group, standard behavior therapy plus experimenter-provided financial incentives for weight loss, standard behavior therapy plus experimenter-provided food, and standard behavior therapy plus food and incentives. Stimulus control strategies (specifically, eating in one place only, shopping from a list, storing food out of sight, and deciding ahead what to eat) were the only variables that predicted weight loss. Additionally, when combined with positive eating behaviors, such as making healthy food choices and limiting portion sizes, stimulus control strategies were the only factors that predicted weight loss and successful maintenance. By encouraging changes in these daily behaviors, new healthier behaviors may be learned and substituted for previously entrenched, unhealthy behavior chains.

Self-Monitoring

Self-monitoring, defined as the systematic observation and recording of one's own specific target behaviors (13), is a critical component of any behavioral treatment for obesity (14). Through daily recording of dietary intake, and the circumstances under which eating occurs, critical information is obtained that allows the therapist to provide more accurate, specific intervention strategies (8,15). Additionally, self-monitoring has not only been found useful in both assessment and treatment phases of weight management, but several studies have documented spontaneous reduction in caloric intake upon initiation of self-monitoring, presumably due to the increased awareness of food intake (10,16).

In a comprehensive investigation of the effectiveness of self-monitoring, Baker et al (17) found monitoring food intake to be positively correlated with weight loss. Further, subjects who monitored more completely (e.g., all food consumed, time of eating, quantity of food eaten, or grams of fat consumed) consistently lost the most weight. Lack of monitoring was negatively correlated with weight loss. These results are consistent with the Sperduto et al (18) finding that behavioral weight loss groups incorporating self-monitoring experienced greater weight reduction, as well as better attendance, than control groups not monitoring their eating and activity levels. Research confirms the need for consistent self-monitoring in behavioral weight reduction programs, not only to produce benefits such as increased awareness of eating behaviors, physical activity patterns, and greater weight loss, but also to prevent failure in self-awareness and self-regulation (17,19). Although there is no doubt that self-monitoring is an effective strategy, adherence can be a problem. Research is needed to uncover effective strategies for maintaining this behavior. Perhaps with the burgeoning of technology, effective tools will be developed. For example, handheld computers could make the task of monitoring food intake more convenient and could also provide prompts to remind individuals to record their intake.

Contingency Management and Self-Reward

Contingency management refers to treatment strategies that attempt to change behavior by modifying its consequences. Contingency management can be a useful and powerful tool in delineating specific target behaviors for change, as well as establishing criteria for success and consequences for both desirable and undesirable outcomes (20,21). Weight loss programs incorporating behavioral contracting have resulted in greater weight loss and lower attrition rates than programs

not incorporating these elements (20,22). Inherent in the use of contingency management are the processes of self-monitoring, self-evaluation, and subsequent self-reward for goals obtained. Mahoney (14) investigated the contribution of self-reward, comparing treatment conditions of self-reward for weight loss, self-reward for habit improvement, self-monitoring without specific instruction in self-reward, and a delayed treatment control group. Results suggested that when self-reward, in the form of a refundable deposit, was added to the process of self-monitoring and self-evaluation, greater weight loss was obtained. Although results of this early study suggest that rewards targeting specific changes in eating habits, as opposed to rewards targeting actual weight loss, are more effective, this is not clearly supported by more recent research (23,24). Additionally, there is some evidence to suggest that subjects self-rewarding for achievement of goals are more likely to maintain their weight loss at 1-year follow-up than those receiving minimal contact or self-monitoring without reward (8,24).

Refundable deposit contracts are a common form of incentive used to facilitate behavior change, whether targeting weight loss, habit change, or group session attendance (20,25). Other types of incentives used include lottery drawings upon completion of group sessions and response-cost procedures involving deduction of moneys for not achieving the specified goals of the contract. In their review of the literature, Brownell et al (8) suggested that behavioral weight control programs incorporating incentives and self-reward, regardless of the type used, have average weight losses 30% greater than those programs not incorporating incentives. Although there is great variation among the types of incentive programs and behaviors targeted in weight management, it is clear that contingency management and self-reward are effective strategies that should continue to be incorporated into behavioral weight management programs.

Cognitive Restructuring

Cognitive restructuring techniques focus on changing the errors in thinking that contribute to maladaptive behaviors (26). Behavioral treatment programs for obesity have incorporated strategies for changes in thought processes among participants (8,27,28). Not only does research suggest that cognitive factors may play a critical role in weight regulation (29), but alteration of these maladaptive cognitions may be related to control over eating and dieting success. Based upon Mahoney et al's (30) early work describing maladaptive cognitions frequently experienced by dieters, common irrational beliefs are identified and modified in order to improve success at weight loss and long-term maintenance. Common irrational beliefs held by overweight individuals include: self-doubt over weight loss ("I've never been able to do it, why would I succeed now?"), establishment of unrealistic goals ("I'll never overeat again"), and punitive self-statements ("I'm a failure because I can't lose weight"). Individuals that hold more of these maladaptive cognitions and disparaging views of self are more likely to experience greater emotional distress and unhealthy eating patterns, which contributes to difficulty losing weight and maintaining a weight loss (10,30,31).

Although cognitive distortions may be commonly experienced in obese individuals, research supporting the utility of specific cognitive restructuring techniques in weight management protocols has been mixed. Studies investigating use of self-instructional training (SIT), a form of cognitive restructuring involving identification of circumstances in which a dieter has poor control and then repeated rehearsal of appropriate self-statements both imaginal and through practice situations (29), suggest no significant differences between SIT and "standard" behavioral treatments in either mean weight loss or alterations in cognitive patterns (27,29,32). Although research to date highlights the importance of cognitive factors in obesity and weight control, identification of specific, clinically effective cognitive techniques is needed. Perhaps incorporating appropriate cognitive outcome measures, rather than focusing on weight loss as a primary outcome, would shed light on the cognitive processes involved in weight loss treatment and how best to manage these.

Social Support

Social support is often described as a critical component of weight management protocols (8,10,33,34) and is commonly included in one of three capacities (35): 1) teaching skills to participants in order to elicit and further enhance their social support networks (11), 2) actively involving significant family members in the weight loss process with the participant, and 3) eliciting social support as part of the group process. Nevertheless, the therapeutic effects of social support in weight management have yet to be investigated independently.

Although involvement of significant family members has generally received mixed support, a meta-analytic review of couples' weight-loss programs (36) found couples' programs to be more effective overall than subject-alone programs. Peer and family social support have been positively correlated with successful weight loss and maintenance, although the mechanism involved in this relationship is unclear. However, Brownell et al (37) caution that the mere presence of a cooperative spouse, or family member, does not guarantee improved weight loss. Brownell et al (37) found that subjects whose spouses attended weight loss sessions and were trained in the specific techniques of modeling, self-monitoring, and reinforcement lost significantly more weight than either subjects with a cooperative spouse who did not attend sessions or subjects with a noncooperative spouse who refused to participate in sessions. The effectiveness of social support may also depend on the gender of the individual trying to lose weight. Wing et al (38) found that women benefited more than men from a weight loss program that included spouses.

Explanations for the positive effects of social support include associations with decreased rates of depression and increased marital adjustment in couples participating together (36), increased instrumental support during the process of weight loss, and assistance with enhancement of self-acceptance and cognitive thought processes (22,39). Further research is needed to discover which types of social support are most helpful for successful weight loss. Retrospective investigations of partners of successful weight reducers, as well as those who are less successful, would provide information on which forms of social support are most effective, as well as which type of individual benefits most from inclusion of social support in a treatment package. Additionally, investigation of the role of social support, whether through extended family or community resources such as a church, may be particularly useful in improving successful weight loss and maintenance in minority populations (40,41).

WEIGHT MAINTENANCE STRATEGIES

It has been well documented that recidivism following weight loss is a serious problem (42). Some estimate that most patients regain all of their weight within 3 to 5 years (43). Although numerous studies have documented high relapse rates for weight control, few investigations have examined innovative maintenance strategies. This section reviews the relevant research on behavioral strategies for weight maintenance.

Maintenance Groups

The foundation of current research into maintenance strategies was established by Perri and colleagues in the 1980s in a series of studies (39,44,45). In these studies, the effects of professional contact, telephone contact, relapse prevention training, social support, exercise, and problem-solving skills were examined. Perri et al (45) examined 26 men and 97 women who were 20% to 100% overweight and who participated in a 20-week group behavior therapy weight management program. During the 20-week program, participants were taught numerous behavioral strategies: self-monitoring, stimulus control, self-reinforcement, cognitive restructuring, and slowing the rate of eating. After 20 weeks, subjects were randomly assigned to follow-up only or to four different 6-month biweekly maintenance programs:

1. A post-treatment contact condition that included weigh-ins, self-monitoring, and therapist-led problem solving of difficulties in maintaining habit changes in eating and exercise behavior. The problem-solving training included four steps: problem identification, brainstorming, decision making, and solution implementation and verification.

2. Post-treatment contact and a social influence program. The social influence program included monetary group contingencies for adherence, participation in lectures, and instructions in peer telephone contact.

3. A post-treatment contact and an aerobic exercise program that combined a new set of exercise goals and therapist-led exercise sessions.

4. A post-treatment contact and a social influence and an aerobic exercise program.

Participation in these behavioral maintenance groups proved highly beneficial. At the 18-month follow-up, the subjects in the four post-treatment programs maintained 82.7% of their weight loss compared to an average sustained weight loss of only 33.3% for the subjects in the no-post-treatment contact condition. Subjects in the combined maintenance condition maintained 99% of their weight loss, suggesting that the combination of high-frequency exercise, coupled with support and problem solving, holds great promise in improving the long-term management of obesity.

Strategies Used by Successful Maintainers

In a recent survey, researchers at the University of Pittsburgh School of Medicine (46) created a National Weight Control

Registry (NWCR) of 629 women and 155 men who lost an average of 30 kg and had maintained a weight loss of at least 13.6 kg for 5 years. The researchers were interested in learning more about the subjects' weight loss and weight maintenance strategies and about what types of behavioral approaches people used. Fifty-five percent of the sample used a formal weight loss program, and 45% lost weight on their own. Most of the subjects (89%) modified both their dietary intake and their physical activity level to lose weight. The three most commonly used strategies to change diet were to limit the intake of certain foods, limit the quantities of food, and to count calories.

During their 5 years of maintenance, most subjects (92%) reported limiting their intake of certain foods. Many also reported relying on self-monitoring techniques for limiting quantities of foods (49%), restricting fat intake (38%), counting calories (36%), or counting fat grams (30%). Subjects also reported using stimulus control techniques. They ate most of their meals at home where food choices are more restricted. Subjects reported engaging in a high level of physical activity, averaging an equivalent of walking 28 miles per week. Subjects engaged in cycling, aerobics, walking, running, and hiking. Thus, these maintainers participated in the type of physical activity that is recommended for weight loss, but the amount of time they reported exercising is more than double what is typically recommended.

Exercise

There is much support for the role of exercise in weight maintenance. For example, Kayman et al (47) found that maintainers were far more likely than regainers to exercise at least three times per week for 30 minutes or more. Maintainers also engaged in more lifestyle activity than relapsers. Since exercise clearly facilitates weight maintenance, research is now focused on how to facilitate the adoption and maintenance of an active lifestyle. One promising approach is home-based exercise programs. Researchers have found that instructing patients in home-based exercise rather than in group clinic–based exercise over a 12-month intervention facilitated weight maintenance at a 3-month follow-up (48). According to the authors, the greater convenience and flexibility of home-based exercise probably contributed to higher exercise adherence. During months 7 through 12, subjects in the home-based condition completed 78% of their exercise sessions compared to 48% in the group condition. Interestingly, subjects in the home-based conditions attended more weight loss group sessions and were more likely to complete food records. Thus, the authors speculate that exercise adherence may promote adherence to other strategies such as group attendance and self-monitoring of eating behavior, both of which facilitate maintenance.

Cognitive Restructuring Strategies

Cognitive restructuring strategies also appear important during the maintenance phase of weight loss. For example, it has been proposed that unrealistic weight loss expectations may contribute to relapse (49). If individuals are disappointed in their ability to reach their goal weight or discouraged with their rate of weight loss, these negative cognitions and emotions may reduce motivation and/or trigger overeating episodes. Recent research examining outcome expectations

reveals the importance of challenging unrealistic outcome expectations (50). In a study of 60 obese women, subjects were asked prior to weight loss to identify their goal weight and four other weights: "dream weight" ("a weight you would choose if you could weigh whatever you wanted"); "happy weight" ("this weight is not as ideal as the first one; it is a weight, however, that you would be happy to achieve"); "acceptable weight" ("a weight that you would not be particularly happy with, but one that you could accept, since it is less than your current weight"); and "disappointed weight" ("a weight that is less than your current weight, but one that you could not view as successful in any way; you would be disappointed if this were your final weight"). Subjects' goal weight averaged a 32% reduction in body weight. Despite a 16-kg weight loss during a 48-week treatment program, only 9% of subjects achieved a "happy weight." Furthermore, although they reported achieving numerous positive physical and psychological effects of weight loss, 47% still had not yet even reached their "disappointed" weight. Cognitive strategies to promote the adoption of a reasonable weight goal need to be identified by future research.

More evidence for the importance of cognitive strategies during the maintenance phase is provided by a study conducted by Kayman et al (47). These investigators found that maintainers incorporated a new eating style but to avoid feelings of deprivation did not completely restrict their intake of problem foods. In contrast, regainers also dieted but did not permit themselves any of their favorite foods, and they viewed their weight loss foods as special foods, different from the foods their family would have and different from the foods they wanted. Thus, classifying foods as "good" and "bad" probably promoted dichotomous thinking and may have contributed to relapse.

Stress Management

Stress management continues to be important as individuals move from the weight loss phase to the weight maintenance phase of weight control. Kayman et al (47) found that regainers and maintainers reported experiencing stressful events at the same rate; however, the two groups differed in how they responded to stress. Maintainers used problem-solving skills or confrontive ways of coping with stress. In contrast, relapsers used emotion-focused or escape-avoidance strategies such as eating, sleeping, or just hoping the problem would go away. A basic component of most stress management interventions is training in problem-solving skills, in which individuals are taught to identify problems, generate solutions, evaluate solutions, implement a solution, and then evaluate the results. Thus stress management strategies, in particular problem-solving skills, may be important for weight maintenance.

Social support has also been identified as a weight loss facilitator (37). A support system can help one to problem-solve, offer emotional support, or be available for practical assistance. Maintainers identify more support systems (51) and are more likely than regainers to seek support when dealing with stress (47).

In summary, continued contact with a professional, consistent exercise, social support, and maintaining dietary intake changes all facilitate weight maintenance (see Table 48-1). Behavioral strategies that have garnered support for their role in weight maintenance include self-monitoring (regular

Table 48-1 Maintenance Strategies
Physical activity
Low-fat diet
Coping skills
Extended treatment
Social support
Reasonable goal weight
Self-monitoring

weighing, measuring, and recording intake), stress management and problem solving, stimulus control, and cognitive restructuring. Although it is clear that there is a relationship between activity level and weight maintenance, it remains unclear how to foster the adoption of a more active lifestyle. Further research is warranted that examines the adoption and maintenance of an active lifestyle in an obese population. Preparing participants and practitioners for adopting a continuous care model of obesity should also be beneficial.

SUMMARY

Twenty years ago Stunkard (52) summarized the literature on the behavioral treatment of obesity in the following manner:

> Although behavior therapy has advanced the treatment of obesity, its results are still of limited clinical significance. Weight losses have been modest and the variability in results large and unexplained. Even long-term maintenance of weight loss, which, it was originally hoped, would be a particular benefit of the behavioral approach, has not yet been established. One possibility of increasing the effectiveness of behavioral treatments is to combine them with other measures—dietary and pharmacological.

Interestingly, the current status of behavioral treatments for obesity could be summarized in much the same manner. For example, in the vein of developing more effective treatments for weight loss, we have witnessed a rebirth of the pharmacologic treatment of obesity. Although there have been some serious recent concerns in this area, new drugs for fighting obesity continue to be developed. Studies have documented the increased effectiveness of treatment programs that combine pharmacologic treatments with behavior therapy when compared to the use of the agent alone (2). A behaviorally focused treatment manual has already been adapted for use with the prescription drug Meridia (53). Behavior therapy will undoubtedly continue to play an integral role in this movement.

Although Stunkard's (52) quotation does still ring true, this is not to say the field has been devoid of innovation and progress. There have been some shifts in conceptualizing the treatment of obesity that will undoubtedly shape its future. The first is a shift from self-management to lifestyle modification. Behavioral treatments of obesity originally focused on self-control procedures, specifically self-monitoring and stimulus control (54). Although self-control procedures are still an integral part of most weight management programs, the focus has begun to shift to a lifestyle modification approach that recognizes that in order to successfully lose weight, the obese individual needs to establish a new lifestyle that supports the maintenance of a healthier and thinner physique (51,55).

Another shift involves goals for weight loss outcome or the evaluation of success. Behavior therapy has been described by Stunkard and other experts in the field as being of "limited clinical significance" because average weight losses are small. However, recent evidence suggests that losing even small amounts of weight (5% to 10% of body weight) can have a significant impact on health (56,57). The Institute of Medicine of the National Academy of Science (58) has defined successful long-term weight loss as a 5% reduction in body weight that is maintained for at least 1 year. Professionals are reaching a consensus that losing 5% to 10% of body weight is a reasonable treatment outcome (22,59). So rather than becoming disillusioned with behavior therapy because we have yet to develop a behavioral treatment that is effective at reducing obese individuals to "normal" weights, we have started to reevaluate what it means to be successful. Although behavior therapy can be evaluated as an effective treatment for achieving modest weight losses, patients may not view a 5% weight loss as a success (50). Thus, more research needs to be conducted so that patients can be convinced to accept smaller weight losses or so that treatments can be developed that produce larger weight losses that can be maintained.

There has also been a movement within the field of obesity treatment toward consideration of individual characteristics and recommending treatments based on those characteristics. Thus, rather than using a single approach with all obese individuals, there is an attempt to tailor or match treatments to individuals. For example, percentage overweight has been used to match individuals to treatment. Treatment recommendations are determined by their likely effectiveness and a risk-benefit analysis (59). Clark et al (60) found greater attrition from a low-intensity weight loss program among individuals with higher levels of obesity. Factors other than level of obesity are also considered important when making treatment decisions. Schwartz et al (61) surveyed experts in weight loss treatment to identify client characteristics important for treatment matching. Five factors were identified by a majority of the experts as important when making treatment decisions: weight, weight loss history, medical condition, eating disorders, and psychiatric comorbidity. Additional matching characteristics may include a history of sexual trauma (62) and a negative body image (63) since both of these factors have been shown to impact obesity treatment outcome. Intuitively, the idea of treatment matching makes sense; however, there has been very little empirical validation of treatment matching models. Research is needed that examines the validity and utility of treatment matching models for obesity.

REFERENCES

1. Kuczmarski RJ, Flegal KM, Campbell SM, et al. Increasing prevalence of overweight among U.S. adults. JAMA 1994;272:205–211.

2. National Task Force on the Prevention and Treatment of Obesity. Long-term pharmacotherapy in the management of obesity. JAMA 1996;276:1907–1915.

3. Foreyt JP, Kondo AT. Advances in behavioral treatment of obesity. Prog Behav Modif 1984;16:231–256.

4. Wadden TA, Stunkard AJ, Liebschutz J. Three-year follow-up of the treatment of obesity by very-low-calorie diet, behavior therapy, and their combination. J Consult Clin Psychol 1988;56:925–928.

5. Mahoney M, Arnkoff DB. Self-management. In: Pomerlau OF, Brady JP, eds. Behavioral medicine: theory and practice. New York: Williams & Wilkins, 1979.

6. Foreyt JP, Cousins JH. Obesity. In: Mash E, Barkley R, eds. Treatment of childhood disorders. New York: Guilford Press, 1989.

7. Ferster CB, Nurnberger JI, Levitt EE. The control of eating. J Mathematics 1962;1:87–109.

8. Brownell KD, Kramer FM. Behavioral management of obesity. Med Clin North Am 1989;73:185–201.

9. Wooley SC, Wooley OW, Dyrenforth SR. Theoretical, practical, and social issues in behavioral treatments of obesity. J Appl Behav Anal 1979;12:3–25.

10. Wadden TA, Bell ST. Obesity. In: Bellack AS, Hersen M, Kazdin AE, eds. International handbook of behavior modification and therapy. 2nd ed. New York: Plenum, 1990.

11. Wadden TA, Foster CD. Behavioral assessment and treatment of markedly obese patients. In: Wadden TA, VanItallie TB, eds. Treatment of the seriously obese patient. New York: Guilford, 1992.

12. French SA, Jeffery RW, Wing RR. Sex differences among participants in a weight-control program. Addict Behav 1994;19(2):147–158.

13. Kanfer FH. Self-monitoring: methodological limitations and clinical applications. J Consul Clin Psychol 1970;35:148–152.

14. Mahoney M. Self-reward and self-monitoring techniques for weight control. Behav Ther 1974;5:48–57.

15. Wilson GT. Behavioral approaches to the treatment of obesity. In: Brownell KD, Fairburn CG, eds. Eating disorders and obesity: a comprehensive handbook, New York: Guilford, 1995.

16. Bellack AS, Rozensky R, Schwartz JS. A comparison of two forms of self-monitoring in a behavioral weight reduction program. Behav Ther 1974;5:523–530.

17. Baker RC, Kirschenbaum DS. Self-monitoring may be necessary for successful weight control. Behav Ther 1993;24:377–394.

18. Sperduto WA, Thompson HS, O'Brien RM. The effect of target behavior monitoring on weight loss and completion rate in a behavioral modification program for weight reduction. Addict Behav 1986;11:337–340.

19. Kirschenbaum DS. Elements of effective weight control programs: implications for exercise and sport psychology. J Appl Sport Psychol 1992;4:77–93.

20. Mavis BE, Stoffelmayr BE. Multidimensional evaluation of monetary incentive strategies for weight control. Psychol Record 1994;44:239–252.

21. Stunkard AJ, Berthold HC. What is behavior therapy: a very short description of behavioral weight control. Am J Clin Nutr 1985;41:821–823.

22. Foreyt JP, Goodrick GK. Factors common to successful therapy for the obese patient. Med Sci Sports Exerc 1991;23:292–297.

23. Jeffery RW, Thompson PD, Wing RR. Effects on weight reduction of strong monetary contracts for caloric restriction or weight loss. Behav Res Ther 1978;16(5):363–369.

24. Kramer FM, Jeffery RW, Snell MK, et al. Maintenance of successful weight loss over 1 year: effects of financial contracts for weight maintenance or participation in skill training. Behav Ther 1986;17:295–301.

25. Sperduto WA, O'Brien RM. Effects of cash deposits on attendance and weight loss in a large-scale clinical program for obesity. Psychol Rep 1983;52:261–262.

26. Beck AT. Cognitive therapy and the emotional disorders. New York: International Universities Press, 1976.

27. DeLucia JL, Kalodner CR. An individualized cognitive intervention: does it increase the efficacy of behavioral interventions for obesity? Addict Behav 1990;15:473–479.

28. Bennett GA. An evaluation of self-instructional training in the treatment of obesity. Addict Behav 1986;11:125–134.

29. Bennett GA. Cognitive-behavioral treatments for obesity. J Psychosom Res 1988;32(6):661–665.

30. Mahoney MJ, Mahoney K. Permanent weight control: a total solution to the dieter's problem. New York: Norton, 1976.

31. Meichenbaum D, Cameron R. The clinical potential of modifying what clients say to themselves. Psychother Theory Res Pract 1974;11:103–117.

32. Yates BT. Cognitive vs. diet vs. exercise components in obesity bibliotherapy: effectiveness as a function of psychological benefits versus psychological costs. South Psychol 1987;3:35–40.

33. Foreyt JP, Goodrick GK. Attributes of successful approaches to weight loss and control. Appl Prev Psychol 1994;3:209–215.

34. Epstein LH, Valoski A, Wing RR, et al. Ten-year outcomes of behav-

ioral family-based treatment for childhood obesity. Health Psychol 1994;13:373–383.

35. Parham ES. Enhancing social support in weight loss management groups. J Am Diet Assoc 1993;93:1152–1156.

36. Black DR, Glesser LJ, Kooyers KJ. A meta-analytic evaluation of couples weight loss programs. Health Psychol 1990;9:330–347.

37. Brownell KD, Heckerman CL, Westlake RJ, et al. The effect of couples training and partner co-operativeness in the behavioral treatment of obesity. Behav Res Ther 1978;16:323–333.

38. Wing RR, Marcus MD, Epstein LH, et al. A family-based approach to the treatment of obese type II diabetic patients. Diabetes Spectrum 1992;5:230.

39. Perri MG, McAdoo WG, McAllister DA, et al. Effects of peer support and therapist contact on long-term weight loss. J Consul Clin Psychol 1987;55:615–617.

40. Foreyt JP. Weight loss programs for minority populations. In: Brownell KD, Fairburn CG, eds. Eating disorders and obesity: a comprehensive handbook. New York: Guilford Press, 1995.

41. Klesges RC, DeBon M, Meyers A. Obesity in African American women: epidemiology, determinants, and treatment issues. In: Thompson JK, ed. Body image, eating disorders, and obesity: an integrative guide for assessment and treatment. Washington D.C.: American Psychological Association, 1996.

42. DePue JD, Clark MM, Ruggiero L, et al. Maintenance of weight loss: a needs assessment. Obes Res 1995;3(3):241–248.

43. Brownell KD, Jeffery RW. Improving long-term weight loss: pushing the limits of treatment. Behav Ther 1987;18:353–374.

44. Perri MG, McAdoo WG, Spevak PA, et al. Effect of a multicomponent maintenance program on long-term weight loss. J Consul Clin Psychol 1984;52(3):480–481.

45. Perri MG, McAllister DA, Gange JJ, et al. Effects of four maintenance programs on the long-term management of obesity. J Consul Clin Psychol 1988;56:529–534.

46. Klem ML, Wing RR, McGuire MT, et al. A descriptive study of individuals successful at long-term maintenance of substantial weight loss. Am J Clin Nutr 1997;66:239–246.

47. Kayman S, Bruvold W, Stern JS. Maintenance and relapse after weight loss in women: behavioral aspects. Am J Clin Nutr 1990;52:800–807.

48. Perri MG, Martin D, Leermakers EA, et al. Effects of group- versus home-based exercise in the treatment of obesity. J Consul Clin Psychol 1997;65(2):278–285.

49. Brownell KD, Wadden TA. Etiology and treatment of obesity: understanding a serious, prevalent, and refractory disorder. J Consul Clin Psychol 1992;60:505–517.

50. Foster GD, Wadden TA, Vogt RA, et al. What is a reasonable weight loss? patients' expectations and evaluations of obesity treatment outcomes. J Consul Clin Psychol 1997;65(1):79–85.

51. Head S, Brookhart A. Lifestyle modification and relapse prevention training during treatment for weight loss. Behav Ther 1997;28:307–321.

52. Stunkard AJ. Behavioral treatment of obesity: the current status. Int J Obes 1978;2(2):237–248.

53. Brownell KD, Wadden TA. The LEARN program for weight control, special medication edition for use with MERIDIA. Dallas: American Health Publishing, 1998.

54. Stuart RB. Behavioral control of overeating. Behav Res Ther 1967; 5:357–365.

55. Perri MG. Improving maintenance of weight loss following treatment by diet and lifestyle modification. In: Wadden TA, VanItallie TB, eds. Treatment of the seriously obese patient. New York: Guilford, 1992.

56. Blackburn GL. Effect of degree of weight loss on health benefits. Obes Res 1995;3:211s–216s.

57. Goldstein DJ. Beneficial effects of modest weight loss. Int J Obes 1991;16:397–416.

58. Institute of Medicine of the National Academy of Sciences. Weighing the options: criteria for evaluating weight management programs. Washington, D.C.: National Academy Press, 1995:139.

59. Brownell KD, Wadden TA. The heterogeneity of obesity: fitting treatments to individuals. Behav Ther 1991;22:153–177.

60. Clark MM, Guise BJ, Niaura RS. Obesity level and attrition: support for patient-treatment matching in obesity treatment. Obes Res 1995; 3(1):63–64.

61. Schwartz MB, Brownel KD. Matching individuals to weight loss treatments: a survey of obesity experts. J Consul Clin Psychol 1995;63(1):149–153.

62. King TK, Clark MM, Pera VP. History of sexual abuse and obesity treatment outcome. Addict Behav 1996;21(3):283–290.

63. Grilo CM. Treatment of obesity: an integrative model. In: Thompson JK, ed. Body image, eating disorders and obesity: an integrative guide for assessment and treatment. Washington, D.C.: American Psychological Association, 1996.

Part IX.

PEDIATRIC MEDICINE

Edited by
Thomas W. Rowland

Introduction to Pediatric Medicine

Thomas W. Rowland

Consider the major causes of morbidity and mortality in the advanced nations of the world: coronary artery disease, hypertension, obesity, type 2 diabetes, and osteoporosis. They all share several characteristics in common. First, they are largely diseases which result from unhealthy behaviors; i.e, these illness to a major extent are a reflection of the way people act (eat, drink, move about). Second, the environment that surrounds individuals plays a significant potentiating role in these behaviors (easy access to cheap, high-calorie food, the expediency of mechanized transportation, the seduction of television and computers). And, third, these diseases, which surface clinically in the adult years, are the end result of life-long pathologic processes (atherosclerosis, low bone density) that have their origins in the pediatric years.

It takes no great insight to synthesize these observations into a sound strategy for diminishing the tragic health impact of these illnesses. Behaviors need to change, environments should be altered, and the approach to prevention must begin in the pediatric years. For this reason, this section stands as one of the most critical of this book, collectively designed to examine and promote the role of exercise and nutrition in the promotion of health. Behavioral changes in what we eat and how we exercise can be expected to have their greatest positive health impact when introduced early in life.

It is also apparent that the benefits of a healthy diet and good exercise habits are expressed in a variety of salutary outcomes. This section will review these outcomes, examining the rationale for a pediatric preventive approach and providing practical advice for early interventions.

In the first chapter, I expand upon the role of the pediatric health provider in introducing long-term preventive health measures in children. There is no question that such an approach is sensible, but it lacks—and probably always will lack—scientific evidence for its justification. That is, considering the difficulty in conducting such an investigation, it is unlikely that a future study will provide proof that the 5-year-old who eats diet A and exercises according to regimin B will have less risk of a myocardial infarction at age 50. It is important to consider, however, that the lack of such evidence does not necessarily preclude an aggressive preventive health approach based on the research information at hand. Indeed, the evidence produced by the authors of all of these chapters is compelling in their identification of the appropriateness of such early interventions.

The next chapter on obesity addresses one of the most pressing health issues in both the pediatric and adult age groups. The extent of adiposity is rising in the population, and efforts to understand the nature of this problem and identify effective means of management are becoming increasingly critical. In Chapter 50, Scott Owens and Bernard Gutin delineate our current state of knowledge and understanding of these issues.

The high incidence of essential hypertension in the adult population is not well understood. It is clear, though, that certain lifestyle behaviors (overeating, sedentary lifestyle) can contribute to the genesis of elevated blood pressure, and that the onset of essential hypertension is often identifiable early in life, particularly during the teenage years. In Chapter 51, I review the issues surrounding early identification of essential hypertension in this age group with a suggested management plan.

In the chapter on substance abuse in children and adolescents, Robert DuRant and Catherine Buchanan outline another issue that bears critical significance for preventive medicine. The devastating impact of smoking and alcoholism on health—and the difficulty of altering these behaviors once established—lend a high sense of immediacy to the role of the pediatric health care provider to the interventions outlined in this chapter.

In the next chapter of this section, Donald Bailey reviews data that provides a strong rationale for prevention of the complications of adult osteoporosis by lifestyles which promote bone accretion during the growing years. This is perhaps the most clearcut scenario that argues for proper diet and exercise in the early years paying health dividends at a much later age.

The importance of maintaining a healthy serum lipid profile with a proper diet in the long-term prevention of atherosclerosis is highlighted in the chapter by Christine Williams. What children eat is one of the most direct control parents have over health behaviors in children and one which may influence future eating habits as well. Parents need to understand the concepts outlined in this chapter, creating an important educational role for health care providers.

The illness outcomes examined in this section are as diverse as they are important in threatening the well-being of the population. It is intriguing, though, that essentially the same interventions in the pediatric years—introduction of a healthy diet and regular exercise—can be expected to have a beneficial effect on all of these disease states. The importance of the pediatric health care provider in preventive medicine rests on this conclusion.

Chapter 49

Pediatric Preventive Medicine: A Window of Opportunity

Thomas W. Rowland

No one is in a better position to spearhead preventive health efforts than the health care provider for children. A full lifetime stretches out before his or her patients, and any intervention resulting in an improvement in health is likely to have long-term beneficial effects. In the primary care setting pediatric patients are seen on a regular basis, allowing reinforcement of health recommendations and monitoring of compliance.

Care of children by necessity involves interaction with parents. The success of health care initiatives often rests on the education and counseling of all members of the family. Office visits thus permit inclusion of family members in health care discussions, which is often critical to effective preventive health management.

It is no surprise, then, that pediatricians and other health professionals caring for children spend much of their time promoting health from a preventive standpoint. They provide immunizations against infectious disease, counsel against the risks of poisoning and accidents, and advocate proper discipline to avoid behavioral disorders. The chapters in this section, though, deal with a preventive role for health care providers in a broader context—interventions that will serve to diminish the risk of chronic disease in adults. Accumulating evidence supports the critical role of early modifications of diet, physical activity, and other lifestyle habits in the prevention of illness in later life, and pediatric health care providers have been thrust into an increasingly important role in these preventive health strategies.

Thirty years ago the idea first took root that pediatricians should take an active role in efforts to decrease the risks of adult cardiovascular disease. This conclusion arose as a natural consequence of scientific data indicating that 1) the process of atherosclerosis—the cause of myocardial infarction, stroke, and peripheral vascular disease—is a lifelong process, beginning during the pediatric years, and 2) risk for atherosclerotic vascular disease is linked to certain coronary risk factors, some of which (including cigarette smoking, hypertension, and hypercholesterolemia) are modifiable by altering behavior. Would it not be logical, it was suggested, that diminishing the incidence of risk factors early in life would have a beneficial effect of reducing the development of atherosclerosis and diminishing cardiovascular complications in later adult years?

The past three decades have witnessed an accumulation of evidence that continues to support this pediatric-based strategy. The pertinence of this issue for children has been underscored by the recognition that coronary risk factors are common in the growing years. Some, in fact, such as obesity, sedentary life style, and salt intake, may be increasing in frequency in the population (1). The importance of reducing these factors has been supported by intervention studies in adults. These investigations have indicated the effectiveness of decreasing specific risk factors (such as hypercholesterolemia) in reducing incidence of cardiovascular disease outcomes. These observations have been coupled with a third: within the United States population, a recent reduction in the incidence of adult cardiovascular disease is likely at least partially due to efforts to reduce unfavorable dietary habits.

The substantiation of a pediatric approach to preventing adult cardiovascular disease has spawned similar ideas for reducing risk of other "adult" diseases. In these concerns the model is similar. Osteoporosis, for example, becomes a serious public health concern in older ages, but the major point of time for bone mineral accretion is in the early years of life.

There exists, then, a strong rationale for efforts to promote bone health through proper diet and activity, particularly during the growing years.

The natural course of obesity follows a similar model. Obese children are more likely to become obese adults; habits that lead to excessive body fat in the pediatric years can be expected to increase the health risks associated with obesity later in life.

THE RATIONALE FOR PEDIATRIC PREVENTIVE MEDICINE

The increasing attention focused on pediatric preventive medicine reflects the gravity and magnitude of its target health problems. The diseases on the "hit list"—coronary artery disease, hypertension, obesity, osteoporosis, and type 2 diabetes mellitus—collectively account for the great majority of death and disability in developed countries of the world. If a pediatric approach to preventing these adult illnesses is effective, the impact on morbidity and mortality in the population will be substantial. It is critical, then, to assess the rationale for the role of preventive efforts during childhood and assess the proper tactics for enacting them.

There is no question that the major diseases causing death and disability in adulthood have their origins much earlier in life (2). Essential hypertension has been identified in children as young as toddlers. The process of atherosclerosis may begin as fatty deposits in blood vessels in the same age group, and raised fibrotic plaques are commonly evident in later adolescence. The critical period for optimization of bone mineralization is in adolescence and early adulthood, and failure to do so increases the risks of osteoporosis in later years. Many overweight adults can trace the origins of their obesity to their childhood years.

There is intriguing evidence, in fact, that the genesis of some of these processes may extend even before birth. Barker et al found that the birthweights of 1586 men born in Sheffield, England, between 1907 and 1925 were correlated with death rates from later cardiovascular disease (3). It was suggested that altered fetal nutrition by some means creates negative affects on cardiac development that might be mediated through hormonal alterations. A similar association between higher systolic and diastolic blood pressure in adulthood and lower birthweight has been reported in Croatia (4). These studies suggest, then, that environmental influences—in this case fetal malnutrition—may have an impact on the development of risk for adult cardiovascular disease from very early stages in life (5).

The lifelong progression of pathologic processes such as atherosclerosis that lead to adult disease is not necessarily inexorable. Indeed, the expectation that such pathogenesis can be ameliorated or even arrested is central to the rationale for a pediatric preventive approach. This conclusion arises from the recognition that certain risk factors are associated with—and are probably causal to—these processes, and that, in many cases, these risk factors are modifiable through alterations in lifestyle behaviors.

Some risk factors, of course, are not alterable. The development of essential hypertension, for example, is strongly influenced by genetic factors. And the risk of myocar-

dial infarction from atherosclerotic vascular disease is much greater if an adult is male rather than female. Changing one's genetic constitution or gender is hardly an appropriate option for reducing the risk of adult chronic disease.

The expectation that risks of adult chronic disease can be favorably modified rests instead with the idea of minimizing those factors—outlined in the following chapters—that can be changed. The role of the health care provider for children in this effort, then, is a reduction of these modifiable risk factors for adult chronic disease at an early time in life. The rationale, albeit not yet proven, behind this approach is that early risk factor reduction has the greatest chance of slowing the pathologic processes that begin during childhood and surface as clinical outcomes (such as myocardial infarction, stroke, and bone fractures) later in the adult years (6).

In summary, then, the rationale for a pediatric approach to prevention of adult chronic disease is based on three established observations: 1) adult diseases such as coronary artery disease, hypertension, and osteoporosis have their origins in childhood and adolescence; 2) certain identifiable factors appear to increase the risks for these diseases; and 3) some of these risk factors are modifiable through changes in lifestyle. It follows, then, that efforts to lessen health risk factors during childhood may pay long-term dividends in preventing or ameliorating chronic diseases of adulthood.

INTERVENTIONS: THE MODIFIABLE RISK FACTORS

The modifiable risk factors for adult chronic disease are all related to behavior—what one eats, how much one exercises, and whether one indulges in high risk activities such as cigarette smoking. Viewed simplistically, the good news is that such behaviors are all very easy to change. To eat a bag of potato chips or not is in direct control of the individual. One has the opportunity to elect to walk to school rather than take the bus. It is not difficult to avoid purchasing cigarettes.

In truth, however, altering human behavior is often extremely difficult. Limiting caloric intake, doing a daily workout, stopping smoking cigarettes are challenging for even the most motivated of patients, and even short-term success often fails in the long run. Habitual behaviors are simply not readily malleable. Efforts at understanding the reasons for behavioral obstacles to reduction of risk factors and identifying strategies for helping patients achieve these goals remains one of preventive medicine's greatest challenges.

At the same time, it is important to note that reduction of risk factors of sufficient degree to strongly affect adult disease morbidity may not involve drastic changes in an individual's habitual lifestyle. Thus, it is possible to make appropriate recommendations to patients for behavioral modification that are not unrealistic.

Diet

Many of the risk factors for adult disease surround dietary habits. Amount of calories, fat consumption, and sodium and calcium intake are the critical issues. A modest reduction of high-fat foods, elimination of salt at the table and in cooking, and regular consumption of low-fat dairy products (skim milk, yogurt) are not difficult changes for most patients to implement. Such dietary adjustments would serve to help protect against obesity, hyperlipidemia, systemic hypertension, and osteoporosis.

Physical Activity

Accumulating research evidence indicates that maintaining regular exercise habits is an effective means of reducing risk factors for many forms of adult chronic disease. Adults who are more physically active can reduce body fat, demonstrate an improved blood lipid profile, lower blood pressure, and improve bone mass. Initially the salutary effects of exercise were connected with aerobic training regimens. It has become clear, however, that regular habits of moderately intense activities can effectively ameliorate health risk factors.

High-Risk Behaviors

Many personal behaviors can increase risk for adult disease (excessive alcohol or drug consumption, frenetic lifestyles). Cigarette smoking, however, stands out in the magnitude of its contribution to deaths from cancer, chronic lung disease, and cardiovascular disease. The difficulties in achieving success in smoking cessation serve to emphasize the public health need to prevent adolescents from starting the smoking habit. The continued high prevalence of smoking in teenagers provides evidence that more effective strategies to achieve this goal are needed.

Intuitively, altering health risk behaviors during childhood might provide a best hope for success in reducing risk for adult disease. That is, personal habits established early in life, at a time when behavior is most malleable, should be expected to persist to the adult years. Getting a 35-year old obese man to suddenly adopt a low-fat, reduced-sodium diet is not likely. But the preschool child who ingests the same diet may be more likely to sustain proper dietary habits later in life.

Any health professional who has attempted such interventions instantly realizes, however, that the child cannot be considered in isolation from the entire family. The young patient's behaviors, access to food, and stimulation to exercise or watch television is controlled by other family members. Efforts to reduce health risk factors in children are unlikely to be successful unless the entire family is joined in the cause. In adolescents the problem is compounded by the fact that in many cases the persons exerting external influence on diet and activity behaviors—the teenager's peers—are not part of the "game plan".

There is yet, in fact, no scientific proof that early childhood habits beget adult behaviors. Nor has it been established that favorable reduction of coronary risk factors in children will in fact diminish the risks of adult cardiovascular disease. But the evidence outlined in the chapters that follow provides a strong rationale for the potential of pediatric interventions to prevent chronic disease in adults by reducing health risk factors.

THE PEDIATRIC APPROACH: WHAT ARE THE ISSUES?

A number of issues surround the appropriate pediatric approach to the prevention of adult disease. In some cases,

these questions have been sufficiently troublesome to cause some skepticism regarding the value of such interventions in the childhood age group. Others surround identifying the most cost-effective means of introducing these measures into primary care practice. Addressing these issues remains a major challenge for those committed to the value of pediatric preventive medicine.

Scientific Evidence

The first issue is whether there is any scientific evidence that pediatric preventive health interventions will lessen the incidence or severity of adult chronic diseases. Unfortunately, no research data exist that demonstrate that reducing health risk factors in a child will diminish the risk of cardiovascular disease or other chronic conditions when he or she becomes an adult. And considering the complexity of such a long-term longitudinal study, with all its confounding variables, it is unlikely that such an investigation will ever be accomplished. Scientific proof of the effectiveness of interventions in childhood to decrease later health risks may never be available.

Based on the rationale outlined above, however, such unequivocal scientific evidence is not necessary to recognize the logical importance of pediatric preventive medicine. Adult health risk factors such as obesity, hypercholesterolemia, and sedentary lifestyle are already common in the pediatric age group. Interventional studies in adults have indicated the effectiveness of reduction of such risk factors on the incidence of adverse health outcomes. For example, improving serum lipid profile in adults has decreased the incidence of cardiovascular events.

A pediatric approach would not, of course, be justified if adverse outcomes were identified that resulted from decreasing health risk factors. Given adherence to recommended guidelines, "side effects" recognized from preventive efforts in children have been unusual. These have included the psychological effects of being identified as at risk for future disease (such as "heart attacks"), side effects of medications, and calorie deprivation by overzealous dietary restriction (7).

Risk Factors and Predictability

A second issue is determining if health risk factors track from childhood to the adult years. There would be little to justify efforts at adult health risk factor identification and intervention in children if the future levels of these factors in the adult years could not be predicted from those in a child or adolescent. If a 5-year old child demonstrates an elevated blood cholesterol level, it would make no sense to lower it if he or she was not expected to demonstrate a high value later on in the adult years.

For this reason, great attention has focused on establishing the trend of health risk factors to retain their rank among groups of individuals as children age into adolescence and young adulthood. Results of those studies are outlined in the different chapters that follow. Whether one can conclude that health risk factors track "well" as a child ages is perhaps open to interpretation (8). For most risk factors there is a good deal of jumping between quintiles of values over time in a given population, so future predictability, although perhaps statistically significant, may not be often high. On the other hand, children who demonstrate a high risk profile (such as systolic blood pressure at the 95th percentile for age) typically have a significantly increased chance of possessing a similar risk on long-term follow-up.

Appropriate Target Groups

Considerable controversy has surrounded the appropriate pediatric target population for risk factor reduction. Should physicians identify only those at high risk or counsel all their patients regarding healthy behavioral changes? Those advocating the latter have noted that 1) most children and adolescents at risk for future disease are not at high risk, and 2) only modest improvements in risk factors among the population can be expected to result in a significant impact on public health (9). On the other hand, overzealous marketing of these preventive health strategies might cause a negative backlash in increasing family anxiety or even creating maladaptive behavioral changes.

It is clear that recommendations that are universally applied to the pediatric population are appropriate—or even necessary—for certain long-term health issues. Advocating increased low-fat dairy products in teenagers to help prevent osteoporosis or promoting a "prudent" diet to improve serum lipid profiles are obvious examples.

However, any strategy that affects the entire pediatric population must be no more than modest in its expectations of altering behavior. Universal recommendations must be acceptable to most families without drastic, unrealistic changes in life style. In addition, no adverse health effects should be expected.

The most reasonable strategy, then, is to institute a combination of these two approaches. General recommendations for improving the quality of the diet and maintaining a physically active lifestyle can be provided that are not difficult to achieve by most families. High-risk patients—those with elevated cholesterol levels, obesity, or sedentary life styles—need to be identified by appropriate history, physical examination, or laboratory measures. These children and adolescents can be highlighted for specific interventions, which in some cases may require more significant dietary alterations or use of medications.

The strategic philosophy for pediatric preventive medicine thus needs to be recognized as twofold. In the following chapters, the specific roles for each of these two approaches will be discussed for the various adult chronic diseases.

Obstacles to Acceptance

Certain aspects of the pediatric approach to long-term health strategies have caused hesitancy, both by physicians and the families of their young patients (10). Concerns regarding future health risk factors in a child lack a sense of immediacy. It may be difficult to convince parents to make significant behavioral changes based on potential adverse health outcomes that may not be apparent until 50 years later. Similarly, physicians may have little confidence in their ability to effect behavioral changes in children and their families.

Physicians are in need of better methods for modifying unhealthy behavior in their young patients. Disillusionment with the ability to alter children's behavior is expected when the means for accomplishing such changes have not been established. How does one get a sedentary child involved in regular physical activity? What strategies hold promise for weight reduction in obese children (and their families)? Are there effective office-based educational strategies for preventing smoking? Additional research and education of physicians on practical means of reducing long-term health risk factors in children are needed if pediatric preventive medicine is to be effective.

Summary

In summary, what began as a concept has grown to become a scientifically supported, logical preventive health initiative: reduction of risk factors for adult chronic disease during the pediatric years is a sound strategy for decreasing mortality and morbidity in the adult years. Consequently, routine interventions to reduce maladaptive health behaviors are warranted in the course of routine pediatric care (11).

Additional research will be important in identifying the most effective means of accomplishing this goal. We need to know more regarding the early identification of children at risk, appropriate means of altering eating and exercise behaviors, and the effective management of high risk patients. Much more insight is necessary, too, in identifying the determinants of health-related behaviors in families. Knowing both what causes and changes risk behaviors is critical to an effective pediatric approach to preventing adult disease.

REFERENCES

1. Bronfin DR, Urbina EM. The role of the pediatrician in the promotion of cardiovascular health. Am J Med Sci 1995;310(suppl):S42–S47.

2. Oalmann MC, Strong JP, Tracy RE, Malcolm GT. Atherosclerosis in youth: are hypertension and other coronary heart disease risk factors already at work? Pediatr Nephrol 1997;11:99–107.

3. Barker DJP, Gluckman PD, Godfrey KM, et al. Fetal nutrition and cardiovascular disease in adult life. Lancet 1993;341:938–941.

4. Kolacek S, Kapetanovic T, Luzar V. Early determinants of cardiovascular risk factors in adults. Acta Paediatr 1993;82:699–704.

5. Rocchini AP. Fetal and pediatric origins of adult cardiovascular disease. Curr Opinion Pediatr 1994;6:591–595.

6. Kwiterovich PO. Prevention of coronary disease starting in childhood: what risk factors should be identified and treated? Coron Artery Dis 1993;4:611–630.

7. Lifschitz F, Moses N. Growth failure: a complication of dietary treatment of hypercholesterolemia. Am J Dis Child 1989;143:537–542.

8. Cunnane SC. Childhood origins of lifestyle-related risk factors for coronary heart disease in adulthood. Nutr Health 1993;9:107–115.

9. Lenfant C, Savage PJ. The early natural history of atherosclerosis and hypertension in the young: National Institutes of Health perspectives. Am J Med Sci 1995; 310(suppl):S3–S7.

10. Rowland TW. Preventive cardiology in children: faith, hope and strategic policy making. Med Exerc Nutr Health 1994;3:178–179.

11. Strong WB, Deckelbaum RJ, Gidding SS, et al. Integrated cardiovascular health promotion in childhood. Circulation 1992;85: 1638–1650.

Chapter 50

Childhood Obesity

Scott Owens
Bernard Gutin

The prevalence of childhood obesity has increased dramatically in the United States and other industrialized nations during the past two to three decades. While the social and psychological burdens often encountered by obese children might seem like challenge enough, there is the additional issue of the short- and long-term medical consequences of their obesity. Since it is likely that pediatricians and other health care professionals will have increasingly frequent treatment opportunities with obese children, it is important to stay abreast of the latest research in the field.

In this chapter we present an overview of the current state of knowledge regarding childhood obesity. Issues related to the definition and prevalence of childhood obesity are discussed first. In the next section, the implications of childhood obesity are presented, emphasizing the notion that many adult diseases have their beginnings in childhood. The etiology of childhood obesity is discussed next, with special emphasis on the importance of the physical activity component of energy expenditure. The final section presents the most recent findings regarding the treatment of childhood obesity, including data that suggest that there is cause for optimism regarding long-term outcomes.

DEFINITION AND PREVALENCE

Defining childhood obesity is difficult, and no generally accepted definition has yet emerged (1,2). Ideally, the definition should reflect adiposity, or the amount of body fat, and be related to morbidity and mortality outcomes. An ideal measure of body fat would be: 1) accurate in its measure of body fat; 2) precise, with a small measurement error; 3) accessible, in terms of simplicity, cost, and ease of use; 4) acceptable to the subject; and 5) have published reference values (3). Unfortunately, no current measure satisfies all these criteria. Highly accurate methods such as isotope dilution or magnetic resonance imaging (MRI) are useful research tools, but are expensive and generally impractical in clinical settings. Underwater densitometry, also widely used in adult research, requires considerable time and subject cooperation, making it less desirable for use with children. These drawbacks have resulted in the continued reliance on anthropometric measurements in the clinical setting. Although not the ideal measures of adiposity for every individual, anthropometric measures tend to satisfy the criteria of simplicity, cost, ease of use, and availability of reference values. Some frequently encountered anthropometric definitions of childhood obesity include body weight greater than 120% of the value predicted from height (4), body mass index (BMI) greater than the 85th percentile (1), triceps skinfold thickness greater than the 85th percentile (5), and a body fat level higher than 25% for boys and 30% girls as estimated from the sum of subscapular and triceps skinfolds (6). Several authors have recommended BMI as the measurement of choice for most clinical settings due to its high reliability and ease of measurement (3,7).

Prevalence data from the third National Health and Nutrition Examination Survey (NHANES III, 1988–1991), which used the 85th percentile of BMI from previous national samples as the reference point, estimated the prevalence of child (age 6 through 11) and adolescent (age 12 through 17) obesity for all race and ethnic groups combined to be 22% (1). Data from this nationally representative cross-sectional survey clearly indicate a dramatic increase in the prevalence of excess body mass in relation to height in children and adolescents in the United States since the mid-1960s. Obesity prevalence increased among all sex and age groups. Similarly, increased ponderosity (weight/height^3) has been reported for cohorts of children examined between 1973 and 1992 in the Bogalusa Heart Study (8). Trends for increased obesity in children also have been observed in other industrialized countries, including France (9) and England and Scotland (10). It is likely, therefore, that pediatricians will encounter the obese child on a routine basis.

IMPLICATIONS

Although obesity-related health problems such as coronary artery disease (CAD), hypertension, and non-insulin dependent diabetes mellitus (NIDDM) tend to present their clinical manifestations in adulthood, evidence indicates these disorders have their beginnings in childhood (11), with obese children tending to have a poorer risk profile for these diseases than their counterparts of normal weight. For example, childhood obesity is associated with elevated levels of triglycerides (8,12) and LDL cholesterol (13), and reduced levels of HDL cholesterol (8,14). Obese children tend to display higher levels of blood pressure (15,16) and insulin (12,13) than non-obese children. In adults, the clustering of risk factors such as dyslipidemia, hypertension, and hyperinsulinemia is often referred to as "syndrome X" or the insulin resistance syndrome; it places an individual at an unusually high risk for CAD and NIDDM (17). For children, data from the Bogalusa Heart Study indicate the clustering of the syndrome X risk factors begins around age 5, that the clustering tracks from childhood into young adulthood, and that it tracks more strongly in obese children (11).

Several other worrisome associations with childhood obesity have been reported recently. In a group of lean and obese children, higher percentages of body fat were associated with increased left ventricular mass and relative wall thickness (the ratio of left ventricular wall thickness to cavity size) and with decreased left ventricular mid-wall fractional shortening (18). In adults, greater left ventricular mass and relative wall thickness are predictive of future cardiovascular morbidity (19). Decreased mid-wall fractional shortening is an index of left ventricular systolic function that identifies individuals at elevated risk for future cardiovascular mortality who are otherwise undetected by conventional endocardial shortening indices (20). Also, in a group of 7- to 13-year-old children, increased body fat was associated with greater endothelial dysfunction as represented by a lower amount of femoral artery dilation in response to the increased blood flow that occurred following the release of a tourniquet (21). Endothelial dysfunction is a relatively early event in atherogenesis (22). More specifically, low levels of endothelium-dependent arterial dilation are associated with various manifestations of cardiovascular disease in adults and children (23). These results support the idea that fatness plays a role in the early stages of the atherogenic process.

In addition to overall adiposity, fat patterning in childhood obesity may have implications. In adults, fat stored in the abdominal region, especially in the visceral compartment, is more clearly associated with syndrome X and the development of CAD and NIDDM than is fat stored in other parts of the body (24–26). Some (27), but not all (12), studies of children have detected an association between fat patterning and risk factors. An important limitation of childhood studies that used anthropometry or dual x-ray absorptiometry (DXA) is that they could not distinguish subcutaneous abdominal adipose tissue from the more deleterious visceral adipose tissue. In adults, various measures of central fat deposition, including the waist/hip ratio or waist circumference alone, may be related to risk factors. However, in children, very little of the abdominal fat is in the visceral adipose tissue compartment relative to the amount in subcutaneous abdominal adipose tissue (28,29). Therefore, at an early stage in the development of syndrome X (i.e., in childhood), it may be necessary to measure visceral adipose tissue directly in order to uncover its relation to other risk factors. In this regard, a study that used MRI in obese children found that visceral adipose tissue, but not subcutaneous abdominal adipose tissue, was significantly related to LDL cholesterol and triglycerides (29). Furthermore, a study involving obese and nonobese adolescent girls found that visceral adipose tissue was significantly correlated with triglycerides, HDL cholesterol, and insulin in the obese girls only (30). On the other hand, a study of nonobese 7- to 10-year-old girls found no significant relationship between visceral adipose tissue and triglycerides, HDL cholesterol, or insulin (31). Therefore, the visceral adipose tissue-risk factor relationship appears to be more pronounced in obese than in lean children. From a clinical perspective, it is not yet clear the extent to which visceral adiposity can be predicted from the anthropometric measurements commonly used in clinical settings.

Not to be overlooked is evidence that childhood obesity is often associated with significant social and psychological problems. In a study of 139 obese and 150 nonobese children aged 9 to 12, the obese children reported more negative physical self-perceptions than their nonobese peers and scored lower on measures of general self-worth (32). Studies show that obese children report more depression and receive more negative peer reactions than nonobese children (33,34). When shown drawings of six children, four with physical disabilities, one with no physical disability, and an obese child, both children and adults rated the obese child as the least likable (35,36). It is likely that the immediacy of the social and psychological implications of obesity are of greater concern to children than the long-term health implications.

ETIOLOGY

Childhood obesity is the result of a complex interaction of genetic and environmental factors. In a recent review of the role of genes in the variation of human body mass, two of the conclusions were: 1) there are good reasons to believe that the genes involved in body mass variation over time in a given individual as well as those responsible for population heterogeneity in body mass eventually will be identified; and 2) there are equally good reasons to believe that environmental conditions and lifestyle characteristics make an even stronger contribution than the genes to intra-individual and inter-individual variation in body mass (37). Regardless of whether the underlying impetus is genetic or environmental, it is understood that obesity results from an imbalance between energy intake and energy expenditure.

Energy Intake

It is evident that accurate and reliable quantitative information about energy and macronutrient intake would be valuable, but such data are difficult to obtain, especially in children. Cross-sectional studies using diet recall methods generally have not found a relationship between body fatness and energy intake (38). These results are counterintuitive, in light of the fact that obese adults and children have relatively high fat-free mass along with their elevated fat mass, and consequently have elevated resting energy expenditure (39), the largest component of 24-hour energy expenditure. Assuming that the energy costs of thermoregulation and growth are small (40), 24-hour energy expenditure must equal energy intake. Using the doubly labeled water procedure (i.e., isotope dilution) to validate self-reported measures of energy intake, it has been found that obese adults (41) and adolescents (42) tend to underreport energy intake to a greater degree than lean people. More objective and expensive means of collecting diet data, such as direct observation, might influence the youth's diet behavior and are very intrusive; thus this methodology is not feasible for most studies. Consequently, methodologic considerations make it difficult to draw any clear conclusions about the role of total free living energy intake in the etiology of obesity.

Perhaps these methodologic difficulties partly explain why it is difficult to find evidence that the increased prevalence of childhood obesity over the past few decades is the result of increased caloric intake. In fact, the reported mean daily energy intakes of 6- to 11-year-olds showed a slight decline (3%) from NHANES II (1976–1980) to NHANES III (1988–1991) (43). In another study, the daily caloric intakes of 1670 (1977–1978) and 1463 (1986–1988) children aged 2 to 10 remained constant over the 10-year period with mean intakes of 1632 kcal in 1978 and 1613 kcal in 1988 (44).

With respect to fat intake, most (45–47), but not all studies (48) support the idea that diets high in fat are associated with body fatness or gain in weight. Lissner et al (49) found that a high-fat diet led to a greater 6-year weight gain in women who were sedentary, but not in those who were physically active. Thus, it may be the synergistic effect of a high-fat diet and sedentary behavior that is a key determinant of obesity. Prospective studies testing this hypothesis have not yet been reported in children.

Energy Expenditure

Total energy expenditure is comprised of resting metabolic rate, the thermic effect of food, and physical activity; resting metabolic rate constitutes 60% to 70% of the total, the thermic effect of food approximately 10%, and physical activity the remainder.

Resting Metabolic Rate

A cross-sectional study found that children of obese parents had relatively low resting metabolic rates (50), suggesting that they were at increased risk for development of obesity. However, when these children were followed up 12 years later (51), the children of the obese parents were not found to be more obese than the children of nonobese parents. Moreover, two larger-scale doubly labeled water studies (40,52) failed to find any evidence that children of obese parents had defects in any aspect of energy expenditure.

Cross-sectional studies comparing obese and nonobese children, in which the influence of body composition was taken into account statistically, have found the groups to have similar resting and 24-hour metabolic rates (42,53,54). However, the cross-sectional nature of these investigations precludes firm conclusions of causality; prospective studies in children of different ages are needed to elucidate the nature of these relationships. In this regard, a recent doubly labeled water study of children (55) failed to show that resting energy expenditure predicted body fatness 2 to 4 years later. Therefore, there is little reason to believe that variation in resting metabolic rate explains the development of childhood obesity.

Thermic Effect of Food

In order to capture most of the thermic effect of food it is necessary to measure postprandial metabolism while the child remains relatively motionless for several hours, a daunting task for both the subjects and investigators. Moreover, the thermic effect of food is the component of energy expenditure that is least reproducible (56). Therefore, it has not been extensively studied and its role in the etiology of childhood obesity is unclear. Although some adult studies suggest that the thermic effect of food may be blunted in obese people (57), cross-sectional studies of children do not provide a consistent picture concerning differences between lean and obese populations (42,53) and no prospective studies in children have been reported.

Physical Activity

Although physical activity constitutes a relatively small portion of total energy expenditure on average, it has potential importance in explaining obesity development for several reasons. First, it is largely volitional. Second, its great individual variability provides an opportunity for it to explain a large portion of the variance in total energy expenditure. Third, activity can increase fat-free mass, the main determinant of resting metabolic rate (56), with long-term consequences on energy balance. Fourth, exercise training can influence substrate utilization, thereby playing a role in how ingested nutrients are partitioned into fat and fat-free mass.

It is problematic to determine from nonexperimental studies whether exercise and body fatness are related because of the difficulty of knowing how to express physical activity. If it is expressed as energy expenditure, then it might be concluded that obese youths are more active than lean youths, as was found in a doubly labeled water study by Bandini et al (42). However, differences in mechanical work done must be considered when interpreting data on energy expenditure during activity; that is, a heavier child uses more energy to move the body a given distance. Thus, if a lean and an obese child display the same free-living activity energy expenditure, it represents less movement in the obese child. Consequently, it is necessary to adjust activity energy expenditure for body weight to determine if variations in movement are associated with fatness. The problem concerns the exponent to use in making this adjustment. If an exponent of one is used—i.e., energy expenditure is simply divided by weight—then an overcorrection may result, automatically creating a negative correlation with fatness (58). Unfortunately, the correction factor varies for different children, depending on how much of their activity involves carrying the body weight (e.g., walking/running) and how much involves activity in which the body weight is supported and most of the work is external (e.g., cycling). The variety of procedures used to try to correct for body weight may account for the discrepant findings of cross-sectional doubly labeled water studies (40,59,60).

Unfortunately, perhaps for some of these same reasons, prospective studies that have used doubly labeled water methodology have not provided a clear picture either. One study (61) suggested that greater activity energy expenditure led to less weight gain during the first year of life in a small group of infants, but a larger-scale study (55) failed to show that activity energy expenditure predicted body fatness 2 to 4 years later.

Time-motion studies, even those that depend on self or parental reporting (which is less objective than energy expenditure measurements), may provide a more direct index of how much actual exercise the child does. Cross-sectional studies of this nature show that active children are less fat (60) even while ingesting more energy (62); however, it is impossible to tell whether the activity caused less fatness or whether lower fatness caused the greater activity. A clearer picture emerges from recent epidemiologic studies in which the exercise levels of children were estimated by the parents in relation to other children of the same age. It was found that lower exercise levels and family history of obesity were principal risk factors for later development of childhood obesity (63) or higher levels of BMI (64). Another recent study, which used the Caltrac movement sensor to measure activity, found that preschoolers who were classified as inactive were 3.8 times as likely as active children to have an increasing triceps skinfold slope during the average of 2.5 years of follow-up (65).

The childhood behavior most frequently cited as contributing to increased physical inactivity is television watching. In a recent study, Gortmaker et al (66) examined the relationship between hours of television viewed and the prevalence of overweight in 1990, and the incidence of overweight from 1986 to 1990 in a nationally representative sample of 746 youths from the ages of 10 to 15. Overweight was defined as BMI greater than the 85th percentile for age and gender. The study reported a strong dose-response relationship between the prevalence of overweight in 1990 and hours of television viewed. After controlling for potentially confounding variables such as previous overweight status, household structure, socioeconomic status, maternal overweight, and ethnicity, the odds of being overweight were 5.3 times greater for youth watching more than 5 hours of television per day compared with those watching 2 hours or fewer. The investigators also examined prospectively the association of variables measured in 1986 with television viewing in 1990. In a multivariate regression predicting television viewing, they found no evidence that causality was running in the opposite than suggested direction, i.e., that being overweight was a cause of television viewing. In a study of younger (aged 3–4) children, on the other hand, television viewing time was not related to fatness (67). A possible explanation for these divergent findings is that the effects of television viewing on weight are likely to

be small in the short term, but to be cumulative across time. By age 10 to 15, the effect of television on increased fatness has had many years to take effect (66).

To the degree that aerobic fitness can be accepted as a proxy for physical activity, recent results of a 3-year longitudinal study of 7- to 12-year olds (68) are pertinent. It was found that those children who increased the most in maximal oxygen consumption were those who increased the most in fat-free mass but increased the least in skinfold fatness.

Another factor to consider is the intensity of the activity. In adults, Tremblay et al (69) found that when total energy expenditure during physical activity was held constant statistically, people who engaged in high-intensity exercise were leaner and had less central fat deposition. However, little is known about the role of different exercise intensities in the etiology of childhood fatness.

Exercise may also influence the accumulation of fat by improving the use of lipids as a substrate for energy (70,71), because fat oxidation has been identified as a risk factor for weight gain in adult Pima Indians (72). People who oxidized less fat than carbohydrate over the course of the day, as indicated by higher respiratory exchange ratios, were more likely to gain weight and fat mass, i.e., the unoxidized fat was more likely to go into storage. This effect was independent of 24-hour energy expenditure measured in the metabolic chamber. However, the ability of lipid oxidation to predict future changes in fatness of children has not yet been elucidated in prospective studies.

In light of the recent discovery in mice that the hormone leptin decreases energy intake and increases energy expenditure, some investigations of these relations have been undertaken in children. Caprio et al (73) found in children and young adults that leptin was closely correlated with subcutaneous abdominal adipose tissue ($r = 0.84$, $p < 0.001$) and somewhat less closely correlated with visceral adipose tissue ($r = 0.59$, $p < 0.001$); in addition, acute increases in insulin concentrations did not affect circulating insulin levels. Lahlou et al (74) found that serum leptin levels were positively correlated with fasting insulin levels, adiposity, and weight gain the previous year, but were not associated with resting energy expenditure. Moreover, leptin was not related to lower energy intake; indeed, the obese children ingested two to three times more energy (measured with self-reports) than the lean children. Salbe et al (75) examined cross-sectional relations among these factors in 5-year-old Pima Indian children. They found that leptin concentrations, which were closely correlated to percent body fat ($r = 0.84$, $P < 0.001$), were also correlated with physical activity level (the ratio of total to resting energy expenditure, measured with doubly labeled water), after adjustment for body fat ($r = .26$, $P < .01$). Nagy et al (76) found black and white girls to have higher leptin levels than black and white boys; however, these differences were no longer significant after controlling for total body composition, visceral adipose tissue, and subcutaneous abdominal adipose tissue. These results indicate that in children leptin is a marker of adiposity, but does not suppress energy intake or halt fat deposition, suggesting some type of leptin resistance. Perhaps the most important lesson to derive is that predictions from mouse studies concerning what relations may exist in humans must be made with great caution.

In brief, the difficulty of measuring activity and diet, compounded by the uncertainty of what is meant by "physical activity," make few definitive conclusions warranted. Perhaps the most reasonable conclusion is similar to one reached in a study of 10-year weight changes in a national cohort of adults (77); i.e., that low physical activity leads to weight gain, while weight gain leads to further diminution of activity. This would imply that interventions that either decrease fatness or increase activity would turn the cycle in the other, more favorable, direction.

Specific Endocrine and Genetic Disorders

Although specific endocrine and genetic disorders appear to be responsible for less than 10% of childhood obesity, it has been suggested that physicians rule them out as causes since they require different modes of therapy (4). Endocrine disorders to consider include Cushing's syndrome, hypothyroidism, and pseudohypoparathyroidism. Syndromes of genetic origin associated with childhood obesity include Prader-Willi, Alstrom, Laurence-Moon-Biedl, Carpenter, and Cohen.

TREATMENT

To begin with, some researchers have cautioned against the use of treatments for obesity in children under age 3 whose parents are not obese (78,79). These children are at low risk of obesity in young adulthood (79). On the other hand, interventions may be warranted in obese children as young as age 1 to 2 if one or both parents are obese. For children who are candidates for treatment, interventions typically include diet and/or exercise. Although dieting alone can result in significant short-term weight loss in obese children, it tends to reduce fat-free mass and resting energy expenditure (80), thereby setting the stage for regain of the lost fat when the diet stops (81). On the other hand, adult studies show that exercise has the potential to reduce the diet-induced loss of fat-free mass (82). In children, the extent to which exercise alone can influence obesity is unclear. School-based interventions, where it is difficult to control and document the exercise stimulus, show mixed results for the effects of exercise on obesity status (83–85). In more highly controlled studies, where the exercise stimulus was well-documented and body fat was measured with DXA, exercise without dietary intervention resulted in significant reductions in body fat (86,87). However, the absolute amount of fat loss attained with exercise alone was modest. Therefore, a combination of exercise and diet seems more sensible for clinical use.

In this regard, one of the more promising treatment models integrates improved nutrition, increased physical activity, and behavioral modification within the context of a parental or family-based intervention. Epstein (88) has outlined the rationale for family-based behavioral interventions for obese children, noting that just as the family environment can contribute to the development of childhood obesity, it can also function as the focal point for the solution. Parenting styles influence the development of food preferences and the ability of the child to regulate intake. Parents and other family members arrange a common environment that may be conducive to overeating or a sedentary lifestyle. They also serve as role models and reinforcers for eating and exercise behaviors.

Components of Family-based Behavioral Interventions

The basic structure of family-based behavioral interventions for childhood obesity tend to be similar, i.e, an initial, short-term treatment phase followed by a longer-term maintenance or continued improvement phase. During initial treatment, children typically meet in group settings once per week for 45 to 90 minutes (89,90) for between 8 (91,92) and 16 weeks (89,90,93). Facilitators for the treatment sessions have included pediatricians, child psychologists, nutritionists, and "trained therapists" (89,94–96). Follow-up sessions usually occur once (89,95) or twice per month (92,93) for 6 months to 1 year. In some cases, parents and children attend the same treatment sessions (89), but more often attend concurrent sessions (92–94). Brownell et al (89) have suggested that in older children and adolescents, having parents and offspring meet concurrently but separately may result in better long-term outcomes. Separate sessions allow for a more open discussion of sensitive issues by both parents and children and help children assume more responsibility for their treatment. Younger children may require more supervision from their parents, and this warrants holding treatment sessions together.

The specific dietary and physical activity interventions vary from study to study, as do the particular behavior modification techniques introduced. Table 50-1 summarizes this information from several family-based behavioral interventions. The variety of behavior modification methods reflects a recognition of the multicomponent nature of obesity treatment and the importance of parental/family involvement.

A number of dietary approaches have been employed; some focus on healthy eating habits rather than energy restriction, while others prescribe significant caloric reduction. As an example of the later, Figueroa-Colon et al (94) utilized a protein-sparing modified fast diet (600–800 kcal/day) for 10 weeks with obese 7- to 11-year-olds on an outpatient basis (with close medical supervision). Subsequently, the subjects transitioned to a hypocaloric balanced diet of 1200 kcal/day for the next 42 months. Although positive results were reported (see Table 50-1), others have suggested that restrictive diets be reserved for massively obese adolescents, or for children and adolescents with morbid complications of obesity, such as hypertension, sleep apnea, or NIDDM (97). Gill (98) recommends only small reductions in energy intake as a part of treatment, suggesting that excessive energy restriction in obese children is unwise and unsafe.

Epstein et al (93) have utilized a nutritional approach labeled the "Traffic Light" Diet. This diet divides food into five categories: fruits and vegetables; grain; milk and dairy; protein and other. Each category is subdivided into red, yellow, and green designations. These colors have the same meaning as they do on a traffic light: stop (red), approach with caution (yellow), and go (green). Red foods are those high in fat or simple carbohydrates, high in calories, and low in nutrient density. Yellow foods are the staples of the diet and supply basic nutrition. Green foods are those that are lower than 20 kcal per average serving, and are represented only in the fruit and vegetable and other (condiments) groups. Children (and overweight parents) are instructed to consume

Table 50-1 Behavior, Diet, and Physical Activity Modifications from Selected Family-based Behavioral Interventions for Childhood Obesity

Study	Year	Ages	Behavior	Diet	Physical activity
Brownell et al (89)	83	12–16	self-monitoring, stimulus control and cue elimination, behavior chains and preplanning, attitude restructuring and cognitive control, engendering family support	nutrition education, emphasis on low sugar, salt and fat	increasing physical activity encouraged
Figueroa-Colon et al (94)	93	7–17	self-monitoring, stimulus control, cue elimination, behavior chains and preplanning, cognitive restructuring, goal setting, parent-child contracting	hypocaloric diets (600–800 kcal/day) for 10 wks); 1200 kcal/day for next 42 wks	gradually increase physical activity using an aerobic points system
Epstein et al (93)	95	8–12	self-monitoring, stimulus control, reinforcement including record keeping for diet and physical activity and reciprocal contracting by parents and children	Traffic Light Diet with target of 1000–1200 kcal/day	subjects reinforced for either increasing physical activity or reducing sedentary behavior
Braet et al (95)	97	7–16	self-instruction, self-observation, self-evaluation, self-reward, behavior rehearsal, contracting, family reinforcement	nutrition education with emphasis on eating healthy rather than eating less; no counting calories	moderate intensity exercise for 30 min/day plus lifestyle changes to increase activity
Johnson et al (90)	97	8–16	cognitive/behavioral approach including contracting, self-monitoring and family support	modified Traffic Light Diet	gradual increase in daily exercise up to 45 min/session, 5–7 days/wk, at 60–80% of max HR

between 1000–1200 kcal/day, to limit "red" foods to seven or fewer per week, and to maintain nutrient balance by eating the recommended servings using the eating-right pyramid or the basic four food groups. Some consider the Traffic Light Diet too structured and limited, however, and instead recommend a "healthy lifestyles" approach to eating habits in which counting calories is not allowed (95).

The nature of the physical activity component covers a considerable range of possibilities. Included here are general recommendations such as exercising for 30 minutes per day in combination with lifestyle changes (taking the stairs, walking instead of going by car, etc.) (95) to the quite specific instruction to increase aerobic exercise according to a graded, 7-week schedule, up to 45 minutes 5 to 7 days per week at 60% to 80% of maximum heart rate (90). A novel approach to physical activity was developed by Epstein et al (93) in which children were reinforced for decreasing sedentary behavior rather than for increasing physical activity per se. Children who were reinforced for decreasing sedentary behavior increased their liking for high-intensity activity and reported lower caloric intake more than did children in the group that was reinforced for increasing physical activity.

Unfortunately, the influence of different types, amounts, and intensities of exercise has not been studied extensively in children. With respect to body fatness and exercise intensity, for example, Bar-Or et al (99) recently concluded that there are too few data available to make a recommendation. In adults, Tremblay et al (100) found that high intensity training was more effective in reducing body fatness than somewhat lower-intensity training. If total energy used during the exercise sessions is the critical parameter, then simply lengthening the low-intensity sessions can allow the youth to use the same amount of energy as would be used in a high-intensity session. Savage et al (101) used this approach with prepubertal boys and found skinfold fat to decline similarly in the low- and high-intensity groups, even though the high-intensity training resulted in a clearer improvement in cardiovascular fitness. Even when the energy expenditure during the training itself is controlled, there are reasons to suspect that higher intensities may be more efficacious in reducing fatness if the intervention continues for a longer period than the typical 2 to 4 months seen in many exercise-only interventions. First, the exponential relationship between exercise intensity and post-exercise metabolism may gradually lead to greater loss of fat as a result of high-intensity training. Second, if high-intensity training increases cardiovascular fitness more effectively, as shown by Savage et al (101), then the youth would be able progressively to use up more energy in a given amount of training time, eventually leading to greater fat loss. On the other hand, it may be that lower-intensity exercise is more agreeable to obese children over the long term, resulting in greater adherence.

Outcomes of Family-based Behavioral Interventions

The optimism associated with family-based behavioral interventions stems from evidence that this treatment approach may

Table 50-2 Outcomes for Family-based Behavioral Interventions for Childhood Obesity

Study	Year	Ages	n	1-year Outcome	5-year Outcome	10-year Outcome
Brownell et al (89)	83	12–16	36	% overweight: −10.7%; blood pressure: −1.9/−1.2 mm Hg		
Mellin et al (96)	87	12–18	34/29	relative weight: −9.9% vs −0.1% in control group		
Figueroa-Colon et al (94)	93	7–17	7/4	% overweight: −23% in protein-sparing diet group vs −20% in hypocaloric diet group; blood pressure: −14/−15 mm Hg when groups combined		
Israel et al (92)	94	8–13	11/9	% above triceps norm: +14.5% in enhanced treatment group vs −1.8% in standard treatment group		
Braet et al (95)	97	7–16	60/49	% overweight: −11% in experimental groups vs +3.5% in control group		
Johnson et al (90)	97	8–16	12/6		% of ideal body weight: −23% in experimental groups vs −11% in control group	
Epstein et al (102)	94	6–12	158 (in 4 studies)			30% of 158 children achieved non-obese status; 34% decreased % overweight by 20% or more

result in long-term benefits to obese children. Table 50-2 summarizes outcomes for family-based behavioral interventions reported at 1, 5, or 10 years after initiating treatment. With the exception of the study by Israel et al (92), meaningful reductions in obesity status were a consistent finding at the 1-year mark. Of even greater interest are the 5-year results from the study by Johnson et al (90) and the combined 10-year results from the four studies of Epstein et al (102). These studies provide the most compelling evidence that the treatment of obesity in children can be successful over extended periods from childhood through adolescence to adulthood (98). From Epstein's perspective, two of the most helpful points to be distilled from their 10-year results are the recommendations that at least one parent be an active participant in the weight loss process and that increasing physical activity is important for the maintenance of long-term weight control (88).

It has been noted, however, that the 10-year follow-up studies were all conducted by the same North American research group and that there is need for other authors to replicate the research, particularly in a non-US setting (103). Another observation is that the family-based behavioral intervention studies have tended to focus on outcomes related to simple anthropometric measurements such as percent overweight or BMI. Left largely unexamined are the effects of

these interventions on more direct measures of body fat and on the risk factors for obesity-related diseases such as CAD and NIDDM. It would be of considerable interest, for example, to know the effects of these interventions on fat patterning, especially visceral adipose tissue. In light of the relationship between visceral adipose tissue CAD risk factors, it is important to clarify how training influences this fat depot. In a recent study of obese 7- to 11-year-olds, children who engaged in 4 months of after-school exercise without dietary intervention or behavior modification declined significantly in visceral fat as compared to the control group (104). Would this favorable result have been enhanced within the context of a long-term, family-based behavioral intervention? Along the same lines, it would be important to know the extent to which a family-based behavioral intervention approach enhances the favorable results (reduced fatness and improved CAD risk factors) obtained in non-family based interventions that utilized exercise alone (83) or diet plus exercise (105,106).

SUMMARY

Childhood obesity is increasing in most modern societies, manifesting both short- and long-term deleterious consequences. The etiology of childhood obesity is complex, with genetic and environmental factors playing contributory roles. There is reason to believe that the long-term treatment of childhood obesity can be successful, however. Family-based behavioral interventions, which integrate dietary change, increased physical activity, and behavior modification within a setting of family support, offer one pathway for achieving this success.

REFERENCES

1. Troiano RP, Flegal KM, Kuczmarski RJ, et al. Overweight prevalence and trends for children and adolescents. Arch Pediatr Adolesc Med 1995;149: 1085–1091.

2. Flegal K. Defining obesity in children and adolescents: epidemiologic approaches. Crit Rev Food Sci Nutr 1993;33:307–312.

3. Power C, Lake J, Cole T. Measurement and long-term health risks of child and adolescent fatness. Int J Obes Rel Metab Disord 1997;21:507–526.

4. Williams CL, Campanaro LA, Squillace M, et al. Management of childhood obesity in pediatric practice. Ann N Y Acad Sci 1997;817:225–240.

5. Must A, Dallal G, Dietz W. Reference data for obesity: 85th and 95th percentiles of body mass index (wt/ht^2) and triceps skinfold thickness. Am J Clin Nutr 1991;53:839–846.

6. Williams D, Going S, Lohman T, et al. Body fatness and risk for elevated blood pressure, total cholesterol, and serum lipoprotein ratios in children and adolescents. Am J Public Health 1992; 82:358–363.

7. Himes JH, Dietz WH. Guidelines for overweight in adolescent preventive services: recommendations from an expert committee. Am J Clin Nutr 1994;59: 307–316.

8. Gidding SS, Bao W, Srinivasan SR, et al. Effects of secular trends in obesity on coronary risk factors in children: the Bogalusa Heart Study. J Pediatr 1995; 127:868–874.

9. Lehingue Y, Picot MC, Millot I, et al. Increase in the prevalence of obesity among children aged 4–5 years in a French district between 1988 and 1993. Revue Epidemiol Sante Publique 1996; 44:37–46.

10. Rona RJ. The national study of health and growth (NSHG): 23 years on the road. Int J Epidemiol 1995;24(suppl):S69–S74.

11. Berenson GS, Srinivasan SR, Bao W. Precursors of cardiovascular risk in young adults from a biracial (black-white) population: the Bogalusa Heart Study. Ann N Y Acad Sci 1997;817: 189–198.

12. Gutin B, Islam S, Manos T, et al. Relation of percentage body fat and maximal aerobic capacity to risk factors for atherosclerosis and diabetes in black and white seven- to eleven-year-old children. J Pediatr 1994;125:847–852.

13. Kikuchi D, Srinivasan S, Harsha D, et al. Relation of serum lipoprotein lipids and apolipoproteins to obesity in children: the Bogalusa Heart Study. Prev Med 1992;21:177–190.

14. Gutin B, Owens S, Treiber F, et al. Weight-independent cardiovascular fitness and coronary risk factors. Arch Pediatr Adolesc Med 1997;151:462–465.

15. Lauer RM, Burns TL, Clarke WR, et al. Childhood predictors of future blood pressure. Hypertension 1991;18(suppl):174–181.

16. McMurray RG, Harrell JS, Levine AA, et al. Childhood obesity elevates blood pressure and total cholesterol independent of physical activity. Int J Obes Relat Metab Disord 1995;19:881–886.

17. Reaven G. Role of insulin resistance in human disease. Diabetes 1988;37:1595–1607.

18. Gutin B, Treiber F, Owens S, Mensah G. Relations of body composition to left ventricular geometry and function in children. J Pediatr 1998;132:1023–1027.

19. Devereux RB, de Simone G, Ganau A, et al. Left ventricular hypertrophy and geometric remodeling in hypertension: stimuli, functional consequences and prognostic implications. J Hypertens 1994;12(suppl): S117–S127.

20. de Simone G, Devereux RB, Mureddu GF, et al. Influence of obesity on left ventricular midwall mechanics in arterial hypertension. Hypertension 1996;28:276–283.

21. Treiber F, Papavassiliou D, Gutin B, et al. Determinants of endothelium-dependent femoral artery vasodilation in youth. Psychosom Med 1997;59:376–381.

22. Meredith IT, Yeung AC, Weidinger FF. Role of impaired endothlium-dependent vasodilation in ischemic manifestations of coronary artery disease. Circulation 1993;87:56–66.

23. Celermajer DS. Endothelial dysfunction: does it matter? is it reversible? J Am Coll Cardiol 1997;30:325–333.

24. Despres JP, Moorjani S, Ferland M, et al. Adipose tissue distribution and plasma lipoprotein levels in obese women: importance of intra-abdominal fat. Arterioscler Thromb 1989;9:203–210.

25. Pouliot MC, Despres JP, Nadeau A, et al. Visceral obesity in men: associations with glucose tolerance, plasma insulin, and lipoprotein levels. Diabetes 1992;41:826–834.

26. Rissanen J, Hudson R, Ross R. Visceral adiposity, androgens, and plasma lipids in obese men. Metabolism 1994;43:1318–1323.

27. Asayama K, Hayashibe H, Dobashi K, et al. Relationships between biochemical abnormalities and anthropometric indices of overweight, adiposity and body fat distribution in Japanese elementary school children. Int J Obes Relat Metab Disord 1995; 19:253–259.

28. Goran MI, Kaskoun M, Shuman WP. Intra-abdominal adipose tissue in young children. Int J Obes Relat Metab Disord 1995; 19:279–283.

29. Brambilla P, Manzoni P, Sironi S, et al. Peripheral and abdominal adiposity in childhood obesity. Int J Obes Relat Metab Disord 1994; 18:795–800.

30. Caprio S, Hyman LD, McCarthy S, et al. Fat distribution and cardiovascular risk factors in obese adolescent girls: importance of the intraabdominal fat depot. Am J Clin Nutr 1996;64:12–17.

31. Yanovski JA, Yanovski SZ, Filmer KM, et al. Differences in body composition of black and white girls. Am J Clin Nutr 1996;64: 833–839.

32. Braet C, Mervielde I, Vandereycken W. Psychological aspects of childhood obesity: a controlled study in a clinical and nonclinical setting. J Pediatr Psychol 1997;22:59–71.

33. Baum CG, Forehand R. Social factors associated with adolescent obesity. J Pediatr Psychol 1984;9:293–302.

34. Strauss CC, Smith K, Frame C, et al. Personal and interpersonal characteristics associated with childhood obesity. J Pediatr Psychol 1985;10:337–343.

35. Richardson SA, Goodman N, Hastorf AH, et al. Cultural uniformity to physical disabilities. Am Sociol Rev 1961;26:241–247.

36. Maddox GL, Back K, Liederman V. Overweight as social deviance and disability. J Health Soc Behav 1968;9:287–298.

37. Bouchard C. Human variation in body mass: evidence for a role of the genes. Nutr Rev 1997; 55(suppl):S21–S30.

38. Miller W, Lindeman A, Wallace J, et al. Diet composition, energy intake, and exercise in relation to body fat in men and women. Am J Clin Nutr 1990;52:426–430.

39. Segal K, Gutin B. Thermic effects of food and exercise in lean and obese women. Metabolism 1983;32:581–589.

40. Davies PS, Wells JC, Fieldhouse CA, et al. Parental body composition and infant energy expenditure. Am J Clin Nutr 1995;61: 1026–1029.

41. Schoeller D, Bandini L, Dietz W. Inaccuracies in self-reported intake identified by comparison with the doubly labeled water method. Can J Physiol Pharmacol 1990;68:941–949.

42. Bandini L, Schoeller D, Cyr H, et al. Validity of reported energy intake in obese and nonobese adolescents. Am J Clin Nutr 1990;52:421–425.

43. Briefel RR, McDowell MA, Alaimo K, et al. Total energy intake of the U.S. population: the third National Health and Nutrition Examination Survey, 1988–1991. Am J Clin Nutr 1995;62(suppl): 1072S–1080S.

44. Albertson AM, Tobelmann RC. Ten-year trend of energy intakes of American children ages 2–10 years. Ann N Y Acad Sci 1993; 699:250–252.

45. Eck L, Klesges R, Hanson C, et al. Children at familial risk for obesity: an examination of dietary intake, physical activity and weight status. Int J Obesity Relat Metab Disord 1992;16:17–18.

46. Nguyen VT, Larson DE, Johnson RK, et al. Fat intake and adiposity in children of lean and obese parents. Am J Clin Nutr 1996; 63:507–513.

47. Maffeis C, Pinelli L, Schutz Y. Fat intake and adiposity in 8 to 11-year-old children. Int J Obes Relat Metab Disord 1996;20: 170–174.

48. Muecke L, Simons-Morton B, Huang I, et al. Is childhood obesity associated with high-fat foods and low physical activity? J Sch Health 1992;62:19–23.

49. Lissner L, Heitman BL, Bengtsson C. Low-fat diets may prevent weight gain in sedentary women: prospective observations from the population study of women in Gothenburg, Sweden. Obes Res 1997;5:43–48.

50. Griffiths M, Payne P. Energy expenditure in small children of obese and non-obese parents. Nature 1976;260:698–700.

51. Griffiths M, Payne AJ, Stunkard JPW, et al. Metabolic rate and physical development in children at risk of obesity. Lancet 1990; 336:76–78.

52. Goran MI, Carpenter WH, McGloin A, et al. Energy expenditure in children of lean and obese parents. Am J Physiol 1995;268:E917–E924.

53. Maffeis C, Schutz Y, Micciolo R, et al. Resting metabolic rate in six- to ten-year-old obese and nonobese children. J Pediatr 1993;122:556–562.

54. Fontvieille A, Dwyer J, Ravussin E. Resting metabolic rate and body composition of Pima Indian and caucasian children. Int J Obes Relat Metab Disord 1992; 16:535–542.

55. Wells JC, Stanley AS, Laidlaw JM, et al. The relationship between components of infant energy expenditure and childhood body fatness. Int J Obes Relat Metab Disord 1996;20:848–853.

56. Ravussin E, Swinburn B. Pathophysiology of obesity. Lancet 1992;350:404–408.

57. Segal K, Gutin B, Albu J, et al. Thermic effects of food and exercise in lean and obese men of similar lean body mass. Am J Physiol 1987;252:E110–E117.

58. Prentice AM, Goldberg GR, Murgatroyd PR, et al. Physical activity and obesity: problems in correcting expenditure for body size. Int J Obes Relat Metab Disord 1996;20:688–691.

59. Davies P, Gregory J, White A. Physical activity and body fatness

in pre-school children. Int J Obes Relat Metab Disord 1995;19:6–11.

60. Goran MI, Hunter G, Johnson R. Physical activity related energy expenditure and fat mass in young children. Int J Obes Relat Metab Disord 1996;20:1–8.

61. Roberts S, Savage J, Coward W, et al. Energy expenditure and intake in infants born to lean and overweight mothers. N Engl J Med 1988;318:461–466.

62. Deheeger M, Rolland-Cachera MF, Fontvieille AM. Physical activity and body composition in 10 year old French children: linkages with nutritional intake. Int J Obes Relat Metab Disord 1997;21:372–379.

63. Mo-suwan L, Geater AF. Risk factors for childhood obesity in a traditional society in Thailand. Int J Obes Relat Metab Disord 1996;20:697–703.

64. Klesges RC, Klesges LM, Eck LH, et al. A longitudinal analysis of accelerated weight gain in preschool children. Pediatrics 1995;95:126–130.

65. Moore LL, Nguyen UDT, Rothman KJ, et al. Preschool physical activity level and change in body fatness in young children. Am J Epidemiol 1995;142:982–988.

66. Gortmaker SL, Must A, Sobol AM, et al. Television viewing as a cause of increasing obesity among children in the United States, 1986–1990. Arch Pediatr Adolesc Med 1996;150:356–362.

67. DuRant RH, Baranowski T, Johnson M, et al. The relationship among television watching, physical activity, and body composition of young children. Pediatrics 1994;94:449–455.

68. Janz KF, Mahoney LT. Three-year follow-up of changes in aerobic fitness during puberty: the Muscatine study. Res Q Exerc Sport 1997;68:1–9.

69. Tremblay A, Despres JP, Leblanc C, et al. Effect of intensity of physical activity on body fatness and fat distribution. Am J Clin Nutr 1990;51:153–157.

70. Mayers N, Gutin B. Physiological characteristics of elite prepubertal cross-country runners. Med Sci Sports Exerc 1979;11:172–176.

71. Saris WH. Effects of energy restriction and exercise on the sympathetic nervous system. Int J Obes Relat Metab Disord 1995;19(suppl):S17–S23.

72. Zurlo F, Ferraro R, Fontvieille A, et al. Spontaneous physical activity and obesity: cross-sectional and longitudinal studies in Pima Indians. Am J Physiol 1992;263:E290–E300.

73. Caprio S, Tamborlane WV, Silver D, et al. Hyperleptinemia: an early sign of juvenile obesity. Relations to body fat depots and insulin concentrations. Am J Physiol 1996;271:E626–E630.

74. Lahlou N, Landais P, De Boissieu D, et al. Circulating leptin in normal children and during the dynamic phase of juvenile obesity: relation to body fatness, energy metabolism, caloric intake, and sexual dimorphism. Diabetes 1997;46:989–993.

75. Salbe AD, Nicolson M, Ravussin E. Total energy expenditure and the level of physical activity correlate with plasma leptin concentrations in five-year-old children. J Clin Inves 1997;99:592–595.

76. Nagy TM, Gower BA, Trowbridge CA, et al. Effects of gender, ethnicity, body composition, and fat distribution on serum leptin concentrations in children. J Clin Endocrinol Metab 1997;82:2148–2152.

77. Williamson DF, Madans J, Anda RF, et al. Recreational physical activity and ten-year weight change in a US national cohort. Int J Obes Relat Metab Disord 1993;17:279–286.

78. Bouchard C. Obesity in adulthood—the importance of childhood and parental obesity. N Engl J Med 1997;337:926–927.

79. Whitaker RC, Wright JA, Pepe MS, et al. Predicting obesity in young adulthood from childhood and parental obesity. N Engl J Med 1997;337:869–873.

80. Maffeis C, Schutz Y, Pinelli L. Effect of weight loss on resting energy expenditure in obese prepubertal children. Int J Obes Relat Metab Disord 1992;16:41–47.

81. Schwingshandl J, Borkenstein M. Changes in lean body mass in obese children during a weight reduction program: effect on short and longterm outcome. Int J Obes Relat Metab Disord 1995;19:752–755.

82. Ballor D, Poehlman E. Exercise-training enhances fat-free mass preservation during diet-induced weight loss: a meta-analytical finding. Int J Obes Relat Metab Disord 1994;18:35–40.

83. Sasaki J, Shindo M, Tanaka H, et al. A long-term aerobic exercise program decreases the obesity index and increases the high density lipoprotein cholesterol concentration in obese children. Int J Obes Relat Metab Disord 1987;11:339–345.

84. Blomquist B, Borjeson M, Larsson Y, et al. The effect of physical activity on the body measurements and work capacity of overweight boys. Acta Paediatr 1965;54:566–572.

85. Seltzer CC, Mayer J. An effective weight control program in a public school. Am J Pub Health 1970;60:679–689.

86. Gutin B, Cucuzzo N, Islam S, et al. Physical training improves body composition of black obese 7–11 year old girls. Obes Res 1995;3:305–312.

87. Gutin B, Owens S, Riggs S, et al. Effect of physical training on cardiovascular health of obese children: Children and Exercise XIX: International Symposium on Pediatric Work Physiology. London: E & FN Spon, 1997:382–389.

88. Epstein LH. Family-based behavioural intervention for obese children. Int J Obes 1996;20(suppl):S14–S21.

89. Brownell KD, Kelman JH, Strunkard AJ. Treatment of obese children with and without their mothers: changes in weight and blood pressure. Pediatrics 1983;71:515–523.

90. Johnson WG, Hinkle LK, Carr RE, et al. Dietary and exercise interventions for juvenile obesity: long-term effect of behavioral and public health models. Obes Res 1997;5:257–261.

91. Epstein LH, Wing RR, Koeske R, et al. Child and parent weight loss in family-based behavior modification programs. J Consult Clin Psychol 1981;49:674–685.

92. Israel AC, Guile CA, Baker JE. An evaluation of enhanced self-regulation training in the treatment of childhood obesity. J Pediatr Psychol 1994;19:737–749.

93. Epstein LH, Valoski AM, Vara LS, et al. Effects of decreasing sedentary behavior and increasing activity on weight change in obese children. Health Psychol 1995;14:109–115.

94. Figueroa-Colon R, Almen K, Franklin F, et al. Comparison of two hypocaloric diets in obese children. Am J Dis Child 1993; 147:160–166.

95. Braet C, van Winckel M, van Leeuwen K. Follow-up results of different treatment programs for obese children. Acta Paediatr 1997;86:397–402.

96. Mellin LM, Slinkard LA, Irwin CE. Adolescent obesity intervention: validation of the SHAPE-DOWN program. J Am Diet Assoc 1987;87:333–338.

97. Dietz WH. Therapeutic strategies in childhood obesity. Horm Res 1993;39(suppl):86–90.

98. Gill TP. Key issues in the prevention of obesity. Br Med Bull 1997;53:359–388.

99. Bar-Or O, Baranowski T. Physical activity, adiposity, and obesity among adolescents. Pediatr Exerc Sci 1994;6:348–360.

100. Tremblay A, Simoneau J-A, Bouchard C. Impact of exercise intensity on body fatness and skeletal muscle metabolism. Metabolism 1994;43:814–818.

101. Savage D, Petratis M, Thomson W, et al. Exercise training effects on serum lipids of prepubescent boys and adult men. Med Sci Sports Exerc 1986;18:197–204.

102. Epstein LH, Valoski A, Wing RR, et al. Ten-year outcomes of behavioral family-based treatment for childhood obesity. Health Psychol 1994;13:373–383.

103. Glenny AM, O'Meara S, Melville A, et al. The treatment and prevention of obesity: a systematic review of the literature. Int J Obes Relat Metab Disord 1997; 21:715–737.

104. Owens S, Allison J, Riggs S, et al. Effect of physical training on visceral adipose tissue and body composition in obese children. Med Sci Sports Exerc 1997;29(suppl):S55. Abstract.

105. Becque MD, Katch VL, Rocchini AP, et al. Coronary risk incidence of obese adolescents: reduction by exercise plus diet interventions. Pediatrics 1988;81:605–612.

106. Rocchini A, Katch V, Schork A, et al. Insulin and blood pressure during weight loss in obese adolescents. Hypertension 1987;10:267–273.

Chapter 51

Essential Hypertension: A Pediatric Perspective

Thomas W. Rowland

The health risks confronting the adult with systemic hypertension have been clearly identified. Men who have a blood pressure higher than 160/95, for example, are three to four times more likely to develop coronary artery disease, congestive heart failure, stroke, and peripheral vascular disease than those with normal blood pressure. Similar risks are apparent for adult women, although the magnitude is less than in men. Consequently, systemic hypertension is a major contributor to death and disability in the general adult population (1).

The risk for cardiovascular complications associated with elevated blood pressure levels appears to be continuous: the higher the pressure, the greater the risk of complications, without a particular safe threshold value. Any intervention that will safely lower blood pressure can be expected to be salutary.

The public health significance of systemic hypertension in adults is underscored by its frequency. It has been estimated that 15% to 25% of individuals in developed nations have elevated blood pressure levels, and this frequency may be much greater in the elderly population. If a value of 160/95 is defined as the threshold for hypertension, approximately 30 million Americans are afflicted. The problem is compounded by the estimation that the majority of adults with hypertension are unaware of their condition.

Although numerous disease states can raise blood pressure, most adults have essential hypertension, or increased blood pressure from no specific identifiable cause. The physiologic mechanisms for essential hypertension are uncertain, but may relate to early stages of increased cardiac output, abnormal renal function, or hormonal changes influencing blood volume and electrolyte concentrations.

What is known is that essential hypertension has a strong genetic basis and is characterized by prominent familial aggregation; tracks to some extent from childhood years into adulthood; and is associated with certain modifiable factors, particularly obesity and dietary salt intake. Moreover, systemic hypertension is often linked in a given individual with a cluster of cardiovascular risk factors such as hyperlipidemia, insulin resistance, poor physical fitness, and obesity (the so-called "metabolic syndrome"), escalating the chances for premature mortality and morbidity from stroke and coronary artery disease.

Given these characteristics, it is reasonable to assume that detection and reduction of modifiable risk factors in the early years of life would reduce the chance of adverse health outcomes of hypertension in the adult years. While no direct proof of the effectiveness of such a strategy is yet at hand, certain evidence is highly supportive. Pharmacologic treatment of adults with systemic hypertension, for instance, clearly reduces their cardiovascular mortality and morbidity.

According to this concept, health care providers for children have an important role in the prevention of adult essential hypertension and its complications. This involves 1) taking steps to detect young patients with systemic hypertension, 2) promoting efforts to reduce risk factors which may contribute to the hypertensive state, and 3) instituting pharmacologic management in those unusual cases in which this becomes necessary. This chapter will assess the rationale for this concept and review appropriate means of diagnosis and management of essential hypertension in the pediatric population.

Although essential hypertension has been reported at very young ages, most cases do not surface clinically until adolescence. Therefore, most hypertension in young children (under age 10) is due to secondary causes, particularly chronic renal disease. As a general rule, the younger the child and the higher the blood pressure, the more likely a causative disease can be identified. The role of the physician in identifying secondary causes of hypertension in children is critical. This chapter, however, will focus only on the roots of adult essential hypertension during the pediatric years as they concern the primary care health provider.

FAMILIAL AGGREGATION OF ESSENTIAL HYPERTENSION

Children who are members of families with essential hypertension are more likely to have higher blood pressures than those who come from normotensive families. Studies assessing blood pressures in twins and adopted children have indicated that much of this familial aggregation of hypertension has a genetic basis. These findings indicate that inheritance strongly influences the physiologic factors that lead to essential hypertension and suggest that such variables might be expressed (and detected) early in life. From a clinical standpoint, too, the familial nature of essential hypertension provides a means of focusing attention on high-risk children, even in a prehypertensive state.

A positive history of hypertension in a child's immediate family members implies increased risk of present or future high blood pressure. Londe et al, for example, reported that 51% of children with hypertension had at least one parent with elevated blood pressure levels, while parental hypertension was observed in only 18% of normotensive children (2). Such familial aggregation of blood pressure has been described in children as young as 2 years old (3).

The Montreal Adoption Survey was conducted to determine the genetic contribution to familial clustering of hypertension (4). Based on findings in 1176 parents, 756 adopted children, and 445 children with their natural parents, the authors concluded that genetic influence accounted for 61% of the variance in blood pressure measurements. Studies of first-degree relatives, however, have suggested a lower genetic contribution to variability in blood pressure (about 30% to 35%) (5).

Studies to examine the effect of heredity on hypertension have also been performed by comparing blood pressure levels in monozygotic and dizygotic twins. An investigation from the National Institutes of Health of 250 monozygotic and 264 dizygotic twin pairs confirmed a high genetic influence (6). The genetic effects on the variability of systolic and diastolic blood pressure in that study were observed to be as high as 82% and 64%, respectively.

It is unclear whether the genetic influence on blood pressure reflects the action of a single gene or is a polygenic effect. In the former case, the presence of the hypertension gene would separate an individual from the normotensive population. In the latter case, one's predisposition to hypertension would depend on the number of such genes inherited. Considering the number of physiologic processes that contribute to blood pressure control, the second mechanism would appear to be more likely. This conclusion is supported by twin studies indicating a prominent genetic influence on renal function, ion transport across cell membranes, and other processes that might influence blood pressure levels.

TRACKING OF BLOOD PRESSURE

The effectiveness of a pediatric approach to preventing adult hypertension is partially contingent upon close tracking of blood pressure levels from childhood to the adult years. Blood pressure measurements taken in a child or adolescent should have predictive value of those that will be obtained in the same individual many years later. Longitudinal studies of blood pressure during the growing years have provided a mixed picture of systolic and diastolic trends, with correlation coefficients ranging from $r = 0.25$ to $r = 0.75$ (7,8). Systolic pressures tend to track better than diastolic pressures, with no significant gender differences in tracking tendencies.

The strength of tracking of blood pressure during childhood thus remains open to interpretation. Some have viewed these findings as indicating that "it is possible to identify groups who appear to be destined for future high blood pressure," (7) while others have contended that "predictions based on single measurements have many limitations." (9) Lauer et al concluded that "these data confirm that there is some consistency of peer rank order of blood pressure during childhood but that many children do not maintain their rank during the period of observation." (7) As a result "whereas for populations early childhood blood pressure elevations are indicative of risk for future high blood pressure, for an individual child there is considerable variability in the prediction." (10)

Few longitudinal investigations have examined the relationship between blood pressure levels in childhood or adolescent years and later on in adulthood. In the Muscatine Study, blood pressures were measured over a 10-year period in schoolchildren aged 7–18 and then again at age 23 or 28 (10). During the childhood years, only 43% of children who had blood pressure in the upper 20th percentile on the initial exam remained in the same quintile as adults. In fact, drop off from the upper quintile occurred early on. Ten percent had blood pressures above the 95th percentile on the first exam, but on the second measurement the frequency fell to 1.7%. A child with an initial blood systolic pressure in the upper quintile had only a 20% chance of his or her reading still being there six years later.

Pearson correlation coefficients between child and adult levels for systolic pressure ranged from $r = 0.21$ to 0.39, and for diastolic pressure the range was $r = 0.11$ to $r = 0.50$. Among the children who had a pressure exceeding the 90th percentile at any time, 24% exhibited pressures above the 90th percentile as adults, 2.4 times the expected number.

Of the adults with high blood pressure, 45% had systolic blood pressure above the 90th percentile at least once as a child; that is, 55% of hypertensive adults had normal systolic blood pressure during childhood. Forty percent of adults with elevated diastolic blood pressure had demonstrated at least one diastolic blood pressure during childhood that was above the 90th percentile.

The findings of this investigation indicated that a 16-year-old who has a systolic blood pressure level exceeding the 90th percentile has triple the risk of having hypertension as an adult than if blood pressure was at the 50th percentile as a teenager. Diastolic blood pressure in adulthood, however, was less predictable from adolescent levels.

In a 24-year follow-up study, Beckett et al found tracking coefficients of $r = 0.23$ and 0.18 for systolic and diastolic blood pressures, respectively, between adolescence and adulthood (11). Rosner et al described the relationships between blood pressure readings at ages 5 to 14 and those repeated 15 years later (12). Coefficients were $r = 0.24$–0.25 for systolic values and $r = 0.30$ to 0.45 for diastolic levels.

These data suggest that, while the hypertensive child carries an increased risk of becoming a hypertensive adult, the predictability of adult blood pressure from a single measurement during childhood is not high. Indeed, as noted by Clarke et al, repeated serial blood pressure recordings would be necessary to identify those at risk for future hypertension (13). The findings in tracking studies also indicate the lack of value of large-scale blood pressure screening programs in children (8).

RACIAL INFLUENCES

In adult populations, the incidence of essential hypertension is clearly related to racial group. African American adults living in the United States have nearly twice the prevalence of essential hypertension as whites. In the National Health Survey, one quarter of adult blacks demonstrated blood pressure readings exceeding 160/95, compared to 14% per cent of whites (14). Thus, adult blacks show both an increased prevalence and severity of systemic hypertension.

In pediatric populations, on the other hand, no consistent influence of race or ethnicity on blood pressure levels has been observed (15). Consequently, published normative blood pressure data accumulated from large population studies do not distinguish between racial groups. It should be noted that this conclusion is based largely on comparisons of measurements in white and African American youth; limited data are available regarding norms in other minority populations, particularly Hispanics and Asian Americans.

While average resting blood pressure measurements are not usually different in black and white children, race may influence other markers of blood pressure control. Black children have been demonstrated to exhibit greater blood pressure responses to maximal exercise testing as well as during the playing of video games (15). These findings imply that black youngsters possess greater vascular reactivity than whites. Black children also demonstrate greater salt sensitivity than whites; given a salt challenge, both normotensive and hypertensive blacks have a greater blood pressure response. Such differences may relate to black-white differences in sodium membrane transport. Thus, while blood pressure levels at rest may not be influenced by race in children, the seeds of physiologic mechanisms that are responsible for the higher prevalence and severity of hypertension in adult blacks may already be at work in the pediatric years.

MODIFIABLE INFLUENCES ON ESSENTIAL HYPERTENSION

The strong genetic influence on essential hypertension implies that to some extent the development of elevated blood pressure levels with age may be inexorable. Still, abundant evidence exists that certain risk factors for hypertension—salt

intake, physical activity, obesity—can be altered by modification of lifestyle. It follows, then, that behavioral interventions to diminish the impact of these factors should prove useful in ameliorating the frequency and severity of adult essential hypertension.

For the pediatric practitioner, such observations suggest that these lifestyle alterations should begin early in life, particularly in children at increased risk for hypertension (based on a positive family history), and changes in diet and physical activity should be helpful management options for patients who demonstrate early essential hypertension. In fact, such behavioral modifications are much more attractive than the alternative use of pharmacologic treatment with its complications and implications for lifelong drug therapy.

Obesity

No single factor influences blood pressure as much as body fat content. This critical observation becomes particularly disturbing given the high prevalence and increasing incidence of obesity in the childhood population. From a more optimistic standpoint, though, it follows that efforts to reduce body fat in children should have a favorable effect on decreasing the risk of developing essential hypertension in adulthood.

The relationship between obesity and blood pressure has been apparent since early studies of the epidemiology of hypertension in children. Among children aged 4 to 15, Londe found that 53% of those with hypertension were obese (weight exceeding the 90th percentile for height and age) (16). Similarly, Lauer et al reported that a quarter of overweight youngsters had blood pressure recordings over the 90th percentile for age (17).

Among 2058 high school students, Levine et al found 110 (5.9%) to be hypertensive. Of these, half had persistence of elevated blood pressure on subsequent recordings. Of the 28 in this group who agreed to have subsequent investigation, 64% were obese (18).

These findings mimicked those in adult populations. Young adults who were initially of normal weight and stayed so had a smaller risk of developing hypertension than those who became obese (19). A 7-year follow-up study by Heyden et al found that increase in weight by adolescents was the only factor that predicted the subsequent development of hypertension (20).

Loss of body fat has been documented to decrease blood pressure. Rocchini described a group of 72 obese adolescents whose blood pressure distribution was skewed to the right compared to that of the normal population (21). After dietary and exercise interventions caused weight loss, the distribution did not differ from the normal teenagers. Decline in blood pressure is typically seen in studies of adults in whom caloric restriction results in weight loss (22).

The influence of obesity on blood pressure is sufficiently strong as to alter commonly used algorithms for diagnosis and management of hypertension in children. For example, since obese children with elevated blood pressure are unlikely to have another cause for their hypertension, institution of weight control is recommended as a first step in their management (23). Children with hypertension who are in the normal weight range, on the other hand, should initially undergo a laboratory investigation for secondary causes of hypertension.

While inappropriately small cuff size can artifactually raise recordings in obese subjects, these individuals have true elevations in blood pressure. The etiology for this obesity-induced hypertension is not clear. Rocchini hypothesized that the most likely mechanism was hyperinsulinemia resulting from selective insulin resistance (21). This in turn would produce renal sodium retention and increased sympathetic nervous activity.

Hypertension is observed to be linked in individuals with not only obesity but also other coronary risk factors, including abnormal serum lipid profile and hyperinsulinemia. That this clustering might have a common etiology has led to the designation of a "metabolic syndrome" or "syndrome X" (24). There is evidence that an underlying mechanism for this grouping of risk factors might involve insulin resistance. In the Bogalusa Heart Study, a 6-year cross-sectional investigation identified a link between plasma insulin and subsequent systolic blood pressure levels, but only in white children (25). Such insights deserve further investigation, as youngsters with the metabolic syndrome carry a high risk for future cardiovascular disease.

In summary, obesity must be considered in the identification of children at risk for hypertension as well as in the diagnostic evaluation and management of those with essential hypertension. Indeed, therapeutic strategies to reduce body fat should be the central focus of treatment of obese children with hypertension, as reduction of fat itself will often result in normalization of blood pressure levels.

Physical Activity

Interest in the role of physical activity in the prevention and management of hypertension in children follows extensive investigation of the exercise-blood pressure relationships in adults. This information indicates that regular physical activity can be important in both directly reducing the risks of essential hypertension and ameliorating other risk factors (obesity, anxiety) for increased blood pressure. Improved exercise habits may be useful as a preventive measure for the development of hypertension as well as a therapeutic strategy in those with established hypertension.

Exercise interventions have been demonstrated to reduce blood pressure levels in both hypertensive and normotensive adults. In the 25 studies of adults with essential hypertension reviewed by Hagberg, 67% and 70% demonstrated a decline in systolic and diastolic pressures, respectively, following a period of endurance exercise training (1). The average reduction was approximately 10 mm Hg. In studies of adults with normal blood pressure, exercise training has lowered average systolic pressure by 4 mm Hg and diastolic pressure by 3 mm Hg (26).

The picture may be somewhat different in children and adolescents. In these age groups significant declines in blood pressure from exercise training have been witnessed in patients with mild essential hypertension but not in those with normal initial blood pressure levels. At least 10 cross-sectional studies have been performed that have demonstrated a negative relationship between blood pressure levels and physical activity or fitness in children who are normotensive (27). In almost all cases, however, this relationship disappeared when body fat was taken into account. That is, the increased body fat in children with low levels of physical fitness and/or activ-

ity has been responsible for the association of these exercise variables with blood pressure.

Of seven longitudinal studies assessing the influence of endurance training in normotensive children on blood pressure, five have shown no effect. In an 8-month training study Hansen et al demonstrated an average 4 mm Hg decrease in systolic pressure in boys but not girls (28). Fisher et al found a 6 mm Hg decline in resting diastolic pressure in children following training (29).

On the other hand, all three training studies in hypertensive adolescents have reported a salutary decline in blood pressure (27). Rowland examined the effects of a 6-month endurance training program on 25 adolescents with borderline hypertension (average blood pressure 137/80) (30). With training, both systolic and diastolic pressures decreased, with an average post-training level of 129/75. No significant changes of blood pressure were observed in a non-training control group. With cessation of training, the blood pressure levels of the hypertensive group returned to pre-training values. The effect was unexpected, since both systolic and diastolic blood pressure levels generally rise significantly during resistance exercise.

All forms of exercise cause an acute rise in blood pressure, and it is of interest, then, to understand why chronic exercise (i.e., a training program) may result in decrease in resting blood pressure levels. Several possible mechanisms exist. First, an acute bout of exercise causes peripheral vasodilation, and this relaxation of peripheral vessels may persist following exercise. This possibility is supported by findings that blood pressure levels in adults with essential hypertension are reduced for as long as 3 hours following a session of endurance exercise.

Second, exercise training results in a decrease in resting sympathetic drive. This is evidenced by a fall in plasma norepinephrine concentration with training, and the magnitude of this decrease has been correlated with declines in resting blood pressure. And, finally, exercise training may cause a reduction in body fat, itself a strong contributor to elevations in systemic blood pressure (see above).

Based on this evidence, a strong rationale exists for increasing physical activity in children and adolescents for both preventing and treating essential hypertension. Regular exercise acts to promote physical fitness, diminish body fat content, and reduce blood pressure by direct mechanisms. The types of activities and forms of training that can be expected to be most efficacious, however, are uncertain. Most studies have utilized programs that conform to criteria that are expected to improve aerobic fitness (maximal oxygen uptake, or Vo_2max): endurance activities, at least three times a week, 20 to 30 minutes per session, at an intensity equivalent to 50% to 70% of maximal heart rate.

Evidence in adults, however, suggests that alterations in blood pressure with training are not related to the magnitude of changes in Vo_2max, and that lower intensity training may be equally effective in blood pressure reduction. This observation is important in managing children and adolescents with hypertension, who may better tolerate lower intensity training with greater program compliance.

Exercise prescriptions for pediatric patients with essential hypertension need to be individualized according to the patient's athletic capabilities, motivation, and body composition. Since any such intervention needs to be long term, the goal must be lifestyle alteration rather than acquiring fitness. As such, the exercise must be acceptable and enjoyable for the patient. Strategies for improving exercise habits of children have been published elsewhere (31).

Salt Intake

The observation that some populations that consume little salt are characterized by low blood pressure initiated interest in the role of limiting dietary salt as a means of decreasing risk of essential hypertension. Not all such population studies have been consistent in this finding, however, and it has been difficult to establish relationships between salt intake and blood pressure levels in developed countries (31). Nonetheless, certain individuals appear to be salt sensitive in regards to blood pressure response; thus for some patients a reduction in salt intake may be effective in diminishing risk for hypertension.

Dietary sodium intake in both American children and adults far exceeds physiologic needs and has been increasing, presumably due to the rise in consumption of processed and restaurant foods (32). Survey studies of older children and adolescents across the United States have indicated a daily sodium intake of approximately 3.8 g per day, almost twice the recommended daily intake.

A modest reduction in dietary salt therefore carries no health risk, and lowering salt intake will cause a decrease in blood pressure in some adults with established hypertension. The evidence for this effect is less compelling in children and adolescents. Cooper et al demonstrated a weak but significant relationship between urinary sodium excretion and blood pressure levels of 11 to 14-year-olds (33). However, Howe et al saw no changes in blood pressure when sodium intake was altered in children in the same age group (34). And Sinaiko et al found no decline in blood pressure when a low-sodium diet was instituted in 13-year-old adolescents with blood pressure above the 85th percentile (35).

A greater frequency of blood pressure sensitivity to increased dietary sodium has been documented in certain high-risk pediatric groups (32). These include children with hypertensive parents, obese adolescents, and African Americans. This observation supports the advocacy for decreasing salt intake as a means of preventing essential hypertension in children and adolescents.

How much salt intake is prudent for children and adolescents? Prineas et al suggested daily sodium intake of 26 mEq per 1000 kcal, a value which is slightly less than half that described in children's usual diets in the United States (36). To reach this goal, no salt should be added either at the table or during cooking, and high-salt snack food should be avoided.

IDENTIFICATION OF THE CHILD AT RISK

Surveillance—identification of children and adolescents with elevated blood pressure—is critical to the role of the physician in identifying and managing young patients with both essential and secondary hypertension. Current recommendations call for yearly determination of blood pressure beginning when a child is 3 years old. When compared to published norms for blood pressure in the pediatric age group, these measurements should allow for detection of youngsters who have either early essential hypertension or blood pressure elevations reflecting underlying disease.

Both systolic and diastolic blood pressure increase with age. Gender differences are small until the age of puberty, when values for males increasingly exceed those for females. At age 8, for example, the 95th percentile of systolic blood pressures for the average-size boy and girl are 116 and 115 mm Hg, respectively. However, the 95th percentile level for the average 17-year-old boy is 136 mm Hg; for a female of the same age, it is 129 mm Hg.

While this effect of age has long been recognized, only recently has it been appreciated that body size is also a critical determinant of blood pressure levels in children and adolescents. The most recent published normative data for the pediatric population, then, consider height as well as age and gender (37). These data define normal blood pressure as a systolic and diastolic pressure below the 90th percentile for height, age, and sex, high normal as between 90th and 95th percentile, and hypertension as readings above the 95th percentile on at least three separate occasions.

Systolic pressure is defined as the onset of Korotkoff sounds as the cuff is being deflated. While controversy has surrounded the definition of diastolic pressure, recent recommendations hold that the fifth Korotkoff sound (K5, actually the disappearance of sound) can be used to define diastolic pressure at all ages. An update from the 1987 Task Force Report on High Blood Pressure in Children and Adolescents uses norms for diastolic pressure in children based on K5 (37).

The 95th percentile values of systolic and diastolic blood pressure in populations of boys and girls according to age and height percentiles are outlined in Tables 51-1 and 51-2 (37). When an individual patient's blood pressures are compared to these published norms it is important to use standardized measurement techniques. Blood pressure should be recorded in the right arm with the subject sitting, preferably after 3 to 5 minutes of rest. The cuff should have a bladder with a width about 75 percent of the length of the upper arm and a length that will cover 80% to 100% of the arm's circumference. During blood pressure determination the deflation rate of the cuff should be approximately 2 to 3 mm Hg per second, as faster or slower rates may cause erroneous readings.

These recommendations, as well as published norms, are based on standard auscultatory techniques using a mercury or aneroid manometer. Automated blood pressure recording devices have become increasingly popular because of their ease of use. However, because of lack of established norms using this type of equipment, plus their need for calibration, the auscultatory method remains the recommended technique.

THE CLINICAL APPROACH

Decision making regarding patients with hypertension is based on a series of questions surrounding appropriate substantiation, amount of laboratory evaluation, and indications for treatment. These issues have been comprehensively discussed in previous publications, to which the reader is referred for

Table 51-1 95th Percentile Blood Pressure Levels for Boys by Height Percentile						
	SYSTOLIC BLOOD PRESSURE (mm Hg) BY HEIGHT PERCENTILE			DIASTOLIC BLOOD PRESSURE (mm Hg) BY HEIGHT PERCENTILE		
AGE	10%	50%	90%	10%	50%	90%
1	99	102	106	55	57	59
2	102	106	109	59	61	63
3	105	109	112	63	65	67
4	107	111	114	67	68	70
5	109	112	115	70	71	73
6	110	114	117	72	74	76
7	111	115	118	74	76	78
8	112	116	119	76	77	79
9	114	117	121	77	79	80
10	115	119	122	78	80	81
11	117	121	124	79	80	82
12	120	123	126	79	81	83
13	122	126	129	80	82	83
14	125	128	132	81	82	84
15	128	131	134	82	83	85
16	130	134	137	83	85	87
17	133	136	140	85	87	89

Data extracted and used by permission from Update on the 1987 Task Force Report on High Blood Pressure in Children and Adolescents. Pediatrics 1998;98:653.

Table 51-2 95th Percentile Blood Pressure for Girls by Height Percentile						
	SYSTOLIC BLOOD PRESSURE (mm Hg) BY HEIGHT PERCENTILE			DIASTOLIC BLOOD PRESSURE (mm Hg) BY HEIGHT PERCENTILE		
AGE	10%	50%	90%	10%	50%	90%
1	102	104	107	57	58	60
2	103	105	108	61	62	64
3	104	107	109	65	66	67
4	106	108	111	67	69	70
5	107	110	112	70	71	72
6	109	111	114	71	73	74
7	110	113	115	73	74	76
8	112	115	117	74	75	77
9	114	117	119	76	77	78
10	116	119	121	77	78	80
11	118	121	123	78	79	81
12	120	123	125	79	80	82
13	122	125	127	80	82	83
14	124	126	129	81	83	84
15	125	128	130	82	83	85
16	126	128	131	83	84	86
17	126	129	131	83	84	86

Data extracted and used by permission from Update on the 1987 Task Force Report on High Blood Pressure in Children and Adolescents. Pediatrics 1998;98:654.

more complete details (37,38). The following discussion of a sample case is based on those recommendations.

The case: a 15-year-old high school freshman has come for a physical examination to clear him for basketball participation. It is noted that his blood pressure is 140/90, a value significantly higher than that recorded on previous office visits. As he is at the 50th percentile for height, the 95th percentile values for his age and gender for systolic and diastolic pressures are 131 and 83 mm Hg, respectively. The appropriate clinical response is dictated by a series of questions.

Does this patient really have hypertension? Since single blood pressure recordings may not be representative of usual blood pressure, hypertension needs to be documented with follow-up measurements. The exception to this recommendation is the child or adolescent who has marked pressure elevations and requires immediate evaluation. In our patient, who is asymptomatic and has mildly elevated blood pressure, the next step is to arrange for at least three follow-up measurements. Preferably this will be performed outside the physician's office, such as by the school nurse, or by a neighbor who has EMT training. Hypertension can be diagnosed by serial follow-up measurements exceeding the 95th percentile.

Ambulatory measurement by automated devices over a 24-hour period may prove useful in documenting hypertension in such patients (39). These are now in common use in adult patients and have been found to be clinically useful.

Their routine use in children awaits further data providing normative values.

Does the patient have any signs or symptoms of hypertension, and is there any evidence of end-organ damage? Complaints of frequent headaches, dizziness, epistaxis, visual problems, or chest pain may reflect elevated blood pressure. The finding of retinal arteriolar narrowing and arteriovenous nicking on funduscopic examination indicates long-standing hypertension. Other indications of end-organ damage, such as cardiomegaly or neurologic deficits, are rare in young patients with hypertension.

Is there any evidence of underlying disease? The list of secondary causes of hypertension is long, and a careful history and physical examination is important in providing clues to underlying disease. Particular attention should be focused on urinary tract symptomatology or past history of urinary tract infection. A neonatal history of umbilical artery catheterization suggests the possibility of renal artery stenosis. A previous illness characterized by joint pain and/or rash might indicate nephritis. Muscle weakness suggests hyperaldosteronism, and spells of flushing and sweating are typical of pheochromocytoma. Questions to the patient regarding therapeutic or recreational drug use (particularly steroids) are important.

On physical examination, attention to peripheral pulses is important in ruling out coarctation of the aorta. An abdominal mass would suggest pheochromocytoma, polycystic kidneys, or Wilms tumor. Renal vascular disease may be manifest by an epigastric bruit. Thyroid enlargement may be seen in hyperthyroidism.

What laboratory workup is indicated? Current recommendations call for a limited laboratory workup in patients with recognized hypertension to screen for secondary causes. This includes complete blood cell count, urinalysis, BUN, electrolytes, and uric acid level. Whether a more comprehensive evaluation is warranted is dependent on one's index of suspicion of a secondary cause. Additional testing should be considered if the patient is young (i.e., preadolescent or of normal weight), the blood pressure elevation is more than mild, the family history is negative for hypertension, and/or there are clues by history or examination of an underlying disease process. This assessment might include echocardiography (to evaluate possible end-organ damage), renal ultrasound and Doppler flow study, and measurement of urine catecholamines, plasma renin activity, and urine and plasma cortisol. As a general statement, a comprehensive laboratory evaluation is warranted in any young patient who is being considered for drug therapy.

What is the best management option? The emphasis in treating hypertension in children and adolescents should be on nonpharmacologic interventions. Drug therapy should be reserved for those with severe hypertension or evidence of end-organ effects.

The adolescent in the present case should be encouraged to continue to participate in regular exercise. A gradual reduction in dietary salt should be recommended, with the goal of eliminating salt at the table and during cooking and limiting salty snack foods. If he was found to be obese, recommendations for lowering caloric intake through decreased fat intake can be advised. Most importantly, planned serial follow-up assessment of blood pressure levels is essential.

SUMMARY

The genetic basis of essential hypertension implies that, at least to some extent, the tendency in certain individuals to experience an abnormal rise of blood pressure with age is inevitable. At the same time, the clear impact of factors such as excess body fat, sedentary lifestyle, and high-salt diet on blood pressure indicate that the risks for essential hypertension can be ameliorated. This calls for early detection and counseling about eating and activity behaviors by the primary care physician. Introducing these strategies early in life provide the optimal approach to preventing adult hypertension and its complications.

REFERENCES

1. Hagberg JM. Exercise, fitness, and hypertension. In: Bouchard C, et al, eds. Exercise, fitness, and health. Champaign, IL: Human Kinetics, 1990:455–466.

2. Londe S, Goldring D, Gollub SW. Blood pressure and hypertension in children: studies, problems, and perspectives. In: New MI, Levine LS, eds. Juvenile hypertension. New York: Raven, 1977:13–21.

3. Zinner FH, Margolius SH, Rosner BR. Does hypertension begin in childhood? studies of the familial aggregation of blood pressure. In: New MI, Levine LS, eds. Juvenile hypertension, New York: Raven, 1977:45–54.

4. Mongeau JG, Biron P, Sing CF. The influence of genetics and household environment upon the variability of normal blood pressure: the Montreal Adoption Survey. Clin Exp Hypertens 1986; 6:647–652.

5. Morton NE, Gulbrandsen DL, Rao DC. Determinants of blood pressure in Japanese-American families. Am J Hum Genet 1980;53:261–270.

6. Feinlieb M, Garrison R, Borhani N. Studies of hypertension in twins. In: Paul O, ed. Epidemiology and control of hypertension. Miami: Symposium Specialists, 1975:3–10.

7. Lauer RM, Clarke WR. Tracking of blood pressure in childhood. In: Children's blood pressure: Eighty-Eighth Ross Conference on Pediatric Research. Columbus, OH: Ross Laboratories, 1985:4–13.

8. Woelk G. Blood pressure tracking from child to adulthood: a review. Centr Afr J Med 1994;40:163–169.

9. Lenfant C, Savage PJ. The early natural history of atherosclerosis and hypertension in the young: National Institutes of Health perspectives. Am J Med Sci 1995; 310(suppl 1):S3–S7.

10. Lauer RM, Clarke WR, Mahoney LT, Witt J. Childhood predictors for high adult blood pressure. Ped Clin N Amer 1993;40:23–39.

11. Beckett LA, Rosner B, Roche AF, Guo S. Serial changes in blood pressure from adolescence into adulthood. Am J Epidemiol 1992; 135:1166–1177.

12. Rosner B, Hennekens CH, Kass EH, Miall WE. Age-specific correlation analysis of longitudinal blood pressure data. Am J Epidemiol 1977;106:306–313.

13. Clarke WR, Schrott HG, Leaverton PE, et al. Tracking of blood lipids and blood pressures in school age children: the Muscatine study. Circulation 1978:58:626–634.

14. National Health Survey: hypertension and hypertensive heart disease in adults, U.S. 1960–1962. Washington DC: US Department of Health, Education, and Welfare, Vital and Health Statistics, 1996. Series 11, No. 13.

15. Alpert BS, Fox ME. Racial aspects of blood pressure in children and adolescents. Pediatr Clin N Am 1993;40:13–21.

16. Londe S, Bourgoignie JJ, Robson AM, et al. Hypertension in apparently normal children. J Pediatr 1971;78:569–575.

17. Lauer RM, Connor WE, Leaverton PE, et al. Coronary heart disease risk factors in school children: the Muscatine study. J Pediatr 1975; 86:697–703.

18. Levine LS, Lewy JE, New MI. Hypertension in high school students: evaluation in New York City. NY State J Med 1976;76:40–44.

19. Stamler J. Lectures in preventive cardiology. New York: Grune & Stratton, 1967.

20. Heyden S, Barte AG, Hames EG, et al. Elevated blood pressure levels in adolescents, Evans County, Georgia. JAMA 1969;209:1683–1690.

21. Rocchini AP. Adolescent obesity and hypertension. Pediatr Clin N Amer 1993;40:81–90.

22. Dustan HP. Obesity and hypertension. In: Lauer RM, Shekelle RB, eds. Childhood prevention of atherosclerosis and hypertension. New York: Raven, 1980:305–312.

23. Report of the Second Task Force on Blood Control in Children—1987. Pediatrics 1987;79:1–25.

24. Schieken RM. New perspectives in childhood blood pressure. Curr Opinion Cardiol 1995;10:87–91.

25. Jiang X, Srinivasan S, Bao W, Berenson G. Association of fasting insulin with longitudinal changes in blood pressure in children and adolescents: the Bogalusa Heart Study. Am J Hypertens 1993;6:564–569.

26. Kelley G, Tran ZV. Aerobic exercise and normotensive adults: a meta-analysis. Med Sci Sports Exerc 1995;27:1371–1377.

27. Alpert BS, Wilmore JH. Physical activity and blood pressure in adolescents. Ped Exerc Science 1994;6:361–380.

28. Hansen H, Froberg K, Hyldebrandt N, Nielsen JR. A controlled study of eight months of physical training and reduction of blood pressure in children: the Odense Schoolchild Study. BMJ 1991;303:682–685.

29. Fisher AG, Brown M. The effects of diet and exercise on selected coronary risk factors in children. Med Sci Sports Exerc 1982;14:171. Abstract.

30. Rowland TW. Exercise and children's health. Champaign, IL: Human Kinetics, 1990.

31. Fixler DE. Epidemiology of childhood hypertension. In: Strong WB, ed. Atherosclerosis: its pediatric aspects. New York: Grune & Stratton, 1987;177–191.

32. Falkner B, Michel S. Blood pressure response to sodium in children and adolescents. Am J Clin Nutr 1997;65(suppl):618S–621S.

33. Cooper R, Soltero J, Liu K, et al. The association between urinary sodium excretion and blood pressure in children. Circulation 1980;62:97–104.

34. Howe PRC, Cobiac L, Smith RM. Lack of effect of short-term changes in sodium intake on blood pressure in adolescent school children. J Hypertens 1991;9:181–186.

35. Sinaiko AR, Gomez-Marin O, Prineas RJ. Effect of low sodium and potassium supplementation on adolescent blood pressure. J Hypertens 1993;21:989–994.

36. Prineas RJ, Gillum RF, Blackburn H. Possibilities for primary prevention of hypertension. In: Lauer RM, Shekelle RB, eds. Childhood prevention of atherosclerosis and hypertension. New York: Raven, 1980:357–366.

37. Update on the 1987 Task Force Report on High Blood Pressure in Children and Adolescents: a working group report from the National High Blood Pressure Education Program. Pediatrics 1996;98:649–658.

38. Report of the Second Task Force on Blood Pressure Control in Children—1987. Pediatrics 1987;79:1–25.

39. Alpert BS, Daniels SR. Twenty-four hour ambulatory blood pressure monitoring: now that technology has come of age—we need to catch up. J Pediatr 1997;130:167–169.

Chapter 52

Tobacco, Alcohol, and Other Substance Use
Among Children and Adolescents

Robert H. DuRant
Catherine Buchanan

EPIDEMIOLOGY OF TOBACCO USE

The use of tobacco by young people remains a substantial threat to the nation's health (1–4). Although more than 50 million Americans have quit smoking since the first Surgeon General's report in 1964, monthly use of tobacco among male high school seniors has not changed much since 1980 and use among females has dropped only slightly (4–6). More than 3 million US adolescents are current smokers and more than 1 million adolescent males use smokeless tobacco (4,7). These children serve as the replacements for the 400,000 American smokers who die and the 1.3 million who quit using tobacco each year (3). Every day approximately 3000 children and teenagers become regular tobacco users (3). In 1995, approximately 22% of high school seniors reported daily smoking, an increase from 17.2% in 1992 (5,8). Among eighth graders, current smoking increased by 30% from 14.3% in 1991 to 18.6% in 1994 (9). Of adults who use tobacco regularly, 37% started by the age of 14 and 89% started by the age of 18 (3). The mean age of initiation is 14.5 years and the mean age of daily use is 17.7 years (4). Rates of regular adolescent smoking have been shown to increase with age, from 11.4% among 12- to 14-year-olds (1) to 38% by the time students have reached the twelfth grade (10). Unfortunately, we are far from the year 2000 goal of a 15% youth initiation rate (11). Moreover, after initiating smoking, the majority of teenagers then try to quit on their own, but are generally unsuccessful (12). Teenagers who attempt to quit typically have withdrawal symptoms comparable to their adult counterparts, and these physiologic symptoms may play a significant role in interfering with attainment of abstinence (13–15).

Data from the National Longitudinal Study on Adoles-cent Health (Add Health) study (16) suggest that frequency of cigarette use was associated with access to cigarettes in the home and a family history of recent suicidal behavior. Less frequent cigarette use was associated with more frequent parental presence in the home, greater shared activities between adolescents and parents, and higher perceived levels of parental expectations related to adolescent school completion. High levels of feelings of school connectedness were also associated with less frequent cigarette use. Youth that appeared older than their peers and had a lower grade-point average smoked cigarettes more often. Among younger adolescents, cigarette use was associated with a high perceived risk of early death and having repeated a grade in school. Among older youth, working 20 or more hours a week was associated with increased frequency of cigarette use. Lower frequency of cigarette use was associated with high levels of personal importance placed on religion and prayer (16).

EPIDEMIOLOGY OF OTHER SUBSTANCE USE

In 1994, the National Household Survey reported that 111 million Americans, or 52% of the population, aged 12 and older had used alcohol in the previous month (17). In 1995 there were 10 million current alcohol users under the age of 21, 4.4 million youth who were binge drinkers, and 1.7 million heavy drinkers (18). About 3% of adolescents in the United States are addicted to alcohol or other drugs (17).

From 1994 to 1995, the rates of adolescent illicit drug use during the previous month increased from 8.2% to 10.9%, which is a doubling of the rate found in 1992. The proportion of eighth-grade students using any illicit drug in the previous 12 months increased from 11% in 1991 to 21% in 1995 (18). Between 1992 and 1995, the percentage of tenth- and twelfth-grade students using any illicit drugs during the previous 12 months increased from 20% to 33% and 27% to 39%, respectively. Examples of the specific illicit drugs used by adolescents are described below. The rates of drug use vary on different surveys of youth.

In the early 1990s marijuana once again began to increase in popularity among adolescents. Marijuana use during the previous 12 months by eighth-grade students increased from 6% in 1991 to 16% in 1995. Among tenth-grade students, the rate of marijuana use increased from 15% in 1992 to 29% in 1995. Among twelfth-grade students, marijuana use increased from 22% in 1992 to 35% in 1995 (18). Recent use (within the preceding 30 days) was reported by 25.3% of ninth- through twelfth-grade students participating in the 1995 CDC Youth Risk Behavior Survey (YRBS) (19). In comparison, among the students participating in the Add Health study in 1994 and 1995, 6.9% of seventh- and eighth-grade students and 15.7% of ninth- to twelfth-grade students reported using marijuana at least once during the previous month (16).

In 1995 nationwide, 7% of high school students had used some form of cocaine during their lifetime and 3.1% of students had used cocaine during the preceding 30 days. The lifetime use of crack of freebase cocaine was lower at 4.5%, but there was a fourfold variation (1.6% to 6.5%) across state YRBS surveys (19).

In 1995, 2% of high school students in the United States reported injecting illegal drugs during their lifetime (18). Also, 16% of the students participating in the YRBS reported to using illegal drugs such as LSD, PCP, ecstasy, mushrooms, speed, ice, or heroin at least once. Inhalant use was reported by 20.3% of students nationwide.

Determining which adolescents are at increased risk of experimenting with illegal drugs and subsequently becoming substance abusers has been an area of research for more than 20 years. Reviews of the literature on risk factors associated with substance abuse indicate that many factors are associated with alcohol and drug use, including childhood personality, hyperactivity, antisocial traits, and stress (20–24). Interpersonal risk factors have also been found to be associated with substance abuse, including family mismanagement, parental substance use, low academic performance, and academic commitment. Finally, a correlation had been found between adolescent substance abuse and associating with substance-using peers (20–24).

As was found with cigarettes, ease of household access to alcohol was associated with more frequent alcohol use by youth in the Add Health Study (16). High levels of connectiveness to parents and family and to school were associated with less frequent alcohol use. Among older adolescents, more frequent parental presence in the home was associated with less frequent use. Increased use of alcohol was correlated with self-reports of appearing older than peers, low grade point average, and low self-esteem. High school students who worked 20 or more hours a week or had same-sex attraction and behavior drank alcohol more often. Among seventh and eighth graders, perceived risk of early death was correlated with more frequent drinking. For both groups, high levels of importance placed on religion and prayer appeared to be a

significant protective factor for alcohol use. The risk factors associated with marijuana use were almost identical to those found for alcohol use (16).

In discussions of substance abuse by adolescents, anabolic-androgenic steroid use is often left out (25). Anabolic-androgenic steroid use by athletes has become a widespread practice throughout the world. In the United States alone, it is estimated that 1 million individuals spend more than $100 million per year on black market anabolic steroids (26–28). Approximately 48% of lifetime anabolic steroid users are 25 or younger (29). Among high school students, between 4% and 15.3% of male adolescents and 0.5% to 6.7% of female adolescents in the United States report having used anabolic steroids (26–29). These differences are largely the result of differences in sampling among the studies. Some of the studies are of students in only one school or school district and vary in the school grades that are sampled. For example, in a study of eleventh-grade students in six high schools in Little Rock, Ark, Johnson et al (40) found that 11% of males and 0.5% of females reported using anabolic steroids. However, in a follow-up study, 7.6% of males and 1.5% of females reported anabolic steroid use. In contrast, DuRant et al (30) found that 5.4% of all ninth-grade males and 1.5% of ninth-grade females in Richmond County, Ga, had ever used anabolic steroids. Among tenth- and twelfth-grade students from 12 schools in Michigan, 12% of males and 4% of females reported previous anabolic steroid use (41). In the first nationally representative sample of adolescents, 0.6% of 12- to 17-year-olds from the National Household Survey on Drug Abuse reported use of anabolic steroids sometime during their life (29). The sex differences for the survey as a whole (ages 12–34) were 0.9% for males and 0.1% for females. The low incidence of use is probably related to the underreporting of drug use behaviors in a household setting (29).

The best estimates to date of anabolic steroid use by high school students were reported by DuRant et al (37), from an analysis of the CDC 1991 YRBS. Nationally, 4.08% of males and 1.2% of females reported having used anabolic steroids during the previous 12 months. Although black students (2.15%) reported a lower prevalence of anabolic steroid use than did students of other races (2.6% to 3.6%), the differences were not statistically significant. No linear trend was found in the prevalence of anabolic steroid use associated with age. Sixteen-year-old (3.48%) and 18-year-old (3.35%) students reported significantly higher prevalences of anabolic steroid use in the previous 12 months than did 15-year-old students (1.54%). In comparison, there were few differences among school grade levels in the prevalence of anabolic steroid use. Students in the South reported a significantly higher rate of anabolic steroid use (3.48%) in the previous 12 months than did students in the Northeast (1.7%) and the West (2.02%). Students in the Midwest (3.0%) were only slightly less likely to use anabolic steroids than were students in the South.

CLUSTERING OF SUBSTANCE USE

There are a number of studies that suggest that there are developmental stages in youth's involvement in the use of drugs (42–48). For example, in an analysis of twelfth-grade students in New York, Kandel et al (43) found that among males, alcohol use preceded marijuana use, marijuana and cigarette smoking preceded the use of cocaine and crack, and cocaine use preceded crack. Among females, alcohol use and cigarette smoking preceded marijuana use, marijuana use precede cocaine, and cocaine use preceded crack use. In a small minority of cases (10%), crack use was initiated before the students had tried marijuana. Because these findings and those from other studies are based on cross-sectional data, the hypothesis of a progression of drug use is not without controversy. Bailey (49) conducted a longitudinal cohort study of sixth- to eighth-graders followed through three rounds of data collection ending when they were in the ninth to eleventh grades. Students who began drinking alcohol and smoking cigarettes earlier, and progressed in frequency of use over time, were more likely to use marijuana and other illicit drugs. However, students who first initiated tobacco and alcohol use at high levels were less likely to use these and other substances subsequently than those who increased their use over time. In other words, the longer students had been using tobacco and alcohol, the more likely they were to progress to using other substances (49).

Regardless of the sequence in the progression of drug use, during adolescence tobacco, alcohol, and other substance use tend to cluster. (1,16,30–32,37,39). An example of this can be seen in the clustering of multiple substance use with anabolic steroid use. DuRant et al (30) examined data from a questionnaire based on the 1989 CDC Secondary School Health Risk Survey and the 1990 CDC Youth Risk Behavior Survey administered to ninth graders. The frequency of anabolic steroid use by ninth graders in Augusta, Ga, was significantly associated with the injection of drugs and the use of cocaine, alcohol, marijuana, cigarettes, and smokeless tobacco. Use of cocaine, shared needles, marijuana, and smokeless tobacco accounted for 33% of the variance in a multiple regression analysis of the frequency of anabolic steroid users among the sample of students studied. When these same youth were studied 4 months later, the relationships between anabolic steroid use and the use of other drugs remained stable (32).

The association between anabolic steroid use and the use of multiple other drugs has also been found to be a nationwide phenomenon with regional variability in the United States. Data from the 1991 CDC Youth Risk Behavior Survey of 12,272 ninth-through twelfth-grade students attending public and private schools in the 50 states and the District of Columbia revealed that students who reported having used alcohol, other drugs, and injecting drugs in the preceding 30 days and having ever used cocaine had significantly higher percentages of anabolic steroid use than did students who did not report these behaviors (37). Logistic repression analysis of lifetime use of anabolic steroids among these high school students found than an injectable drug user had a 17.86 times greater odds ratio (95% confidence interval [CI] = 7.56–42.20) of using anabolic steroids than did a student who did not use injectable drugs. The question did not specifically distinguish between injectable steroid and other injectable drugs; however, "illegal drug use" (odds ratio [OR] = 4.19, 95% CI = 2.32–7.55), male sex (OR = 2.79, CI = 1.62–4.80), alcohol use (OR = 1.83, CI = 1.04–3.20), and engaging in strength exercises (OR = 1.73, CI = 1.07–3.20) were also

significantly positively correlated with anabolic steroid use. In this study, race was not correlated to anabolic steroid use.

DuRant et al (37) also found that the patterns of drug use associated with anabolic steroid use varied regionally. Among adolescents living in the southern United States, where anabolic steroid use was highest, injected drug use was the strongest correlate with anabolic steroid use. Alcohol use and other drug use were the only other variables significantly associated with anabolic steroid use in the South. In the Midwest, injected drug use was also the strongest correlate with steroid use, but the relationship was weaker than that found among students in the South. In addition, male sex, other drug use, engaging in strength-training exercises, participating in school-sponsored sports, and lower academic achievement were associated with an increased likelihood of using anabolic steroids. The relationship between injectable drug use and anabolic steroid use was strongest among students living in the western states. Other significant correlates included other drug use, male sex, smokeless tobacco use, and nonuse of marijuana. The prevalence of anabolic steroid use was lowest in the northeastern states. Among adolescents living in these states, anabolic steroid use was most strongly associated with cocaine use, marijuana use, engaging in strength-training exercises, smokeless tobacco use, and the use of other drugs (37).

As another example of the clustering of drug use, Escobedo et al (1) found that smoking was associated with marijuana use (OR = 3.7, 95% CI = 2.7–5.1), binge drinking (OR = 2.1, CI = 1.6–2.8) and smokeless tobacco use among white male adolescents participating in the 1992 National Health Interview Survey and its YRBS supplement. Among African American males, smoking was associated with marijuana use (OR = 6.4, CI = 3.3–12.1) and binge drinking (OR = 2.1, CI = 1.1–4.2). Among Hispanic males, the relationship between smoking and marijuana use (OR = 2.3, CI = 1.2–4.3) was weaker and the relationship with binge drinking was stronger (OR = 3.4, CI = 2.0–5.6) than was observed among African Americans. Among white females, smoking was associated with other illicit drug use (OR = 1.9, CI = 1.4–2.6), binge drinking (OR = 2.5, CI = 1.9–3.1) and smokeless tobacco use (OR = 2.0, CI = 1.0–4.2). Smoking by African American female adolescents was also associated with marijuana use (OR = 3.7, CI = 1.4–6.5) and binge drinking (OR = 2.8, CI = 1.3–5.7), but the relationships were stronger than those seen among whites. Stronger relationships were found between smoking and marijuana use (OR = 6.4, CI = 3.2–6.5) and binge drinking (OR = 3.4, CI = 2.0–5.6) by Hispanic females than was observed in both whites and African Americans.

Problem-behavior theory provides insight into why substance use behaviors cluster with one another and with other health risk behaviors (50–51). The social ecology of adolescent life provides socially organized opportunities to learn risk and problem behaviors together and normative expectations are that they be performed together (50). Part of the reason that risk and problem behaviors tend to cluster is that different risk behaviors may serve the same social and/or psychological developmental functions for adolescents, such as affirming individuation from parents, trying to achieve adult status, and seeking acceptance from peers. These goals can be fulfilled with healthy risk-taking behaviors such as applying for a part-time job, learning to drive, or asking someone out for a date. However, problem behaviors cluster because they are the manifestations of similar underlying factors (52). For example, peer influences have been found to lead to early cigarette smoking (52), early sexual intercourse (54), marijuana use (55), and criminal behavior (56). Jessor et al posited that a variety of risk and problem behaviors cluster to form a "risk behavior syndrome" that is caused by a general latent variable of unconventionality combined with other "risk domains" (50). The degree of clustering is dependent upon the adolescents' exposure to multiple risk domains from five broad areas: biological, genetics, social environment, perceived environment, personality, and behavior. The level of resiliency is based upon the degree of exposure to protective factors from "protective domains" within these same five areas.

In comparison, social learning theory proposes that different risk and problem behaviors have some influences in common and some influences that are specific, such as one risk behavior serving as a partial cause of another (52). For example, an adolescent who begins to use marijuana regularly may be rejected by conventional peer groups and increase his or her association with peer groups that approve of the health risk and problem behaviors. Social learning from the new group could result in engaging in other problem behaviors and a weakening of bonds to conventional groups. These theories have implications for prevention programs. Jessor (50) has argued that owing to the clustering of health risk and problem behaviors, interventions should target multiple risk behaviors and should address multiple risk factors and protective domains.

TOBACCO, ALCOHOL, AND OTHER DRUG USE AND NUTRITION

Adequate nutrition is particularly important during adolescence, as it is an accelerated period of physical growth and maturity. In a 1995 US national survey of high school students, only 27.7% of students reported eating five or more servings of fruits and vegetables during the day prior to the survey, while 60.5% reported having eaten two or less servings of foods typically high in fat content (18). The identification of factors that may be associated with poor nutrition, such as drug use, would further allow educational efforts to more specifically target those individuals at higher risk.

Little research has been conducted on the relationship between substance use and eating behaviors among adolescents. One study involved 1513 high school students aged 15–18 from the Negev region in Israel, each of whom completed a questionnaire addressing tobacco, alcohol, and other illicit drug use, awareness of the consequences of such usage, and nutrition-related behaviors and attitudes (57). Of the students surveyed, 37% reported use of cigarettes on a regular basis, 41% reported consumption of alcohol, and 4% use of illicit drugs. Compared to those students who reported no cigarette use, students who smoked were more likely not to eat breakfast, not to eat a snack or meal at school, and not to eat three meals a day. Similar significant relationships between these three behaviors and alcohol consumption and illicit drug use were also found, but only when gender was controlled. Among males, drinking alcohol was associated with not eating

breakfast. Among females, alcohol use was associated with not eating a snack or meal at school and not eating three meals per day. Males who used other drugs were less likely to eat breakfast and females who used other drugs were less likely to eat at school. In addition, a greater proportion of those students who smoked and used illicit drugs believed there to be no relation between proper nutrition and health compared to those students who did not smoke or use illicit drugs; no significant difference in opinion was found among those students who used alcohol and those that did not (57).

In a study of 36,284 predominantly white youths aged 12 to 20 in grades 7 to 12 of Minnesota public secondary schools, frequency of fruit and vegetable consumption, dieting frequency, binge eating, frequency of tobacco, alcohol, and marijuana use, weight satisfaction, academic achievement, family connectedness, and sociodemographic and personal variables were measured (58). The variables found to have the strongest association with inadequate fruit and vegetable consumption (defined as eating fruits or vegetables less than once a day) were low socioeconomic status, poor school achievement, and low family connectedness. Use of tobacco, alcohol, and marijuana were associated with inadequate fruit and vegetable consumption, even after controlling for sociodemographic and personal factors.

These studies suggest that smoking, alcohol, and illicit drug use in adolescents may be associated with improper eating behaviors and attitudes. Although generalizations from these results are limited due to their being obtained from a cross-sectional sampling of somewhat homogenous populations, they suggest that a relationship exists between nutrition-related behaviors and attitudes and adolescent drug use that needs to be further explored. A better understanding of such behaviors and attitudes would allow for effective incorporation of nutrition education into substance abuse prevention programs.

DRUG USE AND PHYSICAL ACTIVITY

Research has consistently found a negative association between physical activity and cigarette smoking among adolescents (59–61). A cross-sectional study of 823 students from a suburban public high school in Kentucky found that among the 30% of students reporting participation in school athletics, there were significantly lower rates of current cigarette use (59). Logistic regression analyses controlling for age, sex, race, and grade-point average indicated that nonathletes were four times more likely to smoke cigarettes than athletes. In another cross-sectional study of 1200 male students from seven high schools in northwest Louisiana, medium- and high-intensity athletes were significantly less likely to be heavy smokers than nonathletes and low-intensity athletes; this difference, however, was not significant after controlling for race and grade-point average (60). A 3-year prospective study of 1245 students 12 to 16 years old from two junior high schools in a metropolitan school district near Pittsburgh examined the relationship between baseline leisure-time physical activity, aerobic fitness, and participation in competitive athletics and initiation of substance use among adolescents. High levels of aerobic fitness were found to be associated with a decreased likelihood of initiating cigarette smoking by females when controlling for age, race, and socioeconomic statue, but not among males (61).

Other studies looking at cigarette use and physical activity have been larger in scope and have resulted in similar findings (62–66). A cross-sectional study of 7846 students aged 14 to 18 from 81 South Carolina public schools found that even when controlling for race, gender, and physical education participation, nonathletes were significantly more likely to be smokers than athletes. High activity nonathletes were most likely to be smokers (26.0%), followed closely by sedentary, moderate-, and low-activity nonathletes (23.4%, 22.0%, and 21.8%) (62). In a study of the observations and perceptions of 215 athletic directors/coaches in the state of North Carolina regarding substance use among students, a significantly greater number of athletic directors/coaches believed drug use to be a much bigger or somewhat bigger problem among the general student body than among student athletes (63). Also, more reported a personal awareness and encounter of drug use in the general student body than among student athletes. In terms of cigarette use, 69.2% of athletic directors/coaches believed cigarettes to be a very big or somewhat big problem among the general student body, while 18.4% believed this to be true for student athletes.

Escobedo et al (1) assessed smoking patterns, smoking initiation, and the relationship between participation in interscholastic sports and age at smoking initiation to regular and heavy smoking among adolescents participating in the 1990 YRBS. The study was comprised of 11,248 students in grades 9 to 12 attending public and private schools in the 50 states, the District of Columbia, Puerto Rico, and the Virgin Islands. Seventy-two percent of the students reported smoking at some point (experimental, former, occasional, and regular smokers) while 32% reported being current smokers. Examination of smoking patterns by sports activity showed that those students not participating in interscholastic sports were more likely to be heavy smokers than those students who were involved in interscholastic sports. The prevalence and adjusted odds ratios of regular and heavy smoking decreased considerably with increasing number of sports played. Similarly, in a nationwide random sample of 1200 15- and 16-year-old Icelandic youth, participation in sports was negatively associated with cigarette use (65). A study of 17,251 students from 140 colleges in the United States found that among both males and females, greater degrees of involvement in athletics were associated with decreased use of cigarettes, suggesting that this association may extend beyond high school (66).

Studies examining the association between alcohol use and physical activity among adolescents have reported conflicting findings (54,61–63,65–67). While some studies report physically active adolescents to be at decreased risk for alcohol use, other studies have found these individuals to be at increased risk for both alcohol consumption and binge drinking. In their study of Kentucky youth, Oler et al (59) found significantly lower rates of current alcohol use among school athletes than nonathletes; however, this difference was not significant when controlling for age, sex, race, and grade-point average. In Shields' study (63), 88.2% of athletic directors/coaches reported alcohol to be a very big or somewhat big problem among the general student body, while 60.5% reported alcohol to be a very big or somewhat big problem among student athletes. Among Icelandic youth,

Thorlindsson et al (65) found sports participation to be negatively associated with alcohol use. In contrast, in a 3-year prospective study, Aaron et al (61) reported that participation in competitive sports was associated with an increased likelihood of initiating alcohol consumption among males after controlling for age, race, and socioeconomic status. Males in the high and moderate leisure-time physical activity groups also showed a higher incidence of initiation of alcohol consumption compared with those in the low leisure-time activity group. In a cross-sectional study of students in South Carolina public schools, Rainey et al (62) found that high- and moderate-activity athletes had the highest reports of consuming at least one drink of alcohol within the past 30 days and that high-activity athletes had greater frequencies of alcohol consumption compared to low-activity and sedentary nonathletes after controlling for race, gender, and physical education participation. High-activity athletes also reported the greatest frequency of binge drinking within the past 30 days. Similarly, a study of 257 Canadian youth from five high schools in Saskatoon found a positive association between physical activity and alcohol consumption for highly active males (67). Wechsler et al (66) had comparable findings in their US national study of college students, with more males and females involved in athletics reporting frequent heavy drinking lifestyles than those not involved. Greater degrees of involvement in athletics were also associated with increased reports of binge drinking among both male and female students.

Studies of physical activity and the use of other drugs have mainly concerned smokeless tobacco and marijuana. These studies have generally shown decreased use of marijuana among physically active individuals; however, there have been conflicting findings regarding smokeless tobacco use. Oler et al (59) found that reports of current marijuana use were significantly lower among school athletes than nonathletes and that nonathletes were two times more likely than athletes to use marijuana after controlling for age, sex, race, and grade-point average. No significant difference was found between athletes and nonathletes in terms of smokeless tobacco use. Among athletic directors/coaches participating in Shields' study (63), 34.8% reported marijuana to be a very big or somewhat big problem among the general student body versus 11.7% reporting this to be the case for student athletes: for chewing/dipping tobacco, reports were similar (53.3% vs. 28.6%). In contrast, the analysis of the 1990 YRBS by Escobedo et al (64) revealed that after controlling for race and grade-point average, at every level of sports intensity athletes used chewing tobacco and snuff at significantly higher rates than nonathletes. Similarly, Rainey et al (62) found a positive relationship between smokeless tobacco use and activity level, but this relationship was not significant after controlling for race, gender, and physical education. Wechsler et al (66) demonstrated that greater degrees of involvement in athletics were also associated with increased reports of chewing tobacco use among male students.

Overall, these studies suggest that physically active adolescents are at decreased risk for the use of cigarettes and marijuana, but may also be at increased risk for alcohol consumption and binge drinking as well as smokeless tobacco use. Although several of these studies are cross-sectional in nature, have small sample sizes, and/or consist of ethnically homogenous or geographically limited study populations, the consistent finding of a negative association between physical activity and cigarette and marijuana use support this conclusion. The findings of studies examining physical activity and alcohol consumption among adolescents are not as consistent. However, reports among substance-abusing college students who are involved in athletics that these are behaviors acquired in high school further supports findings of a positive association between physical activity and alcohol use among adolescents. Thus, while physical activity may act as a protective factor against cigarette and marijuana use, it may also place adolescents at increased risk for alcohol and smokeless tobacco use. Further research is needed to investigate the reasons behind abstaining from cigarette and marijuana use but continuing use of alcohol and smokeless tobacco in order to design effective substance abuse prevention programs. Such behaviors could be a result of beliefs that alcohol and smokeless tobacco are less of a detriment to health or less likely to adversely affect one's athletic performance than cigarettes and marijuana. If this is true, then efforts need to be made to encourage physical activity but emphasize the adverse physical effects of these substances among athletes. It is also possible that alcohol use and binge drinking are part of the social aspect of team sports, in which case this type of behavior should be targeted in prevention programs and athletic directors/coaches should be made aware of and instructed to discourage social drinking among student athletes. A combined approach of school-based prevention programs and efforts by coaches to educate students about substance use could potentially be successful in reaching those adolescents at risk.

SCHOOL-BASED TOBACCO–USE PREVENTION PROGRAMS

The Division of Adolescent and School Health (DASH) of the CDC has a program that formally evaluates prevention curricula and/or programs to determine if they should recommend their adoption by schools. A panel of scientists review the evaluations of the curricula in a fashion similar to the way in which a grant application is reviewed by the NIH. If the panel concludes that the research supports the efficacy of a particular curriculum, then a second panel of educators evaluates the curriculum-based established educational criteria.

To date, only two curricula have been selected by DASH to be recommended for adoption by schools. The most comprehensive of these two curricula is Botvin's Life Skills Training Program (68). An advantage of this program is that it not only addresses tobacco use, but also alcohol and other drug use. It consists of 15 units designed primarily for adolescents of middle-school age. There are 10 booster sessions for 14- and 15-year-olds and an additional 5 booster sessions for 15- and 16-year-old. It is designed to target the primary causes of substance use, including tobacco, alcohol, and other drug use, by teaching a combination of health information, general life skills, and tobacco and other drug use resistance skills. Specific topics include self-image and self-improvement, decision making, smoking myths and realities, smoking and biofeedback, alcohol myths and realities, marijuana myths and realities, advertising, coping with anxiety, communication skills, social skills, and assertiveness. The Life Skills Training program includes a variety of teaching methods such as large and small group discussion, worksheets, brainstorming, scripted and unscripted skill practice, demonstrations illustrating the physical effects of cigarette smoking, analysis of advertisements for tobacco and alcohol, and role play.

The program was evaluated among 3597 students from 56 schools in predominately middle-class white suburban and rural communities in three geographic areas of New York. In schools it was found to reduce tobacco, alcohol, and marijuana use between 50% and 75% and its effects lasted up to 6 years (68–71). It has also been found to cut polydrug use up to 66%, reduce pack-a-day smoking by 25% and decrease the use of inhalants, narcotics and hallucinogens. Program effectiveness has been demonstrated among white, African American and Hispanic youth.

The curriculum requires formal training to teach effectively. Life Skills Training is published by Princeton Health Press, which also provides formal training on teaching the curriculum.

The second curriculum recommended by DASH at the CDC is Sussman et al's Project TNT (72–76). Project TNT was designed to target the primary causes of cigarette smoking, smokeless tobacco use, and cigar and pipe smoking among teens. The curriculum provides detailed information about the health consequences of tobacco use and addresses topics including building self-esteem, active listening, effective communication, refusal assertion learning/practice, noncompliance coping (ingratiation and cognitive restructuring) to enhance self-confidence, counteracting advertising images and social activism to change norms, and decision making/public commitment. Project TNT is less comprehensive than the Life Skills Training curriculum described earlier. It consists of 10 sessions of approximately 45 to 50 minutes each and a 2-session booster conducted approximately 1 year after the original curriculum is implemented.

The theoretical basis of Project TNT is that the youth who will be best able to resist using tobacco products are those who 1) are aware of misleading social information that facilitates tobacco use (e.g. advertising, inflating prevalence estimates); 2) have skills that counteract the social pressures to achieve approval by using tobacco; and 3) appreciate the physical consequences that tobacco use may have on their own lives (e.g., the beginnings of addiction). Project TNT counteracts different causes of tobacco use simultaneously because the behavior is determined by multiple causes. This comprehensive approach is well suited to a wide variety of youth who may differ in risk factors that influence their tobacco use.

The curriculum was evaluated among 6716 seventh-grade students in 48 junior high schools. The students were 60% white non-Hispanic, 27% Latino, 7% African American, and 6% Asian American. Schools were randomly assigned to one of four conditions. Three were designed to counteract the effects of separate (single) program components (normative social influence, informational social influence, and physical consequences), whereas a fourth, comprehensive curriculum, Project TNT, was designed to counteract all three effects. One- and 2 year follow-ups of key outcomes were conducted after the core seventh grade intervention was delivered. The "comprehensive social influences plus physical consequences" curriculum showed the largest effects on behavior. Compared to the control condition ("usual school health education"), this program obtained significant effects on initiation and weekly use of smokeless tobacco and cigarettes. The program reduced initiation of cigarettes by approximately 26% over the control group, when 1-year and 2-year follow-up outcomes were averaged together; reduced initiation of smokeless tobacco use by approximately 60%; weekly or more frequent cigarette smoking was reduced by approximately 30%; and weekly or more frequent smokeless tobacco use was eliminated. These data indicate that the same tobacco use prevention program can be delivered to males and females and can be effective over the transitional period from junior to senior high school.

As was discussed earlier, anabolic steroid use is often ignored during discussions of adolescent substance use and prevention. We are aware of only one evaluation of a program to prevent anabolic steroid use. Goldberg et al (77) conducted a randomized trial of a school-based intervention using the ATLAS Program (78) to reduce intent to use anabolic-androgenic steroids among adolescent athletes. The study sample consisted of 1306 football players from 31 different high schools in Portland, Oregon. Schools were paired based on demographic characteristics and then randomly assigned to experimental or control conditions. Seven hundred and two of the students from 15 schools were assigned to the experimental intervention, which consisted of 7 weekly 50-minute class sessions conducted by coaches and trained student peer leaders in addition to 7 weekly weight-room sessions conducted by research staff. Each school was also provided with $3000 of weightlifting equipment prior to beginning the intervention. The classroom sessions gave instruction addressing alternatives to steroid use, side effects of steroid use, sports nutrition, refusal skills to turn down offers to use steroids or other illicit drugs, and analysis of the media in relation to steroid use. Weight-room sessions were geared towards skill training and also sought to keep students in the school environment and away from outside commercial gym influences. Eight hundred and four of the students from 16 schools received the control conditions, which consisted of providing antisteroid informational pamphlets to students but no program intervention. Data were obtained by a 168-item self-report questionnaire completed at school at three different times: just prior to the initial intervention session, just following the final session, and again 9 to 12 months later. Results from data analysis showed significant positive impact on many of the constructs assessed, including significant reductions in adolescent intent to use anabolic steroids and increased knowledge of anabolic steroids and consequences of use compared to individuals in the control group. Positive effects were also seen on student attitudes and beliefs regarding steroid use. Although some of these positive effects were lost in long-term follow-up, the majority persisted, including reduced intent to use anabolic steroids. However, there was no difference between the groups in actual anabolic steroid use. One reason was that actual anabolic steroid use at pretest for both groups and at follow-up for the control group was very low; substantially lower than has been observed in national epidemiologic studies (37). It is quite possible that the ATLAS Program could be more effective in areas where the percent of athletes that use anabolic steroids is higher (30,34,37–39).

School-based prevention curricula also benefit when supplemented with other community-based prevention strategies (79). The public health model takes into consideration the host, agent, and environment, and focuses on the interaction of this triad for the spread of tobacco, alcohol, and other drug-related problems. Mass media campaigns are often used to increase public awareness and to change community norms concerning illegal substance use by youth. Efforts by law enforcement are needed, but often not effectively implemented. For example, in most areas laws preventing children and adolescents from purchasing tobacco products or requiring proof of age to be requested are not enforced. In some communities, neighborhoods characterized by poverty, high unemployment, and minority racial/ethnic residents are "written off" by law enforcement and illegal drugs are easily bought and sold. Efforts by neighborhood and community organizations focusing on changing group norms concerning substance use through both family-based and school-based efforts are crucial to changing the behaviors of law enforcement in their neighborhood (79).

SCREENING AND INTERVENTIONS BY PRIMARY CARE PROVIDERS

Pediatricians and other primary care health care providers have long been aware of the importance of early recognition of drug and alcohol use in their patients. A number of national medical organizations have published guidelines for anticipatory guidance, screening, and referral. Among these are the Guidelines for Adolescent Preventive Services (GAPS) of the American Medical Association (80) and the position paper from the Committee on Substance Abuse of the American Academy of Pediatrics (AAP) (81). More recently, the Maternal and Child Health Bureau (MCHB) has sponsored publication of "Bright Futures: Guidelines for Health Supervision of Infants, Children, and Adolescents" in an effort to set a national standard for screening and early intervention in pediatric practice (82). There is universal agreement that pediatricians should identify, advise, and refer substance-abusing teenagers.

Pediatricians often lack clinical tools that can help them screen, assess, and treat problems within the context of a 30-minute office visit. Among physicians who see adults, the CAGE questions have become a popular screening tool (83). CAGE is both brief and easy to remember. It also has been found to have good sensitivity and specificity for alcohol use disorders among adult medical patients (84). Unfortunately, it has never been formally validated in an adolescent population, and would seem to have poor face validity (e.g., the "eyeopener" question) for adolescents. Riggs et al have suggested another screening mnemonic, RAFFT, with good face validity for adolescents, but these questions have never been formally tested in any population (85). Written questionnaires, such as the Problem Oriented Screening Instrument for Teenagers (POSIT), have been formally tested in adolescents (86–88). Knight et al have found the POSIT to have good reliability in an adolescent medical clinic sample (89). For the alcohol and drug use and abuse screening scale we found a test-retest reliability coefficient of .86 and internal consistency reliabilities of .77

Table 52-1 Alcohol and Drug Use Screening Scale from the POSIT		
1. Do you get into trouble because you use drugs or alcohol at school?	yes	no
2. Have you accidentally hurt yourself or someone else while high on alcohol or drugs?	yes	no
3. Do you miss out on activities because you spend too much money on drugs or alcohol?	yes	no
4. Do you ever feel you are addicted to alcohol or drugs?	yes	no
5. Have you started using more and more drugs and alcohol to get the effect you want?	yes	no
6. Do you ever leave a party because there is no alcohol or drugs?	yes	no
7. Do you have a constant desire for alcohol or drugs?	yes	no
8. Have you had a car accident while high on alcohol or drugs?	yes	no
9. Do you forget things you did while drinking or using drugs?	yes	no
10. During the past month have you driven a car while you were drunk or high?	yes	no
11. Does alcohol or drug use cause your moods to change quickly like from happy to sad or vice versa?	yes	no
12. Do you miss school or arrive late for school because of your alcohol or drug use?	yes	no
13. Do your family or friends ever tell you that you should cut down on your drinking or drug use?	yes	no
14. Do you have serious arguments with friends or family members because of your drinking or drug use?	yes	no
15. Does your alcohol or drug use ever make you do something that you would not normally do—like breaking rules, missing curfew, breaking the law, or having sex with someone?	yes	no
16. Do you have trouble getting along with any of your friends because of your alcohol or drug use?	yes	no
17. Do you ever feel you can't control your alcohol or drug use?	yes	no

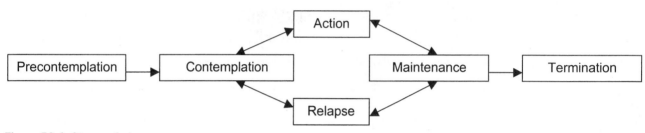

Figure 52-1 Stages of change.

at the initial test and .87 at retest. A list of the 17 questions making up this screening instrument is in Table 52-1. You will notice that tobacco use is not addressed in this screening questionnaire.

If the health care provider determines that a young patient is using substances, it is, in most cases, not necessary to refer the patient to a mental health substance abuse treatment program. Many primary care providers are capable of helping an adolescent change behaviors regarding tobacco, alcohol, and other drug abuse during as few as three to four office visits. The transtheoretical model of how people change addictive behaviors is illustrated in Figure 52-1 (90–92). During each office encounter the health care provider should help the adolescent patient move from one stage of change to the next. The goal of the first office visit is simply to help the patient to start thinking about the problem. This is done by asking appropriate questions, giving feedback and information, and expressing concern. John Knight at Children's Hospital in Boston has developed a tool to help adolescent patients determine where they are in terms of wanting to change their behaviors (Figure 52-2). The contemplation stage begins when an individual considers that they may indeed have a problem, and starts to weigh the "pros and cons" of changing. This stage is characterized by ambivalence. Thus, at the second office visit, the health care provider should ask about the pros and cons of changing behavior, and try to tip the balance in favor of change. The goal of this

encounter is to move the adolescent patient from contemplation to action, and develop a plan for change. Action is defined by an actual change in behavior. The purpose of the third office visit is to check and see how the plan for change is working; offer positive reinforcement if it is, and consider alternatives if it isn't.

"Motivational enhancement therapy" and "motivational interviewing" are largely interchangeable terms for the same therapeutic process that can be used by health care providers to help adolescents change their substance-using behaviors. This approach is based on principles of experimental social psychology (attribution, cognitive dissonance, self-efficacy) that conceptualize motivation as an interpersonal process rather than an intrinsic character trait (93–94). Ambivalence to change in behavior is considered normal and acceptable. Cognitive dissonance is created by contrasting the ongoing problem behavior with changes required to reach individual goals. According to motivational theory, responsibility for change lies entirely with the individual. Pressuring leads to increased resistance to change. Therefore, the health care provider should ask questions that will elicit self-motivational statements (e.g., "How do you think your life would improve if you gave up using drugs?, or "Can you think of any ways that 'safe sex' would help get you closer to your goals?"), and then summarize and support those statements that favor change. This is more likely to lead to initiation, persistence, and compliance with behavior change efforts. As described by Miller et al, there are five basic strate-

For each statement below, please circle the number which best describes how much you agree or disagree right now: the higher the number, the more you agree.

Disagree Strongly 1	Agree Somewhat 2	Unsure 3	Agree Somewhat 4	Agree Strongly 5

1. I don't think I use too much alcohol/drugs.　　　　　　　1 2 3 4 5

2. I am trying to use less alcohol/drugs than I used to.　　　1 2 3 4 5

3. I enjoy alcohol/drugs, but sometimes I use too much.　　　1 2 3 4 5

4. Sometimes I think I should cut down on my alcohol/drug use.　1 2 3 4 5

5. It's a waste of time thinking about my alcohol/drug use.　　1 2 3 4 5

6. I have just recently changed my alcohol/drug use.　　　　1 2 3 4 5

7. Anyone can talk about wanting to do something about alcohol/drug use, but I'm actually doing something about it.　1 2 3 4 5

8. I am at the stage where I should think about using less alcohol/drugs.　1 2 3 4 5

9. My alcohol/drug use is a problem sometimes.　　　　　　1 2 3 4 5

10. There is no need for me to think about changing my alcohol/drug use.　1 2 3 4 5

11. I am actually changing my alcohol/drug use right now.　　1 2 3 4 5

12. Using less alcohol/drugs would be pointless for me.　　　1 2 3 4 5

Figure 52-2 Readiness to change questionnaire.

D	Develop Discrepancy
A	Avoid Arguments
R	Roll with Resistance
E	Express Empathy
S	Support Self-Efficacy

Figure 52-3 Motivational interviewing: basic strategies.

gies underlying this approach, summarized in the DARES mnemonic (Figure 52-3) (94). Miller et al have also described six elements common to effective brief interventions, summarized in another mnemonic known as FRAMES (Figure 52-4) (95). These interviewing strategies form the educational basis for a faculty development project jointly sponsored by the Ambulatory Pediatric Association, the Society for General Internal Medicine, and the Health Resources Services Administration (HRSA). The approach has also been recommended for use in pediatric office practice by Werner (96), Knight (97), and others (98,99).

SUMMARY

Tobacco, alcohol and other illegal drug use by children and adolescents remains a significant public health problem in this country. Research continues to be needed in understanding the causes, prevention, and treatment of illegal substance use by our youth. Pediatricians and other health care professions have a responsibility to advocate for children and adolescents at the local, state, and national level concerning the problem of illegal drug use and to advise legislators, educators, law enforcement officials, and others on what programs have been found to be effective in preventing substance use. Primary health care providers can also successfully screen for substance use among their child and adolescent patients and help them discontinue the use of tobacco, alcohol and other drugs.

Figure 52-4 Effective brief intervention strategies.

F	FEEDBACK on personal risk or impairment
R	Emphasis on personal RESPONSIBILITY for change
A	Clear ADVICE to change
M	A MENU of alternative change options
E	Therapist EMPATHY
S	Facilitation of client SELF-EFFICACY or optimism

REFERENCES

1. Escobedo LG, Reddy M, DuRant RH. Relationship between cigarette smoking and health risk and problem behaviors among US adolescents. Arch Pediatr Adolesc Med 1997;151:66–71.

2. U.S. Department of Health and Human Services. Preventing tobacco use among young people: a report of the Surgeon General. Atlanta: Public Health Service, Centers for Disease Control and Prevention, 1994.

3. Lynch BS, Bonnie RJ. Growing up tobacco free: preventing nicotine addiction in children and youths. Washington, DC: National Academy Press, 1994.

4. US Department of Health and Human Services. Preventing tobacco use among young people: a report of the Surgeon General. Atlanta: Public Health Service, Centers for Disease Control and Prevention, 1994.

5. Giovino GA, Schooley MW, Zhu BP, et al. Surveillance for selected tobacco-use behaviors—United States—1990–1994. MMWR CDC Surveill Summ 1994;43:1–43.

6. Johnston LD, O'Malley PM, Bachman JG. National trends in drug use and related factors among American high school students and young adults, 1975–1992. Rockville, MD: US Department of Health and Human Services, 1993.

7. Cummings KM, Pechacek T, Shopland D. The illegal sale of cigarettes to US minors: estimates by state. Am J Public Health 1994;84:300–302.

8. Johnston LD, O'Malley PM, Bachman JG. National trends in drug use and related factors among American high school students and young adults, 1975–1992. Rockville MD: US Department of Health and Human Services, 1994.

9. Johnston LD. Smoking rates climb among American teenagers, who find smoking increasingly acceptable and seriously underestimate the risks. Ann Arbor: The University of Michigan News and Information Service, 1995.

10. Tobacco use and usual source of cigarettes among high school students—United States, 1995. MMWR Morb Mortal Wkly Rep 1996;45:313–318.

11. McGinnis JM, Lee PR. Healthy people 2000 at mid decade. JAMA 1995;273:1123–1129.

12. Allen K, Moss A, Giovino GA, et al. Teenage tobacco use data: estimates from the teenage attitudes and practices survey, United States, 1989: advance data. Atlanta: Public Health Service, Center for Disease Control and Prevention, National Center for Health Statistics, 1993. Publication No. 224.

13. Hansen WB. Behavioral predictors of abstinence: early indicators of a dependence on tobacco among adolescents. Int J Addict 1983; 18:13–20.

14. Hansen WB, Collins LM, Johnson CA, Graham JW. Self-initiated smoking cessation among high school students. Addict Behav 1985;10:265–271.

15. Ershler J, Levanthal H, Fleming R, Glynn K. The quitting experience for smokers in sixth through twelfth grades. Addict Behav 1989;14:365–378.

16. Resnick MD, Bearman PS, Blum RW, et al. Protecting adolescents from harm: findings from the National Longitudinal Study on Adolescent Health. JAMA 1997; 278:823–832.

17. National Institute on Drug Abuse. National household survey on drug abuse, main findings. Rockville, MD: National Institute on Drug Abuse, 1994.

18. Johnson LD, O'Malley PM, Bachman JG. National survey results on drug use from the Monitoring the Future Study, 1975–1994: vol. 1, secondary school students. Rockville, MD: National Institute on Drug Abuse, 1994. NIH publication no. 95–4026.

19. Kann L, Warren CW, Harris WA, et al. Youth risk behavior surveillance—United States, 1995. MMWR CDC Surveill Summ 1996; 45:1–84.

20. Kaplan H, Johnson R, Bailey C. Explaining adolescent drug use: an elaboration strategy for structural equations modeling. Psychiatry 1988;51:142–163.

21. Maddahia E, Newcomb M, Bentler P. Risk factors for substance abuse: ethnic difference among adolescents. J Subst Abuse 1988; 1:11–23.

22. Croughan JL. The contribution of family studies to understanding drug abuse. In: Robins LN, ed. Series in psychosocial epidemiology, vol. 6: studying drug abuse. New Brunswick, NJ: Rutgers University Press, 1987: 93–116.

23. Catalano R, Hawkins J, Wells E, et al. Evaluation of the effectiveness of adolescent drug abuse

treatment assessment of risks for relapse and promising approaches for relapse prevention. Int J Addict 1991;25:1085–1140, 1990–1991.

24. Coie J, Watt N, West S, et al. The science of prevention: a conceptual framework and some directions for a national research program. Am Psychol 1993;10:1013–1022.

25. DuRant RH, Middleman AB, Spack N. Anabolic-androgenic steroid use by adolescents. Focus and Opinion: Pediatrics 1996;2:245–252.

26. Taylor WN, Black AB. Pervasive anabolic steroid use among health club athletes. Ann Sports Med 1987;3:155–159.

27. Burkett LN, Faldulto MT. Steroid use by athletes in a metropolitan area. Physician Sports Med 1984;12:69–74.

28. Giannini AJ, Miller N, Kocjan DK. Treating steroid abuse: a psychiatric perspective. Clin Pediatr 1991;30:538–542.

29. Yesalis CE, Kennedy NJ, Kopstein AN, et al. Anabolic-androgenic steroid use in the United States. JAMA 1993;270:1217–1221.

30. DuRant RH, Rickert VI, Ashworth CS, et al. Use of multiple drugs among adolescents who use anabolic steroids. N Engl J Med 1993;328:922–926.

31. DuRant Rh, Rickert VI, Ashworth CS. Use of anabolic steroids among adolescents. N Engl J Med 1993;329:889. Letter.

32. DuRant RH, Ashworth CS, Newman C, et al. Stability of the relationships between anabolic steroid use and multiple substance use by young adolescents. J Adolesc Health 1994;15;111–116.

33. Committee on the Judiciary, US Senate. Drug misuse: steroids and human growth hormone: report to the chairman. Washington, DC: Government Printing Office, 1989. Publication no. GAO/HRD-89-109.

34. Komoroski EM, Rickert VI. Adolescent body image and attitudes to anabolic steroid use Am J Dis Child 1992;146:823–828.

35. Buckley WE, Yesalis CE, Freidl KE, et al. Estimated prevalence of anabolic steroid use among male high school seniors. JAMA 1988;260:3441–3445.

36. Yesalis CE, Streit AL, Vicary JR, et al. Anabolic steroid use: indications of habituation among adolescents. J Drug Educ 1989;19:103–116.

37. DuRant RH, Escobedo LG, Heath GW. Anabolic steroid use, strength training and multiple drug use among adolescents in the United States. Pediatrics 1995;96:23–28.

38. Middleman AB, Faulkner AH, Woods ER, et al. High-risk behaviors among high school students in Massachusetts who use anabolic steroids. Pediatrics 1995;96:268–272.

39. DuRant RH, Middleman AB, Faulkner AH, et al. Adolescent anabolic-androgenic steroid use, multiple drug use, and high school sports participation. Ped Exerc Sci 1997;9:150–158.

40. Johnson MD, Jay MS, Shoup B, et al. Anabolic steroid use by male adolescents. Pediatrics 1989;83:921–924.

41. Hubbell N. The use of steroids by Michigan high school students and athletes: an opinion research study of 10th and 12th grade high school students and varsity athletes, November 1989 through January 1990. Lansing: Michigan Department of Public Health, Chronic Disease Advisory Committee, 1990.

42. Torabi MR, Bailey WJ, Majd-Jabbari M. Cigarette smoking as a predictor of alcohol and other drug use by children and adolescents: evidence of the "gateway drugs effect." J Sch Health 1993;63:302–306.

43. Kandel D, Yamaguchi K. From beer to crack: developmental patterns of drug involvement. Am J Public Health 1993;83:851–855.

44. Kandel D, Simcha-Fagan O, Davies M. Risk factors for delinquency and illicit drug use from adolescence to young adulthood. J Drug Issues 1986;16:67–90.

45. Kandel DB, Yamaguchi K, Chen K. Stages of progression in drug involvement from adolescence to adulthood: further evidence for the gateway theory. J Stud Alcohol 1992;53:447–457.

46. Fleming R, Leventhal H, Glynn K, Ershler J. The role of cigarettes in the initiation and progression of early substance use. Addict Behav 1989;14:261–272.

47. O'Donnell JA, Clayton RR. The stepping stone hypothesis: a reappraisal. Chem Dependency 1982;4:229–241.

48. Yamaguchi K, Kandel DB. Patterns of drug use from adolescence to young adulthood: III, sequences of progression. Am J Public Health 1984;74:668–681.

49. Bailey SL. Adolescents' multisubstance use patterns: the role of heavy alcohol and cigarette use. Am J Public Health 1992;82:1220–1224.

50. Jessor R. Risk behavior in adolescence: a psychosocial framework for understanding and action. J Adolesc Health 1992;21:597–605.

51. Jessor R, Donovan JE, Costa FM. Beyond adolescence: problem behavior and young adult development. Cambridge: Cambridge University Press, 1991.

52. Osgood DW, Johnson LD, O'Malley PM, Bachman JG. The generality of deviance in late adolescence and early adulthood. Am Sociol Rev 1988;53:81–93.

53. Krasmick J, Judd CM. Transitions in social influence at adolescence: who induces cigarette smoking. Devel Psychol 1982;18:359–368.

54. Billy JOG, Udry JR. Patterns of adolescent friendship and effects on sexual behavior. Soc Psych Q 1985;48:27–41.

55. Kandel DB. Homaphily, selection, and socialization in adolescent friendships. Am J Soc 1978;84:427–436.

56. Southern EH, Cressey D. Principles of criminology. 5th ed. Philadelphia: JB Lippincott, 1955.

57. Isralowitz RE, Trostler N. Substance use: toward an understanding of its relation to nutrition-related attitudes and behavior among Israeli high school youth. J Adolesc Health 1996;19:184–189.

58. Newmark-Sztainer D, Story M, Resnick MD, Blum RW. Correlates of inadequate fruit and vegetable consumption among adolescents. Prev Med 1996;25:497–505.

59. Oler MJ, Mainous AG, Martin CA, et al. Depression, suicidal ideation, and substance use among adolescents. Arch Fam Med 1994; 3:781–785.

60. Davis TC, Arnold C, Nandy I, et al. Tobacco use among male high school athletes. J Adolesc Health 1997;21:97–101.

61. Aaron DJ, Dearwater SR, Anderson R, et al. Physical activity and the initiation of high-risk health behaviors in adolescents. Med Sci Sports Exerc 1995;27:1639–1645.

62. Rainey CJ, McKeown RE, Sargent RG, Valois RF. Patterns of tobacco and alcohol use among sedentary, exercising, nonathletic, and athletic youth. J Sch Health 1996; 66:27–32.

63. Shields EW. Sociodemographic analysis of drug use among adolescent athletes: observations-perceptions of athletic directors-coaches. Adolescence 1995;30:839–861.

64. Escobedo LG, Marcus SE, Holtzman D, Giovino GA. Sports participation, age at smoking initiation, and the risk of smoking among US high school students. JAMA 1993;269:1391–1395.

65. Thorlindsson T, Vilhjalmsson R, Valgeirsson G. Sport participation and perceived health status: a study of adolescents. Soc Sci Med 1990;31:551–556.

66. Wechsler H, Davenport AE, Dowdall GW, et al. Binge drinking, tobacco, and illicit drug use and involvement in college athletics: a survey of students at 140 American colleges. J Am Coll Health 1997;45:195–200.

67. Faulkner RA, Slattery CM. The relationship of physical activity to alcohol consumption in youth 15–16 years of age. Can J Public Health 1990;81:168–169.

68. Botvin GJ, Baker E, Busenbury L, et al. Long-term follow-up results of a randomized drug abuse prevention trial in a white middle-class population. JAMA 1995; 273:1106–1112.

69. Botvin GJ, Schinke SP, Epstein JA, et al. Effectiveness of culturally-focused and generic skills training approaches to alcohol and drug abuse prevention among minority adolescents: two-year follow-up results. Psychol Addict Behav 1995;9:183–194.

70. Botvin GJ, Schinke SP, Epstein JA, Diaz T. Effectiveness of culturally-focused and generic skills training approaches to alcohol and drug abuse prevention among minority youths. Psychol Addict Behav 1994;8:116–127.

71. Botvin GJ, Busenbury L, Baker E, et al. Smoking prevention among urban minority youth: assessing effects of outcome and mediating variables. Health Psychol 1992; 11:290–299.

72. Sussman S, Dent CW, Stacy AW, et al. Developing school-based tobacco use prevention and cessation programs. Thousand Oaks, CA: Sage, 1995.

73. Sussman S, Dent CW, Stacy AW, et al. Project Towards No Tobacco Use: implementation, process and posttest knowledge evaluation. Health Educ Res 1993;8:109–123.

74. Dent CW, Sussman S, Stacy AW, et al. Two-year behavior outcomes of Project Towards No Tobacco Use. J Clin Consult Psychol 1995;63:676–677.

75. Turner GE, Burciaga C, Sussman S, et al. Which lesson components mediate refusal assertion skill improvement in school-based adolescent tobacco use prevention? Int J Addict 1993;28:749–766.

76. Donaldson SI, Sussman S, Mackinnon DP, et al. Drug abuse prevention programming: do we know what content works? Am Behav Scientist 1996;39:868–883.

77. Goldberg L, Elliott D, Clarke GN, et al. Effects of a multidimensional anabolic steroid prevention intervention: The Adolescent Training and Learning to Avoid Steroids (ATLAS) Program. JAMA 1996; 276:1555–1562.

78. Goldberg L, Elliott DL, Clark GN, et al. The Adolescents' Training and Learning to Avoid Steroids (ATLAS) prevention program. Arch Pediatr Adolesc Med 1996;150: 713–721.

79. Aguirre-Molina M, Garman DM. Community-based approaches for the prevention of alcohol, tobacco and other drug use. Ann Rev Public Health 1996;17:337–358.

80. Elster AB, Kuznets NJ, eds. AMA Guidelines for Adolescent Preventive Services (GAPS). Baltimore: Williams & Wilkins, 1994.

81. Committee on Substance Abuse, American Academy of Pediatrics. Role of the pediatrician in prevention and management of substance abuse. Pediatrics 1993;91:1010–1013.

82. Green M, ed. Bright futures: guidelines for health supervision of infants, children, and adolescents. Arlington, VA: National Center for Education in Maternal and Child Health, 1994.

83. Mayfield D, McLeod G, Hall P. The CAGE questionnaire: validation of a new alcoholism screening instrument. Am J Psychiatry 1974;131: 1121–1123.

84. Bush B, Shaw S, Cleary P, et al. Screening for alcohol abuse using the CAGE questionnaire. Am J Med 1987;82:231–235.

85. Riggs SR, Alario A. RAFFT questions. In: Project ADEPT Manual. Providence, RI: Brown University, 1987.

86. Rahdert ER, ed. The Adolescent Assessment/Referral System Manual. Rockville, MD: National

Institute on Drug Abuse, 1991. DHHS no. (ADM) 91–1735.

87. SAMHSA, CSAT. Screening and assessment of alcohol and other drug abusive adolescents. Rockville, MD: US Department of Health and Human Services, 1993:55–56. DHHS no. 93–2009.

88. McLanly MA, Del Boca F, Babor T. A validation of the problem-oriented screening instrument for teenagers (POSIT). J Ment Health 1994;3:363–376.

89. Knight JR, Goodman E, Pulerwitz T, DuRant RH. Reliability of the problem oriented screening instrument for teenagers (POSIT) in an adolescent medical clinic population. J Adolesc Health 1999 (in press).

90. Prochaska JO, DiClemente CC. Transtheoretical therapy: toward a more integrative model of change. Psychotherapy 1982;19:276–288.

91. Prochaska JO, DiClemente CC. Stages and processes of self-change of smoking: toward an integrative model of change. J Consult Psychol 1983;51:390–395.

92. Miller WR, Benefield RG, Tonigan JS. Enhancing motivation for change in problem drinking: a controlled comparison of two therapist styles. J Consult Psychol 1993;61:455–461.

93. Miller WR. Motivational interviewing with problem drinkers. Behav Psychol 1983;11:147–172.

94. Miller W, Rollnick S. Principles of motivational interviewing. In: Miller W, Rollnick S, eds. Motivational interviewing. New York: Guilford Press 1991:51–63.

95. Miller WR, Sanchez VC. Motivating young adults for treatment and lifestyle change. In: Howard G, ed. Issues in alcohol use and misuse by young adults. Notre Dame IN: Univ Notre Dame Press, 1999 (in press).

96. Werner MJ. Principles of brief intervention for adolescent alcohol, tobacco, and other drug use. Ped Clin North Am 42(2):335–349.

97. Knight JR. Adolescent substance use: screening, assessment, and intervention in medical office practice. Contemp Ped 1997;14:45–72.

98. Rollnick S, Heather N, Bell A. Negotiating behavior change in medical settings: the development of brief motivational interviewing. J Ment Health 1992;1:25–37.

99. Rollnick S, Bell A. Brief motivational interviewing for use by the nonspecialist. In: Miller W, Rollnick S, eds. Motivational interviewing. New York: Guilford Press, 1991:203–213.

Chapter 53

Prevention of Osteoporosis: A Pediatric Concern

Donald A. Bailey

Our understanding of bone mineral loss and skeletal fragility in older adults is limited by our lack of knowledge concerning the determinants of bone mineral acquisition during childhood and adolescence. Prevention of osteoporosis depends not only on reducing the rate of bone loss during adult life, but also on the maximization of bone mineral accrual during the growing years. One of the best predictors of bone mineral status in the elderly is the level of peak bone mass attained by the early adult years (1). In view of this, it has been suggested by a number of investigators that the failure to attain an optimum level of bone mineral during the years of growth is likely to be a significant contributing cause of dangerously low bone-mineral density and fracture risk in older populations (2,3).

While heredity is the prime determinant of peak bone mass, accounting for over 50% of the variance (4), lifestyle and dietary patterns are also involved in a multifactorial state that is a requisite for the maximization of bone mineral during the growing years. Specifically, vigorous weight-bearing physical activity and adequate calcium intake represent the best possibility for enhancing the attainment of an optimum level of bone mineral, within genetic limits.

BONE ADAPTATION PROCESSES

Skeletal tissue is in a constant state of flux throughout life. Changes in the shape, mass, and architecture of bone are controlled by three distinct processes: growth, modeling, and remodeling. During the lifespan, a single process may dominate at certain times, or the three processes may function concurrently at other times. In the immature skeleton all three processes may be active simultaneously, with each having a different function.

Growth is the expression of the genetically programmed, hormonally mediated, process of enlargement of the entire skeleton without regard to concurrent changes in shape that may be occurring regionally in response to local loading factors. In humans, skeletal growth is largely completed before the third decade of life.

Modeling is the process that alters the shape and mass of bones in response to mechanical loading factors. It represents a regional response to specific loading conditions, resulting in the addition of bone, without prior resorption, to surfaces where deformation through high strain is greatest. Since young bone has a greater potential than aging bone for adaptation to loading factors (5), the modeling process occurs primarily during growth and results in a net gain in bone over time. This may result in a reserve of bone beyond that needed for normal activity (6).

Remodeling, although present in young individuals, is the predominant process modifying bone shape and mass in adults. It allows for the replacement of fatigue-damaged bone with new bone. In addition to serving a preservation function, it provides a mechanism for the maintenance of calcium homeostasis. The remodeling cycle begins with an activation phase, followed in sequence by a resorption phase and a formation phase, which are coupled. As new bone never completely replaces the bone that has been resorbed, remodeling results in a net loss of bone over time. This is responsible for the decrease in bone mineral that accompanies old age.

It is important to note that while modeling and remodeling are essentially under the control of mechanical strain

578

levels, they have opposite effects in terms of bone mass. Low strains below a threshold level result in increased remodeling with subsequent loss of bone. Strains above a threshold level will be sufficient to maintain bone, thereby keeping remodeling in a steady state. High strains initiate a modeling response to add more bone to meet the higher strain condition.

BONE MINERAL ACQUISITION DURING THE GROWING YEARS

The establishment of an optimum level of bone mineral during the growing years, when modeling is superimposed on growth, is an important consideration in terms of lifelong skeletal integrity. To explore the possibility of optimizing bone mineral acquisition during the growing years and gain an understanding of modifiable factors that may promote skeletal health, it is first necessary to have an understanding of normal bone mineral accrual rates in growing children.

To investigate how bone mineral is laid down at clinically important sites during the adolescent years, data from an initial sample of 228 children measured annually by dual-energy x-ray absorptiometry (DXA) over a 6-year period were analyzed (7). To address maturational differences between boys and girls of the same chronologic age, bone mineral content (BMC) values were determined at points 2 years on either side of the age of peak height velocity (PHV), which was used as a benchmark of maturity. The results of this study indicate that in the 4 years surrounding PHV, 35% of total body and lumbar spine BMC is laid down, and 27% of femoral neck BMC is accumulated. These values are in agreement with a study by Slemenda et al (8), who reported a 29% increase in BMC at the lumbar spine in the 3 years around the onset of puberty. The clinical significance of these findings can be appreciated by considering the fact that as much bone mineral will be laid down during the 4 adolescent years surrounding PHV as many people will lose during their entire adult life.

Another issue of clinical significance has to do with the observation that during adolescence there is a dissociation between linear growth and bone mineral accrual (9). For all bone sites in both boys and girls, peak velocity in BMC occurs up to one year after PHV. This suggests a transient period of relative bone weakness following the adolescent growth spurt, resulting in a temporary increase in fracture risk. The relationship between fracture incidence in children and the timing of the adolescent growth spurt has been well documented, with fracture rates increasing dramatically during the circumpubertal years (10–12). This research further emphasizes the importance of studying the dynamics of bone mineral changes during the years of growth.

The observation that adolescence is a critical time for bone mineral accumulation should not be surprising. By the time growth ceases, the skeleton should be as strong as it will ever need to be (13). Gains in bone mineral after growth has ceased are probably minimal (8). Since 50% of the variability in bone mass in the very old can be accounted for by peak skeletal mass attained during the growing years (1), it is not unreasonable to assume that fracture risk in the elderly may have childhood antecedents (14). Clearly, more information is needed regarding the precise relationship between modifiable

lifestyle factors like physical activity and nutritional intake and bone mineral accumulation during the growing years.

PHYSICAL ACTIVITY AND BONE MINERAL ACQUISITION

The potential of weight-bearing physical activity to positively influence bone mineral acquisition in children and adolescents is a subject of increasing interest. Although there are still gaps in our understanding of the precise role played by physical activity in bone mineral accumulation during growth, there have been a number of investigators who have studied this topic. The results of one such study suggest that children who are more active physically may emerge from adolescence with a 5% to 10% greater bone mass and density than their less active peers (15).

A recent review up through 1994 has summarized the results of 39 studies of children and adolescents dealing with the topic of exercise and bone mineral status (9). As a result of this review, the authors concluded that more carefully controlled prospective studies were needed to confirm the degree of relationship between physical activity and bone mineral accretion but that the available evidence was strongly supportive, suggesting a significant and positive relationship.

Since the publication of this review, additional studies have provided further evidence as to the importance of physical activity during the growing years (16–20). But the strongest evidence comes from a recent prospective study on children (21) and from two recent preferred limb studies, one on adults who were active as children (22) and one on children exposed to altered loading patterns (23). Preferred limb studies provide a unique experimental model for studying the effect of mechanical loading on bone mineral acquisition. Because genetic, endocrine, and nutritional influences are shared by both limbs, any bilateral disparity in bone mineral accumulation can safely be attributed to differences in mechanical usage.

In a study of 105 elite young adult (aged 18 to 28) female tennis and squash players, the bilateral difference in bone mineral content between the playing and nonplaying arms was measured and compared to similar determinations on 50 healthy control subjects of similar age, height, and weight (22). The young adult athletes who began playing and training for their sport at or before menarche had bilateral differences in BMC of 17 to 24% compared to those who began training after menarche (8 to 14%). In the control group the difference in BMC between limbs was 4%. Clearly, the greater bone mineral in the playing arm can be attributed to the greater strain imposed on this limb by the sport. The starting age appears to be an important consideration, further emphasizing the greater adaptive response to loading of immature bone over mature bone (5).

In another preferred limb study, bone mineral density (BMD) was measured by DXA in regions of the involved and noninvolved proximal femur in 17 children (aged 7 to 14) with unilateral Legg Calve Perthes disease (23). Children with this condition have an altered weight-bearing pattern whereby there is increased mechanical loading on the noninvolved normal hip and reduced loading on the involved painful hip. Thus, these children provide a unique opportunity to study the impact of differential loading on bone mineral acquisition during the growing years while controlling for genetic and other factors. A significantly higher BMD was found for regions of the proximal femur on the noninvolved side over the involved side (4% to 15%), and regions on the noninvolved side were significantly greater than either chronologic or skeletal age-based norms. The results of this study provide further support for the concept than mechanical loading of the skeleton during the growing years is an important factor in bone mineral acquisition.

In one of the few prospective studies on young children, 38 girls (aged 9 to 10) were enrolled in an additional exercise program over and above their regular physical education classes (21). The extra classes of 30 minutes duration were held three times per week for 10 months and involved high impact-loading and strength-building exercises. At the end of the study period, gains in BMC were compared to a control group of 33 girls who had participated only in the regular physical education classes. Bone mineral content for the total body, proximal femur, and lumbar spine increased at a significantly greater rate in the exercise group compared with the controls (7% to 12% vs. 1.5% to 6%). These results suggest that high-impact exercise is beneficial in terms of bone mineral acquisition in children. More important, this study indicates that carefully planned exercise programs can be designed to fulfill the goal of increasing the bone mineral status in children as part of the school curriculum.

Studies that have investigated the response of growing bone in young animals have been reviewed by Forwood et al (5). As a result of this review, these investigators concluded that the animal studies provide incontrovertible evidence that growing bone has a greater capacity to add new bone to the skeleton in response to mechanical loading factors than mature bone. The consistency of the evidence suggests that the animal data have relevance for humans. Considered as a whole, the studies noted above and the animal and human review papers suggest that bone mineral in children can be enhanced by loading factors associated with physical activity.

CALCIUM AND BONE MINERAL ACQUISITION

In assessing the role of physical activity on bone, it is important to recognize that nutritional sufficiency in the form of adequate calcium is a necessary condition for skeletal health and an important enabling factor in terms of activity-related bone mineral maintenance in adults (24). In children, the exact relationship between physical activity, calcium intake, and bone accretion still needs to be studied. It is still unclear whether the bone mineral benefits derived from exercise can be influenced by calcium intakes. While calcium is clearly an essential nutrient for bone health, studies are needed to compare the combined effects of calcium and exercise on the skeleton.

During the adolescent growth spurt some youngsters may show an increase in BMC of over 500 g per year (26). This represents 161 g per year of calcium or 441 mg per day. To retain this amount of calcium would require an intake of 1200 to 1500 mg per day under normal levels of retention. These figures lead to the hypothesis that during phases of rapid growth, bone mineral accumulation may in fact be limited by low dietary intakes of calcium. This in turn has led to a concern that the achievement of an optimal level of bone mineral in adults may be compromised by low calcium intakes during the growing years.

Although there is still controversy concerning the amount of calcium needed to maximize bone mineral accumulation in children and adolescents, there have been a number of studies that have examined the relationship between childhood calcium intake and bone mineral status. These studies have been reviewed in two recent papers (27,28).

Results from cross-sectional studies of childhood calcium intake and bone mineral accumulation are equivocal. Positive associations have been reported at some sites in a number of studies (16,29,30); however, just as many studies report no association (31–34). These inconsistent results may be related to the concept of calcium as a threshold nutrient, whereby a relationship may exist at intakes below a threshold level but disappear at levels above the threshold (35). This hypothesis is supported by two Chinese studies in which mean calcium intakes were very low, in the 250 to 550 mg per day range, and a relationship between calcium intake and bone mineral accretion was observed (36,37). At higher intakes the relationship disappeared.

Retrospective recall studies of childhood nutritional intakes and bone mineral status as adults are more positive. Several studies have reported a relationship between childhood or adolescent milk intake and adult bone density (38–40). A further study compared teenage calcium intakes at ages 13 to 17 with BMD at the hip and forearm in women aged 30 to 39 (41). These investigators concluded that raising teenage dietary calcium intakes into the range of 800 to 1200 mg per day would be associated with a 6% increase in adult bone density at the hip. Another retrospective study reported a trend (although nonsignificant) towards higher bone density at the spine in a group of females with relatively high calcium intakes during the adolescent years compared to a low-intake group (42).

The results of supplementation studies with calcium or dairy products provide further evidence in support of calcium as an important factor in bone mineral accumulation during growth (43–50). The results of these studies are generally consistent. Increments in bone mineral at one or more skeletal sites were greater in supplemented children in comparison to their unsupplemented peers. No evidence of a dose-response relationship was apparent. In those studies in which subjects were followed for a period of time after direct calcium supplementation was withdrawn, the findings were less positive with the differences between groups no longer statistically significant at the end of the follow-up period. As it appears now, the modest gain in bone mass seen in children who are taking calcium or milk supplements is not retained when supplementation is withdrawn. However, when the supplementation is taken in the form of calcium-enriched foods, supplemented children appear to retain their advantage in terms of bone mineral after the follow-up period (49). More evidence is needed to evaluate the long-term sustainability of adolescent calcium supplementation. Nonetheless, given the fact that relatively small differences in bone mass are associated with large differences in fracture rates (51), the modest trends reported in these studies warrant further investigation.

Although the findings of the cross-sectional, retrospective, and supplementation studies are not clearcut as to the beneficial effects of high calcium intakes on bone mineral accumulation in growing children, our knowledge about rates of skeletal bone mineral accretion during growth can be used to generate some recommended calcium intake guidelines for this age group. Martin et al analyzed bone mineral accumulation data from DXA total body scans collected from 228 boys and girls (aged 9.5 to 19.5) measured annually over a four-year period (26). They reported a peak bone mineral accrual rate of 320 g per year in boys and 240 g per year in girls. Using a figure of 32.2% calcium in bone mineral as measured by DXA (25) and a calcium retention efficiency of 20.3% (52), these investigators calculated that a calcium intake of 1355 mg per day for boys and 1005 mg per day for girls would be needed to support adolescent skeletal growth. However, it is well known that estimating rates of change in variables during growth from cross-sectional data results in a flattening of peak values; this is due to intersubject variability reflecting wide differences in maturational status. Thus, the peak values reported in this study are likely to be underestimates for most children. Balancing this with the wide range of calcium absorption efficiency at this age (53), a recommendation of 1200 to 1300 mg per day of calcium during adolescence would seem reasonable. Many children have intakes well below these levels.

CHRONIC ENERGY DEFICITS AND BONE MINERAL ACQUISITION

The bone-promoting effects of mechanical loading and adequate nutrition are modulated by certain hormones. Of particular importance in adolescents are estrogen and testosterone. The protective effect of estrogen on bone has been well established in women; hypoestrogenic states such as menopause, oophorectomy, or prolonged amenorrhea are associated with rapid bone loss, and if the condition is chronic, this can lead to a dangerously low bone mineral density and an increased risk of fracture. Estrogen replacement therapy has been shown to reduce this loss of bone. This has important implications for exercise and nutritional counseling in adolescents. An inadequate energy intake (as in anorexia nervosa), a very high energy expenditure from prolonged intense training, or a combination of the two can lead to a chronic energy deficit. This in turn is associated with disturbances of the normal menstrual cycle. In some cases, this leads to amenorrhea and markedly reduced estrogen levels (54).

It is well established that anorexia nervosa, for which amenorrhea is one of the essential diagnostic criteria, is associated with reduced levels of bone mineral density (55). Further to this, many reports document irregular or absent menses and reduced bone density in girls who train intensely for sports requiring leanness for elite performance. Estimates as to the extent of menstrual dysfunction in elite athletic women range from 2% to 51%, depending on the activity in which they are engaged, as compared to 2% to 5% in nonathletes (56).

Regardless of its origin, prolonged amenorrhea in young females presents a serious potential hazard to the skele-

ton. No study has demonstrated the complete reversibility of bone loss due to anorexia. For example, one study found that values for bone mineral density at four skeletal sites were 56% to 82% below normal in recovered anorectics two years after the resumption of normal menses and the restoration of normal weight (57). To offset the decreased exposure to estrogen it has been suggested that the skeleton must experience greater loads if bone mineral is to be maintained (58). A study on elite gymnasts provides some support for this proposition (59). Although the gymnasts in this study reported a higher incidence of menstrual dysfunction than runners, they had higher bone mineral density values, However, until more studies are completed the preponderance of evidence suggests that the bone-promoting effects of exercise may not be sufficient to compensate for the loss induced by low estrogen unless the magnitude of the loading is very large.

The effect of inadequate energy intakes or prolonged intense training on hormonal status in boys has not been thoroughly investigated, but delayed puberty has been shown to result in reduced bone mineral density values in young adult men. This suggests that the late exposure to increasing testosterone levels has a detrimental effect on bone mineral acquisition in men (60). The effects of exercise on hormonal status in young boys has not been investigated, but a study carried out on young men suggests that serum testosterone may be chronically reduced by intense exercise (61). If this effect is confirmed in adolescents, it is probable that boys face the same skeletal risk as girls in the presence of an endocrine imbalance induced by a chronic energy deficit.

RECOMMENDATIONS

There are still many questions remaining about the complicated mechanisms controlling bone mineral accretion during the growing years and bone mineral loss in the declining years. Longitudinal studies are needed to assess whether the beneficial effects of activity during growth are maintained into later years irrespective of adult activity levels. We need to know more about the threshold levels of physical activity and calcium intake required to elicit a significant bone mineral response. And, from a public health perspective, perhaps the greatest questions have to do with the development of strategies directed at relating a condition of the elderly to a largely disinterested teenage population that will not be at risk for 40 or 50 years.

While there are still more questions than answers, studies of osteoporosis that address not only age-related bone loss but also bone gain during the growing years are clearly needed. The ultimate target population for the prevention of osteoporosis may be the young and not the elderly (62). Taking into account the fact that our knowledge of the complicated mechanisms controlling bone mineral status is still incomplete, on the basis of what we do know it is possible to offer some sound and prudent lifestyle advice to young people.

With regard to exercise programs designed for skeletal health and bone acquisition in the young, the following fundamentals should be kept in mind: a) exercise programs do not elicit benefits that can be generalized to the whole skeleton; b) the skeletal response to exercise is greatest at the site of maximum stress; and c) to cause an adaptive response, the training stimulus must be greater than that habitually encountered. On the basis of these fundamentals and the review of the pertinent literature, the following recommendations can safely be offered to the public at large.

1. An individual should make a lifelong commitment to physical activity at an early age. Growing bones respond to weight-bearing activity by the addition of new bone. The ability to adapt to increases in mechanical loading is much greater in the growing skeleton than in the mature skeleton.

2. Weight-bearing activities that provide impact loading like gymnastics, skipping, aerobics, squash, and basketball are better for the skeleton than weight-supported activities such as swimming or cycling.

3. A variety of vigorous daily activities of short duration that provide a versatile strain distribution throughout the entire skeleton is better for bone health than a prolonged repetitive activity.

4. Activities should be diverse to ensure a varied strain distribution on bone, they should be vigorous enough to ensure impact loading with high strain rates, and they should be progressive in nature.

5. Activities than increase muscle strength and work all large muscle groups should be encouraged as these can be osteogenic; however, static loads applied continuously are not in and of themselves osteogenic.

6. As much as possible, periods of immobility and immobilization should be avoided; when this is not possible because of sickness or injury, even brief periods of daily weight-bearing movements can help to conserve bone mineral.

The responsiveness of the growing skeleton to physical activity is dependent on the sensitivity of bone to circulating hormone levels and nutritional adequacy. This has important implications for exercise prescription in adolescents, which leads to a number of other important recommendations.

1. Children should have a diet of nutritious foods that will meet the recommended dietary intake for calcium, provide adequate but not excessive protein, and limit the intake of sodium and caffeinated beverages (soft drinks, coffee).

2. In girls, abnormal delay of menarche and menstrual dysfunction associated with a chronic energy deficit represents a potential skeletal hazard in terms of bone mineral acquisition and maintenance. A well-balanced diet that is sufficient to meet the energy demands of growth and physical activity should be encouraged. This will facilitate the onset and maintenance of a normal menstrual cycle.

3. Disordered eating habits are destructive to the skeleton at any age; when this occurs during the growing years there may be a permanent deficit in bone mineral status throughout life.

4. Cigarettes should be avoided; they are anti-estrogenic and may interfere with the attainment of an optimum level of bone mineral following skeletal maturation.

REFERENCES

1. Hui SL, Johnston CC, Mazess, RB. Bone mass in normal children and young adults. Growth 1985;49: 34–43.

2. Ott S. Bone density in adolescents. N Engl J Med 1991;325: 1646–1647.

3. Seeman E, Young N, Szmukler G, et al. Risk factors for osteoporosis. Osteoporos Int 1993;3(suppl):40–43.

4. Krall E, Dawson-Hughes B. Heritable and lifestyle determinants of bone mineral density. J Bone Miner Res 1993;8:1–9.

5. Forwood M, Burr D. Physical activity and bone mass: exercise in futility? Bone Miner 1993;21:89–112.

6. Frost H. Mechanical usage, bone mass, bone fragility: a brief overview. In: Kleerekoper M, Krane S, eds. Clinical disorders of bone and mineral metabolism. New York: Mary Ann Liebert, 1989:15–40.

7. Bailey DA. The Saskatchewan pediatric bone mineral accrual study: bone mineral acquisition during the growing years. Int J Sports Med 1997;18(suppl): 191–194.

8. Slemenda CW, Reister TK, Hui SL, et al. Influences on skeletal mineralization in children and adolescents: evidence for varying effects of sexual maturation and physical activity. J Pediatr 1994;125:201–207.

9. Bailey DA, Faulkner RA, McKay HA. Growth, physical activity and bone mineral acquisition. In: Holloszy JO, ed. Exercise and sport sciences review, vol. 24. Baltimore: Williams & Wilkins, 1996; 122–166.

10. Alffram PA, Bauer GCH. Epidemiology of fractures of the forearm. J Bone Joint Surg Am 1962;44: 105–114.

11. Bailey DA, Wedge JH, McCulloch RG, et al. Epidemiology of fractures of the distal end of the radius in children as associated with growth. J Bone Joint Surg Am 1989;71:1225–1231.

12. Blimkie CJR, Levevre J, Beunen GP, et al. Fractures, physical activity, and growth velocity in adolescent Belgian boys. Med Sci Sports Exerc 1993;25:801–808.

13. Parfitt AM. The two faces of growth: benefits and risks to bone integrity. Osteoporos Int 1994;4:-382–398.

14. Bailey DA, McCulloch RG. Osteoporosis: are there childhood antecedents for an adult health

problem? Can J Pediatr 1992;5: 130–134.

15. Slemenda CW, Miller JZ, Hui SL, et al. Role of physical activity in the development of skeletal mass in children. J Bone Miner Res 1991;6:1227–1233.

16. Ruiz JC, Mandel C, Garabedian M. Influence of spontaneous calcium intake and physical exercise on the vertebral and femoral bone mineral density of children and adolescents. J Bone Miner Res 1995;5:675–682.

17. Gunnes M, Lehman E. Physical activity and dietary constituents as predictors of forearm cortical and trabecular bone gain in healthy children and adolescents: a prospective study. Acta Paediatr 1996;85:19–25.

18. Cassell C, Benedict M, Specker B. Bone mineral density in elite 7- to 9-year-old female gymnasts and swimmers. Med Sci Sports Exerc 1996;28:1243–1246.

19. Boot AM, de Ridder MAJ, Pols HAP, et al. Bone mineral density in children and adolescents: relation to puberty, calcium intake and physical activity. J Clin Endocrinol Metab 1997;82:57–62.

20. Dyson K, Blimkie CJR, Davison KS, et al. Gymnastics training and bone density in pre-adolescent females. Med Sci Sports Exerc 1997;29:443–450.

21. Morris F, Naughton G, Gibbs J, et al. Prospective 10-month exercise intervention in pre-menarcheal girls: positive effects on bone and lean mass. J Bone Miner Res 1997;12:1453–1462.

22. Kannus P, Haapasalo H, Sankelo M, et al. Effect of starting age of physical activity on bone mass in the dominant arm of tennis and squash players. Ann Intern Med 1995;123:27–31.

23. Bailey DA, Faulkner RA, Kimber K, et al. Altered loading patterns and femoral bone mineral density in children with unilateral Legg-Calvé-Perthes disease. Med Sci Sports Exerc 1997;29:1395–1399.

24. Specker B. Evidence for an interaction between calcium intake and physical activity on changes in bone mineral density. J Bone Miner Res 1996;11:1539–1544.

25. Ellis KJ, Shypailo RJ, Hergenroeder A, et al. Total body calcium and bone mineral content: comparison of dual-energy X-ray absorptiometry with neutron activation analysis. J Bone Miner Res 1996;11:843–848.

26. Martin AD, Bailey D, McKay HA, Whiting S. Bone mineral and calcium accretion during puberty. Am J Clin Nutr 1997;66:611–615.

27. Blimkie CJ, Chilibeck PD, Davison KS. Bone mineralization patterns: reproductive endocrine, calcium, and physical activity influences during the life span. In: Bar-Or O, Lamb D, Clarkson P, eds. Perspectives in exercise sciences and sports medicine; vol. 3: exercise and the female—a lifespan approach. Carmel, IN: Cooper, 1996;73–141.

28. Barr SI, McKay HA. Nutrition, exercise and bone status in youth. Int J Sport Nutr 1998;8:124–142.

29. Chan GM. Dietary calcium and bone mineral status of children and adolescents. Am J Dis Child 1991;145:631–634.

30. Sentipal JM, Wardlaw GM, Magan J, Matkovic V. Influence of calcium intake and growth indexes on vertebral bone mineral density in young females. Am J Clin Nutr 1991;54:425–428.

31. Grimston SK, Morrison K, Harder JA, Hanley DA. Bone mineral density during puberty in Western Canadian children. Bone Miner 1992;19:85–96.

32. Katzman DK, Bachrach LK, Carter DR, Marcus R. Clinical and anthropometric correlates of bone mineral acquisition in healthy adolescent girls. J Clin Endocrinol Metab 1991;73:1332–1339.

33. Kroger H, Kotaniemi A, Vainio P, Alhava E. Bone densitometry of the spine and femur in children by dual-energy x-ray absorptiometry. Bone Miner 1992;17:75–85.

34. Kroger H, Kotaniemi A, Kroger L, Alhava E. Development of bone mass and bone density of the spine and femoral neck—a prospective study of 65 children and adolescents. Bone Miner 1993;23:171–182.

35. Matkovic V, Heaney RP. Calcium balance during human growth: evidence for threshold behavior. Am J Clin Nutr 1992;55:992–996.

36. Lee WTK, Leung SSF, Lui SSH, Lau J. Relationship between long term calcium intake and bone mineral content of children aged from birth to 5 years. Br J Nutr 1993;70:235–248.

37. Lee WTK, Leung SSF, Ng MY, et al. Bone mineral content of two populations of Chinese children with different calcium intake. Bone Miner 1993;23:195–206.

38. Sandler RB, Slemenda CW, La Porte RE, et al. Postmenopausal bone density and milk consumption in childhood and adolescence. Am J Clin Nutr 1985;42:270–274.

39. Murphy S, Khaw K-T, May H, Compston JE. Milk consumption and bone mineral density in middle aged and elderly women. Br Med J 1994;308:939–941.

40. Matkovic V, Jelic T, Wardlaw GM, et al. Timing of peak bone mass in caucasian females and its implication for the prevention of osteoporosis. J Clin Invest 1994;93:799–808.

41. Nieves JW, Golden AL, Siris E, et al. Teenage and current calcium intake are related to bone mineral density of the hip and forearm in women aged 30–39 years. Am J Epidemiol 1995;141:342–351.

42. Welten DC, Kemper HCG, Post GB, et al. Weight-bearing activity during youth is a more important factor for peak bone mass than calcium intake. J Bone Miner Res 1994;9:1089–1096.

43. Johnston CC, Miller JZ, Slemenda CW, et al. Calcium supplementation and increases in bone mineral density in children. N Engl J Med 1992;327:82–87.

44. Lloyd T, Andon MB, Rollings N, et al. Calcium supplementation and bone mineral density in adolescent girls. JAMA 1993;270:841–844.

45. Andon MB, Lloyd T, Matkovic V. Supplementation trials with calcium citrate malate: evidence in favor of increasing the calcium RDA during childhood and adolescence. J Nutr 1994;124(suppl): 1412S–1417S.

46. Lee WTK, Leung SSF, Wang SH, et al. Double-blind, controlled calcium supplementation and bone mineral accretion in children accustomed to a low-calcium diet. Am J Clin Nutr 1994;60:744–750.

47. Lee WTK, Leung SSF, Leung DMY, et al. A randomized double-blind controlled calcium supplementation trial, and bone and height acquisition in children. Br J Nutr 1995;74:125–139.

48. Chan GM, Hoffman K, McMurry M. Effects of dairy products on bone and body composition in pubertal girls. J Pediatr 1995;126:551–556.

49. Bonjour JP, Carrie A, Ferrari S, et al. Calcium enriched foods and bone mass growth in prepubertal girls: a randomized, double-blind, placebo-controlled trial. J Clin Invest 1997;99:1287–1294.

50. Howson CA, Green R, Hopper J, et al. A co-twin study of the effect of calcium supplementation on bone density during adolescence. Osteoporosis Int 1997;7:219–225.

51. Matkovic V, Kostial K, Simonovic I, et al. Bone status and fracture rates in two regions of Yugoslavia. Am J Clin Nutr 1979;32:540–549.

52. Weaver CM, Martin BR, Plawecki KL, et al. Differences in calcium metabolism between adolescent and adult females. Am J Clin Nutr 1995;61:577–581.

53. O'Brien KA, Abrams S, Liang L, et al. Increased efficiency of calcium absorption during short periods of inadequate calcium intake in girls. Am J Clin Nutr 1996;63:579–583.

54. Yeager K, Agostini R, Nattiv A, Drinkwater B. The female athlete triad: disordered eating, amenorrhea, osteoporosis. Med Sci Sports Exerc 1993;25:775–777.

55. Bachrach LK, Guido D, Katzman DK, et al. Decreased bone density in adolescent girls with anorexia nervosa. Pediatrics 1990;86:440–447.

56. Snow-Harter CM. Bone health and prevention of osteoporosis in active and athletic women. The Athletic Woman 1994;13:389–404.

57. Bachrach LK, Katzman DK, Litt IF. Recovery from osteopenia in adolescent girls with anorexia nervosa. J Clin Endocrinol Metab 1991;72: 602–606.

58. Lanyon LE. Using functional loading to influence bone mass and architecture: objectives, mechanisms and relationship with estrogen of the mechanically adaptive process in bone. Bone 1996; 18(suppl):37S–43S.

59. Robinson TL, Snow-Harter C, Taafee DR, et al. Gymnasts exhibit higher bone mass than runners despite similar prevalence of amenorrhea and oligomenorrhea. J Bone Miner Res 1995;10: 26–35.

60. Finkelstein JS, Neer RM, Biller BMK, et al. Osteopenia in men with a history of delayed puberty. N Engl J Med 325:600–604, 1992.

61. Arce JC, De Souza MJ. Exercise and male infertility. Sports Med 1993;15(3):146–169.

62. Chesnut C. Theoretical overview: bone development, peak bone mass, bone loss, and fracture risk. Am J Med 1991;91(suppl):2S–4S.

Chapter 54

Evaluation and Management of Children with Elevated Cholesterol

Christine L. Williams

The rationale for primary prevention of cardiovascular disease (CVD) in childhood is based on the high prevalence of the disease among adults in most developed countries, its early insidious onset, pathologic evidence that atherosclerosis begins in childhood, and the knowledge that many of the risk factors are lifestyle related and thus potentially preventable.

Elevated cardiovascular risk should be preventable through population-based programs, such as school health curricula, that teach changes in risk-related behavior including nutrition, physical activity, and cigarette smoking. Pediatric population-based interventions have the greatest potential for reducing overall CVD morbidity and mortality. If carried from childhood into adulthood, small decreases in mean serum cholesterol, mean systolic and diastolic blood pressure, and a reduced prevalence of cigarette smoking could significantly reduce CVD mortality.

Approaches to the individual patient at high risk, such as those practiced in the physician's office or clinic, will complement the population approach and are necessary to provide treatment for children with moderately severe to severe elevations in risk factors. In addition, physicians may incorporate general counseling in risk reduction into routine child health assessment as part of population-based prevention.

The following material describes an approach to the evaluation and management of hypercholesterolemia in childhood, within the context of the usual pediatric and family practice clinical office setting.

ATHEROSCLEROSIS IN CHILDHOOD

In the past two decades, it has increasingly been recognized that traditional risk factors for coronary heart disease can be easily identified in childhood, and that they are largely the result of lifestyle habits (cigarette smoking, poor eating habits, and lack of regular physical activity) acquired early in life (1–6). This recognition has stimulated clinical initiatives in pediatric preventive cardiology practice (7–10).

Evidence that the pathologic process of atherosclerosis begins in childhood is also strong. Early support for this view came from autopsy studies of children killed accidentally and of young combat casualties. During the Korean conflict, an autopsy study of 300 soldiers (mean age 22) revealed that 77% of these young men had evidence of coronary atherosclerosis. Fifteen percent had more than 50% stenosis of one or more coronary vessels (11). Similarly, during the Vietnamese conflict, a study of 105 combat casualties (mean age 19) showed that 44% had evidence of coronary atherosclerosis. Remarkably, 1 in 20 of these young soldiers had severe lesions (12). These data suggest that lesions present to such an extensive degree in young men must have been progressing silently throughout childhood.

Additional evidence of childhood onset of atherosclerosis came from the classic studies of Holman et al in New Orleans published in 1958 (13). This group systematically studied aortas from 526 autopsies of children and young adults between the ages of 1 and 40. Fatty streaks were demonstrated in the aortas of all children over the age of 3. Percentage of intimal surface covered with fatty streaks increased slowly through the first decade of life, and then more rapidly during adolescence (occurring sooner in blacks than whites). Fibrous plaques in the aorta began to appear during adolescence, but only increased significantly in the fourth decade of life. Overall there was about a 15-year lag between the development of fatty streaks and fibrous plaques, and in this case whites had a greater extent of intimal involvement than blacks.

Strong et al studied both coronary and aortic lesions in 4737 children and young adults (aged 10 to 39), a subset of the International Atherosclerosis Project sample (14,15). Again almost all aortas had evidence of fatty streak involvement. Coronary fatty streaks were not as frequent, but were detected even in some of the 10- to 15-year-old children. Coronary fibrous plaques were rare before age 20, but increased rapidly between the ages of 20 and 40, more so in men than in women.

Stary studied the left coronary arteries of 422 individuals who died between full-term birth and age 29 (16). He described four types of intimal lesions. The last three types (fatty streaks, pre-atheromas, and atheromas) began during the second decade of life, similar to results of other studies.

The Bogalusa Heart Study recently reported on autopsy specimens from 110 children and young adults, 40% of whom had participated in a study of cardiovascular risk factors in childhood. In a report of 35 subjects (mean age 17.9) with previously measured risk factor levels, these investigators found that aortic fatty streaks covered between 1% and 61% of the intimal surface. Coronary fatty streaks were found in almost all cases but covered only about 1% of the intimal surface (maximal 6.2%). More advanced fibrous plaques were found in six subjects (all male) (17).

Since all of these subjects had previous measurements of coronary risk factors, correlations between the degree of intimal surface coverage and level of risk factors could be determined. Aortic fatty streaks were highly correlated with serum total cholesterol and serum low-density lipoprotein cholesterol (LDL-C) ($r = 0.67$; $P < 0.001$). Coronary fatty streaks as well as fibrous plaques were significantly correlated with very low-density lipoprotein cholesterol (VLDL-C). There was also a general positive association with all of the traditional risk factors (total and LDL-C, triglycerides, systolic and diastolic blood pressure, and ponderal index) as well as a negative association with high-density lipoprotein cholesterol (HDL-C) (17).

CARDIOVASCULAR DISEASE RISK FACTORS IN CHILDREN

Foremost among modifiable risk factors for atherosclerotic cardiovascular disease (CVD) are increased levels of plasma cholesterol, hypertension, and cigarette smoking. These, as well as other contributing factors such as obesity, inactivity, stress, and a family history of premature CVD, hypertension, or dyslipidemia, have been studied in populations of adults and children in the United States and abroad.

Most of the information on CVD risk factor prevalence had been obtained on adult populations. More recently, efforts have been made to extend these observations to children. In the past two decades a great deal has been published on the distribution of CVD risk factors in several populations of children (18–24). In the United States, the New York Know Your Body Study (19,22), the Bogalusa Heart Study (20), the Muscatine Study (21–23), the Cincinnati Lipid Research Clinic Study (24), and others have provided information on thousands of children. Numerous other studies have investigated similar risk factors in other countries (25–31).

Estimates of prevalence of CVD risk factors in pediatric populations vary according to the age, sex, and ethnicity of the children studied. In addition, they vary according to the choice of "at risk" cutoff points for clinical indices such as blood pressure and cholesterol. For example, when total cholesterol levels above 175 mg/dL are considered to be an elevated risk factor, far more children are classified at risk than if a level of 200 mg/dL is utilized. Studies using "adult" cutoff points for high risk therefore have tended to underestimate the magnitude of risk status in children.

In New York, a survey of 3000 children aged 11 to 14 found that 36% had one or more coronary risk factors exclusive of family history (22). The most common risk factors observed in this junior high school population were elevated serum cholesterol (18% were above 180 mg/dL), obesity (16% were more than 20% above ideal weight for height), and cigarette smoking (8% were regular smokers). In a similar study of 95 first-grade students in two New York schools (mean age 6), 21% had one or more risk factors identified. In this age group again, elevated serum cholesterol was common (22% above 180 mg/dL). Obesity was much less prevalent among the 6-year-olds (only 2% were more than 20% above ideal weight for height) (32).

In Wisconsin a survey of 9- to 12-year-old boys found 46% with at least one risk factor for CVD, and 14% with two or more risk factors (33).

Cardiovascular risk factors among children under age 10 will primarily be those of hypercholesterolemia and obesity. Among older children and adolescents these will still be most prevalent, but in addition cigarette smoking and hypertension become more common.

Lipids

Epidemiologic studies have established that elevated levels of serum total and LDL-C (as well as decreased HDL-C) accelerate atherosclerosis and increase the incidence of coronary heart disease. Lipids are essential structural components of animal cells. In addition, they are involved, among other things, in energy metabolism, production of hormones, and development of the myelin sheath around nerves. The liver synthesizes cholesterol itself, so that at any given time about two-thirds of the cholesterol in plasma has been synthesized by the liver and the other third has been contributed by exogenous dietary sources (34). The liver appears capable of synthesizing all of the cholesterol required for body structure and metabolism. Excess plasma LDL-C (resulting either from dietary saturated fat and cholesterol overload, or from genetic abnormalities in cholesterol receptors on cells) contributes to atheromatous buildup in arteries (35–37). In addition, studies have now shown that reduction of plasma LDL-C results in a reduction of mortality and morbidity from CVD, as well as regression of atherosclerotic plaque size (38).

During the past two decades, a large body of literature has emerged describing the distribution of lipid levels in children and adolescents. In adults, risk of CVD rises sharply at total cholesterol levels above 240 mg/dL (approximately the upper quartile of the adult population). The National Institutes of Health Consensus Committee has determined that adult total cholesterol levels between 200 and 239 mg/dL should be considered "borderline high risk" and levels at or above 240 mg/dL should be considered "high risk" (39).

In children in the United States, the upper quartile of total cholesterol levels is generally about 170 mg/dL for 2- to

Table 54-1 Selected Lipid and Lipoprotein Concentrations in Children and Adolescents (mg/dL)

Age	Total Cholesterol Mean	Total Cholesterol 95th%	HDL-C 5th%	HDL-C Mean	HDL-C 95th%	LDL-C Mean	LDL-C 95th%	Triglycerides Mean	Triglycerides 95th%
5–9 yr									
Male	160	203	38	56	75	93	129	56	101
Female	164	205	36	53	73	100	140	60	105
10–14 yr									
Male	158	202	37	55	74	97	133	66	125
Female	160	201	37	52	70	97	136	75	131
15–19 yr									
Male	150	197	30	46	63	94	130	78	148
Female	158	203	35	52	74	96	137	75	132

Adapted from Lipid Research Clinics Program. Population studies data book, vol. I: the prevalance study. Washington, DC: Department of Health and Human Services, 1980. DHHS pub. no. (NIH) 80-1527.

11-year-old children, varying somewhat by age, sex, and race (40–43) (Table 54-1). About 25% to 40% of children in various surveys have total cholesterol levels about 170 mg/dL and between 5% to 15% of children over the age of 2 have total cholesterol levels above 200 mg/dL (a level considered elevated even for adults) (8). The need to reduce cholesterol levels in these children is generally agreed upon, unless the elevation is due to high levels of protective HDL-C, and the LDL-C levels are normal.

Total cholesterol levels are about 70 mg/dL at birth (more than half as HDL-C). Levels increase dramatically by 1 month of age, and are essentially similar to those of 2- to 11-year-olds when table foods are introduced. From age 2 to 11, cholesterol levels are relatively stable, followed by a small dip during puberty (more so in white males). During late adolescence, boys assume more of an adult male lipid pattern with elevated LDL-C and decreased HDL-C. The increasing estrogen levels in maturing girls, on the other hand, helps them maintain their more favorable lipid profile with higher protective HDL-C levels and thus a lower overall risk profile (8,44).

There are many factors that influence cholesterol and lipoprotein levels in childhood including diet, inactivity, obesity, medications, cigarette smoking, inherited conditions, and specific diseases. The majority of children with hypercholesterolemia due to elevated LDL-C are those with both environmental (dietary excess, inactivity, overweight) and genetic components. It is also important to identify the smaller number of children with specific genetic dyslipoproteinemias, such as familial hypercholesterolemia (FH), which occurs in the heterozygous form in about 1 in 200 children (45,46) (Table 54-2). Secondary causes of elevated lipids such as liver, kidney, and thyroid disorders must also be ruled out.

Diet, Obesity, and Lipids

Although obesity does not appear to be as strong an independent risk factor for CVD as hyperlipidemia, its relationship to the development of hypertension and hyperlipidemia, as well as to the development of insulin resistance, make it an impor-

tant variable in the evaluation of CVD risk status as well as in risk-reduction programs.

Environmental causes of obesity including overnutrition and inactivity are important, and these environmental conditions are often shared in family groups (47–49). Overconsumption of energy forces fat cells to enlarge and sometimes to proliferate. Some studies have even shown that highly saturated fat diets increase both size and number of fat cells, whereas diets high in unsaturated fat increase only the size of the fat cells (50).

Inactivity appears to be a major contributor to obesity in children (51). Rose et al reported that large, placid babies actually ate fewer calories than a smaller more active control group of infants (52).

Obesity is common among adults, with studies suggesting that 20% to 30% of US adults are moderately obese, and 3% to 10% are markedly obese (53). Estimates of prevalence among children are also high, with increasing frequency during adolescence. In a study of 3000 junior high school students aged 11 to 14, 16% weighed 120% or more than the mean weight for their height (22). Prevalence of obesity in any population necessarily varies according to the definition of excess body weight or body fatness.

Studies indicate that the prevalence of obesity in US children has been increasing. In the Bogalusa Heart Study, the proportion of 6- to 11-year-olds who were obese increased by more than 50% in the 12 years between 1972 and 1984 (54). More recent comparisons of child and adolescent obesity prevalence in 1976–80 (NHANES II national survey) and subsequently in 1981–91 (NHANES III, Phase 1) show significant increases in obesity among males and females of all groups, even preschool children (55–58).

Obesity in childhood is associated with a higher prevalence of hyperlipidemia, as well as both systolic and diastolic hypertension (59). Because of this association, serious consideration should be given to the possibility that prevention of obesity in childhood could significantly reduce hypertension and cardiovascular disease among adults. Among pediatric studies, the Muscatine study reported on 4000 school-age chil-

Table 54-2 The Genetic Hyperlipidemias

Name	DLP type and Lipid levels	Genetic Mechanism	Comments
Familial hypercholesterolemia (FH)	IIa LDL high CHOL high TRIG normal Clear serum	Autosomal dominant	High risk of early CHD Tendinous xanthomas common Xanthelasma common 0.1–0.5% population frequency 3–6% among MI < 60 population LDL receptor defect Homozygotes/CHD adolescents
Genetic hypercholesterolemia	IIa (IIb) LDL high CHOL high TRIG normal Clear serum	Polygenic	Increased risk of early CHD Rare xanthomas 5% population frequency Increased freq. among MI < 60
Familial combined hyperlipidemia	IIa, IIb, IV rarely V CHOL high TRIG high VLDL high Turbid serum	Autosomal dominant	Increased risk of early CHD Rare xanthomas 1–5% population frequency 11–20% freq. among MI < 60 pop. 1/3rd 1 CHOL; 1/3rd 1 TRIG 1/3rd have high CHOL and TRIG Multiple patterns in 1 family VLDL overproduced in liver
Familial hypertriglyceridemia	IV (V) VLDL high CHOL normal TRIG high	Autosomal dominant	Slight increased risk CHD No xanthomas 1% population frequency 5% frequency among MI < 60 Probably heterogeneous
Broad beta disease (remnant hyperlipidemia)	III IDL CHOL high TRIG high Turbid serum +/–creamy layer	Autosomal recessive	Marked increase early CHD Frequent tuberous xanthomas on palmar creases Rare disease 1% frequency among MI < 60 Peripheral vascular disease Test isolated VLDL
Familial LPL deficiency	I Chylomicrons CHOL sl TRIG very high Cream on serum Clear below	Autosomal recessive	No increase in risk of CHD Eruptive xanthomas common Very rare disease No increase among MI < 60 Disease onset by 2nd decade Abdominal pain/pancreatitis Lipoprotein lipase deficient
Familial type 5 disease	V VLDL CHOL nl/sl high TRIG "sky high" Cream on serum Cloudy below	Autosomal dominant	Variable increase CHD risk Often secondary to disease (diabetes, obesity, ethanol) May be primary genetic disease Adult onset usual Abdominal pain/pancreatitis

dren. They found that of those children with body weight in the upper decile, almost 30% had systolic and diastolic blood pressures above the 90% percentile (21).

Higher mean cholesterol levels are also common among obese children and adolescents. In addition, there is some data to suggest that elevated cholesterol levels in overweight children tend to remain elevated, that is track better, than in children whose weight for height remains lower (60–64).

Diet and Lipids

Many children in the United States consume a diet that falls far short of meeting dietary guidelines recommended by the American Heart Association, and reinforced recently by the National Cholesterol Education Panel, Expert Panel on Cholesterol in Children and Adolescents (65,66).

Information on usual dietary intake of children comes from a variety of sources. The largest national dietary intake database on US children was developed from the National Health and Nutrition Examination Surveys, conducted between 1971 and 1994 (NHANES I,II,III) (67–70). Recent national survey data show that children consume about one-third of their daily calories as snacks, about a half from lunch and dinner, and about one-fifth from breakfast.

Most US children have an excessive intake of high-fat

Table 54-3 NCEP Step I Diet as Compared to Typical Dietary Intake of US Children

Nutrient	NHANES III 1988–91 (% OF TOTAL KCAL)	NCEP STEP I DIET FOR CHILDREN (% OF TOTAL KCAL)
Fat	33–34	30
Saturated	12	— <10
Polyunsaturated	6	— up to 10
Monounsaturated	12	— remaining
Protein	14	15–20
Carbohydrate	50–55	50–55
Cholesterol	194–292 mg/day	100 mg/ 1000 Kcal*

* Up to 300 mg/day (1).
SOURCE: Daily dietary fat and total food energy intakes: National Health and Nutrition Examination Survey (NHANES III), phase I: 1988–1991. MMWR 1994;43:116–117, 123–125, and National Cholesterol Education Program. Report of the Expert Panel on Blood Cholesterol Levels in Children and Adolescents. Washington, DC: National Institutes of Health, National Heart, Lung, and Blood Institute, 1991.

Table 54-4 Milk Composition Comparison Chart

Nutrient	COMMON DESIGNATION OF TYPE OF MILK			
	WHOLE	2% (REDUCED FAT)	1% (LOW FAT)	SKIM (NON FAT)
FAT (g)	8	4.7	2.6	0.4
Saturated fat (g)	5.1	2.9	1.5	0.3
% of calories from fat	48%	35%	23%	4%
Protein (g)	8	8	8	8
Calcium (mg)	288	297	300	302
Total Cal/ 8 oz.	150	125	102	86

foods. On the average they consume 33% to 34% of their calories as fat, compared with the recommended level of 30% or less. This excess intake of dietary fat contributes to adverse health conditions and chronic disease risk factors, such as childhood obesity and hypercholesterolemia.

Data from NHANES III (1988–94) indicates that saturated fat intake (although decreasing gradually over time) is still higher (at 12% of total calories) than the recommended level of less than 10% (Table 54-3). Dairy products are the largest source of saturated fat in children's diets. This is not surprising, since an ounce of full-fat American cheese or an 8 oz glass of whole milk each provide 5 g of saturated fat. The average 10-year-old child following the recommended Step I NCEP diet (see Table 54-3) is usually advised to consume no more than 20 g of saturated fat per day; thus three glasses of whole milk and an ounce of cheese use up the entire day's allotment of saturated fat. Table 54-4 provides a comparison chart for common types of milk and also illustrates the fact that calcium intake is not compromised with use of lower fat milk products.

Americans have gradually switched to buying lower fat milk rather than whole milk. Schools and even fast food chains are now offering low-fat milk as an alternative to whole milk. These same surveys have noted that cheese consumption is increasing, probably because the people who understand that whole milk is almost 50% fat by calories do not understand that full-fat cheese is similar (71).

Consumption of high-fat foods is generally done at the expense of high-fiber foods. American children, like their parents, consume less than optimal amounts of dietary fiber. Mean dietary fiber intake for U.S. children is about 12 g/day (NHANES II) with the majority derived from fruits, vegetables, and cereals. Although there is no RDA for dietary fiber, the American Academy of Pediatrics recommends that children consume 0.5 g/kg/day of dietary fiber, a level which for many children is twice the level of current consumption (72). To increase dietary fiber in children's diets there will need to be more emphasis on consumption of high-fiber breakfast cereals, breads, and crackers, as well as increased intake of fresh fruits and vegetables.

Ellison et al (73) demonstrated that by simply substituting a cereal-based, low-fat breakfast for the usual bacon and egg breakfast, college students could increase their intake of fiber and decrease their intake of dietary fat (from 85 g/day to 70 g/day). Consumption of no breakfast at all, however, often reflects a constellation of negative eating habits. Children and adolescents who skip breakfast have been found to have the highest body mass indices and the highest mean serum cholesterol levels compared with children consuming a variety of other types of breakfast. Children consuming ready-to-eat, high-fiber breakfast cereals were the leanest and had the lowest cholesterol levels in this study (74).

Eating styles of the American family have undergone significant recent change with more and more wives and mothers in the workforce. With 60% of mothers of children under age 6 working, and even a higher percentage of mothers of older children and adolescents, families have turned to the use of ready-made foods and takeout dinners. Frequently, such meals are higher in calories, fat, saturated fat, and sodium than foods prepared from raw ingredients at home. Families with young children now eat out at fast-food and also at sit-down restaurants at increasingly higher numbers. According to surveys by the American Restaurant Association, children under age 6 are one of the fastest growing new consumers of restaurant meals (75).

Parents often have little control over the type and amount of food that children consume away from home. Since one-quarter of calories are usually consumed at lunch (usually at school) and one-third of calories consumed as snacks during the day, this means that almost 60% of the child's daily energy intake, 5 days per week, may be eaten largely outside of the home. This becomes increasingly so for older children and adolescents. This provides another rationale for emphasizing the need for more nutrition education during the preschool period and throughout the school years, with modification of the current lunch program to reflect the AHA/NCEP dietary guidelines.

Lipids and Tobacco Use

Cigarette smoking has been shown to be a major independent risk factor for coronary artery disease. Risk of coronary artery disease increases with the number of cigarettes smoked and the years of smoking. In addition, smoking filter cigarettes provides no protection against the development of coronary artery disease.

It has been estimated that 30% of all deaths from CHD are attributable to smoking, accounting for more than 170,000 deaths each year in the United States alone. Most smokers adopt the habit during adolescence, followed by a lifetime of cigarette consumption. Among young adults of both sexes who are otherwise at low risk of developing coronary artery disease (CAD), up to three quarters of CAD cases may be attributable to cigarette smoking (76–78).

A variety of physiologic changes occur as a result of cigarette smoking and contribute to increased CAD risk. These include altered blood lipid levels, increased carboxyhemoglobin levels, and increased blood viscosity and clotting factor concentrations. In a recent study of child and adolescent smokers (aged 8–19), significant elevations of VLDL, LDL, and triglyceride were found as well as reduction in HDL and total cholesterol (79). Overall, the effect of increased LDL and decreased HDL results in a less favorable lipid profile in terms of CAD risk. In addition, the lipid changes seen in young smokers are greater than that seen in adult smokers.

Even passive smoke has been shown to adversely effect the HDL-C levels of children. In a study of 105 children with at least one smoking parent, the HDL-C was significantly lower in children exposed to passive smoke, primarily maternal smoke. This study suggests that children with long-term exposure to passive smoke may be at elevated risk for the development of CAD (80).

Lipids and Physical Activity

Physical inactivity is an independent risk factor for coronary heart disease, and has assumed increasing importance in preventive cardiology because of its contribution to the development of obesity, abnormal plasma lipids, high blood pressure and hyperglycemia, each of which contributes to risk of coronary heart disease (81).

Studies of physical fitness in pediatric populations have demonstrated that children with higher levels of fitness have higher levels of protective HDL-C. They also have significantly less body fat as measured by skinfold thickness.

The effect of exercise on HDL-C levels appears to be mediated through an increase in muscle lipoprotein lipase (LPL) concentrations. This results in increased triglyceride clearance and HDL-C levels, since free cholesterol produced during triglyceride hydrolysis at the surface of VLDL by LPL is esterified by HDL_3, transforming it into HDL_2 (82).

Health professionals caring for children should emphasize the importance of regular daily physical activity for every member of the family from an early age, and should be active in efforts to increase physical education and sports activities in schools and communities. The goal is to develop in the young child a desire for and an enjoyment of physical activity that will persist throughout adult life. Physical activity should help to maintain a more efficient cardiovascular system, a more favorable lipid profile, an ideal level of body fat, and an avoidance of cigarette smoking (83,84).

Tracking of Lipids and Other Risk Factors

Although there is no doubt that we can identify coronary heart disease risk factors in children, and that they are highly prevalent, the question of how consistently these risk factors track over time has become very important. In this context, "tracking" refers to the degree to which a given measurement retains its rank order over time in a percentile distribution of measures among similarly aged children or adults. Obviously, if the majority of children who have cholesterol or blood pressure values above the 90th or 95th percentiles at an early age continue to have high levels throughout childhood and into adult life, then intervening at an early age is clearly warranted.

Several longitudinal studies of pediatric populations have studied risk factor tracking (61,83,84). Many of these studies are limited by relatively brief periods of follow-up.

The Bogalusa Heart Study, however, has followed a cohort of children for a 12-year period (85–87). Their results show high levels of persistence in rank order for height, weight triceps skinfold, systolic blood pressure, and total cholesterol and LDL-C levels. Tracking correlations are lower for diastolic blood pressure, HDL-C and triglyceride levels. Overall, in this and similar studies, about 70% of children with total cholesterol and LDL-C levels in the top quintile at baseline will still be in the top two quintiles after 12 years of follow-up (61,87,88).

HDL-C levels do not track well until after age 10. In contrast, levels of total cholesterol and LDL-C at 6 months of age are significantly associated with levels at 7 years, and with even higher associations from age 1 to 7 years. Almost two-thirds of the infants with LDL-C levels at or above the 80th percentile level were still in this top quintile at 7 years of age.

It is significant that relative ranking within a peer group tends to stabilize by the age of 2 to 4 years. In addition, even though there are marked lipid changes during puberty, especially for white males, this had little effect on their long-term tracking (89).

A similar study of children aged 8 to 18 who were reevaluated at age 20 to 30 also demonstrated that childhood levels of total cholesterol and LDL-C were good predictors of adult levels, as well as of LDL to HDL ratios (90,91). HDL-C levels in childhood were not good predictors of adult levels. In this study, 62% of the children initially in the top decile (above the 90th percentile) for total cholesterol levels were found to be above the 75th percentile as adults (about 240 mg/dL). In addition, 80% of the children initially in the same top decile for total cholesterol had adult levels above the 50th percentile (about 200 mg/dL). Since the Adult Consensus Panel of the National Heart Lung and Blood Institute of the NIH has established 200 mg/dL to 239 mg/dL as "borderline high risk" and 240 mg/dL and above as "high risk," it would appear that a large proportion of these adults at increased risk can be identified as children.

Similarly, there is a high degree of tracking for blood pressure (systolic more than diastolic) as well as for obesity (86,87,92). Thus there is strong support for treating children with increased risk factors for coronary artery disease, since the weight of evidence suggests that such increased risk status will track over time and lead to disease in adult life if reduction of risk is not achieved.

CLINICAL EVALUATION AND TREATMENT OF HYPERCHOLESTEROLEMIA IN CHILDHOOD

The evaluation and treatment of hypercholesterolemia in childhood includes initial assessment of overall coronary risk status. This includes the presence and degree of elevation of each risk factor, such as blood lipids and lipoproteins, blood pressure, cigarette smoking status, body fatness, diet, and level of physical activity. Normal values and percentile grids are available for interpretation and ranking of pediatric lipid and lipoprotein values, blood pressure, height, weight, and relative weight. Algorithms provide guidance in the stepwise progression of clinical evaluation and treatment. Suggested guidelines for evaluating and treating children with one or more elevated CHD risk actors have only recently begun to be formulated. However, consensus is growing that atherosclerosis begins in childhood and that primary prevention of this insidious, and eventually highly fatal, disease must also begin with children. The potential impact of pediatric interventions could be great. However, risks, costs, and side effects must be carefully and continuously assessed as we gain more experience in this relatively new field of pediatric preventive cardiology.

Risk status in childhood, beginning with assessment of inherited risk based on family history of premature coronary heart disease and other cardiovascular disease, can be easily evaluated, treated, and followed over time. Promotion of health goals through family nutrition counseling, prevention of obesity, avoidance of cigarette smoking, and encouragement of increased daily physical activity are all parts of the prescription for preventing cardiovascular disease in a child's future. These goals are best achieved through a population-wide strategy aimed at reducing cardiovascular risk status in all children over 2 years old, through promoting healthier child and family lifestyles. At the same time, this approach is complemented by strategies to reduce risk status in children with significantly elevated risk factors. The following describes an approach to the clinical evaluation of cardiovascular risk factors in pediatric practice with the goal of identifying and treating children and adolescents at increased risk of developing premature cardiovascular disease in adult life.

Evaluation

The ideal time for clinical evaluation of children's overall CVD risk profile is after the age of 2 years and preferably before entering school at age 5 or 6. The preschool period is preferable because lifestyle habits contributing to development of risk factors are begun during these early years, especially habits related to diet and physical activity. In addition, habits of shorter duration are easier to change than those of long duration; thus interventions aimed at younger children are more likely to succeed. Finally, this is when young parents are eager for advice on child care and visits to the pediatrician are frequent.

Evaluation of risk status should include measurements of blood pressure, height, weight, body fat, and total cholesterol in plasma or serum. In addition, patterns of physical activity, diet,

and cigarette smoking should be assessed for both child and family, since these lifestyles are commonly shared and affect recommendations for treatment. Lipid and lipoprotein measurements should be obtained from parents and siblings, since familial aggregation of hypercholesterolemia is common, reflecting shared heredity, lifestyle, or both.

Detailed initial review and annual update of the family history is essential for the determination of: 1) the familial nature of risk factors, 2) their contribution to the child's risk status, and 3) the degree of aggressiveness of therapy to reduce risk status.

Weight and Lipid Status

Determining weight status for height and estimating (or measuring) degree of body fat is important in evaluating and treating the hyperlipidemic child, since overweight children will need more intensive therapy to reduce caloric intake and increase physical activity.

Height and weight should be plotted on standard NCHS growth charts. Determination of the percentile zones for each measure and comparison of the height percentile with weight percentile gives the first indication if the child is overweight for height. A child whose weight is two or more percentile zones above height may be overweight for height (e.g., a child whose height is in the 10th to 25th percentile and whose weight is in the 75th to 90th percentile for age and sex).

Measurement of subcutaneous fat with skinfold calipers adds valuable information of simple height and weight measures by helping the clinician determine if the overweight child is also overfat. In cases of significant obesity, physical inspection is enough to answer this question; however, skinfold measures are very helpful as baseline determinations and as follow-up measures in subsequent treatment (93).

Lipids and Lipoprotein Profile

Guidelines for screening, evaluation, and treatment of children with hypercholesterolemia in pediatric practice have only recently begun to be formulated (94,95). Recently, the Expert Panel on Blood Cholesterol Levels in Children and Adolescents (95) recommended cholesterol screening of all children over 2 years of age who have a positive family history of premature CHD and other atherosclerotic complications, parental or grandparental history of hypercholesterolemia, or other childhood risk factors (Table 54-5). In the average pediatric practice, this may translate into screening about 50% of children over age 2. Since family history is frequently incomplete or unavailable and is rarely taken in a comprehensive manner or updated annually, and since up to 50% of children with blood cholesterol levels above 200 mg/dL may be missed when screening on the basis of family history alone (93,96–98), others have recommended screening all children over age 2 as part of routine well-child care (94).

The physician who chooses to screen either all patients or only those with a positive family history will still be faced with the decision of what to do next after obtaining that initial cholesterol result. The following is a practical guide for the pediatrician in that situation.

Evaluating the Blood Cholesterol Level

The decision about how to proceed after a single total cholesterol test may be made on the basis of: 1) the degree of

Table 54-5 Sample Cardiovascular Disease Risk Factor "Score Sheet": Children over Age 2

	POTENTIAL RISK OF DEVELOPING HEART DISEASE AS AN ADULT		
	LOW	MODERATE	HIGH
Total blood cholesterol (mg/dL)	170 and below	170–199	200 and above
LDL cholesterol (mg/dL)	Below 110	110–129	130 and above
HDL cholesterol (mg/dL)	45 and above	35–44	below 35
Weight status	Underweight: Below mean for weight for height	Average: 100–119% of ideal weight for height	Overweight: >120% of ideal weight for height
Cigarette smoking	Never smoke	Experiments	Regular smoker
Exercise	Sports regularly	Gym plus play	Gym at school only
Family history[a]	Rare CHD (not in parent or grandparent)	Grandparent, aunt, uncle had CHD before 55	Parent had CHD before 55
Blood pressure[b] (for age/sex)	<75th%	75th–95th%	>95th%

[a] 1st or 2nd-degree relative has high blood pressure or high serum cholesterol (>240 mg/dL).

[b] 95% for SBP (110–130 mm Hg) children age 2–13 years; 95% for DBP (55–85 mm Hg) children age 2–13 years. In older teens, BP > 130/85 is >95th%.

elevation of that single value, 2) the presence of other CVD risk factors in the child, and 3) the nature of the child's family history for premature-onset CVD or major CVD risk factors.

A single low serum cholesterol value (below the 75th percentile, or about 170 mg/dL) in a child with normal blood pressure, normal weight for height, normal activity level, nonsmoking, and with a negative family history does not require further follow-up at this time other than routine care. Cholesterol screening should again be done at the next annual checkup and, if still low, repeated every 3 to 5 years thereafter unless family history or the child's risk status changes. If the child has other risk factors, or if the family history is positive, a fasting lipoprotein profile should be obtained and evaluated (Fig. 54-1).

If there is a single elevated serum cholesterol value in a child, testing should be repeated, preferably within 1 week of the initial test. Variation between the first and second test results could be the result of laboratory technical error, imprecision, lack of accuracy, patient day-to-day variability, or physical state (fever, dehydration). Repeat cholesterol values obtained after 2 or more weeks may reflect dietary changes instituted after the initial result was reported. If the average of the two baseline cholesterol measures is still above the 75th percentile, a complete lipoprotein profile should be determined from a capillary or venous blood sample after a 12-hour fast.

Evaluating the Lipoprotein Profile

The simplest lipoprotein profile consists of a total cholesterol value, a HDL-C value, and a triglyceride value. The physician then may calculate the LDL-C value from Friedewald's formula: LDL-C = TC − HDL-C − TG/5, where TG/5 is an estimate of VLDL-C. Ratios LDL-C/HDL-C (bad to good cholesterol) and TC/HDL-C (total to good cholesterol) may also be calculated. More sophisticated laboratory reports provide the calculated LDL-C, as well as the ratios and population distribution percentiles or "risk scores." Pediatricians

should be wary of extrapolating adult "risk scores" to pediatric age groups, however.

With each of the lipoprotein values available, the next step is to compare the patient's values with a distribution of values from a normal population of children, using age and sex, and race-specific reference values if mean values differ significantly between these groups. Normal values are available in tabular and in grid form from several large epidemiologic studies of children, such as those derived from the Lipid Research Clinics Population Study (see Table 54-1), and the Bogalusa project. General charts for interpretation of children's lipid levels are also helpful for explaining results to parents (Table 54-6).

The most important information desired from the lipoprotein profile may be summarized as follows: 1) Does the child have an LDL-C level above the 75th or 95th percentile? 2) Does the child have an HDL-C level below the 5th or 25th percentile?

It is also important to determine if the triglycerides are elevated above the 95th percentile (and if so, make a mental note to ask if the child was truly fasting) and if the ratio of LDL/HDL is over 3.0 or the TC/HDL ratio is above 4–6 (>4 for adolescents). Higher ratios signal increased risk status.

A small percentage of children will have elevated total cholesterol levels due to high levels of "good" HDL-C. These children do not need dietary intervention unless their LDL-C level is also elevated above the 75th percentile.

Apolipoprotein A1 and B levels may also be measured as part of the lipid evaluation. These may be especially helpful in families with a strong history of premature-onset CVD. In these cases, children with normal levels of LDL-C may have elevated apolipoprotein B, and a diagnosis of hyperapobeta-lipoproteinemia may be made. Such a condition reflects an increased risk of future CVD despite the normal LDL-C levels.

Abnormal Lipoprotein Profiles

By comparing our patient's lipoprotein profile with normal reference values or grids, we are able first to determine if the

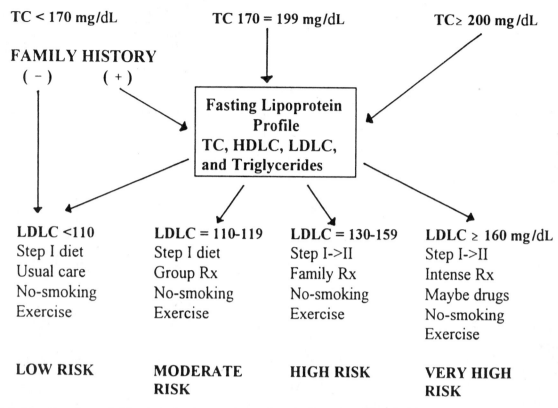

NON-FASTING CHOLESTEROL SCREEN

TC < 170 mg/dL   TC 170 = 199 mg/dL   TC≥ 200 mg/dL

FAMILY HISTORY
(−)   (+)

**Fasting Lipoprotein
Profile
TC, HDLC, LDLC,
and Triglycerides**

LDLC <110
Step I diet
Usual care
No-smoking
Exercise

LDLC = 110-119
Step I diet
Group Rx
No-smoking
Exercise

LDLC = 130-159
Step I->II
Family Rx
No-smoking
Exercise

LDLC ≥ 160 mg/dL
Step I->II
Intense Rx
Maybe drugs
No-smoking
Exercise

LOW RISK   **MODERATE
RISK**   **HIGH RISK**   **VERY HIGH
RISK**

Figure 54-1 Algorithm for pediatric cholesterol screening and evaluation at age 2 and older.

LDL-C or triglycerides are elevated and if the HDL-C is depressed.

Abnormal lipoprotein levels in children and adolescents may be the result of:

- An inherited disorder (single gene or polygenic)
- An underlying disease state
- Medications or drugs (prescriptions/self-administered)
- Overnutrition (high saturated fat diet, with or without obesity)
- Pregnancy

Rule Out Secondary Causes

It is important initially to rule out underlying states such as hypothyroidism, nephrotic syndrome, liver disease, and others outlined in Table 54-7. Physical findings usually suggest such a contributing cause, and laboratory test confirm it. The incidence of asymptomatic liver, kidney, or thyroid disease diagnosed after the lipid abnormality is noted is low; in our clinical population, it is about 1%.

The contribution of medications should be evaluated. Steroids used as anti-inflammatory agents, in oral contraceptives, or illegally in sports are common. Anticonvulsant therapy, thyroid hormone replacement, and tobacco and alcohol use may all alter lipoprotein concentrations.

Familial Dyslipidemias

Children with abnormal lipoprotein profiles may or may not have relatives with similar patterns. Familial aggregation occurs not only because of shared genes but also because of shared environment. Families share diet, exercise routines, and even cigarette smoking habits.

Inherited familial lipid disorders due to a single gene defect (as described earlier in Table 54-2) are usually apparent on taking a family history and determining the lipid profiles of siblings, parents, and grandparents. Premature CVD is often common in relatives if the older relatives affected were male and if they also had one or more of the other major risk factors such as hypertension or cigarette smoking. Often, however, if the older affected relatives were female, nonsmokers, and normotensive, the history of premature CVD may not be present even in the face of total cholesterol levels above 300 mg/dL to 400mg/dL in affected individuals.

In families where 1) the lipid abnormalities clearly run on one side of the family, 2) the lipid levels are very high (two to three times normal), and 3) most of the relatives have had their lipids determined, evaluation of the family and genetic patterns are possible. Often, however, much of the information is not available, and one can only make an educated guess as to whether this is a single-gene familial inherited disorder, a polygenic inherited familial disorder, or familial based on environmental factors.

Table 54-6 Interpretation of Cholesterol and Triglycerides: Children Aged 2–19		
Total Cholesterol		
High	200 or higher	
Borderline high	170–199	
Desirable	below 170	
LDL Cholesterol		
High	130 or higher	
Borderline high	110–129	
Desirable	below 110	
HDL Cholesterol		
Low	below 35	
Borderline low	35–45	
Desirable	above 45	
Triglycerides	<age 10 yrs.	10–19 yrs.
High	100 or higher	130 or higher
Borderline high	75–99	90–120
Desirable	below 75	below 90

Table 54-7 Secondary Causes of Hyperlipoproteinemia		
TYPE	FEATURES	SECONDARY CAUSES
I	⬆chylomicrons	Diabetes mellitus Dysgammaglobulinemia SLE
IIA	⬆LDL	Nephrotic syndrome Hypothyroidism
IIB	⬆LDL ⬆VLDL	Obstructive liver disease Multiple myeloma Porphyria
III	⬆IDL	Hypothyroidism Dysgammaglobulinemia
IV	⬆VLDL	Diabetes mellitus Nephrotic syndrome Pregnancy Hormone use Alcohol excess Glycogen storage disease Gaucher disease Niemann-Pick disease
V	⬆chylomicrons ⬆VLDL	Diabetes mellitus Nephrotic syndrome Alcoholism Myeloma Idiopathic hypercalcemia

Family History

The family history may provide valuable information to the clinician evaluating the child's lipid disorder and risk of premature cardiovascular disease. Family history has been proposed by the NCEP Expert Panel on Blood Cholesterol Levels in Children (95) as a criterion for deciding whether to measure cholesterol in children over 2 years of age (Table 54-8). However, several studies have recently reported that 50% or more of hypercholesterolemic children would be missed if such a criterion were used (93,96–98).

Family history is essential in assessing the familial nature of dyslipidemias and determining the genetic pattern. It also helps us estimate the degree of increased cardiovascular risk for a particular child and therefore guides our decisions regarding treatment. For these reasons, it is essential to obtain as detailed and accurate a family history as possible on all children with elevated cholesterol and/or triglycerides, or isolated low HDL-C. The history should also be updated annually.

In considering the family history, certain questions emerge:

1. Which relative should be surveyed?
2. What diseases and conditions should be ascertained?
3. What age of onset of disease is "premature"?
4. What constitutes a "positive" family history?

Recommendations vary about which relatives should be surveyed, which conditions ascertained, what age of onset of cardiovascular disease should be considered premature, and therefore what should contribute to the positive history designation. A review of family history studies in the literature shows the variety of definitions used and the lack of consensus.

In an ideal situation, both first-degree (parents, siblings) and second-degree (grandparents, blood-related aunts and uncles) relatives would be surveyed. Occurrence of risk factors for atherosclerotic disease would be determined (hypercholesterolemia or other lipid abnormality, hypertension, cigarette smoking, diabetes, obesity, gout); and occurrence and age of

diagnosis/treatment of coronary artery disease and other atherosclerotic complications (myocardial infarction, angina pectoris, sudden cardiac death, stroke, peripheral vascular disease, coronary angioplasty, coronary artery bypass surgery, diagnosis of coronary artery disease) would be assessed.

The definition of "positive" family history varies. The Academy of Pediatrics Committee on Nutrition in their 1989 statement suggests that a myocardial infarction in a first- or second-degree relative younger than age 50 (men) or age 60 (women) or the presence of hypercholesterolemia in such relative(s) be considered a positive family history (99). In their previous 1983 statement, the definition was broader and also included hypertension, obesity, diabetes, and gout (100).

The NCEP Expert Panel on Blood Cholesterol in Children and Adolescents uses age 55 in their definition of premature onset of CHD and related atherosclerotic complications (95) (see Table 54-8). "Premature" coronary artery disease has been variably defined as that occurring before age 60 in either sex, or before age 50 in men and age 60 in women.

The physician's best approach to obtaining a good family history is through a combination of questionnaire and personal interview, and then making a decision about whether the history is significant. A workable definition of positive family history and one used in our Preventive Cardiology Clinic follows: a positive family history is the presence of a first- or second-degree relative who had a major CVD risk factor (total cholesterol ≥240 mg/dL, hypertension treated with medication) or was diagnosed/treated for CHD (heart attack, angina pectoris, sudden cardiac death, cerebrovascular

> **Table 54-8 Summary of Recommendations from the Expert Panel on Blood Cholesterol Levels in Children and Adolescents: National Cholesterol Education Program**
>
> I. **Nutrient recommendations for all children over age 2**
>   A. Nutritional adequacy should be achieved by eating a wide variety of foods.
>   B. Energy (calories) should be adequate to support growth and development and to reach or maintain desirable body weight.
>   C. The following pattern of nutrient intake is recommended:
>   1. Saturated fatty acids: less than 10% of calories
>   2. Total fat: no more than 30% of calories (average)
>   3. Dietary cholesterol: less that 300 mg per day
>   D. School lunch and breakfast programs should increase the availability and encourage the selection of foods that are low in saturated fat, total fat, and cholesterol.
> II. **Cholesterol screening recommendations for all children over age 2**
>   A. Screen children whose parents/grandparents (<55 yrs) had coronary angioplasty or coronary artery bypass surgery or were diagnosed with CHD after coronary arteriography.
>   B. Screen children whose parents/grandparents (<55 yrs) suffered a documented myocardial infarction, angina pectoris, peripheral vascular disease, cerebrovascular disease, or sudden cardiac death.
>   C. Screen the children of parents who have been found to have high blood cholesterol (240 mg/dL or above).
>   D. Screen children whose parental or grandparental medical history is unavailable (at the discretion of the physician).
>   E. Screen children with other risk factors, such as high blood pressure, cigarette smoking, obesity, or who consume excessive amounts of saturated fat, total fat, and cholesterol.
>   F. Blood cholesterol screening should be done as part of routine medical care.

SOURCE: National Cholesterol Education Program. Report of the Expert Panel on Blood Cholesterol Levels in Children and Adolescents. Bethesda, MD: National Institutes of Health, National Heart, Lung, and Blood Institute, 1991. NIH publication no. 91-2732.

accident [CVA], peripheral vascular disease, bypass surgery or angioplasty) with onset before age 55.

Even positive family histories could be further characterized with respect to severity of known family risk factors; numbers of first- and second-degree relatives affected; and early versus later age of onset of clinical cardiovascular disease.

Summary Risk Profile

Based on assessment of the child's lipid profile, in addition to blood pressure, cigarette smoking status, body fatness or weight for height status, usual level of physical activity, and family history, the physician may characterize the child's overall risk profile as normal, borderline high risk, or high risk. Scoring systems have been suggested for such classification; however, it may be a more useful exercise for the physician to go over a risk profile sheet (such as that provided in Table 54-5) with the family and indicate which of the risk factors are elevated and which are not. Both the positive and the negative should be emphasized as a baseline for treatment recommendations. Even children who have seriously abnormal lipid profiles often are nonsmokers and have normal weight and blood pressure, and this should be praised and encouraged while stressing the need to improve the lipid profile.

TREATMENT OF LIPID DISORDERS IN CHILDHOOD

Nutrition Assessment

It is worthwhile and simple for the practicing physician to make an objective assessment of the child's diet by means of

one or two questionnaires that the parent or child can complete before an annual checkup. A simple food frequency check sheet asks the individual to check off how many times per week or month certain foods are eaten. Food frequency questionnaires are usually used to get qualitative information on usual diet; however, some are semiquantitative and can be analyzed to provide quantitative data on dietary intake (101).

Three-day food records are useful and also are used to provide quantitative data on nutrient intake. They may also simply be used as a guide for the pediatrician to review the kinds of meals that are usually served in the child's home. They can be mailed to parents to fill out before the child's appointment, with simple instructions. It should be cautioned that, if the diet record will be analyzed quantitatively, the parent needs a significant amount of instruction for recording everything consumed as well as accurate portion sizes.

These dietary questionnaires can help the pediatrician assess the dietary contributions to problems such as high serum cholesterol or triglycerides, obesity, or borderline hypertension, and begin dietary counseling in the areas most in need of change (i.e., too many fast-food meals, too much cheese, frequent salty snacks, etc.).

Dietary Prescription and Counseling

Diet and exercise are key components in both the prevention and treatment of cardiovascular risk factors in childhood. For children older than 2 years, adherence to a diet that has been variously called the "prudent diet," the American Heart Association or National Cholesterol Education Project "Step I" diet, or the "30% fat" diet will help lower serum total and LDL cholesterol, reduce excess weight gain, and avoid excess sodium intake. The essential elements of the Step I diet are

Table 54-9 Recommended NCEP Step I and II Diets for Reducing Blood Cholesterol Levels in Children over Age 2

NUTRIENT	STEP I[a]	STEP II[a]	PRACTICAL TIPS
Fat: total	<30%	<30%	Reduce all fat intake; use vegetable oils and
Saturated fat	<10%	<7%	margarine; use skim or 1% milk and low-fat dairy
Polyunsaturated	10%	10%	products; avoid fried foods; use lean meats,
Monounsaturated	10–15%	10–15%	fish and poultry
Cholesterol (mg/dL)	<300	<200	Limit eggs to 2 or 3 per week
Carbohydrate	50–60%	50–60%	Eat more whole-grain cereal/breads, fruits, vegetables; eat less sweets
Protein	15–20%	15–20%	Eat less animal protein, more vegetable protein, soy protein
Fiber (g/day)	Age + 5 g/day[b]	Age + 5 g/day[b]	Eat whole grain cereals/bread, fruits/vegetables with peel, oat bran

[a] Percentages are percent of total calories.
[b] "Age + 5" dietary fiber rule: age of child (yrs) + 5 = grams of dietary fiber per day for children >2 years of age (106).
SOURCE: National Cholesterol Education Program. Report of the Expert Panel on Blood Cholesterol Levels in Children and Adolescents. Bethesda, MD: National Institutes of Health, National Heart, Lung, and Blood Institute, 1991. NIH publication no. 91-2732.

listed in Table 54-9. This diet may be further modified to reduce caloric intake if the child is obese (102), to increase caloric intake if the child is underweight, to reduce sodium if indicated, and to increase fiber intake (especially soluble fiber such as that found in oat bran, fruit pectins, and psyllium) to increase satiety and reduce constipation and serum cholesterol.

Dietary Treatment of Dyslipidemia

The vast majority of preadolescent children requiring treatment for a lipid problem will be those with elevated total cholesterol due to a high LDL-C level (above the 75th percentile for age). Elevated triglyceride levels are more commonly seen in adolescence, since even familial hypertriglyceridemic disorders are often not expressed until the second decade. Low HDL-C levels in the 5th to 25th percentile range for age are commonly seen in children with elevated cholesterol levels, especially those with familial dyslipidemias or obesity. A much smaller number will have elevated triglycerides, or low HDL-C alone or in combination. And even fewer will have the rarer lipid disorders, with types I, III, or V. Finally, there will be some children with hyperapobetalipoproteinemia where the LDL-C level will be normal or borderline high, but the apo-B will be above the 95th percentile for age (about >110 mg/dL).

Initial treatment of children with abnormal lipid profiles consists of modifying the child's diet (94,95,103–105). Children with elevated LDL-C, elevated apo-B, and low HDL-C are placed on a Step I diet consisting of normal calories (unless the child is obese), but reduced fat calories as described in Table 54-9. Greatest emphasis is placed on reducing saturated fat intake to less than 10% of calories. Physicians should know the most common sources of saturated fat in children's diets and be able to offer suggestions regarding alternative low-fat foods as the first step in recommending a low-fat diet (Table 54-10).

In some cases, it may be necessary to count grams of saturated fat consumed in order to comply with the goal of 10% or less of calories from saturated fat. A child consuming 1800 calories per day should eat no more than 20 g of saturated fat (1 g of fat = 9 calories; 9 × 20 = 180 calories, which is 10% of the 1800 calorie daily total). Charts of saturated fat content of foods are available so that the parents can see which foods to include in the child's diet and which ones to limit. For example, 8 oz of whole milk contains 5 g of saturated fat (one quarter of the child's allowance for the day), whereas skim milk contains less than 1 g per 8 oz, so that the use of skim milk allows the child more freedom to include other low- to moderately low-fat products in the diet (see Table 54-10).

Consumption of increased amounts of complex carbohydrates and dietary fiber is also stressed. According to the "age + 5" rule, children age 2 and older should consume an amount of total dietary fiber equal to their age (in years) +5 grams per day (106,107). For children with hypercholesterolemia, increasing the soluble fiber content of the diet (e.g., oat bran, pectin, guar gum, psyllium, etc.) has been shown to enhance the cholesterol-lowering effect of the fat-modified Step I diet (108,109). This can be accomplished by encouraging consumption of a moderately high-fiber cereal for breakfast (with low-fat milk), use of whole grain breads and crackers, incorporation of beans in the diet, and consumption of five servings per day of fruits and vegetables.

If the serum triglyceride level is also increased, reduction of simple sugars and achievement of ideal body weight are stressed as well. For most children, limiting intake of simple sugar to less than 10% of daily energy or about 10 to 12 tsps (40 to 44 g) per day is a reasonable goal. Avoid excess sugar intake from beverage sources in the diet (e.g., carbonated beverages, fruit drinks, fruit juices, and sweetened iced teas).

It is essential that caloric intake be maintained to support normal growth. Since fat calories are calorically more dense than protein or carbohydrate, a reduction in dietary fat must be accompanied by an increase in carbohydrate to make up for the loss of fat calories. Most children like complex car-

Table 54-10 Sources of Saturated Fat in Children's Diets

Food Item	Grams of Saturated Fat/Serving
Ice cream, 1 c, 10% fat	9
Hamburger, 3 oz, fast food	8
Hot dog, 2 oz	7
Butter, 1 tbsp	7
Pizza with cheese, 1 slice	6
Cheese, 1 oz American or Swiss	6
Parmesean cheese, 1 tbsp	5
Milk, whole, 1 c	5
Beef, pork, veal, 3 oz Lean	5
Ice milk frozen dessert, 1 c	4
Heavy cream, 1 tbsp	4
Milk, 2% low fat, 1 c	3
Bacon, 2 slices crisp	3
Egg, 1 medium	3
French fries, 10 medium	3
Peanut butter, 2 tbsp	3
Cheese, part-skim mozzarella, 1 oz	3
Cream cheese, 1 tbsp	3
Margarine, 1 tbsp	2
Mayonnaise, 1 tbsp	2
Cupcake, chocolate frosted	2
Brownie, frosted	2
Potato chips, 10	2
Chicken, dark meat, 3 oz	2
Chicken, light meat, 3 oz	1
Milk, 1% low fat, 1 c	1
Bagel, 1 medium	0
Baked potato, 1 medium	0
Marshmallows, 5	0
Milk, skim, 1 c	0
Sorbet, 1 c	0

NOTE: Hamburger, cheeseburger, meatloaf, full-fat dairy products, cheese, beef, hot dogs, ham, lunch meats, eggs, cookies, cakes, doughnuts, butter, pork, white bread and rolls together account for over 60% of the saturated fat in most children's diet. The average 10-year-old child on an 1800-calorie Step I diet should consume less than 20 g saturated fat per day.

bohydrates (potatoes, bread, pasta, rice, etc.), so that this is usually not a problem. Calcium levels are slightly higher in low-fat and skim milk than in regular milk, so that calcium intake need not be compromised on the Step I diet. Intake of other minerals and vitamins will be adequate if a good variety of foods from all food groups is consumed.

Further reduction of saturated fat intake to 7% to calories may be necessary in order to achieve lipid goals. This Step II diet may be prescribed after 6 to 12 months on the Step I diet and should be given an adequate trial before medications are considered. Patients who are not compliant with the Step I diet, however, will be even less compliant on the more restrictive Step II diet. Thus, Step II should be recommended only when compliance to Step I is adequate, but lipid response is insufficient.

Children with normal levels of LDL-C combined with low levels of HDL-C are also treated with a Step I diet if their ratio of LDL/HDL is above 3. The diet will reduce LDL levels so that the ratio will be reduced to a lower risk level. Increased physical activity will also help raise HDL, as will reducing obesity and avoiding cigarette smoking.

Similarly, children with normal to borderline-elevated LDL levels but high apo-B (above 100 mg/dL) are treated with a Step I diet in order to reduce the LDL further and thus reduce the level of apo-B as well.

When a reduced-fat diet is prescribed medically for a child with elevated serum cholesterol or other dyslipidemia, it is important that the parents and child are all adequately counseled with respect to achieving the goal and avoiding problems, specifically, insufficient caloric intake. Parents who are advised simply to cut out fat and cholesterol from the diet are likely to reduce caloric intake without compensating with increased calories from other sources. Case reports have documented such parental dietary overrestrictions and the inadequate growth that can occur as a result (110,111). Regular medical supervision is needed to monitor the progress of children where a low-fat diet has been prescribed in the early phases of treatment.

The goals of dietary treatment should be discussed with parents. For children with baseline LDL-C between 110 and 129 mg/dL, the goal is to reduce it to below 110 mg/dL. For children with baseline LDL-C above 130 mg/dL the goal will be to reduce it initially to below 130 mg/dL and ideally below 110 mg/dL. This may or may not be feasible with dietary intervention alone, depending on the severity of the child's hypercholesterolemia. Gradual achievement of dietary goals over a 6- to 12-month period may be easier for parents and children to accept and may avoid overzealous restrictions.

Follow-up of children with lipid disorders will depend on the nature and severity of the dyslipidemia as well as the presence and need for treatment of other coexisting risk factors. Children on dietary treatment alone should be monitored at least quarterly with repeat lipid measurements and assessment of growth and dietary compliance.

If a reduction of fat intake has resulted in a reduction of caloric intake that has not been compensated for by increasing complex carbohydrate calories, the child will lose weight. This should be corrected through further dietary counseling. In some cases, increasing monounsaturated fat intake will be needed to keep up calories if the child is unable to eat enough complex carbohydrates to compensate. Such situations are not common but must be detected and corrected as soon as possible.

In the usual clinical course, when the patient is compliant with the Step I diet, the total cholesterol and LDL-C will drop 10% to 20%. The subsequent course, however, will be up and down, and long-term monitoring and follow-up are needed to reinforce the diet and maintain the goals.

Parents and child need to understand the natural history of lipid levels through childhood, particularly the pubertal dip seen especially in white adolescent boys and the subsequent increase in total cholesterol and LDL-C and decrease in HDL-C seen later in adolescence and in early adult life.

Parents should be encouraged to reduce their own risk of CVD. Programs that treat families have an advantage in being able to follow and treat both children and parents in a single clinical setting. More than 90% of children with choles-

Table 54-11 Criteria for Initiation of Pharmacologic Therapy for Children and Adolescents with Dyslipidemia

1. LDL cholesterol above 190 mg/dL (or above 160 mg/dL if the child also has two or more other risk factors present) after 1 year of compliance with a reduced-fat diet (progressing from Step I to Step II)
2. Family history of premature onset of CHD (parent, grandparent, or blood-related aunt/uncle with CHD onset before age 55)
3. Child is at least 10 years of age, is otherwise healthy, and shows every evidence of normal growth and development

Adapted from Kwiterovich P. Beyond cholesterol. Baltimore, MD: Johns Hopkins University Press, 1989: 286, and from National Cholesterol Education Program. Report of the Expert Panel on Blood Cholesterol Levels in Children and Adolescents. Bethesda, MD: National Institutes of Health, National Heart, Lung, and Blood Institute, 1991. NIH publication no. 91-2732.

terol levels of 200 mg/dL or above referred to our clinical center have at least one parent who also has hypercholesterolemia. Thus family-oriented screening, counseling, and treatment are preferred.

Pharmacologic Therapy of Dyslipidemia

Medications may be prescribed in the treatment of children and adolescents with lipid abnormalities. Criteria have been suggested for initiating drug therapy in hypercholesterolemic children such as those summarized in Table 54-11. Bile acid sequestrants (e.g., cholestyramine) are presently the drugs of choice for initiating therapy. Although not approved by the Food and Drug Administration (FDA) for treatment of hypercholesterolemia in children, they have been used in severe cases for more than two decades and have been reported to be both effective and safe if monitored carefully. There are also reports of pediatric use of almost all the other cholesterol-lowering drugs that are currently approved by the FDA for use in adults.

Bile acid sequestrants are best begun at a low dose of 2–4 g per day (e.g., one-half to one packet or scoop of cholestyramine or cholestipol powder or 2–4 Cholestid pills per day), and increased slowly to one to two packs (4–8 g) a day. The dose of resin to be used is not related to the body weight of the child but to the levels of total cholesterol and LDL-C. Although dosage schedules indicate up to 4 doses (16 g) of resin, it is rare that a child or adolescent is able to tolerate much more than 2 doses (8 g of cholestyramine) per day. The most common side effects are constipation, gas, and upset stomach. It is important that the patient consume adequate amounts of fluid with each dose (8 oz). Bile acid sequestrants may interfere with the absorption of other medications as well as fat-soluble vitamins, so that vitamin supplementation and attention to the timing of other medication doses may be needed.

For severely affected hypercholesterolemic children, a combination of bile acid sequestrants with an HMG-CoA reductase inhibitor (e.g., lovastatin) is capable of lowering serum cholesterol to almost normal levels. Since there is limited pediatric experience at present with drugs other than the bile acid sequestrants, these agents should be used under the supervision of a lipid specialist and will need more intensive follow-up and monitoring to assess lipid response and side effects. Children with severe lipid disorders may also need assessment of cardiovascular status, i.e., electrocardiogram, exercise treadmill tests, and possibly other measures.

It is important to maintain a supportive atmosphere and avoid creating undue anxiety. Children should be reassured as to their current healthy status, but helped to appreciate the need for preventing future disease to help them live long and healthy lives. In cases of severe lipid abnormalities, however, the risk of CVD onset earlier in adult life (or, in some cases, even in adolescence) will increase the intensity and tempo of treatment and counseling.

Physical Activity in the Treatment of Lipid Disorders

It is important for all children to be physically active, but this is especially true for children with lipid disorders (e.g. low HDL-C), borderline high blood pressure, and/or obesity. These children should be urged to increase their level of regular aerobic physical activity to at least 30 minutes per day at a level that makes the child sweat. Charts can be provided so that children can choose their activities and monitor progress. Appropriate rewards for behaviors can be negotiated through contracts between parent/doctor and child.

The health benefits of regular physical activity in childhood include prevention or reduction of obesity, increased HDL-C, reduced blood pressure in children with early expressions of essential hypertension, improved physical appearance, and greater self-efficacy and self-esteem. It is not uncommon in clinical practice to see HDL-C levels that are higher at the end of an active summer of sports camp and then lower during the more sedentary winter months, especially in cold weather areas.

Treating the Obese Dyslipidemic Child

Since more than one-fourth of US children are currently obese, a significant proportion of dyslipidemic children will also be obese. In this case, the first goal is to implement the NCEP Step I fat-modified diet to reduce LDL-C (and/or triglycerides if elevated). The second goal will be to adjust the diet for weight control. For most children, the goal will be to slow down the rate of weight gain for height. For some extremely obese children (more than 40% above ideal weight for height), some weight loss may be desired. Degree of obesity can be estimated by subtracting the child's actual weight from their desirable weight (mean weight for the child's height). Both actual and desirable weights should be plotted on the child's growth chart and explained to the parents.

It is important for physician, parent, and child (depending on age) to agree on a treatment goal. Whether a physician recommends weight loss, maintenance of the same weight, or a reduced rate of weight gain for each inch grown depends on the age of the child, the severity of the obesity, and the presence of other health problems that are exacerbated by the

Table 54-12 Dietary Prescription for Nutrition Counseling*					
	SERVINGS PER DAY				NOTES
Grains (servings)	5	6	7	8	80 cal/serving
Meat (ounces)	5	5	6	6	60 cal/oz.
Vegetables (servings)	3	3	3	3	<25 cal/serving
Fruit (pieces)	3	3	3	4	60 cal/serving
Milk, skim (glasses)	2	3	3	3	90 cal/serving
Fat (teaspoons)	3	4	4	5	5 gm/tsp
Calories/day	1200	1400	1500	1700	

* Fat: 25–30% calories; carbohydrate 50–55%; protein 15–20%

NOTE: % of calories from fat depends on type of meat served and whether or not skim milk or a higher-fat milk is used. For obese children, choose caloric intake level that is 10–25% below usual intake level, depending on goal of therapy.

obesity (such as high blood pressure or lipid disorders). For superobese children (>40% above ideal weight), some weight loss is usually recommended. For young or mildly obese children, maintenance of weight or reduction of rate of gain may be preferred.

A reasonable goal is to have the child lose 1 lb per week (4 lb per month) until the first goal is reached. To lose 1 lb, 3500 kcal must be eliminated through a combination of decreased caloric intake (diet) and increased caloric expenditure (exercise). The average 9- to 10-year-old child takes in 2000 kcal/day; thus, placing an obese 10-year-old on a 1500-calorie diet should result in a 1 lb/wk weight loss since this represents a 500 kcal/day decrease.

Older teens (especially boys) who have been consuming as much as 3000 kcal/day may have to be brought down gradually to 2500, then 2000, and perhaps even 1500 kcal/day depending on motivation and desire for rapidity of weight loss. Conversely, children under age 10 may need a diet containing fewer than 1500 kcal/day to lose weight.

Implementation of the diet requires an understanding of portion size and allowable food exchanges, and it is most effective when this counseling is provided with the help of a registered dietician. Lists of exchanges can be provided to parents and children, along with the number of exchanges recommended for each food group. An advantage to using this system is that many of the parents will have used it previously if they belonged to Weight Watchers (Table 54-12). Successful implementation of the diet also requires application of behavior modification strategies and parental support.

Not all excess weight in children is fat, however, with up to 50% of excess weight being fat-free mass in some obese individuals. Obese children on the average have increased lean body mass (more muscle and bone is needed to support the excess weight) and increased basal metabolic rate (BMR) compared to lean children and may need increased protein intake during caloric restriction to avoid negative nitrogen balance and loss of lean body mass.

Although it is theoretically possible to achieve weight loss with reduced calorie intake alone, there are compelling reasons for combining caloric reduction with increased caloric expenditure through physical activity. Indeed, the most successful weight-reduction programs appear to be those that combine diet with exercise within a matrix of behavior modification. Twenty minutes of walking, dancing, swimming, or cycling or 10 minutes of running might burn off 100 calories or more, depending on weight. The more calories expended, the less restrictive the diet must be to lose 1 lb per week. The goal of eliminating 500 calories per day can be achieved through any combination of reduced caloric intake and increased physical activity (the "design-it-yourself" diet). Children may be able to lose weight with exercise alone if compensatory caloric increase does not occur.

The best rationale for combining diet and exercise is based on consideration of the metabolic aspects of dieting. Caloric restriction often results in a drop in BMR, making it harder to lose weight. In addition, caloric restriction may result in a loss of lean body mass (as much as 37% of weight lost may be lean body mass). This can be avoided by increasing physical activity, which increases BMR and lean body mass. Basal metabolic rate often remains elevated for several hours after vigorous exercise. Therefore, effective weight reduction is most likely to occur when a combination of diet and exercise is recommended.

SUMMARY

Cardiovascular disease is the leading cause of death in the United States. Although the vast majority of deaths occur in adult life, evidence points to the origins of atherosclerosis in childhood. Atherosclerotic lesions have been demonstrated in the arteries of children at autopsy and are correlated with traditional risk factors for coronary heart disease: cigarette smoking, elevated blood pressure, and abnormal serum lipid levels. More recently, it has been recognized that these coronary heart disease risk factors can be easily identified in children, are highly prevalent in pediatric populations, tend to be persistent and "track" over time, and are largely caused by lifestyle habits acquired early in life, such as a high-fat/low-fiber diet, and lack of regular physical activity. Thus the primary prevention of heart disease must begin in childhood.

Risk status in childhood, beginning with assessment of inherited risk based on family history of premature coronary heart disease and other cardiovascular disease, can be easily evaluated, treated, and followed over time. Promotion of dietary goals through family nutrition counseling, prevention of obesity, avoidance of cigarette smoking, and encouragement of increased daily physical activity are all parts of the prescription needed to prevent cardiovascular disease in a child's future. These goals are best achieved through a population-wide strategy aimed at reducing cardiovascular risk status in all children over 2 years of age through promoting healthier child and family lifestyles. At the same time, this approach would be complemented by strategies to reduce risk status in children with significantly elevated risk factors. Achievement of these goals will require the coordinated efforts of health professionals, schools, mass media, industry, and government. The importance of evaluating and treating CVD risk factors in childhood is based on scientific reports and epidemiologic studies demonstrating that: 1) atherosclerotic lesions begin in childhood, 2) risk factors promoting the development of atherosclerosis are common among children, 3) elevated risk factor levels tend to persist ("track") over time, and 4) lifestyle habits that increase CVD risk are established in childhood (e.g., diet, physical activity, cigarette smoking). Evaluation, treatment, and follow-up of high risk children constitute the core of pediatric preventive cardiology.

Guidelines for evaluating and treating children with one or more elevated CHD risk factors have only recently begun to be formulated. However, consensus is growing that atherosclerosis begins in childhood and that primary prevention of this insidious, and eventually highly fatal, disease must also begin with children. The potential impact of pediatric interventions could be great. Health risks and benefits, as well as economic impact, must all be carefully and continually assessed, however, as we gain more experience in this relatively new field of preventive pediatrics.

REFERENCES

1. Drash A. Atherosclerosis, cholesterol and the pediatrician. J Pediatr 1972;80:693.

2. Kannel WB, Dawber TR. Atherosclerosis as a pediatric problem. J Pediatr 1972;80:544.

3. McMillan GC. Development of arteriosclerosis. Am J Cardiol 1973;31:542.

4. Williams CL, Wynder EL. A blind spot in preventive medicine. JAMA 1976;236:2196–2197.

5. Mitchell SC, ed. Symposium on prevention of atherosclerosis at the pediatric level. Am J Cardiol 1973;31:539.

6. Williams CL. Preventing heart attacks: a pediatric priority. N Y Med Q 1987;7:96–100.

7. Davidson DM, Doyle EJ Jr. Family-directed preventive cardiology. J Fam Pract 1984;18:57.

8. Wynder EL, Berenson GC, Strong WB, et al. Coronary artery disease prevention: cholesterol—A pediatric perspective. Prev Med 1989;18:323–409.

9. Strong WB, Dennison BA. Pediatric preventive cardiology: atherosclerosis and coronary heart disease. Pediatr Rev 1988;9:303–314.

10. Nora JJ. Identifying the child at risk for coronary disease as in an adult: a strategy for prevention. J Pediatr 1980;97:706.

11. Enos WF, Holmes RD, Beyer J. Coronary disease among United States soldiers killed in action in Korea: preliminary report. JAMA 1953;152:1090–1093. [Reprinted as Landmark Article, JAMA 1986;256:2859–2862.]

12. McNamara JJ, Molot MA, Stremple JF. Coronary artery disease in combat casualties in Vietnam. JAMA 1971;216:1185–1187.

13. Holman RL, McGill HC, Strong JP, Geer JC. The natural history of atherosclerosis: the early aortic lesions as seen in New Orleans, in the middle of the 20th century. Am J Pathol 1958;34:209.

14. Strong JP, McGill HC Jr. Pediatric aspects of atherosclerosis. J Atherosclerosis Res 1969;9:251–265.

15. McGill HC Jr, Eggen DA, Strong JP. Atherosclerotic lesions in the aorta and coronary arteries of man. In: Roberts JC Jr, Straus R, eds. Comparative atherosclerosis. New York: Harper & Row, 1965:311–326.

16. Stary HC. Evolution and progression of atherosclerosis in the coronary arteries of children and adults. In: Bates SR, Gangloff EC, eds. Atherosclerosis and aging. New York: Springer-Verlag, 1987:20–36.

17. Newman WP III, Freedman DS, Voors AW, et al. Relation of serum lipoprotein levels and systolic blood pressure to early atherosclerosis: the Bogalusa Heart Study. N Engl J Med 1986;314:138.

18. Berwick DM, Cretin S, Keeler E. Cholesterol, children and heart disease. New York: Oxford Univ Press, 1980.

19. Williams CL. Pediatric risk factors for major chronic disease. St. Louis: Warren Green, 1984.

20. Berenson GS, ed. Causation of cardiovascular risk factors in children: perspectives on cardiovascular risk in early life. New York: Raven, 1986.

21. Lauer RM, Shekelle RB. Childhood prevention of atherosclerosis and hypertension. New York: Raven, 1980.

22. Williams CL, Carter BJ, Wynder EL. Prevalence of selected cardiovascular and cancer risk factors in a pediatric population: the "Know Your Body" Project, New York, USA. Prev Med 1981;10:235–250.

23. Lauer RM, Connor WE, Leaverton PE, et al. Coronary heart disease risk factors in school children: the Muscatine Study. J Pediatr 1975;86:697–706.

24. Morrison JA, Glueck CJ. Pediatric risk factors for adult coronary heart disease: primary atherosclerosis prevention. Cardiovasc Res 1981;2:1269–1275.

25. Golubjatnikov R, Paskey T, Inhorn SL. Serum cholesterol levels of Mexican and Wisconsin school children. Am J Epidemiol 1972;96:36–39.

26. Puska P, Vartianen E, Pallonen U. The North Karelia Youth Project. Prev Med 1981;10:133–148.

27. Kromhout D, Haar F, Hautvast JGAJ. Coronary heart disease risk factors in Dutch school children. Prev Med 1977;6:500–513.

28. Wynder EL, Williams CL, Laakso K, Levenstein M. Screening for risk factors for chronic disease in children from fifteen countries. Prev Med 1981;10:121–132.

29. Kafatos AG, Panagiotakopoulos G, Bastakis N. Cardiovascular risk factor status of Greek adolescents in Athens. Prev Med 1981;10:173–186.

30. Tell GS, Vellar O, Monrad-Hansen HP. Risk factors for chronic diseases in Norwegian school children. Prev Med 1981;10:211–225.

31. Knuiman JT, Hermus RJJ, Hautvast JGAJ. Serum total and high-density lipoprotein cholesterol concentrations in rural and urban boys from 16 countries. Atherosclerosis 1980;36:529–537.

32. Williams CL, Carter BJ, Wynder EL, Blumenfeld TA. Selected chronic disease "Risk Factors" in two elementary school populations: a pilot study. Am J Dis Child 1979;133:704–708.

33. Wilmore JH, McNamara JJ. Prevalence of coronary heart disease risk factors in boys, 9–12 years of age. J Pediatr 1974;84:527–533.

34. Gotto AM Jr, Pownall HJ, Havel RJ. Introduction to the plasma lipoproteins. Methods Enzymol 1986;3:128–135.

35. Brown MS, Goldstein JL. How LDL receptors influence cholesterol and atherosclerosis. Sci Am 1984;25:58–62.

36. Brown MS, Goldstein JL. Lipoprotein receptors in the liver: Control signals for plasma cholesterol traffic. J Clin Invest 1983;72:743–748.

37. Brown MS, Goldstein JL. A receptor-mediated pathway for cholesterol homeostasis. Science 1986;34:232–235.

38. Blankenhorn DH, Nessim SA, Johnson RL, et al. Beneficial effects of combined colestipol niacin therapy on coronary atherosclerosis and coronary venous bypass grafts. JAMA 1987;257:3233–3240.

39. Consensus Conference Panel. Lowering blood cholesterol to prevent heart disease. JAMA 1986;253:2080–2084.

40. Christensen B, Glueck C, Kwiterovich P. Plasma cholesterol and triglyceride distribution in 13,665 children and adolescents: the Prevalence Study of the LRC Program. Pediatr Res 1980;14:194.

41. Cardiovascular profile of 15,000 children of school age in three communities, 1971–1975. Washington, DC: US Dept. of Health and Human Services, Public Health Service, National Institutes of Health, National Heart, Lung, and Blood Institute, 1978. DHEW pub. no. (NIH) 78-1472.

42. Lipid Research Clinics Program. Population studies data book, vol. 1: the prevalence study. Washington, DC: US Dept. of Health and Human Services, Public Health Service, National Institutes of Health, National Heart, Lung, and Blood Institute, 1980. DHHS pub. no. (NIH) 80-1527.

43. Resnicow K, Kotchen JM, Wynder EL. Plasma cholesterol Levels of 6,685 children in the United States. Pediatrics 1989;84:969–976.

44. Berenson GS, Srinivasan SR, Cresanta JL, et al. Dynamic changes of serum lipoproteins in children during adolescence and sexual maturation. Am J Epidemiol 1981;113:157–170.

45. Stanbury JB, Wyngaarden JB, Fredrickson DS, et al, eds. The metabolic basis of inherited disease. 5th ed. New York: McGraw-Hill, 1989.

46. Goldbourt U, Neufeld HN. Genetic aspects of arteriosclerosis. Arteriosclerosis 1986;6:357–363.

47. Garn SM, Clark DC, Guire KE. Growth, body composition and development of obese and lean children. In: Winick M, ed. Childhood obesity. New York: Wiley, 1976.

48. Garn SM, Clark DC. Trends in fatness and the origins of obesity. Pediatrics 1976;57:443–456.

49. Garn SM, Bailey SM, Cole PE. Synchronous fatness changes in husbands and wives. Am J Clin Nutr 1979;32:2375–2377.

50. Martin RJ, Ramsay T, Hausman GJ. Adipocyte development. Pediatr Ann 1984;13:448–452.

51. Dietz WH, Gortmaker SL. Do we fatten our children at the TV set? Pediatrics 1985;75:805–812.

52. Rose HE, Mayer J. Activity, caloric intake, fat storage and the energy balance of infants. Ped 1968;41:18–23.

53. Abram S, Caroll MD, Najjar MF, Robinson MF. Obese and overweight adults in the United States. In: Vital and health statistics. Hyattsville, MD: US Department of Health and Human Services, NCHS Series 11, No. 230, 1982. Pub. No. (PHS) 83-1680.

54. Shear CL, Freedman DS, Burke GL, et al. Secular trends of obesity in early life: the Bogalusa Heart Study. Am J Pub Health 1988;78:75–77.

55. Prevalence of overweight among adolescents—United States, 1988–1991. MMWR 1994;43:818–821.

56. Troiano RP, Flegal KM, Kuczmarski RJ, et al. Overweight prevalence and trends for children and adolescents: the National Health and Nutrition Examination Surveys, 1963 to 1991. Arch Pediatr Adolesc Med 1995;149:1085–1091.

57. Update: prevalence of overweight among children, adolescents and adults—United States, 1988–1994. MMWR 1997;4:199–202.

58. Ogden C, Troiano RP, Briefel R, et al. Prevalence of overweight among preschool children in the United States, 1971 through 1994. Pediatrics 1997;99:e1–e13.

59. Fripp RR, Hodgson JL, Kwiterovich PO. Aerobic capacity, obesity and arteriosclerotic risk factors in male adolescents. Pediatrics 1985;75:813–818.

60. Voors AW, Harsha DW, Webber LS. Clustering of anthropometric parameters, glucose intolerance and serum lipids in children. Atherosclerosis 1982;2:346–355.

61. Orchard TJ, Donahue RP, Kuller LH, et al. Cholesterol screening in childhood: does it predict adult hypercholesterolemia? The Beaver County experience. J Pediatr 1983;103:687–691.

62. Webber LD, Cresanta JL, Voors AW, Berenson GS. Tracking of cardiovascular disease risk factor variables in school-age children. J Chronic Dis 1983;36:647–660.

63. Freedman DS, Shear CL, Srinivasan SR, et al. Tracking of serum lipids and lipoproteins in children over an 8-year period: the Bogalusa Heart Study. Prev Med 1985;14:203–216.

64. Clarke WR, Schrott HG, Leaverton PE, et al. Tracking of blood lipids and blood pressures in school age children: the Muscatine Study. Circulation 1978;58:626–634.

65. Weidman W, Kwiterovich P Jr, Jesse MJ, Nugent E. Task Force Committee of the Nutrition Committee and the Cardiovascular Disease in the Young Council of the American Heart Association: diet in the healthy child. Circulation 1986;74:1411A–1414A.

66. National Cholesterol Education Program. Report of the Expert Panel on Blood Cholesterol Levels in Children and Adolescents. Bethesda, MD: National Heart, Lung, and Blood Institute, 1991. (NIH publication no. 91-2732.)

67. National Center for Health Statistics, Carroll MD, Abraham S, Dresser CM. Dietary intake source data: United States 1976–80. In: Vital and health statistics, series II, no. 231. Hyattsville, MD: U.S. Department of Health and Human Services, Public Health Service, National Center for Health Statistics, 1993. DHHS pub. no. (PHS) 83-1681.

68. Braitman LE, Adkin EV, Stanton JL. Obesity and caloric intake: the National Health and Nutrition Examination Survey of 1971–1975 (NHANES I). J Chron Dis 1985;38:727–732.

69. National Center for Health Statistics, Carroll MD, Abraham S, Dresser CM. Dietary intake source data: United States 1976–80. In: Vital and health statistics, series II, no. 231. Hyattsville, MD: U.S. Department of Health and Human Services, Public Health Service, National Center for Health Statistics, 1993. DHHS pub. no. (PHS) 83-1681.

70. Daily dietary fat and total food energy intakes: National Health and Nutrition Examination Survey (NHANES III), phase 1:1988–1991. MMWR 1994;43:116–117, 123–125.

71. Human Nutrition Information Service. U.S. Dept. of Agriculture, 1991.

72. American Academy of Pediatrics. Carbohydrate and dietary fiber. In: Pediatric nutrition handbook, 3rd ed. Elk Grove Village, IL: American Academy of Pediatrics 1993:100–106.

73. Ellison RC, Morris, Donahue RO, et al. Effects of changing type of breakfast on total dietary fat and cholesterol intake and blood cholesterol. 2nd Int. Conf. on Preventive Cardiology; June 18, 1989: Washington, DC. Abstract.

74. Resnicow KL, Cohn L, Reinhardt J. The relationship between breakfast habits, plasma cholesterol and Quetelet Index in 530 school children. ADA Annual Meeting; October 23, 1989; Kansas City, MO.

75. Crest Special Study. Washington, DC: National Restaurant Association, 1988.

76. The health consequences of smoking: cardiovascular disease; a report of the Surgeon General. Washington, D.C.: U.S. Dept. of Health and Human Services, 1983.

77. Slone D, Shapiro S, Rosenberg L, et al. Relation of cigarette smoking to myocardial infarction in young women. N Engl J Med 1978;298:1273–1276.

78. National Cancer Institute. Smoking and health: a program to reduce the risk of disease in smokers. Washington, DC: US Dept. of Health, Education and Welfare, 1983.

79. Craig WY, Palomaki BS, Johnson AM, Haddow JE. Cigarette smoking-associated changes in blood lipid and lipoprotein levels in the 8- to 19-year old age group: a meta-analysis. Pediatrics 1990;85:155–158.

80. Moskowitz WB, Mosteller M, Schieken RM, et al. Lipoprotein and oxygen transport alterations in passive smoking preadolescent children. Circulation 1990;81:586–592.

81. Frolicher VF, Oberman A. Analysis of epidemiologic studies of physical inactivity as a risk factor for coronary artery disease. Prog Cardiovasc Dis 1972;15:41–65.

82. Thompson PD. What do muscles have to do with lipoproteins. Circulation 1990;81:1428–1430.

83. Strong WB, Wilmore JH. Unfit kids: an office-based approach to physical fitness. Contemp Pediatr 1988;5:33–48.

84. AHA Committee for Atherosclerosis and Hypertension in Childhood. Coronary risk factor modification in children: exercise. Circulation 1986;74:1189A–1191A.

85. Webber LD, Cresanta JL, Voors AW, Berenson GS. Tracking of cardiovascular disease risk factor variables in school-age children. J Chronic Dis 1983;36:647–660.

86. Freedman DS, Shear CL, Srinivasan SR, et al. Tracking of serum lipids and lipoproteins in children over an 8-year period: the Bogalusa Heart Study. Prev Med 1985;14:203–216.

87. Webber LS, Srinivasan SR, Berenson GS. Tracking of serum lipids and lipoproteins over 12 years into young adulthood: the

Bogalusa Heart Study. Circulation 1988;78(suppl 2):481. Abstract.

88. Toda A, Okuni M. Tracking of blood lipids in school age children. J Jap Pediatr Soc 1987; 91:3245.

89. Freedman DS, Srinivasan SR, Cresanta SR, et al. Cardiovascular risk factors from birth to seven years of age: Bogalusa Heart Study. IV. Serum lipids and lipoproteins. Pediatrics 1987; 80(suppl 2):789–796.

90. Clarke WR, Schrott HG, Leaverton PE, et al. Tracking of blood lipids and blood pressures in school age children: the Muscatine Study. Circulation 1978;58:626–634.

91. Lauer RM, Lee J, Clarke WR. Factors affecting the relationship between childhood and adult cholesterol levels: the Muscatine Study. Pediatrics 1988;82:309–318.

92. Lauer RM, Clarke WE, Beaglehole R. Level, trend and variability of blood pressure during childhood: the Muscatine Study. Circulation 1984;69:242–249.

93. Garcia RE, Moodie DS. Routine cholesterol surveillance in childhood. Pediatrics 1989;84:751–755.

94. Wynder EL, Berenson G, Strong WB, Williams CL. Coronary artery disease prevention: cholesterol— A pediatric perspective. Prev Med 1989;18:323–409.

95. National Cholesterol Education Program. Report of the Expert Panel on Blood Cholesterol Levels in Children and Adolescents. Bethesda, MD: National

Heart, Lung, and Blood Institute, 1991. (NIH publication no. 91-2732.)

96. Griffen TC, Cristoffel KK, Binns HJ, MacGuire PA. Family history evaluation as a predictive screen for childhood hypercholesterolemia. Pediatrics 1989;84: 365–373.

97. Davidson DM, Iftner CA, Bradley BJ. Family history predictors of high blood cholesterol levels in 4th grade school children. J Pediatr Health Care 1989;3:3–8.

98. Medici F, Puder D, Williams C. Cholesterol screening in the pediatric office. In: Williams CL, ed. Hyperlipidemia in childhood and the development of atherosclerosis. Ann N Y Acad Sci 1991; 623:248–252.

99. American Academy of Pediatrics, Committee on Nutrition. Indications for cholesterol testing in children. Pediatrics 1989;83: 141–142.

100. American Academy of Pediatrics, Committee on Nutrition. Towards a prudent diet for children. Pediatrics 1983;71:78–80.

101. Willett ML, Reynolds RD, Cotrell-Hoehner S, et al. Validation of a semi-quantitative food frequency questionnaire: comparison with a 1-year diet record. J Am Diet Assoc 1987;87:43–47.

102. Williams CL. Treatment of childhood obesity in pediatric practice. In: Williams CL, Kimm SYS, eds. Prevention and treatment of childhood obesity. Ann N Y Acad Sci 993;699:207–219.

103. Williams CL, Spark A. Guidelines for evaluation and treatment of

children with elevated cholesterol. In: Williams CL, ed. Hyperlipidemia in childhood and the development of atherosclerosis. Ann N Y Acad Sci 1991;623: 239–252.

104. Williams CL. Strategies for implementing an AHA step I diet in children. In: Williams CL, ed. Hyperlipidemia in childhood and the development of atherosclerosis. Ann N Y Acad Sci 1991; 623:253–262.

105. Dwyer J. Diets for children and adolescents that meet dietary goals. Am J Dis Child 1980;134: 1073–1080.

106. Williams CL, Bollella M, Wynder E. A new recommendation for dietary fiber in childhood. Pediatrics 1995;96(suppl):985–988.

107. Williams CL. Importance of dietary fiber in childhood. J Am Diet Assoc 1995;95:1140–1146.

108. Williams CL, Bollella M, Spark A, Puder D. Effectiveness of psyllium fiber in the treatment of children with hypercholesterolemia. J Am Coll Nutr 1995; 14:251–257.

109. Kwiterovich PO. The role of fiber in the treatment of hypercholesterolemia in children and adolescents. Pediatrics 1995; 98(suppl):1005–1009.

110. Pugliese MT, Weyman-Daum M, Moses N, Lifshitz F. Parental beliefs as a cause of nonorganic failure to thrive. Pediatrics 1987; 80:175–178.

111. Lifshitz F, Moses N. Growth failure. Am J Dis Child 1989; 143:537–542.

Part X.

PEDIATRIC FITNESS

Edited by
Patty S. Freedson

Introduction to Pediatric Fitness

Patty S. Freedson

In recent years, the study of children and exercise has become a major topic of interest for researchers and health professionals alike. Exploring children's responses to exercise and the developmental changes that occur during growth and maturation, studying the determinants of physical activity among youth, and examining how children's physical activity and exercise relate to current and future health outcomes are just a few of the areas of inquiry in the area of pediatric fitness. In examining the literature in these areas, one sees that there has been a blurring of the boundaries among the disciplines that are interested in studying children and physical activity. For example, exercise physiologists, exercise epidemiologists, exercise endocrinologists, and health care professionals have all contributed to our expanding body of knowledge related to pediatric exercise. In this section on pediatric fitness, the authors present state of the art reviews on selected topics pertaining to various aspects of children and exercise.

In the first chapter, Betsy Keller reviews the literature on gender differences in the development of fitness. She first examines how body composition, body size, and fitness develop between early childhood and adolescence. She then examines how and when gender differences in these characteristics emerge and what factors have been identified to explain the origins of gender differences in childhood and youth fitness.

William Kraemer, Avery Faigenbaum, Jill Bush, and Bradley Nindl cover the topic of the effects of resistance training in youth and its impact on muscle fitness. The trainability of children with regard to strength is initially discussed to answer the question whether or not children respond to resistance training. This is followed by a discussion of the potential physiologic mechanisms underlying strength development. The effects of resistance training on injury prevention and risk for injury among children and adolescents is presented followed by a summary of what is known regarding the health benefits of resistance training.

In Chapter 57, Stella Volpe and Penny Rosenzweig describe the interaction between iron and endurance performance in adolescents. The first section of their chapter discusses iron metabolism, iron turnover, and iron loss, as well as iron deficiency and its metabolic and physiologic effects. What is known about the effect of iron depletion and iron-deficiency anemia on exercise performance in adolescence and adults is summarized. Strategies to detect and prevent iron-deficiency anemia are presented to conclude the chapter.

In the next chapter, Brian Miller and Mary Jane De Souza explore the impact of exercise on reproductive function and pubertal development. The chapter begins with a review of the basic physiology and endocrinology of reproduction and pubertal development. Current controversies regarding the causes and consequences of late menarche are discussed. The role of nutrition, energy availability, and body composition in pubertal development is followed by a concluding section, which discusses potential health consequences of delayed menarche.

In the last chapter in this section, Stewart Trost and Russell Pate present a descriptive analysis of the physical activity patterns of children and adolescents. Their approach to this topic begins with a summary of current physical activity guidelines and standards for children and youth. This is followed by an analysis of whether or not children and youth satisfy these physical activity participation guidelines. The concluding section of the paper discusses what is known about physical activity tracking between adolescence and adulthood. The notion that children and youth should be physically active is at least partially grounded in the belief that physical activity habits and practices during youth carry over to adulthood when activity has been shown to have a positive effect on numerous health outcomes and reduces the risk for numerous chronic diseases.

The broad scope of the topics covered in this section on pediatric fitness should serve as a foundation of knowledge regarding what is known about various issues regarding children and physical activity. Surveillance of physical activities from an epidemiologic perspective identifies trends in physical activity patterns. Examination of how fitness develops with growth and maturation describes the gender differences in fitness characteristics among children and youth. Current controversies related to the mechanisms underlying reproductive development are discussed in the context of exercise and energy availability. The role of iron and iron deficiency and their effects on endurance performance among adolescent athletes is presented and strategies to detect and prevent this problem are covered. Adaptations to resistance training among children and youth and guidelines for resistance training in this population provide evidence for the benefits of developing muscular fitness in youth.

The physiologic effects of exercise and health implications of various types of physical activity is the common theme among these papers. As we approach the twenty-first century, these issues related to children's physical activity will continue to attract much interest in the research arena and among practitioners who attempt to improve and maintain the health of youth.

Chapter 55

Gender Differences in the Development of Fitness

Betsy Keller

During the developmental years from birth through young adulthood, the cardiovascular, musculoskeletal, endocrine, and nervous systems undergo substantial changes. Consequently, parameters of fitness, including aerobic and anaerobic power, strength, motor performance, and body composition exhibit concomitant changes during this time. In adults, gender differences are typically observed in all of these parameters. It is unclear to what extent the differences are due to inherent, biologic factors as opposed to environmental factors such as physical activity history, training, and/or sociocultural biases that restrict or promote learning and practice of motor activities. It is evident that body size and composition impact physical performance and are responsible for some of the observed gender variation. Thus, the development of gender differences in body size and composition may coincide with the development of gender differences in performance.

Recently, studies have sought to minimize environmental sources of variation between genders (training, physical activity history, etc.) to more accurately quantify true biologic gender differences in performance. However, relatively few longitudinal studies have examined this problem in children, and it is apparent that the period of greatest gender dimorphism occurs at puberty. We have yet to determine the impact of body size differences prior to, during, and following puberty on the magnitude of gender differences in fitness.

This chapter will examine how body size, composition, and parameters of fitness change during the developmental years into late adolescence, and at what point in the development of gender differences these variables appear. The chapter will begin with a discussion of the development of body size and composition so the reader will understand how changes during growth and maturation impact fitness parame-

ters, and the degree to which they may explain the development of gender differences in fitness. The chapter will conclude with a brief examination of sociocultural considerations for gender differences in the development of fitness.

DEVELOPMENTAL AND GENDER DIFFERENCES IN BODY SIZE AND COMPOSITION

Body size and composition necessarily impact physical performance, and the relationship is particularly significant during the developmental years. Body size and composition partially determine several performance related indices such as strength, aerobic capacity, and many measures of motor function during pre-, peri-, and postpubertal years. The manifestation of size-related factors is a function of genes, hormones, nutrition, and environment (1). Throughout adulthood, however, performance is determined to a greater degree by training and practice, whereas size and composition are factors that modify performance. To begin to explain the interrelationships between body size, composition, gender, and fitness, it is important to first understand changes in body composition as a function of growth and development.

Stature

The rate and magnitude of linear growth are determined primarily by genetics and less so by environmental factors. Assuming an energy balance with adequate nutrient composition and normal hormonal development, stature and limb lengths are less influenced by environmental factors such as physical activity than by other body size variables including circumferences, breadths, skinfolds, and weight (1). The rate of linear growth varies throughout childhood and adolescence. It is greatest within the first months of life, increasing at a rate of 30 cm/yr. By age 5, linear growth slows to 7 cm/yr, and is maintained at about 5.5 cm/yr until it decreases briefly, but substantially, shortly before puberty (2).

Gender differences in linear growth become apparent shortly before puberty when the rate of growth accelerates in females at around the age of 10, and peaks (termed peak height velocity, PHV) at 10.5 cm/yr at about age 12. Linear growth correlates fairly well with plasma levels of somatomedin-C (IGF-1) which is characteristically higher in early pubescent females (age 8–10) compared to males (3). Thereafter, the rate of linear growth slows, and stops at around age 15, when epiphyseal fusion is complete. In contrast, the rate of linear growth in males begins to accelerate by 12 years, 2 years later than in females, and PHV of 12 cm/yr occurs around age 14. Linear growth in males is generally completed by age 16 or 17. Although males reach PHV later than females, the greater rate of growth and 2 additional years of growing result in a typical gender difference in stature of about 13 cm (2,4,5). By the end of the PHV growth spurt, the rate of growth decelerates rapidly, with the attainment of 98% of adult height for females at age 14, and males at age 16 (5).

Weight

During the first 2 years of life, the rate of weight gain decreases from 10 kg/yr to 2 kg/yr for females and males. The rate of weight gain increases to about 3 kg/yr throughout childhood until puberty. At puberty, gender differences in the rate of weight gain become evident (2).

Similar to linear growth patterns, females achieve a peak weight velocity (PWV) of 8.5 kg/yr at about age 12, compared to males who reach a greater PWV of 9.5 kg/yr around the age of 14. Thus, females are typically heavier than males at the ages of 12 to 14, before the onset of PWV in males (2). Soon thereafter, PWV decreases to less than 1 kg/yr for females at age 15, and males at age 17 (6).

Skeletal Maturity

Malina defines maturity as the tempo and timing of progress toward the mature state (4). Measures most often used to gauge the degree of maturity include skeletal (skeletal age), pubertal (secondary sex characteristics; e.g., Tanner staging), and/or somatic (age at PHV) indices. In children and adolescents, chronologic age is not a good predictor of maturity, and as such does not adequately indicate the completion of critical growth related to bone, muscle mass, body size, and weight. Thus, when evaluating children for participation in sports and physical activity, chronologic age alone will not sufficiently reveal the degree of bone development, sexual maturation (which is related to development of fat-free mass), and body size. Consequently, children who compete based on chronologic age are not necessarily matched for muscle mass, skeletal maturity, or body weight, and may be at greater risk for injury. However, the aforementioned estimates of maturity are not practical (Tanner staging), involve risk (radiation to determine skeletal age), or cannot be assessed until puberty (age at PHV), thus prompting the development of other noninvasive estimates of maturity (7). The application of a simple, noninvasive measure of maturity would be useful for physical

educators and coaches, particularly for boys, in whom maturity and strength-dependent performance are closely related. For further discussion regarding procedures to assess maturity see Malina (4).

More recently, skeletal maturity has been assessed with dual energy x-ray absorptiometry (DEXA). DEXA provides a safe, noninvasive means to assess whole body and regional bone density and body composition. Total body bone mineral content (TBMC) of girls and boys matched for Tanner stages 1 and 2 (age 5–13) is similar between stages and between genders. In contrast, for Tanner stages 4 and 5 (age 12 to 18), only boys have greater TBMC in stage 5 compared to 4, but in both stages boys have greater TBMC than girls. These data suggest that bone development is similar in females and males prior to puberty, and males continue to increase bone density throughout puberty (8). Others have reported similar findings for prepubertal females and males, and also observed greater prepubertal TBMC in black children compared to white children. However, the racial differences in TBMC appear to be related to body mass and fat-free mass, not ethnicity, gender, or height (9).

It appears that females achieve peak bone mass by age 15 or 16, much earlier than previously thought (10,11), whereas males reach peak bone mass by age 20 (12). Furthermore, cortical bone thickness and bone width increase during and immediately after puberty to a greater extent in males (5), a difference that favors males throughout adulthood (13).

Body Composition

Substantial changes in body composition occur throughout childhood and are most evident around puberty. Methodological problems have impacted the accurate quantification of developmental changes in body composition in young and pubertal children. The two-compartment model used in many studies to assess fat mass and fat-free mass violated some important underlying assumptions when applied to young and prepubertal children. Most notably, tissue density was assumed to be constant across subjects when, in fact, considerable variation occurs prior to adulthood. The prepubertal child has a higher water and lower bone mineral and potassium content compared to an adult, resulting in a characteristically lower density of fat-free mass. The percentage of total body water relative to body weight (%TBW) decreases from approximately 78% at birth to 60% at 1 year of age, where it approximates adult values, and the distribution of body water gradually shifts from extracellular to intracellular with maturation. It appears that %TBW fluctuates during childhood but it is not clear to what extent. However, gender differences in %TBW are evident during puberty when %TBW decreases in females from 61% to 54%, whereas it increases in males from 61% to 65% (14). Thus, changes in density of the fat-free body during growth and maturation are largely a function of changes in fat-free water content. Furthermore, the rate and magnitude of change of fat-free water content varies with gender from before (females, 76%; males, 78%) to after puberty, and may not stabilize at adult values of 71% to 73% until approximately age 15. As discussed previously, the bone mineral content of the fat-free body in prepubertal children is approximately 7% less than in adults, and postpubertal gender differences in BMC would theoretically yield a lower fat-free density in adult females. Since chemical maturity is not attained until mid to late adolescence, estimates of body composition in children and youth must be viewed with caution. Further discussion of body composition assessment and tissue density in children can be found in Houtkooper et al (15), Lohman et al (16), and Slaughter et al (17).

Advances in the development of population and age-specific regression equations, and technology to utilize three- and four-compartment models of body composition (e.g., fat, fat-free minus bone, bone, TBW) have increased the accuracy of body composition assessment in children. However, the interaction of growth, maturation, and physical activity and/or training on body composition make it difficult to isolate normal growth related changes in fat and fat-free mass.

Fat-free mass reflects muscle mass, and in most girls and boys with normal activity patterns (those not training for athletic competition) is similar prior to puberty (5,8,18,19). However, small differences in muscle mass have been reported to favor males as early as age 7 (20). Muscle mass begins to increase in both sexes in early puberty, and gender dimorphism is evident soon thereafter. When grouped according to Tanner stage, gender differences in fat-free mass are small and nonsignificant during Tanner stages 1 and 2 (ages 5 to 13), but are clearly evident during Tanner stages 4 and 5 (age 12 to 18). It is also interesting to note that the increase in total body bone mass in males during Tanner stages 4 and 5 contributes an additional 0.5 kg to the gender differences in the fat-free body (8).

The pattern of accretion of fat-free mass varies by gender as well. A comparison of upper (arm) and lower (calf) body muscle breadths or cross-sectional area (CSA) between genders indicates that the pattern of gain is similar for both genders for the calf, but arm muscle breadth increases at a greater rate in males at and following puberty (20,21,22). Although muscle CSA increases at a greater rate in males, it gradually increases in females as well up to age 17, and then stabilizes. Upon maturity, gender differences in muscle CSA are larger for the upper versus lower extremity, which represents a pattern of muscle growth that has been reported previously (23). Cross-sectional data revealed that by age 6, muscle CSA for females was 94% of muscle CSA for males, but by the twenties was reduced to 55% (21).

Gender differences in body fat are apparent at birth and persist throughout childhood as indicated by greater fat mass in females throughout childhood and puberty (21,24,25). The pattern of fat deposition does not appear to be gender specific prior to puberty, as there is little gender difference in skinfolds at central and peripheral sites (23,26,27). The gender variation in total body fat prior to puberty cannot be accounted for by hormonal differences since they are small in this age range, thus it is difficult to offer a biologic explanation for greater fat mass in preadolescent females. There is some recent cross-sectional evidence, however, of gender-dependent changes in insulin sensitivity during Tanner stages 2 and 3 that are related to body fatness. In girls, insulin sensitivity correlated inversely with body mass index and IGF-1 levels. The relationship was stronger in females who had obese parents. In boys, insulin sensitivity was inversely related to fat mass and Tanner stage (28). Further longitudinal investigation is needed in which growth hormone is studied in conjunction with insulin and IGF-1 to clarify the relationship of gender, insulin, and body fatness during development.

Gender dimorphism in fat mass, relative fat (% fat), and pattern of deposition becomes increasingly evident at puberty, or around age 12 to 13 for girls, and follows a pattern of greater fat gain in the truncal region versus extremities (29). However, fat CSA also increases in the extremities of females, in contrast to a decrease in fat CSA in the extremities of males (21). When categorized by Tanner stage, body fat mass assessed by DEXA increased most between Tanner stages 2 and 4 for both sexes, but when expressed relative to body weight, relative fat increased by 57% in females compared to only 7% in males (8). Following puberty, therefore, females gain body fat at a much greater rate than males, and deposition favors accumulation of fat in the truncal region over the extremities.

Changes in hormone status in females following puberty may explain some of the gender-associated gains in fat, but there remains considerable speculation that a decrease in activity level during puberty contributes to fat accretion. Data from the National Children and Youth Fitness Study (NCYFS) revealed that gender differences in measures of health-related fitness (mile run, chin-ups, and sit-ups) in prepubertal children were explained by differences in physical characteristics (height, weight, skinfolds), whereas following puberty, gender differences were associated with skinfolds and amount of physical activity outside of school (30). Furthermore, a cross-sectional study of body composition and sexual maturation in premenarcheal athletes and nonathletes showed that indices of sexual maturation (height, weight, breast and pubic hair development) were similar between the two groups from ages 7 to 15, whereas relative fat increased in nonathletes and decreased in athletes over this age span (31). Once again, it is difficult to isolate variation in body composition due to genetics, nutrition, training, and environment, but these data are consistent with other reports (4,32,33) that suggest physical activity level to be a confounding factor in the development of adiposity.

DEVELOPMENT OF AEROBIC CAPACITY

Measurement of maximum aerobic power (Vo_2max) is typically achieved with an incremental exercise test. The predominant criteria for evaluating the attainment of Vo_2max is a plateau in oxygen consumption with an increase in workload. However, about 50% of children fail to reach a plateau during an incremental test (34–37). Thus, the term "peak Vo_2" is often discussed in reference to children, and is the highest oxygen uptake measured during a maximal exercise test. Performance on successive maximum graded exercise tests is equally reliable in children (38) compared to adults (39), and peak Vo_2 represents a maximal index of aerobic fitness in children (40,41).

The development of Vo_2max in the mature adult is inextricably tied to the type and degree of physical training (42,43). Vo_2max is most responsive to endurance training (44,45), and has long been considered a marker of endurance capacity in adults (46). However, the relationship between endurance capacity and Vo_2max in children is less clear. Owing in part to the dynamic changes of the cardiopulmonary and musculoskeletal systems, the development of Vo_2max throughout childhood and adolescence is most notably confounded by changes in body size during these periods. Several reports indicate that Vo₂max among prepubertal children is less responsive to aerobic training and is determined to a greater extent by growth related factors (47–51). Others suggest that, in puberty, a critical period or "trigger point" occurs during which hormone activity and sensitivity is maximized. As a result, there is accelerated growth and responsiveness of the cardiovascular stimulus to substantially increase Vo₂max (52). Efforts to document this unique period of endocrine responsiveness suggests such a phenomenon may actually occur, evidenced by increases in linear growth with exercise training during puberty (53), and increases in testosterone and growth hormone levels (54). We have yet, however, to associate the magnitude of endocrine response to a specific critical pubertal stage (55–57). Some studies indicate that training of sufficient intensity and duration can increase Vo₂max in children, probably through enhanced stroke volume (58,59). However, other reports indicate a lack of relationship between Vo₂max (mL/kg per minute) and endurance performance in prepubertal children (60). Improvement in endurance performance without a concomitant increase in Vo₂max may be attributed to increased economy of movement and will be discussed in a subsequent section of this chapter. Independent of body size, absolute Vo₂max (L/min) is determined by several factors that include oxygen delivery variables, peripheral extraction of oxygen, and pulmonary gas exchange. How these factors change in the developing child explain in part the growth-related changes in Vo₂max.

Oxygen Delivery

Oxygen delivery to the muscle is a function of cardiac output (stroke volume × heart rate) and oxygen-carrying capacity. In children, heart rate at a given Vo₂ is higher compared to adults, and implies that cardiac output is compromised by a smaller stroke volume (2). In prepubertal boys between age 11 and 13, stroke volume is highly related to cardiac output and oxygen-carrying capacity (60). The relationship of cardiac dimension, cardiac output, and stroke volume with Vo₂max is largely influenced by body size. As such, chronologic age does not explain satisfactorily the variance in Vo₂ during this phase of maturation. Growth spurts are variable yet contribute to skeletal maturation, therefore it is difficult to predict the age or stage of maturation at which Vo₂max will be greatest. However, peak height velocity generally occurs in males between age 13.5 and 14, and in females between age 11.5 and 12 (61). Because stroke volume is tied closely to body size, it is during these ages that Vo₂max increases at a faster rate compared to the prepubertal stage. The contribution of stroke volume is substantial, as is evident by changes from a preadolescent resting value of 40 mL/beat to 60 mL/beat in an adult male (62). During maximum exercise, young adult males increase resting stroke volume by a factor of 1.99, in contrast to a factor of 1.35 for boys (60). Once again, this change is largely dependent on body and heart size (63) throughout early adolescence and increases fairly linearly with age (61). The rate at which the stroke index (stroke volume related to body surface area) increases from resting to maximum exercise is less in prepubertal children compared to young adults. Potential reasons for this difference may include a reduced myocardial contractility resulting in part from a lower testos-

terone level and/or a reduced sympathetic stimulation in children (60,61). A strong correlation between age and beta-adrenergic receptor density may account for reduced sympathetic stimulation of the ventricular myocardium (64).

Hemoglobin concentration is the primary determinant of oxygen-carrying capacity, and is highly related to peak Vo₂ in children (65). Hemoglobin concentration per unit of body weight increases from childhood and attains adult values late in adolescence (66). Hemoglobin concentration during preadolescence is about 12.9 mg/dL and increases to the average adult value of about 14.0 mg/dL for females and 16.0 mg/dL for males. Consequently, the lower Vo₂max observed in young and prepubertal children relative to late adolescence and adulthood is largely due to a lower hemoglobin concentration, and is tied closely to growth and skeletal maturity (2). Oxygen delivery may be further enhanced in children by higher muscle blood flow compared to adolescents and adults (67,68).

Peripheral Extraction of Oxygen

Oxygen extraction is indicated by arterial-venous oxygen content difference (a-v o₂diff), and is also size and age dependent (69). At near maximal effort, there is little variability in a-v o₂diff across ages. However, age-related changes in submaximal a-v o₂diff are probably related to several factors in older versus younger boys, such as increased oxygen-carrying capacity, skeletal muscle blood flow, oxidative enzymes, myoglobin, and capillary to fiber ratio, all of which are secondary to increasing muscle mass during PHV (69). Peak a-v o₂diff is attained during late adolescence and remains fairly constant into adulthood (70). This growth related change in a-v o₂diff is explained by the increase in slope of the Vo₂/heart rate relationship from pre- to postpubescence. The change in slope varies with body weight and implies that oxygen extraction per heartbeat increases proportionately with body weight in children. Thus in children, regardless of body size, the cardiorespiratory and musculoskeletal systems coordinate during exercise to supply sufficient oxygen for cellular energy requirements. In contrast, oxygen supply during exercise in adults may be mediated to a large degree by training or detraining. For example, cardiac disease diminishes cardiac function. Over time, the heart becomes functionally smaller, and the Vo₂/heart rate relationship becomes characteristically similar to that of young children (71). Therefore, in children, a smaller cardiac output during submaximal and maximal exercise is compensated for with a relatively greater a-v o₂diff (62).

Pulmonary Gas Exchange

In healthy adults, ventilation during submaximal and maximal exercise is generally sufficient to maintain arterial Po₂ and Pco₂ at levels that do not compromise Vo₂ (72). Some work suggests that pulmonary gas exchange during maximal effort in highly trained athletes may compromise Vo₂max due to decreased hemoglobin saturation (73,74). However, this has yet to be demonstrated in children. Alveolar ventilation at a given Vo₂ is similar in both children and adults (75). Changes in maximal ventilation during childhood parallel those observed in absolute Vo₂max (64) and increases with age (72,76) and height (76). Maximal ventilation per kilogram of body weight remains unchanged through adolescence (60), and decreases in early adulthood. Children have less efficient ventilatory responses to exercise as evidenced by a higher ventilatory equivalent for oxygen (Ve/Vo_2) compared to adults (77). This difference may be due to the relative inefficiency observed in children during maximal and submaximal work, thus requiring greater Vo_2 at a given workload (66). It may be that sensitivity to Pco_2 is greater in children resulting in a higher ventilatory response (78), as hyperventilation is often observed in prepubertal children (70).

Dimensional changes in lung capacity and function measured by forced expiratory volume (FEV) and forced expiratory volume in 1 second (FEV_1), correspond to changes in both body size and age (79). Changes in lung volumes increase as the cube of height (80) and are not accounted for by body weight or age alone. Because of the smaller lung volumes in children, tidal volume is also less than that of adults, but to a greater extent than might be predicted based on size (64). This explains in part, why higher respiratory rates are evident in children. Growth-related changes in lung capacity contribute to a decrease in airway resistance (81–84), and decrease the ventilatory work. Maximal effort in children is not limited by ventilation. However, the greater work of ventilation (higher Ve/Vo_2) may limit the intensity of sustained exercise.

Growth-Related Changes in Aerobic Capacity

Maximal aerobic capacity measured in absolute terms (L/min) increases throughout childhood. Prior to puberty it increases 200 mL/min per year due to growth-related changes in components associated with oxygen delivery (blood volume, heart, lung, muscle) (85). When expressed relative to body weight, Vo_2max (mL/kg per minute) is fairly unchanged in early and late prepubescent children. In boys it is about 52 mL/kg per minute and 46 mL/kg per minute in girls. Puberty marks a period of significant change in aerobic capacity that is associated with large changes in body size and composition. Gender differences in the development of Vo_2max are more evident at age 10 to 12 when Vo_2max (mL/kg per minute) stabilizes (in boys) or declines (in girls) through adolescence as body size increases. However, this change is more related to body composition, specifically fat-free mass (FFM), with a decrease in Vo_2 of approximately 5 ml/kg FFM per minute during puberty (62). Endurance performance, measured as treadmill run time, continues to improve during preadolescence, but plateaus in females at about age 10 to 12, and continues to improve in males up to age 16 (60).

Gender Differences in the Development of Aerobic Capacity

As previously discussed, absolute Vo_2max (L/min) in children increases throughout childhood and is largely related to changes in body size. However, gender differences in aerobic capacity are apparent prior to puberty at age 8 to 10 and the onset of gender dimorphism in height, weight, and fat-free mass (19,85–87). A review of numerous cross-sectional and longitudinal studies reveals a progressive increase in Vo_2max (L/min) of males from age 8 to 16, with an annual increase of 11%. In contrast, increases in Vo_2max of females appears to be more variable and occurs from age 8 to 13 at a similar rate. The largest increase occurs between age 11 and 12 for girls (0.24 L/min), and age 12 to 14 for boys (0.32 L/min). Thus, for males the peak rate of increase is greater and persists for 1

additional year compared to females (86). However, the magnitude of gender difference is also due to the continued linear increase in males until age 17, whereas Vo_2max (L/min) in females begins to level off at age 13 (51,86). By age 12, the gender difference in Vo_2max (L/min) is about 12%, and increases to 37% by age 16. Sex differences in hemoglobin and habitual activity level are typically offered to account for gender differences in Vo_2max, however the latter has also been refuted (88). Furthermore, hemoglobin does not differ in young boys and girls and consequently does not explain the gender difference in Vo_2max (L/min) prior to puberty (86). However, the gender differences in left ventricular mass favoring males emerges during pubertal years and is related to increases in body surface area and diastolic blood pressure (an index of arterial resistance). The difference in heart size may partly account for gender differences in Vo_2max (89).

Maximal aerobic speed (MAS) is the minimal running velocity at which Vo_2max occurs, is highly correlated to distance running performance in adults (90,91), and is a function of Vo_2max as well as running economy (92). Evidence suggests that this index of aerobic power follows a similar developmental trend in females and males as described above. Gender differences in MAS are not apparent until age 12, when males exceed females by 11%. MAS continues to increase in males to age 17, when it is almost 60% greater (yearly increase of 0.5 km/hr) than MAS at age 6. In females, MAS increases 0.3 km/hr from age 6 to 12, and remains fairly constant at 11 km/hr thereafter. By age 17, the gender difference in MAS is 24% (93).

When Vo_2max is expressed relative to body mass (mL/kg per minute) the trend is considerably different with respect to gender differences. In males, Vo_2max (mL/kg/min) during treadmill running remains stable prior to puberty, when there is a very slight, if any, increase to age 16. In contrast, females demonstrate a steady decline in relative Vo_2max from age 7 to 16 (86,87). The gender difference in Vo_2max (mL/kg per minute) is generally explained by higher relative body fat development in females during peripubertal years (86). As discussed in the previous section on body composition, there is little gender difference in body weight prior to puberty, however young girls tend to have slightly greater fat mass and less fat-free mass than young boys. The gender difference in fat mass and fat-free mass likely accounts for the declining trend of relative Vo_2max in girls beginning as early as age 7.

Since Vo_2max is also highly related to height (85,87), as well as mass, allometric scaling of Vo_2max to account for height and mass results in the expression of Vo_2max ($mL/kg^{0.67}$ per minute). Studies of adult animals, however, indicate that the scaling exponent of mass should be 0.75. Nevertheless, a 5-year longitudinal study of aerobic power in boys and girls (mean age at beginning of study was 9.2 ± 0.5 yrs) revealed that gender differences in Vo_2max persisted over the 5 years of study when expressed relative to body mass, $mass^{0.67}$, $mass^{0.75}$, or fat-free mass. Additionally, body mass, percent fat, and fat-free mass were similar between genders until the final year of the study. Thus, gender differences in aerobic power were not explained by differences in body fat (86). Similar findings elsewhere (94) suggest that the development of Vo_2max in children is influenced by factors other than body size, and that gender differences in Vo_2max during development are also not accounted for solely by body size or

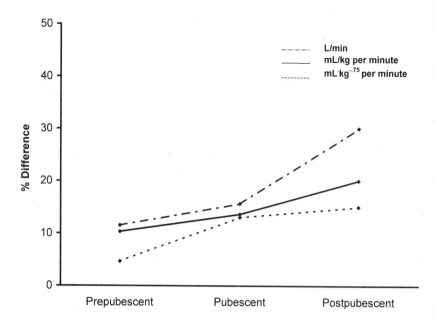

Figure 55-1 Gender differences in prepubescents, pubescents, and postpubescents for three expressions of maximum oxygen consumption (% difference = [males – females/males] × 100).

Legend:
- ·—·— L/min
- ——— mL/kg per minute
- ······ mL·kg$^{-.75}$ per minute

X-axis: Prepubescent, Pubescent, Postpubescent
Y-axis: % Difference (0 to 50)

composition. Figure 55-1 shows gender differences in three expressions of Vo$_2$max from childhood to postpuberty.

It is clear that the absolute measure of Vo$_2$max (L/min) is not appropriate for explaining developmental changes in Vo$_2$max. Because of the strong relationship of mass and height with Vo$_2$max, a measure of absolute Vo$_2$max would not reveal the contribution of growth and development to aerobic power. Until we resolve the use of allometric scaling of body mass, and identify the appropriate power function, Vo$_2$max in children should be expressed relative to body mass. Thus growth, indicated by changes in body mass, is at least partially accounted for in the expression of Vo$_2$.

DEVELOPMENT OF ANAEROBIC PERFORMANCE AND LACTATE THRESHOLD

Characteristic play patterns of children typically involve repeated short bursts of activity followed by periods of inactivity or reduced activity. Rarely do children spontaneously engage in protracted, intense exercise. It stands to reason that the physiologic profile of children may be more consistent with the typical patterns of play. That is, the proportion of physical activity in children accounted for by aerobic and anaerobic metabolism may differ from that of adults. However, little research has focused on the development of anaerobic power and the capacity to do anaerobic work in children even though this index of energy production may better reflect exercise capacity in children than does Vo$_2$max.

In adults, Vo$_2$max has long been considered to be the best sole indicator of aerobic fitness. However, endurance performance appears to be strongly related to lactate threshold (95), as well as aerobic capacity. Studies of anaerobic performance in children have evaluated the contribution of anaerobic performance to aerobic performance (71,96–107). Unfortunately, there are many methodologic inconsistencies (anaerobic power tests, test modalities, measurement of lactic acid) across studies that make direct comparisons not possible.

However, there appears to be a fairly consistent developmental trend in anaerobic performance.

Anaerobic performance is lower in children and adolescents compared to adults (2,97,99,108). When anaerobic power determined during a 30-sec Wingate Anaerobic Test (WAT) or Margaria step running test is expressed in absolute terms or relative to body size, values begin to increase during adolescent years. Falk et al (99) studied anaerobic power in children relative to stages of maturation instead of chronologic age. Absolute peak and mean anaerobic power were lowest in prepubertal (age 10.9) and highest in late pubertal (age 16.2) boys. When expressed relative to body weight, peak anaerobic power increased somewhat with age and tended to be higher in more physically mature males. Peak aerobic power did not differ between groups, thus the ratio of anaerobic/aerobic power increased with age and maturation until the onset of puberty, then stabilized.

The power ratio begins to increase again in early adulthood, and is largely influenced by training (109). In addition, aerobic and anaerobic power are significantly correlated in pre- and midpubertal boys, but not in postpubertal boys. This suggests that younger children (age 14 and younger) lack metabolic specialization of energy production, whereas children in late adolescence begin to demonstrate greater selectivity of energy systems (77).

Anaerobic power increases in children with age and maturity, and exhibits a trend when expressed relative to body or muscle size (99). Thus other factors have been suggested to impact developmental changes in anaerobic power. Serum testosterone levels parallel an increase in lactate production and glycolytic energy production in pubertal boys (110), but testosterone levels do not contribute to body mass, age, and height in accounting for the variance in submaximal lactate levels and peak Vo$_2$ (111). Furthermore, testosterone level in young girls is minimal and presumably does not account for changes in anaerobic power, although this has yet to be examined.

An increase in anaerobic power may be a function of

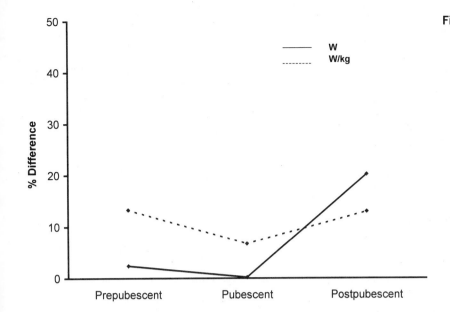

Figure 55-2 Gender differences in prepubescents, pubescents, and postpubescents for absolute (watts) and relative (watts/kg) anaerobic capacity (% difference = [males − females/males] × 100).

enhanced force production. Changes in muscle architecture with increased contractile proteins, myofibrillar density, or connective tissue can increase force production and power output (112). Also, changes in motor unit recruitment patterns to increase force generation have been observed in postpubescent compared to prepubescent boys (20).

The contribution of anaerobic energy production appears to change with age, most notably at puberty (113). Evidence regarding lactate production indicates an increased ability for glycolytic energy production in more mature versus less mature children (99). However, Roemmich et al (2) discuss evidence that indicates other factors or a combination of factors are more likely to contribute to growth-related changes in anaerobic power. The rate-limiting glycolytic enzyme phosphofructokinase (PFK) is higher in adults than children. However, the magnitude of training-related increases in PFK in children do not mirror increases in anaerobic power. Likewise, short term (<5 sec) energy production via stored muscle phosphagens is also only partially responsible for changes in anaerobic power. Adult levels are reached prior to puberty, yet anaerobic power continues to increase into adulthood. Maturational changes in muscle glycogen concentration and rate of glycogen utilization may also explain changes in anaerobic energy production in children but further research is needed to clarify this.

Blood lactate levels are lower in children during exercise, and lactate threshold (LT) is generally higher compared to untrained adults (114). Therefore, children must work at a higher percentage of Vo_2max to achieve LT. This may be a consequence of relatively inefficient movement and gait in children compared to adults, such that stride frequency to sustain a typical "adult" walking velocity is achieved at an increased metabolic cost and aerobic energy demand in children (115,116). In addition, an increase in the volume of active muscle mass with growth (117) and a higher concentration of ATP-recycling and glycolytic enzymes in pubescent versus prepubescent children (118) suggest an increased ability to do anaerobic work in late adolescence.

Lower blood lactate levels in children reflect a smaller amount of active muscle mass. Post Vo_2peak lactate levels are lower in children and tend to peak at about 1 to 2 minutes after exercise, compared to 5 minutes after exercise in adults. Presumably, the faster diffusion of lactate from active muscles to blood is shorter in children due to smaller body size and shorter diffusion distance (86). It has also been suggested that relatively lower sympathetic activity in children decreases vasoconstriction to the liver, which facilitates hepatic clearance of lactic acid (51).

Others have reported lower correlations between LT and Vo_2max in children compared to adults further supporting the lack of energy system specificity in children (77,119). Yet in a study of children aged 11 trained specifically for sprint performance, the power ratio (LT at %Vo_2max) was significantly less than that of endurance trained children and controls (119), which suggests that the measure of LT is sensitive to training in children as well as adults.

Gender Differences in the Development of Anaerobic Performance and Lactate Threshold

Anaerobic peak and mean power vary by gender as a function of maturational stage. Typical gender differences are depicted in Figure 55-2. Gender differences emerge around puberty, and are thought to be related to maturational changes in muscle tissue and neuromuscular function that enhances anaerobic power production per unit of muscle size. In addition, maturity related increases in muscle strength likely contribute to increased anaerobic power observed in postpubertal boys, but additional research is needed to substantiate these theories (2,96).

Gender differences in maximal lactate concentration become evident around puberty when values for girls begin to level off, and boys exhibit larger increases compared to prepubertal changes (2,113). The increase in glycolytic capacity in boys following puberty has been attributed to testosterone levels. However, peak lactate levels are not significantly related

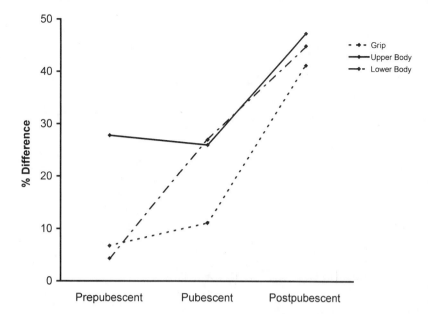

Figure 55-3 Gender differences in prepubescents, pubescents, and postpubescents for grip, upper body, and lower body strength (% difference = [males − females/males] × 100).

Legend:
- - ◆ - - Grip
──◆── Upper Body
- ◆ - Lower Body

Y-axis: % Difference (0, 10, 20, 30, 40, 50)
X-axis: Prepubescent, Pubescent, Postpubescent

to stage of maturation (96,121), but may be a function of chronologic age (113).

DEVELOPMENT OF STRENGTH

In adults, strength is only moderately correlated with weight (r = ~0.50) (122,123). Although it is often expressed as a ratio with weight, it is more highly correlated with muscle cross-sectional area (CSA; r = ~0.75) (124,125). This suggests that strength changes in adults due to training are predominantly associated with increases in muscle CSA. However, in a developing child, strength is related to linear growth and weight, as well as muscle size. Prepubertal strength increases follow a similar trend for many measures including grip, elbow flexion/extension, and knee flexion/extension strength, as well as composite scores consisting of several measures of strength (2). That is, strength increases fairly linearly until puberty, at which point strength continues to increase but at different rates for males and females (126). Peak strength gains in males occur about 6 to 12 months following peak weight and peak height velocities (at around age 12), indicating that factors other than linear growth and weight gain may also contribute to strength increases in children. In fact, strength increases exceed gains in height in prepubertal and pubertal males, indicating that muscle size and maturational factors are involved in strength development prior to and during puberty (2).

While muscle size may be an important determinant of strength in both adults and children, isokinetic strength expressed relative to an index of muscle size (CSA × segment length) is still lower in children than young adults (127,128). However, isometric strength per unit CSA appears constant through adolescence to young adulthood (129). These differences in isometric and isokinetic force production may be due to growth-related changes in neural drive and ability to recruit motor units. For example, it has been suggested that prepubertal children are less able to potentiate muscle activity during the eccentric phase following impact when hopping (130).

Furthermore, initial training-related increases in children's strength is due to neural changes, evidenced by increased integrated EMG amplitude. However, 8 weeks of training did not alter arm anthropometry, further supporting the role of neural drive in the development of children's strength (131).

Other factors including endocrine function and activity level contribute to the effects of height, weight, muscle size, and neural mechanisms on strength development before, during, and following puberty. Maturational changes in key hormones that influence muscle size, including growth hormone, IGF-1, and insulin, as well as adrenal and gonadal hormones, determine the rate and timing of sexual development (2). The importance of chronic physical activity patterns was observed in a study of strength in males and females age 16, and again at age 27. The results indicated that strength, particularly in females, was significantly related to physical activity level at both ages (132). Similarly, a 5-year program of daily physical education resulted in modestly higher isometric strength for children aged 7 to 12. The greatest increase in strength was in 10 to 12 year olds. The lack of changes in muscle girth in these subjects suggested that enhanced strength at this age resulted from improved neuromuscular function (133).

Gender Differences in the Development of Strength

Gender differences in the development of strength are most evident around the age of puberty. Throughout childhood, however, the strength of boys slightly exceeds that of girls and is probably related to the small but consistently greater fat-free mass in males (20). Considerable differences in strength become apparent around age 11 to 13, when strength in females increases slightly then plateaus. In males, the rate of strength gain accelerates at age 12 to 13 and continues to increase throughout the postpubertal years (2). Some of the gender difference in strength following puberty could be attributed to differences in fat-free mass and muscle size; however, males are about 12% stronger than females, whereas their muscles are only about 5% larger (20). Percent gender

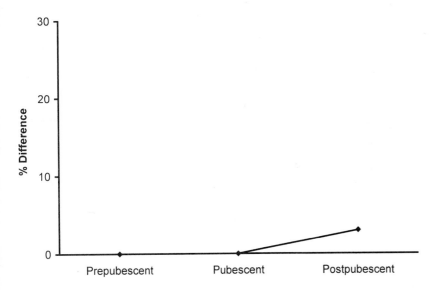

Figure 55-4 Gender differences in prepubescents, pubescents, and postpubescents for leg strength relative to leg size (% difference = [males − females/males] × 100).

differences in strength appear in Figure 55-3 for isometric grip strength, and combined isokinetic and isotonic measures for upper and lower body strength.

Differences in techniques to measure muscle size may account for some of the discrepancy in the strength-muscle size relationship. In adults, muscle cross-sectional area (CSA) assessed by computed tomography was used to normalize strength scores for elbow flexion and knee extension. Absolute strength in females was 52% and 66% of males' strength for upper and lower body, respectively, but there was no gender difference in strength CSA/ratio (134). Likewise, no gender difference occurred between strength-trained adult females and males, or between untrained females and males for maximal isometric torque of the upper and lower body expressed relative to muscle plus bone CSA. However, torque of the trained subjects was greater than that of the untrained subjects of both genders. These results indicate that torque/CSA is similar in males and females, and the strength/CSA response to resistance training is not gender dependent. Furthermore, this study suggests that some of the gender difference in absolute strength may be due to dissimilarity of use, particularly for upper-body strength (135). Greater differences in absolute strength could also be due to gender differences in lean and fat distribution in the upper and lower body (136). Results similar to those in adults were reported in children (aged 9 to 14) for maximal isometric strength of the triceps surae muscle in the lower leg. When expressed relative to muscle plus bone CSA, strength did not differ between genders for 9-, 11-, and 14-year-olds (137).

Others have demonstrated the significance of height or length in the development of strength in children (20,138, 139). Thus, when isometric ankle strength in 7- to 18-year-olds was expressed relative to the product of CSA and leg length, there was no difference between females and males of similar ages (128). However, a study of isokinetic strength in 6- to 9-year old children produced conflicting results (127). There were no gender differences in isokinetic knee extension strength relative to CSA and thigh length at a low velocity of 10.5 rad/sec, but males had greater torque/CSA per thigh

length at a higher speed of 3.14 rad/sec. Gender differences in leg strength expressed relative to measures of limb size are shown in Figure 55-4.

While it appears that some of the gender difference in strength may be accounted for by differences in muscle size, segment length, and degree of use, other differences in muscle contractile characteristics (e.g., fiber area, fiber size, percent fiber distribution) and/or mechanical properties may enable greater isokinetic torque production in males. There is evidence to support these differences in adults (134,137), but further research is needed to evaluate the impact of these factors in children.

Indeed, some of the difference in strength may be accounted for by the expanding influence of sex hormones, primarily testosterone. However, insulin, IGF-1, growth hormone, and thyroid hormones also mediate somatic and muscle tissue growth. It is not clear to what extent these hormones, particularly testosterone, influence age- and sex-associated development of strength and muscle size (20).

Body composition changes in females following puberty clearly contribute to some of the gender differences in strength that increase markedly during the postpubescent years. An increase in relative body fat increases total limb CSA, but does not enhance torque production. However, when strength is expressed as a ratio of muscle plus bone CSA, gender differences are significantly reduced, suggesting that muscle "quality" may be similar between genders. Nevertheless, we must examine further the impact of gender differences in physical activity and/or training as it relates to gender variation in strength, to more precisely determine the extent of true biologic gender differences in strength.

DEVELOPMENT OF MOTOR PERFORMANCE

Motor performance, broadly defined, may encompass performance of a variety of motor tasks, including but not limited to throwing (distance, velocity, kinematics, and accuracy), running (speed and kinematics), jumping (vertical and long),

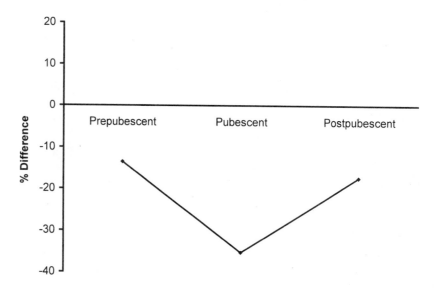

Figure 55-5 Gender differences in prepubescents, pubescents, and postpubescents for flexibility (% difference = [males − females/males] × 100).

agility, flexibility, static and dynamic balance, various measures of strength (e.g., grip strength, flexed arm hang, etc.), and gross and fine motor indices of movement speed (plate tapping) and movement accuracy (pursuit rotor tracking). It is not within the scope of this chapter to discuss mechanisms underlying the developmental aspects of motor control and skill acquisition, but interested readers are directed to Whitall (140).

The development of motor performance increases gradually from early childhood to puberty. Fundamental movement patterns are generally mastered by the age of 5 or 6 (141), after which motor performance is influenced by speed, strength, power, and practice. The performance curves for many of the aforementioned tasks are similar during childhood (142), and the developmental changes in motor performance appear to be related primarily to age (143), and in some measures gender (142,144,145). Gender appears to influence motor performance in children most notably in the task of overhand throwing (145), in which measurable differences occur as early as age 3 (142). Likewise, at this early age performance of flexibility and balance tasks mildly favor females (142), and flexibility in females exceeds that of males throughout life (Figure 55-5) (146). These childhood gender differences have been attributed, in part, to differences in body size. However gender differences in height and weight during childhood are subtle and not likely sufficient to explain differences in motor performance (1).

Puberty, once again, represents a pivotal time in which there is substantial change in various parameters of motor performance. The most dramatic changes in motor performance following puberty are observed in tasks that are most influenced by body size, muscle mass, strength, and power. Changes in body size and composition support the greatest rate of improvement in tasks such as throwing (distance and velocity), running, sit-ups, grip strength, and jumping (vertical and long). Other indices of motor performance that are less dependent on body size and muscle mass demonstrate a slower rate of improvement following puberty, including balance, coordination (plate tapping), and tracking (pursuit rotor) (142).

Gender Differences in the Development of Motor Performance

Gender differences in movement organization and reflexes have been observed in newborns. Newborn females demonstrate a right bias in several distal lower body reflexes in contrast to a left bias in most male newborns. It is not clear if the difference is due to maturity level, since newborn females are more neurologically mature (147). However, the reflex biases observed in newborns parallel gender differences in adults. Thus sex differences in the development of the central nervous system (CNS) may yield persistent differences throughout life. The development of sex differences in CNS organization may be influenced by sex steroids (148).

Assessment of more complex motor skills and performance in children is confounded by several factors. Most research is cross-sectional, thus it is difficult to ascertain the magnitude and origin of gender differences in performance as it relates to growth and development. Additionally, in a meta-analysis of 64 studies, Thomas and French (142) reported that the magnitude of gender differences in some motor tasks (shuttle run and sit-ups) were negatively related to the sex of the first author of the study. That is, the effect sizes were larger, favoring boys, when the first author was female (and presumably the experimenter). This indicates that the experimenter may inadvertently affect motivation or effort, and therefore performance, in subjects of the opposite sex. Furthermore, the effect sizes for shuttle run and dash were larger in published studies, possibly reflecting a bias of journals to publish studies in which differences were significant. There was also a lack of consistency in the types and administration of motor skill tests in various studies. For example, the effect size for sit-ups was larger in studies published prior to 1970. Lack of standardization in early tests, in which sit-ups were done to failure (maximum number of sit-ups), compared to more recent tests with a time limit, may explain, to some degree, the magnitude of reported gender differences.

The meta-analysis of Thomas and French (142) reflects gender comparison data from 31,444 subjects, aged 3 to 20. The gender difference in performance (effect size, expressed

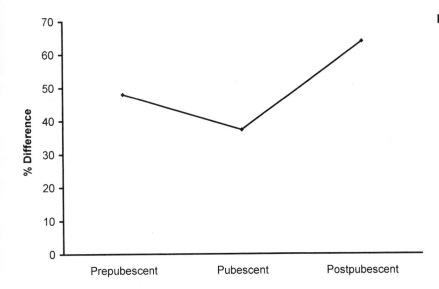

Figure 55-6 Gender differences in prepubescents, pubescents, and postpubescents for throw distance (% difference = [males − females/males] × 100).

in standard deviation units [SD]) was extracted for a total of 702 comparisons of 20 different motor tasks. Age was regressed on effect size and was significant for 12 of the 20 motor tasks. Although this analysis is limited by the use of cross-sectional comparisons, the results are consistent with many previous and subsequent reports.

Prior to puberty, most motor tasks that are dependent on strength, muscle mass, speed, and power (dash, sit-ups, long jump, shuttle run, and grip strength) demonstrate small to moderate effect sizes favoring boys (0.20 SD to 0.50 SD). These small differences vary little throughout childhood to puberty except for sit-ups, in which gender differences favoring males increase by age 7 or 8. This may be due to small but steadily increasing muscle mass development in boys at this age (1). Conversely, tasks related to balance, tracking, and tapping do not differ between genders during childhood, but begin to differentiate in early puberty favoring males around age 11 to 12. Differences at this age are more likely due to environmental causes among boys such as more practice and pressure to excel at these tasks.

Figure 55-6 includes gender differences in throwing during development. Throwing produced the largest effect size of 1.5 SD, which was evident as early as 3 years (for distance and velocity), and increased to 3.5 to 4 SD by the age of 12. It could be argued that young boys practice throwing more frequently, thus resulting in greater gender differences. However, attempts to reduce gender differences in throwing through training and practice have been unsuccessful (149). Others suggest that males achieve a higher level of maturation in throwing skill acquisition, but that form is similar between genders (150,151). Most agree that this magnitude of difference at a very young age cannot be fully accounted for by environmental factors alone, and probably reflect some biologic differences as well (152,153). However, throwing is a specialized skill, the practice of which is largely influenced by sociocultural biases that favor greater activity in males. Thus some insist that the magnitude of gender differences in throwing is more reflective of the degree of engagement, even at a young age, and greater gender differences at puberty are a function of muscle mass and "maturation" of throwing skill

(150,154). Since throwing performance is influenced by power generated from the trunk and legs, it stands to reason that greater fat-free mass in males would generate higher peak velocity and acceleration (154). A recent study reported that somatic characteristics were not highly related to throwing skills in prepubertal girls after controlling for differences in physical activity level (155). Although body size (height and weight) bears little relationship to many motor performances in prepubertal children (1), young boys (age 5) appear to have an advantage in forearm length and arm muscle mass that increases throughout childhood and adolescence (156). Together with a greater biacromial/bicristal ratio in later childhood (1,157), these inherent (genetic) differences may explain some of the gender difference in throwing skill.

There appears to be little gender difference in vertical jump prior to puberty. This is difficult to explain since changes in muscle mass and relative fat, although subtle, should favor boys in performance of this task in late childhood. However, girls reach puberty 1 to 2 years earlier than boys, and in other motor tasks (dash, grip strength, and shuttle run) actually reduce the gender differences until boys reach puberty. If this were the case with vertical jump performance (although it is not for long jump), girls may increase vertical jump at a greater rate than boys at this age, resulting in no change in the effect size until boys reach puberty. When standing long jump (SLJ) distance was expressed as a product with body mass in 12-year-old girls and boys, gender differences disappeared. Similarly, the product of SLJ and body mass expressed relative to lean leg volume was the same for girls and boys. These data suggest that young girls and boys have similar force-generating ability, and that gender differences in SLJ are due to differences in body mass and leg muscle mass (158).

At puberty, gender differences increase substantially in most motor tasks and continue to increase into late adolescence. The effect sizes for jumping, running, sit-ups, and grip strength are generally 1.5 to 2 SD by age 17. However, the magnitude of increase in gender differences is considerably smaller for balance, pursuit rotor tracking, and tapping tasks in which the effect size is less than 1.0 SD at age 17 (142).

There is some discrepancy as to the extent to which females increase motor performance during and following puberty or menarche. Motor and physical (aerobic and anaerobic power) performance was greater in more sexually mature females of the same chronologic age between age 11 and 13. However, maturity level conferred little advantage in performance measures for 10- or 14-year-old females. Thus, the growth period in females from age 11 to 13 may represent a stage of accelerated gains in motor and physical performance (159). While some report that motor performance in females generally plateaus around puberty (160), more recent research indicates that some measures of motor performance continue to increase through late adolescence (161). A study of Flemish girls reported increases in movement speed (plate tapping), shuttle run, and measures of static, dynamic, and explosive strength (vertical jump) until age 16 to 18 (162).

These more recent data may reflect increasing levels of physical activity in young females, suggesting that environmental factors contribute to postpubertal gender differences in motor performance. As indicated previously, this may result in smaller gender differences in these tasks during late adolescence. However, changes in body size, dimension, and composition appear to negatively impact motor performance in postpubertal girls. By age 17, median body weight, lengths, and breadths for girls are at or below the 10th percentile for boys, whereas limb skinfolds are greater than the 90th percentile for boys. Smaller muscle mass and size and greater body fat coincides with poorer motor performance (except flexibility) in postpubescent females (162). Similarly, when menarcheal status is considered, performance in the 1200-m run deteriorates for females after menarche, probably due to an increase in ectomorphy (163).

With the exception of throwing, gender differences in motor performance prior to puberty are small and reasonably attributed to environmental factors that favor development of motor skills in boys. However, given equal emphasis and encouragement in early childhood, motor performance in girls may approach that of boys. Following puberty, changes in body size, composition, strength, and power result in large differences in motor performance of tasks that benefit from these attributes. It is questionable if effect sizes of 1.5 to 2 SD could be explained by environmental factors alone, and we must continue to explore the potential influence of inherent, biologic differences between genders. Yet it is more than likely that motor performance in females could be significantly enhanced by sustained physical activity beginning in early childhood, and thus result in smaller gender differences in motor performance that are due solely to biologic factors.

SOCIOCULTURAL CONSIDERATIONS FOR GENDER DIFFERENCES IN THE DEVELOPMENT OF FITNESS

The fundamental health benefits of regular exercise are well known, particularly as they impact the progression of coronary artery disease. While there is substantial evidence that the deleterious effects of inactivity promote the atherosclerotic process even in young children, we have been relatively ineffective in efforts to counsel children and parents to incorporate regular exercise as a lifestyle behavior (164). A decline of 50% in physical activity levels during adolescence is responsible for the mere 12% of children under age 18 who report a level of physical activity sufficient to promote cardiorespiratory fitness (165). Further examination of this trend of declining physical activity in children reveals evidence that may explain some of the gender differences in the development of fitness discussed in this chapter.

Expectations for behavior begin early in childhood and are molded by sociocultural factors that delineate acceptable gender roles (166). Thus, at an early age, girls and boys behave in a manner that is directed by social norms, cultural biases, and parental influence. These tacit constraints on behavior affect how children interact with each other, and how they learn and acquire knowledge and skills. Gender differences have been observed in preschool children learning fundamental motor skills. Boys emphasized competition and sought validation through competition with same-sex peers. In contrast, girls' social interaction fostered cooperation when learning motor skills. Girls attempted to promote more socially acceptable behaviors and manners when interacting with boys, who in turn exhibited more competitive, aggressive, and physically forward behavior toward girls. As a result, the girls experienced less practice time when learning the motor skills. Of particular interest was the interaction of a small group of Asian children who exhibited cooperative behaviors independent of gender, and thus may illustrate cultural differences in the development of gender roles. How children are socialized to interact, as suggested by these results, may impact on how motor skills are learned and practiced (166).

It is well documented that physical activity levels decrease as children age, with the greatest change occurring around puberty (20,19,167). The change is most noticeable in girls at puberty, when a progressive decline in participation rate begins. Participation in physical activity for young boys is high and remains so throughout adolescence (20). In general, boys engage in more strength and power types of physical activities, whereas girls participate in moderate to light physical activity (167). However, measurable gender differences in physical activity levels and energy expenditure are evident in young girls and boys as well (27,155,168). A study of Swedish children reported that young boys (age 8) were more physically active than young girls, and that VO_2max was significantly correlated to physical activity level in only the young boys. This suggests that aerobic fitness prior to puberty may be influenced by chronic activity level as well as growth and development.

Efforts to explain why there are differences in physical activity levels in children and adolescents must consider the role of social and parental factors. Gender, access to exercise facilities, and perceived benefits of exercise appear to influence exercise behavior (165). Boys are more successful at overcoming barriers to exercise such as time constraints, feelings of fatigue, poor weather, and homework obligations (169). In addition, boys cite support of family and friends as important motivators to be physically active (170). Girls need more family support (171), tend to sustain physical activity if they can do so at home, and need direct parental modeling of physical activity to maintain exercise behaviors. Exercise adherence increases for both boys and girls if they enjoy it, and if their mothers support physical activity in the family (170).

Although there is little physiologic evidence for gender differences in fat-free mass, relative fat, strength, and aerobic capacity prior to puberty, small differences do exist. Likewise, it is unclear why throwing skill is better in young boys. More work is needed to isolate the subtle effects of social and parental differences in how we play with our young daughters and sons, how we teach and to what extent we reinforce motor skill development in each, how educators may or may not bias their teaching based on gender, what we expect of our children in terms of health behaviors, and, most important, what health behaviors we model for our children. For example, children of obese parents tend to be fatter than those of nonobese parents (28). To what extent we attribute that relationship to unalterable, biological factors can only be determined once the aforementioned environmental influences are considered.

At this time we know that childhood inactivity leads to adulthood inactivity. Parental encouragement and modeling of physical activity promotes regular physical activity in children (172). And the strongest predictor of physical activity in adulthood is childhood involvement (173). Other recommendations to promote regular physical activity, particularly in young females, include teaching strategies to overcome barriers to exercise (e.g., issues of self-esteem, peer pressure), facilitate access to community-based activities, and include noncompetitive lifetime activities in physical education classes and recreational activities (169).

SUMMARY

Puberty marks the time of gender differentiation in body size, composition, and indices of fitness. The development of aerobic power is affected greatly by changes in body size and composition. Vo_2max (L/min) continues to increase linearly in males following puberty and throughout adolescence. In females, Vo_2max (L/min) levels off at age 13, and by age 16 there is a difference of 37% between genders. Gender differences in body size and hemoglobin concentration are largely due to differences in testosterone levels following puberty. However, prepubertal body size and hemoglobin is similar between genders and does not account for observed differences in Vo_2max at this age. When expressed relative to body mass, Vo_2max (mL/kg per minute) in males is stable following puberty but declines in females through adolescence, partly as a function of increased body fat.

Anaerobic performance also varies by gender beginning in puberty. Maturational changes in muscle strength, neuromuscular function, and glycolytic capacity are influenced by testosterone levels. Therefore, anaerobic capacity increases in males during adolescence and plateaus in females following puberty.

The rate of strength gain following puberty accelerates in males and increases gradually in females. Gender differences in strength during adolescence are not fully accounted for by differences in muscle size. However, more precise differentiation of fat-free and fat tissue indicates little gender difference in isometric strength per unit CSA. Males produce greater isokinetic torque per unit CSA which may be due to differences in muscle contractile characteristics such as fiber area, fiber size, and percent fiber distribution.

Motor performance in males exceeds that of females following puberty in activities that require strength, power, and speed. At all ages, females exhibit greater flexibility, and males outperform females in overhand throwing.

For all of the aforementioned fitness parameters, small and usually nonsignificant gender differences favoring males are often observed during childhood, prior to puberty (except in flexibility and overhand throwing). With no apparent biologic explanation for these subtle but persistent differences in fitness, the type and level of physical activity behavior that characterizes young girls and boys must be considered. Substantial evidence demonstrates a significant gender difference in physical activity level in young children and adolescents. To accurately delineate the contribution of inherent, biologic factors, more research is needed to quantify the role of physical activity level and other potential environmental factors that impact the development of gender differences in fitness.

REFERENCES

1. Malina RM. Human growth, maturation, and regular physical activity. In: Moritani RA, ed. Advances in pediatric sports sciences, vol 1. Champaign, IL: Human Kinetics, 1984.

2. Roemmich JN, Rogol AD. Physiology of growth and development: its relationship to performance in the young athlete. Clin Sports Med 1995;14:483–502.

3. Denison BA, Ben-Ezra V. Plasma somatomedin-C in 8- to 10-year old swimmers. Pediatr Exerc Sci 1989;1:64–72.

4. Malina RM. Physical growth and biological maturation of young athletes. In: Holloszy J, ed. Exercise and sport sciences review, vol 22. Philadelphia: Williams & Wilkins, 1994.

5. Wheeler MD. Physical changes of puberty. Endocrinol Metab Clin North Am 1991;20:1–14.

6. Tanner JM. Growth at adolescence. Oxford: Blackwell, 1962.

7. Roche AF, Tyleshevski F, Rogers E. Non-invasive measurements of physical maturity in children. Res Q Exerc Sport 1983;54:364–371.

8. Rico H, Reville M, Villa LF, et al. Body composition in children and Tanner's stages: a study with dual-energy x-ray absorptiometry. Metabolism 1993;42:967–970.

9. Nelson DA, Simpson PM, Johnson CC, et al. The accumulation of whole body skeletal mass in third- and fourth-grade children: effects of age, gender, ethnicity, and body composition. Bone 1997;20:73–78.

10. Bonjour JP, Theintz G, Buchs B, et al. Critical years and stages of puberty for spinal and femoral mass accumulation during adolescence. J Clin Endocrinol Metab 1991;73:555–563.

11. Matkovic V, Fontana D, Tominac C, et al. Factors that influence peak bone mass formation: a study of calcium balance and the inheritance of bone mass in adolescent females. Am J Clin Nutr 1990;52:878–888.

12. Theintz G, Buchs B, Rizzoli R, et al. Longitudinal monitoring of bone mass accumulation in healthy adolescents: evidence for a marked reduction after 16 years of age at the levels of lumbar spine and femoral neck in female subjects. J Clin Endocrinol Metab 1992;75:1060–1065.

13. Oyster N. Sex differences in cancellous and cortical bone strength, bone mineral content and bone density. Age Ageing 1992;21:353–356.

14. Malina RM. Adolescent changes in size, build, composition and performance. Hum Biol 1974;46: 117–131.

15. Houtkooper LB, Going SB, Lohman TG, et al. Bioelectrical impedance estimation of fat-free body mass in children and youth: a cross-validation study. J Appl Physiol 1992;72:366–373.

16. Lohman TG, Boileau RA, Slaughter MH. Body composition in children and youth. In: Boileau RA, ed. Advances in pediatric sports sciences, vol 1. Champaign, IL: Human Kinetics, 1984.

17. Slaughter MH, Lohman TG, Boileau RA, et al. Skinfold equations for estimation of body fatness in children and youth. Hum Biol 1988;60:709–723.

18. Brandon LJ, Fillingim J. Body composition and blood pressure in children based on age, race, and sex. Am J Prev Med 1993;9: 34–38.

19. Sunnegårdh J, Bratteby LE. Maximal oxygen uptake, anthropometry and physical activity in a randomly selected sample of 8 and 13 year old children in Sweden. Eur J Appl Physiol 1987;56:266–272.

20. Blimkie JR. Age- and sex-associated variation in strength during childhood: anthropometric, morphologic, neurologic, biomechanical, endocrinologic, genetic, and physical activity correlates. In: Gisolfi CV, Lamb DR, eds. Perspectives in exercise and sports medicine, vol 12. Madison, WI: Brown and Benchmark, 1989.

21. Kanehisa H, Ikegawa S, Tsunoda N, et al. Cross-sectional areas of fat and muscle in limbs during growth and middle age. Int J Sports Med 1994;15:420–425.

22. Malina RM, Johnston FE. Relations between bone, muscle and fat widths of the upper arms and calves of boys and girls studied cross-sectionally at ages 6 to 16 years. Hum Biol 1967;39:211–223.

23. Tanner JM, Hughes PCR, Whitehouse RH. Radiographically determined widths of bone, muscle and fat in the upper arm and calf from age 3–18 years. Ann Hum Biol 1981;8:495–517.

24. McGowan A, Jordan M, MacGregor J. Skinfold thicknesses in neonates. Biol Neonate 1975;25: 66–84.

25. Parizkova J. Body fat and physical fitness, The Hague: Martinus Nijhoff, 1977.

26. Malina RM, Bouchard C. Subcutaneous fat distribution during growth. In: Bouchard C, Johnston FE, eds. Fat distribution during growth and later health outcomes. New York: Liss, 1988.

27. Shepard RJ, Lavallee H. Enhanced physical education and body fat in the primary school child. Am J Hum Biol 1993;5: 697–704.

28. Travers SH, Barrett WJ, Bloch CA. Gender and Tanner stage differences in body composition and insulin sensitivity in early pubertal children. J Clin Endocrinol Metab 1995;80:172–178.

29. Suter E, Hawes MR. Relationship of physical activity, body fat, diet, and blood lipid profile in youths 10–15 yr. Med Sci Sports Exerc 1993;25:748–754.

30. Thomas JR, Nelson JK, Church G. A developmental analysis of gender differences in health related physical fitness. Pediatr Exerc Sci 1991;3:28–42.

31. Plowman SA, Liu NY, Wells CL. Body composition and sexual maturation in premenarcheal athletes and nonathletes. Med Sci Sports Exerc 1991;23:23–29.

32. Nemoto I, Kanehisa H, Miyashita M. The effects of sports training on the age-related changes of body composition and isokinetic peak torque in knee extensors of junior speed skaters. J Sports Med Phys Fitness 1990;30:83–88.

33. Raudsepp L, Jurimae T. Physical activity, fitness, and adiposity of prepubertal girls. Pediatr Exerc Sci 1996;8:259–267.

34. Duncan GE, Mahon AD, Howe CA, et al. Plateau in oxygen uptake at maximal exercise in male children. Pediatr Exerc Sci 1996;8:77–86.

35. Paterson DH, Cunningham DA, Donner A. The effect of different treadmill speeds on the variability of VO_2max in children. Eur J Appl Physiol 1981;47:113–122.

36. Pivarnik JM, Fulton JE, Taylor WE, et al. Aerobic capacity in black adolescent girls. Res Q Exerc Sport 1993;64:202–207.

37. Rivera-Brown AM, Rivera MA, Frontera WR. Achievement of VO_2max criteria in adolescent runners: effects of testing protocol. Pediatr Exerc Sci 1994;6: 236–245.

38. Pivarnik JM, Dwyer MC, Lauderdale MA. The reliability of aerobic capacity (VO_2max) testing in adolescent girls. Res Q Exerc Sport 1996;67:345–348.

39. Katch VL, Sady SP, Freedson P. Biological variability in maximum aerobic power. Med Sci Sports Exerc 1982;14:21–25.

40. Armstrong N, Welsman J, Winsley R. Is peak VO_2 a maximal index of children's aerobic fitness? Int J Sports Med 1996;17:356–359.

41. Rowland TW. Does peak VO_2 reflect VO_2max in children?

evidence from supramaximal testing. Med Sci Sports Exerc 1993;25:689–693.

42. Hickson RC, Bomze HA, Holloszy JO. Linear increase in aerobic power induced by a strenuous program of endurance exercise. J Appl Physiol 1977; 42:372–376.

43. Molloy GN. Varied intensities of training, predicted maximum oxygen uptake and the minimum threshold hypothesis. Percept Mot Skills 1988;67:791–794.

44. Costill DL. The relationship between selected physiological variables and distance running performance. J Sports Med Phys Fitness 1967;7:61–63.

45. Costill DL, Thomason H, Roberts E. Fractional utilization of the aerobic capacity during distance running. Med Sci Sports Exerc 1973;5:248–252.

46. Taylor HL, Buskirk E, Henschel A. Maximal oxygen intake as an objective measure of cardiorespiratory performance. J Appl Physiol 1955;8:73–80.

47. Al-Hazza HM, Sulaiman MA. Maximal oxygen uptake and daily physical activity in 7- to 12-year old boys. Pediatr Exerc Sci 1993;5:357–366.

48. Bar-Or O. Trainability of the prepubescent child. Phys Sports Med 1989;17:65–82.

49. Krahenbuhl GS, Skinner JS, Kohrt WM. Developmental aspects of maximal aerobic power in children. In: Terjung R, ed. Exercise and sport sciences review, vol 13. Philadelphia: Williams & Wilkins, 1985.

50. Sady SP, Katch VL, Berg K, et al. Individual differences in relative endurance and physiological response for prepubescents, adolescents, and adults. Pediatr Exerc Sci 1989;1:54–63.

51. Zwiren LD. Anaerobic and aerobic capacities of children. Pediatr Exerc Sci 1989;1:31–44.

52. Katch VL. Physical conditioning of children. J Adolesc Health Care 1983;3:241–246.

53. Ekblom B. Effect of physical training in adolescent boys. J Appl Physiol 1969;27:35–355.

54. Rowland TW. The "Trigger Hypothesis" for aerobic trainability: a 14-year follow-up. Pediatr Exerc Sci 1997;9:1–9.

55. Fahey TD, Del Valle-Zuris A, Oehlsen G, et al. Pubertal stage differences in hormonal and hematological responses to maximal exercise in males. J Appl Physiol 1979;46:823–827.

56. Knutsson U, Dahlgren J, Marcus C, et al. Circadian cortisol rhythms in healthy boys and girls: relationship with age, growth, body composition, and pubertal development. J Clin Endocrinol Metab 1997;82: 536–540.

57. Weber G, Kartodihardjo W, Klissouras V. Growth and physical training with reference to heredity. J Appl Physiol 1976;40:211–215.

58. Shepard RJ. Effectiveness of training programmes for prepubescent children. Sports Med 1992;13:194–213.

59. Williams JR, Armstrong N, Winter EM, et al. Changes in peak oxygen uptake with age and sexual maturation in boys: physiological fact or statistical anomaly? In: Coudert J, Van Praagh E, eds. Children and Exercise, vol XVI. Paris: Masson, 1992.

60. Rowland TW. Oxygen uptake and endurance fitness in children: a developmental perspective. Pediatr Exerc Sci 1989;1:313–328.

61. Cunningham DA, Paterson DH, Blimkie CJR. The development of the cardiorespiratory system with growth and physical activity. In: Boileau RA, ed. Advances in pediatric sport sciences, vol 1. Champaign, IL: Human Kinetics, 1984.

62. Malina RM, Bouchard C. Growth, maturation, and physical activity. Champaign IL: Human Kinetics, 1991.

63. Seely JE, Guzman CA, Becklake MR. Heart and lung function at rest and during exercise during adolescence. J Appl Physiol 1974;36:34–40.

64. Rowland TW. Exercise and children's health. Champaign, IL: Human Kinetics, 1990.

65. Armstrong N, Williams J, Balding J, et al. The peak oxygen uptake of British children with reference to age, sex, and sexual maturity. Eur J Appl Physiol 1991;62:369.

66. Astrand PO. Experimental studies of physical working capacity in relation to sex and age. Copenhagen: Munksgaard, 1952.

67. Koch G. Aerobic power, lung dimensions, ventilatory capacity, and muscle blood flow in 12-16-year-old boys with high physical activity. In Berg K, Eriksson BO, eds. Children and exercise IX. Baltimore: University Park Press, 1980.

68. Koch G, Fransson L. Essential cardiovascular and respiratory determinants of physical performance at age 12 to 17 years during intensive physical training. In: Rutenfranz J, Mocellin R, Klim F, eds. Children and exercise XII. Champaign, IL: Human Kinetics, 1986.

69. Cunningham DA, Paterson DA, Blimkie AP, et al. Development of cardiorespiratory function in circumpubertal boys: a longitudinal study. J Appl Physiol 1984;56: 302–307.

70. Godfrey S, Davies CTM, Wozniak E, et al. Cardiorespiratory responses to exercise in normal children. Clin Sci 1971;40:419–431.

71. Cooper DM. Development of the oxygen transport system in normal children. In: Bar-Or O, ed. Advances in pediatric sport sciences, vol 3. Champaign, IL: Human Kinetics, 1989.

72. Astrand PO, Rodahl K. Textbook of work physiology. New York: McGraw-Hill, 1977.

73. Caillaud CF, Anselme FM, Prefaut CG. Effects of two successive exercise tests on pulmonary gas exchange in athletes. Eur J Appl Physiol 1996;74:141–147.

74. Pedersen PK, Mandoe H, Jensen K, et al. Reduced arterial O2 saturation during supine exercise in highly trained cyclists. Acta Physiol Scand 1996;158:325–331.

75. Eriksson BO. Physical training, oxygen supply and muscle metabolism in 11–13 year old boys. Acta Physiol Scand 1972;384(suppl):1–48.

76. Chatterjee S, Banerjee PK, Chatterjee P, et al. Aerobic capacity of young girls. Indian J Med Res 1979;69:327–333.

77. Bar-Or O. Pediatric sports medicine for the practitioner. New York: Springer-Verlag, 1983.

78. Cooper DM, Kaplan MR, Baumgarten L, et al. Coupling of ventilation with lung growth. J Appl Physiol 1987;51:699–705.

79. Baxter-Jones ADG, Helms PJ. Effects of training at a young age: a review of the training of young athletes (TOYA) study. Pediatr Exerc Sci 1996;8:31–327.

80. Shepard RJ, Lavallee H. Effects of enhanced physical education on lung volumes of primary school children. J Sports Med Phys Fitness 1996;36:186–194.

81. Armstrong N, Kirby BJ, McManus AM, et al. Prepubescents' ventilatory responses to exercise with reference to sex and body size. Chest 1997;112:1554–1560.

82. Mercier J, Varray A, Ramonatxo M, et al. Influence of anthropometric characteristics on changes in maximal exercise ventilation and breathing patterns during growth in boys. Eur J Appl Physiol 1991;63:235–241.

83. Prioux J, Ramonatxo M, Mercier J, et al. Changes in maximal exercise ventilation and breathing pattern in boys during growth: a mixed cross-sectional longitudinal study. Acta Physiol Scand 1997;161:447–458.

84. Rowland TW, Cunningham LN. Development of ventilatory responses to exercise in normal white children: a longitudinal study. Chest 1997;111:327–332.

85. Rowland T, Vanderburgh P, Cunningham L. Body size and the growth of maximal aerobic power in children: a longitudinal analysis. Ped Exerc Sci 1997;9:262–274.

86. Armstrong N, Welsman JR. Assessment and interpretation of aerobic fitness in children and adolescents. In: Holloszy JO, ed. Exercise and sport sciences reviews, vol 22. Baltimore: Williams and Wilkins, 1994.

87. Krahenbuhl GS, Skinner JS, Kohrt WM. Developmental aspects of maximal aerobic power in children. In: Terjung R, ed. Exercise and sport sciences reviews, vol 13. Baltimore: Williams and Wilkins, 1985.

88. Armstrong N, Balding J, Gentle P, et al. Peak oxygen uptake and physical activity in 11- to 16-year-olds. Pediatr Exerc Sci 1990;2:349–358.

89. Milicevic G, Fabecic-Sabadi V, Rudan P, et al. Sex differences in pubertal growth of the heart. Am J Hum Biol 1997;9:297–302.

90. Lacour JR, Padilla-Magunacelaya S, Chatard JC, et al. Assessment of running velocity at maximal oxygen uptake. Eur J Appl Physiol 1991;62:77–82.

91. Padilla S, Bourdin M, Barhelemy JC, et al. Physiological correlates of middle-distance running performance. Eur J Appl Physiol 1992;62:561–566.

92. di Prampero PE, Atchou G, Bruckner JC, et al. The energetics of endurance running. Eur J Appl Physiol 1986;55:259–266.

93. Berthoin S, Baquet G, Manteca F, et al. Maximal aerobic speed and running time to exhaustion for children 6 to 17 years old. Pediatr Exerc Sci 1996;8:234–244.

94. Kemper HCG, Verschuur R, de Mey L. Longitudinal changes of aerobic fitness in youth ages 12 to 23. Pediatr Exerc Sci 1989;1:257–270.

95. Allen WK, Seals DR, Hurley BF, et al. Lactate threshold and distance-running performance in young and older endurance athletes. J Appl Physiol 1985;58:1281–1284.

96. Armstrong N, Welsman JR, Kirby BJ. Performance on the Wingate anaerobic test and maturation. Pediatr Exerc Sci 1997;9:253–261.

97. Blimkie CJR, Roche P, Hay JT, et al. Anaerobic power of arms in teenage boys and girls: relationship to lean tissue. Eur J Appl Physiol 1988;57:677–683.

98. Berg A, Kim SS, Keul J. Skeletal muscle enzyme activities in healthy young subjects. Int J Sports Med 1986;7:236–239.

99. Falk B, Bar-Or O. Longitudinal changes in peak aerobic and anaerobic mechanical power of circumpubertal boys. Pediatr Exerc Sci 1993;5:318–331.

100. Mero A. Blood lactate production and recovery from anaerobic exercise in trained and untrained boys. Eur J Appl Physiol 1988;57:660–666.

101. Palgi Y, Gutin B, Young J, et al. Physiologic and anthropometric factors underlying endurance performance. Int J Sports Med 1984;5:67–73.

102. Paterson DH, McLellan TM, Stella RS, et al. Longitudinal study of ventilation threshold and maximal O_2 uptake in athletic boys. J Appl Physiol 1987;62:2051–2057.

103. Saavedra C, Lagasse P, Bouchard C, et al. Maximal anaerobic performance of the knee extensor muscles during growth. Med Sci Sports Exerc 1991;23:1083–1089.

104. Vanden Eynde B, Vienne D, Vuylsteke-Wauters M, et al. Aerobic power and pubertal peak height velocity in Belgian boys. Eur J Appl Physiol 1988;57:430–434.

105. Williams JR, Armstrong N, Kirby BJ. The 4 mmol blood lactate level as an index of exercise performance in 11–13 year old

children. J Sport Sci 1990;8: 139–147.

106. Williams JR, Armstrong N. The influence of age and sexual maturation on children's blood lactate responses to exercise. Pediatr Exerc Sci 1991;3:111–120.

107. Wirth A, Trager E, Scheele K, et al. Cardiopulmonary adjustment and metabolic response to maximal and submaximal physical exercise of boys and girls at different stages of maturity. Eur J Appl Physiol 1978;39:229–240.

108. Beneke R, Heck H, Schwarz V, et al. Maximal lactate steady state during the second decade of age. Med Sci Sports Exerc 1996;28: 1474–1478.

109. Blimkie CJR, Roche P, Bar-Or O. The anaerobic-to-aerobic power ratio in adolescent boys and girls. In: Rutenfranz J, Mocellin R, Klimt F, eds. Children and exercise XII. Champaign, IL: Human Kinetics, 1986.

110. Falgairette G, Bedu M, Fellman N, et al. Modifications of aerobic and anaerobic metabolisms in active boys during puberty. In: Beunen G, Ghesquiere J, Reybrouck TM, et al. eds. Children and exercise IX. Stuttgart: Ferdinand Enke, 1990.

111. Welsman JR, Armstrong N, Kirby BJ. Serum testosterone is not related to peak VO2 and submaximal blood lactate responses in 12- to 16-year-old males. Pediatr Exerc Sci 1994;6:120–127.

112. Sale DG. Strength training in children. In: Gisolfi CV, Lamb DR, eds. Perspectives in exercise and sports medicine. Madison, WI: Benchmark, 1989.

113. Pfitzinger P, Freedson P. Blood lactate responses to exercise in children, part 1: peak lactate concentration. Pediatr Exerc Sci 1997;9:210–222.

114. Washington RL, van Gundy JC, Cohen C, et al. Normal aerobic and anaerobic exercise data for North American school-age children. J Pediatr 1988;112:223–233.

115. Forster MA, Hunter GR, Hester DJ, et al. Aerobic capacity and grade-walking economy of children 5–9 years old: a longitudinal study. Pediatr Exerc Sci 1994;6:31–38.

116. Maliszewski AF, Freedson PS. Is running economy different between adults and children? Pediatr Exerc Sci 1996;8:351–360.

117. Atomi Y, Fukunaga T, Hatta H, et al. Lactate threshold: its change with growth and relationship to leg muscle composition in prepubertal children. In: Malina RM, ed. Young athletes. Champaign, IL: Human Kinetics, 1988.

118. Berg A, Keul J. Biochemical changes during exercise in children. In: Malina RM, ed. Young athletes. Champaign, IL: Human Kinetics, 1988.

119. Reybrouck T, Weymans M, Stijns H, et al. Ventilatory anaerobic threshold in healthy children. Eur J Appl Physiol 1985;54:278–284.

120. Reybrouck TM. The use of the anaerobic threshold in pediatric exercise testing. In Bar-Or O, ed. Advances in pediatric sport sciences, vol 3. Champaign, IL: Human Kinetics, 1989.

121. Paterson DH, Cunningham DA. Development of anaerobic capacity in early and late maturing boys. In: Binkhorst RA, Kemper CG, Saris WHM, eds. Children and exercise XI. Champaign, IL: Human Kinetics, 1985.

122. Lamphier DE, Montoye HJ. Muscular strength and body size. Hum Biol 1976;48:147–160.

123. Roberts DF, Provins KA, Morton RJ. Arm strength and body dimensions. Hum Biol 1959;31:334–343.

124. Sale DG, MacDougall JD, Alway SE, et al. Voluntary strength and muscle characteristics in untrained men and women and male bodybuilders. J Appl Physiol 1987;62:1786–1793.

125. Schantz P, Randall-Fox E, Hutchinson W, et al. Muscle fibre type distribution, muscle cross-

sectional area and maximal voluntary strength in humans. Acta Physiol Scand 1983;117:219–226.

126. Miyashita M, Kanehisa H. Dynamic peak torque related to age, sex, and performance. Res Q Exerc Sport 1979;50:249–255.

127. Kanehisa H, Ikegawa S, Tsunoda N, et al. Strength and cross-sectional area of knee extensor muscles in children. Eur J Appl Physiol 1994;68:402–405.

128. Kanehisa H, Yata H, Ikegawa S, et al. A cross-sectional study of the size and strength of the lower leg muscles during growth. Eur J Appl Physiol 1995;72:150–156.

129. Ikai M, Fukunaga T. Calculation of muscle strength per unit cross-sectional area of human muscle by means of ultrasonic measurement. Int Zeit Ange Physiol 1968;26:26–32.

130. Moritani T, Oddson L, Thorstensson A, et al. Neural and biomechanical differences between men and young boys during a variety of motor tasks. Acta Physiol Scand 1989;137: 347–355.

131. Ozmun JC, Mikesky AE, Surburg PR. Neuromuscular adaptations following prepubescent strength training. Med Sci Sports Exerc 1994;26:510–514.

132. Glenmark B, Hedberg G, Kaijser L, et al. Muscle strength from adolescence to adulthood—relationship to muscle fibre types. Eur J Appl Physiol 1994;68:9–19.

133. Shepard RJ, Lavallee H. Impact of enhanced physical education on muscle strength of the prepubescent child. Pediatr Exerc Sci 1994;6:75–87.

134. Miller AEJ, MacDougall JD, Tarnopolsky MA, et al. Gender differences in strength and muscle fiber characteristics. Eur J Appl Physiol 1993;66:254–262.

135. Castro MJ, McCann DJ, Shaffrath JD, et al. Peak torque per unit cross-sectional area differs between strength-trained and

untrained young adults. Med Sci Sports Exerc 1995;27:397–403.

136. Heyward VH, Johannes-Ellis SM, Romer JF. Gender differences in strength. Res Q Exerc Sport 1986;57:154–159.

137. Davies CTM. Strength and mechanical properties of muscle in children and young adults. Scand J Sports Sci 1985;7:11–15.

138. Gilliam TB, Villanacci JF, Freedson PS, et al. Isokinetic torque in boys and girls ages 7 to 13: effect of age, height, and weight. Res Q Exerc Sport 1979; 50:599–609.

139. Sinaki M, Limburg PJ, Wollan PC, et al. Correlation of trunk muscle strength with age in children 5 to 18 years old. Mayo Clinic Proc 1996;71:1047–1054.

140. Whitall J. The evolution of research on motor development: new approaches bringing new insights. In: Holloszy JO, ed. Exercise and sport sciences reviews, vol 23. Baltimore: Williams and Wilkins, 1995.

141. Espenschade AS, Eckert HM. Motor development. 2nd ed. Columbus, OH: Merrill, 1980.

142. Thomas JR, French KE. Gender differences across age in motor performance: a meta-analysis. Psychol Bull 1985;98:260–282.

143. Morris AM, Williams JM, Atwater AE, et al. Age and sex differences in motor performance of 3 through 6-year-old children. Res Q Exerc Sport 1983;53:214–221.

144. Bishop P. Gender differences in motor performance. Nebr Med J 1987;17:19–25.

145. Raudsepp L, Paasuke M. Gender differences in fundamental movement patterns, motor performances, and strength measurements of prepubertal children. Pediatr Exerc Sci 1995; 7:294–304.

146. Bell RD, Hoshizaki TB. Relationships of age and sex with range of motion of seventeen joint

actions in humans. Can J Appl Sport Sci 1981;6:202–206.

147. Tanner J. Fetus into man—physical growth from conception to maturity. Cambridge, MA: Harvard University Press, 1978.

148. Grattan MP, De Vos E, Levy J, et al. Asymmetric action in the human newborn: sex differences in patterns of organization. Child Dev 1992;63:273–289.

149. Halverson LE, Roberton MA, Safrit MJ, et al. Effect of guided practice on overhand-throw ball velocities of kindergarten children. Res Q Exerc Sport 1982; 48:311–318.

150. Nelson KR, Thomas JR, Nelson JK. Longitudinal change in throwing performance: gender differences. Res Q Exerc Sport 1991; 62:105–108.

151. Roberton M. Longitudinal evidence for developmental stages in the forceful overarm throw. J Hum Mov Stud 1978;4:167–175.

152. Nelson JK, Thomas JR, Nelson KR, et al. Gender differences in children's throwing performance: biology and environment. Res Q Exerc Sport 1986;57:280–287.

153. Thomas JR, Marzke MW. The development of gender differences in throwing: is human evolution a factor? In: Enhancing human performance in sport: new concepts and developments, American Academy of Physical Education Papers, no 25. Champaign, IL: Human Kinetics, 1991.

154. Wade MG. Gender differences in throwing: evolutionary evidence of more monkey business? a reaction to Thomas and Marzke. In: Enhancing human performance in sport: new concepts and developments, American Academy of Physical Education Papers, no 25. Champaign, IL: Human Kinetics, 1991.

155. Raudsepp L, Jurimae T. Relationship of physical activity and somatic characteristics with physical fitness and motor skill in

prepubertal girls. Am J Hum Biol 1997;9:513–521.

156. Haubenstricker J, Sapp M. A longitudinal look at physical growth and motor performance: implications for elementary and middle school activity programs. Presented at the Meeting of the American Alliance for Health, Physical Education, Recreation and Dance, Detroit, MI, 1980.

157. Eckert HM. Age changes in motor skills. In: Parick GL, ed. Physical activity: human growth development. New York: Academic Press, 1973.

158. Davies BN. The relationship of lean limb volume to performance in the handgrip and standing long jump tests in boys and girls, aged 11.6–13.2 years. Eur J Appl Physiol 1990;60:139–143.

159. Little NG, Day JAP, Steinke L. Relationship of physical performance to maturation in perimenarchal girls. Am J Hum Biol 1997;9:163–171.

160. Espenschade AS, Meleney HE. Motor performance of adolescent boys and girls of today in comparison with those of 24 years ago. Res Q Exerc Sport 1961;32:186–189.

161. Branta C, Haubenstricker J, Seefeldt V. Age changes in motor skill during childhood and adolescence. In: Terjung RL, ed. Exercise and sport sciences reviews, vol 12. Toronto: DC Heath, 1984.

162. Beunen G, Colla R, Simons J, et al. Sexual dimorphism in somatic and motor characteristics. In: Oseid S, Carlsen K, eds. Children and exercise XIII, vol. 19. Champaign, IL: Human Kinetics, 1989.

163. Frenkl R, Meszaros J, Mohacsi J, et al. Biological maturation and motor performance in 12- to 14-year-old girls. In: Malina RM, ed. Young athletes. Champaign, IL: Human Kinetics, 1988.

164. Rowland TW. Exercise, nutrition, and the prevention of cardiovascular disease: a pediatric perspective. Med Exerc Nutr Health 1992;1:34–41.

165. Garcia AW, Norton Broda MA, Frenn M, et al. Gender and developmental differences in exercise beliefs among youth and prediction of their exercise behavior. J School Health 1995; 65:213–219.

166. Garcia G. Gender differences in young children's interactions when learning fundamental motor skills. Res Q Exerc Sport 1994; 65:213–225.

167. Myers L, Strikmiller PK, Webber LS, et al. Physical and sedentary activity in school children grades 5–8: the Bogalusa heart study. Med Sci Sports Exerc 1996;28: 852–859.

168. Saris WHM. Habitual physical activity in children: methodology and findings in health and disease. Med Sci Sports Exerc 1986;18:253–263.

169. Trost SG, Pate RR, Dowda M, et al. Gender differences in physical activity and determinants of physical activity in rural fifth grade children. J School Health 1996;66:145–150.

170. Stucky-Ropp RC, DiLorenzo TM. Determinants of exercise in children. Prev Med 1993;22:880–889.

171. Treiber FA, Baranowski T, Braden DS, et al. Social support for exercise: relationship to physical activity in young adults. Prev Med 1991;20:737–750.

172. Dennison BA, Straus JH, Mellits D, et al. Childhood physical fitness tests: predictor of adult physical activity levels? Pediatrics 1988;82:324–330.

173. Greendorfer SL. Shaping the female athlete: the impact of the family. In: Boutilier MA, San Giovanni L, eds. The sporting women: feminism and sociological dilemmas. Champaign, IL: Human Kinetics, 1983.

Chapter 56

Resistance Training and Youth: Enhancing Muscle Fitness

William J. Kraemer
Avery D. Faigenbaum
Jill A. Bush
Bradley C. Nindl

Over the past 10 years a greater awareness of the effects of resistance training for youth has been observed (96). However, unfounded fears still exist because of misconceptions about the training modality. It is important that the actual facts related to resistance training and youth are clearly understood as this modality is an important tool in physical conditioning programs for youth. Its benefits are related to: 1) enhanced neuromuscular fitness; 2) prevention of sports injuries; 3) enhanced soft tissue status (especially bone), which may have greater importance in the aging process; and 4) improved sports performance.

EFFECTIVENESS OF YOUTH RESISTANCE TRAINING

It has been previously thought that training-induced strength gains during prepubescence were not feasible due to insufficient concentrations of circulating growth factors and androgens (3). The results from a few studies (38,73,139) were believed to support this contention despite the fact that these studies suffered from methodologic limitations. The majority of the scientific evidence over the last 10 years, however, strongly suggests that children can significantly increase their strength—independent from growth and maturation—providing that the resistance training program is long enough and of high enough intensity (22,36,48–51,57,76,89,103,105,114,118, 119,121,125,145–147).

During childhood, many physiologic changes related to growth and development occur dynamically and rapidly. Muscular strength—defined as the maximal force a muscle or muscle group can generate—normally increases from child-

hood through the early teenage years, at which time there is a striking acceleration of strength in boys and a general plateau of strength in girls (87). Thus strength changes that result from a low-volume (sets × repetitions × load), short-term training program may not be distinguishable from gains due to normal growth and development. In order to delineate training adaptations from those of normal growth and development, a prolonged period of time and an adequate training stimulus are essential.

It appears convincing at this point in time that resistance training is effective in youth. Meta-analyses on resistance training in children (34,51) as well as scientific review papers (13,14,42,54,82,92,115,141,142) and clinical observations (8,94) have reported that properly designed resistance training programs can facilitate the development of the strength of prepubescents and adolescents beyond that which is due to normal growth and development. Children as young as the age of 6 have derived benefits from resistance training (50), and studies have been as long as 9 months (125). To date, there is no clear evidence of any major difference in strength, as measured by selected strength tests, between prepubescent boys and girls (12,115).

A wide variety of progressive resistance training programs appear to work over short periods of training in untrained children; (e.g., from 1 set of 10 repetitions (146) to 5 sets of 15 repetitions (76) have proven to work in eliciting improvements in desired outcome variables. How resistance training programs differentiate over time with training at various ages is still not clear in children nor even in adult populations. Thus the type of resistance training program used may well have an impact on a specific type of training adaptation after initial adaptations are seen at a given age.

This will require longer-term studies in the future. In addition, it appears that training programs will have to be "periodized" or varied over time or boredom could well limit the adherence to a program in an "electronic" culture in which children are conditioned to have short attention spans for a given activity. Studies have used many training modalities and have included a wide variety of equipment, including adult weight machines (36,89,103,105,119,139,147), child-size machines (14,46,48), free weights (21,36,105,114,118), hydraulic machines (143), pneumatic machines (119), isometric contractions (57,73,98), wrestling drills (29), modified pull-ups (9), and calisthenics (50,121).

Comparative Trainability

Muscle strength gains as great as 74% have been reported following 8 weeks of progressive resistance training (48). On average, gains of roughly 30% to 50% are typically observed following short-term (8 to 20 weeks) resistance training programs in children. How much of these gains are related to motor learning effects in the early phase of training remains to be definitively determined. Relative (percentage improvement) strength gains achieved during prepubescence have been reported to be equal to if not greater than the relative gains observed during adolescence (98,103,145). Obviously, the absolute strength gains (e.g., the amount of weight lifted) appear to be greater in adolescents compared to prepubescents (115,139) and adults can make even greater absolute gains than young adolescents (114). The issue of whether training-induced changes observed in prepubescents and adolescents should be compared on a relative or absolute basis remains debatable (115).

Persistence of Training-Induced Strength Gains

The evaluation of strength changes in children with detraining is confounded by the concomitant growth-related strength increases during the same time period (13). Few studies have evaluated the effects of detraining in adults, and relative information on younger populations is not extensive. Nevertheless, limited data suggests that training-induced strength gains in children are impermanent, and tend to regress towards untrained control group values during the detraining period (16,46). The precise mechanisms of the detraining response and the physiologic adapations that occur during this period remain to be fully elucidated, although changes in neuromuscular functioning would appear to play a significant role at least during prepubescence.

A small number of studies have evaluated the effects of training frequency on strength maintenance in children. After 20 weeks of progressive resistance training, a once-weekly maintenance training program was not adequate to maintain the training-induced strength gains in prepubescent boys (12). Conversely, a 1 day/wk maintenance program was just as sufficient as a 2 day/wk maintenance program in retaining the strength gains made after 12 weeks of resistance training in a group of pubescent male athletes (36). Clearly, more information is required before specific maintenance training recommendations can be made. How the young child's body interacts with the specific program stimuli (e.g., amount of adaptation elicited) at different ages, the amount of adaptational advantage trying to be maintained at a given age, and

which types of programs are most effective all would interact on such exercise prescription studies.

Program Evaluation and Testing

Factors such as previous exercise experience, acute program variable design (i.e., number of repetitions/sets, rest between sets, relative repetition maximum load, etc.), specificity of testing and training, choice of equipment, quality of instruction, and whether or not the learning effect was controlled for in the study can directly influence the degree of measured strength increase. In addition, the methods of evaluating changes in muscular strength consequent to training are also important considerations. In several studies the subjects were trained with one modality, but tested using another modality (103,119,142), and in many of the studies strength changes were evaluated by relatively high repetition maximum (RM) values (e.g., 10 RM) (48,146). With the exception of a few studies (36,101,105), strength changes were rarely evaluated by maximal load lifting (i.e., 1 RM testing) on the equipment used in training. Although it is not possible to evaluate 1 RM strength on some types of equipment (e.g., hydraulic machines), this part of the evaluation is potentially problematic.

Many clinicians and researchers have not used 1 RM testing to evaluate training-induced changes in muscular strength because of the unfounded fear that heavy resistance loading may cause structural damage in children. Thus the maximal force production capabilities of children have not been directly evaluated in most studies. It is important to note that no injuries have been reported in prospective studies that utilized adequate warmup periods, appropriate progression of loads, close and experienced supervision, and critically chosen maximal strength tests (1 RM performance lifts, maximal isometric tests, and maximal isokinetic tests) to evaluate resistance training-induced changes in children (36,101,105). Direct strength and power tests are needed in order to evaluate functional changes in children that reflect the physiologic context of the performance variable.

The examination of the relative safety of supervised 1 RM and power testing in laboratory settings performed only to evaluate training-induced changes in muscular strength should be philosophically supported. Most of the forces that children are exposed to in various sports and recreational activities are likely to be greater in both exposure time and magnitude than competently supervised and properly performed maximal strength tests. Conversely, unsupervised and improperly performed 1 RM testing (e.g., inadequate progression of loading and poor lifting technique) and chronic maximum resistance training (e.g., weightlifting training without periodization) should not be performed by children under any circumstances due to the actual risk of injury (108,109,148).

Physiologic Mechanisms for Strength Development

In prepubescents it appears that training-induced strength gains are more related to neural mechanisms (81). In addition, changes in the "quality" of the muscle proteins (e.g., myosin heavy chains) could also explain force production improvements in children. Several training studies (48,89,101,105,114, 143) have reported significant improvements in strength during prepubescence without corresponding increases in gross limb morphology, as compared to a similar control group. Without adequate concentrations of circulating growth factors and androgens to stimulate increases in muscle size, prepubescents appear to experience more difficulty increasing their muscle mass consequent to a resistance training program (up to 20 weeks) as compared to older populations. However, studies have shown the potential for hypertrophy in younger children, so further research is needed to understand the physiologic conditions or program types that cause increases in muscle size (56,93).

Without corresponding increases in fat-free mass, it appears that neural adaptations (i.e., a trend towards increased motor unit activation and changes in motor unit coordination, recruitment, and firing) (101,105) and possibly intrinsic muscle adaptations (as evidenced by increases in twitch torque) (105) appear to be primarily responsible for training-induced strength gains during prepubescence. Enhancements in motor skill performance and the coordination of the involved muscle groups may also play a significant role because measured increases in training-induced strength are typically greater than changes in neuromuscular activation (101,105).

During puberty, testicular testosterone secretion in boys is associated with considerable increases in fat-free mass (82,86). Training-induced strength gains during and after puberty in males may therefore be associated with changes in hypertrophic factors, since hormonal influences on muscle hypertrophy would be imminent (82). Lower levels of androgens in females may limit the absolute magnitude of training-induced increases in muscle hypertrophy (115). Other hormone and growth factors (e.g., growth hormone and insulin-like growth factors) may be at least partly responsible for muscle development in women (80). The growth hormone/insulin-like growth factor-1 axis is recognized as both complex and polymorphic. This axis no doubt is a central one in the endocrine/autocrine interplay between exercise and tissue growth during development and merits future study as related to strength training and youth.

MOTOR FITNESS SKILLS AND SPORTS PERFORMANCE

Improvements in selected motor fitness skills have been reported in children following resistance training programs (50,98,143,147). Several studies have reported increases in the long jump or vertical jump (50,98,143,147) and one study (147) noted increases in 30-meter dash and agility run time. In contrast, two studies (21,48) reported significant increases in strength without concomitant improvements in selected motor performance skills following several weeks of progressive resistance training. Since the effects of resistance training are dependent upon the duration, frequency, speed, and volume of the training stimulus, confounding variables in the program design may partly explain these inconsistent findings. Moreover, the effects of resistance training on motor fitness skills must be distinguished from those associated with growth and maturation.

When evaluating the effects of resistance training on selected motor fitness skills, consideration msut be given to the principle of training specificity. It appears that training adaptations in children, like adults, are specific to the movement pattern, velocity of movement, contraction type, and contraction force (68,116). The specificity of training and possible transfer to related activities was observed in 249 females aged 7 to 19 who participated in a 5-week training program (98). The subjects trained for a particular test (sprint acceleration, vertical jump, or isometric strength) by either running, jumping, or performing isometrics. Independent of age, the greatest improvements were made in the activity for which the subjects trained, although some degree of transfer to nonspecific movements was noted. Again, major training adaptations in children are exercise specific.

That resistance training may enhance sport performance in children seems reasonable because many of the sports in which children participate have a significant strength or power component. Moreover, if stretching exercises are part of the resistance training program, flexibility has been shown to significantly improve (121,143). Anecdotal comments from parents of children who have participated in a resistance training program suggest that resistance training enhances athletic ability (49,143). Scientific evaluations of this observation are difficult because successful athletic performance is the result of many varied factors (i.e., skill, athletic ability, coaching/instruction, psychological, etc.) (82). There have been no long-term studies that have examined the impact of a comprehensive preseason resistance training regimen on improved sports performance in children. Information that would be yielded from such data would be beneficial to fully understand the effects of resistance training on youth sports performance, and to evaluate the potential for carryover into adulthood.

Studies (11,23) have reported improved changes in swimming performance in age-group swimmers. One study (104) demonstrated significant gains in strength and selected gymnastic events in prepubescent girls following a resistance training program. Conversely, one short-term isometric training program did not improve swim speed in 7- to 17-year-old swimmers (2), and a resistance training program compared to basketball practice did not result in any influence on selected basketball skills in 14- and 15-year-old boys (53).

Conclusions regarding the effects of resistance training on sports performance during prepubescence and adolescence are equivocal, primarily due to experimental design problems and limited training time to differentiate performance effects that have high skill components. Collectively, however, limited direct and indirect evidence as well as observations from older populations (52,151) indicate that a commonsense sports-specific resistance training program will result in some degree of improvement in athletic performance. Curtailment of the preseason and inseason practice sessions to allow time for sport preparatory resistance training seems reasonable, providing that the training program is competently supervised, progressive, and of sufficient duration and intensity. In addition, the need for periodized training programs in research designs is needed to optimize programs, especially long-term training programs. Since children can not "play" themselves into shape, one of the greatest benefits of youth resistance training may be its ability to better prepare children for participation in sports and recreational activities, thus reducing injury risk.

PREVENTION OF INJURIES

The popularity of sports participation by American children has grown exponentially over the last two decades. Approximately 30 million American children (roughly 50% of the boys and 25% of the girls) play competitive organized sports, and many others participate in community-based sport programs. With this increase in sports participation have come numerous reports of injuries to the ill-prepared and/or improperly trained youth athlete (28,100). Properly designed and supervised resistance training programs could help to prevent injuries in youth sports and recreational activities.

Resistance training appears to be an effective injury-prevention strategy for adults, and it seems likely that similar mechanisms may be responsible for decreasing the prevalence of injury in youth sports (26,110). The mechanisms by which improving muscle strength may prevent or lessen the severity of an injury include the strengthening of supporting structural tissues (e.g., ligaments, tendons and bones) (31,130); the enhanced ability of a trained muscle to absorb more energy prior to failure (58); and the development of muscle balance and proprioception around a specific joint (72). Not surprisingly, the incidence and recurrence of hamstring injuries in college football players has been shown to decrease when muscle imbalances are corrected (72).

Only a limited number of studies have demonstrated a decreased injury rate in adolescents who have used resistance training (39,71). A preseason conditioning program that included resistance training reduced the number and severity of injuries in high school football players (24). Similarly, resistance training decreased the incidence of shoulder problems in teenage swimmers (39) and older athletes (70).

In one report (71) involving high school boy and girl athletes, the injury rate of athletes who used resistance training was 26.2% versus 72.4% for those who did not. Moreover, the amount of time that each group required for rehabilitation was 2.02 days and 4.82 days, respectively. Even though a motivated athlete who was injured may be more likely to return to practice sooner and endure some pain, this athlete may also spend more time in competition, thereby increasing the risk of injury. Although it may be tempting to generalize these positive findings to prepubescent boys and girls, differences in the quality and quantity of sport training, degrees of aggressiveness and competition, and participation rates in contact and noncontact sports also need to be considered (15).

Furthermore, the inclusion of resistance training to the total exercise dose, which includes free play as well as organized sports, should be carefully considered. Resistance training adds to the chronic, repetitive stress placed upon the immature musculoskeletal system. Some children with relatively immature musculoskeletal systems may not tolerate the same exercise dose that the majority of the children in the same athletic program can tolerate. This biologic uniqueness may result in stress failure syndromes in those children, manifested by a variety of conditions including tendonitis, stress fractures, and juvenile osteochondritis dissecans (28,100).

Due to interindividual variability of stress tolerance, each child must be treated as an individual and observed for signs of incipient stress failure syndromes that would require a modification of the frequency, volume, intensity, and progression of training. With an awareness of this variability in children of the same age to accept and tolerate stress, many of these stress failure syndromes can be prevented through timely intervention.

Resistance training programs should not simply be added onto children's exercise regimens, which may already include several hours of free play and sport-specific training. Rather, youth resistance training programs should ideally be incorporated into a "periodized conditioning program" that varies in volume and intensity throughout the year (128). This means careful attention is paid to planned changes in the exercise intensity, volume, and recovery periods over the year. Correctable risk factors (e.g., muscle imbalances, inflexibility, poor physical condition) should be identified so that coaches and clinicians can address the specific needs of each child. In some instances it may be necessary for young sport specialists to reduce their sport involvement to allow time for preparatory conditioning.

RISK OF INJURY

Many reasons were given for not recommending resistance training for the immature athlete over the past two decades. One of the primary fears was the presumed high risk of injury associated with this type of exercise. This fear of injury associated with youth resistance training was first created by early data gathered by the National Electronic Injury Surveillance System (NEISS) of the United States Consumer Product Safety Commission. NEISS used data from various emergency room departments to make nationwide projections of the total number of injuries related to exercises and equipment. In addition, perception and visions of what weight training looked like from a media and entertainment perspective (adult body builders, weightlifters in competition) also tainted the more mundane activities that actually comprised the supervised training sessions of young people in physical education, YMCA/YWCA, and sports training sessions. Much of the fear was due to the actual lack of experience and familiarity with the modality by most medical and scientific professionals through the 1970s and into the 1980s (e.g., few had every participated in an actual resistance training program themselves).

In 1979 it was reported by the United States Consumer Product Safety Commission (136) that over half of the 35,512 weightlifting injuries requiring emergency room treatment involved 10- to 19-year-olds. In a 1987 report (137), it was revealed that 8590 children under age 14 visited the emergency room because of so-called weightlifting injuries. However, the NEISS reports did not distinguish between injuries associated with resistance training and those associated with the competitive sports of power lifting and weightlifting. This is an important discriminating factor, as any athlete will take greater risks when the upper limits of competition are involved in both training and competition. In reality, the goal of competitive lifting sports is "maximal performance." Thus, separate issues of risk assessment exist (i.e., health and fitness benefits versus competitive sport). This impacts both the training programs needed and the associated risks of competition in sport. Many have confused the assessments of this risk-benefit ratio.

The most common resistance training injuries in the NEISS reports were sprains and strains, although more serious injuries (e.g., epiphyseal fractures and lumbosacral injuries) have been noted in the literature (108,109). However, nationwide projections of emergency room department visits and case series reports of injured young athletes provide limited information on the predisposing factors of these injuries. In fact, many of the reported injuries were actually caused by improper training methods, excessive loading, poorly designed equipment, ready access to the equipment without supervision, or a lack of qualified adult supervision. Although these findings indicate that the unsupervised use of heavy resistive loads in training or competition may be injurious, it is misleading to generalize these findings to properly designed and closely supervised youth resistance training programs.

Generally, the risk of injury associated with resistance training is similar for children and adults. But a traditional area of concern in children is the potential for training-induced damage to the epiphysis, or growth plate, of their long bones (81). The epiphysis is the weak link in the young skeleton because the strength of cartilage is less than that of bone (20). If not properly treated, damage to this area of the bone could cause the epiphysis to seal, resulting in limb deformity and/or the cessation of limb growth (20,92,122). A few retrospective case reports have noted epiphyseal plate fractures during prepubescence (65) and adolescence (10,19,65,79,111,113). However, most of these injuries were due to improper lifting techniques, maximal lifts, or lack of qualified adult supervision. The classic example of a young boy trying to lift a near maximal weight in the basement without supervision or proper understanding of the resistance training techniques or proper programs is the worst-case scenario of increasing the risk of injury to a young person.

Both prepubescents and adolescents are susceptible to growth plate injuries, yet it appears that the potential for this injury in a prepubescent child may be less than in an adolescent child because the growth plates may actually be stronger and more resistant to sheering type forces in the younger child (94). Growth plate fractures have not occurred in any prospective resistance training studies that were characterized by appropriately prescribed training regimens and competent instruction.

The potential for repetitive use soft-tissue injuries is also of concern when children use resistance training. This type of injury often does not always cause children to go to the emergency room or even to see a physician, so the incidence of these injuries is more difficult to determine. Nevertheless, several retrospective studies involving adolescents have associated lower back soft-tissue injuries with resistance training. In fact, lumbosacral pain was the most frequent injury in high school athletes who participated in resistance training programs (19). In one report (19), a majority of the injuries to the lumbar spine may be attributed to the improper use of a device designed to improve vertical jump. A study of adolescent power lifters who presumably trained with maximal or near-maximal resistances revealed that 50% of reported injuries were to the lower back, 18% to the upper extremity, 17% to the lower extremity, and 14% to the trunk (21). Although these studies involved adolescents, the potential for similar injuries in prepubescents should be recognized. Based

on available evidence and clinical observations, training-induced injuries to the lower back seem to pose a noteworthy concern for clinicians and coaches (77,88,115,141).

Prospective studies involving resistance training and children indicate a low risk of injury. In the vast majority of the published studies, no overt clinical injuries having been reported during the resistance training program. Although various training modalities and a variety of training regimens have been used, all the training programs were closely supervised and appropriately prescribed to ensure that the training program was matched to the initial capacity of the child. Only two published studies have reported injuries related to resistance training in children: a shoulder strain that resolved within one week of rest (107) and an undefined "minor" injury (21). In one study (107), there was no evidence of either musculoskeletal injury (measured by biphasic scintigraphy) or muscle necrosis (determined by serum creatine phosphokinase levels) following 14 weeks of progressive resistance training. Generally, the risk of injury consequent to resistance training programs is very low when appropriate training instructions are followed.

Resistance training in children, as with most physical activities, does carry with it some degree of inherent risk of musculoskeletal injury, yet this risk is no greater than many other sports or recreational activities in which children regularly participate. In one prospective study that evaluated the incidence of sports-related injuries in children over a 1-year period, resistance training resulted in 0.7% of 1576 reported injuries, whereas football and basketball resulted in 19% and 15%, respectively, of all injuries (150). When the data were evaluated in terms of 100 participants, football (28.3) and wrestling (16.4) were at the top of the list, but resistance training was not included in this final analysis.

A retrospective evaluation of resistance training and weightlifting injuries incurred by primarily 13- to 16-year-olds revealed that both activities are markedly safer than many other sports and activities (69). Moreover, the results of this study indicated that the rate of injury for weightlifting was lower than that for resistance training. In part, this later finding may be explained by the fact that the sport of weightlifting is typically characterized by knowledgeable coaching and a gradual progression of training loads, which are required to effectively learn the technique of advanced multijoint lifts. In some countries, children as young as the age of 8 are taught advanced multijoint lifts, albeit weight is not added to the bar until age 12 or 13 (83). The potential for injury during the performance of free-weight exercises should not be overlooked, especially accidental drops of weights. (109).

There is the potential for a catastrophic injury if safety standards for youth resistance training (e.g., adult supervision, safe equipment, and age-specific training guidelines) are not followed (63). In one case study report (59), a 9-year-old boy died when a barbell rolled off a bench press support and fell on his chest. This fatality underscores the importance of providing close adult supervision and safe training equipment for all youth resistance training programs, but especially those involving younger children.

Any exercise or activity recommendation for children has risks as well as benefits. Although resistance training injuries will occur, the risk can be minimized by close adult supervision, proper instruction, appropriate program design, and careful selection of training equipment. There are no justifiable safety reasons that preclude prepubescents or adolescents from participating in such a resistance training program.

HEALTH-RELATED BENEFITS

Children should be encouraged to participate in daily physical activity in order to imprint desirable health habits at an early age (60,117). Ideally, at least 50% of a child's time should be devoted to a variety of sport pursuits and physical activities in order to improve various components of physical fitness (i.e., strength, endurance, flexibility, and agility). Although good health habits developed during childhood do not always track into adulthood, the potential positive influence of these habits on the adult lifestyle should be recognized. In order to realize all of the potential positive physical and psychosocial health benefits of youth resistance training, coaches and instructors must appreciate the delicate psychological status and physical uniqueness of children.

Although health should not be defined as simply the absence of disease, an operational definition of health as it applies to children is difficult to define because the knowledge of behaviors and exposures required to achieve optimal health remain debatable. Nevertheless, behaviors and experiences that assimilate health-associated characteristics (e.g., improvements in growth pattern, blood lipid profile, blood pressure, body composition, and psychological well-being) may be deemed desirable for children. The relative impact of differing degrees and combinations of various health-associated characteristics on the overall health of children is not known. Although it is tempting to extrapolate the findings from adult studies to children, caution must be exercised because what is deemed healthy for an adult may not necessarily be so for children.

The extent to which current research supports the utility of youth resistance training in the acquisition of favorable degrees of health-associated characteristics is scant. Nevertheless, limited research supports the contention that the overall health of children is likely to improve rather than be adversely affected by resistance training.

Although the acute blood pressure response to lifting weights is reportedly similar between children and adults (97), blackouts (loss of consciousness) and chronic hypertension—which have been reported in adult competitive weightlifters (30) and adult athletes who overtrain (75)—have not been reported in prepubescents (48,107,118) or adolescents (67) following short-term (8 to 12 weeks) resistance training programs. Submaximal resistance training has actually been shown to decrease the blood pressure of hypertensive adolescents (67), and low-intensity, high-repetition resistance training has been recommended for hypertensive adolescents who want to experience this type of training (149).

Despite the previously held myth that resistance training would stunt the structural growth of children, current observations indicate that youth resistance training (up to 20 weeks) will not have an adverse affect on growth patterns (48,105,114,121,139,143). If age-specific physical activity guidelines as well as nutritional recommendations (e.g., adequate calcium) are followed, physical activity, including resistance training, may favorably influence growth at any stage of development but will not affect the genotypic maximum (7).

Resistance training has enhanced the bone mineral density (BMD) of adults (1,123) and some, but not all (15), evidence indicates that resistance training may be a potent stimulus for bone mineralization in children (31,32,85,138). It seems prudent for children who are at risk for osteopenia or osteoporosis to incorporate some form of resistance training into their regular activity patterns. Although peak bone mass is strongly influenced by genetics, nonhereditary factors such as exercise and proper nutrition are also significant osteogenic stimuli (124). Too much exercise, however, may actually result in the loss of bone and an increased susceptibility to stress fractures (27,140).

As prevalence of childhood obesity in the United States continues to increase (61), the potential influence of resistance training on body composition (the percentage of total body weight that is fat compared to the percentage that is fat free) remains an important health issue. Studies involving prepubescents have reported a decrease in fatness (as measured by skinfold thickness) following resistance training (48,114,121), although a majority of the data suggest that resistance training will not significantly affect the body composition of prepubescent populations without control on dietary intakes. This could, in part, be attributed to the lack of accurate and sensitive methodologies for the detection of changes in body composition. The body composition of adolescent males is more likely to be influenced by resistance training because of hormonal influences on muscle hypertrophy.

Although the issue of childhood obesity is complex (112), a combination of resistance training (e.g., moderate intensities and high repetitions) and aerobic exercise may have the most desirable and long-term effects on fat loss and weight maintenance. Resistance training programs characterized by moderate loads and a high number of repetitions have also favorably influenced the blood lipid profile of prepubescents (143) and similar findings have been reported in adolescents (55).

Psychosocial benefits may be realized from youth resistance training programs. If the program is appropriately designed and supervised by qualified adults who appreciate the importance of having fun, resistance training may offer socialization and related mental health benefits that are comparable to participation in team sports. The instructional period not only affords coaches and instructors the opportunity to educate children about the benefits of a healthy lifestyle (e.g., regular training, good nutrition, adequate sleep), it also increases the likelihood that children will master new skills and techniques. Youth resistance training provides an early opportunity for virtually all participants to be continually challenged and to enhance self-esteem and to achieve set goals.

RECOMMENDED RESISTANCE TRAINING GUIDELINES FOR YOUTH

Prerequisites for the development and administration of safe and effective resistance training programs for youth are an understanding of established training principles and an appreciation for the physical and emotional maturity of children. Although there is no minimum age requirement at which children can begin resistance training, a child must be mentally and emotionally ready to comply with coaching instructions and undergo the stress of a training program. In general, if a child is ready for participation in sport activities, then he or she is ready for some type of resistance training. A medical examination prior to participation is desirable, but is not mandatory for apparently healthy children. Conversely, a medical examination is recommended for children with signs or symptoms suggestive of disease and for children with known disease.

Since the goals of a resistance training program are specific to the individual needs of each child, resistance training programs will differ. Various combinations of acute program variables have proven to be safe and effective for children providing that program developers used scientific information, established training principles, and used common sense (see refs. 81 and 106 for a detailed description of youth resistance training programs). Children must perform all exercises using the correct technique and the exercise stress (e.g., resistance and the rest periods) must be carefully monitored to ensure that each child is tolerating the prescribed training program. The ideal approach is to incorporate resistance training into a periodized conditioning program in which the volume and intensity of training change throughout the year. Instructors must recognize the normal variance of maturation rates of children and be aware of the genetic predispositions for physical development. Children must not be treated as "small adults," nor should adult exercise guidelines and training philosophies be imposed on children.

Trained fitness professionals who have a thorough understanding of youth resistance training and safety procedures must supervise every exercise session. Professional certification specific to the area of strength and conditioning is highly desirable and is available through the National Strength and Conditioning Association (NSCA). An instructor-child ratio of 1:10 is acceptable, but additional supervision may be needed during the first few weeks of the resistance training program. Information should be presented to children in a style and language that is appropriate for their level of understanding. Children should be encouraged to ask questions and freely state their concerns about the program. Charts, posters, and workout cards that promote proper exercise technique and realistic expectations are helpful.

Basic education regarding realistic goals, individual needs, and expected outcomes should be part of the resistance training program. Moreover, the exercise session provides an opportunity for instructors to teach children about their bodies and a healthy lifestyle (e.g., proper nutrition and regular exercise). Instead of competing against each other, children should be encouraged to embrace self-improvement and feel good about their individual performances and improvements (e.g., the ability to correctly perform a multi-joint lift). The focal point of the program should be on learning, proper lifting technique and having fun.

Different resistance training modalities have proven to be equally safe and effective for children. Although resistance training equipment (e.g., free weights and weight machines) is required for many exercises, body-weight resisted and partner-resisted exercises are viable alternatives. Pads and boards may be used to modify certain types of adult-size equipment; however, some exercise machines may not fit a child's limb length. Child-size weight machines that are designed to fit smaller bodies are now available from several manufacturers. Factors such as safety, cost, construction, weight stack increments, and proper fit should be considered when evaluating resistance training equipment for children. In terms of gains in strength/power and motor performance in children, the quality of supervision and the design of the resistance training program appear to be more important than the type of equipment used.

The following guidelines for the design and implementation of youth resistance training programs are recommended (96):

- Each child should be physiologically and psychologically ready to participate in a resistance training program.

- Children should have realistic expectations. Remind children that it takes time to get in shape and learn a new skill.

- The exercise environment should be safe and free of potential hazards.

- The exercise session should include 5 to 10 minutes of warmup and cool-down exercises (e.g., low-intensity aerobic exercise and stretching).

- The exercise equipment should be in good repair and properly sized to fit each child.

- All training sessions must be closely supervised by experienced fitness professionals. Ideally, these fitness professional will possess certifications from nationally recognized organizations (e.g., NSCA).

- Careful and competent instruction regarding exercise technique, training guidelines, and spotting procedures should be given to all children.

- Weight room "etiquette" (e.g., returning weights to proper place and respecting physical differences) should be taught to all children.

- Start with one set of 6 to 8 body-part exercises. Begin with relatively light loads (e.g., 12–15 RM) to allow for appropriate adjustments to be made.

- The resistance should be gradually increased as strength improves. A 5% to 10% increase in overall load is appropriate for most children.

- Progression may also be achieved by gradually increasing the number of sets, exercises, and training sessions per week (i.e., training volume). As a general guideline, 1 to 3 sets of 6 to 15 repetitions on 8 to 10 exercises performed 2 to 3 nonconsecutive days per week is recommended. Throughout the program, observe each child's physical and mental ability to tolerate the prescribed workout.

- Each child should feel comfortable with the prescribed program and should look forward to the next workout. If a child has concerns and/or problems with a training program, the fitness professional is expected to make the appropriate modifications.

- Following 6 to 8 weeks of general resistance training, specific multijoint structural exercises (bench press, squats, leg press) may be introduced into the training program based upon individual needs and competencies. When performing any new exercise, start with a relatively light weight (or even a broomstick) to focus on learning the correct technique while minimizing muscle soreness.

- Following several months of resistance training, advanced multijoint structural exercises (e.g., Olympic lifts and modified cleans, pulls, and presses) may be incorporated into the program, provided that appropriate loads are used and the focus remains on proper form. The purpose of teaching advanced multijoint lifts to children should be to develop neuromuscular coordination and skill technique. Explosive movements with heavy resistance should be avoided during prepubescence, but may be introduced with caution during adolescence.

- If a child seems anxious about trying a new exercise, allow the child to watch a demonstration of the exercise. Teach the child how to perform the exercise and listen to each child's concerns.

- Incorporate the concept of *periodization* into a child's training program by systematically varying the resistance training program throughout the year.

- Discourage interindividual competition and focus on participation with lots of movement and positive reinforcement.

- Make sure that each child enjoys resistance training and is having fun. Do not force a child to participate in a resistance training program.

- Instructors and parents should be good role models. Showing support and encouragement will help to maintain interest.

- Children should be encouraged to drink plenty of fluids before, during, and after exercise.

- Encourage children to participate in a variety of sports and activities.

SUMMARY

Age-specific training guidelines, program variations, and competent supervision will make resistance training programs safe, effective, and fun for children. Instructors must understand the physical and emotional uniqueness of children and, in turn, children must appreciate the potential benefits and risks associated with resistance training. Although the needs, goals, and interests of children will continually change, resistance training should be considered a fundamental and beneficial component of youth fitness and sport programs.

REFERENCES

1. Adams K, Snow-Harter C, Shelley et al. Weightlifters exhibit greater bone density and muscle strength than non-weightlifters. Med Sci Sports Exerc 1993;25: S188.

2. Ainsworth J. The effects of isometric-resistive exercises with the Exer-Genie on strength and speed in swimming [doctoral thesis]. Fayetteville, AK: University of Arkansas, 1970.

3. American Academy of Pediatrics. Strength training, weight and power lifting and bodybuilding by children and adolescents. Pediatrics 1990;86:801–803.

4. American College of Sports Medicine. The prevention of sports injuries of children and adolescents. Med Sci Sports Exerc 1993;25(suppl 8):1–7.

5. American College of Sports Medicine. ACSM'S guidelines for exercise testing and prescription. 5th ed. Baltimore: Williams and Wilkins, 1995.

6. American Orthopaedic Society for Sports Medicine. Proceedings of the conference on strength training and the prepubescent. Chicago: American Orthopaedic Society for Sports Medicine, 1988.

7. Bailey D, Martin A. Physical activity and skeletal health in adolescents. Pediatr Exerc Sci 1994;6(4):330–347.

8. Bar-Or O. Pediatric sports medicine for the practitioner: from physiologic principles to clinical applications. New York: Springer-Verlag, 1983.

9. Baumgartner T, Wood S. Development of shoulder-girdle strength-endurance in elementary children. Res Q Exerc Sport 1984;55:169–171.

10. Benton J. Epiphyseal fractures in sports. Phys Sports Med 1983; 10:63–71.

11. Blanksby B, Gregor J. Anthropometric, strength, and physiological changes in male and female swimmers with progressive resistance training. Aust J Sport Sci 1981;1:3–6.

12. Blimkie C. Age- and sex-associated variation in strength during childhood: Anthropometric, morphologic, neurologic, biomechanical, endocrinologic, genetic, and physical activity correlates. In: Perspectives in exercise science and sports medicine, vol. 2: youth, exercise and sport. Gisolfi CV, Lamb DR, eds. Indianapolis: Benchmark, 1989:99–163.

13. Blimkie C. Resistance training during pre- and early puberty: efficacy, trainability, mechanisms and persistance. Can J Sport Sci 1992;17:264–279.

14. Blimkie C. Resistance training during preadolescence: issues and controversies. Sports Med 1993;15:389–407.

15. Blimkie C. Benefits and risks of resistance training in youth. In: Intensive participation in children's sports. Cahill B, Pearl A, eds. Champaign, IL: Human Kinetics, 1993:133–167.

16. Blimkie C, Martin J, Ramsay D, et al. The effects of detraining and maintenance weight training

on strength development in prepubertal boys. Can J Sport Sci
1989;14:104P.

17. Blimkie C, Ramsay J, Sale D, et
al. Effects of 10 weeks of resistance training on strength development in prepubertal boys. In:
Oseid S, Carlsen K, eds. Children
and exercise XIII. Champaign, IL:
Human Kinetics, 1989:183–197.

18. Blimkie C, Rice S, Webber C,
et al. Effects of resistance training on bone mass and density in
adolescent females. Med Sci
Sports Exerc 1993;25(suppl):
S48.

19. Brady T, Cahill B, Bodnar L.
Weight training related injuries in
the high school athlete. Am J
Sports Med 1982;10:1–5.

20. Bright R, Burstein A, Elmore S.
Epiphyseal-plate cartilage. J
Bone Joint Surg Am 1974;56:
688–703.

21. Brown E, Kimball R. Medical
history associated with adolescent power lifting. Pediatrics
1983;72:636–644.

22. Brown E, Lillegard W, Henderson
R, et al. Efficacy and safety
of strength training with free
weights in prepubescents to early
post pubescents. Med Sci Sports
Exerc 1992;24:S82. Abstract.

23. Bulgakova N, Vorontsov A,
Fomichenko T. Improving the
technical preparedness of young
swimmers by using strength
training. Soviet Sports Rev 1990;
25:102–104.

24. Cahill B, Griffith E. Effect of preseason conditioning on the incidence and severity of high school
football knee injuries. Am J
Sports Med 1978;6:180–184.

25. Calfas K, Taylor W. Effects of
physical activity on psychological
variables in adolescents. Pediatr
Exerc Sci 1994;6:406–423.

26. Chandler T, Kibler W. Muscle
training in injury prevention. In:
Renstron P, ed. The Olympic
book of sports medicine: sports
injuries and their prevention.
Oxford: Blackwell Scientific,
1995:252–261.

27. Caine D, Linder K. Overuse
injuries of growing bones: the
young female gymnast at risk?
Phys Sports Med 1985;13:51–
64.

28. Clain M, Hershman E. Overuse
injuries in children and adolescents. Phys Sports Med 1989;
17:11–123.

29. Clarke D, Vaccaro P, Andresen N.
Physiologic alterations in 7- to 9-
year old boys following a season
of competitive wrestling. Res Q
Exerc Sport 1984;55:318–322.

30. Compton D, Hill P, Sinclair J.
Weight-lifters' blackout. Lancet
1973;2:1234–1237.

31. Conroy B, Kraemer W, Maresh C,
Dalsky G. Adaptative responses of
bone to physical activity. J Med
Exerc Nutr Health 1992;1:64–
74.

32. Conroy B, Kraemer W, Maresh C,
et al. Bone mineral density in
elite junior Olympic weightlifters.
Med Sci Sports Exerc 1993;25:
1103–1109.

33. Cooper DM. New horizons in
pediatric exercise research. In:
Blimkie C, Bar-Or O, eds. New
horizons in pediatric exercise
science. Champaign, IL: Human
Kinetics, 1995:1–24.

34. DeOliveria J, Gallagher J.
Strength training in children: a
meta-analysis. Pediatr Exerc Sci
1995;7:108.

35. Department of Health and
Human Services. Healthy people
2000: national health promotion
and disease prevention objectives. DHHS publication (PHS)
91-50212. Washington, DC: U.S.
Dept. of Health and Human Services, 1991.

36. DeRenne C, Hetzler R, Buxton B,
Ho K. Effects of training frequency on strength maintenance
in pubescent baseball players. J
Strength Cond Res 1996;10:8–
14.

37. Dishman R, Gettman L. Psychological vigor and self-perceptions
of increased strength. Med Sci
Sports Exerc 1981;13:73–74.
Abstract.

38. Docherty D, Wenger H, Collis M,
Quinney H. The effects of variable speed resistance training on
strength development in prepubertal boys. J Hum Movement
Stud 1987;13:377–382.

39. Dominguez R. Shoulder pain in
age group swimmers. In: Erikkson
B, Furberg B, eds. Swimming
medicine IV. Baltimore: University Park Press, 1978:105–109.

40. Ewart C. Psychological effects of
resistive weight training: implications for cardiac patients. Med
Sci Sports Exerc 1989;21:683–
688.

41. Ekblom B. Effects of physical
training in adolescent boys. J
Appl Physiol 1969;27:350–355.

42. Faigenbaum A. Prepubescent
strength training: a guide for
teachers and coaches. Natl
Strength Cond Assoc J 1993;15:
20–29.

43. Faigenbaum A. Psychosocial
benefits of prepubescent strength
training. Strength Cond 1995;17:
28–32.

44. Faigenbaum A, Bradley DF.
Strength training for the young
athlete. Orthop Phys Ther Clin
North Am 1998;7:67–89.

45. Faigenbaum A, Nye-McKeown J,
Morilla C. Coaching athletes with
eating disorders. Strength Cond
1996;18:22–30.

46. Faigenbaum A, Westcott W,
Micheli L, et al. The effects of
strength training and detraining
on children. J Strength Cond Res
1996;10:109–114.

47. Faigenbaum A, Zaichkowsky L,
Gardner D, et al. Anabolic steroid
use by male and female middle
school students. Pediatrics 1998;
101:e6.

48. Faigenbaum A, Zaichkowsky L,
Westcott W, et al. The effects
of a twice per week strength
training program on children.
Pediatr Exerc Sci 1993;5:339–
346.

49. Faigenbaum A, Zaichkowsky L,
Westcott W, et al. Psychological
effects of strength training on

children. J Sport Beh 1997;20: 164–175.

50. Falk B, Mor G. The effects of resistance and martial arts training in 6- to 8-year-old boys. Pediatr Exerc Sci 1996;8:48–56.

51. Falk B, Tenenbaum G. The effectiveness of resistance training in children: a meta-analysis. Sports Med 1996;22:176–186.

52. Fleck S, Kraemer W. Designing resistance training programs. 2nd ed. Champaign, IL: Human Kinetics, 1997.

53. Ford H, Puckett J. Comparative effects of prescribed weight training and basketball programs on basketball skill test scores of ninth grade boys. Percept Mot Skills 1983;56:23–26.

54. Freedson P, Ward A, Rippe J. Resistance training for youth. In: Grana W, Lombardo B, Sharkey J, Stone J, eds. Advances in Sports Medicine and Fitness. Chicago: Yearbook, 1990:57–65.

55. Fripp R, Hodgson J. Effect of resistive training on plasma lipid and lipoprotein levels in male adolescents. J Pediatr 1987;111: 926–931.

56. Fukunga T, Funato K, Ikegawa S. The effects of resistance training on muscle area and strength in prepubescent age. Ann Physiol Anthrop 1992;11:357–364.

57. Funato K, Fukunaga T, Asami T, Ikeda S. Strength training for prepubescent boys and girls. Proceedings of the Department of Sports Science, University of Tokyo, 1987:9–19.

58. Garrett W, Safran M, Seaber A, et al. Biomechanical comparison of stimulated and nonstimulated skeletal muscle pulled to failure. Am J Sports Med 1987;15:448–454.

59. George D, Stakiw K, Wright C. Fatal accident with weight-lifting equipment: implications for safety standards. Can Med Assoc J 1989;140:925–926.

60. Godin G, Valois P, Shephard R, Desharnais R. Prediction of leisure-time exercise behavior: a path analysis (LISREL V model). J Behav Med 1987;10:145–158.

61. Gortmaker S, Dietz W, Sobol A, Wehler C. Increasing pediatric obesity in the United States. Am J Dis Child 1987;141:535–540.

62. Gould D. Intensive sport participation and the prepubescent athlete: competitive stress and burnout. In: Cahill B, Pearl A, eds. Intensive participation in children's sports. Champaign, IL: Human Kinetics, 1993:19–38.

63. Gould J, DeJong A. Injuries to children involving home exercise equipment. Arch Pediatr Adolesc Med 1994;148:1107–1109.

64. Gruber J. Physical activity and self-esteem development in children: a meta-analysis. In: Stull GA, Eckert HM, eds. Effects of physical activity on children. Champaign, IL: Human Kinetics, 1986:30–48.

65. Gumbs V, Segal D, Halligan J, Lower G. Bilateral distal radius and ulnar fractures in adolescent weight lifters. Am J Sports Med 1982;10:375–379.

66. Gutin B, Kasper M. Can vigorous exercise play a role in osteoporosis prevention? a review. Osteoporos Int 1992;2:55–69.

67. Hagberg J, Ehsani A, Goldring D, et al. Effect of weight training on blood pressure and hemodynamics in hypertensive adolescents. J Pediatr 1984;104:147–151.

68. Häkkinen K, Mero A, Kavhanen H. Specificity of endurance, sprint, and strength training on physical performance capacity in young athletes. J Sports Med Phys Fitness 1989;29:27–35.

69. Hamill B. Relative safety of weight lifting and weight training. J Strength Cond Res 1994;8:53–57.

70. Hawkins R, Kennedy J. Impingement syndrome in athletes. Am J Sports Med 1980;8:151–158.

71. Hejna W, Rosenberg A, Buturusis D, Krieger A. The prevention of sports injuries in high school students through strength training. Natl Strength Cond Assoc J 1982;4:28–31.

72. Heiser T, Weber J, Sullivan G, et al. Prophylaxis and management of hamstring muscle injuries in intercollegiate football. Am J Sports Med 1984;12:368–370.

73. Hetherington MR. Effect of isometric training on the elbow flexion force torque of grade five boys. Res Q 1976;47:41–47.

74. Holloway J, Beuter A, Duda J. Self-efficacy and training in adolescent girls. J Appl Soc Psychol 1988;18:699–719.

75. Hunter G, McCarthy J. Pressor response associated with high-intensity anaerobic training. Phys Sports Med 1983;11:151–162.

76. Isaacs L, Pohlman R, Craig B. Effects of resistance training on strength development in prepubescent females. Med Sci Sports Exerc 1994;26:S210. Abstract.

77. Jackson D, Wiltse L, Dingeman R, Hayes M. Stress reactions involving the pars interarticularis in young athletes. Am J Sports Med 1981;9:304–312.

78. James R, Ellsworth E, Oehman S. The effects of weight training on the self-concept of male undergraduates. Memphis State University, Tennessee, 1982.

79. Jenkins N, Mintowt-Czyz W. Bilateral fracture separations of the distal radial epiphyses during weight-lifting. Br J Sports Med 1986;20:72–73.

80. Kraemer W. Endocrine response to resistance exercise. Med Sci Sports Exerc 1988;20(suppl): S152–157.

81. Kraemer W, Fleck S. Strength training for young athletes. Champaign, IL: Human Kinetics, 1993.

82. Kraemer W, Fry A, Frykman P, et al. Resistance training and youth. Pediatr Exerc Sci 1989;1:336–350.

83. Kuland D, Tottossy M. Warm-up, strength and power. Orthop Clin North Am 1983;14:427–448.

84. Lillegard W. Efficacy of strength training in prepubescent to early post pubescent males and females: effects of gender and maturity. Pediatr Rehab 1997;1: 147–157.

85. Loucks A. Osteoporosis prevention begins in childhood. In: Brown E, Brown C, eds. Competitive sports for children and youth. Champaign, IL: Human Kinetics, 1988:213–223.

86. Lowrey G. Growth and development of children. Chicago: Yearbook, 1973.

87. Malina R, Bouchard C. Growth, maturation and physical activity. Champaign, IL: Human Kinetics, 1991.

88. Mason T. Is weight lifting deleterious to the spines of young people? Br J Sports Med 1977;5: 61.

89. McGovern M. Effects of circuit weight training on the physical fitness of prepubescent children. Dissertation Abstracts Int 1984; 45:452A–453A.

90. Melia P, Pipe A, Greenberg G. The use of anabolic androgenic steroids by Canadian students. Clin J Sports Med 1996;6:9–14.

91. Melnick M, Mookerjee S. Effects of advanced weight training on body cathexis and self-esteem. Percept Mot Skills 1991;72: 1335–1345.

92. Metcalf J, Roberts S. Strength training and the immature athlete: an overview. Pediatr Nurs 1993;19:325–332.

93. Mersch F, Stoboy H. Strength training and muscle hypertrophy in children. In: Oseid S, Carlsen K, eds. Children and exercise XIII. Champaign, IL: Human Kinetics, 1989:165–182.

94. Micheli L. Strength training in the young athlete. In: Brown E, Branta C, eds. Competitive sports for children and youth. Champaign, IL: Human Kinetics, 1988:99–105.

95. National Strength and Conditioning Association. Position paper on prepubescent strength training. Natl Strength Cond Assoc J 1985;7:27–31.

96. National Strength and Conditioning Association. Youth resistance training: position paper and literature review. Strength Cond 1996;18:62–75.

97. Nau K, Katch V, Beekman R, Dick M. Acute intraarterial blood pressure response to bench press weight lifting in children. Pediatr Exerc Sci 1990;2:37–45.

98. Nielsen B, Nielsen K, Behrendt-Hansen M, Asmussen E. Training of "functional muscular strength" in girls 7–19 years old. In: Berg K, Eriksson B, eds. Children and exercise IX. Baltimore: University Park Press, 1980:69–77.

99. Nindl BC, Mahar MT, Harman EA, Patton JF. Upper and lower body anaerobic performance: a comparison between male and female adolescent athletes. Med Sci Sports Exerc 1995;27:235–241.

100. Outerbridge A, Micheli L. Overuse injuries in the young athlete. Clin Sports Med 1995; 14:503–516.

101. Ozmun J, Mikesky A, Surburg P. Neuromuscular adaptations following prepubescent strength training. Med Sci Sports Exerc 1994;26:510–514.

102. Payne V, Marrow J, Johnson L, Dalton S. Resistance training in children and youth: a meta-analysis. Res Q Exerc Sport 1997;88:80–89.

103. Pfeiffer R, Francis R. Effects of strength training on muscle development in prepubescent, pubescent and postpubescent males. Phys Sports Med 1986; 14:134–143.

104. Queary J, Laubach L. The effects of muscular strength/endurance training. Technique 1992;12:9–11.

105. Ramsay J, Blimkie C, Smith K, et al. Strength training effects in prepubescent boys. Med Sci Sports Exerc 1990;22:605–614.

106. Roberts S, Weider B. Strength and weight training for young athletes. Chicago: Contemporary Books, 1994.

107. Rians C, Weltman A, Cahill B, et al. Strength training for prepubescent males: is it safe? Am J Sports Med 1987;15:483–489.

108. Risser W. Weight-training injuries in children and adolescents. Am Fam Phys 1991;44:2104–2110.

109. Risser W, Risser J, Preston D. Weight-training injuries in adolescents. Am J Dis Child 1990;144: 1015–1017.

110. Rooks D, Micheli L. Musculoskeletal assessment and training: the young athlete. Clin Sports Med 1988;7:641–677.

111. Rowe PH. Cartilage fracture due to weight lifting. Br J Sports Med 1979;13:130–131.

112. Rowland T. Exercise and children's health. Champaign, IL: Human Kinetics, 1990.

113. Ryan J, Salciccioli G. Fractures of the distal radial epiphysis in adolescent weight lifters. Am J Sports Med 1976;4:26–27.

114. Sailors M, Berg K. Comparison of responses to weight training in pubescent boys and men. J Sports Med 1987;27:30–37.

115. Sale D. Strength training in children. In: Gisolfi GV, Lamb DR, eds. Perspectives in exercise science and sports medicine. Indianapolis: Benchmark Press, 1989:165–216.

116. Sale D, MacDougall D. Specificity in strength training: a review for the coach and athlete. Can J Appl Sports Sci 1981;6:87–92.

117. Sallis J, Patrick K. Physical activity guidelines for adolescents: consensus statement. Pediatr Exerc Sci 1994;6:302–313.

118. Servedio F, Bartels R, Hamlin R, et al. The effects of weight training, using olympic style lifts, on various physiological variables in pre-pubescent boys. Med Sci Sports Exerc 1985;17:288. Abstract.

119. Sewall L, Micheli L. Strength training for children. J Pediatr Orthop 1986;6:143–146.

120. Shepard R. Physical activity and growth. Chicago: Yearbook, 1982: 174.

121. Siegal J, Camaione D, Manfredi T. The effects of upper body resistance training in prepubescent children. Pediatr Exerc Sci 1989;1:145–154.

122. Singer K. Injuries and disorders of the epiphyses in young athletes. In: Weiss M, Gould D, eds. Sport for children and youths. Champaign, IL: Human Kinetics, 1984.

123. Snow-Harter C, Bouxsein M, Lewis B, et al. Effects of resistance and endurance exercise on bone mineral status of young women: a randomized exercise intervention trial. J Bone Miner Res 1992;7:761–769.

124. Snow-Harter C, Marcus R. Exercise, bone mineral density and osteoporosis. In: Holloszy J, ed. Exercise and sport science reviews. vol. 19. Philadelphia: Williams and Wilkins, 1991:351–388.

125. Stahle S, Roberts S, Davis B, Rybicki L. Effect of 2 versus 3 times per week weight training program in boys aged 7 to 16. Med Sci Sports Exerc 1995; 27(suppl):S114. Abstract.

126. Stein P, Motta R. Effects of aerobic and nonaerobic exercise on depression and self-concept. Percept Mot Skills 1992;74:79–89.

127. Staff P. The effect of physical activity on joints, cartilage, tendons and ligaments. Scan J Soc Med 1982;29(suppl):59–63.

128. Stone M, O'Bryant H, Garhammer J. A hypothetical model for strength training. J Sports Med Phys Fitness 1981;21:342–351.

129. Tanner S, Miller D, Alongi C. Anabolic steroid use by adolescents: prevalence, motives, and knowledge of risks. Clin J Sports Med 1995;5:108–115.

130. Tipton C, James S, Mergner W, Tcheng T. Influence of exercise on strength of medial collateral knee ligaments of dogs. Am J Physiol 1970;218:894–902.

131. Tucker L. Weight training experience and psychological well-being. Percept Mot Skills 1982; 55:553–554.

132. Tucker L. Effects of a weight training program on the self-concepts of college males. Percept Mot Skills 1982;54: 1055–1061.

133. Tucker L. Self-concept: a function of self-perceived somatotype. J Psychol 1983;113:123–133.

134. Tucker L. Effect of weight training on self-concept: a profile of those influenced most. Res Q Exerc Sport 1983;54:389–397.

135. Tucker L. Effect of weight training on body attitudes: who benefits most? J Sports Med 1987;27:70–78.

136. United States Consumer Product Safety Commission. National electronic injury surveillance system. Washington, DC. Directorate for Epidemiology, National Injury Information Clearinghouse, 1979.

137. United States Consumer Product Safety Commission. National electronic injury surveillance system. Washington, DC: Directorate for Epidemiology. National Injury Information Clearinghouse, 1987.

138. Virvidakis K, Georgiu E, Korkotsidis A, et al. Bone mineral content of junior competitive weightlifters. Int J Sports Med 1990;11:244–246.

139. Vrijens F. Muscle strength development in the pre- and post-pubescent age. Med Sport 1978; 11:152–158.

140. Warren M, Brooks-Gunn J, Hamilton L, et al. Scoliosis and fractures in young ballet dancers. N Engl J Med 1986;314:1348–1353.

141. Webb D. Strength training in children and adolescents. Pediatr Clin North Am 1990;37:1187–1210.

142. Weltman A. Weight training in prepubertal children: physiologic benefit and potential damage. In: Bar-Or O, ed. Advances in pediatric sport sciences. Champaign, IL: Human Kinetics, 1989:101–129.

143. Weltman A, Janney C, Rians C, et al. The effects of hydraulic resistance strength training in pre-pubertal males. Med Sci Sports Exerc 1986;18:629–638.

144. Weltman A, Janney C, Rians C, et al. Effects of hydraulic-resistance strength training on serum lipid levels in prepubertal boys. Am J Dis Child 1987;141: 777–780.

145. Westcott W. Female response to weight lifting. J Phys Educ 1979; 77:31–33.

146. Westcott W. A new look at youth fitness. Am Fitness Q 1992;11: 16–19.

147. Williams D. The effect of weight training on performance in selected motor activities for preadolescent males. J Appl Sport Sci Res 1991;5:170. Abstract.

148. Wolohan M, Micheli L. Strength training in children. J Musculoskel Med 1990;7:37–52.

149. Zahka K. Adolescent hypertension update. Maryland Med J 1987;36:413–414.

150. Zaricznyj B, Shattuck L, Mast T, et al. Sports-related injuries in school-aged children. Am J Sports Med 1980;8:318–324.

151. Zatsiorsky V. Science and practice of strength training. Champaign, IL: Human Kinetics, 1995.

Chapter 57

Iron and Endurance Performance in Adolescence

Stella L. Volpe
Penny Harris Rosenzweig

Iron deficiency is the most common nutritional deficiency in the world and is most prevalent in older infants (aged 6 months to 24 months), young children, and premenopausal women (1,2). In developing countries it is estimated that 30% to 40% of children and premenopausal women are iron deficient (3). Adolescent females are at an especially high risk for developing iron deficiency due to the onset of menstrual blood loss at a time of rapid growth.

The main focus of this chapter will be on the research performed on the effects of iron depletion and iron deficiency anemia on exercise performance, particularly those studies conducted on adolescents. In addition, absorption and dietary requirements, iron metabolism and function, iron turnover and loss, the stages of iron deficiency, and general physiologic and metabolic effects of iron deficiency will be discussed.

IRON METABOLISM

Dietary Iron Absorption

The main source of iron in humans is dietary (4), the physio-chemical form of which greatly affects iron absorption (5). Iron in pharmaceutical preparations is in the form of non-heme ferrous salts that are readily absorbed in the duodenum, because they remain soluble at near-neutral pH (6). Most dietary non-heme iron, present in eggs, grains, vegetables, and fruits is, however, in the form of ferric iron, which precipitates above pH 2 (5). In order to remain soluble and more available for absorption in the alkaline environment of the duodenum, ferric iron forms complexes with intestinal mucins and un-stable chelates with sugars, ascorbate, and amino acids (5). For example, the inclusion of 75 mg of ascorbic acid (e.g., 5 oz of

orange juice) in a meal of low iron bioavailability can increase the absorption of iron from 5% to approximately 20% in an individual with low iron stores (7). There are, however, other dietary components that decrease iron absorption by precipitating iron or by forming stable chelates that interfere with iron binding to mucins. These components include carbonates, oxalates, phytates, and tannates (5). Assuming iron stores are at normal levels, absorption of non-heme iron varies between 3% and 8%, depending on the presence of these dietary factors (8). The absorption of myoglobin- (Mb) and hemoglobin- (Hb) bound iron (heme iron) found in meat, poultry, and fish can range from 15% to 35%, assuming normal body stores (8). This improvement in absorption can be attributed to the fact that heme iron is soluble in alkaline solutions and is precipitated in an acid milieu, making acid chelation unimportant in facilitating solubility (5).

It appears, however, that the most important factors in iron absorption are not dietary, but related to the status of tissue iron stores and the rate of iron turnover (5). Iron absorption is increased in situations in which there is an increased rate of iron turnover in the plasma, such as during iron deficiency, thalassemia, or sideroblastic anemia. For example, heme iron absorption can range from 15% in an iron-sufficient individual to 35% in an individual with low iron stores (9). Absorption of non-heme iron can range from 2% in an iron-sufficient individual consuming a meal with low bioavailability of iron, to 20% in an individual with low iron stores consuming meal with high bioavailability (9).

Dietary Iron Requirements

Iron requirements for adults are derived from estimates of dietary iron absorption based on experimental measures of iron loss and estimates of total body iron stores. The amount of dietary iron that is absorbed is largely dependent upon the composition of the diet. An individual whose diet consists primarily of cereals and legumes absorbs approximately 5% of the total amount of iron he or she consumes, whereas an individual whose diet is rich in meat, fish, and poultry absorbs approximately 15% of the iron consumed (9).

Average adult iron stores are estimated to be 300 mg and average daily losses are estimated to be approximately 1 mg for men and 1.5 mg for women (10). Estimated daily iron losses for women are higher than for men because of menstruation. However, the estimate of an average daily loss of 1.5 mg in women is not accurate for the 10% of women who lose more than 80 mL of blood every month. Despite iron-rich diets, these women may still need to depend on iron supplementation to prevent depletion of stores (11).

Based on the above estimates, the Recommended Dietary Allowance (RDA) for elemental iron for adults is calculated to be 10 mg/day for men and 15 mg/day for women (10). The RDA for iron in pregnant women is 30 mg/day in order to sustain the growth of both fetal and maternal tissue (10). This level is difficult to attain by diet alone, so iron supplementation during pregnancy is recommended (12).

Lactating women require approximately 0.15– 0.30 mg/day of elemental iron to synthesize breast milk. However, this amount is roughly equivalent to the iron that is saved by cessation of menstrual blood loss during lactation (13). Therefore, lactating women require only 15 mg/day of iron (10).

Iron requirements for growing infants and children are calculated from estimates of average weight gain and estimates of the amount of iron needed to synthesize Hb, Mb, and iron-containing enzymes to sustain this gain (14). To attain the desired storage level of iron of 300 mg by the age of 20 or 25 years, the RDA for iron for children between the ages of 6 months and 10 years is 10 mg/day or 1 mg/kg/day. Between the ages of 10 and 18 years, an additional 2 mg/day of iron is required by males to sustain the pubertal growth spurt. However, from the age of 18 years and throughout adulthood, the RDA for males drops back down to 10 mg/day. Females require an additional 5 mg/day of iron from age 10 to menopause (except during pregnancy) (10). This amount of iron is enough to sustain both pubertal growth and to maintain iron stores during menstruation.

Iron Transport and Function

Once inside the intestinal absorptive cells of the lumen, a small amount of iron may enter circulation via lymphocytes; however, more than 95% of iron enters the blood in mesenteric circulation bound to transferrin (5). Total body iron comprises, on average, 5.0 mg/kg body weight in the adult male and 3.8 mg/kg body weight in the adult female (15). This iron is divided, depending on availability, into that which is essential for normal function and that which is stored for use in times of urgent need.

The majority of essential iron is transported to tissues by the plasma transport protein transferrin. Transferrin delivers iron to the tissues via cell membrane receptors specific for transferrin (15); the body's iron supply is reflected by the degree to which transferrin is saturated by iron. Less than 1% of total body iron is in transit from the intestinal mucosa or reticuloendocytes to tissues with high iron requirements, such as the erythroid bone marrow (15).

Once inside the bone marrow, iron is utilized for Hb synthesis. Hb plays an important role in delivering oxygen from the lungs to the tissues. Several factors affect Hb's affinity for oxygen, as measured by the oxygen dissociation curve. These factors include partial pressure of oxygen, pH, temperature, and organic phosphate content (16). Biochemical adaptations to improve oxygen delivery to tissues occur as a result of the reduced oxygen-carrying capacity of the blood during iron deficiency anemia. However, in severe iron deficiency anemia, the Hb content of the blood is reduced sufficiently to cause chronic tissue hypoxia (16). Mb, which comprises about 10% of total body iron, is also a heme-containing compound. Whereas Hb is present throughout the bloodstream, Mb is present only in muscles, where its primary function is to transport and store oxygen within muscle and to release it to meet increased metabolic needs during muscle contraction (16).

The remainder of essential iron (1% of total body iron) is incorporated into mitochondrial cytochromes, non-heme iron compounds, and other iron-dependent enzymes. Cytochromes are enzymes responsible for both electron transport and the oxidative production of cellular energy in the form of adenosine triphosphate (ATP). For example, cytochromes a and c are present within the cristae of mitochondria in all aerobic cells as well as in other cellular membranes. Cytochrome c is the most easily isolated and best characterized cytochrome. The highest concentrations of cytochrome c are found in cardiac tissue and other tissues that require a high rate of oxygen utilization (17). Cytochrome P-450 aids in the degradation and detoxification of drugs and endogenous substances in the intestinal mucosa and liver cells, respectively (18).

Nicotinamide adenine dinucleotide dehydrogenase (NADH) and succinate dehydrogenase are both non-heme, iron-sulfur complexes involved in oxidative metabolism (17) and are required for the first reaction in the electron transport chain. Hydrogen peroxidases comprise another group of iron-containing enzymes that protect against the highly reactive chemical hydrogen peroxide, which causes lipid peroxidation. Both rat and human erythrocytes show an increase in lipid peroxidative damage with increasing iron deficiency (19,20).

Other enzymes that require iron to function, but do not themselves contain iron, include: aconitase, an enzyme of the tricarboxylic acid cycle; phosphoenolpyruvate carboxykinase, a rate-limiting enzyme involved in gluconeogenesis; and ribonucleotide reductase, an enzyme required for DNA synthesis. Because of iron's major roles in both oxygen transport and ATP formation, a deficiency of this mineral could greatly impair athletic performance, especially in growing adolescents.

Iron Storage

Iron in excess of essential requirements is stored in the form of ferritin and hemosiderin, present primarily in the liver, reticuloendothelial cells, and bone marrow (21,22). Stored iron serves as a reservoir to supply cellular iron needs, mainly for Hb synthesis; however, the iron bound to ferritin is more readily mobilized than iron bound to hemosiderin. With a long-term negative iron balance, iron stores are depleted before iron deficiency is apparent at the tissue level. With a positive iron balance, stores can gradually increase, even if the dietary bioavailability of iron is low. This often occurs in post-menopausal women and with increasing age in men. In the event that iron storage is pathologically increased (hemochromatosis), the only way iron stores can be reduced to avoid tissue damage is via blood letting (12).

Individual iron stores vary throughout the lifecycle. Infants are born with large iron stores proportional to birthweight. Full-term infants have enough stored iron to last until age 6 months (14). However, between the ages of 6 months and 24 months, the growth rate of children is so rapid that iron stores are difficult to accumulate even when dietary intake of iron is adequate. This places young children at a high risk for developing iron deficiency (3), whereas after the age of 2 years, growth rate declines, along with the risk of developing iron deficiency. Consequently, iron stores begin to accumulate. In men, iron stores accumulate gradually throughout adulthood, while in women, iron stores remain low until menopause, at which time they begin to increase (3).

Iron Turnover and Loss

Iron turnover is related to the destruction and production of erythrocytes. Erythrocytes account for approximately two-thirds of total body iron and have a life span of 120 days. This translates into an iron turnover of about 20 mg each day in adults (23). Unlike the turnover rate of erythrocytes, the turnover rate of tissue iron compounds varies widely, and usually corresponds to the rates of turnover of the structures with which they are associated. For example, cytochrome c of rat skeletal muscle has a half-life of 6 days (23).

Small amounts of iron are lost from the body every day as the result of a variety of physiologic functions. The majority of iron loss occurs in bile via the feces (0.6 mg/day), desquamated mucosal cells, and losses of small amounts of blood (24). A much smaller amount of iron is lost daily through sweat and desquamated skin cells (0.2–0.3 mg/day), and a minute amount is lost in the urine (<0.1 mg/day) (25).

Iron loss varies according to gender. Men lose, on average, a total of 1.0 mg/day while premenopausal women lose an average of 1.3 mg/day due to additional losses from menses (average menstrual blood loss totals 30–40 mL/cycle, which translates into 0.4–0.5 mg/day) (25). Some women who experience heavy menstrual flow may lose more than 80 mL of blood in a single cycle, and are therefore unable to maintain positive iron balance (25).

Stages of Iron Deficiency

When left untreated, the severity of iron deficiency increases, eventually leading to the development of iron deficiency anemia. The process by which iron deficiency anemia develops occurs in three overlapping stages. The first stage, known as iron depletion, is manifested only by a decrease in iron storage as measured by serum ferritin (SF) concentration. The normal healthy SF range for adults varies widely between 20 ng/dL and 300 ng/dL (26), and it is generally accepted that a SF concentration below 20 ng/dL is indicative of iron depletion (27). However, the use of this cutoff point varies somewhat among studies, depending on the characteristics of the population under investigation.

The second stage in the development of iron deficiency anemia is called iron deficiency erythropoiesis, or iron deficiency without anemia. The biochemical alterations that occur during this stage reflect the insufficient amount of iron available for Hb synthesis. Although frank anemia is still not present during this stage, there is a decrease in transferrin saturation to below 16% in adults (27) and an increase in erythrocyte protoporphyrin (>0.35 mg/L whole blood or <3.0 μg/g Hb), the precursor to heme (28).

Although with low iron stores there is a compensatory increase in iron absorption to help prevent the progression of iron deficiency to the third stage, this increase in absorption cannot always prevent the onset of frank iron deficiency anemia. A Hb concentration below 12 g/dL in nonpregnant, premenopausal women (normal range = 12–16 g/dL) and below 14 g/dL in men (normal range = 14–18 g/dL), along with evidence of depleted iron stores as measured by a reduced concentration of SF levels, are the criteria for diagnosing iron deficiency anemia in humans (27). The measurement of a decreased Hb concentration alone, however, is not sufficient for diagnosing iron deficiency anemia. Anemia can also be caused by factors completely unrelated to iron deficiency such as infection and mild inflammatory disease (29,30).

Physiologic and Metabolic Effects of Iron Deficiency

Anemia is the best known physical manifestation of iron deficiency. Nonetheless, there are few negative physical consequences of mild anemia (Hb 7–12 g/dL) in sedentary individuals because of compensatory mechanisms that help to maintain an optimal supply of oxygen to the tissues. These mechanisms include: 1) more complete extraction of oxygen from Hb by tissues; 2) redistribution of blood flow to vital organs, such as the heart and brain, at the expense of other tissues; and 3) increased cardiac output (31).

During exercise, these compensatory mechanisms lose their effectiveness due to an increased need for oxygen. Therefore, the physical manifestations of mild iron deficiency anemia are more obvious and are reflected by an impairment in exercise performance. This impairment in exercise performance is related not only to anemia and reduced aerobic capacity, but also to tissue iron depletion and decreased exercise performance (32). Several rat studies have demonstrated that dietary iron deficiency anemia impairs the oxidative production of ATP in skeletal muscle and subsequently impairs the capacity for prolonged exercise (33,34).

Iron deficiency anemia has also been shown to impair psychomotor development, intellectual performance, and elicit changes in behavior in infants and children (35). It is unclear whether the effects of iron deficiency anemia on cognition in children can be corrected. While some studies show evidence of full correction of abnormalities with iron therapy (36), others have not (35).

Thermoregulation in both rats (37) and humans (38) is also affected by iron deficiency anemia by impairing the maintenance of normal body temperature when exposed to cold temperatures. This impairment is related to the decreased production of thyroid hormones and is the result of an enzymatic iron deficiency, rather than anemia (39).

Although anorexia has been observed as a symptom in some studies involving iron-deficient anemic rats (40), Beard et al (41) reported that iron-deficient anemic rats still demonstrated slower growth rates, despite having eaten more than control rats. Therefore, it is plausible that impaired growth in iron-deficient anemic rats arises from an energetic inefficiency. This inefficiency may result from increased rates of glycogenolysis and glycolysis in an attempt to compensate for an impairment in the iron-dependent, enzymatic production of ATP (42).

Henderson et al (43) reported that iron-deficient anemic rats had a significantly higher mean arterial glucose and lactate concentration compared with that of control rats, which reflected the higher rates of glucose turnover and recycling. It appears that major alterations in the glucose metabolism of iron-deficient anemic rats occur as a result of metabolic adaptations to an impairment in the mitochondrial oxidative production of ATP (43,44). Specifically, dietary iron deficiency anemia results in increased blood glucose concentration, glucose recycling, and an increased metabolic rate. Although such adaptations occur in iron-deficient rats during exercise (42,45), the same adaptations have also occurred in rats at rest (43). Thus it is probable that a chronic increase in metabolic rate decreases feed efficiency, leading to slow growth rates in weanling, iron-deficient anemic rats, and possibly even in young growing humans, specifically iron-depleted, adolescent athletes.

In order for iron-deficient anemic rats to maintain the increase in glucose turnover rate proposed to be responsible for this energetic inefficiency (43), an adaptive mechanism would have to be present by which this excess glucose can be taken up into cells. Farrell et al (46) reported that such an adaptation does exist; iron deficiency anemia results in an increase in glucose uptake that is compensated for by an increase in insulin sensitivity.

The three major sites of glucose uptake are skeletal muscle, liver, and adipose tissue (47,48). Farrell et al (46) conjectured that alterations specifically in skeletal muscle sensitivity are responsible for the ability of iron-deficient anemic rats to utilize more glucose than iron-sufficient rats. This hypothesis is based on research by James et al (49) and Kraegen et al (50), who demonstrated that both hepatic and adipose tissue glucose uptake account for a negligible amount of whole-body glucose disposal.

If an increase in glucose turnover and metabolic rate is to result from any physiologic condition, including iron deficiency, it must be triggered by stimulation from the sympathetic nervous system (SNS) (51). Norepinephrine (NE) is the catecholamine that typically facilitates SNS stimulation. Therefore, it follows that a chronic increase in metabolic rate due to iron deficiency would manifest itself by increased levels of NE in the blood and/or urine.

Voorhess et al (52) observed elevated urinary NE levels in iron-deficient anemic children, which returned to normal within 1 week of iron dextran treatment, and before Hb levels had increased substantially. The impairment leading to the elevated levels of urinary NE in the children had to have resulted from an enzymatic iron deficiency, rather than from a Hb deficiency (52).

Based on research by Henderson et al (43) and Brooks et al (44), it is likely that the oxidative enzymes in the mitochondria of the children in Voorhess et al's (52) study were depleted of iron. Such a depletion would have impaired the

production of ATP, resulting in the need for a compensatory response by the SNS. A SNS response would trigger the release of NE in order to increase glycogenolysis and glycolysis, metabolic rate, and hence ATP production. Unfortunately, the occurrence of such a phenomenon in Voorhess et al's study is mere speculation as no measurements were made of mitochondrial enzymatic activity, glucose turnover, or metabolic rate. However, the results of Voorhess et al's study, along with those from Henderson et al and Brooks et al are strong enough to suggest that such a phenomenon could occur as a result of enzymatic iron depletion, pointing to the need for future human research in the area of iron depletion and iron deficiency anemia and their respective impacts on NE, glucose metabolism, resting metabolic rate (RMR), and exercise performance.

IRON DEFICIENCY AND EXERCISE

Incidence and Etiology of Iron Deficiency in Adolescent and Adult Athletes

Because of the major role that iron plays in the delivery of oxygen to body tissues, much research has focused on the incidence and etiology of iron deficiency in athletes. The incidence of iron deficiency anemia among athletes, determined by a Hb concentration below 13.0 g/dL in males and 12.0 g/dL in females is rare (53,54). The incidence of iron depletion, marked by normal Hb levels, but reduced iron stores, is a relatively common occurrence among athletes. The incidence of iron depletion has been reported to range between 30% and 50%, especially among female athletes and those athletes, both male and female, who participate in endurance sports such as cross-country running and cross-country skiing (53,55–57). The range varies, possibly due to the different criteria established by researchers to define iron deficiency anemia. Additionally, because a number of studies include subjects comprising a wide range of ages, the incidence of iron deficiency in both adolescents and adult athletes will be discussed in this section.

A large study conducted by Schena et al (57) is an example of research indicating a high rate of iron depletion specifically among athletes who participate in endurance sports. Of the 326 male athletes and 85 sedentary controls, aged 17 to 26, Schena et al reported that iron depletion, as indicated by a SF level below 20 ng/dL, is more widespread among both aerobic and anaerobic athletes than among sedentary subjects. Among athletes in different sports, Schena et al reported a higher percentage of iron depletion (SF < 20 ng/dL) in those participating in the endurance disciplines, in comparison with those whose activities were primarily anaerobic in nature. However, despite a high incidence of iron depletion among athletes, only 5.5% demonstrated the presence or near presence of iron deficiency anemia (Hb < 14 g/dL).

Because of this apparent predisposition of endurance athletes to iron depletion, many researchers have focused on the relationship between iron deficiency and distance running. Balaban et al (53) investigated the frequency of both iron depletion and iron deficiency anemia in a group of 35 male and 37 female adult nationally ranked, or otherwise highly competitive, runners. About 33% of the male runners and

Table 57-1 Serum Ferritin Concentration and Hemoglobin at Onset and Completion of Competitive Running Season

	Males (n = 17)		Females (n = 9)	
Week	Serum Ferritin (ng/mL) ± SD	Hemoglobin (g/dL) ± SD	Serum Ferritin (ng/mL) ± SD	Hemoglobin (g/dL) ± SD
0	29.4 ± 17.8	14.7 ± 1.0	26.6 ± 11.4	13.3 ± 0.4
11	23.9 ± 11.9	14.8 ± 0.9	14.0 ± 6.8	13.7 ± 0.4

Reprinted by permission of Elsevier Science from Rowland TW, Black SA, Kelleher JF. Iron deficiency in adolescent athletes. J Adolesc Health 1987;8:322–326. Copyright 1987 by the Society of Adolescent Medicine.

Table 57-2 Number of Girls Deficient in Each Category

	Hemoglobin	Percent Transferrin Saturation	Serum Ferritin
Athletes (n = 32)	4 (12.5%)	17 (53%)[a]	14 (44%)
Nonathletes (n = 31)	1 (3%)	5 (16%)[a]	11 (35%)
Blacks (n = 37)	2 (5%)	16 (43%)	19 (51%)[b]
Whites (n = 26)	3 (12%)	6 (23%)	6 (23%)[b]

Lower limits of normal: hemoglobin–whites 12.2 gm/dL; blacks 11.38 gm/dL; percent transferrin saturation—16%; serum ferrition—12 µg/L

[a,b] Same superscript denotes significant difference between the values; $p < 0.05$

Reprinted by permission of Elsevier Science from Brown RT, McIntosh SM, Seabolt VR, et al. Iron status of adolescent female athletes. J Adolesc Health 1985;6:349–352. Copyright 1985 by the Society of Adolescent Medicine.

62% of the female runners were using iron supplements, several male and female runners were taking aspirin or non-steroidal anti-inflammatory drugs (NSAIDS), and some female runners reported having been diagnosed with disordered eating and having irregular menses. Even after the iron supplementation among some of the athletes had been accounted for, Balaban et al concluded that iron deficiency anemia is not a statistically common condition in either male or female runners, and that the incidence of iron depletion in runners appears to be no more common than in non-runners. These conclusions are strikingly different from those made by Schena et al (57), who determined that iron depletion is more common among male athletes, especially endurance athletes such as runners, compared with nonathlete controls. If Balaban et al subdivided their subjects according to running specialty, it is possible that the incidence of iron depletion among long-distance runners would have been higher than that among sedentary individuals, especially considering the results Schena et al presented, which indicated that iron depletion is more prevalent among endurance athletes. Addi-

tionally, although Balaban et al did account for differences in iron supplementation among groups, they did not account for the reported inequalities of aspirin and NSAID use, menstrual irregularities, oral contraceptive use, disordered eating, or dietary intake between groups, all of which can have an affect on iron stores (11,25,58–60).

Others have reported a higher incidence of iron deficiency anemia and/or iron depletion in female athletes compared with sedentary female controls (55,56). Plowman et al (56) examined the incidence of iron deficiency anemia and iron depletion specifically among female high school and collage cross-country runners, aged 14 to 22. Iron status measurements indicated a higher incidence of iron depletion among runners compared with sedentary subjects.

Rowland et al (61) specifically studied a group of high school male and female cross-country runners to assess the incidence of iron depletion, determine gender differences of iron deficiency, and to evaluate iron status changes over the course of the cross-country season. At the beginning of the season, only 1 of the 30 male athletes and 8 of the 20 female athletes had iron deficiency, based upon their serum ferritin levels (defined as ≤ 12 ng/mL). However, by the end of the cross-country season, 4 more male athletes and 1 more female athlete became iron deficient (Table 57-1). Rowland et al concluded that iron deficiency without anemia frequently occurs in high school cross-country runners, more so in the female athletes, and that preseason screening is not sufficient due to a drop in serum ferritin during training. Brown et al (62) also reported that female track athletes had significantly lower SF levels and transferrin saturation than their nonathletic counterparts. Furthermore, they reported a greater incidence of iron deficiency in African American adolescents compared with Caucasian adolescents (Table 57-2) (62).

It appears that endurance sports and sports with more emphasis on body weight and aesthetics have a higher prevalence of iron deficiency than other sports. For example, Mahlamaki et al (63) reported that none of their control subjects had iron deficiency anemia; however, 15% of the dancers in their study had iron deficiency anemia. Although the subjects took iron supplements for 10 weeks, this time frame was not long enough to increase iron stores. It is imperative that individuals with iron deficiency anemia take supplements for a period of time sufficient to increase their iron stores (shown by an increase in SF levels). Even when iron stores are increased, supplementation needs to continue until

Table 57-3 Incidence of Iron Deficiency During the Running Season

STUDY GROUP	No. of SUBJECTS	IRON DEFICIENT RUNNERS			
		TEST 2 (DAY 40)	TEST 3 (DAY 75)	TOTAL NO.	%
Female runners (n = 41)					
Iron treatment group	14	1	4	5	35
Diet treatment group	13	3	2	5	37
Control subjects	14	4	0	4	28
Total	41	8	6	14	34
Male runners (n = 25)					
Iron treatment group	9	0	0	0	
Diet treatment group	8	0	2	2	
Control subjects	8	0	0	0	
Total	25	0	2	2	8

SOURCE: Nickerson HJ, Holubets MC, Weiler BR, et al. Causes of iron deficiency in adolescent athletes. J Pediatr 1989;114:657–663.

the individual can maintain these stores without supplementation. Additionally, Nickerson et al (64) reported that 34% of female cross-country runners and 8% of male cross-country runners were diagnosed with iron deficiency (Table 57-3). Some causes of this high incidence, especially in female athletes, include low iron stores and gastrointestinal bleeding (64).

The previous investigations provide a basic overview of the incidence of iron depletion and iron deficiency anemia in both male and female athletes. Whereas iron deficiency anemia appears to be less common among all athletes of both genders (53,55,57), iron depletion occurs with greater frequency among certain types of athletes. In general, endurance athletes of both sexes who participate in aerobic sports such as cross-country running and cross-country skiing have a higher incidence of iron depletion than those athletes who participate in anaerobic sports (57,61). This phenomenon is thought to result from losses of iron-containing substances in the urine and feces of these athletes due to gastrointestinal bleeding, as well as from myoglobinuria due to myofibrillar stress and hemoglobinuria due to intravascular hemolysis (65–67).

Female athletes are susceptible to these same losses, and they additionally experience iron loss as a result of menstruation (11) and possibly because of an inadequate dietary intake of iron. As a result of these factors, female athletes have an especially high risk of developing iron depletion. The effects of iron depletion or iron deficiency anemia can be even more devastating in the growing adolescent athlete, in whom not only athletic performance but overall growth can be impaired.

Effects of Iron Deficiency Anemia and Iron Depletion on Athletic Performance in Adolescents and Adults

The realization that endurance athletes are particularly susceptible to iron depletion led to a flood of research focused on the effects of iron depletion on exercise performance and the potential for improving exercise performance with iron supplementation. Although it is well documented that the third and final stage, iron deficiency anemia, impairs exercise performance as measured by a reduction in maximal oxygen con-

sumption (Vo_2max) (68,69), the evidence is inconclusive as to the effects of iron depletion on exercise performance.

There are two major components to exercise performance: aerobic capacity and endurance. Based on both physiologic and biochemical evidence from rat studies (42,45), it appears that these two components differ in the way they are affected by iron depletion and iron deficiency anemia. Aerobic capacity, measured by Vo_2max, is based upon the ability of red blood cells to efficiently deliver oxygen to tissues (42). Therefore, the maintenance of aerobic capacity is dependent upon an adequate supply of Hb to red blood cells and is not impaired until iron deficiency is severe enough for anemia to be present (42,45,70–72). The degree of iron deficiency that is necessary to impair exercise endurance is, however, much less clear. Exercise endurance is contingent upon the ability of enzymes inside the mitochondria of the muscles to generate ATP. Many of these mitochondral enzymes require iron as a cofactor. Therefore, exercise endurance is dependent upon an adequate supply of iron for these enzymes to function. Additionally, because mitochondrial enzymes generate ATP aerobically, an adequate supply of oxygen is also required if they are to function optimally. Considering that these enzymes require both an adequate supply of iron as well as an adequate supply of oxygen to function, it seems logical that their ability to generate ATP would be impaired if either of these requirements are not met.

Serum iron (SI) concentration reflects the amount of iron available for transport to places in the body such as the mitochondrial enzymes. Because iron stores are depleted in the early stages of iron deficiency, it follows that the amount of iron available for transport would then decrease and, subsequently, exercise endurance would be impaired. Indeed, some researchers have observed significant decreases in exercise endurance in individuals who are iron depleted, but not anemic (71); however, others have not (70,72,73). While several researchers have also observed significant decreases in exercise endurance in iron deficient rats in the absence of anemia (45), other researchers have observed a decrease in exercise endurance in rats only in the presence of iron deficiency anemia (42). Physiologic differences between rats and humans and/or differences between biologic age and maturity among subjects from different studies may be responsible for conflicting results.

One of the first studies to investigate both physiologic and biochemical differences in the ways in which iron deficiency anemia affects exercise endurance and aerobic capacity in 21-day-old Sprague Dawley rats was conducted by Davies et al (42). They reported that anemia in the iron-deficient rats was manifested by a 48% decrease in Vo_2max and a 50% lower Vo_2max workload compared with that of control rats. Large increases in both Vo_2max and Vo_2max workload were observed in the iron-deficient anemic rats who had erythrocyte-transfusions; however, despite these marked improvements, the Vo_2max and Vo_2max workload of the iron-deficient anemic, erythrocyte-transfused rats remained lower than the control rats (42).

Davies et al (42) also reported that iron deficiency was present in these animals at an enzymatic level. Although oxidative phosphorylation was not inhibited, decreased muscle oxidase activities in anemic animals resulted in a decreased muscular potential for mitochondrial ATP synthesis. This decrease in potential for ATP synthesis was reflected in a 93% decrease in endurance capacity in iron-deficient anemic animals compared with controls. Interestingly, maximal endurance times were not increased at all by exchange transfusion in the iron-deficient anemic animals.

In order to maintain performance during submaximal exercise bouts, in the face of a reduced muscle mitochondrial capacity, iron-deficient rats could be expected to supplement oxidative phosphorylation with increased rates of glycogenolysis and glycolysis. Acidosis created by high rates of glycolysis in iron-deficient rats would be buffered by bicarbonates, leading to a higher ratio of expired carbon dioxide to oxygen consumed. Indeed, this phenomenon was indicated by significantly higher R values measured for iron-deficient rats compared with controls, during Vo_2max testing. Further evidence for increased rates of glycogenolysis and glycolysis was indicated by very large increases in blood lactate concentrations after endurance tests in iron-deficient anemic, sham-transfused rats. This increase was partially alleviated by exchange transfusion of erythrocytes (42).

Resting blood glucose and blood lactate levels were also higher in the iron-deficient anemic animals than in the controls. Additionally, after exhaustive endurance exercise, the control rats' glycogen and glucose levels were substantially decreased, whereas those of the iron-deficient anemic rats were much less affected; blood transfusion did not affect this pattern. These differences are most likely due to the fact that iron-deficient anemic rats were not able to run long enough to deplete glucose and glycogen stores (42).

Upon examination of these results, it is evident that the effects of iron deficiency anemia (low Hb levels) on exercise performance are quite distinct from the effects of iron deficiency (low cellular iron stores) on exercise performance. A decrease in oxygen delivery due to reduced Hb levels appears to result in a decrease in Vo_2max. This hypothesis is supported by the observation that a partial correction of Hb levels by exchange transfusion in the iron-deficient anemic rats significantly improved both Vo_2max and Vo_2 workload in the rats (42). However, Hb correction resulted in no significant improvement in the substantially lower exercise endurance times observed in the rats with iron deficiency anemia, com-

pared with iron-sufficient controls. Therefore, instead of being restricted by oxygen delivery, exercise endurance is apparently restricted by oxidative capacity, as the iron-deficient anemic rats had significantly lower mitochondrial oxidase specific activities and lower concentrations of muscle mitochondria than the controls. Furthermore, the ratios of expired carbon dioxide to inspired oxygen and blood lactate levels were higher in the iron-deficient anemic rats compared with controls. These increases are indicative of an increase in the rate of glycogenolysis and glycolysis, which would help to compensate for an impairment in the ability of the mitochondrial oxidative enzymes to produce ATP.

It is also interesting to note that exchange transfusions did not completely correct Vo_2max to levels observed in the plasma- and sham-transfused control rats. It is conceivable that this remaining deficit was due to a reduction in oxidative capacity, and that the affect of iron deficiency anemia on oxidative capacity is not exclusive to exercise endurance. Additionally, there may be a threshold Hb value above which Vo_2max is not altered by either oxidative capacity or oxygen delivery. This hypothesis is based on the observation that a reduction in Hb to 10 g/dL in the plasma-transfused control rats had no effect on Vo_2max (42). Further research to determine how various levels of severity of iron deficiency affect Vo_2max, exercise endurance, and oxidative capacity is warranted by these results.

Such an experiment was undertaken by Perkkio et al (45). As in Davies et al's (42) study, male Sprague-Dawley rats at age 21 days were used as subjects. The rats were divided into four groups, each of which received a diet with an iron content (ferric citrate) of either 9, 15, 30, or 50 mg/kg of body weight. Mean blood Hb concentration ranged from 13.9 ± 0.4 g/dL in the animals receiving 50 mg/kg iron daily to 6.1 ± 0.2 g/dL in the animals receiving only 9 mg/kg iron daily. Impairment of Vo_2max and endurance capacity due to these varying degrees of iron deficiency differed markedly. Endurance capacity did not decrease significantly at Hb concentrations between 14 g/dL and 10 g/dL, but declined by over 70% at Hb concentrations between 10 g/dL and 8 g/dL. Comparatively, Vo_2max decreased only 16% at a Hb concentration between 14 g/dL and 8 g/dL, but then decreased significantly below a Hb concentration of 7 g/dL.

These results suggest that endurance capacity is much more sensitive to the severity of iron deficiency than Vo_2max and, therefore, rats are better able to compensate for decrements in oxygen transport and uptake (due to low Hb levels) than for decrements in mitochondrial oxygen utilization (due to enzymatic iron depletion). The compensatory mechanisms identified in previous research (74) that would enable an animal to maintain a normal or near-normal Vo_2max, despite decreased Hb concentrations, include a shift of the Hb-oxygen dissociation curve to the right, and more complete extraction of oxygen from blood as it crosses the capillary bed.

The less effective compensatory mechanism stimulated in response to an enzymatic level of iron deficiency appears to involve an increase in glycogenolysis and glycolysis to supplement an impairment in the oxidative production of ATP. In a study by Perkkio et al (45), this mechanism was suggested by a strong inverse relationship between blood lactate levels and Hb concentration following a 2-minute run test, as well

Table 57-4 Hematologic Parameters in Both Controls and Iron-Deficient Subjects Before and After Iron therapy

	Hgb (gm/dL)	Saturation (%) (Fe/TIBC)	Ferritin (ng/mL)	Transferrin (mg/mL)
Controls (n = 6)				
Before therapy	13.8 ± 1.1	25.3 ± 9.7	19.8 ± 4.9	2.28 ± 0.31
After therapy	14.3 ± 0.9	27.2 ± 7.9	13.7 ± 4.3	2.11 ± 0.25
Iron deficients (n = 9)				
Before therapy	12.2 ± 0.4[a]	12.1 ± 4.8[a]	10.0 ± 2.0[b]	2.30 ± 0.22
After therapy	12.7 ± 0.5[d]	32.8 ± 11.9[f]	22.1 ± 7.8[e]	2.45 ± 0.18[c]

Values are means ± SD. P values for controls vs. iron deficient—before therapy: [a]$P < 0.02$, [b]$P < 0.005$; after therapy: [c]$P < 0.02$. P values for before vs. after therapy—controls: no significant differences; iron-deficients [d]$P < 0.05$, [e]$P < 0.002$, [f]$P < 0.001$. Reprinted by permission from Schoene RB, Escourrou P, Robertson T, et al. Iron repletion decreases maximal exercise lactate concentrations in female athletes with minimal iron-deficiency anemia. J Lab Clin Med 1983;102:306–312.

as by significantly reduced exercise endurance times and cytochrome c concentrations in rats with Hb concentrations below 10 g/dL.

It is apparent that iron deficiency without anemia and iron deficiency in the presence of anemia impair exercise performance via two distinct mechanisms: by reducing mitochondrial oxygen utilization and/or by reducing oxygen transport via Hb (42,45). These reductions manifest themselves by decreases in exercise endurance and oxygen consumption, respectively. Mitochondrial oxidative capacity appears to be more sensitive to the severity of iron deficiency anemia than oxygen transport because of more effective compensatory mechanisms that exist to maintain SI at near normal levels, despite a reduction in Hb concentration (45). However, neither exercise endurance nor Vo₂max seem to be significantly impaired in rats unless Hb concentrations are below 10 g/dL (45). This leads to the conclusion that, in rats, iron deficiency must be quite severe and anemia must be present before any measurable impairment in either exercise endurance or aerobic capacity is evident.

The severity of iron deficiency critical to an impairment in either measure of exercise performance in humans is questionable. Schoene et al (72) studied the effects of 2 weeks of iron therapy on exercise performance and exercise-induced lactate production in trained female athletes, aged 18 to 35, with iron deficiency anemia. After 2 weeks of iron supplementation, a significant improvement in both Hb and SF levels was noted in the iron-deficient anemic group who had received iron therapy, but this did not correspond to significant changes in Vo₂max (Table 57-4). Interestingly, lactate concentration at 1 minute after exercise did decrease significantly in the iron-deficient anemic group after therapy. None of the iron-deficient anemic participants who received the placebo demonstrated significant changes in any of the above parameters.

The results of Schoene et al's (72) study may appear to conflict with the findings of Perkkio et al's (45) study, in that Perkkio et al observed significant decreases in their iron deficient subjects' Vo₂max, whereas Schoene et al did not. However, upon closer examination, although there are no means by which to directly compare the degree of tissue iron depletion of women athletes with that of rats, it does seem evident that the severity of iron deficiency in the women in

Schoene et al's study was considerably less than that of the rats in Perkkio et al's study. The participants in the experimental group in Schoene et al's study were iron depleted (initial mean SF concentration 10.0 ± 1.8 ng/dL), but only borderline anemic (initial mean Hb concentration 12.3 ± 0.4 g/dL), whereas the majority of the rats in Perkkio et al's study were severely anemic (mean Hb concentrations between 13.9 ± 0.4 g/dL and 6.1 ± 0.2 g/dL). Furthermore, Perkkio et al found no major impairment in Vo₂max in rats with Hb concentrations above 10 g/dL.

Post-exercise lactate levels did improve in the iron-deficient anemic women in Schoene et al's (72) study following iron therapy. Davies et al (42) and Perkkio et al (45) correlated low lactate levels with impairments in muscle oxidative capacity. Therefore, it is possible that the iron-depleted women in Schoene et al's study did have an impairment in mitochondrial oxidative capacity. However, there is no direct evidence for this as neither exercise endurance nor mitochondrial oxidative capacity were measured. Nonetheless, if these women did have an impairment in oxidative capacity, this suggests that the severity of iron deficiency necessary for such an impairment to occur is less in humans than it is in rats.

To more directly determine if iron depletion in the absence of anemia impairs endurance capacity in humans, Rowland et al (71) studied 30 high school female cross-country runners who were randomized in a double-blind fashion to iron therapy or placebo groups for 4 weeks. SF levels fell progressively from baseline to midpoint testing in both groups and continued to drop at the end of the season in the placebo group. Runners who underwent iron therapy showed a significant rise in SF at the final testing when compared with levels at midpoint or with the values for the placebo-treated runners at the final testing time (71). Treadmill endurance time decreased from midpoint in the placebo-treated participants compared to an increase in endurance time in the iron-treated subjects. Although iron therapy did not improve treadmill endurance times more than might be expected by a training effect, the decrement in endurance time from midpoint to final point in the placebo group was significantly different from the improvement during the same period in the iron-treated runners. Furthermore, a direct relationship was observed between individual SF levels at the time

Table 57-5 Physical Performance Factors in Study Groups[1]

FACTOR	IRON-DEPLETED GROUP (*n* = 15)	IRON-SUFFICIENT GROUP (*n* = 15)
Vo_2max (L/min)	2.2 ± 0.39	2.5 ± 0.40
Vo_2max by weight (mL/kg per min)	37.7 ± 7.0	42.3 ± 6.6
Vo_2max by fat-free mass (mL/kg per min)	46.3 ± 8.3	53.2 ± 7.5[2]
δ-Efficiency (%)	25.1 ± 3.3	25.3 ± 2.6
Respiratory exchange ratio at ventilatory threshold	0.89 ± 0.07	0.91 ± 0.06
Vo_2 at ventilatory threshold (% of Vo_2max)[3]	58.9 ± 8.3	56.0 ± 10.4

[1] x ± SD; Vo_2max, maximal oxygen consumption; Vo_2, oxygen uptake.
[2] Significantly different from iron-depleted group, $P < 0.05$.
[3] Oxygen consumption expressed as a percentage of Vo_2max at ventilatory threshold.
Reprinted by permission from Zhu YI, Haas JD. Iron depletion without anemia and physical performance in young women. Am J Clin Nutr 1997;66:334–341. © American Society for Clinical Nutrition.

of the final testing and change in treadmill endurance time ($r = 0.74$; $P < 0.05$). This indicates that iron therapy prevented the decrement in endurance time that occurred in the placebo group from also occurring in the iron-treated group. Perhaps more significant improvements in endurance time to exhaustion would have been noted with a larger sample size and if menstrual loss and dietary iron intake had been controlled.

Nevertheless, Rowland et al (71) demonstrated that iron depletion in the absence of anemia (SF below 10 ng/dL, Hb > 12 g/dL) impairs exercise performance in humans by decreasing endurance time to exhaustion. Unfortunately, measures of blood lactate and mitochondrial enzymatic activity were not made to confirm mitochondrial enzymatic depletion of iron.

However, muscle biopsies to determine mitochondrial enzymatic activity were collected in another human study by Newhouse et al (70), in which the effect of iron depletion without anemia and subsequent repletion on exercise performance was measured. Forty female recreational runners, aged 18 to 40, were selected (SF < 20 ng/dL; Hb > 12 g/dL) and either given oral iron supplementation or a placebo (double-blind). Subject selection criteria, such as no use of NSAIDS, were strictly enforced. Muscle biopsies, from the lateral portion of the right quadriceps muscle, were analyzed for citrate synthase activity and cytoplasmic α-glycerophosphate dehydrogenase (α-GPDH) activity to estimate oxidative capacity of the muscle.

As a result of the 8 weeks of iron supplementation, the mean SF level of the iron group was significantly higher than that of the placebo group (37.7 ± 19.7 ng/dL vs. 17.2 ± 8.9 ng/dL). Although this improvement was statistically significant, it is still modest considering that the normal range for SF levels in females extends to 160 ng/mL. The mean SF level of a large screening ($N = 1104$) of US female non-runners was 69.6 ng/dL (75). The lack of statistical significance reported by Newhouse et al (70) is actually not surprising given that iron deficiency anemia impairs exercise endurance, but not aerobic capacity (42,45,71). Both the Wingate test and the anaerobic speed test used by Newhouse et al are too short to be measures of endurance.

Considering the results from both Schoene et al's (72) study and Rowland et al's (71) study, it is surprising that in Newhouse et al's (70) study no significant differences between groups were observed in either of the two enzymes representative of oxidative capacity. However, it is possible that significant differences were not apparent because the particular oxidative enzymes measured in Newhouse et al's study are not iron dependent. It is also possible that the participants in Newhouse et al's study were not sufficiently iron depleted to influence endurance capacity. The iron-depleted participants in both Schoene et al's study and Rowland et al's study had mean SF levels below 10 ng/dL. Conversely, the iron-depleted participants in Newhouse et al's study had a mean SF below 12 ng/dL, but the cut-off for being included in the iron depleted group in Newhouse et al's study was a SF below 20 ng/dL.

An investigation conducted by Lamanca et al (73), in which more appropriate measures of endurance capacity were made, revealed similar results as Newhouse et al (70): no significant differences in Vo_2max, intensity, heart rate, time to exhaustion, or postexercise lactate levels were reported between the eight athletic iron depleted women and the eight controls, aged 21 to 35. Time to exhaustion on the endurance test was 14% less for the iron-depleted group, but this difference was not statistically significant between groups. Nonetheless, the difference in endurance of 3.8 minutes is of considerable practical importance, especially during competition.

More recently, Zhu et al (76) assessed if iron depletion, without anemia, affected athletic performance in women aged 19 to 36. Their results showed some enlightening evidence, which must be further studied. The iron-depleted group had a significantly lower Vo_2max compared with the iron-sufficient group (Table 57-5). However, the decreased Vo_2max in the iron-depleted group was significantly associated with SF levels, not Hb levels, as has been previously reported. These authors concluded that, "…reduction in VO_2max in non-anemic women with iron depletion was likely caused by factors related to reduced body iron storage but was unrelated to decreased oxygen-transport capacity of the blood" (76).

Comparison of the Effects of Iron Deficiency on Adolescents and Adults

Despite the different mechanisms by which aerobic capacity and exercise endurance are affected by iron deficiency, it is evident from animal studies (42,45) that iron deficiency anemia must be present in rats before either of these measurements are impaired. Whether such a severe stage of iron deficiency must be present in humans before both aerobic capacity and exercise endurance is impaired is unclear. Whereas the results from some human studies have indicated diminished exercise endurance in subjects who are iron depleted but not anemic (71), results from other studies have reported no significant impairment in exercise endurance in iron-depleted (non-anemic) humans (70,73). Although it is probable that differences in physiology may account for conflicting results between rat and human studies (42,45,71), it is likely that differences in biological age and development may explain discrepancies among human studies (70–73).

The human studies that did not find significant differences in the endurance capacity of iron-depleted athletes used adults (70,72,73), while the human study that did find significant reductions in endurance capacity due to iron depletion used adolescents (71). Hallberg et al (77) determined that an extra 0.38 mg/day of iron above normal adult requirements is required during adolescent growth for blood volume expansion and iron-containing tissue compounds such as myoglobin and cytochromes in growing muscle; during adolescence, the individual will gain about 20% of adult height and 50% of adult weight (78). Furthermore, the onset of menses in adolescent girls increases iron loss, putting an even greater strain on iron stores (78).

The important physiologic need iron serves during growth is clearly apparent by comparing the results of an animal study that used weanling rats to another animal study which used adult rats. Perkkio et al (45) reported significant reductions in endurance capacity in animals fed iron-deficient diets from the time they were weaned. Furthermore, these reductions were linked to a reduced Mb content, cytochrome levels, and mitochondrial enzyme activity. Comparatively, in another study in which fully grown adult rats were fed an iron-deficient diet for 300 days, no significant reductions in Mb content or cytochrome oxidase activity were observed (79). Therefore, it seems likely that young individuals (weanling rats, children, or adolescents) are more vulnerable than adults to negative consequences arising from iron deficiency, even in its early stages. This is because young individuals are in the process of rapid growth and therefore have greater relative needs for energy and iron, for its incorporation into the iron-dependent oxidative enzymes in the mitochondria of newly forming lean body mass. Even increasing rates of glycogenolysis and glycolysis to supplement the subsequent impairment in the oxidative generation of ATP (42) does not appear to be sufficient to maintain exercise endurance capacity at normal levels (42,45,71). Additionally, this enzymatic iron deficiency may actually impair growth and development in young individuals as evidenced by the significantly lower body weights of the iron deficient rats compared with iron-sufficient controls in both Davies et al's study (42) and Perkkio et al's study (45).

PREVENTION OF IRON DEFICIENCY

Dietary iron deficiency can be prevented in two major ways: by increasing iron content and bioavailability in the diet, and by supplementing the diet with iron in the form of tablets or liquid. Factors such as education, lifestyle, cost, food availability, ethnicity, as well as political and religious beliefs will determine if and how prevention will occur.

Dietary iron content and bioavailability can be increased most effectively by consuming a diet rich in meat, fish, and poultry because these foods contain heme iron. Heme iron is absorbed two to three times more readily than the non-heme iron found in cereals and grains (12). As an added benefit, there are other factors in meat, fish, and poultry that promote the absorption of non-heme iron from the entire meal.

There are many individuals, however, who cannot afford the expense of a meat-based diet, or who do not consume animal products for religious, ethnic, political, or environmental reasons. Such individuals must depend solely on less absorbable, non-heme sources of iron. Fortunately, ascorbic acid effectively promotes the absorption of non-heme iron (12). Therefore, consuming citrus fruits and fruit juices along with a meal will greatly increase iron bioavailability.

Consuming foods that are fortified with iron is also an effective way by which to increase iron content in the diet (80). Ferrous sulfate is a highly soluble form of iron commonly used in the fortification of canned and jarred food and foods with a short shelf-life such as bread, bakery products, and infant formula (80).

Individuals who cannot effectively meet their needs for iron through food have the option of supplementing their diet with iron in the form of tablets or liquid. The efficacy of supplemental iron is influenced by several factors, including dose; iron stores of the recipient; whether iron supplementation is taken between meals; and whether iron is consumed alone or in combination with a vitamin-mineral supplement (81).

Iron in supplemental form is better absorbed by individuals who have either low iron stores or iron deficiency erythropoiesis, and those who are anemic (82). In fact, iron absorption can be as high as 50% in individuals with iron deficiency anemia. Additionally, iron in supplemental form is absorbed twice as well when taken between meals rather than with meals. It is also better to take an iron supplement alone, rather than in combination with a daily vitamin-mineral tablet, because most of these tablets contain calcium carbonate and magnesium oxide that inhibit iron absorption (83).

If iron supplementation in combination with a vitamin-mineral tablet is unavoidable because of added expense or inconvenience, iron absorption can be maximized by choosing a tablet that contains at least 60 mg of elemental iron and no more than 250 mg of calcium carbonate (83).

Assessment of Anemia in the Adolescent Athlete

As discussed, there are a number of reasons why an athlete may become iron depleted or iron-deficient anemic. These possibilities, including low dietary intake of iron, should all be assessed carefully in the adolescent athlete, since low levels of serum iron and ferritin can result in impaired performance and health, including cognitive ability. Regardless of the athlete's abilities and competitiveness in his/her sport, screening for anemia in adolescent athletes is necessary and should not be overlooked.

Raunikar et al (84) have listed a number of points that should be taken into consideration when assessing the adolescent athlete for iron deficiency anemia. These include a meticulous medical history and physical examination. They identified some clues that may assist the clinician in identifying the risk of the adolescent for developing iron deficiency anemia: lower socioeconomic status, inadequate nutrition, intensive physical training, use of NSAIDS or other gastric irritants, family history of anemia or chronic disease that may cause anemia, and, for female athletes, menstrual cycle history. Raunikar et al (84) also list some clinical manifestations of iron deficiency anemia, e.g., cheilosis, glossitis, pallor, and koilonychia.

Often adolescent athletes are required to have a preparticipation physical exam from their own physician or their school's physician. This is an opportune time to screen the athlete for iron deficiency anemia. Screening can allow for intervention, if required, and provide a good reference point for all other physical examinations (84).

A number of biochemical tests can be used to determine if an adolescent athlete suffers from iron deficiency anemia. Usually, Hct and Hb are the first line of biochemical tests used; if these values are not within normal limits, more specific tests to determine the type of anemia, if present, will be required. Raunikar et al (84) state the following instances when laboratory screening for iron deficiency anemia should be performed in the adolescent athlete: if there is a clinical suspicion of anemia, if the adolescent athlete is in a high risk group for anemia (e.g., heavy menstrual cycles, intense physical activity, inadequate dietary intake), or if a biochemical test was not done at the physical exam.

If an adolescent athlete is diagnosed with iron deficiency anemia, the appropriate course is oral iron therapy at a dose of 6 mg of elemental iron/kg body weight per day. This same course of action is necessary for iron-deficient athletes without anemia in order to prevent anemia from occurring. Finally, consultation with a registered dietitian is necessary in order to ensure that the adolescent athlete is practicing healthy dietary habits, and, if not, that the athlete's habits are altered to ensure proper growth, iron storage, health, and athletic performance. NSAIDS and other gastric irritants should be avoided, unless absolutely necessary (84).

Iron depletion or iron deficiency anemia does not require that adolescent or adult athletes terminate participation in their respective sports. It is important that the anemia is curtailed by supplementation, proper dietary intakes, and balanced physical training. Iron deficiency anemia resulting from other diseases, however, may warrant that the athlete discontinue participation in his/her respective sport until the underlying cause is determined or cured (84). Iron deficiency anemia is a disease that can be easily treated. Early detection is the key. Coaches and clinicians must look for the warning signs of iron deficiency anemia, such as fatigue, pallor, and improper dietary intakes, and take appropriate action as soon as possible so that health and performance are not impaired.

TREATMENT OF IRON DEFICIENCY

For individuals who are diagnosed with iron deficiency anemia, iron supplementation is the most expedient way to increase iron stores and prevent adverse physiologic effects (12). Ferrous sulfate is the least expensive and most widely used form of iron supplementation (12). Although therapy with ferrous sulfate may result in gastrointestinal side effects such as stomach upset and constipation, the occurrence and severity of these adverse side effects are directly proportional to dose and usually only occur when the dose is larger than necessary. Slow-release iron supplementation will result in fewer side effects than ferrous sulfate when a large dose of iron is required. However, slow-release iron is more expensive than either ferrous sulfate, ferrous gluconate, or ferrous fumarate. Slow-release iron is also better absorbed with meals rather than between meals (85).

For adults who are diagnosed with iron deficiency anemia, a daily dose of at least 60 mg of elemental iron (300 mg ferrous sulfate) taken between meals is recommended (12,86). A daily dose of 30 mg (2–3 mg/kg) elemental iron is recommended for infants and children with iron deficiency anemia (12). In general, the smaller the dose of iron and the more severe the anemia, the more iron is absorbed. A response to iron therapy in individuals with iron deficiency anemia should be evident within 1 month, manifested by an increase in Hb concentration by at least 1 g/dL (12). Even if Hb is within the normal range after only 1 month of therapy, supplementation should be continued for an additional 2 to 3 months to ensure the development of adequate iron stores. If no improvement in Hb concentration is evident after 1 month of therapy, further tests are necessary to determine if there is some other cause related to the presence of anemia (12).

SUMMARY

Iron depletion and iron deficiency anemia do occur in adolescent and adult athletes. Prevention is imperative, and will minimize the impairments in growth, overall health, and exercise performance observed with this deficiency. Nonetheless, if iron depletion or iron deficiency anemia occur, supplementation with the appropriate amount of iron as well as consultation with a registered dietitian usually results in improvement of iron status and allows the athlete to continue his/her sport, unless other problems exist.

REFERENCES

1. Dallman PR, Yip R, Johnson L. Prevalence and causes of anemia in the United States, 1976–1980. Am J Clin Nutr 1984;38:302–316.

2. Pilch SM, Senti FR, eds. Assessment of the iron nutritional status of the U.S. population based on data collected in the Second National Health and Nutrition Examination Survey, 1976–1980. Bethesda, MD: Life Sciences Research Office, Federation of the American Societies for Experimental Biology, 1984.

3. Yip R. Age related changes in iron metabolism. In: Brock JH, Halliday JW, Pippard MJ, eds. Iron metabolism in health and

disease. London: WB Saunders, 1994.

4. Fontecave M, Pierre JL. Iron: metabolism, toxicity and therapy. Societe Francaise de Biochimie et biologie moleculaire 1993;75: 767–773.

5. Conrad ME. Regulation of iron absorption. In: Essential and toxic trace elements in human health: an update. New York: Wiley-Liss, 1993.

6. Benjamin EL, Cortell S, Conrad ME. Bicarbonate induced iron complexes and iron absorption: one effect of pancreatic secretions. Gastroenterology 1967;53:389–396.

7. Monsen E, Balintfy J. Calculating dietary iron bioavailability: refinement and computerization. J Am Diet Assoc 1982;30:307–311.

8. Czajka-Narins DM. Minerals. In: Mahan KL, Arlin M, eds. Krause's food, nutrition & diet therapy. 8th ed. Philadelphia: WB Saunders, 1992.

9. Monsen ER, Hallberg L, Layrisse M, et al. Estimation of available dietary iron. Am J Clin Nutr 1978; 31:134–141.

10. National Research Council recommended dietary allowances. 10th ed. Washington, DC: National Academy Press, 1989.

11. Hallberg L, Hogdahl AM, Nilsson L. Menstrual blood loss and iron deficiency. Acta Med Scand 1966; 180:639–650.

12. Yip R, Dallman PR. Iron. In: Ziegler EE, Filer LJ, eds. Present knowledge in nutrition. 7th ed. Washington, DC: IL SI Press, 1996.

13. Lonnerdal B, Keen CL, Hurley LS. Iron, copper, zinc, and manganese in milk. Ann Rev Nutr 1981;1: 149–174.

14. Dallman PR, Siimes MA, Stekel A. Iron deficiency in infancy and childhood. Am J Clin Nutr 1980; 33:86–118.

15. Huebers H, Finch CA. Transferrin: physiologic behavior and clinical

implications. Blood 1987;64:763–767.

16. Finch CA, Lenfant L. Oxygen transport in men. N Engl J Med 1972; 286:407–410.

17. Dallman PR. Biochemical basis for the manifestations of iron deficiency. Ann Rev Nutr 1986;6: 13–40.

18. Dallman PR. Tissue effects of iron deficiency. In: Jacobs A, Worwood M, eds. Iron in biochemistry and medicine. London: Academic Press 1974.

19. Jain SK, Yip R, Hoesch RM, et al. Evidence of peroxidative damage to the erythrocyte membrane in iron deficiency. Am J Clin Nutr 1983;37:26–30.

20. Yip R, Mohandus N, Jain SK. Red cell deformability in iron deficiency. In: Saltman P, Hegenauer J, eds. The biochemistry and physiology of iron. Amsterdam: Elsevier, 1982.

21. Deiss A. Iron metabolism in reticuloendothelial cells. Semin Hemat 1983;20:81–90.

22. Hershko C. Storage iron regulation. Prog Hemat 1977;10:105–148.

23. Booth FW, Holloszy JO. Cytochrome c turnover in rat skeletal muscles. J Biochem 1977;252: 416–419.

24. Green R, Charlton RW, Seftel H, et al. Body iron excretion in man: a collaborative study. Am J Med 1968;45:336–353.

25. Hallberg L, Hogdahl AM, Nilsson L, et al. Menstrual blood loss—a population study: variation at different ages and attempts to define normality. Acta Obstet Gynecol Scand 1966a;45:320–351.

26. Cook JD, Skikne BS. Serum ferritin: a possible model for the assessment of nutrient stores. Am J Clin Nutr 1982;35:1180–1185.

27. Zeman FJ, Ney DM. In: Shustak MB, eds. Applications of clinical nutrition. Englewood Cliffs, NJ: Prentice Hall, 1988.

28. Dallman PR, Yip R, Oski FA. Iron deficiency and related nutritional

anemias. In: Nathan DG, Oski FA, eds. Hematology of infancy and childhood. Philadelphia: WB Saunders, 1992.

29. Reeves JD, Yip R, Kiley VA, et al. Iron deficiency in infants: the influence of mild antecedent infections. J Pediatr 1984;105:874–879.

30. Yip R, Dallman PR. The role of inflammation and iron deficiency as causes of anemia. Am J Clin Nutr 1988;48:1295–1300.

31. Varat MA, Adolph RJ, Fowler NO. Cardiovascular effects of anemia. Am Heart J 1972;83:416–426.

32. Viteri FE, Torun B. Anemia and physical work capacity. Clin Hematol 1974;3:609–626.

33. Finch CA, Miller LR, Inamdar A, et al. Iron deficiency in the rat: physiological and biochemical studies of muscle dysfunction. J Clin Invest 1976;58:447–453.

34. McLane JA, Fell RD, McKay RH, et al. Physiological and biochemical effects of iron deficiency on rat skeletal muscle function. Am J Physiol 1981;241:C47–C54.

35. Lozoff B. Behavioral alterations in iron deficiency. Adv Pediatr 1988; 35:331–359.

36. Idjradinata P, Pollitt E. Reversal of developmental delays in iron-deficient anemic infants treated with iron. Lancet 1993;341:1–4.

37. Beard JL, Green W, Miller L, et al. Effects of anemia and iron deficiency on thyroid hormone levels and thermoregulation during acute cold exposure. Am J Physiol 1984;247:R114–R119.

38. Beard JL, Borel MJ, Derr J. Impaired thermoregulation and thyroid function in iron-deficiency anemia. Am J Clin Nutr 1990;52: 813–819.

39. Beard J, Tobin B, Green W. Evidence for thyroid hormone deficiency in iron-deficient anemic rats. J Nutr 1989;119: 772–778.

40. Gibson RS. Principles of nutritional assessment. New York: Oxford University Press, 1990.

41. Beard J, Tobin B. Feed efficiency and norepinephrine turnover in iron deficiency. Proc Soc Exp Biol Med 1987;184:337–344.

42. Davies JK, Donovan CM, Refino CJ, et al. Distinguishing effects of anemia and muscle iron deficiency on exercise bioenergetics in the rat. Am J Physiol 1984;246: E535–E543.

43. Henderson SA, Dallman PR, Brooks GA. Glucose turnover and oxidation are increased in the iron-deficient anemic rat. Am J Physiol 1986;250:E414–E421.

44. Brooks GA, Henderson SA, Dallman PR. Increased glucose dependence in iron deficient rats. Am J Physiol 1987;250:E414–E421.

45. Perkkio MV, Jansson LT, Brooks GA, et al. Work performance in iron deficiency of increasing severity. J Appl Physiol 1985;58:1477–1480.

46. Farrell PA, Beard JL, Druckenmiller M. Increasing insulin sensitivity in iron-deficient rats. J Nutr 1988;118:1104–1109.

47. Bjorntorp P, Sjostrom L. Carbohydrate storage in man: speculations and some quantitative considerations. Metabolism 1978;27:1853–1865.

48. Curtis-Prior PB, Trethewey J, Stewart GA, et al. The contribution of different organs and tissues of the rat to assimilation of glucose. Diabetologia 1969;5:384–391.

49. James DE, Kraegen EW, Chrisholm DJ. Effects of exercise training on in vivo insulin action in individual tissues of the rat. J Clin Invest 1985;76:657–666.

50. Kraegen EW, James DE, Jenkins AB, et al. Dose response curves for in vivo insulin sensitivity in individual tissues in rats. Am J Physiol 1985;148:E353–E362.

51. Tortora GJ, Grabowski SR. The endocrine system. In: Roesch B, Muskin MRG, Farrell TR, eds. Principles of anatomy and physiology. New York: Harper Collins, 1993.

52. Voorhess ML, Stuart MJ, Stockman JA, et al. Iron deficiency anemia and increased urinary norepinephrine excretion. J Pediatr 1975;86: 542–547.

53. Balaban EP, Cox JV, Snell P, et al. The frequency of anemia and iron deficiency in the runner. Med Sci Sports Exerc 1989;21:643–648.

54. Fogelholm GM, Himber JJ, Alopaeus K, et al. Dietary and biochemical indices of nutritional status in male athletes and controls. J Am Coll Nutr 1992;11: 181–191.

55. Parr RB, Bachman LA, Moss RA. Iron deficiency in female athletes. Phys Sportsmed 1984;12:81–86.

56. Plowman SA, McSwegin PC. The effects of iron supplementation on female cross country runners. J Sports Med 1981;21: 407–416.

57. Schena F, Pattini A, Mantovanelli S. Iron status in athletes involved in endurance and in prevalently anaerobic sports. In: Sports nutrition: minerals and electrolytes. Philadelphia: CRC Press, 1995.

58. Diagnostic and statistical manual of mental disorders. Washington, DC: American Psychiatric Association, 1980.

59. Harris SS. Helping active women avoid anemia. Phys Sportsmed 1995;23:35–46.

60. Rees JM. Minerals. In: Mahan KL, Arlin M, eds. Krause's food, nutrition & diet therapy. 8th ed. Philadelphia: WB Saunders, 1992.

61. Rowland TW, Black SA, Kelleher JF. Iron deficiency in adolescent endurance athletes. J Adolesc Health 1987;8:322–326.

62. Brown RT, McIntosh SM, Seabolt VR, et al. Iron status of adolescent female athletes. J Adolesc Health 1985;6:349–352.

63. Mahlamaki E, Mahlamaki S. Iron deficiency in adolescent female dancers. Br J Sports Med 1988; 22:55–56.

64. Nickerson HJ, Holubets MC, Weiler BR, et al. Causes of iron deficiency in adolescent athletes. J Pediatr 1989;114:657–663.

65. Bank WJ. Myoglobinuria in marathon runners: possible relationship to carbohydrate and lipid metabolism. Annals NY Acad Sci 1977;301:942–950.

66. Ben BT, Motley CP. Myoglobinemia and endurance exercise: a study on 25 participants in a triathlon competition. Am J Sports Med 1984;12:113–118.

67. Miller BJ, Pate RR, Burgess W. Foot impact force and intravascular hemolysis during distance running. Int J Sports Med 1988;9: 56–60.

68. Haymes EM. Nutritional concerns: need for iron. Med Sci Sports Exerc 1987;19:S197–S200.

69. Sherman AR, Kramer B. Iron nutrition and exercise. In: Hickson JE, Wolinsky I, eds. Nutrition in exercise and sport. Boca Raton, FL: CRC Press, 1989.

70. Newhouse IJ, Douglas B, Clement DB, et al. The effects of prelatent/latent iron deficiency on physical work capacity. Med Sci Sports Exerc 1989;21:263–268.

71. Rowland TW, Deisroth MB, Green MG, et al. The effect of iron therapy on the exercise capacity of nonanemic iron deficient adolescent runners. Am J Dis Child 1988;142:165–169.

72. Schoene R, Escourrou P, Robertson H, et al. Iron repletion decreases maximal exercise lactate concentrations in female athletes with minimal iron deficiency anemia. J Lab Clin Med 1983; 102:306–312.

73. Lamanca JJ, Haymes EM. Effects of iron repletion on Vo_2max, endurance, and blood lactate in women. Med Sci Sports Exerc 1993;25:1386–1392.

74. Schwartz SR, Frantz RA, Shoemaker WC. Sequential hemodynamic and oxygen transport responses in hypovolemia, anemia, and hypoxia. AM J Physiol 1981; 241:H863–H871.

75. Nickerson HJ, Tripp AD. Iron deficiency in adolescent cross-country runners. Phys Sportsmed 1983;11:60–66.

76. Zhu YI, Haas JD. Iron depletion without anemia and physical performance in young women. Am J Clin Nutr 1997;66:334–341.

77. Hallberg L, Rossander-Hulten L. Iron requirements in menstruating women. Am J Clin Nutr 1991;54:1047–1058.

78. Tanner JM. Foetus into man. Cambridge, MA: Harvard University Press, 1978.

79. Koziol BJ, Ohira Y, Simpson DR, et al. Biochemical skeletal muscle and hematological profiles of moderate and severely iron deficient and anemic adult rats. J Nutr 1978;108:306–1314.

80. Bothwell TH, Macphail P. Prevention of iron deficiency by food fortification. In: Fomon SJ, Zlotkin S, eds. Nutritional anemias. New York: Raven Press, 1992.

81. Earl R, Woeteki L, eds. Iron deficiency anemia: recommended guidelines for prevention, determination and management among U.S. children and women of childbearing age. Washington, DC: National Academy Press, 1993.

82. Skikne B, Baynes RD. Iron absorption. In: Brock JH, Halliday JW, Pippard MJ, Powell LW, eds. Iron metabolism in health and disease. London: WB Saunders, 1994.

83. Babior BM, Peters WA, Briden PM, et al. Pregnant women's absorption of iron from prenatal supplements. J Repro Med 1985;30:355–357.

84. Raunikar RA, Sabio H. Anemia in the adolescent athlete. Am J Dis Child 1992;146:1201–1205.

85. Solvell L. Oral iron therapy—side effects. In: Hallber L, ed. Iron deficiency: pathogenesis, clinical aspects, therapy. London: Academic Press, 1970.

86. Yoshida T, Udo M, Chida M, et al. Dietary iron supplement during severe physical training in competitive female distance runners. Sports Training, Med, Rehab 1990;1:279–285.

Chapter 58

Physical Activity and Pubertal Development in Girls: Impact of Exercise and Energy Availability on the Reproductive System

Brian E. Miller

Mary Jane De Souza

The normal function of the reproductive system in both animals and humans relies on complex interactions between feedback mechanisms of several endocrine systems. During puberty, exercise training has been implicated as a contributing factor for disturbances in pubertal development, such as the age of menarche. Late menarche, which is common to some elite athletic groups, may not be caused by exercise training itself, but may be related to a deficit in the availability of energy. Unfortunately, research on reproductive function throughout puberty is limited and most work has been cross-sectional or retrospective in design. However, there is an abundance of data available in studies of both animals and women that supports the role of energy availability in modulating reproductive function. However, the precise mechanism(s) responsible for a later menarcheal age in some athletes remains unknown. This chapter, consequently, reviews past (body fat, body weight, exercise stress) and present (energy availability, leptin) concepts and hypotheses that have been postulated as contributory factors in the onset of menarche.

PHYSIOLOGY AND ENDOCRINOLOGY OF REPRODUCTION AND PUBERTY: A BRIEF REVIEW

The Hypothalamic-Pituitary-Ovarian (H-P-O) Axis

The normal function of the hypothalamus, pituitary, and ovary are a prerequisite for the maintenance of normal menstrual function in mature women and also for the initiation of menstruation and other pubertal events in young girls. A normal H-P-O axis is dependent upon a complex system of negative and positive feedback interactions between the hypo-

thalamus, pituitary, and ovary. There are five primary hormones involved in the H-P-O axis. The hypothalamus, which can be viewed as the pacemaker of the system, releases gonadotropin-releasing hormone (GnRH) in pulses that occur at a frequency of one pulse every 60 to 120 minutes. Normal pulsatile release of GnRH is required for normal reproductive function and disturbances such as a shorter or longer pulse frequency result in abnormal release of the pituitary hormones and, subsequently, disturbed ovarian function. In fact, it has been demonstrated, via exogenous administration of GnRH to monkeys, that the pituitary release of luteinizing hormone (LH) and follicle-stimulating hormone (FSH) require a very precise pattern of pulsatile release of GnRH (1).

LH and FSH are also released in a pulsatile manner and stimulate the ovary, resulting in follicular recruitment and development, ovulation, and production of the ovarian steroids (estradiol and progesterone). The ovarian steroids, in turn, are responsible for the initiation and maintenance of secondary sex characteristics, maintenance of bone mineral density, and preparation of the endometrium for implantation of an embryo. If the interactions of the hypothalamus, pituitary, and ovary are disrupted at any level in the feedback loop, disturbances can occur that may lead to menstrual dysfunction and hypoestrogenemia (2,3). It should be noted that the regulation of the H-P-O axis and normal reproductive function is much more complex than discussed here. In addition to GnRH, LH, FSH, estradiol, and progesterone, there are numerous other peptides and neurotransmitters that are also involved in control of the menstrual cycle (e.g., follicular recruitment and ovulation). The function of these peptides and neurotransmitters have been reviewed in detail elsewhere (4,5).

Table 58-1 Summary of Pubertal Events

TERM	TYPE OF EVENT	EVENT MONITORED
Adrenarche	Endocrinologic	Increased adrenal androgens
Pubarche	Physical	Tanner stages of pubic hair
Gonadarche	Endocrinologic	Increased estrogens
Thelarche	Physical	Tanner stages of breast development
Menarche	Physical	First menstruation
Ovulation	Endocrinologic	Mid-cycle LH surge

As stated, the hypothalamus acts as the pacemaker, or the pulse generator, for the H-P-O axis in that it controls the function of the entire reproductive axis. Control of the pulsatile release of GnRH from the GnRH-producing neurons, which are primarily located in the arcuate nucleus of the hypothalamus, is not completely understood. It does appear, however, that GnRH neurons are modulated by other neurons from higher brain centers, which integrate and transmit external and internal information from a variety of sources. Moreover, the autonomic nervous system and hormones from other nonreproductive endocrine glands, such as the adrenal and thyroid glands, can modulate the GnRH-producing neurons.

Prior to the onset of pubertal changes, the hypothalamus is in a relative state of quiescence, with very low levels of GnRH being released. The maturation of the H-P-O axis over several years leads to the development of regular ovulatory cycles (6,7). The initial stages of puberty, however, occur well before the initiation of reproductive function and include events that extend over many years.

Physiology of Puberty

Puberty is a continuous process comprised of a series of endocrine and physical events that occur in a successive and overlapping manner. While adrenarche is the first event signaling the onset of puberty, the establishment of consistent and cyclic ovulatory cycles is the endpoint of puberty (8). Each hormonal event that occurs during the course of the pubertal transition produces a significant but separate transformation in the physical characteristics of the maturing girl. A summary of the physical and endocrinologic events of puberty are provided in Table 58-1.

The hypothalamic-pituitary-ovarian (H-P-O) axis is relatively quiescent from birth to about age 6. Between the ages of 6 and 8, however, there is a gradual increase in the production of the adrenal androgens (androstenedione, dehydroepiandrosterone, and dehydroepiandrosterone-sulfate [DHEA-S]) that continues until age 13 to 15 (6,7). This first event of puberty is adrenarche. Adrenarche results in the first physical sign of the ensuing chain of events leading to puberty, including the development of pubic hair, axillary hair, and sebaceous glands. The second and predominant endocrine event of puberty is the progressive maturation in the functional level of the H-P-O axis that leads, over several years, to the development of gonadarche, thelarche, menarche, and eventually to regular ovulatory cycles.

It is not until the age of 8 to 10 that the CNS begins to mature and the hypothalamic GnRH pulse generator becomes gradually less sensitive to gonadal steroids. Erratic bursts of GnRH release initially occur during sleep. Gradually, over a period of several years, the pulses become more regular at night and over time, extend throughout the day (6,7). This diurnal GnRH activity corresponds to an increase in pituitary gonadotropin reserve and the pulsatile release of LH and FSH, which stimulate the production of estrogens from the ovary (9). In fact, in female monkeys, it has been demonstrated that exogenous administration of GnRH in a pulsatile manner stimulates reproductive hormone release and initiates ovulatory cycles (10). Additionally, in humans with delayed puberty, exogenous administration of GnRH can initiate development of the H-P-O axis (11). This pubertal event, i.e., the production of the ovarian steroids, is gonadarche (6,7).

Also by the age of 8 to 10, the increasingly apparent estrogen levels coincident with gonadarche promote breast development, which is the pubertal event called thelarche. By the age of 12 and 14, the continued increase in ovarian estrogen concentration stimulates the endometrium, producing the first menstruation, called menarche (6). Menarche is a pubertal event that occurs at a time largely determined by genetic factors (12) and modified, to a certain extent, by environmental factors (13,14).

It should be noted that the appearance of menarche does not imply that the reproduction system is functionally mature. Anovulatory cycles, which lack the production of progesterone and an adequate LH surge, are frequent in the years following menarche (15). The hypothalamic GnRH pulse generator is still erratic at times and unless the hypothalamus can maintain consistent pulses every 60 to 120 minutes, oligo-ovulatory or anovulatory cycles predominate (8). Moreover, the positive feedback of estrogens on hypothalamic GnRH and pituitary LH and FSH release requires several years of maturation before this feedback effect is present consistently during each cycle, resulting in regular and ovulatory menstrual cyclicity. When all of these physiologic changes have taken place and the system has stabilized, we can assume that the transition of the reproductive system from childhood to adulthood has been completed. The adult reproductive system, however, is not static; it is a dynamic system that is responsive to a wide array of influential factors, particularly energy intake and energy expenditure.

EFFECTS OF EXERCISE ON PUBERTAL DEVELOPMENT

While several studies have provided evidence that a later age of menarche is associated with intensive exercise training, it is still unclear if other specific events of puberty are affected. A primary issue to be addressed when reviewing the published investigations on this topic is the semantic difference between the expressions "delayed puberty" and "later age of puberty." Studies on exercising adolescents reported a later age for the occurrence of some pubertal events; however, these studies have not been able to clearly establish whether this difference represents a trend towards sports participation by "late" maturing girls, or whether exercise produces a "delay" in the

Table 58-2 Age of Menarche in Different Athletic Populations	
POPULATION	AGE OF MENARCHE (YEARS)
Sedentary controls	12.7
High school athletes	13.1
College athletes	13.0
Olympic athletes	13.7
Ballet dancers	15.4
Athletes trained before menarche	15.0
Athletes trained after menarche	12.6

appearance and progression of pubertal events (14,16,17). In fact, it has been suggested that when referring to exercise training and the onset of puberty, the term "later age of puberty" should be used, since "delayed" can be interpreted as causative, that is, training delays menarche (18).

As previously described, the increase in adrenal androgens is the initial physiologic change associated with puberty. In an attempt to determine if adrenarche is affected by exercise training, investigators compared DHEA-S levels in female gymnasts and age-matched untrained girls and found that the physiologic increase in DHEA-S levels was delayed about 1.5 years in the gymnasts (19). Peltenburg et al (16), however, did not find any difference in DHEA-S levels between female gymnasts and swimmers and concluded that adrenarche occurs at a similar age in these two trained groups. In relation to pubarche, as assessed by the age of appearance and development of pubic hair, researchers found that exercising and nonexercising girls had parallel pubarcheal development (17,20). In contrast, other investigators reported a lower public hair maturation stage in female gymnasts than in swimmers or controls (16). Thus, the onset of adrenarche in athletic girls may occur an average of 1 to 1.5 years later when compared to untrained girls and these effects are independent of the mode of exercise training (16,19). However, it appears that the physical manifestation of adrenal androgen activity, pubarche, is unaltered in exercising girls (17,20).

There is contradictory data regarding the timing of thelarche (breast development) in trained adolescent girls. Some investigators reported less maturity in breast development of female gymnasts and ballet dancers compared to swimmers and controls (16,17). In contrast, other authors have found either no delay in breast development (20) or a stimulatory effect of exercise training on breast development (21).

Menarche, considered the culmination of events during the pubertal process and indicative of the advanced maturational state of the reproductive system, is the pubertal event most extensively studied in trained adolescents. Data does indicate that menarche occurs at a later age in exercising girls (14,22,23). A later age of menarche has also been reported in exercising girls of several different national origins participating in various sport activities (14,24,25). Table 58-2 describes the age of menarche in adolescent girls from different exercising populations. Thus it appears that exercise training results in a later age of menarche in adolescents. It is interesting to note that the age of menarche seems to be directly related to

the competitive level and years of intensive training prior to menarche (25,26).

Animal data has provided stronger evidence in support of an exercise-related alteration in pubertal development (27). Studies in rats have demonstrated that prolonged exercise delays growth and normal development of the reproductive axis (28,29). Bronson et al (30) have shown that prolonged exercise in rats almost entirely blocked the pulsatile release of LH (2 pulses/24 hr in the exercise rats versus 1 pulse/hr in the ad lib feed rats). Caution must be taken when interpreting these results (28,29), since the rats were given food rewards in order to prompt exercise activity, which may confound the independent effects of exercise and diet (27). In fact, Bronson et al explain that the rats in their experiment run in a cage system that forces the animal to perform bouts of exercise on a running wheel in order to trigger a food dispenser, and that the rats only receive an amount of food that a young animal would require under ad lib conditions, but not working conditions. Thus an increased energy expenditure occurs without commensurate compensation of energy intake to meet the metabolic demands of the prolonged exercise.

The pubertal growth spurt may also be compromised in female athletes. Theintz et al (31) demonstrated that young gymnasts advanced through puberty without a normal growth spurt. This pubertal growth spurt is dependent upon normal circulating levels of growth hormone (GH), insulin-like growth factor I (IGF-I), thyroid hormones, ovarian steroids, the ability of the bones to respond to the hormones involved with longitudinal growth, and an adequate supply of energy in the form of oxidizable fuels (32–35). As we will see in a later section, nutrition and energy availability may not only be involved in normal growth and skeletal development, but may also play a critical role in the initiation of puberty and the maintenance of the H-P-O axis. More detailed reviews are available on the physiology of growth and development and the influence of exercise training (36,37).

Proposed Models for Later Age of Menarche in Athletes

Two models have been proposed to explain the later age of menarche in athletes. The first model is the theory proposed by Frisch et al, who attempted to identify a minimal weight and body fat as critical requirements for the onset of menstruation (38–42). Applying this theoretical model to exercising adolescents, Frisch (38) suggested that intense exercise training delays menarche by decreasing body fat and the fat/lean ratio. While it is clear that exercise training during adolescence results in changes in body composition and, most likely, in a later age of menarche, these two factors may be independent and unrelated. Therefore, the appearance of menarche associated with a specific or minimal percentage of body fat in these trained girls may be purely coincidental. Additionally, Frisch's theories and conclusions have been challenged since the equations used to develop the theories have statistical errors associated with them (43,44). Moreover, Frisch et al did not perform direct measurements of body fat, but instead made indirect assessments using height and weight equations that were used to predict total body water (45). The regression equation used by Mellits et al has also been shown to overestimate body fatness in lean female athletes (46).

The second model is the two-part hypothesis proposed by Malina (14) that excludes physical activity as a delaying factor for menarche. Malina proposed inherited "physique" as the first factor explaining the later age of menarche in exercise trained girls. In other words, athletes are already genetically predisposed to be late maturers, which is a physical advantage for success in sport and athletic competition. The second factor is called the "socialization process," in which late maturers tend to be socially involved in sports because of their "biologic lateness." More recently, Malina et al (47) has suggested, based on retrospective analysis of age of menarche in athletes and their mothers and sisters, that the later age of menarche in athletes is largely determined by a familial factor. Also in support of Malina's original hypothesis, Baxter-Jones et al (18) found a significant correlation between menarcheal age of mothers and their athletic daughters. In addition, the authors found that the maternal menarcheal age and the type of sport (gymnastics, tennis, and swimming) were the best predictors of the athlete's menarcheal age. Since the gymnasts had the latest age of menarche and the amount of training did not appear to have any effect on menarcheal age in the other athletes studied, it was concluded that late maturation in girls may contribute to a young girl's decision to continue participation in gymnastics. That is, predisposition to a somatotype or physique appropriate for sports performance and a slower maturation process will direct these girls towards sports involvement. These two theories were helpful as they identified physiologic and psychosocial data associated with the later age of menarche in athletes; however, both models appear incomplete in their approach to this issue. It should also be noted that these studies relied on retrospective recall data by the athletes, their mothers, and their sisters.

There is limited data on the occurrence of menstrual irregularities in adolescents during the immediate years following menarche. Marker (23) studied the immediate postmenarcheal years in exercising adolescents and did not observe a menstrual dysfunction attributable to intensive prepubescent exercise training. Bonen et al (48), however, did find a higher incidence of anovulatory menstrual cycles in trained girls associated with a hormone profile that differed significantly from controls. The trained adolescents had lower FSH concentrations and lower FSH/LH ratios during the follicular phase than nonexercising adolescents, changes which result in inadequate follicular maturation and anovulatory cycles (48). It is unknown whether or not these altered hormonal profiles and menstrual cycle characteristics of exercising adolescents early in the postmenarcheal years are related to a higher prevalence of shortened luteal phase lengths, anovulatory cycles, oligomenorrhea, exercise-related amenorrhea, and infertility later in life.

Current Hypotheses: the Stress of Exercise or the Availability of Energy?

Recently, there have been reports in sedentary and exercising women that indicate energy availability, and not the stress of exercise, may be responsible for the variety of menstrual disturbances observed in exercising postmenarcheal women (49,50). Although prospective data in chronically exercising women is lacking, Loucks et al have shown that sedentary women placed in a state of low energy availability for 4 days have low-triiodothyronine syndrome (51) and altered LH

pulsatility (49). Moreover, it has been suggested that the low energy availability and not the stress of exercise is responsible for the observed changes in thyroid status and disrupted LH pulsatility. Data from our own lab also suggests that energy availability may be involved in the development of anovulatory cycles in recreational women runners. Perhaps the so-called "exercise-related" changes in pubertal development are not related to exercise itself, but rather to the energy status of the exercising individual. As discussed in the next section, nutrition and energy intake have profound effects on the reproductive system and pubertal events.

NUTRITION AND PUBERTAL DEVELOPMENT

There is an abundance of data that has targeted nutrition, and more specifically the availability of oxidizable metabolic fuels, in the regulation and function of the H-P-O axis. Although epidemiologic evidence has shown that the timing of puberty is earlier in nourished girls and later in malnourished girls (52–54), stronger evidence for the role of nutrition in pubertal development has come from studies in animals. In animals that are undernourished, pubertal events and the maturation of the reproductive axis are delayed and remain delayed for the duration of the malnourished state (55,56). As we will see in the next section, only when energy intake is increased will puberty progress and the H-P-O axis mature. Similarly, in humans, there is strong evidence to support the animal literature. In both men and women who are undernourished, there are decreases in pituitary gonadotropin secretion as well as suppressed ovarian and gonadal function (57,58). These observed disturbances are not the result of a failure at the level of the pituitary or gonads, but rather a result of a suppressed drive from the GnRH pulse generator (59).

As stated previously, energy availability appears to play a critical role in normal reproductive function. The question, therefore, is "Does energy availability or the stress of exercise modulate pubertal development?"

Low Energy Availability

Operationally, energy availability can be defined as dietary energy intake minus energy expenditure due to exercise (49), whereas, energy balance is defined as dietary energy intake minus 24-hour total energy expenditure (i.e., basal metabolic rate, thermogenic effect of a meal, and physical activity). For our purposes, we will utilize the term energy availability. Detailed reviews are available that provide evidence that reproductive function in mammals is dependent upon energy availability (60,61). In rats that have had puberty delayed by chronic malnutrition, an increase in food intake is rapidly followed by an increase in LH pulsatility (56). Cameron et al (62) provided strong support for the energy availability hypothesis when the authors found that exercised-related amenorrhea in monkeys could be reversed following an increase in food intake. Most important, the reversal of amenorrhea resulted even when the exercise regimen was maintained.

Although there are no prospective data available that specifically examine the role of exercise stress, dietary energy intake, and energy availability, short-term experiments have been completed. In a series of experiments in habitually sedentary women in which subjects were placed into groups of varying energy availability (accomplished via manipulation of increased exercise expenditure and controlled dietary energy intake), the women in a state of low energy availability (i.e., <25 kcal per kg lean body mass (LBM) per day) had suppressed LH pulsatility (49). This effect was independent of exercise training, but dependent upon reduced dietary energy intake and low energy availability (50). It has been suggested that any external perturbation that decreases circulating energy has the potential to dampen the central drive to the H-P-O axis (63).

Unfortunately, there are no similar studies in children with delayed puberty or a later age of menarche, although Lindholm et al (64) found that juvenile elite gymnasts had a lower mean daily energy intake and expended more calories than a reference group of healthy girls of comparable age. The authors speculate that the later age of menarche in the gymnasts may be explained, in part, by their increased expenditure and lower energy intake. It has also been shown that the incidence of onset of menarche increased in dancers with delayed puberty following an injury that prevented training (17). Based on the energy availability data discussed thus far, it appears that the observed increase in the incidence of menarche associated with a decrease in training may have been due to an increase in energy availability and not to the decrease in exercise training itself. Clearly, there is much more prospective research needed to clarify the relative role of exercise expenditure and dietary energy intake in modulating pubertal development.

Body Fat Revisited: the Role of Leptin

Previously, we have discussed the critical weight hypothesis and the proposal of a critical amount of body fat necessary for the onset of menarche. Although these theories have been criticized extensively, it appears that body fat may indeed be somewhat involved in the initiation of puberty. Recently, leptin, a hormonal product of adipocytes, has received much attention in the literature with respect to reproductive function in both animals and humans. Data has supported a role for leptin in a complex feedback system between adipocytes and the hypothalamus, specifically, reproductive function (65–67), appetite control, and energy balance (68–70). The precise mechanism through which leptin mediates its action remains unknown, although leptin receptors have been isolated in the human hypothalamus and ovary (71–72).

The initial interest for leptin's role in reproductive function has come from studies in mice with a mutation in the *ob* gene, which is responsible for leptin production. In these *ob/ob* mice that lack leptin production from adipocytes, there is a decreased energy expenditure, an increase in food intake, obesity, and also infertility (68–70). Interestingly, exogenous administration of leptin reverses these aforementioned atypical changes (65,67). In humans, a potential role for leptin in modulating the reproductive axis in exercising women has also been demonstrated. Laughlin et al (73) concluded that in their group of exercising women, leptin levels were significantly reduced regardless of menstrual status, but in amenorrheic athletes, a diurnal rhythm was absent when compared to cyclic athletes. In addition, the lower leptin levels were associated with metabolic changes in response to chronic energy deficits, such as hypoinsulinemia and hypercortisolemia.

Animal data has indicated that leptin may be involved in the initiation of puberty. Normal prepubertal mice receiving exogenous leptin can have puberty advanced by several days (74). Additional data in mice suggest that although leptin is associated with an earlier puberty, leptin may not be the primary signal, but rather act in a permissive fashion to allow pubertal maturation to progress (75). Cheung et al (75) have speculated that circulating levels of leptin rise over the course of development and permit the reproductive system to become active at a given level of circulating leptin. Since it appears that leptin acts as a potential link between metabolic status and reproductive function in mature animals (65), it is not surprising that leptin may also be involved in the initiation of puberty.

Human data have also been consistent with the animal findings, in that there appears to be a link between circulating leptin levels and pubertal development. Prospective data in boys demonstrated that leptin levels are low during prepuberty, increase during the initiation of puberty, and gradually decline until postpuberty (76). Similarly, prospective data in girls showed that serum leptin levels were related to menarcheal age (77). How exercise, energy availability, and leptin interact during puberty remains to seen.

Collectively, these data would logically support a complex interaction among exercise, energy availability, low body fat, and leptin. We can speculate that strenuous exercise, not compensated by increased dietary energy intake, would result in a state of low energy availability, lower body fat, and thus lower leptin levels, which may adversely affect the H-P-O axis. The originally proposed hypothesis (38) that a critical body weight or body fat percentage is a prerequisite for menarche lacked a mechanism linking body fat and reproductive function. Although leptin now appears to be an attractive mechanism, Rogol (78) states that the role of body fat and weight is not as simple as Frisch's original proposal. Additionally, Rogol (78) brings attention to the fact that the longitudinal assessment of body composition during pubertal development is difficult, since puberty is a time of rapid changes in body composition. Indirect measurements of body composition need to account for the changing chemical composition of the compartments and equations need to account for the degree of physical maturity (79). Clearly, this is an exciting area that requires much more well-controlled, prospective research.

INFLUENCE OF DELAYED/LATER AGE OF MENARCHE ON BONE DENSITY AND BREAST CANCER RISK

Bone Mineral Density

Physical activity has been advocated to contribute to the prevention of osteoporosis and fractures. Bone may be the most responsive to the osteogenic stimulus of exercise during periods of growth (80–83). More important, the largest gains in bone mineral density (BMD) may occur during the year prior to menarche and during the first few years following menarche (84–86). In fact, increases in BMD during perimenarcheal years are highly dependent upon sex hormones (87). Although data are limited with respect to the long-term consequences of vigorous training during puberty, Warren et al

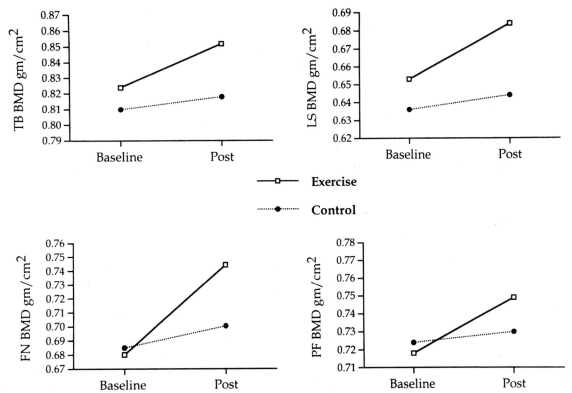

Figure 58-1 Absolute change in BMD at various sites across 10 months (mean ± SD). (Reproduced by permission from Morris FI, Naughton GA, Gibbs JL, et al. Prospective ten-month exercise intervention in premenarcheal girls: positive effects on bone and lean mass. J Bone Miner Res 1997;12:1453–1462.)

(88) did report the occurrence of stress fractures in young ballet dancers. Recent data, however, suggests that weight-bearing exercise during the pubertal years results in a significant increase in BMD when compared to controls (89,90). In young girls (age 9.5 ± 0.9), 10 months of a controlled, weight-bearing exercise regimen resulted in significant increases in BMD (Fig. 58-1) when compared to a control group (89). Similarly, active prepubertal gymnasts also had higher BMDs than controls at all sites except the skull (90). In fact, even the BMD of former gymnasts is similar to (91) or greater than (Fig. 58-2) normal controls (90). Collectively these data support the notion that exercise during this critical time of development is a potent stimulus for the accretion of bone mass.

It is not clear at this time whether a later age of menarche in athletes is detrimental to the attainment of bone mass and a resultant increase in fracture risk later in life. It has been reported that age of menarche is negatively correlated with total body, femoral neck, and lumbar spine BMD in gymnasts (92). In contrast, a positive correlation was seen in the running and control groups (92). In that investigation, the age of menarche for the gymnasts was 16.2 years, the runners 14.4 years, and the controls 13.0 years. The menarcheal age of the gymnasts in the aforementioned studies (90,91) was also significantly later (≈14.6 years) than the control groups (≈12.7 years). In both studies, however, the group of former gymnasts exhibited a similar or greater BMD than the controls. Perhaps the negative correlation seen in the Robinson et al (92) data set was attributed to a much later menarcheal age

(16.2 years) of their gymnasts, compared to the gymnasts in the Lindholm et al (91) and Bass et al (90) studies. Thus, the much later age of menarche and the subsequent hypoestrogenemic environment for a longer period of time during this critical time of bone mineral accrual may be detrimental to the achievement of peak bone mass. Caution must be taken when interpreting some of these data, since many of the former gymnasts in one study (91) began using oral contraceptives between 2 to 4 years prior to their BMD assessment at the age of ≈21 years. The effect of the oral contraceptive use following participation in gymnastics and prior to their BMD assessment may confound the influence of the later menarcheal age. In contrast, Bass et al (90) stated that exposure to oral contraceptives was an exclusionary factor in their group of women. Since BMD of the retired gymnasts was significantly higher than the controls, it appears that the later age of menarche had little influence on BMD at the age of assessment (≈25.0 years) in that study.

Although it appears that vigorous physical activity during the years preceding menarche is a potent stimulus for bone accretion, the impact of later menarcheal age is still unclear. Prospective studies are needed that assess BMD, in conjunction with sex steroids, in various athletic populations across the pubertal years, with specific attention to age of menarche. Although gymnastics may represent an extreme in exercise training that will not apply to most youth, other data do support a role of moderate physical activity in promoting bone density (81,82,93,94). It is clear, though, that weight-bearing physical activity is the appropriate osteogenic stimulus

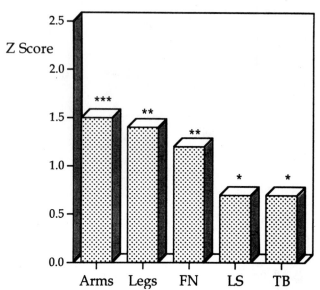

Figure 58-2 Cross-sectional data showing regional areal bone density expressed as *z* scores in retired gymnasts. The *z* scores are higher than the predicted mean value in controls (represented by zero) at each site (except skull). *$P < 0.05$, **$P < 0.01$, ***$P < 0.001$ compared with zero. (Reproduced by permission from Bass S, Pearce G, Bradney M, et al. Exercise before puberty may confer residual benefits in bone density in adulthood: studies in active prepubertal and retired gymnasts. J Bone Miner Res 1998;13:500–507.)

since it has been shown that nonweight-bearing exercise, such as swimming, does not have the same beneficial effect on bone mass gain (95–97).

Breast Cancer Risk

Up to this point, the discussion on exercise, nutrition, and a later age of menarche in athletes has focused on the adverse alteration in the H-P-O axis and the potential for a hypoestrogenemic environment that affects bone accretion during critical periods of skeletal maturation. A later menarcheal age, however, may be a favorable event in reducing the risk of

breast cancer development later in life. Apter (98) has stated that an earlier age of menarche that is associated with increased ovarian steroid production may induce a higher degree of breast epithelial proliferation. Epidemiologic evidence does suggest that the total number of ovulatory cycles and the cumulative exposure to ovarian steroids may be determinants of breast cancer risk (99,100). Other evidence has also shown that the younger a women's age at menarche, the higher the risk of breast cancer (101–105). Exercise throughout life, however, appears to be associated with a decreased risk of breast cancer (106). Clearly, although a causative relationship cannot be discerned from these epidemiologic data, exercise throughout a women's life does appear to reduce her risk of breast cancer development. More detailed reviews are available that focus on breast cancer and reproductive factors (107) and endogenous steroids (108).

SUMMARY

Exercise is an important part of a healthy lifestyle and undoubtedly contributes to improved health throughout life. The effect of physical activity during puberty, however, remains to be an area that requires additional research. Most studies have focused on the age of menarche, while few have examined other pubertal events, such as adrenarche, thelarche, and pubarche. There is also limited data available that focuses on the endocrine response of the H-P-O axis to exercise training and energy availability during pubertal development. Until these topics are investigated in greater detail with well-controlled, prospective studies, our understanding of the relationship between exercise and pubertal development will remain speculative at best.

Epidemiologic evidence is suggestive of a reduction in breast cancer risk in women that had a later or delayed menarcheal age. In contrast, we might expect a negative association between menarcheal age and BMD because of the potential failure to attain peak bone mass. Results from studies in young athletes suggests that weight-bearing exercise is a potent stimulus for skeletal development during this critical time of bone deposition. Moreover, prepubertal and retired gymnasts have higher BMD than their sedentary or normally active counterparts. It is still very unclear, however, how the longer hypoestrogenemic environment associated with a later age of menarche affects bone accretion and the risk of low bone mass and osteoporosis later in life.

REFERENCES

1. Wildt L, Hausler A, Marshall G, et al. Frequency and amplitude of gonadotropin-releasing hormone stimulation and gonadotropin secretion in the Rhesus monkey. Endocrinology 1981;109:376.

2. Yen SSC. Chronic anovulation due to CNS-hypothalamic-pituitary dysfunction. In: Yen SSC, Jaffe RB, eds. Reproductive endocrinology. 2nd ed. Philadel-phia: WB Saunders, 1986:500–545.

3. Yen SSC. The human menstrual cycle: neuroendocrine regulation. In: Yen SSC, Jaffe RB, eds. Reproductive endocrinology. 3rd ed. Philadelphia: WB Saunders, 1991:273–308.

4. Kalra SP. Modulatory neuropeptide-steroid signaling for the preovulatory luteinizing hormone-releasing hormone discharge. Endocr Rev 1993;14:507–538.

5. Gougen A. Regulation of ovarian follicular development in primates: facts and hypotheses. Endocr Rev 1996;17:121–155.

6. Apter D. Serum steroids and pituitary hormones in female

puberty: a partly longitudinal study. Clin Endocrinol 1980;12: 107–120.

7. Ducharme JR, Forest M, De Peretti E, et al. Plasma adrenal and gonadal sex steroids in human pubertal development. J Clin Endocrinol Metab 1976;42: 468–476.

8. Styne DM, Grumbach MM. Puberty in the male and female: its physiology and disorders. In Yen SSC, Jaffe RB, eds. Reproductive endocrinology. Philadelphia: WB Saunders, 1986:313–384.

9. Apter D, Butzow TL, Laughlin GA, et al. Gonadotropin-releasing hormone pulse generator activity during pubertal transition in girls: pulsatile and diurnal patterns of circulating gonadotropins. J Clin Endocrinol Metab 1993;76:940–949.

10. Wildt L, Marshall G, Knobil E. Experimental induction of puberty in the female Rhesus monkey. Science 1980;207: 1373–1375.

11. Crowley WF, McArthur JW. Simulation of the normal menstrual cycle in Kallman's syndrome by pulsatile administration of luteinizing hormone-releasing hormone (LHRH). J Clin Endocrinol Metab 1980;51:173–175.

12. Treolar SA, Martin NG. Age at menarche as a fitness trait: non-additive genetic variance detected in a large twin sample. Am J Human Gene 1990;47: 137–148.

13. Brooks-Gunn J, Warren MP. Mother-daughter differences in menarcheal age in adolescent girls attending national dance company schools and non-dancers. Ann Hum Biol 1988;15: 35–44.

14. Malina PM. Menarche in athletes: a synthesis and hypothesis. Ann Hum Biol 1983;10:1–24.

15. Borsos A, Lampe LG, Balogh A, et al. Ovarian function immediately after the menarche. Int J Gynaecol Obstet 1986;24:239–242.

16. Peltenburg AL, Erich WBM, Bernink MJE, et al. Biological maturation, body composition, and growth of female gymnasts and control group of school girls and girls swimmers, aged 8 to 14 years: a cross-sectional survey of 1064 girls. Int J Sports Med 1984;5:36–42.

17. Warren MP. The effects of exercise on pubertal progression and reproductive function in girls. J Clin Endocrinol Metab 1980;5: 1150–1157.

18. Baxter-Jones A, Helms P, Preece M. Age at menarche. Lancet 1984;343:423–424.

19. Brisson GR, Ledoux M, Dulac S, et al. Dysadrenarche as a possible explanation for delayed onset of menarche in gymnasts. In: Knuttgen HG, et al, eds. Biochemistry of exercise. Champaign, IL: Human Kinetics, 1983:631–636.

20. Plowman SA, Liu NY, Wells CL. Body composition and sexual maturation in premenarcheal athletes and nonathletes. Med Sci Sports Exerc 1991;23:23–29.

21. Bar-Or O. Predicting athletic performance. Phys Sportsmed 1975; 3:80–85.

22. Lindholm C, Hagenfeldt K, Ringertz B-M. Pubertal development in elite juvenile gymnasts: effects of physical training. Acta Obstet Gynecol Scand 1994;73:269–273.

23. Marker K. Influence of athletic training on the maturity process of girls. Med Sport 1981;15: 117–126.

24. Malina RM, Bouchard C, Shoup RF, et al. Age at menarche, family size, and birth order in athletes at the Montreal Olympic Games, 1976. Med Sci Sports Exerc 1979;11:354–358.

25. Mokha R, Sidhu LS. Age of menarche in Indian female basketball and volleyball players at different competitive levels. Br J Sports Med 1989;23:237–238.

26. Malina RM, Spirduso WW, Tate C, et al. Age at menarche and selected menstrual characteristics in athletes at different competitive levels and in different sports. Med Sci Sports Exerc 1978;10:218–222.

27. Loucks AB. The reproductive system and physical activity in adolescents. In: Blimkie CJR, Bar-Or O, eds. New horizons in pediatric exercise science. Champaign, IL: Human Kinetics, 1991:27–37.

28. Manning JM, Bronson FH. Effects of prolonged exercise on puberty and luteinizing hormone secretion in female rats. Am J Physiol 1989;257:R1359–1364.

29. Manning JM, Bronson FH. Suppression of puberty in rats by exercise: effects on hormone levels and reversal with GnRH infusion. Am J Physiol 1991; 260:R717–723.

30. Bronson FH, Manning JM. Food consumption, prolonged exercise, and LH secretion in the peripubertal female rat. In: Pirke KM, Wuttke W, Schweiger U, eds. The menstrual cycle and its disorders. Berlin: Springer-Verlag, 1989: 42–49.

31. Theintz GE, Howald H, Weiss U, et al. Evidence for a reduction of growth potential in adolescent female gymnasts. J Pediatr 1993;122:306–313.

32. Mansfield MJ, Emans SJ. Growth in female gymnasts: should training decrease during puberty? J Pediatr 1993;122:237–240.

33. Lifshitz F. Nutritional dwarfing in adolescents. Growth Genet Horm 1987;3:1–5.

34. Theintz GE. Endocrine adaptation to intensive physical training during growth. Clin Endocrinol 1994;41:267–272.

35. Jahreis G. Influence of intensive exercise on insulin-like growth factor I, thyroid and steroid hormones in female gymnasts. Growth Regul 1991;1:95–99.

36. Borer KT. The effects of exercise on growth. Sports Med 1995;20: 375–397.

37. Roemmich JM, Rogol AD. Physiology of growth and development:

its relationship to performance in the young athlete. Clin Sports Med 1995;14:483–502.

38. Frisch RE, McArthur JW. Menstrual cycles: fatness as a determinant of minimum weight for height necessary for their maintenance or onset. Science 1974; 185:S949–951.

39. Frisch RE, Revelle R. Height and weight at menarche and a hypothesis of critical body weights and adolescent events. Science 1970;169:397–399.

40. Frisch RE, Revelle R. The height and weight of girls and boys at the time of initiation of the adolescent growth spurt in height and weight and the relationship to menarche. Hum Biol 1971a; 43:140–159.

41. Frisch RE, Revelle R. Height and weight at menarche and a hypothesis of menarche. Arch Disease Child 1971b;46:695–701.

42. Frisch RE. The right weight: body fat, menarche, and fertility. Proc Nutr Soc 1994;53:113–129.

43. Reeves J. Estimating fatness. Science 1979;204:881.

44. Trussell J. Statistical flaws in evidence for the Frisch hypothesis that fatness triggers menarche. Hum Biol 1980;52:711–720.

45. Mellits ED, Cheek DB. The assessment of body water and fatness from infancy to adulthood. Monogr Soc Res Child Dev 1970;35:12–26.

46. Loucks AB, Horvath SM, Freedson PS. Menstrual status and validation of body fat prediction in athletes. Hum Biol 1984; 56:383–392.

47. Malina RM, Ryan RC, Bonci CM. Age at menarche in athletes and their mothers and sisters. Ann Hum Biol 1994;21:417–422.

48. Bonen A, Belcastro AN, Ling W, et al. Profiles of selected hormones during menstrual cycles of teenage athletes. J Appl Physiol 1981;50:545–548.

49. Loucks AB, Heath EM. Dietary restriction reduces luteinizing hormone (LH) pulse frequency during waking hours and increases LH pulse amplitude during sleep in young menstruating women. J Clin Endocrinol Metab 1994;78:910–915.

50. Loucks AB, Verdun M, Heath EM. Low energy availability, not stress of exercise, alters LH pulsatility in exercising women. J Appl Physiol 1998;84:37–46.

51. Loucks AB, Callister R. Induction and prevention of low-T3 syndrome in exercising women. Am J Physiol 1993;264:R924–930.

52. Frisch RE. Weight at menarche: similarity for well-nourished and under-nourished girls at differing ages, and evidence for historical constancy. Pediatrics 1972;50:445–450.

53. Bhalla M, Shrivastava JR. A prospective study of the age of menarche in Kanpur girls. Indian Pediatr 1976;11:486–493.

54. Meyer F, Moisan J, Marcoux D, Bouchard C. Dietary and physical determinants of menarche. Epidemiology 1990;1:377–381.

55. Foster DL, Olster DH. Effect of restricted nutrition on puberty in the lamb: patterns of tonic luteinizing hormone (LH) secretion and competency of the LH surge system. Endocrinology 1985;116:375–381.

56. Bronson FH. Food-restricted, prepubertal, female rats: rapid recovery of luteinizing hormone pulsing with excess food, and full recovery of pubertal development with gonadotropin-releasing hormone. Endocrinology 1986; 118:2483–2487.

57. Warren MP, Van de Wiele RL. Clinical and metabolic features of anorexia nervosa. Am J Obstet Gynecol 1973;117:435–449.

58. Smith SR, Chetri MK, Johanson AJ, et al. The pituitary-gonadal axis in men with protein-calorie malnutrition. J Clin Endocrinol Metab 1975;41:60–69.

59. Marshall JC, Kelch RP. Low dose pulsatile gonadotropin-releasing hormone in anorexia nervosa. J Clin Endocrinol Metab 1979;49: 712–718.

60. Bronson FH. Seasonal regulation of reproduction in mammals. In: Knobil E, Neil J, eds. The physiology of reproduction. Vol. 2. New York: Raven Press, 1988: 1831–1871.

61. Wade GN, Schneider JE. Metabolic fuels and reproduction in female mammals. Neurosci Biobehav Rev 1992;16:235–272.

62. Cameron JL, Nosbisch C, Helmreich DL, et al. Reversal of exercise-induced amenorrhea in female Cynomolgus monkeys (Macaca fascicularis) by increased food intake. Seventy-Second Annual Meeting of The Endocrine Society, 1990. Abstract 1042.

63. Cameron JL. Nutritional determinants of puberty. Nutr Rev 1996; 54:S17–S22.

64. Lindholm C, Hagenfeldt K, Hagman U. A nutrition study in juvenile elite gymnasts. Acta Paediatr 1995;84:273–277.

65. Baresh IA, Cheung CC, Weigle DS, et al. Leptin is a metabolic signal to the reproductive system. Endocrinology 1996;137:3144–3147.

66. Ahima RS, Prabakaran D, Mantzoros C, et al. Role of leptin in the neuroendocrine response to fasting. Nature 1996;382: 250–252.

67. Chehab FF, Lim ME, Lu R. Correction of the sterility defect in homozygous female mice by treatment with recombinant leptin. Nature Genetics 1996;12: 318–320.

68. Pelleymounter M, Cullen M, Baker M, et al. Effects of the obese gene product on body weight regulation in ob/ob mice. Science 1995;268:540–543.

69. Halaas J, Gajiwala K, Maffei M, et al. Weight reducing effects of the plasma protein encoded by the obese gene. Science 1995; 269:543–546.

70. Weigle D, Bukowski T, Foster D, et al. Recombinant ob protein

reduces feeding and body weight in the *ob/ob* mouse. J Clin Invest 1995;96:2065–2070.

71. Considine RV, Considine EL, Williams CJ, et al. The hypothalamic leptin receptor in humans: identification of incidental sequence polymorphisms and absence of the *db/db* mouse and *fa/fa* rat mutations. Diabetes 1996;19:922–994.

72. Cioffi J, Shafer A, Zupanic T, et al. Novel B219/OB receptor isoforms: possible role of leptin in hematopoieses and reproduction. Nature Med 1996;2:585–588.

73. Laughlin GA, Yen SSC. Hypoleptinemia in women athletes: absence of a diurnal rhythm with amenorrhea. J Clin Endocrinol Metab 1997;82:318–321.

74. Ahima RS, Dushay, J, Flier SAN, et al. Leptin accelerates the onset of puberty in normal female mice. J Clin Invest 1997; 99:391–395.

75. Cheung CC, Thornton JE, Kuijper JL, et al. Leptin is a metabolic gate for the onset of puberty in the female rat. Endocrinology 1997;138:855–858.

76. Mantzoros CS, Flier JS, Rogol AD. A longitudinal assessment of hormonal and physical alteration during normal puberty in boys: V: rising leptin levels may signal the onset of puberty. J Clin Endocrinol Metab 1997;82: 1066–1070.

77. Matkovic V, Ilich JZ, Skugor M, et al. Leptin is inversely related to age at menarche in human females. J Clin Endocrinol Metab 1997;82:3239–3245.

78. Rogol AD. Leptin and puberty. J Clin Endocrinol Metab 1998;83: 1089–1090. Editorial.

79. Roemmich JN, Clark PA, Weltman A, et al. Alterations in growth and body composition during puberty: I: comparing multi-compartment body composition. J Appl Physiol 1997;83: 927–935.

80. Haapasalo H, Kannus P, Sievanen H, et al. Long-term unilateral loading and bone mineral density and content in female squash players. Calcif Tissue Int 1994; 54:249–255.

81. Welten DC, Kemper HCG, Post GB, et al. Weight-bearing activity during youth is a more important factor for peak bone mass than calcium intake. J Bone Miner Res 1994;9:1089–1096.

82. Slemenda CW, Reister TK, Hui SL, et al. Influences of skeletal mineralization in children and adolescents: evidence for varying effects of sexual maturation and physical activity. J Pediatr 1994; 125:201–207.

83. Kannus P, Haapasalo H, Sankelo M, et al. Effect of starting age of physical activity on bone mass in the dominant arm of tennis and squash players. Ann Intern Med 1995;123:27–31.

84. Gunnes M. Bone mineral density in the cortical and trabecular distal forearm in healthy children and adolescents. Acta Paediatr 1994;83:463–467.

85. Kroger H, Kotaniemi A, Kroger L, et al. Development of bone mass and bone density of the spine and femoral neck—a prospective study of 65 children and adolescents. Bone Miner 1993;23: 171–182.

86. Bonjour J-P, Theintz G, Buchs B, et al. Critical years and stages of puberty for spinal and femoral bone mass accumulation during adolescence. J Clin Endocrinol Metab 1991;73:555–563.

87. Theintz G, Buchs B, Rizzoli D, et al. Longitudinal monitoring of bone mass accumulation in healthy adolescents: evidence for a marked reduction after 16 years of age at the levels of lumbar spine and femoral neck in female subjects. J Clin Endocrinol Metab 1992;75:1060–1065.

88. Warren MP, Brooks-Gunn J, Hamilton LH, et al. Scoliosis and fractures in young ballet dancers: relation to delayed menarche and secondary amenorrhea. N Engl J Med 1986;314:1348–1353.

89. Morris FI, Naughton GA, Gibbs JL, et al. Prospective ten-month exercise intervention in premenarcheal girls: positive effects on bone and lean mass. J Bone Miner Res 1997;12:1453–1462.

90. Bass S, Pearce G, Bradney M, et al. Exercise before puberty may confer residual benefits in bone density in adulthood: studies in active prepubertal and retired gymnasts. J Bone Miner Res 1998;13:500–507.

91. Lindholm C, Hagenfeldt K, Ringertz H. Bone mineral content of young female former gymnasts. Acta Paediatr 1995;84:1109–1112.

92. Robinson TL, Snow-Harter C, Taaffe DR, et al. Gymnasts exhibit higher bone mass than runners despite similar prevalence of amenorrhea and oligomenorrhea. J Bone Miner Res 1995;10:2635.

93. Gunnes M, Lehman EH. Physical activity and dietary constituents as predictors of forearm cortical and trabecular bone gain in healthy children and adolescents: a prospective study. Acta Paediatr 1996;85:19–25.

94. Cooper C, Cawley M, Bhalla A, et al. Childhood growth, physical activity, and peak bone mass in women. J Bone Miner Res 1995; 10:940–947.

95. Taaffe DR, Snow-Harter C, Connolly DA, et al. Differential effects of swimming versus weight-bearing activity on bone mineral status of eumenorrhiec athletes. J Bone Miner Res 1995;10:586–593.

96. Cassell C, Benedict M, Specker B. Bone mineral density in elite 7- to 9-yr-old female gymnasts and swimmers. Med Sci Sports Exerc 1996;28:1243–1246.

97. Crimston SK, Willows ND, Hanley DA. Mechanical loading regime and its relationship to bone mineral density in children. Med Sci Sports Exerc 1993;25:1203–1210.

98. Apter D. Hormonal events during female puberty in relation to breast cancer risk. Eur J Cancer Prev 1996;5:476–482.

99. Henderson BE, Ross RK, Judd HL, et al. Do regular ovulatory cycles increase breast cancer risk? Cancer 1985;56:1206–1208.

100. Henderson BE, Ross RK, Bernstein L. Estrogens as a cause of human cancer: the Richard and Hinda Rosenthal Foundation Award Lecture. Cancer Res 1998;48:246–253.

101. Hsieh C-C, Trichopoulos D, Katsouyanni K, et al. Age at menarche, age at menopause, height, and obesity as risk factors for breast cancer: association and interactions in an international case-control study. Int J Cancer 1990;46:796–800.

102. Paffenbarger RS Jr, Kampert JB, Chang H-G. Characteristics that predict risk of breast cancer before and after menopause. 1980;112:258–268.

103. Brinton LA, Schairer C, Hoover RN, et al. Menstrual factors and risk of breast cancer. Cancer Invest 1988;6:245–254.

104. Kampert JB, Whittemore AS, Paffenbarger RS Jr. Combined effect of childbearing, menstrual events, and body size on age-specific breast cancer risk. Am J Epidemiol 1988;128:962–979.

105. Helmrich SP, Shapiro S, Rosenberg L, et al. Risk factors for breast cancer. Am J Epidemiol 1983;117:35–45.

106. Bernstein L, Henderson BE, Hanisch R, et al. Physical exercise and reduced risk of breast cancer in women. J Natl Cancer Inst 1994;86:1403–1408.

107. Kelsey JL, Gammon MD, John EM. Reproductive factors and breast cancer. Epidemiol Rev 1993;15:36–47.

108. Bernstein L, Ross RK. Endogenous hormones and breast cancer risk. Epidemiol Rev 1993;15:48–65.

Chapter 59

Physical Activity in Children and Youth

Stewart G. Trost
Russell R. Pate

Regular participation in physical activity is an important component of a healthy lifestyle. Among adults, higher levels of physical activity are associated with reduced risk of coronary heart disease (1), hypertension (2), type II diabetes mellitus (3), obesity (4), certain cancers (5), and some mental health problems (6). Moreover, long-term prospective studies have consistently demonstrated that the risk of all-cause mortality is significantly lower in physically active and/or fit adults relative to their sedentary counterparts (7,8) and that midlife increases in physical activity or fitness are associated with significant reductions in risk for all-cause mortality (9,10). This scientific evidence has prompted several medical and public health organizations to issue position statements and official recommendations endorsing promotion of physical activity for enhancement of public health (11–13).

Physical activity is also beneficial to the health of children and adolescents. Among youth, physical activity is inversely associated with a number of cardiovascular disease risk factors, including elevated blood lipids (14), hypertension (15), obesity (16), and cigarette smoking (17), while positively associated with physical fitness (18), HDL cholesterol (14), bone mass (19), and psychological well-being (20). Importantly, because physical activity habits developed early in life may persist into adulthood (21), adequate participation in physical activity during childhood and adolescence may be of critical importance in the prevention of chronic disease later in life. The purpose of this chapter is to review the descriptive epidemiology of physical activity in children and adolescents. Specifically, we will examine three primary questions: 1) What guidelines/recommendations are there for youth participation in physical activity? 2) To what extent do children and adolescents meet existing guidelines for participation in physical

activity? and 3) What evidence, if any, is there to support the notion that physical activity behavior "tracks" from childhood and adolescence into adulthood?

PHYSICAL ACTIVITY GUIDELINES FOR CHILDREN AND ADOLESCENTS

Although a number of medical and public health organizations have issued position statements endorsing the promotion of lifetime physical activity in youth (22–26), the type and amount of physical activity required by young people to gain health benefits remains poorly understood. Nevertheless, several recommendations or guidelines for youth physical activity have been published.

Healthy People 2000 (27), which describes the health promotion and disease prevention goals for Americans in the year 2000, includes a number of objectives pertinent to physical activity in young people. Of the nine objectives related to physical activity, objectives 1.3 and 1.4 serve as "guidelines" as to the amount and type of physical activity in which youngsters should participate.

1.3 Increase to at least 30% the proportion of people aged 6 and older who engage regularly, preferably daily, in light to moderate physical activity for at least 30 minutes per day.

1.4 Increase to at least 20% the proportion of people aged 18 and older and to at least 75% the proportion of children and adolescents aged 6 through 17 who engage in vigorous physical activity that promotes the development and maintenance of cardiorespiratory fitness 3 or more days per week for 20 or more minutes per occasion.

Blair et al (28) took an alternative approach to formulating a guideline for youth physical activity. Working from the epidemiologic literature linking physical activity to health benefits in adults, Blair estimated that a daily energy expenditure in physical activity of 12.6 kJ/kg of body weight (3 kcals/kg per day) was an appropriate target. This level of activity, when extrapolated to children, corresponds to 20 to 40 minutes of moderate to vigorous physical activity. To account for the hypothesized decline in physical activity between childhood and adulthood, the authors suggested applying a 33% adjustment, yielding an activity recommendation of 16.8 kJ/kg of body weight (4 kcals/kg per day). In similar fashion, Corbin et al (29) proposed a "lifetime physical activity" guideline based on daily energy expenditure. It recommended that, at a minimum, children and adolescents accumulate 30 minutes of moderate physical activity daily (3–4 kcal/kg per day). For optimal benefit, the authors recommended an accumulation of 60 minutes of moderate to vigorous physical activity daily (6–8 kcal/kg per day). The emphasis on the accumulation of moderate to vigorous physical activity throughout the day differs from traditional prescription-based activity guidelines that stress the importance of continuous bouts of physical activity.

To date, the most extensive effort to develop guidelines on the types and amounts of physical activity needed by young people has been the 1994 International Consensus Conference on Physical Activity Guidelines for Adolescents (30). After an extensive review of the pertinent scientific literature, a panel of leading scientists, health care providers, and public health officials issued the following recommendations for physical activity participation during adolescence.

- All adolescents should be physically active daily, or nearly every day, as part of play games, sports, work, transportation, recreation, physical education, or planned exercise, in the context of family, school, and community activities.

- Adolescents should engage in three or more sessions per week of activities that last 20 minutes or more at a time and that require moderate to vigorous levels of exertion.

DESCRIPTIVE EPIDEMIOLOGY OF PHYSICAL ACTIVITY IN CHILDREN AND ADOLESCENTS

Information regarding the percentage of children and adolescents meeting the above recommendations for participation in physical activity is available from two major sources: large-scale population-based surveys utilizing self-report measures of physical activity and small group studies employing more burdensome measures of physical activity such as direct observation and heart rate monitors.

Population-based Surveys

The National Children and Youth Fitness Study

The National Children and Youth Fitness Study (NCYFS) assessed physical activity in a national probability sample of youths aged 10 to 18 (31). Students provided detailed information about the types, frequency, and duration of physical activity engaged in during the previous 12-month period. On average, students reported being engaged in sports, active games, and exercise for 760 minutes per week, with boys reporting approximately 10% greater participation in physical activity than girls. Defining appropriate physical activity as exercise involving large muscle groups in dynamic movements for 20 minutes or longer, three or more time weekly, at an intensity requiring 60% of maximal aerobic capacity, NCYFS estimated that approximately half of boys and girls in grades 5 through 12 were achieving at least the minimum weekly requirement. In a secondary analysis of NCYFS-I data, Pate et al (32) combined estimated physical activity during physical education with physical activity performed outside the school. Using a conservative estimate of one-third of class time engaged in physical activity, it was estimated that youngsters spent an average of 1.8 hours per day engaged in physical activity. It was noted, however, that the standard deviation was considerable (50% to 60% of the mean), underscoring the notion that there was considerable variability in the physical activity habits of US adolescents.

Phase II of the NCYFS examined the physical activity habits and physical fitness of a representative sample of US children aged 6 to 9 (33). In contrast to NCYFS-I, which utilized self-report data from students, physical activity information for NCYFS II was provided by parents and teachers. Items pertinent to children's participation in physical activity included: 1) the parent's and teacher's rating of the child's physical activity level relative to same-sex peers; 2) involvement in community organizations through which the child engaged in physical activity at least three times a week in the past year; 3) the child's five most frequent physical activities in these community organizations; and 4) the number of days per week that each parent exercised with the child for 20 minutes or more. Unfortunately these items did not allow the investigators to estimate time spent in moderate to vigorous physical activity.

Relative to their same-sex peers, parents and guardians rated males above average in physical activity level and females as average. Teachers rated boys as much more active than girls. Among all children aged 6 through 9, nearly all (84.3%) reported participation in at least one community organization in the previous year. These organizations included public parks and recreation programs (65.3%), community-based sports programs (31.9%), churches and other places of worship (24.2%), private health clubs and spas (18.9%), and scouting groups (14.6%). Activities that were most frequently performed in these community organizations were swimming, running/sprinting, baseball/softball, bicycling, and soccer. On average, parents and guardians reported exercising with their children less than 1 day per week (34).

Youth Risk Behavior Surveillance System

In 1990, the US Centers for Disease Control and Prevention (CDC) initiated Youth Risk Behavior Surveillance System (YRBSS). The national school-based survey includes several items to measure physical activity behaviors relevant to national health objectives. These include participation in structured vigorous physical activity, participation in light to moderate physical activity, participation in physical activity to promote strength and flexibility, participation in school and

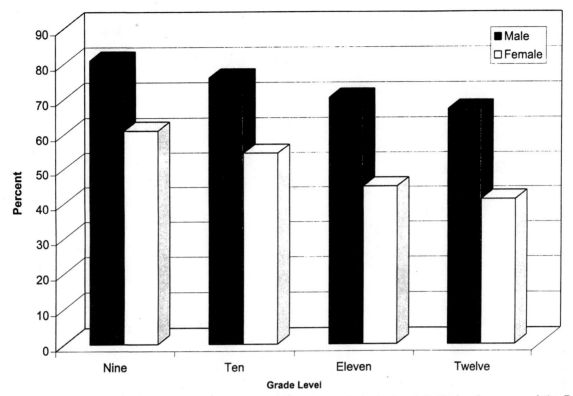

Figure 59-1 Percentage of young people reporting participation in vigorous physical activity during 3 or more of the 7 days preceding the survey. (Source: Department of Health and Human Services. Physical activity and health: a report of the Surgeon General. Atlanta, GA: U.S. Department of Health and Human Services, Centers for Disease Control and Prevention, National Center for Chronic Disease Prevention and Health Promotion, 1996.)

community-based sports teams, and participation in school physical education. Physical activity data from the 1995 school-based survey and the 1992 NHIS home-based survey are summarized below.

In the 1995 school-based survey (35), 63.7% of all students reported participation in vigorous physical activity during 3 or more of the 7 days preceding the survey. Consistent with earlier surveys, male students (74.4%) were significantly more likely to be vigorously active than female students (52.1%). Across sex and grade-level groups, white students (67.0%) were more likely than African American (53.2%) and Hispanic students (57.3%) to report participation in sustained vigorous physical activity. As shown in Figure 59-1, participation in vigorous physical activity declined with grade level. Notably, this decline was more pronounced among female than male students, dropping from 60.9% in ninth grade to 41.0% in twelfth grade. With respect to moderate physical activity, 21.0% of students in grades 9 through 12 reported walking or riding a bicycle for 30 minutes or more during 5 or more of the 7 days preceding the survey. Across all sex and grade level groups, African American (26.8%) and Hispanic students (27.0%) were more likely than white students (18.3%) to report walking or bicycling for 30 minutes or more during the previous week. Across all racial/ethnic groups, the percentage of students reporting bicycling and walking declined with grade level. By the twelfth grade, the percentage of male and female students reporting bicycling and walking for 30 minutes or more on at least 5 or more of the previous 7 days was 17.7% and 16.1%, respectively.

Overall, 50.3% of students reported engaging in strengthening activities during 3 or more of the 7 days preceding the survey. The prevalence of strength-promoting activities was higher in male students (59.1%) than female students (41.0%), and was higher among white (52.8%) and Hispanic students (47.4%) than among African American students (41.4%). Fifty-three percent of students reported performing stretching activities during 3 or more of the 7 days preceding the survey. Participation in activities to promote strength and flexibility declined with grade level, with the decline being greater in female than male students.

Approximately half (50.3%) of students reported participation in one or more sport teams run by a school in the 12 months preceding the survey, with approximately 37% of students reporting participation in community-based sports teams. Participation in team sports was more prevalent among male students than female students and was more likely among white students than it was among African American and Hispanic students. Overall, 59.6% of students reported being enrolled in school physical education programs, with approximately half of that number (25.4%) reporting enrollment in daily physical education. Among those enrolled in physical education programs, 69.7% reported participation in exercise or sport for 20 minutes or more during a typical class.

The 1992 household-based NHIS-YRBS (12) examined physical activity behavior in 10,695 young people aged 12 to 21. Participation in vigorous physical activity, bicycling and walking, and strengthening and stretching activities were

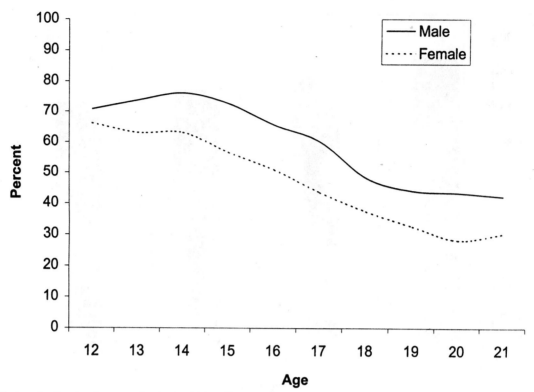

Figure 59-2 Age decline in vigorous physical activity. (Source: Department of Health and Human Services. Physical activity and health: a report of the Surgeon General. Atlanta, GA: U.S. Department of Health and Human Services, Centers for Disease Control and Prevention, National Center for Chronic Disease Prevention and Health Promotion, 1996.)

assessed by items appearing on the school-based survey. Across the entire sample, 53.7% reported participation in vigorous physical activity during 3 or more of the 7 days preceding the survey. Consistent with data obtained in the school-based surveys, the prevalence of vigorous physical activity was higher in males (60.2%) than females (47.2%), and was higher in whites (54.6%) that African Americans (52.6%) and Hispanics (49.5%). As shown in Figure 59-2, participation in vigorous physical activity across all racial/ethnic and sex groups declined with age, with the decline being larger in females than males. Approximately 27% of the sample reported participation in walking or bicycling for 30 minutes or more during 5 of the 7 days preceding the survey. Similar to vigorous physical activity, participation in moderate-intensity activities such as walking and bicycling declined with age.

Forty-eight percent of the sample reported participation in stretching activities during 3 or more of the 7 days preceding the survey, with 45.6% reporting participation in strength-promoting activities on 3 or more days during the same period. Males (54.6%) were significantly more likely than females (36.4%) to report participation in strength-promoting activities. Across all racial/ethnic groups, participation in stretching and strengthening activities declined with age.

1988 Campbell's Survey on Well-being

The 1988 Campbell's survey (36) examined leisuretime physical activity in a national probability sample of Canadian youth aged 10 to 14 and 15 to 19, respectively. Respondents

were asked about the frequency of participation in a extensive number of leisuretime activities over the previous 12 months. These data were used to derive an estimate of weekly time spent in leisuretime physical activity, weekly energy expenditure in leisuretime physical activity, and weekly participation in sustained aerobic activity. Seventy-two percent of males aged 10 to 14 and 69% of males aged 15 to 19 reported an energy expenditure in leisuretime physical activity of 3 kcal/kg or more per day. In comparison, 49% of females aged 10 to 14 and 39% of females aged 15 to 19 reported an energy expenditure in leisuretime physical activity of 3 kcal/kg or more per day. More than 90% of males and 85% of females reported participation in leisuretime physical activity for 3 or more hours a week for at least 9 out of the 12 previous months. Defining adequate aerobic activity as participation in 30 or more minutes of moderate intensity activity ($\geq$50% of age-predicted aerobic capacity) every other day, only 16% of males aged 10 to 19 reported adequate participation in aerobic activity. Less than 15% of females aged 10 to 14 and less than 10% of females aged 15 to 19 reported adequate aerobic activity.

Allied Dunbar National Fitness Survey

The Allied Dunbar National Fitness Survey (37) examined the patterns of physical activity and level of physical fitness in a population-representative sample of English young people aged 16 to 24. Detailed information was collected via interview about the type, intensity, duration, and frequency of physical activity performed in the previous four weeks. Data were reduced to the frequency and intensity of 20-minute activity bouts in the previous 4 weeks. Those who reported no 20-minute bouts of physical activity in the past 4 weeks were assigned to level zero. Those who reported 1 to 4 20-minute bouts mixed between moderate and vigorous physical activity were assigned to level one. Those who reported 5 to 11 20-minute bouts mixed between moderate and vigorous activity were assigned to level two. Those reporting 12 or more 20-minute bouts of physical activity were assigned to level three, four, or five, depending on whether bouts were moderate only, mixed between moderate and vigorous, or vigorous only. Approximately 30% of males and 64% of females were assigned to level zero, one, or two. Among males, 30% were assigned to level five, 23% to level four, and 15% to level three. Among females, 9% were assigned to level five, 16% to level four, and 22% to level three. Collectively, the data indicated that substantial proportions of English young people, in particular females, do not engage in regular, sustained moderate to vigorous physical activity.

The Amsterdam Growth Study

Van Mechelen et al (38) evaluated physical activity behavior in a cohort of Dutch youth over a 15-year period. Baseline assessments were conducted at age 13 with follow-up assessments performed at age 14, 15, 16, 21, and 27. Physical activity during the preceding 3-month period was assessed via a semistructured interview and expressed as total weekly physical activity (≥ 4 METs), weekly light physical activity (4 to 7 METs), weekly medium to heavy physical activity (7 to 10 METs), and weekly heavy physical activity (≥ 10 METs). Among females, total physical activity time decreased from 9.1 hr/wk at age 13 to 8.4 hr/wk at age 27. Among males, total physical activity time declined from 10.6 hr/wk at age 13 to 7.3 hr/wk at age 27. For both males and females, reported participation in light activities increased up to age 21, declining thereafter. At each assessment, females reported significantly greater participation in light physical activities. Over time, males and females reported similar participation in medium to heavy activities, beginning at just under 4 hr/wk at age 13 and declining to just over 1 hr/wk at age 21. At age 13, males reported nearly five times as much heavy physical activity (~2.5 hr/wk) as females (~0.5 hr/wk). Over the 15-year follow-up period, the participation of females in heavy physical activity remained virtually unchanged. However, among males, participation in heavy physical activity declined markedly. By age 21, males averaged less than 1 hr/wk of heavy physical activity.

The Berlin-Bremen Study

Fuchs et al (39) longitudinally examined physical activity behavior in a sample of 932 German children in grades six and seven. Physical activity was assessed via self-report questionnaire on five occasions (waves) over a 2- to 3-year period. From wave one to wave five, time spent in moderate physical activity (3–6 METs) declined from 6.5 to 5.9 hr/wk. Over the same period, time spent in vigorous physical activity (≥ 7 METs) declined from 2.4 to 2.1 hr/wk. Males reported approximately 3 hr/wk more total physical activity than

females, primarily because of their greater participation in vigorous physical activity.

Child and Adolescent Trial for Cardiovascular Health (CATCH)

Simons-Morton et al (40) performed structured physical activity interviews in 2410 third-grade students from 96 schools in four distinct regions in the United States. On average, students reported 89.9 minutes of moderate to vigorous physical activity daily and 34.7 minutes of vigorous physical activity daily. Approximately 37% of third graders reported less than 60 minutes of moderate to vigorous physical activity, with 12.8% reporting less than 30 minutes. Boys reported significantly greater participation in physical activity than girls and white children reported more physical activity than African American or Hispanic children. The prevalence of moderate to vigorous physical activity was highest in California and lowest in Louisiana. The results indicated that, as early as the third grade, many children are in need of intervention programs to increase physical activity.

Summary of Population-based Surveys

Population-based studies conducted in North America and Europe indicate that substantial numbers of children and adolescents participate in adequate amounts of moderate to vigorous physical activity. In the studies that examined participation in sustained bouts of vigorous physical activity, estimates of the percentage of youth meeting prescription-based vigorous activity guidelines range from 50% to 70%. Across studies there is consistent evidence that males are more active than females, and physical activity declines with age, with the decline being greater in females than males.

Studies Employing Objective Measures of Physical Activity

Given the limitations associated with self-reported measures of physical activity in children and adolescents (41), a preferable approach is to assess physical activity using objective monitoring techniques. Direct observation techniques or devices such as heart rate monitors and accelerometers can be used, with minimal subject reactivity, to quantify accumulated participation in physical activity at selected intensity levels. This section summarizes the studies employing objective monitoring techniques to quantify physical activity behavior among children and adolescents. A general limitation of these studies is that they involve relatively small, non-representative samples of youth. Yet, despite this limitation, they provide a valuable opportunity for researchers to assess, in an indirect manner, the validity of self-report data obtained in population surveys. Moreover, they provide valuable physical activity data in populations of youth for whom self-report methods are not feasible, i.e., young children.

Direct Observation

Baranowski et al (42) employed direct observation to examine structured aerobic activity among children in grades three through six. Twenty-four students (10 males, 14 females) were observed for approximately 12 hours per day for 2 consecutive days. Aerobic activity was defined as 20 minutes in which rapid trunk movements through space were maintained without stopping. Over the 2-day monitoring period, no aerobic activity, according to the above criteria, was observed. Applying the less stringent criterion of trunk movements sustained for 14 minutes with one stop of 2 minutes or less, approximately half of the children were judged to have participated in daily aerobic activity. The average daily time engaged in aerobic activity was 80 minutes for boys and 55 minutes for girls. Activity time also decreased with grade level. For third to fourth graders and fifth to sixth graders, the average daily time engaged in aerobic activity was 80 and 41 minutes, respectively.

Sleap et al (43) utilized direct observation to quantify physical activity behavior in 179 English school students. Observations were performed during school breaks, physical education class, and free time outside of school. On average, students were engaged in moderate to vigorous physical activity (MVPA) for 122.3 minutes per day. Only 21% of students engaged in one or more sustained 20-minute periods of MVPA; however, nearly all students (95%) demonstrated one or more sustained 5-minute period of MVPA.

Bailey et al (44) developed an intensive observation protocol to quantify the level and tempo of physical activity in 15 children aged 6 to 10. Observations were recorded every 3 seconds during 4-hour time blocks beginning at 8:00 AM and ending at 8:00 PM. Based on laboratory measurements of oxygen consumption, recorded activities were classified as low ($<11\,mL \cdot kg^{-1} \cdot min^{-1}$), moderate ($11$–$24.5\,mL \cdot kg^{-1} \cdot min^{-1}$), or high intensity ($>24.5\,mL \cdot kg^{-1} \cdot min^{-1}$). Children were found to engage in low and moderate activities 77.1% and 19.8% of the time, respectively. Subjects engaged in very little high intensity activity (3.1%). The median duration of low and medium activities was 6 seconds, with high intensity activities lasting, on average, 3 seconds. The results suggested that children accumulate appreciable amounts of light to moderate activity throughout the day, but do so in an intermittent rather than continuous manner.

Heart Rate Monitoring

Seliger et al (45) utilized heart rate monitoring over a 24-hour period to quantify the habitual physical activity of eleven 12-year-old boys. On average, boys spent 34% of the time engaged in mild intensity activities (~3 METs), and only 3% of the time in moderate intensity activities (~5–6 METs). At no time did the boys engage in heavy intensity activity (~10 METs).

Gilliam et al (46) utilized heart rate monitoring to characterize the physical activity patterns of 40 children aged 6 to 7. Over the 12-hour monitoring period (8:00 AM to 8:00 PM) the number of vigorous physical activity minutes (heart rate >160 beats/min) was 20.9 and 9.4 for boys (n = 22) and girls (n = 18), respectively. On average, the number of minutes with heart rate > 140 was 56.2 and 29.6 for boys and girls, respectively.

Sallo et al (47) utilized daily heart rate monitoring to examine the pattern of physical activity and time spent in MVPA in kindergarten and first-grade school children in Estonia. Children were observed over a 4-day monitoring period that included 2 weekdays and 2 weekend days. Participation in MVPA was defined as the number of minutes with a heart rate between 140 and 157 beats/min. On average, boys exhibited 40 and 34 minutes of MVPA on weekdays and

weekend days, respectively. Girls exhibited similar participation in physical activity, exhibiting 43 and 32 minutes of MVPA on weekdays and weekends, respectively. Participation in vigorous physical activity was defined as the number of minutes with a heart rate greater than 157 beats/min. On average, boys exhibited 17 and 14 minutes of vigorous activity on weekdays and weekend days, respectively. Girls, on average, exhibited 11 and 10 minutes of vigorous activity on weekdays and weekends, respectively. Only 20% of boys and 17% of girls engaged in sustained periods of MVPA for 20 minutes or greater. In contrast, all participants exhibited 1-minute, 2-minute, and 5-minute periods of sustained MVPA. Eighty percent of boys and 90% of girls exhibited 5- to 9-minute periods of sustained MVPA.

Gilbey et al (48) utilized continuous heart rate monitioring to assess the physical activity patterns of Singapore school children aged 9 to 10. Fifty boys and 64 girls were monitored for three 14-hour periods during normal school days. Additionally, 43 boys and 53 girls were monitored for 14 hours on a Saturday. Participation in MVPA was defined as the number of daily minutes with a heart rate of more than 139 beats/min. On weekdays, the mean accumulated time engaged in MVPA was 47.3 and 29.6 minutes for boys and girls, respectively. On weekend days, mean accumulated time engaged in MVPA was 42.4 and 33.3 minutes for boys and girls, respectively. Participation in vigorous physical activity was defined as the number of daily minutes with a heart rate of more than 159 beats/min. On weekdays, the mean accumulated time engaged in vigorous physical activity was 15.4 and 10 minutes for boys and girls, respectively. On weekend days, mean accumulated time engaged in vigorous physical activity was 13.1 and 9.5 minutes for boys and girls, respectively. Notably, 20% of boys and more than 50% of girls never exhibited a single 10-minute period of sustained MVPA. Conversely, all boys and approximately 86% of girls demonstrated at least one 5-minute period of sustained MVPA.

Janz et al (49) performed whole day heart monitoring in 76 children and adolescents aged 16 to 17. Participation in aerobic activity was defined as the total number of minutes spent at or above 60% heart rate reserve. Among prepubescent males and females, respectively, the average time spent in aerobic activity was 23.6 and 29.1 minutes. Among pubescent males and females, respectively, the average daily time spent in aerobic activity was 10.9 and 8.2 minutes.

Sallis et al (50) performed continuous heart rate monitoring in a sample of fifth (n = 36), eighth (n = 36), and eleventh (n = 30) grade students. Students were monitored from approximately 7:30 AM to 11:30 PM. Among fifth grade students, the average number of minutes with a heart rate of more than 139 beats/min was 44.9 and 42.7 for males and females, respectively. Among eighth grade students, the average number of minutes with a heart rate of more than 139 beats/min was 27.6 and 28.8 for males and females, respectively. Among twelfth grade students, the average number of minutes with a heart rate of more than 139 beats/min was 41.7 and 13.2 for males and females, respectively.

Armstrong et al (51) utilized continuous heart rate monitoring to assess the physical activity patterns of British school children aged 11 to 16. Students were monitored over three normal weekdays and one Saturday from 9:00 AM to 9:00 PM. Boys had heart rates greater than 139 beats/min for a significantly higher percentage of time than girls during the weekday (6.2% vs. 4.3%) and on Saturday (5.6% vs. 2.6%). On weekdays and on Saturday, boys had significantly more 5- and 10-minute periods of sustained periods of a heart rate of more than 139 beats/min. On weekdays, approximately 77% of boys and 88% of girls demonstrated no 20-minute periods with heart rate greater than 139 beats/min, with this percentage increasing to 88% and 96.7%, respectively, on Saturday. In agreement with other monitoring studies, it was concluded that few British children and adolescents participate in sustained periods of MVPA.

Summary of Objective Monitoring Studies

Results from the objective monitoring studies are summarized in Table 59-1. Estimates of daily participation in moderate to vigorous physical activity range from 8 to 122 minutes, with an average approximating 40 minutes per day. These studies consistently show that only a small percentage (<20%) of children and adolescents engage in sustained 20-minute bouts of moderate to vigorous physical activity. However, it appears that relatively large percentages of children and adolescents engage in moderate to vigorous physical activity for 5- and 10-minute periods.

TRACKING OF PHYSICAL ACTIVITY BEHAVIOR

Tracking refers to the maintenance of relative rank or position within a group over time. From a public health perspective, the concept of tracking is of considerable importance as it implies that health behaviors established early in life are carried through into adulthood. The notion that physical activity behavior tracks from childhood into adolescence provides a strong rationale for the promotion of physical activity in children and adolescents. To date, however, relatively few studies have investigated the extent to which physical activity behavior tracks during childhood and adolescence.

Saris et al (52) examined the stability of physical activity behavior in a cohort of 217 boys and 189 girls. Data were collected every 2 years beginning at age 6 and ending at age 12. Total energy expenditure and energy expenditure in activities above 50% of aerobic capacity was estimated from 24-hour heart rate monitoring using the individual regression equation between heart rate and oxygen consumption. Interperiod correlation coefficients for total energy expenditure ranged from 0.30 to 0.42. Interperiod correlation coefficients for energy expenditure in activities above 50% of aerobic capacity were less than 0.20.

Pate et al (53) investigated the tracking of physical activity in 47 3- to 4-year-old children. Physical activity was assessed via continuous heart rate monitoring on at least 2 and up to 4 days per year. Participation in physical activity was quantified as the percentage of observed minutes between 3:00 PM and 6:00 PM during which the heart rate was 50% or more above individual resting level (PAHR-50 index). The Spearman rank order correlation between the PAHR-50 index in year one and year three was 0.57 ($P < .001$).

Sallis et al (54) examined the tracking of physical activ-

ity at home and recess in 351 children (mean age 4.4 years). Physical activity was directly observed over a 2-year period. Measurement waves occurred every 6 months, with each wave consisting of 2 days of observation within 1 week. Children were observed for up to 60 minutes at home on a weekday evening and up to 30 minutes during recess at preschool or school. Tracking coefficients (Pearson r) for physical activity performed at home were 0.16 (based on 1 day of observation) and 0.27 (mean of 2 days observation). Tracking coefficients for activity at recess were 0.04 (1 day of observation) and 0.12 (mean of 2 days observation).

Kelder et al (55) studied the tracking of physical activity in adolescents residing in two communities participating in the Minnesota Heart Health Program study. Physical activity was assessed via self-report questionnaire on an annual basis, beginning in seventh grade and ending in twelfth grade. Tracking was analyzed by 1) dividing baseline physical activity values into quintiles; 2) computing the mean in each quintile; and 3) ascertaining the mean for each activity quintile maintained its relative position over time. Tracking was most apparent in the extremes of the physical activity distribution, i.e., those with the highest (>6 hr) and the lowest (<1 hr) weekly exercise time.

As part of the Cardiovascular Risk in Young Finns Study, Raitakari et al (56) examined the stability of physical activity behavior in Finnish youth. Leisuretime physical activity was assessed via self-report questionnaire in randomly selected population-representative samples of youth aged 3 to 19. Baseline assessments were performed in 1980, with follow-up assessments performed in 3-year intervals in 1983 and 1986. Rank order correlations between physical activity at baseline and 3-year follow-up were statistically significant and ranged from 0.33 to 0.54. Rank order correlations between physical activity at baseline and 6-year follow-up, while statistically significant, were smaller in magnitude, ranging from 0.17 to 0.43. Tracking coefficients were generally stronger among males and older age groups. To examine the stability of active and sedentary behavior, participants were classified as active or sedentary. Forty-one percent of males and 29% females classified as active at age 12 remained active at age 18. Conversely, 56% of males and 63% of females classified as sedentary at age 12 remained sedentary at age 18.

In the 15-year Amsterdam Growth Study, van Mechelen and Kemper (38) calculated interperiod correlation coefficients for total weekly energy expenditure and energy expenditure in organized sports. For time periods of approximately 5 years, there was suggestive evidence of tracking for total energy expenditure in both males ($r = 0.32 - 0.44$) and females ($r = 0.25 - 0.58$). For weekly energy expenditure in organized sports, short-term (~5 year) interperiod correlations were higher at 0.53 and 0.59 for males and females, respectively. For longer periods of follow-up (10 to 15 years), there was little evidence of tracking for any of the physical activity variables ($r < 0.20$). The investigators also examined the stability of membership in the highest and lowest quintile for total weekly energy expenditure. Among males, 9 out of the 21 participants (42.8%) in the highest quintile for weekly energy expenditure at baseline (age 13) remained in the highest quintile at 4-year follow-up (age 16). Similarly, 12 of the 21 males (57.1%) in the lowest quintile for weekly energy expenditure at baseline remained in the lowest quintile at 4-year follow-up.

Table 59-1 Summary of Descriptive Studies Utilizing Objective Measures of Physical Activity

Study	Sample	Method Used	Minutes of Moderate to Vigorous Physical Activity Daily	Minutes of Vigorous Physical Activity Daily
Baranowski et al (42)	N = 24 3rd and 4th graders Males and females USA	Direct observation	Males = 80 Females = 55 Grades 3–4 = 80 Grades 5–6 = 41	
Sleap et al (43)	N = 179 Ages 5–11 Males and females England	Direct observation	All children = 122.3	
Bailey et al (44)	N = 15 Ages 6–10 Males and females USA	Direct observation	All children = 43.7	All children = 5.9
Seliger et al (45)	N = 11 Age 12 Males only Czechoslovakia	Heart rate monitoring	Males = 74	Males = 0
Gilliam et al (46)	N = 40 Ages 6–7 Males and females USA	Heart rate monitoring	Males = 35.3 Females = 20.2	Males = 20.9 Females = 9.4
Sallo et al (47)	N = 54 Preschool and first grade Males and females Estonia	Heart rate monitoring	*Weekday:* Males = 40 Females = 43 *Weekend:* Males = 34 Females = 32	*Weekday:* Males = 17 Females = 11 *Weekend:* Males = 14 Females = 10
Gilbey et al (48)	N = 105 Ages 9–10 Males and females Singapore	Heart rate monitoring	*Weekday:* Males = 47.3 Females = 29.6 *Weekend:* Males = 42.4 Females = 33.3	*Weekday:* Males = 15.4 Females = 10.0 *Weekend:* Males = 13.1 Females = 9.5
Janz et al (49)	N = 76 Ages 6–17 Males and females USA	Heart rate monitoring	*Prepubescent:* Males = 23.6 Females = 29.1 *Pubescent:* Males = 10.9 Females = 8.2	
Sallis et al (50)	N = 102 Grades 5, 8, and 11 Males and females USA	Heart rate monitoring	*Grade 5:* Males = 44.9 Females = 42.7 *Grade 8:* Males = 27.6 Females = 28.8 *Grade 11:* Males = 40.3 Females = 16.4	
Armstrong et al (51)	N = 266 Ages 11–16 Males and females England	Heart rate monitoring	*Weekday:* Males = 45 Females = 31 *Weekend:* Males = 40 Females = 19	

Among females, 7 out of the 24 participants (29.2%) in the highest quintile for weekly energy expenditure at baseline (age 13) remained in the highest quintile at 4-year follow-up (age 16). Seven of the 24 females (29.2%) in the lowest quintile for weekly energy expenditure at baseline remained in the lowest quintile at 4-year follow-up.

SUMMARY

This review examined evidence from large population-based surveys using self-report methods and smaller group studies using objective measures of physical activity. Both study types indicate that a large percentage of children and adolescents meet accepted guidelines for daily participation in moderate intensity physical activity. There is also consistent evidence that males are more active than females and that participation in physical activity declines with age, more so in females than males. However, there is considerable disagreement between study types regarding the percentage of youth meeting guidelines for moderate to vigorous physical activity. Results from population-based studies conducted in the United States indicate that approximately two-thirds of adolescent youth engage in three or more 20-minute sessions of vigorous physical activity per week. However, evidence from studies using objective measures of physical activity indicates that children and adolescents tend to perform activity on an intermittent rather than continuous basis, and that a relatively small percentage of children and adolescents (<20%) engage in sustained 20-minute bouts of moderate to vigorous physical activity. This suggests that the self-report questionnaires employed in population-based surveillance studies may be insensitive to intermittently performed physical activity, and as a result, may be providing overestimates of the percentage of youth meeting traditional prescription-based guidelines for moderate to vigorous physical activity.

Clearly, population-based surveillance studies using objective measures of physical activity are warranted, particularly among adolescent youth. Relatively few studies have examined the tracking of physical activity during childhood and adolescence. Although studies vary considerably with respect to length, age group studied, measurement of physical activity, and method used to assess tracking, there is some evidence that, over short time periods (3 to 5 years), physical activity behavior tracks. Over longer periods of follow-up (6 to 10 years) there is little evidence that physical activity behavior tracks during childhood and adolescence.

REFERENCES

1. Powell KE, Thompson PD, Caspersen CJ, et al. Physical activity and the incidence of coronary heart disease. Ann Rev Public Health 1987;8:253–287.

2. Faggard RH, Tipton CM. Physical activity, fitness, and hypertension. In: Bouchard C, Shephard RJ, Stephens T, eds. Physical activity, fitness, and health. Champaign, IL: Human Kinetics, 1994.

3. Helmrich SP, Ragland DR, Leung RW, et al. Physical activity and reduced occurrence of non-insulin dependent diabetes mellitus. N Engl J Med 1991;325:147–152.

4. Trembley A, Despres J-P, Leblanc C, et al. Effects of intensity of physical activity on body fatness and fat distribution. Am J Clin Nutr 1990;51:153–157.

5. Kohl HW, LaPorte RE, Blair SN. Physical activity and cancer: an epidemiological perspective. Sports Med 1988;6:222-237.

6. King AC, Taylor CB, Haskell WL, et al. Influence of regular aerobic exercise on psychological health. Health Psychol 1989;8:305–324.

7. Blair SN, Kohl HW, Paffenbarger RS, et al. Physical fitness and all-cause mortality. JAMA 1989;262:2395–2401.

8. Paffenbarger RS, Hyde RT, Wing AL, et al. Physical activity, all-cause mortality and longevity of college alumni. N Engl Med 1986;314:605–613.

9. Blair SN, Kohl HW, Barlow CE, et al. Changes in physical fitness and all-cause mortality. JAMA 1995;273:1093–1098.

10. Paffenbarger RS, Kampert JB, Lee I-M, et al. Changes in physical activity and other lifeway patterns influencing longevity. Med Sci Sports Exerc 1994;26:857–865.

11. Pate RR, Pratt M, Blair SN, et al. Physical activity and public health: a joint recommendation from the Centers for Disease Control and Prevention and the American College of Sports Medicine. JAMA 1995;273:402–407.

12. Department of Health and Human Services. Physical activity and health: a report of the Surgeon General. Atlanta, GA: U.S. Department of Health and Human Services, Centers for Disease Control and Prevention, National Center for Chronic Disease Prevention and Health Promotion, 1996.

13. NIH Consensus Development Panel on Physical Activity and Cardiovascular Health. Physical activity and cardiovascular health. JAMA 1996;276:241–246.

14. Armstrong N, Simons-Morton B. Physical activity and blood lipids in adolescents. Pediatr Exerc Sci 1994:6:381–405.

15. Alpert BS, Wilmore JH. Physical activity and blood pressure in adolescents. Pediatr Exerc Sci 1994;6:361–380.

16. Ward DS, Evans R. Physical activity, aerobic fitness, and obesity in children. Med Exerc Nutr Health 1995;4:3–16.

17. Escobedo LG, Marcus SE, Holtzman E, Giovino GA. Sports participation, age at smoking initiation, and the risk of smoking among US high school students. JAMA 1993;269:1391–1395.

18. Malina RM. Physical activity and fitness of children and youth: questions and implications. Med Exerc Nutr Health 1995;4:123–135.

19. Bailey DA, Martin AD. Physical activity and skeletal health in adolescents. Pediatr Exerc Sci 1994; 6:330–347,1994.

20. Calfas KJ, Taylor WC. Effects of physical activity on psychological variables in adolescents. Pediatr Exerc Sci 1994;6:406–423.

21. Malina RM. Tracking of physical activity and physical fitness across the lifespan. Res Q Exerc Sport 1996;67:48–57.

22. American Academy of Pediatrics Committees on Sports Medicine and School Health. Physical fitness and the schools. Pediatrics 1987;80:449–450.

23. American Medical Association. AMA guidelines for adolescent preventive services (GAPS): recommendations and rationale. Baltimore: Williams and Wilkins, 1994.

24. American College of Sports Medicine. Opinion statement on physical fitness in children and youth. Med Sci Sports Exerc 1988;20: 422–423.

25. Riopel RA, Boerth RC, Coates TJ, et al. Coronary risk factor modification in children: exercise: a statement for physicians by the committee on atherosclerosis and hypertension in childhood of the Council on Cardiovascular Disease in the Young, American Heart Association. Circulation 1986;74: 1189A–1191A.

26. Center for Disease Control and Prevention. Guidelines for school and community programs to promote lifelong physical activity among young people. MMWR 1997;46(no. RR-6).

27. Public Health Service. Healthy people 2000: national health promotion and disease prevention objectives. Washington, DC: U.S. Department of Health and Human Services, 1990. DHHS publication no. PHS 91-50212.

28. Blair SN, Clark DG, Cureton KJ, Powell KE. Exercise and fitness in childhood: implications for a lifetime of health. In: Gisolfi CV, Lamb DR, eds. Perspectives in exercise science and sports

medicine. Indianapolis: Benchmark Press, 1989:401–430.

29. Corbin CB, Pargrazi RP, Welk GJ. Toward an understanding of appropriate physical activity levels for youth. Phys Act Fitness Res Dig 1994;1:1–8.

30. Sallis JF, Patrick K. Physical activity guidelines for adolescents: consensus statement. Pediatr Exerc Sci 1994;6:302–314.

31. Ross JG, Gilbert GG. The national children and youth fitness study: a summary of findings. J Phys Educ Recreation Dance 1985;56,45–50.

32. Pate RR, Long BJ, Heath GW. Descriptive epidemiology of physical activity in adolescents. Pediatr Exerc Sci 1994;6:434–447.

33. Ross JG, Pate RR. The national children and youth fitness study II: a summary of findings. J Phys Educ Recreation Dance 1987;58: 51–56.

34. Ross JG, Pate RR, Caspersen CJ, et al. The national children and youth fitness study II: home and community in children's exercise habits. J Phys Educ Recreation Dance 1987;58:85–92.

35. Kann L, Warren W, Harris WA, et al. Youth risk behavior surveillance—United States, 1995. J Sch Health 1996;66:365–377.

36. Stephens T, Craig CL. The wellbeing of Canadians: highlights of the 1988 Campbell's Survey. Ottawa: Canadian Fitness and Lifestyle Institute, 1990.

37. Sports Council and Health Education Authority. Allied Dunbar National Fitness Survey. London: Belmont Press, 1993.

38. van Mechelen W, Kemper HCG. Habitual physical activity in longitudinal perspective. In: Kemper HCG ed. The Amsterdam Growth Study: a longitudinal analysis of health, fitness, and lifestyle. Champaign, IL: Human Kinetics, 1995:135–158.

39. Fuchs et al. Patterns of physical activity among German adolescents: the Berlin-Bremen Study. Prev Med 1988;17:746–763.

40. Simons-Morton BG, McKenzie TJ, Stone E, et al. Physical activity in a multiethnic population of third graders in four states. Am J Public Health 1997;87:45–50.

41. Pate RR. Physical activity assessment in children and adolescents. Crit Rev Food Sci Nutr 1993;33: 321–326.

42. Baranowski T, Hooks P, Tsong Y, et al. Aerobic physical activity among third- to sixth-grade children. J Dev Behav Pediatr 1987;8:203–206.

43. Sleap M, Warburton P. Physical activity levels of 5–11-year old children in England: cumulative evidence from three direct observation studies. Int J Sports Med 1996;17:248–253.

44. Bailey RC, Olson J, Pepper SL, et al. The level and tempo of children's physical activities: an observational study. Med Sci Sports Exerc 1995;27:1033–1041.

45. Seliger V, Trefny Z, Bartunkova S, Pauer M. The habitual activity and physical fitness of 12 year old boys. Acta Paediatr Belg 1974; 28(suppl):54–59.

46. Gilliam TB, Freedson PS, Geenen DL, Shahraray B. Physical activity patterns determined by heart rate monitoring in 6–7 year-old children. Med Sci Sports Exerc 1981; 13:65–67.

47. Sallo M, Silla R. Physical activity with moderate to vigorous intensity in preschool and first-grade schoolchildren. Pediatr Exerc Sci 1997; 9:44–54.

48. Gilbey, Gilbey. The physical activity of Singapore primary school children as estimated by heart rate monitoring. Pediatr Exerc Sci 1995;7:26–35.

49. Janz KF, Golden JC, Hansen JR, Mahoney LT. Heart rate monitoring of physical activity in children and adolescents: the Muscatine study. Pediatrics 1992;89:256–261.

50. Sallis JF, Buono MJ, Roby JJ, Micale FG, Nelson JA. Seven-day recall and other physical activity self-reports in children and adolescents. Med Sci Sports Exerc 1993;25:99–108.

51. Armstrong N, et al. Patterns of physical activity among 11 to 16 year old British children BMJ 1990;301:203–205.

52. Saris WHM, Elvers JWH, van't Hof MA, Binkhorst RA. Changes in physical activity of children aged 6 to 12 years. In: Rutenfranz F, Mocellin R, Klimmt F, eds. Children and exercise XII. Champaign, IL: Human Kinetics, 1980.

53. Pate RR, Baranowski T, Dowda M, Trost SG. Tracking of physical activity in young children. Med Sci Sports Exerc 1996:28:92–96.

54. Sallis JF, Berry CC, Broyles SL, et al. Variability and tracking of physical activity over 2 yr in young children. Med Sci Sports Exerc 1995;27:1042–1049.

55. Kelder SH, Perry CL, Klepp K-I, Lytle LL. Longitudinal tracking of adolescent smoking, physical activity and food choice behaviors. Am J Public Health 1994:84: 1121–1126.

56. Raitakari OT, Porkka KVK, Taimela S, et al. Effects of persistent physical activity and inactivity on coronary risk factors in children and young adults: the cardiovascular risk in young Finns study. Am J Epidemiol 1994;140:195–205.

Part XI.

FAMILY PRACTICE

Edited by
Charles B. Eaton

Introduction to Family Medicine

Charles B. Eaton

This section is written for generalist physicians (family physicians, internists, pediatricians, general practitioners), nurse practitioners, and other health care providers to address the needs of physical activity counseling and other lifestyle counseling issues in the context of a busy, primary care office setting. When necessary, it reiterates topics explored in more depth in other sections of the book, not from the viewpoint of an exercise physiologist, clinical psychologist, nutritionist, or medical specialist but from the perspective of a generalist.

In the first chapter, Kevin Burroughs et al focus on the preparticipation evaluation of the collegiate or high school athlete. Since the majority of children and adolescents who participate in sports are examined by primary care physicians, this chapters details the elements of a preparticipation examination based upon an evolving body of research that are effective in preventing injury and improving the safety of athletes. Specific components of the history and physical exam are reviewed in detail, with excellent up-to-date references enumerating the prevalence of abnormal findings. A step-based approach that allows for a cost-effective workup of common problems found in young athletes such as a systolic murmur and the concern of hypertrophic cardiomyopathy is presented. A detailed table of medical conditions affecting sports participation adapted from the American Academy of Pediatrics Committee on Sports Medicine and Fitness is given that is very helpful in providing medical clearance to athletes.

The next chapter, by Michael Goldstein et al, reviews office-based physical activity counseling in healthy adults. The authors discuss the importance of such an intervention and barriers to providing this service. An extensive review of the trials in primary care that focus on the efficacy of physical activity counseling and the lessons learned from such trials is given. The authors then address in detail a useful model of physical activity counseling based upon the transtheoretical model of behavior change that has been tested in several clinical trials in primary care office practices.

Carol Garber addresses physical activity counseling in patients with chronic disease within the office setting in the next chapter. Criteria for screening high-risk patients who will benefit from increased levels of supervision while exercising, indications for exercise stress testing, contraindications to exercise training, and risk stratification for appropriate supervision of exercise training are reviewed. Exercise prescriptions for improving cardiovascular fitness and body composition are clearly described, along with information-packed tables that allow for appropriate exercise intensity and special considerations for many common chronic diseases to be incorporated in the exercise counseling recommendations. An appendix listing Internet resources is particularly helpful.

The next chapter of this section focuses on exercise counseling in the fastest growing segment of the population, namely the elderly. This chapter, by Daniel Forman et al, highlights the need for exercise counseling in this age group, discusses some of the health risks to be considered in the elderly before initiating exercise, and details an exercise prescription best suited for the elderly, including aerobic training, muscle strength and endurance training, and stretching exercises.

The last chapter focuses on providing lifestyle-oriented counseling services within the context of a busy office practice. Highlights of this chapter include a discussion of primordial prevention, helpful tips regarding setting up and maintaining an office-based system for lifestyle intervention, and a review of the 5 A's of lifestyle counseling. Several patient care tools available for reproduction are found in this chapter that should help practices with lifestyle-oriented counseling.

Chapter 60

Preparticipation Evaluation of the Collegiate or High School Athlete

Kevin Burroughs
Mike Hilts
Karl Fields

The preparticipation examination (PPE), or "sports physical," was introduced following the publication of "the Bill of Rights for the School and College Athlete" in 1970 (1). This document was developed by the American Medical Association's Committee on Medical Aspects of Sports to promote safety in athletics. The PPE, a brief evaluation to determine whether a potential athlete can participate in sport, was devised as a good-faith effort to protect athletes. While the PPE quickly grew to become one of the most common office visits to physicians, at the time of implementation no convincing literature supported the efficacy of this preventive screening. Ongoing research continues to try to clarify which components of the PPE actually lessen risk for the athlete. The modern PPE consists of variable components of the history (general and specific), the physical examination, and laboratory testing.

HISTORY

The history portion of the PPE identifies up to 70% of the significant abnormalities detected by the PPE (2). This appears to be the most important aspect of the evaluation and positive responses to certain questions often help guide the physical examination. The quality of the historical information varies greatly. Effort is required to confirm that information obtained is valid. To help ensure this, questions should be reviewed with a parent/guardian, or at minimum the parent must sign the form to indicate that they have reviewed the answers.

Generally the history can focus on questions that are most pertinent to sports activity and incumbent risks. Unfortunately, as many as 78% of high school athletes consider the PPE to be their annual health assessment (3). This implies that, whenever possible, general health maintenance issues should be addressed. The utility of addressing general health concerns is minimal, however, unless a parent/guardian can help provide accurate health information; follow-up of medical issues can be arranged with the athlete's primary physician; and concerns are communicated to both the athlete and the parent/guardian. The examiner ultimately can best determine the value of a more comprehensive evaluation.

Determining why an athlete wants to participate in sports may influence the type of questions asked on the PPE as different age groups have separate risks, concerns, and goals. For example, prepubescent athletes (ages 6 to 10) generally feel that having fun is the most important aspect of sports and thus a question asking if exercise is enjoyable may be needed. In this youngest group, previous significant injury is uncommon, but undiagnosed congenital problems are more likely to be identified. Pubescent athletes (ages 11 to 15) are more likely to have more general health concerns, such as weight loss, sexual activity, or drugs. A history exploring this may uncover adolescent health issues that could also affect participation. Most elite athletes are in the postpubescent age group (ages 16 to 30), and thus the PPE needs to consider the athlete's skill level. History of previous injury is especially important in this group, to determine if adequate rehabilitation has occurred. Evidence of incomplete recovery and rehabilitation correlates with increased injury risk in sports. Higher level sport participation requires more comprehensive rehabilitation before the athlete resumes activity.

While many approaches to the PPE have been developed, consensus exists on specific areas that should be covered in the history. These are discussed in more detail in the following sections.

Cardiovascular

Cardiovascular problems pose the greatest risk of sudden death and as such, specific queries seek to determine whether anything in the athlete's history should arouse concern. Specific cardiovascular questions often included in PPEs are:

- Have you ever been dizzy during or after exercise?
- Have you ever had chest pain during exercise?
- Do you tire more quickly than your friends?
- Have you ever had high blood pressure?
- Have you ever had a heart murmur?
- Have you ever felt that your heart skipped beats, or felt your heart racing for no reason?
- Has any family member died of heart problems?
- Did anyone in your family die suddenly before age 50? (Sudden death is defined as less than 24 hours from onset of symptoms.)

These questions potentially can identify cardiac conditions that cause sudden cardiac death. Since only 1 in 200,000 athletes would be expected to die suddenly while participating in a sport, a very sensitive tool is needed to identify the at-risk individual. Unfortunately, the PPE has not proven to be effective in identifying these rare cardiovascular abnormalities. In one study, 158 cases of sudden death were reviewed; of the 115 athletes who had a standard PPE, only 3% were suspected of having cardiovascular disease (4).

PPEs often detect the most prevalent cardiovascular disorder: hypertension. Adjustment of blood pressure levels to account for age and size norms helps determine affected individuals. In addition, blood pressure measurements should be obtained by individuals with appropriate skills. A history of elevated blood pressure or of hypertension in immediate family members may require a more careful follow-up. No direct association has been found between hypertension and sudden cardiac death, but it has been shown that echocardiographic evidence of diastolic dysfunction occurs within 10 years of diagnosis in young hypertensives. Therefore, early detection and treatment focuses on preventing end organ damage.

Less common but serious cardiovascular problems in young athletes include hypertrophic cardiomyopathy (HCM), concentric left ventricular hypertrophy (LVH), Marfan's syndrome (risk of aortic rupture), congenital coronary artery anomalies, and myocarditis. Arrhythmias, mitral valve prolapse, arrythmogenic right ventricular dysplasia, and prolonged QT syndrome are among other potential causes of morbidity and mortality. Use of illicit drugs and ergogenic substances, such as cocaine and anabolic steroids, are relatively common causes of acquired cardiac disease that should be evaluated.

Syncope, exertional chest pain, dyspnea, or excessive fatigue, or a family history of sudden premature cardiac death are historical clues to significant underlying disease. The nature of the specific complaint may help guide the clinician. For example a history of syncope during vigorous exercise suggests a congenital structural anomaly, whereas syncope after exercise is more typical of conditions like hyperventilation (5). Although exertional chest pain alone is a nonspecific symptom and exercise-induced asthma often causes such discomfort, exertional chest pain can be a sign of significant pathology in a young athlete when associated with other findings. It may occur with HCM, Marfan syndrome, valve problems, or coronary artery anomalies. A family history of early cardiac death may suggest autosomal dominant disorders such as Marfan syndrome, familial hyperlipidemia, the Romano-Ward form of prolonged QT syndrome, or hypertrophic cardiomyopathy.

Musculoskeletal

The second area of concern on the PPE is the musculoskeletal system. Specific questions that help predict potential problems are:

- Have you ever had a fracture or broken bone?
- Have you ever worn a cast or had x-rays?
- Have you had a sprain, strain, or swelling after injury?

Orthopedic injuries are the most frequent reason for disqualification from sports participation. The above questions screen for serious injuries that may have had inadequate therapy or rehabilitation. Further questioning should determine what activities the athlete has been able to do without difficulty. Unresolved pain and swelling after an injury may warrant radiographic imaging to rule out growth plate abnormalities, occult fracture, or osteochondritis dessicans. Recurrent joint swelling without trauma should alert the examiner to a possible rheumatologic disorder.

Problematic musculoskeletal areas include the knee, ankle, and shoulder. Unstable knees account for most of the chronic musculoskeletal instability that ultimately leads to disqualification. However, in the absence of symptoms or a history of trauma, the presence of joint laxity or tightness on physical exam, and its contribution to athletic injury, is presently unknown. Common acute knee injuries are collateral ligament sprains, meniscal damage, cruciate ligament sprains, and patellar subluxation or dislocation. Persistent swelling with activity or mechanical symptoms warrant a more thorough examination to see if any of these injuries has been ignored.

Chronic shoulder problems usually arise from repetitive microtrauma, resulting in anterior instability and secondary impingement. Athletes who repeatedly throw or use overhead motions, such as in tennis, are the most prone to these disorders. Any athlete who has persistent pain with these activities or has had a dislocation should be questioned about recurrent symptoms and about their specific rehabilitation program.

Chronic ankle pain, swelling, or recurrent sprains may indicate ankle instability. Since ankle sprains are common in most running and jumping sports, an athlete with these symptoms may need a functional assessment along with the standard ankle examination. A thorough ankle exam will help determine whether strengthening or bracing is needed.

Pulmonary

Cough is the most common pulmonary symptom in athletes and often is symptomatic of asthma. Questions to screen for this include:

- Do you cough persistently after exercise?
- Have you had wheezing/asthma in the past?
- Do you have any allergies or allergic rhinitis?
- Is there a family history of asthma or allergy-related problems?

Exercise-induced asthma (EIA) is present in up to 15–20% of adolescent and high school athletes. EIA patients may need additional treatment during conditions such as allergy seasons or cold weather. A history of persistent coughing with exercise leads to a diagnosis of EIA in 60% to 70% of these individuals. In addition, athletes who have allergic rhinitis have a 50% chance of experiencing EIA at some time. A classic history, a successful trial of inhaled bronchodilators, or a positive exercise challenge can confirm the diagnosis. Positive responses to the pulmonary questions warrant a screening test measured by peak expiratory flow rates (PEFR), first before running outdoors for 6 to 12 minutes, and then again at regular intervals for 15 to 20 minutes after exercise. The classic positive response is a 15% or greater drop in PEFR at 6 to 8 minutes after stopping exercise (6). A positive response on the history directs a more specific evaluation to confirm the diagnosis because the physical examination rarely yields a positive finding.

Neurologic

Neurologic injuries typically occur in contact and collision sports and may pose the risk of catastrophic injury. Screening questions for previous neurologic problems include:

- Have you ever had a head injury?
- Have you ever been knocked out or unconscious?
- Have you ever had a seizure?
- Have you ever had a stinger, burner, or pinched nerve?

Questions regarding previous concussion are included in an effort to prevent "second impact" catastrophic head injuries. A single concussion increases risk of subsequent occurrence by fourfold. Questions should be asked about persistent symptoms because symptomatic individuals may have had a more serious initial injury than suspected and should be protected from further head trauma.

More than one episode of transient brachial plexus injury, or persistent weakness or numbness, warrants imaging studies such as flexion and extension cervical spine x-rays and/or MRI to rule out serious underlying conditions that may include cervical instability, cervical spine stenosis, congenital fusion, or intervertebral disc protrusion. Proper neck and upper extremity strengthening should be encouraged, and proper sports techniques taught, such as in tackling.

An athlete with epilepsy must be well controlled to participate in any collision/contact sport. In addition, certain sports activities raise greater risks for patients with seizure disorders. For this reason water sports, climbing sports, and vehicular sports rarely are considered safe for these individuals. A neurologic consultation should be considered when questions arise concerning diagnosis and/or the effect of sport on seizure control.

Heat Illness

One of the avoidable causes of death in sport is hyperthermia. The questions on the PPE that address this risk are:

- Have you ever fainted or almost fainted during exercise?
- Do you get frequent muscle cramps?
- Do you become fatigued more quickly than your friends?

Prior problems with heat increase the risk for future events; likewise, poor conditioning, obesity, medical illnesses, dehydration, and certain medications (antihistamines, caffeine) magnify the risk. Participants who have experienced heat illness need special monitoring. Near-syncope during exercise, frequent muscle cramps, and inordinate weakness may be clues to impending problems. Recording the athlete's body weight before and after a workout or practice can help detect loss of body fluids, which should then be rapidly replaced. A loss of 5% or more of body weight over several days should be medically evaluated.

Approximately 8% to 10% of African Americans in the United States have sickle cell trait, which is possibly linked to exercise-related rhabdomyolysis during heat injuries. However, routine screening for sickle cell trait is not currently recommended, and unwarranted restrictions or limitations should not be placed on the athlete with the trait. Nevertheless, a known history of sickle trait justifies cautious advice for the athlete competing in hot environs or at extreme altitude.

Cold exposure can likewise impair performance and affect the athlete's well-being. Hypothermia and frostbite are the most common conditions encountered. Athletes participating in outdoor sports during fall and winter months should be instructed on proper dress, such as wearing several thin layers rather than one heavy garment, covering the head and neck (up to 50% of heat loss occurs there), and protecting hands to avoid frostbite. Perspiration or rain will significantly increase body heat loss, so appropriate clothing material is essential to maximize dryness.

Skin

The major reason for reviewing skin problems is because of the risk of contagion to other athletes. In addition, chronic skin diseases can be worsened by sports participation. One question that can help determine this risk is: Do you have any skin problems, such as itching, rashes, acne, warts, fungus, or blisters?

Infectious skin conditions that should delay participation in contact sports until proper treatment is underway or completed include scabies, herpes simplex virus infection, active impetigo, tinea corporis, and molluscum contagiosum.

Epidemics of tinea corporis have occurred among wrestlers. To prevent contagion, lesions must be treated with antifungals and covered with a gas-permeable membrane, such as ProWrap.

Wrestlers and other athletes who are prone to frequent skin abrasions are at risk for cutaneous herpes simplex. Fomites can transmit the virus, as evidenced by an outbreak of HSV-1 among kayakers who developed lesions in the lumbosacral area, probably due to inoculation via an infected spray skirt. High attack rates have led the NCAA Wrestling Committee to recommend that the athlete not participate until free of new lesions for 3 days and the lesions are crusted; the athlete must also be on acyclovir (or another appropriate antiviral) at tournament time.

Spread of impetigo has been reported both in soccer and football. Lesions spread quickly to multiple areas of the body. Typical guidelines require completion of at least 3 days of antibiotics and/or no new lesions in the 48 hours prior to competition. Lesions must be covered for competition.

Sports-related spread of molluscum contagiosum has been well documented. Skin trauma probably plays a role, as boxers and wrestlers typically develop lesions on hands, face, and upper body locations. Less logical spread has been reported in sports such as cross-country running. Without treatment, lesions can last 6 to 9 months, or longer. Athletes in close-contact sports should have the lesions curetted or covered with a gas-permeable membrane, such as Op-site.

General Medical Problems

Certain aspects of an athlete's general health may affect participation. The examiner should review chronic illnesses and their required medications. Immunizations should be updated, especially tetanus, measles-mumps-rubella, and hepatitis B. Allergy status, including hypersensitivity or anaphylaxis to bee stings or medications, should be determined so that proper anticipatory measures can be taken.

Noting the use of mouth, ear, or eyewear is of added importance in the case of the athlete who becomes injured or unconscious. Special problems may occur in the athlete who has lost one of a paired organ. These athletes may still participate in certain activities, depending on the organ and sport.

Diabetic athletes require careful management, but should be encouraged to participate in regular physical activity. Lipid profiles as well as respiratory and cardiac fitness parameters are improved in diabetics who exercise, just as in the rest of the population. Athletes must understand that caloric intake should increase in proportion to activity intensity and that the timing of intake is crucial. Injecting insulin into more actively used body parts will cause more rapid absorption. These factors all must be considered when preparing the diabetetic athlete for participation.

Special Questions for Female Athletes

Some specific questions should be added to the evaluation of female athletes:

- First menstrual period?
- Last menstrual period?
- Longest time between periods last year?
- How much would you like to weigh?
- Have you ever tried diet or weight loss techniques?
- How much do you exercise?
- Do you have a history of a stress fracture?

Normal menstrual cycles occur regularly every 25 to 38 days. Oligomenorrhea is the term for cycles occurring inconsistently (fewer than 9 per year). Amenorrhea is the cessation of the reproductive cycle for 4 months or longer. Before amenorrhea can be diagnosed, pregnancy must be excluded. Up to one third of competitive college long-distance runners have significant menstrual disorders. Some of the many factors that effect menstrual function are decreased body fat, lower body weight, nutrient imbalance, physical and emotional stress, and alterations of hormone concentrations from disturbance of the hypothalamic-pituitary axis. Although there are typically no lasting or irreversible effects of amenorrhea on fertility,

there is a problem with skeletal demineralization in hypoestrogenic women. The loss of bone mass resulting from this condition is not completely reversible. An increased incidence of stress fractures of long bones and feet has been reported, but an exact causal relationship has not yet been defined. Menstrual disorders may serve as a clue to concomitant eating disorders, as can a large discrepancy between the athlete's desired weight and actual weight. Athletes competing in endurance sports, activities with weight classes, or in which judging may be influenced by appearance are at higher risk for developing the female athlete triad, which involves interrelated disordered eating, amenorrhea, and osteopenia. This is discussed in more detail in Chapter 17.

Drug Use, Psychological Problems, and Confidential Matters

The PPE may not allow time for discussion of sensitive matters. However, since athletes in the adolescent age range may participate in a number of high-risk behaviors, the physician with adequate rapport should make appropriate inquiries about lifestyle. Alcohol is the most commonly abused substance, followed by marijuana, cocaine, amphetamines, and anabolic steroids. Both cigarettes and smokeless tobacco are known to cause lung and oral cancer, as well as many other significant problems, and their use should be discouraged. Steroid use causes many side effects including liver damage, testicular atrophy, menstrual cycle irregularities, and increased LDL cholesterol; it has also been associated with sudden cardiac death.

Unstable home situations can be discovered through careful questioning, and, when extreme, follow-up evaluation should be arranged with social service agencies. Many athletes have questions about common medical subjects, such as acne or obesity. These remain sensitive issues to teenagers and are more easily addressed at a single-examiner PPE, rather than in a group setting. In general, the more significant psychological and personal issues are more likely to be brought to the team physician, who is with the athletes frequently enough to gain their confidence, rather than to a physician performing a one-time PPE. The history can include the question: Is there anything you would like to discuss with the doctor?

THE PHYSICAL EXAMINATION

Two primary formats have been used for performing the physical examination, the "station" method and the "private office" setting. The station method uses several examiners, each focusing on a specific aspect of the physical evaluation. Although there are advantages and disadvantages for both settings, the end result of evaluation is the same: a disqualification rate of approximately 1%. For this reason physicians may choose a personal examination if they are hoping to establish rapport and follow the athlete during the season, or a station format if they wish to efficiently screen large numbers of athletes. Ultimately, the type of format used will be based on the availability of resources in the community and the preference of the individual physicians.

The scope of the examination varies by the intent of the examiner. The physician who is also the athlete's primary care physician may often perform a comprehensive physical examination as part of an overall health screening. Since the primary reason for a PPE is to allow safe sports activity, physicians with limited ongoing contact with the athlete should generally choose a screening exam that focuses on detecting the main problems that might interfere with participation or make participation unwise. No data in the under-21 age group suggests that a comprehensive exam provides any greater reduction in injury or death (7). Whatever the scope of the physical examination, areas of concern identified in the history merit more careful assessment.

General Appearance

Overall body habitus can be a predictor of abnormalities for the examiner. For example, particularly tall, thin individuals may encourage the examiner to consider Marfan's syndrome. Marfan's is an autosomal dominant inherited connective tissue disorder that may not present fully until adolescence or early adulthood. One of the manifestations of this disease is an increased risk of aortic dissection, which may be missed unless aortic regurgitation is present on auscultation (8). Thus, if two of the following features are noted, further evaluation should be undertaken: family history of Marfan's, a cardiovascular abnormality, arm span greater than height, or ocular abnormality (dislocated or ectopic lens).

If an athlete looks particularly thin, the physician may look for stigmata that suggest an eating disorder. This is particularly true in sports in which physical shape and size are part of the judging of competition, such as gymnastics, diving, and figure skating. Studies have shown a 15% to 62% prevalence of pathologic eating disorders in female athletes (9). Affect should also be noted, as gross aberrancies might signify depression or drug use (cocaine, steroids, etc.).

Vital Signs

While elevations in blood pressure may be due to anxiety regarding the exam, these heightened levels should return to within normal after a brief period of quiet rest. Repeated elevations in blood pressure warrant follow-up and evaluation. Improper cuff size can lead to inaccurate measurements, particularly in large individuals. Upper limits of blood pressure should be adjusted for age and size to determine the levels that require further evaluation. For example, a blood pressure of 135/91 qualifies as severe hypertension for a 10- to 12-year old and 145/93 exceeds the 99th percentile for a 13- to 15-year-old (10). The blood pressure should be obtained in the right arm with the antecubital fossa at the level of the heart to best correspond with standardized tables. Elevation of temperature, pulse, or respirations might raise suspicion of current illness or use of certain medications.

Eyes, Nose, Throat

Snellen charts can be used to screen visual acuity. While poor acuity is not necessarily a disqualifying condition, it may explain poor performance in many sports. Similarly, noting the use of glasses or contacts may be of value as poor vision could place an athlete at risk in sports such as baseball where the ball could strike the individual's head. Athletes rendered unconscious may need contacts removed.

Unless dictated by a history of concussion or other neurologic condition, the only other essential components of the eye exam include appearance and pupil equality. Anisocoria (unequal pupil size) may be either pathologic or physiologic. Awareness of baseline anisocoria is important in the event of a head injury and, if present, this information should be made available to the trainer and/or coach for use in onfield assessment. In an athlete with a history of long-standing diabetes mellitus, a more extensive ocular evaluation, including fundoscopy, is warranted.

Screening of the nose or throat is not a routine part of the physical evaluation of athletes. However, dental problems are among the leading reasons that athletes miss training, as well as seek care at major competitions like the Olympic Games. When time allows, a brief examination of the mouth may identify treatable problems. Similarly, nasal examination may help detect stigmata of allergic rhinitis, and in the individual with breathing difficulties, the exam may reveal a deviated septum. Concerns revealed by the history would lead to the inclusion of either of these examinations.

Cardiovascular Examination

Sudden cardiac death (SCD) is estimated to occur 10 to 25 times per year in the United States in individuals under the age of 30 (11) and represents 85% of all sudden deaths in athletes (4). Major causes of SCD are often divided into those occurring in young athletes (less than age 30) versus those in older athletes. Anatomic abnormalities are the primary etiology in those less than age 30, with hypertrophic cardiomyopathy causing 36% to 50% of deaths (the number of black athletes in this group is disproportionately larger: 48% vs 26% of deaths, $P = 0.01$) (4,12,13). And even though studies point out that a cardiac examination does not efficiently or accurately identify individuals at risk of SCD, a thorough cardiac examination is one of the key aspects of the physical examination and should be included regardless of the format. (12,13). Table 60-1 shows a list of common causes of SCD in young athletes (14).

Many athletes show changes related to conditioning that lead to what has been termed "athletic heart." This manifests on examination as physical, electrocardiographic, radiographic, and echocardiographic evidence of enlargement.

Table 60-1 Causes of Sudden Death During Exertion in Young Subjects	
COMMON	**UNCOMMON**
Hypertrophic cardiomyopathy	Myocarditis
Anomalous coronary artery origin and course	Aortic stenosis
	Mitral valve prolapse
Atherosclerotic coronary artery disease	Right ventricular dysplasia
Aortic rupture (Marfan's syndrome)	Conduction system abnormalities
Idiopathic concentric left ventricular hypertrophy	Amyloidosis
	Sarcoidosis
	Cardiac tumors

Furthermore, endurance athletes may show effects of increased vagal tone as evidenced by resting bradycardia and first degree and second degree AV block. ST segment changes typical of early repolarization and precordial T wave inversion are frequent. Systolic ejection murmurs may result from the increase in stroke volume associated with bradycardia. Benign murmurs tend to be accentuated in the supine position, so evaluation is best done in the sitting position. Inspection, palpation, and auscultation should be performed, with auscultation taking place in a quiet room.

Identification of pathologic murmurs is the goal of auscultation during the PPE. Systolic murmurs louder than grade 3 and any diastolic murmur are considered abnormal. A murmur suggestive of HCM requires specific physical examination approaches. The murmur of HCM may be variable, but is characterized as systolic, heard best at the left sternal border, sometimes intermittent in character, and increased with Valsalva and standing while decreased with squatting. These changes can be explained by the murmur, which is accentuated when the left ventricular end diastolic volume (LVEDV) is decreased (standing, Valsalva) but becomes softer with increased return and elevated LVEDV (squatting, lying). In murmurs of aortic stenosis as well as benign murmurs, the converse is true. If these changes are observed, further workup including an electrocardiogram (ECG) and chest X-ray are warranted.

ECG criteria that suggest HCM but that are absent in the athletic heart syndrome include: superior QRS complex axis deviation; anterior displacement of electrical forces; absence of normal septal Q waves; presence of deep Q waves, or a QS pattern, and deeply inverted T waves in the precordial leads; and exercise-reversible ST elevation and T wave changes (15). Abnormalities on ECG or chest x-ray suggest the need for echocardiography. Diagnostic criteria for HCM include: 1) an LV that is hypertrophied but not dilated in absence of systemic disease, 2) an intraventricular septum or left free wall thickness of >15 mm, and 3) a septal to LV free wall ratio greater than 1.3.

Gender and racial differences may influence the response of the myocardium to athletic training (16). Female athletes show marked increases in LV thickness when compared with sedentary individuals of the same sex (17), but not to the same degree as the change seen in men (18). Because the pathologic changes in HCM are similar for women and men, differentiation of pathologic changes versus athletic heart in women is not clinically as difficult (19). No clinical outcome studies to date indicate that the echocardiogram should be used as a screening tool and as such testing remains reserved for those who appear to be at higher risk.

A midsystolic click, particularly if associated with a midsystolic murmur, increases the likelihood of mitral valve prolapse. Absence of a femoral pulse or asymmetry when compared to the radial pulse is a good screen for coarctation of the aorta. A fixed, split S2 raises the concern for atrial septal defect.

Musculoskeletal Examination

The orthopedic evaluation arguably is the most important aspect of the examination portion of the PPE (7), and yields the highest number of abnormalities (20). Garrick et al have proposed the "2-minute musculoskeletal screening exam" or the 13-point musculoskeletal screening exam (21). Critical evaluation of the 2-minute exam has shown the overall sensitivity to be approximately 50% (22) when compared with thorough orthopedic evaluations. Considering the high risk of orthopedic injury in many sports, a joint-specific exam with sport-specific emphasis seems more appropriate. This exam, with practice, can be completed in a short time. Given that evidence shows that most injuries are actually reinjuries, and that joint laxity or instability leads to an increased risk of further injury, a thorough assessment of joints most commonly injured seems warranted. Specifically recommended are evaluation of the shoulder, knee, and ankle, as these are the most commonly injured areas and are pertinent to all sports.

Shoulder

The most common sports problems of the shoulder are: acromio-clavicular (AC) joint injury; instability from prior dislocation or subluxation; and rotator cuff tendonitis, impingement, or tear. The rotator cuff is a musculotendinous unit comprised of the supraspinatus, infraspinatus, teres minor, and subscapularis muscles (23). Assessment of the shoulder should begin with inspection, looking for deltoid atrophy and/or other asymmetry as the patient faces the examiner. The patient then, with elbows at sides, flexes the elbows 90° with the hands in the neutral position. The patient is then instructed to internally rotate (subscapularis), externally rotate (infraspinatus and teres minor), flex (biceps strength), and extend (triceps strength) against resistance. The three heads of the deltoid can also be assessed in this position by resisted shoulder motions of forward flexion, abduction, and extension.

The patient then performs the "empty the can" maneuver to assess the supraspinatus (abduction of the shoulder to 90°, forward flexion to 45°, and internal rotation). The supraspinatus tendon is the most frequently injured aspect of the rotator cuff. This can primarily be attributed to the anatomy of the area, as the tendon travels through the supraspinatus fossa of the scapula through a "tunnel" with the acromion above, coracoid below, and the coracoacromial ligament spanning the gap. Additionally, the tendon has a "critical zone" created by an area of hypovascularization near the humeral insertion of the supraspinatus. During overhead movements of the arm, this outlet is considerably narrowed and can cause impingement and repetitive microtrauma, particularly to a swollen tendon. Pain on this screening maneuver suggests clinical problems. In addition, significant weakness to elevation or the initiation of abduction may suggest a true rotator cuff tear (rare in younger athletes).

Shoulder instability and specifically anterior laxity can be assessed by the "bye-bye" test. This is performed by having the patient abduct to 90°, then externally rotate the arm as anterior pressure is applied to the posterior surface of the humeral head. A positive test consists of apprehension or pain with this maneuver. This is more sensitive for anterior instability, and the yield is increased when the anterior force is applied while in the 90/90 position (24). Downward traction and notation of a "dimple" just beneath the acromion suggests inferior laxity.

The AC joint is palpable and direct tenderness or pain on a cross-over test may indicate AC joint pathology. A previous AC joint dislocation may lead one AC joint to appear asymetrically elevated.

Knee

The knee is the most frequently injured joint in athletics. (7,25) Evaluation of the knee begins with visual inspection of the quadriceps with the patient in the supine position. Muscle atrophy can be a sign of significant knee pathology, and specifically wasting of the vastus medialis oblique can be a contributor to lateral knee pain and patellar tracking problems. Ballottement of the patella indicates effusion, and contraction of the quadriceps with compression of the patella can indicate patellofemoral syndrome pain.

Stress applied to the varus and valgus to assess the collateral ligaments should be performed with the knee in full extension and at 20° to 30° of flexion to assess the superficial and deep bands of the ligaments. Lachman's test can then be performed to assess the integrity/laxity of the anterior cruciate ligament (ACL). Pathology of this ligament is the most common cause of serious problems. While the Lachman's test is more sensitive and specific of ACL laxity or disruption, many still perform the anterior drawer test. When used, the anterior drawer should be performed with the knee in 30° of flexion so as not to give a false-negative result secondary to restraint of anterior translation by the hamstrings. While finding serious pathology in an asymptotic athlete with no history of knee trauma is rare, many conditions such as patellofemoral syndrome (PFSS), iliotibial band syndrome (ITBS), or structural ligament laxity can be referred to a trainer or physical therapist for appropriate strengthening and conditioning.

Ankle

The ankle is the most commonly injured joint in soccer and basketball and the second most commonly injured joint in all sports. The mechanism of injury is the key to many athletic injury diagnoses and this is particularly true in the ankle. In general, a "rule of 80s" applies to the ankle: 80% of ankle injuries are sprains, 80% of sprains are inversion, and 80% of inversion sprains affect the anterior talofibular (ATF) ligament. Assessment of complete disruption or laxity of this ligament can be done by performing the drawer test. The principal is the same as that of the anterior drawer for the knee, in which an attempt is made to "slide" the foot forward with respect to the shin. The drawer test has been found to have a low positive predictive value. The talar tilt test can also be performed but is much more difficult for those not used to performing the maneuver. Essentially, a varus stress of one ankle may reveal significantly more tilting of the talus than is noted on the opposite side. A functional assessment can be made by having the athlete stand and walk on "tiptoes" and then walk on the lateral edge of the feet. Pain or apprehension of either of these warrants more specific testing.

When a player sprains his or her ankle, a loss of proprioception takes place along with the ligamentous disruption. This "position sense" is important in causing muscular "bracing" of the ankle when placed in positions that can lead to injury. The best means of assessing this is by having the patient stand on one foot with his or her eyes closed, and watching for inability to maintain the position. If this is found, ankle strengthening and proprioceptive training should

be undertaken, and the degree of instability should guide the physician in the use of prophylactic bracing.

Additional Musculoskeletal Assessment

Additional musculoskeletal assessment can be used for sport-specific emphasis. For example, evaluation of the elbow and wrist may need to be performed on gymnasts. The necks of divers and football players should be assessed for stability and strength (also atlantoaxial instability is noted in 10% to 20% of patients with Down's syndrome). The back should be checked for scoliosis, particularly in young girls presenting for their first athletic evaluation. In addition to back inspection, extension and flexion should be assessed in gymnasts, as there is an increased risk of spondylolysis/spondylolisthesis in these athletes. Running athletes need more careful assessment of the foot to assess arch height, Morton's foot, and other anatomic changes associated with overpronation such as forefoot varus and hell valgus.

Lungs, Abdomen, Genitourinary Tract, Skin and Neurologic Examination

These components have a limited role in the PPE unless specifically indicated by the athlete's history. Clearly, the athlete with concussion in the past 12 months merits a thorough neurologic examination. An athlete with a history of hemoglobinopathy or recent mononucleosis might have splenomegaly, which can sometimes be found on examination. Wrestlers need a skin examination as infectious rashes affect participation. Screening for a single testicle or testicular mass could prove embarassing for the athlete, but in appropriately chaperoned and private settings may be included in an examination in which the examiner thinks this is needed. Studies of PPEs have not demonstrated the utility of testicular examination in detecting testicular cancer even though this seems like a logical preventive health service.

Tanner Staging

Age has been the stratifying criteria for athletes for many years. However, there are several studies that support using maturity assessment in the PPE (26). Proponents of maturity assessment believe that it more accurately reflects physical potential, and thus matching athletes of the same maturity level will decrease the incidence of injury and allow more psychological benefit for the immature athlete. Conversely, other studies have shown that in several sports there is actually an increase in the number of injuries with increasing age and thus Tanner stage. Because there is no definitive data supporting the use of Tanner staging, this type of classification to stratify athletes is not currently used. Physicians may wish to use this information to counsel athletes in choosing a sport, but should not use it as a disqualifier from competition.

If Tanner staging is to be used, there is evidence that athletes need not be subjected to the embarrassment of physician assessment of development especially when the exam is conducted in an open "station" manner. Duke et al (27) examined the ability of 43 girls, aged 9 to 17, and 23 boys, aged 11 to 18, to assess themselves according to the Tanner stages. The self-ratings correlated well with ratings by an examining physician. Kreipe et al investigated handgrip strength and the ability to self-assess Tanner stages in 364 male adolescents. They reported a moderately high correlation ($r = .788$) between self-assessed and physician-assessed Tanner staging. A grip strength of less than 55 lb (24.9 kg) was used to denote immaturity. A high correlation ($r = .803$) between grip strength and physician-assessed Tanner stage was recorded.

LABORATORY AND OTHER SCREENING TESTING

For high school athletes, screening tests such as urinalysis, and complete blood count have not been shown to be cost effective in the PPE (28,29). The urinalysis often shows protein-uria, but the workup of this in the PPE population has not led to detection of serious renal pathology. Anemia, an essential component of the "female triad," is best followed by the athlete's regular physician, and screening should thus be performed during an annual exam. If the athlete complains of fatigue or excessively heavy menstruation, a complete blood count would be appropriate as a directed test.

For collegiate athletes, who typically are away from their usual primary care physician, complete blood counts and urinalysis may be part of their yearly evaluation and used to monitor other general health concerns.

The role of other laboratory screening has yet to be defined. Lipid profiles in individuals with a family history of early cardiovascular disease or fasting glucose levels in overweight athletes with a positive family history of diabetes mellitus may ultimately prove reasonable tests, but no data supports this currently. More debate exists over the use of urine drug screens, and testing HIV and hepatitis B. The risk of spreading HIV through sports contact remains infinitessimally small. Hepatitis B virus spread through contact sport poses minimal risk, although the disease is more contagious than HIV and one case of sports-related spread has occurred. Current efforts focus on encouraging athletes to receive hepatitis B immunization. Drug use, on the other hand, is common, but the ethical consideration of random testing raises serious medical, legal, and confidentiality issues. Drug testing at championship competitions now commonly occurs, but few high schools or colleges mandate testing.

Extensive work has been done to review the cost effectiveness and benefit of both ECG and echocardiography in the screening exam (12,30,31). While very sensitive for LVH and arrhythmias, the number of significant findings on ECG is minimal. Echocardiography is both sensitive and specific in diagnosing HCM. Drawbacks to echocardiography are cost and studies that have found no increased number of athletes who would be disqualified when echocardiography is used as a screening exam.

Exercise-induced asthma is a common medical condition in athletes. Exercise challenges with serial peak flows combined with history effectively identify many affected athletes. Mass screening tests for this condition do take time to perform, so unless a study shows utility and cost effectiveness in evaluating all athletes, screening will likely remain selective for those individuals with a suggestive history.

Strength and flexibility testing as well as Vo_2 max and even gait analysis may all provide useful information to coaches and trainers. However, none of these measures would likely influence whether an athlete could compete. Thus, while some mass screens may include stations for performing these measures, they do not constitute a core evaluation needed for the PPE.

CLEARANCE FOR SPORTS PARTICIPATION

At the conclusion of the examination process the physician must make a determination as to whether the athlete can compete without restriction; after specific therapy; or should not participate at all. For the vast majority of athletes this decision is straightforward. In fact, the disqualification rate in this young, physically active group of individuals averages approximately 1%. With this in mind, if the physician thinks an athlete needs disqualification, careful review of the situation seems appropriate. In most instances, referral for specialty evaluation or a second opinion may help make the athlete comfortable with the decision or may point out alternatives short of complete removal from sport.

Typically only approximately 10% of athletes require rehabilitation or medical therapy to compete effectively. Decision making in this group requires knowledge of the demands of the sport and the physiologic consequences of the particular injury or disease. In general, the physician determines if a given injury is likely to worsen by participation or whether the problem makes the athlete prone to a secondary, perhaps more serious injury. In case of illness the considerations include whether the sport places the athlete at undue risk or the activity could worsen control of the disease. Another important concern is the likelihood of spread of a contagious disease and the protection of other athletes from harm.

In most cases, athletes can continue modified activity until adequate rehabilitation or treatment allows them to return safely to full participation. Sports are classified by intensity, static and dynamic demand as well as by contact and collision risk. Classification of these can be found in tables in the preparticipation monographs produced by several governing medical associations (32,33). Using these, the athlete can choose viable options enabling continued participation at some level. The lifetime benefits of physical conditioning and the psychological benefits to this age group merit every effort to promote ongoing participation rather than disqualification.

SUMMARY

The PPE focuses on promoting safe participation for athletes. Whatever the format of the examination, key components are a careful history (particularly as this relates to sport), an appropriate examination that at minimum gives careful attention to the cardiovascular and musculoskeletal system, and a rational assessment for clearance to participate. A significant number of athletes can be given rehabilitation to help them compete more safely. A small number of individuals, approximately 1%, require disqualification, but more comprehensive evaluation should follow the PPE before finally excluding them from sports activity. Data has not shown that this process results in superior outcomes for athletes. Ongoing research is focused on determining the scope, content, and utility of this process with the hope that we can achieve safer sports participation in the future.

REFERENCES

1. O'Donoghue DH. Treatment of injuries to athletes. Philadelphia: WB Saunders, 1970.

2. Fields KB. Clearing athletes for participation in sports: the North Carolina Medical Society Sports Medicine Committee's recommended examination. North Carolina Med J 1994;55:116–119.

3. Goldberg B, Saraniti A, Witman P, Gavin M, Nicholas JA. Preparticipation sports assessment: an objective evaluation. Pediatrics 1980;66:736–744.

4. Marion BJ, Shirani J, Poliac LC, et al. Sudden death in young competitive athletes. JAMA 1996;276:199–204.

5. Strauss RH. Sports medicine. 2nd ed. Philadelphia: WB Saunders, 1991.

6. Fields KB, Reimer CD. Pulmonary problems in athletes. In: Fields KB, Fricker PA, eds. Medical problems in athletes. Malden, MA: Blackwell Science, 1997:136–150.

7. DuRant RH, Seymore C, Linder CW, Jay S. The preparticipation examination of athletes: comparison of single and multiple examiners. AM J Dis Child 1985;139:657–661.

8. Cantwell JD. Marfan's syndrome: detection and management. Phys Sports Med 1986;14:51–55.

9. Joy E Clark N, Ireland ML, et al. Team management of the female athlete triad. Phys Sports Med 1997;25:95–110.

10. Kaplan NM, Deveraux RB, Miller HS. Task force 4: systemic hypertension. J Am Coll Cardiol 1994;24:845–899.

11. Van Camp SP. Sudden death. Clin Sports Med 1992;11:273.

12. McCaffrey FM, Braden DS, Strong WB. Sudden cardiac death in young athletes. Am J Dis Child 1991;145:177–183.

13. Maron BJ, Roberts WC, McAllister HA. Sudden death in young athletes. Circulation 1980;62:218.

14. Fahrenbach MC, Thompson PD. The preparticipation sports examination: cardiovascular considerations for screening. Cardiol Clin 1992;10:319–328.

15. Oakley GDG. The athletic heart. Cardiol Clin 1987;5:319–329.

16. Lewis JF. Considerations for racial differences in the athlete's heart. Cardiol Clin 1992;10:329–333.

17. Bjornstad H, Smith G, Storstein L, et al. Electrocardiographic and echocardiographic findings in top athletes, athletic students and sedentary controls. Cardiology 1993;82:66–74.

18. George KP, Wolfe LA, Burggraf GW, Norman R. Electrocardiographic and echocardiographic characteristics of female athletes. Med Sci Sports Exerc 1995;27:1326–1370.

19. Pelliccia A, Maron BJ, Culasso F, et al. Athlete's heart in women: echocardiographic characterization of highly trained elite female athletes. JAMA 1996;276:211–215.

20. Rifat SF, Ruffin MT, Gorenflo DW. Disqualifying criteria in a preparticipation sports evaluation. J Fam Pract 1995;41:42–50.

21. Tanji JL. Tracking of elevated blood pressure values in adolescent athletes at a 1-year follow-up. Am J Dis Child 1991;145:665–667.

22. Gomez JE, Landry GL, Bernhart DT. Critical evaluation of the 2-minute orthopedic screening examination. AM J Dis Child 1993;147:1109–1113.

23. Rodgers JA, Crosby LA. Rotator cuff disorders. Am Fam Physician 1996;54:127–134.

24. Speer KP, Hannafin JA, Altchek DW, Warren RF. An evaluation of the shoulder relocation test. Am J Sports Med 1994;22:177–183.

25. Hulse E, Strong WB. Preparticipation for athletics. Pediatr Rev 1987;9:173–182.

26. Caine DJ, Broekhoff J. Maturity assessment: a viable preventative measure against physical and psychological insult to the young athlete? Phys Sports Med 1987;15:67–79.

27. Duke RM, Litt IF, Gross RT. Adolescent's self-assessment of sexual maturation. Pediatrics 1980;66:918–920.

28. Peggs JF, Reinhardt RW, O'Brien JM. Proteinuria in adolescent sports physical examinations. J Fam Pract 1986;22:80–81.

29. Taylor WC III, Lombardo JA. Preparticipation screening of college athletes: value of complete blood count. Phys Sports Med 1990;18:106–118.

30. Weidenbener EJ, et al. Incorporation of screening echocardiography in the preparticipation exam. Clin J Sport Med 1995;5:86–89.

31. Lewis JF, et al. Preparticipation echocardiographic screening for cardiovascular disease in a large, predominantly black population of collegiate athletes. Am J Cardiol 1989;64:1029–1033.

32. AAP Committee on Sports Medicine and Fitness. Medical conditions affecting sports participation. Pediatrics 1994;94:757–760.

33. AAFP, AAP, AMSSM, AOSSM, AOASM. Preparticipation physical evaluation, 2nd ed. Minneapolis, MN: The Physician and Sportsmedicine, 1997:1–49.

Chapter 61

Office-Based Physical Activity Counseling in Healthy Adults

Michael G. Goldstein

Bernardine M. Pinto

Bess H. Marcus

Charles B. Eaton

Lisa M. Menard

Felise Milan

Primary care providers in office-based practice have the potential to play an important role in reducing health risks related to their patients' physical inactivity. This chapter will review: the rationale for promoting physical activity counseling by primary care providers; barriers to the delivery of physical activity counseling by health care providers; results of studies on physical activity counseling in primary care settings; and a recommended approach to patient-centered physical activity counseling in primary care settings.

PHYSICAL ACTIVITY COUNSELING: THE ROLE OF PRIMARY CARE PROVIDERS

Health care settings offer a potentially attractive vehicle for making changes in the levels of physical activity of sedentary individuals because patients visit physicians and other health care providers frequently. Approximately 76% of the US population visit a physician in the course of a year, with an average of 5.3 visits per year (1). Moreover, patients look to physicians for advice regarding preventive behavior. Wallace et al, in a large survey of British patients, reported that 61% of men and 53% of women thought physicians should be definitely or probably interested in their patients' level of exercise (2). Older adults, who are most likely to be sedentary, are especially likely to express a preference for receiving help for exercise adoption from a health professional (3).

In 1996, the United States Preventive Services Task Force (USPSTF) recommended that clinicians counsel all patients to incorporate regular physical activity into their daily routines (4). Though the evidence that clinician counseling can increase physical activity of asymptomatic patients is limited (see discussion below), the recommendation of the USPSTF was based on the proven efficacy of regular physical activity in reducing the risk for coronary heart disease, diabetes, hypertension, and obesity, and the potential impact of physician counseling on patients' levels of physical activity (4). After reviewing the evidence linking moderate physical activity to improved health status, the US Centers for Disease Control and Prevention (CDC) and the American College of Sports Medicine (ACSM) recently recommended that every American adult should accumulate at least 30 minutes of moderate physical activity (e.g., brisk walking, gardening) over the course of most days of the week (5). The USPSTF also recommends that clinicians counsel sedentary patients to engage in moderate-intensity physical activity as an initial goal (4). One of the US Public Health Service's Health Objectives for the Year 2000 is to increase to at least 50% the percentage of primary care providers who appropriately assess and counsel their patients about physical activity (6).

Despite these recommendations and the potential benefits of clinician-delivered counseling, the rate of physical activity counseling in clinical settings is generally low (2,7–10). A survey of a random national sample of 1349 internists found that 48% counseled all their patients about exercise, but only 15% counseled inactive patients for at least 5 minutes at every visit (10). A more recent survey indicated that only 49% of primary care physicians believed that regular daily physical activity was very important for the average patient (11). Moreover, even when providers deliver a message about physical activity, the content and intensity of the counseling is rather limited. In a survey of physicians in Alabama, while 91% of the respondents "encouraged" their patients to participate in regular exercise, 70% did not develop exercise prescriptions and only 23% were familiar with the American College of Sports Medicine guidelines for exercise prescriptions (12). Physicians appear to be even less likely to provide physical activity counseling for asymptomatic patients (29%) than for high-risk patients (64%) (7). Research studies that have surveyed patients report even lower rates of exercise counseling by physicians than those utilizing data from physician self-report (2,9).

BARRIERS TO PHYSICAL ACTIVITY COUNSELING

Barriers to provider involvement in physical activity counseling can be categorized as deficits in knowledge, deficits in skill, attitudinal barriers, and organizational barriers (see Table 61-1) (13,14). While most physicians recognize the importance of health promotion and risk factor reduction, they may not be fully aware of the risks associated with sedentary behavior and the health benefits of increasing physical activity. Moreover, physicians have limited knowledge of behavior change principles and interventions, and they lack knowledge about patient education materials and other resources (15,16). Many physicians rely on simply providing advice because they have inadequate knowledge of effective counseling techniques, including how to enhance motivation and negotiate a specific physical activity plan (15,17–19). Knowledge deficits are accompanied by lack of skills in effective counseling techniques, including assessment skills to make an adequate assessment of the patient's needs, skills to motivate and to assist the patient to change their level of physical activity, and skills to help the patient maintain physical activity over time (19).

Attitudinal barriers to counseling about physical activity among physicians include beliefs that patients don't want to change and a lack of confidence that they can influence patient behavior (15). Lack of confidence is also a function of a tendency to measure success by final outcomes, rather than recognizing that lasting behavior change occurs only after multiple trials and through intermediate steps. Provider attitudes are also shaped by the prevailing model in medicine, the biomedical model, which emphasizes a focus on diagnosis and treatment of disease and undervalues the influence of behavior on health and disease. Medical education for physicians has generally neglected training in patient education and counseling skills, and traditional medical training has not yet adopted a systems-based biopsychosocial model that embraces the role of the patient, family, community, and other social forces in shaping health and illness (20). Finally, providers with negative personal health practices are less likely to counsel patients regarding prevention (10,21).

Organizational barriers to provider involvement in physical activity counseling include limited use of reminder systems and other office systems that enhance the delivery of preventive services, limited reimbursement for counseling and preventive care services, and limited availability of patient education materials and other resources to assist the provider in delivering physical activity counseling (14,16,21–23). Many medical offices are not organized to provide patient education or preventive care services, amidst the competing demands of an office full of sick patients.

These knowledge, skill, attitudinal, and organizational

Table 61-1 Barriers to Health Care Provider Involvement in Physical Activity Counseling

PHYSICIAN BARRIERS
Knowledge Deficit
Risk of sedentary behavior on morbidity and mortality
Guidelines for physical activity counseling
Behavior change theory and principles
Specific physical activity counseling strategies
Resources for patients—materials and programs
Skill Deficit
Interviewing/assessment skills
Patient education skills
Behavioral counseling skills
Maintenance/relapse prevention skills
Beliefs and Attitudes
Patients don't want to change or can't change
Perceived ineffectiveness/lack of confidence in helping patients adhere to change
Emphasis on final outcomes
Disease-oriented biomedical approach
Provider-centered, directive style
Moralistic view of behavior problems
Poor personal health habits
Dearth of role models practicing preventive care
ORGANIZATIONAL BARRIERS
Limited use of office systems/reminders that enhance delivery of preventive counseling
Limited reimbursement for patient education and preventive counseling
Poor coordination with self-help and behavioral treatment programs
Limited involvement of office staff in patient education/ health promotion activities

Adapted from Goldstein MG, Ruggiero L, Guise BJ, Abrams DB. Behavioral medicine strategies for medical patients. In: Stoudemire A, ed. Clinical psychiatry for medical students. Philadelphia: JB Lippincott, 1994: 671–693, and Goldstein MG, DePue J, Kazura A, Niaura R. Models for provider-patient interaction: applications to health behavior change. In: Shumaker SA, Scheon EB, Ockene JK, McBee WL, eds. The handbook of health behavior change. 2nd ed. New York: Springer, 1998:85–113.

---

barriers need to be addressed in efforts to enhance the delivery of physical activity interventions in primary care settings.

RESULTS OF STUDIES ON PHYSICAL ACTIVITY COUNSELING IN PRIMARY CARE SETTINGS

To date, only a few studies have tested whether clinical counseling can improve patients' activity levels. Several studies have examined the effects of a multiple risk factor intervention that included physical activity among the targets for counseling. In the INSURE study, activity counseling was delivered in the context of a multiple risk-factor, physician-delivered intervention (24). In this study, 33.8% of the intervention vs. 24.1% of control patients ($p < .05$) reported starting to exercise (comparisons adjusted for age, gender and location). Though these results are encouraging (i.e., a 40% greater rate of starting to exercise in the intervention group), maintenance of physical activity over time was not assessed.

In a controlled study conducted in a single family medicine practice in Ohio, Kelly et al found improvements in physical activity at 1 month follow-up among patients who received counseling to change several risk behaviors including sedentary behavior (defined as exercising less than two times per week) when compared to patients who did not participate in the study due to scheduling problems (25). The short follow-up and the non-randomized nature of this study limit the importance of these findings. The Johns Hopkins Medicare Preventive Services Demonstration Project evaluated the effects of preventive examinations on smoking, excess alcohol intake, and sedentary lifestyle over 2 years in a sample of over 3000 elderly patients from 3 hospital clinics, 13 community group practices, and 103 office practices (26). Despite adequate compliance (>70% of those who received a preventive exam received counseling on each of the risk behaviors), no significant changes in physical activity occurred in the intervention group when compared to control group after adjusting for several relevant demographic variables.

In a randomized controlled trial conducted by the OXCHECK Study Group in the United Kingdom, the effects of a "general health check" was evaluated. The intervention in the OXCHECK study was provided by nurses trained to use a patient-centered communication model to address cardiovascular disease and cancer risk behaviors including vigorous exercise (27). Evaluation of 2205 intervention patients and 1916 control patients at a 3-year follow-up showed that 70.9% of the control group and 67.6% of the intervention group self-reported vigorous exercise less than once per month. Though the results from this well-designed clinical trial were statistically significant, the clinical relevance of a 3.5% absolute difference in performing vigorous exercise more than once per month is quite limited.

Using a quasi-experimental design to assess the effects of a "health check" by British general practitioners aimed at changing multiple risk factors for prevention of stroke and heart disease, Dowell et al found no effects on self-reported vigorous exercise at 1-year follow-up and actually reported a significant decrease in exercise at the 2-year follow-up in the group that received the health check (28).

In summary, the results of studies that included physical activity counseling by clinicians within a multiple risk-factor intervention suggest some limited short-term effects on physical activity and disappointing long-term benefits.

Several other studies have tested the impact of interventions that focused on physical activity alone. Lewis et al reported that brief physician advice produced an increase in minutes of exercise, but frequency of exercise was not assessed and follow-up was limited to 1 month (29). In a randomized clinical trial known as the Green Prescription trial, the effects of the combination of a written prescription and patient education materials vs. verbal advice alone was evaluated in a convenience sample of 446 sedentary patients from 37 general practices in New Zealand (30). Results at a 6-week follow-up showed significant increases in physical activity in the group that received written advice when compared to the group that received advice alone. At an 11-month follow-up of patients who reported increased activity at 6 weeks, 59% had maintained the increase in physical activity.

In Project PACE (Provider-based Assessment and Counseling for Exercise), 12 physicians provided 3 to 5 minutes of physical activity counseling tailored to the patient's level of activity and readiness to become active (31). Activity counseling was based on the stages of change theory and social cognitive theory. A health educator made a brief booster phone call to patients (mean age = 39) 2 weeks after the initial physician counseling. Ten control physicians were trained in hepatitis B detection. Self-reported physical activity and readiness to adopt/maintain activity were collected at baseline and at 4- and 6-week follow-ups. When compared to patients in the control condition, patients in the intervention condition reported significantly increased minutes walking per week (+40 min/wk vs. +10 min/wk in the control group), and increased readiness to adopt activity (31). Objective activity monitoring (Caltrac electronic accelerometers) on a subsample of subjects confirmed a significant treatment effect. However, the PACE trial had several limitations: physicians were not randomly assigned to conditions; the sample was made up of relatively young patients (mean age = 39); a subsample of the original sample was included in the analyses; and a short-term outcome (6 weeks) was reported.

Using concepts from the transtheoretical model of change, social cognitive theory, and a patient-centered model of provider-delivered counseling (13,14,19), Marcus et al conducted a pilot study that examined the efficacy and feasibility of a physician-delivered physical activity intervention that included counseling, the provision of an exercise prescription, and a physical activity manual that was designed to provide information that was matched to the patient's stage of motivational readiness to engage in regular physical activity (32). Participating physicians were trained in physical activity counseling and reported providing counseling for approximately 5 minutes to eligible patients. The efficacy of the physician-delivered counseling intervention was evaluated by examining self-reports of physical activity using the Physical Activity Scale for the Elderly (PASE) (33) among patients who received counseling vs. a control group of patients who received usual care. Regression analysis showed that at post-treatment, patients in the intervention vs. the control group reported 20% increase in PASE scores. When the dose of the counseling intervention was entered as a variable in a regression model, results showed a significant difference in PASE scores (maximum difference of 31 points) between patients who received all five components of the counseling intervention vs. those who did not receive any counseling (32).

The results of this pilot study led Goldstein et al to test the efficacy of the intervention in patients aged 50 and over in a recently completed randomized controlled trial, Physically Active for Life (PAL) (34). Physicians in 12 intervention practices received training in the delivery of brief physical activity counseling. Subjects in the intervention practices ($n = 181$) received brief activity counseling matched to their stage of motivational readiness, a prescription for physical activity, a patient manual, a follow-up appointment with their physician to discuss activity counseling, and three newsletter mailings. Subjects in the 12 control practices (n = 174) received usual care. Measures of motivational readiness for physical activity and level of physical activity were administered to subjects in both conditions at baseline, 6 weeks after their initial appointment, and at 8 months.

Results of the PAL trial indicate that the intervention was feasible and acceptable to both patients and physicians (35). Intervention physicians evaluated the training session as quite useful and rated the PAL program materials favorably. Intervention physicians also considered that the PAL training and materials improved their ability to provide exercise counseling to their older patients. Comparisons between the two groups showed significant improvements in physician confidence regarding counseling patients about physical activity for intervention group physicians, compared to control physicians ($p < .05$) (35). Process data collected from participating offices indicated that 99% of intervention group patients (n = 181) received counseling at their initial office visit and 77% of these patients returned for a follow-up counseling visit (35). Patient evaluations of the exercise counseling and support materials were also obtained. Ninety-three percent (141/151) of the patients in the intervention group who provided process data at 6 weeks reported receiving activity counseling from their physician during the initial visit and indicated that the physician spent an average of 8.9 minutes (SD 0.19) counseling them about exercise (35). At the 8 month follow-up, patients were asked about the effect of their doctor's attention to physical activity on their satisfaction with care received at the doctor's office. Patients in the intervention group were significantly more likely to report an increase in satisfaction with care compared with the control group ($t = 4.55$, $df = 255$, $p < .01$) (35). Thus, physicians and patients indicated the PAL project offered an acceptable and feasible approach to promote physical activity in older adults. Evaluation of the efficacy of the PAL intervention suggests promising short-term effects on levels of motivational readiness, particularly among those subjects who were least motivated to engage in regular physical activity at baseline (34). However, when compared to usual care, the PAL intervention did not produce significant short-term or long-term increases in levels of physical activity (34). In summary, findings from the PAL study indicate that the intervention was feasible and acceptable to both providers and patients and produced short-term effects on levels of motivational readiness (34). However, these effects did not translate into significant increases in levels of physical activity (34).

Taken together, the results of trials testing the impact of physical activity interventions in primary care settings suggest that these interventions are feasibile and acceptable. Generally, the trials suggest promising short-term effects on levels of physical activity, but no maintenance of these effects. However, both the PACE and PAL trials, which utilized interventions based on the transtheoretical model of change and social cognitive theory, demonstrated positive effects on motivational readiness to engage in regular physical activity. These findings suggest that more comprehensive and intensive interventions may be necessary to achieve lasting physical activity behavior change among sedentary individuals. Such interventions should be based on proven behavior change models and might include: the delivery of counseling by trained ancillary staff; use of written exercise prescriptions and other patient education materials; use of expert computer systems to deliver tailored messages consistent with the patient's stage of motiva-

tional readiness; multiple personal follow-up contacts; and resources to help overcome barriers to adopting regular physical activity (e.g., access to supervised exercise programs).

AN APPROACH TO PATIENT-CENTERED PHYSICAL ACTIVITY COUNSELING IN PRIMARY CARE

Table 61-2 presents an approach to physical activity counseling in primary care that is based on an integration of a generic patient-centered counseling approach (13,14,19), and the application of the transtheoretical model and social cognitive theory to the adoption of regular physical activity (18,36). Cognitive, attitudinal, instrumental, behavioral, and social levels of the counseling process are addressed through a series of questions and statements. This version of the "5A" approach was also adapted from a physician-delivered counseling strategy developed by the Smoking, Tobacco and Cancer Program, Division of Cancer Prevention and Control, National Cancer Institute (37). Though full implementation of this counseling approach would take several minutes, physicians can also utilize a subset of the questions and statements listed in the table if time is limited.

Address the Agenda

The first step is to "Address the agenda." This is done by bringing up the issue of physical activity, but only after the patient's agenda for the visit has been addressed. Patients are more likely to be receptive to discussing physical activity when their specific concerns and questions have already been addressed by the clinician. As noted in the section on barriers earlier in this chapter, physicians and other primary care providers may not be inclined to address physical activity routinely. Even when they plan to bring up physical activity, health care providers may forget to do so. Use of prompts and other office systems (e.g., assessment forms, posters, monitoring forms) can help motivated providers to remember to bring up the issue of physical activity during routine office visits.

Assess

The next step is to determine the patient's current level of physical activity and motivational readiness to become active. Five stages of motivational readiness are identified in the transtheoretical model: precontemplation, contemplation, preparation, action, and maintenance (36,38). The descriptions of the stages of motivational readiness as applied to physical activity are listed in Table 61-3. The results of the assessment of stage of motivational readiness will determine the focus of the clinician's subsequent efforts and establish goals for the outcome of the counseling session. For individuals in the precontemplation or contemplation stage, the goal for the "assist" phase of the counseling is to motivate them to consider increasing their levels of physical activity, while for those in preparation or action, the goal is to provide specific behavioral interventions to assist them to achieve and maintain desired levels of regular physical activity.

If the patient is found to be in the precontemplation or contemplation stage, further assessment of the patient's knowledge, attitudes, beliefs, and fears about making changes

Table 61-2 Physical Activity Counseling Based on a Patient-Centered Approach and the Transtheoretical Model

Address the Agenda
- Attend to patient's agenda
- Express desire to talk about risk factors:
  "I'd like to talk to you about your level of physical activity."
- Define problem:
  "You are ____" (e.g., not physically active)
  "This means ____"

Assess
- Assess patient's current level of physical activity
- Assess and clarify patient's knowledge, beliefs and concerns:
  "What do you know about the benefits of physical activity?"
- Assess and clarify patient's feelings about risk and change in behavior:
  "How do you feel about becoming more physically active?"
- Assess patient's previous experience with change:
  "What have you tried in the past?"
- Assess stage of change and clarify patient's goals:
  "Are you willing to increase your level of activity now?"
  "Are you considering changing your level of activity in a few weeks?"
- Assess pros and cons for change:
  "What reasons do you have for wanting (or not wanting) to become more physically active?"
  "What might get in the way of your becoming physically active?"

Advise
- Provide personalized information regarding risk and benefits of change
- Provide physiologic feedback, when available:
  "Your test results (physical findings, etc.) indicate that ____ is affecting your health. This could be improved by increased levels of physical activity."
- Tell patient that you strongly advise engaging in regular physical activity

Assist
- Provide support, understanding, praise and reinforcement:
  "I can help you by ____"
  "It's often difficult to change from inactivity to activity."
  "I can understand why you might be concerned about injury."

"It's great that you're considering becoming active."
- Describe intervention options
- Negotiate an intervention plan; match intervention to stage of change

For Patients in Precontemplation
- Provide personalized information on health benefits of activity
- Provide personalized messages about risk
- Address feeling and provide support

For Patients in Contemplation
- Praise interest in thinking about becoming active
- Acknowledge and reinforce patient's reasons for wanting to exercise
- Identify remaining barriers to activity
- Help to overcome barriers
- Elicit patient's preferences and negotiate initial steps towards exercise
- Identify available resources and supports
- Write exercise prescription

For Patients in Preparation
- Praise current level of activity
- Reinforce benefits of activity that patient has noted and suggest others
- Identify remaining barriers to activity
- Help to overcome barriers
- Negotiate steps towards achieving a regular exercise program
- Identify available resources and supports
- Write exercise prescription
- Identify potential triggers for relapse and plan response

For Patients in Action and Maintenance
- Praise current level of activity
- Reinforce benefits patient has noted and suggest others
- Encourage self-monitoring and self-reward
- Identify barriers to continued activity
- Problem solve to overcome barriers
- Reinforce use of resources and supports
- Write new exercise prescription

For Follow-Ups
- Assess progress
- Identify barriers, if any
- Negotiate new goals
- Write new exercise prescription

Arrange Follow-up
- Establish time for follow-up visit or call
- Reaffirm plan

Adapted from Pinto B, Goldstein M, Marcus B. Activity counseling by primary care physicians. Prev Med 1998;27:506–513.

in levels of physical activity is quite useful. Assessment of these domains will allow the physician or health care provider to clarify the benefits of physical activity for the patient and correct any misconceptions that the patient might have. For example, if a patient states that she believes that vigorous exercise is necessary to receive health benefits, the clinician could inform the patient about the benefits of moderate levels of physical activity. Patients who express exaggerated fears about injury might be reassured about the safety of a slow, graduated approach to a physical activity program.

Clarification, legitimization, and expressions of support and respect may help the patient to feel understood when fears or concerns are expressed. Examples of these are listed in Table 61-2. When patients express interest in increasing their levels of physical activity, praise and encouragement from the clinician can be quite effective. Provision of empathic responses may help the patient to feel more comfortable talking to the health care provider about his or her behavior and may increase receptivity to offers to help him or her to change (39).

Table 61-3 Stages of Motivational Readiness for Physical Activity

Precontemplation	No physical activity and does not intend to start
Contemplation	No physical activity but intends to start
Preparation	Irregular physical activity
Action	Regular physical activity* for < six months
Maintenance	Regular physical activity for > six months

* Regular physical activity is defined as three or more times per week for at least 20 minutes each time.
Adapted from Marcus BH, Rakowski W, Rossi JS. Assessing motivational readiness and decision-making for exercise. Health Psychol 1992;11:257–261.

Advise

All patients should receive advice. Personalized messages, based on the patient's symptoms and his or her medical and family history, may increase the patient's awareness about the personal hazards of sedentary behavior (cons) and the relevance of the benefits of physical activity (pros). Personalized messages are more likely to move patients closer to action than mini-lectures about the negative health effects of a sedentary lifestyle. Specific feedback on the impact of sedentary behavior on their symptoms, disease state, or risk for future illness may be helpful to enhance motivation to change (39). For example, results from an assessment of bone density may be used to help patients understand their risk for osteoporosis and provide an opportunity to link increased physical activity with reduction in risk.

Assist

"Assist" involves providing further stage-matched interventions (see Table 61-2) for the precontemplator or contemplator, and identification of barriers to change enables the health care provider to explore potential solutions that might then free the patient to seriously consider change. As noted above, an appropriate goal for a patient in precontemplation is to seriously consider increasing their level of physical activity. For contemplation, an appropriate goal is to take small steps toward change. For example, a patient who is not willing to engage in daily 30-minute walks might be willing to park his car a 5-minute walk from the entrance to his workplace. He might also be willing to use stairs rather than an elevator whenever possible. By negotiating intermediate steps toward achieving regular physical activity, the clinician and the patient become engaged in the process of change. At subsequent visits, the clinician can reinforce achievement of these limited goals, and encourage further increases in activity. Primary care providers have the advantage of providing follow-up on interventions over repeated routine visits. When the patient is finally ready to become physically active, appropriate action-oriented strategies can be prescribed. Identification and use of other supports and resources, such as inexpensive, effective self-help manuals, educational materials, and community resources, may also facilitate movement of a precontemplator or contemplator toward change.

Interventions for assisting patients in the preparation or action stage are also listed in Table 61-2. A specific plan is developed by first reviewing options for initiating change and then negotiating with the patient to choose among these options. It is important to elicit the patient's preferences for initial steps toward change. For example, if a patient is willing to begin a program of increased physical activity, the provider may ask the patient to identify those physical activities that the patient has most enjoyed in the past (e.g., bike rides with family members). The provider can then ask the patient to consider resuming this activity while also asking the patient what led them to discontinue it. Problem-solving strategies are utilized to identify and address problems in the implementation of the plan. Patients in the preparation or action stage may benefit from behavioral interventions such as setting a specific target date for beginning a physical activity program, writing a prescription or contract, providing written instructional materials, teaching behavioral skills (e.g., self-monitoring, goal setting, self-reward), and enhancing social support for physical activity. Individuals are likely to be most successful when multiple cognitive and behavioral strategies are utilized when attempting to change behavior (40). Behavioral strategies to enhance adoption of new behaviors are described in detail elsewhere (41). The use of a physical activity or exercise prescription is described in a separate section below.

When physicians and office staff are not able to spend the time necessary to teach specific behavioral skills to patients, self-help materials (provided by government or voluntary agencies) can be used by motivated individuals to learn these techniques. The PACE project has developed self-help materials that are matched to patients' stage of motivational readiness and can be used as self-help material (Project PACE, San Diego State University, 619-594-5949), and the PAL project has developed a patient manual that was specifically developed for older persons. (The PAL manual is not available for dissemination presently. Anyone who is interested in more information can contact the lead author of this chapter for its availability.) The health care provider can also provide motivated patients with referrals to an exercise physiologist, a health educator, or a multidisciplinary behavioral medicine program.

Arrange Follow-up

Arranging follow-up is an essential component to an effective counseling intervention. Once the clinician and patient have developed a plan for addressing physical activity, it is useful to take some time to ask the patient to reaffirm their commitment to the plan and establish a specific time for a follow-up visit or phone call. Patients should also be encouraged to call the provider or a designated office staff person if they develop any problems or new symptoms related to physical activity.

At the follow-up visit, the clinician can again utilize the "5A" approach to assess the patient's adherence to the plan and work with the patient to solve problems and overcome any barriers that have arisen. For patients who were previously in early stages of motivational readiness, reassessment may reveal that they are now ready to take initial steps toward increasing their level of physical activity. Assessment for those who have developed a specific physical activity plan may expose slips or relapses. Relapses or slips, often viewed as failures by the patient, can be reframed as an opportunity for learning and corrective action (42). It is useful for the provider to remind the patient that successful behavior change almost always requires multiple trials. Most importantly, follow-up visits provide an opportunity for the provider to review, reinforce, and praise the patient for his/her efforts and for achieving any of his or her initial goals. At the end of the follow-up session, new goals should be identified and affirmed and a new physical activity prescription can be provided.

USING A PHYSICAL ACTIVITY PRESCRIPTION TO ENHANCE ADOPTION OF PHYSICAL ACTIVITY

As noted in the "Assist" section in the "5A" counseling strategy above, providing the patient with a written physical activity prescription can be a useful way to specify a plan for initiating, changing, or maintaining physical activity. A copy of the prescription, signed by the clinician, can also be saved for the medical record to facilitate monitoring of the physical activity plan. Having the patient sign the prescription may further enhance their commitment. An example of an exercise prescription form is depicted in Table 61-4. Each prescription should specify four components of the physical activity plan: intensity, type, frequency, and time (or duration). These four components can be easily remembered by both providers and patients when the mnemonic FITT is used (43).

Determining the appropriate level of intensity of physical activity is usually the first step in completing the prescription. Physical activity has been defined as "any bodily movement produced by skeletal muscles that results in energy expenditure," (5) while moderate physical activity refers to any activity performed at an intensity of 3 to 6 METS (work metabolic rate/resting metabolic rate) or 4 to 7 kcal/min (5). This level of physical activity can be achieved by most healthy adults by walking briskly (3–4 mph), cycling for pleasure (<10 mph), swimming with moderate effort, pulling a golf cart, mowing the lawn with a power mower, painting, or performing general cleaning at home (5). Moderate activity has also been defined as activity at 50% to 70% of maximum heart rate (220 − age) (44).

In contrast, vigorous activity has been defined as more than 6.0 METs, more than 7 kcal/min, or more than 70% maximum heart rate. For most sedentary patients, a moderate level of physical activity is an appropriate initial goal, especially if they have not engaged in vigorous physical activity in the recent past or if they have a medical condition that would preclude their participation in vigorous activity or require formal exercise testing (5,43,44). As a public health message for the nation, the American College of Sports Medicine, the Centers for Disease Control and Prevention (5), a National Institutes of Health Consensus Panel (45), the US Preventive Services Task Force (4), and the Recent Surgeon Generals' Report on Physical Activity and Health have all recommended that each individual accumulate 30 minutes or more of *moderate*-intensity physical activity on most days of the week. For individuals already engaged in moderate activity, advancement to vigorous activity may be an appropriate goal, while those individuals who have been totally sedentary might be best off starting out with a goal of activity that falls below the level of moderate intensity (e.g., walking slowly, light stationary cycling, or light stretching). As noted in the section above on counseling individuals who are in early stages of motivational readiness, starting out with a low level of intensity of activity can be an effective strategy to motivate an individual to adopt regular physical activity as an eventual goal.

Patients can be taught to monitor the level of intensity of physical activity in several ways, including determining their desired heart rate zone and instructing them to take their pulse rate while exercising using a perceived exertion scale, such as the Borg Perceived Exertion Scale. If patients are able to talk comfortably but get a little sweaty while exercising, this usually indicates that they are within 50% to 75% of their maximum heart rate.

Once the level of intensity of physical activity is decided upon, the other elements of the FITT exercise prescription can be completed. To meet the recommendations of the CDC, ACSM, and USPSTF, the goal for moderate-intensity activity should be five or more days a week and the duration of activity each day should be 30 minutes; for vigorous levels of activity, the goals are 3 sessions of 20 minutes or more (4,5). However, as noted previously, for patients who are not willing to meet the goal for moderate-intensity activity, an appropriate initial goal might be to engage in very short bouts (e.g., 5 to 10 minutes) of activity a few times per week. Such patients might be encouraged to gradually increase the time spent during each session of activity so that they eventually accumulate at least 30 minutes per day. Patients who choose to engage in activities meeting criteria for moderate or vigorous intensity should also be encouraged to spend a few minutes to warm up with stretching exercises or light activity, especially if they are older adults or have been very sedentary. Finally, the type of activity chosen for the exercise prescription should be based on several criteria: something the patient enjoys; an activity that was previously engaged in on a regular basis; an activity that can be easily integrated into daily routine (e.g., walking during lunch break, housework, yard work); an activity that meets social or recreational needs or goals (e.g., sports, dancing); and an activity that can be performed safely or under supervision (e.g., walking clubs, use of a fitness facility).

Table 61-4 Exercise Prescription

Suggested Program (FITT)

Frequency: _____ times per week

Intensity: _____ moderate _____ vigorous

Type: _____ activity type

Time: _____ minutes per session

Comments:
_____

_____   _____
          Signature   Date

The prescription plan may also specify a variety of activities that can be combined to meet the overall goal for frequency and duration.

The use of an exercise or physical activity prescription facilitates the behavior change process in a number of ways. First, it sets a specific physical activity goal for the patient. Second, like other prescriptions written by the health provider, it conveys the importance of physical activity to the patient and builds on the influence and authority of the health care provider. Third, it gives the health care provider something concrete and tangible to do to address the problem of sedentary behavior. Fourth, the process of completing the prescription facilitates the development of a mutually agreed-upon plan for addressing physical activity. The prescription, if also signed by the patient, serves as a written contract between patient and provider that may enhance the patient's adherence to the plan. Finally, if a copy of the prescription is saved in the chart, it can be used during subsequent visits to review the patient's progress.

REFERENCES

1. National Center for Health Statistics. Health, United States, 1989. Washington, DC: U.S. Department of Health and Human Services, 1990.

2. Wallace P, Brennan P, Haines A. Are general pactitioners doing enough to promote health lifestyle? findings of the Medical Research Council's general practice research framework study on lifestyle and health. BMJ 1987;294:940–942.

3. Booth M, Bauman A, Owen N, Gore C. Physical activity preferences, preferred sources of assistance, and perceived barriers to increased activity among physically inactive Australians. Prev Med 1997;26:131–137.

4. U.S. Preventive Services Task Force. Guide to clinical preventive services, 2nd ed. Baltimore: Williams and Wilkins, 1996.

5. Pate R, Pratt M, Blair S, et al. Physical activity and public health: a recommendation from the Centers for Disease Control and Prevention, and the American College of Sports Medicine. JAMA 1995;271:402–407.

6. US Department of Health and Human Services. Healthy people 2000: national health promotion and disease prevention objectives. Washington, DC: US Department of Health and Human Services, Public Health Service, 1990.

7. Rosen M, Logson D, Demak M. Prevention and health promotion in primary care: baseline results on physicians from the INSURE project on lifecycle preventive health services. Prev Med 1984; 13:535–548.

8. Lewis C, Wells K, Ware J. A model for predicting the counseling practices of physicians. J Gen Intern Med 1986;1:14–19.

9. Lewis CE. Disease prevention and health promotion practices of primary care physicians in the United States. Am J Prev Med 1988;4:9–16.

10. Lewis CE, Clancy C, Leake B, Schwartz JS. The counseling practices of internists [see comments]. Ann Intern Med 1991; 114:54–58.

11. Wechsler H, Gevine S, Idelson R, et al. The physician's role in health promotion revisited—a survey of primary care practitioners. N Engl J Med 1996; 334:996–998.

12. Williford H, Barfield B, Lazenby R, Olson M. A survey of physicians' attitudes and practices related to exercise promotion. Prev Med 1992;21:630–636.

13. Goldstein M, DePue J, Kazura A, Niaura R. Models for provider-patient interaction: applications to health behavior change. In: Shumaker SA, Scheon EB, Ockene JK, McBee WL, eds. The handbook of health behavior change. 2nd ed. New York: Springer, 1998:85–113.

14. Goldstein MG, Ruggiero L, Guise BJ, Abrams DB. Behavioral medicine strategies for medical patients. In: Stoudemire A, ed. Clinical psychiatry for medical students. Philadelphia: JB Lippincott, 1994:671–693.

15. Orleans CT, George LK, Houpt JL, Brodie KH. Health promotion in primary care: a survey of U.S. family practitioners. Prev Med 1985;14:636–647.

16. Kottke TE, Blackburn H, Brekke ML, Solberg LI. The systematic practice of preventive cardiology. Am J Cardiol 1987;59:690–694.

17. Lazare A, Putnam S, Lipkin MJ. Three functions of the medical interview. In: Lipkin MJ, Putnam S, Lazare A, eds. The medical interview: clinical care, education, research. New York: Springer-Verlag, 1995:3–19.

18. Pinto B, Goldstein M, Marcus B. Activity counseling by primary care physicians. Prev Med 1998;27: 506–513.

19. Grueninger U, Duffy F, Goldstein M. Patient education in the medical encounter: how to facilitate learning, behavior change and coping. In: Lipkin MJ, Putnam S, Lazare A, eds. The medical interview: clinical care, education, research. New York: Springer-Verlag, 1995:122–133.

20. Taylor VM, Taplin SH, Urban N, et al. Medical community involvement in a breast cancer screening promotional project. Public Health Rep 1994;109:491–499.

21. Frank E, Kunovich-Frieze T. Physicians' prevention counseling behaviors: current status and future directions. Prev Med 1995; 24:543–545.

22. McPhee SJ, Detmer WM. Office-based interventions to improve delivery of cancer prevention services by primary care physicians. Cancer 1993;72:1100–1112.

23. Pommerenke FA, Dietrich A. Improving and maintaining preven-

tive services: part 1: applying the patient path model [published erratum appears in J Fam Pract 1992;34:398]. J Fam Pract 1992; 34:86–91.

24. Logsdon D, Lazaro C, Meier R. The feasibility of behavioral risk reduction in primary care. Am J Prev Med 1989;22:110–121.

25. Kelly R. Controlled trial of a time-efficient method of health promotion. Am J Prev Med 1988;4: 200–207.

26. Burton L, Paglia M, German P, et al. The effect among older persons of a general preventive visit on three health behaviors: smoking, excessive alcohol drinking, and sedentary lifestyle. Prev Med 1995;24:492–497.

27. Imperial Cancer Research Fund OXCHECK Study Group. Effectiveness of health checks conducted by nurses in primary care: final results of the OXCHECK study. BMJ 1995;310:1099–1104.

28. Dowell A, Ochera J, Hilton S, et al. Prevention in practice: results of a 2-year follow-up of routine health promotion interventions in general practice. Fam Pract 1996; 13:357–362.

29. Lewis B, Lynch W. The effect of physician advice on exercise behavior. Prev Med 1993;22:110–121.

30. Swinburn B, Walter L, Arroll B, et al. The Green Prescription Study: a randomized controlled trial of exer-

cise prescription in general practice. Am J Public Health 1998; 88:288–291.

31. Calfas K, Long B, Sallis J, et al. A controlled trial of physician counseling to promote the adoption of physical activity. Prev Med 1996; 25:225–233.

32. Marcus B, Goldstein M, Jette A, et al. Training physicians to conduct physical activity counseling. Prev Med 1997;26:382–388.

33. Washburn R, Smith K, Jette A, Janney C. The physical activity scale for the elderly (PASE): development and evaluation. J Clin Epidemiol 1993;48:153–162.

34. Goldstein M, Pinto B, Marcus B, et al. Physician-based activity counseling for middle-aged and older adults: a randomized trial. Ann Behav Med 1999 (in press).

35. Pinto B, Goldstein M, DePue J, Milan F. Acceptability and feasibility of physician-based counseling: The PAL Project. Am J Prev Med 1998;15:95–102.

36. Marcus B, Simkin L. The stages of exercise behavior. J Sports Med 1993;33:83–88.

37. Glynn TJ, Manley MW. How to help your patients stop smoking: a National Cancer Institute manual for physicians. Bethesda, MD: Smoking, Tobacco and Cancer Program, Division of Cancer Prevention and Control, National Cancer Institute, 1989. NIH publication no. 89–3064.

38. Marcus B, Rakowski, Rossi J. Assessing motivational readiness and decision-making for exercise. Health Psychol 1992;11:257–261.

39. Miller WR, Rolnick S, Motivational interviewing: preparing people to change addictive behavior. New York: Guilford, 1991.

40. Marcus B, Rossi J, Selby V, et al. The stages and processes of exercise adoption and maintenance in a worksite sample. Health Psychol 1992;11:386–395.

41. Russell M. Behavioral counseling in medicine: strategies for modifying at-risk behavior. New York: Oxford University Press, 1986.

42. Marlatt G, Gordon J. Relapse prevention. New York: Guilford, 1985.

43. American College of Sports Medicine. Guidelines for exercise testing and prescription. 4th ed. Philadelphia: Lea and Febiger, 1991.

44. U.S. Department of Health and Human Services. Physical activity and health: a report of the Surgeon General. Atlanta, GA: U.S. Department of Health and Human Services, Centers for Disease Control and Prevention, National Center for Chronic Disease Prevention and Promotion, 1996.

45. NIH Consensus Development Panel on Physical Activity and Cardiovascular Health. Physical activity and cardiovascular health. JAMA 1996;276:241–246.

Chapter 62

Exercise Prescription for Patients with Chronic Health Problems

Carol Ewing Garber

Most patients can benefit significantly from a program of regular physical activity, and physician attention to this important heart disease risk factor can greatly influence patient behavior and health outcomes (1). While referral to a clinical exercise physiologist or a medically based exercise rehabilitation program may be optimal for most patients with chronic disease, this is often not possible due to lack of reimbursement or unavailability of trained personnel or facilities. This chapter will present some background information concerning exercise prescription followed by a simple approach for providing physician-delivered exercise prescription within the office setting.

RECOMMENDATIONS FOR PHYSICAL ACTIVITY

Public health experts recommend 30 minutes or more of physical activity of at least moderate intensity on most days of the week for most adults (2–4). The public health emphasis on daily moderate activity for all has been advocated because adherence to moderate activity is higher and because of the numerous health benefits associated with regular participation in moderate activity, including the reduction of cardiovascular disease (CVD) risk and CVD risk factors (hypertension, obesity, HDL cholesterol) and other important health benefits (5–7). Since more than 50% of American adults are sedentary, there are many reasons to utilize this approach to improving physical activity (2).

The health and fitness benefits attained by participation in physical activity are dose related (2). Thus, many additional benefits can be realized by adding a program of vigorous physical activity that will result in improvements in physical fitness (2–4,8).

Improving physical fitness should be considered an eventual goal for most patients (8–10). Guidelines for improving fitness are discussed in more detail below (8–10). The best approach for a particular patient will be determined by the patient's health status, attitudes about physical activity, current and previous history of physical activity, and personal goals for a program of physical activity.

SCREENING FOR EXERCISE

Prior to initiating a program of regular exercise, it is important to screen for contraindications to exercise and to obtain clinical information relevant to developing the exercise prescription. Patients who are not medically stable or whose condition can be exacerbated by exercise should delay embarking on an exercise-training program. Contraindications to exercise training are listed in Table 62-1. Patients who present with any relative contraindications may exercise if the benefits of physical activity outweigh the risks. These patients may require increased levels of supervision to assure safety. Indications for a medically based exercise program include the following:

- Coronary artery disease
- Myocardial infarction
- Coronary artery bypass surgery
- Cardiac transplantation
- Heart failure
- Hypertension
- Chronic obstructive pulmonary disease

Table 62-1 Contraindications for Exercise Training	

ABSOLUTE CONTRAINDICATIONS

Acute myocardial infarction
Unstable angina
Uncontrolled cardiac arrhythmias causing symptoms or
  hemodynamic compromise
Acute systemic or pulmonary embolus
Acute pulmonary infarction
Acute myocarditis or pericarditis
Acute aortic dissection
Uncontrolled symptomatic heart failure
Uncontrolled diabetes mellitus (glucose > 400) or other
  metabolic disease
Thrombophlebitis or intracardiac thrombi
Acute systemic illness or fever

RELATIVE CONTRAINDICATIONS

Left main coronary stenosis
Moderate stenotic valvular disease
Electrolyte abnormalities
Tachyarrhythmias or bradyarrhythmias
Severe arterial hypertension (systolic BP > 200 mm Hg
  or diastolic BP > 110)
High-degree arterioventricular block
Hypertrophic cardiomyopathy or other forms of outflow
  tract obstruction
Neuromuscular, muskulosketal or rheumatoid disorders
  exacerbated by exercise
Uncontrolled sinus tachycardia (>120 bpm)
Advanced or complicated pregnancy
Symptomatic orthostatic hypotension

Adapted from American College of Sports Medicine. ACSM's
guidelines for exercise testing and prescription. 5th ed.
Baltimore: Williams and Wilkins, 1995; and Gibbons RJ, Balady
GJ, Beasley JW et al. ACC/AHS guidelines for exercise testing:
a report of the American College of Cardiology/American Heart
Association Task Force on Practice Guidelines (Committee on
Exercise Testing). J Am Coll Cardiol 1997;30:260–315.

Table 62-2 Medical Screening for Physical Activity	
Medical history	Past history
	Current health status
	Current medications
	Family history
Lifestyle information	Smoking
	Nutrition and weight
	Physical activity
	Substance abuse
	Past experience with lifestyle change
Psychosocial history	Home situation
	Mental status/outlook
	Religious/cultural factors
Physical examination	Vital signs
	Review of systems
Laboratory tests (as indicated)	ECG
	Exercise stress test
	X-Ray
	Hemoglobin
	Glucose
	TSH
	Urinalysis
	Other

Adapted from American College of Sports Medicine. ACSM's
exercise management for persons with chronic diseases and
disabilities. Champaign, IL: Human Kinetics, 1997; and
American College of Sports Medicine. ACSM's guidelines for
exercise testing and prescription. 5th ed. Baltimore: Williams
and Wilkins, 1995.

rately. Table 62-2 lists the information recommended prior to writing an exercise prescription. Indications for stress testing are shown in Table 62-3 and a scheme for stratifying a patient's risk of cardiovascular events is shown in Table 62-4. A physical activity assessment questionnaire is found in Table 62-5.

- Chronic renal failure
- Renal transplant
- Diabetes mellitus
- Limiting arthritis or rheumatoid disease
- Percutaneous transluminal coronary angioplasty
- Obesity
- Valvular surgery
- Orthopedic or neuromuscular limitations to exercise
- Peripheral vascular disease

Middle-aged and older patients and those with chronic illnesses, including those with or at high risk for coronary artery disease, should undergo a comprehensive physical examination prior to starting vigorous activity or significantly increasing a program of physical activity. For some patients, additional laboratory data such as an exercise stress test may be needed to evaluate exercise safety and assess risk more accu-

PHYSICAL FITNESS

There are four components of physical fitness: aerobic or cardiovascular fitness, musculoskeletal fitness, flexibility, and body composition. Cardiovascular fitness represents the interface between several body systems that support sustained physical effort involving repetitive contraction of large muscle groups. Cardiovascular fitness, most often measured by maximal oxygen uptake (Vo_2max), represents the ability of the cardiovascular and pulmonary systems to deliver oxygen and nutrients to the working muscles and the muscles to extract and utilize oxygen and nutrients.

Musculoskeletal fitness is the product of the strength and endurance of the muscles, bones, and connective tissue and is an important determinant of the ability of the musculoskeletal system to perform work. Muscular strength is the maximal force that can be generated by a particular muscle group, and muscular endurance is the ability of a muscle group to perform repeated, sustained work. Muscular strength

Table 62-3 Indications for Exercise Stress Testing Before Starting Exercise Training

PATIENT STATUS	Iᵃ	IIAᵇ	IIBᶜ	IIIᵈ
Post-MI	Submaximal at 4–7 days Symptom limited (>2 weeks)	Post MI with revascularization after discharge	Periodic monitoring of post MI patients continuing to exercise	None
Suspected or known CVD	Patients with suspected or known CVD	None	Patients with WPW, ST segment abnormalities, left bundle-branch block	None
Post-revascularization	Patients with recurrent symptoms	After discharge	None	None
Asymptomatic	None	Sedentary men >40 and women >50 years Patients at high risk for CAD	None	Routine screening of asymptomatic men and women

ᵃ Class I: Conditions for which there is evidence and/or general agreement that a given procedure is useful and effective.
ᵇ,ᶜ Class II: Conditions for which there is conflicting evidence and/or a divergence of opinion about the usefulness/efficacy of a procedure or treatment.
ᵇ Class IIa: Weight of evidence is in favor of usefulness/efficacy.
ᶜ Class IIb: Evidence is less established regarding efficacy.
ᵈ Class III: Conditions for which there is no evidence for efficacy.
Adapted from American College of Sports Medicine. ACSM's guidelines for exercise testing and prescription. 5th ed. Baltimore: Williams and Wilkins, 1995; and Gibbons RJ, Balady GJ, Beasley JW et al. ACC/AHS guidelines for exercise testing: a report of the American College of Cardiology/American Heart Association Task Force on Practice Guidelines (Committee on Exercise Testing). J Am Coll Cardiol 1997;30:260–315.

Table 62-4 Risk Stratification

LOW RISK	MODERATE RISK	HIGH RISK
Uncomplicated MI	MI complicated by shock or CHF (within previous 6 months)	MI complicated by CHF, shock, or complex ventricular arrhythmias
Functional capacity >8 METs 3 weeks after clinical event	Functional capacity <8 METs 3 weeks after clinical event	Survivor of cardiac arrest
No ischemia	Exercise-induced ischemia (ST depression 1–2 mm)	Exercise-Induced myocardial ischemia (ST depression >2 mm)
No ventricular dysfunction	Mild to moderate LV dysfunction (EF 30–50%)	Severely depressed LV function (EF <30%)
No complex arrhythmias	Inability to monitor exercise intensity	Resting complex ventricular arrhythmias
Asymptomatic at rest and exercise with capacity adequate for most occupational and recreational activities	Unwilling or unable to comply with exercise prescription	Exertional hypotension

Adapted from American College of Sports Medicine. ACSM's guidelines for exercise testing and prescription. 5th ed. Baltimore: Williams and Wilkins, 1995.

can be measured using several devices, including isokinetic devices, dynomometers, and weights. It is frequently reported as the maximal voluntary contraction (MVC) or the one-repetition maximum (1-RM), which refers to the maximal weight or force that can be lifted or generated one time by a muscle group. Testing of muscular endurance is often done by repeated calisthenics tests, such as pushups and situps.

Flexibility is the range of motion of a joint and can be measured using goniometers or by functional tests such as stretching exercises. Body composition is the proportion of fat and lean tissue in the body. It can be estimated in several ways including body mass index, skinfold measures, bioelectrical impedance, and hydrostatic weighing.

Table 62-5 Physical Activity Assessment

1. Do you currently participate in any regular physical activity that causes your breathing to increase, your heart to beat faster, and/or you to work up a sweat?
   Yes   No
   If yes, determine the following for each activity:
   What kind of activity?
   For how long do you do this activity each time?
   How many days per week?
   How long have you been doing this activity?
2. Do you do any walking on regular basis?
   Yes   No
   If yes: How many days per week?
3. How far do you walk?
4. How long does it take you to complete this walk?
5. Do you consider your walk to be brisk or leisurely?
6. How long have you been walking?
7. How much time do you spend each day on your feet moving around doing things? (list number of hours per day)
   i)   None
   ii)   Less than 1 hour per day
   iii)   1–2 hours per day
   iv)   3–5 hours per day
   v)   More than 6 hours per day
8. Do you do any heavy (hard) physical activity as part of your job or around your home? (This would include lifting or carrying heavy objects, carrying groceries or other heavy objects upstairs, carpentry, chopping wood, digging dirt, heavy gardening, scrubbing floors on hands and knees, heavy housework or similar activities.)
   If yes:
   What kind of activity do you do?
   How often do you do it?
   For how long do you do this activity?
9. Do you consider your activity level to be more, less or about the same as others your age?
10. Does your activity level change during different seasons?
    Yes   No
    If yes, Which season are you most active?
    The least?
    Why does your activity level change?
11. Does your health limit your physical activity in any way?
    Yes   No
    If so, how?
    For what reason?

THE EXERCISE SESSION

The exercise session usually has three phases: a warmup, a conditioning phase, and a cool down. The warmup and cool-down consist of 5 to 15 minutes of low intensity activity and stretching. The conditioning phase may last 10 to 60 minutes, depending on the activity, the fitness level of the participant, and the fitness goals. Aerobic training and/or muscular strength and endurance activities are performed during the conditioning phase of the activity session.

FACTORS IN THE EXERCISE PRESCRIPTION

Several factors can be manipulated in order to improve physical fitness: exercise mode, intensity, duration, frequency, and the rate of progression of exercise. The manner in which these factors are manipulated is determined by the patient's physical conditioning level and the desired outcomes.

Exercise Mode

A variety of activities ordinarily considered "exercise" and those done as part of home or occupational tasks or for recreation can be chosen for a program of physical activity. These activities share several characteristics: they are rhythmic in nature, are done for a sustained period of time (10 minutes or more), and involve one or more large muscle groups. Table 62-6 lists examples of activities within these categories that can be considered for a physical activity program.

A program of physical activity can contain one or more of these activities and include both moderate and vigorous activities to allow for a daily schedule of physical activity. Two or more vigorous activities may be done on alternating days to minimize joint stress and the potential for injury. An exercise program is most effective when the activities chosen are performed at least two to three times per week because many of the physiologic effects of training are specific to the muscles involved in the activity.

Exercise Intensity

Exercise intensity is assessed in several ways: energy expenditure (oxygen uptake; Vo_2), heart rate (HR), or ratings of perceived exertion (RPE). Metabolic equivalents (MET) are an index used to express energy expenditure, with 1 MET representing resting energy expenditure and higher numbers representing multiples of the resting level. For example, 2 MET is double the resting energy expenditure, 3 MET is three times the resting level, and so forth.

The measured or predicted oxygen uptake or MET level can be used to prescribe exercise. This method requires exercise testing with measurement of oxygen uptake or the estimation of oxygen uptake using prediction formulas and exercise workload, heart rate, and/or exercise duration. When oxygen uptake is measured, it is most accurate to use the oxygen uptake reserve for the development of the exercise prescription (11). To calculate the oxygen uptake reserve, a percentage of the difference between maximal oxygen uptake and resting oxygen uptake is added to the resting oxygen uptake. More simply, a percentage of the maximal oxygen uptake can be used, although this can underestimate or overestimate the actual exercise intensity by as much as 20% (4).

The target heart rate for exercise is determined by use of the measured or estimated maximal heart rate. The estimated heart rate, calculated as 220 − age, is frequently used since exercise testing may not be available. The intensity of exercise is prescribed using the heart rate reserve method, in which a percentage of the difference between the maximal heart rate and the resting heart rate is taken and then added to the resting heart rate. A straight percentage of the maximal heart rate can be used, but this generally underestimates the exercise intensity.

The ratings of perceived exertion (RPE) is a scale used to rate the intensity of effort, based on the perception of the

Table 62-6 Physical Activities

ACTIVITY TYPE	ACTIVITIES
Exercise	Walking, bicycling, aerobic dance, swimming, tennis, racquetball, soccer, calisthenics, jogging, running, exercise machines, basketball, volleyball, badminton
Occupational	Delivering mail, house painting, truck driving (making deliveries, carrying, and lifting), heavy carpentry, construction work, physical labor
Household	Raking the lawn, sweeping and mopping, mowing the lawn with a stand-up mower, cleaning windows, scrubbing floors, chopping wood, moving moderate to heavy objects, home repair, car maintenance.
Recreational	Dancing, sightseeing on foot, hunting, playing the drums, canoeing, skin diving, snorkeling, hiking, horseback riding, skiing, skating, golf (if on foot), ping-pong

Adapted from U.S. Department of Health and Human Services. Physical activity and health: a report of the Surgeon General. Atlanta, GA: U.S. Department of Health and Human Services, Centers for Disease Control and Prevention, National Center for Chronic Disease Prevention and Health Promotion, 1996; and American College of Sports Medicine. ACSM's guidelines for exercise testing and prescription. 5th ed. Baltimore: Williams and Wilkins, 1995.

Table 62-7 Determining Exercise Intensity

INTENSITY	RPE	% MAXIMAL HEART RATE	% VO$_2$ MAX OR MAXIMAL METS	% VO$_2$ RESERVE OR HEART RATE RESERVE	% MAXIMAL VOLUNTARY CONTRACTION (RESISTANCE EXERCISE)
Very light	<10	<35	<25	<20	<30
Light	10–11	35–54	25–44	20–39	30–49
Moderate	12–13	55–69	45–59	40–59	50–69
Hard	14–16	70–89	60–84	60–84	70–84
Very hard	17–19	>90	>85	>85	>85
Maximal	20	100	100	100	100

Adapted from American College of Sports Medicine. ACSM position stand: the recommended quantity and quality of exercise for developing and maintaining cardiorespiratory and muscular fitness in healthy adults. Med Sci Sports Exerc 1990;22:265–274; and U.S. Department of Health and Human Services. Physical activity and health: a report of the Surgeon General. Atlanta, GA: U.S. Department of Health and Human Services, Centers for Disease Control and Prevention, National Center for Chronic Disease Prevention and Health Promotion, 1996.

physical sensations during exertion (12,13). This scale has been validated against physiologic measures of exercise intensity such as blood lactate concentrations, heart rate, and oxygen uptake (13).

The exercise intensity recommended for improvement in cardiovascular fitness can be prescribed using any of these methods (8–10). To achieve improvements in fitness, the exercise intensity should be set in the following ranges:

- RPE: 12 to 16

- Heart rate reserve or oxygen uptake reserve: 40% to 85%

- Maximal heart rate: 55% to 90%

- Vo$_2$max or Maximum METs: 50% to 85%

Individuals who are fit will not achieve much of an increase in cardiorespiratory fitness when exercising at the lower end of the intensity range. On the other hand, very deconditioned individuals will realize substantial improvements in cardiorespiratory fitness and may benefit from intensities lower than these listed. In the earliest phases of an

exercise-training program, exercise toward the lower end of the range is best tolerated in patients who are sedentary, while exercise in the midrange is suggested for those of average conditioning. Only the highly fit will be able to sustain exercise in the highest range for a sufficient amount of time. Table 62-7 compares the various methods at several levels of intensity.

Exercise Frequency and Duration

Vigorous exercise should be performed 3 to 5 days per week, with exercise on most days per week recommended for moderate intensity exercise. Daily activity is optimal for the greatest health benefit and to assist in developing a regular habit of activity. However, this may be too frequent in the early phases of an exercise program.

For the improvement of cardiovascular fitness, vigorous exercise performed for 20 to 60 minutes is recommended (8–10). Although activity performed continuously is most efficacious, intermittent activity done for 10 continuous minutes with an interspersed rest or done several times per day for a total of 20 minutes or more can result in significant gains in fitness, particularly in those who are very deconditioned (8,9). The suggested level for most people is 30 to 45 minutes of activity per day, and this can be continuous or intermittent depending on the fitness level of the individual and the goals of the activity program (2–4,8,9).

Exercise Progression

For most people, it takes 3 to 6 months or longer to reach a goal for exercise duration, intensity, and frequency. It is often helpful in sedentary individuals to start with a short duration (10 to 20 minutes) of activity at a moderate intensity repeated one or more times per day on 3 or more days per week. The patient can gradually work up to 30 to 45 minutes of continuous moderate to vigorous activity done daily over several months. In general, in sedentary individuals it is best to work on exercise duration first until 30 to 45 minutes are achieved, then increase frequency until exercise is done daily, and then increase the intensity of the exertion.

EXERCISE PRESCRIPTION FOR RESISTANCE TRAINING

Resistance training for improved muscular strength and conditioning is recommended 2 to 3 days per week for most adults (8–10). For adults under age 50, 1 set of 8 to 12 repetitions of exercises for each of the major muscle groups is suggested. For those over age 50, increased repetitions of the exercises (10 to 15) is recommended to reduce the possibility of injury. The reader is referred elsewhere for detailed recommendations and rationale for exercise prescription for improving muscular strength and endurance (8–10).

EXERCISE PRESCRIPTION FOR FLEXIBILITY TRAINING

Range of motion exercises for each of the major muscle groups are suggested 2 to 3 times per week to maintain flexibility of the joints and to reduce injury (1,8,9). These exercises should be repeated four or more times and can be done as static or dynamic stretches. Static stretches should be held at the point of mild discomfort for 10 to 30 seconds. Proprioceptive neuromuscular facilitation (PNF) techniques involve an isometric contraction followed by passive stretching through a range of motion. The contraction should last about 6 seconds followed by a 10 to 30 second assisted stretch. Ballistic stretching with repetitive bouncing motions can also be used, although these may result in injury if not done correctly.

EXERCISE PRESCRIPTION FOR PATIENTS WITH CHRONIC DISEASE

Exercise prescription for patients with chronic disease follows the same general principles that are used for healthy individuals, with modifications made as necessary to accommodate the disease pathology and to attain treatment and disease prevention goals. Table 62-8 summarizes the special considerations for patients with a variety of chronic diseases. Most of these

patients can exercise safely, but some may benefit from increased supervision, particularly in the early phases of training. An algorithm for exercise prescription is shown in Figure 62-1.

The goals of exercise training in these patients usually includes several of the following:

- Increase cardiovascular fitness
- Improve muscular strength and endurance
- Improve range of motion
- Improve body composition and body weight
- Increase functional capacity and physical activity endurance
- Improve or maintain activities of daily living
- Decrease heart rate, blood pressure, and myocardial oxygen demand at submaximal exertion
- Increase lactate and ventilatory threshold
- Decrease cardiovascular disease risk factors
- Reduce sensitivity to dyspnea
- Reduce stress and anxiety
- Improve mood
- Improve sleep
- Improve feelings of well-being and self-esteem
- Improve quality of life

Cardiac Patients

Exercise is prescribed for cardiac patients from an exercise test that has been administered with the patient on his/her usual medications, because many of the anti-ischemic drugs affect the heart rate, blood pressure, and electrocardiographic responses to exercise (6,8,10,14). If this is not possible, exercise can be prescribed using the RPE or a heart rate of 20 beats per minute (bpm) greater than the resting heart rate (6,8–10,14). When there is symptomatic or asymptomatic myocardial ischemia, the target heart rate may be set about 10 to 25 bpm less than onset of myocardial ischemia. Exercise

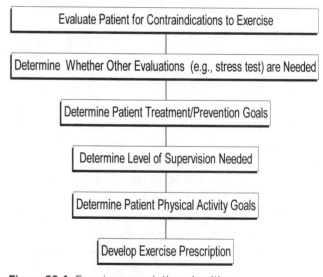

Figure 62-1 Exercise prescription algorithm.

Table 62-8 Considerations for Patients with Chronic Diseases

DISEASE	SPECIAL CONSIDERATIONS

Myocardial infarction/ angina pectoris/ silent myocardial ischemia	Most can benefit from a cardiac rehabilitation program
	Medical supervision for moderate and high risk patients is recommended
	Very deconditioned patients can train at a lower intensity and may benefit >2 shorter exercise sessions (5–15 min)
	Monitor for abnormal signs and symptoms
	Monitor for anginal symptoms/ ECG changes
	Avoid Valsalva maneuvers
	Exercise Intensity:
	  40–85% of heart rate reserve measured while on usual cardiac medications
	  HR of 10–25 BPM less than onset of myocardial ischemia
	Increase warm-up and cool down to 10 minutes in patients with myocardial ischemia (with or without symptoms)

Revascularization (coronary artery bypass surgery, percutaneous transluminal coronary angioplasty)	Most can benefit from a cardiac rehabilitation program Usually can start exercise earlier than MI patients and have more rapid progression of exercise program Upper extremity ROM exercises for CABGs patients CABGs patients should start with 1–2 lb weights and increase after 6–10 weeks or when sternum has healed Monitor for signs and symptoms of restenosis or graft occlusion
Pacemakers	Most can benefit from a cardiac rehabilitation program Exercise below ischemic threshold Pacemaker may limit range of motion of upper extremities
Implantable defibrillators	Most can benefit from a cardiac rehabilitation program Exercise below activation threshold for implantable defibrillator Defibrillator may limit range of motion of upper extremities May have ventricular arrhythmias
Congestive heart failure	Most can benefit from a cardiac rehabilitation program May have low exercise tolerance Can benefit from lower intensity exercise May benefit from interval training with interspersed rest periods or several short exercise periods per day if very deconditioned May have prolonged fatigue following exercise Monitor signs and symptoms of decompensation (increased dyspnea and weight gain)
Cardiac transplant	Most can benefit from a cardiac rehabilitation program Upper body range of motion limited for 6–10 weeks Monitor exercise intensity using ratings of perceived exertion May have silent ischemia Delayed heart rate recovery Avoid high-resistance exercise in those with history of corticosteroid use (high fracture risk) Strength training: start with 1–2 lb weights and increase after 6–10 weeks or when sternum has healed Avoid Valsalva maneuvers
Hypertension	Defer exercise if systolic BP >200 or diastolic BP >110 Exercise intensity: 40–85% of heart rate reserve measured while on usual medications Avoid Valsalva maneuvers
Peripheral artery disease	Exercise limited by claudication pain May increase claudication threshold by exercising to significant claudication May benefit from interval training with rest periods interspersed Monitor for signs and symptoms of myocardial ischemia
Pulmonary disease	Avoid early morning exercise when symptoms are worst May improve compliance by exercising at lower intensities May benefit from interval training with rest interspersed or several shorter exercise sessions per day Maintain oxygen saturation >90% Exercise intensity: RPE of somewhat hard (11–13 on 6–20 scale) Dyspnea <2/4 (moderate, but can continue exercise) Monitor for signs and symptoms of CVD

Table 62-8 continues

Chapter 62   **Exercise Prescription for Patients with Chronic Health Problems**   **701**

Table 62-8 *Continued*

DISEASE	SPECIAL CONSIDERATIONS
Diabetes mellitus	May need a CHO snack before exercise if BG <80–100
	CHO snack every 30 min with prolonged exercise
	Insulin dose may need reduction
	Delay exercise if blood glucose >260 or ketones in urine
	Watch for signs and symptoms of hypoglycemia
	Hypoglycemia may be delayed after exercise
	Avoid injecting insulin in areas over exercising muscles
	Monitor for signs and symptoms of CHD
Obesity	Low impact activity will reduce risk of injury
	Emphasize duration of activity over intensity
	May need equipment modification
	Increased risk of hyperthermia
	Monitor for signs and symptoms of CHD
	For patients with CHD, diabetes, hypertension, follow appropriate guidelines
Renal failure	Hemodialysis patients may not tolerate exercise on hemodialysis days
	Peritoneal dialysis patients may be more comfortable without full abdomen
	Spontaneous tendon repture can occur in patients with long-term renal failure
	Fatigue is often limiting factor
	Monitor for signs and symptoms of CVD
	If diabetic, follow diabetic guidelines
Frailty	Monitor for balance difficulties
	May benefit from exercise done while sitting and/or use of assistive devices
	May benefit from interval training with rest interspersed or several shorter exercise sessions per day
	Increase risk of hyperthermia
	Monitor for signs and symptoms of CHD
	May have difficulty in following directions due to cognitive deficits
	Emphasize exercise duration
Osteoporosis	Avoid forward flexion of spine
	Patients with kyphosis may have increased fatigue due to impaired pulmonary function
	Patients with kyphosis need to exercise while sitting or with assistive devices
	Monitor for balance difficulties
	Monitor for signs and symptoms of CHD
Arthritis	Avoid overstretching affected joints
	Avoid high-impact, high-repetition, high-resistance exercise
	May be susceptible to stress fractures if on steroids
Parkinson's disease	Autonomic dysfunction may alter heart rate response to exercise
	Monitor for balance difficulties and orthostatic hypotension
	May be prone to hyperthermia
	Monitor for signs and symptoms of CHD
Stroke/head injury	Monitor for balance difficulties
	May benefit from exercise while sitting or with assistive devices
	May need to perform unilateral exercise
	May have visual deficits
	May have cognitive and communication deficits
	Monitor for signs and symptoms of CHD and arthritis
Mental illness	Monitor for dizziness, hypertension, hypotension, tachycardia, ECG changes, gait disturbances secondary to medications
	May need more time for familiarization
Low back syndrome	Avoid high-impact exercise
	Avoid trunk exercises during first 2 weeks

Adapted from American College of Sports Medicine. ACSM's exercise management for persons with chronic diseases and disabilities. Champaign, IL: Human Kinetics, 1997.

should be prescribed by RPE in patients with cardiac transplantation due to the cardiac denervation. Transplant patients will have a delayed heart rate recovery following exercise (14,15).

Patients with myocardial ischemia or compensated heart failure, and those who are very deconditioned, often benefit from lengthening the warmup and the cool-down phase to 10–15 minutes. Those with angina pectoris that occurs regularly with exercise may eliminate or reduce anginal episodes by taking sublingual nitroglycerine before starting exercise (14,15).

Patients with heart failure, a low ischemic threshold, significant deconditioning, and/or with orthopedic or neuromuscular limitations can benefit from intermittent exercise in which exercise is performed at a moderate to vigorous intensity for 5 to 10 minutes followed by rest or slow exercise for 1 to 5 minutes, and then repeating the sequence one or more times. This approach often makes it possible for a patient to complete 30 minutes or more of moderate to vigorous exercise, although they are unable to perform it continuously. Another approach that can be helpful for symptomatic and debilitated patients is to engage in several short exercise sessions completed over the course of the day. For example, a patient might walk for 10 minutes in the morning, afternoon, and early evening, for a total of 30 minutes per day.

Most patients can safely engage in resistance exercises as long as they avoid Valsalva maneuvers and keep their exercise intensity below the ischemic threshold. Patients recovering from coronary artery bypass grafting and cardiac transplantation should use very light (1 to 2 lb) weights for the first 6 to 10 weeks until the sternum has healed. Patients with pacemakers or implantable defibrillators may have limited range of motion in the upper extremities (6,9,10,15).

All patients with coronary heart disease should be monitored for angina pectoris, dyspnea, weight gain, or prolonged fatigue. They should be instructed about symptoms, including chest discomfort or pain and shortness of breath, that should be reported to their physician, particularly if there is a change in their usual symptoms.

Hypertension

Hypertensive patients can realize significant improvement in their blood pressure control by engaging in regular physical activity. Lifestyle activity including physical activity is recommended for reducing blood pressure (16). An acute bout of aerobic exercise can result in 10 to 20 mm Hg reductions in blood pressure that persist for as long as 9 hours following exercise (7,17,18). When exercise is performed chronically, an average reduction in systolic blood pressure of 10 mm Hg and diastolic blood pressure of 8 mm Hg may be realized (7,17).

Patients with uncontrolled hypertension (stage 2 or 3: SBP > 160, DBP > 100) should begin pharmacologic therapy prior to embarking on an exercise program (14,16). Exercise should be prescribed in the recommended manner for adults. Hypertensive patients should avoid heavy resistance exercise or Valsalva' maneuver (7,14,17,18).

Peripheral Artery Disease

Patients with peripheral artery disease can benefit from walking or other weight-bearing exercise until they experience severe claudication pain (19–21). They should rest until the pain subsides and then resume their activity. Exercising in this manner can increase the claudication (ischemic) threshold and walking duration (14,19–21).

Some non-weight bearing activity such as cycling can be beneficial in a program for peripheral vascular disease patients because claudication often limits exercise intensity. Often patients with peripheral artery disease can work at higher exercise intensity during non-weight bearing activity and, therefore, attain greater improvement in cardiovascular fitness and body composition.

Pulmonary Disease

Exercise can result in significant improvement in the pulmonary patient's tolerance to exercise and in their ability to carry out activities of daily living (14,24,25). Intermittent exercise is often prescribed due to dyspnea in these patients. Exercise is usually prescribed based on RPE and level of dyspnea. Patients can exercise up to a moderate level of dyspnea and may benefit from learning techniques such as pursed lip breathing.

Patients with pulmonary disease generally do better if they exercise later in the day and if they exercise intermittently. Patients who experience oxygen desaturation during exercise should exercise while on oxygen. Patients with exercise-induced asthma may benefit from using inhalers prior to exercise, avoiding exercise in the cold, and exercising in a warm, moist environment (14,22,23).

Diabetes Mellitus

Diabetic patients can improve their glucose control and reduce their risk of cardiovascular disease (14,24,25). It is best for diabetics to exercise daily on a consistent schedule. Checking blood glucose before and after exercise is recommended for all diabetic patients, particularly in the early stages of an exercise program. Patients should be observant for hypoglycemia, which can occur several hours after exercise. Blood glucose should generally be below 200 mg/dL before starting exercise, although patients with a blood glucose level of 200 to 400 mg/dL may exercise under medical supervision. Patients with ketones should delay exercise. A CHO snack is recommended if blood sugar levels are below 80 to 100 mg/dL. When engaging in physical activity lasting more than 60 minutes, a carbohydrate snack should be taken every hour (24–27).

Exercise should be avoided during the peak action of insulin and patients may need to adjust or omit their dose of insulin according to the type of insulin and their exercise schedule. Patients should avoid injecting insulin over the working muscles since exercise may facilitate absorption of insulin. Patients taking oral hypoglycemic agents may need to decrease their dose of medication, if they exercise on a regular basis (24–27).

Proper footwear, including socks, must be encouraged in all diabetic patients and they should be instructed to check their feet before and after exercise. Patients with retinopathy should avoid bouncing or jarring exercise and those with neuropathies should be cautious about exercising in areas with rough surfaces and in extremes of temperature. (24–27).

Renal Disease and Renal Transplant

Exercise training can help renal failure patients maintain adequate fitness to perform activities of daily living. Exercise tolerance in renal failure patients is usually limited by fatigue. These patients can benefit from intermittent exercise and exercise sessions spread out through the day. Patients may be unable to tolerate exercise on hemodialysis days, although benefit has been shown when patients exercise during hemodialysis. Peritoneal dialysis patients may find it easier to exercise when their abdomen is not full. Since CHD is prevalent in this patient population, careful monitoring for signs and symptoms of CHD is important. Patients with diabetes need to follow guidelines for diabetic patients (14,28,29).

Obesity and Overweight

Regular physical activity is an important component of a successful program of weight loss or weight management. The goal with overweight or obese patients is to increase their daily caloric expenditure by approximately 200–300 kilocalories. This can be accomplished by prescribing exercise of moderate intensity that is done either continuously or intermittently throughout the day. The latter approach may improve adherence in patients who have been sedentary (9,14,30).

Weight bearing exercise should be avoided in patients who are obese because of an increased risk of joint injury. Hyperthermia is also a risk for these patients, so exercise should be performed with adequate environmental control. Obese patients are at increased risk for CHD, diabetes, and hypertension, and should be monitored for signs and symptoms of those diseases (9,14,30).

Arthritis, Osteoporosis, and Lower Back Pain

Physical activity is important in the management of arthritis and osteoporosis. Flexibility and resistance training are particularly important for patients with arthritis or osteoporosis in order to maintain range of motion and muscular strength. Patients should avoid overstretching and extreme flexion of the spine. These patients can engage in aerobic exercise, but do best with non-weight bearing and water exercise (5,9,31–34). Patients with low back pain should avoid trunk exercises during the first 2 weeks after the onset of symptoms (14). Osteoporotic patients with kyphosis may have impaired pulmonary function and may need to perform exercise while sitting or with the use of assistive devices. Patients taking steroids are susceptible to fractures and tendon rupture, and should be particularly careful to avoid excessive stress on the joints (14).

Frailty and Old Age

Older patients can benefit greatly from exercise. Studies of the elderly have shown similar improvements in fitness in older and younger men and women (8,35). The main considerations in prescribing exercise for elderly patients are their comorbidities and problems with balance and cognition. Patients with balance problems should exercise in a sitting position or with the use of assistive devices. Those with cognitive deficits will need closer supervision and frequent repetition of instruction. Elderly patients may be significantly deconditioned and can benefit from interval training or shorter, frequent exercise sessions performed throughout the day (14,35). Because of their higher risk of CVD and other diseases, elderly patients should be closely monitored for signs and symptoms of disease.

Parkinson's Disease

The role of exercise training in patients with Parkinson's disease has not been well studied. However, it is believed that exercise training is beneficial in reducing the risk of CHD and in maintaining activities of daily living. Parkinson's disease patients may have difficulty with balance and orthostatic hypertension, and so may need to exercise in a sitting position or with use of assistive devices. They often have autonomic dysfunction and thus altered heart rates, and are prone to hyperthermia with exercise. Exercise should be monitored by RPE and is best done in a climate-controlled environment (14).

Stroke/Head Injury

Exercise training is important in this patient group to reduce the risk of CHD and to maintain activities of daily living. Balance difficulties are prevalent in this population and they may need to use assistive devices or perform exercise in a sitting position. Unilateral exercise may be necessary for these patients. Increased monitoring may be needed due to cognitive and visual deficits (14).

SUMMARY

Patients need a lot of encouragement to initiate and to continue a program of regular exercise, particularly if they are suffering from a chronic disease. They need to understand the importance of regular physical activity in maintaining and/or improving their health. Careful instruction about the types, intensity, frequency, and duration of activity is important, and the patient needs to be able to recognize signs and symptoms for discontinuing exercise and for contacting their physician. Considerable information for health professionals and laypersons are available on the Internet or by contacting several organizations. These contacts are listed in Table 62-9. While giving this advice is time consuming when a clinical exercise physiologist is not available, the health benefits to the patient can be substantial.

Table 62-9 Suggested Internet Resources

American Heart Association
http://www.amhrt.org/index.html *or* call 1-800 AHA-USA1

American Diabetes Association
http://www.diabetes.org/ *or* call 1-800-232-6733

American Alliance of Health Physical Education Recreation and Dance
http://www.aahperd.org/ *or* call 1-800-213-7193

American College of Sports Medicine
http:/www.acsm.org/sportsmed/ *or* call: (317) 637–9200

American Association of Cardiovascular and Pulmonary Rehabilitation
http://128.220.112.180/aacvpr/aacvpr.html *or* call 608-831-6989

President's Council on Physical Fitness and Sports
http://www.indiana.edu/~preschal/council.html *or* call 202-690-9000

American Arthritis Foundation
http://www.arthritis.org/ *or* call 404-872-7100

Centers for Disease Control
http://www.cdc.gov/nccdphp/phyactiv.htm *or* call 404-639-3311

REFERENCES

1. Fletcher GF. How to implement physical activity in primary and secondary prevention: a statement for healthcare professionals from the Task Force on Risk Reduction, American Heart Association. Circulation 1997; 96:355–357.

2. U.S. Department of Health and Human Services. Physical activity and health: a report of the Surgeon General. Atlanta, GA: U.S. Department of Health and Human Services. Centers for Disease Control and Prevention, National Center for Chronic Disease Prevention and Health Promotion, 1996.

3. National Institutes of Health. Physical activity and cardiovascular health. NIH Consens Statement. 1995;13:1–33.

4. Pate RR, Pratt M, Blair SN, et al. Physical activity and public health: a recommendation from the Centers For Disease Control And Prevention and the American College Of Sports Medicine. JAMA 1995;273:402–407.

5. American College of Sports Medicine ACSM position stand on osteoporosis and exercise. Med Sci Sports Exerc 1995;27: i–vii.

6. American College of Sports Medicine. ACSM position stand: exercise for patients with coronary artery disease. Med Sci Sports Exerc 1994;26:i–v.

7. American College of Sports Medicine. ACSM position stand: physical activity, physical fitness, and hypertension. Med Sci Sports Exerc 1993;25:i–x.

8. American College of Sports Medicine. ACSM position stand: the recommended quantity and quality of exercise for developing and maintaining cardiorespiratory and muscular fitness in healthy adults. Med Sci Sports Exerc 1990;22: 265–274.

9. American College of Sports Medicine. ACSM's guidelines for exercise testing and prescription. 5th ed. Baltimore: Williams and Wilkins, 1995.

10. Fletcher GF, Balady G, Froelicher VF, et al. Exercise standards: a statement for healthcare professionals from the American Heart Association. Circulation 1995; 91:580–615.

11. Swain DP, Leutholtz BC. Heart rate reserve is equivalent to %VO$_2$ reserve, not to %VO$_2$max. Med Sci Sports Med 1997;29:410–414.

12. Borg G. Psychophysical bases of perceived exertion. Med Sci Sports Exerc 1982;14:377–381.

13. Noble BJ, Borg GA, Jacobs I, et al. A category-ratio perceived exertion scale: relationship to blood and muscle lactates and heart rate. Med Sci Sports Exerc 1983;15: 523–528.

14. American College of Sports Medicine. ACSM's exercise management for persons with chronic diseases and disabilities. Champaign, IL: Human Kinetics, 1997.

15. Shephard RJ. Responses of the cardiac transplant patient to exercise and training. Exerc Sports Sci Rev 1992;20:297–321.

16. National Institutes of Health, Heart Lung Blood Institute. Sixth Report of the Joint National Committee on the Prevention, Detection and Treatment of High Blood Pressure. NIH publication no. 93-1088.

17. Tipton CM. Exercise training and hypertension: an update. Exerc Sports Sci Rev 1991;19:447–450.

18. Gordon NF, Scott CB, Wilkinson WJ, et al. Exercise and mild essential hypertension: recommendations for adults. Sports Med 1990;10:390–404.

19. Patterson RB, Pinto B, Marcus B, et al. Value of a supervised exercise program for the therapy of arterial claudication. J Vasc Surg 1997;25:312–318.

20. Gardner AW, Poehlman ET. Exercise rehabilitation programs for the treatment of claudication pain: a

meta-analysis. JAMA 1995;274: 975–980.

21. Regensteiner JG, Hiatt WR. Exercise rehabilitation for patients with peripheral arterial disease. Exerc Sports Sci Rev 1995;23: 1–24.

22. Olopade CO, Beck KC, Viggiano RW, Staats BA. Exercise limitation and pulmonary rehabilitation in chronic obstructive pulmonary disease. Mayo Clin Proc 1992; 67:144–157.

23. Cooper CB. Determining the role of exercise in patients with chronic pulmonary disease. Med Sci Sports Exerc 1995;27:147–157.

24. Ruderman N, Devlin JT, eds. Health professional's guide to diabetes and exercise. Alexandria, VA: American Diabetes Association, 1995.

25. Bell DS. Exercise for patients with diabetes. Postgrad Med 1992;92: 195–198.

26. American Diabetes Association. Medical management of insulin-dependent (type I) diabetes. 3rd ed. Alexandria, VA: American Diabetes Association, 1997.

27. American Diabetes Association. Medical management of non-insulin-dependent (type II) diabetes. 4th ed. Alexandria, VA: American Diabetes Association, 1997.

28. Painter P. The importance of exercise in rehabilitation of patients with end-stage renal disease. Am J Kidney Dis 1994; 24:S2–9.

29. Harter HR. Exercise in the dialysis patient. Semin Dial 1994;7: 192–198.

30. Stefanik ML. Exercise and weight control. Exerc Sports Sci Rev 1993;21:363–396.

31. Minor MA, Lane NE. Recreational exercise in arthritis. Rheum Dis Clin North Am 1996;22:563–577.

32. Ytterberg SR, Mahowald ML, Krug HE. Exercise for arthritis. Bail-

lieres Clin Rheumatol 1994;8: 161–189.

33. Prior JC, Barr SI, Chow R, Faulkner RA. Prevention and management of osteoporosis: consensus statements from the Scientific Advisory Board Of The Osteoporosis Society Of Canada: 5: physical activity as therapy for osteoporosis. Can Med Assoc J 1996;155: 940–944.

34. Mosekilde L. Osteoporosis and exercise. Bone 1995;17:193–195.

35. Shephard RJ. The scientific basis for exercise prescribing for the very old. J Am Geriatri Soc 1990;38: 62–70.

Chapter 63

Exercise Counseling in the Elderly

Daniel E. Forman
Charles T. Pu
Carol Ewing Garber

Although aging is associated with functional decline and illness, many of the typical impediments to healthy living are modifiable. Properly performed exercise may allay and even reverse customary "age-related" patterns of clinical deterioration (1–3). Physicians have the potential to delay and possibly even prevent enfeeblement and disease by providing their patients with clear advice and encouragement to exercise.

Exercise programs for the elderly must speak to the needs of a broad spectrum of older adults in order to be effective. Frail, dependent elderly need techniques and environments to safely regain strength, function, and independence. Vigorous elderly need strategies to maintain health and to minimize injury in the course of more intense training. Between these extremes are the majority of older adults, those who are still relatively healthy and independent but who nevertheless are becoming more sedentary with an associated progression of disease and frailty. These adults need approaches to preserve their vitality, function, and well-being, as well as strategies to adhere to exercise behaviors.

Both intrinsic and extrinsic barriers to exercise are highly prevalent among the elderly. Many older adults fear they will hurt themselves with exercise, and they often cling to outdated ideas that sedentary lifestyles are safer. Ironically, well-meaning families and doctors may heighten their anxieties about exercise, further undermining inclinations for regular activity. In fact, such non-intended disinclinations to exercise typically define a path towards fraility. Studies indicate that few older adults who become sedentary see themselves as ever again becoming active. Even among elderly who exercise occasionally it is rarely considered a routine health-preserving priority.

Logistic hurdles often add to disinclinations to exercise. Time constrictions in doctor-patient interactions increasingly limit opportunities to discuss exercise meaningfully. Unaffordable costs and unworkable transportation requirements for facility-based exercise programs may be prohibitive. Caregiving responsibilities to an infirmed spouse or relative also frequently limit exercise options. In addition, comorbid illnesses among elderly are common, and exercise recommendations are often complicated by musculoskeletal limitations and overall debility. Additionally, pharmacologic regimens often effect balance, metabolism, body temperature, thirst, continence, mood, and other functions. All these factors must be considered as integral parts of an effective exercise program for elders.

THE LINK BETWEEN FUNCTION AND HEALTH IN THE ELDERLY

Cardiovascular fitness is often quantified by measuring peak Vo_2 (oxygen uptake) or functional tests of cardiovascular endurance such as the 6-minute walk test. In patients with heart failure and coronary heart disease, the most common health conditions among the elderly, prognosis correlates more to exercise performance (Vo_2 peak and the 6-minute walk distance) than to ejection fraction, coronary anatomy, and/or other central mechanisms of cardiac function (4,5). Given that such measures of exercise performance provide critical assessments of health and prognosis, exercise training (which improves exercise performance) is a logical health care priority.

Peak Vo_2 typically diminishes 9% to 13% per decade after age 35, but this decline may be attenuated by regular activity (6). Some of the age-related decline of Vo_2 is unavoidable, such as that accrued by down-regulation of cardiac beta-1 responses, i.e., senescent autonomic changes occur independently of lifestyle or disease states. However, decreases in skeletal muscle mass and performance as well as changes in vasomotor function are at least partially attributable to decreased physical activity. Therefore, senescent muscle and vascular physiology with significant functional correlates can be modified with regular exercise.

Thus while Framingham data and other epidemiologic studies show reductions in mobility and increasing frailty with age, such patterns are not inevitable. Likewise, while Jette et al show that 66% of women over age 85 are unable to lift 10 pounds and morphologic analyses show customary atrophy in senescent skeletal muscle (7), other studies show that strength training can generate muscle mass and improved function (8–11).

Similarly, vascular senescence is typically associated with morphologic stiffening, with resultant increases in afterload, and hypertension (12,13). Clinical implications include detrimental effects on cardiac function and impaired vasodilatory responses (14,15) (with demand ischemia and claudication). However, with exercise and other healthful lifestyle interventions, afterload can be reduced, stroke volume increased, and vasomotor performance improved.

Even beyond these specific cardiovascular and skeletal muscle benefits, exercise is known to exert a multitude of other salutary effects. Metabolic function, bone strength, respiration, gastrointestinal motility, sleep patterns, mood, and cognition are among the many functional and health parameters that improve with exercise. Rather than acquiescing passively to decline, proactive management with exercise provides an opportunity to preserve health and to transcend some of the otherwise typical tolls of time.

HEALTH CONSIDERATIONS BEFORE INITIATING EXERCISE

Prior to initiating exercise, a complete physical evaluation is essential. However, the need for exercise stress testing for all older adults remains controversial. Exercise testing is useful to clarify issues of blood pressure responses, coronary ischemia, arrhythmias, and other potential clinical instability (16). Its value is unequivocal among patients with known coronary heart disease (CHD) or significant cardiac risk factors. However, in adults whose physical examination and history suggest that they are healthy, embarking on a *low-intensity* exercise program is considered safe without additional testing at any age.

Another significant aspect of exercise testing for older adults involves the choice of testing modality and protocol. Many elderly are simply channeled into Bruce treadmill protocols, i.e., protocols designed primarily for younger adults. The experience of a treadmill itself, especially when coupled to the arduous Bruce protocol, may overwhelm older adults, often leading to foreshortened studies that are nondiagnostic and detrimental to exercise adherence due to patient anxiety. Consequently, many physicians opt to assess their older patients using pharmacologic stress tests. The tests often involve use of dipyridamole (Persantine), a vasodilator, used in

combination with a nuclear isotope (thallium or Sestamibi), while the patient lies supine. However, while dipyridamole stress testing sensitively diagnoses ischemia in the elderly, the procedure provides no quantification of exercise performance in terms of exercise duration, heart rate, or blood pressure, factors that are critical for effective exercise guidance.

Therefore, a better option when planning an exercise program for older adults is exercise stress testing using modalities, protocols, and intensities tailored to the limited capacities of the patient. Treadmill protocols such as the modified Naughton that use slow walking speeds may be better suited to frail adults. Bicycle testing with low increments of resistance progression may be preferable for adults with walking impairments. Although heart rate and blood pressure responses are reduced with such low-intensity protocols (blunting their diagnostic sensitivity for ischemia), nuclear isotopes (thallium or Sestamibi) can be incorporated into the tests to offset this deficiency. Unfortunately, concerns about aging, variable modalities, low-intensity protocols, and the importance of exercise guidance may not be a priority in exercise stress test laboratories.

The pre-exercise physical examination often reveals other signs that warrant additional testing and therapy prior to an exercise program. Coronary heart disease, hypertension, congestive heart failure, and valvular heart disease are common and have a direct impact on management choices. Similarly, orthostatic hypotension, gait abnormalities, joint instability, arthritis, neuropathy, chronic obstructive pulmonary disease, anemia, diabetes, and other conditions must be incorporated into an integrated assessment with appropriate medications, timing, diet, footware, monitoring, as well as exercise prescription. Iatrogenic medication effects must also be considered to ensure that incontinence, somnolence, or other problems are not inadvertent side effects of diuretics, sedative agents, and other medications that might better be discontinued, especially in the context of an exercise program.

EXERCISE PRESCRIPTION BEST SUITED TO THE NEEDS OF THE ELDERLY

Exercise prescription should be individualized and incorporate specific recommendations for frequency, duration, and mode of training based on the results of physical exam and exercise testing. Cardiovascular benefits of greater intensity and duration, while having theoretical advantages, are often offset by greater susceptibility to injury, complications, as well as decreased adherence.

Therefore, exercise of moderate or low intensity is generally safer and more sustainable for the elderly. Daily sessions of light to moderate exercise intensity (50% to 69% of predicted maximal heart rate) for 15 to 30 minutes are typically well tolerated and effective in achieving physiologic/clinical benefits among older adults. Some adults, typically those who are more feeble, do better with shorter exercise sessions (10 to 20 minutes) that are repeated two or more times per day. For those who are particularly deconditioned and/or frail, sometimes only very short exercise periods can be tolerated. An appropriate regimen might then be 5 minutes of low-intensity exercise (e.g., walking) followed by 2 minutes of rest, with this sequence then repeated three to five times a day for a total of 15 to 30 minutes of exercise.

The use of heart rate to gauge the goals of exercise intensity is often difficult for the elderly. A simpler alternative is to rely on the Borg (17) rating scale of perceived exertion (a scale of 6 to 20, i.e., "very, very light" to "very, very hard;" Table 63-1). A rating of 10 to 13 ("fairly light" to "somewhat hard") corresponds to an exercise intensity of 50% to 69% of the maximum predicted heart rate, a level that will typically yield improvements in physical fitness and health among older adults.

Among those elderly who exercise, many participate in large group exercise sessions with uniformly very low-intensity training goals. The logic for very low-intensity training is usually based on the goal of insuring a common denominator of safety. Unfortunately, these training goals may also diminish potential for maximal physiologic benefit. Therefore, more ideal programs should incorporate individualized training goals, with progression of exercise duration and intensities that may garner greater functional benefits. Safety could still be preserved by greater emphasis on proper form, careful rotation of exercise modalities (to avoid overuse of a particular joint or muscle), and vigilant monitoring.

For most adults, adherence is best achieved using exercises that are readily available, economical, enjoyable, safe, and unintimidating. Some adults find the ambience of an exercise center stimulating and enticing, but to others it may seem overwhelming and foreign. For some adults, line dancing in an empty room may be the only type of exercise that is palatable. Likewise, logistic issues like weather (e.g., snow or heat), transportation, time of day, spousal care, and the availability of medical oversight may constitute key differences between successful and ineffective exercise programming. Recently, novel exercise programs have successfully used two-way transtelephonic communications and even closed circuit television to achieve medical supervision of exercise while still overcoming barriers of distance, weather, and spousal caregiving responsibilities (18).

Table 63-1 Borg Perceived Exertion Scale

6	
7	very, very light
8	
9	very light
10	
11	fairly light
12	
13	somewhat hard
14	
15	hard
16	
17	very hard
18	
19	very, very hard
20	

SOURCE: Borg G. Perceived exertion as an indicator of somatic stress. Scand J Rehabil Med 1970;2:92–98.

AEROBIC TRAINING

Aerobic training involves many repetitive contractions of large muscle groups with a force production that is relatively low (less than 40%) and constant. Prospective studies have demonstrated that young men and women respond to aerobic training with improvements in Vo_2, cardiovascular flow reserve, ventricular filling, afterload reduction, and other measures of central cardiovascular performance. Other studies show similar cardiovascular gains among septuagenarians participating in aerobic training, as well as reduced decline of Vo_2 among adults aged 80 and older compared to sedentary, age-matched controls.

Given that the normal loss of aerobic capacity is about 1% per year among sedentary elderly, even routine activities of daily living (ADLs) like stair climbing and carrying groceries will eventually constitute close to 100% of a sedentary adult's remaining aerobic capacity. Thus, to some sedentary elderly with declining Vo_2, ADLs become high-intensity burdens. A vicious cycle towards frailty becomes likely as many of these weakened adults discontinue some activities as the physiologic costs become too severe. Progressive inactivity begets increasing weakness and activity intolerance, which escalates inactivity and further decline. By slowing loss of Vo_2, aerobic training preserves the capacity and inclination to stay active and independent.

Warmup is critical prior to aerobic training to increase blood flow, muscle temperature, and vasodilation, as well as ventilatory and metabolic responses. Warmup exercises typically consist of low-intensity dynamic activity using the same muscles to be used during the exercise. Aerobic exercises usually begin at lower intensities for 2 to 6 weeks, and then gradually increase in duration and intensity. Increasing duration as little as 5 minutes every 3 to 4 weeks may be sufficient for older and/or frail adults. Ultimately, aerobic goals plateau on a maintenance level based on the individual's desired level of fitness or health.

Alternating or rotating different types of aerobic exercise such as walking, cycling, stepping, dancing, swimming, and aquatic aerobics will use different muscle groups, minimizing injury and increasing the likelihood of compliance. Supervision is critical, not only for monitoring intensity, timing, position, and general safety but in helping those with cognitive impairment to navigate the regimens and equipment.

Equipment should also be selected carefully to best accommodate the needs and limitations of older adults. Only certain brands of treadmills have the capacity to perform at the very low speeds required by some elderly. Recumbent cycles and recumbent steppers may be better tolerated by older adults, many of whom are shrunken with osteoporosis, as well as suffering from diminished flexibility and reduced balance. Similarly, arm ergometers may be especially appealing to those with lower extremity impairments. In general, guard rails, safety belts, and harnesses provide critical components for safety and patient confidence. Likewise, stop buttons, non-slip flooring, and optimal lighting are important.

When available, use of water aerobics and/or swimming are also options for exercise that can result in excellent training effects with minimal joint strain. In contrast, activities such as running, jumping rope, and high-impact aerobics are best avoided.

After aerobic exercises are completed, cool down with light activities such as walking is crucial. Cooling down activity allows for continued venous return despite exercise-induced peripheral vasodilation. Nonetheless, hypotension (especially in adults using antihypertensive medications), overheating (especially in adults using anticholinergic medications), and arrhythmias (especially in patients with CHD) are all common during cool down, and close monitoring is essential.

MUSCLE STRENGTH AND ENDURANCE TRAINING

Strength training entails either static (isometric) and dynamic contractions of a muscle group against a resistance. Older men and women have been shown to gain strength and endurance in response to strength training, with associated gains in muscle mass and improved neural recruitment patterns. Furthermore, gains in muscle mass only accrue with strength training; while aerobic training has prominent benefits, there is added benefit from a composite program that combines aerobic and strength training. This is particularly true among the elderly, since senescent skeletal atrophy is otherwise pervasive and devastating.

Muscle strength and endurance are critical parameters for the elderly, particularly in maintaining functional independence. Hand strength is necessary for opening doors, containers, and faucets. Upper body strength is essential for lifting. Quadriceps strength has been identified as the single most important factor in a person's ability to walk, sit, stand, and climb stairs. Not only does diminished lower body strength predict nursing home placement, but it plays a key role in susceptibility to falls, especially in context of other typical changes associated with aging, such as diminished balance, flexibility, gait, baroreceptor sensitivity, proprioception, and vision.

Priorities at the onset of a strength training program are proper form and breathing. The initial sessions should involve strength-training maneuvers using little or no resistance. Proper form is emphasized to minimize injury. It is similarly important to avoid breath holding or Valsalva, which can lead to dangerous fluctuations in blood pressure and even syncope. In general, it is best to exhale during flexion (positive or concentric contraction), and to inhale during extension (negative or eccentric contraction). Proper warmup is also crucial. Very low-intensity aerobic movement and gentle range of motion exercises help prepare the joint and limb.

Once form, breathing, and warmup are secure, small weights (typically 0.5 to 1.0 lb) are added. In addition to light dumbells, common dynamic training tools include weighted balls, bars, rubberized tubing, and bands. The choices of weight increments and modes must be carefully selected relative to the specific joint and its musculoskeletal limitations, and the patient's exercise goals.

Current recommendations for adults aged 50 and older are initial use of light weights in sets of 10 to 15 repetitions for each muscle group. The repetitions should proceed to an endpoint of fatigue. Joint pain should be avoided. If the patient cannot tolerate at least 10 repetitions, lowering the weights should be considered.

Once 10 to 15 repetitions are comfortably tolerated, weights may be gradually increased, commonly using 0.5- to 1.0-lb increments. With each advancement, the number of repetitions are typically decreased to 6 to 8 repetitions before advancing towards 10 to 15. Strength training is usually administered only two to three times a week on nonconsecutive days.

Compared to free weights, exercise machines have the advantage of better controlling body and limb position, and theoretically the potential for greater safety. Still, not only are many of these machines intimidating, but some lack the capacity for the small increments of progression that are critical for older adults. Moreover, some of the machines (Nautilus and Universal) place resistive stresses on a joint that vary as the weight is moved through a range of motion. Such fluctuations may be harmful, and consequently certain machines have been designed to generate dynamic resistance with more constant stresses (such as Keiser pneumatic exercise machines) that may be safer. While conceptually appealing, such pneumatic exercise equipment is expensive and its availability is limited.

Resistance training can also be accomplished using isometric exercise, such as lifting or pushing against an immovable object, e.g., squeezing a ball between one's knees. This has the advantage of added safety, since stresses on joints are constant. However, overall training stimulus is restricted to one joint angle, and therefore the training benefits are more limited.

STRETCHING EXERCISES

Flexibility involves the range of motion around a joint as well its intrinsic ease of movement. With sedentary aging, muscles have a natural tendency to shorten and contract, connective tissue to stiffen and weaken, and joints to become stiff and restricted. Posture, balance, and gait all deteriorate. Stretching exercises help maintain and improve flexibility, with reduced joint instability, falls, and frailty.

To initiate safe and effective stretching exercises, adequate muscle warmup is critical. The rhythmic movements of aerobic exercise are an effective means to prepare muscles and joints for stretching, and so many programs incorporate stretching into the latter part of an aerobic training session. Stretching may also be completed separately or at the onset of a training session as long as adequate warmup is first completed. In fact, many value stretching prior to strength training as an important means to prepare the joint and muscle for the resistance stresses.

Static stretching, i.e., stretching the muscle group to the point of tension and then holding, is preferable over ballistic training (repetitive bouncing movements), which has a greater chance of causing injury. Optimal stretching usually means that specific joints and muscles are stretched and held 10 to 13 seconds. Typically, such stretching routines should be performed about two to three times a week, with four repetitions at each joint/muscle per session (depending on the stage of training).

EXERCISE SAFETY AND INTERCURRENT ILLNESS

While well-supervised exercise programs help insure optimal safety and give an incentive to exercise, many adults still prefer to exercise more independently. However, the possibilities of complications and/or injury must be weighed against the choice to exercise in isolation. Therefore, simple advice for elderly is that one exercise with or near to a friend, thereby ensuring safety and confidence even among those for whom larger exercise programs seem undesirable.

Among older adults, the likelihood of intercurrent illness is always high, with high potential to hamper exercise routines. As little as 2 weeks of bedrest is known to cause marked detraining, and may quickly wipe out years of exercise advantages. Therefore, it is important that an exercise pattern be maintained in the midst of an illness at whatever level is tolerated. For example, in a bedridden patient, range of motion exercises may help allay the progression of detraining. Bedridden patients may also be able to continue limited weight training, which helps to preserve strength and function.

Arthritis is another factor that becomes a rationalization not to exercise for many of the elderly. However, exercise often helps alleviate some of the effects of arthritis, improving cartilage and increasing muscle mass that help dissipate joint stresses and trauma. Therefore, even in the midst of a flareup of arthritis, it is important that exercise regimens continue, often on a modified basis and then slowly advancing as tolerated.

SUMMARY

Exercise guidance for older adults has the potential to improve health and independence. A composite program of aerobic, resistance, and stretching exercises will promote strength, aerobic capacity, and joint stability, all critical components in health and well-being. However, there is no absolute, standardized exercise prescription for all. The capacities and limitations of each patient determine an optimal regimen.

A frail and deconditioned adult might, for example, benefit particularly from an exercise program that prioritizes strength training. In fact, many deconditioned elderly are too weak initially to even consider aerobic training activities. Therefore, the exercise program may consist of only low-

intensity strength training for several weeks before sufficient strength and flexibility for aerobic training has accrued. Similarly, while 10 to 15 repetitions are usually the goal in strength training programs for the elderly, the number of repetitions may initially need to be reduced in those who are unusually deconditioned. Eventually, aerobic training should be added to training programs for the frail; recumbent steppers or recumbent bicycles may provide added security and safety compared to upright exercises. Furthermore, upper body training often produces disproportionate strain and hypertension, and isolated lower body exercises may be preferable.

Exercise guidance for robust older elderly must address different priorities. Many of these adults may be inclined to exercise intensely, leading to an entirely different set of concerns, e.g., the need for pretraining stress testing, and the need to set guidelines for strength, aerobic, and stretching training that are safe and sustainable. Even among such robust elderly, aerobic and strength training at mild to moderate intensities are likely to achieve maximum benefit with a minimum of risk. Low-to moderate-intensity daily aerobic exercises can be combined with daily stretching and moderate-intensity strength training (10 to 15 repetitions twice weekly). Emphasis needs to be placed on consistency and gentle progression to alleviate the greater susceptibility to complications and injury. Exercise programs should ideally include aspects of personal monitoring and guidance to best attain optimal exercise form and strategy for health and safety.

Among the principles distinguishing exercise training for all types of elderly patients is the value of prudence. Starting each exercise with low intensity and advancing slowly provides maximal safety and efficacy. Also particularly important in the elderly are periods of stretching, warmup, and cooldown activity. Since vasomotor responses and joint stability are both intrinsically limited by age, the extra time and care to complete these steps provide crucial elements of safety. Proper form and monitoring also have added importance in minimizing mishaps among the exercising elderly.

Using the simple guidelines outlined in this review, exercise has the potential to significantly improve the health status of older adults. Despite the fundamental and well-known benefits of exercise, it still is commonly eclipsed by other clinical concerns and therapies for the elderly. Thus, amidst the many advances in modern geriatric medicine, exercise is still novel therapy waiting to be implemented.

REFERENCES

1. U.S. Department of Health and Human Services. Physical activity and health: a report of the Surgeon General. Atlanta, GA: U.S. Department of Health and Human Services, Center for Disease Control and Prevention, National Center for Chronic Disease Prevention and Health Promotion, 1996:1–33.

2. Shephard RJ. The scientific basis for exercise prescribing for the very old. J Am Geriatr Soc 1990;38:62–70.

3. Mosekilde L. Osteoporosis and exercise. Bone 1995;17:193–195.

4. Chua TP, Ponikowski P, Harrington D, et al. Clinical correlates and prognostic significance of the ventilatory response to exercise in chronic heart failure. J Am Coll Cardiol 1997;29:1585–1590.

5. Bittner V, Weiner DH, Rodgers WJ, et al. Prediction of mortality and morbidity with a 6-minute walk test in patients with left ventricular dysfunction: SOLVD investigators. JAMA 1993;270:1702–1707.

6. Rogers MA, Hagberg JM, Martin WH III, et al. Decline in Vo$_2$ max with aging in master athletes and sedentary men. J Appl Physiol 1990;68:2195–2199.

7. Jette AM, Branch LG. The Framingham Disability Study: physical

disability among the aging. Am J Public Health 1981;71: 1211–1216.

8. Fiatarone MA, O'Neill EF, Ryan ND, et al. Exercise training and nutritional supplementation for physical fraility in very elderly people. N Engl J Med 1994; 330:1769–1775.

9. Fiatarone MA, Marks EC, Ryan ND, et al. High intensity strength training in nonagenarians: effects on skeletal muscle. JAMA 1990; 263:3029–3034.

10. Frontera WR, Merideth CN, O'Reilly KP, et al. Strength conditioning in older men: skeletal muscle hypertrophy and improved function. Palo Alto, CA: American Physiological Society, 1988.

11. Grimby G, Aniansson A, Hedberg M, Henning GB. Training can improve muscle strength and endurance in 78- to 84-year-old men. J Appl Physiol 1992;73: 2517–2523.

12. Rosenthal J. Aging and the cardio-vascular system. Gerontology 1987;33:3–8.

13. Kelly R, Hayward C, Avolio A, O'Rourke M. Noninvasive determination of age-related changes in the human arterial pulse. Circulation 1989;80: 1652–1659.

14. Gerhard M, Roddy MA, Creager SJ, Creager MA. Aging progressively impairs endothelium-dependent vasodilation in forearm resistance vessels of humans. Hypertension 1996;27:849–853.

15. Hornig B, Maier V, Drexler H. Physical training improves endothelial function in patients with chronic heart failure. Circulation 1996;93:210–214.

16. Gibbons RJ, Balady GJ, Beasley JW, et al. ACC/AHS guidelines for exercise testing: a report of the American College of Cardiology/American Heart Association Task Force on Practice Guidelines (Committee on Exercise Testing). J Am Coll Cardiol 1997;30: 260–315.

17. Borg G. Psychophysical bases of perceived exertion. Med Sci Sports Exerc 1982;14:377–381.

18. Sparks KD, Shaw DK, Eddy D, et al. Alternatives for cardiac rehabilitation patients unable to return to a hospital-based program. Heart Lung 1993;22:298–303.

Chapter 64

Lifestyle-Oriented Family Practice

Charles B. Eaton

Family physicians as primary care physicians have the opportunity to provide preventive care and lifestyle-oriented counseling as well as give therapeutic care to patients with diseases and undifferentiated problems. The degree to which family physicians provide lifestyle counseling will vary from practice to practice and clinician to clinician.

Which preventive services or what type of lifestyle counseling should be offered? A review of the leading causes of death by age group and the modifiable risk factors associated with each major cause of mortality is useful in identifying those lifestyle issues that should be considered as targets for counseling intervention. The leading causes of death vary by age, but most can be prevented or their morbidity can be significantly modified through lifestyle changes. Table 64-1 lists the top 10 causes of death for three age groups based upon Healthy People 2000 report (1).

CHILDHOOD

Lifestyle-oriented counseling should begin in childhood. The No. 1 cause of death in childhood is injury. Nearly half of all injuries in childhood and early adulthood are unintentional, and the majority are related to motor vehicle accidents. Lack of use of seat belts and safety seats in childhood and excess alcohol consumption in early adulthood are the leading causes of fatality from motor vehicle accidents. Homicides and suicides are also leading causes of death in children, adolescents, and young adults, and are often related to the use of firearms and alcohol. Alcohol consumption among teenagers and young adults is a significant problem. In a 1987 national survey, 28% of eighth graders and 38% of tenth graders reported heavy drinking (2).

Cigarette smoking is an important risk factor in cancer, heart disease, and use of illicit drugs. It is estimated that 30% of all cancer and 85% of lung cancer is linked to cigarette smoking (3). Although the chronic diseases caused by cigarette smoking occur in adulthood, their roots are in adolescence. The earlier a cigarette smoker begins, the less likely he or she is to quit. Three-fourths of high school seniors who smoke report that they smoked their first cigarette by grade 9.

It is estimated that 78% of adolescent girls and 86% of adolescent boys have engaged in sexual intercourse by age 20 (4). Early sexual activity increases the risk of unwanted pregnancy, as well as that of HIV and other sexually transmitted diseases. Teenage pregnancies are associated with significant psychosocial problems including unemployment, low birthweight infants, and inadequate parenting skills. While delaying sexual activity is one obvious solution, teenage sexual activity is a complex problem with important family, social, and economic factors. Successful interventions have been limited, and appear to need the full support of parents, other advisors, and peer role models.

The nutritional and exercise habits of adults appear to be developed in childhood and adolescence. Many chronic diseases or risk factors for chronic disease such as obesity, hypertension, diabetes mellitus, coronary heart disease, and probably some cancers can be prevented by developing healthy lifestyles that involve adoption of low-fat, low-salt dietary patterns and regular moderate or vigorous physical activity.

For high-risk youths, it appears that comprehensive programs are needed to provide indepth counseling and positive alternatives to alcohol, drug abuse, teenage pregnancy, and violence. Developing comprehensive programs for

713

Table 64-1 Top Ten Causes of Death by Age Group

Age 1–14	Age 15–24	Age 25–65
Injuries	Injuries	Cancer
Cancer	Homicide	Heart disease
Congenital anomalies	Suicide	Injuries
Homicide	Cancer	Stroke
Heart disease	Heart disease	Suicide
Pneumonia/ influenza	Congenital anomalies	Liver disease
Suicide	HIV infection	Chronic lung disease
Meningitis	Pneumonia/ influenza	Homicide
Chronic lung disease	Stroke	HIV infection
HIV infection	Chronic lung disease	Diabetes

problem adolescents is beyond the scope of most primary care practices. However, programs for adolescent obesity and smoking cessation can be implemented in a family practice setting and are particularly successful when done in conjunction with family members. The prevention of the development of risk factors (primordial prevention) through counseling regarding the adoption of regular exercise, appropriate eating habits, and abstinence from cigarette smoking, alcohol, and substance use are the interventions most likely to be successful in late childhood and adolescence. Primordial prevention (i.e., adoption of regular physical activity, eating three nutritionally balanced meals daily including five to seven servings of fruits and vegetables daily) can more effectively be implemented through collaboration with community organizations such as schools, churches, scouts, clubs, and other civic organizations. Family physicians, as community leaders, can work with local health department officials, school nurses, nutritionists, recreation department heads, coaches, and others to be sure that regular physical activity and appropriate balanced nutrition is provided in schools, recreation programs, and at civic events.

Table 64-2 Coronary Heart Disease Risk Factor Prediction Chart

1. FIND POINTS FOR EACH RISK FACTOR

Age (If Female)				Age (If Male)				HDL-Cholesterol		Total-Cholesterol		Systolic Blood Pressure		Other	
Age	Pts.	Age	Pts.	Age	Pts.	Age	Pts.	HDL-C	Pts.	Total-C	Pts.	SBP	Pts	Other	Pts.
30	–12	47–48	5	30	02	57–59	13	25–26	7	139–151	–3	98–104	–2	Cigarettes	4
31	–11	49–50	6	31	–1	60–61	14	27–29	6	152–166	–2	105–112	–1	Diabetic-male	3
32	–9	51–52	7	32–33	0	62–64	15	30–32	5	167–182	–1	113–120	0	Diabetic-female	6
33	–8	53–55	8	34	1	65–67	16	33–35	4	183–199	0	121–129	1	ECG-LVH	9
34	–6	56–60	9	35–36	2	68–70	17	36–38	3	200–219	1	130–139	2		
35	–5	61–67	10	37–38	3	71–73	18	39–42	2	220–239	2	140–149	3	0 pts for	
36	–4	68–74	11	39	4	74	19	43–46	1	240–262	3	150–160	4	each NO	
37	–3			40–41	5			47–50	0	263–288	4	161–172	5		
38	–2			42–43	6			51–55	–1	289–315	5	173–185	6		
39	–1			44–45	7			56–60	–2	316–330	6				
40	0			46–47	8			61–66	–3						
41	1			48–49	9			67–73	–4						
42–43	2			50–51	10			74–80	–5						
44	3			52–54	11			81–87	–6						
45–46	4			55–56	12			88–96	–7						

2. SUM POINTS FOR ALL RISK FACTORS

$$\overline{\text{Age}} + \overline{\text{HDL-C}} + \overline{\text{Total-C}} + \overline{\text{SBP}} + \overline{\text{Smoker}} + \overline{\text{Diabetes}} + \overline{\text{ECG-LVH}} = \overline{\text{Point Total}}$$

NOTE: MINUS POINT SUBTRACT FROM TOTAL

3. LOOK UP RISK CORRESPONDING TO POINT TOTAL

	Probability			Probability			Probability			Probability			Probability	
Pts.	5 Yr.	10 Yr.	Pts.	5 Yr.	10 Yr.	Pts.	5 Yr.	10 Yr.	Pts.	5 Yr.	10 Yr.	Age	Women	Men
≤1	<1%	<2%	10	2%	6%	19	8%	16%	28	19%	33%	30–34	<1%	3%
2	1%	2%	11	3%	6%	20	8%	18%	29	20%	36%	35–39	<1%	5%
3	1%	2%	12	3%	7%	21	9%	19%	30	22%	38%	40–44	2%	6%
4	1%	2%	13	3%	8%	22	11%	21%	31	24%	40%	45–49	5%	10%
5	1%	3%	14	4%	9%	23	12%	23%	32	25%	42%	50–54	8%	14%
6	1%	3%	15	5%	10%	24	13%	25%				55–59	12%	16%
7	1%	4%	16	5%	12%	25	14%	27%				60–64	13%	21%
8	2%	4%	17	6%	13%	26	16%	29%				65–69	9%	30%
9	2%	5%	18	7%	14%	27	17%	31%				70–74	12%	24%

These charts were prepared with the help of William B. Kannel, M.D., Professor of Medicine and Public Health and Ralph D'Agostino, Ph.D., Head, Department of Mathematics, both at Boston University, Keaven Anderson, Ph.D., Statistician, NHLBI, Framingham Study; Daniel McGee, Ph.D., Associate Professor, University of Arizona.

ADULTHOOD

Adults have the opportunity to assume personal responsibility for their health and are candidates for lifestyle-oriented counseling and medical care. Seven major lifestyle issues (excess alcohol, excess calories, excess dietary fat, excess dietary salt, cigarette smoking, physical inactivity, and obesity) are associated with five of the major causes of death for this age group (cancer, heart disease, stroke, injury, chronic lung disease).

OFFICE-BASED SYSTEM

An effective lifestyle-oriented family practice requires screening and labeling at-risk patients, a physician reminder system, a patient-centered physician message to change risky lifestyles, prevention team assistance, and systematic follow-up. Since patients come to physicians with a variety of complaints, many related to acute symptoms, an effective screening and labeling system needs to be developed. One approach is to use stickers on the front of the chart or prevention cards (5) (Fig. 64-1) to trigger the physician to address these lifestyle issues. Another effective system that we have utilized in our primary care office is to change the routine vital sign protocol to include weight, blood pressure, smoking, and physical activity status, and eliminate pulse, respiration, and temperature unless specifically requested by the physician. This simple change allows for all adult patients to be assessed for hypertension, obesity, smoking, and sedentary lifestyle at every patient visit. Some offices determine high-risk patients by using computer-based health risk appraisals or the Framingham risk equation (6) for estimating CHD risk (Table 64-2).

Physician reminders can be of several types. Some investigators have tried computer-generated prevention lists either clipped to paper charts or as a screen in an electronic medical record. Other projects have used touch screen technology in the waiting room of the physician's office to obtain patient input used to develop screening and risk factor counseling profiles for each patient. Another method is to have the medical assistants, on the day prior to the visit, attach reminders to the chart based upon a chart audit. Still others have used flow sheets, patient-initiated reminders, or stage of change questionnaires (Table 64-3).

The physician's message needs to be tailored to the patient's needs and the time commitment available for lifestyle changes. This time commitment will vary based upon reimbursement issues and the physician's personal interest and training. Other chapters in this text focus on smoking cessation, nutritional assessment and counseling, physical activity counseling, and other interventions in more detail.

A physician-based counseling program called the "5 As," adopted by the National Cancer Institute for smoking cessation, is a useful model that appears to be applicable to most lifestyle counseling sessions. The elements of this program are: 1) address the agenda, 2) assess, 3) advise, 4) assist, and 5) arrange follow-up."

Addressing the agenda can be prompted by a prevention checklist, tickler system, or vital sign stamp that includes lifestyle issues or other methods mentioned above. A statements such as, "As your personal physician, I am interested in preventing disease as much as treating illness. I am concerned about your ____ (smoking, lack of physical activity, high fat diet, etc.) and wondered how you feel about this?" is one way in which the topic can be addressed.

Assessing the patient's psychological state, stage of change, motivational state, and barriers to change is the next step. Figure 64-2 outlines the stages of change for smoking cessation, and similar paradigms have been proposed for physical activity, high-fat diet, and other lifestyle risk factors (7). The patient's previous experience with the lifestyle change suggested, previous attempts to change, environmental and social factors, and perceived confidence in the ability to make changes (self-efficacy) are all helpful pieces of information in tailoring counseling advice for lifestyle changes. Another important aspect of the assessment is to determine which of several lifestyle behaviors that may be unhealthy should be the focus of the advice and counseling session. A discussion of the patient's priorities and a shared agreement of the most important change to make is essential. Behavioral research has shown that patients attempting to make multiple changes are far less likely to succeed than those who make sequential changes, one at a time.

Advice should be personalized and, when possible, linked to the patient's present health problems or family history. This personalization by the patient's primary care physician appears to empower the behavior change message. Linkage by the physician of the health behavior to the patient's present or future health problems increases the likelihood that the patient will attempt lifestyle change over the short term.

Assistance in designing a specific behavioral program for a lifestyle change is the next step in the counseling process. A stage-matched approach has been found helpful in office-based practice. For patients in the pre-contemplative or contemplative stage, referral or in-depth counseling efforts are not appropriate; instead the role of the physician is to readdress the issue at the next visit. For those patients in the action stage, in-depth counseling is appropriate. This can be done by the physician or may be delegated to an office team member or a specialty clinic. Establishing an assistance program for each risk factor is an important aspect of a lifestyle-oriented family practice. This may include training one or a combination of providers, such as nurses, nutritionists, social workers, exercise physiologists, pharmacists, and health educators, to focus on smoking cessation, substance abuse, nutritional counseling, physical activity counseling, weight loss, and enhanced medication compliance. It is important that whoever does the counseling does more than just transmit knowledge about a particular subject matter; the counselor should also focus on problem solving, skill building, and reinforcement. Self-help guides, a list of support groups in the community, referrals to preventive cardiology clinics, cardiac rehabilitation programs, nutritionists, clinical psychologists, and substance abuse counselors, should be made available to all who desire or need their services.

In assisting patients in making a specific behavior change, identifying problem areas or barriers to overcome is important. Eliciting patients' preferences, detailing plans for lifestyle change and explaining the rationale for the plans is the next step. Negotiating short-term and long-term goals are important. Communicating the importance of the tasks and

NAME ——————————————————————————

©NOKOMIS CLINIC, Ltd.

——— PREVENTION CARD ———

ITEM	FREQ.	STATUS									
		Prior	1987	1988	1989	1990	1991	1992	1993	1994	1995
√ Health Evaluation											
Risk Appraisal											
Tobacco (#/day)	yearly										
Alcohol (#/day)	yearly										
Exercise (#/wk)	yearly										
Seat Belts (%)	yearly										
√ Td	10 yrs										
Flu	yr. 65+										
√ Blood Pressure	yearly										
√ Weight	yearly										
Breast	yearly										
Pelvic											
Cholesterol											
Stool Blood											
Pap											
Sigmoidoscopy											
Mammogram											

Figure 64-1 Prevention card for patient chart. (Reprinted by permission from Solberg LI, Kottke LE, Brekke ML. The prevention-oriented practice. In: Ockene IS, Ockene JK, eds. Prevention of coronary heart disease. Boston: Little, Brown, 1992.)

Current Physical Activity Status
Circle one number only

1. I do not exercise or walk regularly now, and I do not intend to start in the near future.
2. I do not exercise or walk regularly, but I have been thinking of starting.
3. I am trying to start to exercise or walk. (or) During the last month I have started to exercise or walk on occasion (or on weekends only).
4. I have exercised or walked infrequently (or on weekends only) for over one month.
5. I am doing vigorous or moderate exercise, less than 3 times per week (or moderate exercise less than 2 hours per week).
6. I have been doing moderate exercise, 3 or more times per week (or more than 2 hours per week) for the last 1–6 months.
7. I have been doing moderate exercise, 3 or more times per week (or more than 2 hours per week) for 7 months or more
8. I have been doing vigorous exercise, 3–5 times per week for 1–6 months.
9. I have been doing vigorous exercise, 3–5 times per week for 7–12 months.
10. I have been doing vigorous exercise, 3–5 times per week for 12 months.
11. I do vigorous exercise 6 or more times per week.

SOURCE: Centers for Disease Control, Cardiovascular Health Branch. Project PACE: physician manual. Atlanta: Centers for Disease Control, 1992.

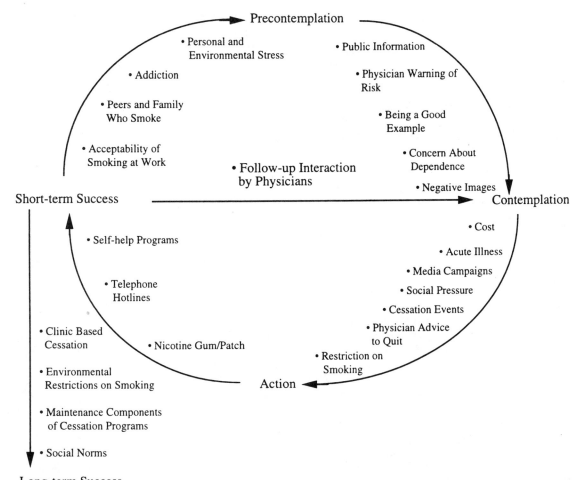

Figure 64-2 The stages of change process for smoking cessation. (Reprinted by permission from Houston TP, et al. How to help patients stop smoking: guidelines for diagnosis and treatment of nicotine dependence. Chicago: American Medical Association, 1994.

Activity Record

the active way to health

On this form, check the days you do the activity prescribed for you. Then take it back to your doctor.

What activity did your doctor prescribe?

For how long?   And how often?

	1	2	3	4	5	6	7	8	9	10	11	12	13	14	15	16	17	18	19	20	21	22	23	24	25	26	27	28	29	30	31
January																															
February																															
March																															
April																															
May																															
June																															
July																															
August																															
September																															
October																															
November																															
December																															

Notes

This form may be reproduced or modified for use in patient care by an individual medical practice without permission. However, it may not be distributed or sold without the express written permission of Charles B. Eaton, M.D., Memorial Hospital of Rhode Island.

Figure 64-3 Sample physical activity log for patient use.

goals set by writing them down is important. A written prescription or written behavioral contract have both been used with some success. Self-monitoring by the use of a daily log is critical for most difficult lifestyle changes. Figure 64-3 is a log for physical activity that we have adopted in our lifestyle-oriented family practice. Having the patient use their own words to describe in detail the steps they are going to take to make a lifestyle change will ensure that the patient has incorporated your suggestions into a plan. Be sure to summarize major points and anticipate problematic situations. Use patient education and self-help materials sparingly so as to not overwhelm the patient with new knowledge.

Arranging follow-up is the critical final step. Since behavioral or lifestyle changes occur in the context of a social setting, most patients will relapse or become non-adherent. Therefore, patients need a supportive system of follow-up that may include phone calls, office visits, mailings near crucial dates (i.e. quit dates for smoking), and computerized tracking systems. Figure 64-4 is a schema of the post-hospitalization feedback system for patients with CHD initiated by our Heart Disease Prevention Center. Prior to leaving the counseling session, agreeing on a means to evaluate progress and the time period for evaluation, is critical to insure appropriate follow-up. We have found e-mail to be a nearly ideal method for timely, inexpensive feedback for those patients who have Internet access.

DEVELOPING AN OFFICE-BASED SYSTEM

A successful lifestyle-oriented family practice cannot exist in a vacuum but needs a supportive office system. Using business principles, eight elements have been found to be required for such a system. These include policy establishment, staff endorsement, coordination, an implementation plan, orientation and training, resource allocation, chart audits, and a maintenance program. The office management needs to clearly state its commitment to the treatment of lifestyle-modified risk factors. A single individual should be made accountable and given the authority and responsibility to implement the program. The support staff needs to understand the need for the system and help develop the office-based system so that all elements are incorporated. Coordination of the system usually relies upon effective communication between the nurse manager and the physician director. An implementation plan needs to be developed that identifies role definitions, determines job descrip-

718   Part XI   Family Practice

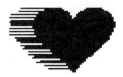

RIASS
RI Atherosclerosis Surveillance System

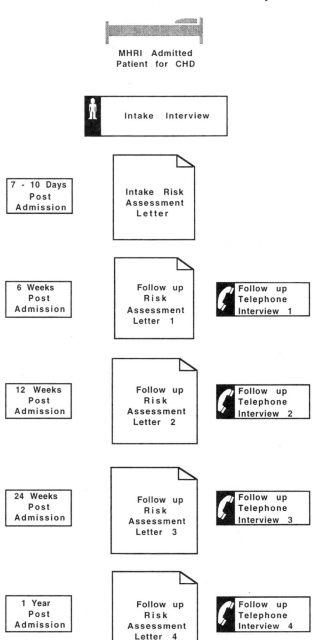

MHRI Admitted
Patient for CHD

Intake Interview

7 - 10 Days Post Admission — Intake Risk Assessment Letter

6 Weeks Post Admission — Follow up Risk Assessment Letter 1 — Follow up Telephone Interview 1

12 Weeks Post Admission — Follow up Risk Assessment Letter 2 — Follow up Telephone Interview 2

24 Weeks Post Admission — Follow up Risk Assessment Letter 3 — Follow up Telephone Interview 3

1 Year Post Admission — Follow up Risk Assessment Letter 4 — Follow up Telephone Interview 4

Figure 64-4 Post-hospitalization feedback system for CHD patients.

tions, performs financial impact analyses, arranges scheduling plans, and plots a timetable for initiation. Each staff member (physician, nurse, secretary and others) needs to be informed of the implementation plan, given the opportunity to feel involved, and trained in the tasks required to implement the plan.

The necessary resource allocations include development of materials or purchase of self-help materials such as those available from the American Heart Association, American Lung Association, and National Cancer Institute for each risk factor. In addition, providing patients with a list of referral sources in their communities is most beneficial.

Periodic chart audits or a comparable evaluation tool are critical in determining whether a program is successful. Formal feedback to providers about their success, problem solving concerning lack of progress, and a reward system are important elements of a maintenance system to encourage continued interest by physicians and staff. Without such maintenance programs, physicians and staff lose interest in providing lifestyle counseling, because most providers recall their failures and not their successes. Feedback activities may include a graph of the number of patients who have successfully quit smoking with the program or the posting of pictures of all successful patients who quit smoking. Other examples, would be a graph of the average LDL cholesterol decline in patients that are in the program, or a global map with the cumulative miles walked by patients in your practice, going across the country or around the world.

SUMMARY

A lifestyle-oriented family practice can be developed in a busy family practice setting when business and organizational principles are applied to help prevent disease and promote lifestyle changes. Identifying high risk-individuals and providing comprehensive services using a team-based approach to those patients who are motivated and in a psychological state predicting successful lifestyle change allows for time-efficient management of lifestyle issues. For those patients at low risk or who are not currently motivated to make changes, continued follow-up and feedback related to these lifestyle issues is critical. Even among those patients who make significant lifestyle changes, the majority relapse or experience short-term lapses. The continued follow-up of these patients is most important for continued success. Just as patients lose interest if they do not experience success with lifestyle changes, so do practitioners lose interest in lifestyle counseling if they fail to understand the cyclical nature of behavior change and the need for reinforcement. For example, a 10% quit rate in smoking needs to be viewed as a success, and the need for as many as seven short-term quit attempts prior to complete cessation is not unusual. Use of medications in conjunction with behavioral approaches to help manage risk factors when behavioral approaches alone are not successful should be incorporated into disease management systems and should not be seen as failures but rather quality medical care.

REFERENCES

1. U.S. Department of Health and Human Services. Healthy people 2000: national health promotion and disease prevention objectives. DHHS publication no. (PHS) 91-50212. Washington, DC: US. Department of Health and Human Services, 1991.

2. American School Health Association, Association of the Advancement of Health Education and Society for Public Health Education. National adolescent student health survey. Oakland, CA: Third Party Press, 1989.

3. Doll R. and Peto R. The causes of cancer: quantitative estimates of available risks of cancer in the United States today. J Natl Cancer Inst 1981;66:1111–1308.

4. National Research Council. Risking the future: adolescent sexuality, pregnancy and child bearing. Washington, DC: National Academy Press, 1987.

5. Solberg LI, Kottke TE, Brekke ML. The prevention-oriented practice. In: Prevention of coronary heart disease. Ockene IS, Ockene JK, eds. Boston: Little, Brown, 1992.

6. Kannel WB, D'Agostino R, Anderson K, McGee D. Coronary heart disease risk factor prediction chart, In: Goroll AH, May LA, Mulley AG, eds. Primary care medicine: office evaluation and management of the adult patient. 3rd ed. Philadelphia: JB Lippincott, 1995.

7. Houston TP, et al. How to help patients stop smoking: guidelines for diagnosis and treatment of nicotine dependence. Chicago: American Medical Association, 1994.

Part XII.

CARDIOVASCULAR REHABILITATION AND SECONDARY PREVENTION

Edited by
Barry A. Franklin

Introduction to Cardiovascular Rehabilitation and Secondary Prevention

Barry A. Franklin

The potential value of exercise therapy in cardiac patients was recognized as early as the clinical description of coronary heart disease itself. In 1772, Herberden noted that one of his symptomatic patients was "nearly cured" after 6 months of sawing wood on a regular basis. Until the mid-1980s, secondary prevention of coronary atherosclerosis focused primarily on exercise training and a prudent diet. These regimens generally resulted in improved functional capacity, reduced myocardial demands at submaximal work rates, and modest decreases in cardiovascular mortality. However, reinfarction rates and the course of atherosclerotic heart disease remained largely unchanged.

Today, exercise training continues to play an important role in the medical management and rehabilitation of patients with cardiovascular disease. Although hypertension, hyperlipidemia, obesity, and diabetes mellitus may be favorably affected by regular physical activity, exercise alone should not be expected to alter global coronary risk status. Contemporary cardiovascular rehabilitation programs have further improved health-related outcomes by complementing exercise with education and counseling, medical surveillance and emergency support (when appropriate), pharmacotherapy, and interventions to enhance psychosocial functioning and long-term adherence to lifestyle changes. These interventions include assessing the patient's "readiness" for change, providing services that are designed to circumvent or attenuate common barriers to enrollment and adherence (e.g., offering group and home-based programs), keeping goals short-term and attainable, using motivational incentives accruing to periodic exercise testing and risk factor assessment, recruiting spouse and family support of the intervention, and archiving goal achievements.

The traditional paradigm suggested that the degree of coronary artery stenosis determined the risk of acute coronary events. Accordingly, revascularization procedures were viewed as the only effective approach to improving prognosis. However, intensive measures to control hyperlipidemia with diet, drugs, and exercise, especially in combination, have now been shown to stabilize and even reverse the otherwise inexorable progression of atherosclerotic coronary artery disease. Added benefits include a reduction in anginal symptoms, decreases in exercise-induced myocardial ischemia, fewer recurrent cardiac events, and diminished need for coronary artery bypass surgery and percutaneous transluminal coronary angioplasty. These findings suggest a new paradigm in the treatment of patients with coronary artery disease, including therapeutic measures to promote plaque stabilization and normalization of endothelial function.

The authors of this section represent a prestigious group of scientists, clinicians, and researchers, whose contributions over the years have profoundly influenced the field of cardiac rehabilitation as it exists today. Each painstakingly worked to summarize, in a clear and concise manner, the latest research findings in their respective areas, with specific reference to patient care and application. The author of the first chapter in this section, Victor Froelicher, details the role of exercise testing in the evaluation of clinically stable coronary patients, with specific reference to methodology, new American College of Cardiology/American Heart Association guidelines, status postrevascularization or anginal therapy, functional capacity, cardiac rhythm disorders, valvular heart disease, and exercise programming. The remaining chapters in this section review a variety of clinically relevant topics, including clinical practice guidelines on cardiac rehabilitation, outcomes achieved with multifactorial risk factor reduction, exercise for the coronary patient and its associated risk, psychosocial considerations, evaluating and treating peripheral vascular disease, and future directions.

L. Kent Smith summarizes the clinical practice guidelines on cardiac rehabilitation, which were derived from an extensive and critical review of 334 references in the scientific literature. The most substantial benefits included improvements in exercise tolerance, symptoms, blood lipid levels, psychosocial well-being, and reductions in cigarette smoking and mortality. Patients with heart failure and after cardiac transplantation, as well as elderly patients, were also addressed.

William Haskell and Joseph Carlson meticulously review the methodology and results of major clinical trials of multifactorial risk factor modification, emphasizing randomized studies that evaluated changes in coronary atherosclerotic lesions by quantitative angiography and subsequent fatal and nonfatal cardiac events. Mechanisms by which these interventions might provide benefit are briefly discussed and include partial (albeit small) anatomic regression of coronary artery stenoses, a reduced incidence of plaque rupture, and improved coronary artery vasomotor function.

Barry A. Franklin and associates summarize the physiologic and clinical bases for the prescription of exercise in patients with coronary artery disease, with particular emphasis on the optimal exercise dosage, upper body and resistance training, exercise trainability, aerobic and myocardial demands of common leisure activities, risk of exercise training, and special patient populations.

Roy J. Shephard describes the pathophysiologic mechanisms underlying exercise-related cardiovascular complications, as well as the risks and benefits of exercise in the older, coronary-prone individual and in those with established atherosclerotic heart disease. Although the risk of cardiac arrest and acute myocardial infarction appears to increase transiently during strenuous exercise compared with the risk at other times, especially among those with heart disease who are habitually sedentary, the overall risk of a cardiovascular event appears to be reduced in persons who are regular exercisers.

Elizabeth Gullette and James Blumenthal discuss psychosocial variables associated with the development and clinical manifestations of heart disease, contextual factors that may moderate coronary risk status, and potential mechanisms by which psychosocial variables increase the risk of cardiac events in patients with heart disease. Training in behavior modification, stress management, and relaxation techniques is discussed in relation to lowering indices of self-reported emotional stress, modifying Type-A behavior and attenuating levels of depression, social isolation, and anger and hostility.

Andrew Gardner extends the continuum of care by describing the significance and classification of peripheral arterial occlusive disease, associated cardiovascular complications and their sequelae, acute exercise responses in afflicted patients, appropriate exercise rehabilitation, and methods to evaluate the effectiveness of an exercise program. Notably, the value of the ankle-brachial index for detecting peripheral vascular disease is detailed.

Finally, Nanette Wenger elegantly forecasts how rehabilitation of the cardiac patient in the next millennium may differ from that undertaken today, emphasizing changes in the clinical spectrum of coronary heart disease and of heart failure, expansion of the populations considered eligible for rehabilitative care, and an escalating emphasis on preventive interventions.

Chapter 65

The Role of Exercise Testing in the Evaluation of the Patient with Stable Heart Disease

Victor Froelicher

The indications for exercise testing in patients with stable heart disease that are discussed in this chapter include prognostic assessment in stable coronary disease patients, evaluation of treatments and therapeutic interventions, evaluation of arrhythmias and valvular disease, and as part of the preoperative work up for noncardiac surgery. This chapter begins with some methodologic considerations for testing patients for the above-mentioned reasons. This information is evidence-based by following the ACC (American College of Cardiology)/AHA (American Heart Association) Guidelines for Exercise Testing (1).

METHODOLOGY

The large number of different exercise protocols in use has led to some confusion regarding how physicians compare tests between patients and serial tests in the same patient. The most common protocols, their stages, and the predicted oxygen cost of each stage are illustrated in Figure 65-1. When the treadmill was first introduced into clinical practice, practitioners adopted protocols used by major researchers (2–5). In 1980, Stuart et al (6) surveyed 1375 exercise laboratories in North America and reported that of those performing treadmill testing, 65.5% use the Bruce protocol for routine clinical testing. This protocol uses relatively large and unequal 2- to 3-MET (metabolic equivalent term) increments in work every 3 minutes. Large and uneven work increments such as these have been shown to result in a tendency to overestimate exercise capacity (7). Investigators have since recommended protocols with smaller and more equal increments (8,9). Currently the guidelines suggest that more graduated protocols be used

and have urged physicians to consider METs not minutes of exercise.

Redwood et al (10) performed serial testing in patients with angina and reported that work rate increments that were too rapid resulted in a reduced exercise capacity, and could not be reliably used for studying the effects of therapy. Smokler et al (11) reported that among 40 pairs of treadmill tests conducted within a 6-month period, tests that were less than 10 minutes in duration showed a much greater percentage of variation than those that were greater than 10 minutes in duration. Buchfuhrer et al (12) performed repeated maximal exercise testing in five normal subjects while varying the work rate increment. Maximal oxygen uptake varied with the increment in work; the highest values were observed when intermediate increments were used. Lipkin et al (13), on the other hand, observed that among patients with chronic heart failure, small work increments yielding a long test duration (31 ± 15 minutes) resulted in reduced values for maximal oxygen uptake, minute ventilation, and arterial lactate compared with tests using more standard increments. These observations have led a number of investigators to suggest that protocols should be individualized for each patient such that test duration is approximately 8 to 12 minutes.

Ramp Testing

An approach to exercise testing that has gained interest in recent years is the ramp protocol, in which work increases constantly and continuously (Figure 65-2). The guideline for "optimizing" exercise testing would appear to be facilitated by the ramp approach, since work increments are small, and since it allows for increases in work to be individualized, a given test duration can be targeted.

Figure 65-1 Treadmill protocols.

FUNCTIONAL CLASS	CLINICAL STATUS	O₂ COST ml/kg/min	METS	BICYCLE ERGOMETER	BRUCE 3 MIN STAGES MPH	BRUCE %GR	BALKE-WARE % GRADE AT 3.3 MPH 1 MIN STAGES	USAFSAM MPH	USAFSAM %GR	"SLOW" USAFSAM MPH	"SLOW" USAFSAM %GR	McHENRY MPH	McHENRY %GR	STANFORD % GRADE AT 3 MPH	STANFORD % GRADE AT 2 MPH	ACIP MPH	ACIP %GR	CHF MPH	CHF %GR	METS
NORMAL AND I	HEALTHY, DEPENDENT ON AGE, ACTIVITY			1 WATT = 6.1 Kpm/min	5.5	20														
				FOR 70 KG BODY WEIGHT Kpm/min	5.0	18														
		56.0	16				26													16
		52.5	15	1500			25	3.3	25							3.4	24.0			15
		49.0	14				24 23					3.3	21			3.1	24.0			14
		45.5	13	1350	4.2	16	22 21													13
		42.0	12				20 19	3.3	20			3.3	18	22.5		3.0	21.0			12
		38.5	11	1200			18 17							20.0				3.4	14.0	11
	SEDENTARY HEALTHY	35.0	10	1050	3.4	14	16 15	3.3	15	2	25	3.3	15	17.5		3.0	17.5	3.0	15.0	10
		31.5	9	900			14 13					3.3	12	15.0		3.0	14.0	3.0	12.5	9
		28.0	8	750			12 11	3.3	10	2	20			12.5		3.0	10.5	3.0	10.0	8
		24.5	7		2.5	12	10 9					3.3	9	10.0	17.5					7
II		21.0	6	600			8 7	3.3	5	2	15	3.3	6	7.5	14.0	3.0	7.0	3.0	7.5	6
		17.5	5	450	1.7	10	6 5			2	10			5.0	10.5			2.0	10.5	5
III	LIMITED SYMPTOMATIC	14.0	4	300	1.7	5	4 3			2	5			2.5	7.0	3.0	3.0	2.0	7.0	4
		10.5	3	150	1.7	0	2	3.3	0			2.0	3	0	3.5	2.5	2.0	2.0	3.5	3
		7.0	2				1	2.0	0	2	0					2.0	0.0	1.5	0.0	2
IV		3.5	1															1.0	0.0	1

Key: ACIP, asymptomatic cardiac ischemia pilot; CHF, congestive heart failure (modified Naughton); Kpm/min, kilopond meters per minute; METS, metabolic equivalents; MPH, miles per hour; %GR, percent grade; USAFSAM, United States Air Force School of Aerospace Medicine.

EXERCISE PROTOCOLS

Figure 65-2 Ramp protocol.

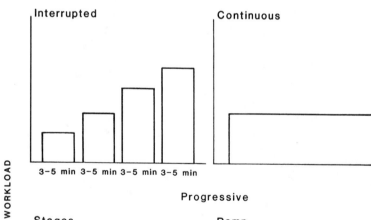

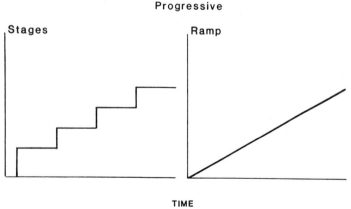

To investigate this, we compared ramp treadmill and bicycle tests to protocols more commonly used clinically. Ten patients with chronic heart failure, 10 with coronary artery disease (CAD) who were limited by angina during exercise, 10 with coronary artery disease who were asymptomatic during exercise, and 10 age-matched normal subjects performed three bicycle tests and three treadmill tests (Bruce, Balke, and ramp) in randomized order on different days. For the ramp tests, ramp rates on the bicycle and treadmill were individualized to yield a test duration of approximately 10 minutes for each subject. Maximal oxygen uptake was significantly higher (18%) on the treadmill protocols versus the bicycle protocols collectively, confirming previous observations. Only minor differences in maximal oxygen uptake, however, were observed between the treadmill protocols themselves or between the cycle ergometer protocols themselves. We observed that: 1) Oxygen uptake is overestimated from tests that contain large increments in work, and 2) the variability in estimating oxygen uptake from work rate is markedly greater on these tests than for an individualized ramp treadmill test. Because this approach appears to offer several advantages, we presently perform all our clinical and research testing using the ramp.

Blood Pressure Measurement

In patients with heart disease, careful measurement of systolic blood pressure (SBP) is critical. Although numerous clever devices have been developed to automate blood pressure measurement during exercise, none can be recommended. The time-proven method of the examiner holding the patient's arm with a stethoscope placed over the brachial artery remains the most reliable. A mercury manometer is preferred to an aneroid manometer. The patient's arm should be free of the hand rails so that noise is not transmitted up the arm. It is sometimes helpful to mark the brachial artery. If SBP appears to be increasing sluggishly or decreasing, it should be taken again immediately. Also, with the onset or worsening of chest pain, ST shifts, or arrhythmias, blood pressure should be taken immediately. If a drop in SBP of 20 mm Hg or more occurs after a normal rise or if it drops below the value obtained in the standing position prior to testing, the test should be stopped in patients with congestive heart failure or a prior myocardial infarction or who are exhibiting signs or symptoms of ischemia. So-called exertional hypotension is associated with cardiac arrests in the exercise laboratory and with a poor prognosis (14).

ST segment analysis is beyond the scope of this chapter and is not covered here. Please refer to the guidelines or a standard text.

PROGNOSTIC USE OF THE EXERCISE TEST

There are two principal reasons for estimating prognosis. The first is to provide accurate answers to patients' questions regarding the probable outcome of their illness. Although discussion of prognosis is inherently delicate and probability statements can be misunderstood, most patients find this information useful in planning their affairs regarding work, recreational activities, personal estate, and finances. The second reason to determine prognosis is to identify those patients in whom interventions might improve outcome.

Although improved prognosis equates with increased quantity of life, quality-of-life issues must also be taken into account. In that regard, it is apparent that in certain clinical settings, catheter or surgical interventions provide better therapy than medication. However, these interventions, when misapplied, can have a negative impact on the quality of life (inconvenience, complications, and discomfort), as well as creating a financial burden to the individual and to society.

The ACC/AHA Guidelines for the Prognostic Use of the Standard Exercise Test

Indications for Exercise Testing to Assess Risk and prognosis in patients with symptoms or a prior history of coronary artery disease:

Class I. Conditions for which there is evidence and/or general agreement that the standard exercise test is useful and helpful to assess risk and prognosis in patients with symptoms or a prior history of coronary artery disease.

- Patients undergoing initial evaluation with suspected or known CAD. Specific exceptions are noted below in Class IIb.
- Patients with suspected or known CAD previously evaluated with significant change in clinical status.

Class IIb. Conditions for which there is conflicting evidence and/or a divergence of opinion that the standard exercise test is useful and helpful to assess risk and prognosis in patients with symptoms or a prior history of coronary artery disease but the usefulness/efficacy is less well established.

- Patients who demonstrate the following ECG abnormalities:
  - Pre-excitation (Wolff-Parkinson White) syndrome;
  - Electronically paced ventricular rhythm;
  - More than one millimeter of resting ST depression; and
  - Complete left bundle branch block.
- Patients with a stable clinical course who undergo periodic monitoring to guide management

Class III. Conditions for which there is evidence and/or general agreement that the standard exercise test is not useful and helpful to assess risk and prognosis in patients with symptoms or a prior history of coronary artery disease and in some cases may be harmful.

- Patients with severe comorbidity likely to limit life expectancy and/or candidacy for revascularization.

The evidence supporting these guidelines is presented throughout this chapter.

Part of the Basic Patient Evaluation

Per the published guidelines, patients with known or suspected coronary disease are usually evaluated initially after a careful cardiac history and physical examination with an exercise test. It can be performed safely and inexpensively and even accomplished in the physician's office. In addition to diagnostic information, the test gives practical and clinically valuable information regarding exercise capacity and response to therapy. Patients with clinical data and exercise test responses considered abnormal or associated with a high enough proba-

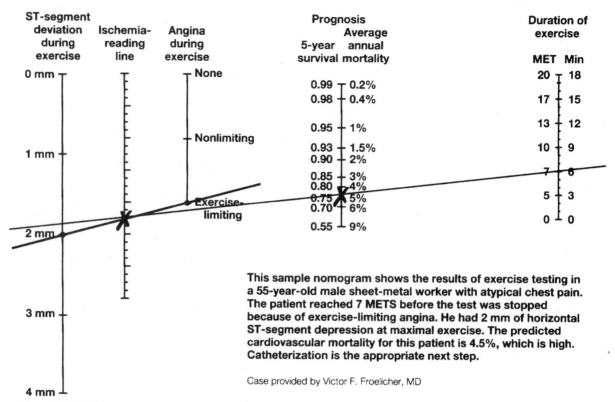

ST-segment deviation during exercise	Ischemia-reading line	Angina during exercise	Prognosis 5-year survival	Average annual mortality		Duration of exercise MET Min

This sample nomogram shows the results of exercise testing in a 55-year-old male sheet-metal worker with atypical chest pain. The patient reached 7 METS before the test was stopped because of exercise-limiting angina. He had 2 mm of horizontal ST-segment depression at maximal exercise. The predicted cardiovascular mortality for this patient is 4.5%, which is high. Catheterization is the appropriate next step.

Case provided by Victor F. Froelicher, MD

Figure 65-3 The DUKE nomogram.

bility for cardiac events or of having severe coronary disease are frequently evaluated further by coronary angiography. A study evaluating the appropriateness of the performance of coronary angiography in clinical practice considered angiography to be inappropriate nearly a quarter of the time because of the failure to obtain an exercise test (15).

The Duke Nomogram

Mark et al studied 2842 consecutive patients who underwent cardiac catheterization and exercise testing and whose data was entered into the Duke computerized medical information system (16). The median follow-up for the study population was 5 years and 98% complete. All patients underwent a Bruce protocol exercise test and had standard ECG measurements recorded. A treadmill angina index was assigned a value of 0 if angina was absent, 1 if typical angina occurred during exercise, and 2 if angina was the reason the patient stopped exercising. To make the score apply to other treadmill protocols, it is necessary to convert minutes in the Bruce protocol to METs with the equation: METs equals 1.3 (minutes) −2.2 or minutes in the Bruce protocol equals METs +2.2 divided by 1.3.

A score was calculated as: exercise time − (5 × ST maximum net deviation) − (4 × angina index), where exercise time is measured in minutes and ST deviation in millimeters. Patients at high risk with a score of −11 or lower had a 5-year survival of 72%. Patients at moderate risk with a score of −10 to +4 had a 5-year survival of 91%, and patients with a low-risk score of +5 or greater had a 5-year survival rate of 97%. When total cardiac events were considered, the

high-risk group had a 5-year survival rate of 65%, the moderate-risk group 86%, and the low-risk group 93%. The treadmill score contained prognostically important information even after the information provided by clinical and catheterization data was considered. The score can be expressed as a nomogram (Figure 65-3). This nomogram is considered by many to be the major advance in exercise testing in the past 10 years, as is demonstrated by its inclusion in all of the major guidelines.

EVALUATION OF TREATMENTS

The exercise test can be used to evaluate the effects of both medical and surgical treatment. The effects of various medications including nitrates, digitalis, and antihypertensive agents have been evaluated by exercise testing. Although exercise testing has been used to evaluate patients before and after coronary artery bypass surgery and coronary angioplasty, a definitive comparison between the procedures has not been possible. One problem with using treadmill time or work load rather than measuring maximal oxygen uptake in serial studies is that people learn to perform treadmill walking more efficiently. Treadmill time or work load can increase during serial studies without any improvement in cardiovascular function. Thus, it is important to include the measurement of ventilatory oxygen uptaken when the effects of medical or surgical treatment are being evaluated by treadmill testing. It is important to differentiate ventilatory oxygen consumption from myocardial oxygen consumption, but the distinction between peak and maximal oxygen consumption is artificial and meaningless. Ventilatory anaerobic threshold has not fulfilled its promise as a means to evaluate submaximal exercise tolerance.

Evaluation of Antianginal Agents

Reproducibility

Since studies using standard exercise testing are required by the Federal Drug Administration (FDA) prior to approval of antianginal agents, it is important to know the reproducibility of exercise variables in angina patients. To evaluate reproducibility, Sullivan et al studied 14 angina patients with 3 consecutive days of treadmill testing (17). Prior studies evaluating the changes of work performance in patients with angina pectoris concentrated on improvements in total exercise time. Sklar et al, using moderately severe angina as an endpoint, observed coefficients of variation (standard deviation divided by the mean $\times$ 100) of approximately 5% for total treadmill time (18). Similarly, Sullivan found a coefficient of variation of 6% for peak time. However, when the interclass coefficient (ICC) was determined to test for reproducibility, a rather low value of $r = .70$ was obtained. During sequential exercise testing, many investigators have noted an increase in total treadmill time in normals, angina patients, and congestive heart failure (CHF) patients. In the study by Sullivan et al, we observed better reproducibility for oxygen uptake when compared to time at each analysis point.

The ability to reproducibly determine anginal pain during exercise testing is critical to the evaluation of therapeutic interventions. Previous investigations have included a baseline exercise test in which the patient becomes familiar with the exercise testing equipment and staff. Studies by Redwood (19) and others have stressed the importance of a properly designed exercise test protocol when evaluating patients with stable angina pectoris. In the study by Sullivan et al, the baseline test familiarized the patient with the equipment and staff and evaluated his or her exercise capacity. From this, an individualized protocol was designed to allow the patient sufficient time on the treadmill before stopping because of anginal pain. The advantage of the individualized protocol over one protocol for all patients is that it provides a gradual increase in work and is specific for each patient's exercise capacity.

Conclusions from the study of Sullivan et al include: 1) Measured oxygen uptake should be used instead of total exercise time because it is a more accurate and reproducible measure of aerobic exercise capacity; 2) the ventilatory threshold is a reproducible submaximal exercise variable at which to evaluate myocardial ischemia and myocardial oxygen demand; 3) a pretrial exercise test allows the patient to become familiar with the exercise testing staff, the equipment, and the nature of his or her anginal endpoints; 4) the treadmill protocol should be designed for the patient's exercise capacity with 2-MET or less increments per stage; 5) computerized techniques for ECG analysis provide reproducible measurement of ST segment displacement; and 6) statistical methods based on the estimate of the measurement error associated with a particular variable can be used by the clinician and/or investigator to better plan and evaluate an intervention.

Evaluation of Long-Acting Nitrates for Angina Therapy

It has been difficult to demonstrate the efficacy of long-acting nitrate preparations in the treatment of angina pectoris. More objective measurements during exercise testing are available that could make this possible, but they rarely have been applied. Key questions that we have tried to answer are (20): Can gas exchange variables and computerized ST segment analysis accurately and reproducibly detect beneficial changes during exercise in angina patients treated acutely with sublingual nitrates or after treatment with long-acting nitrate preparations? Do these beneficial changes persist after chronic administration of the long-acting agents for 2 weeks?

Why do the controversy and disparate results exist with clinical studies of the use of the long-acting nitrates? Some of the explanations for this include the following: (1) Acute (single-dose) effects can be demonstrated for the long-acting preparations but when the agents are given chronically, tolerance can develop; (2) there is a definite placebo effect involved in the treatment of angina; (3) nitrate blood levels are difficult to measure, but some modes of delivery clearly do not result in effective blood levels; (4) acute peaks of nitrates in the blood may be more effective than a chronic level; (5) treadmill time or workload is not a reproducible measurement; and (6) more objective measurements using expired gases and computerized ST segment analysis rarely have been used.

The response to a drug differs according to its administration between when given only on the day of the test versus when given for days (chronic administration as in clinical practice) preceding the first day of exercise testing. Parker et al have demonstrated partial tolerance to the hemodynamic effects of isosorbide dinitrate within 48 hours of initiating therapy (21). Thadani et al demonstrated that acute resting hemodynamics and exercise variables in angina patients are attenuated during chronic therapy (22). Resting hemodynamic changes that persisted for 8 hours during acute therapy were demonstrable for only 4 hours during chronic therapy. Similarly, significant increases in exercise capacity were observed for 8 hours after acute and only 2 hours during chronic therapy.

Evaluation of Transdermal Nitroglycerin

Transdermal nitroglycerin (TDN) systems are advertised to offer 24-hour relief from angina pectoris. The basis for this extended therapeutic effect was inferred from studies documenting constant plasma nitroglycerin levels 24 hours after transdermal application and from preliminary studies in patients with angina pectoris. However, recent controlled studies have produced conflicting results as to the efficacy of TDN systems in patients with angina (23). Sullivan et al studied 16 patients with stable angina pectoris in a double-blind crossover manner utilizing treadmill exercise testing with the direct measurement of ventilatory oxygen uptake, 1 and 24 hours after application of a 20-cm^2 TDN system and identical placebo (24). Testing was performed after a 3-day lead in period on either an active patch or placebo. No statistically significant differences were observed between TDN and placebo in any of the resting hemodynamic or peak angina variables at 1 or 24 hours. A significant increase in the double product at the submaximal workload was observed 1 hour after TDN relative to placebo. However, no significant differences were observed in any of the other measured variables at the submaximal work load, 1 or 24 hours post-TDN.

Correlation of Changes in Resting Systolic Blood Pressure with Exercise Capacity

Although the effectiveness of nitrates for the long-term prophylaxis of exertional angina is controversial, investigations utilizing large dosages have demonstrated persistent physiologic effects. During a titration period, the observation of a 10-mm Hg decrease in resting SBP and/or a 10-beat/min increase in resting heart rate has been utilized in studies attempting to demonstrate an increase in exercise capacity following nitrate administration. These criteria have served a dual purpose of documenting physiologic changes in variables known to affect myocardial oxygen demand and to identify subjects nonresponsive to nitrates prior to inclusion in a study. If after nitrate administration changes in blood pressure and/or heart rate are correlated with changes in exercise capacity, the utilization of these variables by the clinician could identify patients expected to improve exercise tolerance during nitrate therapy.

In order to determine if these practical criteria could predict improved exercise capacity in angina pectoris patients treated with nitrates, both nitrate-responsive and nonresponsive subjects were included. Nineteen patients with stable angina pectoris were studied in a double-blind placebo-controlled manner. Significant increases in resting heart rate and peak oxygen uptake and decreases in resting SBP were observed 1 hour postnitrate relative to placebo. Changes in peak oxygen uptake and total treadmill time during nitrate administration relative to placebo correlated to changes in resting supine SBP and diastolic blood pressure (DBP) ($r = -.54$ to $-.62$) but not to changes in resting heart rate. These results suggest that during administration of nitrates, a decrease in resting SBP and DBP is essential to ensure increases in exercise capacity. Conversely, a lack of blood pressure response to nitrates is indicative of no improvement in exercise tolerance. Improvement in oxygen uptake and treadmill time was noted in 10 of 11 patients with a greater than 5-mm Hg drop in supine SBP. In contrast, in five of the remaining seven patients without a greater than 5-mm Hg drop in supine SBP there was no improvement in exercise capacity.

Safety of Placebo in Studying Angina

Because the safety of withholding standard therapy and enrolling patients with stable angina in placebo-controlled trials was not known, Glasser et al identified all events leading to the dropout from trials of 12 antianginal drugs submitted in support of new drug applications to the FDA (25). Persons who dropped out of the trials had adverse cardiovascular events or other causes without knowledge of drug assignment. There were 3161 subjects who entered any randomized, double-blind phase of placebo-controlled protocols; 197 (6.2%) withdrew because of cardiovascular events. There was no difference in risk of adverse events between drug and placebo groups. A prospectively defined subgroup analysis showed that groups who received calcium antagonists were at an increased risk of dropout compared with placebo groups, primarily because of a disproportionate number of adverse events in studies of one drug. In conclusion, there were few adverse experiences associated with short-term placebo use. Withholding active treatment of angina does not increase the risk of serious cardiac events.

Pre- and Postrevascularization

The following summarizes the ACC/AHA Guidelines for recommendations regarding exercise testing of patients pre– and post–revascularization procedures (PTCA, stenting, and other techniques).

Class I. Conditions for which there is evidence and/or general agreement that the standard exercise test is useful and helpful for evaluating patients pre- and postrevascularization. *Definitely use the exercise test:*

1. To demonstrate the presence of myocardial ischemia (ST depression, angina) in patients prior to revascularization.
2. To evaluate patients with recurrent symptoms suggesting myocardial ischemia after revascularization.

Class II a. Conditions for which there is conflicting evidence and/or a divergence of opinion that the standard exercise test is useful and helpful for evaluating patients pre- and postrevascularization but the weight of evidence for usefulness or efficacy is in favor of the exercise test. *Probably use the exercise test:*

> After discharge for activity counseling and/or exercise training as part of cardiac rehabilitation in patients who have undergone coronary revascularization. There are no data to support redoing the testing without a change in symptomatology.

Class II b. Conditions for which there is conflicting evidence and/or a divergence of opinion that the standard exercise test is useful and helpful for evaluating patients pre- and postrevascularization but the usefulness/efficacy is less well established. *Maybe use the exercise test for:*

1. Detection of restenosis in asymptomatic patients within the first months after angioplasty or stenting.
2. Routine monitoring on a periodic basis of asymptomatic patients after revascularization for restenosis, graft occlusion, or disease progression.

Class III. Conditions for which there is evidence and/or general agreement that the standard exercise test is not useful and helpful for evaluating patients pre- and postrevascularization and in some cases may be harmful. *Do not use the standard exercise ECG test:*

> To localize ischemia for determination of the site for intervention (which is better done with an imaging study).

Patients who are to undergo myocardial revascularization should have documented ischemic or viable myocardium, especially if they are asymptomatic; otherwise the procedure serves no purpose. The exercise ECG is useful in these circumstances, particularly if the patient has multivessel disease and the culprit vessel does not need to be defined. However, in the setting of single-vessel disease, the sensitivity of the exercise ECG is frequently suboptimal, especially if the revascularized vessel supplies the posterior wall.

In symptomatic patients after coronary artery bypass surgery (CABS), exercise testing may be used to discriminate cardiac and noncardiac causes of recurrent chest pain, which is often atypical after surgery. If a management decision is to be based on the presence of ischemia, the exercise ECG is sufficient. However, if a management decision is to be based on the site and extent of ischemia, perfusion stress testing (nuclear or echocardiographic) is preferred. In asymptomatic patients after CABS, the development of silent graft disease, especially with venous conduits, is clearly a major concern. In symptomatic patients after PTCA or stenting, a positive exercise test is predictive of restenosis. However, the value of a negative exercise test is reduced by the limited sensitivity of exercise testing, particularly for single-vessel disease.

Evaluation of PTCA

Berger et al reported follow-up data in 183 patients who had undergone PTCA at least 1 year earlier (26). Vandormael et al reported the safety and short-term benefit of multilesion PTCA in 135 patients, 66 of whom had a minimum of 6 months' follow-up (27). Rosing et al reported that exercise testing after successful PTCA exhibited improved ECG and symptomatic responses, as well as improved myocardial perfusion and global and regional left ventricular function (28). Ernst et al in The Netherlands described the results of functional and anatomic follow-up of 25 patients who underwent PTCA (29). These and other studies were summarized by Dubach (see below).

Prediction of Restenosis with the Exercise Test

Honan et al performed a study to demonstrate whether a treadmill test could predict restenosis in 289 patients 6 months after a successful emergency angioplasty of the infarct-related artery for acute myocardial infarction (MI) (30). After excluding those with interim interventions, medical events, or medical contraindications to follow-up testing, both a treadmill test and a cardiac catheterization were completed in 144 patients, 88% of those eligible for this assessment. Of six follow-up clinical and treadmill variables examined by multivariable logistic regression analysis, only exercise ST depression was independently correlated with restenosis at follow-up. The sensitivity of ST depression of 0.10 mV or greater for detecting restenosis was only 24% (13 of 55 patients), and the specificity was 88% (75 of 85 patients). Angina symptoms and exercise treadmill test results in this population had limited value for predicting anatomic restenosis 6 months after emergency angioplasty for acute MI.

Bengtson et al studied 303 consecutive patients with successful PTCA and without a recent MI (31). Among the 228 patients without interval cardiac events, early repeat revascularization, or contraindications to treadmill testing, 209 (92%) underwent follow-up angiography, and 200 also had a follow-up treadmill test and formed the study population. Restenosis occurred in 50 patients (25%). Five variables were individually associated with a higher risk of restenosis: recurrent angina, exercise-induced angina, a positive treadmill test, more exercise ST deviation, and a lower maximum exercise heart rate. However, only exercise-induced angina, recurrent angina, and a positive treadmill test were independent predictors of restenosis.

Wijns et al evaluated exercise testing and thallium scintigraphy in predicting recurrence of angina pectoris and restenosis after a primary successful PTCA (32). In 89

patients, a symptom-limited exercise ECG and thallium scintigraphy were performed 4 weeks after they had undergone successful PTCA. The ability of the thallium scintigram to predict recurrence of angina was 66% versus 38% for the exercise ECG. Restenosis was predicted in 74% of patients by thallium but only in 50% of patients by the exercise ECG. Thallium was highly predictive but the ECG was not. Restenosis had occurred to some extent already at 4 weeks after the PTCA in most patients in whom it was going to occur.

Evaluation of CABS Patients

Hultgren et al analyzed the 5-year effect of medical versus surgical treatment on symptoms and exercise performance in patients with stable angina who entered the Veterans Administration Cooperative Study from 1972 to 1974 (33). Ryan and the coronary artery surgery study (CASS) group reported the results of exercise testing performed in 81% of the 780 patients randomized at entry (34). Gohlke et al evaluated exercise responses in patients with different angiographically defined degrees of revascularization with serial exercise tests in 435 patients 1 to 6 years after CABS (35).

To determine whether preoperative exercise testing adds important independent prognostic information in patients undergoing CABS, Weiner and the CASS group analyzed 35 variables in 1241 enrolled patients. All patients underwent a treadmill test before CABS and were followed for 7 years. Survival in this surgical cohort was 90.6%. Multivariate stepwise discriminant analysis identified the left ventricular score and the final exercise stage achieved as the two most important independent predictors of postoperative survival. In a subgroup of 416 patients with three-vessel coronary disease and preserved left ventricular function, the probability of postoperative survival at 7 years ranged from 95% for those patients able to exercise to 10 METs to 83% for those whose exercise capacity was less than 5 METs. Exercise capacity was found to be an important independent predictor of postoperative survival.

Comparison of PTCA and CABS

Dubach performed a retrospective assessment of veterans being treated at Long Beach VA Medical Center (36). All patients identified as having undergone exercise testing before and after PTCA and CABS were considered for selection according to medication status and timing of exercise tests. Twenty-eight patients formed the CABS group and 38 patients formed the PTCA group. Since the timing of the tests was according to usual clinical practices, the exercise tests were performed an average of 2.5 weeks after PTCA and 5 months after CABS. The medication status was comparable, but there were significantly more patients with multivessel disease in the CABS group than in the PTCA group. CABS was found to be significantly more effective in decreasing signs and symptoms of ischemia than PTCA, but there was no significant difference in estimated aerobic capacity.

Dubach reviewed 27 studies reporting exercise testing both before and after revascularization with CABS or PTCA (36). Medication status, percentage with multivessel disease, and methods of exercise capacity measurement differed between studies. More than twice as many patients had multivessel disease in the CABS studies as in the PTCA studies. Hemodynamic improvements and lessening of ischemia during exercise testing were comparable in both groups. CABS and PTCA result in a similar decrease in the signs and symptoms of exercise-induced ischemia. However, the severity of coronary disease was milder in those who underwent PTCA.

Despite the much lower percentage of patients with multivessel disease included in the PTCA group (28% versus 80% in CABS group), the average reduction in angina pectoris and in ST segment depression in the pooled studies is similar: 49% in angina and 40% in ST segment depression after PTCA and 50% and 35% after CABS, respectively. Meier et al have provided the only data comparing the exercise test results in patients who have undergone PTCA to those who have undergone CABS (37). However, their CABS group was composed of patients in whom PTCA failed. Thus, the patients were not primarily assigned to CABS. Those patients who underwent PTCA had a higher work capacity 1, 2, and 3 years after revascularization compared with the CABS group.

Ideally, exercise test variables should be obtained immediately after CABS or PTCA in order to have comparable situations. It has been demonstrated that within 5 to 6 months after PTCA 30% to 35% of the dilated vessels restenose (38). After CABS, about 10% to 15% of the grafts are occluded in the first 6 months. But whereas patients after PTCA will be able to perform a symptom-limited exercise test within days after the procedure (39), patients after CABS will only be able to do so weeks after the operation, during which time the highest rate of early graft occlusions is reported (40). An interesting report suggested, however, that testing within a day after PTCA seems safe, but a reported 5% incidence of acute occlusion in patients with intimal dissection makes it prudent to wait in these patients (41).

ACC/AHA GUIDELINES FOR PERIOPERATIVE CARDIOVASCULAR EVALUATION FOR NONCARDIAC SURGERY

The following is a summary of the ACC/AHA guidelines providing a framework for considering cardiac risk of noncardiac surgery in a variety of patient and surgical situations (42). The overriding message from the guidelines is that intervention is rarely necessary simply to lower the risk of surgery unless such intervention is indicated irrespective of the preoperative context. A careful history is crucial to the discovery of cardiac and associated diseases that would place the patient in a high-surgical-risk category. The history should also seek to determine the patient's exercise capacity using specific questions. The importance of an appropriate medical history is apparent from a prospective study of 878 consecutive patients (43). A preoperative clinical index (diabetes mellitus, prior MI, angina, age >70 years, congestive heart failure) was used to stratify patients. A gradient of risk for severe disease was seen with increasing numbers of clinical markers. The following prediction rules were developed: The absence of severe coronary disease was predicted with a positive predictive value of 96% for patients who had no (1) history of diabetes, (2) prior angina, (3) previous MI, or (4) history of congestive heart failure; the absence of critical coronary disease was predicted with a positive predictive value of 94% for those who had no

(1) prior angina, (2) previous MI, or (3) history of congestive heart failure.

Carliner et al reported abnormal exercise-induced ST segment depression in 16% of 200 patients older than 40 years (mean age, 59 years) being considered for elective surgery (44). Their prospective study was in a general population of patients in whom less than a third had peripheral vascular disease and were undergoing noncardiac surgery. Only two patients (1%) had a markedly abnormal exercise test. Of the 32 patients with an abnormal exercise test, five (16%) died or had a nonfatal MI. Of 168 patients with a negative test, 157 (93%) did not die or have an MI. In this series, however, the results of preoperative exercise testing were not statistically significant independent predictors of cardiac risk. Endpoint events were more common in patients aged 70 years or older. Endpoint events were also more common in patients with an abnormal (positive or equivocal) exercise test response than in those with a negative response (27% versus 14%); however, preoperative exercise results were not statistically significant independent predictors of cardiac risk. Using multivariate analysis, the only statistically significant independent predictor of risk was the preoperative ECG. The finding that endpoint events were more common in patients with an abnormal ECG than in those with a normal ECG (23% versus 7%) is consistent with another study of the resting ECG (45).

Who Should Undergo an Exercise Test Prior to Noncardiac Surgery?

- Is the non-cardiac surgery emergent? If emergent, there is not time for further evaluation and the patient should proceed to surgery. Exercise testing is not indicated!

- Has the patient undergone coronary revascularization in the past 5 years? If the patient has had complete surgical revascularization in the past 5 years or coronary angioplasty from 6 months to 5 years ago, and if his or her clinical status has remained stable without recurrent signs or symptoms of ischemia in the interim, the likelihood of perioperative cardiac death or MI is extremely low and exercise testing would not lead to another intervention. Exercise testing is not indicated!

- Has the patient undergone a coronary evaluation in the past 2 years? If an individual has undergone extensive coronary evaluation with either noninvasive or invasive techniques within 2 years and if the findings indicate that coronary risk has been adequately assessed with favorable findings, repeat stress testing is usually unnecessary. An exception to this rule is the patient who has experienced a definite change or new symptoms of coronary ischemia since the prior coronary evaluation. Exercise testing is not indicated!

- Does the patient have one of the unstable coronary syndromes or major clinical predictors of risk (unstable coronary disease or decompensated CHF, hemodynamically significant arrhythmias, and/or severe valvular heart disease)? Stabilization followed by noninvasive evaluation (possibly exercise testing) or invasive testing is required prior to surgery.

- Does the patient have intermediate clinical predictors of risk (angina pectoris, prior MI by history or ECG, compensated or prior CHF, or diabetes mellitus)? If such a patient has an estimated exercise capacity of less than 4 METs (unable to do normal activities) or if a high-risk surgical procedure is to be done, then an exercise test or another stress test is indicated. The first choice for noninvasive testing is the standard exercise test. If the patient cannot exercise, then a nonexercise stress test is indicated.

- Does the patient have none of or only the minor clinical predictors of risk? Noncardiac surgery is generally safe for patients with minor or none of the clinical predictors of clinical risk who exhibit moderate or excellent exercise capacity (equal to or greater than 4 METs), regardless of surgical type. Patients with poor exercise capacity facing higher-risk operations (vascular, anticipated long and complicated thoracic, abdominal, and head and neck) should be considered for an exercise or another stress test. The first choice for testing is the standard exercise test. It is almost never appropriate to recommend coronary bypass surgery or other invasive interventions such as coronary angioplasty that would not otherwise be indicated in an effort to reduce the risk of noncardiac surgery.

- Is the patient scheduled for a high-risk surgical procedure? All patients with intermediate clinical predictors and all patients with no or minor predictors with a low estimated exercise capacity should undergo an exercise or nonexercise stress (pharmacologic) test. The first choice for testing is the standard exercise test. The results of noninvasive testing can then be used to determine further perioperative management. Such management may include intensified medical therapy or cardiac catheterization, which may lead to coronary revascularization or potential cancellation or delay of the elective noncardiac operation. Alternatively, results of the noninvasive test (usually a standard exercise test) may lead to a recommendation to proceed directly with surgery. In some patients, the risk of coronary angioplasty or corrective cardiac surgery may approach or even exceed the risk of the proposed noncardiac surgery.

Clinical Predictors of Increased Perioperative Cardiovascular Risk

Major Predictors

These predictors mandate intensive management, which may result in delay or cancellation of surgery unless it is emergent. Consider coronary angiography and/or exercise or nonexercise stress testing when stabilized.

- Unstable coronary syndromes
- Recent MI (>7 days but less than 1 month) with evidence of important ischemic risk by clinical symptoms or noninvasive study
- Unstable or severe angina (Canadian class III or IV)
- Decompensated congestive heart failure
- Significant arrhythmias
  - High-grade atrioventricular block
  - Symptomatic ventricular arrhythmias with underlying heart disease

- Supraventricular arrhythmias with uncontrolled ventricular rate
- Severe valvular disease

Intermediate Predictors

These are validated markers of risk of perioperative cardiac complications that justify careful assessment of the patient's current status. If the patient with intermediate predictors has an estimated exercise capacity of 4 METs or less, then exercise or nonexercise stress testing is indicated. If the patient's estimated exercise capacity is greater than 4 METs, stress testing is only indicated in those who are undergoing high-risk surgery (aortic and other major vascular, peripheral vascular, or prolonged surgical procedures associated with large fluid shifts and/or blood loss).

- Mild angina pectoris (Canadian class I or II) (46)
- Prior MI by history or pathological Q waves
- Compensated or prior congestive heart failure
- Diabetes mellitus

Minor Predictors

Minor predictors are recognized markers for cardiovascular disease that have not been proven to independently increase perioperative risk. Patients with or without these features with an estimated exercise capacity less than 4 METs who are to undergo high-risk surgery (aortic and other major vascular, peripheral vascular, or prolonged surgical procedures with extreme alterations in volume status) should undergo an exercise or a nonexercise stress test. Otherwise no testing is indicated.

- Advanced age
- Abnormal ECG (left ventricular hypertrophy, left bundle branch block, ST-T abnormalities)
- Rhythm other than sinus (e.g., atrial fibrillation)
- Low functional capacity (e.g., inability to climb one flight of stairs with a bag of groceries)
- History of stroke
- Uncontrolled systemic hypertension

Note that patients with minor clinical predictors are treated in the same manner as patients with no clinical predictors.

Myocardial Infarction

A history of MI or pathological Q waves by ECG is listed as an intermediate predictor, whereas a recent MI is a major predictor. In this way the separation of MI into the traditional 3- and 6-month intervals has been avoided (47). If a recent stress test does not suggest residual myocardium at risk, the likelihood of reinfarction after noncardiac surgery is low. Although there are no adequate clinical trials on which to base firm recommendations, it is reasonable to wait at least 1 month after MI to perform elective surgery.

Surgical Procedures

The risk stratification of various types of noncardiac surgical procedures is based on several studies (48). It is clear that major emergent operations in the elderly (those opening a visceral cavity and those likely to be accompanied by major bleeding or fluid shifts) place patients at highest risk. Vascular procedures appear particularly risky, and, primarily because of the likelihood of associated coronary disease, justify careful preoperative screening for myocardial ischemia in many instances. Patients undergoing minor surgical procedures do not require stress testing.

EVALUATION OF EXERCISE CAPACITY

The exercise test can be used to evaluate the exercise capacity of asymptomatic individuals or of patients with various forms of heart disease. Patients who exaggerate their symptoms or who mainly have a psychological impairment often can be identified. Exercise testing can more accurately measure the degree of cardiac impairment than can a physician's assessment of exercise capacity. As previously described, maximal oxygen uptake, either directly measured or estimated, is the best noninvasive measurement of the functional capacity of the cardiovascular system and has a major impact in predicting prognosis. The determination of a patient's exercise capacity affords an objective measurement of the degree of cardiac impairment and can be useful in patient management. Exercise testing can also be used as part of an athletic program, a fitness program, or a rehabilitation program. Following a patient's progress in an exercise program with serial exercise testing can optimize the training program and provides a good way to encourage adherence.

EVALUATION OF CARDIAC RHYTHM DISORDERS

The following is a summary of the ACC/AHA guidelines regarding recommendations for use of exercise testing in patients with cardiac rhythm disorders.
Class I. Conditions for which there is evidence and/or general agreement that the standard exercise test is useful and helpful for evaluating patients with cardiac rhythm disorders. A standard exercise test is definitely appropriate for the following patients:
Identification of optimal pacemaker settings in patients with rate-adaptive pacemakers.

Class II a. Conditions for which there is conflicting evidence and/or a divergence of opinion that the standard exercise test is useful and helpful for patients with cardiac rhythm disorders but the weight of evidence for usefulness or efficacy is in favor of the exercise test. A standard exercise test is probably appropriate for the following patients:
1. Patients with known or suspected exercise-induced arrhythmia.
2. Medical, surgical, or ablative therapy in patients with exercise-induced arrhythmia (including atrial fibrillation).

Class II b. Conditions for which there is conflicting evidence and/or a divergence of opinion that the standard exercise test is useful and helpful for evaluating patients with cardiac rhythm disorders but the usefulness/efficacy is less well established. A standard exercise test may be appropriate for the following patients:

Isolated ventricular premature beats in middle-aged patients without other evidence of coronary artery disease.
Class III. Conditions for which there is evidence and/or general agreement that the standard exercise test is not useful and helpful for patients with cardiac rhythm disorders and in some cases may be harmful. A standard exercise test is definitely not appropriate for the following patients:
Investigation of isolated premature beats in patients less than 40 years of age.

Exercise testing has a well-established role in the identification of the appropriate settings for adaptive-rate pacemakers using various physiologic sensors. A number of studies have compared different pacing modes with respect to their influence on exercise capacity. A formal exercise test may not always be necessary since the required data can be obtained using a simple walk.
Exercise testing may be employed in the evaluation of patients with symptoms that suggest exercise-induced arrhythmias, such as exercise-induced syncope. The utility of exercise testing in such patients is variable, depending on the arrhythmia in question. Exercise testing may also be used to evaluate medical therapy in patients with exercise-induced arrhythmias.

Evaluation of Ventricular Arrhythmias

Because few reports document the safety of exercise testing in patients with malignant ventricular arrhythmias, Young et al reviewed the complications of symptom-limited exercise tests in 263 patients with such arrhythmias who underwent a total of 1377 maximal treadmill tests (49). Seventy-four percent of the population studied had a history of ventricular fibrillation or hemodynamically compromising ventricular tachycardia, and the remainder had experienced ventricular tachycardia in the setting of either recent MI or poor left ventricular function. Complications were noted in 24 patients (9.1%) during 32 tests (2.3%), whereas 239 patients (90.9%) were free of complications during 1345 tests (97.7%). There were no deaths, MIs, or lasting morbid events. Clinical descriptors associated with complications included male sex, presence of coronary artery disease, and a history of exertional arrhythmia. Clinical variables previously considered to confer increased risk during exercise, such as poor left ventricular function, high-grade ventricular arrhythmias before or during exercise, exertional hypotension, and ST depression, were not predictive of complications. Occurrence of a complication was also unaffected by the use of antiarrhythmic drugs at the time of exercise. Complication frequency in their study group was compared with that in a reference population of 3444 cardiac patients without histories of symptomatic arrhythmia who underwent 8221 exercise tests. Of these, four subjects (0.12%) developed ventricular fibrillation (0.05% of tests) without fatality or lasting morbidity.
Woelfel et al studied 14 patients with exercise-induced ventricular tachycardia (VT) with serial treadmill testing (50). Those with reproducible VT were treated with a beta-blocking agent and later with verapamil. In 11 patients (79%), VT of similar rate, morphologic characteristics, and duration was reproduced on two consecutive treadmill tests performed 1 to 14 days apart. Beta blockade prevented recurrent VT during acute testing in 10 of 11 patients and during chronic therapy in 9. Eight patients had an consistent relation between a critical

sinus rate and the onset of VT. In these patients, successful therapy correlated with preventing achievement of the critical sinus rate during maximal exercise. The researchers also found verapamil to be effective in this group.

Sami et al performed a retrospective study to examine the prognostic significance of exercise-induced ventricular arrhythmia in patients with stable CAD who were included in the multicenter patient registry of the CASS (51). The 5-year event-free survival was not influenced by the presence of exercise-induced arrythmias. Using a regression analysis of selected clinical and angiographic risk factors, the only independent significant risk factors that were found for cardiac events were the number of coronary arteries diseased and the ejection fraction (EF).

Califf et al at Duke studied the prognostic information provided by ventricular arrhythmias associated with treadmill testing in 1293 consecutive nonsurgically treated patients undergoing an exercise test within 6 weeks of cardiac catheterization (52). The 236 patients with simple ventricular arrhythmias (at least one premature ventricular contraction [PVC], but without paired complexes or ventricular tachycardia) had a higher prevalence of significant CAD (57% versus 44%), three-vessel disease (31% versus 17%), and abnormal left ventricular function (43% versus 24%) than did patients without ventricular arrhythmias. Patients with paired complexes or ventricular tachycardia had an even higher prevalence of significant coronary artery disease (75%), three-vessel disease (39%), and abnormal left venticular function (54%). In the 620 patients with significant CAD, patients with paired complexes or ventricular tachycardia had a lower 3-year survival rate (75%) than did patients with simple ventricular arrhythmias (83%) and patients with no ventricular arrhythmias (90%). Ventricular arrhythmias were found to add independent prognostic information to the noninvasive evaluation, including history, physical examination, chest x-ray, ECG, and other exercise test variables ($p = .03$). Ventricular arrhythmias made no independent contribution once the cardiac catheterization data were known. In patients without significant CAD, no relation between ventricular arrhythmias and survival was found.

Weiner et al investigated the determinants and prognostic significance of ventricular arrhythmias during exercise testing (53). Eighty-six patients with such arrhythmias were identified from a consecutive series of 446 patients who underwent treadmill testing and cardiac catheterization. At a mean follow-up period of 5.3 years, the presence of exercise-induced ventricular arrhythmias was not associated with increased cardiac mortality in the medically treated patients. We have not even found technical ventricular tachycardia induced by exercise to be predictive of adverse events (54).

The Effect Of Drugs on Exercise Performance in Chronic Atrial Fibrillation

In patients with chronic atrial fibrillation (AF), the primary goal of therapy is to control the rapid heart rate response at rest and during exercise. Digoxin has been the drug of choice to control resting heart rate. However, digoxin has limited effectiveness in controlling heart rates during exercise or other stresses. The concomitant use of beta-adrenergic or calcium channel blocking agents with digoxin has been recommended as a better means of controlling heart rate.

Nine male patients with chronic AF, eight treated with digoxin, underwent a randomized, double-blind maximal-dose celiprolol/placebo study using exercise testing with measured ventilatory parameters to assess the effect of beta-adrenergic blockade on exercise capacity (55). Celiprolol did not alter gas exchange variables such as minute ventilation, oxygen uptake, and respiratory exchange ratio; this is consistent with studies in normal subjects. A significant decrease in heart rate and SBP occurred at the anaerobic threshold during celiprolol therapy.

Treatment with Diltiazem

Since a calcium antagonist may offer chronotropic control but less negative inotropic effect, it could be more advantageous in the treatment of atrial fibrillation. Therefore, Atwood et al tested these patients after stabilizing them on diltiazem (56). They exhibited an improvement in treadmill time and no decrease in $\dot{V}o_2$ max with good heart rate control. This suggests that diltiazem is the agent of choice for these patients. Clinically, the decrease in the gas exchange aerobic threshold (ATge) and reduction in oxygen uptake at higher workloads becomes important in patients who desire an active lifestyle.

EVALUATION OF VALVULAR HEART DISEASE

The following is a summary of the ACC/AHA guidelines regarding recommendations for exercise testing of adults with valvular heart disease.

Class I. Conditions for which there is evidence and/or general agreement that the standard exercise test is useful and helpful for evaluating patients with valvular heart disease. *The standard exercise test is not definitely recommended for evaluating any patient with valvular heart disease.*

None

Class II a. Conditions for which there is conflicting evidence and/or a divergence of opinion that the standard exercise test is useful and helpful for evaluating adults with valvular heart disease but the weight of evidence for usefulness or efficacy is in favor of the exercise test.

None

Class II b. Conditions for which there is conflicting evidence and/or a divergence of opinion that the standard exercise test is useful and helpful for evaluating adults with valvular heart disease but the usefulness/efficacy is less well established. *The standard exercise test may be used for evaluating exercise capacity in patients with valvular heart disease.*

Evaluation of exercise capacity

Class III. Conditions for which there is evidence and/or general agreement that the standard exercise test is not useful and helpful for evaluating adults with valvular heart disease and in some cases may be harmful. *Do not use the standard exercise test to evaluate patients with symptomatic, severe critical aortic stenosis.*

In symptomatic patients with documented valvular disease, the course of treatment is usually clear and exercise testing is not required. However, Doppler echocardiography has greatly increased the number of asymptomatic patients with defined valvular abnormalities. The primary value of exercise testing in valvular heart disease is to objectively assess exercise capacity and the extent of patient disability, both of which may have implications for clinical decision making. This is particularly important in the elderly, who may not have symptoms because of their limited activity. The use of the exercise ECG for the diagnosis of coronary artery disease in these situations is limited by false-positive responses caused by left ventricular hypertrophy and baseline ECG abnormalities. In patients with aortic stenosis, the test should be directly supervised by a physician using a slowly progressive protocol with frequent manual BP determinations. Exercise should be terminated in the absence of an appropriate increase in SBP, slowing of the heart rate with increasing exercise, and frequent premature beats (57,58).

EVALUATION FOR AN INDIVIDUALIZED EXERCISE PROGRAM

The exercise test can be used to evaluate the safety of participating in an exercise program and can help formulate an exercise prescription. Because of the wide scatter of maximal heart rate when plotted against age, it is advantageous to determine an individual's maximal heart rate, in order to assign a target for training, rather than give a predicted value. In certain individuals, it can be helpful to objectively evaluate their response to exercise in a monitored situation prior to embarking on an exercise program. In adult fitness or cardiac rehabilitation programs, an exercise test can be used to safely progress an individual to a higher level of performance. Also, the improvement in exercise performance secondary to training demonstrated by an exercise test can be an effective incentive and encouragement to people in such programs.

REFERENCES

1. Gibbons RJ, Balady GJ, Beasley JW, et al. ACC/AHA Guidelines for Exercise Testing. A report of the American College of Cardiology/American Heart Association Task Force on Practice Guidelines (Committee on Exercise Testing). J Am Coll Cardiol 1997; 30(1):260–311.

2. Balke B, Ware R. An experimental study of physical fitness of air force personnel. US Armed Forces Med J 1959;10:675–688.

3. Astrand PO, Rodahl K. Textbook of work physiology. New York: McGraw-Hill, 1986:331–365.

4. Bruce RA. Exercise testing of patients with coronary heart disease. Ann Clin Res 1971;3: 323–330.

5. Ellestad MH, Allen W, Wan MCK, Kemp G. Maximal treadmill stress testing for cardiovascular evaluation. Circulation 1969;39: 517–522.

6. Stuart RJ, Ellestad MH. National survey of exercise stress testing facilities. Chest 1980;77: 94–97.

7. Sullivan M, McKirnan MD. Errors in predicting functional capacity for postmyocardial infarction patients using a modified Bruce protocol. Am Heart J 1984;107: 486–491.

8. Webster MWI, Sharpe DN. Exercise testing in angina pectoris: the importance of protocol design in clinical trials. Am Heart J 1989; 117:505–508.

9. Panza JA, Quyyumi AA, Diodati JG, et al. Prediction of the frequency and duration of ambulatory myocardial ischemia in patients with stable coronary artery disease by determination of the ischemic threshold from exercise testing: importance of the exercise protocol. J Am Coll Cardiol 1991;17: 657–663.

10. Redwood DR, Rosing DR, Goldstein RE, et al. Importance of the design of an exercise protocol in the evaluation of patients with angina pectoris. Circulation 1971; 43:618–628.

11. Smokler PE, MacAlpin RN, Alvaro A, Kattus AA. Reproducibility of a multi-stage near maximal treadmill test for exercise tolerance in angina pectoris. Circulation 1973; 48:346–351.

12. Buchfuhrer MJ, Hansen JE, Robinson TE, et al. Optimizing the exercise protocol for cardiopulmonary assessment. J Appl Physiol 1983; 55(5):1558–1564.

13. Lipkin DP, Canepa-Anson R, Stephens MR, Poole-Wilson PA. Factors determining symptoms in heart failure: comparison of fast and slow exercise tests. Br Heart J 1986;55:439–445.

14. Dubach P, Froelicher VF, Klein J, et al. Exercise-induced hypotension in a male population—criteria, causes, and prognosis. Circulation 1988;78:1380–1387.

15. Chassin MR, Kosecoff J, Solomon DH, Brook RH. How coronary angiography is used: clinical determinants of appropriateness. JAMA 1987;258:2543–2547.

16. Mark DB, Hlatky MA, Harrell FE, et al. Exercise treadmill score for predicting prognosis in coronary artery disease. Ann Intern Med 1987;106:793–800.

17. Sullivan M, Genter F, Savvides M, et al. The reproducibility of hemodynamic, electrocardiographic, and gas exchange data during treadmill exercise in patients with stable angina pectoris. Chest 1984;86:375–382.

18. Sklar J, Johnston GD, Overlie P, et.al. The effects of a cardioselective (metoprolol) and a nonselective (propranolol) beta-adrenergic blocker on the response to dynamic exercise in normal men. Circulation 1982;65:894–899.

19. Redwood DR, Rosing DR, Goldstein RE, et al. Importance of the design of an exercise protocol

in the evaluation of patients with angina pectoris. Circulation 1971; 43:618–628.

20. Abrams J. The mystery of nitrate resistance. Am J Cardiol 1991; 68:1393–1396.

21. Parker JO, VanKoughnett KA, Fung HL. Transdermal isosorbide dinitrate in angina pectoris: effect of acute and sustained therapy. Am J Cardiol 1984;54:8–13.

22. Thadani U, Manyari D, Parker JO, Fung HL. Tolerance to the circulatory effects of isosorbide dinitrate: rate of development and cross tolerance to glyceral trinitrate. Circulation 1980;61:526–535.

23. Thompson RH. The clinical use of transdermal delivery devices with nitroglycerin. Angiology 1983;34: 23–31.

24. Sullivan MA, Savvides M, Abouantoun S, et al. Failure of transdermal nitroglycerin to improve exercise capacity in patients with angina pectoris. J Am Coll Cardiol 1985;5:1220–1223.

25. Glasser SP, Clark PI, Lipicky RJ, et al. Exposing patients with chronic, stable, exertional angina to placebo periods in drug trials. JAMA 1991;265:1550–1554.

26. Berger E, Williams DO, Reinert S, Most AS. Sustained efficacy of percutaneous transluminal coronary angioplasty. Am Heart J 1986;111:233–236.

27. Vandormael MG, Chaitman BR, Ischinger T, et al. Immediate and short-term benefit of multilesion coronary angioplasty: influence of degree of revascularization. J Am Coll Cardiol 1985;6: 983–991.

28. Rosing DR, Van Raden MJ, Mincemoyer RM, et al. Exercise, electrocardiographic and functional responses after percutaneous transluminal coronary angioplasty. Am J Cardiol 1984;53:36C–41C.

29. Ernst S, Hillebrand FA, Klein B, et al. The value of exercise tests in the follow-up of patients who underwent transluminal coronary angioplasty. Int J Cardiol 1985;7: 267–279.

30. Honan MB, Bengtson JR, Pryor DB, et al. Exercise treadmill testing is a poor predictor of anatomic restenosis after angioplasty for acute myocardial infarction. Circulation 1989;80:1585–1594.

31. Bengtson JR, Mark DB, Honan MB, et al. Detection of restenosis after elective percutaneous transluminal coronary angioplasty using the exercise treadmill test. Am J Cardiol 1990;65:28–34.

32. Wijns W, Serruys PW, Simoons ML, et al. Predictive value of early maximal exercise test and thallium scintigraphy after successful percutaneous transluminal coronary angioplasty. Br Heart J 1985;53: 194–200.

33. Hultgren HN, Peduzzik P, Ketre K, Takoro T. The 5 year effect of bypass surgery on relief of angina and exercise performance. Circulation 1985;72:V79–V83.

34. Ryan TJ, Weiner DA, McCabe CH, et al. Exercise testing in the coronary artery surgery study randomized population. Circulation 1985; 72:V31–V36.

35. Gohlke H, Gohlke-Barwolf C, Samek L, et al. Serial exercise testing up to 6 years after coronary bypass surgery: behavior of exercise parameters in groups with different degrees of revascularization determined by postoperative angiography. Am J Cardiol 1983; 51:1301–1306.

36. Dubach P, Froelicher V, Atwood JE, et al. A comparison of the exercise test responses pre/post revascularization: does coronary artery bypass surgery produce better results than percutaneous transluminal coronary angioplasty? J Cardiac Rehab 1990;10:120–125.

37. Meier B, Gruentzig AR, Siegenthaler WE, Schlumpf M. Long-term exercise performance after percutaneous transluminal coronary angioplasty and coronary artery bypass grafting. Circulation 1983;68:796–802.

38. King SB, Talley JD. Coronary arteriography and percutaneous transluminal coronary angioplasty: changing patterns of use and results. Circulation 1989;79(suppl I):I-19–I-23.

39. Deligonul U, Vandormael MG, Younis LT, Chaitman BR. Prognostic significance of silent myocardial ischemia detected by early treadmill exercise after coronary angioplasty. Am J Cardiol 1989; 64:1–5.

40. Grondin CM, Campeau L, Thornton JC, et al. Coronary artery bypass grafting with saphenous vein. Circulation 1989;79(suppl I): I-I-4–I-29.

41. Sionis D, Vrolix M, Glazier J, et al. Early exercise testing after successful PTCA: a word of caution. Am Heart J 1992:123:530–532.

42. Eagle KA, Brundage BH, Chaitman BR, et al. Guidelines for perioperative cardiovascular evaluation for noncardiac surgery. Report of the American College of Cardiology/American Heart Association Task Force on Practice Guidelines. Committee on Perioperative Cardiovascular Evaluation for Noncardiac Surgery. Circulation 1996;15;93(6):1278–1317.

43. Paul SD, Eagle KA, Kuntz KM, et al. Concordance of preoperative clinical risk with angiographic severity of coronary artery disease in patients undergoing vascular surgery. Circulation 1996;94(7): 1561–1566.

44. Carliner NH, Fisher ML, Plotnick GD, et al. Routine preoperative exercise testing in patients undergoing major noncardiac surgery. Am J Cardiol 1985;56: 51–58.

45. Goldberger AL, O'Konski M. Utility of the routine elecrocardiogram before surgery and on general hospital admission. Ann Intern Med 1986;105:552–557.

46. Campeau L. Grading of angina pectoris. Circulation 1976;54: 522–523.

47. Goldman L, Caldera DL, Nussbaum SR, et al. Multifactorial index of cardiac risk in noncardiac surgical procedures. N Engl J Med 1977;297:845–850.

48. Rao TL, Jacobs KH, El-Etr AA. Reinfarction following anesthesia in patients with myocardial infarction. Anesthesiology 1983;59: 499–505.

49. Young DZ, Lampert S, Graboys TB, Lown B. Safety of maximal exercise testing in patients at high risk for ventricuar arrhythmia. Circulation 1984;70:184–191.

50. Woelfel A, Foster JR, McAllister RG, et al. Efficacy of verapamil in exercise-induced ventricular tachycardia. Am J Cardiol 1985;56:292–297.

51. Sami M, Chaitman B, Fisher L, et al. Significance of exercise-induced ventricular arrhythmia in stable coronary artery disease: a coronary artery surgery study project. Am J Cardiol 1984;54:1182.

52. Califf RM, McKinnis RA, McNeer M, et al. Prognostic value of ventricular arrhythmias associated with treadmill exercise testing in patients studied with cardiac catheterization for suspected ischemic heart disease. J Am Coll Cardiol 1983;2:1060–1067.

53. Weiner DA, Levine SR, Klein MD, Ryan TJ. Ventricular arrhythmias during exercise testing: mechanism, response to coronary bypass surgery and prognostic significance. Am J Cardiol 1984;53:1553.

54. Yang JC, Wesley RC, Froelicher VF. Ventricular tachycardia during routine treadmill testing: risk and prognosis. Arch Intern Med 1991;151:349–353.

55. Atwood JE, Sullivan M, Forbes S, et al. The effect of beta-adrenergic blockade on exercise performance in patients with chronic atrial fibrillation. J Am Coll Cardiol 1987;10:314–320.

56. Atwood JE, Myers JN, Sullivan MJ, et al. Diltiazem and exercise performance in patients with chronic atrial fibrillation. Chest 1988;93:20–25.

57. Areskog NH. Exercise testing in the evaluation of patients with valvular aortic stenosis. Clin Physiol 1984;4:201–208.

58. Atwood JE, Kawanishi S, Myers J, Froelicher VF. Exercise and the heart: exercise testing in patients with aortic stenosis. Chest 1988;93:1083–1087.

Chapter 66

New Clinical Practice Guidelines for Cardiac Rehabilitation: What Have We Learned?

L. Kent Smith

The final decade of the twentieth century has witnessed the evolution of the concept and the development and publication of clinical practice guidelines. This evermore commonly used term has several definitions in both common usage and, most particularly, in medical or professional usage. In the medical arena, guidelines have been defined by several major organizations including the American Medical Association, the Institute of Medicine, the Joint Commission on Accreditation of Healthcare Organizations, the Physician Payment Review Commission, and the United States Preventive Services Task Force. When the U.S. Congress mandated in the Budget Resolution Act of 1989 that the Agency for Health Care Policy and Research (AHCPR) of the Pubic Health Service develop "cinically relevant guidelines," the definition chosen was as follows:

> Practice guidelines are systematically developed statements to assist practitioner and patient decisions about appropriate health care for specific clinical circumstances.

As AHCPR fulfilled the mission of developing clinical practice guidelines, emphasis was placed upon basing the recommendations in the guidelines on scientific evidence (1). The AHCPR-supported clinical practice guideline on the topic of cardiac rehabilitation (Clinical Practice Guideline No. 17) was published in October of 1995 and carefully adhered to the principles of basing conclusions or recommendations regarding the benefits of exercise training on firm scientific evidence. The methodologist consultant to the cardiac rehabilitation guideline development group provided the rationale that was followed in the development of the guideline; namely, "evidence-based guideline development links recommendations directly to scientific evidence of effectiveness; rules of evidence are emphasized over expert opinion in

making recommendations" (2). The degree to which this goal was achieved and the high level of professional acceptance of the Clinical Practice Guideline for Cardiac Rehabilitation was underscored by the document's endorsement by the American Heart Association and the American College of Cardiology plus several other relevant professional societies (3).

GUIDELINE DEVELOPMENT PROCESS

The development of the AHCPR Clinical Practice Guideline for Cardiac Rehabilitation (4) was a 3-year endeavor. It was initiated in 1992 and was completed with the publication of the guideline in October of 1995. The work of the guideline development was undertaken by a panel of experts that included consumer members as well as professional members from both clinical and academic perspectives, including cardiology, internal medicine, family medicine, nursing, behavioral science, dietetics, physical therapy, and exercise physiology. The guideline principally focused on patients with coronary heart disease as well as heart failure but could be applied to patients with a broader range of cardiovascular conditions. The guideline broadly approached the wide array of services provided in the rehabilitative setting to patients with cardiovascular disease in the areas of exercise training and the areas of education, counseling, and behavioral interventions. However, throughout the development and with the publication of the guideline, the document emphasized the interrelated nature of these various healthcare services and the mutually reinforcing benefits of an integrated and comprehensive program of rehabilitation. The guideline clearly stated the strength of the scientific evidence upon which each of the 34 specific recommendations were based (21 recommendations pertaining to the exercise training component, 10 related to education, counseling, and behavioral interventions, and an additional 3 recommendations regarding organizational issues).

For the major topics covered by the Clinical Practice Guideline, the document provided detailed tables of evidence (a total of 17) that specified the scientific studies pertaining to the recommendation and provided sufficient detail for the reader to review the strength and consistency of the scientific evidence regarding the specific recommendation. The evidence tables listed the various specific scientific references, described the patients involved in the specific study, described the intervention process, and documented the outcome of interest, including specification of the statistical significance. The evidence tables primarily feature the randomized controlled trials that pertain to a specific outcome. These trials are summarized in the text of the guideline, and other evidence pertaining to the specific outcome is also reviewed (the nonrandomized controlled trials as well as observational studies); together, they constitute the evidence base for the guideline recommendation. Table 66-1 summarizes the evidence base regarding the various outcomes resulting from exercise training in the setting of cardiac rehabilitation. Table 66-2 enumerates the scientific evidence regarding the education, counseling, and behavioral intervention components of cardiac rehabilitation.

CARDIAC REHABILITATION AS SECONDARY PREVENTION

As the extensive review of the scientific literature pertaining to cardiac rehabilitation took place in the course of development of the Clinical Practice Guideline, it became very clear that the evolving concepts of secondary prevention of atherosclerotic cardiovascular disease and cardiac rehabilitation were synonymous. Because of this, the abbreviated version of the guideline, the Quick Reference Guide for Clinicians, was entitled Cardiac Rehabilitation as Secondary Prevention (5). The comprehensive approach to the management of patients with established atherosclerotic vascular disease is incorporated in modern-day cardiac rehabilitation; this approach, as the guideline documents detail, constitutes secondary prevention. The essential interrelated components of cardiac rehabilitation services to provide secondary prevention are illustrated in the decision tree (Figure 66-1) taken from the Clinical Practice Guideline for Cardiac Rehabilitation.

PATIENT CATEGORIES COVERED BY THE GUIDELINE

Cardiovascular disease is the leading cause of morbidity and mortality in the United States, accounting for over 50% of all deaths. Coronary heart disease (CHD), with its clinical manifestations of stable angina pectoris, unstable angina, acute myocardial infarction, and sudden cardiac death, affects 13.5 million Americans. The almost 1 million annual survivors of myocardial infarction and the 7 million patients with stable angina pectoris are candidates for cardiac rehabilitation, as are the more than 300,000 patients who undergo coronary artery bypass graft (CABG) surgery and the 360,000 patients

who undergo percutaneous transluminal coronary angioplasty (PTCA) and other transcatheter procedures each year. An estimated 4.7 million patients with heart failure may also be eligible. Although beneficial outcomes from cardiac rehabilitation services can be expected in most of these patients, only about 20% of such patients currently participate in cardiac rehabilitation programs (6).

DEFINITION

The U.S. Public Health Service definition of cardiac rehabilitation, used by the guideline, states that "cardiac rehabilitation services are comprehensive, long-term programs involving medical evaluation, prescribed exercise, cardiac risk factor modification, education and counseling. These programs are designed to limit the physiologic and psychological effects of cardiac illness, reduce the risk for sudden death or reinfarction, control cardiac symptoms, stabilize or reverse the atherosclerotic process, and enhance the psychosocial and vocational status of selected patients." This guideline provides recommendations for cardiac rehabilitation services for patients with CHD and heart failure, including those following cardiac transplantation.

PURPOSE OF THE GUIDELINE

This guideline is designed for use by health practitioners who provide care to patients with cardiovascular disease. This includes physicians (primary care, cardiologists, and cardiovascular surgeons), nurses, exercise physiologists, dietitians, behavioral medicine specialists, psychologists, and physical and occupational therapists. The information can guide clinical decision making regarding referral and follow-up of patients for cardiac rehabilitation services as well as administrative decisions regarding the availability of and access to cardiac rehabilitation services. The guideline details the outcomes that result from cardiac rehabilitation services. The interventions examined involve two parallel applications: 1) exercise training, and 2) education, counseling, and behavioral interventions. The guideline emphasizes the added effectiveness of multifactorial cardiac rehabilitation services integrated in a comprehensive approach.

OUTCOMES OF CARDIAC REHABILITATION SERVICES

Exercise Tolerance
Cardiac rehabilitation exercise training consistently improves objective measures of exercise tolerance, without significant cardiovascular complications or other adverse outcomes. Appropriately prescribed and conducted exercise training is recommended as an integral component of cardiac rehabilitation services, particularly for patients with decreased exercise tolerance. Continued exercise training is required to sustain improved exercise tolerance (7).

Strength Training
Strength training improves skeletal muscle strength and endurance in clinically stable coronary patients. Training

Table 66-1 Summary of Evidence for Cardiac Rehabilitation Outcomes: Effects of Exercise Training

	Evidence Base[a]				Strength of Evidence[b]
Outcome	Total Number of Studies	Randomized Studies	Nonrandomized Studies	Observational Studies	
Exercise Tolerance	114	46	25	43	A
Exercise Tolerance (Strength Training)	7	4	3	0	B
Exercise Habits	15	10	2	3	B
Symptoms	26	12	7	7	B
Smoking	24	12	8	4	B
Lipids	37	18	6	13	B
Body Weight	34	11	7	16	C
Blood Pressure	18	9	6	3	B
Psychological Well-being	20	9	8	3	B
Social Adjustment and Functioning	6	2	2	2	B
Return to Work	28	10	9	9	A
Morbidity	42 (+2 survey reports)	15	14	13	A
Mortality	31 (+2 survey reports)	17	8	6	B
Pathophysiologic Measures:					
Changes in atherosclerosis	9	5	1	3	A/B
Changes in hemodynamic measurements	5	0	0	5	B
Changes in myocardial perfusion/ myocardial ischemia	11	6	2	3	B
Changes in myocardial contractility, ventricular wall motion abnormalities, and/or ventricular ejection fraction	22	9	5	8	B
Changes in cardiac arrhythmias	5	4	0	1	B
Heart Failure Patients	12	5	3	4	A
Cardiac Transplantation Patients	5	0	1	4	B
Elderly Patients	7	0	1	6	B

[a] Number of studies from scientific literature by type of study design.

[b] Rating for strength of evidence:

A Scientific evidence from well-designed and well-conducted controlled trials (randomized and nonrandomized) provides statistically significant results that consistently support the guideline statement.

B Scientific evidence is provided by observational studies or by controlled trials with less consistent results.

C Guideline statement supported by expert opinion; the available scientific evidence did not present consistent results or controlled trials were lacking.

Table 66-2 Summary of Evidence for Cardiac Rehabilitation Outcomes: Effects of Education, Counseling, and Behavioral Interventions

OUTCOME	EVIDENCE BASE[a]				STRENGTH OF EVIDENCE[b]
	TOTAL NUMBER OF STUDIES	RANDOMIZED STUDIES	NONRANDOMIZED STUDIES	OBSERVATIONAL STUDIES	
Smoking	7	5	1	1	B
Lipids	18	12	3	3	B
Weight	5	3	1	1	B
Blood Pressure	2	0	2	0	B
Exercise Tolerance	3	1	1	1	C
Symptoms	4	2	1	1	B
Return to Work	3	2	0	1	C
Stress/Psychological Well-being	14	7	5	2	A
Morbidity	3	3	0	0	B
Mortality	8	8	0	0	B

[a] Number of studies from scientific literature by type of study design.
[b] Rating for strength of evidence:
   A Scientific evidence from well-designed and well-conducted controlled trials (randomized and nonrandomized) provides statistically significant results that consistently support the guideline statement.
   B Scientific evidence is provided by observational studies or by controlled trials with less consistent results.
   C Guideline statement supported by expert opinion; the available scientific evidence did not present consistent results or controlled trials were lacking.

measures designed to increase skeletal muscle strength can safely be included in the exercise-based rehabilitation of clinically stable coronary patients, when appropriate instruction and surveillance are provided (8).

Exercise Habits

Cardiac rehabilitation exercise training promotes increased participation in exercise by patients after myocardial infarction and coronary artery bypass surgery. This effect does not persist long-term after completion of exercise rehabilitation. Long-term exercise training is recommended to provide the benefit of enhanced exercise tolerance and exercise habits (9).

Symptoms

Exercise rehabilitation decreases angina pectoris in patients with CHD and decreases symptoms of heart failure in patients with left ventricular systolic dysfunction (10). Exercise training is recommended as an integral component of the symptomatic management of these patients. Symptoms of angina pectoris are also reduced by cardiac rehabilitation education, counseling, and behavioral interventions alone or as a component of multifactorial cardiac rehabilitation.

Smoking

A combined approach of cardiac rehabilitation education, counseling, and behavioral interventions results in smoking cessation and relapse prevention (11). Smoking cessation and relapse prevention programs should be offered to patients who are smokers to reduce their risk of subsequent coronary events. Smoking cessation is achieved by specific smoking cessation strategies.

Lipids

Intensive nutrition education, counseling, and behavioral interventions improve dietary fat and cholesterol intake. Education, counseling, and behavioral interventions about nutrition—with and without pharmacologic lipid-lowering therapy—result in significant improvement in blood lipid levels and are recommended as a component of cardiac rehabilitation. Optimal lipid management requires specifically directed dietary and, as medically indicated, pharmacologic management, in addition to cardiac rehabilitation exercise training (12).

Body Weight

Multifactorial cardiac rehabilitation that combines dietary education, counseling, and behavioral interventions designed to reduce body weight can help patients lose weight. Education or cardiac rehabilitation exercise training as sole interventions are unlikely to achieve and maintain weight loss. The optimal management for overweight patients to promote maintenance of weight loss requires multifactorial rehabilitation including nutrition education and counseling and behavioral modification, in addition to exercise training (13).

Blood Pressure

Expert opinion supports a multifactorial education, counseling, behavioral, and pharmacologic approach as the recommended strategy for the control of hypertension. This approach is documented to be effective in nonrehabilitation populations. Neither education, counseling and behavioral interventions nor cardiac rehabilitation exercise training as sole interventions has been shown to control elevated blood pressure levels.

Psychological Well-Being

Education, counseling, and/or psychosocial interventions, either alone or as components of multifactorial cardiac rehabilitation, result in improved psychological well-being and are recommended to complement the psychosocial benefits of exercise training (14).

Social Adjustment and Functioning

Cardiac rehabilitation exercise training improves social adjustment and functioning and is recommended to improve social outcomes.

Return to Work

Cardiac rehabilitation exercise training exerts less of an influence on rates of return to work than many nonexercise variables including employer attitudes, prior employment status, economic incentives, and the like. Exercise training as a sole intervention is not recommended to facilitate return to work. Nor have education, counseling, and behavioral interventions resulted in improvement rates of return to work. Many patients return to work without formal interventions. However, in selected patients, formal cardiac rehabilitation vocational counseling may improve rates of return to work.

Morbidity and Safety Issues

The safety of exercise rehabilitation is well established; rates of myocardial infarction and cardiovascular complications during exercise training are very low (15). Cardiac rehabilitation exercise training does not change rates of nonfatal reinfarction (16). Education, counseling, and behavioral interventions, as components of multifactorial cardiac rehabilitation, may decrease progression of coronary atherosclerosis and lower recurrent coronary event rates.

Mortality and Safety Issues

Based on meta-analyses, total and cardiovascular mortality are reduced following myocardial infarction in patients who participate in cardiac rehabilitation exercise training, especially as a component of multifactorial rehabilitation. Education, counseling, and behavioral interventions reduce cardiac and overall mortality rates and are recommended in the multifactorial rehabilitation of patients with CHD (17).

PATHOPHYSIOLOGIC MEASURES

Coronary Atherosclerosis

Cardiac rehabilitation exercise training as a sole intervention does not result in regression or limitation of progression of angiographically documented coronary atherosclerosis. Exer-

cise training, combined with intensive dietary intervention, with and without lipid-lowering drugs, results in regression or limitation of progression of angiographically documented coronary atherosclerosis and is recommended (7).

Hemodynamic Measurements

Cardiac rehabilitation exercise training has no apparent effect on development of coronary collateral circulation and produces no consistent changes in cardiac hemodynamic measurements at cardiac catheterization. Exercise training in patients with heart failure and a decreased ventricular ejection fraction produces favorable hemodynamic changes in the skeletal musculature and is recommended to improve skeletal muscle functioning.

Myocardial Perfusion and/or Evidence of Myocardial Ischemia

Cardiac rehabilitation exercise training decreases myocardial ischemia as measured by exercise ECG, ambulatory ECG recording, and radionuclide perfusion imaging and is recommended to improve these measure of myocardial ischemia (18).

Myocardial Contractility, Ventricular Wall Motion Abnormalities, and/or Ventricular Ejection Fraction

Cardiac rehabilitation exercise training has little effect on ventricular ejection fraction and regional wall motion abnormalities and is not recommended to improve measures of ventricular systolic function. The effect of exercise training on left ventricular function in patients after anterior Q wave myocardial infarction with left ventricular dysfunction is inconsistent.

Occurrence of Cardiac Arrhythmias

Cardiac rehabilitation exercise training has inconsistent effects on ventricular arrhythmias.

EFFECTS OF CARDIAC REHABILITATION SERVICES ON SPECIAL POPULATIONS

Patients with Heart Failure and Cardiac Transplantation

Cardiac rehabilitation exercise training in patients with heart failure and moderate to severe left ventricular systolic dysfunction improves functional capacity and symptoms, without changes in left ventricular function (19). Cardiac rehabilitation exercise training is recommended to attain functional and symptomatic improvement.

Cardiac rehabilitation exercise training in patients following cardiac transplantation improves measures of exercise tolerance and is recommended for this purpose.

Elderly Patients

Elderly coronary patients have exercise trainability comparable to younger patients participating in similar cardiac rehabiliation exercise training (20). Elderly female and male patients show comparable improvement. Referral to and participation in exercise rehabilitation is less frequent at an elderly age, especially for elderly females. No complications or

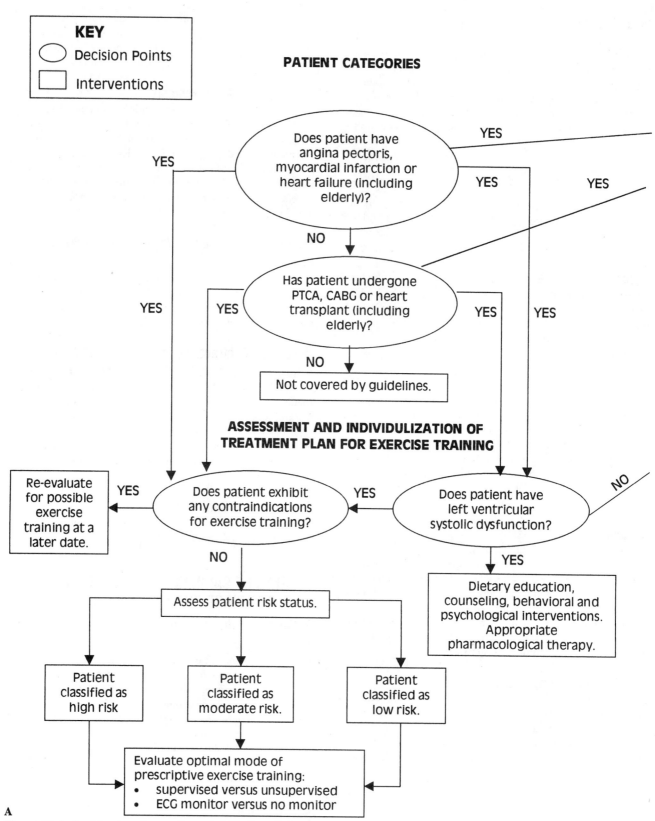

KEY
- ⬭ Decision Points
- ▭ Interventions

PATIENT CATEGORIES

Does patient have angina pectoris, myocardial infarction or heart failure (including elderly)? — YES / YES / YES

NO ↓

Has patient undergone PTCA, CABG or heart transplant (including elderly? — YES / YES / YES / YES

NO ↓

Not covered by guidelines.

ASSESSMENT AND INDIVIDULIZATION OF TREATMENT PLAN FOR EXERCISE TRAINING

Does patient exhibit any contraindications for exercise training? ← YES — Does patient have left ventricular systolic dysfunction? — NO

YES → Re-evaluate for possible exercise training at a later date.

NO ↓

Assess patient risk status.

Does patient have left ventricular systolic dysfunction? — YES ↓

Dietary education, counseling, behavioral and psychological interventions. Appropriate pharmacological therapy.

Patient classified as high risk

Patient classified as moderate risk.

Patient classified as low risk.

Evaluate optimal mode of prescriptive exercise training:
- supervised versus unsupervised
- ECG monitor versus no monitor

A

Figure 66-1 Decision tree for cardiac rehabilitation. (Adapted from: Cardiac rehabilitation: clinical practice guideline no. 17. Rockville, MD: Agency for Health Care Policy and Research, 1995. Publication no. 96-0672.)

ASSESSMENT AND INDIVIDUALIZATION OF TREATMENT PLAN FOR RISK FACTOR MODIFICATION, PSYCHOSOCIAL STATUS

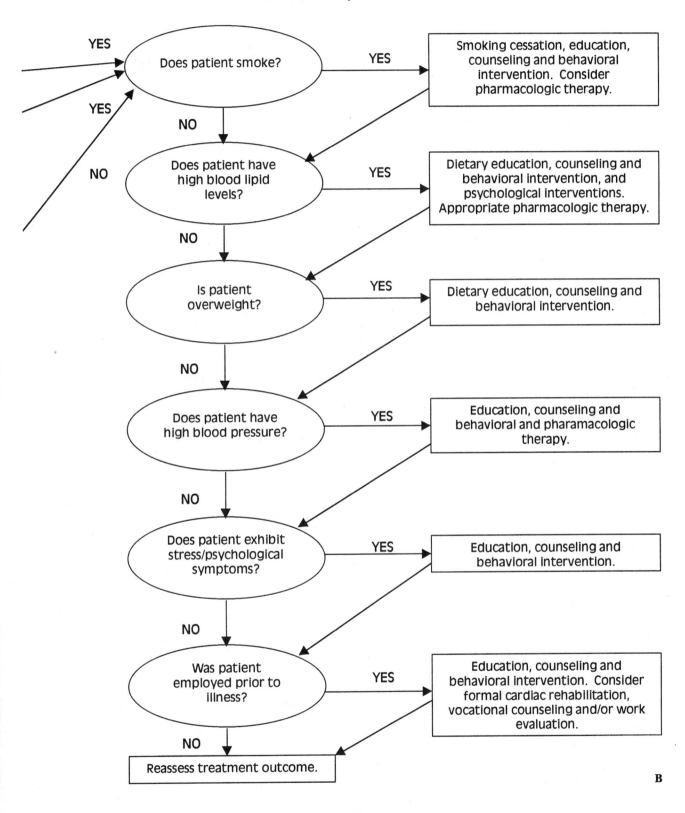

adverse outcomes of exercise training at an elderly age were described in any study. Elderly patients of both genders should be strongly encouraged to participate in exercise-based cardiac rehabilitation.

ALTERNATE APPROACHES TO THE DELIVERY OF CARDIAC REHABILITATION SERVICES

Alternate approaches to the delivery of cardiac rehabilitation services, other than traditional supervised group interventions, can be implemented effectively and safely for carefully selected clinically stable patients (12). Transtelephonic and other means of monitoring and surveillance of patients can extend cardiac rehabilitation services beyond the setting of supervised, structured, group-based rehabilitation. These alternative approaches have the potential to provide cardiac rehabilitation services to low- and moderate-risk patients who comprise the majority of patients with stable CHD, most of whom do not currently participate in structured supervised cardiac rehabilitation.

COST OUTCOMES

The Clinical Practice Guideline addressed the issue of cost-effectiveness of cardiac rehabilitation programs. As with other outcomes covered in the guideline, this issue was based upon scientific evidence in the medical literature. There were a limited number of studies of cardiac rehabilitation services, including randomized controlled trials and nonrandomized controlled trials, that addressed the cost-effectiveness issue. Although variation was noted, the average cost of a 12-week

cardiac rehabilitation program was approximately $1000 per patient. Regarding the issue of cost-effectiveness or actual savings of medical care costs, several points were addressed and conclusions made.

It is difficult to estimate the savings that widespread use of cardiac rehabilitation will reap. This is an area that needs greater study. However, from the limited trials that have been conducted there are indications that the potential for cost savings is great.

In a randomized trial of an 8-week comprehensive cardiac rehabilitation program, the incremental cost (subtracting the cost of usual care) of services was $480 per patient (21). The results of a second trial estimated that cardiac rehabilitation saved $739 per patient in reduced hospital admissions after 21 months (22).

Comparing the estimated $480 per patient cost with the conservative savings estimate of $739 in reduced hospital admissions, the net saving is $259 per patient. If an additional 50% of the 2.4 million Americans annually who have recognized heart disease receive effective cardiac rehabilitation, the American health system would save more than $310 million in hospital costs alone over about a 2-year period.

GUIDELINE AVAILABILITY

The Clinical Practice Guideline for Cardiac Rehabilitation, AHCPR Publication No. 96-0672, and the Quick Reference Guide for Clinicians, Cardiac Rehabilitation as Secondary Prevention, AHCPR Publication No. 96-0673, are available from the AHCPR Publications Clearinghouse; call toll-free 800-358-9295 or write to P.O. Box 8547, Silver Spring, MD 20907.

REFERENCES

1. Institute of Medicine. Clinical practice guidelines: directions for a new program. Washington, D.C.: National Academy Press, 1990.

2. Woolf SH. Practice guidelines, a new reality in medicine: methods of developing guidelines. Arch Intern Med 1992;152:946–952.

3. Smith SC. Guidelines for Cardiac Rehabilitation. National Press Release. Washington, D.C.: American Heart Association National Center, Office of Communications for Agency for Health Care Policy and Research, 1995.

4. Wenger NK, Froelicher ES, Smith LK. Cardiac rehabilitation. Clinical Practice Guideline No. 17. AHCPR Publication No. 96-0672. Rockville, MD: U.S. Department of Health and Human Services,

Public Health Service, Agency for Health Care Policy and Research and the National Heart, Lung, and Blood Institute, 1995.

5. Wenger NK, Froelicher ES, Smith LK. Cardiac rehabilitation as secondary prevention. Clinical Practice Guideline. Quick Reference Guide for Clinicians, No. 17. AHCPR Publication No. 96-0673. Rockville, MD: U.S. Department of Health and Human Services, Public Health Service, Agency for Health Care Policy and Research and the National Heart, Lung, and Blood Institute, 1995.

6. Leon AS, Certo C, Comoss P. Scientific evidence of the value of cardiac rehabilitation services with emphasis on patients following myocardial infarction— Section I: exercise conditioning component. J Cardiopulm Rehabil 1990;10:79–87. Position paper.

7. Haskell WL, Alderman EL, Fair JM. Effects of intensive multiple risk factor reduction on coronary atherosclerosis and clinical cardiac events in men and women with coronary artery disease: the Stanford Coronary Risk Intervention Project (SCRIP). Circulation 1994;89:975–990.

8. McCartney N, McKelvie RS, Haslam DR. Usefulness of weightlifting training in improving strength and maximal power output in coronary artery disease. Am J Cardiol 1991;67:939–945.

9. Todd IC, Ballatyne D. Effect of exercise training on the total ischaemic burden: an assessment by 24 hour ambulatory electrocardiographic monitoring. Br Heart J 1992;68:560–566.

10. Meyer TR, Casadei B, Coats AJ. Angiotensin-converting enzyme

inhibition and physical training in heart failure. J Intern Med 1991; 230:407–413.

11. Taylor CB, Houston-Miller N, Killen JD. Smoking cessation after acute myocardial infarction: effects of a nurse-managed intervention. Ann Intern Med 1990;113:118–123.

12. DeBusk RF, Houson-Miller N, Superko HR. A case-management system for coronary risk factor modification after acute myocardial infarction. Ann Intern Med 1994; 120:721–729.

13. Karvetti RL, Hamalainen H. Long-term effect of nutrition education on myocardial infarction patients: A 10-year follow-up study. Nutr Metab Cardiovasc Dis 1993;3: 185–192.

14. Oldridge NB, Guyatt G, Jones N. Effects on quality of life with com-prehensive rehabilitation after acute myocardial infarction. Am J Cardiol 1991;67:1084–1089.

15. Van Camp SP, Peterson RA. Cardiovascular complications of out-patient cardiac rehabilitation programs. JAMA 1986;256:1160–1163.

16. O'Connor GT, Buring JE, Yusuf S. An overview of randomized trials of rehabilitation with exercise after myocardial infarction. Circulation 1989;80:234–244.

17. Oldridge NB, Guyatt GH, Fischer ME. Cardiac rehabilitation after myocardial infarction: combined experience of randomized clinical trials. JAMA 1988;260:945–950.

18. Sebrechts CP, Klein JL, Ahnve S. Myocardial perfusion changes following 1 year of exercise training assessed by thallium-201 circumferential count profiles. Am Heart J 1986;112:1217–1226.

19. Meyer TR, Casadei B, Coats AJ. Angiotensin-converting enzyme inhibition and physical training in heart failure. J Intern Med 1991; 230:407–413.

20. Ades PA, Waldmann ML, Gillespie C. A controlled trial of exercise training in older coronary patients. J Gerontol 1995;50A:M7–M11.

21. Oldridge N, Furlong W, Feeny D. Economic evaluation of cardiac rehabilitation soon after acute myocardial infarction. Am J Cardiol 1993;72:154–161.

22. Ades PA, Huang D, Weaver SO. Cardiac rehabilitation participation predicts lower rehospitalization costs. Am Heart J 1992;123:916–921.

Chapter 67

Delayed Progression or Regression of Coronary Atherosclerosis with Intensive Risk Factor Modification

William L. Haskell
Joseph J. Carlson

Among many patients with documented coronary heart disease (CHD) and their physicians, there has been substantial interest in whether or not intensive medical or risk factor management can either halt the progression or produce regression of existing altherosclerosis in coronary arteries. Of particular interest has been the idea that intensive risk factor management might cause disease regression and thus restore the patient's cardiac health and avoid the need for invasive procedures such as percutaneous transluminal angioplasty (PTCA) or coronary artery bypass graft (CABG) surgery. This interest in the medical or lifestyle management of atherosclerosis, and especially regression of disease, was initially fueled by animal experimentation showing that atherosclerosis induced by a high-fat and high-cholesterol diet could be reversed by return to the plant-based diet typically consumed by these animals (1,44). Many clinicians doubted that this atherosclerosis and its reversal, which could be achieved within 12 to 36 months in monkeys, was similar to the process that occurred over years or decades in humans. Also, interest was stimulated by unsubstantiated claims of regression being achieved by various approaches such as vegetarian diets (53) or ethylenediaminetetraacetic acid (EDTA) chelation therapy (28) and published case reports demonstrating probable disease regression but without good evidence as to its causation (34).

Over the past 2 decades published data from a wide variety of randomized clinical trials have demonstrated that intensive single or multiple risk factor reduction in patients with established CHD can decrease the rate of coronary atherosclerosis progression, enhance disease regression in selected patients, and significantly reduce clinical cardiac events, including hospitalizations involving expensive invasive diag-

nostic and treatment procedures. During this same period, basic research in vascular wall biology has redefined much of the atherosclerotic-thrombotic process that leads to clinical events as well as new mechanisms of disease such as plaque disruption, endothelial erosion, local stimulation of thrombosis, and the loss of dilation responses in coronary arteries that may be favorably modified via risk factor and medical management (15,16,24,39).

This chapter provides a brief review of the major clinical trials that contributed to the current recommendations by the American Heart Association (63) and the American College of Cardiology (24a) for the intensive multifactor management of patients with established atherosclerotic vascular disease. The primary focus will be on those randomized trials that evaluated coronary artery disease progression and regression by quantitative coronary arteriography or documented fatal and nonfatal clinical cardiac events. Mechanisms by which these interventions might provide benefit are briefly discussed, and the clinical implications based on this research are presented.

RANDOMIZED CLINICAL TRIALS OF ATHEROSCLEROSIS AND CLINICAL CARDIAC EVENTS IN PATIENTS WITH CORONARY HEART DISEASE

It became clear in the mid-1980s during implementation of randomized clinical trials of CHD primary prevention with initial clinical cardiac events as the major outcome, such as the Lipid Research Clinics Coronary Primary Prevention Trial

(41) and the Multifactor Risk Factor Intervention Trial (47), that because of their high cost in dollars and resources, other research designs were necessary to test a variety of therapeutic approaches. With advancements in computer-based quantitative coronary arteriography during the late 1970s and early 1980s, it became possible to accurately and reliably measure very small changes in the lumen diameter of epicardial coronary arteries (7). These procedures allowed for the first time the systematic evaluation of the effects of specific "antiatherosclerotic therapies" on changes in artery lumen diameter. Using variations of this quantitative angiographic technique, a number of randomized clinical trials have been completed in patients with CHD, testing a variety of different risk reduction approaches. Interventions have included intensive lipoprotein management using single or multiple drug regimens (3–6,9,12, 33,35,36,43,52,56,66), single or multiple changes in lifestyle, including diet, exercise, smoking cessation, and stress management (27,30,48,49,51,59,60,69), multifactor interventions incorporating both changes in lifestyle plus lipid lowering medications (31,45,54,69), and ileal bypass surgery (11). In addition to these angiographically based studies, other randomized trials with clinical events as the major outcome have demonstrated that both pharmacologic (13,22,57,58) and lifestyle (23,42,62) interventions decrease cardiovascular morbidity and mortality in patients with existing CHD (secondary prevention) as well as in patients without clinical evidence of disease (17,41,61). Other interventions that have been tested in randomized, controlled trials that have not significantly modified disease progression but appear to possibly reduce new lesion formation include calcium channel blockade (40,67).

Angiographic Trials: Hypolipidemic Drugs

The greatest amount of data demonstrating that improvements in the cardiovascular risk profile of patients with CHD can slow the rate of disease progression, and in some cases enhance regression, comes from double-blind, randomized trials with patients assigned to either lipid lowering medication or a placebo. Prior to these studies, which used quantitative coronary arteriography in randomized controlled trials, several studies had demonstrated that a decrease in the rate of coronary artery disease (CAD) progression might be possible using cholesterol lowering medications and/or a low-saturated-fat diet (2,14,29,38,50). Although some decrease in disease progression was indicted in most of these studies, they all were limited by lack of either a control group, a small sample size, or small changes in plasma lipid concentrations.

The more recent randomized studies have typically lasted for 2 to 4 years, some have included both men and women, and patient ages have ranged from 40 to 74 years at study entry. All of these studies have used quantitative coronary angiographic techniques, but the actual recording and analysis procedures have varied from study to study, eliminating the possibility of actually pooling the angiographic data across studies and making direct comparisons among the different studies difficult. For example, it is not possible to say that one intervention had a greater or better angiographic effect than another intervention because of these measurement differences, but also because of differences in patient selection criteria and study duration.

The primary angiographic results achieved by these cholesterol lowering drug studies are summarized in Table 67-1 (section A) and have been extensively reviewed by others (8,26,65). In all of the studies, except for the NHLBI Type II Study (6), MARS (4), and HARP (56), the authors reported a significant reduction in the rate of lumen narrowing or disease progression in the treatment group as compared to the placebo group for their primary angiographic endpoint. Although the absolute magnitude of this change in lumen size is small, if continued over a decade or more it would have a major effect on coronary flow reserve. Of the 14 lipid lowering drug studies listed in Table 67-1, only the SCOR project (37) reported a net enlargement in lumen size in the treatment group (regression) using the study primary angiographic endpoint (percentage of area stenosis). All of the other studies reporting discrete changes in lumen size observed a reduction in lumen size in both the treatment and control groups (progression). More importantly, these relatively small reductions in disease progression are associated with several mechanisms that may lead to a reduction in clinical cardiac events (15,21).

Variation in progression/regression rates among studies probably is contributed to by differences in the study length and the overall risk status for disease progression of the patents. For example, different rates of cigarette smoking by both the treatment and control groups could have influenced the rates of progression or regression (68). Other major risk factors, such as hypertension, diabetes, or low HDL-C concentrations, as well as patients' degree of depression or hopelessness (20), could contribute to interstudy differences in the rate of lumen narrowing and clinical cardiovascular events.

Angiographic Trials: Multifactor Lifestyle Interventions

Since the atherosclerotic-thrombotic process leading to clinical cardiac events is influenced by a number of factors, a multifactor approach to cardiovascular disease (CVD) prevention and management is the basis for current national guidelines (24a,63). Multifactor interventions evaluated in clinical trials using coronary angiography have included lifestyle changes only [LHT (27,51), STARS (69), and Heidelberg (30,48,49,59,60)] and lifestyle changes plus the use of cholesterol lowering medications [STARS (69) and SCRIP (31)] (see Table 67-1, sections B and C). The control groups in these studies are patients randomly assigned to "usual care" provided by their own physicians. All of these studies report significant reductions in the rate of epicardial artery lumen narrowing in the treatment group versus the control group, with more patients in the treatment groups demonstrating disease regression and less progression. It is interesting to note that in three of these four studies (LHT, STARS, and Heidelberg), the treatment groups had an increase in lumen size (regression), whereas the control groups had a decrease in lumen size (progression).

The Lifestyle Heart Trial (51) evaluated an intensive 1-year multifactor treatment program consisting of a low-fat vegetarian diet, mild- to moderate-intensity physical activity, stress reduction/relaxation, smoking cessation, and social support. After recruitment into the study and baseline clinical, risk factor, and angiographic evaluations, the authors state that 94 eligible patients were randomly assigned to treatment (N = 53) or usual care (N = 43) (Note: this is 96 not 94 as reported in the article). However, of the 53 patients assigned

Table 67-1 Randomized Clinical Trials Using Angiography to Assess Progression and Regression of Coronary Atherosclerosis

STUDY	TOTAL N	PT. TYPE	THERAPY	DURATION (months)	Δ LUMEN T/C	% PROGRES. T/C	% REGRES. T/C	% NO CHANGE T/C	% DIFFERENCE CVD EVENTS
A. Lipid Lowering Medications									
NHLBI Type-II (6)	116	CAD + High LDL-C	Chole.	60	NA	32/49	7/7	53/42	33 D + NF MI
CLAS (5)	162	CABG + TC = 165–300	Col. + N	24	+0.3/+0.8ᵃ global change score	39/61	16/2	45/37	0 All CVD
FATS (9)	106	High Apo B	Col. + N / Col + Lovastatin	30	-0.002/-0.05ᵃ / -0.002/-0.05ᵃ mm. Δ min. dia.	25/46 / 21/46	39/11 / 32/11	36/43 / 47/43	73* F = NF CHD
SCOR (37)	72	FH	Col. + N + Lovastatin	24	+0.80/-1.53ᵃ % area stenosis	20/41	33/13	NA	T = 0%; C = 3%
MARS (4)	247	CAD + TC = 190–285	Lovastatin	24	+1.6/+2.2 % dia. stenosis	29/41	23/12	48/47	28
CCAIT (66)	299	CAD + TC = 220–300	Lovastatin	24	-0.05/-0.09ᵃ mm. Δ min. dia.	33/50	19/13	NA	21
MAAS (43)	345	CAD	Simvastatin	48	-0.04/-0.83ᵃ mm. Δ min. dia.	23/33	19/12	53/43	30* All CHD
HARP (56)	79	CAD + TC = 180–250	Prava. + N + Chole. + Gemfibrozil	30	-0.14/-0.15 mm. Δ min. dia	23/28	13/13	NA	33 All CHD
PLAC I (52)	408	CAD + LDL-C = 130–190	Pravastatin	36	0.06 difference* mm. Δ min. dia.	NA	NA	NA	60* All CHD
BECAIT (18,19)	81	Post MI <45 y + dyslipidemia	Bezafibrate	60	-0.06/-0.17* mm. Δ min. dia.	74/85	21/13	5/3	73*
CIS (3)	203	CAD +	Lovastatin TC = 207–350	28	-0.02/-0.10ᵃ mm. Δ min. dia.	NA	NA	NA	24
Post CABG (12)	1192	CABG + LDL = 130–175	Lovastatin + Chole.	52	-0.197/-0.379ᵃ mm. Δ min. dia.	24/35	5/4	NA	29 revascularization
LCAS (33)	340	CAD	Fluva. / Fluva. + Chole.	30	-0.024/-0.094* / -0.041/-0.117* mm. Δ min. dia	29/36 / 29/39	14/8 / 15/8	NA / 57/53	33 All CHD
REGRESS (35)	653	CAD + TC = 155–310	Pravastatin	24	-0.06/-0.10* mm. Δ mean dia.	44/55	17/9	37/35	38ᵃ
B. Lifestyle Only Intervention									
LHT (12 months) (51)	41	CAD	Diet + Exercise + Relax + Support	12	-2.2/+3.4ᵃ Δ% dia. stenosis	18/53	82/42	0/0	NA
Heidelberg (59)	62	CAD	Diet + Exercise	12	-1/+3* Δ % rel. dia. reduction	20/42	30/4	50/54	-20
STARS (69)	50	CAD + High TC	Low-Fat Diet	39	+0.030/-0.232ᵃ mm. Δ min. width	15/46	38/4	47/50	69*
C. Lifestyle Plus Lipid Lowering Medications									
SCRIP (31)	246	CAD	Diet + Weight Exercise + Smoke + Relax + Drugs	48	-0.10/-0.18* mm. Δ min. dia.	50/50	21/10	20/18	40*
STARS (69)	48	CAD + High TC	Chole. + Low-Fat Diet	39	+0.117/-0.232ᵃ mm. Δ min. width	12/46	33/4	55/50	89ᵃ
D. Surgery									
POSCH (5 years) (11)	634	Post MI + LDL-C > 140	Ileal Bypass	60	NA	38/65	13/5	50/36	35ᵃ

Total N = sample size contributing to primary angiographic results; Δ lumen = change in lumen size for primary angiographic endpoint; % progres. = % of patients demonstrating disease progression (lumen narrowing); % regres. = % of patients demonstrating disease regression (lumen enlargement); % no change = % of patients demonstrating no significant change in lumen size; % difference CVD events = difference in CVD event rate between treatment and control groups divided by the rate in the control group × 100; T = treatment group; C = control or placebo group; Col. = colestid; N = niacin; Chole. = cholestyramine; Prava. = pravastatin; Fluva. = fluvastatin; min. = minimum; dia. = diameter; FH = familial hypercholesterolemia; D = death; NF = nonfatal; F = fatal; MI = myocardial infarction; NA = not available; CHD = coronary heart disease; CVD = cardiovascular disease.

* = $p < .05$.
ᵃ = $p < .01$.

to the treatment group, only 28 entered the program (53%) of the 43 assigned to the control group, only 20 (42%) agreed to participate. This loss of subjects is important when considering the generalizability of the results. Treatment consisted of a week-long intensive introduction to the program in which patients lived in a hotel and received instruction and practice on various components of the intervention. For the remainder of the year, treatment patients met twice a week for approximately 4 hours for group support sessions at which they received instruction regarding diet, exercise, and relaxation and were provided food they were to eat during the week (how much of their food was provided is not stated). Patients were instructed to exercise 3 hours per week and to practice relaxation techniques for at least 1 hour per day. The one treatment group patient who smoked at baseline stopped. Clinical, risk factor, and angiographic measurements were repeated after 1 year on 41 subjects (43% of those subjects randomized and 85% of those who accepted entry into the study).

Adherence to the intensive lifestyle treatment program was reported to be excellent, with highly significant reductions in total cholesterol, low-density lipoprotein (LDL) cholesterol, apolipoprotein B, and body weight as compared to 1-year changes in patients assigned to the control group. Plasma triglyceride concentration increased by 22% and high-density lipoprotein (HDL) cholesterol fell slightly in the treatment group (frequently the result of very low fat diets). Reported chest pain frequency and duration was significantly less in the treatment patients, and this benefit appeared to occur within 1 month of starting the intervention.

Small but significant improvements were reported for the main angiographic measurements, with the average percentage of diameter stenosis decreasing from 40.0% to 37.8% in the treatment group and increasing in the control group from 42.7% to 46.1% (p for differences in the changes between groups = .001). Disease regression as defined by any decrease in percentage of stenosis was observed in 82% of the treatment patients, but it was also observed in 42% of control patients. This is a high rate of "spontaneous regression" and likely reflects the analysis methods for this measurement, which do not take into account day-to-day measurement variation. Using these data, the ratio of the rate of regression in the treatment to control group is 1.95, which is similar to that reported in many other angiographic trials even though the absolute rate of regression reported in the angiographically based risk reduction trials typically is much lower.

After 5 years of follow-up, patients remaining in the treatment group (n = 20) still demonstrated improved coronary artery stenosis scores as compared to control patients (n = 15), and they had a significant decrease in the size and severity of myocardial perfusion abnormalities as determined by positron emission tomography (27). However, the only risk factors in which the change between baseline and 5 years was greater in the treatment group than the control group were body weight (p < .001) and plasma cholesterol (p = .04).

The other major angiographically based clinical trial that limited its interventions to multiple changes in lifestyle was a combined low-fat and low-cholesterol diet and aerobic exercise training program conducted in Heidelberg, Germany (48,49,59). Patients (N = 113; men aged 53.5 years) with stable angina pectoris performed clinical, risk factor, and angiographic measurements prior to participation in a program of intensive aerobic exercise and a low-fat and low-cholesterol diet. The treatment program was initiated with a 3-week stay on a metabolic ward in the hospital during which patients were provided a low-fat and low-cholesterol diet and instructed on how to prepare a diet that met American Heart Association phase 3 guidelines (total fat <20% of calories, cholesterol < 200 mg/day, polyunsaturated fat/saturated fat ratio >1.0). The exercise program consisted of two 60-minute sessions per week of supervised training (intensity = 75% of measured maximal heart rate) and 30 minutes per day at home using a stationary cycle ergometer. Compliance to the supervised exercise program was calculated at 68% (range = 39% to 92%).

Cardiovascular drugs were prescribed by the patient's personal physician as indicated, but lipid lowering drugs were not part of the regimen. Informational sessions were conducted four times per year for patients and spouses to discuss dietary, psychosocial, and exercise-related problems. Also, patients were offered the opportunity to discuss personal problems after each exercise training session. The control group members (N = 57) spent 1 week on the metabolic ward where they received identical instructions about the value of regular exercise and a low-fat diet and were served a low-fat diet (American Heart Association phase 1). Adherence to these guidelines was left up to their own initiative.

The 12-month program of exercise and diet produced significantly greater improvements in physical working capacity (p < .0005), maximal oxygen uptake (p < .05), and maximal rate-pressure product (p < .05) compared to changes in the control patients. The treatment program also reduced indicators of myocardial ischemia during maximal exercise testing (e.g., progressive angina and ST segment depression). Using a 24-hour recall questionnaire, significant reductions were reported in the treatment group for intake of calories (−27% versus −19%; p < .05), total fat (−53% versus −25%; p < .05), and cholesterol (−62% versus −35%; p < .05). The reductions in body mass index, total cholesterol, LDL cholesterol, total to HDL cholesterol ratio, and triglycerides over the 1 year were significantly greater in the treatment group compared to controls (all p < .05).

Overall, the changes in coronary artery morphology after one year (N = 92) were more favorable in the treatment group, demonstrating no real change in minimum segment diameter (0.92 ± 0.72 mm to 0.91 ± 0.67 mm), whereas a small decrease (progression) was observed in the control group (1.00 ± 0.87 mm to 0.87 ± 0.79 mm; p for difference in changes between groups <.05). When percentage change in relative diameter reduction is used as the endpoint, the treatment group demonstrated a small increase in lumen size (regression) compared to a small decrease (progression) for the control group (65 ± 24% to 64 ± 23% in the treatment group and 63% ± 29% to 66% ± 28% in the control group; p < .05). More patients in the treatment group demonstrated regression (30%) than in the control group (4%). Disease progression was noted in 20% of the treatment group and 42% in the control group, with no significant angiographic change reported for 50% in the treatment group and 54% in the control group.

The patients in this study also had follow-up arteriograms after a mean of 6 years of follow-up (48,49). Patients were continued in their assigned groups, with the treatment

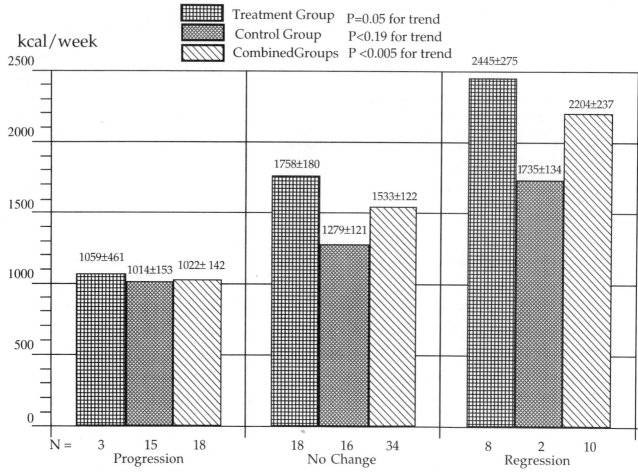

kcal/week

Figure 67-1 Relation between level of energy expenditure during physical activity and change in coronary artery lumen size in patients completing 1 year in the Heidelberg Coronary Atherosclerosis Study (Source: Hambrecht R, Nieubauer J, Marburger C, et al. Various intensities of leisure time physical activity in patients with coronary artery disease: effects on cardiorespiratory fitness and progression of coronary atherosclerotic lesions. J Am Coll Cardiol 1993;22:468–477.)

group instructed to participate in at least two group exercise sessions per week and continue with at least two home exercise session per week and to maintain a low-fat and low-cholesterol diet. Adherence to the exercise program was 68% for the first year and averaged 33% for the next 5 years. Control group patients remained in "usual care." At an average follow-up of 6.1 ± 1.7 years, a total of 90 patients had quantitative coronary arteriography repeated (treatment group = 40, control group = 50). There were no significant between group differences in the changes between baseline and 6 years for smoking, body mass, or any plasma lipoprotein concentrations, whereas maximal exercise capacity increased in the treatment group ($p < .05$). Relative stenosis diameter demonstrated modest but nonsignificant progression in the treatment group (58.9% ± 34.7% to 62.0% ± 25.9%) and a significant worsening in the control group (54.7% ± 34.7% to 66.6% ± 30.2%; $p < .0005$). In the treatment group, 59% of patients showed progression, 22% no change, and 19% regression, whereas in the control group 74% showed progression, 26% no change, and regression was not observed (significant difference in rate of retardation of lesion progres-

sion; $p < .0001$). Over the 6 years, none of the metabolic variables were significantly related to disease progression, with only physical work capacity contributing independently to changes in relative diameter reduction.

For a subset of the patients randomized in this study, Hambrecht et al (30) reported on the relation between intensity and amount of physical activity performed over the first year to changes in cardiorespiratory fitness and progression of coronary atherosclerotic lesions (N = 29 in the treatment group and 33 in the control group). Figure 67-1 displays the relation between level of exercise-induced energy expenditure and change in coronary morphology expressed as progression, no change, and regression separately for the treatment and control groups and for the two groups combined. The trend for the combined analysis was highly significant ($p < .005$). On average, a subject who demonstrated disease regression expended about 2200 kcal/week in nonwork activity, whereas those with disease progression expended about 1000 kcal/week.

In addition to this randomized trial, Schuler et al (60) reported a smaller study in nonrandomized patients (N = 36), with angiographic measurements performed at baseline and 1 year. Patients were assigned to treatment if they lived near the hospital and to control if they lived farther away. The diet and exercise regimens for the treatment and controls groups were the same as for the larger randomized study. Changes in coronary artery lumen size are not reported, but more treatment patients demonstrated regression (7 versus 1), fewer treatment patients had no change (6 versus 11), and a similar number of patients had progression (5 versus 6). The overall trend for the treatment improving disease status was significant ($p = .048$).

Angiographic Trials: Lifestyle Plus Cholesterol Lowering Medications

Only two major angiographic trials have been published that have systematically evaluated the effects of a treatment program combining lifestyle and lipid lowering medications: the St. Thomas Atherosclerosis Regression Study (STARS) (69) and the Stanford Coronary Risk Intervention Project (SCRIP) (31,46,54).

STARS evaluated the effects of a cholesterol lowering medication (8 mg of cholestyramine twice daily) plus a plant-based reduced fat and cholesterol diet (total fat 27% of calories, saturated fat 8% to 10% of calories, cholesterol 100 mg per 1000 calories, polyunsaturated fat 8% of calories, and increased water-soluble dietary fiber) or a diet only group versus usual care on angiographic and clinical outcomes. Patients consisted of 90 men with CHD (mean age of 51.5 years) randomized to the three groups, but with 74 of them completing baseline and follow-up arteriograms at a mean of 39 ± 3.5 months. Both treatments resulted in highly significant reductions in total cholesterol, LDL cholesterol, and total cholesterol to HDL cholesterol ratio, with triglycerides being reduced only in the diet only group. The diet plus drug group had a 36% reduction in LDL cholesterol, and in the diet only group the reduction was 16%. No significant changes were reported for body weight, blood pressure, or cigarette smoking. Mean diameter of the measured epicardial coronary artery segments decreased in patients randomized to usual care (-0.201 ± 0.062 mm) but increased slightly for patients in either the diet only ($+0.003 \pm 0.087$ mm) or diet plus drug group ($+0.103 \pm 0.051$). The magnitude of changes in artery diameter for the usual care group was significantly different from the two treatments.

Similar results were seen for other angiographic measures, with overall progression observed in 46% of usual care patients, 15% of diet only patients, and 12% in the diet plus drug group. Regression was reported for 4% of usual care patients, 38% of diet only patients, and 33% of diet plus drug patients. One of the most interesting aspects of this study is that a plant-based diet that produced a reduction in LDL cholesterol of 16% had nearly as much of an effect on improving the angiographic measurements as a similar diet plus cholestyramine, which decreased LDL cholesterol by 36%. These results are consistent with the idea that plant-based diets may influence disease progression/regression and clinical cardiac events by mechanisms other than LDL cholesterol lowering.

SCRIP has been the only major, large-scale randomized trial to determine the effects of a multifactor risk reduction program using both multiple lifestyle changes plus cholesterol lowering medications on the progression and regression of coronary atherosclerosis and clinical cardiac events in men and women with established heart disease. This study was unique compared to other angiographic trials in that it: 1) included attempts to manage all of the major risk factors for atherosclerosis, 2) included both men and women with risk factor profiles that represent most adults who present with CHD, and 3) retained more than 90% of randomized patients in the study for 4 years.

The SCRIP risk reduction program was designed to be practical for all participants and generalizable to most adults. Patients (N = 300 randomized) were recruited who had mild to moderate atherosclerosis and lived within a 6-hour driving time of Stanford University Medical Center. After completion of baseline medical/risk factor evaluations and computer-assisted quantitative coronary arteriography, patients were randomized to the usual care of their own physician (n = 155) or to an intensive multifactor risk reduction program (n = 145) conducted by the SCRIP staff. All patients were scheduled for medical/risk factor evaluations annually for 4 years and repeat quantitative coronary arteriogram after 4 years. The risk reduction program consisted of lifestyle interventions including a low-fat, low-cholesterol, and low-sodium diet, regular exercise, stress management, smoking cessation, and weight loss. When indicated, the research team used a combination drug regimen for lowering LDL cholesterol and triglycerides and raising HDL cholesterol. The risk reduction program was based on a "physician-supervised, nurse-manager model" using other health professionals to assist with the intervention. Treatment patients visited the clinic approximately once every 2 months over the 4 years for an average of slightly less than six visits per year, and the intervention program required no special facilities. Of the 300 patients that were randomized into the trial, follow-up arteriograms were obtained on 274 (92%).

Once the necessary clinical and risk factor data were available, a preliminary "risk management plan" was designed by the SCRIP nurse in consultation with the project physician and other team members. This plan included short- and long-term goals for relevant risk factors. This preliminary plan was then reviewed by the nurse with the patient, and modifications were made as needed. The follow-up contact schedule was individualized based on each patient's needs and available resources. The normal priority for risk modification was to assist smokers to stop smoking; reduce LDL cholesterol by diet, weight loss, and medications; increase HDL cholesterol by stopping smoking, exercise, weight loss, and medications; reduce triglycerides by exercise, diet, weight loss, and medications; normalize plasma glucose and insulin by exercise, diet, weight loss, and medications; reduce adiposity by diet and exercise; and reduce psychological stress using various stress management techniques. In addition to the diet being low in saturated fat and cholesterol, it emphasized the consumption of vegetables, grains, fruits, and fish. Cholesterol lowering medications were prescribed based on National Cholesterol Education Program adult treatment guidelines, except that the goal for LDL cholesterol was set at 110 mg/dL rather the 130 mg/dL (later reduced to ≤100 mg/dL in the National Cholesterol Treatment Program II adult treatment guidelines).

Table 67-2 Risk Factor Changes in the Special Intervention and Usual Care Groups in the Stanford Coronary Risk Intervention Project

VARIABLE	USUAL CARE (N = 127)			RISK REDUCTION (N = 118)			$p^\dagger$
	BASELINE	ON-STUDY*	ABSOLUTE CHANGE	BASELINE	ON-STUDY*	ABSOLUTE CHANGE	
Cigarette Smoking							
Current smokers	17.3% (n = 22)	18.1% (n = 23)	+0.8%	10.1% (n = 12)	10.1% (n = 12)	0.0%	0.47
Body Composition							
Weight (kgs)	84.6 ± 14.5	85.5 ± 15.0	+0.9 ± 3.6[b]	80.4 ± 12.7	77.4 ± 11.9	−3.0 ± 4.0[d]	.0001
Body mass index (kg/m²)	27.1 ± 3.6	27.4 ± 3.9	+0.3 ± 1.2[b]	26.8 ± 3.4	25.8 ± 3.3	−1.0 ± 1.3	.0001
Sum of skinfolds (mm)	52.7 ± 17.1	53.2 ± 16.4	+0.5 ± 13.1	52.8 ± 17.9	46.4 ± 14.7	−6.4 ± 13.6	.0001
Blood pressure (mmHg)							
Systolic blood pressure	118.1 ± 14.7	121.2 ± 13.3	+3.1 ± 10.5[c]	121.1 ± 16.5	120.5 ± 14.1	−0.6 ± 11.1	.008
Diastolic blood pressure	72.0 ± 8.	72.4 ± 7.6	+0.4 ± 6.6	70.9 ± 9.2	69.6 ± 7.9	+1.3 ± 7.1[a]	.066
Graded Exercise Test							
Maximum MET level	9.1 ± 2.9	9.9 ± 3.	+0.7 ± 2.1[d]	8.6 ± 3.4	10.3 ± 3.5	+1.7 ± 2.4[d]	.001
Heart rate at 4METs (b/min)	98.6 ± 16.6	94.4 ± 12.9	−4.2 ± 11.5[d]	101.6 ± 18.6	96.1 ± 14.9	−5.5 ± 15.0[c]	.680
Lipoprotein Profile							
Total cholesterol (mmol/L)	5.87 ± 0.96	5.79 ± 0.75	−0.09 ± 0.63	6.03 ± 1.05	5.03 ± 0.73	−0.99 ± 0.83[d]	.0001
LDL cholesterol (mmol/L)	4.04 ± 0.87	3.89 ± 0.67	−0.16 ± 0.59	4.07 ± 0.93	3.12 ± 0.60	−0.95 ± 0.81[d]	.0001
HDL cholesterol (mmol/L)	1.10 ± 0.28	1.16 ± 0.29	0.06 ± 0.17[d]	1.19 ± 1.49	1.33 ± 0.38	0.14 ± 0.23[d]	.001
TC/HDL-C	5.60 ± 1.46	5.28 ± 1.31	−0.32 ± 0.98	5.36 ± 1.49	4.08 ± 1.15	−1.27 ± 1.04[d]	.0001
Triglycerides (mmol/L)	1.75 ± 1.41	1.76 ± 0.91	0.01 ± 0.97	1.77 ± 1.22	1.42 ± 0.69	−0.34 ± 0.87[d]	.002
Lp (a) (mg/dL) (n = 98,97)[e]	19.8 ± 21.4	19.9 ± 25.4	0.14 ± 12.1	19.2 ± 27.3	18.1 ± 27.8	−1.06 ± 13.4	.51
Apolipoprotein B (mg/dL) (n = 99,97)[e]	112.2 ± 32.1	105.1 ± 38.6	−7.0 ± 43.0	116.5 ± 35.1	90.3 ± 33.5	−26.2 ± 34.8[d]	.0008
Glucose Tolerance Test (n for fasting = 125,116; n for nonfasting = 112,104)							
Fasting glucose (mmol/L)	5.79 ± 2.02	6.16 ± 1.80	0.37 ± 1.73[a]	5.79 ± 1.36	5.62 ± 1.36	−0.17 ± 1.15	.005
1-hour post-load glucose (mmol/L)	8.82 ± 3.18	9.03 ± 3.63	0.20 ± 2.71	8.66 ± 3.21	7.64 ± 2.67	−1.03 ± 2.38[d]	.0005
Fasting insulin (pmol/L)	123 ± 83	126 ± 91	3 ± 85	130 ± 191	101 ± 87	−30 ± 133[a]	.033
1-hour post-load insulin (pmol/L)	947 ± 579	959 ± 745	11 ± 641	916 ± 570	823 ± 749	−93 ± 667	.084
Revised Framingham Coronary Heart Disease Risk Score	15 ± 7	14 ± 6	−.5 ± 3	15 ± 7	11 ± .06	−4.0 ± .04[d]	.0001

* On-study values are the mean ± SD for measurements recorded annually over the 4 years patients were assigned to the special intervention or usual care groups.
† p represents the comparison of usual care versus risk reduction group for the change from baseline to on-study values.
Within group comparison for the change from baseline to on-study values: ([a] $p < .05$, [b] $p < .01$, [c] $p < .001$, [d] $p < .0001$).
[e] For Lp (a) and apolipoprotein B on-study sample measured only at year 4.

Selected educational materials were provided the participant and family, and a follow-up contact schedule for the next 6 months was made. This contact schedule included clinic or laboratory visits, enrollment in risk reduction classes, phone calls, and mailings. As many low-cost or free community services were used as possible (for stopping smoking, exercise, weight loss, nutrition education, cardiac rehabilitation, etc.). Direct referrals were made to these programs, or the patient was provided information on how to enroll.

This project was very successful with highly significant reductions occurring in many major risk factors in the risk reduction group but not in the usual care group (Table 67-2). Significant improvements were seen in dietary intake of saturated fat and cholesterol, all the lipid and lipoprotein measurements, fasting glucose, body weight, exercise capacity, and Framingham risk score. Most risk factors were significantly improved by the end of the first year, and this improvement was retained or enhanced over the next 3 years. An exception was body weight, which was reduced by an average of 11 pounds at the end of first year, but then became less each of the following years with the mean reduction from baseline being 5.6 pounds at year 4.

The main angiographic outcome for SCRIP was the rate of change in the minimum diameter of diseased segments. Secondary angiographic measures included mean diameter of diseased and nondiseased segments, new lesion formation, and measurements of net progression and regression. The risk reduction group showed a rate of narrowing of diseased coronary artery segments that was 47% less than subjects in the usual care group (change in minimum diameter of −0.024 ± 0.066 mm/year versus −0.045 ± 0.073 mm/year; $p < .02$). Net disease regression occurred in approximately twice as many risk reduction as usual care patients (20.2% versus 10.3%; $p = .07$), and the number of new lesions per patient tended to be less in the risk reduction group (0.30 versus 0.47; $p = .06$) (54). The number of hospitalizations for primary cardiac events was significantly less in the risk reduction patients (n = 25) compared to those assigned to usual care (n = 44; $p < .05$).

Comparison of Angiographic Changes Among Studies

Most of the studies using angiographic endpoints were initiated with the goal of testing the potential for reductions in disease progression and not necessarily to demonstrate disease regression. But given the interest by the public and healthcare professionals in regression, much of the focus in considering the results of these studies has been on the achievement of regression. Increased regression of disease as a result of the therapy is reported in a number of the angiographic trials based on the number of patients showing some increase in

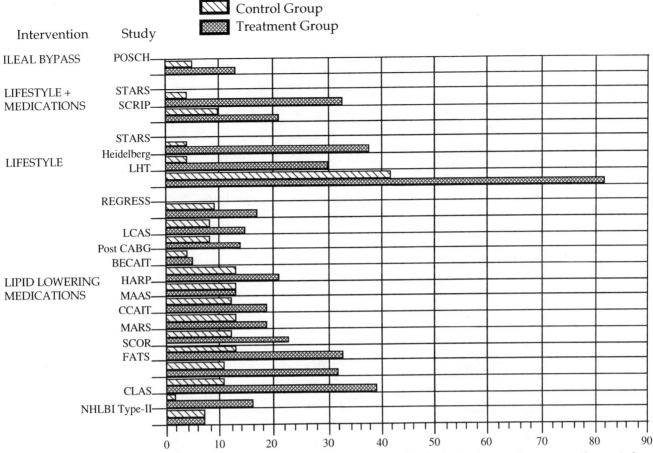

Figure 67-2 The percentage of patients demonstrating coronary artery regression in the treatment group versus the control group in studies using arteriography to determine the effects of risk factor modification. (See Table 67-1 for abbreviations and references and the text for discussion.)

artery lumen diameter. Since angiography allows only visualization of the open lumen and not of the artery wall or plaque mass, it has been assumed in these studies that a larger lumen is due to regression of a plaque. However, using quantitative arteriography, there is no way to be sure if the increase in lumen size is due to a reduction in atherosclerotic mass (regression), a decrease in thrombosis mass, or an increase in artery size due to vasodilatation or angiogenesis. Although some therapies, like cholesterol lowering drugs, might work primarily on reducing atherosclerotic mass, other therapies like diet (omega-3 fatty acids) or aspirin might influence blood clotting/fibrinolytic mechanisms and exercise might change artery diameter by flow-mediated vascular remodeling (32).

The reported rate of regression in the treatment group (percentage of patients demonstrating regression) in the various studies ranges from a low of 5% in the Post CABG Trial and 7% in the NHLBI Type-II Study to 82% in the Lifestyle Heart Study (Figure 67-2). The rate of progression in the treatment groups ranges from 10% in the Heidelberg Heart Study to 50% in SCRIP (Figure 67-3). These differences in progression or regression rates are probably due more to differences in measurement methodology and subject selection than the effectiveness of the intervention.

In many of the studies, the day-to-day variation of the angiographic measurement procedure was taken into account so that subjects who did not have a change in artery diameter greater than the estimated measurement error were classified as not changing (9,31). In other studies, such as the Lifestyle Heart Study, subjects were classified as having either disease progression or regression and the studies did not take into account the issue of measurement variation (51). Also, some studies only considered a subject to have shown regression if one or more artery segments had an increase in diameter (beyond that considered to be measurement error) and no other eligible segment showed significant narrowing (disease progression). If the subjects had artery segments that showed both progression and regression, they were reported as "mixed" in some studies and nonchangers in other studies.

If one considers that the effect of measurement methodology on classifying patients as having disease progression or regression should have a reasonably similar effect on measurements in both the treatment and control groups, then this effect can be "normalized" by contrasting the rate of disease progression or regression within each study. One way to do this is to divide the rate of progression or regression in the treatment group by the rate in the control

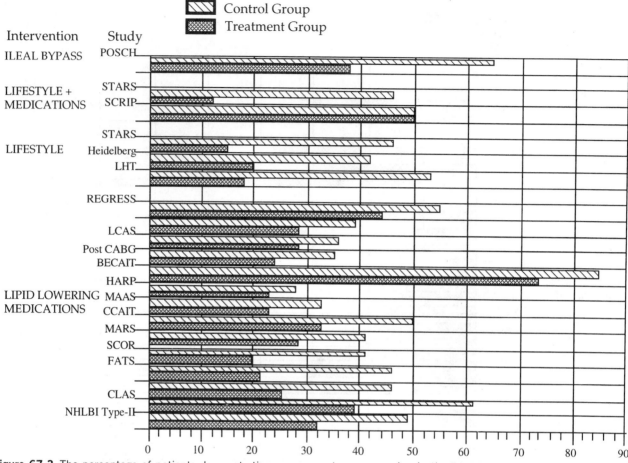

Figure 67-3 The percentage of patients demonstrating coronary artery progression in the treatment group versus the control group in studies using arteriography to determine the effects of risk factor modification. (See Table 67-1 for abbreviations and references and the text for discussion.)

group. Based on the data in Table 67-1 and Figure 67-2, the ratio for the percentage of patients in the treatment group as compared to the percentage of patients in the control group reported to show regression for a study ranges from a high of 9.5 in STARS to a low of 1.0 in the NHLBI Type-II Trial and HARP, with a median ratio of 1.9, a mean ratio of 3.4, and 13 of the studies having a ratio in the range of 1.5 to 3.5. Thus, on average, patients in the treatment groups demonstrated disease regression 2.0 to 3.5 times more frequently than the control groups. High ratios are primarily due to very low rates of regression in the control group.

When rates of progression are compared between the treatment and control groups in the studies listed in Table 67-1 and Figure 67-3, there is a lower rate in the treatment group in all the studies except for SCRIP, in which the ratio was 1.0. For a majority of the studies, the ratio of treatment group to control group progression ranges from 0.26 to 1.0 with the mean and median at 0.66. Thus, on average, there was approximately a 34% reduction in the number of patients showing progression in the treatment groups as compared to the control groups. There lower rates of progression, when expressed as the percentage of patients demonstrating pro-

gression, were not significant between groups in all of the studies, and as a secondary endpoint the results of statistical analyses were not always reported.

Effects on Clinical Cardiovascular Events

Even though most of the angiographically based clinical trials were not designed with the power to detect significant reductions in fatal or nonfatal clinical cardiac events (based on intervention effectiveness and intervention adherence data from prior studies such as the Lipid Research Clinics Coronary Primary Prevention Trial and the Multiple Risk Factor Intervention Trial), many of these studies carefully documented hospitalizations and deaths in the treatment and control groups (Table 67-1, last column). Out of the 19 different angiographic trials reported in Table 67-1, 18 studies reported CVD events, with 8 of these reporting a significantly lower event rate for the treatment group as compared to the control group. Another eight studies reported nonsignificant lower rates in the treatment groups. The Heidelberg study is the only one to report a nonsignificant higher event rate in the treatment group. In most cases these are *post hoc* comparisons and need to be viewed as preliminary data. However, the magnitude of the reductions achieved in many studies and

Table 67-3 Clinical Events in Treatment and Control Groups in Randomized Clinical Trials Directed at Cardiovascular Risk Factor Reduction Published Since 1990

STUDY	TOTAL N	SUBJECTS	DURATION (months)	INTERVENTION	FATAL CHD	N-F MI	F + NF CHD	FATAL CVD	ALL-CAUSE DEATH
					EVENTS (T/C)				
Primary Prevention									
WOSCPOS (61)	6595	M LDL-C > 155	59	Pravastatin	38/52 p = .13	143/204 p < .001	150/218 p < .001	50/73 p = .03	106/135 p = .05
AF/TEX CAPS (17)	5608	M + W TC & LDL-C average HDL-C low	58	Lovastatin	15/11 too small a number	NA	116/183 p < .0008	17/25 too small a number	77/80 NS
Secondary Prevention									
4S(58)	4444	M + W AP or MI	65	Simvastatin	111/189 p = .0003	279/418 p < .001	431/632 p < .00001	136/207 p < .001 Stroke	182/256 p = .0003
CARE (57)	4159	M + W MI + TC < 240	60	Pravastatin	96/119 p = .10	135/173 p = .02	212/274 p = .003	54/78 p = .03 Stroke	180/196 p = .37
IEIS (62)	406	AMI	12	Fruit and vegetable diet	20/34 p < .01	30/48 p < .05	50/82 p < .001	1/2 NS All CVD	21/38 p < .01
Lyon Heart Study (42)	605	AMI	27	Mediterranean diet	3/16 NA	5/17 NA	8/33 p = .001	14/59 p < .0001	8/20 p = .02

Total N = number of subjects that contributed to calculation of event rates; CHD = coronary heart disease; N-F = nonfatal; MI = myocardial infarction; F = fatal; CVD = cardiovascular disease; TC = total cholesterol; M = men; W = women; AP = angina pectoris; AMI = acute myocardial infarction; NA = not available; NS = not significant.
* These studies did not include angiographic measurements and were designed to test the effect of lipid lowering agents or dietary changes with clinical events as the primary endpoint.

their consistency with larger randomized trials with reductions in clinical events as the primary prestated outcome make for a very compelling argument that intensive single or multifactor risk reduction can significantly reduce clinical cardiovascular events in a wide range of patients with CHD (57,58) or without CHD (17,61).

Summarized in Table 67-3 are the clinical cardiovascular events reported in randomized clinical trials of CHD risk reduction that included people with and without CHD at entry. Although most of the data are on men, when women are included they appear to benefit as much as men, and older persons and patients with diabetes also show benefit. Accompanying reductions in fatal and nonfatal myocardial infarctions and angina pectoris are reductions in PTCA and CABG surgery. In addition to the reduction in CHD fatal and nonfatal events, substantial reductions (25% to 40%) in LDL cholesterol concentration by statin drugs have been shown to reduce the risk of stroke by 24% in a meta-analysis of seven studies (10).

Two nonangiographic studies cited in Table 67-3 are worth special note in that they are diet only trials in post–myocardial infarction patients that report large reductions in clinical cardiac events (42,62). Both studies have significant design problems, but the results should be of major interest given the increased likelihood that various micronutrients like antioxidant vitamins or nonnutrients like fiber and phytoestrogens might have a highly favorable effect on the atherosclerotic-thrombotic process (16). These data are consistent with the three angiographic studies (51,59,69) that included a lifestyle only intervention with diet being a major or sole component of the intervention and demonstrated significant reductions in disease progression and myocardial ischemia.

CLINICAL IMPLICATIONS AND RECOMMENDATIONS

It now appears that many clinical cardiac events, including myocardial infarction, cardiac arrest, and unstable angina pectoris, occur when a plaque ruptures or there is erosion of the endothelium, allowing blood in the lumen to come in contact with platelet aggregation factors in the plaque, which stimulates the formation of a blood clot that can rapidly occlude the artery (15,24). These so-called "culprit lesions" that rupture tend to be the early lipid-filled plaques rather than the more advanced complex lesions. Thus, prevention of clinical cardiac events may be achieved by the reduction of new lesion formation, stabilization of existing lesions, reduction in the rate of existing lesion growth or progression, decrease in lesion size or regression, and the reduction of platelet aggregation or an increase in fibrinolysis.

Given the complex and multifactorial nature of the pathobiology of the events that contribute to the development, progression, regression, and stabilization of atherosclerotic lesions and thrombosis, there are a variety of mechanisms by which therapies could cause a reduction in CHD morbidity and mortality. Also, it is possible that selected therapies might reduce the occurrence or severity of clinical cardiac events by their effects on the myocardium instead of the coronary arteries, including reduction of myocardial work at rest and during exercise, an increase in myocardial electrical stability, or an enhancement of intrinsic myocardial contractility.

The effectiveness of secondary prevention programs is achieved by establishing individualized goals for optimal risk factor status, carefully instructing the patient about what will need to be done to achieve these goals, educating the patient on how to achieve the behavior change required, identifying resources to be used, and frequent monitoring of progress and feedback. The failure of many secondary prevention programs is due to the lack of mutual goal setting, commitment to the process on the part of all of the staff and patient, and frequent patient contact or follow-up. For example, only 20% of men and 14% of women patients with CHD being managed in academic medical centers in North America in 1996 were being treated to achieve an LDL cholesterol goal of 100mg/dL at 6 months after hospitalization (46). Also, many patients are provided inadequate instruction on what lifestyle changes need to be made and how to effectively achieve these changes.

Results from the angiographic and clinical endpoint studies are exceedingly encouraging and indicate that the medical and lifestyle management of existing coronary artery disease may be an effective alternative to invasive interventions such as CABG surgery or PTCA. Of even more importance is the increasing possibility that the process of atherosclerosis might be mostly preventable, slowed, or even reversed so that it becomes a disease of clinical importance in only the very elderly. Although the results from these studies are very encouraging and provide substantial evidence that men and women at high risk for clinical cardiac events may be able to prevent the progression of atherosclerosis and its sequelae, many major questions on how to effectively implement such programs for much of the population are still unresolved. This is especially true of a number of questions related to the generalizability and relative cost-effectiveness of these interventions. These questions will only be answered by projects designed to test these interventions in a variety of real-life settings.

A new comprehensive risk reduction program is needed based on successful clinical research programs such as the Stanford Coronary Risk Intervention Project or the Lifestyle Heart Trial that have demonstrated significant benefits using new integrated models of intervention. The program needs to maximize the efficient use of physicians and nonphysician personnel; provide effective communication via mail, telephone, fax, and electronic mail; include cost-effective participant and program tracking and feedback using a computer-based participant management system; incorporate the use of printed, audio, and video educational materials; and take advantage of existing corporate and community resources. The program should be designed for use in various medical/healthcare delivery settings and be independent of any specific reimbursement scheme. The guidelines for patient management in such a program have been published by the American Heart Association (63) and the American College of Cardiology (24a). Also, new models for risk stratification and the delivery of risk reduction programs are being developed and evaluated (25,55).

Demonstration of the health benefits and cost-effectiveness, as well as the generalizability, of an approach that successfully produces a significant decrease in coronary artery disease progression and clinical cardiac events, including PTCA and CABG surgery, will provide the scientific and organizational basis for the effective implementation of such a program by healthcare delivery organizations. Even a modest reduction in the use of invasive evaluation procedures and hospitalizations for myocardial infarction, cardiac arrest, or congestive heart failure would substantially reduce healthcare costs in many technologically advanced societies.

REFERENCES

1. Armstrong ML, Megan MB. Lipid depletion in atheromatous coronary arteries in rhesus monkeys after regressive diets. Circ Res 1972; 30:675–680.

2. Arntzenius AC, Kromhout D, Barth JD, et al. Diet, lipoproteins and the progression of coronary atherosclerosis: the Leiden Intervention Trial. N Engl J Med 1985;312: 805–811.

3. Bestchorn HP, Rensing UFE, Roskamm H, et al. The effect of simvastatin on progression of coronary artery disease: the Multicenter Coronary Intervention Study (CIS). Eur Heart J 1997;18:226–234.

4. Blankenhorn DH, Azen SP, Kramsch DM, et al. Coronary angiographic changes with lovastatin therapy: the Monitored Atherosclerosis Study (MARS). Ann Intern Med 1993;119:969–976.

5. Blankenhorn DH, Nessim SA, Johnson RL, et al. Beneficial effects of combined colestipol-niacin therapy on coronary atherosclerosis and coronary venous bypass grafts. JAMA 1987;257: 3233–3240.

6. Brensike JF, Levy RI, Kelsey SF, et al. Effects of therapy with cholestyramine on progression of coronary atherosclerosis: results of the NHLBI Type II Coronary Intervention Study. Circulation 1984;69:313–324.

7. Brown BG, Bolson EL, Frimer M, et al. Quantitative coronary arteriography: Estimation of dimensions, hemodynamic resistance and atheroma mass of coronary artery lesions using the arteriogram and computer digital computation. Circulation 1977; 55:329–337.

8. Brown BG, Zaho X-Q, Sacco DE, et al. Lipid lowering and plaque rergression: New insights into prevention of plaque disruption and clinical events in coronary disease. Circulation 1993;87: 1781–1791.

9. Brown G, Alberts JJ, Fisher LD, et al. Regression of coronary artery disease as a result of intensive lipid-lowering therapy in men with high levels of apolipoprotein B. N Engl J Med 1990;323:1289–1298.

10. Bucher HC, Griffith LE, Guyatt GH. Effect of HMG-CoA reductose inhibitors on stroke: A meta-analysis of randomized, controlled trials. Ann Intern Med 1998;128:89–95.

11. Buchwald H, Matts JP, Fitch LL, et al. For the Program on the Surgical Control of the Hyperlipidemias (POSCH) Group: changes in sequential coronary arteriograms and subsequent coronary events. JAMA 1992;268:1429–1433.

12. Campeau L, Knatterud GL, Domanski M, et al. The effect of aggressive lowering of low-density lipoprotein cholesterol levels and low-dose anticoagulation on obstructive changes in saphenous-vein coronary-artery bypass grafts. N Engl J Med 1997; 336(3):153–162.

13. Carlson LA, Rosenhamer G. Reduction in mortality in the Stockholm Ischemic Heart Disease Secondary Prevention Study by combined treatment with clofibrate and nicotinic Acid. Acta Med Scand 1988;223:403–418.

14. Cohn K, Sakai FJ, Langston MF. Effect of clofibrate on progression of coronary disease: A prospective angiographic study in man. Am Heart J 1975;89:591–598.

15. Davies MJ. Stability and instability: two faces of coronary atherosclerosis. Circulation 1996;94: 2013–2020.

16. Diaz MN, Frei B, Vita J, et al. Antioxidants and atherosclerotic heart disease. N Engl J Med 1997;337:408–416.

17. Downs JR, Clearfield M, Wels S, et al. Final results of the Air Force/ Texas Coronary Atherosclerosis Prevention Study. JAMA 1998;279: 1615–1622.

18. Ericsson CG, Hamsten A, Nilsson J, et al. Angiographic assessment of effects of bezafibrate on progression of coronary artery disease in young male postinfarction patients. Lancet 1996;347:849–853.

19. Ericsson CG, Nilsson J, Grip L, et al. Effect of bezafibrate treatment over five years on coronary plaques causing 20% to 50% diameter narrowing (the Bezafibrate Coronary Atherosclerosis Intervention Trial [BECAIT]). Am J Cardiol 1997;80:1125–1129.

20. Everson SA, Kaplan GA, Goldberg DE, et al. Hopelessness and 4-year progressing carotid atherosclerosis: the Kuopio Ischemic Heart Disease Risk Factor Study. Arterioscler Thromb Vasc Biol 1997;17:1490–1495.

21. Falk E, Shah PK, Fuster V. Coronary plaque disruption. Circulation 1995;92:657–671.

22. Frick MH, Elo O, Happa K, et al. Helsinki Heart Study: primary prevention trial with gemfibrozil in middle-aged men with dyslipidemia. N Engl J Med 1987;317:1237–1245.

23. Friedman M, Thoresen CE, Gill JJ, et al. Alteration in type A behavior and its effect on cardiac recurrences in post-myocardial infarction patients: summary results of the Recurrent Coronary Prevention Project. Am Heart J 1986;12:653–665.

24. Fuster V, Lewis A. Conner Memorial Lecture: mechanisms leading to myocordial infarction: insights from studies of vascular biology. Circulation 1995;91: 2126–2146.

24a. Fuster V, Pearson T. 27th Bethesda Conference: matching the intensity of risk factor management with the hazard for coronary disease events. J Am Coll Cardiol 1996;27:958–1047.

25. Gordon NF, Haskell WL. Comprehensive cardiovascular disease risk reduction in a cardiac rehabilitation setting. Am J Cardiol 1997;80:69H–73H.

26. Gould AL, Rossouw JE, Santanello NC, et al. Cholesterol reduction yields clinical benefit. Circulation 1998;97:946–952.

27. Gould KL, Ornish D, Scherwitz L, et al. Changes in myocardial perfusion abnormalities by positron emission tomography after long-term, intense risk factor modification. JAMA 1995;274:894–901.

28. Grier MT, Meyers DG. So much writing, so little science: a review of 37 years of literature on edetate sodium chelation therapy. Ann Pharmacother 1993;27:1504–1509.

29. Hahnmann HW, Bunte T, Hellwig N, et al. Progression and regression of minor coronary arterial narrowings by quantitative angiography after fenofibrate therapy. Am J Cardiol 1991;67: 957–961.

30. Hambrecht R, Niebauer J, Marburger C, et al. Various intensities of leisure time physical activity in patients with coronary artery disease: effects on cardiorespiratory fitness and progression of coronary atheroscleortic lesions. J Am Coll Cardiol 1993;22:468–477.

31. Haskell W, Aldermann AL, Fair JM, et al. Effects of intensive multiple risk factor reduction on coronary atherosclerosis and clinical cardiac events in men and women with coronary artery disease: the Stanford Coronary Risk Intervention Project (SCRIP). Circulation 1994; 89:975–990.

32. Haskell W, Sims C, Myll J, et al. Coronary artery size and dieting capacity in ultradistance runners. Circulation 1993;87:1076–1082.

33. Herd AJ, Ballantyne CM, Farmer J, et al. Effects of fluvastatin on coronary atherosclerosis in patients with mild to moderate cholesterol elevations (Lipoprotein and Coronary Atherosclerosis Study [LCAS]). Am J Cardiol 1997;80: 278–286.

34. Hubbard JD, Inkeles S, Barnard RJ. Nathan Pritikin's heart. N Engl J Med 1985;313:52. Letter.

35. Jukema JW, Bruschke AVG, Van Boven AJ, et al. Effects of lipid lowering by pravastatin on progression and regression of coronary artery disease in symptomatic men with normal to moderately elevated serum cholesterol levels. Circulation 1995;91:2528–2540.

36. Jukema JW, Bruschke AVG, Van Boven AJ, et al. Effects of lipid lowering by pravastatin on progression and regression of coronary artery disease in symptomatic men with normal to moderately elevated serum cholesterol levels. Circulation 1995;91:2528–2540.

37. Kane JP, Malloy MJ, Ports TA, et al. Regression of coronary atherosclerosis during treatment of familial hypercholesterolemia with combined drug regimens. JAMA 1990;264:3007–3012.

38. Kuo PT, Hayase K, Kostis JB, et al. Use of combined diet and colestipol in long-term (7-7$\frac{1}{2}$ yr) treatment of patients with type II hyperlipoproteinemia. Circulation 1979;59(2):199–211.

39. Libby P. Molecular basis of the acute coronary syndrome. Circulation 1995;91:2844–2850.

40. Lichtlen PR, Hugenholtz PG, Rafflenbeul W, et al. Retardation of

angiographic progression of coronary artery disease by nifedipine. Lancet 1990;335:1109–1113.

41. Lipid Research Clinics Program. The Lipid Research Clinics Coronary Primary Prevention Program: I. reduction in the incidence of coronary heart disease. JAMA 1984;251:351–364.

42. Logeril DE, Renaud MD, Mamelle N, et al. Mediterranean alpha-linolenic acid-rich diet, in secondary prevention of coronary heart disease. Lancet 1994;343:1454–1459.

43. MAAS Investigators. Effect of simvastatin on coronary atheroma: the Multicentre Anti-Atheroma Study (MAAS). Lancet 1994;344:633–638.

44. Mann GV, Andrus SB, McNally A, et al. Xanthomatosis and atherosclerosis produced by diet in an adult rhesus monkey. J Lab Clin Med 1956;48:533–550.

45. Miller BD, Alderman EL, Haskell W, et al. Predominance of dense low-density lipoprotein particles predicts angiographic benefit of therapy in the Stanford Coronary Risk Intervention Project. Circulation 1996;94:2146–2153.

46. Miller M, Byington RP, Hunninghake D, et al. Lipid lowering therapy in CHD patients at academic medical centers: undertreatment and evidence of a gender gap. J Am Coll Cardiol 1998;31:186A. Abstract.

47. Multiple Risk Factor Intervention Trial Research Group. Multiple Risk Factor Intervention Trial: risk factor changes and mortality results. JAMA 1982;248:1465–1477.

48. Niebauer J, Hambrecht R, Schlierf G, et al. Five years of exercise and low fat diet: Effects on progression of coronary artery disease. J Cardiopulm Rehabil 1994;15:47–64.

49. Niebauer J, Hambrecht R, Velich T, et al. Attenuated progression of coronary artery disease after 6 years of multifactorial risk intervention. Circulation 1997;96:2534–2541.

50. Nikkila EA, Viiknikoski P, Valle M, et al. Prevention of progression of coronary atherosclerosis by treat-

ment of hyperlipidaemia: a seven year prospective angiographic study. Br Med J 1984;289:220–223.

51. Ornish D, Brown SE, Scherwitz LW, et al. Can lifestyle changes reverse coronary heart disease? Lancet 1990;336:129–133.

52. Pitt B, Mancini GBJ, Ellis SG, et al. Pravastatin limitation of atherosclerosis in the coronary arteries (PLAC I). J Am Coll Cardiol 1994;23:131A.

53. Pritikin N, McGrady P. The Pritikin program for diet and exercise. New York: Grosset and Dunlap, 1979.

54. Quinn TG, Aldermann AL, Haskell W. Development of new coronary atherosclerotic lesions during a 4-year risk reduction program: the Stanford Coronary Risk Intervention Project (SCRIP). J Am Coll Cardiol 1994;24:900–908.

55. Roitman JL, LaFontaine T, Drimmer AM. A new model for risk stratification and delivery of cardiovascular rehabilitation services in the long-term clinical management of patients with coronary artery disease. J Cardiopulm Rehabil 1998;18:113–123.

56. Sacks FM, Pasternak RC, Gibson CM, et al. Effect on coronary atherosclerosis of decrease in plasma cholesterol concentrations in normocholesterolaemic patients. Lancet 1994;344:1182–1186.

57. Sacks FM, Pasternak RC, Move LA, et al. The effect of pravastatin on coronary events after myocardiac infarction in patients with average cholesterol levels. N Engl J Med 1996;335:1001–1009.

58. Scandinavian Simvastatin Survival Study Group. Randomized trial of cholesterol lowering in 4444 patients with coronary artery disease: the Scandinavian Simvastatin Survival Study (4S). Lancet 1994;344:1383–1389.

59. Schuler G, Hambrecht R, Schlierf G, et al. Regular physical exercise and low-fat diet: Effects on progression of coronary artery disease. Circulation 1992;86:1–11.

60. Schuler G, Hambrecht R, Schlierf G, et al. Myocardial perfusion and

regression of coronary artery disease in patients on a regimen of intensive physical exercise and low fat diet. J Am Coll Cardiol 1992;19:34–42.

61. Shepherd J, Cobbe SM, Ford I, et al. Prevention of coronary heart disease with pravastatin in men with hypercholesterolmeia. N Engl J Med 1995;333:1301–1307.

62. Singh RB, Rastogi SS, Verma R, et al. An Indian experiment with nutritional modulation in acute myocardial infarction. Am J Cardiol 1992;69:879–885.

63. Smith SC, Blair SN, Criqui MH, et al. Preventing heart attack and death in patients with coronary disease. Circulation 1995;92:2–4.

64. Standberg TE, Salomaa VV, Nau VA, et al. Long-term mortality after 5-year multifactorial primary prevention of cardiovascular diseases in middle-aged men. JAMA 1991;266:1225–1229.

65. Superko RH, Krauss RM. Coronary artery disease regression: convincing evidence for the benefit of aggressive lipoprotein management. Circulation 1994;90:1056–1069.

66. Waters D, Higginson L, Gladstone, et al. Effects of monotherapy with an HMG-CoA reductase inhibitor on the progression of coronary atherosclerosis as assessed by serial quantitative arteriography. Circulation 1994;89:959–968.

67. Waters D, Lespérance J, Francetich M, et al. A controlled clinical trial to assess the effect of a calcium channel blocker on the progression of coronary atherosclerosis. Circulation 1990;82:1940–1953.

68. Waters D, Lespérance J, Gladstone P, et al. Effects of cigarette smoking on the angiographic evolution of coronary atherosclerosis. Circulation 1996;97:614–621.

69. Watts GF, Lewis B, Brunt JNH, et al. Effects on coronary artery disease of lipid-lowering diet or diet plus cholestyramine in the St. Thomas Atherosclerosis Regression Study. Lancet 1992;339:563–569.

Chapter 68

Exercise Prescription for the Coronary Patient: An Update

Barry A. Franklin
Kimberly Bonzheim
Adam deJong
Andrea Watson

When formulating exercise prescriptions for cardiac patients, it is critical to provide a sufficient exercise dosage to elicit beneficial training effects, yet provide a program that the patient perceives as enjoyable and rewarding to enhance long-term compliance. Although it is important to follow established exercise guidelines, these cannot be applied in an overly rigid manner that ignores individual preferences or comorbid conditions.

Ideally, the exercise prescription should be based on the results of a symptom-limited exercise test. The test provides valuable information regarding the ischemic electrocardiographic (ECG) threshold, symptoms, hemodynamics, perceived exertion, supraventricular and ventricular arrhythmias, and functional capacity. Moreover, the results can aid in promoting confidence and self-efficacy and in risk-stratifying patients to determine the appropriate level of medical supervision and monitoring. This chapter reviews the physiologic and clinical bases for the prescription of exercise in patients with coronary artery disease (CAD), with specific reference to the optimal exercise dosage (intensity, frequency, and duration), upper body and resistance training, exercise trainability, aerobic and myocardial demands of common leisure activities, risk of exercise training, and special patient populations.

INTENSITY

The prescribed exercise intensity should be above a minimal level to induce favorable adaptation and improvement in aerobic fitness, yet below the metabolic rate that evokes abnormal signs or symptoms. For most deconditioned cardiac patients, the threshold intensity for exercise training probably lies between 40% and 60% of the aerobic capacity ($\dot{V}o_2max$); however, considerable evidence indicates that it increases in direct proportion to the pretraining $\dot{V}o_2max$ (Figure 68-1) (1). Improvement in aerobic capacity with low to moderate training intensities suggests that the interrelation among the training intensity, frequency, and duration may permit a decrease in the intensity to be partially or totally compensated for by increases in the exercise duration, frequency, or both.

Because heart rate and oxygen consumption are linearly related during dynamic exercise involving large muscle groups, a predetermined training or target heart rate (THR) has become widely used as an index of exercise intensity (2). Prescribed heart rates for aerobic conditioning are generally determined by one of two methods from data obtained during peak or symptom-limited exercise testing: the maximal heart rate reserve method of Karvonen et al (3), in which THR = (maximal heart rate − resting heart rate) × 50% to 80% + resting heart rate, or the percentage of maximal heart rate method (4). The former more closely approximates the same percentage of the maximum oxygen uptake "reserve" (5,6), rather than the percentage of $\dot{V}o_2max$ (7). For example, a patient with a functional capacity of 5 metabolic equivalents (METs) would have a 4-MET "reserve," considering resting metabolism as 1 MET. If the patient were exercising at 60% of his or her heart rate reserve, he or she would be working at 4 METs × 60% = 2.4 METs + 1 MET = 3.4 METs, rather than 3 METs. This terminology is preferred because it is incorrect to relate heart rate reserve to a level of metabolism that starts from zero rather than a resting level (8). Additional advantages include increased accuracy in the prescribed THR, relative exercise intensity, and calculation of the net

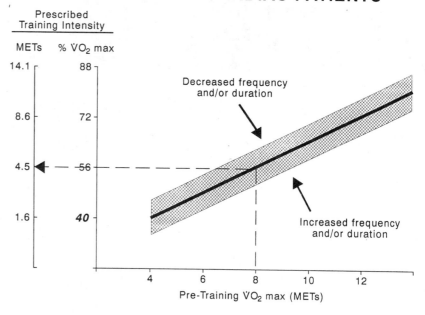

Figure 68-1 Theoretical relation between aerobic capacity (METs) and the minimal intensity for exercise training, expressed as a percentage of the maximal oxygen uptake ($\dot{V}O_2$max). The threshold intensity for training increases in direct proportion to the $\dot{V}O_2$max before training; however, it can be modulated by altering the exercise duration, frequency, or both. For example, a patient with a peak capacity of 8 METs would exercise at approximately 56% of his or her $\dot{V}O_2$max, or 4.5 ± 0.5 METs, to further increase his or her functional capacity.

THEORETICAL THRESHOLD INTENSITIES FOR TRAINING CARDIAC PATIENTS

caloric expenditure (6). On the other hand, computing the THR as a fixed percentage of the measured peak heart rate has been shown to yield remarkably similar regressions of percentage of maximum oxygen uptake reserve (percentage of $\dot{V}O_2$R) on relative heart rate (percentage of maximum heart rate), regardless of the subject's age, gender, medications, or clinical status (4). However, this method underestimates the percentage of $\dot{V}O_2$R by 10% to 15%, especially during light to moderate exercise intensities (8).

The rating of perceived exertion also provides a useful and important adjunct to heart rate as an intensity guide for cardiac exercise training (9). Exercise rated as 11 to 13 (6 to 20 scale), between "fairly light" and "somewhat hard," generally corresponds to the upper limit of prescribed training heart rates during the early stages of outpatient cardiac rehabilitation (e.g., phase II). For higher levels of training (phases III or IV), ratings of 12 to 14 may be appropriate, which is equivalent to approximately 60% to 80% $\dot{V}O_2$R. Although perceived exertion correlates well with exercise intensity, even in patients taking beta-blockers (10), ischemic ST segment depression and serious ventricular arrhythmias (e.g., recurring couplets, salvos, or paroxysms of sustained ventricular tachycardia) can occur at low ratings of perceived effort (11).

Determining Exercise Intensity Without a Preliminary Exercise Test

In some instances it may not be feasible to conduct a symptom-limited exercise test prior to starting a cardiac rehabilitation program. The patient's health insurance may not fully cover a stress test, especially if one has been recently performed. Symptom-limited exercise testing may be contraindicated immediately after hospital discharge, yet the referring physician may request an accelerated rehabilitation regimen. Other patient subsets that may be inappropriate for exercise testing include those with extreme debilitation or orthopedic

limitations, or those with left ventricular dysfunction who are limited by shortness of breath (12). In such patients, a period of continuous ECG telemetry monitoring is highly recommended. The THR can be initially set at 20 beats/min above rest, and gradually increased to a perceived exertion of "somewhat hard" in the absence of symptoms, abnormal hemodynamics, threatening ventricular arrhythmias, or ECG changes signifying myocardial ischemia. If telemetry monitoring suggests new-onset ischemic ST segment depression, this should be confirmed with 12-lead electrocardiography during a simulated exercise session.

Pharmacologic stress tests are commonly used in patients whose inability to exercise may compromise the predictive accuracy of the exercise test, including those with neurologic, vascular, or orthopedic impairment of the lower extremities. These tests may include dipyridamole or adenosine studies with concomitant myocardial perfusion imaging or dobutamine echocardiography. Although these tests are associated with an increased sensitivity and specificity (>85%), they do not provide an assessment of functional capacity, hemodynamic responses to progressive work, or an ischemic ECG threshold.

A dobutamine stress test may, in some instances, increase the cardiac demands to equal to or greater than 85% of the age-predicted maximal heart rate. If the echocardiogram or myocardial perfusion imaging results are negative for ischemia, the highest heart rate obtained can be used as a guide to determine the initial THR. On the other hand, an abnormal test may not necessarily define the ischemic ECG threshold, and other complementary methods (e.g., symptoms, perceived exertion, ECG telemetry) should be used in conjunction with conservative heart rate guidelines to determine the exercise intensity.

Recently, investigators compared the rehabilitation outcomes in 229 post–myocardial infarction and coronary artery

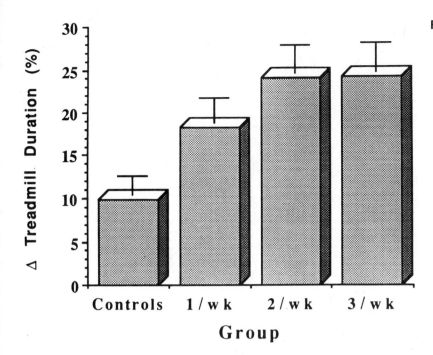

Figure 68-2 Percentage increases (mean ± SE) in treadmill duration in response to varied frequencies of training. The 2-exercise session per week group showed identical improvement to the 3 session per week group, that is, 24%.

bypass patients who had undergone preliminary symptom-limited exercise testing with 271 matched patients who did not (13). All subjects underwent a 12-week exercise-based cardiac rehabilitation program, including ECG-telemetry monitoring for the first 3 to 6 weeks. The group with no preliminary exercise test started at a training intensity of 2 to 3 METs and progressed using heart rate and perceived exertion. Both groups showed similar physiologic improvements and there were no cardiovascular complications in either group.

Influence of Beta-blockers on Prescribed Heart Rates For Training

Experience in our cardiac rehabilitation program revealed a discordance between prescribed and achieved exercise training heart rates among coronary patients receiving a single morning dose of atenolol, a long-acting cardioselective beta-blocker. We hypothesized that the ECG and hemodynamic responses to morning exercise might be modulated by therapy more than those evoked in the late afternoon or early evening. Accordingly, we studied the diurnal variation in heart rate, blood pressure, symptoms, and ischemic ECG responses to morning and late afternoon exercise testing and training (i.e., via Holter monitoring) in 18 men with CAD who were taking a single morning dose of atenolol (14).

Although mean exercise time for morning versus afternoon testing was not significantly different, 11.2 versus 11.5 minutes, peak exercise heart rates during afternoon exercise testing were uniformly higher (range, 5 to 35 beats/min; $\bar{x} =$ 20 beats/min; $p < .001$), as were the double products 272 versus 208 mm Hg × (beats per minute) × 10^{-2}. There were no ischemic ECGs during morning exercise testing. In contrast, 5 of the 18 patients (28%) demonstrated significant ST segment depression (≥1.0 mm horizontal or downsloping) during afternoon testing; one of these patients had concomitant angina.

Analysis of the hourly summaries and corresponding histograms generated by ambulatory ECG monitoring revealed that two patients demonstrated significant ST segment depression during morning exercise bouts, whereas four patients had ischemic ECGs during exercise training in the afternoon. These findings have implications for exercise safety in light of studies suggesting a causal relationship between silent ischemia and malignant ventricular arrhythmias in patients with clinically stable CAD (15). Thus, prescribed heart rates for training should be based on an exercise test conducted under conditions as similar as possible, with respect to the timing of medications, to those under which the patient will be exercising (16).

FREQUENCY

The amount of improvement in $\dot{V}o_2$max increases as a function of the frequency of training. Increases in aerobic fitness, however, tend to plateau when the frequency of training exceeds 3 days/week, and the incidence of injury increases disproportionately (17). Moreover, recent studies suggest that two exercise sessions are as effective as three per week for cardiorespiratory conditioning in the early weeks of phase II cardiac rehabilitation (18). The training regimens of two and three sessions per week produced similar increases in treadmill time (Figure 68-2) and aerobic capacity, with associated decreases in submaximal heart rate.

DURATION

The duration of exercise required to elicit a significant training effect varies inversely with the intensity; the greater the intensity, the shorter is the duration of exercise necessary to achieve favorable adaptation and improvement in cardiorespiratory fitness. Exercise sessions lasting only 10 to 15 minutes

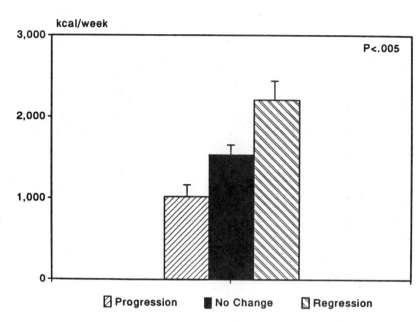

Figure 68-3 Effects of leisure time physical activity on coronary morphology in intervention and control groups combined. The lowest activity level was noted in patients with progression of coronary artery disease (1022 ± 142 kcal/week) compared with patients with no change (1533 ± 122 kcal/week) or regression (2204 ± 237 kcal/week) (*p* < .005). (Adapted from Hambrecht R, Nieubauer J, Marburger C, et al. Various intensities of leisure time physical activity in patients with coronary artery disease: effects on cardiorespiratory fitness and progression of coronary atherosclerotic lesions. J Am Coll Cardiol 1993;22:468–477.)

may improve aerobic fitness, and 30- to 45-minute sessions are even more effective (19). Moreover, recent studies suggest that longer exercise sessions can be *accumulated* in shorter periods of activity (i.e., three 10- or 15-minute exercise bouts), yielding similar physiologic improvements provided that the total volume of training (kilocalorie expenditure) is comparable (20–23). For some patients, this exercise regimen may fit better into a busy schedule than a single long bout.

EXERCISE DOSAGE FOR HALTING AND REVERSING HEART DISEASE?

Physical conditioning does not necessarily halt the progression of CAD or, for that matter, prevent restenosis or reinfarction (24). Conventional exercise training does little to improve left ventricular ejection fraction, regional wall motion abnormalities, resting hemodynamics, and collateral circulation. Studies describing changes in ventricular arrhythmias following exercise rehabilitation have also produced inconsistent results (25). However, intensive multifactorial interventions (including exercise) can result in regression or limitation of progression of angiographically documented coronary atherosclerosis (26–28).

To determine the amount of physical activity (in kilocalories per week) required to retard the progression of coronary atherosclerotic lesions, Hambrecht et al (28) studied the effects of exercise training and a low-fat diet (fat <20% of energy, cholesterol <200 mg/day, polyunsaturated-to-saturated fatty acids ratio >1), without concomitant lipid lowering agents, on coronary morphology in patients with baseline coronary angiography and stable angina pectoris. An exercise-diet intervention group (n = 29) was compared with a control group (n = 33) receiving usual care. After 12 months, repeat angiography showed regression of CAD or no change in coronary morphology in 26 intervention patients (90%) compared with 18 patients (55%) in the control group. Higher levels of leisure time physical activity were associated with

either no change or reversal of coronary atherosclerotic lesions (Figure 68-3). These findings suggest that a minimum of 1600 kcal/week of physical activity may halt the progression of CAD, whereas regression may be achieved with an energy expenditure of 2200 kcal/week. For many patients, these goals would require walking 24 and 32 km (15 and 20 miles) per week, respectively.

In summary, a recent consensus statement on preventing heart attack and death in patients with coronary disease extolled the importance of a minimum of 30 to 60 minutes of moderate-intensity activity 3 or 4 times weekly supplemented by an increase in daily lifestyle activities (e.g., walking breaks at work, using stairs, gardening, household work); 5 to 6 hours a week was suggested for maximum cardioprotective benefits (29). Increasing physical activity in daily living can be helpful in this regard (Figure 68-4).

UPPER BODY TRAINING

The cardiovascular adaptations to exercise training appear to be largely specific to the muscle groups that have been trained (Figure 68-5) (30). Similar muscle-specific adaptations have been shown for blood lactate (31) and pulmonary ventilation (32). The lack of interchangeability of training benefits from the legs to the arms, and vice versa, appears to discredit the general practice of prescribing exercise for the legs alone. Consequently, cardiac patients who rely on their upper extremities for occupational and leisure-time activities should be advised to train the arms as well as the legs, with the expectation of improved cardiorespiratory and hemodynamic responses to both forms of effort.

Although upper extremity exercise training for cardiac patients has been traditionally proscribed, at a given heart rate, arm exercise elicits no greater incidence of arrhythmias, ischemic ST segment depression, or angina pectoris than does leg exercise (33). Moreover, recent studies suggest that the arms respond to aerobic exercise conditioning in the same

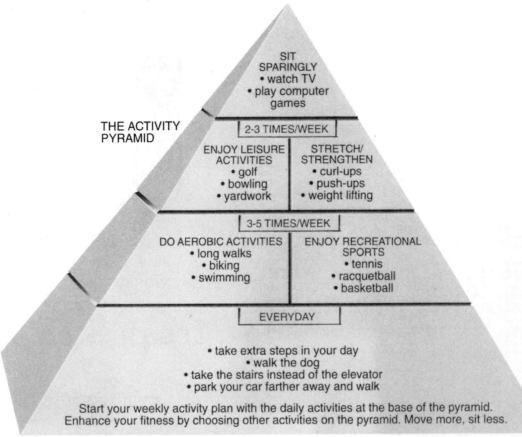

THE ACTIVITY PYRAMID

SIT SPARINGLY
• watch TV
• play computer games

2-3 TIMES/WEEK

ENJOY LEISURE ACTIVITIES
• golf
• bowling
• yardwork

STRETCH/ STRENGTHEN
• curl-ups
• push-ups
• weight lifting

3-5 TIMES/WEEK

DO AEROBIC ACTIVITIES
• long walks
• biking
• swimming

ENJOY RECREATIONAL SPORTS
• tennis
• racquetball
• basketball

EVERYDAY

• take extra steps in your day
• walk the dog
• take the stairs instead of the elevator
• park your car farther away and walk

Start your weekly activity plan with the daily activities at the base of the pyramid. Enhance your fitness by choosing other activities on the pyramid. Move more, sit less.

Figure 68-4 The Activity Pyramid, analogous to the USDA's Food Guide Pyramid, has been suggested as a model to facilitate public and patient education for the adoption of a progressively more active lifestyle. (Copyright © 1996, Park Nicollet Health Source® Institute for Research and Education. Reprinted by permission.)

qualitative and quantitative manner as the legs, showing comparable relative decreases in submaximal rate-pressure product and increases in peak power output and aerobic fitness (Figure 68-6) for both sets of limbs when the same frequency, intensity, and duration are used for the upper and lower extremities (34).

Arm Exercise Prescription

Guidelines for arm exercise prescription (Table 68-1) should include recommendations regarding three variables (35): the appropriate exercise heart rate; the work rate or power output (e.g., in kilogram meters per minute) that will elicit a sufficient metabolic load for training (36); and the proper training equipment or modalities.

RESISTANCE TRAINING

Traditionally, rehabilitation programs have emphasized dynamic aerobic exercise to physically condition individuals with cardiovascular disease. However, complementary resistance training has now been shown to increase muscular strength and endurance, facilitate activities of daily living, expedite return-to-work rates, and partially offset the adverse

psychological effects of coronary disease. Because many occupational and recreational activities involve lifting, pushing, or pulling movements of the upper extremities, increases in muscular strength and endurance should be highly beneficial. Moreover, increasing evidence now suggests that resistance training has favorable effects on health and fitness variables (37). This section reviews the role of resistance training in cardiac rehabilitation, with specific reference to its physiologic basis and rationale, implementation, safety, and efficacy. Participation criteria and prescriptive guidelines are also provided.

Rationale for Resistance Training

Considerable data seem to support resistance exercise as an adjunct to conventional aerobic training in cardiac rehabilitation. Resistance training is highly effective in developing and maintaining muscular strength and endurance, muscle mass, and physical function. It is of value in the treatment of low back pain, osteoporosis, diabetes, obesity, and orthopedic injuries (37), and may be helpful in reducing the susceptibility to falls in elderly patients (38). Regular progressive resistance exercise training may also have a favorable effect on resting blood pressure (in mildly hypertensive patients) (39) and lipid and lipoprotein levels (40).

Figure 68-5 *A.* Arm training using a cycle ergometer markedly decreased the heart rate response during arm exercise at low and high workloads, whereas the heart rate reduction during leg work was small. *B.* Similarly, leg training markedly decreased the heart rate during leg work, whereas the heart rate reduction during arm work was minimal. (Adapted from Clausen JP, Trap-Jensen J, Lassen NA. The effects of training on the heart rate during arm and leg exercise. Scan J Clin Lab Invest 1970;26:295–301.)

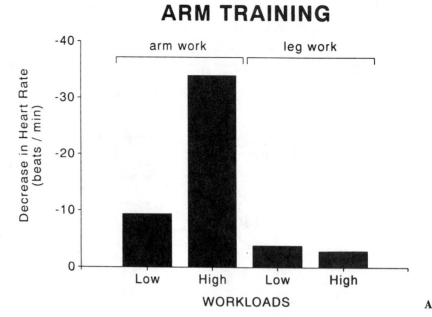

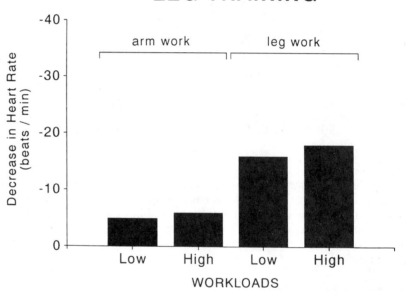

Although previous studies have suggested that resistance training programs offer little or no benefit to cardiovascular function, these studies generally evaluated the conditioning response with treadmill or cycle ergometer testing using $\dot{V}o_2$max as the criterion measure. When comparing cardiovascular responses to a standardized lifting (41) or isometric test (42) before and after strength training, decreases in heart rate and blood pressure have been reported. There are also intriguing data to suggest that resistance training can increase muscular endurance with modest or no improvement in aerobic capacity (43). Thus, it appears that resistance training can decrease cardiac demands during daily activities like carrying groceries or lifting moderate to heavy objects, while simultaneously increasing the capacity to sustain these endeavors.

Eligibility and Exclusion Criteria
The clinician should consider previously published risk stratification criteria when recommending a resistance training program for patients with coronary disease (25). Many low- to moderate-risk patients should be encouraged to incorporate resistance training in their physical conditioning program, especially those who rely on their upper extremities for work or recreational pursuits. On the other hand, the safety of strength training in high-risk patients has not been well studied.

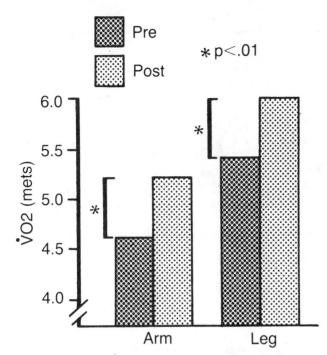

Pre
Post
*p<.01

Figure 68-6 Mean V̇o₂max values, expressed as METs, during arm and leg exercise testing before and after upper and lower extremity training in men with previous myocardial infarction. (Adapted from Franklin BA, Vander L, Wrisley D, et al. Trainability of arms versus legs in men with previous myocardial infarction. Chest 1994;105:262–264.)

Table 68-1 Guidelines for Arm Exercise Prescription	
VARIABLE	**COMMENT**
Target Heart Rate	~10–15 beats per minute lower than for leg training
Work Rate	~50% of the power output (kgm/min) used for leg training
Equipment	Arm ergometer, combined arm-leg ergometer, rowing machine, wall pulleys, simulated cross-country skiing devices

Exclusion criteria for resistance training are similar to or slightly more cautious than those used for any outpatient cardiac exercise program (i.e., phase III to IV) (44). Patients are generally excluded from participation for any of the following reasons: left ventricular dysfunction (ejection fraction <30%); evidence of myocardial ischemia during exercise testing, manifested as significant ST segment depression (>0.1 mV), angina pectoris, or reversible defects on myocardial perfusion imaging (i.e., thallium or Cardiolite); uncontrolled hypertension (systolic blood pressure >160 mm Hg or diastolic blood pressure >100 mm Hg); acute congestive heart failure; threatening ventricular arrhythmias; aortic stenosis (severe or symptomatic); or a functional capacity less than 5 METs. It should be emphasized that these include both absolute and relative contraindications, and that a patient's participation in resistance training should be contingent upon approval of the medical director and/or his or her personal physician. For example, deconditioned patients at low risk may safely participate in resistance training if modest weight loads are employed.

Certain patient subsets may derive added benefits from resistance training and should be strongly encouraged to participate. Older patients often demonstrate dramatic improvements in muscular strength and endurance, gait speed (45), and bone mineral density, thus reducing the potential for debilitating osteoporosis and falls. Similarly, cardiac transplant recipients who participate in resistance training may offset

the deleterious effects of prednisone therapy on lean body mass (46). Women may also experience remarkable improvements in physical function following a resistance training program. Indeed, the Framingham study recently revealed that half of all women over 65 years of age were unable to lift a 10-pound plate!

Time Course to Resistance Training

It has been suggested that cardiac patients who wish to initiate resistance training should have participated in a traditional aerobic exercise program for at least 3 months (47). This time period permits sufficient observation of the patient in a supervised setting and allows for the cardiorespiratory and musculoskeletal adaptations needed to progress to more intense exercise. Nevertheless, recent studies have shown that for selected patients, mild to moderate resistance training can be safely implemented even sooner, with beneficial results (48). Current national guidelines recommend that post–myocardial infarction and coronary artery bypass patients undergo 3 to 6 weeks of supervised aerobic exercise before initiating resistance training (49,50). Those patients undergoing percutaneous transluminal coronary angioplasty need wait only 1 to 2 weeks postintervention.

Prescriptive Guidelines

Low-level resistance exercise using light dumbbells (e.g., 1 to 3- or 5-pound weights), hand-wrist weights, mild calisthenics, or low-tension elastic bands may be used in phase I and II exercise programs in patients who are clinically stable. These activities should be performed throughout the entire range of motion, and patients should be cautioned to avoid the Valsalva maneuver. For phases III and IV, resistance training may be performed using weight machines. These provide a wider variety of exercises and reduce the isometric component often associated with free weights. Weight machines also allow the patient to easily titrate training loads, eliminating the need for a "spotter."

Numerous studies have reported on the efficacy of resistance training in patients with coronary disease (51–54). In these studies, circuit weight training was added to the physical conditioning regimens of cardiac patients who were already involved in regular aerobic exercise, generally for 3 months or more. Three 30- to 60-minute exercise sessions were offered

Figure 68-7 Classification of resistance training intensity. Using weight loads that permit 8 to 15 repetitions will generally facilitate improvements in muscular strength and endurance, regardless of age or health status.

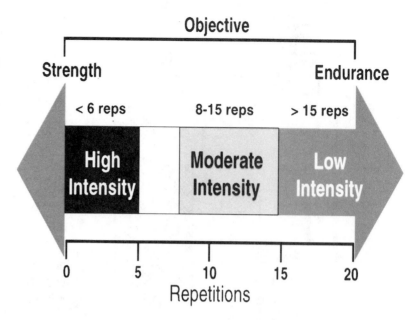

each week, and the duration of the training programs ranged from 10 to 156 weeks. Although intensity prescriptions ranged from 30% to 40% (51) to 80% of the one-repetition maximum (1 RM) (53), both regimens yielded similar relative improvements in strength (~25%). These findings suggest that heavy resistance training, which may disproportionately increase cardiac demands, offers little additional benefit in strength to this population (25).

Although the traditional strength training prescription has involved performing each exercise three times (e.g., three sets of 10 to 15 repetitions per set), recent studies suggest that one set provides similar improvements in muscular strength and endurance (55). Consequently, for the average patient beginning a strength training regimen, single-set programs performed a minimum of two times per week are recommended over multiple-set programs because they are highly effective and less time-consuming. Such regimens should include 8 to 10 different exercises at a load that permits 10 to 15 repetitions per set (Figure 68-7) (55). Heart rates should not exceed those prescribed for aerobic exercise training, and perceived exertion should range from 11 to 14 ("fairly light" to "somewhat hard") on the Borg category scale.

Safety of Resistance Training

Recently, application of resistance testing or training in the rehabilitation of patients with coronary disease was reviewed from 12 different studies that involved 242 patients (25). In most of these studies, circuit weight training was added to the physical conditioning regimens of coronary patients who had already participated in endurance exercise training, generally for 3 months or more. The frequency, intensity, and duration of these resistance training programs varied from three 30- to 60-minute sessions per week at 25% to 80% of 1 RM for 6 to 26 weeks. All studies reported significant improvements in weight carrying tolerance (time) or increases in muscular strength. The absence of signs or symptoms of myocardial ischemia, abnormal hemodynamic responses, and untoward

events in these studies, with one possible exception of an uncomplicated myocardial infarction that occurred 1.5 hours after resistance training and a vigorous game of basketball (53), respectively, suggests that strength training is safe for aerobically trained patients who are clinically stable.

EVALUATING THE RESPONSE TO TRAINING

We have employed both maximal and submaximal exercise testing to assess serial changes in cardiovascular fitness. However, in the era of managed health care, the latter may be preferred as it provides a simple and cost-effective alternative to assess the training response. Submaximal testing is easy to administer and requires no physician supervision. The baseline exercise test protocol is followed, facilitating a comparison of the heart rate, blood pressure, and rating of perceived exertion at standard submaximal workloads. The endpoint of the test is that work load at which the upper limit of the prescribed THR has been achieved. Aerobic capacity can be estimated by plotting the submaximal or minitest heart rate versus work load relationship; the latter is expressed in METs, extrapolated to the maximum heart rate attained on initial exercise testing (Figure 68-8).

Failure to Respond to Training

Determinants of the magnitude of the conditioning response may include the patient's clinical status and underlying CAD, response to graded exercise testing, medications, exercise prescription, time from the acute cardiac event, and compliance with the exercise prescription. Arvan (56) reported that post–myocardial infarction patients who have both significant left ventricular dysfunction and myocardial ischemia were unlikely to demonstrate an adequate training response, at least within the first 12 weeks of rehabilitation. Moreover, patients who have poor rehabilitation potential often show reduced inotropic and/or chronotropic reserves, limiting angina pec-

Workloads	Mini-Test			Initial Test (Pre-conditioning)		
	Heart Rate	Blood Pressure	RPE	Heart Rate	Blood Pressure	RPE
Rest	64	106/74		59	120/78	
2.0 mph 0% grade	68	122/70	6	94	130/78	11
3.0 mph 0% grade	76	132/74	7	113	158/78	14
3.0 mph 2.5% grade	80	136/80	9	120	170/78	15-16
3.0 mph 5.0% grade	86	142/78	9-10	125	182/78	17
3.0 mph 7.5% grade	98	146/82	12			
3.0 mph 10% grade	106	148/80	13-14			

Estimated Peak Mets After Phase II Exercise Program – From mini test results

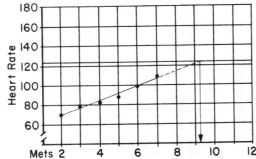

Maximum METS before exercise program

5

Maximum METS after exercise program

9 - 10

Figure 68-8 Comparison of heart rate, blood pressure, and rating of perceived exertion (RPE) to identical submaximal workloads during "mini-testing" versus initial (baseline) exercise testing. Extrapolation of the "mini-test" heart rate–workload relationship permits estimation of the aerobic capacity, expressed in METs.

toris, threatening ventricular arrhythmias, or marked ST segment depression during or after exercise (57). Despite demonstration of a significant correlation ($r = -.68$) between aerobic capacity and infarct size, the latter has proved to be a poor predictor of the subject's ability to increase aerobic power with physical conditioning (58).

The severity or progression of underlying CAD may also represent a major obstacle to improvement. Approximately 15% of myocardial infarction patients show minimal or no cardiovascular improvement, despite faithful attendance and sustained participation (5 years) in an exercise-based rehabilitation program (59). Coronary arteriograms in these patients typically revealed diffuse disease with 90% or more stenosis of two arteries. In such patients, the preferred therapy may include coronary revascularization, more aggressive medical management (e.g., drug therapy), or both, prior to initiation of a cardiac exercise training program.

A suboptimal training response may also be due to intercurrent illness or injury (e.g., concomitant disease, surgery, orthopedic complications), inadequate adherence to the exercise prescription, exercising below the thresholds necessary for favorable adaptation and improvement, failure of supervision, or poor motivation. Although it has been suggested that patients taking beta-blockers have impaired exer-cise trainability (60), numerous reports have shown that appropriately selected patients may derive considerable physiologic benefit from an exercise training program in the presence of long-term beta-blockade therapy, despite therapeutic dosages and a reduced training heart rate (61–63). Moreover, there is also no physiologic or metabolic basis to suggest a blunted training response in patients taking calcium channel blockers (64).

AEROBIC AND MYOCARDIAL DEMANDS OF COMMON LEISURE TIME ACTIVITIES

Because snow shoveling and lawn mowing are common activities for home owners, patients often seek medical advice on their ability to undertake these tasks after recovery from an acute myocardial infarction, coronary revascularization surgery, or percutaneous transluminal coronary angioplasty. A concern in recommending moderate to vigorous physical activity for patients with cardiovascular disease is the precipitation of cardiovascular complications. Untoward events have been reported in both the medical literature and lay press after snow shoveling (65) and lawn mowing (66). Until recently, few controlled investigations have addressed the

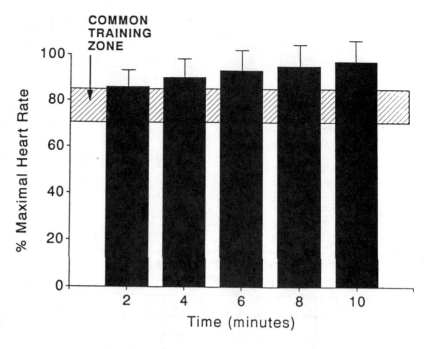

Figure 68-9 Percentage of maximal heart rate (mean ± SD) attained with self-paced, lift-throw shoveling over time (10-minute work bout) in healthy untrained men. The common training zone represents the relative heart rate range (70% to 85% of maximal heart rate) generally prescribed for aerobic exercise training.

aerobic and myocardial demands of these activities in persons with and without heart disease.

Snow Shoveling

Recent studies suggest that shoveling light snow is safe and approximates the work intensity commonly prescribed for aerobic exercise training (70% to 85% of maximal heart rate) (67). However, excess cardiac deaths have been primarily associated with "heavy snowfalls" (68). To assess the physiologic responses to manual snow shoveling in the cold (2°C), we studied 10 healthy untrained men ($\bar{x} \pm SD$ age = 32.4 ± 2.1 years) who were asked to clear a 10-cm high tract of heavy, wet snow using a lightweight plastic shovel (1.4 kg) on concrete pavement (69). The men were instructed to repetitively lift and throw snow at a rate at which they removed snow at home, which averaged 12 ± 2 loads per minute at approximately 7.3 kg per load (including the weight of the shovel).

The highest observed values for heart rate, oxygen consumption, systolic blood pressure, and perceived exertion (6 to 20 scale) during snow shoveling and treadmill testing were compared. Oxygen consumption during snow shoveling (5.7 METs) was 39% lower than the energy expenditure of these subjects during maximal treadmill testing (9.3 METs). During snow shoveling, the peak heart rate, blood pressure, and perceived exertion of our subjects increased to extremely high levels, averaging 175 beats/min, 198 mm Hg, and 16.7 ("very hard" effort), respectively. These values were comparable to or higher than the maximum values achieved by the same subjects during maximal treadmill testing. After only 2 minutes of shoveling, the heart rates of most of our subjects exceeded the upper limit commonly prescribed for aerobic exercise training, that is, 85% of the maximal heart rate attained during treadmill testing. Moreover, the subjects' heart rates continued to increase throughout the 10-minute bout of work, failing to plateau (Figure 68-9) (70). During this period, the average subject lifted and threw nearly a ton of snow (12 lifts/min ×

7.3 kg/lift × 10 minutes = 876 kg or 1927 lb), which is equivalent to the weight of a mid-size automobile! It was concluded that heavy snow shoveling elicits myocardial demands that rival maximal treadmill testing in sedentary men. These responses may contribute to the plethora of cardiovascular complications commonly reported in middle-aged and elderly persons after heavy snowfalls.

Lawn Mowing

The notion that lawn mowing can trigger cardiac arrest or acute myocardial infarction, particularly among habitually sedentary persons with heart disease, has been substantiated by several recent reports (66,71,72). To clarify the cardiorespiratory requirements of manual (hand-push-operated) versus automated (self-propelled) grass cutting, we studied 10 low-risk men with heart disease ($\bar{x} \pm SD$ age = 60.5 ± 7.1 years) who cut two 4 ± 1-cm-high, 25-m-long tracts of grass, using manual and automated methods, in random order, with 15-minute rest periods between each 10-minute bout of work (73). Heart rate, oxygen consumption, blood pressure, and perceived exertion were measured and compared with values obtained during maximal exercise testing.

The highest observed heart rate values for each subject during manual and automated grass cutting ranged from 71% to 109% and 51% to 86%, respectively, of the peak heart rate achieved during treadmill exercise testing. Oxygen uptake during manual and self-propelled mowing averaged 20.3 and 15.4 mL/kg/min, corresponding to 5.8 and 4.4 METs, respectively. Blood pressure and rating of perceived exertion were also reduced during automated grass cutting. It was concluded that manual lawn mowers may evoke heart rate and systolic blood pressure responses that approach and exceed those attained during maximal exercise testing. The excessive cardiac demands may be deceptively camouflaged by the moderate aerobic requirements and perceived effort ("fairly light" exertion).

Table 68-2 Summary of Contemporary Exercise-Based Cardiac Rehabilitation Complication Rates

Investigator	Year	Patient Exercise Hours	Cardiac Arrest	Myocardial Infarction	Fatal Events	Major Complications*
Van Camp et al (77)	1980–1984	2,351,916	1:111,996[a]	1:293,990	1:783,972	1:81,101
Digenio et al (78)	1982–1988	480,000	1:120,000[b]		1:160,000	1:120,000
Vongvanich et al (79)	1986–1995	268,503	1:89,501[c]	1:268,503[c]	0:268,503	1:67,126
Franklin et al (80)	1982–1998	292,254	1:146,127[c]	1:97,418[c]	0:292,254	1:58,451

* MI and cardiac arrest; [a] fatal 14%; [b] fatal 75%; [c] fatal 0%.

RISK OF EXERCISE TRAINING

Cardiovascular events during exercise training are more likely to occur among cardiac patients than among presumably healthy adults. For patients with CAD, the relative risk of developing cardiac arrest during vigorous exercise is estimated to be 6 to 164 times greater than at rest or during light activity (74). More recent studies have shown that the risk of acute myocardial infarction after strenuous exercise is two to six times greater than what might be expected to occur spontaneously (75,76).

By increasing myocardial oxygen demands and simultaneously shortening diastole, and thus coronary perfusion time, exercise may evoke a transient oxygen deficiency at the subendocardial level, which can be exacerbated by a decreased venous return secondary to abrupt cessation of activity. Symptomatic or silent myocardial ischemia can alter depolarization, repolarization, and conduction velocity, triggering threatening ventricular arrhythmias that may degenerate into ventricular tachycardia or fibrillation (15). In addition, sodium-potassium imbalance, increased catecholamine excretion, and circulating free fatty acids all may be arrhythmogenic. Thus, special care should be taken for patients who, on their most recent exercise stress test, demonstrated signs and/or symptoms of myocardial ischemia, which may be harbingers of malignant ventricular arrhythmias. Such patients should be restricted to training intensities that are approximately 10 to 15 beats/min below the heart rate heralding the ischemic ECG (≥1.0 mm ST segment displacement) or anginal thresholds during exercise testing (50).

Contemporary estimates of major cardiovascular complications (acute myocardial infarction or cardiac arrest) in exercise-based cardiac rehabilitation programs range from approximately 1:100,000 to 1:300,000 patient exercise hours (Table 68-2) (77–80). Further analysis of the most recent cardiac rehabilitation program survey revealed that 18 of 21 cardiac arrest patients (86%) were successfully resuscitated (77). Thus, exercise rehabilitation has been shown to be relatively safe with nonfatal and fatal events being rare. Nevertheless, a profile of the high-risk patient has emerged (Table 68-3). Although it has been suggested that a variety of pathophysiologic mechanisms for acute cardiac events are more likely to be operative during the early morning hours, two studies (80,81) that compared morning with afternoon exercise have reported no difference in overall cardiovascular complication rates.

Table 68-3 Patient Characteristics Associated with Exercise-Related Cardiovascular Complications

Clinical Status
Multiple myocardial infarctions
Impaired left ventricular function (ejection fraction <25%)
Rest or unstable angina pectoris
Serious dysrhythmias at rest
High-grade left anterior descending lesions and/or significant (≥75% occlusion) multivessel atherosclerosis on angiography
Low serum potassium

Exercise Training Participation
Disregard for appropriate warm-up and cool-down
Consistently exceeds prescribed training heart rate (i.e., intensity violators)

Exercise Test Data
Low or high exercise tolerance (≤4 METs or ≥10 METs)
Chronotropic impairment off drugs (<120 beats/min)
Inotropic impairment (exertional hypotension with increasing workloads)
Myocardial ischemia (angina and/or ST depression ≥0.2 mV)
Malignant cardiac dysrhythmias (especially in patients with impaired left ventricular function)

Other
Cigarette smoker
Male gender

Recommendations to Reduce the Incidence of Cardiovascular Complications

Recommendations to increase surveillance and reduce the incidence of cardiovascular complications during exercise-based cardiac rehabilitation programs include the following:

- *Ensure medical clearance and follow-up, including serial exercise testing.* If possible, patients entering a cardiac rehabilitation program should be evaluated via exercise testing. Thereafter, exercise testing once a year is usually considered adequate (82), although more frequent tests may be

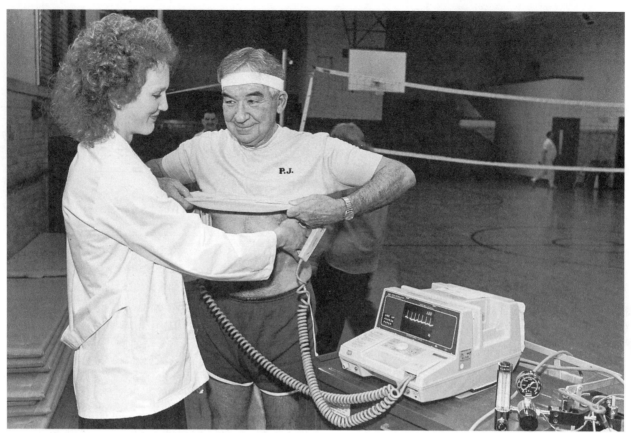

Figure 68-10 Technique of obtaining instantaneous electrocardiographic rhythm strips with defibrillator paddle electrodes during outpatient cardiac exercise programs.

necessary if the patient demonstrates signs or symptoms suggestive of a deterioration in clinical status.

- *Provide on-site medical supervision and establish an emergency plan.* Cardiac rehabilitation programs should be medically supervised and equipped with a defibrillator and appropriate emergency drugs. Our 16-year experience (80) and the results of others (79) suggest that acute cardiac events can be successfully treated by nursing staff, assisted by exercise physiologists/technologists and emergency medical service backup, without direct gymnasium supervision by a physician (i.e., in the exercise room).

- *Promote patient education.* Patients should know their THR for exercise training and how to take their pulse accurately. They should also be strongly encouraged to remain at or below their prescribed intensity and counseled to discontinue exercise and seek medical advice if they experience major warning signs or symptoms (i.e., chest pain, lightheadedness, palpitations) that may suggest a deterioration in their clinical status and/or impending cardiovascular complications. Rehabilitation staff should be alerted as to changes in their medication regimen since an updated THR may be warranted.

- *Advocate a mild to moderate exercise intensity.* Victims of exercise-related sudden cardiac death often have a history of poor compliance with the prescribed training heart rate range (i.e., exercise intensity violators) (83,84).

These and other recent data (85) suggest that unconventionally vigorous exercise is associated with an increased risk of cardiovascular complications in patients with CAD. The lower the intensity, the less likely it is that an exercise-related complication will occur. Fortunately, a reduced exercise intensity may be partially or totally compensated for by adopting more frequent or longer training sessions (1), or both.

- *Use continuous or instantaneous ECG monitoring for selected patients.* The degree of ECG surveillance should be linked inversely with cardiac stability of the patient. As an alternative to costly continuous or transtelephonic ECG monitoring, we have employed instantaneous electrocardiography (recording ECG rate, rhythm, and repolarization through defibrillator paddles; see Figure 68-10) to screen for ST segment displacement, threatening ventricular arrhythmias (Figure 68-11), and exercise intensity violators (86).

- *Emphasize appropriate warm-up and cool-down procedures.* A disproportionate number of cardiovascular complications have been reported during the warm-up and cool-down phases of exercise (87). A gradual warm-up (e.g., brisk walking or mild resistance cycle ergometry) serves to decrease the occurrence of ECG (88) and wall motion abnormalities (89) that are suggestive of myocardial ischemia and/or ventricular irritability—abnormalities

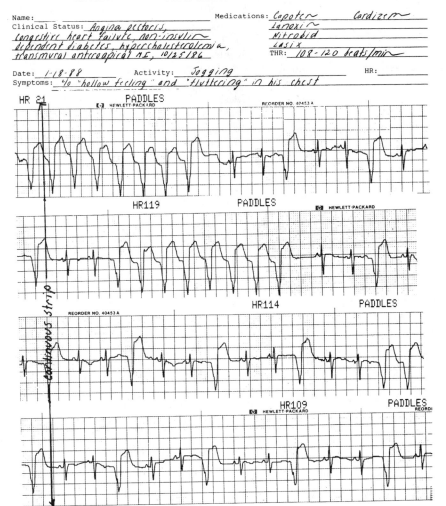

WILLIAM BEAUMONT HOSPITAL
Department of Medicine
Division of Cardiovascular Diseases - Cardiac Rehabilitation

Name: _____
Clinical Status: *Angina pectoris,*
congestive heart failure, non-insulin
dependent diabetes, hypercholesterolemia,
transmural anteroapical MI, 10/25/86

Medications: *Capoten   Cardizem*
Lanoxin
Nitrobid
Lasix
THR: *108-120 beats/min*

Date: *1-18-88*   Activity: *Jogging*   HR: _____
Symptoms: *c/o "hollow feeling" and "fluttering" in his chest*

HR 21   PADDLES
HEWLETT-PACKARD   REORDER NO. 40453 A

HR119   PADDLES
HEWLETT-PACKARD

continuous strip

REORDER NO. 40453 A   HR114   PADDLES

HR109   PADDLES
HEWLETT-PACKARD   REORD

Figure 68-11 Ventricular tachycardia documented by instantaneous electrocardiography in a symptomatic patient during a phase III gymnasium exercise session.

that may be provoked by sudden strenuous exertion. A cool-down enhances venous return during recovery, reducing the possibility of postexercise hypotension and related sequelae. Moreover, it attenuates the potential, deleterious effects of the postexercise rise in plasma catecholamines (90).

- *Modify recreational game rules and minimize competition.* Myocardial and aerobic demands during recreational activities are influenced, to a large extent, by team members and opponent expertise. Also, the excitement of competition may increase sympathetic activity and catecholamine excretion and lower the threshold to malignant ventricular arrhythmias. Exercise leaders should minimize competition and modify game rules to decrease the myocardial and aerobic requirements of recreational activities. For example, conventional volleyball rules may be modified to include one or more bounces of the ball per side.

- *Take precautions in the cold.* Dynamic exercise in cold weather is relatively safe if proper clothing is worn and the wind chill factor is considered. Nevertheless, inhala-

tion of or exposure to cold air may increase stroke volume and cardiac work, activate the thermoregulatory reflex causing cutaneous systemic vasoconstriction to conserve body heat, and trigger reflex spasm or constriction of the coronary arteries (91). The consequent increases in peripheral vascular resistance and arterial pressure coupled with a reduction in coronary blood flow may precipitate symptomatic or silent myocardial ischemia. For those who suffer from angina when inhaling cold air, discomfort can be reduced or alleviated by wearing a face mask to warm the inspired air (92).

- *Consider added cardiac demands in the heat.* Exercise in hot and humid weather may constitute an even greater hazard for the exerciser with coronary disease. Heart rate and myocardial oxygen demands increase disproportionately to keep up with increasing aerobic requirements. Patients who are not acclimated to heat and who are exposed to temperatures higher than 24°C experience added heart rate increases of 1 beat/min/°C while exercising (Figure 68-12) and 2 to 4 beats/min/°C with concomitant increased humidity (93). Specific suggestions for

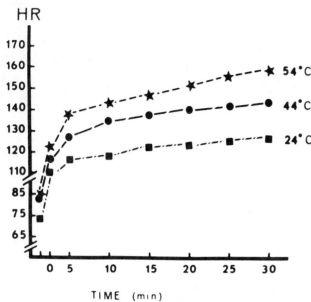

Figure 68-12 Influence of environmental temperature on heart rate responses at a constant exercise workload. Heart rate increases approximately 1 beat/min for each °C increment in ambient temperature above 24°C. (Adapted from Pandolf KB, Cafarelli E, Noble BJ, et al. Hyperthermia: effect on exercise prescription. Arch Phys Med Rehabil 1975;56:524–526.)

exercising in warm weather include: drinking fluids before, during, and after physical activity; decreasing the exercise dosage (e.g., speed, duration, resistance) at temperatures higher than 27°C and/or relative humidity higher than 75%; and wearing light clothing and shorts to facilitate cooling by evaporation.

SPECIAL PATIENT POPULATIONS

The exercise prescription uses objective information derived from a recent stress test such as heart rate, blood pressure, perceived exertion, symptoms, ECG changes, and functional capacity. This approach is adequate for most cardiac patients; however, patients who have specific needs to consider when formulating the exercise prescription include those with permanent pacemakers, implantable cardioverter defibrillators (ICDs) (94), and congestive heart failure (95), and women (96) and the elderly (97).

Permanent Pacemakers

Permanent pacemakers consist of a pulse generator and a lead system. Many newer pacemakers also have a rate-responsive component for patients with chronotropic impairment. There is a standardized code used to define all pacemakers:

- The first letter represents the chamber or chambers with pacing capabilities.
- The second letter represents the chamber or chambers with sensing capabilities.

- The third letter represents the response elicited when intrinsic rhythm is sensed.
- The fourth letter represents rate-responsive properties.

For example, a VVIR pacemaker indicates that *V* (the ventricle can be paced), *V* (the ventricle can be sensed), *I* (inhibition will take place if intrinsic rhythm is sensed), and *R* (rate response to activity is programmed). Another common setting is the DDD system. The *D*s represents dual control for both atria and ventricles. The DDDR pacemaker most closely resembles the heart's electrical system because it provides atrioventricular synchrony.

Exercise prescriptions for pacemaker patients should be based on a recent stress test, with specific reference to the workload achieved, pacemaker response, hemodynamics, perceived exertion, and symptoms (94). In these patients, ST segment changes may be uninterpretable with respect to myocardial ischemia. Alternative stress tests that utilize myocardial perfusion imaging such as Cardiolite or thallium, or exercise echocardiography, may be helpful in this regard. Moreover, the use of target MET levels or upper heart rate limits should be considered for pacemaker-dependent patients because of the nonlinear relationship between oxygen consumption and heart rate.

There is a 6-week period following implantation during which the patient should avoid raising the arm on the affected side above the shoulder. Thereafter, patients may participate in physical activities that are compatible with their functional capacity. Nevertheless, contact sports and vigorous upper body activities should be avoided. Initial ECG telemetry monitoring is recommended to ensure proper functioning of the pacemaker during progressive physical activity.

Implantable Cardioverter Defibrillator

An implantable cardioverter defibrillator (ICD) consists of a cardioverter device and a lead system. The device is usually implanted in the lower left or right quadrant of the abdomen or in the pectoral region; it is programmed to recognize rapid rhythms and respond in a tiered fashion. The first tier is usually an overdrive or burst pacing to terminate threatening arrhythmias. If the rapid rhythm continues, the second tier is usually a small shock, about 5 J. If this is not successful, the next tiers are a series of shocks, about 30 J, until the rhythm terminates. Because the device is programmed to detect arrhythmias using heart rate as the main criteria, it is critical to know the cutoff rate. The upper limit for exercise training should be at least 20 beats/min below this value.

Many patients with ICDs also have concomitant left ventricular dysfunction. These patients should be closely monitored using continuous or instantaneous ECG telemetry, perceived exertion, blood pressure, and astute clinical assessment to titrate a safe and effective exercise dosage (94). All staff members should be familiar with ICDs and comfortable working with this challenging patient subset. A magnet should be readily available to inactivate the device should it malfunction.

Heart Failure

Heart failure is often associated with exercise intolerance secondary to impairment in cardiac output, left ventricular sys-

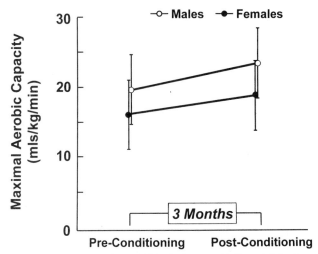

Figure 68-13 Aerobic capacity before and after physical conditioning in older (≥62 years) men and women with coronary heart disease. Maximal oxygen consumption (mL/kg/min) increased by 19% and 17% in the men and women, respectively (both *p* < .001). (Adapted from Ades PA, Waldman ML, Polk DM, et al. Referral patterns and exercise response in the rehabilitation of female coronary patients aged ≥62 years. Am J Cardiol 1992;69: 1422–1425.)

tolic dysfunction, reduced muscle endurance, abnormal pulmonary function, or combinations thereof. Traditionally, heart failure was treated with bed rest and restricted physical activity. Although this treatment is still appropriate for acute or unstable conditions, exercise can be safe and beneficial for those with chronic heart failure. Physical conditioning in patients with heart failure and moderate to severe left ventricular dysfunction results in improved functional capacity and reduced symptoms (98–102). Peripheral (skeletal muscle) adaptations are largely responsible for the increase in exercise tolerance (103).

Careful consideration is necessary when developing an exercise prescription for patients with heart failure. Those with an ejection fraction less than 30% should be carefully monitored for signs and symptoms of myocardial ischemia and worrisome ventricular arrhythmias. An electrolyte imbalance should be corrected prior to initiating an exercise training program. Moreover, supervisory staff should be vigilant for signs and/or symptoms suggesting a deterioration in clinical status: increasing fatigue, unusual shortness of breath, edema, sudden weight gain, and cyanosis.

The exercise intensity should be based on a symptom-limited treadmill or cycle ergometer evaluation, using a target heart rate range corresponding to approximately 50% to 75% $\dot{V}o_2max$ (100). Warm-up and cool-down periods should be lengthened to a minimum of 10 to 15 minutes each, and patients should be advised to avoid isometric exertion and extremes in temperature and/or humidity. Walking, stationary cycling and other aerobic activities, including arm exercise training (101), are recommended; however, modest initial workloads should be gradually increased over time. Ratings of

perceived exertion and dyspnea may be preferentially used over more conventional methods of exercise intensity regulation (e.g., heart rate or workload targets). Exercise sessions should initially be brief (e.g., 10 to 15 minutes), increasing as patients' tolerance improves.

Women

The effects of exercise rehabilitation in women with CAD have not been as well studied as those in men. Only 3% of the 4500 patients evaluated in a meta-analysis of randomized trials of cardiac rehabilitation after myocardial infarction were women (104). Nevertheless, recent studies suggest that women with and without CAD respond to aerobic training in much the same way as men when subjected to comparable programs in terms of frequency, intensity, and duration of exercise (Figure 68-13) (105,106).

As women become increasingly involved in comprehensive cardiac rehabilitation programs, consideration of gender-specific variables must be realized and incorporated into their therapeutic regimens. Relevant concerns include their older age upon program entry, decreased muscle mass and bone mineral density, menopausal or postmenopausal symptoms, hormone replacement therapy, the potential for increased musculoskeletal complications, and stress urinary incontinence (107). The challenge is to enroll increasing numbers of women, at an earlier stage of their disease, in home-based or group cardiac rehabilitation programs that are designed to circumvent or attenuate common barriers to participation and adherence (e.g., lack of transportation), so that many more women may realize the benefits that secondary prevention can provide.

Elderly Patients

Older coronary patients show similar improvements to younger patients participating in exercise-based rehabilitation programs (108). Elderly women and men also demonstrate comparable exercise trainability (109). However, referral to and participation in exercise rehabilitation is less frequent in older adults, especially women (105).

A major goal for the elderly population is to maintain functional independence. An exercise program that enhances aerobic fitness, flexibility, and muscular strength and endurance is an effective way to accomplish this goal. To reduce the potential for musculoskeletal injury, warm-up should be extended to 10 to 15 minutes and include stretching, calisthenics, and low-level activities. The aerobic phase of the exercise should *accumulate* 30 minutes or more of endurance activities on most and preferably all days of the week (110). Walking, swimming, cycling, rowing, and dancing are often employed in programs for older adults. Training zones can be prescribed using heart rate and perceived exertion at metabolic loads corresponding to 50% to 80% $\dot{V}o_2max$. Heart rate monitors are recommended for patients who have difficulty palpating their pulse. It is generally suggested that older persons begin at mild to moderate workloads for a longer duration, increasing the intensity as favorable adaptation and improvement occurs. Adjunctive resistance training should also be used to enhance muscular strength and endurance, which may reduce the potential for falls (38).

SUMMARY

The prescription of medications and exercise should, in many ways, be managed similarly. Both have a dose-response relationship with therapeutic levels, a potential for overdose, indications and contraindications, side effects, and special precautions. The salutary effects of each are relatively short-lived, and both types of therapy are associated with poor long-term compliance.

To simply tell a cardiac patient to "get more exercise" is analogous to saying "take more medicine" without providing specific instructions. For optimal outcomes, the exercise prescription should be individualized and periodically adjusted so that the overload principle is continually evoked. If exercise guidelines were approached with the same precision and respect as when any pharmacologic agent is prescribed, fewer complications and greater benefits would undoubtedly occur.

REFERENCES

1. Franklin BA, Gordon S, Timmis GC. Amount of exercise necessary for the patient with coronary artery disease. Am J Cardiol 1992;69:1426–1432.

2. Wilmore JH. Exercise prescription: role of the physiatrist and allied health professional. Arch Phys Med Rehabil 1976;57:315–319.

3. Karvonen M, Kentala K, Mustala O. The effects of training on heart rate: a longitudinal study. Ann Med Exp Biol Fenniae 1957;35:307–315.

4. American Heart Association. Exercise testing and training of individuals with heart disease or at high risk for its development: a handbook for physicians. Dallas: American Heart Association, 1975.

5. Swain DP, Abernathy KS, Smith CS, et al. Target heart rates for the development of cardiorespiratory fitness. Med Sci Sports Exerc 1994;26:112–116.

6. Swain DP, Leutholtz BC. Heart rate reserve is equivalent to $\dot{V}O_2$ reserve, not to % $\dot{V}O_2$ max. Med Sci Sports Exerc 1997;29:837–843.

7. Davis JA, Convertino VA. A comparison of heart rate methods for predicting endurance training intensity. Med Sci Sports Exerc 1975;7:295–298.

8. Pollock ML, Gaesser GA, Butcher JD, et al. The recommended quantity and quality of exercise for developing and maintaining cardiorespiratory and muscular fitness, and flexibility in healthy adults. Med Sci Sports Exerc 1998;30:975–991.

9. Borg GAV. Psychophysical bases of perceived exertion. Med Sci Sports Exerc 1982;14:377–381.

10. Pollock ML, Lowenthal DT, Foster C, et al. Acute and chronic responses to exercise in patients treated with beta-blockers. J Cardiopulm Rehabil 1991;11:132–144.

11. Williams MA, Fardy PS. Limitations in prescribing exercise. J Cardiovasc Pulm Techn 1980;8:36–38.

12. McConnell TR. Exercise prescription: when the guidelines do not work. J Cardiopulm Rehabil 1996;16:34–37.

13. McConnell TR, Klinger TA, Gardner JK, et al. Cardiac rehabilitation without exercise tests for post-myocardial infarction and post-bypass surgery patients. J Cardiopulm Rehabil 1998;18:458–463.

14. Franklin BA, Gordon S, Timmis GC. Diurnal variation of ischemic response to exercise in patients receiving a once-daily dose of beta-blockers. Chest 1996;109:253–257.

15. Hoberg E, Schuler G, Kunze B, et al. Silent myocardial ischemia as a potential link between lack of premonitoring symptoms and increased risk of cardiac arrest during physical stress. Am J Cardiol 1990;65:583–589.

16. Wilmore JH, Freund BJ, Joyner MJ, et al. Acute response to submaximal and maximal exercise consequent to beta-adrenergic blockade: implications for the prescription of exercise. Am J Cardiol 1985;55:135D–141D.

17. Pollock ML, Gettman LR, Milesis CA, et al. Effects of frequency and duration of training on attrition and incidence of injury. Med Sci Sports Exerc 1977;9:31–36.

18. Dressendorfer RH, Franklin BA, Cameron JL, et al. Exercise training frequency in early post-infarction cardiac rehabilitation: influence on aerobic conditioning. J Cardiopulm Rehabil 1995;15:269–276.

19. Pollock ML, Wilmore JH. Exercise in health and disease. 2nd ed. Philadelphia: W.B. Saunders, 1990.

20. DeBusk RF, Stenestrand U, Sheehan M, et al. Training effects of long versus short bouts of exercise in healthy subjects. Am J Cardiol 1990;65:1010–1013.

21. Ebisu T. Splitting the distance of endurance training: on cardiovascular endurance and blood lipids. Jpn J Phys Educ 1985;30:37–43.

22. Jakicic JM, Wing RR, Butler BA, et al. Prescribing exercise in multiple short bouts versus one continuous bout: effects on adherence, cardiorespiratory fitness, and weight loss in overweight women. Int J Obes 1995;19:893–901.

23. Murphy MH, Hardman AE. Training effects of short and long bouts of brisk walking in sedentary women. Med Sci Sports Exerc 1998;30:152–157.

24. Gamble P, Froelicher VF. Can an exercise program worsen heart disease? Physician Sports Med 1982;10:69–77.

25. Wenger NK, Froelicher ES, Smith LK, et al. Cardiac rehabilitation. Clinical Practice Guideline No. 17. AHCPR Publication No. 96-0672. Rockville, MD: U.S. Department of Health and Human Services, Public Health Service, Agency for Health Care Policy and Research and the National Heart, Lung, and Blood Institute, 1995.

26. Haskell WL, Alderman EL, Fair JM, et al. Effects of intensive multiple risk factor reduction on coronary atherosclerosis and clinical cardiac events in men and women with coronary artery disease: the Stanford Coronary Risk Intervention Project (SCRIP). Circulation 1994;89:975–990.

27. Ornish D, Brown SE, Scherwitz LW, et al. Can lifestyle changes reverse coronary heart disease? Lancet 1990;336:129–133.

28. Hambrecht R, Niebauer J, Marburger C, et al. Various intensities of leisure time physical activity in patients with coronary artery disease: effects on cardiorespiratory fitness and progression of coronary atherosclerotic lesions. J Am Coll Cardiol 1993;22:468–477.

29. Smith SC, Blair SN, Criqui MH, et al. Preventing heart attack and death in patients with coronary disease. Circulation 1995;92:2–4.

30. Clausen JP, Trap-Jensen J, Lassen NA. The effects of training on the heart rate during arm and leg exercise. Scand J Clin Lab Invest 1970;26:295–301.

31. Klausen K, Rasmussen B, Clausen JP, et al. Blood lactate from exercising extremities before and after arm or leg training. Am J Physiol 1974;227:67–72.

32. Rasmussen B, Klausen K, Clausen JP, et al. Pulmonary ventilation, blood gases and blood pH after training of the arms or the legs. J Appl Physiol 1975;38:250–256.

33. Fardy PS, Doll NE, Reitz NL, et al. Prevalence of dysrhythmias during upper, lower and combined upper and lower extremity exercise in cardiac patients. Med Sci Sports Exerc 1981;13:137. Abstract.

34. Franklin BA, Vander L, Wrisley D, et al. Trainability of arms versus legs in men with previous myocardial infarction. Chest 1994;105:262–264.

35. Franklin BA. Exercise testing, training and arm ergometry. Sports Med 1985;2:100–119.

36. Wetherbee S, Franklin BA, Hollingsworth V, et al. Relationship between arm and leg training work loads in men with heart disease: implications for exercise prescription. Chest 1991;99:1271–1273.

37. Pollock ML, Vincent KR. Resistance training for health. President's Council Phys Fitness Sports Res Digest 1996;2(8).

38. Fiatarone MA, Evans WJ. The etiology and reversibility of muscle dysfunction in the aged. J Gerontol 1993;48:77–83.

39. Franklin BA, Gordon S, Timmis GC. Exercise prescription for hypertensive patients. Ann Med 1991;23:279–287.

40. Goldberg L, Elliot DL, Schutz RW, et al. Changes in lipid and lipoprotein levels after weight training. JAMA 1984;252:504–506.

41. McCartney N, McKelvie RS, Martin J, et al. Weight-training-induced attenuation of the circulatory response of older males to weight lifting. J Appl Physiol 1993;74:1056–1060.

42. Lewis S, Nygaard E, Sanchez J, et al. Static contraction of the quadriceps muscle in man: cardiovascular control and responses to one-legged strength training. Acta Physiol Scand 1984;122:341–353.

43. Hickson RC, Rosenkoetter MA, Brown MM. Strength training effects on aerobic power and short-term endurance. Med Sci Sports Exerc 1980;12:336–339.

44. Franklin BA, Bonzheim K, Gordon S, et al. Resistance training in cardiac rehabilitation. J Cardiopulm Rehabil 1991;11:99–107.

45. Fiatarone MA, Marks EC, Ryan ND, et al. High-intensity strength training in nonagenarians. JAMA 1990;263:3029–3034.

46. Verrill DE, Ribisl PM. Resistive exercise training in cardiac rehabilitation: an update. Sports Med 1996;21:347–383.

47. Kelemen MH. Resistive training safety and assessment guidelines for cardiac and coronary prone patients. Med Sci Sports Exerc 1989;21:675–677.

48. Squires RW, Muri AJ, Anderson LJ, et al. Weight training during phase II (early outpatient) cardiac rehabilitation. J Cardiopulm Rehabil 1991;11:360–364.

49. American Association of Cardiovascular and Pulmonary Rehabilitation. Guidelines for cardiac rehabilitation programs. 2nd ed. Champaign, IL: Human Kinetics, 1995.

50. American College of Sports Medicine. Guidelines for graded exercise testing and exercise prescription. 5th ed. Baltimore: Williams and Wilkins, 1995.

51. Kelemen MH, Stewart KJ, Gillilan RE, et al. Circuit weight training in cardiac patients. J Am Coll Cardiol 1986;7:38–42.

52. Stewart KJ, Mason M, Kelemen MH. Three-year participation in circuit weight training improves muscular strength and self-efficacy in cardiac patients. J Cardiopulm Rehabil 1988;8:292–296.

53. Ghilarducci LEC, Holly RG, Amsterdam EA. Effects of high resistance training in coronary artery disease. Am J Cardiol 1989;64:866–870.

54. Sparling PB, Cantwell JD, Dolan CM, et al. Strength training in a cardiac rehabilitation program: a six-month follow-up. Arch Phys Med Rehabil 1990;71:148–152.

55. Feigenbaum MS, Pollock ML. Strength training: rationale for current guidelines for adult

fitness programs. Physician Sports Med 1997;25:44–64.

56. Arvan S. Exercise performance of the high risk acute myocardoal infarction patient after cardiac rehabilitation. Am J Cardiol 1988;62:197–201.

57. Pyfer HR, Mead WF, Frederick RC, et al. Exercise rehabilitation in coronary heart disease: community group programs. Arch Phys Med Rehabil 1976;57:335–342.

58. Carter CL, Amundsen LR. Infarct size and exercise capacity after myocardial infarction. J Appl Physiol 1977;42:782–785.

59. Hellerstein HK. Anatomic factors influencing effects of exercise therapy of ASHD subjects. In: Roskamm H, Reindell H, eds. Das Chronisch Kranke Herz. Stuttgart: F.K. Shattauer Verlag, 1973.

60. Zohman LR. Exercise stress test interpretation for cardiac diagnosis and functional evaluation. Arch Phys Med Rehabil 1977;58:235–240.

61. Gordon NF, Kruger PE, Hons BA, et al. Improved exercise ventilatory responses after training in coronary heart disease during long-term beta-adrenergic blockade. Am J Cardiol 1983;51:755–758.

62. Laslett LJ, Paumer L, Scott-Baier P, et al. Efficacy of exercise training in patients with coronary artery disease who are taking propranolol. Circulation 1983;68:1029–1034.

63. Pratt CM, Welton DE, Squires WG, et al. Demonstration of training effect during chronic beta-adrenergic blockade in patients with coronary artery disease. Circulation 1981;64:1125–1129.

64. Hossack KF, Bruce RA. Improved exercise performance of persons with stable angina pectoris receiving diltiazem. Am J Cardiol 1981;47:95–101.

65. Heppell R, Hawley SK, Channer KS. Snow shoveler's infarction. BMJ 1991;302:469–470.

66. Cooke CT, Margolius KA. Sudden death while lawnmowing. Med J Aust 1992;157:720. Letter.

67. Sheldahl LM, Wilke NA, Dougherty SM, et al. Effect of age and coronary artery disease on response to snow shoveling. J Am Coll Cardiol 1992;20:1111–1117.

68. Glass RI, Zack MM. Increase in deaths from ischemic heart disease after blizzards. Lancet 1979;1:485–487.

69. Franklin BA, Hogan P, Bonzheim K, et al. Cardiac demands of heavy snow shoveling. JAMA 1995;273:880–882.

70. Franklin BA, Bonzheim K, Gordon S, et al. Snow shoveling: a trigger for acute myocardial infarction and sudden coronary death. Am J Cardiol 1996;77:855–858.

71. Freeman Z. Sudden death while lawnmowing. Med J Aust 1992;158:216. Letter.

72. Graham CE. Sudden death while lawnmowing. Med J Aust 1992;158:216. Letter.

73. Haskin-Popp C, Nazareno D, Wegner J, et al. Aerobic and myocardial demands of lawn mowing in patients with coronary artery disease. Am J Cardiol 1998;81:1243–1245.

74. Cobb LA, Weaver WD. Exercise: a risk for sudden death in patients with coronary heart disease. J Am Coll Cardiol 1986;7:215–219.

75. Mittleman MA, Maclure M, Tofler GH, et al. Triggering of acute myocardial infarction by heavy physical exertion: protection against triggering by regular exertion. N Engl J Med 1993;329:1677–1683.

76. Willich SN, Lewis M, Löwel H, et al. Physical exertion as a trigger of acute myocardial infarction. N Engl J Med 1993;329:1684–1690.

77. Van Camp SP, Peterson RA. Cardiovascular complications of outpatient cardiac rehabilitation programs. JAMA 1986;256:1160–1163.

78. Digenio AG, Sim JGM, Dowdeswell RJ, et al. Exercise-related cardiac arrest in cardiac rehabilitation: the Johannesburg experience. S Afr Med J 1991;79:188–191.

79. Vongvanich P, Paul-Labrador MJ, Merz CNB. Safety of medically supervised exercise in a cardiac rehabilitation center. Am J Cardiol 1996;77:1383–1385.

80. Franklin BA, Bonzheim K, Gordon S, et al. Safety of medically supervised outpatient cardiac rehabilitation exercise therapy: a 16-year follow-up. Chest 1998;114:902–906.

81. Murray PM, Herrington DM, Pettus CW, et al. Should patients with heart disease exercise in the morning or afternoon? Arch Intern Med 1993;153:833–836.

82. Fletcher GF, Balady G, Froelicher VF, et al. Exercise standards: a statement for healthcare professionals from the American Heart Association. Circulation 1995;91:580–615.

83. Mead WF, Pyfer HR, Trombold JC, et al. Successful resuscitation of two near simultaneous cases of cardiac arrest with a review of fifteen cases occurring during supervised exercise. Circulation 1976;53:187–189.

84. Hossack KF, Hartwig R. Cardiac arrest associated with supervised cardiac rehabilitation. J Cardiac Rehabil 1982;2:402–408.

85. Friedwald VE Jr, Spence DW. Sudden cardiac death associated with exercise: the risk-benefit issue. Am J Cardiol 1990;66:183–188.

86. Franklin BA, Reed PS, Gordon S, et al. Instantaneous electrocardiography: a simple screening technique for cardiac exercise programs. Chest 1989;96:174–177.

87. Haskell WL. Cardiovascular complications during exercise training of cardiac patients. Circulation 1978;57:920–924.

88. Barnard RJ, MacAlpin R, Kattus AA, et al. Ischemic response to sudden strenuous exercise in

healthy men. Circulation 1973; 48:936–942.

89. Foster C, Anholm JD, Hellman CK, et al. Left ventricular function during sudden strenuous exercise. Circulation 1981;63: 592–596.

90. Dimsdale JE, Hartley H, Guiney T, et al. Postexercise peril: plasma catecholamines and exercise. JAMA 1984;251:630–632.

91. Hattenhauer M, Neill WA. The effect of cold air on angina pectoris and myocardial oxygen supply. Circulation 1975;51: 1053–1058.

92. Kavanagh T. A cold weather "jogging mask" for angina patients. Can Med Assoc J 1970; 103:1290–1291.

93. Pandolf KB, Cafarelli E, Noble BJ, et al. Hyperthermia: effect on exercise prescription. Arch Phys Med Rehabil 1975;56:524–526.

94. West M, Johnson T, Roberts SO. Pacemakers and implantable cardioverter defibrillators. In: Durstine JL, ed. ACSM's exercise management for persons with chronic diseases and disabilities. Champaign IL: Human Kinetics, 1997:37–41.

95. Myers J. Congestive heart failure. In: Durstine JL, ed. ACSM's exercise management for persons with chronic diseases and disabilities. Champaign, IL: Human Kinetics, 1997:48–53.

96. Williford HN, Scharff-Olson M, Blessing DL. Exercise prescription for women. Sports Med 1993;15:299–311.

97. Pollock M, Graves J, Swart D, et al. Exercise training and prescription for the elderly. South Med J 1994;87:S88–S95.

98. Belaardinelli R, Georgiou D, Socco V, et al. Low intensity exercise training in patients with chronic heart failure. Am J Cardiol 1995;26:975–982.

99. Kao W, Jessup M. Exercise testing and training in patients with congestive heart failure. J Heart Lung Transplant 1994;13: S117–S121.

100. Keteyian S, Browner C, Schairer J. Exercise testing and training of patients with heat failure due to left ventricular systolic dysfunction. J Cardiopulm Rehabil 1997; 17:19–28.

101. Kellermann JJ, Shemesh J, Fisman EZ, et al. Arm exercise training in the rehabilitation of patients with impaired ventricular function and heart failure. Cardiology 1990;77:130–138.

102. Sullivan MJ, Higginbotham NB, Cobb FR. Exercise training in patients with severe left ventricular dysfunction: hemodynamic and metabolic effects. Circulation 1988;78:506–515.

103. Balady GJ, Fletcher BJ, Froelicher ES, et al. Cardiac rehabilitation programs: a statement for healthcare professionals from the American Heart Association. Circulation 1994;90:1602–1610.

104. O'Connor GT, Buring JE, Yusuf S, et al. An overview of randomized trials of rehabilitation with exercise after myocardial infarction. Circulation 1989;80:234–244.

105. Ades PA, Waldman ML, Polk DM, et al. Referral patterns and exercise response in the rehabilitation of female coronary patients aged ≥62 years. Am J Cardiol 1992;69:1422–1425.

106. Cannistra LB, Balady GJ, O'Malley CJ, et al. Comparison of the clinical profile and outcome of women and men in cardiac rehabilitation. Am J Cardiol 1992;69:1274–1279.

107. Franklin BA, Bonzheim K, Berg T. Gender differences in rehabilitation. In: Julian DG, Wenger NK, eds. Women and heart disease. London: Martin Dunitz, 1997: 151–171.

108. Ades PA, Hanson JS, Gunther PG, et al. Exercise conditioning in the elderly coronary patient. J Am Geriatr Soc 1987;35:121–124.

109. Ades PA, Grunvald MH. Cardiopulmonary exercise testing before and after conditioning in older coronary patients. Am Heart J 1990;120:585–589.

110. Pate RR, Pratt M, Blair SN, et al. Physical activity and public health: a recommendation from the Centers for Disease Control and Prevention and the American College of Sports Medicine. JAMA 1995;273:402–407.

Chapter 69

Clarifying the Risks and Benefits of Exercise Training for Patients with Heart Disease

Roy J. Shephard

Some early investigators regarded both myocardial infarction and sudden cardiovascular death as essentially random and unpredictable events (1,2). Others recognized that unaccustomed, intensive physical activity and severe emotional stress were common precipitants of "heart attacks" (3–7), raising the issue of the risks of heavy exercise relative to its health benefits (8,9).

In the young adult, sudden, exercise-related death often reflects either an anomalous origin in the coronary arteries or a congenital cardiomyopathy (10–13). Because of limitations of space, comment on such problems is limited to three observations: Exercise-induced deaths are extremely rare in young adults; correct diagnosis is equally rare even when the individual has undergone extensive screening; and the exercise participation of many healthy young people has been jeopardized by the overenthusiastic misdiagnosis of "abnormalities" (12,13).

In older adults, exercise-related deaths are usually due to coronary vascular narrowing. During and immediately following exercise, there is a 5- to 50-fold increase in the risk of a cardiac catastrophe relative to sedentary rest (5,7,14). Moreover, a similar order of risk persists if exercise is undertaken following a nonfatal myocardial infarction (15). After a brief discussion of the underlying pathology, we thus evaluate the risks and benefits of both preventive exercise in the older, coronary-prone individual (the process of secondary prevention) and exercise rehabilitation for those who have already sustained a heart attack (the process of tertiary prevention).

PATHOLOGIC MECHANISMS

Coronary atherosclerosis is the most commonly reported pathological finding when an older adult dies suddenly either during or immediately following a bout of vigorous physical activity (16–18). Nevertheless, the postmortem diagnosis is reached by a process of elimination, and given the high prevalence of coronary atherosclerosis in older members of the general population, the published total probably includes a proportion of individuals who have some coronary vascular narrowing, but have died from other, unidentified causes. If those who die within 24 hours of the onset of symptoms are included in calculations, about 60% of all sudden deaths (rest and exercise combined) are attributed to coronary vascular disease (16). Coronary atherosclerosis is the dominant pathology even in older athletes who die while they are exercising (19). Other potential mechanisms increasing the vulnerability of the aging myocardium to vigorous physical activity include infections (viral or sarcoid), exposure to industrial chemicals, and the abuse of substances such as alcohol, cocaine, or solvents.

Myocarditis

Controversy continues as to whether acute viral myocarditis is a common trigger of a cardiac catastrophe. Personal experience includes a 14-year-old student who died suddenly immediately following an attack of influenza and a "postcoronary" runner from the Toronto Rehabilitation Centre who was apparently in good physical condition, but died after completing the first 8 km of a marathon run. Lay colleagues subsequently suggested that the latter individual had developed a "flu-like illness" some 3 weeks before his death, although he had failed to report this to his physician. There thus seems a distinct possibility that an influenzal myocarditis contributed to the demise of this man, although it also remains possible that his unreported symptoms were part of the vague malaise that is one of the few warning signs of an impending infarction or reinfarction (20).

Animal studies support the view that exhausting exercise increases the probability that circulating viruses will locate in the myocardium. Gatmaitan et al (21) found that after viral inoculation, enforced exercise increased the virulence of the resulting Coxsackie B myocarditis. Exhausting exercise increases viral load, disease severity, myocyte necrosis, and mortality (22–28).

A number of human studies have linked the death of athletes or physically active individuals to an acute myocarditis (29–33). Although some authors maintain that viral myocarditis is only rarely a cause of sudden cardiac death, others have found that fever (34) and myocarditis (35) precede as many as 8% to 12% of cases of sudden cardiac death in young adults. Infecting organisms include the Coxsackie viruses (36) and *Chlamydia pneumoniae* (37). Functional studies of infected individuals may reveal diagnostically helpful changes in the averaged electrocardiogram (38), surface potentials, and echocardiogram (39).

Drug Abuse

The abuse of various drugs can also be a factor contributing to sudden cardiac death (16). Alcohol abuse may cause sudden death either directly (from a lethal overdose, cardiac arrhythmia, or sleep apnea), or indirectly (because of vomiting-induced electrolyte disturbances, chronic nutritional deficiencies, and resulting alcoholic cardiomyopathy).

Cocaine abuse may provoke sudden cardiac death by causing coronary vascular spasm, an alpha-adrenergic receptor-activated increase of myocardial oxygen consumption, or thrombosis. In a few instances, cocaine abusers may also show a contraction band necrosis, although it is still debated how much this contributes to their death (10).

Volatile substance abuse (particularly toluene sniffing) can precipitate sudden cardiac death by causing an AV block or sinus bradycardia.

Occupational Factors

Hazardous occupations can occasionally precipitate sudden death (16). Workers at a dynamite factory showed a propensity to die on Monday mornings. These employees had been exposed to high levels of nitrate fumes while they were working on the shop floor. There was thus a reactive spasm of the coronary vessels when exposure was withdrawn over the weekend, and an increased susceptibility to sudden cardiac death when physically demanding work was resumed on Monday mornings; the reactive coronary vascular spasm exacerbated the usual morning prevalence of coronary attacks (40).

RISKS AND BENEFITS OF EXERCISE IN SECONDARY PREVENTION

The risk that vigorous physical activity will provoke a cardiac catastrophe was highlighted in retrospective questioning of patients who were recovering from nonfatal myocardial infarctions (41). Individually matched controls were drawn from the worksites of affected individuals. Relative to the matched controls, a high proportion of heart attack victims reported that

Table 69-1 The Timing of Attacks of Nonfatal Infarction: Data from 98 Successive Primary Incidents		
	NUMBER OF CASES	
TYPE OF ACTIVITY	**ACTUAL**	**PREDICTED FROM FRACTION OF DAY NORMALLY ALLOCATED TO ACTIVITY**
Sleeping	17	33
Working	11	29
Relaxing at Home	21	16
Driving	8	5
Dining	7	5
Personal Toilet	3	4
Odd Jobs	10	2
Sport and Vigorous Physical Activity	9	2
Walking	8	1
Other	4	1

Based upon data published by Shephard RJ. Sudden death: a significant hazard of exercise. Br J Sports Med 1974;8:101–110.

they had been engaged in sport or vigorous physical activity at the time of their cardiac incident. In contrast, less than the expected proportion of victims had been engaged in sedentary pursuits (Table 69-1).

Vuori (7) estimated the risk of a fatality at 1 in 11.7 million sessions of walking and 1 in 6.7 million sessions of jogging. These figures may be compared with the risk of a half hour of sedentary middle-aged life, when there is about a 1 in 35 million chance of sustaining a myocardial infarction.

The precise level of risk depends on the type of physical activity that is undertaken, on the fitness of the individual relative to task demands, and on the immediate environmental circumstances: time of day, weather conditions, and any associated competitive or psychosocial stress (20,42). Other factors with a potential influence on risk include the individual's age and gender, the period of attribution, and (in retrospective analyses) a selective recall of unusual events by the victims themselves or (in the case of fatalities) by their immediate relatives.

Influence of Age

The incidence of ischemic heart disease rises steeply with age. There is also some increase in the incidence of exercise-related deaths to 50 years of age, but a plateauing of incidents thereafter; indeed, the relative risk of sport-related deaths is less in the elderly than in middle-aged individuals (Table 69-2) (7,43). Presumably, the age-related increase of coronary vascular disease is offset by a decrease in participation and a more cautious approach to the sports under examination; an elderly person may be more willing than a middle-aged man to admit that he or she is becoming tired and that a heavy physical task exceeds his or her current strength.

In the very old (>80 years), there is some evidence that lifespan may be shortened by continued participation in vigorous physical activity (44).

Influence of Gender

An early report (45) noted that exercise-related sudden death was much less common in women than in men; subsequent studies have found almost no cases in women older than 30. One reason for this is the lower prevalence of ischemic heart disease in women (7,46,47). Moreover, women have traditionally undertaken fewer heavy physical tasks, and even when they have engaged in demanding physical activity, they have been less likely to persist with it in the face of severe fatigue or other warning signs of overexertion (42).

Influence of Training

Training lowers the relative intensity of a given activity, and thus decreases the risk that it will provoke a cardiac catastrophe. In experimental animals, a training program also increases the threshold electrical shock needed to induce ventricular fibrillation (48).

The heart rate and blood pressure of a fit individual are lower at any given power output, thus reducing myocardial oxygen consumption (49). Coronary vascular perfusion is also enhanced by a lengthening of the diastolic phase of the cardiac cycle, and there is an increase of vagal tone, as shown by analyses of R–R intervals. A strengthening of the skeletal muscles may contribute to the reduction in risk, since the trained individual can perform heavy lifting at a smaller fraction of maximal voluntary force, and there is a correspondingly smaller rise of systemic blood pressure during the bout of activity (49).

If protection is to be gained, it seems particularly important that training be pursued on a regular basis. Willich et al (50) found the relative risk of a cardiac catastrophe during strenuous exercise increased from 1.3 times the resting level in those who exercised 4 or more days per week to 6.9 in those who exercised less than 4 times per week. Likewise, Mittleman et al (51) found an increase of relative risk from 2.4 in those who were active at least 5 times a week to 107 in those who were active less than once per week.

Influence of Attribution Period

Some studies have attributed a cardiac catastrophe to physical activity only when the two events were concurrent. Others have considered the possible contribution of exercise to all events occurring over the next 1, 6, or even 24 hours (52), accepting those incidents in which there were bridging symptoms between the bout of physical activity and the cardiac incident. The latter approach sets an upper limit to the cardiac risks associated with vigorous exercise, but inevitably it tends to add in randomly occurring cardiac events, thus augmenting the apparent danger of exercise.

Average Risk Ratios

Shephard (41) estimated that the concurrent risk of a cardiac incident was increased about fivefold when a middle-aged or older apparently healthy man engaged in a sustained bout of vigorous physical activity. Subsequent analyses have been more elegant, but have not greatly changed the overall perception of risk (Table 69-2) (7).

Table 69-2 Analysis of 248 Cases of Sudden Death During Sport in Relation to Age		
AGE GROUP	NUMBER OF CASES	PERCENTAGE OF CASES
5–20	54	21.8
20–30	43	17.3
30–40	45	18.1
40–50	47	19.0
Over 50	59	23.8

Based on material published by Kabisch D, Funk S. Tödesfällen im organisierten und angleiteten Sport (Deaths in organized and supervised sports). Dtsche Z Sportmed 1991;42:464–470.

Wendt et al (53) found no complications when 385,000 exercise tests were performed on athletes. In Germany, soccer is the sport most commonly implicated in sudden cardiac death (43), but this probably reflects the popularity of soccer in Europe. Elsewhere, squash and distance running have been suggested as dominant precipitants of sudden death (10,54); again, this may be because of their popularity rather than because of any unusual risks inherent in such pursuits.

Implications for Health Policy

Given that vigorous physical activity appreciably increases the immediate risk of sudden cardiac death, a sedentary individual might well ask why he or she should adopt an exercise program. Shephard (41) examined this issue, and estimated that the immediate adverse consequences of a bout of vigorous physical activity were more than outweighed by an enhanced cardiovascular prognosis in the intervals between exercise sessions. The same concept has since been developed by Kohl et al (55) and Siscovick (14). It can also be inferred from the extensive meta-analyses of Powell et al (56) and Berlin et al (57), both of which have shown a two- to three-fold reduction of cardiovascular mortality among exercisers. Nevertheless, benefit is contingent on the regularity of physical activity, and as noted above, the acute risk of exercise is substantially increased if it is pursued only occasionally.

On current evidence, the benefits of regular physical activity substantially outweigh the risks, even if analysis is restricted simply to the data for sudden cardiovascular deaths. If account is taken also of the beneficial effects of exercise on other chronic diseases, mood state, psychological health, and functional capacity in advanced old age, the arguments in favor of an active lifestyle become very strong. However, certain precautions can be taken to reduce further the already remote risk of an exercise-induced cardiac catastrophe.

Environmental Factors

The risk of sudden cardiac death is increased by unaccustomed exertion, particularly if the subject is ill-prepared for the required intensity of effort. Excitement and competitive pressure also seem to be precipitants of a cardiac emergency (41). Older adults should thus avoid prolonged and/or intense bouts of sport and physical activity if they have not been active recently.

Willich (40) has also found that the risk of sudden death is greater in the morning. Other considerations (such as high afternoon temperatures) may make it desirable to exercise in the early morning, but such considerations must be balanced carefully against the greater inherent cardiac risk of morning exercise.

Type of Exercise

It is difficult to compare the risks associated with various sports and pastimes, because the popularity of a particular sport and the level of competition that is reached vary widely from one country to another (7). However, activities that increase circulating catecholamines because they are exciting or dangerous seem to carry a greater risk than an equivalent intensity of exercise performed on a treadmill or a cycle ergometer (58).

Other factors being equal, prolonged isometric exercise is likely to induce a larger increase of blood pressure, and therefore a greater increase of cardiac work rate, than an equivalent dose of rhythmic endurance exercise. Older adults should thus be careful to avoid prolonged straining against a closed glottis when undertaking isometric activity.

Warning Signs

The individual who is vulnerable to an exercise-induced cardiac catastrophe may have a family history of premature sudden death. Often, they also have one or more major cardiac risk factors such as cigarette smoking, hypertension, hypercholesterolemia, and obesity. They may show persistent abnormalities of the resting electrocardiogram or ST segmental depression during exercise (20,59). However, all of these factors merely increase the individual's statistical risk of an incident, and an exercise-induced cardiac death remains quite possible in a person who shows none of these signs and symptoms.

There are few immediate warning signs, other than a vague malaise in the final 6 hours before the incident (41). This malaise may reflect an exacerbation of existing coronary atherosclerosis. It is wise for older adults to avoid strenuous physical activity if they feel unwell, have a cold or viral infection, or note frank chest pain or an irregular heart rhythm (59).

Older adults should avoid prolonged, unaccustomed, and heavy physical activity of any type, particularly if it involves isometric straining, or persistence in sport or household chores when these are causing symptoms. An appropriately graded bout of physical activity should not leave the person more than pleasantly tired a few hours later. Specific reasons to moderate the intensity of an exercise regimen include outdoor activity when the weather is extremely hot or cold, and all types of vigorous physical activity when the individual concerned faces business or social problems or time pressures.

Age Ceiling

Survival curves for exercisers and nonexercisers appear to converge around the age of 80 years (60). The calculation of specific risk ratios suggests that vigorous exercise ceases to augment lifespan around 80 years of age, and even moderate exercise may increase the likelihood of death in those who are over the age of 90 years (44,61). However, in those over the age of 80 years, it is probably an error to weigh the risks and benefits of exercise simply in terms of changes in longevity. Quality-adjusted life expectancy is more important than mere survival (62); relative to the person who has become sedentary, an individual who remains physically active is much more likely to keep his or her independence and to enjoy a good quality of life.

Drug Therapy

There seems to be no justification for using specific antiarrhythmic drugs as a preventive measure in the general population. However, it may be useful to check for evidence of a serum deficiency of magnesium, particularly in "hard water" areas of the country; it may be prudent to offer magnesium supplements to older individuals who live in such regions during bouts of warm weather.

Screening and Supervision

Given the risks detailed above, what level of preliminary medical screening and exercise supervision is needed to minimize the danger that exercise will induce a sudden cardiac death? Is it necessary for every exercise candidate over the age of 30 years to have a resting electrocardiogram and a full clinical examination, further supplemented by a stress electrocardiogram if the person is over the age of 35 years (63)? Or is it acceptable for paramedical health professionals and even the lay public to make an initial triage of risk, using a simple, self-administered questionnaire such as the Revised PAR-Q test (64)? Application of Bayes' theorem shows that because of the low prevalence of abnormalities in the general population, widespread ECG stress testing yields a high proportion of false-positive test results—possibly as many as two thirds of those who are examined (20). Although the majority of the false diagnoses can be resolved by additional laboratory examinations (echocardiography, scintigraphy, and angiography), a large segment of the population is exposed to much unnecessary anxiety and expense.

Debate continues on the optimal scale of screening and supervision when providing exercise programs for the general population (65,66). Factors modifying the recommendation have included the recent concept that moderate rather than vigorous activity is needed (67,68), and increasing attempts to use the ordinary daily routine as a means of obtaining the necessary activity. However, the American College of Sports Medicine (69) has now gone far toward accepting the Canadian concept that screening and subsequent medical supervision are unnecessary for the healthy adult who is free of cardiac risk factors and is contemplating no more than a modest increase in habitual physical activity.

RISKS AND BENEFITS OF EXERCISE IN TERTIARY PREVENTION

Given that vigorous physical activity can substantially augment the risk of a cardiac catastrophe in an apparently healthy adult, an even greater risk might be anticipated following myocardial infarction.

Shephard (15) noted that over a 20-month follow-up period, 4.1% of a sample of postcoronary patients had sustained a recurrence of their infarction; 24% of these episodes were closely associated with various types of physical activity, and a further 24% of those affected reported vigorous physical activity (sometimes of an unusual nature) in the previous few hours. Some early cardiac rehabilitation programs experienced a very high risk of cardiac arrest and/or ventricular fibrillation; for instance, Pyfer et al (70) encountered 13 such episodes in 90,000 hours of gymnasium exercise. More recent assessments of risk come from both laboratory exercise testing and programs of tertiary rehabilitation.

Risks of Exercise Testing

Data on the risks of exercise testing have been collected largely from cardiac departments, but in some cases the statistics are hard to interpret because they are for unspecified mixtures of "coronary-prone" and "postcoronary" patients.

Rochmis et al (71) surveyed 73 North American laboratories, finding one fatal episode per 10,000 exercise tests. Stuart et al (72) noted as many as 8.9 complications per 10,000 exercise stress tests, although not all of the incidents resulted in death. Atterhog et al (73) obtained similar results in a prospective study of 20 Swedish exercise testing centers; they reported 24 complications, including 2 deaths, in 50,000 exercise tests. Gibbons et al (74), likewise, had an overall complication rate of 0.8 per 10,000 exercise tests, although given the absence of problems in the most recent 45,000 evaluations, they argued that the risk of testing had diminished as the experience of the investigators had increased.

Risks of Tertiary Rehabilitation

The risk of exercise-induced death in a well-designed medically supervised program of tertiary rehabilitation is quite low relative to laboratory testing, in part because the intensity of effort is lower, and in part because the participants are less anxious. Values range from 1 in 60,000 hours (75) to 1 in 300,000 hours of supervised exercise (76).

The risk is apparently a little greater when vigorous physical activity is undertaken without direct medical supervision (1 in 110,000 hours) (76). Evidence that continuous electrocardiographic monitoring increases program safety remains equivocal. Haskell (75) found fewer complications in programs that offered continuous telemetry monitoring, but this may reflect a lower staff-patient ratio in the institutions concerned. Van Camp et al (77) found similar frequencies of myocardial infarction, cardiac arrest, and death in groups that were stratified by the extent of telemetric monitoring, although again interpretation of the findings is limited by a nonrandom assignment of patients to the various options.

Factors Modifying Risk
Characteristics of Primary Attack

Reinfarction is a little more likely if the patient has a history of multiple infarctions, but recurrences seem unrelated to many traditional markers of the severity of the initial infarct (such as the extent of symptoms and ECG abnormalities, the magnitude of enzyme changes, episodes of cardiac arrest and arrhythmia, or the extent of the decrease in blood pressure during the acute episode) (78). However, warning features on entry to a rehabilitation program include the extent of continuing disability, shortness of breath and angina of effort, a low

peak cardiac output, and a compensating widening of the arteriovenous oxygen difference. Unfortunately, none of these findings are sufficiently consistent to gauge prognosis in the individual patient.

Type of Exercise

In about a half of patients, the recurrence comes about while the patient is participating in the normal rehabilitation program, since this is the main type of vigorous activity in which the post-coronary patients engage (78). However, in our series, 3 of 19 episodes occurred while patients were playing golf, and one while playing tennis; other incidents involved the frequent climbing of ladders, chopping ice "all the morning," "several hours" of raking a lawn, and "four hours" of earth moving.

Risk Factors

Current smoking, angina, hypertension, and hypercholesterolemia did not distinguish effectively between those patients who sustained a recurrence while they were exercising and those who were affected at other times (78). However, there were trends linking an increased risk of an exercise-induced incident with poor exercise compliance and with both resting and exercise-induced ECG abnormalities.

Pattern of Rehabilitation

There has been much discussion concerning the merits of low- versus high-intensity rehabilitation programs following myocardial infarction. The early data of Paterson et al (79), subsequently confirmed by Ehsani et al (80) and by Quaglietti et al (81), show that with higher intensities of activity it is possible to induce gains in myocardial function, as opposed to merely peripheral vascular adaptations. There is no evidence that within the levels of activity adopted by rehabilitation centers a high-intensity program has greater danger than a low-intensity program, even while the exercise is being performed. Moreover, by improving myocardial function and lengthening the diastolic phase, high-intensity programs probably reduce risks outside of formal rehabilitation classes. In one center, a substantial group of postcoronary patients brought themselves to a level of training at which they were able to run a marathon distance; although this group was self-selected, their mortality was as low as if not lower than that of the average patient attending the Toronto Rehabilitation Centre (76).

Age of Patient

There is evidence that the older patient responds less well to cardiac rehabilitation, but this may be because greater caution keeps the older person from an effective dose of exercise (82). There are no specific data to suggest that the danger of rehabilitation is any greater in older individuals.

Drug Therapy

It is now widely accepted that beta-blocking agents have a favorable impact on prognosis following myocardial infarction (83–85). In our study of patients who had entered a rehabilitation program, reinfarction and death were only half as common in those individuals who were receiving some type of beta-blocking medication (84). Peters (86) has emphasized that such treatment is particularly effective in protecting postcoronary patients against early morning surges of sympathetic activity.

Risks and Benefits

Our early data suggested that the exercising postcoronary patient had about a sixfold increase in the immediate risk of a recurrence relative to rest (15). A more recent paper reported that the risk of cardiac arrest for an exercising patient with coronary vascular disease was 6 to 164 times greater than the spontaneous incidence (87).

Despite this risk, various meta-analyses confirm that the overall mortality is reduced by 20% to 30% in patients who follow a program of progressive rehabilitation following myocardial infarction (88,89). Certainly, the danger of provoking an exercise-induced catastrophe is not a valid argument against a policy of active rehabilitation following myocardial infarction.

Screening and Supervision

There has been considerable discussion of the need for various forms of screening and supervision of rehabilitation programs following myocardial infarction (75,77). Most insuring agencies in the United States have now concluded that for the average patient, the risks of a recurrence are extremely low, and after hospital discharge such individuals have little or no need for supervised exercise (90). Those who need closer attention can be determined by a preliminary triage, including an exercise test at hospital discharge. The counterargument favoring a supervised program for all postcoronary patients is that the individual then obtains added advice, together with encouragement of regular exercise and a healthy lifestyle; there may also be an earlier detection of any adverse changes in clinical condition. All of these factors could have a favorable influence upon prognosis (91).

SUMMARY

The overall benefits of a physically active lifestyle substantially outweigh the danger that an acute bout of vigorous physical activity may provoke myocardial infarction and/or sudden cardiac death. Cardiac catastrophes are hard to predict, and for this reason complicated screening procedures are not warranted. Nevertheless, there are a few simple precautions that can reduce the dangers of both secondary and tertiary rehabilitation, and these procedures should be observed, particularly by older individuals who already have a number of major cardiac risk factors.

Dr. Shephard's research is supported in part by a research grant from Canadian Tire Acceptance Limited.

REFERENCES

1. Master AM. The role of effort and occupation (including physicians) in coronary occlusion. JAMA 1960;174:942–948.

2. Parkinson J, Bedford DE. Cardiac infarction and coronary thrombosis. Lancet 1928;1:4–11.

3. Fitzhugh G, Hamilton BE. Coronary occlusion and fatal angina pectoris. Study of the immediate causes and their prevention. JAMA 1933;100:475–480.

4. Phipps C. Contributory causes of coronary thrombosis. JAMA 1936; 106:761–762.

5. Shephard RJ. Ischemic heart disease and exercise. London: Croom Helm, 1981.

6. Shephard RJ. Exercise and sudden death: an overview. Sport Sci Rev 1995;4(2):1–13.

7. Vuori IM. Sudden death and exercise: effects of age and type of activity. Sport Sci Rev 1995;4(2): 46–84.

8. Bouchard C, Shephard RJ, Stephens T, et al. Exercise, fitness and health. Champaign, IL: Human Kinetics, 1990.

9. Bouchard C, Shephard RJ, Stephens T. Physical activity, fitness and health. Champaign, IL: Human Kinetics, 1994.

10. Goodman J. Exercise and sudden cardiac death: etiology in apparently healthy individuals. Sport Sci Rev 1995;4(2):14–30.

11. Maron B. Asymmetry in hypertrophic cardiomyopathy: the septal to free wall thickness revisited. Am J Cardiol 1985;55:835–838.

12. Maron BJ (Chair). Cardiovascular preparticipation screening of competitive athletes. Med Sci Sports Exerc 1996;28:1445–1452.

13. Shephard RJ. The athlete's heart: is big beautiful? Br J Sports Med 1996;30:5–10.

14. Siscovick DS. Risks of exercising: sudden death and injuries. In:

Bouchard C, Shephard RJ, Stephens T, et al, eds. Exercise, fitness and health. Champaign, IL: Human Kinetics, 1990:707–713.

15. Shephard RJ. Recurrence of myocardial infarction: observations on patients participating in the Ontario multicentre exercise-heart trial. Eur J Cardiol 1980;11:147–157.

16. Hackel D, Reimer KA. Sudden death: Cardiac and other causes. Durham, NC: Carolina Academic Press, 1994.

17. Manninen V, Halonen PI. Sudden coronary death. Basel: S. Karger, 1978.

18. Vinolas X, Guindo J, Homs E, et al. Precursors of sudden death. In: Brouset JP, ed. Proceedings of the Fifth World Congress on Cardiac Rehabilitation. Andover, Hants (UK): Intercept Publications, 1993:163–172.

19. Torg J. Sudden cardiac death in the athlete. In: Torg J, Shephard

RJ, eds. Current therapy in sports medicine 3. Philadelphia: Mosby–Year Book, 1995:8–10.

20. Shephard RJ. Ischemic heart disease and exercise. London: Croom Helm, 1981.

21. Gatmaitan BG, Chason JL, Lerner AM. Augmentation of the virulence of murine Coxsackie virus B3 myocardiopathy by exercise. J Exp Med 1970;131:1121–1136.

22. Cabinian AE, Kiel RJ, Smith F, et al. Modification of exercise-aggravated Coxsackie virus B3 murine myocarditis by T lymphocyte suppression in an inhibited model. J Lab Clin Med 1990;115:454–462.

23. Ilbäck NG, Friman G, Beisel WR, et al. Modifying effects of exercise on the clinical course and biochemical responses of the myocardium in influenza and tularemia in mice. Infect Immun 1984;45:498–504.

24. Ilbäck NG, Fohlman J, Friman G. Exercise in Coxsackie B3 myocarditis: effects on heart lymphocyte subpopulations and the inflammatory reaction. Am Heart J 1989;117:1298–1302.

25. Kiel RJ, Smith FE, Chason J, et al. Coxsackie virus B3 myocarditis in C3H/HeJ mice: description of an inbred model and the effect of exercise on virulence. Eur J Epidemiol 1989;5:348–350.

26. Lerner AM, Wilson FM. Virus cardiomyopathy. Progr Med Virol 1973;15:63–78.

27. Reyes MP, Lerner AM. Interferon and neutralizing antibody in sera of exercised mice with Coxsackie B3 myocarditis. Proc Soc Exper Biol Med 1976;151:333–338.

28. Tilles JG, Elson RH, Shaka JA, et al. Effect of exercise on Coxsackie A9 myocarditis in adult mice. Proc Soc Exper Biol Med 1964;117:777–782.

29. Bouhour JB, Borgat C. Sudden death and myocarditis during activities and sports performance. Int J Sports Cardiol 1985;2:81–85.

30. Koskenvuo K. Sudden deaths among Finnish conscripts. Br Med J 1976;2:1413–1415.

31. Phillips M, Robinowitz M, Higgins JR, et al. Sudden cardiac death in Air Force recruits: a 20-year review. JAMA 1986;256:2696–2699.

32. Topaz O, Edwards JE. Pathologic features of sudden death in children, adolescents and young adults. Chest 1985;87:476–482.

33. Wentworth P, Jentz LA, Croal AE. Analysis of sudden unexpected death in Southern Ontario with emphasis on myocarditis. Can Med Assoc J 1979;120:676–680, 706.

34. Drory Y, Kramer MR, Lev B. Exertional sudden death in soldiers. Med Sci Sports Exerc 1991;23:147–151.

35. McCaffrey FM, Braden DS, Strong WB. Sudden cardiac death in young athletes: a review. Am J Dis Children 1991;145;177–183.

36. Sutton GC, Harding HB, Truehart RP, Clark HB. Coxsackie B4 myocarditis in an adult: successful isolation of virus from ventricular myocardium. Aerospace Med 1967;20:66–69.

37. Wesslen L, Pahlson C, Friman G, et al. Myocarditis caused by Chlamydia pneumoniae (TWAR) and sudden unexpected death in a Swedish elite orienteer. Lancet 1992;340:427–428. Letter.

38. Vacek JL, Smith S. The effects of exercise during viraemia on the single averaged electrocardiogram. Am Heart J 1990;119:702–705.

39. Montague TJ, Marrie TJ, Bewick DJ, et al. Cardiac effects of common viral illnesses. Chest 1988;94:919–925.

40. Willich SN. Circadian influences and possible triggers of sudden cardiac death. Sport Sci Rev 1995;4(2):31–45.

41. Shephard RJ. Sudden death: a significant hazard of exercise. Br J Sports Med 1974;8:101–110.

42. Tofler GH, Stone PH, MacClure M, et al and the MILIS group. Analysis of possible triggers of acute myocardial infarction (the MILIS study). Am J Cardiol 1990;66:22–27.

43. Kabisch D, Funk D. Todesfälle im organisierten und angeleiten Sport. Dtsche Z Sportmed 1991;42:464–470.

44. Linsted KD, Tonstad S, Kuzma JW. Self-report of physical activity and patterns of mortality in Seventh-Day Adventist men. J Clin Epidemiol 1991;44:355–364.

45. Romo M. Factors relating to sudden death in acute ischaemic heart disease: a community study in Helsinki. Acta Med Scand 1972;547(suppl):7–92.

46. Fechner, G, Püchsel K. Pathologisch-anatomische Untersuchungsbefunde von Todesfällen beim Sport (Pathological-anatomical examination results of fatalities in sports). Dtsche Z Sportmed 1986;37(2):35–40.

47. LaHarpe R, Rostan A, Frye C. La mort subite lors de la pratique d'un sport: l'éclairage de la médecine légale (Sudden deaths in sports: findings in forensic examinations). Schweiz Z Sportmed 1992;40:65–70.

48. Hull SS, Vanoli E, Adamson PB, et al. Exercise training confers anticipatory protection from sudden death during acute myocardial ischemia. Circulation 1994;89:548–552.

49. Shephard RJ. Physiology and biochemistry of exercise. New York: Praeger, 1982.

50. Willich SN, Lewis M, Löwel H, et al. Physical exertion as a trigger of acute myocardial infarction. N Engl J Med 1993;329:1684–1690.

51. Mittelman MA, Maclure M, Tofler GH, et al. Triggering of acute myocardial infarction by heavy physical exertion: protection against triggering by regular exertion. N Engl J Med 1993;329:1677–1683.

52. Rochmis P, Blackburn H. Exercise tests: a survey of procedures, safety and litigation experience in approximately 170,000 tests. JAMA 1971;217:1061–1066.

53. Wendt T, Scherer WD, Kaltenbach M. Life-threatening complications in 1741106 ergometries. Dtsche Med Wochenschrift 1984;109:123–127.

54. Northcote RJ, Flannigan C, Ballantyne D. Sudden death and vigorous exercise—a study of 60 deaths associated with squash. Br Heart J 1986;55:198–203.

55. Kohl HW, Powell KE, Gordon NF, et al. Physical activity, physical fitness and sudden death. Epidemiol Rev 1992;14:37–58.

56. Powell KE, Thompson PD, Caspersen CJ, Kendrick JS. Physical activity and the incidence of coronary heart disease. Ann Rev Public Health 1987;8:253–287.

57. Berlin JA, Coldlitz GA. A meta-analysis of physical activity in the prevention of coronary heart disease. Am J Epidemiol 1990;132:612–628.

58. Blimkie CJ, Cunningham DA, Leung FY. Urinary catecholamine excretion and lactate concentrations in competitive hockey players aged 11 to 23 years. In: Lavallée H, Shephard RJ, eds. Frontiers of activity and child health. Québec: Editions du Pélican, 1977:313–321.

59. Shephard RJ. Can we identify those for whom exercise is hazardous? Sports Med 1984;1:75–86.

60. Pekkanen J, Martti B, Nissinen A, et al. Reduction of premature mortality by high physical activity: a 20-year follow-up of middle-aged Finnish men. Lancet 1987;(i):1473–1477.

61. Paffenbarger RS, Hyde RT, Wing AL, et al. Some interrelationships of physical activity, physiological fitness, health and longevity. In: Bouchard C, Shephard RJ, Stephens T, eds. Physical activity, fitness and health. Champaign, IL: Human Kinetics Publishers, 1994:119–133.

62. Shephard RJ. Physical activity and quality of life. Quest 1996;48:354–365.

63. Cooper KH. Guidelines in the management of the exercising patient. JAMA 1970;211:1663–1667.

64. Shephard RJ, Thomas S, Weller I. The Canadian Home Fitness Test: 1991 update. Sports Med 1991;11:358–366.

65. Franklin BA, Kahn JK. Detecting the individual prone to exercise-related sudden cardiac death. Sport Sci Rev 1995;4(2):85–105.

66. Pratt M. Exercise and sudden death: implications for health policy. Sport Sci Rev 1995;4(2):106–122.

67. Pate RR, Pratt M, Blair SN, et al. Physical activity and public health: a recommendation from the Centers for Disease Control and Prevention and the American College of Sports Medicine. JAMA 1995;273:402–407.

68. U.S. Surgeon General. Physical activity and health. Washington, D.C.: U.S. Department of Health and Human Services, 1996.

69. American College of Sports Medicine. Guidelines for graded exercise testing and prescription. 5th ed. Philadelphia: Lea & Febiger, 1995.

70. Pyfer HR, Mead WF, Frederick RC. Cardiac arrest during medically supervised exercise training—a report of 13 successful defibrillations. Med Sci Sports Exerc 1975;7:72.

71. Rochmis P, Blackburn H. Exercise tests: a survey of procedures, safety and litigation experience in approximately 170,000 tests. JAMA 1971;217:1061–1066.

72. Stuart RJ, Ellestad MH. National survey of exercise stress testing facilities. Chest 1980;77:94–97.

73. Atterhog JH, Jonsson B, Samuelsson R. Exercise testing: a prospective study of complication rates. Am Heart J 1979;98:572–579.

74. Gibbons L, Blair SN, Kohl HW, Cooper K. The safety of maximal exercise testing. Circulation 1989;80:846–852.

75. Haskell WL. The efficacy and safety of exercise programs in cardiac rehabilitation. Med Sci Sports Exerc 1994;26:815–823.

76. Shephard RJ, Kavanagh T, Tuck J, Kennedy J. Marathon jogging in post-myocardial infarction patients. J Cardiopulm Rehabil 1983;3:321–329.

77. Van Camp SP, Peterson RA. Cardiovascular complications of outpatient cardiac rehabilitation programs. JAMA 1986;256:1160–1163.

78. Shephard RJ. Recurrence of myocardial infarction in an exercising population. Br Heart J 1979;41:133–138.

79. Paterson DH, Shephard RJ, Cunningham DA, et al. Effects of physical training upon cardiovascular function following myocardial infarction. J Appl Physiol 1979;47:482–489.

80. Ehsani AA, Martin WH, Heath GW, Coyle EF. Cardiac effects of prolonged and intense exercise training in patients with coronary artery disease. Am J Cardiol 1982;50:246–254.

81. Quaglietti S, Froelicher VF. Physical activity and cardiac rehabilitation for patients with coronary artery disease. In: Bouchard C, Shephard RJ, Stephens T, eds. Physical activity, fitness and health. Champaign, IL: Human Kinetics, 1994:591–608.

82. Kavanagh T, Shephard RJ, Doney H, Pandit V. Intensive exercise in coronary rehabilitation. Med Sci Sports Exerc 1973;5:34–39.

83. Beta-blocker Heart Attack Trial Research Group. A randomized trial of propranolol in patients with acute myocardial infarction: mortality results. JAMA 1982;247:1707–1714.

84. Kavanagh T, Shephard RJ, Chisholm AW, et al. Prognostic indexes for patients with ischemic heart disease enrolled in an exercise-centered rehabilitation program. Am J Cardiol 1979;44:1230–1240.

85. Norwegian Multicenter Group. Timolol-induced reduction in mortality and reinfarction in patients surviving acute myocardial infarction. N Engl J Med 1981;304:801–807.

86. Peters RW. Propranolol and the morning increase in sudden cardiac death: the beta-blocker heart attack trial experience. Am J Cardiol 1990;66:57G–59G.

87. Cobb LA, Weaver WD. Exercise: a risk for sudden death in patients with coronary heart disease. J Am Coll Cardiol 1986;7:215–219.

88. Oldridge NB, Guyatt G, Fischer M, Rimm RA. Randomized clinical trials of cardiac rehabilitation: combined experience of randomized clinical trials. JAMA 1988; 260:945–950.

89. Shephard RJ. Exercise in the tertiary prevention of ischemic heart disease. Can J Sport Sci 1989;14: 74–84.

90. Franklin BA, Bonzheim K, Berg T, Bonzheim S. Hospital- and home-based cardiac rehabilitation outpatient programs. In: Pollock ML, Schmidt DH, eds. Heart disease and rehabilitation. 3rd ed. Champaign, IL: Human Kinetics, 1995: 209–228.

91. Vongvanich P, Merz CNB. Supervised exercise and electrocardiographic monitoring during cardiac rehabilitation: impact on patient care. J Cardiopulm Rehabil 1996; 16:233–238.

Chapter 70

Psychosocial Considerations in Coronary Heart Disease: Implications for Rehabilitation

Elizabeth C.D. Gullette
James A. Blumenthal

A steadily growing body of research has provided evidence for the adverse effects of psychosocial factors on prognosis in patients with established coronary heart disease (CHD). Furthermore, a number of intervention studies, while limited in scale and methodology, provide encouraging evidence for the clinical efficacy of psychosocial interventions aimed at ameliorating this adverse impact. This chapter provides an overview of psychosocial factors associated with the development and clinical manifestations of CHD, discusses contextual factors that may moderate this risk, and suggests potential mechanisms by which psychosocial factors increase the risk of adverse events in patients with CHD. In addition, the chapter provides a select review of psychosocial interventions in patients with CHD and concludes with suggestions for future research in the area.

PSYCHOSOCIAL RISK FACTORS

Type A Behavior Pattern and Hostility

Early observations by Friedman et al (1) suggested that a large proportion of patients with CHD displayed a particular constellation of behaviors and personality traits, characterized by a hard-driving, competitive nature, a strong need for recognition and achievement, a sense of time urgency, and free-floating hostility. These attributes are termed the *Type A behavior pattern* (TABP). Early retrospective studies supporting Friedman et al's initial observations found that patients with CHD were more likely to exhibit TABP than Type B behavior (2). Likewise, several prospective studies found TABP to be predictive of CHD events in initially healthy individuals, most notably the Western Collaborative Group Study (WCGS) (3).

Based on a critical review of such studies, an expert panel of biomedical and behavioral scientists convened by the National Heart, Lung, and Blood Institute concluded that TABP indeed contributed to CHD, conferring a twofold increased risk, which was of the same order of magnitude as cigarette smoking, hypertension, and elevated serum cholesterol. Furthermore, this risk was independent of traditional risk factors (4).

More recently, studies investigating the relationship between TABP and various clinical endpoints have provided inconsistent results. For example, a 22-year follow-up study of the WCGS did not support the earlier findings of a relationship between CHD and TABP (5). Several other more recent studies also have raised questions regarding the association between TABP and CHD, including the Multiple Risk Factor Intervention Trial (6) and the Aspirin Myocardial Infarction Study (7). Thus, recent reviews of the research have qualified the TABP-CHD relationship (8–10). TABP is a multidimensional construct best represented by component measures (11), and it is clear that not all aspects of TABP are pathogenic.

Based on these considerations, many investigators have narrowed their focus and refined their analyses of Type A components. Hostility has been the most extensively studied of these components (12). Interview ratings of hostility have been associated with CHD in cross-sectional studies (13,14). Similarly, prospective studies have shown behavioral ratings of hostility to predict initial CHD events and further development of CHD (15). Along these lines, Goodman et al (16) found that patients undergoing percutaneous transluminal angioplasty (PTCA) with high hostility ratings were 2.5 times more likely to have subsequent restenosis compared to low-hostility patients. Furthermore, hostility scores were positively correlated with the number of restenosed arteries. Although the follow-up of the WCGS failed to support the earlier findings of a relationship between global TABP and clinical events, analysis of these data indicated increased mortality rates among those highest in hostility (17), and further analysis of the 8½-year follow-up data showed hostility to be a significant risk factor for CHD (18).

Self-reporting measures also have been used to investigate the relationship between hostility and coronary artery disease (CAD). In an early cross-sectional study of 424 patients undergoing diagnostic coronary arteriography, Williams et al (19) found that hostility, as measured by the Cook-Medley Scale, and TABP were both independently related to atherosclerosis. However, hostility scores were more strongly associated with atherosclerosis than was TABP. These findings have been strengthened by studies that have found similar results with other indicators of disease activity, such as frequency and severity of myocardial ischemia (20). In addition, prospective studies also have shown Cook-Medley hostility scores to predict CHD morbidity and overall mortality (21,22).

Recent reviews of the literature support the role of hostility in CHD (12,23–25). Thus, hostility has been shown to be a robust independent risk factor for CHD morbidity and mortality across numerous studies, despite differences in measurement tools, subject populations, and outcomes studied, and is therefore a target for many interventional studies in cardiac patients.

Depression and Anxiety

In addition to personality traits such as TABP and hostility that have been identified as risk factors for adverse cardiac events, it has been observed that myocardial infarction (MI) and sudden death may be preceded by excessive fatigue, lack of energy, hopelessness, and other symptoms of general distress (26). Depression in particular has been found to be a relatively common psychiatric disorder among individuals with CAD and constitutes an important risk factor for cardiac morbidity and mortality (27,28). Carney et al (29), for instance, found major depressive disorder to be the best predictor of major cardiac events over a 12-month follow-up period of patients found to have CHD determined by cardiac catheterization. Furthermore, the relationship was independent of disease severity or smoking status.

Depression is particularly common among patients following an MI or cardiac surgery. Prevalence estimates of depression in this group are as high as 45% or more (30,31), and nearly 20% of patients meet criteria for major depression, compared to only about 3% of comparable members of the general population (32). Depression is a significant factor in relation both to patients' adjustment after a cardiac event and to future morbidity and mortality (33,34). In one study, for example, Frasure-Smith et al (28) found depression to be significantly related to cardiac mortality at 6- and at 12-month follow-up and to be a significant predictor of mortality even after controlling for other important predictors, including previous MI, Killip class, and premature ventricular contractions (PVCs) of 10 or more per hour.

Vital exhaustion is a condition that resembles depression but occurs without feelings of sadness and other symptoms such as feelings of worthlessness or guilt. Several studies have shown that vital exhaustion is related to cardiac events and CHD severity (35–37). Kop et al (35) found vital exhaustion to predict new cardiac events in 127 post-PTCA patients during 1.5 years of follow-up (odds ratio = 2.7). Multiple logistic regression showed the predictive value of vital exhaustion to be independent of traditional risk factors and initial disease severity.

Anxiety also is a risk factor for CHD events. In a meta-analytic review of 14 studies that investigated the relationship between anxiety and coronary disease, Friedman et al (38) found anxiety to be a significant predictor of cardiac events, including both MI and angina. More recent studies have supported these findings and in particular point to a relationship between anxiety and sudden cardiac death (39). In one prospective study evaluating the association between symptoms of anxiety and risk of CHD using data from the Normative Aging Study, Kawachi et al (40) found that, over 32 years of follow-up, the multivariate adjusted odds ratio for men reporting two or more anxiety symptoms was 1.94 for fatal coronary heart disease and 4.46 for sudden cardiac death.

As with depression, prevalence rates of moderate to severe anxiety among MI patients in the hospital are relatively high, with estimates as high as 40% or more (41). Moreover, about 15% to 20% of patients still report anxiety 1 year after hospital discharge. Frasure-Smith (42) evaluated 461 post-MI men in the hospital and followed them for over 5 years. A high level of psychological distress in the hospital was found to confer a threefold increase in cardiac mortality over the 5 years of follow-up. In addition, highly stressed patients had 1.5 times the risk of recurrent MI over follow-up. In a related study, anxiety was associated with an adjusted odds ratio of 2.21 for a later cardiac event (43). Similar studies of post-MI patients also have found anxiety to have prognostic significance for future problems, including the occurrence of cardiac arrhythmias (44).

Acute Emotional Distress

Acute emotional distress, in addition to chronic traits, also has been implicated in the occurrence of cardiac events in CHD patients. For example, Kark et al (45) examined the association between a life-threatening stressor, Iraqi missile attacks on Israel during the Gulf War in 1991, and subsequent mortality. The number of daily deaths during the 4-month period surrounding the war increased from December through January and subsequently declined through mid-March. In particular, there was an abrupt, significant increase in the number of deaths on January 18, the day of the first strike on Israeli cities, with a significant 58% increase in mortality risk on the first day of attacks. This increase was mainly due to CHD, other cardiovascular diseases, and a group of unknown causes, most probably representing sudden cardiac death.

In a naturalistic study of severe stress—a catastrophic natural disaster—Leor et al (46) reviewed the county coroner's records from the time surrounding the massive Los Angeles earthquake in January 1994. Results indicated that the number of sudden cardiac deaths rose sharply from a daily average of 4.6 in the preceding week to 24 on the day of the earthquake, only 3 of which could be attributed to physical exertion. Because the number of sudden cardiac deaths declined during the 6 days following the earthquake, to a daily average of only 2.7, the authors concluded that the earthquake itself was a significant trigger of sudden cardiac death, and based on the fact that sudden deaths due to cardiac causes declined in the week after the earthquake, that emotional stress precipitated cardiac events in predisposed individuals.

In addition to extreme emotional stress, everyday stressors have been shown to have potentially damaging health consequences. Mental stress, for example, has been shown to provoke myocardial ischemia in the laboratory in 50% to 66% of cardiac patients with prior evidence of exercise-induced ischemia (47–50). Moreover, stress during daily life has been associated with an increased incidence of ischemia measured by ambulatory monitoring (51–53), as well as with the occurrence of MI (54). Using the recently developed case-crossover design, Mittleman et al (54) reported a relative risk of 2.3 for MI in the 2 hours following an episode of anger, indicating that anger was a trigger that doubled the risk of MI.

CONTEXTUAL OR ENVIRONMENTAL FACTORS

Social Support

A lack of social support and social isolation have been implicated as risk factors for both cardiac morbidity and mortality. Prospective studies have found initially healthy individuals as well as post-MI patients who live alone or who lack adequate social support to be at increased risk of future cardiac events, independent of other known risk factors. Case et al (55) observed a 6-month mortality of 15.8% among post-MI patients living alone (16.4% of total sample) versus only 8.8% among those living with others. In a follow-up study of patients with angiographically documented CAD, Williams et al (56) observed a 5-year mortality rate of 50% among those who were most socially isolated (unmarried with no confidant; 2.6% of total sample) versus only 17% among those not so isolated. Given their large sample sizes (1234 and 1368, respectively), strong effects, and ability to statistically control for known biomedical predictors, these studies provide strong evidence for the important contribution of social isolation to poor outcomes in patients with established CAD. In a study of 194 elderly post-MI patients, Berkman et al (57) reported that the presence of emotional support prior to the MI was the post powerful and significant predictor of survival after the MI. At 1-year follow-up, 55% of patients without support had died, compared to only 27% with two or more sources of support. In all of these studies the impact of social isolation on prognosis was independent of left ventricular ejection fraction and other potent biomedical prognostic factors. Although an insufficient number of minority patients were included to ascertain the impact of social isolation upon their prognosis, these studies did include enough women to show that social isolation led to poorer prognosis in both genders.

Low Socioeconomic Status

It has long been known that low socioeconomic status (SES) is a significant contributor to increased CHD risk in healthy persons and to poor prognosis in CHD patients (58). Ruberman et al (59) found low education level to be a potent predictor of mortality, although not independently of social isolation. Williams et al (56) found that the 5-year mortality

rate of CAD patients with incomes less than $10,000/year was 1.9 times higher than that among patients with incomes greater than $40,000/year. This effect was independent of social isolation and disease severity. Case et al (55) also found SES, as documented by less than a twelfth grade education, to predict increased first recurrent events, independently of social isolation or physical risk factors. Taken altogether, these findings make a convincing case that low SES does contribute to poor prognosis in established CAD. The evidence suggests that SES has an impact over and above that conveyed by social isolation, but it is plausible to suggest that at least some of the adverse effects of low SES are mediated by its associations with depression and social isolation. Depressive symptoms are inversely related to SES in the general population (60), so that SES may interact with psychosocial risk factors and potentially produce an additive effect.

Job Strain

Certain job characteristics, either by themselves or in combination, also have been implicated as psychosocial risk factors for coronary disease, in particular psychological workload and decision latitude (61). Job strain, which involves a combination of these two factors, has been the subject of intensive research in recent years. The job strain model characterizes exposure to psychosocial job stressors along the two dimensions of *demand* (psychological workload) and *control* (decision latitude). In a prospective study of CAD risk among Swedish men, Karasek et al (61) found that high job demands were associated with disease. Low decision latitude on the job, characterized by low intellectual discretion and low personal schedule freedom, was associated with the development of cardiac symptoms, and the job strain combination of low personal control over schedules and high job demands was associated with a fourfold increase in risk of cardiovascular-related death. These relationships remained significant after controlling for age, education, and overweight. Subsequent research has supported this relationship between the combination of high job demand and low control and increased risk of both CAD (62–64) and risk factors for CAD including hypertension and increased left ventricular mass (65).

POTENTIAL MECHANISMS LINKING PSYCHOSOCIAL VARIABLES AND CORONARY HEART DISEASE

Several hypotheses have been proposed regarding the mechanisms whereby psychosocial variables may increase the risk for the development of CAD and the occurrence of clinical CHD events. It is widely believed that the relationship between psychosocial variables and CHD is mediated by activity of the sympathetic-adrenomedullary system, as reflected by heightened cardiovascular and neuroendocrine responses to behavioral stimuli including mental stress.

Cardiovascular and Neuroendocrine Reactivity

Exaggerated cardiovascular and neuroendocrine responses to psychosocial stressors have been proposed as one mechanism for promoting the progression of CAD and clinical CHD events. Animal studies have shown a relationship between enhanced cardiovascular responses and atherosclerosis (66). In addition, heightened responses to behavioral challenges in humans have been associated with increased cardiac mortality (67) and with the occurrence of myocardial ischemia (47), as well as with risk factors for CAD, including hypertension and dyslipidemia (68,69).

The process by which recurrent activation of the sympathetic nervous system, involving exaggerated heart rate and blood pressure responses to stress, may contribute to atherosclerosis is likely through its contribution to endothelial injury. Among the possible causes of such injury are mechanical forces, such as turbulence and sheer stress. In addition, chronic neuroendocrine hyperreactivity producing increased levels of circulating catecholamines, corticosteroids, and reproductive hormones may promote endothelial dysfunction, as well as other physiologic changes. Stress may also affect clotting factors, and may acutely promote plaque rupture.

Not all individuals respond to stress in the same way, however, and psychophysiologic studies of humans have shown significant variability in cardiovascular and neuroendocrine reactivity to laboratory stressors. Exaggerated responsivity to stress may be considered an individual difference characteristic, and investigators have sought to associate psychosocial variables, including personality traits (e.g., TABP), mood (e.g., anger), and contextual variables (e.g., harassment or competition), that distinguish high and low reactors (70).

Heart Rate Variability

In addition to the contribution of heightened sympathetic and neuroendocrine activity, the antagonism of the parasympathetic nervous system on sympathetic activity also may influence the pathogenesis of CAD. The balance between sympathetic and parasympathetic (vagal) activity can be assessed using analysis of heart rate variability (HRV), in which decreased variability is an independent risk factor for mortality among patients with CAD. Research has shown that laboratory challenges can disrupt the sympathovagal balance, such that sympathetic nervous system activity becomes dominant under stress (71), suggesting that chronic negative arousal may be associated with decreased HRV. Indeed, research has shown decreased HRV to be associated with TABP (72,73), as well as with anxiety (74) and depression (75). Alternatively, the mechanism by which such psychological traits or states impact HRV also may be behavioral, for example, through nonadherence to regimens that affect sympathovagal balance, including regular physical activity and use of cardiac medications.

Myocardial Ischemia

Recent research has examined the relationship between stress and myocardial ischemia. Laboratory studies (47,49) have shown that exercise testing produces significant increases in heart rate and blood pressure, and that the double product, an indicator of myocardial oxygen demand, is consequently significantly elevated. Although mental stress is also associated with increases in blood pressure and heart rate, it generally does not produce as great an increase in heart rate as exercise, but may be associated with greater diastolic blood pressure responses. The double product associated with mental stress, therefore, is considerably less than the double product associated with exercise. This suggests that increased myocardial

oxygen demand is not the only determinant of mental stress–induced ischemia and that myocardial oxygen supply also may be restricted during mental stress ischemia.

The possibility that a reduction in myocardial oxygen supply may be at least partially responsible for mental stress ischemia has been investigated in studies of both animals (76) and humans (77). Such research has indicated differential vasomotor responses in stenosed versus nonstenosed coronary arteries; whereas vasodilation occurs in normal segments of coronary arteries during mental stress, paradoxical vasoconstriction leading to myocardial ischemia occurs in atherosclerotic segments. Although the precise substances responsible for such vasoconstriction have not been identified, it is known that several neurohumoral substances, such as catecholamines, are released during mental stress and may be responsible for abnormal vasoconstriction.

PSYCHOSOCIAL INTERVENTIONS: IMPACT ON PROGNOSIS

More than a half-dozen clinical trials of CHD patients have evaluated the efficacy of interventions aimed at reducing the adverse impact of psychosocial factors on the prognosis of CHD patients, and offer encouragement that psychosocial interventions have the potential to reduce morbidity and mortality associated with adverse psychosocial risk profiles in CHD patients. Other studies, including both inpatients and outpatients, have demonstrated that psychosocial interventions can reduce distress and improve quality of life.

In-Hospital Psychosocial Intervention Programs

Several in-hospital psychosocial interventional studies have been conducted in post-MI patients in an effort to enhance their quality of life and improve their long-term survival. Brief interventions have been implemented as early as immediately following MI or surgery, during a patient's hospital stay, and have been associated with improvements in psychosocial and physical functioning. In an early evaluation of such an intervention, Gruen (78) studied the effects of brief supportive psychotherapy during hospitalization on the recovery of 70 MI patients. Results indicated that patients improved significantly on a variety of measures, including psychosocial functioning (depression, anxiety, and fear), return to normal activity, length of hospitalization, and number of days in intensive care.

Besides the medical benefits of such an intervention, reduced length of hospitalization and time spent in intensive care indicate that these programs also may be cost-effective. Such treatments may have a positive impact on patients' productivity, for example, in terms of how soon they return to work. Thockcloth et al (79) studied the effects on return-to-work rates of an intervention by a social worker and occupational therapist who saw cardiac patients within the first few days of admission to the hospital. Results of this study showed that the intervention patients returned to work significantly earlier than control patients.

Other studies of inpatient psychological therapies support these findings of improved psychosocial and physical functioning (80,81). To evaluate the overall efficacy of such programs across studies, Mumford et al (82) reviewed 34 controlled studies of in-hospital interventions consisting of informational or emotional support provided to surgical or MI patients. These authors found that patients receiving such support did better on average compared to patients who received ordinary care. Specifically, treated patients reported less anxiety, pain, and distress than controls, and they cooperated more with treatment, had fewer complications, and recovered more quickly. In fact, those patients receiving psychological treatment, as evaluated by 13 of these studies, were released from the hospital on average more than 2 days before control patients. Thus such interventions, although nonspecific and brief, are not only beneficial to the patient's psychological and physical well-being but are also cost-effective. In this era of managed care and cost containment, however, it remains to be seen if psychosocial interventions affect the length of hospital stays.

Outpatient Psychosocial Intervention Programs

Intervention programs specifically targeting psychosocial factors shown to play a role in coronary disease also have been implemented after hospitalization as part of more comprehensive and longer-term rehabilitation programs, both to reduce distress during rehabilitation and potentially to impact cardiac morbidity and mortality. This approach is based on research with both healthy individuals and CHD patients that has generally shown such psychosocial variables to be modifiable. Research has demonstrated, for example, that interventions for healthy TABP individuals result in reduced Type A behavior (83,84). Likewise, Type A behavior has been modified, to varying degrees, in patients with heart disease (85–87).

In one of the earliest psychosocial interventional studies, Adsett et al (88) observed that coronary patients lacking close family relationships and the support of friends had more difficulty adjusting after an MI. Their study assessed the efficacy of short-term group psychotherapy for six male post-MI patients having trouble adjusting to their situation, with treatment including their spouses. Results showed improved psychosocial adaptation for both patients and their spouses, although there was no control group. Similarly, Trzcieniecka-Green et al (89) studied the effects of a 12-week relaxation-based stress management program on a variety of psychosocial variables in 78 patients following MI, coronary artery bypass graft (CABG), or PTCA. After treatment and at follow-up, subjects showed significant improvements in anxiety, depression, general psychological well-being, activities of daily living, social activity, quality of interactions, and satisfaction with sexual relationships. Because there was no control group, however, conclusive statements about the results are not possible.

There have been a number of randomized, controlled trials assessing improvements in psychosocial factors in CAD patients, however, that support these findings. These studies have used a variety of therapeutic techniques, from relaxation training and cognitive-behavioral treatment to group counseling. Stern et al (90) evaluated the effects of group counseling versus exercise therapy in 160 MI patients who exhibited a low functional capacity on treadmill testing, were anxious and/or depressed, or both. Subjects were randomly assigned to 12 weeks of an exercise program, group counseling, or a control group. Both active groups showed improvements in

psychological functioning as compared to the control group. Specifically, the subjects who underwent group counseling substantially reduced their level of depression and interpersonal friction and increased their sense of friendliness, independence, and sociability, whereas the control group showed no changes.

Van Dixhoorn et al (91) evaluated the impact of adding relaxation training to a traditional physical conditioning program in 69 MI patients who were randomly assigned to an exercise and relaxation group or an exercise-only control group. Patients in the relaxation training group showed significant improvements in well-being and feelings of invalidism, whereas those in the exercise-only group did not show psychological improvements. Additionally, in this study patients with coronary-prone (Type A) behavior patterns showed the greatest improvements resulting from relaxation training. Van Dixhoorn et al have replicated these results and other research supports these findings as well (92). Using an alternative approach, Lewin et al (93) implemented a home-based psychosocial self-help program for post-MI patients. These authors found that psychological adjustment, as assessed by the Hospital Anxiety and Depression Scale, was better in the treatment group compared to the control group. Moreover, those in the treatment group had significantly fewer hospital readmissions during the first 6 months, and they had significantly less contact with their doctors over the next year. As in many of these studies, the greatest improvements were seen in those patients who were clinically anxious or depressed at baseline.

A limited number of studies have extended this research using cardiac morbidity and mortality as clinical outcomes. In a controlled trial of brief group psychotherapy for post-MI patients, for example, Rahe et al (94) randomly assigned 44 patients to either a control condition or a supportive, educational group therapy condition with a modest emphasis on modification of coronary-prone behaviors. All patients were followed for 3 years. Patients in the treatment condition showed significantly less coronary morbidity, including arrhythmias, mild to moderate congestive heart failure, and angina pectoris, as well as lower mortality at follow-up compared to control patients, and this was not explained by changes in conventional coronary risk factors. Therapy patients, however, did show changes in certain coronary-prone behaviors. Because educational information presented in the therapy sessions was largely forgotten over follow-up, the authors concluded that it was primarily the general support provided by the therapy that explained the outcome differences.

In the Ischemic Heart Disease (IHD) Life Stress Monitoring program (95,96), 461 post-MI men patients were assigned to either a usual care condition or an experimental intervention in which a monitor would call once a month and administer Goldberg's General Health Questionnaire (GHQ). Whenever a patient's responses generated a GHQ score of 5 or more, the monitor informed the nurse assigned to that patient, who would then schedule a home visit to work with the patient until the patient's problems were resolved or he or she was able to deal with them alone and the GHQ score had returned to normal. No single theory or approach to stress reduction was used; rather, the nurses' "mandate was to try and lower the stress levels of their patients using whatever strategies and interventions seemed appropriate for each patient." This intervention can best be characterized as one that provided patients with added social support, both instrumental in terms of dealing with problems and emotional in terms of providing a caring human being to listen to the patient describe his or her problems.

The monitoring group began to exhibit reduced mortality relative to the usual care group after 4 months. By the end of the first 12 months of follow-up, the monitoring group experienced a 47% reduction in cardiac mortality relative to the usual care group. Interestingly, of the patients on beta-blockers, 11% of the controls died compared to only 3% of the treated group, suggesting that stress management might further complement medical therapy. Long-term follow-up revealed that the group with high distress (GHQ $\geq$ 5) assigned to stress monitoring/nurse intervention experienced significant reductions in both recurrent MI ($p = .004$) and cardiac mortality ($p = .006$) over 5 years. Whether in usual care or monitoring intervention groups, the low-distress group (GHQ < 5) experienced lower mortality than the high-distress group assigned to usual care. Thus, it was only in those with high distress that the psychosocial intervention in this study led to improved prognosis.

The IHD Life Stress Monitoring study had several methodologic limitations. First, no women were included in the sample. Because women are as susceptible to psychosocial factors following MI as men (55,59) and have an even poorer overall prognosis than men following MI, it is essential that future intervention trials include women in numbers sufficient to evaluate the impact of the intervention upon their prognosis. Because minority groups have not been present in any of the studies in sufficient numbers to evaluate the impact of psychosocial factors upon their prognosis following MI, it will also be essential to include them in any future intervention trials, both to document whether psychosocial factors affect their prognosis and to show whether such effects, if present, can be ameliorated by the interventions used.

A second problem in the IHD Life Stress Monitoring study was that patients were asked for their consent after randomization had occurred. Differences in refusal rates between the two conditions led to several imbalances between the groups; for example, the control group contained a significantly larger proportion of low-SES patients than the monitoring group, indicating a bias whereby low-SES patients were less likely to volunteer for the monitoring condition if randomized to it. *Post hoc* analyses of the response of subgroups to the monitoring intervention suggested that even though underrepresented in the monitoring group, low-SES patients' prognosis was more positively affected by the intervention than that of high-SES patients. Moreover, after control for the SES differences between control and treatment groups using Cox proportional hazards regression, the group assignment was still significantly associated with survival. Given the known impact of low SES on survival following MI, however, it will be essential in future intervention studies to include adequate numbers of low-SES patients and to ensure that they are adequately represented in treatment and control groups.

A third limitation of the IHD Life Stress Monitoring study was the absence of any process variables (e.g., adherence to regimens, myocardial ischemia, or arrhythmias

assessed with ambulatory ECG), apart from the GHQ, that might have helped explain why the intervention worked or for whom.

Recently, Frasure-Smith et al (97) attempted to replicate their findings in a new sample of 1376 post-MI men and women. Patients completed a baseline interview that included assessment of anxiety and depression. Patients were then randomized to either an intervention condition or to a usual care control group. As in the earlier study, patients randomly assigned to the intervention were telephoned 1 week after discharge, and then every month for 1 year. If a patient scored 5 or more on the 20-item GHQ scale or he or she was readmitted to the hospital, the research assistant contacted the study nurse who then arranged for an initial 1-hour visit at the patient's home or at another convenient location. After the first visit, the nurse then arranged for a second visit within a month, and subsequent visits were arranged as needed.

The intervention had no overall survival impact (the overall odds ratios were 1.44 and 1.41 for cardiac and all-cause mortality, respectively). Moreover, there was a higher cardiac (9.4% versus 5.0%) and all-cause mortality (10.3% versus 5.4%) among women in the intervention group. There was no evidence of either benefit or harm among men. However, this study had a major flaw: There was no evidence that the intervention successfully reduced the patients' distress levels. Indeed, patients apparently were more distressed than in the previous study, but the nurses failed to successfully lower their subjective distress. Because the intervention failed to significantly reduce distress, it is not surprising that the intervention had no beneficial impact on clinical outcomes.

In a large-scale study of post-MI patients, the Recurrent Coronary Prevention Project (RCPP) (98) randomized 1035 men and women who had suffered an MI within the past 6 months to cardiologic counseling (n = 270) or to an intervention that included cardiac counseling but also included a behavioral program designed to reduce Type A behavior (n = 592). A third group, who refused randomization, formed an additional usual care control group. The intervention consisted of weekly group meetings in which cognitive behavior therapy and behavior therapy principles were applied to train patients in skills and strategies to reduce Type A behavior, including both the time urgency and hostility components. Subjects were given "drills" to practice as homework between group meetings, and the results of their efforts were shared with other group members at the meetings. The intervention was successful in reducing both time urgency and hostility, using behavioral observation to assess these components. At 3-year follow-up, statistically significant reductions in Type A behaviors were observed in those assigned to the Type A counseling treatment group. In addition, CHD recurrence rates were significantly lower (7.2%) among the treatment group compared with the control group (13%). This pattern continued at the 4½-year assessment, marking the end of treatment, with 35.1% of treatment group participants showing a marked reduction in Type A behaviors compared to 9.8% in the control group, and a cardiac recurrence rate of 12.9% in the treatment group versus 21.1% in the control group and 28.2% in the nonrandom comparison group (87).

As a further evaluation of the efficacy of Type A counseling in this cohort, at the end of the 4½-year study, Friedman et al switched 300 of the treatment subjects into a no-treatment control group and 114 of the former control subjects into a Type A counseling group and followed them for 1 year. The formerly treated controls were found to have maintained their reduced Type A behavior and their relatively low cardiac recurrence rate. Moreover, those former controls who underwent 1 year of treatment significantly reduced their Type A behavior and showed a similar significant reduction in cardiac morbidity. Altogether, these results demonstrated a significant benefit of Type A counseling in reducing both Type A behavior and recurrent cardiac events. Furthermore, this benefit persisted well after the cessation of treatment. Mendes de Leon et al (99) reported on the specific behavioral and psychosocial changes that occurred as a result of the Type A treatment program in the RCCP. They found that patients in the treatment group showed significant reductions not only in global TABP, but also in the components of hostility, time urgency, and impatience. Furthermore, they had reduced depression and anger and improvements in self-efficacy, social support, and well-being. As with the initial IHD Life Stress Monitoring study, the RCPP enrolled mostly men and too few minority group members to evaluate its impact upon them. Another omission was the absence of any reports of process variables that might be mediators of the treatment benefits.

Another intervention study was that of Ornish et al (100) in which 48 patients with angiographically documented CAD were assigned to usual care (n = 20) or a comprehensive lifestyle change program (n = 28) incorporating exercise, low-fat vegetarian diet, stopping smoking, and stress management training, with twice-weekly group support meetings. Adherence to all aspects of the program was carefully monitored. Compared to the usual care group, patients in the intervention group were more likely to show regression of angiographically documented lesions after 1 year in the program. The patients who were most adherent to the overall program showed the most pronounced regression of their coronary stenoses.

Given the comprehensive and extensive nature of the intervention in this study, it is not possible to identify which aspects of the program were responsible for the regression of arterial lesions. Certainly social support was provided by the twice-weekly group meetings and may have played an important part, but in the absence of a controlled design that permits evaluation of the impact of the various components, it is only possible to say that the "package" was responsible for whatever benefits were observed. The observation that those most adherent to the overall program experienced the greatest decrease in arterial stenoses is useful in guiding future trials to assess adherence to the intervention regimen. The Ornish et al study also obtained consent after patients were informed of their group assignment, so that strict randomization procedures were not followed. Moreover, the sample size was too small to determine if changes in the extent of CAD were associated with reductions in clinical CHD events.

Other clinical studies also have examined the effect of behavioral interactions on morbidity and mortality but lacked adequate power to detect group differences (101,102). One study that was adequately powered, however, failed to show significant benefits for the psychosocially treated group (103). In this large-scale clinical trial conducted in Great Britain, 2328 patients discharged home from the hospital within 28 days from a confirmed MI participated in a randomized clini-

cal trial comparing usual care to a comprehensive rehabilitation program comprising psychological therapy, counseling, relaxation training, and stress management training over seven weekly group outpatient sessions for patients and their spouses. At 6 months' follow-up, there were no significant differences between rehabilitation patients and controls in reported anxiety and depression. Rehabilitation patients reported less angina and medication. At 12 months there were no differences in clinical complications, clinical sequelae, health service use, return to work, or mortality. It was concluded that rehabilitation programs offered little objective benefit to post-MI patients. However, the short duration of the intervention and the failure to document treatment effectiveness were major limitations of the study. Indeed, the prevalence of clinical anxiety and depression remained high (33% and 19%, respectively), which suggests that the intervention failed to effectively modify those relevant psychosocial risk factors that are thought to affect clinical prognosis. Therefore, like the Frasure-Smith et al study (97), it is not surprising that the interventions that were unable to alter psychosocial risk factors would also fail to reduce clinical cardiac events.

A recent Duke study of patients with mental stress–induced myocardial ischemia reported that patients who underwent 16 weeks of stress management training exhibited a relative risk of further cardiac events of only 0.26 compared to usual care controls (104). In this study, 107 men and women with documented coronary disease and evidence of either ambulatory ischemia or mental stress–induced ischemia were assigned to stress management or exercise training or to a usual care control group. Although the Duke study had several methodologic shortcomings, including a nonrandom control group, the findings demonstrated that stress management was effective in reducing stress-induced ischemia and ambulatory ischemia. Moreover, the 74% reduction in clinical events including MI, death, and revascularization procedures because of progressive angina was highly significant. Exercise training also was associated with a 32% reduction in risk for cardiac events, although this reduction did not achieve statistical significance.

The intervention trials reviewed above have several features in common. All included some aspect—whether regular group meetings or nurse home visits—that *directly* provided patients with added social support, over and above whatever support systems they had access to on their own. This suggests that providing social support has considerable promise as an intervention that will improve prognosis in patients with established CAD. The Ornish et al study, the RCPP, and the Duke study also included instruction in what can be broadly characterized as stress management techniques—relaxation skills, cognitive strategies to decrease anger and hurrying, communication and assertion skills, time management, and the like. In addition to whatever direct benefits these components of the intervention provided (e.g., decreased sympathetic activation caused by relaxation and anger control), they also have the potential to increase social support *indirectly* (i.e., if one is not hostile toward one's family and friends, they may be more likely to provide social support). Another useful aspect of Frasure-Smith et al's intervention was the use of a tailored, stepped-care approach in which the patient got help only when a threshold (GHQ ≥ 5) was exceeded, and then the help was continued until the problem was resolved.

As reviewed above, the extant research on psychosocial interventions in post-MI patients suggests that programs that provide the patient with social support may be beneficial. Randomized trials that specify or target particular patients (e.g., patients with high levels of psychological distress, depression, or social isolation) are needed to determine whether these interventions are effective in reducing mortality and morbidity among these patients at increased psychosocial risk.

An important point to keep in mind is the fact that the vast majority of studies have focused on white, middle-class men. The most effective interventions will most likely be those that are specifically targeted at psychosocial issues of relevance to individual patients or groups of patients. It is therefore essential to determine the generalizabililty of research thus far and to explore the psychosocial factors that may be more or less salient for other ethnic groups and for women. One of the few studies looking at such differences between men and women (105), for example, found that women reported poorer quality of life than men, especially regarding psychosocial functioning and emotional behavior, and this was independent of functional capacity. Women in this study had a higher incidence of other comorbid conditions, especially arthritis, and were more likely than men to be widowed, thereby making them more vulnerable to the negative impact of social isolation.

In an attempt to quantify the efficacy of psychosocial interventions within cardiac rehabilitation programs and to determine whether or not the addition of such treatments to traditional drug and exercise interventions improves patient outcomes, Linden et al (106) performed a meta-analysis of 23 randomized controlled trials that included data on anxiety, depression, biological risk factors, mortality, and recurrence of cardiac events. The total subject pool included 2024 patients in psychosocial treatment compared to 1156 control patients. Results of the analysis showed improvements in psychological distress, systolic blood pressure, heart rate, and cholesterol levels for those patients in the psychosocial intervention groups. Furthermore, control patients experienced higher mortality and cardiac event recurrence rates during the first 2 years of follow-up, with log-adjusted odds ratios of 1.70 for mortality and 1.84 for recurrence, representing a 41% reduction in cardiac all-cause mortality and a 46% reduction in nonfatal cardiac events for psychosocially treated patients.

CONCLUSIONS

Psychosocial variables play an important role in the development and clinical manifestations of CHD, and contribute to

adjustment and quality of life following MI and cardiac surgery. Future research should be to determine the generalizability of findings. In particular, studies should target minorities and women, both to determine whether or not the same pychosocial factors relevant to white men play a similar role in the development of CHD in these groups, and to determine the efficacy of psychosocial interventions in their treatment. Not all therapies may be helpful to all patients, depending on a variety of individual and environmental factors. For example, in the recent study by Frasure-Smith et al (97), older women actually had higher mortality rates in the treated group relative to controls. It will also be important, therefore, to assess the appropriateness of various approaches for different patients and to evaluate the benefits of implementing more individualized programs. SES, age, gender, coping style, type and level of distress, social support, and disease severity, among others, are all relevant factors that may influence the psychosocial adjustment of patients with CAD as well as the effectiveness of treatment. Lower-SES patients, for example, may face a variety of daily stressors that differ from those experienced by more affluent patients, and these stressors must be taken into account in any effort to reduce these patients' distress levels.

More research is needed to identify other factors that distinguish those who could potentially benefit from such interventions and those who do not so that high-risk patients can be targeted for psychosocial treatment. One large-scale study that has recently begun specifically targets such high-risk individuals. The Enhancing Recovery in Coronary Heart Disease (ENRICHD) Study is a multicenter clinical trial to determine the effects of psychosocial intervention, aimed at increasing social support and reducing depression, in post-MI patients who are at high psychosocial risk because of depression or low perceived social support. Primary endpoints in this study include all-cause mortality and recurrent MI; secondary endpoints include revascularization procedures, cardiovascular hospitalizations, and changes in risk factors, as well as changes in the severity of depression, degree of social support, and health-related quality of life. More such clinical trials are needed because there is currently a paucity of randomized clinical trials of psychosocial interventions for CHD patients. Lastly, research is clearly needed to determine the mechanisms underlying the detrimental effects of psychosocial variables on cardiovascular health as well as those responsible for the improvements resulting from successful psychosocial interventions.

REFERENCES

1. Friedman M, Rosenman RH. Association of specific overt behavior pattern with blood and cardiovascular findings. JAMA 1959;169:1286–1296.

2. Dembroski TM, Weiss SM, Shields JL, eds. Coronary prone

behavior. New York: Springer-Verlag, 1978.

3. Rosenman RH, Brand RJ, Jenkins D, et al. Coronary heart disease in the Western Collaborative Group Study: final follow-up experience of 8½ years. JAMA 1975;233:872–877.

4. Review Panel on Coronary-Prone Behavior and Coronary Heart Disease. Coronary-prone behavior and coronary heart disease: a critical review. Circulation 1981; 63:1199–1215.

5. Ragland DR, Brand RJ. Type A behavior and mortality from coro-

nary heart disease. N Engl J Med 1988;318:65–69.

6. Shekelle RB, Hulley SB, Neaton JD, et al. The MRFIT Behavior Pattern Study, II: type A behavior and incidence of coronary heart disease. Am J Epidemiol 1985; 122:559–570.

7. Shekelle RB, Gale M, Norusis M. Type A score (Jenkins Activity Survey) and risk of recurrent coronary heart disease in the Aspirin Myocardial Infarction Study. Am J Cardiol 1985;56: 221–225.

8. Manuck SB, Kaplan JR, Matthews KA. Behavioral antecedents of coronary heart disease and atherosclerosis. Arteriosclerosis 1986;6:2–14.

9. Matthews KA, Haynes SG. Type A behavior pattern and coronary risk: update and critical evaluation. Am J Epidemiol 1986;123: 923–960.

10. Miller TQ, Turner CW, Tindale RS, et al. Reasons for the trend toward null findings in research on Type A behavior. Psychol Bull 1991;110:469–485.

11. Edwards JR, Baglioni AJ Jr. Relationship between Type A behavior pattern and mental and physical symptoms: a comparison of global and component measures. J Appl Psychol 1991;76(2):276–290.

12. Smith TW. Hostility and health: current status of a psychosomatic hypothesis. Health Psychol 1992; 11(3):139–150.

13. Dembroski TM, MacDougall JM, Williams RB, et al. Components of Type A, hostility, and anger in relationship to angiographic findings. Psychosom Med 1985; 47(3):219–233.

14. MacDougall JM, Dembroski TM, Dimsdale JE, Hackett TP. Components of Type A, hostility, and anger-in: further relationships to angiographic findings. Health Psychol 1985;4:137–152.

15. Matthews KA, Glass DC, Rosenman RH, Bortner RW. Competitive drive, pattern A, and coronary heart disease: a further analysis of some data from the Western Collaborative Group Study. J Chron Dis 1977;30: 489–498.

16. Goodman M, Quigley J, Moran G, et al. Hostility predicts restenosis after percutaneous transluminal coronary angioplasty. Mayo Clin Proc 1996;71(8):729–734.

17. Carmelli D, Halpern J, Swan GE, et al. 27-year mortality in the Western Collaborative Group Study: construction of risk groups by recursive partitioning. J Clin Epidemiol 1991;44(12):1341–1351.

18. Hecker MH, Chesney MA, Black GW, et al. Coronary-prone behaviors in the Western Collaborative Group Study. Psychosom Med 1988;50:153–164.

19. Williams RB Jr, Haney TL, Lee KL, et al. Type A behavior, hostility, and coronary atherosclerosis. Psychosom Med 1980;42:539–549.

20. Helmers KF, Krantz DS, Merz CN, et al. Defensive hostility: relationship to multiple markers of cardiac ischemia in patients with coronary disease. Health Psychol 1995;14:202–209.

21. Barefoot JC, Dahlstrom WG, Williams RB. Hostility, CHD incidence, and total mortality: a 25-year follow-up study of 255 physicians. Psychosom Med 1983;45(1):59–63.

22. Shekelle RB, Gale M, Ostfeld AM, Paul O. Hostility, risk of coronary heart disease, and mortality. Psychosom Med 1983;45: 109–114.

23. Booth-Kewley S, Friedman HS. Psychological predictors of heart disease: a quantitative review. Psychol Bull 1987;101(3):343–362.

24. Matthews KA. Coronary heart disease and type A behaviors: update on and alternative to the Booth-Kewley and Friedman (1987) quantitative review. Psychol Bull 1988;104:373–380.

25. Miller TQ, Smith TW, Turner CW, et al. A meta-analytic review of research on hostility and physical health. Psychol Bull 1996; 119(2):322–348.

26. Van Diest R, Appels A. Vital exhaustion and depression: a conceptual study. J Psychosom Res 1991;35:535–544.

27. Frasure-Smith N, Lespérance F, Talajic M. Depression following myocardial infarction: impact on 6-month survival. JAMA 1993; 270(15):1819–1825.

28. Frasure-Smith N, Lespérance F, Talajic M. Depression and 18-month prognosis after myocardial infarction. Circulation 1995; 91(4):999–1005.

29. Carney RM, Rich MW, Freedland KE, et al. Major depressive disorder predicts cardiac events in patients with coronary artery disease. Psychosom Med 1988; 50(6):627–633.

30. Burker EJ, Blumenthal JA, Feldman M, et al. Depression in male and female patients undergoing cardiac surgery. Br J Clin Psychol 1995;34(pt 1):119–128.

31. Trelawney-Ross C, Russell O. Social and psychological responses to myocardial infarction: multiple determinants of outcome at six months. J Psychosom Res 1987;31:125–130.

32. Carney RM, Rich M, teVelde A, et al. Major depressive disorder in coronary artery disease. Am J Cardiol 1987;60(16):1273–1275.

33. Ahern DK, Gorkin L, Anderson JL, et al. Biobehavioral variables and mortality or cardiac arrest in the Cardiac Arrhythmia Pilot Study (CAPS). Am J Cardiol 1990;66(1):59–62.

34. Barefoot JC, Helms MJ, Mark DB, et al. Depression and long-term mortality risk in patients with coronary artery disease. Am J Cardiol 1996; 78(6):613–617.

35. Kop WJ, Appels APWM, de Leon CFM, et al. Vital exhaustion predicts new cardiac events after successful coronary angioplasty. Psychosom Med 1994;56:281–287.

36. Falger PR, Schouten EG. Exhaustion, psychological stressors in the work environment, and acute myocardial infarction, in adult men. J Psychosom Res 1992; 36(8):777–786.

37. Appels A, Mulder P. Excess fatigue as a precursor of myocardial infarction. Eur Heart J 1988; 9(7):758–764.

38. Friedman HS, Booth-Kewley S. The "disease-prone personality": a meta-analytic view of the construct. Am J Psychol 1987; 42(6):539–555.

39. Kawachi I, Colditz GA, Ascherio A, et al. Prospective study of phobic anxiety and risk of coronary heart disease in men. Circulation 1994;89:1992–1997.

40. Kawachi I, Sparrow D, Vokonas PS, Weiss ST. Symptoms of anxiety and risk of coronary heart disease: the Normative Aging Study. Circulation 1994;90: 2225–2229.

41. Stern MJ, Pascale L, McLoone JB. Psychosocial adaptation following an acute myocardial infarction. J Chron Dis 1976;29: 523–526.

42. Frasure-Smith N. In-hospital symptoms of psychological stress as predictors of long-term outcome after acute myocardial infarction in men. Am J Cardiol 1991;67(2):121–127.

43. Frasure-Smith N, Lespérance F, Talajic M. The impact of negative emotions on prognosis following myocardial infarction: is it more than depression? Health Psychol 1995;14(5):388–398.

44. Follick MJ, Gorkin L, Capone FJ, et al. Psychological distress as a predictor of ventricular arrhythmias in a post-myocardial infarction population. Am Heart J 1988;116(1 pt 1):32–36.

45. Kark JD, Goldman S, Epstein L. Iraqi missile attacks on Israel: the association of mortality with a life-threatening stressor. JAMA 1995;273:1208–1210.

46. Leor J, Poole WK, Kloner RA. Sudden cardiac death triggered by an earthquake. N Engl J Med 1996;334:413–419.

47. Blumenthal JA, Jiang W, Waugh RA, et al. Mental stress-induced ischemia in the laboratory and ambulatory ischemia during daily life: association and hemodynamic features. Circulation 1995;92(8):2102–2108.

48. Deanfield JE, Shea M, Kensett M, et al. Silent myocardial ischemia due to mental stress. Lancet 1984;2(8410):1001–1005.

49. Rozanski A, Bairey CN, Krantz DS, et al. Mental stress and the induction of silent myocardial ischemia in patients with coronary artery disease. N Engl J Med 1988;318:1005–1012.

50. Tavazzi L, Bosimini E, Giubbini R, et al. Silent ischemia during mental stress: scintigraphic evidence and electrocardiographic patterns. Adv Cardiol 1990;37: 53–66.

51. Barry J, Selwyn AP, Nabel EG, et al. Frequency of ST-segment depression produced by mental stress in stable angina pectoris from coronary artery disease. Am J Cardiol 1988;61(13):989–993.

52. Gabbay FH, Krantz DS, Kop WJ, et al. Triggers of myocardial ischemia during daily life in patients with coronary artery disease: physical and mental activities, anger, and smoking. J Am Coll Cardiol 1996;27(3): 585–592.

53. Gullette ECD, Blumenthal JA, Babyak M, et al. Effects of mental stress on myocardial ischemia during daily life. JAMA 1997;277(19):1521–1526.

54. Mittleman MA, Maclure M, Sherwood JB, et al for the Determinants of Myocardial Infarction Onset Study Investigators. Triggering of acute myocardial infarction onset by episodes of anger. Circulation 1995;92:1720–1725.

55. Case RB, Moss AJ, Case N, et al. Living alone after myocardial infarction: impact on prognosis. JAMA 1992;267(4):515–519.

56. Williams RB, Barefoot JC, Cliff RM, et al. Prognostic importance of social and economic resources among medically treated patients with angiographically documented coronary artery disease. JAMA 1992;267:520–524.

57. Berkman LF, Leo-Summer L, Horowitz R. Emotional support and survival after myocardial infarction. Ann Intern Med 1992; 117:1009–1013.

58. Kaplan GA, Kiel JE. Socioeconomic factors and cardiovascular disease: a review of the literature. Circulation 1993;88:1973–1993.

59. Ruberman W, Weinblatt E, Chaudhary JD, et al. Psychosocial influences on mortality after myocardial infarction. N Engl J Med 1984;311:552–559.

60. Adler NE, Boyce T, Chesney MA, et al. Socioeconomic status and health: the challenge of the gradient. Am Psychol 1994;49: 308–315.

61. Karasek RA, Baker D, Marxer F, et al. Job decision latitude, job demands, and cardiovascular disease: a prospective study of Swedish men. Am J Public Health 1981;71:694–705.

62. Karasek RA, Theorell TG, Schwartz JE, et al. Job characteristics in relation to the prevalence of myocardial infarction in the US Health Examination Survey (HES) and the Health and Nutrition Examination Survey (HANES). Am J Public Health 1988;78:910–918.

63. Karasek RA, Theorell TG, Schwartz JE, et al. Job, psychological factors and coronary heart disease: Swedish prospective findings and U.S. prevalence findings using a new occupational inference method. Adv Cardiol 1982;29: 62–67.

64. Tyroler A, Haynes SG, Cobb LA, et al. Environmental risk factors in coronary heart disease. Circulation 1987;76(suppl I):139–144.

65. Schnall PL, Peiper C, Schwartz JE, et al. The relationship

between 'job strain,' workplace diastolic blood pressure, and left ventricular mass index: results of a case-control study. JAMA 1990;263:1929–1935.

66. Manuck SB, Kaplan JR, Clarkson TB. Behaviorally induced heart rate reactivity and atherosclerosis in cynomolgus monkeys. Psychosom Med 1983;45:95–108.

67. Keys A, Taylor HL, Blackburn H, et al. Mortality and coronary heart disease among men studied for 23 years. Arch Intern Med 1971;128:201–214.

68. Barnett PH, Hines EA, Schirger A, et al. Blood pressure and vascular reactivity to the cold pressor test. JAMA 1963;183: 845–848.

69. Burker EJ, Fredrikson M, Rifai N, et al. Serum lipids, neuroendocrine and cardiovascular responses to stress in men and women with mild hypertension. Behav Med 1994;19(4):155–161.

70. Krantz DS, Manuck SB. Acute psychophysiologic reactivity and risk of cardiovascular disease: a review and methodologic critique. Psychol Bull 1984;96:435–464.

71. Pagani M, Mazzuero G, Ferrari A, et al. Sympathovagal interaction during mental stress: a study using spectral analysis of heart rate variability in healthy control subjects and patients with a prior myocardial infarction. Circulation 1991;83(suppl 4):II43–II51.

72. Kamada T, Miyake S, Kumashiro M, et al. Power spectral analysis of heart rate variability in Type As and Type Bs during mental workload. Psychosom Med 1992;54: 462–470.

73. Kamada T, Sato N, Miyake S, et al. Power spectral analysis of heart rate variability in Type As during solo and competitive mental arithmetic task. J Psychosom Res 1992;36:543–551.

74. Kawachi I, Sparrow D, Vokonas PS, Weiss ST. Decreased heart rate variability in men with phobic anxiety (data from the Normative Aging Study). Am J Cardiol 1995;75:882–885.

75. Carney RM, Saunders RD, Freedland KE, et al. Association of depression with reduced heart rate variability in coronary artery disease. Am J Cardiol 1995; 76(8):562–564.

76. Verrier RL, Hagestad EL, Lown B. Delayed myocardial ischemia induced by anger. Circulation 1987;75:249–254.

77. Yeung AC, Vekshtein VI, Krantz DS, et al. The effect of atherosclerosis on the vasomotor response of coronary arteries to mental stress. N Engl J Med 1991;325:1551–1556.

78. Gruen W. Effects of brief psychotherapy during the hospitalization period on the recovery process in heart attacks. J Consult Clin Psychol 1975;43(2): 223–232.

79. Thockcloth RM, Ho SO, Wright W. Is cardiac rehabilitation really necessary? Med J Aust 1973;2: 669–674.

80. Langosch W, Seer P, Brodner G, et al. Behavior therapy with coronary heart disease patients: results of a comparative study. J Psychosom Res 1982;26(5): 475–484.

81. Oldenburg B, Perkins RJ, Andrews G. Controlled trial of psychological intervention in myocardial infarction. J Consult Clin Psychol 1985;53:852–859.

82. Mumford E, Schlesinger H, Glass G. The effects of psychological intervention on recovery from surgery and heart attacks: an analysis of the literature. Am J Public Health 1982;72:141–151.

83. Jenni M, Wollersheim J. Cognitive therapy, stress management training, and the Type A behavior pattern. Cognitive Ther Res 1979;3:61–73.

84. Roskies E, Kearney H, Spevack M, et al. Generalizability and durability of treatment effects in an intervention program for coronary-prone (Type A) managers. J Behav Med 1979;2:195–207.

85. Burrell G, Sundin O, Strom G, et al. Heart and lifestyle: a Type A treatment program for myocardial infarction patients. Scand J Behav Ther 1986;15:87–93.

86. Razin AM, Swencionis C, Zohman LR. Reduction of physiological, behavioral, and self-report responses in Type A behavior: a preliminary report. Int J Psychiatry Med 1986;16:31–47.

87. Friedman M, Thoresen CE, Gill JJ, et al. Alteration of Type A behavior and its effect on cardiac recurrences in postmyocardial infarction patients: summary results of the recurrent coronary prevention project. Am Heart J 1986;112(4):653–665.

88. Adsett CA, Bruhn JG. Short-term group psychotherapy for postmyocardial infarction patients and their wives. Can Med Assoc J 1968;99(12):577–584.

89. Trzcieniecka-Green A, Steptoe A. Stress management in cardiac patients: a preliminary study of the predictors of improvement in quality of life. J Psychosom Res 1994;38:267–280.

90. Stern MJ, Gorman PA, Kaslow L. The group counseling v exercise therapy study: a controlled intervention with subjects following myocardial infarction. Arch Intern Med 1983;143:1719–1725.

91. Van Dixhoorn J, de Loos J, Duivenvoorden HJ. Contribution of relaxation training to the rehabilitation of myocardial infarction patients. Psychother Psychosom 1983;40:137–147.

92. Van Dixhoorn J, Duivenvoorden HJ, Pool J, Verhage F. Psychic effects of physical training and relaxation therapy after myocardial infarction. J Psychosom Res 1990;34:327–337.

93. Lewin B, Robertson IH, Cay EL, et al. Effect of self-help postmyocardial infarction rehabilitation on psychological adjustment and use of health services. Lancet 1992;339:1036–1040.

94. Rahe RH, Ward HW, Hayes V. Brief group therapy in myocardial infarction rehabilitation: three- to four-year follow-up of a controlled trial. Psychosom Med 1979;41: 229–242.

95. Frasure-Smith N, Prince R. The ischemic heart disease life stress monitoring program: impact on mortality. Psychosom Med 1985; 47:431–445.

96. Frasure-Smith N, Prince R. Long-term follow-up of the ischemic heart disease life stress monitoring program. Psychosom Med 1989;51:485–513.

97. Frasure-Smith N, Lespérance F, Prince R, et al. Randomised trial of home-based psychosocial nursing intervention for patients recovering from myocardial infarction. Lancet 1997;350: 473–479.

98. Friedman M, Thoreson CD, Gill JJ, et al. Feasibility of altering Type A behavior after myocardial infarction: Recurrent Coronary Prevention Project Study: methods, baseline results and preliminary findings. Circulation 1982;66:83–92.

99. Mendes de Leon CF, Powell LH, Kaplan BH. Change in coronary-prone behaviors in the Recurrent Coronary Prevention Project. Psychosom Med 1991; 53:407–419.

100. Ornish D, Brown SE, Scherwitz LW, et al. Can lifestyle changes reverse coronary heart disease? the lifestyle heart trial. Lancet 1990;336:129–133.

101. Dracup K. A controlled trial of couples group counseling in cardiac rehabilitation. J Cardiac Rehabil 1985;5(9):436–442.

102. van Dixhoorn J, et al. Cardiac events after myocardial infarction: possible effects of relaxation therapy. Eur Heart J 1987;8: 1210–1214.

103. Jones DA, West RR. Psychological rehabilitation after myocardial infarction: multicentre randomized controlled trial. Br Med J 1996;313:1517–1521.

104. Blumenthal JA, Jiang W, Babyak M, et al. Stress management and exercise training in cardiac patients with myocardial ischemia: effects on prognosis and evaluation of mechanisms. Arch Intern Med 1997;157: 2213–2223.

105. Loose MS, Fernhall B. Differences in quality of life among male and female cardiac rehabilitation participants. J Cardiopulm Rehabil 1995;15:225–231.

106. Linden W, Stossel C, Maurice J. Psychosocial interventions for patients with coronary artery disease: a meta analysis. Arch Intern Med 1996;156:745–752.

Chapter 71

Peripheral Vascular Disease Rehabilitation

Andrew W. Gardner

Atherosclerotic cardiovascular disease is the most significant health problem in the United States; heart and cerebrovascular diseases were the first and fourth leading causes of death in 1990, respectively (1). Atherosclerosis in the arteries of the lower extremities (peripheral vascular disease) is also an important medical concern because there is a high risk that concomitant coronary and cerebral artery disease is present (2), and because ischemic pain in the leg musculature severely limits daily physical activities. One of the more common forms of peripheral vascular disease is peripheral arterial occlusive disease (PAOD), resulting from atherosclerosis of the arteries of the lower extremities. Although the majority of the research literature on PAOD has come from the discipline of vascular surgery, the field of exercise physiology is growing in importance because of the need to rehabilitate this patient population with a program of regular exercise. The synergistic collaboration between these two disciplines is particularly important for the clinical management of PAOD patients, because the primary goal for the vascular surgeon is to improve circulation and limb viability, while the primary concern of the exercise physiologist is to regain function that was lost through the years of having this chronic disease. This chapter will concentrate on the following topics: significance of PAOD, definition and classification of PAOD, cardiovascular risk associated with PAOD, risk factors for PAOD, acute exercise responses in PAOD patients, exercise rehabilitation programs for PAOD patients, and methods to evaluate the effectiveness of an exercise program.

DEFINITION AND CLASSIFICATION

Peripheral arterial occlusive disease occurs from lesions that develop in the abdominal aorta, iliac, femoral, popliteal, and tibial arteries. Consequently, blood flow distal to the arterial lesions is reduced, which ultimately has a negative impact on ambulation and functional independence of elderly patients with PAOD. The hallmark clinical measure for detecting PAOD is the ankle/brachial index (ABI), which is the ratio of systolic blood pressure measured in the ankle and in the arm (3). In PAOD patients, the reduction in leg blood flow results in a low ankle pressure and a low ABI value. The prevalence of PAOD is highly dependent on the exact ABI cutpoint used to detect inadequate peripheral circulation. Based on the literature, the definition of an abnormal ABI has ranged from 0.80 to 0.97 (4–7), with a value of 0.90 or lower generally considered to be the best reference standard (8). The normal range of ABI is widely accepted as a value of 1.00 or higher, with values between 0.91 and 1.00 considered to represent borderline PAOD (8). The prevalence of PAOD is 10% in the general population above age 55 when an ABI value of 0.90 or lower is used as the definition of PAOD (8).

In the early stages of PAOD, the reduction in blood flow does not result in any noticeable symptoms, and is defined as stage I (asymptomatic PAOD) according to the widely accepted Fontaine classification system (Table 71-1) (9). As PAOD progresses, ischemic pain in the leg musculature occurs when patients walk, and is classified as stage II (intermittent claudication). Stage II patients can be further classified as having mild intermittent claudication (pain-free walking distance >200 m) or severe intermittent claudication (pain-free walking distance <200 m). In more advanced stages of disease, blood flow is reduced to such an extent that pain is experienced even while at rest (stage III, rest pain). Further progression of the disease leads to ischemic ulcerations on the lower extremities and gangrene (stage IV, gangrene/tissue loss). Patients with stage III or stage IV PAOD have critical

Table 71-1 Fontaine Classification of Peripheral Arterial Occlusive Disease	
STAGE	**SYMPTOMS**
I	Asymptomatic
II	Intermittent claudication
IIa	Pain-free, claudication walking >200 m
IIb	Pain-free, claudication walking <200 m
III	Rest pain
IV	Gangrene, tissue loss

leg ischemia in which the ischemic process endangers part or all of the lower extremity. These patients usually are candidates for aggressive intervention such as surgery, and are managed clinically by vascular surgeons.

Clinicians clearly have their greatest impact on the clinical management of mildly affected patients with stage I and stage II PAOD, and in revascularized patients who typically have significant hemodynamic improvements but who may remain functionally dependent due to the extreme deconditioning process that occurs with critical leg ischemia. These patients usually are good candidates for more conservative treatments such as exercise rehabilitation and/or medication therapy. It should be noted that if asymptomatic PAOD patients (stage I) can be identified, they probably are ideal candidates for exercise rehabilitation because the atherosclerotic process has not advanced enough to interfere with the ability to exercise. The focus of the remainder of this chapter will center on the evaluation and treatment of patients with stage I and stage II PAOD.

EPIDEMIOLOGY AND ECONOMICS

Peripheral arterial occlusive disease is a slowly progressive disease manifest by lesions in the arteries of the lower extremities. Due to its progressive nature, PAOD is highly prevalent in the elderly population. The annual incidence of PAOD increases sharply with age; the rate increases 342% from 26 cases per 20,000 men and women between the ages of 45 and 54 to 115 cases per 20,000 men and women between the ages of 65 and 74 (9). Given that the number of people over age 65 in the United States is projected to grow to 67 million by the year 2040 (10), as many as 400,000 people will develop PAOD every year over the next 40 years. Consequently, PAOD is emerging as a significant cause of disability in the American population.

The economic impact of PAOD is substantial. The standard medical care has primarily consisted of drug treatment for patients with mild PAOD, and surgery for patients with more severe disease. Altogether, PAOD accounts for 267,000 hospitalizations, 2.7 million office visits, and 42,500 deaths in the United States annually (11). The estimated 1994 national health care cost for PAOD surgical procedures alone was over $3.3 billion per year (12). The combination of a 69% growth rate in the elderly population by the year 2020 (13), and the 107% to 132% increase in the cost and number

of PAOD-related surgical procedures (12) indicates that the health care and financial burden of PAOD will escalate over the next few decades.

CARDIOVASCULAR RISK

The presence of PAOD is associated with a poor prognosis of long-term survival (14–19). Compared to subjects without PAOD, the relative risk for all-cause mortality associated with PAOD ranges between 1.8 and 3.1 (16–18), indicating that the mortality rate is 80% to 210% higher in patients with abnormally low ABI values of 0.85 or lower (16) or 0.90 or lower (17–18). McKenna et al (16) report a 5-year survival estimate for PAOD patients and non-PAOD controls of 63% and 90%, respectively, while the 10-year survival was 46% and 77%. Vogt et al (18) report an even lower 10-year survival estimate of 39% and 35% in older men and women with PAOD, respectively.

The prognosis of PAOD patients worsens as the severity of PAOD increases (14–18). For example, patients with ABI values of 0.30 or lower had a relative risk of death of 1.8 compared to patients with ABI values between 0.50 and 0.91 (15), and patients with ABI values of 0.40 or lower had a 3.35 relative risk for mortality compared to patients with ABI values above 0.85 (16). Additionally, the cardiovascular mortality in symptomatic PAOD patients (stages II, III, and IV) was 11 times higher than in non-PAOD controls (20), while in asymptomatic PAOD patients (stage I), the mortality rate was only 5 times higher.

The relationship between the presence and severity of PAOD with subsequent mortality is stronger than in many other medical conditions known to reduce survival. The adjusted relative risk for mortality associated with PAOD (2.36) was higher than the risk of diabetes (1.64) or stroke (1.88), and was second only to congestive heart failure (2.38) (16). However, PAOD patients with severe disease (ABI ≤ 0.30) had a greater relative risk than congestive heart failure patients (15). These data suggest that PAOD is of substantial medical concern and that, once identified, patients with PAOD should undergo interventions designed to improve their cardiovascular disease risk factor profile and to increase their functional capacity to prevent complications from the disease.

RISK FACTORS FOR PAOD

Risk factors for PAOD are typical of those for coronary artery disease, including cigarette smoking, race (non-Caucasian), diabetes, age, systolic blood pressure, body mass index (BMI), high density lipoprotein cholesterol (HDL-C), total cholesterol, creatinine, and forced vital capacity (21–23). In addition, properties of blood rheology and coagulation also play a role in the development of arterial occlusive disease. Increased blood viscosity and plasma fibrinogen are associated with the clinical course of PAOD (24) and with higher risks of coronary artery disease and recurrent myocardial infarction (25–26). Elevated levels of plasminogen activator inhibitor-1 activity and tissue plasminogen activator antigen also are related to the progression and complications of atherosclerosis

(27–30). Finally, preliminary evidence shows that physical inactivity is independently associated with a lower ABI in men and women who have ABI values in the normal range (31), supporting the notion that activity level may be a factor contributing to the development of PAOD (32).

Exercise training has a beneficial effect in reducing blood viscosity and red cell aggregation in PAOD patients (33), as well as improving the fibrinolytic profile in young and old healthy subjects (34), patients who have experienced myocardial infarction (35), and patients with type II diabetes (36). Thus, exercise rehabilitation may improve the clinical outcomes of PAOD patients by altering the more traditionally accepted risk factors (e.g., blood lipids, blood pressure, obesity) as well as measures of blood rheology and coagulation. Furthermore, exercise rehabilitation is the method of choice to improve functional outcomes in PAOD patients who have ambulatory disability due to intermittent claudication (37).

EXERCISE REHABILITATION PROGRAMS FOR PAOD PATIENTS

Improvements in Claudication Measurements

Significant improvements in claudication pain occur following exercise rehabilitation. For example, a recent meta-analysis (37) demonstrates that in 21 exercise rehabilitation studies (33,38–57) conducted between 1966 and 1993, the average distance walked on a treadmill to onset of claudication pain increased 179% from 126 ± 57 m (mean ± standard deviation) to 351 ± 189 m following rehabilitation, and the average distance walked to maximal claudication pain increased 122% from 326 ± 148 m to 723 ± 592 m.

Potential Mechanisms for the Improvement in Claudication Measurements

Numerous mechanisms have been proposed to explain the improvement in walking distances to the onset and to maximal claudication pain following exercise rehabilitation. The mechanisms primarily center on hemodynamic and enzymatic adaptations within the exercising musculature of the symptomatic leg(s). Specifically, these mechanisms include an increased blood flow (38,47,56,58) to the exercising leg musculature, a more favorable redistribution of blood flow (57,59), greater utilization of oxygen (60) due to a higher concentration of oxidative enzymes (41), improved hemorheological properties of the blood (33), a decreased reliance upon anaerobic metabolism (55,60), and an improvement in the efficiency of walking (61,62). It may be that no one particular mechanism is primarily responsible for the improvement in claudication pain symptoms with exercise rehabilitation. Rather, it may be that a combination of changes in these factors contributes to the improved waking distances. Improvements in psychosocial attitude due to accomplishments that are achieved during exercise rehabilitation may further enhance this effect.

To address the peripheral hemodynamic mechanism, a number of studies have assessed ABI and calf blood flow both before and after a program of exercise. On average, calf blood flow under resting and maximal conditions increases by approximately 19% (41–44,47,48,50–52,57,60,63–66) and

ABI increases by approximately 7% (45,49–52,55,58,59,65–67) following exercise rehabilitation. Only a few studies have examined the change in redistribution of peripheral blood flow, blood viscosity, leg arteriovenous oxygen difference, concentration of oxidative enzymes, and efficiency of walking. Consequently, the changes in these variables following exercise rehabilitation are not well established in PAOD patients. Since the magnitude of change in calf blood flow and ABI does not approach that of the changes in the walking distances to onset (179%) and to maximal (122%) claudication pain (37), either small changes in peripheral blood flow yield exponential improvements in claudication pain symptoms, or the other mechanisms mentioned above also contribute to the improved outcome.

Exercise Program Components Predicting Improved Claudication Measurements

Although substantial increases in the average distances to onset and to maximal claudication pain during treadmill walking are noted in the above studies, considerable variability among the studies exists. For example, the increased distance to onset of pain ranges between 72% and 746%, and the increased distance to maximal pain ranges between 61% and 739% (37). Differences in the components of exercise programs (e.g., intensity, duration, and frequency of exercise sessions) may largely account for these widely divergent responses. Although the previous exercise programs are generally effective in the treatment of intermittent claudication, none of the studies compared different components of exercise to determine an optimal exercise rehabilitation program.

Because no experimental study can systematically examine the effects of all of the components of an exercise rehabilitation program, the literature was analyzed by meta-analysis techniques to identify the most important exercise components for eliciting optimal improvements in claudication pain distances. Six of the following components were examined: 1) frequency of exercise (sessions per week); 2) duration of exercise (minutes per session); 3) mode of exercise (walking vs. a combination of exercises); 4) length of the program (weeks); 5) claudication pain endpoint used in the program (onset vs. near maximal pain); and 6) level of supervision (supervised vs. supervised plus home-based exercise). All of the exercise rehabilitation components had a significant effect on the magnitude of change in the claudication distances except for the level of supervision. For example, programs that exercised patients to near-maximal claudication pain were more effective than programs that exercised patients to only the onset of pain (Fig. 71-1). Additionally, programs consisting of higher exercise duration, higher frequency, greater program length (Fig. 71-2), and walking as the only mode of exercise (Fig. 71-3) were more effective than programs consisting of lower exercise duration, lower frequency, shorter program length, and having patients train by a variety of exercise modes. The addition of home exercise to supplement the amount of exercise performed in a supervised setting did not result in additional ambulatory benefit.

Of the five components that had an effect on the change in the claudicaton distances, only three were found to have an independent effect through multivariate analyses. These components were the claudication pain endpoint used

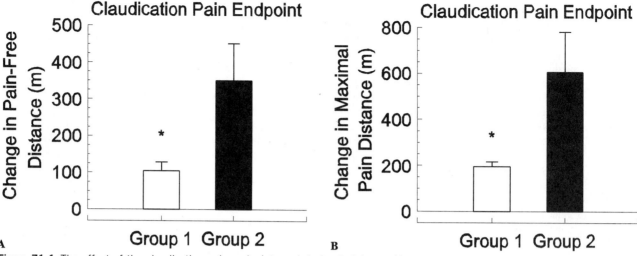

Figure 71-1 The effect of the claudication pain endpoint used during training sessions on changes in claudication pain distances from 21 studies (37). Group 1 = studies that had patients exercise to onset of claudication, Group 2 = studies that had patients exercise to near-maximal claudication. Values are adjusted means ± standard errors of the change in the pain-free (A) and maximal pain (B) distances after statistically controlling for the other five exercise program components. (*Significantly lower than group 2 [$p < 0.01$].)

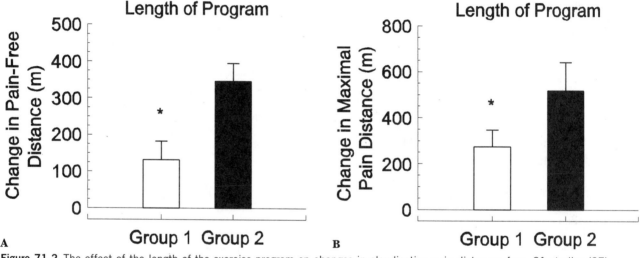

Figure 71-2 The effect of the length of the exercise program on changes in claudication pain distances from 21 studies (37). Group 1 = studies that had patients exercise less than 6 months, Group 2 = studies that had patients exercise at least 6 months. Values are adjusted means ± standard errors of the change in the pain-free (A) and maximal pain (B) distances after statistically controlling for the other five exercise program components. (*Significantly lower than group 2 [$p < 0.01$].)

in the program, the length of the program, and the mode of exercise (37). The combination of these components explained nearly 90% of the variance in the increase in the walking distances following exercise rehabilitation (37). Although the duration and frequency of the exercise sessions are not independent predictors of the change in claudication pain times, programs should have the patients walk for at least 30 minutes per session and for at least three sessions per week, as these amounts were more beneficial than programs using a lower exercise duration and frequency. Finally, it should be noted that the appropriate exercise intensity to use during training cannot be determined at this time because no study

has addressed this issue. There is a common misconception that walking beyond the onset of pain to near maximal pain is an increase in intensity when, in fact, it is merely an increase in duration. The rate of work performed while walking, regardless of the duration, is the important consideration when setting the appropriate exercise intensity. Since heart rate is commonly used as a means to adjust the intensity of exercise, a conservative recommendation for claudicants who are beginning rehabilitation is to walk at an appropriate speed and grade on a treadmill to elicit an intensity of approximately 50% of their heart rate reserve, and to gradually increase the intensity to 70% to 80% by completion of

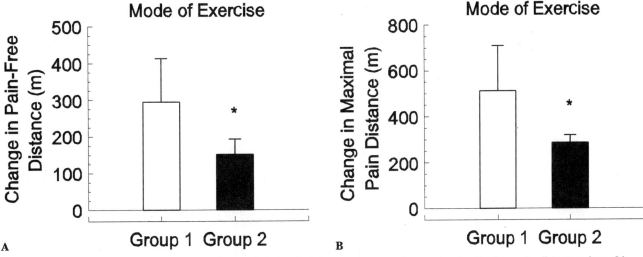

Figure 71-3 The effect of the mode of exercise used during training sessions on changes in claudication pain distances from 21 studies (37). Group 1 = studies that had patients train solely by walking, Group 2 = studies that had patients train using a combination of exercises. Values are adjusted means ± standard errors of the change in the pain-free (A) and maximal pain (B) distances after statistically controlling for the other five exercise program components. (*Significantly lower than group 1 [$p < 0.05$].)

Table 71-2 Recommended Exercise Program for Patients with Peripheral Arterial Occlusive Disease

EXERCISE COMPONENT	COMMENT
Frequency	3 exercise sessions per week
Intensity	Progression from 50% of peak exercise capacity to 80% by the end of the program
Duration	Progression from 15 min of exercise per session to more than 30 min by the end of the program
Mode	Weight bearing (e.g., walking, stair climbing). Non-weight bearing tasks (e.g., bicycling) may be used for warming up and cooling down
Type of Exercise	Intermittent walking to near maximal claudication pain
Program Length	At least 6 mos

the program. Recommendations for an exercise program for patients with PAOD are summarized in Table 71-2.

METHODS TO EVALUATE THE EFFECTIVENESS OF AN EXERCISE PROGRAM

The main effect that PAOD has on acute exercise is the development of claudication pain in the leg musculature due to insufficient blood flow. As a result, claudication and peripheral hemodynamic measurements obtained from a treadmill test are the primary criteria to assess the effectiveness of an exercise program (68). The specific claudication variables that are measured to assess the functional severity of PAOD include the distances (or times) to onset and to maximal claudication pain. Peripheral hemodynamic measurements are obtained in conjunction with claudication measurements to provide a more objective assessment of disease severity. The most accepted variable is the ankle systolic blood pressure measured before and after the treadmill test, which is needed to calculate ABI values.

The primary objective of a treadmill test for patients with PAOD is to obtain reliable measures of 1) the rate of claudication pain development, 2) the peripheral hemodynamic responses to exercise, and 3) the presence of coexisting coronary heart disease. The test should be a progressive test with gradual increments in grade. By having a test with small increases in exercise intensity, claudication distances of patients can be stratified according to disease severity. Highly reliable treadmill protocols for patients with PAOD utilize a constant walking speed of 2 mph and gradual increases in grade of either 2.0% or 3.5% every 2 minutes beginning at 0% grade (69,70). Typical distances to onset of pain and to maximal pain are approximately 170 m and 360 m, respectively (71). This protocol also is effective in documenting the inadequacy of the circulation in the lower extremities with exercise, as the ABI typically drops from a resting value of 0.6 to approximately 0.2 immediately following the treadmill test (69). Gas exchange measures during the treadmill test show that PAOD patients with intermittent claudication have peak oxygen consumption values in the range of 12 to 15 mL/kg per minute (72), which is approximately 50% of age-matched controls. Favorable changes following a program of exercise rehabilitation should include greater walking distances covered before the occurrence of the onset and maximal claudication pain, an increase in peak oxygen consumption, and possibly a blunted drop in ABI and a faster recovery of ABI to the resting baseline value.

Claudication and ABI are the most common measurements obtained in patients with intermittent claudication because the literature has primarily taken a vascular perspective on this population. However, further contributions to the literature concerning the improvement in function of PAOD patients following exercise rehabilitation may be best accomplished by taking more of a gerontologic perspective in the future, which goes beyond the measurement of claudication distances and ABI. Since the typical profile of a PAOD patient is that of an elderly person with chronic ambulatory disability, the decline in physical functioning with aging may be accelerated in this population due to the extreme deconditioning brought about from the disease process. Consequently, performance on a 6-minute walk test as well as measures of gait, walking economy, balance, flexibility, and lower extremity strength may be expected to be worse in PAOD patients than in age-matched controls, which may improve through a program of exercise rehabilitation. However, to date information on these measures in the PAOD population is sparse (73).

In addition to the above mentioned laboratory measures of physical function, assessment of the impact that ambulatory and functional limitations have on routine activities performed in the community setting may provide a truer measure of disability. The free-living daily physical activity measured by an accelerometer is one such measure because it quantifies the amount of movement done over an extended period of time. The free-living daily physical activity as measured by an accelerometer is approximately 33% lower in PAOD patients than in non-PAOD subjects of similar age, and it becomes progressively lower in claudicants with worsening disease severity as measured by ABI (74). Furthermore, cigarette smoking, which is common in the PAOD population, decreases the free-living daily physical activity by an additional 30% (75). Thus, PAOD patients with intermittent clau-

dication are at the extreme low end of the physical activity spectrum. It is not clear whether the typical improvements in claudication distances following exercise rehabilitation translate into increases in free-living daily physical activity in the community setting. Further research is needed to examine this issue as well as to determine whether functional improvements are related to enhanced quality of life in this elderly, disabled population.

SUMMARY

Peripheral arterial occlusive disease is a significant health concern in the elderly population that will continue to increase in future years. Conservative management of patients with asymptomatic PAOD and patients with intermittent claudication is recommended to modify risk factors and improve ambulatory ability, while patients with more severe PAOD typically require revascularization of the lower extremities. Exercise rehabilitation is a highly effective, conservative treatment to improve ambulation in patients with intermittent claudication. To date, the primary focus of attention on the benefits of exercise rehabilitation has centered on the increase in walking distances to onset and to maximal claudication pain during a treadmill test. Future research should focus on the improvement in other functional outcomes commonly reported in the geriatric literature that may be more representative of everyday activities such as submaximal exercise performance, walking economy, balance, flexibility, and lower extremity strength. Until these measures are obtained, the full benefit of exercise rehabilitation for PAOD patients remains unclear.

Dr. Gardner is supported by a Special Emphasis Research Career Award from the National Institute on Aging (NIA) (K01-AG-00657), by a Geriatric Leadership Academic Award from NIA (K07-AG00608), and by a Claude D. Pepper Older American Independence Center (OAIC) from NIA (P60-AG12583).

REFERENCES

1. U.S. health trends. J NIH Res 1992;4:95.

2. Kannel WB. Some lessons in cardiovascular epidemiology from Framingham. Am J Cardiol 1976; 37:269–282.

3. Carter SA. Clinical measurement of systolic pressures in limbs with arterial occlusive disease. JAMA 1969;207:1869–1874.

4. Crique MH, Fronek A, Barrett-Connor, et al. The prevalence of peripheral arterial disease in a defined population. Circulation 1985;71:510–515.

5. Hiatt WR, Marshall JA, Baxter J, et al. Diagnostic methods for peripheral arterial disease in the San Luis Valley Diabetes Study. J Clin Epidemiol 1990;43:597–606.

6. Carter SA. Indirect systolic pressures and pulse waves in arterial occlusive disease of the lower extremities. Circulation 1968;37:624–637.

7. Ouriel K, McDonnell AE, Metz CE, et al. A critical evaluation of stress testing in the diagnosis of peripheral vascular disease. Surgery 1982;91:686–693.

8. Weitz JI, Byrne J, Clagett P, et al. Diagnosis and treatment of chronic arterial insufficiency of the lower extremities: a critical review. Circulation 1996;94:3026–3049.

9. Pentecost MJ, Criqui MH, Dorros G, et al. Guidelines for peripheral percutaneous transluminal angioplasty of the abdominal aorta and lower extremity vessels. Circulation 1994;89:511–531.

10. Vogt MT, Wolfson SK, Kuller LH. Lower extremity arterial disease and the aging process: a review. J Clin Epidemiol 1992;45:529–542.

11. Kannel WB. The demographics of claudication and the aging of the American population. Vasc Med 1996;1:60–64.

12. Tunis SR, Bass EB, Steinberg EP. The use of angioplasty, bypass surgery, and amputation in the management of peripheral vascular disease. N Engl J Med 1991;325:556–562.

13. U.S. Department of Commerce, Economics and Statistics Administration Bureau of the Census. Global aging—comparative indicators and future trends. Washington DC: US Census Bureau, 1991.

14. Howell MA, Colgan MP, Seeger RW, et al. Relationship of severity of lower limb peripheral vascular disease to mortality and morbidity: a six-year follow-up study. J Vasc Surg 1989;9:691–697.

15. McGrae-McDermott M, Feinglass J, Slavensky R, et al. The ankle-brachial index as a predictor of survival in patients with peripheral vascular disease. J Gen Intern Med 1994;9:445–449.

16. McKenna M, Wolfson S, Kuller L. The ratio of ankle and arm arterial pressure as an independent predictor of mortality. Atherosclerosis 1991;87:119–128.

17. Vogt MT, Cauley JA, Newman AB, et al. Decreased ankle/arm blood pressure index and mortality in elderly women. JAMA 1993;270:465–469.

18. Vogt MT, McKenna M, Anderson SJ, et al. The relationship between ankle-arm index and mortality in older men and women. J Am Geriatr Soc 1993;41:523–530.

19. Vogt MT, Wolfson SK, Kuller LH. Segmental arterial disease in the lower extremities: correlates of disease and relationship to mortality. J Clin Epidemiol 1993;46:1267–1276.

20. Criqui MH, Langer RD, Fronek A, et al. Mortality over a period of 10 years in patients with peripheral arterial disease. N Engl J Med 1992;326:381–386.

21. Newman AB, Sutton-Tyrell K, Rutan GH, et al. Lower extremity arterial disease in elderly subjects with systolic hypertension. J Clin Epidemiol 1991;1:15–20.

22. Newman AB, Siscovick DS, Manolio TA, et al. Ankle-arm index as a marker of atherosclerosis in the cardiovascular health study. Circulation 1993;88:837–845.

23. Newman AB, Sutton-Tyrell K, Kuller LH. Lower-extremity arterial disease in older hypertensive adults. Arterioscler Thromb 1993;13:555–562.

24. Dormandy JA, Hoare E, Khattab AH, et al. Prognostic significance of rheological and biochemical findings in patients with intermittent claudication. BMJ 1973;4:581–583.

25. Kannel WB, Wolf PA, Castelli WP, et al. Fibrinogen and risk of cardiovascular disease: the Framingham study. JAMA 1987;258:1183–1186.

26. Benderly M, Graff E, Reicher-Reiss H, et al. Fibrinogen is a predictor of mortality in coronary heart disease patients. Arterioscler Thromb 1996;16:351–356.

27. Hamsten A, Wiman B, DeFaire U, et al. Increased plasma levels of a rapid inhibitor of tissue plasminogen activator in young survivors of myocardial infarction. N Engl J Med 1985;313:1557–1563.

28. Huber K, Jorg M, Probst P, et al. A decrease in plasminogen activator inhibitor 1 activity is associated with a significantly reduced risk for coronary restenosis. Thromb Haemost 1992;67:209–213.

29. Jansson JH, Nilsson TK, Olofsson BO. Tissue plasminogen activator and other risk factors as predictors of cardiovascular events in patients with severe angina pectoris. Eur Heart J 1991;12:157–161.

30. Lindgren A, Lindoff C, Norrving B, et al. Tissue plasminogen activator and plasminogen activator inhibitor-1 in stroke patients. Stroke 1996;27:1066–1071.

31. Gardner AW, Sieminski DJ, Montgomery PS. Physical activity is related to ankle/brachial index in subjects without peripheral arterial occlusive disease. Angiology 1997;48:883.

32. Housley E, Leng GC, Donnan PT, et al. Physical activity and risk of peripheral arterial disease in the general population: Edinburgh artery study. J Epidemiol Community Health 1993;47:475–480.

33. Ernst EEW, Matrai A. Intermittent claudication, exercise, and blood rheology. Circulation 1987;76:1110–1114.

34. Stratton JR, Chandler WL, Schwartz RS, et al. Effects of physical conditioning on fibrinolytic variables and fibrinogen in young and old healthy adults. Circulation 1991;83:1692–1697.

35. Estelles A, Aznar J, Tormo G, et al. Influence of a rehabilitation sports programme on the fibrinolytic activity of patients after myocardial infarction. Thrombosis Res 1989;55:203–212.

36. Schneider SH, Kim HC, Khachadurian AK, et al. Impaired fibrinolytic response to exercise in type II diabetes: effects of exercise and physical training. Metabolism 1988;37:924–929.

37. Gardner AW, Poehlman ET. Exercise rehabilitation programs for the treatment of claudication pain: a meta-analysis. JAMA 1995;274:975–980.

38. Alpert JS, Larsen A, Lassen NA. Exercise and intermittent claudication: blood flow in the calf muscle during walking studied by the Xenon-133 clearance method. Circulation 1969;39:353–359.

39. Carter SA, Hamel ER, Paterson JM, et al. Walking ability and ankle systolic pressures: observations in patients with intermittent claudication in a short-term walking exercise program. J Vasc Surg 1989;10:642–649.

40. Clifford PC, Davies PW, Hayne JA, et al. Intermittent claudication: is a supervised exercise class worth while? BMJ 1980;281:1503–1505.

41. Dahllof AG, Bjorntorp P, Holm J, et al. Metabolic activity of skeletal muscle in patients with peripheral arterial insufficiency: effect of physical training. Eur J Clin Invest 1974;4:9–15.

42. Dahllof AG, Holm J, Schersten T, et al. Peripheral arterial insufficiency: effect of physical training on walking tolerance, calf blood flow, and blood flow resistance. Scand J Rehab Med 1976;8:19–26.

43. Ekroth R, Dahllof AG, Gundevall B, et al. Physical training of patients with intermittent claudication: indications, methods, and results. Surgery 1978;84:640–643.

44. Ericsson B, Haeger K, Lindell SE. Effect of physical training on intermittent claudication. Angiology 1970;21:188-192.

45. Feinberg RL, Gregory RT, Wheeler JR, et al. The ischemic window: a method for the objective quantitation of the training effect in exercise therapy for intermittent claudication. J Vasc Surg 1992;16:244–250.

46. Holm J, Dahllof AG, Bjorntorp P, et al. Enzyme studies in muscles of patients with intermittent claudication: effect of training. Scand J Clin Lab Invest 1973;31(suppl):201–205.

47. Jonason T, Ringqvist I. Effect of training on the post-exercise ankle blood pressure reaction in patients with intermittent claudication. Clin Physiol 1987;7:63–69.

48. Larsen OA, Lassen NA. Effect of daily muscular exercise in patients with intermittent claudication. Lancet 1966;2:1093–1096.

49. Lepantalo M, Sundberg S, Gordin A. The effects of physical training and flunarizine on walking capacity in intermittent claudication. Scand J Rehab Med 1984;16:159–162.

50. Lundgren F, Dahllof AG, Schersten T, et al. Muscle enzyme adaptation in patients with peripheral arterial insufficiency: spontaneous adaptation, effect of different treatments and consequences on walking performance. Clin Sci 1989;77:485–493.

51. Mannarino E, Pasqualini L, Menna M, et al. Effects of physical training on peripheral vascular disease: a controlled study. Angiology 1989;40:5–10.

52. Mannarino E, Pasqualini L, Innocente S, et al. Physical training and antiplatelet treatment in stage II peripheral arterial occlusive disease: alone or combined? Angiology 1991;42:513–521.

53. Rosetzsky A, Struckmann J, Mathiesen FR. Minimal walking distance following exercise treatment in patients with arterial occlusive disease. Ann Chir Gynaecol 1985;74:261–264.

54. Rosfors S, Bygdeman S, Arnetz BB, et al. Longterm neuroendocrine and metabolic effects of physical training in intermittent claudication. Scand J Rehab Med 1989;21:7–11.

55. Ruell PA, Imperial ES, Bonar FJ, et al. Intermittent claudication: the effect of physical training on walking tolerance and venous lactate concentration. Eur J Appl Physiol 1984;52:420–425.

56. Skinner JS, Strandness DE Jr. Exercise and intermittent claudication: II. effect of physical training. Circulation 1967;36:23–29.

57. Zetterquist S. The effect of active training on the nutritive blood flow in exercising ischemic legs. Scand J Lab Invest 1970;25:101–111.

58. Hall JA, Barnard RJ. The effects of an intensive 26-day program of diet and exercise on patients with peripheral vascular disease. J Cardiac Rehabil 1982;2:569–574.

59. Jonason T, Ringqvist I. Prediction of the effect of training on the walking tolerance in patients with intermittent claudication. Scand J Rehab Med 1987;19:47–50.

60. Sorlie D, Myhre K. Effects of physical training in intermittent claudication. Scand J Clin Lab Invest 1978;38;217–222.

61. Ernst E. Physical exercise for peripheral vascular disease: a review. Vasa 1987;16:227–231.

62. Womack CJ, Sieminski DJ, Katzel LI, et al. Improved walking economy in patients with peripheral arterial occlusive disease. Med Sci Sports Exerc 1997;29:1286–1290.

63. Jonason T, Ringqvist I, Oman-Rydberg A. Home-training of patients with intermittent claudication. Scand J Rehab Med 1981;13:137–141.

64. Fitzgerald DE, Keates JS, MacMillan D. Angiographic and plethysmographic assessment of graduated physical exercise in the treatment of chronic occlusive arterial disease of the leg. Angiology 1971;22:99–106.

65. Hiatt WR, Regensteiner JG, Hargarten ME, et al. Benefit of exercise conditioning for patients with peripheral arterial disease. Circulation 1990;81:602–609.

66. Lundgren F, Dahllof AG, Lundholm K, et al. Intermittent claudication—surgical reconstruction or physical training? a prospective randomized trial of treatment efficiency. Ann Surg 1989;209:346–355.

67. Williams LR, Ekers MA, Collins PS, et al. Vascular rehabilitation: benefits of a structured exercise/risk modification program. J Vas Surg 1991;14:320–326.

68. Hiatt WR, Hirsch AT, Regensteiner JG, et al. Clinical trials for claudication: assessment of exercise performance, functional status, and clinical end points. Circulation 1995;92:614.

69. Gardner AW, Skinner JS, Cantwell BW, et al. Progressive versus single-stage treadmill tests for evaluation of claudication. Med Sci Sports Exerc 1991;23:402.

70. Hiatt WR, Nawaz D, Regensteiner JG, et al. The evaluation of exercise performance in patients with peripheral vascular disease. J Cardiopulmonary Rehabil 1988;12:525–532.

71. Gardner AW, Ricci MR, Pilcher DB, et al. Practical equations to predict claudication pain distances from a graded treadmill test. Vasc Med 1996;1:91–96.

72. Gardner AW. The effect of cigarette smoking on exercise capacity in patients with intermittent claudi-

cation. Vasc Med 1996;1:181–186.

73. Montgomery PS, Gardner AW. The clinical utility of a 6-minute walk test in peripheral arterial occlusive disease patients. J Am Geriatr Soc 1998;46:706–771.

74. Sieminski DJ, Gardner AW. The relationship between daily physical activity and the severity of peripheral arterial occlusive disease. Vasc Med 1997;2:174–178.

75. Gardner AW, Sieminski DJ, Killewich LA. The effect of cigarette smoking on free-living daily physical activity in older claudication patients. Angiology 1997;48:947–955.

Chapter 72

Contemporary Cardiac Rehabilitation: The Next Millennium

Nanette K. Wenger

Rehabilitation of the cardiac patient in the next millennium will likely differ substantially from that undertaken today, owing to a number of interrelated variables. Among these are changes in the demography of the population of the United States; changes in the demography of cardiovascular disease, and in particular changes in the clinical spectrum of coronary heart disease and of heart failure; a substantial expansion of the populations considered eligible for cardiac rehabilitative care; and an escalating emphasis on preventive interventions, with the boundaries between primary and secondary prevention tending to blur. Each of these issues is addressed in turn.

The Clinical Practice Guideline *Cardiac Rehabilitation*, released by the U.S. Agency for Health Care Policy and Research and cosponsored by the National Heart, Lung, and Blood Institute, highlighted that cardiac rehabilitation services, despite their proven benefits, are widely underutilized in the United States (1). Barriers to the use of cardiac rehabilitation services include a lack of physician referral, a lack of access to such services, a lack of insurance reimbursement for cardiac rehabilitative care, and personal reluctance to alter lifestyle habits. Remediation of these barriers remains an unmet need in the rehabilitation of the cardiac patient that hopefully will be progressively addressed in the next millennium.

CONTRIBUTORS TO THE CHANGING SPECTRUM OF CARDIAC REHABILITATION

Changes in the Demography of the U.S. Population

As is the case worldwide, there has been progressive aging of the U.S. population, with the subset of patients aged 80 years and older being the component with the greatest expansion in size. Half of 1.5 million episodes of myocardial infarction that occur annually affect patients older than 65 years of age. Based on 1993 data, 55% of the more than 300,000 U.S. patients who underwent coronary artery bypass graft (CABG) surgery were 65 years of age and older, as were 45% of the patients who had percutaneous transluminal coronary angioplasty (PTCA) or other transcatheter interventional procedures. Elderly patients are also at higher risk of disability following a coronary event than are their younger counterparts. Further, heart failure is the most common discharge diagnosis for hospitalized Medicare patients and the fourth most common discharge diagnosis for all patients hospitalized in the United States; heart failure of multiple and multifactorial etiologies may be the entry point to cardiac rehabilitation for many patients at elderly age. However, current rates of entry into cardiac rehabilitation in the United States are substantially lower for elderly than for younger patients (2,3), with elderly women even less likely to be referred than elderly men (4). Nonetheless, cardiac rehabilitation in the next millennium will, of necessity, include larger numbers of elderly and very elderly patients.

Changes in the Demography of Cardiovascular Disease in the United States

Coronary heart disease deaths increased sharply in the United States during the first half of the twentieth century, with mortality rates peaking in the mid-1960s and continuously declining in subsequent years. Whether this decline will persist remains conjectural, given the aging of the population. The decline in coronary mortality has been attributed to a variety of interventions, particularly those addressing acute coronary heart disease events and chronic manifestations of coronary heart disease. Included are the improved prehospital care of acute coronary events, improvement of pharmacologic therapies and of both transcatheter and surgical revascularization procedures, and progressively intensive efforts to reduce traditional coronary risk factors, both before and following an initial coronary event.

By contrast, heart failure has become the new cardiac epidemic, with heart failure the only cardiovascular diagnosis that continues to increase in prevalence. This likely reflects the success in managing a broad variety of underlying cardiovascular illnesses and prolonging survival, with heart failure the final common pathway for patients with multiple presentations of coronary heart disease, of hypertension, and of valvular heart disease, among others, particularly at elderly age (5). Not only has the prevalence of heart failure increased steadily with aging of the U.S. population, but the improved rates of survival attendant on the use of newer therapies for a variety of cardiovascular disease events have engendered an expanding population with residual ventricular dysfunction. It is currently estimated that 4.7 million patients in the United States with heart failure are potential candidates for cardiac rehabilitation. Many of these patients with end-stage heart failure of a variety of etiologies become candidates for cardiac transplantation. Cardiac rehabilitation is now an intrinsic component of both the preoperative and postoperative management of heart failure patients undergoing cardiac transplantation, owing to the documentation of its benefits and safety (1,6).

Expansion of the Population Considered Eligible for Cardiac Rehabilitation

In the early years of cardiac rehabilitation, the 1950s to the 1970s, the major innovative intervention was exercise training, which was applied predominantly to patients recovering from an uncomplicated myocardial infarction. Early criteria developed by the American Heart Association identified as unsuitable for exercise rehabilitation patients older than 65 years of age, patients with complications of myocardial infarction, patients with cardiac enlargement or heart failure, patients with serious arrhythmias, and patients with a variety of other complicating or comorbid illnesses. By the end of the twentieth century, many categories of patients who were initially arbitrarily excluded from exercise rehabilitation began to constitute a substantial percentage of the enrollees in structured exercise rehabilitation programs. Currently, among the newer categories of patients considered eligible for cardiac rehabilitation in general and exercise rehabilitation in particular are elderly coronary patients (2,3,7–10); intermediate- to high-risk coronary patients with combinations of residual myocardial ischemia, cardiac arrhythmias, and/or compensated heart failure (11–14); and a variety of other medically complex cardiac patients (15–21). Since coronary heart disease predominantly affects women at older age, a greater proportion of women with coronary disease are likely to require cardiac rehabilitative care as the population ages. As well, the increased spectrum of eligible patients includes those with compensated heart failure (22), and those after cardiac transplantation are now considered candidates for rehabilitative care (23). A number of recent studies have shown both that patients with compensated heart failure or severe left ventricular dysfunction of many etiologies can exercise with safety and that modest improvement in their functional capacity can enable prolongation of an independent lifestyle. Cardiac rehabilitation is also currently recommended for patients after heart valve surgery and those with implanted pacemakers and cardioverter defibrillators (24).

Whereas in the early years of cardiac rehabilitation one of the major goals of an exercise regimen was return to remunerative employment, for contemporary elderly and medically complicated cardiac patients there is often a different goal—an improvement in functional status designed to enable the attainment and maintenance of independent living. This component of clinical care is an outcome that is valued personally by elderly patients and is also valued by society in that it may have far-ranging cost-saving implications, averting or delaying the need for expensive long-term institutional care.

Based on the recommendations of a recent World Health Organization Expert Committee (25), all patients with cardiac disease are considered appropriate for cardiac rehabilitation services, with the varying applications of exercise training, education, and counseling differing with the underlying disease, the severity of such disease, and the goals of the rehabilitative interventions.

Contemporary Emphasis on Preventive Intervention

The latter half of the twentieth century has been characterized by continuing documentation of the benefits of preventive interventions for risk reduction, particularly for coronary heart disease. Randomized clinical trials in patients with coronary heart disease have provided convincing evidence that risk factor modification is beneficial in decreasing all-cause mortality as well as cardiovascular morbidity and mortality, with multifactorial coronary risk reduction providing the most substantial benefit. Coronary risk factors are documented as particularly deleterious for patients with coronary heart disease, those who are at the highest risk for coronary events, disability, and death. It is the combination of the need for secondary prevention and the context of rising healthcare costs that render it essential to select those interventions for coronary risk reduction that are of proven value in the secondary prevention of coronary heart disease (26). The recent 27th Bethesda Conference of the American College of Cardiology (27) displayed a hierarchy of benefits of preventive interventions, defining patients known to have cardiovascular disease as those most likely to derive benefit from such preventive approaches, and outlined the preventive interventions documented to improve outcomes as those most intensively recommended (Table 72-1). Thus these aspects are most likely to be incorporated into the educational and counseling components of cardiac rehabilitation in the twenty-first century.

Barriers to the Delivery of Cardiac Rehabilitation Services and Their Potential Remediation

The recommendations of the Clinical Practice Guideline *Cardiac Rehabilitation* (1), as well as those of the World Health Organization Expert Committee (25), are likely to influence physician practices in the referral for cardiac rehabilitation, as well as to favorably change insurance reimbursement for such

Table 72-1 Cardiovascular Risk Factors: The Evidence Supporting Their Association with Disease, the Usefulness of Measuring Them, and Their Responsiveness to Intervention

Risk Factor	Evidence for Association with CVD		Clinical Measurement	Response to	
	Epidemiologic	Clinical Trials	Useful?	Nonpharmacologic Therapy	Pharmacologic Therapy
Category I (risk factors for which interventions have been proved to lower CVD risk)					
Cigarette Smoking	+++	++	+++	+++	++
LDL Cholesterol	+++	+++	+++	++	+++
High-Fat/Cholesterol Diet	+++	++	++	++	—
Hypertension	+++	+++ (stroke)	+++	+	+++
Left Ventricular Hypertrophy	+++	+	++	—	++
Thrombogenic Factors	+++ (fibrinogen)	+++ (aspirin, warfarin)	+ (fibrinogen)	+	+++ (aspirin, warfarin)
Category II (risk factors for which interventions are likely to lower CVD risk)					
Diabetes Mellitus	+++	+	+++	++	+++
Physical Inactivity	+++	++	++	++	—
HDL Cholesterol	+++	+	+++	++	+
Triglycerides; Small, Dense LDL	++	++	+++	++	+++
Obesity	+++	—	+++	++	+
Postmenopausal Status (Women)	+++	—	+++	—	+++
Category III (risk factors associated with increased CVD risk that, if modified, might lower risk)					
Psychosocial Factors	++	+	+++	+	—
Lipoprotein(a)	+	—	+	—	+
Homocysteine	++	—	+	++	++
Oxidative Stress	+	—	—	+	++
No Alcohol Consumption	+++	—	++	++	—
Category IV (risk factors associated with increased CVD risk, but which cannot be modified)					
Age	+++	—	+++	—	—
Male Gender	+++	—	+++	—	—
Low Socioeconomic Status	+++	—	+++	—	—
Family History of Early-Onset CVD	+++	—	+++	—	—

CVD = cardiovascular disease; HDL = high-density lipoprotein; LDL = low-density lipoprotein; + = weak, somewhat consistent evidence; ++ = moderately strong, rather consistent evidence; +++ = very strong, consistent evidence; — = evidence poor or nonexistent.
Reprinted with permission from the American College of Cardiology from Fuster V, Pearson TA. 27th Bethesda Conference: matching the intensity of risk factor management with the hazard for coronary disease events. J Am Coll Cardiol 1996;27:957–1047.

services. These latter changes have begun to be evident in the governmental insurance programs in the 1990s (6).

The message of the Clinical Practice Guideline *Cardiac Rehabilitation* is that cardiac rehabilitation is a combination of services that help patients with heart disease improve their functional ability, particularly their tolerance for physical activity; decrease their symptoms; and, through a variety of educational and counseling activities, achieve and maintain optimal health. In the current era of evidenced-based medicine, the guideline is the first to comprehensively and objectively examine the specific outcomes of the delivery of cardiac rehabilitation services; highlighted and referenced in the guideline is that the most substantial benefits documented in the scientific literature include improvement in exercise toler-

ance, amelioration of symptoms, improvement in blood lipid levels, reduction in cigarette smoking, improvement in psychosocial well-being, reduction of stress, and reduction in mortality (1). The scientific database for cardiac rehabilitation, developed during the past 2 or 3 decades and displayed in the guideline, should enable the restructuring and expansion of rehabilitative care.

Currently, for governmental healthcare insurance programs, and likely to be adopted by private insurers as well, the discharge planning for patients with an acute coronary event must include the application of secondary preventive interventions, with specific components that address the identified coronary risk characteristics of an individual patient. The cardiac rehabilitation setting can provide an

Table 72-2 Minimal Guidelines for Risk Stratification

RISK LEVEL	CHARACTERISTICS
Low	No significant left ventricular dysfunction (i.e., ejection fraction ≥50%)
	No resting or exercise-induced myocardial ischemia manifested as angina and/or ST segment displacement
	No resting or exercise-induced complex arrhythmias
	Uncomplicated myocardial infarction, coronary artery bypass surgery, angioplasty, or atherectomy
	Functional capacity ≥6 METs on graded exercise test 3 or more weeks after clinical event
Intermediate	Mild to moderately depressed left ventricular function (ejection fraction 31% to 49%)
	Functional capacity <5 to 6 METs on graded exercise test 3 or more weeks after clinical event
	Failure to comply with exercise intensity prescription
	Exercise-induced myocardial ischemia (1 to 2 mm ST segment depression) or reversible ischemic defects (echocardiographic or nuclear radiography)
High	Severely depressed left ventricular function (ejection fraction ≤30%)
	Complex ventricular arrhythmias at rest or appearing or increasing with exercise
	Decrease in systolic blood pressure of >15 mm Hg during exercise or failure to rise with increasing exercise workloads
	Survivor of sudden cardiac death
	Myocardial infarction complicated by congestive heart failure, cardiogenic shock, and/or complex ventricular arrhythmias
	Severe coronary artery disease and marked exercise-induced myocardial ischemia (>2 mm ST segment depression)

NOTE: MET = metabolic equivalent units.
Reprinted by permission from American Association of Cardiovascular and Pulmonary Rehabilitation. Guidelines for rehabilitation programs. Champaign, IL: Human Kinetics, 1995:14. Copyright 1995 by American Association of Cardiovascular and Pulmonary Rehabilitation.

optimal venue for the delivery of multifactorial secondary preventive services.

An innovative component of the guideline *Cardiac Rehabilitation* is the iteration of alternative approaches to the delivery of cardiac rehabilitation services, other than the traditional supervised group and individual programs. These alternative approaches are often home-based and have been shown to be effectively and safely implemented for carefully selected, clinically stable cardiac patients. Home-based rehabilitation can extend cardiac rehabilitation beyond the traditional supervised setting and broaden the availability of such services, as well as likely decreasing their cost (28–32).

The emphasis of cardiac rehabilitation at the end of the twentieth century is the tailoring of rehabilitative care to the needs of the individual, such that the delivery of rehabilitative care is based on the patient's clinical status, personal desires, and requirements for specific interventions. This approach is likely to prove both more successful and more cost-effective than the prior indiscriminate application of multiple components of rehabilitative care, and is likely to be further refined in the next millennium.

COMPONENTS OF CARDIAC REHABILITATION
Exercise Training
In the early years of exercise rehabilitation, although the exercise training was supervised, continuous ECG monitoring was not a routine component of care, as these early exercise rehabilitation programs antedated the widespread availability of ECG telemetry. ECG telemetry achieved widespread use in

the 1970s and 1980s, and substantially added to the cost and complexity of exercise rehabilitation. Current data suggest that continuous ECG monitoring did not provide added safety during supervised exercise for low-risk coronary patients (33,34). ECG monitoring is currently generally recommended only for high-risk patients and for selected patients who have problems in exercising (25, 35–38). Controversy still exists as to whether more extensive ECG monitoring is warranted (39).

A major contributor to the increased safety of exercise training, allowing for the stratification of patients by risk status for exercise, is the routine clinical application of risk stratification procedures for patients known to have coronary heart disease and particularly following a coronary event. These procedures are designed, initially, to guide the need for additional invasive testing during or following the hospitalization, as well as to guide the need for additional medications. However, such exercise test data, identifying patients who have residual myocardial ischemia, can also help gauge their risk for exercise training (Tables 72-2 and 72-3). Low-risk patients can perform reasonable levels of physical activity without adverse consequences; on the other hand, high-risk patients have a low peak exercise capacity and often have the early onset of myocardial ischemia, serious arrhythmias, ventricular dysfunction, or combinations of these problems with exercise. About half of all contemporary survivors of myocardial infarction are considered as low risk, in part related to the application of newer therapies, as are many patients following successful myocardial revascularization procedures. This low-risk status enables added options for the implementation of exercise training. Additionally, goals of exercise training may differ for these low-risk patients; although, in the early years

| Table 72-3 | Criteria for Electrocardiographic Monitoring |

1. Severely depressed left ventricular function (ejection fraction below 30%)
2. Resting complex ventricular arrhythmia
3. Ventricular arrhythmias appearing or increasing with exercise
4. Decrease in systolic blood pressure with exercise
5. Survivors of sudden cardiac death
6. Survivors of myocardial infarction complicated by congestive heart failure, cardiogenic shock, serious ventricular arrhythmias, or some combination of the three
7. Severe coronary artery disease and marked exercise-induced ischemia (ST segment depression ≥ 2 mm)
8. Inability to self-monitor heart rate because of physical or intellectual impairment

Reprinted with permission from the American College of Cardiology from Parmley WW. Position report on cardiac rehabilitation: recommendations of the American College of Cardiology on cardiovascular rehabilitation. J Am Coll Cardiol 1986;7:451–453.

of exercise rehabilitation, rehabilitative care was shown to effect an improvement in survival, such benefit is less likely to be demonstrable in contemporary low-risk coronary patients. Thus, the goal of most low-risk patients in undertaking a physical activity regimen and of their physicians in recommending exercise training is more likely to be an improvement in functional status and a limitation of activity-related symptoms (i.e., improvement in life quality).

Risk stratification data are limited for noncoronary patients, although patients with heart failure are generally considered to be at increased risk, predominantly owing to their frequent sudden death. This concept has been challenged by the apparent low risk of unsupervised exercise training for patients with heart failure in a number of reported studies (12,14,40–42). There has been vast improvement in the pharmacologic management of patients with heart failure caused by left ventricular systolic dysfunction; the newer pharmacotherapies, particularly angiotensin-converting enzyme inhibitor drugs (with the potential addition of beta-blockade as well), may enable increased exercise training in this population and may alter their risk status as well. A study of unsupervised exercise training of moderate intensity for patients with compensated heart failure of a severity to be listed for cardiac transplantation (42), with documented benefit and safety, attests to the changing spectrum of risk status.

In addition to the contributions of risk stratification to the safety of exercise training, the patterns of exercise training have changed as well. In the mid-twentieth century, the traditional exercise regimen was of higher intensity—70% to 85% of the highest level safely achieved at exercise testing. Contemporary data have shown that exercise training of low to moderate intensity, in the 50% to 70% heart rate range, can effect comparable improvements in functional capacity and endurance to those produced by high-intensity exercise. An increase in exercise frequency and/or duration compensates for the decrease in exercise intensity. The application of lower-intensity exercise training likely provides greater safety during unsupervised exercise (because patients no longer approach their ischemic threshold) as well as potentially promoting improved adherence to exercise training (because of the greater comfort and fewer musculoskeletal complications during exercise), which thus makes exercise more enjoyable. Lower-intensity training increases the applicability of unsupervised exercise as well as the acceptance of exercise training by larger numbers of patients, particularly unfit patients, those with low exercise capacity, and elderly patients (25,43,44). Additionally, although isometric exercise was traditionally considered contraindicated for cardiac patients, particularly patients with coronary heart disease, recent studies have documented that mild to moderate resistive exercise training can safely and effectively improve both skeletal muscle strength and cardiovascular endurance in low-risk cardiac patients who have demonstrated their ability to perform adequate levels of aerobic exercise (7 to 8 METs) (45–49). The benefits of resistive or strength exercise training, a modality likely to be increasingly employed in the next millennium, include its capacity to improve the ability to perform a variety of tasks of daily living, tasks in the workplace, and tasks of leisure activities that require a combination of physical strength and muscular exertion. Additionally, the diversity of an exercise regimen that incorporates resistance training may increase patient acceptability and adherence.

The traditional supervised exercise training regimen, predominantly for coronary patients in the 1960s through the 1980s, began with an in-hospital early ambulation component, initially called a phase I program. This was followed by posthospital supervised therapeutic exercise training, termed a phase II component. The subsequent phase III component involved lesser degrees of supervision and electrocardiographic monitoring. Many coronary patients currently discharged from the hospital, particularly those following myocardial revascularization procedures, are of low-risk status and directly enter a phase III program; for others, medically directed home exercise may be a suitable alternative. Variations to this approach include home-based exercise guided by television communication, by computer-guided systems, or by other forms of interactive communications.

In the next millennium, outpatient exercise rehabilitation will likely be described by the characteristics of the exercise training and the requirement, duration, and complexity of the surveillance, based on the patient's clinical and risk factor status, rather than by the traditional phases of earlier years that typically had fixed durations and compositions. This is concordant with responding to an individual patient's needs for exercise training, rather than requiring the patient to conform to program phases or requirements (50).

Particularly to be highlighted are the benefits of home-based exercise; these include improved accessibility, improved flexibility of time, lesser cost, and the fostering of greater independence in exercising. The unknowns of this approach need to be ascertained, since there is increased application of home-based exercise in a clinical rather than a research setting, relate to adherence, to long-term efficacy, and to safety for patients at intermediate to high risk. Benefits of supervised or group exercise training include the enhanced ability to implement and monitor risk reduction, the availability of a peer support group, and the availability of both professional support and a social support system. This variability in the application of exercise training has reinforced the importance of individualization of the rehabilitation plan to meet the needs of specific patients.

The areas of exercise training to be studied more carefully in the next millennium involve patients with severe cardiovascular disease; elderly patients; those with significant comorbidity; those with residual myocardial ischemia, compensated heart failure, or serious arrhythmias; those with complications of medical or surgical therapies; those with severe angina pectoris; and the like. Whether these patients require closer surveillance and/or ECG monitoring of their exercise training for extended time periods remains uncertain (35,36,39).

An improvement in exercise tolerance was among the most prominent benefits of cardiac rehabilitation exercise training identified in the Clinical Practice Guideline *Cardiac Rehabilitation* (1). This improvement in objective measures of exercise tolerance, effected without significant cardiovascular complications or other adverse outcomes, was evident in patients with angina pectoris and myocardial infarction, those patients who had undergone CABG surgery and PTCA, patients with compensated heart failure or with a decreased ventricular ejection fraction, and patients who had undergone cardiac transplantation. The improvement in exercise tolerance was evident for both women and men and occurred in elderly patients as well. Patients with decreased functional capacity at baseline appeared to benefit most (51). For severely disabled cardiac patients, even small improvements in physical work capacity may have a major impact on the quality of their lives, enabling them to maintain a reasonably independent lifestyle.

Education and Counseling

The current emphasis on secondary prevention requires that intensive education and counseling be undertaken to provide patients with cardiovascular disease with the information, the skills, and the motivation to undertake and maintain coronary and other cardiac risk reduction across the life span. The major focus is on lifestyle changes, as well as adherence to medication regimens if such are required. Although measures for the secondary prevention of coronary heart disease must be maintained over the long term to be effective, almost half of all patients receiving risk reduction therapy discontinue all these interventions within a year (52); the challenge for the next millennium is to institute those behavioral interventions that will encourage adherence to risk reduction over the long term. A combined education, counseling, and behavioral intervention strategy seems the most effective in promoting health, reducing risk, and favorably altering lifestyles (1,32,53,54). Risk reduction has been shown to be feasible and appears warranted at elderly age as well, given the greater prevalence and severity of coronary disease in the elderly population. Whether the same interventions are equally effec-

tive for men and women and across the life span remains currently unanswered, because few studies have enrolled patients over 70 years of age or included women; these issues will require ascertainment in the next millennium.

Because of the frequent clustering of coronary risk factors, risk reduction in clinical practice is optimally multifactorial, an approach likely to be increasingly effective in a cardiac rehabilitation setting. Meta-analysis of randomized controlled trials of cardiac rehabilitation demonstrated a 26% greater reduction in total mortality rate with multifactorial cardiac rehabilitation than when exercise training was the sole intervention (55).

Comprehensive coronary risk reduction remains the cornerstone of the continuing care of the coronary patient, since this approach reduces reinfarction, decreases the need for myocardial revascularization procedures, reduces cardiovascular-related hospital admissions, improves quality of life, and decreases cardiovascular and overall mortality rates (56). Among the recent advances likely to be expanded in the next millennium is the behavioral approach to reducing coronary risk. This comprises not only the transmission of information, but practical training in the skills needed for adoption of a healthy lifestyle, and provision of the opportunity to practice and reinforce these skills.

In the early years of cardiac rehabilitation education and counseling, most of the initial educational programs were conducted in the hospital; as well, education and counseling were often done on an individual basis, or at best in small groups, entailing a considerable demand on health provider resources. Contemporary early discharge from the hospital after a coronary event limits or precludes comprehensive hospital-based education and counseling, such that this must be deferred to an ambulatory care setting. Both patients and their families must be provided adequate information and confidence to assume personal responsibility for their long-term cardiovascular care. Whereas there is good documentation of the success of education and counseling in supervised structured cardiac rehabilitation settings, very recent, although limited, studies suggest that a specialized cardiac nurse management approach, with periodic clinic assessments, may be equally effective (30,32).

Home-based approaches will likely be substantially expanded in the next millennium, buttressed by the more generalized availability of relevant new technologies (57) for interactive teacher-learner communication. Newer technologies may help deliver effective, uniform, high-quality educational messages to patients and their families, both at lower cost and at times convenient for the learner, as well as permit repetition of the teaching if desired. Among the options currently being explored are interactive television teaching at home, with the educational focus being scheduled medical center presentations and discussions. Computer-based learning is increasingly applied, again in the interactive mode. Issues of patient education and counseling in the workplace may be undertaken by employers. The benefits to employers of rehabilitative care for their patient-employees include an earlier return to work, less disability, less absenteeism, reduced financial commitment to sickness and disability payments, reduced training costs for replacement of personnel, and greater productivity (25); employers may thus encourage coronary rehabilitative care as a component of their managed care plans.

Psychosocial and Vocational Aspects

The importance of psychosocial variables in the prognosis of patients with established coronary heart disease has received increasing attention toward the end of the twentieth century. The Type A behavior pattern and its subset of hostility, with intervention for its correction, has received attention as a coronary preventive strategy. As well, depression has been associated with unfavorable outcomes, particularly following myocardial infarction, with the impact of major depression equivalent to that of prior infarction and of left ventricular dysfunction (58). Social isolation is increasingly being studied for effectiveness of interventions, based on documentation that socially isolated patients with coronary disease had far less favorable outcomes than did their non–socially isolated counterparts (59); the impact of social isolation on prognosis was independent of physiologic prognostic factors, including left ventricular function. Although the contribution of peer support in a structured rehabilitation setting has not been ascertained, it may be helpful given the predictive power of social isolation for coronary mortality (60). Emotional support, also, is an independent risk factor for mortality following a coronary event (61).

There is substantial correlation between the perception of health status and return to usual family and community activities, as well as to recreational and occupational pursuits, following a cardiac event; importantly, this perception has been shown to be favorably altered by education and counseling.

Since coronary disease is the leading diagnosis in the United States for which patients receive premature disability benefits under the Social Security system, and almost one fourth of men and women receiving Social Security disability allowance are considered permanently disabled because of a diagnosis of coronary heart disease (62), cardiac rehabilitation services (including exercise training and education and counseling), as well as specific vocational rehabilitation interventions, are likely to receive increased attention in the next millennium. The high cost of disability and failure to return to work must be included when the cost-effectiveness of rehabilitative care is ascertained; as well, the indirect healthcare costs of disability, including lessened productivity, loss of income, unemployment insurance costs, and public welfare costs, must be included in the equation. Return to work is likely to be both an economic and a psychosocial imperative for many cardiac patients.

Few studies of return to work in the supervised structured cardiac rehabilitation setting have included specific vocational interventions; whether these will improve the rates of return to work and maintenance of employment remains to be ascertained. Psychological problems, predominantly anxiety and depression, appear to be greater obstacles to the resumption of preillness activities by coronary patients than physical incapacity. Return to work is increasingly recognized as an outcome measure that is economically, physically, and socially relevant to a wide variety of cardiac patients, but one that may relate poorly to restoration of functional capacity. Currently, symptomatic and functional improvements in survivors of myocardial infarction and myocardial revascularization procedures correlate poorly with return to work, as well

as with the general resumption of preillness lifestyle; psychosocial status appears to be a more important determinant that limits occupational and social reintegration (63).

The application and assessment of the role of vocational rehabilitation is a major challenge for the twenty-first century.

WHAT WE MUST LEARN IN THE NEXT MILLENNIUM

Much of the data related to the outcomes of the application of cardiac rehabilitation services to patients with coronary heart disease derive from the prethrombolytic era and do not include patients who received current medical or revascularization therapies. The outcomes of exercise training and education and counseling must be ascertained for patients treated with current medical and surgical therapies. Additionally, very limited information is available for elderly patients, for women of all ages, for populations of low educational and socioeconomic levels, and for patients of ethnic minorities. Whether the application of exercise training and education and counseling differs in these subsets of patients must be determined.

Of particular importance is the outcome of rehabilitative exercise training with and without supervision and with and without electrocardiographic monitoring in patients of higher risk status; this includes patients with heart failure, elderly patients, and patients with complex cardiovascular diseases. These data are needed to guide the exercise training recommendations for such subpopulations of patients. As well, the safety and efficacy of strength or resistance training must be ascertained in higher-risk patients, particularly elderly patients, women, unfit cardiac patients, and others at moderate to high cardiovascular risk. There must be further prospective evaluation of the safety and benefits of exercise rehabilitation in patients with compensated heart failure and impaired ventricular systolic function, as well as delineation of the degree of supervision required for these patients.

Because of the need for cost-effective interventions, evaluation is needed of the cost-effectiveness of various modes of delivery of cardiac rehabilitation services. Included in this approach is ascertainment of the optimal education and counseling strategies for coronary risk reduction and other preventive strategies.

The development and assessment of measures to ascertain changes in psychosocial functioning and quality of life in patients undergoing cardiac rehabilitation must be undertaken; current measures may not have relevance to or may be insensitive in nonpsychiatric populations. As well, features must be identified that enhance adherence to cardiac rehabilitation services, both exercise training and risk reduction. Behavioral interventions for lifestyle changes must be developed that are applicable to large populations of coronary and other cardiac patients, as well as evaluation of their efficacy in subsets of patients related to gender, age, and ethnic differences (1).

SUMMARY

The challenge to the delivery of cardiac rehabilitation services in the next millennium will be to select, develop, and provide appropriate rehabilitative care for an individual cardiac patient and to tailor the method of delivery of these services based on medical needs, cost concerns, patient preferences, and health provider recommendations. During the past two decades, research on effective interventions for coronary risk factor modification has identified that these are well accepted and well tolerated by high-risk patients with identified coronary disease; importantly, regardless of the initial cost, this approach often has an attractive longer-term cost-effectiveness ratio. Vigorous attention to cost-effective strategies to improve established coronary risk factors remains the major focus of most clinicians; well-designed cardiac rehabilitation is likely to deliver this cost-effective strategy. Incorporating the combination of healthcare provider recommendations and patient preferences is likely to both facilitate independence in cardiac rehabilitation and to encourage adherence to rehabilitative care.

This evolving pattern of rehabilitative care, related to the selection of specific rehabilitative services appropriate for an individual patient's characteristics, requirements, and/or preferences, will include choices of individual versus group physical activity programs, education and counseling sessions, and the like, designed to address the diversity of the cardiac population, diverse as to age, severity of illness, comorbidity, and expectations of outcome. The goal for the next millennium is that all approaches must be designed to encourage progressive independence in rehabilitative care, which is the basis for the adoption of a lifetime healthy lifestyle. This concept should be attractive to patients, to their healthcare providers, and to those responsible for the cost of rehabilitative cardiac care (1).

REFERENCES

1. Wenger NK, Froelicher ES, Smith LK, et al. Cardiac rehabilitation. Clinical Practice Guideline No. 17. AHCPR Publication No. 96-0672. Rockville, MD: U.S. Department of Health and Human Service, Public Health Service, Agency for Health Care Policy and Research and the National Heart, Lung, and Blood Institute, 1995.

2. Ades PA, Hanson JS, Gunther PG, et al. Exercise conditioning in the elderly coronary patient. J Am Geriatr Soc 1987;35:121–124.

3. Lavie CJ, Milani RV, Littman AB. Benefits of cardiac rehabilitation and exercise training in secondary coronary prevention in the elderly. J Am Coll Cardiol 1993;22:678–683.

4. Ades PA, Waldmann ML, Polk D, et al. Referral patterns and exercise response in the rehabilitation of female coronary patients aged ≥62 years. Am J Cardiol 1992;69:1422–1425.

5. American Heart Association. AHA Heart and Stroke Statistical Update. Dallas: American Heart Association, 1998.

6. Agency for Health Care Policy and Research. Cardiac rehabilitation programs. Health Technology Assessment Reports, 1991, No. 3. DHHS Publication No. AHCPR 92-0015. Rockville, MD: U.S. Department of Health and Human Services, Public Health Service,

Agency for Health Care Policy and Research, 1991.

7. Ades PA, Grunvald MH. Cardiopulmonary exercise testing before and after conditioning in older coronary patients. Am Heart J 1990;120:585–589.

8. Ades PA, Huang D, Weaver SO. Cardiac rehabilitation participation predicts lower rehospitalization costs. Am Heart J 1992;123:916–921.

9. Ades PA, Waldmann ML, Gillespie C. A controlled trial of exercise training in older coronary patients. J Gerontol 1995;50A:M7–M11.

10. Williams MA, Maresh CM, Esterbrooks DJ, et al. Early exercise training in patients older than age 65 years compared with that in younger patients after acute myocardial infarction or coronary artery bypass grafting. Am J Cardiol 1985;55:263–266.

11. Meyer TR, Casadei B, Coats AJ, et al. Angiotensin-converting enzyme inhibition and physical training in heart failure. J Intern Med 1991;230:407–413.

12. Giannuzzi P, Temporelli PL, Tavazzi L, et al. EAMI—Exercise training in anterior myocardial infarction: an ongoing multicenter randomized study; preliminary results on left ventricular function and remodeling. Chest 1992;101(suppl 5):315S–321S.

13. Grodzinski E, Jette M, Blumchen G, et al. Effects of a four-week training program on left ventricular function as assessed by radionuclide ventriculography. J Cardiopulm Rehabil 1987;7:518–524.

14. Giannuzzi P, Tavazzi L, Temporelli PL, et al. Long-term physical training and left ventricular remodeling after anterior myocardial infarction: results of the Exercise in Anterior Myocardial Infarction (EAMI) Trial. J Am Coll Cardiol 1993;22:1821–1829.

15. Arvan S. Exercise performance of the high risk acute myocardial infarction patient after cardiac rehabilitation. Am J Cardiol 1988;62:197–201.

16. Ehrman J, Keteyian S, Fedel F, et al. Ventilatory threshold after exercise training in orthotopic heart transplant recipients. J Cardiopulm Rehabil 1992;12:126–130.

17. Hertzeanu HL, Shemesh J, Aron LA, et al. Ventricular arrhythmias in rehabilitated and nonrehabilitated post-myocardial infarction patients with left ventricular dysfunction. Am J Cardiol 1993;71:24–27.

18. Kavanagh T, Yacoub MH, Mertens DJ, et al. Cardiorespiratory responses to exercise training after orthotopic cardiac transplantation. Circulation 1988;77:162–171.

19. Kavanagh T, Yacoub MH, Merterns DJ, et al. Exercise rehabilitation after heterotopic cardiac transplantation. J Cardiopulm Rehabil 1989;9:303–310.

20. Kellermann JJ, Shemesh J, Fisman EZ, et al. Arm exercise training in the rehabilitation of patients with impaired ventricular function and heart failure. Cardiology 1990;77:130–138.

21. Sullivan MJ, Higginbotham NB, Cobb FR. Exercise training in patients with severe left ventricular dysfunction: hemodynamic and metabolic effects. Circulation 1988;78:506–515.

22. World Health Organization/Council on Geriatric Cardiology Task Force on Heart Failure Education, Gyarfas I, Wenger NK (Co-chairs). Concise guide to the management of heart failure. Geneva: World Health Organization, 1995.

23. Wenger NK, Haskell WL, Kanter K, et al. Ad hoc Task Force on Cardiac Rehabilitation: Cardiac rehabilitation services after cardiac transplantation: Guidelines for use. Cardiology 1991;20:4–5.

24. Wenger NK, Balady GK, Cohn LH, et al. Ad hoc Task Force on Cardiac Rehabilitation: Cardiac rehabilitation services following PTCA and valvular surgery: Guidelines for use. Cardiology 1990;19:4–5.

25. World Health Organization Expert Committee. Rehabilitation after cardiovascular diseases, with special emphasis on developing countries. Technical Report Series No. 831. Geneva: World Health Organization, 1993.

26. Ryan TJ, Anderson JL, Antman EM, et al. ACC/AHA guidelines for the management of patients with acute myocardial infarction: executive summary. A report of the American College of Cardiology/American Heart Association Task Force on Practice Guidelines (Committee on Management of Acute Myocardial Infarction). Circulation 1996;94:2341–2350.

27. Fuster V, Pearson TA. 27th Bethesda Conference: matching the intensity of risk factor management with the hazard for coronary disease events. J Am Coll Cardiol 1996;27:957–1047.

28. Miller NH, Haskell WL, Berra K, et al. Home versus group exercise training for increasing functional capacity after myocardial infarction. Circulation 1984;70:645–649.

29. DeBusk RF, Haskell WL, Miller NH, et al. Medically directed at-home rehabilitation soon after uncomplicated acute myocardial infarction: a new model for patient care. Am J Cardiol 1985;55:251–257.

30. Haskell WL, Alderman EL, Fair JM, et al. Effects of intensive multiple risk factor reduction on coronary atherosclerosis and clinical cardiac events in men and women with coronary artery disease: the Stanford Coronary Risk Intervention Project (SCRIP). Circulation 1994;89:975–990.

31. Fletcher BJ, Dunbar SB, Felner JM, et al. Exercise testing and training in physically disabled men with clinical evidence of coronary artery disease. Am J Cardiol 1994;73:170–174.

32. DeBusk RF, Houston Miller N, Superko HR, et al. A case-management system for coronary risk factor modification after acute myocardial infarction. Ann Intern Med 1994;120:721–729.

33. Fagan ET, Wayne VS, McConachy DL. Serious ventricular arrhythmias in a cardiac rehabilitation programme. Med J Aust 1984;141:421–424.

34. Van Camp SP, Peterson RA. Cardiovascular complications of outpatient cardiac rehabilitation programs. JAMA 1986;256:1160–1163.

35. Parmley WW. Position report on cardiac rehabilitation: recommendations of the American College of Cardiology on cardiovascular rehabilitation. J Am Coll Cardiol 1986;7:451–452.

36. American College of Physicians, Health and Policy Committee. Cardiac rehabilitation services. Ann Intern Med 1988;109:671–673. Position paper.

37. DeBusk RF, Blomqvist CG, Kouchoukos NT, et al. Identification and treatment of low-risk patients after acute myocardial infarction and coronary-artery bypass graft surgery. N Engl J Med 1986;314:161–166.

38. Wenger NK. Rehabilitation after cardiovascular diseases: report and recommendations of a World Health Organization Expert Committee (October 1991). Int J Sports Cardiol 1992;1:101–103.

39. Fletcher GF, Balady G, Froelicher VF, et al. Exercise standards: a statement for healthcare professionals from the American Heart Association. Circulation 1995;91:580–615. Special report.

40. Squires RW, Lavie CJ, Brandt TR, et al. Cardiac rehabilitation in patients with severe ischemic left ventricular dysfunction. Mayo Clin Proc 1987;62:997–1002.

41. Williams RS. Exercise training of patients with ventricular dysfunction and heart failure. In: Wenger NK, ed. Exercise and the heart. 2nd ed. Philadelphia: FA Davis, 1985:219–231.

42. Stevenson LW, Steimle AE, Fonarow G, et al. Improvement in exercise capacity of candidates awaiting heart transplantation. J Am Coll Cardiol 1995;25:163–170.

43. Blumenthal JA, Rejeski WJ, Walsh-Riddle M, et al. Comparison of high- and low-intensity exercise training early after acute myocardial infarction. Am J Cardiol 1988;61:26–30.

44. Goble AJ, Hare DL, Macdonald PS, et al. Effect of early programmes of high and low intensity exercise on physical performance after transmural myocardial infarction. Br Med J 1991;65:126–131.

45. Kelemen MH. Resistance training safety and essential guidelines for cardiac and coronary prone patients. Med Sci Sports Exerc 1989;21:675–677.

46. Sparling PB, Cantwell JD, Dolan CM, et al. Strength training in a cardiac rehabilitation program: a six-month follow-up. Arch Phys Med Rehabil 1990;71:148–152.

47. Stewart KJ, Mason M, Kelemen MH. Three-year participation in circuit weight training improves muscular strength and self-efficacy in cardiac patients. J Cardiopulm Rehabil 1988;8:292–296.

48. Wilke NA, Sheldahl LM, Levandoski SG, et al. Transfer effect of upper extremity training to weight carrying in men with ischemic heart disease. J Cardiopulm Rehabil 1991;11:365–372.

49. Franklin BA, Bonzheim K, Gordon S, et al. Resistance training in cardiac rehabilitation. J Cardiopulm Rehabil 1991;11:99–107.

50. Wenger NK. Rehabilitation of the patient with coronary heart disease. In: Alexander WA, Schlant RC, Fuster V, et al, ed. The heart. 9th ed. New York: McGraw-Hill, 1998:1619–1631.

51. Balady GJ, Jette D, Scheer J, et al, and the Massachusetts Association of Cardiovascular and Pulmonary Rehabilitation Database Investigators. Changes in exercise capacity following cardiac rehabilitation in patients stratified according to age and gender: results of the Massachusetts Association of Cardiovascular and Pulmonary Rehabilitation Multicenter Database. J Cardiopulm Rehabil 1996; 16:38–46.

52. Smith SC Jr. Risk-reduction therapy: the challenge to change. Circulation 1996;93:2201–2211.

53. Blumenthal JA, Levenson RM. Behavioral approaches to secondary prevention of coronary heart disease. Circulation 1987; 76(suppl I):I-130–I-137.

54. Newton KM, Sivarajan ES, Clark JL. Patient perceptions of risk factor changes and cardiac rehabilitation outcomes after myocardial infarction. J Cardiopulm Rehabil 1985;5:159–168.

55. Oldridge N, Guyatt GH, Fischer ME, et al. Cardiac rehabilitation after myocardial infarction: combined experience of randomized clinical trials. JAMA 1988;260: 945–950.

56. Zafari AM, Wenger NK. Secondary prevention of coronary heart disease. Arch Phys Med Rehabil 1998;79:1006–1017.

57. Wenger NK, ed. The education of the patient with cardiac disease in the twenty-first century. New York: LeJacq Publishing, 1986.

58. Frasure-Smith N, Lesperance F, Talajic M. Depression and 18-month prognosis after myocardial infarction. Circulation 1995;91: 999–1005.

59. Appels A. Mental precursors of myocardial infarction. Br J Psychiatry 1990;156:465–471.

60. Orth-Gomer K, Unden A-L, Edwards M-E. Social isolation and mortality in ischemic heart disease: a 10-year follow-up study of 150 middle-aged men. Acta Med Scand 1988;224:205–215.

61. Berkman LF, Leo-Summers L, Horwitz RI. Emotional support and survival after myocardial infarction: a prospective, population-based study of the elderly. Ann Intern Med 1992;117:1003–1009.

62. Wenger NK. Impairment, disability, and the cardiac patient. Qual Life Cardiovasc Care 1987;3:56. Editorial.

63. Walter PJ, ed. Return to work after coronary artery bypass surgery: psychosocial and economic aspects. Berlin: Springer-Verlag, 1985.

Part XIII.

EPIDEMIOLOGY

Edited by
Harold W. Kohl, III

Introduction to Epidemiology

Harold W. Kohl, III

Population-based studies have provided much of the evidence of the role that physical inactivity and dietary practices play in prominent chronic diseases. Indeed, many policy decisions for national health guidelines have been based on scientific evidence provided from population-based studies in the absence of the traditional randomized controlled trial. One need look only as far as the literature on the effects of cigarette smoking on health to realize the impact that population-based studies, in the absence of the "ultimate" randomized controlled trial, can have.

At the heart of this population-based evidence are epidemiologic study designs and methods that allow prospective, concurrent, and retrospective observations in large populations to be translated into quantitative measures of disease incidence, relative risks, and attributable risks. By allowing comparisons and contrasts among various population subgroups such as exposed versus unexposed, young versus old, male versus female, active versus inactive, and others, clear pictures regarding disease burdens and factors influencing those burdens can be found. Although each of the chapters in this section could arguably be included within other sections dealing with specific clinical problems, the substantial contributions of epidemiologic studies in these areas seem to warrant a separate section.

As the basis for epidemiologic study of disease and risk factors, surveillance data provide us not only with baseline prevalence information, but also trends in prevalence over time. The chapter by Carl Caspersen and Aaron Folsom, originally printed in the landmark 1995 United States Surgeon General's Report on Physical Activity and Health, provides an excellent and authoritative source of patterns and trends in physical activity using all sources of nationally representative data in the United States. It clearly helps identify possible trends and differences in activity and inactivity among population subgroups.

Many excellent reviews are available detailing the relationship between physical inactivity and the risk of cardiovascular disease, cancer, and diabetes mellitus. Aspects of dietary intake as related to risk of these diseases have also been more than adequately presented in the literature. However, because physical inactivity and aspects of dietary intake are likely interrelated and interactive in their relations with disease processes and disease outcomes, it follows that evaluations of one without the other presents an incomplete picture. With this realization in mind, three authors in this section have expertly and elegantly reviewed studies that have concomitantly evaluated physical activity and aspects of dietary intake as related to three major disease outcomes.

Mark A. Pereira has contributed a thoughtful chapter on the independent and interactive effects of diet and physical activity in the prevention of cardiovascular disease. The roots of the entire field of the epidemiology of physical activity can be traced to initial interest in its role in cardiovascular disease. In addition to observational studies, this chapter includes a critical review of randomized clinical trials designed to compare the effects of diet and physical activity on cardiovascular disease risk factors. The difficult task of wading through literally hundreds of studies over decades was expertly accomplished in this clearly written and organized chapter.

The chapter with Janet E. Fulton as the lead author tackles the broad topic of physical activity, diet, and type II diabetes mellitus. Since obesity is a well-established risk factor for type II diabetes, and is also the primary manifestation of an imbalance between energy intake and expenditure, this chapter necessarily includes a brief treatment of body fat distribution, weight gain, and weight loss. The roles that physical activity and diet play in the risk of these body composition measures is discussed as is the potential link through obesity toward the development of diabetes.

Finally, Christine Friedenreich, in her chapter evaluating the association of physical activity, diet, and cancer, systematically reviews evidence linking physical activity and diet to risk of cancers of the breast, colon, and prostate. In addition to a comprehensive review, a useful section on current methodologic limitations in existing studies as well as suggestions for future research are also provided.

All authors have made a substantial effort in making recommendations for future studies. As we have many years of study of physical activity as it relates to disease outcomes and many years of study of diet as it relates to disease outcomes, a future effort in epidemiology must be a more concerted effort toward integrating the study of the two risk factors simultaneously. Without the simultaneous information on each, the canvas is only half complete.

Chapter 73

Patterns and Trends in Physical Activity

Carl J. Caspersen
Aaron R. Folsom

INTRODUCTION

This chapter documents patterns and trends of reported leisure-time physical activity of adults and adolescents in the United States and compares the findings to the goals set by *Healthy People 2000* (U.S. Department of Health and Human Services [USDHHS] 1990). The information presented here is based on cross-sectional data from national- and state-based surveillance systems, sponsored by the Centers for Disease Control and Prevention (CDC), that track health behaviors including leisure-time physical activity. Although self-reported survey information about physical activity is likely to contain errors of overreporting, there is no other feasible way to estimate physical activity patterns of a population. Moreover, there is no widely accepted "gold standard" methodology for measuring physical activity.

Editor's Note: A fundamental aspect of the science of epidemiology and public health is surveillance. Surveillance accomplishes many goals, including benchmarking, tracking trends, and identifying potential groups and subgroups as targets for interventions. This chapter was originally published in the landmark 1995 publication, *Physical Activity and Health: A Report of the Surgeon General*. Using five sources of existing nationally representative data, the original authors, Carl Caspersen and Aaron Folsom compiled a definitive work detailing the physical activity patterns over time for various population subgroups, by geographic region, by state, and by other factors. It is the most complete work available and is included here in its entirety as it was orignally published rather than attempt a new chapter that most certainly would not be definitive. Not only does the chapter provide the surveillance data, it allows the reader an understanding of the strengths and limitations of national surveillance data. (Harold W. Kohl III, Section Editor)

Occupational and most domestic physical activities are not presented because such information is not available. Most national goals address leisure-time rather than occupational physical activity because people have more personal control over how they spend their leisure time and because most people do not have jobs that require regular physical exertion. Nonetheless, measuring only leisure-time physical activity leads to an underestimate of total physical activity, especially for those people with physically demanding jobs.

Five surveys provided data on physical activity for this review: 1) the National Health Interview Survey (NHIS), which included questions on physical activity among adults in 1985, 1990, and 1991; 2) the Behavioral Risk Factor Surveillance System (BRFSS), a state-based survey of adults that was conducted monthly by state health departments, in collaboration with the CDC, and included questions on physical activity from 1986 through 1992 and in 1994; 3) the Third National Health and Nutrition Examination Survey (NHANES III) of U.S. adults from 1988 through 1994 (data from Phase I, 1988–1991, were available for presentation in this report); 4) the 1992 household-based NHIS Youth Risk Behavior Survey (NHIS-YRBS) of 12- through 21-year-olds; and 5) the national school-based Youth Risk Behavior Survey (YRBS), which was conducted in 1991, 1993, and 1995 among students in grades 9–12. The methodologies of these surveys are summarized in Table 73-1 and are described in detail in Appendices A and B of this chapter.

When adult data from the NHIS, BRFSS, and NHANES III are presented for comparison, they are shown from the most nearly contemporaneous survey years. Otherwise, the most recent data are presented. For determining

Survey Title	Abbreviated Title	Sponsor	Mode of Survey Administration	Years	Population, Age	Response Rate	Sample Size	Physical Activity Measure[b]
Adults								
National Health Interview Survey	NHIS	National Center for Health Statistics (NCHS), Centers for Disease Control and Prevention (CDC)	Household interview	1985, 1990, 1991	US, 18+ years	83–88%	36,399 in 1985, 41,104 in 1990, 43,732 in 1991	F/I/T/D over past 2 weeks
Behavioral Risk Factor Surveillance System	BRFSS	National Center for Chronic Disease Prevention and Health Promotion (NCCDPHP), CDC	Telephone interview	1986–1991	25 states[c] and D.C., 18+ years	62–71%	Approx. 35,000–50,000	F/I/T/D over past month
				1992	48 states and D.C. 18+ years	71%	96,343	
				1994	49 states and D.C. 18+ years	70%	106,030	
Third National Health and Nutrition Examination Survey	NHANES III	NCHS, CDC	Household interview	1988–91 (Phase I)	US, 18+ years	82%	9,901	F/T over past month
Youths								
Youth Risk Behavior Survey	YRBS	NCCDPHP, CDC	Self-administered in school	1991, 1993, 1995	US, 9th–12th grades (approximately 15–18 years)	70–78% of selected schools; 86–90% of students	12,272 in 1991, 16,296 in 1993, 10,904 in 1995	F/I/T/D over past week
National Health Interview Survey-Youth Risk Behavior Survey	NHIS-YRBS	NCHS, CDC	Household administration via audiotape and self-completed answer sheets	1992	US, 12–21 years	74%	10,645	F/I/T over past week

[a] Available at the time this report was compiled.
[b] F = frequency; I = intensity; T = type; D = duration.
[c] Alabama, Arizona, California, Florida, Georgia, Hawaii, Idaho, Illinois, Indiana, Kentucky, Massachusetts, Minnesota, Missouri, Montana, New Mexico, New York, North Carolina, North Dakota, Ohio, Rhode Island, South Carolina, Tennessee, Utah, West Virginia, and Wisconsin.

trends, BRFSS data are restricted to those states that collected physical activity information each year.

Responses to questions included in the surveys were compiled (see Appendix B) into categories approximately corresponding to the *Healthy People 2000* physical activity objectives. These objectives are based on the health-related physical activity dimensions of caloric expenditure, aerobic intensity, flexibility, and muscle strength (Caspersen 1994). Thus the "regular, sustained physical activity" category used here pertains to total caloric expenditure and includes a summation of activities of any intensity, whereas the "regular, vigorous" category pertains to aerobic intensity and therefore includes only activities of vigorous intensity. Because some activities (e.g., vigorous activity of 30 minutes duration) fall into both of these categories, the categories are not mutually exclusive. Adding together the proportion of people in each category thus yields an overestimate of the proportion of people who are regularly physically active. More clear-cut is the category of inactivity, which is considered to be the most detrimental to health and is thus important to monitor as an indicator of need for intervention. Measures of stretching and strength training are also derived, when possible, from the survey responses.

The various surveys differ in the means by which they are conducted, in the wording of questions, in the time of year, in population sampling frames, in response rates, and in definitions of physical activity—all of which may cause differences in the resulting physical activity estimates. However, even with these differences, the data from the several data collection systems reveal a number of consistencies in patterns and trends in self-reported leisure-time physical activity.

PHYSICAL ACTIVITY AMONG ADULTS IN THE UNITED STATES

Recent Patterns of Leisure-Time Physical Activity

Physical Inactivity during Leisure Time

Physical inactivity during leisure time is one of the easiest measures to define in population surveys. Inactivity was conceptualized in the NHIS, BRFSS, and NHANES III as no reported leisure-time physical activity in the previous 2 to 4 weeks. *Healthy People 2000* objective 1.5 states that the proportion of leisure-time physical inactivity among people aged 6 years and older should be no more than 15 percent by the year 2000 (USDHHS 1990).

The proportion of U.S. adults aged 18 years and older who were classified as physically inactive during leisure time varied somewhat among the three recent surveys (Table 73-2). In the 1991 NHIS, 24.3 percent reported no activity in the

previous 2 weeks. In the 1992 BRFSS, 28.7 percent of adults reported no activity during the previous month. In the 1988–1991 NHANES III, in which for operational reasons participants tended to be surveyed in the North in the summer and the South in the winter, the prevalence of inactivity during the previous month was somewhat lower—21.7 percent.

Thus, despite minor differences, the surveys are consistent in finding that about one-fourth of U.S. adults do not engage in any leisure-time physical activity, a proportion far from the 15 percent target of *Healthy People 2000* objective 1.5. Also evident across the surveys in that more women than men are physically inactive (Figure 73-1). The ratio of physical inactivity prevalence for women relative to that for men ranged from 1.2 to 1.7 across the three surveys. Findings for racial and ethnic groups, unadjusted for socioeconomic differences, were generally in accord across the surveys (Table 73-2): whites had a lower prevalence of leisure-time inactivity than blacks, Hispanics, and persons categorized as "other."

Among the sex-specific racial and ethnic groups, white men were the least likely to be inactive (<26 percent). White women had a prevalence of inactivity (23.1–29.0 percent) similar to that among black men and lower than that among Hispanic men. At least one-third of black women and Hispanic women reported no physical activity in their leisure time.

In all three surveys, the prevalence of physical inactivity was higher in older groups (Figure 73-1). Fewer than one in four adults aged 18–29 years engaged in no physical activity, whereas about one in three men and one in two women over 74 years of age were inactive (Table 73-2). For the most part,

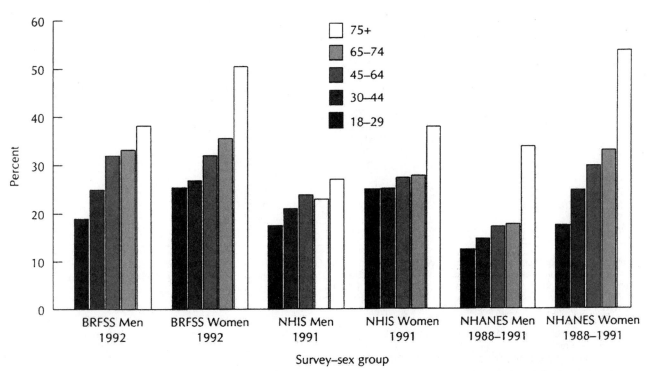

Figure 73-1 Percentage of adults aged 18+ years reporting no participation in leisure-time physical activity by sex and age.

Table 73-2 Percentage of Adults Aged 18+ Years Reporting No Participation in Leisure-time Physical Activity, by Various Demographic Characteristics, National Health Interview Survey (NHIS), Third National Health and Nutrition Examination Survey (NHANES III), and Behavioral Risk Factor Surveillance System (BRFSS), United States

DEMOGRAPHIC GROUP	1991 NHIS[a]	1988–1991 NHANES III[a]	1992 BRFSS[a,b]
Overall	**24.3** (23.2, 25.3)[c]	**21.7** (19.0, 24.5)	**28.7** (28.3, 29.1)
Sex			
Males	**21.4** (20.2, 22.6)	**15.8** (12.4, 19.2)	**26.5** (25.9, 27.1)
Females	**26.9** (25.8, 28.0)	**27.1** (23.0, 31.3)	**30.7** (30.1, 31.3)
Race/Ethnicity			
White, non-Hispanic	**22.5** (21.4, 23.7)	**18.2** (15.6, 20.8)	**26.8** (26.4, 27.2)
Males	**20.3** (19.0, 21.6)	**12.9** (9.6, 16.1)	**25.3** (24.7, 25.9)
Females	**24.6** (23.4, 25.8)	**23.1** (19.0, 27.1)	**28.2** (27.6, 28.8)
Black, non-Hispanic	**28.4** (26.4, 30.4)	**30.4** (25.6, 35.3)	**38.5** (36.9, 40.1)
Males	**22.5** (20.0, 25.0)	**20.6** (14.5, 26.8)	**33.1** (30.9, 35.3)
Females	**33.2** (30.8, 35.6)	**38.1** (30.9, 45.2)	**42.7** (40.7, 44.7)
Hispanic[d]	**33.6** (31.0, 36.3)	**36.0** (32.5, 39.5)	**34.8** (32.8, 36.8)
Males	**29.6** (26.0, 33.2)	**29.1** (24.3, 33.9)	**30.2** (27.3, 33.1)
Females	**37.4** (34.1, 40.8)	**43.8** (38.5, 49.1)	**39.0** (36.5, 41.5)
Other	**26.7** (23.4, 30.0)		**31.4** (28.9, 33.9)
Males	**22.8** (18.2, 27.3)	[e]	**27.6** (24.1, 31.1)
Females	**30.8** (27.0, 34.7)		**35.8** (32.3, 39.3)
Age (years)			
Males			
18–29	**17.6** (15.8, 19.4)	**12.5** (9.0, 16.0)	**18.9** (17.7, 20.1)
30–44	**21.1** (19.8, 22.5)	**14.5** (10.9, 18.1)	**25.0** (24.0, 26.0)
45–64	**23.9** (22.1, 25.7)	**16.9** (13.0, 20.8)	**32.0** (30.8, 33.2)
65–74	**23.0** (20.4, 25.6)	**17.5** (12.2, 22.8)	**33.2** (31.2, 35.2)
75+	**27.1** (23.8, 30.4)	**34.5** (28.0, 41.1)	**38.2** (35.3, 41.1)
Females			
18–29	**25.0** (23.4, 26.6)	**17.4** (13.4, 21.4)	**25.4** (24.2, 26.6)
30–44	**25.2** (23.8, 26.6)	**24.9** (20.6, 29.3)	**26.9** (25.9, 27.9)
45–64	**27.4** (25.9, 28.9)	**29.4** (24.6, 34.2)	**32.1** (30.9, 33.3)
65–74	**27.8** (25.7, 29.9)	**32.5** (25.9, 39.2)	**36.6** (34.8, 38.4)
75+	**37.9** (35.3, 40.6)	**54.3** (47.9, 60.6)	**50.5** (48.5, 52.5)
Education			
<12 yrs	**37.1** (35.3, 38.9)	**34.5** (31.2, 37.8)	**46.5** (45.3, 47.7)
12 yrs	**25.9** (24.7, 27.1)	**20.8** (17.4, 24.3)	**32.8** (32.1, 33.6)
Some college (13–15 yrs)	**19.0** (17.8, 20.2)	**15.7** (11.4, 19.9)	**22.6** (21.9, 23.4)
College (16+ yrs)	**14.2** (13.1, 15.3)	**11.1** (6.9, 15.4)	**17.8** (17.0, 18.5)
Income[f]			
<$10,000	**30.3** (28.4, 32.2)	**34.5** (30.3, 38.7)	**41.5** (40.1, 42.9)
$10,000–19,999	**30.2** (28.5, 32.0)	**28.5** (24.5, 32.6)	**34.6** (33.6, 35.6)
$20,000–34,999	**24.3** (22.9, 25.7)	**18.7** (14.8, 22.6)	**26.9** (26.1, 27.7)
$35,000–49,999	**19.5** (18.1, 20.9)	**15.9** (10.9, 20.9)	**23.0** (22.0, 24.0)
$50,000+	**14.4** (13.2, 15.6)	**10.9** (6.7, 15.1)	**17.7** (16.9, 18.5)
Geographic region			
Northeast	**25.9** (24.5, 27.3)	**21.6** (8.5, 34.6)	**29.5** (28.5, 30.5)
North Central	**20.8** (18.7, 22.9)	**16.7** (7.6, 25.8)	**28.6** (27.8, 29.4)
South	**27.0** (25.2, 28.8)	**24.8** (18.4, 31.1)	**32.4** (31.6, 33.2)
West	**22.5** (19.5, 25.5)	**22.6** (14.8, 30.5)	**22.0** (21.0, 23.0)

SOURCES: Centers for Disease Control and Prevention, National Center for Health Statistics, NHIS, public use data tapes, 1991; Centers for Disease Control and Prevention, National Center for Health Statistics, NHANES, public use data tapes, 1988–1991; Centers for Disease Control and Prevention, National Center for Chronic Disease Prevention and Health Promotion, BRFSS, 1992.
[a] NHIS asked about the prior 2 weeks; BRFSS asked about the prior month.
[b] Based on data from 48 states and the District of Columbia.
[c] 95% confidence intervals.
[d] Hispanic reflects Mexican-Americans in NHANES III.
[e] Estimates unreliable.
[f] Annual income per family (NHIS) or household (BRFSS).

the prevalence of physical inactivity was greater among persons with lower levels of education and income. For example, there was twofold to threefold more inactivity from lowest to highest income categories: only 10.9 to 17.8 percent of participants with an annual family income of $50,000 or more reported no leisure-time physical activities, whereas 30.3 to 41.5 percent of those with an income less than $10,000 reported this.

The prevalence of inactivity among adults tended to be lower in the north central and western states than in the northeastern and southern states (Table 73-2). Participants surveyed in the winter months reported being physically inactive substantially more often than did those surveyed during the summer months (Figure 73-2). In the 1994 BRFSS, state-specific prevalences of physical inactivity from 49 states and the District of Columbia ranged from 17.2 to 48.6 (Table 73-3).

Regular, Sustained Physical Activity during Leisure Time

Healthy People 2000 objective 1.3 proposes that at least 30 percent of people aged 6 years and older should engage regularly, preferably daily, in light to moderate physical activity requiring sustained, rhythmic muscular movements for at least 30 minutes per day (USDHHS 1990). Regular, sustained activity derived from the NHIS and the BRFSS was defined as any type or intensity of activity that occurs 5 times or more per week and 30 minutes or more per occasion (see Appendix B). This definition approximates the activity goal of the *Healthy People 2000* objective but includes vigorous activity of at least 30 minutes duration as well. Comparable information was unavailable in the NHANES III. The percentage of U.S.

adults meeting this definition of regular, sustained activity during leisure time was about 22 percent in the two surveys (23.5 in the NHIS and 20.1 in the BRFSS; see Table 73-4)—8 percentage points lower than the *Healthy People 2000* target.

The prevalence of regular, sustained activity was somewhat higher among men than women; male:female ratios were 1.1:1.3. The two surveys found no consistent association between racial/ethnic groups and participation in regular, sustained activity. The prevalence of regular, sustained activity tended to be higher among 18- through 29-year-olds than among other age groups, and it was lowest (≤15 percent) among women aged 75 years and older. Education and income levels were associated positively with regular, sustained activity. For example, adults with a college education had an approximately 50 percent higher prevalence of regular, sustained activity than those with fewer than 12 years of education. Among the regions of the United States, the West tended to have the highest prevalence of adults participating in regular, sustained activity (Table 73-4). Regular, sustained activity, which comprises many outdoor activities, was most prevalent in the summer. In the 1994 BRFSS, state-specific prevalences of regular, sustained activity ranged from 11.6 to 28.3 (Table 73-3).

Regular, Vigorous Physical Activity during Leisure Time

People who exercise both regularly and vigorously would be expected to improve cardiovascular fitness the most. The NHIS and the BRFSS defined regular, vigorous physical activity as rhythmic contraction of large muscle groups, performed at 50 percent or more of estimated age- and sex-specific

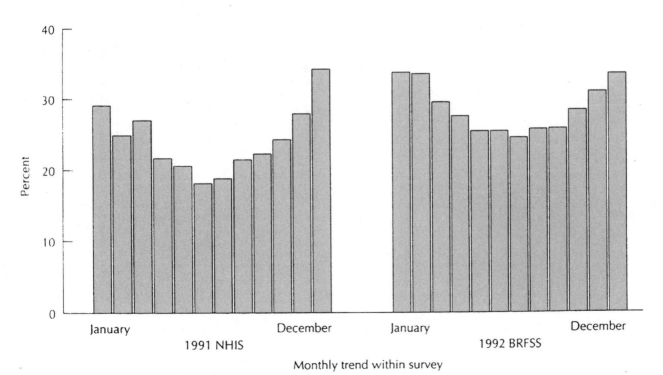

Figure 73-2 Percentage of adults aged 18+ years reporting no participation in leisure-time physical activity by month.

Table 73-3 Percentage of Adults Aged 18+ Years Reporting Participation in No Activity; Regular, Sustained Activity; and Regular, Vigorous Activity, by State,[a] Behavioral Risk Factor Surveillance System (BRFSS), 1994, United States

	No Activity	Regular, Sustained Activity	Regular, Vigorous Activity
Overall	**29.4** (29.0, 29.8)[b]	**19.7** (19.3, 20.1)	**14.0** (13.6, 14.4)
Alabama	**45.9** (43.2, 48.6)	**17.1** (14.9, 19.3)	**11.2** (9.4, 13.0)
Alaska	**22.8** (19.9, 25.7)	**28.3** (24.8, 31.8)	**15.1** (12.4, 17.8)
Arizona	**23.7** (21.2, 26.2)	**17.8** (15.4, 20.2)	**17.9** (15.4, 20.4)
Arkansas	**35.1** (32.6, 37.6)	**17.2** (15.0, 19.4)	**10.7** (9.1, 12.3)
California	**21.8** (20.2, 23.4)	**21.9** (20.3, 23.5)	**15.7** (14.5, 16.9)
Colorado	**17.2** (15.0, 19.4)	**26.5** (24.1, 28.9)	**15.9** (14.1, 17.7)
Connecticut	**22.1** (19.9, 24.3)	**26.9** (24.5, 29.3)	**16.9** (14.9, 18.9)
Delaware	**36.4** (34.0, 38.8)	**17.7** (15.7, 19.7)	**14.1** (12.5, 15.7)
D.C.	**48.6** (45.3, 51.9)	**11.6** (9.4, 13.8)	**8.7** (6.9, 10.5)
Florida	**28.0** (26.2, 29.8)	**23.8** (22.2, 25.4)	**20.0** (18.6, 21.4)
Georgia	**33.0** (30.6, 35.4)	**18.0** (16.0, 20.0)	**13.5** (11.9, 15.1)
Hawaii	**20.8** (18.6, 23.0)	**25.5** (23.3, 27.7)	**18.3** (16.3, 20.3)
Idaho	**21.9** (19.7, 24.1)	**26.3** (23.8, 28.8)	**15.7** (13.7, 17.7)
Illinois	**33.5** (31.1, 35.9)	**15.7** (13.9, 17.5)	**14.6** (12.8, 16.4)
Indiana	**29.7** (27.7, 31.7)	**18.8** (17.0, 20.6)	**13.0** (11.4, 14.6)
Iowa	**33.2** (31.2, 35.2)	**15.9** (14.3, 17.5)	**13.3** (11.9, 14.7)
Kansas	**34.5** (31.8, 37.2)	**16.8** (14.6, 19.0)	**13.9** (11.9, 15.9)
Kentucky	**45.9** (43.5, 48.3)	**13.2** (11.6, 14.8)	**11.3** (9.9, 12.7)
Louisiana	**33.5** (30.8, 36.2)	**16.8** (14.8, 18.8)	**11.3** (9.5, 13.1)
Maine	**40.7** (37.8, 43.6)	**13.0** (11.0, 15.0)	**11.3** (9.5, 13.1)
Maryland	**30.5** (28.9, 32.1)	**17.6** (16.2, 19.0)	**14.5** (13.3, 15.7)
Massachusetts	**24.0** (21.6, 26.4)	**23.2** (21.0, 25.4)	**17.4** (15.4, 19.4)
Michigan	**23.1** (21.1, 25.1)	**21.8** (19.8, 23.8)	**14.5** (12.9, 16.1)
Minnesota	**21.8** (20.4, 23.2)	**20.1** (18.7, 21.5)	**15.4** (14.2, 16.6)
Mississippi	**38.5** (35.6, 41.4)	**14.0** (12.0, 16.0)	**9.8** (8.2, 11.4)
Missouri	**32.0** (29.3, 34.7)	**18.0** (15.8, 20.2)	**10.8** (9.0, 12.6)
Montana	**21.0** (18.6, 23.4)	**21.8** (19.3, 24.3)	**15.0** (12.6, 17.4)
Nebraska	**24.3** (22.1, 26.5)	**16.7** (14.7, 18.7)	**14.7** (12.9, 16.5)
Nevada	**21.7** (19.5, 23.9)	**25.3** (22.9, 27.7)	**14.1** (12.3, 15.9)
New Hampshire	**25.8** (23.3, 28.3)	**21.2** (19.0, 23.4)	**17.0** (14.8, 19.2)
New Jersey	**30.9** (28.2, 33.6)	**20.7** (18.3, 23.1)	**11.6** (9.8, 13.4)
New Mexico	**19.8** (17.3, 22.3)	**25.5** (22.6, 28.4)	**18.4** (16.0, 20.8)
New York	**37.1** (34.7, 39.5)	**14.8** (13.2, 16.4)	**10.6** (9.2, 12.0)
North Carolina	**42.8** (40.3, 45.3)	**12.7** (11.1, 14.3)	**9.3** (7.9, 10.7)
North Dakota	**32.0** (29.6, 34.4)	**20.2** (18.0, 22.4)	**13.9** (12.1, 15.7)
Ohio	**38.0** (35.1, 40.9)	**15.9** (13.7, 18.1)	**12.4** (10.4, 14.4)
Oklahoma	**30.4** (28.0, 32.8)	**23.0** (20.8, 25.2)	**11.1** (9.5, 12.7)
Oregon	**20.8** (19.2, 22.4)	**27.3** (25.3, 29.3)	**18.7** (17.1, 20.3)
Pennsylvania	**26.5** (24.9, 28.1)	**21.2** (19.6, 22.8)	**14.5** (13.3, 15.7)
South Carolina	**31.4** (29.2, 33.6)	**15.1** (13.3, 16.9)	**11.9** (10.3, 13.5)
South Dakota	**30.8** (28.4, 33.2)	**19.4** (17.4, 21.4)	**11.9** (10.3, 13.5)
Tennessee	**39.7** (37.7, 41.7)	**15.0** (13.6, 16.4)	**12.7** (11.3, 14.1)
Texas	**27.8** (25.1, 30.5)	**20.7** (18.2, 23.2)	**13.0** (11.0, 15.0)
Utah	**21.0** (18.8, 23.2)	**21.6** (19.4, 23.8)	**14.3** (12.5, 16.1)
Vermont	**23.3** (21.5, 25.1)	**25.7** (23.7, 27.7)	**18.4** (16.6, 20.2)
Virginia	**23.0** (20.6, 25.4)	**24.6** (22.2, 27.0)	**14.6** (12.8, 16.4)
Washington	**18.2** (16.8, 19.6)	**25.7** (24.1, 27.3)	**16.8** (15.4, 18.2)
West Virginia	**45.3** (43.1, 47.5)	**14.3** (12.7, 15.9)	**9.8** (8.4, 11.2)
Wisconsin	**25.9** (23.2, 28.6)	**22.7** (20.2, 25.2)	**12.7** (10.7, 14.7)
Wyoming	**20.9** (18.4, 23.4)	**27.9** (24.8, 31.0)	**16.3** (13.9, 18.7)

SOURCE: Centers for Disease Control and Prevention, National Center for Chronic Disease Prevention and Health Promotion, BRFSS, 1994.

[a] Includes 49 states and the District of Columbia. Data for Rhode Island were unavailable.
[b] 95% confidence intervals.

Table 73-4 Percentage of Adults Aged 18+ Years Reporting Participation in Regular, Sustained Physical Activity (5+ times per week for 30+ minutes per occasion),by Various Demographic Characteristics, National Health Interview Survey (NHIS) and Behavioral Risk Factor Surveillance System (BRFSS), United States

DEMOGRAPHIC GROUP	1991 NHIS[a]	1992 BRFSS[a,b]
Overall	23.5 (22.9, 24.1)[c]	20.1 (19.7, 20.5)
Sex		
Males	26.6 (25.7, 27.5)	21.5 (20.9, 22.1)
Females	20.7 (19.9, 21.5)	18.9 (18.4, 19.3)
Race/Ethnicity		
White, non-Hispanic	24.0 (23.2, 24.7)	20.8 (20.4, 21.2)
Males	26.7 (25.7, 27.6)	21.9 (21.3, 22.5)
Females	21.5 (20.6, 22.4)	19.8 (19.2, 20.4)
Black, non-Hispanic	22.9 (21.4, 24.4)	15.2 (14.0, 16.4)
Males	28.9 (26.6, 31.3)	18.5 (16.5, 20.5)
Females	18.0 (16.2, 19.8)	12.6 (11.4, 13.8)
Hispanic	20.0 (18.1, 21.9)	20.1 (18.5, 21.7)
Males	23.7 (20.6, 26.7)	21.4 (18.9, 23.9)
Females	16.5 (14.3, 18.7)	18.9 (16.7, 21.1)
Other	23.4 (20.5, 26.2)	17.3 (15.1, 19.5)
Males	25.5 (21.0, 30.0)	19.7 (16.6, 22.8)
Females	21.1 (17.7, 24.6)	14.5 (12.0, 17.0)
Age (years)		
Males		
18–29	32.0 (30.2, 33.7)	26.8 (25.4, 28.2)
30–44	24.1 (22.8, 25.3)	17.4 (16.6, 18.2)
45–64	24.2 (22.8, 25.6)	18.9 (17.7, 20.1)
65–74	29.2 (27.0, 31.4)	26.8 (24.8, 28.8)
75+	24.6 (21.8, 27.4)	23.2 (20.5, 25.9)
Females		
18–29	23.2 (21.6, 24.8)	19.9 (18.7, 21.1)
30–44	20.4 (19.4, 21.4)	18.5 (17.7, 19.3)
45–64	20.6 (19.4, 21.8)	19.4 (18.4, 20.4)
65–74	21.3 (19.5, 23.0)	19.0 (17.6, 20.4)
75+	13.8 (12.2, 15.4)	15.0 (13.4, 16.6)
Education		
<12 yrs	18.1 (17.0, 19.2)	15.6 (14.6, 16.6)
12 yrs	21.9 (21.0, 22.7)	17.8 (17.2, 18.4)
Some college (13–15 yrs)	26.8 (25.7, 28.0)	22.7 (21.9, 23.5)
College (16+ yrs)	28.5 (27.3, 29.6)	23.5 (22.7, 24.3)
Income[d]		
<$10,000	23.6 (21.8, 25.5)	17.6 (16.6, 18.6)
$10,000–19,999	20.4 (19.3, 21.4)	18.7 (17.9, 19.5)
$20,000–34,999	23.2 (22.2, 24.2)	20.3 (19.5, 21.1)
$35,000–49,999	23.9 (22.7, 25.1)	20.9 (19.9, 21.9)
$50,000+	28.0 (26.8, 29.2)	23.5 (22.5, 24.5)
Geographic region		
Northeast	23.9 (22.8, 25.0)	20.2 (19.2, 21.2)
North Central	24.2 (22.7, 25.6)	18.2 (17.4, 19.0)
South	21.1 (19.9, 22.2)	19.0 (18.4, 19.6)
West	26.1 (24.6, 27.5)	24.0 (23.0, 25.0)

SOURCES: Centers for Disease Control and Prevention, National Center for Health Statistics, NHIS, public use data tapes, 1991; Centers for Disease Control and Prevention, National Center for Chronic Disease Prevention and Health Promotion, BRFSS, 1992.
[a] Based on data from 48 states and the District of Columbia.
[b] NHIS asked about the prior 2 weeks; BRFSS asked about the prior month.
[c] 95% confidence intervals.
[d] Annual income per family (NHIS) or household (BRFSS).

maximum cardiorespiratory capacity, 3 times per week or more for at least 20 minutes per occasion (see Appendix B). The prevalence of regular, vigorous leisure-time activity reported by U.S. adults was about 15 percent (16.4 percent in the 1991 NHIS and 14.2 percent in the 1992 BRFSS; see Table 73-5). This prevalence is lower than the goal stated in *Healthy People 2000* objective 1.4, which is to have at least 20 percent of people aged 18 years and older engage in vigorous physical activity at 50 percent or more of individual cardiorespiratory capacity 3 days or more per week for 20 minutes or more per occasion (USDHHS 1990).

The proportion performing regular, vigorous activity was 3 percentage points higher among men than women in the NHIS, but it was 3 percentage points higher among women than men in the BRFSS. This difference between sexes in the surveys may be related to the BRFSS's use of a correction procedure (based on speeds of activities like walking, jogging, and swimming) to create intensity coding (Appendix B; Caspersen and Powell [unpublished technical monograph] 1986; Caspersen and Merritt 1995). Regular, vigorous activity tended to be more prevalent among whites than among blacks and Hispanics (Table 73-5). These racial and ethnic patterns were somewhat more striking among women than among men.

The relationship between regular, vigorous physical activity and age varied somewhat between the two surveys. In the NHIS, the prevalence of regular, vigorous activity was higher for men and women aged 18–29 years than for those aged 30–64 years, but it was highest among men and women aged 65 years and older. Among men participating in the BRFSS, regular, vigorous activity increased with age from those 18–29 years old to those ≥65 years old. Among women participating in the BRFSS, the prevalence of regular, vigorous activity was higher for those aged 30–74 years than for those aged 18–29 years and ≥75 years.

The finding of generally lower prevalences of regular, vigorous activity among younger than older adults (Table 73-5) may seem unexpected. It is explained partly by both the greater leisure time of older adults and the use of an age-related relative intensity classification (Caspersen, Pollard, Pratt 1987; Stephens and Caspersen 1994; Caspersen and Merritt 1995). Because cardiorespiratory capacity declines with age, activities that would be moderately intense for young adults, such as walking, become more vigorous for older people. If the two surveys had instead used an absolute intensity classification, the estimated prevalence of people engaging in regular, vigorous physical activity would have fallen dramatically with age. (This age-related drop in activities of high absolute intensity is shown in Table 73-6 and described in the next section.) Likewise, the male:female ratio of vigorous activity prevalence in Table 73-5 would rise if an absolute intensity classification were used, because women have a lower average cardiorespiratory capacity than men.

In both surveys, the proportion of adults reporting regular, vigorous activity was higher in each successive educational category (Table 73-5). Adults who had college degrees reported regular, vigorous activity approximately two to three times more often than those who had not completed high school. In the NHIS, a similar positive association was seen between income and regular, vigorous physical activity.

In the BRFSS, the prevalence of regular, vigorous physical activity was highest at the highest income level. The prevalence of regular, vigorous physical activity was not consistently related to employment status or marital status in the two surveys. It was higher in the West than in other regions of the United States and in warmer than in colder months. In the 1994 BRFSS, state-specific prevalences of regular, vigorous activity ranged from 6.7 to 16.9 (Table 73-3).

Participation in Specific Physical Activities

NHIS participants reported specific activities in the previous 2 weeks (Table 73-6). By far, walking was the most commonly reported leisure-time physical activity, followed by gardening or yard work, stretching exercises, bicycling, strengthening exercises, stair climbing, jogging or running, aerobics or aerobic dancing, and swimming. Because these percentages are based on all participants in the year-round NHIS, they underestimate the overall prevalence of participation in seasonal activities, such as skiing.

Substantial differences exist between the sexes for many activities. Gardening or yard work, strengthening exercises, jogging or running, and vigorous or contact sports were more commonly reported by men than women. Women reported walking and aerobics or aerobic dancing more often than men and reported participation in stretching exercises, bicycling, stair climbing, and swimming about as often as men. Participation in most activities, especially weight lifting and vigorous or contact sports, declined substantially with age (Table 73-6). The prevalence of walking, gardening or yard work, and golf tended to remain stable or increase with age. Among adults aged 65 years and older, walking (>40 percent prevalence) and gardening or yard work (>20 percent prevalence) were by far the most popular activities.

Healthy People 2000 objective 1.6 recommends that at least 40 percent of people aged 6 years and older should regularly perform physical activities that enhance and maintain muscular strength, muscular endurance, and flexibility (USDHHS 1990). National surveys have not quantified all these activities but have inquired about specific sentinel activities, such as weight lifting and stretching. In the 1991 NHIS, 14.1 percent of adults reported "weight lifting and other exercises to increase muscle strength" in the previous 2 weeks (Table 73-7). Participation in strengthening activities was more than twice as prevalent among men than women. Black men tended to have the highest participation (26.2 percent) and black women the lowest (6.9 percent). Participation was much higher among younger than older adults, among the more affluent than the less affluent, and in the West than in other regions of the United States.

Of special concern, given the promising evidence that strengthening exercises provide substantial benefit to the elderly (see Chapter 4), is the low prevalence of strengthening activities among those aged 65 or older (≤6.4 percent in men and ≤2.8 percent in women; see Table 73-7).

Adult participation in stretching activity over the previous 2 weeks was 25.5 percent in the NHIS (Table 73-7). Stretching participation declined with age and tended to be associated positively with levels of education and income and to be lower in the South than in other regions of the United States.

Table 73-5 Percentage of Adults Aged 18+ Years Participating in Regular, Vigorous Physical Activity (3+ times per week for 20+ minutes per occasion at 50+ percent of estimated age- and sex-specific maximum cardiorespiratory capacity), by Various Demographic Characteristics, National Health Interview Survey (NHIS) and Behavioral Risk Factor Surveillance System (BRFSS), United States

Demographic Group	1991 NHIS[a]	1992 BRFSS[a,b]
Overall	**16.4** (15.9, 16.9)[c]	**14.4** (14.0, 14.8)
Sex		
Males	**18.1** (17.4, 18.8)	**12.9** (12.5, 13.3)
Females	**14.9** (14.3, 15.5)	**15.8** (15.4, 16.2)
Race/Ethnicity		
White, non-Hispanic	**17.2** (16.6, 17.7)	**15.3** (14.9, 15.7)
Males	**18.6** (17.9, 19.3)	**13.3** (12.7, 13.9)
Females	**15.9** (15.2, 16.6)	**17.1** (16.5, 17.7)
Black, non-Hispanic	**12.9** (11.7, 14.0)	**9.4** (8.6, 10.2)
Males	**16.0** (13.9, 18.0)	**9.5** (8.1, 10.9)
Females	**10.4** (9.0, 11.7)	**9.4** (8.4, 10.4)
Hispanic	**13.6** (11.9, 15.2)	**11.9** (10.5, 13.3)
Males	**15.6** (12.9, 18.3)	**12.4** (10.2, 14.6)
Females	**11.7** (9.9, 13.4)	**11.4** (9.8, 13.0)
Other	**16.8** (14.5, 19.1)	**11.8** (10.0, 13.6)
Males	**18.8** (15.2, 22.3)	**11.5** (9.0, 14.0)
Females	**14.8** (11.9, 17.8)	**12.2** (10.0, 14.4)
Age (years)		
Males		
18–29	**19.7** (18.3, 21.1)	**8.0** (7.2, 8.8)
30–44	**13.7** (12.8, 14.6)	**11.1** (10.3, 11.9)
45–64	**14.9** (13.7, 16.1)	**16.3** (15.3, 17.3)
65–74	**27.3** (25.2, 29.5)	**20.6** (18.8, 22.4)
75+	**38.3** (35.2, 41.5)	**20.6** (18.1, 23.1)
Females		
18–29	**16.0** (14.7, 17.3)	**11.4** (10.6, 12.2)
30–44	**13.3** (12.4, 14.1)	**18.0** (17.2, 18.8)
45–64	**12.1** (11.1, 13.0)	**17.7** (16.7, 18.7)
65–74	**18.5** (16.9, 20.1)	**16.5** (15.1, 17.9)
75+	**22.6** (20.5, 24.7)	**12.8** (11.4, 14.2)
Education		
<12 yrs	**11.9** (11.1, 12.8)	**8.2** (7.4, 9.0)
12 yrs	**13.6** (13.0, 14.3)	**11.5** (10.9, 12.1)
Some college (13–15 yrs)	**18.9** (17.9, 19.9)	**14.9** (14.3, 15.5)
College (16+ yrs)	**23.5** (22.4, 24.6)	**21.9** (21.1, 22.7)
Income[d]		
<$10,000	**15.5** (14.1, 17.0)	**9.0** (8.2, 9.8)
$10,000–19,999	**14.4** (13.5, 15.4)	**10.8** (10.2, 11.4)
$20,000–34,999	**15.5** (14.6, 16.4)	**14.2** (13.6, 14.8)
$35,000–49,999	**16.0** (14.9, 17.0)	**16.3** (15.5, 17.1)
$50,000+	**21.5** (20.4, 22.6)	**20.5** (19.5, 21.5)
Geographic region		
Northeast	**16.1** (15.2, 16.9)	**13.8** (13.0, 14.6)
North Central	**16.5** (15.5, 17.5)	**13.7** (13.1, 14.3)
South	**14.7** (13.9, 15.5)	**13.8** (13.2, 14.4)
West	**19.2** (17.9, 20.5)	**16.8** (16.0, 17.6)

SOURCES: Centers for Disease Control and Prevention, National Center for Health Statistics, NHIS, 1991; Centers for Disease Control and Prevention, National Center for Chronic Disease Prevention and Health Promotion, BRFSS, 1992.
[a] NHIS asked about the prior 2 weeks; BRFSS asked about the prior month.
[b] Based on data from 48 states and the District of Columbia.
[c] 95% confidence intervals.
[d] Annual income per family (NHIS) or household (BRFSS).

Activity Category	Males						Females						All Ages and Sexes
	18–29	30–44	45–64	65–74	75+	All	18–29	30–44	45–64	65–74	75+	All	
Walking for exercise	32.8	37.6	43.3	50.1	47.1	39.4	47.4	49.1	49.4	50.1	40.5	48.3	44.1
Gardening or yard work	22.2	36.0	39.8	42.6	38.4	34.2	15.4	28.6	29.6	28.2	21.5	25.1	29.4
Stretching exercises	32.1	27.2	20.0	15.5	15.7	25.0	32.5	27.7	21.4	21.9	17.9	26.0	25.5
Weight lifting or other exercise to increase muscle strength	33.6	21.2	12.2	6.4	4.7	20.0	14.5	10.6	5.1	2.8	1.1	8.8	14.1
Jogging or running	22.6	14.1	7.7	1.4	0.5	12.8	11.6	6.5	2.5	0.8	0.4	5.7	9.1
Aerobics or aerobic dance	3.4	3.3	2.1	1.6	1.0	2.8	19.3	12.3	6.6	4.2	1.6	11.1	7.1
Riding a bicycle or exercise bike	18.7	18.5	14.0	10.8	8.4	16.2	17.4	16.9	12.6	11.4	6.0	14.6	15.4
Stair climbing	10.5	11.4	9.6	6.0	4.0	9.9	14.6	12.8	10.3	7.3	5.6	11.6	10.8
Swimming for exercise	10.1	7.6	5.3	3.1	1.4	6.9	8.0	7.5	4.6	4.2	1.5	6.2	6.5
Tennis	5.7	3.3	2.9	1.1	0.4	3.5	3.1	2.4	1.3	0.6	0.1	2.0	2.7
Bowling	7.0	5.2	3.0	2.8	1.6	4.7	4.8	4.2	2.8	2.5	1.1	3.6	4.1
Golf	7.9	8.6	7.9	9.7	4.9	8.2	1.4	1.7	2.2	3.3	0.7	1.8	4.9
Baseball or softball	11.0	6.9	1.8	0.4	—	5.8	3.2	1.7	0.3	0.2	—	1.4	3.5
Handball, racquetball, or squash	5.2	2.8	1.5	0.3	—	2.7	1.0	0.4	0.4	0.1	—	0.5	1.6
Skiing	1.5	1.0	0.4	0.1	—	0.9	0.9	0.6	0.3	0.0	—	0.5	0.7
Cross country skiing	0.1	0.5	0.5	0.2	0.4	0.4	0.3	0.4	0.6	0.2	0.2	0.4	0.4
Water skiing	1.5	0.7	0.3	—	—	0.7	0.7	0.5	0.1	0.0	—	0.4	0.5
Basketball	24.2	10.5	2.4	0.1	0.1	10.5	3.1	1.7	0.4	—	0.2	1.5	5.8
Volleyball	6.8	3.0	1.1	0.2	0.2	3.1	4.4	1.9	0.5	0.0	0.1	1.8	2.5
Soccer	3.3	1.4	0.3	0.1	—	1.4	0.9	0.4	0.1	—	—	0.4	0.9
Football	7.6	1.8	0.4	0.2	—	2.7	0.7	0.4	0.0	—	—	0.3	1.5
Other sports	8.6	7.9	6.0	6.2	5.2	7.3	4.5	4.5	3.6	4.3	2.8	4.1	5.7

NOTE: 0.0 = quantity less than 0.05 but greater than zero; — = quantity is equal to zero.
SOURCE: Centers for Disease Control and Prevention, National Center for Health Statistics, NHIS, 1991.

Leisure-Time Physical Activity among Adults with Disabilities

Although little information is available on physical activity patterns among people with disabilities, one recent analysis was based on the special NHIS Health Promotion and Disease Prevention Supplement from 1991. Heath and colleagues (1995) compared physical activity patterns among people with disabilities (i.e., activity limitations due to a chronic health problem or impairment) to those among people without disabilities. People with disabilities were less likely to report engaging in regular moderate physical activity (27.2 percent) than were people without disabilities (37.4 percent). People with disabilities were also less likely to report engaging in regular vigorous physical activity (9.6 percent vs. 14.2 percent). Correspondingly, people with disabilities were more likely to report being inactive (32 percent vs. 27 percent).

Trends in Leisure-Time Physical Activity

Until the 20th century, people performed most physical activity as part of their occupations or in subsistence activities. In Western populations, occupation-related physical demands have declined, and the availability of leisure time has grown. It is generally believed that over the past 30 years, as both the popularity of sports and public awareness of the role of physical activity in maintaining health have increased, physical activity performed during leisure time has increased (Stephens 1987; Jacobs et al 1991). Stephens concluded that the increase was greater among women than men and among older than younger adults and that the rate of increase probably was more pronounced in the 1970s than between 1980 and 1985 (Stephens 1987). However, no systematic data were collected on physical activity among U.S. adults until the 1980s.

Even now, few national data are available on consistently measured trends in physical activity. The NHIS has data from 1985, 1990, and 1991, and the BRFSS has consistent data from the same 25 states and the District of Columbia for each year between 1986 and 1992 and for 1994. According to the NHIS, participation in leisure-time physical activity among adults changed very little between the mid-1980s and the early 1990s (Table 73-8 and Figure 73-3). Similarly, in the BRFSS (Table 73-8 and Figure 73-4), little improvement was evident from 1986 through 1994.

Table 73-7 Percentage of Adults Aged 18+ Years Reporting Participation in Any Strengthening Activities[a] or Stretching Exercises in the Prior 2 Weeks, by Various Demographic Characteristics, National Health Interview Survey (NHIS), United States, 1991

DEMOGRAPHIC GROUP	STRENGTHENING ACTIVITIES	STRETCHING EXERCISES
Overall	**14.1** (13.6, 14.6)[b]	**25.5** (24.7, 26.4)
Sex		
Males	**20.0** (19.2, 20.7)	**25.0** (24.0, 26.1)
Females	**8.8** (8.3, 9.2)	**26.0** (25.1, 27.0)
Race/Ethnicity		
White, non-Hispanic	**13.7** (13.2, 14.2)	**25.9** (24.9, 26.8)
Males	**18.8** (18.0, 19.6)	**24.9** (23.8, 26.0)
Females	**9.0** (8.5, 9.6)	**26.7** (25.7, 27.8)
Black, non-Hispanic	**15.5** (14.2, 16.9)	**24.2** (22.5, 26.0)
Males	**26.2** (23.7, 28.7)	**24.7** (22.1, 27.3)
Females	**6.9** (5.8, 8.0)	**23.9** (21.7, 26.0)
Hispanic	**15.8** (13.9, 17.6)	**22.4** (19.9, 24.9)
Males	**23.4** (20.3, 26.5)	**23.6** (20.4, 26.7)
Females	**8.6** (7.0, 10.3)	**21.3** (18.3, 24.3)
Other	**14.9** (12.3, 17.5)	**30.0** (26.2, 33.8)
Males	**20.3** (16.0, 24.7)	**31.4** (26.0, 36.8)
Females	**9.2** (6.6, 11.7)	**28.5** (24.3, 32.7)
Age (years)		
Males		
18–29	**33.6** (31.7, 35.5)	**32.1** (30.1, 34.2)
30–44	**21.2** (20.1, 22.3)	**27.2** (25.8, 28.6)
45–64	**12.2** (11.1, 13.4)	**20.0** (18.6, 21.5)
65–74	**6.4** (5.1, 7.7)	**15.5** (13.4, 17.6)
75+	**4.7** (3.1, 6.3)	**15.7** (13.2, 18.3)
Females		
18–29	**14.5** (13.3, 15.6)	**32.5** (30.7, 34.2)
30–44	**10.6** (9.9, 11.4)	**27.7** (26.3, 29.0)
45–64	**5.1** (4.5, 5.8)	**21.4** (20.1, 22.8)
65–74	**2.8** (2.0, 3.7)	**21.9** (20.0, 23.8)
75+	**1.1** (0.7, 1.6)	**17.9** (16.0, 19.9)
Education		
<12 yrs	**7.4** (6.6, 8.1)	**14.7** (13.5, 15.8)
12 yrs	**12.3** (11.7, 13.0)	**22.6** (21.7, 23.6)
Some college (13–15 yrs)	**18.3** (17.3, 19.2)	**31.3** (29.9, 32.7)
College (16+ yrs)	**19.6** (18.6, 20.6)	**35.4** (34.0, 36.9)
Income[c]		
<$10,000	**12.9** (11.4, 14.4)	**23.4** (21.7, 25.1)
$10,000–$19,999	**10.7** (9.8, 11.6)	**21.0** (19.7, 22.3)
$20,000–$34,999	**14.3** (13.4, 15.1)	**25.6** (24.4, 26.9)
$35,000–$49,999	**15.3** (14.3, 16.3)	**28.9** (27.4, 30.4)
$50,000+	**19.1** (18.1, 20.2)	**33.5** (32.1, 34.9)
Geographic region		
Northeast	**13.8** (12.9, 14.8)	**24.9** (23.6, 26.2)
North Central	**14.5** (13.6, 15.3)	**28.5** (26.5, 30.6)
South	**12.4** (11.6, 13.3)	**20.8** (19.2, 22.4)
West	**16.5** (15.4, 17.7)	**29.9** (28.1, 31.7)

SOURCE: Centers for Disease Control and Prevention, National Center for Health Statistics, NHIS, 1991.
[a] Strengthening activities include weight lifting and other exercises to increase muscle strength.
[b] 95% confidence intervals.
[c] Annual income per family.

PHYSICAL ACTIVITY AMONG ADOLESCENTS AND YOUNG ADULTS IN THE UNITED STATES

The most recent U.S. data on the prevalence of physical activity among young people are from the 1992 household-based NHIS-YRBS, which sampled all young people aged 12–21 years, and the 1995 school-based YRBS, which included students in grades 9–12. Variations in estimates between the NHIS-YRBS and the YRBS may be due not only to the distinct populations represented in each survey but

Table 73-8 Trends in the Percentage of Adults Aged 18+ Years Reporting Participation in No Activity; Regular, Sustained Activity; and Regular, Vigorous Activity, by Sex, National Health Interview Survey (NHIS) and Behavioral Risk Factor Surveillance System (BRFSS), United States, from 1985–1994

	1985, 1990, 1991 NHIS			1986–1994 BRFSS[a]		
	MALES	FEMALES	TOTAL	MALES	FEMALES	TOTAL
No activity						
1985	19.9 (18.8, 20.9)[b]	26.3 (25.3, 27.3)	23.2 (22.3, 24.1)			
1986				31.2 (30.0, 32.4)	34.3 (33.3, 35.3)	32.8 (32.0, 33.6)
1987				29.6 (28.4, 30.8)	33.9 (32.9, 34.9)	31.8 (31.0, 32.6)
1988				27.5 (26.5, 28.5)	31.5 (30.5, 32.5)	29.6 (28.8, 30.4)
1989				28.8 (27.8, 29.8)	33.6 (32.6, 34.6)	31.3 (30.5, 32.1)
1990	24.9 (23.9, 25.9)	32.4 (31.4, 33.4)	28.3 (28.0, 29.7)	28.6 (27.6, 29.6)	32.3 (31.3, 33.3)	30.5 (29.7, 31.3)
1991	21.4 (20.2, 22.6)	26.9 (25.8, 28.0)	24.3 (23.2, 25.3)	29.0 (28.0, 30.0)	32.8 (32.0, 33.6)	31.0 (30.4, 31.6)
1992				26.7 (25.9, 27.5)	31.4 (30.6, 32.2)	29.2 (28.6, 29.8)
1993						
1994				28.7 (27.9, 29.5)	33.0 (32.2, 33.8)	30.9 (30.3, 31.5)
Regular, sustained activity						
1985	27.5 (26.6, 28.4)	22.5 (21.7, 23.3)	24.9 (24.2, 25.5)			
1986				19.5 (18.5, 20.5)	18.1 (17.3, 18.9)	18.8 (18.2, 19.4)
1987				20.0 (18.8, 21.2)	17.6 (16.8, 18.4)	18.8 (18.2, 19.4)
1988				20.5 (19.5, 21.5)	19.6 (18.8, 20.4)	20.0 (19.4, 20.6)
1989				20.0 (19.0, 21.0)	18.0 (17.2, 18.8)	19.0 (18.4, 19.6)
1990	29.0 (28.1, 29.9)	22.7 (22.0, 23.4)	25.7 (25.1, 26.3)	20.5 (19.5, 21.5)	18.5 (17.7, 19.3)	19.4 (18.8, 20.0)
1991	26.6 (25.7, 27.5)	20.7 (19.9, 21.5)	23.5 (22.9, 24.1)	19.5 (18.7, 20.3)	18.3 (17.5, 19.1)	18.9 (18.3, 19.5)
1992				21.0 (20.2, 21.8)	18.4 (17.8, 19.0)	19.7 (19.1, 20.3)
1993						
1994				19.3 (18.5, 20.1)	18.1 (17.5, 18.7)	18.7 (18.1, 19.3)
Regular, vigorous activity						
1985	17.2 (16.1, 18.3)	15.1 (14.3, 15.8)	16.1 (15.3, 16.8)			
1986				11.2 (10.4, 12.0)	10.3 (9.7, 10.9)	10.7 (10.1, 11.3)
1987				10.7 (9.9, 11.5)	10.6 (10.0, 11.2)	10.7 (10.1, 11.3)
1988				11.1 (10.3, 11.9)	12.3 (11.5, 13.1)	11.7 (11.1, 12.3)
1989				11.3 (10.5, 12.1)	11.9 (11.3, 12.5)	11.6 (11.2, 12.0)
1990	18.9 (18.1, 19.7)	15.9 (15.3, 16.4)	17.3 (16.8, 17.8)	11.0 (10.2, 11.8)	12.9 (12.3, 13.5)	12.0 (11.6, 12.4)
1991	18.1 (17.4, 18.8)	14.9 (14.3, 15.5)	16.4 (15.9, 16.9)	11.2 (10.6, 11.8)	12.6 (12.0, 13.2)	11.9 (11.5, 12.3)
1992				11.8 (11.2, 12.4)	12.2 (11.6, 12.8)	12.0 (11.6, 12.4)
1993						
1994				11.4 (10.8, 12.0)	11.4 (10.8, 12.0)	11.4 (11.0, 11.8)

SOURCES: Centers for Disease Control and Prevention, National Center for Health Statistics, NHIS, 1985, 1990, 1991; Centers for Disease Control and Prevention, National Center for Chronic Disease Prevention and Health Promotion, BRFSS, 1986–1992 and 1994.
[a] 25 states and the District of Columbia.
[b] 95% confidence intervals.

also to the time of year each survey was conducted, the mode of administration, the specific wording of questions, and the age of respondents. Trends over time can be monitored only with the YRBS, which was conducted in 1991 and 1993 as well as in 1995. An assessment of the test-retest reliability of the YRBS indicated that the four physical activity items included in the study had a kappa value (an indicator of reliability) in the "substantial" (i.e., 61–80) or "almost perfect" (i.e., 81–100) range (Brener et al 1995).

Physical Inactivity

Healthy People 2000 objective 1.5 calls for reducing to no more than 15 percent the proportion of people aged 6 years and older who are inactive (USDHHS 1990). For this report, inactivity was defined as performing no vigorous activity (exercise or sports participation that made the respondent "sweat or breathe hard" for at least 20 minutes) and performing no light to moderate activity (walking or bicycling for at least 30

minutes) during any of the 7 days preceding the survey. Among 12- through 21-year-olds surveyed in the 1992 NHIS-YRBS, the prevalence of inactivity in the previous week was 13.7 percent and was higher among females than males (15.3 percent vs. 12.1 percent) (Table 73-9). Overall, there was no difference among racial and ethnic groups, but black females had a higher prevalence than white females (20.2 percent vs. 13.7 percent). For both males and females, inactivity increased with age.

Similarly, in the 1995 school-based YRBS, the prevalence of inactivity in the previous week was 10.4 percent (Table 73-9) and was higher among females than males (13.8 percent vs. 7.3 percent). The prevalence was higher among black students than white students (15.3 percent vs. 9.3 percent) and among black females than white females (21.4 percent vs. 11.6 percent). Among female high school students, a substantial increase in inactivity was reported in the upper grades.

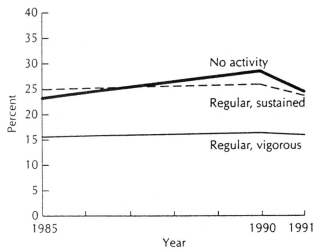

Figure 73-3 Trends in leisure-time physical activity of adults aged 18+ years, NHIS.

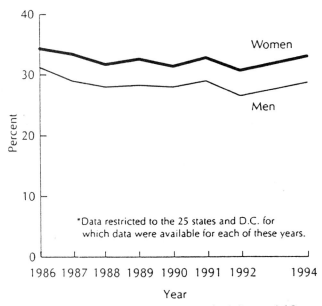

Figure 73-4 Trends in the percentage of adults aged 18+ years participating in no leisure-time activity, BRFSS.*

Thus the *Healthy People 2000* goal for inactivity has been met for adolescents overall but not for black females or for young adults.

Vigorous Physical Activity

Healthy People 2000 objective 1.4 (USDHHS 1990) proposes to increase to at least 75 percent the proportion of children and adolescents aged 6–17 years who engage in vigorous physical activity that promotes cardiorespiratory fitness 3 days or more per week for 20 minutes or more per occasion. In the 1992 NHIS-YRBS, 53.7 percent of 12- through 21-year-olds reported having exercised or taken part in sports that made them "sweat and breathe hard" during 3 or more of the 7 days preceding the survey (Table 73-10). However, one-fourth

reported no vigorous activity during the same time period. Prevalences of vigorous activity were higher among males than females (60.2 percent vs. 47.2 percent) and among white youths than Hispanic youths (54.6 percent vs. 49.5 percent) (Table 73-10). Vigorous physical activity declined with age. Among males, the prevalence of vigorous activity was at least 60 percent for those aged 12–17 years but was lower at older ages (e.g., 42.2 percent among 21-year-olds). Among females aged 12–14 years, the prevalence was at least 60 percent but was lower at older ages (e.g., 30.2 percent among 21-year-olds). The prevalence of vigorous activity was associated positively with income and was higher during the spring than during other seasons.

In the 1995 YRBS, 63.7 percent of students in grades 9–12 reported having exercised or taken part in sports that made them "sweat and breathe hard" for at least 20 minutes during 3 or more of the 7 days preceding the survey (Table 73-10). However, 16.0 percent reported no vigorous physical activity during the same time period. Subgroup patterns were similar to those reported for the NHIS-YRBS. Vigorous physical activity was more common among male than female students (74.4 percent vs. 52.1 percent) and among white than black or Hispanic students (67 percent vs. 53.2 percent and 57.3 percent, respectively). Among both male and female students, vigorous activity was less common in the upper grades. From 1991 through 1995, the overall prevalence did not change significantly among students in grades 9–12 (data not shown).

NHIS-YRBS and YRBS data clearly show that the prevalence of vigorous physical activity among young people falls short of the *Healthy People 2000* goal of 75 percent.

Other Physical Activity

Healthy People 2000 objective 1.6 (USDHHS 1990) aims for at least 40 percent of people aged 6 and older to regularly perform physical activities that enhance and maintain muscular strength, muscular endurance, and flexibility. The 1992 NHIS-YRBS indicated that 45.6 percent of 12- through 21-year-olds had participated in strengthening or toning activities (e.g., push-ups, sit-ups, or weight lifting) during at least 3 of the 7 days preceding the survey (Table 73-11). These activities were more common among males than females (54.6 percent vs. 36.4 percent) and among white and Hispanic youths than black youths (46.4 percent and 45.4 percent, respectively, vs. 39.8 percent). Among both males and females, the prevalence of strengthening or toning activities decreased as age increased and was greater among young people living in households with higher incomes.

Similar to the NHIS-YRBS, the 1995 YRBS indicated that 50.3 percent of students in grades 9–12 had participated in strengthening or toning activities during at least 3 of the 7 days preceding the survey (Table 73-11). Subgroup patterns were similar to those reported for the 1992 NHIS-YRBS. Male students were more likely than female students to participate in strengthening or toning activities (59.1 percent vs. 41.0 percent), and white students were more likely than black students to do so (52.8 percent vs. 41.4 percent). Among female students, participation was greater among those in lower grades, but this practice did not vary by grade among male students. Between 1991 and 1995, the overall prevalence

Table 73-9 Percentage of Young People Reporting No Participation in Vigorous or Moderate Physical Activity during Any of the 7 days Preceding the Survey, by Demographic Group, 1992 National Health Interview Survey-Youth Risk Behavior Survey (NHIS-YRBS) and 1995 Youth Risk Behavior Survey (YRBS), United States

DEMOGRAPHIC GROUP	1992 NHIS-YRBS[a]		1995 YRBS[b]
Overall	**13.7** (12.9, 14.5)[c]		**10.4** (9.0, 11.9)
Sex			
Males	**12.1** (11.0, 13.2)		**7.3** (6.5, 8.1)
Females	**15.3** (14.1, 16.5)		**13.8** (11.2, 16.3)
Race/Ethnicity			
White, non-Hispanic	**13.4** (12.4, 14.5)		**9.3** (7.9, 10.7)
Males	**13.1** (11.7, 14.6)		**7.3** (6.4, 8.1)
Females	**13.7** (12.4, 15.1)		**11.6** (8.7, 14.4)
Black, non-Hispanic	**14.7** (12.7, 16.6)		**15.3** (12.4, 18.2)
Males	**9.2** (6.9, 11.5)		**8.1** (5.4, 10.7)
Females	**20.2** (17.0, 23.5)		**21.4** (16.9, 25.8)
Hispanic	**14.3** (12.4, 16.3)		**11.3** (8.6, 14.1)
Males	**11.1** (8.4, 13.8)		**7.5** (5.1, 9.9)
Females	**17.8** (14.9, 20.7)		**15.0** (10.6, 19.5)
Age (years)		**Grade in school**	
Males		**Males**	
12	**7.7** (5.1, 10.2)		
13	**6.0** (3.6, 8.3)		
14	**3.6** (2.1, 5.1)		
15	**6.3** (3.7, 8.9)	9	**6.0** (3.4, 8.7)
16	**9.6** (6.8, 12.4)	10	**5.2** (3.0, 7.4)
17	**10.5** (7.2, 13.9)	11	**7.9** (4.3, 11.4)
18	**18.8** (14.4, 23.3)	12	**10.0** (7.4, 12.5)
19	**18.6** (14.7, 22.5)		
20	**22.3** (17.9, 26.8)		
21	**18.1** (14.3, 21.9)		
Females		**Females**	
12	**8.4** (5.2, 11.5)		
13	**6.8** (4.4, 9.2)		
14	**8.3** (5.1, 11.5)		
15	**9.8** (7.0, 12.6)	9	**8.7** (6.1, 11.3)
16	**14.4** (10.9, 17.9)	10	**9.2** (7.3, 11.0)
17	**16.8** (13.2, 20.3)	11	**17.8** (13.6, 22.0)
18	**18.7** (14.5, 22.8)	12	**18.5** (13.3, 23.7)
19	**22.3** (18.1, 26.5)		
20	**25.0** (21.0, 28.9)		
21	**19.6** (16.4, 22.9)		
Annual family income			
<$10,000	**14.9** (12.6, 17.3)		
$10,000–19,999	**16.0** (14.1, 17.9)		
$20,000–34,999	**12.2** (10.6, 13.8)		
$35,000–49,999	**13.8** (11.6, 15.9)		
$50,000+	**11.2** (9.8, 12.7)		

SOURCES: Centers for Disease Control and Prevention, National Center for Health Statistics, NHIS-YRBS, 1992 machine readable data file and documentation, 1993; Centers for Disease Control and Prevention, National Center for Chronic Disease Prevention and Health Promotion, YRBS 1995 data tape (in press).
[a] A national household-based survey of youths aged 12–21 years.
[b] A national school-based survey of students in grades 9–12.
[c] 95% confidence intervals.

of strengthening or toning activities among students in grades 9–12 did not change (data not shown).

In the 1992 NHIS-YRBS, 48.0 percent of 12- through 21-year-olds reported having participated in stretching activities (e.g., toe touching, knee bending, or leg stretching) during at least 3 of the 7 days preceding the survey. White and Hispanic youths were more likely than black youths to report this (49.2 percent and 48.5 percent, respectively, vs. 40.7 percent). Overall, the prevalence of stretching activities did not differ by sex, although these activities were more common among

Table 73-10 Percentage of Young People Reporting Participation in Vigorous Physical Activity during 3 or More of the 7 Days Preceding the Survey, by Demographic Group, 1992 National Health Interview Survey-Youth Risk Behavior Survey (NHIS-YRBS) and 1995 Youth Risk Behavior Survey (YRBS), United States

DEMOGRAPHIC GROUP	1992 NHIS-YRBS[a]	1995 YRBS[b]
Overall	**53.7** (52.5, 54.9)[c]	**63.7** (60.4, 66.9)
Sex		
Males	**60.2** (58.6, 61.8)	**74.4** (72.1, 76.6)
Females	**47.2** (45.6, 48.8)	**52.1** (47.5, 56.8)
Race/Ethnicity		
White, non-Hispanic	**54.6** (53.2, 56.0)	**67.0** (62.6, 71.4)
Males	**60.2** (58.4, 62.0)	**76.0** (73.0, 78.9)
Females	**49.0** (46.8, 51.2)	**56.7** (50.0, 63.4)
Black, non-Hispanic	**52.6** (49.9, 55.3)	**53.2** (49.6, 56.8)
Males	**62.7** (58.8, 66.6)	**68.1** (62.8, 73.4)
Females	**42.3** (38.6, 46.0)	**41.3** (33.5, 42.1)
Hispanic	**49.5** (46.6, 52.4)	**57.3** (53.7, 60.9)
Males	**56.7** (52.6, 60.8)	**69.7** (64.9, 74.5)
Females	**41.7** (38.2, 45.2)	**45.2** (39.9, 50.6)

Age (years)		**Grade in school**	
Males		**Males**	
12	**70.8** (66.7, 74.9)		
13	**73.7** (69.4, 78.0)		
14	**76.1** (72.2, 80.0)		
15	**72.6** (68.1, 71.1)	9	**80.8** (75.9, 85.6)
16	**65.6** (60.3, 70.9)	10	**75.9** (72.5, 79.3)
17	**60.2** (54.7, 65.7)	11	**70.2** (67.5, 72.9)
18	**48.4** (43.1, 53.7)	12	**66.9** (63.0, 70.7)
19	**44.1** (38.4, 49.8)		
20	**43.4** (38.5, 48.3)		
21	**42.2** (37.1, 47.3)		
Females		**Females**	
12	**66.2** (62.1, 70.3)		
13	**63.1** (58.0, 68.2)		
14	**63.1** (58.4, 67.8)		
15	**56.6** (51.9, 61.3)	9	**60.9** (54.8, 67.0)
16	**50.9** (45.6, 56.2)	10	**54.4** (47.6, 61.3)
17	**43.6** (38.1, 49.1)	11	**44.7** (40.6, 48.9)
18	**37.5** (32.2, 42.8)	12	**41.0** (34.6, 47.5)
19	**32.6** (27.3, 37.9)		
20	**28.2** (23.9, 32.5)		
21	**30.2** (25.5, 34.9)		
Annual family income			
<$10,000	**46.7** (43.2, 50.2)		
$10,000–19,999	**48.5** (46.0, 51.1)		
$20,000–34,999	**55.0** (52.5, 57.6)		
$35,000–49,999	**58.4** (55.5, 61.3)		
$50,000+	**60.2** (57.9, 62.6)		

SOURCES: Centers for Disease Control and Prevention, National Center for Health Statistics, NHIS-YRBS, 1992 machine readable data file and documentation, 1993; Centers for Disease Control and Prevention, National Center for Chronic Disease Prevention and Health Promotion, YRBS 1995 data tape (in press).

[a] A national household-based survey of youths aged 12–21 years.
[b] A national school-based survey of students in grades 9–12.
[c] 95% confidence intervals.

black males than among black females (44.9 percent vs. 36.5 percent). Among both males and females, the prevalence was higher in the younger age categories. Participation was also higher with higher family income.

In the 1995 YRBS, 53.0 percent of students in grades 9–12 reported having participated in stretching activities during at least 3 of the 7 days preceding the survey (Table 73-12). Subgroup patterns were generally similar to those reported for the NHIS-YRBS. Similar proportions of male and female students participated in stretching activities (55.5 percent and 50.4 percent, respectively), and white students were more likely than black students to do so (55.1 percent vs.

Table 73-11 Percentage of Young People Reporting Participation in Strengthening or Toning Activities during 3 or More of the 7 Days Preceding the Survey, by Demographic Group, 1992 National Health Interview Survey-Youth Risk Behavior Survey (NHIS-YRBS) and 1995 Youth Risk Behavior Survey (YRBS), United States

DEMOGRAPHIC GROUP	1992 NHIS-YRBS[a]	Grade in school	1995 YRBS[b]
Overall	**45.6** (44.4, 46.8)[c]		**50.3** (46.6, 54.0)
Sex			
Males	**54.6** (53.0, 56.2)		**59.1** (56.1, 62.1)
Females	**36.4** (34.8, 38.0)		**41.0** (36.0, 46.0)
Race/Ethnicity			
White, non-Hispanic	**46.4** (45.0, 47.8)		**52.8** (47.2, 58.4)
Males	**54.4** (52.6, 56.2)		**60.3** (56.4, 64.2)
Females	**38.4** (36.4, 40.4)		**44.4** (36.4, 52.4)
Black, non-Hispanic	**39.8** (37.5, 42.2)		**41.4** (37.9, 45.0)
Males	**53.2** (49.3, 57.1)		**54.2** (49.7, 58.6)
Females	**26.2** (23.1, 29.3)		**31.3** (26.7, 35.9)
Hispanic	**45.4** (42.5, 48.3)		**47.4** (41.8, 53.1)
Males	**53.3** (49.4, 57.2)		**57.8** (51.9, 63.8)
Females	**36.9** (33.2, 40.6)		**37.4** (29.6, 45.2)
Age (years)			
Males		**Males**	
12	**59.4** (54.7, 64.1)		
13	**66.3** (62.2, 70.4)		
14	**61.1** (56.0, 66.2)		
15	**66.6** (61.9, 71.3)	9	**65.3** (58.0, 72.5)
16	**61.3** (56.0, 66.6)	10	**60.0** (55.8, 64.2)
17	**53.9** (48.6, 59.2)	11	**55.9** (52.5, 59.2)
18	**46.0** (41.3, 50.7)	12	**54.7** (49.7, 59.7)
19	**45.2** (39.7, 50.7)		
20	**42.0** (37.5, 46.5)		
21	**40.5** (35.8, 45.2)		
Females		**Females**	
12	**43.9** (39.6, 48.2)		
13	**46.9** (41.6, 52.2)		
14	**47.6** (42.7, 52.5)		
15	**44.0** (39.1, 48.9)	9	**51.3** (42.9, 59.8)
16	**38.1** (33.6, 42.6)	10	**45.6** (38.3, 53.0)
17	**37.1** (32.0, 42.2)	11	**31.0** (27.6, 34.3)
18	**31.1** (25.6, 36.6)	12	**30.0** (25.1, 34.9)
19	**26.4** (22.1, 30.7)		
20	**26.3** (22.0, 30.6)		
21	**23.2** (19.3, 27.1)		
Annual family income			
<$10,000	**36.4** (33.7, 39.1)		
$10,000–$19,999	**44.6** (41.9, 47.3)		
$20,000–$34,999	**46.5** (44.0, 49.1)		
$35,000–$49,999	**49.6** (46.7, 52.5)		
$50,000+	**51.4** (49.1, 53.8)		

SOURCES: Centers for Disease Control and Prevention, National Center for Health Statistics, NHIS-YRBS, 1992 machine readable data file and documentation, 1993; Centers for Disease Control and Prevention, National Center for Chronic Disease Prevention and Health Promotion, YRBS 1995 data tape (in press).
[a] A national household-based survey of youths aged 12–21 years.
[b] A national school-based survey of students in grades 9–12.
[c] 95% confidence intervals.

45.4 percent). Participation in stretching activities declined across grades for both male and female students. Between 1991 and 1995, the overall prevalence among students in grades 9–12 did not change significantly (data not shown).

Thus the *Healthy People 2000* objective for strengthening and stretching activities has been met overall among adolescents and young adults but not among all subgroups.

Healthy People 2000 objective 1.3 (USDHHS 1990)

Table 73-12 Percentage of Young People Reporting Participation in Stretching Activities during 3 or More of the 7 Days Preceding the Survey, by Demographic Group, 1992 National Health Interview Survey-Youth Risk Behavior Survey (NHIS-YRBS) and 1995 Youth Risk Behavior Survey (YRBS), United States

Demographic Group	1992 NHIS-YRBS[a]		1995 YRBS[b]
Overall	**48.0** (46.8, 49.2)[c]		**53.0** (49.9, 56.2)
Sex			
Males	**48.2** (46.6, 49.8)		**55.5** (52.3, 58.7)
Females	**47.9** (46.3, 49.5)		**50.4** (46.6, 54.3)
Race/Ethnicity			
White, non-Hispanic	**49.2** (47.8, 50.6)		**55.1** (50.8, 59.3)
Males	**48.0** (46.0, 50.0)		**56.1** (52.1, 60.1)
Females	**50.4** (48.4, 52.4)		**53.9** (48.2, 59.5)
Black, non-Hispanic	**40.7** (38.0, 43.4)		**45.4** (41.7, 49.0)
Males	**44.9** (41.0, 48.8)		**50.5** (45.0, 55.9)
Females	**36.5** (32.8, 40.2)		**41.5** (36.6, 46.3)
Hispanic	**48.5** (45.8, 51.2)		**49.1** (45.0, 53.2)
Males	**49.9** (46.0, 53.8)		**54.8** (50.1, 59.6)
Females	**47.0** (43.3, 50.7)		**43.5** (37.6, 49.5)
Age (years)		**Grade in school**	
Males		**Males**	
12	**55.4** (50.5, 60.3)		
13	**62.0** (57.3, 66.7)		
14	**57.9** (53.2, 62.6)		
15	**56.1** (51.0, 61.2)	9	**65.7** (58.9, 72.6)
16	**54.0** (48.7, 59.3)	10	**51.1** (47.8, 54.4)
17	**48.2** (42.9, 53.5)	11	**52.9** (48.1, 57.6)
18	**36.2** (31.1, 41.3)	12	**49.8** (42.0, 57.7)
19	**36.7** (32.0, 41.4)		
20	**32.9** (28.4, 37.4)		
21	**38.5** (33.4, 43.6)		
Females		**Females**	
12	**62.5** (58.0, 67.0)		
13	**62.5** (57.2, 67.8)		
14	**61.6** (56.7, 66.5)		
15	**57.9** (53.0, 62.8)	9	**59.9** (52.8, 67.0)
16	**52.0** (47.1, 56.9)	10	**55.8** (49.6, 61.9)
17	**42.0** (37.1, 46.9)	11	**39.5** (33.7, 45.3)
18	**38.5** (33.0, 44.0)	12	**38.4** (32.7, 44.1)
19	**33.1** (28.0, 38.2)		
20	**33.9** (29.6, 38.2)		
21	**35.0** (30.9, 39.1)		
Annual family income			
<$10,000	**40.8** (37.7, 43.9)		
$10,000–$19,999	**44.5** (41.8, 47.2)		
$20,000–$34,999	**48.2** (45.9, 50.6)		
$35,000–$49,999	**51.9** (49.2, 54.6)		
$50,000+	**54.2** (51.7, 56.8)		

SOURCES: Centers for Disease Control and Prevention, National Center for Health Statistics, NHIS-YRBS, 1992 machine readable data file and documentation, 1993; Centers for Disease Control and Prevention, National Center for Chronic Disease Prevention and Health Promotion, YRBS 1995 data tape (in press).

[a] A national household-based survey of youths aged 12–21 years.
[b] A national school-based survey of students in grades 9–12.
[c] 95% confidence intervals.

proposes to increase to at least 30 percent the proportion of people aged 6 and older who engage regularly, preferably daily, in light to moderate physical activity for at least 30 minutes per day. Walking and bicycling can be used to measure light to moderate physical activity among young people. In the 1992 NHIS-YRBS, 26.4 percent of 12- through 21-year-olds reported having walked or bicycled for 30 minutes or more on at least 5 of the 7 days preceding

Table 73-13 Percentage of Young People Reporting Participation in Walking or Bicycling for 30 Minutes or More during 5 or More of the 7 days Preceding the Survey, by Demographic Group, 1992 National Health Interview Survey-Youth Risk Behavior Survey (NHIS-YRBS) and 1995 Youth Risk Behavior Survey (YRBS), United States

DEMOGRAPHIC GROUP	1992 NHIS-YRBS[a]		1995 YRBS[b]
Overall	26.4 (25.4, 27.4)[c]		21.1 (18.7, 23.5)
Sex			
Males	29.1 (27.5, 30.7)		21.6 (18.4, 24.8)
Females	23.7 (22.3, 25.1)		20.5 (17.8, 23.2)
Race/Ethnicity			
White, non-Hispanic	25.1 (23.9, 26.3)		18.3 (15.0, 21.6)
Males	27.5 (25.7, 29.3)		19.7 (15.5, 23.8)
Females	22.7 (21.1, 24.3)		16.8 (13.9, 19.8)
Black, non-Hispanic	26.9 (24.6, 29.2)		27.0 (23.2, 30.9)
Males	29.8 (26.7, 32.9)		27.2 (23.2, 31.2)
Females	23.9 (20.2, 27.6)		26.4 (20.8, 32.0)
Hispanic	32.3 (29.8, 34.9)		26.8 (22.6, 31.0)
Males	35.5 (31.6, 39.4)		26.0 (19.9, 32.1)
Females	28.8 (25.5, 32.1)		27.6 (23.8, 31.5)
Age (years)		**Grade in school**	
Males		**Males**	
12	38.9 (34.6, 43.2)		
13	37.3 (32.4, 42.2)		
14	35.3 (31.2, 39.4)		
15	33.9 (29.0, 38.8)	9	27.9 (22.1, 33.7)
16	29.9 (25.6, 34.2)	10	21.7 (17.8, 25.6)
17	22.2 (17.7, 26.7)	11	19.2 (16.2, 22.1)
18	23.3 (18.6, 28.0)	12	17.7 (13.1, 22.3)
19	21.3 (17.2, 25.4)		
20	22.0 (17.9, 26.1)		
21	23.3 (19.0, 27.6)		
Females		**Females**	
12	32.2 (28.1, 36.3)		
13	28.5 (24.0, 33.0)		
14	28.7 (23.8, 33.6)		
15	22.9 (18.8, 27.0)	9	22.5 (18.5, 26.5)
16	22.9 (18.8, 27.0)	10	22.8 (18.5, 27.2)
17	19.4 (15.5, 23.3)	11	16.8 (13.3, 20.3)
18	20.1 (16.0, 24.2)	12	16.1 (11.6, 20.6)
19	18.8 (14.5, 23.1)		
20	20.8 (16.7, 24.9)		
21	22.1 (18.4, 25.8)		
Annual family income			
<$10,000	27.8 (25.1, 30.5)		
$10,000–$19,999	29.5 (26.8, 32.2)		
$20,000–$34,999	27.6 (25.2, 30.0)		
$35,000–$49,999	25.5 (23.2, 27.9)		
$50,000+	23.5 (21.5, 25.5)		

SOURCES: Centers for Disease Control and Prevention, National Center for Health Statistics, NHIS-YRBS, 1992 machine readable data file and documentation, 1993; Centers for Disease Control and Prevention, National Center for Chronic Disease Prevention and Health Promotion, YRBS 1995 data tape (in press).
[a] A national household-based survey of youths aged 12–21 years.
[b] A national school-based survey of students in grades 9–12.
[c] 95% confidence intervals.

the survey (Table 73-13). These activities were more common among males than females (29.1 percent vs. 23.7 percent) and among Hispanic youths than white or black youths (32.3 percent vs. 25.1 percent and 26.9 percent, respectively). Walking or bicycling decreased as age increased and was more prevalent in the fall than in other seasons.

In the 1995 YRBS, 21.1 percent of students in grades

9–12 reported having walked or bicycled for 30 minutes or more on at least 5 of the 7 days preceding the survey (Table 73-13). Male and female students reported similar prevalences of these activities. Black and Hispanic students were more likely than white students to have walked or bicycled (27.0 percent and 26.8 percent, respectively, vs. 18.3 percent). Between 1993 and 1995, the overall prevalence among students in grades 9–12 did not change significantly (data not shown).

It thus appears that the *Healthy People 2000* objective for light to moderate physical activity has not been attained by adolescents and young adults.

The 1992 NHIS-YRBS provided information on participation in seven additional types of physical activity during 1 or more of the 7 days preceding the survey: aerobics or dancing; baseball, softball, or Frisbee®[1]; basketball, football, or soccer; house cleaning or yard work for at least 30 minutes; running, jogging, or swimming for exercise; skating, skiing, or skateboarding; and tennis, racquetball, or squash (Table 73-14). Among 12- through 21-year-olds, males were more likely than females to participate in baseball, softball, or Frisbee®; in basketball, football, or soccer; in running, jogging, or swimming for exercise; in skating, skiing, or skateboarding; and in tennis, racquetball, or squash. Females were more likely than males to participate in aerobics or dancing and in house cleaning or yard work for at least 30 minutes. White youths were more likely than black or Hispanic youths to participate in skating, skiing, or skateboarding and in tennis, racquetball, or squash. For both males and females, increasing age was associated with decreasing participation in baseball, softball, or Frisbee®; in basketball, football, or soccer; in running, jogging, or swimming for exercise; and in skating, skiing, or skateboarding. For females, participation in aerobics or dancing and in tennis, racquetball, or squash also decreased by age.

Physical Education in High School

The YRBS provides data on enrollment and daily attendance in school physical education for students in grades 9–12. (See Chapter 6 for a discussion of the availability of physical education programs.) In 1995, 59.6 percent of students in grades 9–12 were enrolled in physical education (Table 73-15). Enrollment did not vary by sex or race/ethnicity, but it decreased by grade. Between 1991 and 1995, overall enrollment in physical education among students in grades 9–12 did not change significantly (data not shown).

Healthy People 2000 objective 1.8 (USDHHS 1990) recommends increasing to at least 50 percent the proportion of children and adolescents in grades 1–12 who participate in daily school physical education. The 1995 YRBS indicated that daily attendance in physical education among high school students was 25.4 percent and did not vary by sex or race/ethnicity (Table 73-15). Daily attendance decreased with increasing grade for both male and female students.

Between 1991 and 1995, overall daily attendance in physical education classes in grades 9–12 decreased significantly, from 41.6 percent to 25.4 percent (data not shown). Current trend data thus indicate that the *Healthy People 2000* goal of 50 percent has not been attained and is also becoming more distant.

Healthy People 2000 objective 1.9 (USDHHS 1990) recommends that students be active for at least 50 percent of the class time they spend in physical education. In 1995, 69.7 percent of students in grades 9–12 who were taking physical education reported being physically active for at least 20 minutes, which is about half of a typical class period (Table 73-15). This active participation was more common among male students than female students (74.8 percent vs. 63.7 percent) and among white students than black students (71.3 percent vs. 59.0 percent). Between 1991 and 1995, the overall percentage of students in grades 9–12 taking physical education who reported being physically active for at least 20 minutes decreased from 80.7 percent to 69.7 percent (data not shown). Decreases between 1991 or 1993 and 1995 occurred for students in all grades. Thus a decreasing proportion of the high school students who are enrolled in physical education classes are meeting the *Healthy People 2000* goal for time spent being physically active in class.

Only 18.6 percent of all high school students were physically active for at least 20 minutes on a daily basis in physical education classes (data not shown).

Sports Team Participation

The YRBS provides data on participation on sports teams during the 12 months preceding the survey for students in grades 9–12. In 1995, 50.3 percent of students participated on sports teams run by a school, and 36.9 percent participated on sports teams run by other organizations (Table 73-16). Participation on sports teams run by a school was more common among male students than female students (57.8 percent vs. 42.4 percent) and among white students than Hispanic students (53.9 percent vs. 37.8 percent). Between 1991 and 1995, participation on sports teams run by a school increased significantly among high school students overall, from 43.5 percent to 50.3 percent (data not shown). Specific increases were identified among female students, white and black students, and students in grades 11 and 12.

Participation on sports teams run by other organizations besides a school was more common among male students than female students (46.4 percent vs. 26.8 percent) and among white students than Hispanic students (39.1 percent vs. 32.0 percent). Between 1991 and 1995, overall participation among students in grades 9–12 on sports teams run by other organizations did not change significantly (data not shown).

CONCLUSIONS
Adults
1. Approximately 15 percent of U.S. adults engage regularly (3 times a week for at least 20 minutes) in vigorous physical activity during leisure time.

---

[1] Use of trade names is for identification only and does not imply endorsement by the U.S. Department of Health and Human Services.

Table 73-14 Percentage of Young People Reporting Participation in Selected Physical Activities during 1 or More of the 7 Days Preceding the Survey, by Demographic Group, 1992 National Health Interview Survey-Youth Risk Behavior Survey (NHIS-YRBS)[a], United States

Demographic Group	Aerobics or Dancing	Baseball, Softball, or Frisbee®	Basketball, Football, or Soccer	House Cleaning or Yard Work for ≥30 Minutes	Running, Jogging, or Swimming	Skating, Skiing, or Skateboarding	Tennis, Raquetball, or Squash
Overall	38.2 (37.1, 39.2)[b]	22.4 (21.4, 23.4)	45.8 (44.6, 47.1)	82.8 (81.7, 83.8)	55.3 (54.1, 56.6)	13.3 (12.5, 14.0)	10.5 (9.8, 11.2)
Sex							
Males	22.6 (21.3, 24.0)	27.2 (25.7, 28.8)	61.7 (60.1, 63.3)	78.1 (76.6, 79.5)	57.6 (55.9, 59.3)	15.9 (14.8, 17.0)	11.7 (10.7, 12.8)
Females	53.9 (52.4, 55.5)	17.5 (16.4, 18.7)	29.7 (28.2, 31.3)	87.5 (86.3, 88.7)	53.0 (51.4, 54.7)	10.6 (9.6, 11.5)	9.3 (8.4, 10.2)
Race/Ethnicity							
White, non-Hispanic	35.0 (33.7, 36.2)	23.6 (22.3, 24.9)	44.7 (43.1, 46.2)	83.1 (81.9, 84.3)	55.8 (54.3, 57.3)	15.2 (14.2, 16.2)	11.4 (10.6, 12.3)
Black, non-Hispanic	49.4 (46.6, 52.1)	16.6 (14.3, 18.9)	49.5 (46.7, 52.3)	84.2 (81.9, 86.5)	52.4 (49.5, 55.3)	9.0 (7.3, 10.8)	5.4 (4.2, 6.6)
Hispanic	42.0 (39.0, 45.0)	23.4 (21.1, 25.7)	47.1 (44.4, 49.8)	80.1 (77.9, 82.4)	53.6 (50.9, 56.4)	9.8 (8.2, 11.5)	8.0 (6.7, 9.4)
Age (years)							
Males							
12	26.9 (22.5, 31.2)	46.4 (41.6, 51.3)	81.2 (77.4, 85.0)	76.9 (72.9, 81.0)	72.8 (68.3, 77.3)	32.5 (27.8, 37.3)	14.4 (10.8, 18.0)
13	23.4 (19.6, 27.3)	40.6 (35.8, 45.3)	84.3 (80.8, 87.9)	83.3 (80.1, 86.5)	74.3 (70.1, 78.4)	26.2 (22.1, 30.3)	13.3 (10.3, 16.4)
14	22.0 (18.4, 25.7)	40.9 (36.6, 45.2)	78.5 (74.3, 82.6)	79.4 (75.5, 83.4)	71.2 (66.8, 75.6)	20.7 (16.9, 24.5)	14.5 (11.3, 17.8)
15	21.9 (17.7, 26.1)	25.6 (21.0, 30.3)	76.7 (72.5, 81.0)	82.9 (79.3, 86.5)	70.8 (66.5, 75.1)	19.9 (15.9, 23.9)	15.3 (11.7, 18.9)
16	24.5 (20.2, 28.9)	27.4 (22.9, 31.9)	69.6 (64.5, 74.6)	79.6 (75.7, 83.6)	63.4 (58.8, 68.1)	13.4 (10.0, 16.8)	10.4 (7.4, 13.3)
17	20.8 (16.8, 24.6)	22.5 (18.1, 26.9)	59.3 (54.2, 64.3)	78.7 (74.5, 82.9)	55.3 (49.9, 60.7)	12.2 (8.6, 15.7)	11.3 (8.0, 14.6)
18	19.0 (14.9, 23.1)	20.8 (16.3, 25.2)	54.6 (49.1, 60.0)	70.9 (65.9, 75.9)	47.4 (42.2, 52.5)	9.4 (6.3, 12.4)	11.6 (8.3, 14.9)
19	24.0 (19.6, 28.4)	17.5 (13.8, 21.2)	43.8 (38.5, 49.0)	75.0 (69.6, 80.4)	46.3 (41.3, 51.2)	10.8 (7.7, 14.0)	9.9 (6.9, 12.8)
20	21.2 (17.2, 25.2)	17.0 (13.3, 20.8)	38.5 (33.9, 43.2)	74.4 (70.3, 78.5)	34.4 (29.9, 38.9)	8.6 (6.1, 11.2)	8.2 (5.5, 10.8)
21	21.4 (17.2, 25.7)	15.6 (12.1, 19.1)	32.4 (27.6, 37.1)	77.6 (73.7, 81.5)	39.8 (34.1, 45.5)	5.9 (3.8, 7.9)	9.5 (6.5, 12.5)
Females							
12	63.1 (58.7, 67.5)	37.9 (33.4, 42.5)	62.6 (57.6, 67.6)	88.0 (84.8, 91.2)	80.5 (76.4, 84.5)	24.9 (20.5, 29.3)	13.9 (10.5, 17.3)
13	63.7 (59.5, 67.9)	30.3 (26.2, 34.3)	61.6 (56.9, 66.3)	88.1 (85.1, 91.1)	76.2 (72.1, 80.3)	19.7 (16.1, 23.4)	12.4 (9.2, 15.6)
14	63.7 (59.0, 68.3)	29.1 (24.7, 33.5)	51.9 (46.8, 57.1)	87.2 (83.9, 90.4)	72.9 (68.6, 77.2)	14.8 (11.6, 18.0)	13.0 (10.0, 15.9)
15	62.0 (57.5, 66.4)	22.6 (18.3, 26.9)	41.6 (37.2, 46.1)	88.5 (85.3, 91.7)	65.4 (60.7, 70.1)	10.0 (7.0, 12.9)	16.1 (12.6, 19.6)
16	55.7 (50.5, 60.9)	16.0 (12.3, 19.6)	28.0 (23.3, 32.6)	89.1 (85.7, 92.5)	59.7 (54.8, 64.6)	8.9 (6.2, 11.7)	11.1 (8.0, 14.2)
17	54.0 (48.8, 59.2)	10.2 (7.4, 13.1)	23.4 (19.0, 27.7)	86.0 (82.6, 89.4)	49.0 (43.5, 54.4)	4.8 (2.7, 6.8)	8.0 (5.4, 10.5)
18	50.3 (45.2, 55.5)	11.4 (7.3, 15.4)	13.8 (10.2, 17.4)	87.0 (83.4, 90.5)	41.5 (35.8, 47.3)	8.1 (5.5, 10.7)	6.9 (4.4, 9.5)
19	44.8 (39.1, 50.4)	6.9 (4.4, 9.3)	8.5 (6.0, 11.0)	82.6 (78.1, 87.1)	32.9 (27.8, 38.0)	6.6 (4.1, 9.1)	3.8 (2.1, 5.4)
20	40.7 (36.2, 45.2)	7.6 (4.8, 10.4)	6.9 (4.7, 9.1)	87.1 (83.0, 91.2)	30.8 (25.8, 35.7)	5.8 (3.5, 8.0)	5.8 (3.6, 8.0)
21	45.6 (41.0, 50.2)	8.4 (5.9, 10.9)	7.5 (5.2, 9.8)	89.8 (86.2, 93.4)	30.3 (26.0, 34.6)	4.8 (3.1, 6.6)	4.1 (2.2, 5.9)

source: Centers for Disease Control and Prevention, National Center for Health Statistics, NHIS-YRBS, 1992 machine readable data file and documentation, 1993.
[a] A national household-based survey of youths aged 12–21 years.
[b] 95% confidence intervals.

Table 73-15 Percentage of Students in Grades 9–12 Reporting Enrollment in Physical Education Class, Daily Attendance in Physical Education Class, and Participation in Exercise or Sports for at Least 20 Minutes During an Average Physical Education Class, by Demographic Group, 1995 Youth Risk Behavior Survey (YRBS),[a] United States

Demographic Group	Enrolled in Physical Education	Attended Physical Education Daily	Exercised or Played Sports ≥20 Minutes per Class[b]
Overall	**59.6** (48.6, 70.5)[c]	**25.4** (15.8, 34.9)	**69.7** (66.4, 72.9)
Sex			
Males	**62.2** (52.5, 71.8)	**27.0** (16.8, 37.2)	**74.8** (71.8, 77.8)
Females	**56.8** (44.1, 69.6)	**23.5** (14.5, 32.4)	**63.7** (59.3, 68.1)
Race/Ethnicity			
White, non-Hispanic	**62.9** (49.8, 76.1)	**21.7** (9.9, 33.5)	**71.3** (67.0, 75.6)
Males	**64.2** (52.6, 75.8)	**23.3** (11.2, 35.3)	**74.8** (71.1, 78.5)
Females	**61.7** (46.4, 77.0)	**19.9** (8.0, 31.8)	**67.1** (60.5, 73.8)
Black, non-Hispanic	**50.2** (45.1, 55.3)	**33.8** (29.9, 37.8)	**59.0** (54.6, 63.3)
Males	**56.8** (50.6, 62.9)	**37.7** (32.3, 43.0)	**71.8** (65.9, 77.8)
Females	**44.4** (37.3, 51.5)	**30.1** (25.8, 34.5)	**46.6** (39.3, 53.8)
Hispanic	**51.0** (40.9, 61.2)	**33.1** (24.5, 41.8)	**68.5** (62.8, 74.1)
Males	**57.6** (48.6, 66.6)	**36.2** (28.8, 43.6)	**76.0** (67.0, 85.0)
Females	**44.6** (31.2, 58.0)	**30.1** (18.7, 41.5)	**59.0** (52.5, 65.6)
Grade in school			
Males			
9	**80.5** (75.1, 85.9)	**42.1** (23.3, 60.8)	**76.5** (72.2, 80.9)
10	**72.6** (62.3, 82.8)	**34.8** (18.9, 50.8)	**73.1** (67.9, 78.3)
11	**51.5** (32.8, 70.1)	**17.4** (9.3, 25.6)	**75.8** (70.3, 81.2)
12	**45.4** (29.0, 61.9)	**14.8** (9.2, 20.4)	**73.7** (68.1, 79.3)
Females			
9	**80.8** (73.8, 87.8)	**39.7** (21.5, 58.0)	**65.6** (57.2, 74.1)
10	**71.4** (59.3, 83.5)	**33.8** (17.4, 50.3)	**63.9** (58.8, 68.9)
11	**41.2** (22.8, 59.6)	**12.3** (7.6, 17.1)	**57.2** (48.4, 66.0)
12	**39.1** (20.9, 57.2)	**11.1** (6.5, 15.7)	**66.0** (59.7, 72.4)

SOURCE: Centers for Disease Control and Prevention, National Center for Chronic Disease Prevention and Health Promotion, YRBS 1995 data tape (in press).
[a] A national school-based survey of students in grades 9–12.
[b] Among students enrolled in physical education.
[c] 95% confidence intervals.

2. Approximately 22 percent of adults engage regularly (5 times a week for at least 30 minutes) in sustained physical activity of any intensity during leisure time.

3. About 25 percent of adults report no physical activity in their leisure time.

4. Physical inactivity is more prevalent among women than men, among blacks and Hispanics than whites, among older than younger adults, and among the less affluent than the more affluent.

5. The most popular leisure-time physical activities among adults are walking and gardening or yard work.

Adolescents and Young Adults

1. Only about one-half of U.S. young people (ages 12–21 years) regularly participate in vigorous physical activity. One-fourth report no vigorous physical activity.

2. Approximately one-fourth of young people walk or bicycle (i.e., engage in light to moderate activity) nearly every day.

3. About 14 percent of young people report no recent vigorous or light to moderate physical activity. This indicator of inactivity is higher among females than males and among black females than white females.

4. Males are more likely than females to participate in vigorous physical activity, strengthening activities, and walking or bicycling.

5. Participation in all types of physical activity declines strikingly as age or grade in school increases.

6. Among high school students, enrollment in physical education remained unchanged during the first half of the 1990s. However, daily attendance in physical education declined from approximately 42 percent to 25 percent.

Table 73-16 Percentage of Students in Grades 9–12 Reporting Participation on at least One Sports Team Run by a School or by Other Organizations during the Year Preceding the Survey, by Demographic Group, 1995 Youth Risk Behavior Survey (YRBS),[a] United States

DEMOGRAPHIC GROUP	PARTICIPATION ON SPORTS TEAM RUN BY A SCHOOL	PARTICIPATION ON SPORTS TEAM RUN BY OTHER ORGANIZATION
Overall	**50.3** (46.6, 54.0)[b]	**36.9** (34.4, 39.4)
Sex		
Males	**57.8** (53.7, 62.0)	**46.4** (43.4, 49.3)
Females	**42.4** (38.6, 46.2)	**26.8** (24.2, 29.4)
Race/Ethnicity		
White, non-Hispanic	**53.9** (49.6, 58.2)	**39.1** (35.7, 42.5)
Males	**59.9** (54.8, 65.0)	**47.2** (43.0, 51.4)
Females	**47.1** (43.0, 51.2)	**29.9** (26.8, 32.9)
Black, non-Hispanic	**45.0** (39.9, 50.2)	**32.4** (29.0, 35.9)
Males	**57.9** (52.6, 63.2)	**46.8** (42.4, 51.1)
Females	**34.9** (28.2, 41.7)	**21.1** (16.5, 25.8)
Hispanic	**37.8** (33.6, 42.0)	**32.0** (28.5, 35.6)
Males	**48.6** (44.0, 53.2)	**43.2** (37.9, 48.4)
Females	**27.3** (21.9, 32.7)	**21.2** (16.5, 25.9)
Grade in school		
Males		
9	**61.7** (54.0, 69.4)	**52.8** (47.0, 58.7)
10	**55.6** (50.1, 61.1)	**46.9** (42.4, 51.4)
11	**56.0** (49.7, 62.4)	**43.1** (40.6, 45.7)
12	**58.3** (52.0, 64.6)	**42.8** (39.2, 46.3)
Females		
9	**43.7** (39.2, 48.2)	**32.0** (28.2, 35.9)
10	**47.9** (42.8, 53.0)	**32.4** (26.8, 38.0)
11	**39.4** (32.1, 46.7)	**23.8** (19.9, 27.6)
12	**38.8** (32.4, 45.1)	**19.8** (15.2, 24.3)

SOURCE: Centers for Disease Control and Prevention, National Center for Chronic Disease Prevention and Health Promotion, YRBS 1995 data tape (in press).
[a] A national school-based survey of students in grades 9–12.
[b] 95% confidence intervals.

7. The percentage of high school students who were enrolled in physical education and who reported being physically active for at least 20 minutes in physical education classes declined from approximately 81 percent to 70 percent during the first half of this decade.

8. Only 19 percent of all high school students report being physically active for 20 minutes or more in daily physical education classes.

Research Needs

1. Develop methods to monitor patterns of regular, moderate physical activity.

2. Improve the validity and comparability of self-reported physical activity in national surveys.

3. Improve methods for identifying and tracking physical activity patterns among people with disabilities.

4. Routinely monitor the prevalence of physical activity among children under age 12.

5. Routinely monitor school policy requirements and of students' participation in physical education classes in elementary, middle, and high schools.

APPENDIX A: SOURCES OF NATIONAL SURVEY DATA

National Health Interview Survey (NHIS)

This analysis used data from the 1991 NHIS to determine current prevalences of physical activity, and from 1985, 1990, and 1991 to determine physical activity trends, among U.S. adults aged 18 years and older (National Center for Health Statistics [NCHS] 1988, 1993; NCHS unpublished data). Since 1957, NCHS has been collecting year-round health data from a probability sample of the civilian, noninstitutionalized adult population of the United States. The design included oversampling of blacks to provide more precise estimates. For the 1985, 1990, and 1991 special supplement on health promotion and disease prevention, one adult aged 18 years or older was randomly selected from each family for participation from the total NHIS sample. Interviews were conducted in the homes; self-response was required for this special supplement, and callbacks were made as necessary. The sample was poststratified by the age, sex, and racial distribution of the U.S. population for the survey year and weighted to provide national estimates. The overall response rate for the NHIS has been 83 to 88 percent.

Behavioral Risk Factor Surveillance System (BRFSS)

The Centers for Disease Control and Prevention (CDC) initiated the BRFSS in 1981 to help states obtain prevalence estimates of health behaviors, including physical activity, that were associated with chronic disease. The BRFSS conducts monthly, year-round, telephone interviews of adults aged 18 years of age and older sampled by random-digit dialing (Remington et al 1988; Siegel et al 1991; Frazier, Franks, Sanderson 1992). Physical activity questions have been consistent since 1986, except for a minor change from 1986 to 1987. In 1994, the most recent survey available, 49 states and the District of Columbia participated. Only 25 states and the District of Columbia have participated continuously since 1986. For 1986–1991, sample sizes ranged from approximately 35,000 to 50,000, and response rates from 62 to 71 percent; for 1992, the sample size was 96,343, and the response rate 71 percent; for 1994, the sample size was 106,030, and the response rate 70 percent. For examination of trends, analysis was restricted to the 25 states and the District of Columbia, that had consistently participated from 1986 through 1994. For 1992 cross-sectional analyses, data were included from all 48 states that had participated that year and from the District of Columbia. For 1994 cross-sectional analyses, data were included from the 49 participating states and from the District of Columbia.

Third National Health and Nutrition Examination Survey (NHANES III)

NHANES III is the seventh in a series of national health examination surveys that began in the 1960s. The sample for NHANES III (NCHS 1994a) was selected from 81 counties across the United States. The survey period covered 1988–1994 and consisted of two phases of equal length and sample size. Both Phase I (1988–1991) and Phase II (1992–1994) used probability samples of the U.S. civilian non-institutionalized population. Black and Mexican American populations were oversampled to obtain statistically reliable estimates for these minority groups. Phase II data were not available at the time this report was prepared. In Phase I, the selected population was 12,138 adults 18 years of age or older, of which 82 percent (9,901) underwent a home interview that included questions on physical activity. Participants in NHANES III also underwent a detailed medical examination in a mobile examination center. NHANES III data were weighted to the 1990 U.S. civilian noninstitutionalized population to provide national estimates.

Youth Risk Behavior Survey (YRBS)

The CDC developed the YRBS (Kolbe 1990; Kolbe, Kann, Collins 1993) to measure six categories of priority health-risk behaviors among adolescents: 1) behaviors that contribute to intentional and unintentional injuries; 2) tobacco use; 3) alcohol and other drug use; 4) sexual behaviors that result in unintended pregnancy and sexually transmitted diseases, including HIV infection; 5) unhealthy dietary behaviors; and 6) physical inactivity. Data were collected through national, state, and local school-based surveys of high school students in grades 9–12 during the spring of odd-numbered years and through a 1992 national household-based survey of young people aged 12–21 years. The 1991, 1993, and 1995 national

school-based YRBS (Kann et al 1993; CDC unpublished data) used three-stage cluster sample designs. The targeted population consisted of all public and private school students in grades 9–12 in the 50 states and the District of Columbia. Schools with substantial numbers of black and Hispanic students were sampled at relatively higher rates than all other schools.

Survey procedures were designed to protect student privacy and allow anonymous participation. The questionnaire was administered in the classroom by trained data collectors, and students recorded their responses on answer sheets designed for scanning by computer. The school response rates ranged from 70 to 78 percent, and the student response rate ranged from 86 to 90 percent. The total number of students who completed questionnaires was 12,272 in 1991, 16,296 in 1993, and 10,904 in 1995. The data were weighted to account for nonresponse and for oversampling of black and Hispanic students.

National Health Interview Survey-Youth Risk Behavior Survey (NHIS-YRBS)

To provide more information about risk behaviors among young people, including those who do not attend school, the CDC added a youth risk behavior survey to the 1992 National Health Interview Survey (CDC 1993; NCHS 1994b). The survey was conducted as a follow-back from April 1992 through March 1993 among 12- through 21-year-olds from a national probability sample of households. School-aged youths not attending school were oversampled. NHIS-YRBS interviews were completed for 10,645 young people, representing an overall response rate of 74 percent.

The questionnaire for this survey was administered through individual portable cassette players with earphones. After listening to questions, respondents marked their answers on standardized answer sheets. This methodology was designed to help young people with reading problems complete the survey and to enhance confidentiality during household administration. Data from this report were weighted to represent the U.S. population of 12- through 21-year-olds.

APPENDIX B: MEASURES OF PHYSICAL ACTIVITY IN POPULATION SURVEYS

There is no uniformly accepted method of assessing physical activity. Various methods have been used (Stephens 1989); unfortunately, estimates of physical activity are highly dependent on the survey instrument. The specific problems associated with using national surveillance systems—such as those employed here—to monitor leisure-time physical activity have been reviewed previously (Caspersen, Merritt, Stephens 1994).

All of the population surveys cited have employed a short-term recall of the frequency, and in some cases the duration and intensity, of activities that either were listed for the participant to respond to or were probed for in an open-ended manner. The validity of these questions is not rigorously established. Estimates of prevalence of participation are influenced by sampling errors, seasons covered, and the number and wording of such questions; generally, the more activities offered, the more likely a participant will report some activity. Besides defining participation in any activity or in individual activities, many researchers have found it useful to define summary indices of regular participation in vigorous activity or moderate activity (Caspersen 1994; Caspersen, Merritt, Stephens 1994). These summary measures often require assumptions about the intensity of reported activities and the frequency and duration of physical activity required for health benefits.

National Health Interview Survey (NHIS)

Participants in the NHIS were asked in a standardized interview whether they did any of 22 exercises, sports, or physically active hobbies in the previous 2 weeks: walking for exercise, jogging or running, hiking, gardening or yard work, aerobics or aerobic dancing, other dancing, calisthenics or general exercise, golf, tennis, bowling, bicycling, swimming or water exercises, yoga, weight lifting or training, basketball, baseball or softball, football, soccer, volleyball, handball or racquetball or squash, skating, and skiing (National Center for Health Statistics [NCHS] 1992). They were also asked, in an open-ended fashion, for other unmentioned activities performed in the previous 2 weeks. For each activity, the interviewer asked the number of times, the average minutes duration, and the perceived degree to which heart rate or breathing increased (i.e., none or small, moderate, or large).

The physical activity patterns were scored by using data for frequency and duration derived directly from the NHIS. To estimate the regular, vigorous physical activity pattern, a previously proposed convention was followed (Caspersen, Pollard, Pratt 1987). One of two sex-specific regression equations was used to estimate the respondent's maximum cardiorespiratory capacity (expressed in metabolic equivalents [METs]) (Jones and Campbell 1982): [60−0.55 • age (years)]/3.5 for men, and [48−0.37 • age (years)]/3.5 for women. One MET is the value of resting oxygen uptake relative to total body mass and is generally ascribed the value of 3.5 milliliters of oxygen per kilogram of body mass per minute (for example, 3 METs equals 3 times the resting level; walking at 3 miles per hour on a level surface would be at about that intensity). Individual activity intensity was based on reported values (Taylor et al 1978; Folsom et al 1985; Stephens and Craig 1989).

The final activity intensity code for a specific activity was found by selecting one of three conditions corresponding to the perceived level of effort associated with usual participation. The perceived effort was associated with none or small, moderate, or large perceived increases in heart rate or breathing. For example, the activity intensity code for three levels of volleyball participation would be 5, 6, and 8 METs as the perceived effort progressed from none or small to large increases in heart rate or breathing. In some cases, a single intensity code was averaged for several types of activity participation that were not distinguished in the NHIS. This averaging was done for such activities as golf, calisthenics or general exercise, swimming or water exercises, skating, and skiing. To determine if an activity would qualify a person to meet the intensity criterion of vigorous physical activity, each intensity code

had to meet or exceed 50 percent of the estimated age- and sex-specific maximum cardiorespiratory capacity.

For this report, three patterns of leisure-time activity were defined (Caspersen 1994):

- *No physical activity:* No reported activity during the previous 2 weeks.

- *Regular, sustained activity:* ≥5 times per week and ≥30 minutes per occasion of physical activity of any type and at any intensity.

- *Regular, vigorous activity:* ≥3 times per week and ≥20 minutes per occasion of physical activity involving rhythmic contractions of large muscle groups (e.g., jogging or running, racquet sports, competitive group sports) performed at ≥50 percent of estimated age- and sex-specific maximum cardiorespiratory capacity.

Behavioral Risk Factor Surveillance System (BRFSS)

The BRFSS questionnaire first asks, "During the past month, did you participate in any physical activities or exercises such as running, calisthenics, golf, gardening, or walking for exercise?" If yes, participants were asked to identify their two most common physical activities and to indicate the frequency in the previous month and duration per occasion (Caspersen and Powell 1986; Caspersen and Merritt 1995). If running, jogging, walking, or swimming were mentioned, participants were also asked the usual distance covered.

The reported frequency and duration of activity were used for scoring. Intensity of physical activity was assigned by using the same intensity codes as the NHIS, and a correction procedure (explained later in this section) based on speeds of activities was used to create intensity codes for walking, running/jogging, and swimming (Caspersen and Powell 1986; Caspersen and Merritt 1995).

The estimate of speed was made by dividing the self-reported distance in miles by the duration in hours. The speed estimate was entered into specific regression equations to refine the intensity code for these four activities, because the application of a single intensity code is likely to underestimate or overestimate the intensity. Based on previously published formulae (American College of Sports Medicine 1988), five equations were constructed for predicting metabolic intensity of walking, jogging, and running at various calculated speeds:

Equation 1 METs = 1.80
(Speeds < 0.93 mph)

Equation 2 METs = 0.72 × mph + 1.13
(Speeds ≥ 0.93 but <3.75 mph)

Equation 3 METs = 3.76 × mph − 10.20
(Speeds ≥ 3.75 but <5.00 mph)

Equation 4 METs = 1.53 × mph + 1.03
(Speeds ≥ 5.00 but <12.00 mph)

Equation 5 METs = 7.0 or 8.0
(Speeds ≥ 12.00 mph)

Below 0.93 mph, an intensity code of 1.8 METs (Equation 1) was used, to be consistent with Montoye's intensity code for residual activities like those associated with slow movements (Montoye 1975). Equation 2 is extrapolated to include speeds as slow as 0.93 mph—the point at which metabolic cost was set at 1.8 METs. Persons whose calculated speeds fell between 0.93 and 12.0 mph were assigned an intensity from equations 2, 3, or 4, regardless of whether they said they walked, jogged, or ran. Equation 3 was created by simply connecting with a straight line the last point of equation 2 and the first point of equation 4. This interpolation was seen as a reasonable way to determine intensity within the range of speed where walking or jogging might equally occur. This assignment method was considered to be more objective, specific, and generally conservative than assigning an intensity code based solely on the self-reported type of activity performed. Thus, as a correction procedure for self-reported speeds judged likely to be erroneously high, an intensity of 2.5 METs was assigned for walking speeds above 5.0 mph, 7.0 METs for jogging speeds above 12.0 mph, and 8.0 METs for running speeds above 12.0 mph.

Another set of regression equations predicted metabolic intensity from swimming velocity:

Equation 6 METs = 1.80
            (Speeds < 0.26 mph)

Equation 7 METs = 4.19 × mph − 0.69
            (Speeds ≥ 0.26 but <2.11 mph)

Equation 8 METs = 8.81 × mph − 9.08
            (Speeds ≥ 2.11 but <3.12 mph)

Equation 9 METs = 5.50
            (Speeds ≥ 3.12 mph)

These equations were set forth in a Canadian monograph of energy expenditure for recreational activities (Groupe d'étude de Kino-Quebec sur le système de quantification de la dépense énergétique 1984). However, swimming speeds up to 3.12 mph for the crawl and backstroke, in the derivation of equations 7 and 8, were obtained from published research (Holmer 1974a; Holmer 1974b; Passmore and Durnin 1955). Default intensity codes were assigned as follows: 1.8 METs for swimming speeds less than 0.26 mph, and 5.5 METs for velocities greater than 3.12 mph, because such speeds are improbable and likely reflected errors in self-report.

Definitions used for leisure-time physical activity were the same as those described for the NHIS earlier in this appendix.

Third National Health and Nutrition Examination Survey (NHANES III)

The NHANES III questions that addressed leisure-time physical activity (NCHS 1994a) were adapted from the NHIS. Participants first were asked how often they had walked a mile or more at one time in the previous month. They were then asked to specify their frequency of leisure-time physical activity during the previous month for the following eight activities: jogging or running, riding a bicycle or an exercise bicycle, swimming, aerobics or aerobic dancing, other dancing, calisthenics or exercises, gardening or yard work, and weight lifting. An open-ended question asked for information on up to four physical activities not previously listed. Information on duration of physical activity was not collected.

Northern sites selected for NHANES III tended to be surveyed in warm rather than cold months, which might have led to a greater prevalence of reported physical activity than would otherwise be obtained from a year-round survey. No physical activity was defined as no reported leisure-time physical activity in the previous month. Regular, sustained activity and regular, vigorous activity were not defined for NHANES III because of the lack of information on activity duration.

Youth Risk Behavior Survey (YRBS)

In the YRBS questionnaire (Kann et al 1993), students in grades 9–12 were asked eight questions about physical activity. The question on vigorous physical activity asked, "On how many of the past 7 days did you exercise or participate in sports activities for at least 20 minutes that made you sweat and breathe hard, such as basketball, jogging, fast dancing, swimming laps, tennis, fast bicycling, or similar aerobic activities?" The questionnaire asked separately about the frequency of three specific activities in the previous 7 days: 1) stretching exercises, such as toe touching, knee bending, or leg stretching; 2) exercises to strengthen or tone the muscles, such as push-ups, sit-ups, or weight lifting; and 3) walking or bicycling for at least 30 minutes at a time. Participants were asked about physical education, "In an average week when you are in school, on how many days do you go to physical education (PE) classes?" and "During an average physical education (PE) class, how many minutes do you spend actually exercising or playing sports?" Students were also asked, "During the past 12 months, on how many sports teams run by your school did you play? (Do not include PE classes.)" and "During the past 12 months, on how many sports teams run by organizations outside of your school did you play?"

National Health Interview Survey-Youth Risk Behavior Survey (NHIS-YRBS)

The NHIS-YRBS questionnaire (NCHS 1994b) ascertained the frequency of vigorous physical activity among U.S. young people aged 12–21 years by asking, "On how many of the past 7 days did you exercise or take part in sports that made you sweat and breathe hard, such as basketball, jogging, fast dancing, swimming laps, tennis, fast bicycling, or other aerobic activities?" Ten other questions asked about the previous 7 days' frequency of participating in the following specific activities: 1) stretching exercises, such as toe touching, knee bending, or leg stretching; 2) exercises to strengthen or tone muscles, such as push-ups, sit-ups, or weight lifting; 3) house cleaning or yard work for ≥30 minutes at a time; 4) walking or bicycling for ≥30 minutes at a time; 5) baseball, softball, or Frisbee[1]; 6) basketball, football, or soccer; 7) roller skating, ice skating, skiing, or skate-boarding; 8) running, jogging, or swimming for exercise; 9) tennis, racquetball, or squash; and 10) aerobics or dance. Questions about duration and intensity were not asked.

---

[1] Use of trade names is for identification only and does not imply endorsement by the U.S. Department of Health and Human Services.

REFERENCES

American College of Sports Medicine. *Guidelines for exercise testing and prescription*. 3rd ed. Philadelphia: Lea and Febiger, 1988:168–169.

Brener ND, Collins JL, Kann L, Warren CW, Williams BI. Reliability of the Youth Risk Behavior Survey questionnaire. *American Journal of Epidemiology* 1995;141:575–580.

Caspersen CJ. What are the lessons from the U.S. approach for setting targets. In: Killoran AJ, Fentem P, Caspersen C, editors. *Moving on: international perspectives on promoting physical activity*. London: Health Education Authority, 1994:35–55.

Caspersen CJ, Merritt RK. Physical activity trends among 26 states, 1986–1990. *Medicine and Science in Sports and Exercise* 1995;27:713–720.

Caspersen CJ, Merritt RK, Stephens T. International physical activity patterns: a methodological perspective. In: Dishman RK, editor. *Advances in exercise adherence*. Champaign, IL: Human Kinetics, 1994:73–110.

Caspersen CJ, Pollard RA, Pratt SO. Scoring physical activity data with special consideration for elderly populations. In: Data for an aging population. *Proceedings of the 21st national meeting of the Public Health Conference on Records and Statistics*. Washington, DC: U.S. Government Printing Office, 1987:30–4. DHHS Publication No. (PHS)88–1214.

Centers for Disease Control. *1992 BRFSS Summary Prevalence Report*. Atlanta: U.S. Department of Health and Human Services, Public Health Service, Centers for Disease Control, National Center for Chronic Disease Prevention and Health Promotion, 1992.

Centers for Disease Control. Youth Risk Behavior Survey, 1991 data tape. Atlanta: U.S. Department of Health and Human Services, Public Health Service, Centers for Disease Control, National Center for Chronic Disease Prevention and Health Promotion, 1991. National Technical Information Service Order No. PB94–500121.

Centers for Disease Control and Prevention. *1994 BRFSS Summary Prevalence Report*. Atlanta: U.S. Department of Health and Human Services, Public Health Service, Centers for Disease Control and Prevention, National Center for Chronic Disease Prevention and Health Promotion, 1994.

Centers for Disease Control and Prevention. National Health Interview Survey—Youth Risk Behavior Survey, 1992 machine readable data file and documentation. Atlanta: U.S. Department of Health and Human Services, Public Health Service, Centers for Disease Control and Prevention, National Center for Health Statistics, 1993.

Centers for Disease Control and Prevention. Youth Risk Behavior Survey, 1993 data tape. Atlanta: U.S. Department of Health and Human Services, Public Health Service, Centers for Disease Control and Prevention, National Center for Chronic Disease Prevention and Health Promotion, 1993. National Technical Information Service Order No. PB95–503363.

Centers for Disease Control and Prevention. Youth Risk Behavior Survey, 1995 data tape. Atlanta: U.S. Department of Health and Human Services, Public Health Service, Centers for Disease Control and Prevention, National Center for Chronic Disease Prevention and Health Promotion (in press).

Folsom AR, Caspersen CJ, Taylor HL, Jacobs DR Jr, Luepker RV, Gomez-Marin O, et al. Leisure-time physical activity and its relationship to coronary risk factors in a population-based sample: the Minnesota Heart Survey. *American Journal of Epidemiology* 1985;121:570–579.

Frazier EL, Franks AL, Sanderson LM. Behavioral risk factor data. In: *Using chronic disease data: a handbook for public health practitioners*. Atlanta: U.S. Department of Health and Human Services, Public Health Service, Centers for Disease Control, National Center for Chronic Disease Prevention and Health Promotion, 1992:4-1–4-17.

Groupe d'étude de Kino-Quebec sur le système de quantification de la dépense énergétique (GSQ). Rapport final. Québec: Government du Québec, 1984.

Heath GW, Chang MH, Barker ND. Physical activity among persons with limitations—United States, 1991. Paper presented at the annual meeting of the Society for Disability Studies, June 17–19, 1995, Oakland, California.

Holmer I. Energy cost of arm stroke, leg kick, and the whole stroke in competitive swimming styles. *European Journal of Applied Physiology* 1974a; 33:105–118.

Holmer I. Propulsive efficiency of breaststroke and freestyle swimming. *European Journal of Applied Physiology* 1974b;33:95–103.

Jacobs DR Jr, Hahn LP, Folsom AR, Hannan PJ, Sprafka JM, Burke GL. Time trends in leisure-time physical activity in the upper Midwest, 1957–1987: University of Minnesota Studies. *Epidemiology* 1991;2:8–15.

Jones NL, Campbell EJM. *Clinical exercise testing*. 2nd ed. Philadelphia: W.B. Saunders, 1982:249.

Kann L, Warren W, Collins JL, Ross J, Collins B, Kolbe LJ. Results from the national school-based 1991 Youth Risk Behavior Survey and progress toward achieving related health objectives for the nation. *Public Health Reports* 1993;108(Suppl 1): 47–67.

Kolbe LJ. An epidemiological surveillance system to monitor the prevalence of youth behaviors that most affect health. *Health Education* 1990;21:44–48.

Kolbe LJ, Kann L, Collins JL. Overview of the Youth Risk Behavior Surveillance System. *Public Health Reports* 1993; 108(Suppl 1):2–10.

Montoye HJ. *Physical activity and health: an epidemiologic study of an entire community*. Englewood Cliffs, NJ: Prentice Hall, 1975.

National Center for Health Statistics. *Plan and operation of the Third National Health and Nutrition Examination Survey, 1988–94*. Vital and Health Statistics, Series 1, No. 32. Hyattsville, MD: U.S. Department of Health and Human Services, Public Health Service, Centers for Disease Control and Prevention, National Center for Health Statistics, 1994a. DHHS Publication No. (PHS)94–1308.

National Center for Health Statistics, Adams PF, Benson V. *Current estimates from the National Health Interview Survey, 1990.* Vital and Health Statistics, Series 10, No. 181. Hyattsville, MD: U.S. Department of Health and Human Services, Public Health Service, Centers for Disease Control, National Center for Health Statistics, 1991. DHHS Publication No. (PHS) 92–1509.

National Center for Health Statistics, Benson V, Marano MA. *Current estimates from the National Health Interview Survey, 1992.* Vital and Health Statistics, Series 10, No. 189. Hyattsville, MD: U.S. Department of Health and Human Services, Public Health Service, Centers for Disease Control and Prevention, National Center for Health Statistics, 1994b. DHHS Publication No. (PHS)94–1517.

National Center for Health Statistics, Piani AL, Schoenborn CA. *Health promotion and disease prevention: United States, 1990.* Vital and Health Statistics, Series 10, No. 185. Hyattsville, MD: U.S. Department of Health and Human Services, Public Health Service, Centers for Disease Control and Prevention, National Center for Health Statistics, 1993. DHHS Publication No. (PHS)93–1513.

National Center for Health Statistics, Schoenborn CA. *Health promotion and disease prevention: United States, 1985.* Vital and Health Statistics, Series 10, No. 163. Hyattsville, MD: U.S. Department of Health and Human Services, Public Health Service, Centers for Disease Control, National Center for Health Statistics, 1988. DHHS Publication No. (PHS) 88–1591.

Passmore R, Durnin JVGA. Human energy expenditure. *Physiological Reviews* 1955;35:801–840.

Remington PL, Smith MY, Williamson DF, Anda RF, Gentry EM, Hogelin GC. Design, characteristics, and usefulness of state-based behavioral risk factor surveillance: 1981–87. *Public Health Reports* 1988;103:366–375.

Siegel PZ, Brackbill RM, Frazier EL, Mariolis P, Sanderson LM, Waller MN. Behavior Risk Factor Surveillance, 1986–1990. *Morbidity and Mortality Weekly Report* 1991;40(No. SS–4): 1–23.

Stephens T. Design issues and alternatives in assessing physical activity in general population surveys. In: Drury TF, editor. *Assessing physical fitness and physical activity in population-based surveys.* Hyattsville, MD: U.S. Department of Health and Human Services, Public Health Service, Centers for Disease Control, National Center for Health Statistics, 1989: 197–210. DHHS Publication No. (PHS)89–1253.

Stephens T. Secular trends in adult physical activity: exercise boom or bust? *Research Quarterly for Exercise and Sport* 1987;58:94–105.

Stephens T, Caspersen CJ. The demography of physical activity. In: Bouchard C, Shephard RJ, Stephens T, editors. *Physical activity, fitness, and health: international proceedings and consensus statement.* Champaign, IL: Human Kinetics, 1994:204–213.

Stephens T, Craig CL. Fitness and activity measurement in the 1981 Canada Fitness Survey. In: Drury TF, editor. *Assessing physical fitness and physical activity in population-based surveys.* Hyattsville, MD: U.S. Department of Health and Human Services, Public Health Service, Centers for Disease Control, National Center for Health Statistics, 1989:401–32. DHHS Publication No. (PHS)89–1253.

Taylor HL, Jacobs DR Jr, Schucker B, Knudsen J, Leon AS, DeBacker G. A questionnaire for the assessment of leisure-time physical activities. *Journal of Chronic Diseases* 1978; 31:741–755.

U.S. Department of Health and Human Services. *Healthy People 2000: national health promotion and disease prevention objectives—full report, with commentary.* Washington, DC: U.S. Department of Health and Human Services, Public Health Service, 1990. DHHS Publication No. (PHS)91–50212.

Chapter 74

Independent and Interactive Effects of Diet and Physical Activity in the Prevention of Cardiovascular Disease

Mark A. Pereira

The purpose of this chapter is to review the scientific evidence for independent and interactive effects of diet and physical activity in the prevention of cardiovascular disease (CVD). Initially, an overview of the public health burden of cardiovascular disease and a discussion of lifestyle changes associated with the epidemiologic transition from communicable to noncommunicable disease is presented. A synopsis of the epidemiologic literature pertaining to the independent roles of diet and physical activity in the prevention of CVD is provided next. The final section is a critical review of randomized clinical trials comparing the effects of diet, exercise, and combinations of both on CVD risk factors. The summary includes future research needs.

THE BURDEN OF CARDIOVASCULAR DISEASE: PAST, PRESENT, AND FUTURE

Lifestyle changes throughout the 20th century have resulted in a steady increase in deaths from noncommunicable diseases. With the exception of 1918, CVD has been the most common cause of death in the United States in every year since the turn of the century (1). In 1995, there were more deaths in both males (455,152, or 47.4% of all deaths) and females (505,440, or 52.6% of all deaths) from CVD than from the combined total of deaths attributed to cancer, accidents, chronic obstructive pulmonary disease, pneumonia/influenza, and diabetes mellitus (1). It is estimated that 58.2 million Americans (more than 1 in 5) have at least one type of CVD; on average, CVD causes a death every 33 seconds (1).

Cardiovascular diseases could be referred to as "diseases of choice" because of the level of control that individuals have over many of the risk factors, such as tobacco use, diet, and physical activity. The combination of poor diet and lack of physical activity has been estimated to cause 300,000 deaths annually; this makes these factors second only to tobacco use as the most important "external" cause of death in the United States (2). This mortality estimate was a conservative one due to the complexity of these behaviors and the difficulty in disentangling their independent relationships to disease outcomes at the population level. It is important to realize that although *rates* of CVD have been declining, the population is aging to the extent that the actual CVD burden on society has remained relatively constant and the epidemic is likely to continue well into the next century. In contrast to a decline in the CVD death rate of 22.0% from 1985 to 1995, the total number of CVD deaths in the United States declined only 2.8% (1). In 1959, 8% of the US population was over the age of 65 years; it has been projected that this age group will comprise 13% of the US population by the year 2000, and this percentage is expected to double by the year 2020 (3).

In addition to the increasing lifespan resulting in the continued burden of CVD, most westernized countries are in the midst of an obesity epidemic. From 1976 to 1991 the prevalence of overweight adults in the United States increased from 25.4% to 33.3%, and the average body weight increased by 8 pounds (4). Although obesity is clearly the result of a gene-environment interaction, such a profound change in body weight over the course of only a few decades clearly rules out any purely genetic phenomenon responsible for the obesity epidemic. There is little question about the pernicious impact of excess weight on the risk for chronic diseases among many populations (5–7). However, there is much debate about the actual magnitude of the increased risk for CVD, morbidity, and mortality due to excess weight (8).

Surveillance systems have demonstrated a decline in the percentage of calories from dietary fat and saturated fat, and there is some evidence, although not as clear, that total caloric intake has remained relatively constant over the second half of the century (9). As such, increased caloric intake is probably not driving the obesity epidemic. Since leisuretime physical activity appears to have remained relatively constant over the past decade in the United States, with an estimated 60% of US adults reporting little or no leisuretime physical activity and 25% to 30% reporting no leisure-time activity at all (10), most of the decrease in energy expenditure appears to be coming from nonleisure activity, such as activities of daily living, activity on the job, and other activity around the home. The current obesity epidemic has likely arisen from subtle shifts in the steady state condition induced by changes in physical activity too diffuse to permit quantitative assessment (11). Therefore, the most likely causes for the obesity epidemic are the technologic advances throughout this century that have eliminated a considerable proportion of energy expenditure from our daily regimen. Telephones, cars, televisions, remote control devices, power tools and machines, computers, and the plethora of other automated devices have drastically changed the way Americans spend their time and have resulted in chronic positive energy balance within individuals over time and among individuals over generations, leading to the steady accumulation of adiposity.

The declining age-standardized rates of coronary heart disease in the United States since approximately 1970 (1) may be partly attributed to some success at the population level in dietary changes over the course of the century (i.e., improved methods of food preparation and storage have resulted in a downward trend in the consumption of dietary saturated fat and sodium [9], leading to lower levels of serum cholesterol and blood pressure [12]). However, although there are no surveillance data for occupational physical activity, there is little doubt that industrialization and technologic advances have resulted in decreased energy expenditure at work (more machines and computers and less walking and labor) and commuting to work (more cars and buses and less walking and cycling). In their review of physical activity and coronary heart disease, Powell et al (13) noted that 20 of 24 studies conducted prior to 1969 assessed occupational activity in contrast to 3 of 19 studies after 1970. Furthermore, in the San Francisco Longshoreman study, the proportion of men in the highest category of energy expenditure decreased from 40% to 5% (14), prohibiting follow-up analyses of occupational activity in this population. This downward slope of occupational activity runs counter to the sharp increase in deaths due to heart disease. Figure 74-1 depicts the tracking of trends in deaths from diseases of the heart (1), prevalence of overweight estimated from three surveys since 1960 (4), miles per person traveled in motor vehicles (15), and televisions per household over the course of the 20th century (16). Given the apparent steady decline in energy expenditure during non-leisure time due to technologic advances, the aging of the population, and the obesity epidemic, it becomes discouragingly clear that the prevention of cardiovascular disease will continue to be a tremendous public health challenge in the next century.

THE EPIDEMIOLOGY OF DIET AND PHYSICAL ACTIVITY IN THE PREVENTION OF CVD

Over the course of the 20th century a wealth of information has accumulated supporting the role of physical activity and diet in the development of CVD. Although we understand the general characteristics of an optimal lifestyle for cardiovascular health, there is much debate concerning the specific components and doses of exercise (17–20) and diet (21,22) that are critical for optimal cardiovascular health. Much of the problem is the inability of epidemiologic studies to accurately measure the complexity of physical activity and dietary behaviors, and to analyze both of these with sufficient methodologic and statistical consideration for potential confounders of the hypothesized associations. The well-known clustering of lifestyle behaviors among individuals within populations (23–28) makes it difficult to tease out independent effects on CVD risk factors, morbidity, and mortality. For example, Ursin et al (28) reported a correlation of −0.40 between leisuretime physical activity and dietary fat from an analysis of the data in NHANES, and others have reported similar findings (25,27).

Although total dietary fat is not necessarily atherogenic independent of the proportions of specific fatty acids (29–33), it is important to realize in interpreting epidemiologic research that the correlation between total dietary fat and saturated fat is strong. Furthermore, there are many other components of diet related to CVD risk that are not typically measured in epidemiologic studies or considered as confounders, such as the amount of dietary fiber and relative levels of the intake of whole plant foods, meats, and dairy products. As such, the potential for confounding is often underestimated in the design and interpretation of epidemiologic studies. All too often there is ample reason to suspect insufficient control for characteristics and behaviors that covary with the exposure of interest (physical activity or diet) and that may be causally associated with CVD.

These methodologic limitations of observational epidemiologic studies should be borne in mind when reviewing the literature. Figure 74-2 illustrates the complexity of potential interactions among diet, physical activity, and other behaviors and characteristics. These interrelationships make the design and interpretation of nonrandomized observational epidemiologic studies challenging. Such a picture is actually a simplistic perspective in that each component of risk consists of many subcomponents (e.g., multiallelic genes or types of fatty acids) that interact with the other facets of the paradigm. Many of the factors also interact with psychosocial and societal influences that are often beyond the control of the individual and the investigator. Ultimately, what needs to be demonstrated is consistency of results across various study designs examining similar biologically coherent hypotheses among many populations. In fact, consistency among many study designs and populations is a strength of clinical and epidemiologic population-based research on physical activity and diet in the prevention of CVD. However, only the randomized controlled clinical trial is suited to formally test

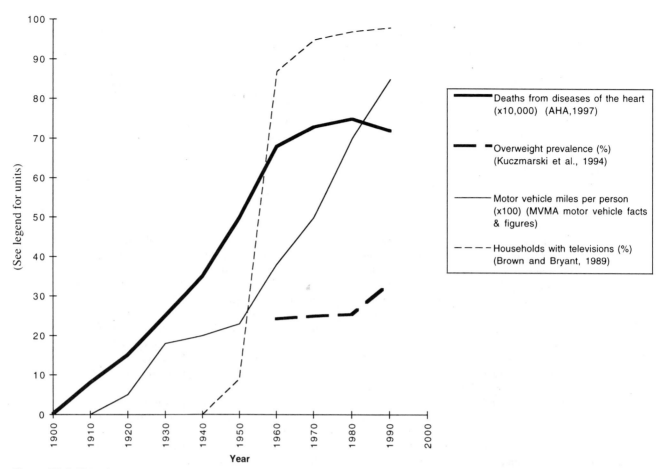

Figure 74-1 Twentieth century trends in deaths from diseases of the heart, prevalence of overweight adults, motor vehicle miles per person, and percentage of households with televisions. (*Adapted from American Heart Association. 1998 Heart and Stroke Statistical Update. Dallas, TX: American Heart Association, 1997. Source: National Center for Health Statistics and the American Heart Association. Total CVD rates are not available for most of the century. "Diseases of the heart" represents about three-fourths of total CVD mortality.)

hypotheses of causal effects between the behavioral modification and the specific health parameter under study.

DEFINITIONS AND MEASUREMENT ISSUES

Physical Activity

In conveying the basic concepts used in physical activity epidemiology, Caspersen et al (34) defined physical activity as "any bodily movement produced by skeletal muscles that results in energy expenditure." Exercise was defined as a component of physical activity "that is planned, structured, and repetitive, with the purpose of improving or maintaining one or more components of physical fitness" (34). For most adults exercise contributes minimally to total daily energy expenditure or daily physical activity (35,36); depending on the individual's leisure habits and occupation, exercise may contribute anywhere from 0% in a sedentary individual to 50% or more of daily energy expenditure in endurance athletes or lumberjacks. Limiting the scope of study to exercise would leave out most of the energy expenditure above and beyond resting metabolic rate for most middle-aged and older individuals. However, in order to manipulate energy expenditure to a

sufficient degree to stimulate a detectable physiologic response on fitness or CVD risk factors, clinical studies generally focus on exercise as the mutable exposure variable.

As discussed in detail elsewhere, the questionnaire is the method of choice for assessing physical activity in epidemiologic studies due to its nonreactiveness, practicality in terms of time and cost, applicability, and acceptable validity (37,38). However, more precise measurements of energy expenditure, such as doubly labeled water or activity monitors, may be used in smaller studies to validate the questionnaires or to measure exercise compliance in intervention studies (37–39). Because there is little physical activity in the workplace in today's society (13), most questionnaires in recent epidemiologic research focus on leisuretime exercise behavior. However, depending on the characteristics of the study population, there still may be a need to assess work or home-related activity. Therefore, many of the questionnaires used to measure physical activity in the population include not only leisuretime exercise habits, but occupational physical activity and activities such as household chores that do not satisfy the definition of exercise (40). In older or sick populations it may be particularly important to ask about activities of daily living, which may differentiate among activity levels or functional ability (41,42).

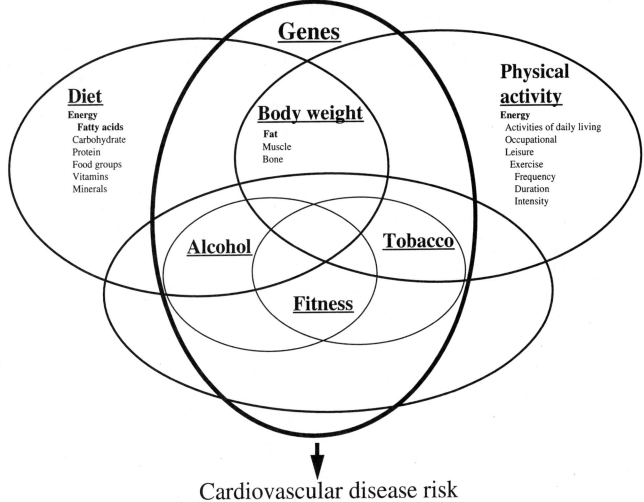

Figure 74-2 Environmental and genetic interactions of diet and physical activity on cardiovascular disease risk.

Diet

Diet is a complex behavior with an overwhelming array of components with potential for independent and interactive effects with other dietary constituents and other lifestyle behaviors on CVD risk. As with the components of physical activity, knowledge of nutrients in the diet is essential in understanding the biologic mechanisms whereby certain dietary behaviors may modify the CVD risk factor profile. Dietary intake is partitioned into macronutrients, consisting of fat, protein, and carbohydrate, and micronutrients, including water-soluble and fat-soluble vitamins and minerals. Although of no energy value due to its resistance to digestive enzymes, dietary fiber is another important dietary constituent related to chronic disease risk (43,44). Good dietary sources of soluble fiber include certain fruits and vegetables, oats, and beans, whereas insoluble fiber is more ubiquitous in plant foods and is especially concentrated in wheat bran (43,44).

The vast majority of research on dietary interventions aimed at reducing CVD risk have focused on reducing energy intake to promote weight loss and concomitant risk factor reduction, as well as decreasing saturated fatty acid intake and increasing dietary fiber through consumption of whole plant

foods. Although there are many other dietary components that are purported to have etiologic roles in CVD, such as antioxidants, flavonoids, and alcohol, in-depth discussion of these nutrients is beyond the scope of this chapter.

As with physical activity, the complexity of diet makes its measurement for epidemiologic study very challenging. There are many different ways of assessing diet in epidemiologic research, the most common being the food frequency questionnaire. More specific and labor-intensive methods, such as dietary records and 24-hour recalls, are commonly used in small clinical studies or to validate food frequency questionnaires for use in epidemiologic research. For detailed discussion of nutritional assessment in epidemiologic research, the reader is referred to publications by Thompson et al (45) and Willett (46).

RELATION TO CARDIOVASCULAR HEALTH

Physical Activity

For a more comprehensive review, the reader is referred to the Surgeon General's Report on Physical Activity and Health

(10); this report is reprinted in Chapter 73. Physical activity has been shown to be favorably associated with a wide array of metabolic factors related to CVD risk, most notably HDL cholesterol (47–49) and blood pressure (50–52). Exercise may indirectly effect CVD risk through favorable effects on body composition (53,54). The reduction in adiposity in particular is usually associated with reduction in blood pressure, LDL cholesterol and other potential atherogenic blood lipoproteins, and an increase in HDL cholesterol. There is good scientific evidence that exercise can lower blood pressure and raise HDL cholesterol independent of effects on body weight. The suspected biologic mechanism through which exercise is thought to raise HDL is an augmentation of lipoprotein lipase activity associated with an increase in HDL and a decrease in triglycerides (55). Exercise has also been shown to lower blood pressure independent of body weight changes via attenuating sympathetic activity, norepinephrine spillover, and total peripheral resistance (50,56). As such, the propensity for lowering CVD risk through a physically active lifestyle is underscored by the different indirect and direct pathways through which physical activity operates.

Regular physical activity may also improve myocardial vascularization and the oxidative capacity of skeletal muscles (47,57), improve insulin sensitivity and glucose control (58,59), reduce triglyceride levels (49), and reduce platelet aggregation through beneficial effects on hemostatic factors such as fibrinogen (60). Although these factors are not traditionally used to evaluate CVD risk, they hare all been demonstrated in varying degrees to be directly or indirectly related to the risk of developing CVD.

The beneficial effects of physical activity may depend on the type, frequency, duration, and intensity of the activity as well as the risk factor or specific clinical condition of interest. In general, it becomes apparent that there is much overlap among the components comprising the spectrum of physical activity in the prevention of CVD. For example, total energy expenditure is a critical component for body weight maintenance and therefore important in the prevention of such conditions as hypertension, low HDL cholesterol, high LDL cholesterol, and hyperinsulinemia, all of which have potential atherogenic affects. Therefore, exercise type (endurance activities with large muscle groups as walking and jogging), frequency (daily), and duration (at least 20 minutes), are all probably important for preventing CVD through various mechanistic pathways related to energy balance and prevention of adipose accumulation and blood lipid and blood pressure control.

Blood pressure is one CVD risk factor that may have an intensity threshold in its relationship to physical activity. Independent of weight loss, randomized clinical studies have consistently demonstrated that low-to moderate-intensity activities are equally as effective, and perhaps more effective, in reducing blood pressure as compared to high-intensity physical activities (61–64). These findings are consistent with some animal models reviewed by Tipton (50). Although such clear inferences cannot be drawn from population-based studies, some prospective epidemiologic studies have corroborated these clinical findings (65,66).

The epidemiologic study of physical activity and CVD was pioneered by two scientists in the middle of this century: Dr. Jeremy N. Morris from the London School of Hygiene and Tropical Medicine (67–70) and Dr. Ralph S. Paffenbarger, Jr., from the Stanford University School of Medicine (71–73). Following Morris and Paffenbarger, observational epidemiologic investigations of the relationship between physical activity and coronary heart disease have consistently demonstrated a reduced risk for coronary heart disease in both men and women across many populations (10,13,74). Powell et al (13) have provided a comprehensive review of articles in the English language providing data to estimate the risk for coronary heart disease at various activity levels. These authors concluded that the literature supports an inverse and causal relationship between physical activity and coronary heart disease, and the magnitude of the relative risk appears to be similar to the relative risks from hypertension, hypercholesterolemia, and smoking. Their estimate associated with a physically inactive lifestyle of an approximate twofold increase in the relative risk (1.9) of coronary heart disease was replicated 3 years later in the formal meta-analysis conducted by Berlin et al (74). It should be noted that at the time of these reviews many studies did not include older individuals or women, and therefore the results pertain primarily to middle-aged men. However, studies with women and older adults have since been accumulating (75–77) and suggest that the benefit in these populations is similar.

Caspersen (78) has discussed the concept of the population attributable risk, which takes into account both the relative risk and the prevalence of the risk factor in question. Because of the high prevalence of physical inactivity (60%) compared to the other risk factors, it was estimated that 16.1% of all-cause mortality is due to physical inactivity in comparison to 22.5% for cigarette smoking (which has a lower prevalence but a somewhat higher relative risk), 10.3% for weight gain, and 6.4% for hypertension. Although these estimates were compiled approximately 10 years ago, they are still quite relevant today as the prevalence and relative risks of these factors in the population have not changed appreciably.

The nature of the dose-response relationship between physical activity and CVD is an area in need of further research using careful clinical studies. The difficulty is that the epidemiologic data are not precise enough to tease out the independent effects of different types and quantities of activity. Epidemiologic studies are limited by the difficulty in recall of physical activities of low to moderate intensity. Therefore, there is a need for more appropriately designed clinical trials to determine the specific components of exercise programs and the optimal doses of exercise for favorable effects on CVD risk. Given the complexity of physical activity, the overlapping importance of the various components that may affect the outcome of interest, and the dependence of the measured associations on the distribution of physical activity and the risk factor in the population of interest, it is not surprising that there is no consensus from the epidemiologic literature on the optimal type, duration, frequency, and intensity necessary to achieve health benefits. It has been suggested that the literature on the epidemiology of physical activity supports the notion that most of the reduction in risk for chronic diseases and all-cause mortality may be observed at the low end of the physical activity spectrum, between the least active and low to moderately active individuals, with more but proportionally less health benefit conferred by moving from a moderated level of activity to a higher level (79). However, not all studies support this dose-response relationship between physical activity and health (80–82), and there is much debate in the scientific community regarding this issue and the physical activity recommendations set forth by the American College of Sports Medicine and the Centers for Disease Control and Prevention (17–20).

Figure 74-3 shows the medians of pooled relative risks for various heart disease endpoints computed in the meta-analysis of Berlin et al (74). For epidemiologic studies that enabled an evaluation of the dose-response relationship by having at least three categories of activity (sedentary, moderate activity, high activity), the median pooled relative risk of heart disease was 1.4 (40% increased risk) for those in the moderate-activity category compared to those in the high-activity category. When comparing the risk for heart disease in the sedentary individuals compared to the high-activity category, the median pooled relative risk further increased to 1.8 (80% increased risk). The figure also shows the range in pooled relative risks across the various heart disease endpoints reported by Berlin et al (74). These pooled estimates computed in a carefully executed meta-analysis appear to indicate that the relationship between physical activity and heart disease is linear. It should be kept in mind that this conclusion is a tenuous one due to the limited number of activity categories and the inconsistent methodologies across studies.

Diet

Much of what is known about diet and CVD comes from the work of Dr. Ancel Keys and his pioneering efforts in the Seven Countries Study (83,84). Ancel Keys' experiments, which began over 40 years ago at the Laboratory of Physiological Hygiene at the University of Minnesota, revealed that the proportions of dietary saturated and polyunsaturated fatty acids are directly related to the concentration of serum cholesterol (29–32). Keys' Score was developed to predict how much of a change in dietary cholesterol can be expected from dietary changes of saturated and polyunsaturated fatty acids dependent upon the individual's current usual diet (29). Determined to "prove" the cholesterol hypothesis at the population level, Keys established the Seven Countries Study along with colleagues in Japan, Greece, Yugoslavia, Italy, the Netherlands, Finland, and the United States. In the Seven Countries Study, dietary fatty acids were directly related to serum cholesterol at the population level and, after taking measurement error into account, the individual level (85). The reader is encouraged to refer to other sources for more detail on the methodology and results of the Seven Countries Study (83,84).

The findings of the Seven Countries Study continue to be supported in many other populations, such as Framingham, Mass. Commenced in 1948, the Framingham Study is the oldest population-based longitudinal epidemiologic study of CVD, and is the origin of the term "risk factor." The Framingham Risk Score was developed to estimate the risk for coronary heart disease based on age, HDL cholesterol, total cholesterol, systolic blood pressure, smoking, diabetes, and left ventricular hypertrophy measured by electrocardiography (86). As lifestyle interventions are more likely to affect various lifestyle habits (e.g., smoking) and physiologic parameters (body weight, LDL cholesterol, blood pressure), the Framingham Risk Score may be particularly useful in behavioral interventions as opposed to pharmaceutical studies aimed at

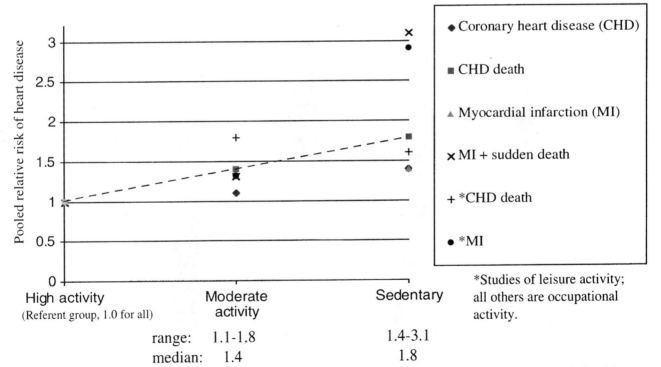

Figure 74-3 Dose-response relationship between physical activity and heart disease endpoints from pooled relative risks computed by Berlin et al (74).

lowering LDL cholesterol with limited potential to affect other behavioral or biologic CVD risk factors.

There is much current debate on the issue of the optimal type and quantity of dietary fat to minimize risk for CVD (21,22). The National Cholesterol Education Program (NCEP) recommended a dietary fat intake below 30% of total calories and saturated fat below 10% of calories (Step 1), and eventually 7% (Step 2), in order to lower LDL cholesterol and reduce risk for future CVD events (87,88). However, recent studies appear to question the validity of these dietary guidelines. As shown in Figure 74-4, Knopp et al (89) have demonstrated no further LDL cholesterol reduction by decreasing fat intake below 28% of calories over the course of 1 year in hypercholesterolemic patients. In fact, patients consuming less than 26% of calories from fat demonstrated statistically significant reductions in HDL cholesterol (89). The Nurses' Health Study compared 14-year relative risks for nonfatal myocardial infarction and coronary heart disease from various dietary fatty acid intake levels in 80,082 women (33). As Ancel Keys had proposed 40 years earlier, replacing saturated fatty acids and trans-fatty acids with poly- and monounsaturated fatty acids is more effective in preventing coronary heart disease than is the reduction of overall fat intake.

The US Health Professionals follow-up study of 43,757 men demonstrated a 22% increase in the risk for myocardial infarction for individuals in the top quintile of saturated fat intake compared with the bottom quintile (90). However, this risk estimate was completely attenuated after adjustment for dietary fiber, demonstrating essentially no independent relationship between dietary saturated fat and incidence of myocardial infarction. This study demonstrated many lifestyle and dietary characteristics, including physical activity, that were strongly associated with the level of saturated fat intake (90). Therefore, one must consider the plethora of dietary components other than fatty acids that have potential causal associations with CVD risk factors and, ultimately, endpoints. For example, epidemiologic studies have demonstrated reductions in risk for CVD (91) and diabetes (92,93) for individuals with relatively high consumption of dietary fiber, which may have beneficial effects on slowing dietary cholesterol and carbohydrate absorption, thereby controlling the concentrations of glucose and cholesterol in the blood (43,44,94,95).

There is good evidence for the role of dietary sodium and potassium in the regulation of blood pressure and risk for hypertension (96,97). Although the magnitude of the effects on blood pressure have been modest (98,99), such small downward shifts in the population distribution of blood pressure may have a substantial public health impact by decreasing the prevalence of high values for the risk factor in question (100,101).

The study of diet can focus on 1) specific nutrients— the "magic bullet" approach, such as saturated fat or vitamin E intake; 2) specific foods, such as cruciferous vegetables; or 3) more generally on the frequency of consumption of foods from specified food group categories, such as meat, dairy, or vegetable. The problem with the magic bullet approach is its lack of relevance to dietary guidelines geared towards the consumption of naturally occurring and available foods. It is difficult epidemiologically, and even clinically, to tease out causal effects of single nutrients, such as minerals or antioxidant vitamins. It is also challenging to make public health recommendations about these specific nutrients, especially if the

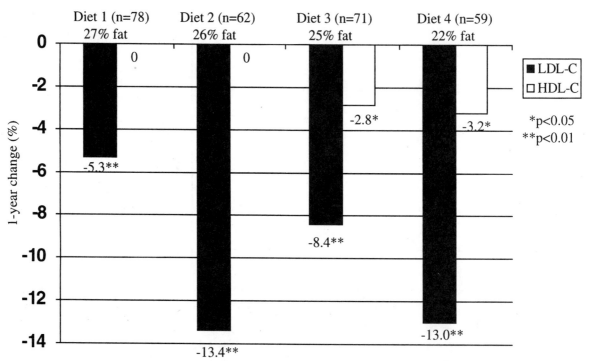

Figure 74-4 Changes in LDL and HDL cholesterol from four different low-fat diets in hypercholesterolemic patients. (Adapted from Knopp CH, Waldon CE, Retzlaff BM, et al. Long-term cholesterol-lowering effects of 4 fat-restricted diets in hypercholesterolemic and combined hyperlipidemic men. JAMA 1997;278:1509–1515.)

biologic effects of naturally occurring dietary vs. unnatural supplement forms may not be similar (102) or if the latter may be harmful in some forms or doses (103). Potter has discussed this issue in a commentary in the *American Journal of Epidemiology* regarding diet and colorectal cancer:

> . . . there will be very few magic bullets. Therefore, formulating pills to match a risk that is defined as [cancer site by sex by metabolic profile . . . and so forth] will be much more problematic than encouraging a general increase in the consumption of plant foods. This is a step we can take right now and enjoy the built-in redundancy of multiple agents with independent, overlapping, and perhaps interactive mechanisms. Besides, well-prepared food tastes better (104).

As with physical activity, dietary modification may confer effects on CVD risk through changes in body weight (energy consumption less than energy expenditure) and subsequent changes in blood pressure or lipids. As such, the most profound reductions in risk are in initially overweight individuals who have a lot to "gain" by modifying their lifestyle. Still, there are other direct physiologic pathways through which diet and exercise can independently or jointly alter CVD risk. The following sections will discuss studies examining the effectiveness of both diet and exercise interventions on CVD risk factors. Few studies have implemented the appropriate study design to evaluate potential interactive effects of diet and exercise. Both the benefits and potential risks from behavioral interventions on CVD risk will be considered in reviewing these studies.

INTERACTIONS OF PHYSICAL ACTIVITY AND DIET
Mechanisms

Discussed below are the biologic bases for the experimental study of independent and interactive effects of diet and exercise on CVD risk. Following this brief discussion of mechanisms will be a thorough review of relevant randomized clinical trials.

Body Weight and Composition

Both diet and exercise have the propensity to reduce body weight or to attenuate weight gain through their effects on energy balance. However, the independent effects of these behaviors on body weight and composition may be quite different. The loss of adipose tissue from caloric restriction without exercise may be accompanied by a loss of lean tissue (105,106,136). Loss of lean tissue is not a desirable physiologic effect, especially in populations such as young adults who are at a critical life period with respect to the development of peak bone mass or in postmenopausal women who are at particular risk for rapid bone loss due to aging and declining levels of endogenous estrogen (107,108). Furthermore, this loss in lean tissue may be accompanied by decreases in resting energy expenditure (109), which may lower total energy expenditure, thereby deterring the long-term maintenance of weight loss. Exercise, especially of a weight-bearing nature using the large muscle groups (brisk waking, aerobic dance, resistance training, etc.) has been shown to result in maintenance of lean tissue and favorable losses of body fat (53). As

expected, the combination of diet and exercise tend to result in optimal fat loss, lean tissue maintenance or gain, and long-term maintenance of weight loss (105,110,111,136). An abundance of clinical studies have been conducted comparing the independent and interactive effects of diet and exercise on change in body weight and composition. The reader is referred to several comprehensive reviews on this topic (53,105,111). Only those clinical studies of diet and exercise that have evaluated blood lipids and/or blood pressure in addition to body weight and/or composition will be included in the review of randomized clinical trials in the next section.

Lipids

Diet and exercise programs have both been shown to lower LDL and to raise HDL cholesterol. The primary mechanisms are reductions in dietary saturated fat intake, which will lower LDL (89), and reductions in adiposity, which may lower LDL and raise HDL (53,112). Whereas diet may result in LDL reduction through both direct effects on saturated fatty acid reduction and indirect effects on adiposity reduction through decreased energy intake, exercise will lower LDL primarily through the indirect pathway of reduced adiposity (53,113). A potential adverse consequence of lowering dietary fat intake is that HDL cholesterol may be concomitantly lowered with LDL (89,114). Exercise may be more effective than diet alone at decreasing the lipogenically active visceral body fat, thereby further potentiating favorable effects on LDL and HDL (53,112). Also, an increase in the particularly anti-atherogenic HDL subfraction HDL_2 may be an exercise-specific response (115). Polyunsaturated and monounsaturated fatty acids may have favorable effects on LDL and HDL when consumed in moderation and in place of saturated fatty acids in the diet, but there is still much to learn about the physiologic effects of manipulating dietary fatty acids (116,117).

Blood Pressure

Body weight is a strong independent determinant of blood pressure (96). Therefore, as discussed above, diet and physical activity may interact to confer beneficial effects on body weight, and these two interventions can also be expected to interact favorably on blood pressure. As reviewed earlier, the separate and direct effects of exercise (through attenuation of sympathetic activity and total peripheral resistance) and diet (through decreased intake of sodium, potassium, and fat) on blood pressure, which are independent of the indirect effects through adiposity, provide substantial biologic plausibility for an interactive effect of these behaviors on the control of blood pressure.

Other Mechanisms Related to CVD Risk

There are several other potential mechanisms through which diet and exercise may interact to improve the CVD risk factor profile, although these do not necessarily involve established traditional risk factors for CVD. Although more studies are needed to learn about the interaction of diet and exercise, these theoretical mechanistic interactions on CVD risk may be appreciated from favorable physiologic and biochemical effects of optimal consumption of macronutrients, vitamins, and minerals in conjunction with regular aerobic-type exercise of a weight-bearing nature using the large muscle groups.

Mechanisms could include lowering serum triglyceride concentrations, direct effects on the myocardium and its vasculature, improved cardiac output and skeletal muscle oxygen metabolic capacity, favorable effects on the oxygen-carrying capacity of the blood, improved insulin and glucose metabolism and insulin sensitivity in skeletal muscle, and improvements in hemostatic factors leading to a reduced propensity for platelet aggregation and thrombogenesis.

Given the number of potential biologic mechanisms, the complexity of diet and exercise, and the various populations of study, it is only through randomized controlled trials that we can attempt to examine the potential additive interactive effects of diet and exercise. The trials completed to date that have examined both diet and exercise on CVD risk factors will now be reviewed.

Randomized Trials of Diet and Exercise on CVD Risk Factors

There have been many studies examining the combined effects of exercise and diet on the primary or secondary prevention of CVD (98,114,118–120). Although these studies are important applications of interventions and many have demonstrated favorable results, it is not possible to evaluate the independent or interactive effects of the diet and exercise intervention components. There are even potential deleterious effects of weight loss by diet alone, which, as discussed earlier, may be especially relevant to perimenopausal women who are at high risk for bone loss leading to osteoporosis. Another potential deleterious effect of dietary interventions without exercise is the decrease in HDL cholesterol which, as demonstrated earlier (89), may accompany a decrease in fat intake (see Fig. 74-4).

The studies reviewed below are those that randomized participants and included measures of body weight and/or body composition as well as cholesterol and/or blood pressure. Since there were not a large number of studies satisfying these criteria, those studies that did not use a control group are also included. In order to evaluate the independent and possibly interactive effects of diet and exercise, the necessary design must include four arms: 1) control (C), 2) diet (D), 3) exercise (E), and 4) diet + exercise (DE). Unfortunately, only five studies were found that incorporated this design. Comparisons and effects described as statistically significant are based on $p < .05$. All 16 studies reviewed used some type of aerobic exercise for at least 3 days per week for at least 30 minutes per occasion. The most popular exercise intervention was walking or walking/jogging (10 studies). Diets were aimed at losing weight and/or improving blood lipid levels and were therefore reduced calorie and/or reduced fat diets. Several studies tested the NCEP Step 1 or Step 2 diets aimed at reducing the amount of dietary fat and decreasing the ratio of saturated fat to polyunsaturated fat and monounsaturated fat (87,88). Participants tended to be middle-aged overweight men and/or women often having an elevated risk for CVD, such as high LDL cholesterol or low HDL cholesterol.

Two studies of the independent effects of diet and exercise (121,122), as well as several follow-up studies to Wood et al (122) (109,115,123,124), indicate that diet and exercise are both effective in overall weight reduction and lipid changes. However, exercise may have several advantages over diet

along by 1) maintaining lean mass (121,122), 2) attenuating the depression of energy expenditure (109), 3) having a greater propensity to increase HDL_2 cholesterol and apolipoprotein A-I (Apo-AI) (115,121), and 4) enhancing long-term maintenance of weight loss (123).

Eight randomized studies compared a combined diet and exercise intervention to a diet intervention alone on body weight and lipid changes. Several of these studies were limited by lack of a control group (110,125–128), short duration of less than 6 months (110,125,127–128,136), and/or poor intervention compliance (110,128,129). As summarized in Figure 74-5, it appears from this limited body of evidence that the maximum benefit from adding exercise to a dietary intervention is seen in body fat loss and HDL cholesterol changes. Because the study by Wood et al (130) provided results separately for men and women, the maximum number of contrasts summarized in Figure 74-5 is nine. Also, for some measures the number is less than nine because some studies did not report all measures (e.g., only three studies reported HDL_2 cholesterol). Four of seven contrasts reported more fat loss from DE than from D and six of 9 reported more favorable HDL changes for DE than for D. Three HDL_2 contrasts demonstrated greater increases in DE than D. Only one of seven LDL cholesterol contrasts and one of five diastolic blood pressure contrasts demonstrated a greater decrease for DE than for D. It is also important to note that none of the studies showed a more favorable effect for D compared to DE for any of the risk factors examined. In addition, other potential interactive effects of diet and exercise were reported by Nolte et al (125,136), who found increased resting metabolic rate for DE, and Wood et al (130), who reported an increase Apo-AI and a decrease in the estimated 12-year risk for coronary heart disease for DE compared to D or C.

The six randomized trials summarized in Table 74-1 all implemented appropriate study designs to examine the interactive effects of diet and exercise on CVD risk factors, with the exception of the study by Hughes et al (131), which lacked a control group (C). It is difficult to draw conclusions about the potential interaction of diet and exercise on CVD risk due to the limited number of studies and their methodologic flaws and inconsistencies. Three of the six studies were only 12 weeks in duration and the study by Hellénius et al (132) appeared to have poor compliance to the interventions. Although the study by Wing et al (133) had good compliance to diet and exercise over the first 6 months, the compliance over the remaining 18 months was poor. Probably as a result of this poor compliance, the physiologic benefits noted at 6 months were not observed at the end of the 24 month study (133). Reid et al (56) did not report LDL cholesterol and Hagan et al (134) and Hughes et al (131) did not report blood pressure. The best evidence from these limited data for additive effects of diet and exercise appears to be for body weight and LDL cholesterol. Two studies reported more weight loss for DE than for D or E alone and five studies reported significant decreases in body weight for DE. Five studies reported significant weight loss for D, while only one reported significant weight loss for E. Four studies demonstrated significant decreases in LDL for DE compared to two studies for D and none for E.

Unfortunately, only three studies reported results for body composition; one revealing more fat loss for DE than

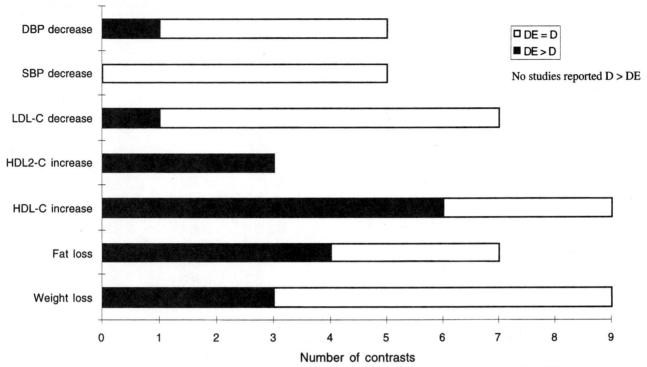

Figure 74-5 Summary of studies comparing the effects of diet (D) to the interaction of diet and exercise (DE) on cardiovascular risk factors. The figure includes a total of nine possible contrasts from eight studies (Wood et al [122] reported sex-stratified results). Since all variables were not reported in all studies, the total number of contrasts varies. (DBP = diastolic blood pressure; SBP = systolic blood pressure.)

for D or E and two revealing more fat loss for D than for E. Hagan et al (134) reported more lean tissue loss for DE and D compared to E. For HDL cholesterol three studies demonstrated no change in any groups and two studies demonstrated decreases in D and mixed findings for E (increase and no change) and DE (decrease and no change). Of the three studies reporting blood pressure findings, Reid et al (56) and Hellénius et al (132) reported decreases across all groups for systolic and diastolic blood pressure, with Reid et al (56) also demonstrated a clear interaction of these two interventions on systolic and diastolic blood pressure. Stefanick et al (135) found a decrease for diastolic blood pressure in women of the DE group only. Reid et al (56) was the only study of the five to compute an estimate of risk for coronary heart disease and reported a greater reduction in risk for DE compared to D or E.

Table 74-2 summarizes the independent and interactive effects of diet and exercise as estimated from the 16 randomized clinical trials of diet and exercise reviewed above. Double arrows indicate additive interactions of diet and exercise. Double arrows are not shown for lean mass, resting energy expenditure, or HDL cholesterol because the independent effects of diet and exercise work in opposite directions, with the independent effects of diet being unfavorable and exercise being favorable. However, it is important to note that the interventions tested were primarily low-fat and/or low-calorie diets and/or aerobic exercise. The potential interaction for these parameters is that exercise may attenuate the decrease in resting energy expenditure, lean mass, and HDL cholesterol that may be accompanied by weight loss through diet (especially low-fat diets) alone. Furthermore, the combination of diet and exercise may induce more body fat loss, lower LDL

cholesterol and blood pressure, and reduce overall CVD risk to a greater degree than either intervention alone.

SUMMARY

It is suggested from limited studies (both in number and methodology) that, particularly in individuals with elevated CVD risk, the combination of diet and exercise may work to preserve or increase lean mass, promote fat loss or attenuate adipose accumulation over time, lower LDL cholesterol and blood pressure, and raise or maintain HDL concentrations more than either intervention accomplishes alone. Other benefits may be gained through a combination of diet and exercise that relate to non-traditional CVD risk factors. However, more and better studies are needed to precisely quantify the magnitude of the combined effects of diet and exercise and to evaluate the optimal combinations of dietary and exercise components and their doses depending on the population and risk factor of interest.

Diet and physical activity are analogous to automobile maintenance. For the best performance we buy the best fuel, which is the cleanest and most efficient; analogous to a diet with moderate amounts and optimal proportions of fatty acids, ample high-quality lean protein, and plenty of high-quality non-refined carbohydrates in the form of whole fruits, vegetables, and grains. For best performance we also maintain engine parts through regularly scheduled preventive maintenance, which is analogous to a daily physical activity routine with emphasis on the large muscle groups for cardiovascular and musculoskeletal fitness.

Table 74-1 Summary of Randomized Trials Comparing the Independent and Combined Effects of Diet and Exercise on Cardiovascular Disease Risk Factors

Study	Population	Treatments (n)				Duration	Compliance	Result[a]				
		Control (C)	Diet (D)	Exercise (E)	Diet + Exercise (DE)			Body Mass	HDL-C	LDL-C	Total:HDL	Blood Pressure
Hagan et al (134)	Overweight men and women, age ~37 ± 7	(24)	↓Fat, ↓cal (24)	Walk/jog 30 min/d 5 d/wk (24)	(24)	12 wk	Appeared to be good based on logs and diaries	**Total & Fat** DE↓>D,E,C D↓>E,C **Lean** DE↓>E,C D↓>E,C	All ↔	All ↔	DE↓>E,C, for men only	NR
Hellénius et al (132)	Men at increased risk for CVD, age 35–60	(40)	↓Cal ↓Fat (40)	Walk, jog other, 30–45 min/d, 2–3 d/wk (39)	(39)	6 mo	44%E and 26%DE participated in all sessions; 80%E and 44%DE kept activity logs	**Total** DE↓>E,D E,D↓>C	**Total** ↔ all	D,DE↓	NR	**SBP&DBP** E,D↓
Hughes et al (131)	Women and men with impaired glucose tolerance, age 50–78	None	↓Fat ↑Fiber (4 M, 5 W)	Cycle ergometry 45 min/d, 4 d/wk (7 M, 10 W)	(4 M, 6 W)	12 wk	Food was provided and exercise was supervised	**Total** E,DE↓ D↔ **Fat** All↔	**Total** D,DE↓ E↔	D,DE↓ E↔	DE↑	NR
Reid et al (56)	Overweight women and men at↑ risk for CHD, age 19–60	(23)[b]	↓Cal ↓Fat (9)	Cycle ergometry 40 min/d, 3 d/wk (7)	(7)	12 wk	5/8 W, 18/22 M completed the program; ≥95% of exercise sessions completed	**Total** D,DE↓ **Fat** D,DE↓	**Total** E↑ D↓ DE↔	NR	NR	**SBP&DBP** DE↓>D,E D,E↓>C
Stefanick et al (135)	Women (age 45–64) and men (age 30–64 yrs) with↓HDL & ↑LDL	(46 M) (45 W)	↓Fat ↓Cal (49 M) (46 W)	Walk/jog ≥10 miles/wk (47 W) (43 M)	(48 M) (43 W)	1 yr	Appeared to be good based on dietary and fitness changes	**Total (M&W)** DE,D↓>E,C	**Total (M&W)** All ↔	(W) DE↓>C (M) DE↓>E,C	All ↔	**DBP** (W) DE↓>C
Wing et al (133)	Overweight women (~80%) and men at ↑ risk for diabetes, age 40–55	(40)	↓Cal ↓Fat (37)	Gradually increase to 1500 kcal/wk; e.g., brisk walking (37)	(40)	2 yr	Good for first 6 months and poor thereafter	**6 & 12 mo** D,DE↓ >E,C **24 mo** All ↔	**6 mo** D↓ **12 mo** All ↑ **24 mo** All ↔	**6 mo** D↓ **12 mo** All ↔ **24 mo** All ↔	NR	**SBP&DBP** D,DE↓ >E,C **24 mo** All ↔

LDL = low density lipoprotein cholesterol; HDL = high density lipoprotein cholesterol; total:HDL = ratio of total cholesterol to high density lipoprotein cholesterol; SBP = systolic blood pressure; DBP = diastolic blood pressure; M = men; W = women.
[a] Significant ($p < 0.05$) change (↑ or ↓) or no change (↔) compared to (>) C, D, or E.
[b] Subjects served as own controls in cross-over design.

	Diet	Exercise	Exercise + Diet
Table 74-2 Summary of Independent and Interactive Effects of Diet and Exercise on Cardiovascular Disease Risk Factors and Physiologic Parameters			
Body mass	↓	↓ or ↔	↓↓
Fat mass	↓	↓	↓↓
Lean mass	↓ or ↔	↑ or ↔	↔
Resting energy expenditure	↓ or ↔	↑ or ↔	↔
LDL cholesterol	↓	↓ or ↔	↓↓
HDL cholesterol	↓ or ↔	↑	↔
Blood pressure	↓	↓	↓↓
Overall CVD risk	↓	↓	↓↓

↓ = Independent lowering effect; ↑ = Independent increasing effect; ↔ = No effect; ↓↓ = Additive interactive lowering effect.

There is a need for more controlled randomized clinical studies using state-of-the-art methods of measurement of diet and exercise. To maximize compliance, diet should be manipulated by providing meals and the exercise should be supervised over a sufficient duration with follow-up contacts to monitor postprogram compliance and CVD risk factors. Issues of particular interest are the amounts and types of fatty acids and whole plant foods in conjunction with varying types of exercise programs. Most studies have tested reduced-calorie low-fat diets aimed at weight loss and LDL cholesterol reduction, with few interventions of diet and exercise implementing diets aimed at increasing the consumption of nutrient-rich whole plant foods. The caloric intake and expenditure should be manipulated through the design as well as the proportion of nutrients and the nature of the exercise program in terms of duration, frequency, and intensity.

Scientists have been continuing to debate such unanswered questions as: How much fat should we eat? What proportions of fatty acids are optimal? How much exercise is enough? What types, durations, intensities, and frequencies of exercise are optimal? We know that modifying fat intake is important if one is starting at a fat intake of 37% of calories or becoming active is a good idea if a person is sedentary, but what is the long-term goal and how should it be achieved? Also, how much is potentially too much in terms not only of CVD risk but other factors related to quality of life? The answers to these questions are not forthcoming because of the absence of carefully designed trials demonstrating consistency among studies in various populations. Nonetheless, the totality of epidemiologic and clinical evidence is sufficiently strong regarding the benefits of fat–modified diets with abundant plant foods and regular physical activity that, given ample economic and political latitude, failure to promote such healthy lifestyles in schools, workplaces, and communities is inexcusable.

Acknowledgments: The helpful comments on drafts of this chapter from Dr. Anne G. Pemberton and Dr. M. Kathryn H. Schmitz are greatly appreciated.

REFERENCES

1. American Heart Association. 1998 heart and stroke statistical update. Dallas, TX: American Heart Association, 1997.

2. McGinnis JM, Foege WH. Actual causes of death in the United States. JAMA 1993;270:2207–2212.

3. Schneider EL, Guralnik JM. The aging of America: impact on health care costs. JAMA 1990;263:2335–2340.

4. Kuczmarski RJ, Flegal KM, Campbell SM, et al. Increasing prevalence of overweight among US adults. JAMA 1994;272:205–211.

5. Stevens J, Cai J, Pamuk E, et al. The effect of age on the association between body mass index and mortality. N Engl J Med 1998;338:1–7.

6. Lindsted KD, Singh PN. Body mass and 26-year risk of mortality among women who never smoked: findings from the Adventist Mortality Study. Am J Epidemiol 1997;146:1–11.

7. Manson JE, Willett WC, Stampfer MJ, et al. Body weight and mortality among women. N Engl J Med 1995;333:677–685.

8. Kassirer JP, Angell M. Losing weight—an ill-fated new year's resolution. N Engl J Med 1998;338:52–54.

9. Popkin BM, Siega-Riz AM, Haines PS. A comparison of dietary trends among racial and socioeconomic groups in the United States. N Engl J Med 1996;335:716–720.

10. U.S. Department of Health and Human Services. Physical activity and health: a report from the Surgeon General. Atlanta, GA: U.S. Department of Health and Human Services, Centers for Disease Control and Prevention, National Center for Chronic Disease Prevention and Health Promotion, 1996.

11. Flatt JP. McCollum Award Lecture, 1995: diet, lifestyle, and weight maintenance. Am J Clin Nutr 1995;62:820–836.

12. National Center for Health Statistics. Health, United States, 1995. Hyattsville, MD: Public Health Service, 1996.

13. Powell KE, Thompson PD, Caspersen CJ, et al. Physical activity and the incidence of coronary heart disease. Ann Rev Public Health 1987;8:253–287.

14. Brand RJ, Paffenbarger RS Jr, Sholtz RI, Kampert JB. Work activity and fatal heart attack studied by multiple logistic risk analysis. Am J Epidemiol 1979; 110:52–62.

15. MVMA Motor Vehicle Facts & Figures [various years]. Motor Vehicle Manufacturers Association of the United States, Inc.

16. Brown D, Bryant J. An annotated statistical abstract of the United States. In: Media use in the information age: emerging patterns of adoption and consumer use. Bryant J, Salvaggio JL, eds. Hillsdale, NJ: Lawrence Erlbaum Associates, 1989:259–302.

17. Barinaga M. How much pain for cardiac gain? Science 1997; 276:1324–1327.

18. McDonald KA. U. of California scientist takes issue with government guidelines for exercise. Chronicles of Higher Education 1997;44:A15–A16.

19. Williams PT. Letter to the editor. JAMA 1995;274:533–534.

20. Winett RA. Letter to the editor. JAMA 1995;274:534–535.

21. Connor WE, Connor SL. Should a low-fat, high carbohydrate diet be recommended for everyone? N Engl J Med 1997;337:562–563.

22. Katan MB, Grundy SM, Willett WC. Should a low-fat, high carbohydrate diet be recommended for everyone? N Engl J Med 1997; 337:563–566.

23. Steptoe A, Wardle J, Fuller R, et al. Leisure-time physical exercise: prevalence, attitudinal correlates, and behavioral correlates among young Europeans from 21 countries. Prev Med 1997;26:845–854.

24. Serdula MK, Byers T, Mokdad AH, et al. The association between fruit and vegetable intake and chronic disease risk factors. Epidemiology 1996;7:161–165.

25. Eaton C, McPhillips J, Gans K, et al. Cross-sectional relationship between diet and physical activity in two southeastern New England communities. Am J Prev Med 1995;11:238–244.

26. Johnson NA, Boyle CA, Heller RF. Leisure-time physical activity and other health behaviours: are they related? Aust J Pub Health 1995;19:69–75.

27. Simoes E, Byers T, Coates R, et al. The association between leisure-time physical activity and dietary fat in American adults. Am J Pub Health 1995;85:240–244.

28. Ursin G, Zieglar RG, Subar AF, et al. Dietary patterns associated with a low-fat diet in the national health examination follow-up study: identification of potential confounders for epidemiologic analyses. Am J Epidemiol 1993;137:916–927.

29. Keys A, Andersen JT, Grande F. Serum cholesterol response to dietary fat. Lancet 1957;1:787.

30. Keys A, Andersen JT, Grande F. Prediction of serum cholesterol responses of man to changes of fats in the diet. Lancet 1957;2:959.

31. Keys A, Andersen JT, Grande F. Serum cholesterol in man: dietary fat and intrinsic responsiveness. Circulation 1959;19:201–214.

32. Keys A, Anderson JT, Grande F. Serum cholesterol response to changes in the diet: IV: particular saturated fatty acids in the diet. Metabolism 1965;14:776–787.

33. Hu FB, Stampfer MJ, Manson JE, et al. Dietary fat intake and the risk of coronary heart disease in women. N Engl J Med 1997; 337:1491–1499.

34. Caspersen CJ, Powell KE, Christenson GM. Physical activity, exercise, and physical fitness. Public Health Reports 1985;100:126–131.

35. Ravussin E, Rising R. Daily energy expenditure in humans: measurements in a respiratory chamber and by doubly labeled water. In: Energy metabolism: tissue determinants and cellular corollaries. Kinney JM, Tucker HN, eds. New York: Raven Press, 1992.

36. Ravussin E, Bogardus C. A brief overview of human energy metabolism and its relationship to essential obesity. Am J Clin Nutr 1992;55(suppl):242S–245S.

37. Montoye HJ, Taylor HL. Measurement of physical activity in population studies: a review. Hum Biol 1984;56:195–216.

38. LaPorte RE, Montoye HJ, Caspersen CJ. Assessment of physical activity in epidemiologic research: problems and prospects. Public Health Reports 1985;100:131–146.

39. Ainsworth BE, Montoye HJ, Leon AS. Methods of assessing physical activity during leisure and work. In: Bouchard C, Shephard RJ, Stephens T, eds. Physical activity, fitness, and health: International Proceedings and Consensus Statement. Champaign, IL: Human Kinetics, 1994:145–159.

40. Pereira MA, FitzGerald SJ, Gregg EW, et al. A collection of physical activity questionnaires for health-related research. Kriska AM, Caspersen CJ, eds. Med Sci Sports Exerc 1997;29:S1–S205.

41. Voorips LE, Revelli ACJ, Dongelmans PCA, et al. A physical activity questionnaire for the elderly. Med Sci Sports Exerc 1991;23:974–979.

42. LaPorte RE, Adams LL, Savage DD, et al. The spectrum of physical activity, cardiovascular disease and health: an epidemiological perspective. Amer J Epidemiol 1984;120:507–517.

43. Anderson JW, Story L, Sieling B, Chen W-JL. Hypocholesterolemic effects of high-fiber diets rich in water-soluble plant fibers: long-term studies with oat-bran and bean-supplemented diets for hypercholestrolemic men. J Can Diet Assoc 1984;45:140–149.

44. Anderson JW, Smith BM, Gustafson NJ. Health benefits and practical aspects of high-fiber diets. Am J Clin Nutr 1994;59(suppl):1242S–1247S.

45. Thompson FE, Byers T. Dietary assessment resource manual. J Nutr 1994;124(11S):2245S–2317S.

46. Willett W. Nutritional Epidemiology. New York: Oxford University Press, 1998.

47. Leon AS. Effects of exercise conditioning on physiologic precursors of coronary heart disease. J Cardiopulmon Res 1991;11:46–57.

48. Stefanick ML, Wood PD. Physical activity, lipid and lipoprotein metabolism, and lipid transport. In: Bouchard C, Shephard RJ, Stephens T, eds. Physical activity, fitness, and health: International Proceedings and Consensus Statement. Champaign, IL: Human Kinetics, 1994:417–431.

49. Durstine JL, Haskell WL. Effects of exercise training on plasma lipids and lipoproteins. In: Holloszy JO, ed. Exercise and sport science reviews. Vol. 22. Baltimore: Williams & Wilkins, 1994:477–521.

50. Tipton CM. Exercise training and hypertension: an update. In: Holloszy JO, ed. Exercise and sports science reviews. Vol. 19. Baltimore: Williams & Wilkins, 1991:447–504.

51. Arakawa K. Antihypertensive mechanism of exercise. J Hypertens 1993;11:223–229.

52. Kelley G, McClellan P. Antihypertensive effects of aerobic exercise: a brief meta-analytical review of randomized controlled trials. Am J Hypertens 1994;7:115–119.

53. Bouchard C, Deprés J-P, Tremblay A. Exercise and obesity. Obes Res 1993;1:133–147.

54. Buemann B, Tremblay A. Effects of exercise training on abdominal obesity and related metabolic complications. Sports Med 1996;21:191–212.

55. Sady SP, Thompson PD, Cullinane EM, et al. Prolonged exercise augments plasma triglyceride clearance. JAMA 1986;256:2552-2555.

56. Reid CM, Dart AM, Dewar WM, et al. Interactions between the effects of exercise and weight loss on risk factors, cardiovascular haemodynamics and left ventricular structure in overweight subjects. J Hypertension 1994;12:291–301.

57. Haskell WL, Alderman EL, Fair JM, et al. Effects of intensive multiple risk factor reduction on coronary atherosclerosis and clinical cardiac events in men and women with coronary artery disease: the Stanford Coronary Risk Intervention Project (SCRIP). Circulation 1994;89:975–990.

58. Holloszy JO, Schultz J, Kusnierkiewicz J, et al. Effects of exercise on glucose tolerance and insulin resistance. Acta Med Scand 1986;711(suppl):55–65.

59. Koivisto VA, Yki-Jarvinen H, DeFronzo RA. Physical training and insulin sensitivity. Diabetes Metab Rev 1986;1:445–481.

60. Leon AS. Physical activity and risk for ischemic heart disease: an update, 1990. In: Oja P, Telama R, eds. Sport for all. New York: Elsevier, 1991:251–264.

61. Hagberg JM, Montain SJ, Martin WH III, et al. Effect of exercise training in 60- to 69-year old persons with essential hypertension. Am J Cardiol 1989;64:348–353.

62. Matsusaki M, Ikeda M, Tashiro E, et al. Influence of workload on the antihypertensive effect of exercise. Clin Exp Pharmacol Physiol 1992;19:471–479.

63. Marceau M, Kouame N, Lacourciere Y, Cleroux J. Effects of different training intensities on 24 hour blood pressure in hypertensive subjects. Circulation 1993;88:2803–2811.

64. Braith RW, Pollock ML, Lowenthal DT, et al. Moderate- and high-intensity exercise lowers blood pressure in normotensive subjects 60 to 79 years of age. Am J Cardiol 1994;73:1124–1128.

65. Paffenbarger RS Jr, Jung DL, Leung RW, Hyde RT. Physical activity and hypertension: an epidemiological view. Ann Med 1991;23:319–327.

66. Haapanen N, Milunpalo S, Vuori I, Oja P, Pasanen M. Association of leisure time physical activity with the risk of coronary heart disease, hypertension and diabetes in middle-aged men and women. Int J Epidemiol 1997;26:739–747.

67. Morris JN, Heady JA, Raffle PAB, et al. Coronary heart disease and physical activity of work. Lancet 1953;2:1053–1056.

68. Morris JN, Heady JA, Raffle PAB, et al. Coronary heart disease and physical activity of work. Lancet 1953;2:1111–1120.

69. Morris JN, Kagan A, Pattison DC, et al. Incidence and prediction of ischemic heart disease in London busmen. Lancet 1966;2:553–559.

70. Morris JN, Chave SPW, Adam C, et al. Vigorous exercise in leisure-time and the incidence of coronary heart disease. Lancet 1973;1:333–339.

71. Paffenbarger RS, Laughlin ME, Gima AS, et al. Work activity of longshoremen as related to death from disease and stroke. N Engl J Med 1970;282:1109–1114.

72. Paffenbarger RS Jr, Hale WE. Work activity and coronary heart mortality. N Engl J Med 1975;292:545–550.

73. Paffenbarger RS Jr, Wing AL, Hyde RT. Physical activity as an index of heart attack risk in college alumni. Am J Epidemiol 1978;108:161–175.

74. Berlin JA, Colditz GA. A meta-analysis of physical activity in the prevention of coronary heart disease. Am J Epidemiol 1990;132:612–628.

75. Kushi LH, Fee RM, Folsom AR, et al. Physical activity and mortality in postmenopausal women. JAMA 1997;277:1287–1292.

76. Hakim AA, Petrovitch H, Burchfiel CM, et al. Effects of walking on mortality among nonsmoking retired men. N Engl J Med 1998;338:94–99.

77. LaCroix AZ, Leveille SG, Hecht JA, e al. Does walking decrease

the risk of cardiovascular disease hospitalizations and death in older adults? J Am Geriatr Soc 1996;44:113–120.

78. Caspersen CJ. Physical inactivity and coronary heart disease (guest editorial). Phys Sportsmed 1987; 15:43–44.

79. Pate RR, Pratt M, Blair SN, et al. Physical activity and public health: a recommendation from the Centers for Disease Control and Prevention and the American College of Sports Medicine. JAMA 1995;273:402–407.

80. Lee I-M, Hsieh C-C, Paffenbarger RS Jr. Exercise intensity and longevity in men. JAMA 1995; 273:1179–1184.

81. Paffenbarger RS Jr, Hyde RT, Wing AL, et al. A natural history of athleticism and cardiovascular health. JAMA 1984;252:491–495.

82. Kannel WB, Sorlie P. Some health benefits of physical activity: the Framingham Study. Arch Int Med 1979;139:857–861.

83. Keys A. Seven Countries: a multivariable analysis of death and coronary heart disease. Cambridge, MA: Harvard University Press, 1980.

84. Toshima H, Koga Y, Blackburn H, Keys A, eds. Lessons for science from the Seven Countries Study. Tokyo: Springer-Verlag, 1994.

85. Kromhout D, Bloemberg BPM. Dietary saturated fatty acids serum cholesterol, and coronary heart disease. In: Toshima H, Yoga Y, Blackburn H, Keys A, eds. Lessons for science from the Seven Countries Study. Tokyo: Springer-Verlag, 1994.

86. Anderson KM, Wilson PWF, Odell PM, et al. An updated coronary risk profile: a statement for health professionals. Circulation 1991;83:356–362.

87. The Expert Panel. Report of the National Cholesterol Education Program Expert Panel on detection, evaluation, and treatment of high blood cholesterol in adults. Arch Intern Med 1988;148:36–39.

88. The Expert Panel. Summary of the Second Report of the National Cholesterol Education Program (NCEP) Expert Panel on detection, evaluation, and treatment of high blood cholesterol in adults (Adult Treatment Panel II). JAMA 1993;269:3015–3023.

89. Knopp KH, Walden CE, Retzlaff BM, et al. Long-term cholesterol-lowering effects of 4 fat-restricted diets in hypercholesterolemic and combined hyperlipidemic men. JAMA 1997;278:1509–1515.

90. Ascherio A, Rimm E, Giovannucci EL, et al. Dietary fat and risk of coronary heart disease in men: cohort follow up study in the United States. BMJ 1996;313:84–90.

91. Pietinen P, Rimm EB, Korhonen P, et al. Intake of dietary fiber and risk of coronary heart disease in a cohort of Finnish men: the Alpha-Tocopherol, Beta-Carotene Cancer Prevention Study. Circulation 1996;94:2720–2727.

92. Salmerón J, Ascherio A, Rimm EB, et al. Dietary fiber, glycemic load, and risk of NIDDM in men. Diabetes Care 1997;20:545–550.

93. Salmerón J, Manson JE, Stampfer MJ, et al. Dietary fiber, glycemic load, and risk of non-insulin-dependent diabetes mellitus in women. JAMA 1997;277:472–477.

94. Ripsin CM, Keenan JM, Jacobs DR Jr, et al. Oat products and lipid lowering: a meta-analysis. JAMA 1992;267:3317–3325.

95. Mekki N, Dubois C, Charbonnier M, et al. Effects of lowering fat and increasing dietary fiber on fasting and postprandial plasma lipids in hypercholesterolemic subjects consuming a mixed Mediterranean-Western diet. Am J Clin Nutr 1997;66:1443–1451.

96. Stamler R. The primary prevention of hypertension and the population blood pressure problem. In: Marmot M, Elliot P, eds. Coronary heart disease epidemiology. New York: Oxford University Press, 1992.

97. National Institutes of Health, National Heart, Lung, and Blood Institute. The fifth report of the Joint National Committee on Detection, Evaluation, and Treatment of High Blood Pressure (JNC V). Arch Intern Med 1993;153:154–183.

98. The Trials of Hypertension Prevention Collaborative Research Group. Effects of weight loss and sodium reduction intervention on blood pressure and hypertension incidence in overweight people with high-normal blood pressure: The Trials of Hypertension Prevention, Phase II. Arch Intern Med 1997;157:657–667.

99. Whelton PK, He J, Cutler JA, et al. Effects of oral potassium on blood pressure: meta-analysis of randomized controlled clinical trials. JAMA 1997;277:1624–1632.

100. Rose G. Ancel Keys Lecture. Circulation 1981;84:1405–1409.

101. Rose G. Sick individuals and sick populations. Int J Epidemiol 1985;14:32–38.

102. Kushi LH, Folsom AR, Prineas RJ, et al. Dietary antioxidant vitamins and death from coronary heart disease in postmenopausal women. N Engl J Med 1996;334:1156–1162.

103. The Alpha-Tocopherol, Beta Carotene Cancer Prevention Study Group. The effect of vitamin E and beta carotene on the incidence of lung cancer and other cancers in male smokers. N Engl J Med 1994;330:1029–1035.

104. Potter JD. Food and phytochemicals, magic bullets and measurement error: a commentary. Am J Epidemiol 1996;144:1026–1027.

105. Ballor DL, Poehlman ET. Exercise-training enhances fat-free mass preservation during diet-induced weight loss: a meta-analytical finding. Int J Obesity 1994;18:35–40.

106. Pritchard JE, Nowson CA, Wark JD. Bone loss accompanying diet-induced or exercise-induced weight loss: a randomized con-

trolled study. Int J Obesity 1996; 20:513–520.

107. Sowers MR, Galuska DA. Epidemiology of bone mass in premenopausal women. Epidemiol Rev 1993;15:374–398.

108. Hansen MA, Overgaard K, Christiansen C. Spontaneous postmenopausal bone loss in different skeletal areas—followed up for 15 years. J Bone Min Res 1995;10:205–210.

109. Frey-Hewitt B, Vranizan KM, Dreon DM, et al. The effect of weight loss by dieting or exercise on resting metabolic rate in overweight men. Int J Obesity 1990; 14:327–334.

110. Pavlou KN, Krey S, Steffee WP. Exercise as an adjunct to weight loss and maintenance in moderately obese subjects. Am J Clin Nutr 1989;49:1115–1123.

111. Pronk NP, Wing RR. Physical activity and long-term maintenance of weight loss. Obes Res 1994;2:587–599.

112. Pouliot MC, Després JP, Lemieux S, et al. Waist circumference and abdominal sagittal diameter: best simple anthropometric indexes of abdominal visceral adipose tissue accumulation and related cardiovascular risk in men and women. Am J Cardiol 1994; 73:460–468.

113. Tran ZV, Weltman A. Differential effects of exercise on serum lipid levels seen with changes in body weight. JAMA 1985;254:919–924.

114. Simkin-Silverman L, Wing RR, Hansen DH, et al. Prevention of cardiovascular risk factor elevations in healthy premenopausal women. Prev Med 1995;24:509–517.

115. Williams PT, Krauss RM, Vranizan KM, et al. Changes in lipoprotein subfractions during diet-induced and exercise-induced weight loss in moderately overweight men. Circulation 1990;81:1293–1304.

116. Schaeffer EJ. Effects of dietary fatty acids on lipoproteins and cardiovascular disease risk: summary. Am J Clin Nutr 1997;65(suppl):1655S–1656S.

117. Caggiula AW, Mustad VA. Effects of dietary fat and fatty acids on coronary artery disease risk and total and lipoprotein cholesterol concentrations: epidemiological associations. Am J Clin Nutr 1997;65(suppl):1597S–1610S.

118. Whelton PK, Appel LJ, Espeland MA, et al. Sodium reduction and weight loss in the treatment of hypertension in older persons. JAMA 1998;279:839–846.

119. Oldridge NB. Cardiac rehabilitation and risk factor management after myocardial infarction: clinical and economic evaluation. Wiener Klinische Wochenschrift 1997;2(suppl):6–16.

120. Ornish D, Brown SE, Scherwitz LW, et al. Can lifestyle changes reverse coronary heart disease? The Lifestyle Heart Trial. Lancet 1990;336:129–133.

121. Schwartz RS. The independent effects of dietary weight loss and aerobic training on high density lipoprotein and apolipoprotein A-I concentrations in obese men. Metabolism 1987;36:165–171.

122. Wood PD, Stefanick M, Dreon DM, et al. Changes in plasma lipids and lipoproteins in overweight men during weight loss through dieting as compared with exercise. N Engl J Med 1988; 319:1173–1179.

123. King AC, Frey-Hewitt B, Dreon DM, et al. Diet vs exercise in weight maintenance. Arch Intern Med 1989;149:2741–2746.

124. Williams PT, Stefanick ML, Vranizan KM, et al. The effects of weight loss by exercise or by dieting on plasma high-density lipoprotein (HDL) levels in men with low, intermediate, and normal-to-high HDL at baseline. Metabolism 1994;43:917–924.

125. Nolte LJ, Nowson CA, Dyke AC. Effect of dietary fat reduction and increased aerobic exercise on cardiovascular risk factors. Clin Exp Pharmacol Physiol 1997;24:901–903.

126. Leighton RF, Repka FJ, Birk TJ, et al. The Toledo exercise and diet study. Arch Intern Med 1990;150:1016–1020.

127. Nieman DC, Haig JL, Fairchild KS, et al. Reducing-diet and exercise-training effects on serum lipids and lipoproteins in mildly obese women. Am J Clin Nutr 1990;52:640–645.

128. Pavlou KN, Whatley JE, Jannace PW, et al. Physical activity as a supplement to a weight-loss dietary regimen. Am J Clin Nutr 1989;49:1110–1114.

129. Sopko G, Leon AS, Jacobs JR Jr., et al. The effects of exercise and weight loss on plasma lipids in young obese men. Metabolism 1985;34:227–236.

130. Wood PD, Stefanick ML, Williams PT, et al. The effects of plasma lipoproteins of a prudent weight-reducing diet, with or without exercise, in overweight men and women. N Engl J Med 1991; 325:461–466.

131. Hughes VA, Fiatarone MA, Ferrara CM, et al. Lipoprotein response to exercise training and a low-fat diet in older subjects with glucose intolerance. Am J Clin Nutr 1994;59:820–826.

132. Hellénius M-L, Faire Ud, Berglund B, et al. Diet and exercise are equally effective in reducing risk for cardiovascular disease: results of a randomized controlled study in men with slightly to moderately raised cardiovascular risk factors. Atherosclerosis 1993;103:81–91.

133. Wing RR, Venditti E, Jakicic JM, et al. Lifestyle intervention in overweight individuals with a family history of diabetes. Diabetes Care 1998;21:350–359.

134. Hagan RD, Upton SJ, Wong L, et al. The effects of aerobic conditioning and/or caloric restriction in overweight men and women. Med Sci Sports Exerc 1986; 18:87–94.

135. Stefanick ML, Mackey S, Sheehan M, et al. Effects of the NCEP step 2 diet and aerobic exercise on plasma lipoproteins in postmenopausal women and

men with low HDL-cholesterol combined with moderately elevated LDL-cholesterol. N Engl J Med 1998;339:12–20.

136. Svendsen OL, Hassager C, Christiansen C. Effect of an energy-restrictive diet, with or without exercise, on lean tissue mass, resting metabolic rate, cardiovascular risk factors, and bone in overweight postmenopausal women. Am J Med 1993;95: 131–140.

Chapter 75

The Epidemiology of Obesity, Physical Activity, Diet, and Type 2 Diabetes Mellitus

Janet E. Fulton
Harold W. Kohl, III

The purpose of this chapter is to provide the reader with an overview and a description of the epidemiologic studies examining the associations between obesity, physical activity, dietary intake, and type 2 diabetes mellitus. In doing so, we will answer the following questions:

1. Is obesity independently associated with the development of type 2 diabetes?

2. Is physical activity independently associated with the development of type 2 diabetes?

3. Are the components of dietary intake (macro- and micronutrients) independently associated with the development of type 2 diabetes?

We have included a brief section on obesity because it is a well-established risk factor for development of type 2 diabetes and is a manifestation of the imbalance between energy intake and energy expenditure. We have chiefly limited our presentation to investigations that study type 2 diabetes as the outcome, although some studies we examine measure the intermediate disease processes of type 2 diabetes—insulin resistance and impaired glucose tolerance.

EPIDEMIOLOGY

The field of epidemiology is defined by Hennekens et al as the study of the distribution and determinants of disease frequency in human populations (1). Epidemiologists seek to understand the etiology of disease and discern the degree to which an exposure affects the risk of disease. Several epidemiologic study designs are used to investigate the association between risk factors (i.e., exposures) and diseases. These study designs are often dichotomized into descriptive studies (including correlational, case reports, case series, or cross-sectional designs) and analytic strategies (such as case-comparison, cohort, or intervention studies). Descriptive studies describe the general characteristics of the distribution of a disease, particularly in relation to person, place, and time (1), whereas analytic strategies determine whether or not the risk of disease is different for persons exposed or not exposed to the factor of interest (1). Epidemiologic hypotheses are tested with analytic designs. In this chapter, we will investigate the association between three potentially modifiable risk factors for type 2 diabetes mellitus: obesity, physical activity, and dietary intake. Further, we will evaluate the scientific evidence within the context of the study design because it is a critical factor to determine the relative contribution of the study to the evidence for causality. In doing so, we will attempt to determine if the associations between the risk factors and disease are causal.

CAUSALITY

Obtaining knowledge about the distribution of disease and its risk factors from descriptive epidemiology leads to the development of hypotheses concerning disease causation. The development and testing of hypotheses, using analytic strategies, help us understand disease causation and are crucial to the development of preventive measures (2).

How do we determine if an exposure (i.e., risk factor) "causes" a disease? A causal association has been described as one in which the change in frequency of the exposure results in a corresponding change in the frequency of the outcome or disease of interest (1). Causation is not determined by examining an individual study, but by examining the totality of the evidence. Causation is determined by evaluating a logical sequence of events to determine whether: 1) the observed association between an exposure and disease is valid and 2) the totality of evidence taken from a number of sources (i.e., studies) supports a causal association. In individual studies, the validity of a statistical association is evaluated to determine the likelihood that the results are not due to chance, bias, or confounding. If chance, bias, or confounding are unlikely explanations for the observed finding, then we may conclude that the observed association is statistically and, thus, internally valid. Once the validity of the statistical association is determined, then we must evaluate whether the totality of evidence supports a cause and effect association. Several epidemiologic criteria are used to determine causality. These criteria include but are not limited to the strength of the association (the magnitude of the odds ratio or relative risk), biologic plausibility to support the hypothesis, consistency of the findings with other investigations, compatibility of the time sequence (the exposure precedes the occurrence of disease), and evidence of a dose-response relationship (the observation of a gradient of risk associated with the degree of exposure) (1). In this chapter, we will present studies that examined the association between obesity, physical activity, dietary intake, and type 2 diabetes mellitus and, in doing so, will present evidence about the causal nature of each of these associations.

DISEASE DEFINITION

Type 2 diabetes mellitus (previously known as non–insulin-dependent diabetes or adult-onset diabetes) is characterized by a deficiency of insulin or a decreased ability of the body to use insulin (a hormone secreted by the pancreas). Insulin allows glucose to enter body cells and be converted into energy. Insulin is also needed by the body to synthesize protein and store fats. In uncontrolled diabetes, glucose and lipids remain in the bloodstream and, in time, damage the body's organs and contribute to heart disease (3,4).

Type 2 diabetes is usually diagnosed among middle-aged people who are overweight or obese. Onset of type 2 diabetes is often gradual, resulting in mild symptoms (e.g., polydipsia, polyuria, weight loss) over extended periods of time or no symptoms at all. Often the condition is diagnosed

when elevated fasting glucose levels are detected during a routine physical examination of a person with no noticeable symptoms (3,4).

Table 75-1 shows the recently modified diagnostic criteria for type 2 diabetes. The American Diabetes Association lowered the diagnostic criterion for type 2 diabetes from a fasting plasma glucose level of 140 mg/dL or higher to a level of 126 mg/dL or higher, and eliminated routine clinical use of oral glucose tolerance tests, which are more difficult and expensive to perform than fasting glucose tests (4). When symptoms of diabetes are present, a confirmed non-fasting plasma glucose value of 200 mg/dL or higher indicates a diagnosis of type 2 diabetes. If a physician determines an oral glucose tolerance test is warranted, then a confirmed 2-hour plasma glucose value of 200 mg/dL or higher indicates a diagnosis of diabetes. Plasma glucose values from 110 mg/dL to less than 126 mg/dL indicate impaired fasting glucose, a pre-diabetic condition that is often predictive of type 2 diabetes.

ECONOMIC BURDEN

Diabetes mellitus is a devastating disease. Diabetes is the seventh leading cause of death in the United States and contributes to thousands of deaths each year (3). Individuals with diabetes are at increased risk for heart disease, blindness, kidney failure, and lower extremity amputations unrelated to injury. In 1997, an estimated $98 billion in direct ($44 billion) and indirect costs ($54 billion) were spent on diabetes in the United States (5).

NATURAL HISTORY

The natural history of type 2 diabetes follows a series of progressive physiologic events, culminating in overt manifestation of symptoms and disease often only in the final stages of the disease (6). Progression from insulin resistance to type 2 diabetes follows what has been labeled a "two-step model" (7). Figure 75-1 shows the course of progressive events from insulin resistance to impaired glucose tolerance culminating in insulin secretory failure and overt type 2 diabetes. As shown, age, obesity, and physical inactivity are risk factors for developing insulin resistance. According to the model, hypothesized risk factors for progression from insulin resistance to impaired

---

Table 75-1 American Diabetes Association Criteria for the Diagnosis of Diabetes Mellitus

1. Symptoms of diabetes plus casual plasma glucose concentration ≥ 200 mg/dL (11.1 mmol/L). Casual is defined as any time of day without regard to time since last meal. The classic symptoms of diabetes include polyuria (excessive urination), polydipsia (excessive thirst), and unexplained weight loss.
   OR
2. Fasting plasma glucose ≥ 126 mg/dL (7.0 mmol/L). Fasting is defined as no caloric intake for at least 8 hours.
   OR
3. 2-hour plasma glucose ≥ 200 mg/dL during an oral glucose tolerance test. The test should be performed as described by WHO (9), using a glucose load containing the equivalent of 75 g of anhydrous glucose dissolved in water. (This measure is not recommended for routine clinical use.)

Adapted with permission from American Diabetes Association. Report of the expert committee on the diagnosis and classification of diabetes mellitus. Diabetes Care 1997;20:1183–1197.

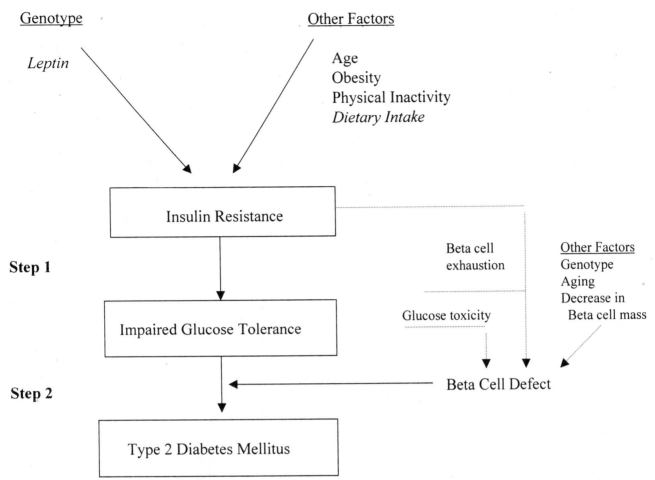

Genotype   Other Factors

Leptin   Age
                                            Obesity
                                            Physical Inactivity
                                            Dietary Intake

Step 1   Insulin Resistance

                                                    Beta cell   Other Factors
                                                    exhaustion   Genotype
                                                                       Aging
                                                                       Decrease in
                                                    Glucose toxicity   Beta cell mass

                    Impaired Glucose Tolerance

Step 2   Beta Cell Defect

                    Type 2 Diabetes Mellitus

Figure 75-1 Two-step model to describe the development of type 2 diabetes. Italicized words (i.e., leptin and dietary intake) and dotted lines are hypothesized contributory factors. (Adapted from Saad MF, Knowler WC, Pettitt DJ, et al. A two-step model for development of non-insulin-dependent diabetes. Am J Med 1991:90:229–235. Used by permission from Exerpta Medica Inc.)

glucose tolerance or type 2 diabetes may include pancreatic beta cell exhaustion, glucose toxicity, and genotype.

Type 2 diabetes is a syndrome of impaired insulin sensitivity and relative insulin deficiency. Insulin regulates the transport of glucose to cells, prompts glucose metabolism and synthesis of proteins, and suppresses lipolysis (8). Glucose is the key regulator of the pancreatic islet system because it regulates not only insulin and glucagon secretion directly but also adjusts responses to other substrates, free fatty acids, and amino acids, as well as other hormones and neural factors. Many factors affect regulation of the glucose homeostatic mechanism. Interpretation of any aspect of the glucose homeostatic mechanism should take into account the interrelationships of islet cell secretory function, hepatic glucose output, and peripheral glucose uptake at the respective hormone and substrate levels (8).

EPIDEMIOLOGY

Prevalence and Incidence in the United States

In the United States, an estimated 15.6 million adults have type 2 diabetes mellitus and approximately one half of the cases are undiagnosed, suggesting a much higher prevalence of this disease. Recent national estimates from analysis of the National Health and Nutrition Examination Survey population show that the prevalence (proportion of the population with type 2 diabetes) of diagnosed type 2 diabetes in 1988–1994 was 5.1% (10.2 million people) in the US population aged 20 to 74. The prevalence of undiagnosed type 2 diabetes was 2.7% (5.4 million people). The prevalence of impaired fasting glucose (110 mg/dL to <126 mg/dL) was 6.9% (13.4 million people). Similar prevalences were observed in men and women; however, prevalence for non-Hispanic blacks and Mexican Americans were 1.6 and 1.9 times that for non-Hispanic whites. Prevalence of type 2 diabetes in the total US population aged 40 to 74 increased from 8.9% in 1976–1980 to 12.3% in 1988–1994, using American Diabetes Association criteria for determining type 2 diabetes. Similar increases in prevalence were observed using World Health Organization criteria (casual plasma glucose ≥200 mg/dl) (9) and there was an increase from 11.4% in 1976–1980 to 14.3% in 1988–1994. In most populations of European origin, type 2 diabetes accounts for 90% to 95% of all cases of diabetes (10).

In the United States, the incidence (number of new cases) of type 2 diabetes continues to increase. The incidence of diabetes increased in the early 1980s, leveled off in the middle of the decade, and then increased sharply in the 1990s. In 1994, the age-adjusted incidence of diabetes (3.51 per 1000) was 49% higher than the incidence in 1980 (2.36 per 1000). In the 1990s, the number of new cases of diabetes averaged 748,000 per year, and increased from 629,000 new cases in 1990 to 939,000 new cases in 1994 (11,12).

Prevalence in Other Countries

The prevalence of type 2 diabetes varies throughout populations of the world. Prevalence of type 2 diabetes among middle-aged adults is less than 3% in rural or traditional communities in developing countries throughout the world, although their counterparts in urban or nontraditional communities have five to ten times higher prevalence of the disease (13). Current prevalence estimates of type 2 diabetes in populations of European origin range from 3% to 15% (13).

Certain populations are at especially high risk for type 2 diabetes. The prevalence of type 2 diabetes among men and women aged 30–64 is especially high among the Pima Indians of Arizona (age-adjusted prevalence among men = 49% and women = 51%), the Chinese living on Mauritius (age-adjusted prevalence among men = 16% and women = 10%), and the Nauruans of Micronesia (age-adjusted prevalence among men = 41% and women = 42%) (14). Clearly, both environmental and genetic factors play a role in the development of type 2 diabetes (13,15).

OBESITY AND TYPE 2 DIABETES

Defining Obesity in Epidemiologic Studies

In epidemiologic studies, obesity is typically defined as some combination of height and weight because measurement or self-reported estimates of height and weight are relatively easily obtained in large populations. Historically, Quetelet's index, most commonly referred to as the body mass index (weight in kilograms divided by the square of height in meters) and the percentage of desirable weight (most often based on the 1959 Metropolitan Life Insurance tables), have been used to estimate obesity in epidemiologic studies of type 2 diabetes (16). A small number of studies have used skinfold thicknesses (17). The body mass index (BMI) provides an estimate of general obesity that is relatively inexpensive to obtain in a large population. Validity of the BMI has been shown as BMI is independent of height and is inversely correlated with body density estimated from hydrostatic weighing in adults ($r = -0.67$ to -0.85) (18). To determine risk of type 2 diabetes associated with various levels of obesity, investigators most often compare individuals in the highest to those in the lowest proportion of the distribution (e.g., using tertiles, quartiles, or quintiles).

Etiology

Both obesity and type 2 diabetes are considered to be heterogeneous diseases comprising multiple etiologies. As many as 90% of individuals with type 2 diabetes are classified as overweight or obese (3). However, not all overweight or obese individuals develop type 2 diabetes (2,19). The exact mechanism(s) underlying the association between obesity and type 2 diabetes remains to be identified, although there is a strong positive association between obesity and the development of type 2 diabetes (20). Obesity is associated with insulin resistance (21) and with a reduced number of insulin receptors (22). Recent biochemical and genetic developments in obesity research include the discoveries of the protein leptin (a hormone secreted by fat cells that affects the control of energy balance) (23) and its receptor (24) and the mutations causing some forms of obesity in rodents (23–25). In mice, leptin acts as a feedback signal to the centers in the hypothalamus controlling food intake, energy expenditure, and the hormonal axes controlling adrenal and gonadal function. Most obese people have a normal leptin gene sequence and, in general, obese people have higher plasma leptin levels than nonobese people (26). Unfortunately, we do not yet know what will be the relevance of these discoveries to the etiology of human obesity and its association with type 2 diabetes (20).

Energy Balance

Energy balance is classically defined by the equation: change in energy stores equals energy intake minus energy expenditure (27). During stable weight periods, energy intake equals energy expenditure, and the equation is accurate because only a limited change in body composition can occur without a change in body weight. Some have suggested that obesity may originate not from small changes in energy intake or energy expenditure, but in the chronic imbalance between energy intake and energy expenditure (27).

Since obesity is an established risk factor for development of type 2 diabetes, understanding the components and factors that control energy balance may be the key to understanding the causes of type 2 diabetes (2,28). Gaining further knowledge about the relationships between obesity, physical activity, and dietary intake and type 2 diabetes, considered alone and in combination, may help to determine the risk factors most likely to lead to type 2 diabetes.

Many excellent reviews (16,19,20,29) have been written on the epidemiology of obesity and type 2 diabetes; thus, a comprehensive review of the topic is not presented in this chapter. Herein, we will briefly summarize the large body of research describing the relationship between obesity and the development of type 2 diabetes.

Cross-sectional Studies

Obesity promotes disease in the genetically susceptible, but obesity is neither a sufficient nor a necessary cause for developing type 2 diabetes (2,19). In general, findings from cross-sectional studies show greater risk of type 2 diabetes among persons with higher body mass index or percentage desirable weight, although results have varied across populations. In their review of obesity and type 2 diabetes, Manson et al (16) compared the highest to the lowest weight categories and showed estimates of relative risks that ranged from no association to a sixfold increased risk of type 2 diabetes. These results may be confounded, however, because people with diabetes often lose weight just prior to clinical diagnosis, which may explain why some investigators have not observed a cross-sectional association between obesity and type 2 diabetes. A limitation of cross-sectional studies is the inability to assess the temporal association between the exposure and the disease (i.e., it is not possible to tell whether obesity preceded or followed the occurrence of diabetes).

Cohort Studies

In a cohort study, a group of individuals (free from the disease under investigation) is defined on the basis of the presence or absence of an exposure. Eligible participants are then followed over a period of time to assess the occurrence of the outcome (1). Because the exposure precedes the outcome in this study design, investigators can make statements about the temporality of the association. That is, the exposure causes the development of the outcome, not vice versa. However, prospective cohort studies are very time-consuming and expensive to conduct because they often entail following a large number of individuals for many years (1).

In prospective studies, where exposure status is not affected by the disease condition, baseline obesity status is consistently associated with development of type 2 diabetes (17,30–32). In a combined analysis of six prospective cohort studies, investigators found a 13% increase in risk of developing type 2 diabetes for every $4\,kg/m^2$ increase in body mass index (about 25 lb), independent of fasting and 2-hour post challenge glucose levels (33). Further, another review of 10 prospective studies showed that relative risks of type 2 diabetes ranged from 1.4 to 60.9, and the median relative risk from the reported studies was 3.5 (16). Some, but not all, of the studies were controlled for the potential confounding variables of age, sex and ethnicity (where appropriate), blood lipids, blood glucose, blood pressure, cigarette smoking, and family history of diabetes (16). Specifically, among 841 middle-aged men living in the Netherlands, subscapular skinfold thickness (comparing the highest to the lowest quartile) was associated with a 3.2-fold increase in 25-year incidence of type 2 diabetes (95% CI = 1.7–6.1) (17). Among 82,609 women aged 30 to 55 participating in the Nurses' Health Study, increasing risk of diabetes was observed with increasing decile of body mass index (RR ranged from 2.1 to 58.2). Among women of average BMI ($23.0–23.9\,kg/m^2$), the relative risk was 3.5 times that of women having a BMI less than $22.0\,kg/m^2$. In summary, obesity is an independent risk factor for development of type 2 diabetes in men and women and the risk of type 2 diabetes increases with the extent of obesity.

Body Fat Distribution

Besides general obesity, the upper body or central distribution of body fat induces an additional risk for the development of type 2 diabetes (29). Body fat distribution is most often defined as a ratio of circumferences (waist to hip) or a ratio of subcutaneous skinfold thicknesses (subscapular to triceps). Insulin resistance has been shown to increase with increasing abdominal or visceral obesity (34), although the exact location of fat stores that contribute to insulin resistance are currently under investigation (35). Body fat distribution may be even more closely correlated with development of type 2 diabetes than with relative weight or BMI (19). These observations are not new. In 1956, Vague (36) observed that among persons with diabetes the male pattern of subcutaneous fat (android or upper-body obesity) was found more often than the female fat pattern.

In the review by Manson et al, in prospective cohort studies, according to indices of body fat distribution (i.e., centrality index, waist to hip ratio, and subscapular skinfold) the age-adjusted relative risk of type 2 diabetes ranged from 1.8 to 13.6 (16,29,37,38). Recent findings from the Nurses' Health Study showed among 43,581 women followed for 8 years, the relative risk of type 2 diabetes was 3.1 (95% CI = 2.3–4.1; controlled for BMI, age, family history of diabetes, exercise, cigarette smoking, intakes of saturated fat, calcium, potassium, magnesium, and glycemic index) when comparing the highest to the lowest decile of waist to hip ratio (39). Among 51,529 men participating in the Health Professionals Study, investigators showed a 1.7-fold (95% CI = 1.1–2.7) increase in risk (controlled for BMI, age, family history of diabetes, and smoking status) of type 2 diabetes when comparing the fifth to the first quintile of waist to hip ratio (40).

Weight Gain

The duration and magnitude of obesity may create further deterioration in the glucose homeostatic mechanisms that may lead to glucose intolerance and clinical diabetes (41). Several recent prospective studies indicate that weight gain, independent of initial obesity, is associated with development of type 2 diabetes. Among a nationally representative group of 8545 men and women participating in the National Health and Nutrition Examination Survey I, investigators evaluated the change in weight from the periods 1971–1975 to 1982–1984 on the association with incident type 2 diabetes diagnosed from 1982–1984 to 1992. Among all participants, relative risks of type 2 diabetes associated with gaining 5–<8, 8–<11, 11–<20, and ≥20 kg were 2.1, 1.2, 2.7, and 3.8, respectively (42). Analysis of men participating in the Health Professionals Study showed that gains in weight of 4.5 to 13.6 and, 13.6 or more kg were associated with relative risks of type 2 diabetes of 1.7 and 4.5, respectively (40). Among Pima Indians, rate of weight (kg) gain per year was associated with incidence of type 2 diabetes in men (RR = 1.24; 95% CI = 1.04–1.49) and in women who were not initially overweight (RR not reported, p for trend = 0.01) (43).

Weight Loss

Weight loss improves the insulin resistance characteristic of obesity and type 2 diabetes (44,45). Weight loss amplifies the action of insulin whereby it acts to suppress hepatic glucose output and to improve uptake of glucose into peripheral tissues (44). Nearly all aspects of peripheral glucose uptake show improvement with weight loss and only small weight loss (5% to 10% of initial weight) is necessary to improve insulin resistance, although the exact mechanism has not yet been identified (45,46).

Weight loss interventions have been the traditional mode of therapy for obese patients with type 2 diabetes (20). Investigators have generally used dietary weight-loss strategies to promote moderate caloric restriction, alteration of macronutrients in the diet (i.e., low-fat or high-monounsaturated-fat diets), or very low calorie diets (400–800 kcal/day). Unfortunately, the current dietary strategies are usually not effective for achieving long-term weight loss (47). Among persons with type 2 diabetes, available data show that weight loss is difficult to achieve and even more difficult to maintain. With moderate caloric restriction diets, individuals generally lose about

10% of their initial body weight; however, an average of one third of the lost weight is usually regained in the year following treatment (20). Evidence suggests that prolonged weight loss may be achieved among non-diabetic persons when weight-loss therapy is provided on a long-term basis (20,48).

Exercise interventions have been shown to improve lipid and insulin levels, even in the absence of weight loss (20). Investigators generally observe a 2 to 3 kg weight loss with exercise compared with control groups (49). When exercise is combined with a dietary intervention, the average additional weight loss is 1.8 kg in addition to weight loss with diet alone. Although exercise does not contribute to large differences in the absolute additional weight loss, cross-sectional studies have shown that individuals who exercise may maintain their weight losses better than those who do not exercise (50,51).

Causality

Evidence exists to support a causal association between obesity and the development of type 2 diabetes (Table 75-2). Evidence to date, from several large prospective cohort studies, indicates a consistently strong association between obesity and type 2 diabetes. A dose-response gradient has been observed in studies of weight gain and weight loss and type 2 diabetes. The weakest evidence concerns the biologic plausibility of the association; the exact mechanism has not yet been identified. Hopefully, rapid advancements in the fields of molecular biology and genetics research will identify the specific biologic mechanism(s) in the near future.

Summary

Obesity (as defined by BMI) is a risk factor for development of type 2 diabetes among adults in many populations. Findings from prospective cohort studies show that the relative risk for development of type 2 diabetes increases as the extent of obesity increases. An android body fat pattern (upper body fat patterning) also appears to be independently associated with development of type 2 diabetes. Gaining weight over the course of adulthood appears to be positively associated with the development of diabetes, and losing weight improves the insulin resistance associated with type 2 diabetes. However, weight loss is typically difficult to maintain over time (i.e., more than one year). The addition of an exercise component to dietary intervention strategies may increase maintenance of weight loss, although prospective studies need to be conducted to test this hypothesis.

PHYSICAL ACTIVITY AND TYPE 2 DIABETES

Measurement of Physical Activity in Epidemiologic Studies

Physical activity is a complex behavior that has been defined as "any bodily movement produced by skeletal muscles that results in energy expenditure" (52). Exercise is a subcategory of physical activity that is "planned, structured, repetitive, and purposive" (52). Measurement of physical activity, especially for epidemiologic research, is an arduous and often challenging task. Accurate assessment of physical activity is critical to determine its effect on the risk of disease.

Although it is possible to measure physical activity using laboratory methods such as doubly-labeled water or calorimetry, in most epidemiologic studies physical activity is assessed indirectly using questionnaires. Because epidemiologic studies often require participation from a large group of individuals, it is neither cost-effective nor time-efficient to use methodologies other than questionnaires. Questionnaires can be administered in many ways (self-administered, interviewer-administered, or mailed to the respondent) and typically have been designed to assess leisure-time, transportational, or occupational physical

Table 75-2 Evaluation of Causal Criteria to Support the Association Between Obesity and Type 2 Diabetes Mellitus

CAUSAL CRITERIA	EVIDENCE
Biologic plausibility	• Obesity is associated with insulin resistance. • Obesity is associated with a reduced number of insulin receptors.
Strength of the association	• In a combined analysis of six prospective studies, there was a 13% increase in risk of type 2 diabetes with each 4 kg/m² increase in BMI. • Difficult to determine an overall estimate of relative risk, although in one review, the median relative risk of type 2 diabetes was 3.5, when comparing the highest to the lowest portions of the distribution.
Consistency with other studies	• Most cross-sectional studies show a positive association between obesity and type 2 diabetes, although some cross-sectional studies have not found an association, presumably due to weight loss associated with development of type 2 diabetes. • A positive association between obesity and type 2 diabetes is consistently observed in prospective studies although findings may be influenced by positive paper bias (bias toward acceptance of papers with positive findings).
Temporality	• Prospective studies consistently show a positive association between obesity and type 2 diabetes.
Dose-response	• As obesity increases, the risk of developing type 2 diabetes increases. • Weight loss reduces symptoms of type 2 diabetes (i.e., insulin resistance) and reduces the need for hypoglycemic medications.

activity (53). Measurement typically requires determining the frequency, intensity, duration, and mode of physical activity, but can also be assessed using a global estimate of the level of physical activity. Time frames for recall of physical activity are generally either recent (e.g., yesterday, during the past 7 days), or historical (e.g., over the past year, or during one's lifetime). A complete review of questionnaires used in epidemiologic studies to assess physical activity that provides reliability and validity information is found in a resource edited by Kriska et al (54).

Epidemiologic Evidence

Biologically, physical activity appears to have short- and long-term effects on carbohydrate metabolism and glucose tolerance. During a single bout of physical activity, glucose uptake is increased by contracting skeletal muscle and enhanced glucose uptake into the cells that appears to be related to increased blood flow to the muscle and enhanced glucose transport into the muscle cell. These physiologic changes may persist for 24 hours or more as glycogen is being replenished in the muscle (55,56). Long-term adaptations to exercise training show that physical activity increases sensitivity to insulin and thus helps to prevent the development of type 2 diabetes. Long-term adaptations may prevent the development of insulin resistance (and impaired glucose tolerance) and thus may prevent the cascade of events leading to a relative deficiency in the amount of circulating insulin and development of overt type 2 diabetes (57).

Many authors have reviewed the epidemiologic literature to determine the association between physical activity and type 2 diabetes (8,15,56,58). Available evidence supports an inverse association between physical activity and type 2 diabetes. Recent findings from one clinical trial to examine the effects of physical activity and diet in preventing type 2 diabetes will also be presented. In this section, we provide an overview of epidemiologic studies of the association between physical activity and type 2 diabetes, but will not present an exhaustive review of the literature. A more comprehensive review of the literature may be found in other sources (15,16,58).

Migration Studies

Early observations of the association between physical activity and type 2 diabetes were shown in migration studies where populations abandon their native (often agrarian) lifestyles and migrate to different (often more industrialized) environments. Generally, migration studies show that groups who abandon their native culture experience greater prevalence of chronic disease risk factors than when living their traditional lifestyle. The prevalence of diabetes was two times higher among Japanese men and women living in Hawaii than among Japanese living in Hiroshima (59). This phenomenon has been observed in other cultures as well. O'Dea (60) observed that Australian aborigines who change their traditional hunter-gatherer lifestyle to a more industrialized lifestyle develop higher prevalence of type 2 diabetes, obesity, impaired glucose tolerance, hypertriglyceridemia, hypertension, and hyperinsulinemia. Because migration or ecologic studies report the change or correlation of group data (change in prevalence when moving from hunter-gatherer to industrialized lifestyle), findings from migration or ecologic studies are useful to

develop and generate hypotheses but are not appropriate designs to test specific hypotheses because sufficient data on individuals are lacking.

Cross-sectional Studies

Most cross-sectional studies show that individuals with type 2 diabetes are less physically active than their non-diabetic counterparts (15,61), although some cross-sectional studies have found that physical activity was not associated with type 2 diabetes (62–70).

Among 384 male and 680 female Pima Indians, aged 15 to 59, Kriska et al (71) showed, in males, that current levels of physical activity were inversely associated (non-standardized regression coefficient = −0.01, $p = 0.005$) with fasting and 2-hour plasma glucose after controlling for age, obesity, and fat distribution. Historical physical activity during ages 12 to 18 (OR = 0.45, 95% CI = 0.27–0.75) and 19 to 34 (OR = 0.47, 95% CI = 0.28–0.78) were also inversely associated with type 2 diabetes. A strength of this study is that type 2 diabetes was not self-reported, but diagnosed using oral glucose tolerance tests. In the Zutphen Elderly Study, Feskens et al (72) examined 389 men aged 70 to 89 and observed that insulin levels were lowest among men with the highest physical activity, obtained from minutes per week spent in leisure physical activity (physical activity and fasting insulin, $r = −0.13$; and 2-hour insulin, $r = −0.19$, $p < 0.05$ for both correlations, controlling for age, BMI, subscapular-triceps skinfold ratio, cigarette smoking, and energy intake). One recent cross-sectional study investigated the effect of frequency and intensity of physical activity on insulin sensitivity among African American, Hispanic, and non-Hispanic white men and women aged 40 to 69 participating in the Insulin Resistance Atherosclerosis Study. In this study, Mayer-Davis et al (73) observed a positive association between frequency of participation in categories of vigorous physical activity (rarely or never, 1–3 times/month, 1 time/wk, 2–4 times/wk, 5 times/wk) and insulin sensitivity (adjusted regression coefficients to corresponding physical activity categories: 0.90, 1.12, 1.38, 1.43, and 1.59) and an inverse association between frequency of participation in vigorous physical activity and fasting insulin values (adjusted regression coefficients to corresponding physical activity categories: 113.86, 109.34, 101.66, 92.98, and 83.87) (p for trend not reported). Regression coefficients were adjusted for age, race, sex, alcohol intake, cigarette smoking, percentage of calories from dietary fat, and hypertension status. Nonvigorous energy expenditure was positively associated with insulin sensitivity ($p < 0.05$), but was not associated with fasting insulin.

Cohort Studies

In a retrospective cohort study (i.e., the cohort is investigated at a later point in time, following occurrence of the outcome), investigators classified 5398 survivors of 7559 female college alumni as former athletes (n = 2622) or nonathletes (n = 2772) based on their collegiate sport participation (74). Type 2 diabetes was determined from self-reported responses to a mail questionnaire. The prevalence of type 2 diabetes among athletes was 0.57% and among non-athletes it was 1.30%; RR was 2.2 (95% CI, 1.2–4.7), Unfortunately, it was not possible to adequately separate type 1 from type 2 diabetes, but using onset above age 40 as indicative of type 2 diabetes and eliminating cases of gestational diabetes, the relative risk of type 2 diabetes increased to 3.4 (95% CI, 1.3–8.7). Several potential biases may have influenced the findings of this study, the most notable being that nonathletes were fatter than athletes; thus, detection of diabetes may have been more likely among nonathletes (75).

Table 75-3 presents a description of nine prospective cohort studies to investigate the association between physical activity and risk of type 2 diabetes. Sample sizes ranged from 127 to 87,253. The largest studies (76,77) were conducted among nurses and physicians enrolled in ongoing clinical trials to test the effects of estrogen and aspirin on the prevention of cardiovascular diseases in women and men, respectively. All studies used self-report methodologies, either in-person or through the mail, to assess physical activity. Type 2 diabetes was ascertained from self-reports (76–79), medical records or death certificates (80,81), and laboratory measures (82–84). Length of follow-up ranged from 2 to 14 years. All studies reported a protective effect of physical activity on the risk of type 2 diabetes; relative risk and odds ratios ranged from 0.94 to 0.41. One study showed no association among women (83), whereas another study reported a nonsignificant odds ratio after adjusting for BMI (84). Five of the nine studies observed a dose-response gradient as the risk of type 2 diabetes decreased with increasing levels of physical activity. In a detailed analysis conducted by Helmrich et al, the authors showed a dose-response effect among all reported physical activities and also when restricting the analysis to vigorous activities only (Table 75-3). An additional protective effect of vigorous physical activity was noted when the data were analyzed separately. A threshold of physical activity (i.e., 40 minutes of activity at 5.5 METs) has been proposed at which a reduced risk of type 2 diabetes is observed (84). Thus, independent of age and BMI, the data in Table 75-3 support the hypothesis that participation in physical activity is a protective risk factor for development of type 2 diabetes. Levels of increasing caloric expenditure in physical activity and increased participation in vigorous physical activity appear to provide additional protection against development of type 2 diabetes.

Intervention Studies

To date, two intervention studies have investigated the effect of lifestyle interventions, including physical activity, on the prevention of type 2 diabetes. Eriksson et al (85) conducted a nonrandomized trial to test the effect of lifestyle interventions on progression and development of type 2 diabetes. Participants were male (aged 48.1 ± 0.7) residents of Malmo, Sweden. Men were assigned (nonrandomly) to two treatment groups (group 1 included 41 patients with newly detected type 2 diabetes; group 2 included 181 patients with impaired glucose tolerance) and two comparison groups (group 3 included 79 men with impaired glucose tolerance; group 4 included 114 randomly selected men with normal glucose tolerance). Groups 1 and 2 received dietary and physical activity interventions through a "borderline diabetes clinic." After 6 years, BMI was reduced by 2.3% to 3.7% among treated individuals, whereas BMI increased by 0.5% to 1.7% in nonintervention men. Glucose tolerance was normalized in more than half of men in group 2 with impaired glucose tolerance and

incidence of diabetes was 10.6%. Relative risk of diabetes development in group 2 compared with group 3 was 0.37 (95% CI 0.20–0.68). Less than 10% of participants dropped out during the trial. Although treatment was not randomized in this trial, findings did show that a large group of sedentary and overweight glucose-intolerant and diabetic men could successfully complete a 5-year intervention program.

Pan et al (86) randomized 530 (M = 283, F = 247) individuals from Da Qing, China, with impaired glucose tolerance into four treatment groups (by clinical site): 1) control, 2) diet only, 3) exercise only, or 4) diet and exercise. Dietary interventions promoted eating a diet of 55% to 65% carbohydrates, 25% to 30% fat, and 10% to 15% protein. Participants who had a BMI higher than $25 \, kg/m^2$ were encouraged to reduce calorie intake to gradually lose 0.5 kg to 1.0 kg per month. Exercise interventions promoted increasing daily amounts of leisure physical activity by at least one unit of activity each day, defined as 30 minutes of mild activity, 20 minutes of moderate activity, 10 minutes of strenuous activity, or 5 minutes of very strenuous activity. Participants received individual and group counseling at various intervals throughout the trial. Findings showed a 31% to 46% reduction in risk of diabetes among all treatment groups (adjusted for baseline BMI and fasting plasma glucose); relative risk of diabetes for diet, exercise, and diet plus exercise were 0.69, 0.54, and 0.58 (p < 0.05 for all), respectively.

Causality

Evidence exists to support a causal association between physical activity and type 2 diabetes (Table 75-4). The association between physical activity and type 2 diabetes is biologically plausible; physical activity has been shown to enhance uptake of glucose into cells and increase sensitivity to insulin. Independent of age and BMI, prospective cohort studies show a consistent protective effect to physical activity, with relative risks that have ranged from 0.94 to 0.41. A dose-response gradient was observed in five of the nine prospective studies presented.

Summary

In summary, physical inactivity is an independent risk factor for development of type 2 diabetes. Prospective cohort studies consistently show an inverse association between physical activity and development of type 2 diabetes, independent of age and BMI, although the minimal dose of physical activity commensurate with a decreased incidence of diabetes has not yet been determined. Findings from one randomized clinical trial indicates that treatment with exercise is comparable to treatment with diet or diet plus exercise in the prevention of progression from impaired glucose tolerance to type 2 diabetes.

The ability to obtain accurate estimates of an individual's physical activity behavior is a limitation in many epidemiologic studies. Thus, improving the validity of existing instruments and developing new instruments to measure the physical activity of large groups of individuals are important areas of research. In addition, research is needed to determine the minimal (and perhaps maximal) doses of the frequency and intensity of physical activity that reduces the incidence of type 2 diabetes.

DIETARY INTAKE AND TYPE 2 DIABETES
Measurement of Dietary Intake in Epidemiologic Studies

As with physical activity, measurement of dietary intake is a challenging endeavor. For a comprehensive description of

nutritional assessment methods, refer to other sources (87–89).

In general, three methodologies are used in epidemiologic studies to assess components of dietary intake: 1) dietary record; 2) 24-hour recall; and 3) food frequency (89). Dietary records require the respondent to record all food and bever-

Table 75-3 Prospective Cohort Studies of Physical Activity and Type 2 Diabetes Mellitus

Reference	Characteristics of Study Participants	Physical Activity Assessment Method	Assessment of Type 2 Diabetes	Period of Follow-up	Number of Cases of Type 2 Diabetes	Main Findings			Dose-Response Observed
Helmrich et al (78)	5990 Univ. Pa. men, aged 39–69	Mail questionnaire to assess weekly energy expenditure in leisure-time physical activity, vigorous sports, moderate sports, and number of flights of stairs climbed and blocks walked each week	Self-reported using mail questionnaire to assess whether participant had a "history of diabetes"	1962–1976	202	*kcal/week* <500 500–999 1000–1499 1500–1999 2000–2499 2500–2999 3000–3499 ≥3500 *p* for trend *age adjusted	All activities *RR** 1.00 0.94 0.79 0.78 0.68 0.90 0.86 *0.52* 0.01	Vigorous sports *RR** 1.00 0.69 — 0.53 0.86 0.56 0.40 *0.46* 0.05	Yes
Manson et al (76)	87,253 female nurses participating in Nurses' Health Study, aged 34–59, 98% Caucasian	Mail questionnaire in 1980: "At least once a week do you engage in any regular activity similar to brisk walking, jogging, bicycling, etc. long enough to work up a sweat? If yes, how many times per week? What activity is this?"	Self-reported in response to: "Have you ever had diabetes mellitus diagnosed?"	1976–1984	1267	Women who exercised vigorously: *Times/week* 0 1 2 3 4+ *p* for trend *age and BMI adjusted	*RR** 1.00 0.89 0.71 0.93 *0.86* >0.05		No
Schranz et al (82)	127 men and women, ≥15 years of age, living in Malta	Self-reported usual hr/d (or per wk) spent in light (≥3 and <6 METs) and heavy activity (≥6 METs) during work, leisuretime, or for transportation. Physical activity index calculated by weighting number of hours spent in light and heavy activity.	Diabetes and impaired glucose tolerance classified according to 1980 WHO criteria	1981–1983	22	Cumulative incidence (inc) of impaired glucose tolerance and type 2 diabetes *Physical activity Inc** low 7.9 moderate 17.8 *high* *21.7* *p* for trend 0.01 *age adjusted			Yes, based on two cases in high-activity group
Manson et al (77)	21,271 US male physicians participating in Physicians' Health Study, aged 40–84	Mail questionnaire to assess "How often do you exercise vigorously enough to work up a sweat?"	Self-reported on mail questionnaire	1982–1988 (mean = 5 years)	285	Men who exercised vigorously: *Times/week* 0 1 2–4 ≥5 *p* for trend *age and BMI adjusted	*RR** 1.00 0.78 0.68 *0.71* 0.009		Yes
Lipton et al (80)	11,097 white and black participants in NHANES I epidemiologic follow-up study, aged 25–70	Self-reported global assessment of physical activity during work and leisuretime	Sources: (1) self- or proxy-reported at follow-up, (2) by diagnosis listed on hospital or nursing home report, (3) diabetes reported on death certificate	1971–1987	880	Among all men and women: low compared to high level of physical activity OR* = 1.28, (*p* < 0.05) *adjusted for age, race, sex, BMI, subscapular:triceps skinfold ratio, systolic blood pressure, and education			No

Table 75-3 continues

Table 75-3 (*Continued*)

Reference	Characteristics of Study Participants	Physical Activity Assessment Method	Assessment of Type 2 Diabetes	Period of Follow-up	Number of Cases of Type 2 Diabetes	Main Findings	Dose-response Observed
Burchfiel et al (79)	6815 Japanese-American men in the Honolulu Heart Program living on the island of Oahu, aged 45–68	Self-reported number of hours spent per 24-hour period in basal, sedentary, slight, moderate, and heavy intensity activities. Index created by weighting intensity categories by estimated oxygen consumption.	Self-reported history of taking insulin or oral hypoglycemic agents at second or third examinations	1968–1974	All men, n = 391; Among men with non-fasting glucose <225 mg/dL, n = 250	Among all men: OR* = 0.50 (95% CI = 0.34–0.73) Among men with non-fasting glucose <225: OR* = 0.48 (95% CI = 0.30–0.77) *adjusted for age, BMI, CHD risk factors, and restricted to men free of CVD	Yes, among men in lower four quintiles of BMI
Monterrosa et al (83)	353 Mexican American men and 491 Mexican American women in the San Antonio Heart Study; aged 25–64	Self-reported average times/wk during past year engaged in leisure-time physical activity	Laboratory determined by WHO criteria or currently taking insulin or oral antidiabetic drugs	1982–1990	Men, n = 20 Women, n = 37	Among men: Leisuretime physical activity inversely associated with diabetes OR* = 0.41 (95% CI = 0.18–0.93) *adjusted for age, SES, and structural assimilation Among women: OR* = 1.43, (95% CI = 0.85–2.41)	No
Perry et al (81)	7097 British men aged 40–59	Self-reported derived score based on frequency and intensity of activities. Grouped into inactive, light, moderate, moderately vigorous, and vigorous categories.	Sources: (1) self-reported by mail questionnaires in 1983 and 1992, (2) medical record review, (3) death certificate review	1978–1991 (mean = 12.8 years)	178	Moderate versus inactive, OR* = 0.40, (95% CI = 0.20–0.80) *adjusted for age, BMI, prevalent CHD, cigarette smoking, systolic blood pressure, HDL cholesterol, heart rate, and uric acid p for linear trend = 0.003, but did not report ORs by physical activity level.	Yes, but did not report ORs
Lynch et al (84)	751 men residing in Kuopio, Finland, aged 42–60	Minnesota Leisure Time Physical Activity Questionnaire: 12-month history of 15 most common leisure-time physical activities of middle-aged Finnish men	Type 2 diabetes diagnosed if: (1) fasting blood glucose ≥120 mg/dL or, (2) 2-hour oral glucose tolerance test ≥180 mg/dL or, (3) history of treatment for type 2 diabetes	1984–88 to 1991–93 (median = 4.2 years)	46	Reduced risk of type 2 diabetes seen at ≥5.5 METs intensity and 40 min duration: OR* = 0.44 (95% CI = 0.22–0.88) compared with those not meeting this threshold *adjusted for age, baseline glucose, and CHD risk factors After adjustment for BMI, OR = 0.77 (95% CI = 0.38–1.53).	No

ages and the amounts of each consumed over a period of days. Dietary records are often considered a validation standard by which other dietary assessment methods are compared. Three to four days of recordkeeping are considered optimal because more than this may be burdensome to the participant. Underreporting on food records may occur because of either incomplete recording or the impact of the recording process on dietary choices (89).

During a 24-hour recall, the respondent is queried by an interviewer to name all foods and beverages consumed during the past 24 hours. The interview is usually conducted in a structured format, with specific probes from the interviewer. Respondent burden is low because the 24-hour recall interview usually lasts about 20 minutes and the interviewer

records all responses. Because an individual's diet may vary from day to day, 24-hour recalls are most useful to describe the average dietary intake of a group (89).

The food frequency approach involves asking respondents to report their usual frequency of consumption of food from a list of foods for a specific time period. Information on the frequency of listed foods eaten is obtained. A semi-quantitative food frequency interview involves requesting respondents to specify the portion size of the food. Quantification of dietary intake is not as accurate as with records or recalls; however, the food frequency methodology is designed to estimate the respondent's usual intake of foods and has become a common way to estimate usual dietary intake (89).

Table 75-4 Evaluation of Causal Criteria to Support the Association Between Physical Activity and Type 2 Diabetes Mellitus

CAUSAL CRITERIA	EVIDENCE
Biologic plausibility	• Physical activity has short and long-term effects on carbohydrate metabolism and glucose tolerance. • Physical activity in combination with insulin may enhance glucose uptake into cells. • Exercise training studies show that physical activity may increase sensitivity to insulin.
Strength of the association	• Based on findings from nine prospective cohort studies and one clinical trial, with varying levels of physical activity, relative risks of type 2 diabetes ranged from 0.94 to 0.41.
Consistency with other studies	• Some cross-sectional studies did not show that physical activity was associated with type 2 diabetes. • Consistent protective effect of physical activity on risk of type 2 diabetes observed in cohort studies although findings may be influenced by positive paper bias (bias toward acceptance of papers with positive findings).
Temporality	• Nine prospective cohort studies and one clinical trial show protective effect of physical activity on risk of developing type 2 diabetes. Length of follow-up ranged from 2 to 16 years.
Dose-response	• Five of nine prospective studies show evidence of a dose-response effect, although one study had only two cases in the "high" activity group (81) and another study observed a dose-response gradient only among men in the lower four quintiles of body mass index (78).

Epidemiologic Evidence

Dietary intake is thought to be associated with type 2 diabetes mainly through its association with overweight or obesity (29,90). Specific nutritional components have been hypothesized to be associated with risk of type 2 diabetes including fat consumption, especially saturated fat intake, low intake of dietary fiber, and high intake of carbohydrates (resulting in a high glycemic index). Elements such as chromium, zinc, potassium, calcium, and magnesium, and vitamins such as vitamin E may also be associated with insulin resistance or development of type 2 diabetes.

Energy Intake

Energy intake, independent of obesity, has not been shown to be associated with type 2 diabetes. In cross-sectional (72) and prospective cohort studies (30), energy intake was not associated with insulin sensitivity or incidence of type 2 diabetes, respectively.

Macronutrients

Dietary Fat

Consumption of a high-fat diet has been hypothesized to be associated with development of type 2 diabetes. In 1935, Himsworth noted that populations with high dietary fat intake also had higher diabetes mortality rates (91). Whether intake of dietary fat intake leads to the development of diabetes, independent of obesity, is still unknown. However, consumption of high-fat diets have been shown to cause insulin resistance in rats and may alter cell membrane function and, thus, insulin receptor activity even apart from effects on body fatness (92).

The association between dietary fat intake and development of diabetes in the epidemiologic literature is equivocal. In a study of 9494 Israeli men who underwent extensive dietary assessments using a method similar to the Burke interview (30), univariate analysis indicated no association between total dietary intake or other dietary variables with type 2 diabetes after 5 years of follow-up. Similarly, among 277 female Pima Indians aged 25 to 44 who underwent a modified Burke interview, among the 87 cases that developed, there was no association between baseline fat consumption and incidence of diabetes (2).

In contrast, two recent studies by Marshall et al (93,94) lend support for the dietary fat-type 2 diabetes association. In a cross-sectional study, 24-hour recall of diet was used to determine the association between dietary fat intake and type 2 diabetes and glucose intolerance among 1317 US men and women residing in the San Luis valley. After adjustment for age, sex, ethnicity, calories, and BMI, a 40 g/d increase in fat intake was associated with type 2 diabetes (OR = 1.51, 95% CI = 0.85–2.67) and impaired glucose tolerance (OR = 1.62, 95% CI = 1.09–2.41) (93). Subjects with impaired glucose tolerance (n = 134) from the same population were then followed prospectively for 1 to 3 years (between 1984 and 1988). Twenty incident cases of diabetes were ascertained. Following adjustment for age, sex, ethnicity, obesity, and energy intake, a 40 g/d increase in fat intake was associated with a 3.4-fold increase in development of type 2 diabetes (95% CI = 0.8–13.6). Following additional adjustment for fasting glucose, insulin, and 1-hour insulin, the odds ratio was 6.0 (95% CI = 1.2–29.8) (94). Further, among 84,360 nurses enrolled in a prospective cohort study, independent of BMI or previous weight change, intake of vegetable fat (but not saturated fat) was associated with development of self-reported diabetes (95).

Sucrose

Although sucrose intake may modify liver function and impair insulin action (96), studies to date have not consistently associated sucrose intake with the development of type 2 diabetes or progression from impaired glucose tolerance to type 2 diabetes (97). In a prospective cohort study of 9494 Israeli men, intake of sucrose was inversely related to subsequent diabetes incidence, but the result was not independent of energy intake and body fatness (30). Findings from a prospective cohort study of 84,360 female nurses showed that sucrose intake obtained from a semiquantitative food-frequency questionnaire was not associated with 6-year risk of diabetes (95). In one clinical trial to test the effect of a high-carbohydrate, low-sucrose diet and drug treatment with phenformin on progression to type 2 diabetes, 204 men with impaired glucose tolerance were randomized to receive combinations of a 120 g/d carbohydrate diet, limited sucrose intake, and 50 mg of phenformin. After 5 years of follow-up, there were no differences in progression to diabetes by treatment group. Fasting and 2-hour blood glucose were significantly associated with development of diabetes (97).

Carbohydrates

Carbohydrates are known to be strong potentiators of beta cell activity and therefore may influence glucose tolerance and diabetes (29). In his classic work, Himsworth observed an inverse association with the energy density from carbohydrates and national diabetes mortality rates (91). In addition, he noticed a decrease in national diabetic mortality rates during periods of food rationing (during the First World War) that resulted in increased relative contribution of carbohydrates to the diet (29,91).

Prospective cohort studies conducted to date do not support the association between intake of carbohydrate and development of diabetes. Dietary intake using the cross-check dietary history method was assessed among 841 men in the Zutphen Study. After 25 years of follow-up, no association was observed between carbohydrate intake or any other dietary component and onset of diabetes (17). Similarly, among 84,360 female nurses, carbohydrate intake was not associated with development of self-reported diabetes (95). Because the intake of different carbohydrate-rich foods results in different glycemic responses, it may be necessary to examine the effects of carbohydrate-rich foods separately. Furthermore, dietary intake may be most associated with progression to insulin resistance rather than beta cell failure and the onset of diabetes (Figure 75-1) (29).

Glycemic Index

Diminished ingestion of dietary fiber and increased usage of dietary carbohydrates (i.e., a high glycemic index) has been associated with increased incidence of diabetes in two recent prospective cohort studies (90). Among 65,173 female nurses participating in the Nurses' Health Study, investigators observed a positive association between the glycemic index and the 6-year risk of developing diabetes (RR = 1.37; 95% CI = 1.09 − 1.71, p for trend = 0.005) comparing women in the highest with women in the lowest glycemic index quintile following adjustment for age, BMI, smoking, physical activity, family history of diabetes, alcohol consumption, cereal fiber intake, and total energy intake (98). Similar findings were observed among 42,759 male health professionals (RR = 1.37; 95% CI = 1.02 − 1.83, p for trend = 0.003) (99). In both studies, the combination of a high glycemic load and a low cereal fiber intake were associated with an increased risk of type 2 diabetes (RRs were 2.50 in women [95% CI = 1.14 − 5.51] and 2.17 in men [95% CI = 1.04 − 4.54]).

Micronutrients

Potassium, Calcium, and Magnesium

Potassium, calcium, and magnesium have been shown to increase insulin secretion and reduce blood glucose concentrations in animal and human models (100–102). In one prospective cohort study among 84,360 female nurses, potassium, calcium, and magnesium were inversely associated with 6-year risk of diabetes. Comparing women in the highest with women in the lowest quintile, relative risks of diabetes for potassium, calcium, and magnesium were 0.62 (p for trend = 0.008), 0.70 (p for trend = 0.005), and 0.68 (p for trend = 0.02), respectively (95).

Chromium

Chromium is an essential nutrient required for normal metabolism of carbohydrates and lipids (103). One randomized trial of 180 adults with type 2 diabetes showed favorable effects of a 1000 µg dose compared with participants taking 200 µg of chromium and a placebo group. Fasting glucose was lower in the 1000 µg group after 2 and 4 months (4-month results for 1000 µg group = 7.1 ± 0.2 mmol/L; placebo group = 8.8 ± 0.3 mmol/L) (104). Although these findings require considerable validation, the beneficial effects of chromium supplementation on type 2 diabetes may deserve further scientific investigation.

Zinc

The trace element zinc plays a fundamental role in the storage, antigenicity, and regulation of insulin and thus is directly involved in the physiologic function of insulin (105). Zinc-insulin crystals are present in the beta cells of the pancreas, and there is evidence supporting the hypothesis that zinc is utilized by these cells in the storage and regulation of insulin secretion (105). The association between zinc intake and type 2 diabetes has yet to be explored in the epidemiologic literature.

Vitamin E

Vitamin E may be associated with diabetes because pancreatic islet cells with low oxidative enzyme activities may be sensitive to free radical injury. As an antioxidant, vitamin E is hypothesized to provide protection from oxidative stress that could result in free radical tissue damage, leading to diabetes (106). Preliminary evidence from one prospective cohort study supports this hypothesis. Salonen et al (106) showed that, among 944 Finnish men aged 42 to 60, low plasma vitamin E (below the median) was associated with a 3.9-fold risk of incident diabetes (95% CI = 1.8 − 8.6) after 4 years of follow-up (RRs were adjusted for age, BMI, and CHD risk factors).

Causality

Compared with the number and quality of studies regarding obesity and physical activity, investigations concerning dietary intake and the development of type 2 diabetes require considerable validation (90). Available data do not support the evidence for a causal association between dietary intake of macronutrients or micronutrients and development of type 2 diabetes.

Summary

Energy intake and sucrose intake, independent of obesity, do not appear to be associated with development of type 2 diabetes. Similarly, independent of dietary fat intake, intake of carbohydrates are not associated with development of type 2 diabetes. Independent of obesity, intake of dietary fat may be associated with development of type 2 diabetes, although the evidence presented to date has been inconsistent. Additional evidence from prospective studies is needed to confirm this hypothesized association. Low-fat diets (National Cholesterol Education Program Step 1 or Step 2 diets) are recommended for individuals with type 2 diabetes or for those individuals who are at high risk for diabetes for purposes of weight reduction. Glycemic index (low dietary fiber and high carbohydrate intake) was associated with development of type 2 diabetes in two prospective cohort studies among male physicians and female nurses, although more studies are needed to confirm this finding. Micronutrients such as potassium, calcium, magnesium, chromium, and zinc, and vitamins such as vitamin E deserve further investigation because they may be possible contributory factors to the development of type 2 diabetes.

ONGOING PRIMARY PREVENTION TRIALS

In June 1996, the National Institutes of Health launched the Diabetes Prevention Program (DPP) for type 2 diabetes at 25 centers across the United States. This 6-year trial was designed to determine if the onset of type 2 diabetes can be prevented or delayed among persons with impaired glucose tolerance using diet and exercise or the medications metformin or troglitazone. Four treatment arms were included in the original study design: 1) usual care control group, 2) metformin treatment group, 3) troglitazone treatment group, and 4) lifestyle intervention group (including nutrition and physical activity counseling) (107). The troglitazone arm was recently terminated due to complications from liver toxicity (personal communication, Sanford Garfield, Project Coordinator, DPP, National Institute of Diabetes and Digestive and Kidney Diseases) (108). The medical community eagerly awaits the findings from this important long-term study (107).

PHYSICAL ACTIVITY AND NUTRITIONAL RECOMMENDATIONS FOR PERSONS WITH TYPE 2 DIABETES

Control of blood glucose is the critical component to prevent complications from diabetes. The Diabetes Complications and Control Trial (DCCT) (109), a national 10-year study that involved 1441 volunteers with type 1 diabetes, demonstrated that control of blood glucose prevented the onset or delayed the progression of eye, kidney, and nerve damage by at least 50% (109).

Treatment for type 2 diabetes typically includes physical activity, diet control, home blood glucose testing, and, in some cases, oral medication and/or insulin. About 40% of people with type 2 diabetes require insulin (3,4).

Physical activity treatment for persons with type 2 diabetes requires the prescription of an appropriate activity program for each individual. Prior to initiating an exercise program, an evaluation should be performed to detect hypertension, neuropathy, and silent cardiac ischemia (107,110). All elderly patients or those with longstanding diabetes should have a stress electrocardiogram before undertaking a strenuous exercise program to prevent angina, elevated blood pressure, arrhythmias, or sudden death.

Because most persons with type 2 diabetes have excess body fat, the primary dietary treatment is to reduce weight by caloric restriction (4,112). Specific primary dietary goals for treatment of persons with type 2 diabetes are to 1) reduce blood glucose levels to normal; 2) achieve optimal serum lipid levels; 3) provide adequate calories to maintain or attain a reasonable weight; and 4) improve overall health through optimal nutrition. The Dietary Guidelines for Americans and the Food Guide Pyramid summarize these nutritional guidelines (112).

SUMMARY

Development of type 2 diabetes is clearly associated with obesity and, to a lesser extent, with physical activity. Data from prospective cohort studies of men and women confirm these findings. From our review, dietary intake has not been independently associated with development of type 2 diabetes.

The prevalence and incidence of type 2 diabetes are increasing in the U.S. population and are especially high among adult minority populations. Type 2 diabetes represents a substantial burden on public health. Improvements to public health will require that the scientific community gain a better understanding of the biochemical and environmental factors that influence the development of and progression to type 2 diabetes and that this knowledge be translated into effective intervention programs.

Acknowledgments: The authors sincerely thank Maria P. Alexander, MPH, for editorial assistance.

REFERENCES

1. Hennekens CH, Buring JE. Epidemiology in medicine. Boston: Little, Brown, 1987.

2. Bennett PH. Epidemiology of diabetes mellitus. In: Rifkin H, Porte D Jr, eds. Diabetes mellitus: theory and practice. 4th ed, New York: Elsevier, 1990:357–377.

3. Centers for Disease Control and Prevention diabetes home page. Centers for Disease Control and Prevention Web site. Available at: http://www.cdc.gov/nccdphp/ddt/

dbspot.htm#article1. Accessed April 29, 1998.

4. American Diabetes Association. Report of the expert committee on the diagnosis and classification of diabetes mellitus. Diabetes Care 1997;20: 1183–1197.

5. American Diabetes Association. Economic consequences of diabetes mellitus in the U.S. in 1997. Diabetes Care 1998;21: 296–307.

6. Bennett PH. Primary prevention of NIDDM: a practical reality. Diabetes Metab Rev 1997;13: 105–111.

7. Saad MF, Knowler WC, Pettitt DJ, et al. A two-step model for development of non-insulin-dependent diabetes. Am J Med 1991;90: 229–235.

8. Gudat U, Berger M, Lefebvre PJ. Physical activity, fitness, and non-insulin-dependent (type II) diabetes mellitus. In: Bouchard C, Shephard RJ, Stephens T, eds. Proceedings of the Second International Conference on Physical Activity, Fitness, and Health; 1992 May 5–9; Toronto, Ontario, Champaign, IL: Human Kinetics, 1994.

9. World Health Organization. Diabetes mellitus: report of a WHO Study Group. Geneva: World Heath Organization, 1985. Tech. Rep. Series, No. 727.

10. Harris MI, Flegal KM, Cowie CC, et al. Prevalence of diabetes, impaired fasting glucose, and impaired glucose tolerance in U.S. adults: the Third National Health and Nutrition Examination Survey, 1988–94. Diabetes Care 1998;21:518–524.

11. Centers for Disease Control and Prevention. Diabetes surveillance, 1997. Atlanta: U.S. Department of Health and Human Services, 1997.

12. Centers for Disease Control and Prevention. Trends in the prevalence and incidence of self-reported diabetes mellitus—United States, 1980–1994. MMWR 1997;46: 1013–1018.

13. Harris MI. Epidemiological studies on the pathogenesis of non-insulin-dependent diabetes mellitus (NIDDM). Clin Invest Med 1995;18:231–239.

14. World Health Organization. World Health Organization Web site. Available at: URL: http://www.who.ch/ncd/dia/tables1.htm#t1. Accessed April 29, 1998.

15. Kriska AM, Blair SN, Pereira MA. The potential role of physical activity in the prevention of non-insulin-dependent diabetes mellitus: the epidemiological evidence. Exerc Sport Sci Rev 1994;22:121–143.

16. Manson JE, Spelsberg A. Primary prevention of non-insulin-dependent diabetes mellitus. Am J Prev Med 1994;10:172–184.

17. Feskens EJM, Kromhout D. Cardiovascular risk factors and the 25-year incidence of diabetes mellitus in middle-aged men. Am J Epidemiol 1989;130:1101–1108.

18. Keys A. Overweight, obesity, coronary heart disease and mortality. Nutr Rev 1980;38:297–307.

19. Barrett-Connor E. Epidemiology, obesity, and non-insulin-dependent diabetes mellitus. Epidemiol Rev 1989;11:172–181.

20. Maggio CA, Pi-Sunyer FX. The prevention and treatment of obesity: application to type 2 diabetes. Diabetes Care 1997;20: 1744–1766.

21. DeFronzo RA, Ferrannini E. Insulin resistance: a multifaceted syndrome responsible for NIDDM, obesity, hypertension, dyslipidemia, and atherosclerotic cardiovascular disease. Diabetes Care 1991;14:173–194.

22. DeFronzo RA, Bonadonna RC, Ferrannini E. Pathogenesis of NIDDM: a balanced overview. Diabetes Care 1992;15:318–368.

23. Zhang Y, Proenca R, Maffei M, et al. Positional cloning of the mouse obese gene and its human homologue. Nature 1994;372: 425–432.

24. Chua SC, Chung WK, Wu-Peng S, et al. Phenotypes of mouse *diabetes* and rat *fatty* due to mutations in the OB (leptin) receptor. Science 1996;271: 994–996.

25. Fan W, Boston BA, Kesterson RA, et al. Role of melanocortinergic neurons in feeding and the *agouti* obesity syndrome. Nature 1997; 385:165–168.

26. O'Rahilly S. Non-insulin dependent diabetes mellitus: the gathering storm. BMJ 1997;314: 955–959.

27. Ravussin E, Swinburn BA. Pathophysiology of obesity. Lancet 1992;340:404–408.

28. Blair SN, Horton E, Leon AS, et al. Physical activity, nutrition, and chronic disease. Med Sci Sports Exerc 1996;28:335–349.

29. Feskens EJM. Nutritional factors and the etiology of non-insulin-dependent diabetes mellitus: an epidemiological overview. World Rev Nutr Diet 1992;69:1–39.

30. Medalie JH, Papier C, Herman JB, et al. Diabetes mellitus among 10,000 adult men. Israel J Med Sci 1974;10:681–697.

31. Colditz GA, Willett WC, Stampfer MJ, et al. Weight as a risk factor for clinical diabetes in women. Am J Epidemiol 1990;132:501–513.

32. Ohlson LO, Larsson B, Bjorntorp P, et al. Risk factors for type 2 (non-insulin-dependent) diabetes mellitus: thirteen and one-half years of follow-up of the participants in a study of Swedish men born in 1913. Diabetologia 1988;31:798–805.

33. Edelstein SL, Knowler WC, Bain RP, et al. Predictors of progression from impaired glucose tolerance to NIDDM: an analysis of six prospective studies. Diabetes 1997;46:701–710.

34. Despres JP. Abdominal obesity as important component of insulin-resistance syndrome. Nutrition 1993;9:452–459.

35. Abate N. Insulin resistance and obesity: the role of fat distribu-

tion pattern. Diabetes Care 1996;19:292–294.

36. Vague J. The degree of masculine differentiation of obesities: a factor determining predisposition to diabetes, atherosclerosis, gout, and uric calculous disease. Am J Clin Nutr 1956;4:20–34.

37. Haffner SM, Stern MP, Hazuda HP, et al. Role of obesity and fat distribution in non-insulin-dependent diabetes mellitus in Mexican Americans and non-Hispanic whites. Diabetes Care 1986;13:1099–1105.

38. Lundgren H, Bengtsson C, Blohme G, et al. Adiposity and adipose tissue distribution in relation to incidence of diabetes in women: results from a prospective population study in Gothenburg, Sweden. Int J Obes 1989;13:413–423.

39. Carey VJ, Walters EE, Colditz GA, et al. Body fat distribution and risk of non-insulin-dependent diabetes mellitus in women; the Nurses' Health Study. Am J Epidemiol 1997;145:614–619.

40. Chan JM, Rimm EB, Colditz GA, et al. Obesity, fat distribution, and weight gain as risk factors for clinical diabetes in men. Diabetes Care 1994;17:961–969.

41. Felber JP, Acheson KJ, Tappy L, eds. From obesity to diabetes. Chichester, England: John Wiley, 1993.

42. Ford ES, Williamson DF, Liu S. Weight change and diabetes incidence: findings from a national cohort of US adults. Am J Epidemiol 1997;146:214–222.

43. Hanson RL, Narayan KM, McCance DR, et al. Rate of weight gain, weight fluctuation, and incidence of NIDDM. Diabetes 1995;44:261–266.

44. Henry RR, Wiest-Kent TA, Scheaffer L, et al. Metabolic consequences of very-low-calorie diet therapy in obese non-insulin-dependent diabetic and nondiabetic subjects. Diabetes 1986;35:155–164.

45. National Institutes of Health, National Heart, Lung, and Blood Institute. Clinical guidelines on the identification, evaluation, and treatment of overweight and obesity in adults: the evidence report. Washington, DC: National Institutes of Health, 1998.

46. Albu J, Konnarides C, Pi-Sunyer FX. Weight control: metabolic and cardiovascular effects. Diabetes Rev 1995;3:335–347.

47. American Diabetes Association. Nutrition recommendations and principles for people with diabetes mellitus. Diabetes Care 1996;19(suppl 1):S16–S19.

48. Perri MG, Sears SF, Clark JE. Strategies for improving maintenance of weight loss: toward a continuous care model of obesity management. Diabetes Care 1993;16:200–209.

49. King AC, Tribble DL. The role of exercise in weight regulation in nonathletes. Sports Med 1991;11:331–349.

50. Gormally J, Rardin D, Black S. Correlates of successful response to a behavioral weight control clinic. J Counsel Psychol 1980;27:179–191.

51. Kayman S, Bruvold W, Stern JS. Maintenance and relapse after weight loss in women: behavioral aspects. Am J Clin Nutr 1990;52:800–807.

52. Caspersen CJ, Powell KE, Christenson GM. Physical activity, exercise, and physical fitness: definitions and distinctions for health-related research. Public Health Rep 1985;100:126–131.

53. Ainsworth BE, Montoye HJ, Leon AS. Methods of assessing physical activity during leisure and work. In: Bouchard C, Shephard RJ, Stephens T, eds. Proceedings of the Second International Conference on Physical Activity, Fitness, and Health; 1992 May 5–9; Toronto, Ontario. Champaign, IL: Human Kinetics, 1994.

54. Kriska AM, Caspersen CJ, eds. A collection of physical activity questionnaires for health-related research. Med Sci Sports Exerc 1997;29(suppl):S1–S205.

55. Harris MI, Hadden WC, Knowler WC, et al. Prevalence of diabetes and impaired glucose levels in U.S. population aged 20–74 yr. Diabetes 1987;36:523–534.

56. U.S. Department of Health and Human Services. Physical activity and health: a report of the Surgeon General. Atlanta: U.S. Department of Health and Human Services, Centers for Disease Control and Prevention and Health Promotion, 1996.

57. Holloszy JO, Schultz J, Kusnierkiewicz J, et al. Effects of exercise on glucose tolerance and insulin resistance: brief review and some preliminary results. Acta Med Scan Suppl 1986;711:55–65.

58. Kriska AM, Bennett PH. An epidemiological perspective of the relationship between physical activity and NIDDM: from activity assessment to intervention. Diabetes Metab Rev 1992;8:355–372.

59. Kawate R, Yamakido M, Nishimoto Y, et al. Diabetes mellitus and its vascular complications in Japanese migrants on the island of Hawaii. Diabetes Care 1979;2:161–170.

60. O'Dea K. Westernization and non-insulin-dependent diabetes in Australian Aborigines. Ethn Dis 1991;1:171–187.

61. James SA, Jamjoum L, Raghunathan TE, et al. Physical activity and NIDDM in African Americans. Diabetes Care 1998;21:555–562.

62. King H, Taylor R, Zimmet P, et al. Non-insulin-dependent diabetes (NIDDM) in a newly independent Pacific nation: the Republic of Kiribati. Diabetes Care 1984;7:409–415.

63. Dowse GK, Zimmet PZ, Gareeboo H, et al. Abdominal obesity and physical inactivity as risk factors for NIDDM and impaired glucose tolerance in Indian, Creole, and Chinese Mauritians. Diabetes Care 1991;14:271–282.

64. Kriska AM, Gregg EW, Utter AC, et al. Association of physical activity and plasma insulin levels

in a population at high risk for NIDDM. Med Sci Sports Exerc 1993;26(suppl):S121.

65. Montoye HJ, Block WD, Metzner H, et al. Habitual physical activity and glucose tolerance: males age 16–64 in a total community. Diabetes 1977;26:172–176.

66. Taylor RJ, Bennett PH, LeGonidec G, et al. The prevalence of diabetes mellitus in a traditional-living Polynesian population: the Wallis Island Survey. Diabetes Care 1983;6:334–340.

67. Fisch A, Pichard E, Prazuck T, et al. Prevalence and risk factors of diabetes mellitus in the rural region of Mali (West Africa): a practical approach. Diabetologia 1987;30:859–862.

68. Jarrett RJ, Shipley MJ, Hunt R. Physical activity, glucose tolerance, and diabetes mellitus: the Whitehall Study. Diabetic Med 1986;3:549–551.

69. Levitt NS, Katzenellenbogen JM, Bradshaw D, et al. The prevalence and identification of risk factors for NIDDM in urban Africans in Cape Town, South Africa. Diabetes Care 1993;16:601–607.

70. Harris MI. Epidemiological correlates of NIDDM in Hispanics, whites, and blacks in the U.S. population. Diabetes Care 1991;14(suppl):639–648.

71. Kriska AM, LaPorte RE, Pettit DJ, et al. The association of physical activity, with obesity, fat distribution and glucose intolerance in Pima Indians. Diabetologia 1993;36:863–869.

72. Feskens EJM, Loeber JG, Kromhout D. Diet and physical activity as determinants of hyperinsulinemia: the Zutphen Elderly Study. Am J Epidemiol 1994;140:350–360.

73. Mayer-Davis EJ, D'Agostino R Jr, Karter AJ, et al. Intensity and amount of physical activity in relation to insulin sensitivity: the Insulin Resistance Atherosclerosis Study. JAMA 1998;279:669–674.

74. Frisch RE, Wyshak G, Albright TE, et al. Lower prevalence of diabetes in female former college athletes compared with nonathletes. Diabetes 1986;35:1101–1105.

75. Jarrett RJ. Epidemiology and public health aspects of non-insulin-dependent diabetes mellitus. Epidemil Rev 1989;11:151–171.

76. Manson JE, Rimm EB, Stampfer MJ, et al. Physical activity and incidence of non-insulin-dependent diabetes mellitus in women. Lancet 1991;338:774–777.

77. Manson JE, Nathan DM, Krolewski AS, et al. A prospective study of exercise and incidence of diabetes among US male physicians. JAMA 1992;268:63–67.

78. Helmrich SP, Ragland DR, Leung R, et al. Physical activity and reduced occurrence of NIDDM. N Engl J Med 1991;325:147–152.

79. Burchfiel CM, Sharp DS, Curb JD, et al. Physical activity and incidence of diabetes: the Honolulu Heart Program. Am J Epidemiol 1995;141:360–368.

80. Lipton RB, Liao Y, Cao G, et al. Determinants of incident non-insulin-dependent diabetes mellitus among blacks and whites in a national study: the NHANES I epidemiologic follow-up study. Am J Epidemiol 1993;138:826–839.

81. Perry IJ, Wannamethee SG, Walker MK, et al. Prospective study of risk factors for development of non-insulin dependent diabetes in middle-aged British men. BMJ 1995;310:560–564.

82. Schranz A, Tuomilehto J, Marti B, et al. Low physical activity and worsening of glucose tolerance: results from a 2-year follow-up of a population sample in Malta. Diabetes Res Clin Pract 1991;11:127–136.

83. Monterrosa AE, Haffner SM, Stern MP, et al. Sex differences in lifestyle factors predictive of diabetes in Mexican-Americans. Diabetes Care 1995;18:448–456.

84. Lynch J, Helmrich SP, Lakka TA, et al. Moderately intense physical activities and high levels of cardiorespiratory fitness reduce the risk of non-insulin-dependent diabetes mellitus in middle-aged men. Arch Inter Med 1996;156:1307–1314.

85. Eriksson KF, Lindgarde F. Prevention of type 2 (non-insulin-dependent) diabetes mellitus by diet and physical exercise. Diabetologia 1991;34:891–898.

86. Pan XR, Li GW, Hu YH, et al. Effects of diet and exercise in preventing NIDDM in people with impaired glucose tolerance. Diabetes Care 1997;20:537–544.

87. Willett WC. Nutritional epidemiology. New York: Oxford University Press, 1990.

88. Margetts BM, Nelson M. Design concepts in nutritional epidemiology. New York: Oxford University Press, 1991.

89. Thompson FE, Byers T. Dietary assessment resource manual. J Nutr 1994;124(suppl):245S–317S.

90. Vinicor F. Primary prevention of type II diabetes mellitus 1998 (in press).

91. Himsworth HP. Diet and the incidence of diabetes mellitus. Clin Sci Mol Med 1935;2:117–148.

92. Clandinin MT, Cheema S, Field CJ, et al. Dietary lipids influence insulin action. Ann N Y Acad Sci 1993;683:151–163.

93. Marshall JA, Hamman RF, Baxter J. High-fat, low-carbohydrate diet and the etiology of non-insulin-dependent diabetes mellitus: the San Luis Valley Diabetes Study. Am J Epidemiol 1991;134:590–603.

94. Marshall JA, Hoag S, Shetterly S, et al. Dietary fat predicts conversion from impaired glucose tolerance to NIDDM: the San Luis Valley Diabetes Study. Diabetes Care 1994;17:50–56.

95. Colditz GA, Manson JE, Stampfer MJ, et al. Diet and risk of clinical diabetes in women. Am J Clin Nutr 1992;55:1018–1023.

96. Storlien LH, Kraegen EW, Jenkins AB, et al. Effects of sucrose vs starch diets on in vivo insulin action, thermogenesis, and obesity in rats. Am J Clin Nutr 1988;47:420–427.

97. Jarrett RJ, Keen H, Fuller JH, et al. Worsening to diabetes in men with impaired glucose tolerance ("borderline diabetes"). Diabetologia 1979;16:25–30.

98. Salmeron J, Manson JE, Stampfer MJ, et al. Dietary fiber, glycemic load, and risk of non-insulin-dependent diabetes mellitus in women. JAMA 1997;277:472–477.

99. Salmeron J, Ascherio A, Rimm EB, et al. Dietary fiber, glycemic load, and risk of NIDDM in men. Diabetes Care 1997;20:545–550.

100. Sjogren A, Floren CH, Nilsson A. Oral administration of magnesium hydroxide to subjects with insulin-dependent diabetes mellitus: effects on magnesium and potassium levels and on insulin requirements. Magnesium 1988;7:117–122.

101. Durlach J, Collery P. Magnesium and potassium in diabetes and carbohydrate metabolism: review of the present status and recent results. Magnesium 1984;3:315–323.

102. Karolyi G. Serum calcium and magnesium in diabetes control. Eur J Pediatr 1987;146:621–622.

103. Critchfield TS, Burris A. Chromium supplements: what's the story? Diabetes Forecast 1996;49:24–26.

104. Anderson R, Cheng N, Bryden N, et al. Beneficial effects of chromium for people with Type II diabetes. Diabetes 1996;45(suppl):S124A.

105. Wahid MA, Fathi SAH, Aboul-Khair MR. Zinc in human health and disease. La Ricerca Clin Lab 1988;18:9–16.

106. Salonen JT, Nyyssonen K, Tuomainen TP, et al. Increased risk of non-insulin dependent diabetes mellitus at low plasma vitamin E concentrations: a four year follow-up study in men. BMJ 1995;311:1124–1127.

107. Feuerstein BL, Weinstock RS. Diet and exercise in type 2 diabetes mellitus. Nutrition 1997;13:95–99.

108. Gitlin N, Julie NL, Spurr CL, et al. Two cases of severe clinical and histologic hepatotoxicity associated with troglitazone. Ann Int Med 1998;129:36–38.

109. Anonymous. The effect of intensive treatment of diabetes on the development and progression of long-term complications in insulin-dependent diabetes mellitus: the Diabetes Control and Complications Trial Research Group. N Engl J Med 1993;329:977–986.

110. Zierath JR, Wallberg-Henriksson H. Exercise training in obese diabetic patients. Sports Med 1992;14:171–189.

111. National Institutes of Health. Diet and exercise in non-insulin-dependent diabetes mellitus. NIH Consensus Statement Online 1986 Dec 8–10;6:1–21. Available at: http://text.nlm.nih.gov/nih/cdc/www/60txt.htm. Accessed April 29, 1998.

112. American Diabetes Association. Nutrition recommendations and principles for people with diabetes mellitus. Diabetes Care 1994;17:519–522.

Chapter 76

The Association of Physical Activity, Diet, and Cancer

Christine M. Friedenreich

Over the past fifteen years, mounting evidence has indicated that physical activity and dietary intake may influence the risk of developing certain types of cancer. The most prevalent malignancies in the developed world (other than lung cancer, which is mainly attributable to smoking) are cancers of the colon, rectum, breast, and prostate. These cancers appear to be associated with low levels of physical activity and high-fat or high-calorie diets (1). Physical activity and dietary intake influence many metabolic processes and levels of various endogenous hormones, some of which may be related to specific cancers; hence, it is biologically plausible that these lifestyle factors influence the risk of developing cancer. The etiology of cancer is complex and there is still little understanding of the underlying biologic and pathogenic mechanisms that are operative in cancer causation. The best evidence that currently exists for the role of physical activity and diet in relation to cancer risk comes from epidemiologic studies that have directly examined these associations.

The purpose of this chapter is to review systematically the epidemiologic literature on the association between physical activity, dietary intake, and cancers of the breast, colon, and prostate. This review has two main components. First, the evidence accumulated to date on these associations is presented. Second, the methodologic limitations of previous research are described. Directions for future research are provided throughout. Only those epidemiologic studies that have measured both physical activity and dietary intake in relation to cancer outcomes are included in this review. For the purposes of this review, physical activity is considered the main lifestyle risk factor, while the influence of dietary intake is restricted to its role as a potential confounder or effect modifier of the association between physical activity and cancer.

METHODS

A computerized literature search of MEDLINE was undertaken and supplemented with manual searches of the recent literature for all studies that examined the association between physical activity and cancer. From this set of studies, all those that had measured dietary intake in addition to physical activity were selected. For inclusion in this review, a study had to have measured total caloric intake, since the focus of this chapter is on energy intake and expenditure as measured, respectively, by total caloric intake and by physical activities. Studies that measured only alcohol intake or some components of dietary intake, such as micronutrients, were excluded.

Each study's methods and results were tabulated to include the study design, data collection methods for physical activity and diet assessment, the main results, and comments on the type of adjustment for confounding and assessment of effect modification that was done in the analysis. The strengths and weaknesses of each study were examined and are reported. No quantitative synthesis of this literature was attempted because of the differences among the samples, designs, measurement of physical activity and dietary intake, and analytic methods of the studies. Based on this review, the gaps in knowledge of the association between diet and physical activity and these cancers were delineated. These gaps are used to suggest directions for future research in this area.

REVIEW OF THE EPIDEMIOLOGIC EVIDENCE

The majority of epidemiologic research on the relation of physical activity and dietary intake to cancer outcomes has focused on colon cancer. The first evidence that lifestyle factors might be implicated in the etiology of this cancer was found by Tannenbaum in 1945, who observed that high caloric intake potentiated the incidence of tumors induced by a carcinogen (2). A large body of epidemiologic evidence has since accumulated that permits public health recommendations to be made regarding the changes in dietary intake and levels of physical activity needed for a reduction in the risk of colon cancer. A smaller but steadily growing literature on physical activity and breast cancer is emerging. The evidence for an association between physical activity and breast cancer is strongly suggestive but in need of further delineation. Much more research attention has focused on dietary intake and its role in the etiology of breast cancer. However, few strong associations have been found other than an increased risk with moderate to high alcohol intake (3). Very few studies have examined both of these risk factors simultaneously in relation to breast cancer. For prostate cancer, a growing number of investigations have been conducted on either dietary intake or physical activity, but very few have considered both factors. The evidence for an association for either of these lifestyle factors is somewhat suggestive but still poorly delineated. This section reviews each of these major cancer sites and the epidemiologic evidence that has accumulated for the role of physical activity and dietary intake in the etiology of these cancers.

Colon Cancer

A total of 40 studies have been published that have examined the association between physical activity and colon cancer (4). Of these 40 studies, 13 have assessed physical activity and total caloric intake (5–17). The study designs, population samples, and data collection methods used for the assessment of physical activity and dietary intake have varied considerably across these investigations (Table 76-1).

Three studies reviewed here examined colorectal cancer (7–9), seven included only colon cancer (5,6,12,13,15,16), and the remaining three studies investigated the effect of physical activity separately for colon and rectal cancers (9,11,14). Since an association with physical activity has been observed mainly for colon cancer and not for rectal cancers, the possibility of observing any association was decreased in those studies that combined the two sites. All of the studies reviewed here used population-based designs (either case-control or prospective cohorts), histologically confirmed incident cases, and population controls. The study by Benito et al (9) from Spain also included hospital controls as a separate comparison group.

Physical activity was assessed by occupational activity alone in two studies (6,9), by recreational activity alone in two studies (13,15), by occupational and recreational activity in seven studies (5,6,10–12,14), and by occupational, recreational, and household activity in three studies (8,16,17). The assessment was for current activity in seven studies (5,6,9,11–13,15), lifetime occupational activity in two studies (6,14), and for some time periods during the life of the study participants (e.g., 10, 20 years before the interview) in three studies (8,16,17). Only one study (10) assessed activity for different ages. The frequency, intensity, and duration of activity was recorded in seven studies (5,8,11,14–17). The other studies used a simple assessment of activity that included only

one or two of the parameters of activity. Six of these studies (5,6,8,9,11,17) used interview-administered food frequency questionnaires and six others had self-administered instruments (10,11,13–16). The remaining study by Albanes et al (7) used a 24-hour recall method for assessing dietary intake in the NHANES cohort.

Despite the heterogeneity of the methods used in these studies, they provide strong and consistent evidence for a decrease in risk of colon cancer with increased levels of physical activity. Specifically, a decrease in colon cancer is observed in individuals who are physically active as measured in their occupations (6,9), their recreational activities (15), their occupational and recreational activities (5,10–12,14), or all activities (16,17). Three studies found no relation between activity and colon cancer (13) or colorectal cancer risk (7,8). The magnitude of the risk reduction is up to 50% for those individuals who are categorized as the most physically active compared to those who are inactive. This risk reduction was statistically significant in 6 studies (5,10,11,14,15,17). A consistent dose-response relation has been found in 8 of these 13 studies (5,6,9,10,11,15–17), indicating that the risk reduction becomes greater with increasing levels of physical activity. No threshold effect was seen in these studies between physical activity levels and risk of colon cancer.

The confounding effects of dietary intake as well as body mass index (BMI), alcohol intake, and other colon cancer risk factors have been assessed, to some extent, in all of the studies reviewed here. The exception is the study by Benito et al (9), which did measure dietary intake but in which only adjustment for age was made and no assessment of confounding or any other risk factors was undertaken. Examining confounding by these lifestyle and personal factors is important to ensure that the association between physical activity and colon cancer is independent of other factors. From these studies, it appears that there is little confounding by total caloric intake or other components of diet including dietary fat and fiber intake. No confounding by BMI, alcohol intake, or other more minor risk factors was found. The one exception is the study by Whittemore et al (11) in which a stronger association was observed for physical activity after controlling for dietary intake in the North American study population. Such an increase in the strength of the association was not observed for the Chinese study subjects.

Effect modification of the association between physical activity and colon cancer by dietary intake was examined in four studies (5,10,11,17). Physical activity and dietary intake appear to modify jointly their respective effects on colon cancer. Slattery et al (5) found caloric intake increased as the level of activity increased in cases and controls. They also found a trend toward decreased colon cancer risk from high levels of dietary intake when high levels of physical activity are present. Gerhardsson et al (10) found a positive interaction between physical activity and intake of total energy, protein, total fat, and browned meat surface, and a negative interaction with dietary fiber. The results for fiber are noteworthy as they suggest that a high fiber intake may only be protective in individuals who are physically active and may even increase the risk in subjects who are sedentary. Whittemore et al (11) observed a positive interaction between saturated fat intake and physical activity. For both men and women in that study, risk among the sedentary Chinese American population

Table 76-1 Summary of Epidemiologic Studies of Physical Activity, Dietary Intake, and Colon Cancer

Reference, Country	Study Design	Study Sample	No. of Cases/ Controls	Physical Activity Measurement/ Definition	Dietary Assessment Method	Results	Comments
Slattery et al (5), USA	Population-based case-control study	Utah Cancer Registry, RDD controls	M: 110/180 C F: 119/204 C	Interview-administered questionnaire. Detailed questions on occupational and recreational activity for 2 years prior to diagnosis.	Interview-administered FFQ	RR (90% CI) for high vs. low total activity: M: 0.7 (0.4–1.3), F: 0.5 (0.3–0.9) Dose-response relation. Statistically significant results for intense activity.	Protective effect. Adjusted for age, BMI, fiber, total caloric intake. No confounding of association by dietary intake. Effect modification by gender (greater decrease in risk for females). Joint effects of physical activity and diet on colon cancer risk.
Peters et al (6), USA	Population-based case-control study	LA County Cancer Surveillance Program and neighborhood controls	147 case-control pairs	Interview-administered questionnaire. Lifetime occupational titles used to classify subjects into sedentary, moderate and high-activity groups.	Interview-administered FFQ	RR for all cases for very active at job vs. sedentary: 1.1 (0.5–2.3) Right side: 1.0 (0.3–3.2) Transverse/descending: 0.8 (0.2–2.7) Sigmoid: 1.6 (0.5–5.1) Rectum: 0.7 (0.2–2.5) Dose-response for transverse/descending colon cancers only.	No effect. No confounding by diet, occupational exposures, BMI. Adjusted for education only.
Albanes et al (7), USA	Prospective cohort	NHANES 1 follow-up, 5138 men, 7407 women	128 CR	Self-administered questionnaire. Two questions on current recreational (R) and non-recreational (O) activity.	24-hour recall	RR for active vs. inactive non-recreational activity: M: 0.6 (0.3–1.4), F: 1.4 (0.5–3.3) Much vs. little exercise: M: 1.0 (0.5–1.9), F: 0.8 (0.4–1.7)	Protective effect for males, occupational activity only. Results for colon and rectum combined. Adjusted for age only as no confounding found for dietary fat, total caloric intake, BMI, in addition to other non-dietary factors.
Kune et al (8), Australia	Population-based case-control study	All incident cases from Melbourne and population register for controls	M: 388/398 CR F: 327/329 CR	Interview-administered questionnaire. Previous 20 years of occupational and recreational activity combined	Interview-administered diet history	RR for most active vs. totally inactive: M: 1.5 (0.8–2.7), F: 0.9 (0.3–2.8)	No effect. Adjusted for age, BMI and diet.
Benito et al (9), Spain	Population- and hospital-based case-control study	Cases identified through pathology labs in Majorca, population controls from census, hospital controls from two hospitals	M: 151/158 population and 103 hospital CR F: 135/137 population and 100 hospital CR	Interview-administered questionnaire. Current occupational activity rated into four categories from sedentary to exhausting.	Interview-administered FFQ	RR for exhausting work vs. sedentary work (M and F combined, no CI given): Pop'n: 0.7, Hospital: 0.5 Dose-response for hospital controls only.	Protective effect. Results for colon and rectum combined. Adjusted for age. No adjustment for diet or any other confounders.

Reference, location	Study design	Population	Cases/controls	Activity assessment	Diet assessment	Relative risk (RR)	Comments
Gerhardsson et al (10), Sweden	Population-based case-referent study	All incident cases from Stockholm County and population controls from register	M: 163 C, 107 R F: 189 C, 110 R 512 controls	Self-administered questionnaire. Lifetime occupational and recreational activities rated as sedentary, fairly active and very active for every five years from 1950 to 1985.	Self-administered FFQ	RR for very active vs. sedentary: Right colon: M: 1.3 (0.3–5.0), F: 0.7 (0.2–2.5) Left colon: M: 0.3 (0.1–1), F: 0.2 (0.1–0.8) Rectum: M: 1.1 (0.4–3.3), F: 0.7 (0.2–2.0) Dose-response relation.	Protective effect. Adjusted for age, gender, BMI, energy, protein, fat, fiber, browned meat. All not confounders. Interaction with fiber intake found.
Whittemore et al (11), USA, Canada, and China	Multicenter population-based case-control study	Cancer registries in British Columbia, Los Angeles, San Francisco-Oakland, 17 hospitals in China	M: 274/1376 C,R F: 192/1112 C,R	Interview-administered questionnaire. Current occupational activity, time spent sleeping, sitting, in light, moderate, vigorous activity, and distance walked or cycled.	Interview-administered diet history	RR for active vs. sedentary occupations: North America: M: 0.4 (0.2–0.9), F: 0.8 (0.3–2.3) China: M: 0.7 (0.3–1.7), F: 0.6 (0.2–1.8) Recreational activities: North America: M: 0.6 (0.4–0.9), F: 0.5 (0.3–0.8) China: M: 1.2 (0.5–2.6), F: 0.4 (0.2–1.0) Dose-response relation.	Protective effect. Rectal cancer not related to occupational activity. Increased risk for saturated fat. Stronger association between saturated fat and colorectal cancer in sedentary than in active (effect modification).
Thun et al (12), USA	Nested case-control within a prospective cohort	Cancer Prevention Study II (764,343 adults). Used 5746 controls sampled from population	M: 611/3051 C F: 539/2695 C	Self-administered questionnaire. Current recreational and occupational activity (none, slight, moderate, heavy).	Short self-administered FFQ	RR for heavy exercise vs. none: M: 0.6 (0.3–1.3), F: 0.9 (0.4–2.0)	Protective effect. Adjusted for vegetables, fruits, grains, total fat, BMI, family history of colon cancer, aspirin use.
Bostick et al (13), USA	Prospective cohort	Iowa Women's Health Study, 35,215 women	212 C	Self-administered questionnaire. Two questions on current moderate and vigorous recreational activity.	Self-administered FFQ	RR for vigorous vs. low activity: 0.95 (0.7–1.4)	No effect. Adjusted for age, total caloric intake, height, parity, vitamin E intake, combined effect of vitamin E and age, vitamin A.
Longnecker et al (14), USA	Population-based case-control study	Cases from hospitals and registries in five US states, controls from population lists	163 C 242 R 703 community controls	Telephone-administered questionnaire. Three measures of occupation: 5 years ago, 20 years ago and most representative of	Self-administered FFQ	RR for occupational activity "more than light" vs. light work, right colon: 0.7 (0.3–1.5) RR for 2+ hours/week recreational activity vs. none: 0.6 (0.3–0.97)	Protective effect. Adjusted for energy intake, fat, fiber, calcium, alcohol intake, BMI, family history of colorectal cancer, smoking, race, income, respondent status. All not confounders.

Table 76–1 continues

Table 76-1 (Continued)

Reference, Country	Study Design	Study Sample	No. of Cases/ Controls	Physical Activity Measurement/ Definition	Dietary Assessment Method	Results	Comments
				lifetime occupation and time spent in six current recreational activities.		RR for highest categories of occupational and recreational activity vs. lowest: 0.4 (0.2–1.1)	
Giovannucci et al (15), USA	Prospective cohort study	Health Professionals Follow-up Study: 47,723 men	203 C	Self-administered questionnaire. Average time/week over past year in walking, moderate and vigorous activity, stairs climbed.	Self-administered FFQ	RR for highest vs. lowest quintile of total MET-hours of activity 0.5 (0.3–0.9)	Protective effect. Adjusted for age, dietary components (methione, folate, fiber, red meat, energy), alcohol, BMI, family history of colon cancer, history of screening for colon cancer or polyp diagnosis, smoking, aspirin use.
White et al (16), USA	Population-based case-control study	Seattle-Puget Sound Surveillance, Epidemiology, and End Results registry, RDD controls	M: 251/233 C F: 193/194 C	Telephone-administered questionnaire. Lifetime occupational activity. Recreational and household activity over 10 years prior to the 2 years before diagnosis	Self-administered FFQ	RR for highest vs. lowest quartiles recreational activity (METS/wk): M: 0.7 (0.4–1.1), F: 0.7 (0.4–1.3) Occupational activity (METS/wk): M: 0.9 (0.5–1.5), F: 1.0 (0.6–1.7) Household activity (hr/wk): M: 0.9 (0.5–1.6), F: 0.8 (0.4–1.4) Dose-response relation.	Protective effect. Adjusted for age, not confounded by BMI, diet or other health behaviors. Trend in risk significant.
Slattery et al (17), USA	Population-based case-control study	Kaiser Permanente Program in California, eight counties in Utah, Twin Cities in Minnesota; population controls identified with RDD and population lists	M: 1099/1290 C F: 889/1120 C	Interview-administered questionnaire. Occupational, recreational and household activity for the referent year and 10 and 20 years ago	Interview-administered diet history	RR for high vs. no physical activity: M: 0.6 (0.5–0.8), F: 0.6 (0.5–0.8) Dose-response relation.	Protective effect. Adjusted for age, energy intake, fiber, calcium, BMI, family history of cancer, aspirin. Effect modification by BMI and energy intake.

C = colon cancer; R = rectal cancer; CR = colorectal cancer; RR = relative risk (95% CI unless otherwise indicated); NHANES = U.S. National Health and Nutrition Examination Survey; NHEFS = NHANES I Epidemiologic Follow-up Study; RDD = random digit dialing; FFQ = food frequency questionnaire; BMI = body mass index.

increased more than fourfold from the lowest to the highest category of saturated fat intake. For active study participants, the risk of colon cancer increased with fat intake for men but not for women. In contrast to these three studies, in the most recent study by Slattery et al (17), participants with higher activity levels were at lower risk irrespective of their energy intake and this pattern was more marked in men than women. These findings suggest that among those who are physically active, energy intake presents no risk and is, in fact, protective for women (17).

Some effect modification by gender is seen for the association between physical activity and colon cancer. The study by Slattery et al (5) found a 52% decrease in risk of colon cancer in women but only a 30% decrease in men. Likewise, in the study by Gerhardsson et al (10), a 60% risk reduction was found for women and only a 40% reduction for men. The larger risk reduction for women was not, however, consistently found in these studies. Thun et al (12) noted a larger risk reduction in men than in women for recreational activity as did Albanes et al (7) for nonrecreational activity. These two latter studies had very crude physical activity assessments and, therefore, their results need to be interpreted more cautiously since some misclassification was likely.

Effect modification by anatomic site of the colon cancer is also possible. Three of these studies (6,10,17) examined the association by tumour site and, in two of these studies, a greater risk reduction was found for cancers of the transverse/descending or left colon (6,10). Slattery et al (17) found no differences in risk according to anatomic site of the tumour.

The modifying effect of age was examined in the study by Slattery et al (17) and no difference in effect was observed across different age groups. Two studies (10,17) that examined effect modification by BMI found a positive interaction between physical activity and BMI. Gerhardsson et al (10) noted that the excess relative risk of both high BMI and low physical activity was 3.6 and that 24% of left colon cancer among these study subjects was attributable to the interaction of physical activity and BMI. Slattery et al (17) also found positive interaction between BMI and physical activity that was particularly evident for men in their sample.

Only one study examined the combined effects of more than two risk factors on colon cancer risk (17). Slattery et al (17) found that study participants who reported no vigorous activity and had high caloric intakes and a large BMI were at higher risk than those who were active and had low caloric intakes and low BMI. An unfavorable energy balance had more effect in men than in women, with a relative risk of over 7 found for men who were in the high-BMI, high-energy, and low physical activity category and a risk of less than 2 noted for women in this same category. Slattery et al (17) concluded that, at high levels of physical activity, risk of colon cancer is not influenced by body mass for both sexes or by higher energy intake among women. They noted that two things change among those who are not physically active: BMI becomes a more important indicator of risk, and the risk associated with higher energy intake increases.

From these investigations, there appears to be no important confounding of physical activity by other risk factors. Some effect modification by dietary intake, gender, tumour site, and BMI has been found. However, since few studies have examined interactions between physical activity

and other factors and because these interactions are still unclear, more studies are needed that delineate the joint effects of these factors. In so doing, a better understanding of the biologic effects of these risk factors can be obtained.

Breast Cancer

A total of 21 studies have been published that have examined the association between physical activity and breast cancer (18). Of these 21 studies, 7 have included measurements of dietary intake as well as physical activity (7,19–24). As with colon cancer, these studies have varied widely in their designs, samples, and methods used for assessing physical activity and dietary intake (Table 76-2). All but one of these investigations were population based; the exception was a hospital-based case-control study from Japan (20). Physical activity was assessed for recreational activity alone in 3 studies (19,20,22); the remaining 4 studies all measured some aspects of occupational and recreational activity (7,21,23,24). Two of the 7 studies assessed activity over different time periods in life (21,22) and the others examined current activity only. The frequency, intensity, and duration of activity was measured directly in 3 studies (21,22,24), while the other studies assessed only one or two of the components of physical activity. One study (7) used a 24-hour recall to measure dietary intake and the remaining studies used self-administered food frequency questionnaires (19,23,24), interview-administered diet history (20), or food frequency questionnaires (21,22).

The evidence for an association between physical activity and breast cancer risk is not as consistent as has been shown for colon cancer. Overall, there is a reduction in breast cancer risk with increased levels of occupational and recreational activity. The magnitude of the risk reduction is in the order of 10% to 30%. The overall or subgroup results associated with high levels of physical activity were statistically significantly reduced in five of these seven studies (20–24). There is some evidence for a dose-response relation from the few studies that have examined it (19,21–24). No confounding by dietary intake has been found in any of these studies. Indeed, no confounding by any established breast cancer risk factors has been shown. Some evidence for effect modification was, however, found in these studies. The risk reduction associated with increased levels of physical activity is more evident in women who are younger at diagnosis (21,24), premenopausal (24), lean (24), and parous (24). The results regarding interactions between breast cancer risk factors and physical activity are based on very few studies and require confirmation in future studies.

Prostate Cancer

A total of 15 published studies have examined the association between physical activity and the risk of developing prostate cancer (25). Of these studies, only 4 have measured both physical activity and dietary intake (7,26–28). As with the studies of other cancer sites, the methods used in these studies have varied (Table 76-3). These four studies were population-based and used interview-administered questionnaires to measure physical activity. Dietary intake was assessed with a 24-hour recall (7), a self-administered food frequency questionnaire (27), and interview-administered diet histories (26,28). The results from these studies were inconsistent, with 1 study finding an increased risk of prostate cancer for active

Table 76-2 Summary of Epidemiologic Studies of Physical Activity, Dietary Intake, and Breast Cancer

Reference, Country	Study Design	Study Sample	No. of Cases/ Controls	Physical Activity Measurement/ Definition	Dietary Assessment Method	Results	Comments
Albanes et al (7), USA	Prospective cohort	NHANES I and NHEFS 7413 women	122	Interview-administered questionnaire. Two questions on current recreational (R) and non-recreational (O) activity	24-hour recall	RR for quite inactive vs. very active: R: 1.0 (0.6–1.6), O: 1.1 (0.6–2.0) Premenopausal women: R: 0.6 (0.3–1.2), O: 0.4 (0.1–1.8) Postmenopausal women: R: 1.7 (0.8–2.9), O: 1.5 (0.7–2.8)	No overall effect, protective effect in premenopausal women. Adjusted for age, dietary fat, age at FFTP, parity, menopausal status, family history of breast cancer, BMI, smoking. No confounding by these factors or for total energy intake.
Friedenreich et al (19), Australia	Population-based case-control study	Cancer registry in Adelaide and controls selected from electoral roll	444/444	Self-administered questionnaire. Current recreational physical activity converted into kcal/wk.	Self-administered FFQ	RR for low vs. highest quartile overall: 0.7 (0.5–1.1) Premenopausal: 0.6 (0.3–1.2) Postmenopausal: 0.7 (0.4–1.2) Some indication of dose-response (N.S.)	Protective effect. Adjusted for age, energy intake and BMI. No confounding for these factors or for: age at menarche, age at FFTP, parity, menopausal status, history of bilateral oophorectomy, OC and HRT use, family history of breast cancer, BBD, smoking, education.
Hirose et al (20), Japan	Hospital-based case-control study	Aichi Cancer Center Hospital—one center source for cases and controls	1186/ 23,163	Self-administered questionnaire. Frequency of current recreational activity.	Interview-administered diet history	RR for none vs. ≥2 times/week: Premenopausal: 0.7 (0.6–1.0) Postmenopausal: 0.7 (0.5–1.0)	Protective effect. Adjusted for age, several dietary components (e.g. meats, vegetables), alcohol intake, age at menarche, age at FFTP, breastfeeding, BMI, height, smoking.
D'Avanzo et al (21), Italy	Multi-center population-based	Hospitals in six geographic areas were sources for cases and controls	2569/ 2588	Interview-administered questionnaire. Occupational and recreational activity at ages: 15–19, 30–39, 50–59	Interview-administered FFQ	15–19 years: R: 0.9 (0.8–1.2), O: 0.8 (0.5–1.4) 30–39 years: R: 0.8 (0.6–1.1), O: 0.6 (0.4–1.0) 50–59 years: R: 0.7 (0.4–1.1), O: 0.8 (0.4–1.5) Dose-response relation.	Protective effect. Adjusted for age, caloric intake, age at menarche, age at FFTP, parity, age at menopause, menopausal status, calorie intake, family history of breast cancer, BBD, BMI, smoking, education, center. BMI not a confounder. Stronger inverse association for younger age (<60) at diagnosis.

Study	Design	Population	N	Exposure assessment	Results	Comments
McTiernan et al (22), USA	Population-based case-control study	Washington State Cancer Registry and RDD controls	537/492	Interview-administered questionnaire. Recreational activity between ages 12 to 21 and two years before interview.	RR for no exercise vs. ≥3 hours/week in high intensity exercise: 0.6 (0.4–1.0) Postmenopausal: 0.6 (0.3–0.9) Dose-response relation.	Protective effect. Adjusted for age, education. Other factors considered were not confounders: dietary fat intake, age at menarche, age at FFTP, parity, menopausal status, OC and HRT use, family history of breast cancer, BBD, BMI, education, mammography screening history.
Fraser et al (23), USA	Prospective cohort	Adventist Health Study, 20,341 women	218	Self-administered questionnaire. Two questions on frequency of current vigorous recreational and occupational activity.	RR for high vs. low level of total physical activity: 0.7 (0.5–0.9)	Protective effect. Adjusted for age, energy and fat intake, age at FFTP, OC and HRT use, family history of breast cancer, BBD, BMI. No confounding.
Thune et al (24), Norway	Population surveys	Three counties surveyed in 1974–1978 and 1977–1983 (n = 25, 624 women)	351	Self-administered questionnaire. Occupational (O), recreational (R), and total activity (Tot) in years preceding surveys. Repeated assessments (Rep)	RR for sedentary vs. consistently active: R: 0.6 (0.4–0.95), O: 0.5 (0.3–0.9), Tot: 0.5 (0.4–1.1), Rep: 0.7 (0.4–1.1) Age at entry, recreational: <45: 0.4 (0.2–0.8), ≥45: 0.8 (0.5–1.4) BMI, recreational: <22.8: 0.3 (0.11–0.70), 22.8–25.7: 0.9 (0.5–2.0), >25.7: 0.8 (0.5–1.5) Dose-response relation.	Protective effect. Adjusted for age at entry, parity, BMI, height, county of residence. No evidence of confounding for these factors. Also considered confounding by energy intake, fat intake, serum lipids/ glucose, age at FFTP, menopausal status, smoking. Stratified by age, menopausal status, BMI. Found greater effect in women <45 years, premenopausal and BMI <22.8.

RR = relative risk 95% (CI unless otherwise indicated); NHANES = U.S. National Health and Nutrition Examination Survey; NHEFS = NHANES I Epidemiologic Follow-up Study; RDD = random digit dialing; BBD = benign breast disease; FFQ = food frequency questionnaire; FFTP = first full term pregnancy; BMI = body mass index; OC = oral contraceptives; HRT = hormone replacement therapy.

892

Table 76-3 Summary of Epidemiologic Studies of Physical Activity, Dietary Intake, and Prostate Cancer

Reference, Country	Study Design	Study Sample	No. of Cases/ Controls	Physical Activity Measurement/ Definition	Dietary Assessment Method	Results	Comments
Albanes et al (7), USA	Prospective cohort	NHANES I and NHEFS 5138 women	95	Interview-administered questionnaire. Two questions on current recreational (R) and non-recreational (O) activity.	24-hour recall	RR for very active vs. inactive: O: 0.8 (0.4–1.4), R: 0.6 (0.3–1.0) Dose response relation.	Protective effect. Adjusted for age. No confounding by energy intake, BMI, smoking, SES, race.
West et al (26), USA	Population-based case-control	Utah Cancer Registry, RDD controls	362/685	Interview-administered questionnaire. Time spent in current (3 years prior to diagnosis) moderate and vigorous activities converted to calories expended.	Interview-administered diet history	RR for active vs. inactive: 2.0 (0.8–5.2) for men aged 45–67 with aggressive tumors.	Increased risk. Assessed confounding and interaction and none found. Crude risk estimates, not age-adjusted. No other association between physical activity and prostate cancer.
Andersson et al (27), Norway	Population-based case-control study	Örebro, Norway county hospital and population register for controls who were screened with PSA and DRE tests before selection	256/252	Interview-administered questionnaire. Physical activity during puberty as compared to classmates.	Self-administered FFQ for current diet and diet 20 years ago, short interview-administered FFQ for diet in adolescence	RR for higher vs. lower physical activity during puberty: 0.7 (0.4–1.1)	Protective effect. Adjusted for age, grade of urbanization, adult farming. No adjustment for dietary intake. No association for adolescent diet.
Whittemore et al (28), USA, Canada	Multicenter population-based case-control study	Black (B), white (W), Japanese (J) and Chinese (C) American controls selected from population lists or by RDD	1655/1645	Interview-administered questionnaire. 24-hour daily activity and occupational activity for activity at ages 20–29, 40–49 and current (prediagnosis) activity	Interview-administered diet history	RR for highest vs. lowest tertiles of hours per day spent in any activity B: 1.2 p(trend) = 0.9, W: 0.92 p = 0.62, J: 0.84 p = 0.76, C: 0.70 p = 0.11	No effect. Adjusted for energy and fat intake. No other assessment of confounding done.

RR = relative risk (95% CI unless otherwise indicated); NHANES = U.S. National Health and Nutrition Examination Survey; NHEFS = NHANES I Epidemiologic Follow-up Study; RDD = random digit dialing; SES = socioeconomic status; BBD = benign breast disease; FFQ = food frequency questionnaire; BMI = body mass index; PSA = prostate specific antigen test; DRE = digital rectal examination.

men (26), 1 finding no effect associated with increased recreational and occupational activity (28) and 2 finding a decreased risk with increased levels of physical activity in puberty (27) or in adult life (7). The magnitude of the association ranged from a twofold increased risk (26) to a 40% decreased risk (7). A dose-response relation was noted in the study by Albanes et al (7), but no other studies found any dose-response. No confounding by dietary intake or other prostate cancer risk factors has been found in these studies. Effect modification of physical activity by dietary intake or other risk factors has not been examined in these studies.

Other Cancer Sites

Very few epidemiologic studies have been conducted that have examined the association between physical activity and other cancer outcomes. In total, four studies have examined the association between physical activity and endometrial cancer (29–32), two have been conducted on testicular cancer (33,34), one each on lung cancer (35) and ovarian cancer (36). A few cohort studies examined the association between physical activity and several sites (37–39). None of these studies measured dietary intake as well as physical activity.

METHODOLOGIC LIMITATIONS OF PREVIOUS RESEARCH

A number of important methodologic limitations of previous research need to be considered when reviewing the epidemiologic evidence. These include the lack of understanding of the underlying biologic mechanisms that are operative for the associations between physical activity and dietary intake and these cancers, the difficulty in measuring these complex exposures, and the problems of unidentified and uncontrolled residual confounding and effect modification. This section addresses each of these limitations individually.

Biologic Mechanisms

A number of biologic mechanisms have been postulated for the role of physical activity in reducing colon, breast, and prostate cancers, but no single underlying biologic model for each cancer site has been identified. For colon cancer, several biologic mechanisms have been suggested that involve colonic transit time, endogenous hormones, antioxidant enzymes, and insulin resistance. Physical activity may reduce colon cancer risk by decreasing the time that potential carcinogens in the fecal matter are in contact with the colonic mucosa (40–42). Physical activity may also increase prostaglandin levels that increase intestinal motility (43) and that inhibit colon cell proliferation (44). Antioxidant levels increase with exercise in experimental models (45) and antioxidants may protect against colon cancer (42). One recent hypothesis that unifies the roles of energy intake, body mass, and physical activity has strong plausibility. McKeown-Eyssen (46) has proposed that these risk factors (i.e. high-fat diets, obesity, physical inactivity) may operate through influences on serum triglycerides and insulin resistance that have been more commonly associated with coronary heart disease and diabetes mellitus than colon cancer. She argues this type of metabolic profile could

act as a growth-promoting milieu that is particularly beneficial for neoplastic cells.

For breast cancer, the postulated mechanisms by which physical activity influences risk include alterations in endogenous hormones, energy balance, and immune function. First, breast cancer risk is influenced by factors that are related to endogenous hormone profiles (47) and physical activity may modify breast cancer risk via a hormone-related pathway, for example, by reducing the cumulative exposure to ovarian hormones, by delaying menarche, or by reducing the number of ovulatory cycles (48). Second, physical activity may affect breast cancer risk through its observed influence on energy balance and the prevention of obesity and weight gain. Obesity during postmenopausal years and weight gain during life have been shown to increase breast cancer risk (49,50). However, obesity is associated with a decreased risk of breast cancer among premenopausal women (51,52). In premenopausal years, fat stores may affect the balance between pituitary and ovarian hormones, while in postmenopausal women, endogenous ovarian production of estrogens is reduced, which increases the importance of their synthesis in peripheral adipose tissue (53). Thus, in overweight postmenopausal women, it is hypothesized that there may be increased conversion of precursor substrates to estrogens in adipose tissue (54). The third plausible biologic mechanism is that physical activity may enhance the immune system by improving the capacity and numbers of natural killer cells (55) that may influence breast carcinogenesis.

For prostate cancer, the biologic mechanism that is operating may also involve endogenous hormones. It is possible that higher levels of physical activity may affect male sex hormone metabolism by decreasing circulating testosterone. Athletes have been shown to have lower basal levels of testosterone and individuals who exercise may have a temporary decrease in postexercise levels of testosterone (56–59). However, the impact of changes in serum androgen concentrations on the risk of prostate cancer remains unclear.

An understanding of the underlying biologic model would answer questions regarding the appropriate induction period for the effect of physical activity, i.e., when should an individual be physically active to experience a benefit from this activity? To determine when the induction period is for cancer, physical activity needs to be assessed over several time periods, or ideally across the entire lifetime of each respondent. Another aspect of the physical activity-cancer association that would be better understood with knowledge of the underlying biology of the relation is what type of activity, and what intensity, duration, and frequency of activity are needed for a risk reduction.

Physical Activity Assessment

No methods have been developed to measure physical activity that are entirely valid, reliable, practical, noninterfering, and noninvasive (60). Each method that has been developed has some major limitations (61). For epidemiologic studies, the most frequently used method has been the questionnaire or survey method. Commonly, respondents are asked to complete either a self-administered or an interview-administered questionnaire that covers their occupational and/or recreational activities. Some questionnaires have been developed that also measure other aspects of daily living including household activities, walking, stair climbing, and bicycling done for transportation. The time period for exposure measurement is generally short term: the previous week, month, or year. The parameters that are measured usually include the frequency and duration of the activity, although sometimes the intensity is also recorded. Frequently, respondents report the frequency and duration of activities that are categorized into set intensity levels (e.g., light, moderate, heavy).

The studies reviewed here have had imprecise measurements of physical activity. For example, one study (6) used occupational title to infer the amount of activity; thus a group rather than individual assessment of activity was made. Other studies (7,9,12,13,19,20,23,27) assessed physical activity using a few simple questions that required a subjective interpretation of the amount of activity actually performed. Group assignment of activity levels or classification of study subjects into a few broad categories results in exposure misclassification, which leads to an underestimation of the true impact of physical activity on cancer. Such nondifferential misclassification bias is a concern for the sites where little (e.g. rectal cancer), or inconsistent (e.g. prostate) effects have been observed for association of physical activity with cancer.

Another major limitation of previous epidemiologic studies of physical activity and cancer outcomes is that a single assessment of exposure was used that may not have accurately reflected individuals' true activity levels over their lifetimes. Very few studies have tried to combine activity information from different time periods; rather, they measured activity at one time point. The specific timeframe during which physical activity might influence cancer risk is unknown; thus, in those studies with discrepant findings, it is unclear whether physical activity was assessed at the appropriate time. Furthermore, a lag period between activity assessment and ascertainment of cancer may be important. Most investigators did not allow for a lag period in their assessment of physical activity. A spurious inverse association may arise if individuals with as yet undiagnosed disease had decreased their activity levels. These individuals might also transfer to a less physically demanding job with the onset of illness; thus relating occupational activity at the time of diagnosis to cancer risk may reflect illness instead. At present, it is unclear how much lag time is required.

As noted above, most studies assessed one or two types of physical activity; very few have measured total activity (i.e., occupational, recreational, and household activity) with all components of activity (i.e. duration, frequency, and intensity). Most questionnaires were developed for a white male population and consequently do not capture some of the activities commonly performed by women or by other ethnic groups or minorities. Hence, numerous aspects of the measurement of physical activity need to be improved to permit a more complete assessment of the association with cancer outcomes to be made.

Dietary Assessment

To understand the complex interrelationship of energy intake, energy expenditure, and cancer outcomes, valid and reliable measures of lifetime exposures are needed. For etiologic investigations of diet and its association with cancer, the time periods of interest are usually a few decades before the occurrence of cancer, given the long latency period for cancer. In the studies reviewed here, the most commonly used dietary assessment methods were food frequency questionnaires or diet histories. Both of these methods assess current or recent dietary intake in a comprehensive manner and permit a relatively valid and reliable estimation of total caloric intake as well as macro- and micronutrient intakes. One study used a 24-hour recall (7), which is a notably less reliable and valid dietary assessment method since one day's intake is not representative of an individual's usual dietary intake.

Although considerable research effort has been given to developing these dietary assessment methods, they provide only an approximation of an individual's diet over his/her lifetime since the assessment is restricted to, at most, one year of intake and because they are based on a list of foods that may not capture the dietary intake of the respondent, particularly if the respondent belongs to a different ethnic or minority group. Only one investigation (27) reviewed here attempted to measure dietary intake during childhood and adolescence and to relate this intake to prostate cancer risk later in life. Very little research effort has focused on measuring lifetime dietary intake and examining the risk for different time periods. Researchers have restricted themselves to current or recent consumption, although methods to improve the recall ability of study subjects are being developed and could be used to improve retrospective reporting (62).

Half of the studies included here used self-administered questionnaires, which are usually chosen as they are cost-effective and efficient. For the remaining studies, which used interview-administered questionnaires, more accurate reporting of dietary intake was possible since the interviewers can clarify any questions for the respondents. Self-administered food frequency questionnaires require a high level of literacy and the ability to estimate usual dietary intake over a long time period (generally a year); hence, they are of limited value for certain members of the study population (e.g., elderly, illiterate or poorly educated, very ill). Even for the literate and educated participant, reporting usual dietary habits can be challenging as it requires a good awareness of the constituents of one's diet.

Since the dietary assessment methods of these studies provided only an approximation of energy intake for a respondent's lifetime, a full examination of the association between physical activity, dietary intake, and cancer outcomes was not possible. To overcome these limitations, new dietary assessment methods are needed that measure lifetime dietary patterns.

Control for Confounding and Effect Modification

Without a clear understanding of the underlying biologic models and mechanisms that are operative in the putative associations of physical activity and cancer risk, it is difficult to know which factors are potential confounders and which are effect modifiers. Residual confounding may have influenced some of the previously conducted studies, since several studies did not assess confounding completely. The main confounder that was considered in this review is dietary intake, which, as noted above, was only measured and controlled for in 30% of the published studies identified for review.

The challenge in epidemiologic research is to differentiate between confounders, effect modifiers, and those factors that are on the causal pathway, since bias can be introduced into a study when adjustment is made for a factor that is a consequence of the exposure of interest (63,64). Obesity is an example of a risk factor that may be a confounder or an effect modifier, or may be on the causal pathway between physical activity and cancer risk. Exercise reduces body fatness (65) and therefore physical activity may reduce cancer risk by its influence on obesity. Another challenge is to determine the relative importance of different risk factors in cancer etiology. Slattery et al (17) has postulated that physical activity is the strongest determinant of risk for colon cancer and that the associations for energy intake and BMI are dependent on the level of physical activity of the population. Thus, the greatest colon cancer risk reduction, they suggest, may result from increasing levels of physical activity rather than reducing caloric intake.

Some of the discrepancies in study results may be due to underlying differences in characteristics of subjects included. Thus it is important to consider modifying effects of physical activity according to other patient characteristics. It would be useful for future studies to examine carefully effects of physical activity within defined strata of dietary intake and other cancer risk factors, especially since such analyses may provide insights into etiologic mechanisms. Examples of other risk factors would include body size, body fat distribution patterns, and, for breast cancer, exogenous hormone use histories, especially given recent findings of substantial interactive effects on breast cancer risk of body size and use of estrogen replacement therapy (50). Studies of interactive effects, however, will need to assure that there is sufficient statistical power within the subgroups to enable meaningful interpretations.

SUMMARY

Strong and consistent epidemiologic evidence exists that increased physical activity confers a protective effect for colon cancer and some evidence suggests that dietary intake may be an effect modifier, but not a confounder, of this association. Other important risk factors that modify the association between physical activity and colon cancer are gender, anatomic site of the tumor, and BMI. Physical activity may be the most important determinant of colon cancer risk and the key component of colon cancer prevention strategies along with weight maintenance through caloric restriction. The evidence for a protective effect of physical activity on breast cancer is not as strong as found for colon cancer, but it is still highly suggestive and worth further investigation to clarify the magnitude and nature of the association. The evidence for an association between prostate cancer and physical activity is still quite inconsistent and requires further study. Dietary intake does not appear to be an important confounder of the association between physical activity and these two latter cancer sites. However, since total caloric intake may be related to obesity and because obesity is a risk factor for breast cancer, future studies should make an effort to measure dietary intake and examine its relationship with physical activity more completely.

Research effort should be directed at new studies that are designed to address specifically the current gaps in our understanding of the underlying biologic models, the components of physical activity that are required for an effect, and the influence of confounding and effect modification on this relation. An understanding of how dietary intake and physical activity interact at a physiologic level, what mechanisms are involved, and which type of metabolic milieu influences neoplastic activity is needed. Some of the biologic mechanisms that combine the influence of diet, physical activity, and obesity have been postulated and need to be directly investigated in molecular epidemiologic studies. Future physical activity questionnaires need to be designed for different population groups and should measure all types of activity (i.e., occupational, recreational and household), for all time periods (i.e., across entire lifetimes) and including all parameters (i.e., frequency, duration, and intensity) of physical activity. Dietary questionnaires are needed that assess lifetime dietary intake. Larger sample sizes are necessary to assess the interactive effects on risk of cancer at each level of physical activity and dietary intake. Once the results of past studies are confirmed and the relationship between physical activity, dietary intake, and cancer outcomes are more fully elucidated, public health recommendations can be made that clearly outline the patterns of physical activity that are needed for cancer prevention.

Acknowledgement: While working on this chapter, Dr. Friedenreich was supported by a National Health Research Scholar Award from Health Canada.

REFERENCES

1. World Cancer Research Fund. Nutrition and the prevention of cancer: a global perspective. Washington, DC: American Institute for Cancer Research, 1997.

2. Tannenbaum A. The dependence of tumor formation on the degree of caloric restriction. Cancer Res 1945;5:609–615.

3. Hunter DJ, Willett WC. Diet, body build, and breast cancer. Ann Rev Nutr 1994;14:393–418.

4. Colditz GA, Cannuscio CC, Frazier AL. Physical activity and reduced risk of colon cancer: implications for prevention. Cancer Causes Control 1997;8:649–667.

5. Slattery ML, Schumacher MC, Smith KR, et al. Physical activity, diet, and risk of colon cancer in Utah. Am J Epidemiol 1988;128:989–999.

6. Peters RK, Garabrandt DH, Yu MC, et al. A case-control study of occupational and dietary factors in colorectal cancer in young men by subsite. Cancer Res 1989;49:5459–5468.

7. Albanes D, Blair AA, Taylor PR. Physical activity and risk of cancer in the NHANES I population. Am J Public Health 1989; 79:744–750.

8. Kune G, Kune S, Watson L. Body weight and physical activity as predictors of colorectal cancer risk. Nutr Cancer 1990;13: 9–17.

9. Benito E, Obrador A, Stiggelbout A, et al. A population-based case-control study of colorectal cancer in Majorca: I: dietary factors. Int J Cancer 1990;45:69–76.

10. Gerhardsson de Verdier M, Steineck G, Hagman U, et al. Physical activity and colon cancer: a case-referent study in Stockholm. Int J Cancer 1990;46:985–989.

11. Whittemore AS, Wu-Williams AH, Lee M, et al. Diet, physical activity and colorectal cancer among Chinese in North America and China. J Natl Cancer Inst 1990; 82:915–926.

12. Thun MJ, Calle EE, Namboodiri MM, et al. Risk factors for fatal colon cancer in a large prospective study. J Natl Cancer Inst 1992;84: 1491–1500.

13. Bostick R, Potter J, Kushi L, et al. Sugar, meat, fat intake, and non-dietary risk factors for colon cancer incidence in Iowa women (United States). Cancer Causes Control 1994;5:38–52.

14. Longnecker M, Gerhardsson de Verdier M, Frumkin H, et al. A case-control study of physical activity in relation to risk of cancer of the right colon and rectum. Int J Epidemiol 1995;24:42–50.

15. Giovannucci E, Ascherio A, Rimm EB, et al. Physical activity, obesity, and risk of colon cancer and adenoma in men. Ann Intern Med 1995;122:327–334.

16. White E, Jacobs E, Daling J. Physical activity in relation to colon cancer in middle-aged men and women. Am J Epidemiol 1996;144:42–50.

17. Slattery ML, Potter J, Caan B, et al. Energy balance and colon cancer—beyond physical activity. Cancer Res 1997;57:75–80.

18. Friedenreich CM, Thune I, Brinton LA, et al. Epidemiologic issues related to the association between physical activity and breast cancer. Cancer 1998;83: 600-610.

19. Friedenreich CM, Rohan TE. Physical activity and risk of breast cancer. Eur J Cancer Prev 1995;4:145–151.

20. Hirose K, Tajima K, Hamajima N, et al. A large-scale, hospital-based, case-control study of risk factors of breast cancer according to menopausal status. Jpn J Cancer Res 1995;86:146–154.

21. D'Avanzo B, Nanni O, La Vecchia C, et al. Physical activity and breast cancer risk. Cancer Epidemiol Biomark Prev 1996;5:155–160.

22. McTiernan A, Stanford JL, Weiss NS, et al. Occurrence of breast cancer in relation to recreational exercise in women age 50–64 years. Epidemiology 1996;7:598–604.

23. Fraser GE, Shavlik D. Risk factors, lifetime risk, and age at onset of breast cancer. Ann Epidemiol 1997;7:375–382.

24. Thune I, Brenn T, Lund E, et al. Physical activity and the risk of breast cancer. N Engl J Med 1997;336:1269–1275.

25. Oliveria SA, Lee I-M. Is exercise beneficial in the prevention of prostate cancer? Sports Med 1997;23:271–278.

26. West DW, Slattery ML, Robison LM, et al. Adult dietary intake and prostate cancer risk in Utah: a case-control study with special emphasis on aggressive tumors. Cancer Causes Control 1991;2: 85–94.

27. Andersson S-O, Baron J, Wolk A, et al. Early life risk factors for prostate cancer: a population-based case-control study in Sweden. Cancer Epidemiol Biomark Prev 1995;4:187–192.

28. Whittemore AS, Kolonel LN, Wu AH, et al. Prostate cancer in relation to diet, physical activity, and body size in blacks, whites, and Asians in the United States

and Canada. J Natl Cancer Inst 1995;87:652–661.

29. Shu XO, Hatch MC, Zheng W, et al. Physical activity and risk of endometrial cancer. Epidemiology 1993;4:342–349.

30. Levi F, La Vecchia C, Negri E, et al. Selected physical activities and the risk of endometrial cancer. Br J Cancer 1993;67: 846–851.

31. Sturgeon SR, Brinton LA, Berman ML, et al. Past and present physical activity and endometrial cancer risk. Br J Cancer 1993;68:584–589.

32. Olson SH, Vena JE, Dorn JP, et al. Exercise, occupational activity, and risk of endometrial cancer. Ann Epidemiol 1997;7:46–53.

33. Gallagher RP, Huchcroft S, Phillips N, et al. Physical activity, medical history, and risk of testicular cancer (Alberta and British Columbia, Canada). Cancer Causes Control 1995;6:398–406.

34. Thune I, Lund E. Physical activity and the risk of prostate and testicular cancer: a cohort study of 53,000 Norwegian men. Cancer Causes Control 1994;5: 549–556.

35. Thune I, Lund E. The influence of physical activity on lung-cancer risk: a prospective study of 81,516 men and women. Int J Cancer 1997;70:57–62.

36. Mink PH, Folsom AR, Sellers TA, et al. Physical activity, waist-to-hip ratio, and other risk factors for ovarian cancer: a follow-up study of older women. Epidemiology 1996;7:38–45.

37. Lee IM, Paffenbarger RS Jr. Physical activity and its relation to cancer risk: a prospective study of college alumni. Med Sci Sports Exerc 1994;26:831–837.

38. Pukkla E, Poskiparta M, Apter D, et al. Life-long physical activity and cancer risk among Finnish female teachers. Eur J Cancer Prev 1993;2:369–376.

39. Dosemeci M, Hayes RB, Vetter R, et al. Occupational physical activity, socioeconomic status, and risk

of 15 cancer sites in Turkey. Cancer Causes Control 1993;4: 313–323.

40. Cordain L, Latin R, Behnke J. The effects of aerobic running program on bowel transit time. J Sports Med 1986;26:101–104.

41. Reddy BS, Wynder EL. Metabolic epidemiology of colon cancer: fecal bile acids and neutral sterols in colon cancer patients and patients with adenomatous polyps. Cancer 1977;39:2533–2539.

42. Zaridze DG. Environmental etiology of large-bowel cancer. J Natl Cancer Inst 1983;70:389–400.

43. Thor P, Konturek JW, Konturek SJ, Anderson JH. Role of prostaglandins in control of intestinal motility. Am J Physiol 1985;248: G353–G359.

44. Reddy BS, Maruyama H, Kelloff G. Dose-related inhibition of colon carcinogenesis by dietary piroxicam, a nonsteroidal anti-inflammatory drug, during stages of rat colon tumor development. Cancer Res 1987;47:5340–5346.

45. Kanter MM, Hamlin RL, Unverferth DV, et al. Effect of exercise training on antioxidant enzymes and cardiotoxicity of doxorubicin. J Appl Physiol 1985;59: 1298–1303.

46. McKeown-Eyssen G. Epidemiology of colorectal cancer revisited: are serum triglycerides and/or plasma glucose associated with risk? Cancer Epidemiol Biomark Prev 1994;3:687–695.

47. Kelsey L, Gammon MD, John EM. Reproductive factors and breast cancer. Epidemiol Rev 1993;15: 36–47.

48. Bernstein L, Ross RK, Lobo RA, et al. The effects of moderate physical activity on menstrual cycle patterns in adolescence: implications for breast cancer prevention. Br J Cancer 1987;55:681–685.

49. Ziegler RG, Hoover RN, Nomura AMY, et al. Relative weight, weight change, height, and breast cancer risk in Asian-American women. J Natl Cancer Inst 1996;88:650–660.

50. Huang Z, Hankinson SE, Colditz GA, et al. Dual effects of weight and weight gain on breast cancer risk. JAMA 1997;278:1407–1411.

51. Ursin G, Longnecker MP, Haile RW, et al. A meta-analysis of body mass index and risk of premenopausal breast cancer. Epidemiology 1995;6:137–141.

52. Swanson CA, Coates RJ, Schoenberg JB, et al. Body size and breast cancer risk among women under age 45 years. Am J Epidemiol 1996;143:698–706.

53. Sherman BM, Korenman SG. Inadequate corpus luteum function: a pathophysiological interpretation of human breast cancer epidemiology. Cancer 1974;33:1306–1312.

54. Siiteri PK. Adipose tissue as a source of hormones. Am J Clin Nutr 1987;45(suppl):277–282.

55. Shephard RJ, Shek PN. Heavy exercise, nutrition and immune function: is there a connection? Int J Sports Med 1995;16:491–497.

56. Hackney AC, Sinning WE, Bruot BC. Reproductive hormonal profiles of endurance-trained and untrained males. Med Sci Sports Exerc 1988;20:60–65.

57. Hackney AC, Sinning WE, Bruot BC. Hypothalamic-pituitary-testicular axis function in endurance-trained males. Int J Sports Med 1990;11:298–303.

58. Morville R, Pesquies PC, Guezennec CY, et al. Plasma variations in testicular and adrenal androgens during prolonged physical exercise in man. Ann Endocrinol 1979;40:501–510.

59. Wheeler GD, Wall SR, Belcastro AN, et al. Reduced serum testosterone and prolactin levels in male distance runners. JAMA 1984; 252:514–516.

60. Kriska AM, Caspersen CJ. Introduction to a collection of physical activity questionnaires. Med Sci Sports Exerc 1997;29: S5–9.

61. LaPorte RE, Montoye HJ, Caspersen CJ. Assessment of physical activity in epidemiologic research: problems and prospects. Public Health Rep 1985;100: 131–146.

62. Friedenreich CM. Improving long term recall in epidemiologic studies. Epidemiology 1994;5:1–4.

63. Robbins JM, Greenland S. Identifiability and exchangeability for direct and indirect effects. Epidemiology 1992;3:143–155.

64. Weinberg CR. Toward a clearer definition of confounding. Am J Epidemiol 1993;137:1–8.

65. Williamson DF, Madans J, Anda RF, et al. Recreational physical activity and ten-year weight change in a US national cohort. Int J Obes 1993;17:279-286.

Part XIV.

HEALTH PROMOTION

Edited by
Michael P. O'Donnell

Introduction to Health Promotion

James M. Rippe

The field of health promotion has yielded important public health understandings as well as new scientific advances in the field of lifestyle medicine. This section provides a comprehensive overview of modern health promotion in a variety of settings.

The section starts with a chapter by Mark Wilson on "Health Promotion in the Workplace." It is perhaps at the worksite where health promotion programs have flourished most dramatically. The chapter provides an historical overview to worksite health promotion as well as documenting various areas where worksite health promotion programs have yielded important public health benefits.

The subsequent chapter by Larry Chapman shows how health promotion programs have grown within managed care settings. As managed care has become more prevalent within medicine, health promotion programs have flourished as cost-effective means of both lowering cost and improving outcome for a variety of conditions.

The chapter by Michael O'Donnell provides an authoritative look at currently available research literature in health promotion and assesses the strength of this literature in various areas. The author concludes that progress has been made in the methodologic quality of research and in assessment of the impact of today's health promotion programs, but he also cautions that there is still significant room for improvement.

Steven Aldana assesses the important topic of the financial effects of health promotion programs in his chapter. As the author points out, for health promotion programs to be considered a legitimate part of corporate business plans, they must demonstrate a positive financial effect on the bottom line. The author reviews evidence relating to this issue.

The section concludes with a chapter by Jonathan Fielding envisioning the future of health promotion. Fielding points out that the entire field of health is in a state of evolution. He postulates that health promotion will increasingly become "population-based" and also suggests that focusing attention on interventions early in life will provide a very important area of future growth for health promotion.

Chapter 77

Health Promotion in the Workplace

Mark G. Wilson

In the last three decades, worksite disease prevention and health promotion programs have grown exponentially, probably faster than in any other setting. Worksite programs have progressed from individual interventions devised to address one risk factor or target group to multicomponent programs designed to affect major health problems with multiple causes, such as cardiovascular disease and cancer (1). This chapter provides an overview of worksite disease prevention and health promotion programs as part of the corporate health strategy. It begins by reviewing the evolution of disease prevention and health promotion efforts and its tremendous growth in the last half century. Next, it carries this theme into the workplace and discusses the evolution of disease prevention and health promotion in corporate health programs. The chapter then documents the prevalence of worksite disease prevention and health promotion activities in the United States and the benefits of such activities to the health and well-being of the employees and the organizations involved. Finally, the chapter will examine worksite trends and consider the role of disease prevention and health promotion in corporate health programs over the next decade.

EVOLUTION OF DISEASE PREVENTION AND HEALTH PROMOTION

The changes in health and illness that have occurred in the twentieth century are well-known. While these changes are a tribute to advancements in the health care and public health systems, they also reflect a fundamental shift in the nature and provision of health care services. This shift transcends the current debate about the provision of and payment for

medical care to scrutinize the fundamental nature of health and health care. Our increased ability to prolong life has forced us to examine issues related to the quality of life and the extent to which health affects that quality of life. Consequently, our definition of health and health care has changed. It is now evident that good health comes from reducing unnecessary suffering, illness, and disability and improving quality of life. Good health means preventing premature death, preventing disability, promoting an environment that supports human life, cultivating family and community support, enhancing an individual's ability to respond and to take action, and assuring that all people achieve and maintain a maximum level of functioning (2). Improvements in the health status of the nation depend on continued progression in the quality of and access to health care services and the ability to prevent, or at least delay, the onset of disease and disability. Clearly, the health of the nation will be improved to the extent that medical care and disease prevention strategies can be better integrated (3).

The shift toward placing more emphasis on the prevention of disease and the promotion of health is reflected by the goals for the nation developed by the Department of Health and Human Services and outlined in the publication *Healthy People 2000* (2), which challenges the nation to 1) increase the span of healthy life, 2) reduce health disparities, and 3) achieve access to preventive services for all. It targets 21 priority areas within three broad categories: health promotion, health protection, and preventive services. Within each priority area, *Healthy People* specifies objectives for improving health status, reducing risk, and providing services and protection for the population and specific subgroups disproportionally affected by the problem in question (2).

A common theme that runs through the objectives is one of shared responsibility. Accomplishment of these goals and objectives starts with the individual's sharing responsibility for his or her health. Success also depends on organizations, communities, and governments acting responsibly by providing a support structure for these voluntary actions. Finally, achieving these objectives hinges on a collaborative effort by medical and health professionals at all levels, sharing equal responsibility for the health of the individual. This collaboration can be accomplished by providing support for primary preventive actions when the individual is largely healthy, secondary preventive interventions to identify problems early to minimize long-term damage, and tertiary preventive strategies to treat illness or disability after it has occurred.

One avenue for achieving these objectives is through disease prevention and health promotion programs offered at worksites. In the United States, 110 million adults spend approximately one-third of their lives at the worksite and an additional 100 million of their dependents are potentially affected by worksite activities (3,4). Our employment impacts our economic status, geographic location, social network, family structure, political convictions, lifestyle, and personality. It naturally follows that the workplace, with its captive audience, social support structure, facilities, convenience, and communication structure, is a potentially effective setting for reaching individuals and their families (4). Furthermore, work organizations are playing an increasingly larger role in the national health care debate, because they are funding a large share of health care costs and seeking alternatives for managing their increasing employee health care costs (3).

EVOLUTION OF DISEASE PREVENTION AND HEALTH PROMOTION IN THE WORKPLACE

The evolution of worksite disease prevention and health promotion programs has been characterized as progressing through a series of generations (5). First-generation programs were those primarily offered for reasons unrelated to health. For example, a number of companies that have had no-smoking policies for a century or more instituted those policies for quality control or safety reasons, because the health hazards of smoking were largely unknown at that time. For decades, companies have sponsored softball teams and bowling leagues largely as a means of improving employee morale rather than as a means of reducing the risk for cardiovascular disease by increasing cardiorespiratory fitness.

Second-generation programs were characterized by a focus on a single intervention designed to impact a single risk factor or behavior and targeted toward one specific group. Many of the earlier worksite fitness facilities were open only to executives as a "perk" or were set up because of concern over losing key personnel as a result of myocardial infarction or coronary artery disease (6–8). Other companies have offered annual physical examinations to their executives for decades.

Third-generation programs were devised to offer a variety of interventions aimed at a variety of risk factors. "Cafeteria" programs were common in organizations in this group. These programs allow employees to choose from a variety of activities, some of which were designed to lower risk of disease while others were developed to increase awareness or improve morale. Many early third-generation programs targeted cardiovascular disease and its multiple risk factors (9–12) while recent efforts have focused on cancer (13–15).

Fourth-generation programs were designed to provide a comprehensive approach to worker health. These programs transcend the individual or group behavior change approach to include 1) environmental supports conducive to health, such as modifying company cafeteria menus and eliminating cigarette vending machines from the worksite, 2) organizational interventions, such as no-smoking policies or mandatory use of seat belts in company vehicles, and 3) interventions designed to affect employees' families and the communities in which they reside, such as providing child care centers, sponsorship of community events, or "adopt a school" programs.

Although fourth-generation programs are the gold standard, disease prevention and health promotion programs currently being conducted at work sites across the country more often fall into the second- or third-generation categories. Striving for a fourth-generation program requires considerable commitment on the part of the organization and a willingness to view each employee as a complete person who is a key to the company's success. In this philosophy, the long-term viability of the organization depends considerably on the health and well-being of its employees.

The evolution from second to fourth generation requires the acceptance of certain principles (5). These principles include:

- A true health benefit package should include a balanced mix of health promotion programs and medical resources.
- Quality of care can be improved by better management of health care resources.
- The organization should manage the purchase and provision of health care.
- Better management would lead to cost savings, which should be shared by employees and the organization.
- The organization should develop a strategy that would involve short-term and long-term objectives.
- The strategy should include dependents and retirees as well as employees.
- Significant leadership, commitment, and investment on the part of the organization is necessary to achieve these goals.
- Programs should not be used to hide real health and medical problems caused by the work setting.
- Programs require involvement of the community in which they operate.

The adoption of these principles requires more than just formalizing them in company documents. It requires a fundamental shift in the organization's approach to the health and well-being of its employees. At the same time, success requires the direct participation and support of the health care system outside the workplace. In fact, with the United States health care system rapidly changing into a managed care system, increased emphasis will be placed on cost containment strategies and the development of community-wide partnerships among physicians, hospitals, insurers, employers, and individuals (3). These changes provide a unique opportunity to fully integrate worksite disease prevention and health promotion programs with community-based medical care services.

PREVALENCE OF DISEASE PREVENTION AND HEALTH PROMOTION PROGRAMS IN THE WORKPLACE

The interest in worksite disease prevention and health promotion activities has grown significantly in the past two decades and has been documented through a series of national surveys (16–20). This growth has been fueled by employers' concern over escalating health care costs and their increasing share of those costs, by growing competition in the marketplace and the need to attract and retain the best and the brightest workers, and by trends toward corporate downsizing, increased use of part-time employees, and outsourcing of services, all of which demand higher levels of productivity from fewer workers.

In 1985, the Office of Disease Prevention and Health Promotion of the U. S. Public Health Service conducted a national survey to determine the prevalence of disease prevention and health promotion activities being offered by employers (16). The survey was a stratified, random sample of private sector worksites in the United States with 50 or more employees. The survey was designed to assess the prevalence of worksite disease prevention and health promotion activities and describe the nature of those activities. The final sample consisted of 1358 worksites with 320 of those classified as small worksites (50 to 99 employees) (16).

The results indicated that 65.8% of worksites offered some type of disease prevention and health promotion activity to their employees. Smoking control activities were the most prevalent (35.6%), followed by health risk assessment (29.5%), back care (28.6%), stress management (26.6%), and exercise and fitness programs (22.1%) (Figure 77-1). The prevalence of activities varied significantly by the size of the worksite, i.e.,

larger worksites were more likely to offer disease prevention and health promotion activities than small worksites (88% versus 56%, respectively), and also varied considerably by industry type (17). The data also showed that 85% of worksites reported that all permanent employees were eligible to participate, 30% reported that dependents were eligible, and 30% indicated that retirees were eligible to participate in the activities (16).

In 1992, the Office of Disease Prevention and Health Promotion (ODPHP) repeated the national survey on 1507 worksites. The methods and criteria for inclusion in the survey were similar to the 1985 survey; the difference was the extent of information gathered by the survey. The 1992 survey expanded the number of disease prevention and health promotion activities that were covered from 9 to 18 and assessed various aspects of program administration, ranging from program coordination to evaluation (18).

The survey results indicated that the size of the worksite was the strongest predictor of the quantity and type of disease prevention and health promotion activity offered. Ninety-nine percent of large worksites (more than 750 employees) offered at least one activity to their employees, while 75% of small worksites (50 to 99 employees) offered at least one activity (18). Using categories comparable with the 1985 survey, 81% of worksites offered at least one disease prevention and health promotion activity (19). The most prevalent activities included job hazards and injury prevention (64%), exercise and fitness (41%), smoking control (40%), and stress management (37%) (Figure 77-2).

In 90% of worksites surveyed, all employees were eligible to participate in disease prevention and health promotion activities; this figure was higher than in 1985. However, the 1992 survey found reductions in the proportion of worksites that indicated the dependents (22%) and retirees (16%) were eligible to participate as well. The most common reasons for initiating disease prevention and health promotion activities were to improve employee health (41%), to reduce health insurance costs (27%), and to improve employee morale (17%) (18). Finally, there has been an overall increase from the 1985 survey in preventive services offered. Specifically, 52% of worksites in 1992 offered activities to measure employee

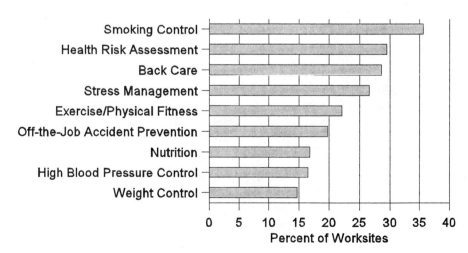

Figure 77-1 Prevalence of worksite disease prevention and health promotion activities in 1985. (Reproduced from U.S. Department of Health and Human Services. National survey of worksite health promotion activities. Washington, DC: Government Printing Office, 1987.)

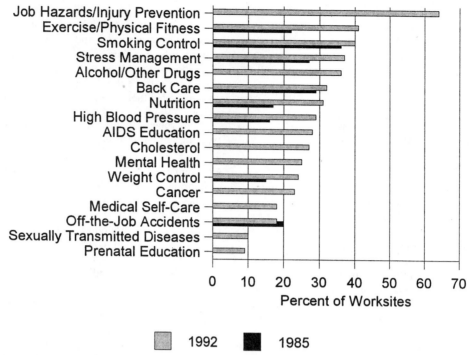

0   10   20   30   40   50   60   70
Percent of Worksites

□ 1992   ■ 1985

Figure 77-2 Worksite disease prevention health promotion in or activities offered by subject, 1985 and 1992. (Reproduced from U.S. Department of Health and Human Services. National survey of workplace health promotion activities. Washington, DC: Government Printing Office, 1992.)

health status and health risk, compared with 30% in 1985. In particular, 32% offered periodic examinations; 14%, questionnaires to measure employee health status; 32%, blood pressure screening; 20%, cholesterol screening; 16%, blood sugar screening; and 12%, cancer screening (19).

In 1995, the U.S. Centers for Disease Control and Prevention (CDC), to better understand how worksites were engaged in disease prevention and health promotion efforts, conducted a national probability survey to track progress since the 1992 survey. The primary purpose of the survey was to acquire a more comprehensive picture of HIV/AIDS activities in the workplace. However, a secondary objective of the survey was to track progress of other health promotion efforts in order to understand how general workplace trends might affect HIV/AIDS issues in the workplace. Consequently, the survey included a substantive number of questions designed to track trends in worksite policies, screening programs, and disease prevention and health promotion activities (20).

Comparison of the 1992 ODPHP survey and the 1995 CDC survey showed an increased prevalence of worksite policies requiring the use of occupant protection systems (28%), opposing the use of illegal drugs (7%), and providing protection for persons with HIV/AIDS (21%) (20). The prevalence of alcohol and smoking policies remained approximately the same, probably because of their high prevalence on the 1992 survey. Between 1992 and 1995, there was little change in the overall percentage of worksites offering disease prevention and health promotion classes or activities. Of the eight content areas measured in the 1992 survey, only smoking cessation classes showed decreases (8% overall). The prevalence of screenings offered by worksites declined overall: a decrease of

15% in high blood pressure, 7% in cholesterol, and 6% in cancer screenings was reported (20).

An important limitation of the 1985 and 1992 surveys was that they did not sample very small worksites, namely those with fewer than 50 employees. Approximately 95% of all worksites have fewer than 50 employees and 43% of all employees in the U.S. work in these organizations (21). The ultimate impact of the workplace as a setting for health promotion may be limited to the extent that the small worksite segment of the working population can be reached. Consequently, the CDC survey included worksites ranging from 15 to 49 employees.

An analysis of the data comparing small worksites (15 to 49 and 50 to 99 employees) to large worksites (more than 100 employees) showed that small worksites were offering disease prevention and health promotion activities to their employees but generally less often than large worksites (22). The most common type of programs offered by small worksites tended to involve worker protection (occupational safety and health, back injury prevention, hazard notification, and CPR training) rather than health promotion. Small worksites also had alcohol, illegal drug, smoking, occupant protection, and HIV/AIDS policies, but at lower levels than large worksites. A surprising percentage of small worksites provided health insurance to their employees: 91% of worksites with 15 to 49 employees and 96% of worksites with 50 to 99 employees offered insurance. This compares favorably to the percentage of large worksites (98%) that reported offering health insurance to their employees.

These data support the growing prevalence of worksite disease prevention and health promotion activities. More worksites than even before have been implementing health-related policies; offering multiple activities designed to decrease multiple health risks; providing incentives, such as flexible spending accounts or subsidizing participation in community programs; allowing employees to participate on company time; and collaborating with individuals and organizations outside the worksite to provide services.

THE BENEFITS OF WORKSITE DISEASE PREVENTION AND HEALTH PROMOTION PROGRAMS

Since worksites became a viable setting for public health interventions, a number of hypotheses about the value to the organization of disease prevention and health promotion activities have been promulgated. The most commonly cited benefits include a decrease in absenteeism, turnover, accidents, and worker's compensation claims; improved productivity; decreased health care costs; increased employee morale; enhanced community relations and organizational image; and an improvement in health behaviors, health risk reduction, and health status (23–26).

Surveys conducted over the last two decades have asked employers to report why they offered disease prevention and health promotion programs to their employees and what the benefits were. The most commonly cited responses to both questions included improved employee health, reduced health care costs, increased productivity, and improved employee morale (16,18). However, what scientific evidence is there to support such claims?

The scientific evidence supporting the effectiveness of disease prevention and health promotion programs conducted in clinical and community settings for reducing risks of premature morbidity and mortality has existed for decades (27–31). Disease prevention and health promotion interventions have become increasingly sophisticated in terms of the scholarly refinement and testing of theoretical concepts and the methodologic quality of the research. It has only been recently, however, that similar strategies have been tested in worksite settings. The most complete evidence examining the effectiveness of worksite programs was reported in a series of reviews published in the *American Journal of Health Promotion* (32–40). The foundation for those reviews was a comprehensive review of the literature that was conducted by the CDC, which was designed to provide a state-of-the-science look at the effectiveness of worksite disease prevention and health promotion activities. The CDC searched nine health-related databases from 1968 to 1994, conducted a reference search of articles retrieved, followed through with a manual search of key sources not covered in the databases, and asked a recognized expert in the particular area to review their respective area of expertise (41,42). Each author summarized the identified studies, provided a research rating for each study, and provided a rating for their respective literature as a whole. These reviews of over 350 worksite studies document the growing scientific evidence for the effectiveness of worksite disease prevention and health promotion programs. This evidence is presented in detail in Chapter 79.

Not only is the magnitude of evidence growing, but the quality of that evidence is also increasing. One analysis of all

the studies cited in the reviews showed that 34% of the studies used an experimental design (randomized with a control group) while 29% used a quasi-experimental design (comparison group only), 26% tracked subjects for longer than 1 year, and 64% included more than 100 subjects in the study (43).

The evidence supporting the financial impact of worksite disease prevention and health promotion programs is also growing. This evidence has been summarized in a series of reviews over the past decade (44–47) and is reviewed in Chapter 80. Generally speaking, empirical evidence exists to support the effectiveness of worksite programs for reducing health care costs and absenteeism and the cost-effectiveness of health promotion activities.

Whether from a research or organizational perspective, the evidence supporting the benefits of disease prevention and health promotion programs is robust. However, the value of worksite disease prevention and health promotion programs is not a result of their effects on any individual variable, such as health care costs. The value of worksite programs lies in their ability to affect multiple variables, some of which are financial, organizational, and health-related. It is this multiplicative effect that assures worksite programs are a cornerstone of an organization's efforts to positively affect the health and well-being of their employees.

STATE OF THE ART IN WORKPLACE HEALTH

Despite the evidence demonstrating the effectiveness of worksite disease prevention and health promotion programs for changing individual behaviors, even the best designed and implemented programs only reach a small proportion of the total workforce (48). Program participation rates generally range from 10% to 75%, and the majority of these individuals are the "working well," or those who are healthier and have higher levels of interest and motivation (49,50). What is needed is a shift from individually focused interventions to more comprehensive strategies integrating environmental, organizational, and community level strategies (48).

This integrative perspective on worker health has generated considerable discussion in the worksite literature (1,42,51–53) and is currently the gold standard of worksite programs. The concept is delineated in an integrative model of worker health (53). The model features three interactive components that all have the potential to affect worker health. The components include job demands and worker characteristics at the individual level, work environment at the organizational level, and extraorganizational factors at the community level (Figure 77-3). Job demands consist of physical and psychological demands of a particular job, while worker characteristics include health risk factors and health-related behaviors such as hypertension, smoking, and alcohol consumption. These individual factors are commonly addressed through medical departments, occupational safety and health, health promotion, and employee assistance programs. The majority of the worksite health studies conducted to date have examined these individual level variables (41,42).

The work environment component takes a broad view of the total work environment and includes both physical and social factors not specific to any particular job (53). The

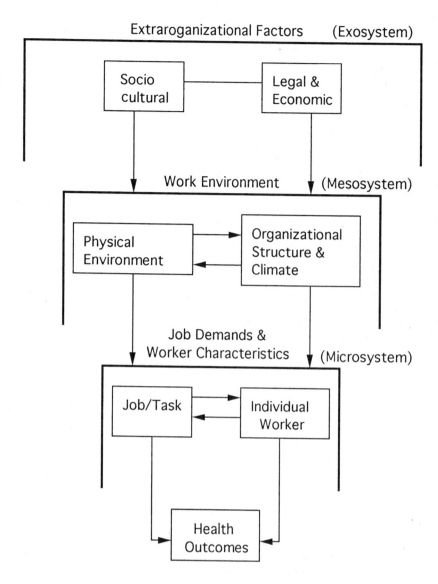

Figure 77-3 Integrative model of worker health. (Reproduced by permission from DeJoy DM, Southern DJ. An integrated perspective on worksite health promotion. J Occup Med 1993;35:1211–1230.)

physical work environment typically falls under Occupational Safety and Health Administration (OSHA) jurisdiction and thus is carefully monitored and regulated. The social environment is related to the organization's structure and culture. Although there is little agreement on the specific tenets of organizational culture, there is consensus among researchers and practitioners alike that this culture has a significant influence on the health of the organization (54–59).

Baker et al have proposed an integrated model that delineates psychosocial-environmental conditions that are precursors to stress (52). They propose a combination of worksite health promotion and occupational safety and health interventions to address the psychosocial factors influencing worker health. Some organizations are forming "health management teams," involving medical, health promotion, employee assistance, occupational safety and health, and benefits departments, in a effort to address employee health from a organization-wide perspective and to develop and implement intervention strategies across organizational lines.

Extraorganizational factors include sociocultural, legal, and economic factors that are usually external to an organiza-

tion and out of its direct control (53). Day care needs for dual career families and legislation regulating family leave are examples of extraorganizational factors that affect organizations and workers. Stokols et al maintain that state-of-the-art programs create healthier worksites through comprehensive programs responsive to community needs (3). They argue that practitioners should be developing more comprehensive approaches to worksite disease prevention and health promotion that are designed to improve workers' health habits, the environmental quality of their worksite, the social climates of their organization, and the communities in which they reside. A key element of this extraorganizational component is the medical care community. It is essential that physicians, hospitals, clinics, and managed care organizations work together to foster an integrative approach to worker health, one that transcends the workplace (51). Some organizations are already developing partnerships with managed care organizations that provide a "win-win" situation for all involved (60,61).

Recently, social ecologic theory has been proposed to provide a framework for developing comprehensive strategies for promoting employee health (51). The social ecologic paradigm postulates that the individual's health status is affected by multiple personal and environmental factors; that environments have multiple physical, social, and cultural dimensions that influence a variety of health outcomes; and that linkages exist between both work and nonwork environments (51,62,63). The social ecologic approach attempts to combine biomedical, behavioral, educational, environmental, and regulatory interventions at all levels (individual, organizational, and community), using an interdisciplinary, multimethod approach to positively affect worker health and well-being (Figure 77-4) (62–64). The social ecologic approach has been successful in some community applications (65,66) but has yet to be tested in a work site setting.

In summary, the state of the art worksite disease prevention and health promotion program incorporates a comprehensive perspective on worker health and well-being. It uses both passive and active strategies at individual, organizational, and community levels to affect physiologic and psychosocial factors related to health. The state-of-the-art program employs a coalition of intraorganizational and extra-organizational health professionals dedicated to a comprehensive approach to worker health and well-being and is positioned to create a healthy workforce and, in turn, a healthy organization.

FUTURE DIRECTIONS

The future of worksite disease prevention and health programs will rely on their ability to adapt to ever changing business and health care climates. This adaptation will propel practitioners away from their traditional approaches to disease prevention, health promotion, and activities that have primarily been designed to decrease individual health risks. The nucleus of the new approach will entail activities that are integrated with the medical care community and designed to create a healthy organization.

The integration of worksite disease prevention and health promotion programs with medical care services may be fostered through a number of avenues (3). One approach

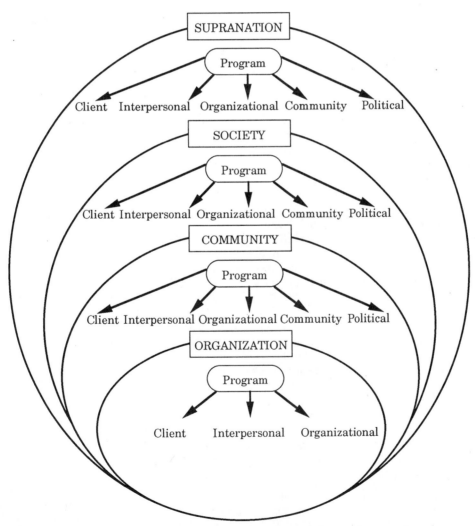

Figure 77-4 Schematic representation of the model of the ecologic approach in health promotion programs. (Reproduced by permission from Richard L, Potvin L, Kishchuk N, et al. Assessment of the integration of the ecological approach in health promotion programs. Am J Health Prom 1996;10:318–328.)

involves the synthesis of primary, secondary, and tertiary prevention strategies that complement and reinforce medical services being provided by physicians working in nonoccupational settings. Already, companies that routinely provide medical surveillance and health risk assessments are referring those at high risk to their physician (9,67–70). This approach will also allow physicians to continue to monitor the individual's recovery after they have returned to work and enable the physician and worksite professional to implement a coordinated rehabilitation program.

A second avenue includes the development of innovative applications of new technologies for providing cost-effective health management programs. This strategy will increase the cost-effectiveness of disease prevention and health promotion and health care programs by allowing the monitoring and follow-up of patients on a continuous basis in a fashion that does not require considerable physician time. It can also be used to encourage modifications in an individual's health behavior with activities delivered through their computer at work or their television at home. A third approach involves improving access to populations that are difficult to reach. These populations include small companies, mobile workers, retirees, uninsured employees, or those working in rural or hard-to-reach locations, such as oil platforms. Many times, these individuals' only link to health services is through community-based organizations and clinics. Deliberate coordination between the employer and these community-based organizations can make these organizations the provider of choice rather than the provider of last resort for primary as well as tertiary preventive services.

Another approach integrates disease prevention and health promotion programs and clinical preventive services into corporate benefit plans. Health benefit plans should routinely cover preventive clinical services and health promotion programs for which effectiveness has been documented (3). Finally, a fifth approach includes developing worksite disease prevention and health promotion interventions that are consistent with, and have the potential to improve, managed care approaches to health care delivery. More and more employers will develop partnerships with managed care organizations to better integrate disease prevention and health promotion services into changing medical service modalities. These partnerships can benefit all involved parties by mutually sharing the risk relative to capitated health programs (3).

This coordinated effort between disease prevention and health promotion practitioners and medical care providers should be integrated with organizational strategies for the purpose of creating a healthy organization. For decades, work

organizations have been interested in worker productivity and its effect on the organizational bottom line. Considerable research has been conducted to establish the link between specific organizational, environmental, and individual factors and productivity. Studies have examined the relationship between productivity and social support (71), job demands (71–73), job characteristics (74), decision latitude (73), organizational commitment (75), quality of working life (76), role autonomy (77), role ambiguity, organizational ethics (78), and organizational climate (79,80).

More recently organizations have been pursuing activities designed to improve worker health in an attempt to enhance productivity and affect the bottom line through reduced health care costs. The concept of a healthy work organization centers on the premise that organizations that foster employee health and well-being are also profitable and competitive in the marketplace. This premise acknowledges that the work experience can have important positive effects on employee self-esteem, satisfaction, and health, which, in turn, are critical to the overall effectiveness of the organization. Although empirical evidence is scarce for this new approach, considerable discussion and some descriptive evidence have been used to support the viability of these concepts (68,81,82).

Increasingly, organizations will adopt a proactive approach to increase worker health, satisfaction, and productivity with the understanding that it will affect their bottom line. Disease prevention and health promotion practitioners can play a central role in this approach, because it will require assessment, coalition building, intervention development, implementation, communication, and evaluation strategies similar to those that they have been trained to employ. In addition, since workers only spend a portion of their day at the worksite, a healthy organization cannot become a reality without the strong support of the community in which it resides. This support can take a variety of forms but must be continuous and integrated with healthy organization strategies.

The challenge will be to move worksite health programs beyond the narrow confines of individual behavior change or reducing health insurance costs and toward embracing quality of work issues and, eventually, a leadership role for improving quality of life for the entire community (4). Successful organizations will be those that will be able to maximize their human capital. High-quality service and products are only as good as the people that are producing and performing them. Employee health services integrated with other business functions and community health services will be a key to enhancing human capital and maximizing the competitiveness and success of the organization (81).

REFERENCES

1. DeJoy DM, Wilson MG, Huddy DC. Health behavior change in the workplace. In: DeJoy DM, Wilson MG, eds. Critical issues in worksite health promotion. Boston: Allyn & Bacon, 1995:97–122.

2. U.S. Department of Health and Human Services. Healthy people

2000. Washington, DC: Government Printing Office, 1991.

3. Stokols D, Pelletier KR, Fielding JE. Integration of medical care and worksite health promotion. JAMA 1995;273:1136–1142.

4. DeJoy DM, Wilson MG, eds. Critical issues in worksite health

promotion. Boston: Allyn & Bacon, 1995.

5. O'Donnell MP, Ainsworth T, eds. Health promotion in the workplace. New York: Wiley Medical, 1984:vii.

6. Shephard RJ. Exercise and employee-wellness initiatives.

Health Educ Res 1989;4:233–243.

7. Pauly JT, Palmer JA, Wright CC, et al. The effect of a 14-week employee fitness program on selected physiological and psychological parameters. J Occup Med 1982;24:457–463.

8. Durbeck DC, Heinzelmann F, Schacter J, et al. The National Aeronautics and Space Administration-U.S. Public Health Service Health evaluation and enhancement program: summary of results. Am J Cardiol 1972;30:784–790.

9. Erfurt JC, Foote A, Heirich MA. Worksite wellness programs: incremental comparison of screening and referral alone, health education, follow-up counseling, and plant organization. Am J Health Prom 1991;5:438–448.

10. Bauer RL, Heller RF, Challah S. United Kingdom Heart disease prevention project: 12-year follow-up of risk factors. Am J Epidemiol 1985;121:563–569.

11. Rose G, Heller RF, Pedoe HT, et al. Heart disease prevention project: a randomised controlled trial in industry. Br Med J 1980; 1:747–751.

12. Bjurstrom LA, Alexiou NG. A program of heart disease intervention for public employees. J Occup Med 1978;20:521–531.

13. Tilley BC, Vernon SW, Glanz K, et al. Worksite cancer screening and nutrition intervention for high-risk auto workers: design and baseline findings of the Next Step trial. Prev Med 1997;26:227–235.

14. Abrams DB, Boutwell WB, Grizzle J, et al. Cancer control at the workplace: the Working Well trial. Prev Med 1994;23:15–27.

15. Sorensen G, Morris DM, Hunt MK, et al. Work-site nutrition intervention and employees' dietary habits: the Treatwell program. Am J Public Health 1992;82:877–880.

16. U.S. Department of Health and Human Services. National survey of worksite health promotion activities: a summary. Washington, DC: USDHHS, 1987:1–10.

17. Fielding JE, Piserchia PV. Frequency of worksite health promotion activities. Am J Public Health 1989;79:16–20.

18. U.S. Department of Health and Human Services. 1992 national survey of worksite health promotion activities: final report. Washington, DC: Government Printing Office, 1992:29–41.

19. U.S. Department of Health and Human Services. 1992 national survey of worksite health promotion activities: summary. Amer J Health Prom 1993;7:452–464.

20. Centers for Disease Control and Prevention. Business responds to AIDS benchmark study: final report. Atlanta: CDC, 1996:1–30.

21. Chenoweth DM. Health promotion in small businesses. In: DeJoy DM, Wilson MG, eds. Critical issues in worksite health promotion. Boston: Allyn & Bacon, 1995: 273–294.

22. Wilson MG, DeJoy DM, Jorgensen CM, et al. Prevalence of health promotion programs in small worksites. Am J Health Prom 1999 (in press).

23. O'Donnell MP, Harris JS, eds. Health promotion in the workplace. 2nd ed. Albany: Delmar, 1994: 41–65.

24. Eddy JM, Gold RS, Zimmerli WH. Evaluation of worksite health enhancement programs. Health Values 1989;13:3–9.

25. Chenoweth DH. Planning health promotion at the worksite. Indianapolis: Benchmark, 1987:3–10.

26. Parkinson, RS, ed. Managing health promotion in the workplace. Palo Alto: Mayfield, 1982:7–12.

27. National Cancer Institute. Changes in cigarette-related disease risks and their implication for prevention and control. Washington, DC: Government Printing Office, 1997: 477–565.

28. World Cancer Research Fund. Food, nutrition, and the prevention of cancer: a global perspective. Washington, DC: American Institute for Cancer Research, 1997:72–90.

29. U.S. Department of Health and Human Services. Physical activity and health: a report of the Surgeon General. Atlanta: Centers for Disease Control and Prevention, 1996:81–172.

30. National Cancer Institute. Tobacco and the clinician: interventions for medical and dental practice. Washington, DC: Government Printing Office, 1994:3–37.

31. U.S. Department of Health and Human Services. The Surgeon General's report on nutrition and health. Washington: Government Printing Office, 1988:1–20.

32. Eddy JM, Fitzhugh EC, Wojtowicz GG, et al. The impact of worksite-based safety belt programs: a review of the literature. Am J Health Prom 1997;11:281–289.

33. Heaney CA, Goetzel RZ. A review of health-related outcomes of multi-component worksite health promotion programs. Am J Health Prom 1997;11:290–307.

34. Murphy LR. Stress management in work settings: a critical review of the health effects. Am J Health Prom 1996;11:112–135.

35. Roman PM, Blum TC. Alcohol: a review of the impact of worksite interventions on health and behavioral outcomes. Am J Health Prom 1996;11:136–149.

36. Wilson MG, Jorgensen C, Cole G. The health effects of worksite HIV/AIDS interventions: a review of the research literature. Am J Health Prom 1996;11:150–157.

37. Anderson DR, Staufacker MJ. The impact of worksite-based health risk appraisal on health-related outcomes: a review of the literature. Am J Health Prom 1996;10: 499–508.

38. Glanz K, Sorensen G, Farmer A. The health impact of worksite nutrition and cholesterol intervention programs. Am J Health Prom 1996;10:453–470.

39. Hennrikus DJ, Jeffery RW. Worksite intervention for weight control: a review of the literature. Am J Health Prom 1996;10:471–498.

40. Shephard RJ. Worksite fitness and exercise programs: a review of methodology and health impact. Am J Health Prom 1996;10:436–452.

41. Wlson MG. A comprehensive review of the effects of worksite health promotion on health-related outcomes: an update. Am J Health Prom 1996;11:107–108.

42. Wilson MG, Holman PB, Hammock A. A comprehensive review of the effects of worksite health promotion on health-related outcomes. Am J Health Prom 1996;10:429–435.

43. Wilson MG. The status of evaluation in worksite health promotion. Presented at American Evaluation Association annual conference, Atlanta, GA, 1996.

44. Pelletier KR. A review and analysis of the health and cost-effective outcome studies of comprehensive health promotion and disease prevention programs at the worksite: 1993–1995 update. Am J Health Prom 1996;10:380–388.

45. Pelletier KR. A review and analysis of the health and cost-effective outcome studies of comprehensive health promotion and disease prevention programs at the worksite: 1991–1993 update. Am J Health Prom 1993;8:50–62.

46. Pelletier KR. A review and analysis of the health and cost-effective outcome studies of comprehensive health promotion and disease prevention programs. Am J Health Prom 1991;5:311–313.

47. Warner KE, Wickizer TM, Wolfe RA, et al. Economic implications of workplace health promotion programs: review of the literature. J Occup Med 1988;30:106–112.

48. Stokols D, Allen JR, Bellingham RL. The social ecology of health promotion: implications for research and practice. Am J Health Prom 1996;10:247–251.

49. Wilson MG, DeJoy DM. Maximizing participation and adherence in health promotion programs. In: DeJoy DM, Wilson MG, eds. Critical issues in worksite health promotion. Boston: Allyn & Bacon, 1995:123–142.

50. Wilson MG. Factors associated with, issues related to, and suggestions for increasing participation in workplace health promotion programs. Health Values 1990;14:29–36.

51. Stokols D, Pelletier KR, Fielding JE. The ecology of work and health: research and policy directions for the promotion of employee health. Health Educ Q 1996;23:137–158.

52. Baker E, Israel BA, Schurman S. The integrated model: implications for worksite health promotion and occupational health and safety practice. Health Educ Q 1996;23:175–190.

53. DeJoy DM, Southern DJ. An integrative perspective on worksite health promotion. J Occup Med 1993;35:1211–1230.

54. Baun WB. Culture change in worksite health promotion. In: DeJoy DM, Wilson MG, eds. Critical issues in worksite health promotion. Boston: Allyn & Bacon, 1995:29–49.

55. Allen JR. Breaking the cycle of broken promises: the role of supportive cultural environments in successful health promotion. Am J Health Prom 1993;7:323–324.

56. Schein EH. Organizational culture. Am Psychol 1990;45:109–119.

57. Rudman WJ, Steinhardt M. Fitness in the workplace: the effects of a corporate health and fitness program on work culture. Health Values 1988;12:4–17.

58. Allen RF, Allen JR. A sense of community, a shared vision and a positive culture: core enabling factors in successful culture-based health promotion. Am J Health Prom 1987;1:40–47.

59. Allen JR, Allen RF. Achieving health promotion objectives through cultural change. systems. Am J Health Prom 1986;1:42–49.

60. Leutzinger J, Wilkie S. Working together toward a healthier population: partnering with managed-care organizations. Worksite Health 1997;4:15–19.

61. Kirchhofer A, Wilkerson J. Partners for better health: linking managed care and health promotion. Presented at the Association for Worksite Health Promotion Region III Conference, Atlanta, GA 1997.

62. Stokols D. Translating social ecological theory into guidelines for community health promotion. Am J Health Prom 1996;10:282–298.

63. Richard L, Potvin L, Kishchuk N, et al. Assessment of the integration of the ecological appraoch in health promotion programs. Am J Health Prom 1996;10:318–328.

64. McLeroy KR, Bibeau D, Steckler A, et al. An ecological perspective on health promotion programs. Health Educ Q 1988;15:351–377.

65. Buchanan DR. Building academic-community linkages for health promotion: a case study in Massachusetts. Am J Health Prom 1996;10:262–269.

66. Duhl LJ. An ecohistory of health: the role of "Healthy Cities". Am J Health Prom 1996;10:258–261.

67. Harvey MR, Whitmer RW, Hilyer JC, et al. The impact of a comprehensive medical benefit cost management program for the city of Birmingham: results at five years. Am J Health Prom 1993;7:296–303.

68. Henritze J, Brammell HL, McGloin J. LIFECHECK: A successful, low touch, low tech, in-plant, cardiovascular disease risk identification and modification program. Am J Health Prom 1992;7:129–136.

69. Dalton BA, Harris JS. A comprehensive approach to corporate health management. J Occup Med 1991;33:338–348.

70. Bertera TL. Planning and implementing health promotion in the workplace: a case study of the Du Pont Company experience. Health Educ Q 1990;17:307–327.

71. House JS, Cottington EM. Health and the workplace. In: Aiken LA, ed. Applications of social science to clinical medicine and health policy. New Brunswick:

Rutgers University Press, 1986: 392–416.

72. Johansson G, Johnson JV, Hall EM. Smoking and sedentary behavior as related to work organization. Soc Sci Med 1991;32: 837–846.

73. Karasek R, Baker D, Marxer F, et al. Job decision latitude, job demands, and cardiovascular disease: a prospective study of Swedish men. Am J Health Prom 1981;71:694–705.

74. Karasek RA, Theorell T, Schwartz JE, et al. Job characteristics in relation to the prevalence of myocardial infarction in the U.S. Health Examination Survey (HES) and the Health and Nutrition Examination Survey (HANES). Am J Public Health 1988;78:910–918.

75. Jamal M. Relationship of job stress and type-A behavior to employees' job satisfaction, organizational commitment, psychosomatic health problems, and turnover motivation. Human Relations 1990;43:727–738.

76. Cook J, Wall T. New work attitude measures of trust, organizational commitment, and personal need non-fulfillment. J Occup Psychol 1980;53:39–52.

77. Lysonski S, Andrews JC. Effects of moderating variables on product managers' behavior. Psychol Reports 1990;66:295–306.

78. Froelich KS, Kottke JL. Measuring individual beliefs about organizational ethics. Educ Psychol Measurement 1991;51: 377–383.

79. DeJoy DM, Gershon RRM, Murphy LR, et al. A work-systems analysis of compliance with universal precautions among health care workers. Health Educ Q 1996;23: 159–174.

80. DeJoy DM, Murphy L, Gershon RM. The influence of employee job/task, and organizational factors on adherence to universal precautions among nurses. Int J Indus Ergonomics 1995;16:43–55.

81. Bellingham R, Pelletier KR. Health promotion in business and industry: an overview and status report. In: DeJoy DM, Wilson MG, eds. Critical issues in worksite health promotion. Boston: Allyn & Bacon, 1995:3–27.

82. Rosen RH, Berger L. The healthy company: eight strategies to develop people, productivity, and profits. New York: G.P. Putnam, 1991:1–12.

Chapter 78

Health Promotion in Managed Care

Larry S. Chapman

This chapter provides an overview of managed care and health promotion. An historical perspective is first presented, followed by the identification of many of the major forces that are shaping health promotion and disease prevention in managed care settings. Next, the most typical forms of organized health promotion in managed care settings are described along with the major pitfalls, hindrances, and challenges associated with programming efforts. After this, an optimal design for health promotion and disease prevention in managed care settings is explored along with evaluation strategies that can be used to assess the effectiveness and efficiency of such efforts. Finally, a few concluding comments are offered, along with identification of some of the major issues that will shape the future of health promotion and disease prevention in managed care.

PERSPECTIVES ON MANAGED CARE

The history of managed care in the U.S. can be characterized as long and with many important watershed events. Some of the major landmarks include: the beginning roots of managed care in the form of prepaid group practices developed in the early 1930s, the establishment of the Kaiser Foundation Health Plans and Permanente Medical Groups in the 1940s, and the founding of Group Health Cooperative in Seattle in the mid-1940s and Group Health Association in Washington, DC, in the 1950s. In 1973, the federal Health Maintenance Organization (HMO) Act was passed, which formally launched the present day managed care movement. In the 25 years since the passage of the act, managed care has undergone significant diversification, propelled by pressures created

by the rapid increase in health costs during the eighties and early nineties. A central concept of managed care resides in the movement, reaching from informal patterns and systems of referral and patient flow through the health care system to the formalization of those patterns of referral and patient movement.

The various major alternative health care financing or delivery arrangements such as health maintenance organizations (HMOs), preferred provider organizations (PPOs), point-of-service (POS) plans, exclusive provider organizations (EPOs), and managed indemnity plans are the most typical organizational forms represented in the health care marketplace, all of which use clinical oversight or contracting and discounting strategies as part of an effort to more efficiently manage the delivery of health care services. One working definition of "managed care" is the following:

> The formal organization of health care financing and delivery characterized by active review and oversight of health care provision through the use of clinically derived criteria and/or peer review combined with contracting, direct employment of providers, and/or discounting, which is intended to result in cost-effective, high-quality patient care. Managed care may also include various types and forms of economic risk-sharing and delivery of service arrangements (1).

The literature concerning HMOs, PPOs, and EPOs as examples of different organizational expressions of managed care is expanding at a rapid pace, and a variety of forces are now guiding the evolution of these various organizational forms of health care financing and delivery.

Newer forms of the "alphabet soup" of managed care

include: integrated delivery systems (IDS), physician hospital organizations (PHOs), and direct service organizations (DSOs). Because of the dynamic nature of the marketplace and the pressure for innovation, the rapid proliferation of these new managed care forms is not likely to slow in the near term (2). The term "managed care" is frequently associated with more rigorous applications of utilization management within indemnity plan environments, so that the operative definition of managed care always should be carefully clarified. To more clearly explain the context for health promotion and disease prevention efforts within managed care, some of the fundamental issues shaping current day forms of managed care are described below.

The original conceptualization of health maintenance organizations (HMOs) by Paul Ellwood et al (3) included a strong focus on the provision of "health maintenance" and prevention services and on capabilities that were seen as clearly proactive in their approach to personal health management, rather than simply as a reactive response to expressed patient needs.

From a practical vantage point, the extent to which health promotion and disease prevention are addressed in managed care settings is often dependent on the economic incentives that drive the health care being provided (4). If greater economic benefit accrues to individual providers and to managed care organizations from the delivery of more health services, it is unlikely that a large programmatic investment will be made in prevention efforts. If greater economic returns accrue from increased efficiency in health care delivery aided by such things as the use of proven preventive interventions, it is more likely that significant levels of investment in programming will occur. Another axiom that appears to apply to health care at large is that the more highly organized and vertically integrated the health care delivery structure, the more likelihood that health promotion and disease prevention will be formally addressed (5).

Traditionally, indemnity health insurance (i.e., indemnification or payment for the financial liability associated with health care use) has allowed the beneficiary to enter the marketplace and engage any willing provider to meet their needs by delivering services (i.e., making a diagnosis, providing treatment, and monitoring the results) and be reimbursed. This freedom of choice, when combined with limited reason or motivation to use these "insurance dollars" wisely, generally leads to more expensive health care and to economic inefficiency (6). As a consequence, employers, who on a national basis pay the bulk of health benefit costs for employees and their family members, have pursued managed care as a primary strategy for attaining better value and greater economic efficiency from their benefit dollars (7).

The organizational form of managed care usually follows one of three basic patterns. First, indemnity plans allow relative freedom of provider choice but can be more tightly "managed." This approach has the advantage of minimal restriction of the employee's freedom of choice of provider, while more closely monitoring utilization and costs. This first form is generally the least "managed" and is usually less efficient than the other two major patterns. The second major pattern involves the use of preferred provider organizations (PPOs). These managed care plans generally restrict the range of provider choice that consumers have by providing

positive and negative incentives (a.k.a., "steerage") to encourage use of the "preferred providers." The types of "steerage" used include higher or lower payroll contributions for coverage, increased or eliminated deductibles, differential co-insurance, benefit enrichments, lower or higher annual maximum out-of-pocket levels, less claim submission hassle, and others. The basic issue in this organizational form is that the preferred providers generally charge a "wholesale" price rather than a "retail" price and do not assume the collective risk for health care of health plan members. The third major form is the health maintenance organization (HMO) model, which generally operates on a capitation basis with all the risk of health care utilization by health plan beneficiaries transferred to the HMO organization. There are many variants on the HMO model (i.e., network model, staff model, individual practice arrangement (IPA) model, open-ended model, and POS variations) but the major attribute of this form of managed care is the capitated financing of the liability for health care utilization for a defined group of people. To somewhat confuse the situation, many HMOs, to gain increased market share, have begun to offer large employers the return of the economic risk for their beneficiary populations, resulting in a hybrid HMO delivery system that provides coverage on a self-insured or experience-rated basis for purchasers. Supposedly, this provides the greatest efficiency in health care delivery while the purchaser maintains full control over the economic risk of utilization for the group.

Also inherent in the general concept of managed care are several additional defining characteristics. These include:

- Formal systems of conducting clinical supervision of health care utilization under the plan
- Formal screening, selection, and referral networks for providers
- Prior negotiation with providers about fees or sharing of economic risk
- Provision and use of on-going utilization and cost information to manage the plan
- Ongoing monitoring of provider performance
- Significant diversity in health promotion and disease prevention programming

Even with the ongoing emergence of a consumer backlash, the dominant role and position of managed care in our health care system is not likely to be reversed in the years ahead. The ever expanding mainstream presence of managed care along with increased competitive pressures are likely to provide fertile ground for the expansion and evolution of health promotion and disease prevention efforts.

MAJOR FORCES SHAPING HEALTH PROMOTION AND PREVENTION IN MANAGED CARE

The changing pattern of health promotion and disease prevention programming in managed care is being influenced by a number of major forces (8). These major forces work to either restrain or enhance the expansion of health promotion and disease prevention efforts in managed care. Table 78-1 contains two lists of the major forces affecting prevention programming in managed care settings, with a few words of

Table 78-1 Major Forces Shaping Prevention Efforts in Managed Care

Factors Likely to Restrain Prevention Efforts

"Free-rider" economic principle	If others provide preventive services and purchasers can benefit without having to, they will.
Severe price competition	Exceptionally tight margins may eliminate investment in prevention, particularly for those who are likely to leave the plan in the near term.
Managed care backlash	If consumers avoid managed care plans because of the backlash against managed care, it will lead to less managed care and less preventive activity.
Growth of "virtual" networks	These "virtual" networks, with limited organizational resources, generally have a lower level of investment in prevention.
Significant disenrollment levels	If disenrollment is high, prevention with a long lead time is less economically defensible, leading to lower investment.
Absence of regulatory requirements	Without specific legislative requirements, managed care plans may not invest uniformly in prevention.
Removal of cost-sharing incentive for health care	With lower point-of-use consumer cost-sharing, there is less of a consumer demand for prevention and demand management.

Factors Likely to Enhance Prevention Efforts

Need for product differentiation	Pressure to differentiate health plans will likely result in increased prevention investment and capability.
Greater consumer interest in prevention	Market demand expressed by individual consumers will likely increase the amount of prevention in managed care.
Purchaser interest in prevention	Specific demands of purchasers will likely increase the amount of prevention.
Increasing scientific evidence for prevention	As more scientific evidence mounts regarding prevention, more will be desired and performed.
Technologic developments	Newer technology that can be used to deliver preventive services more efficiently and effectively can increase the amount of prevention performed by managed care plans.
Increased capitation and risk transfer	The greater the proportion of the population under capitation the greater the investment in prevention.
Expansion of HEDIS requirements	The heavier the reliance by purchasers on prevention-related HEDIS indicators as a proxy measure of quality of care, the more prevention will be carried out by managed care organizations.
Use of financial wellness incentives	As more employers and MCOs use financial wellness incentives, health promotion and disease prevention efforts will increase.
Expansion of the transtheoretical model (stages of change)	As broader application of the transtheoretical model occurs, resulting in more effective programs, more health promotion and disease prevention efforts will likely result.

HEDIS, Health Plan Employer Data Information Set.

explanation, based on whether they are likely to restrain or enhance prevention efforts in managed care settings.

TYPICAL HEALTH PROMOTION OFFERINGS IN MANAGED CARE SETTINGS

There is no central information source that has information on all the primary, secondary, and tertiary prevention activity currently provided by the more than 700 managed care organizations (MCOs), but an older article (9) examined the health promotion activity of more than 300 HMOs. More recently, another article published in the *American Journal of Health Promotion* examined 20 HMOs serving one large employer and found a very wide range of health promotion and disease prevention activities (10). Table 78-2 reflects a summary of the findings in this article regarding the primary, secondary, and tertiary prevention targets and modalities offered by at least 40% of the 20 HMOs surveyed. Many additional prevention targets and intervention modalities can be included in a managed care–based health promotion and disease prevention program. Again, these proposed prevention activities constitute a possible minimum approach for an MCO.

PITFALLS AND CHALLENGES

There are a number of major pitfalls and challenges to the delivery of health promotion and disease prevention efforts in managed care settings. These pitfalls appear to be more significant in selected forms of MCOs than in others (11). Some of the major challenges include:

Table 78-2 Typical Health Promotion and Disease Prevention Components of Managed Care Organizations

Prevention Targets	In-Facility Group Education	Worksite-Based Education or Screening	Printed Materials	Video Materials
Smoking cessation	X	X	X	
Weight management	X	X	X	X
Nutrition education	X	X	X	X
Stress management	X	X	X	X
General wellness	X		X	
Physical activity		X	X	
Health risk appraisal		X	X	
Cholesterol testing	X	X	X	
Blood pressure screening		X	X	
Mammography		X	X	
Childbirth education	X		X	
Diabetes education	X		X	X
Asthma management	X		X	X
Medical self-care	X	X	X	X
Parenting and childcare	X		X	X
High-risk pregnancy intervention	X		X	

SOURCE: Reproduced by permission from Chapman L. Worksite health promotion in the managed care era. The Art of Health Promotion (newsletter) 1998;1(6):6.

Program Design Limitations

- Inadequately or poorly designed programs and activities
- Overemphasis on preventive targets with long lead times for improvements in health and reduction in health care utilization
- Fragmentation or lack of integration of preventive efforts
- Confusion of consumers regarding preventive interventions and expectations about prevention
- Unwillingness for MCOs to work in cooperation with employers
- Conflict with revenue production objectives

Program Implementation Difficulties

- Poorly implemented programs that were initially well designed
- Lack of a balanced set of incentives for prevention among practitioners, patients, and MCOs
- Overt or covert bias against prevention on the part of practitioners
- Insufficient technical and clinical knowledge about preventive interventions and newer prevention methods
- Absence of adequate administrative structure for follow-up and programming

Program Evaluation Weaknesses

- Difficulty associated with measuring "what does not occur" (i.e., the prevention of morbidity)
- Inadequate linkage of clinical information between program and practitioners
- Fragmentation of clinical information on prevention procedures

- Expansive information requirements under Health Plan Employer Data Information Set (HEDIS)

Each of these potential pitfalls has specific countermeasures to assure that they do not lead to less than optimal interventions or program efforts. Many of these countermeasures and counterresponses can be observed in the design of the more optimal forms of programming that follow.

OPTIMAL DESIGN OF HEALTH PROMOTION PROGRAMS IN MANAGED CARE

Optimal health promotion and disease prevention programming in managed care are certainly possible, but they require a very clear commitment and strong leadership from health plan senior managers. The term "optimal" also has to take into consideration the size of the population base served by the organization and the financial resources available for use in providing a full range of health promotion and disease prevention efforts. In addition to these general considerations, a companion set of issues are of significant concern in the development of an optimal health promotion and disease prevention program. These include:

- The need to recognize restraining and enhancing forces that are unique to the specific managed care environment
- The need to determine and summarize the prevention needs of the population involved
- The need to recognize what interventions should fit into each of the three program intervention levels contained in Figure 78-1.

In accordance with the program pyramid model, which defines the mix of interventions that are relevant for the population-at-large, as well as for groups within the popula-

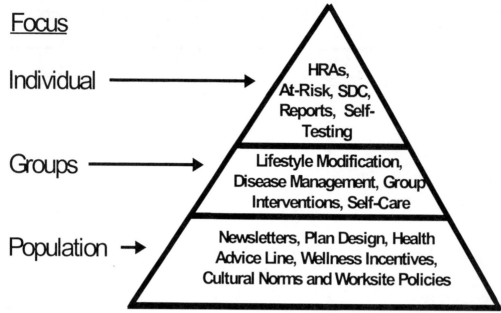

Focus

Individual ⟶

Groups ⟶

Population →

(Pyramid contents:)

HRAs, At-Risk, SDC, Reports, Self-Testing

Lifestyle Modification, Disease Management, Group Interventions, Self-Care

Newsletters, Plan Design, Health Advice Line, Wellness Incentives, Cultural Norms and Worksite Policies

Figure 78-1 Program pyramid for population health management (HRA, health risk appraisal; SDC, self-directed change materials).

tion (including the needs of individuals), the previously identified considerations help determine the unique health promotion and disease prevention needs for these defined populations. Needs can usually be addressed through a core set of interventions or technology (12–16). This core technology has been integrated and is identified as the proactive prevention model (PPM) (17). The major characteristics of this model are as follows:

1. Require the completion of a morbidity-based health risk appraisal (HRA) as a part of initial enrollment or annual re-enrollment. This may require the establishment of an incentive for completion if it is not possible to use an enrollment disincentive (annual survey).

2. Provide a personalized feedback report to each individual completing the survey (report).

3. Conduct a proactive phone-based or mail-based intervention with those individuals who have excess risk for cardiovascular disease, selected cancers, or selected chronic conditions and have not completed some basic preventive screening examinations according to their need (at-risk intervention).

4. Offer access for individuals to request a variety of different self-directed change materials in the survey report package and at the point of contact during the at-risk intervention process (materials).

5. Mail a monthly wellness newsletter to each home (newsletter).

6. Mail to each home a general medical self-care text with an option to call and order an accompanying explanatory video or complete a self-test on the book with a mail-back incentive provision (text).

7. Promote the use of a toll-free health advice line that can provide a broad range of information on health education topics, consumer coaching, and other health

issues; information on program offerings available through your MCO staff or from other community agencies; and access to pre-recorded audio messages on a large number of health and wellness topics (health advice line).

8. Develop and offer a set of educational interventions that address the needs and interests of the population group involved (program interventions).

9. Possible addition of an incentive dimension with a merchandise catalog for selected wellness achievements linked to the annual HRA (incentive).

This core set of interventions and prevention technology, when combined with tailored educational interventions, represents one of the most efficient approaches to the management of health for geographically concentrated or dispersed populations. This technology allows the tailoring of the intervention to fit the organizational and clinical objectives of the managed care organization, while providing a working platform for population health management.

EVALUATION STRATEGIES FOR MANAGED CARE SETTINGS

All health promotion and disease prevention activities should have an evaluation and metrics strategy. Without it, the outcome and value of prevention is neither documented nor validated (18,19). It is critical that a valid and credible process be used for evaluating the prevention efforts that are directed at defined population groups within a managed care plan. In this section, a variety of evaluation and metric strategies are suggested.

There are nine major recommended evaluation strategies for health promotion and disease prevention efforts that are focused on defined populations.

Accomplishment of Formal Objectives

This evaluation strategy requires the adoption of measurable objectives for the health management initiative, which are used as reference points for the comparison of actual accomplishments versus desired accomplishments. These objectives can take many different forms, from purely operational objectives (i.e., provide a health questionnaire to all adult health plan members by March 15th) to outcome-oriented objectives (i.e., reduce the number of adults within the high-risk level for total serum cholesterol in the target population by 25% by July 1). This constitutes a very flexible component of an overall program evaluation plan and can meet many different technical, programmatic, and political objectives, if designed carefully.

Common Form of Metrics

- Percent of objective accomplished
- Classification of objective as fully achieved, partially achieved, or not achieved
- The specific form depends on the type and format of the objectives that are used

HEDIS Indicators

This evaluation strategy involves the measurement and collection of HEDIS indicators, including more than 50 prevention-oriented indicators within HEDIS version 3.0, released in 1997. These indicators provide normative references for evaluating performance across entire health plan populations. Some of the types of issues included in HEDIS are: immunization rates, prenatal care, otitis media treatment patterns, flu shots to at-risk populations, asthmatic treatment patterns, retinal exams for diabetic patients, pap smear rates, cesarean section rates, and vaginal birth after casarean (VBAC) rates (20).

Common Form of Metrics

- Rates for specific indicators
- Age- and sex-adjusted indicator scores
- Positional ranking with other MCOs

Participation Levels

This evaluation strategy involves the measurement of the size of the eligible population, the proportion at-risk for the specific prevention issue or target being addressed, and the number and proportion that have taken part in the appropriate health management activity to date. If the health management effort being evaluated has multiple sessions or multiple interventions, the participation measures can include the percent of planned activities that were completed. The purpose of this evaluation strategy is to determine the overall effectiveness of the program in meeting the needs of the population involved and to help determine the magnitude of interventions used by the population.

Common Form of Metrics

- Number of individuals in the defined population
- Number and percent of individuals at-risk
- Number and percent of individuals at-risk who participate in the program
- Number of individuals completing each level of program

Participant Feedback

This evaluation strategy uses direct feedback on a range of issues from individual participants. Some of the major types of participant feedback include: perceptions about strengths, weaknesses, and quality of the program; perceptions about satisfaction with the program or activity; perceptions about the role of the program in supporting behavior change; and the perception of participants about what would be most helpful as a follow-up. The purpose of this evaluation strategy is to provide information that will help evaluate the relevance of the program to observed behavioral change and to enhance the effectiveness of the health management activity involved.

Common Form of Metrics

- Number and proportion of participants indicating particular levels of quality of the program (quantitative or qualitative scales)
- Number and proportion of participants indicating particular levels of satisfaction with the program
- Number and proportion of participants indicating particular levels of perceived importance of the program to personal behavior change associated with the program
- Number and proportion of participants requesting various follow-up intervention modalities or activities

Health Risk Prevalence Changes

This evaluation strategy includes data on risk factors and health behavior from the participant or target population, usually collected from health questionnaires or from biometric screening results. Risk prevalence data are often portrayed as percentages of a base population group. Changes in health risk prevalence are significant outcome measures to monitor in virtually all health management initiatives. The concept of prevalence in an epidemiologic sense reflects the innate burden of risk existing within a defined population at any point in time. For evaluation validity, consistent time intervals and times of the year for measurement are recommended. The aging of populations should also be examined and adjusted for in the context of the total population. Gender correction is also recommended. If individuals are used as their own controls in providing health-risk prevalence comparisons, then the aging or maturation in the population sample should be considered for adjustment of the population data. Typical health-risk prevalence comparisons may include percent of tobacco users (smoking and smokeless), average serum cholesterol level, and percent not wearing safety restraints in motor vehicles.

Common Form of Metrics

- Number and proportion with an identified risk factor
- Average score for the selected risk factor before and after the intervention for the population and the comparison group

Changes in Stage of Readiness

This evaluation strategy involves the categorization of subjects in the population according to their stage of change regarding a specific health behavior. For example, if regular moderate exercise were the behavioral focus, the number and percent of individuals in each of the following five categories would be determined at a specific point in time (21,22):

- Those not considering moderate (or vigorous) exercise
- Those considering beginning exercise but with no plans to do so within 30 days
- Those who have made a decision to start exercising within the next 30 days
- Those who have been exercising but have not been consistently at it for a minimum of 2 years
- Those who have been exercising regularly on a consistent basis for a period of more than 2 years

Movements in stages of change are based on comparing each individual's stage of readiness at intervals and then comparing the percent of individuals who have progressed to the next stage or regressed to earlier stages and measuring the percent in each of the major stages. These evaluation parameters are useful in reviewing the extent to which the intervention is resulting in the desired behavior and the movement of the stage of readiness to change in the population.

Common Form of Metrics:

- Percent of persons in each stage of change, at baseline, for a specific health behavior
- Percent in each stage of change at follow-up for that specific health behavior
- Percent of change in number of persons in each stage of change before and after the program or intervention
- Percent of target population in first three stages of change at baseline and follow-up
- Percent of target population in last two stages of change at baseline and follow-up

Risk Status Changes

This next evaluation strategy requires the capability to categorize each individual in the population or group as at low, medium, or high risk for a specific outcome. In the case of specific risks that are not measured in a quantitative manner, each individual may be viewed as at risk, not at risk, or potentially at risk with the passage of time. An example of the quantitatively defined risk is serum cholesterol levels as recommended by the National Heart, Lung, and Blood Institute of the National Institutes of Health National Cholesterol Education Program. A low-risk serum cholesterol level would be less than 200 mg/dL, a medium-risk level would be 200 to 239 mg/dL, and a high-risk level would be more than 240 mg/dL. Similar examples exist for high-density lipoprotein (HDL) level and ratio, low-density lipoprotein (LDL) level, and triglyceride level. The proportion or percent of an adult population in each of the three categories can then be determined at baseline and at consistent future points in time. An example of a nonquantitative risk status change would be the number or percent of individuals in a defined population that are at risk from the lack of seat belt use. This evaluation strategy is limited to subjects as their own comparisons, if the same population is examined before and after the implementation of the program.

Common Forms of Metrics

- Percent of subjects in each risk category at baseline
- Percent of subjects in each risk category at follow-up

- Number of subjects in entire population that could theoretically be at risk (extrapolated from sample data)
- Percent of subjects potentially at risk who are actually at risk

Utilization and Cost Effects

This evaluation strategy is profoundly important because it has the potential of providing the economic justification for expenditures on prevention and health management. Utilization of health care services is one of the major areas of focus within this evaluation area. The conventional approach to measuring utilization of health care includes: hospital admission or discharge rates, days of hospitalization, average length of stay, physician visit rates, prescriptions filled, specialty referral rates, and dental visit rates. Utilization generally drives the cost of health care for the population involved and, therefore, is exceedingly important in arriving at an assessment of the economic impact of the health management initiative. Cost effects are generally related to the health care costs associated with the group but can also include lost time costs (sick leave, absenteeism, and management of disability salary/wage replacement) and worker compensation costs (both medical reimbursement and salary continuation).

Common Form of Metrics

- Rate of use of a specific type of health care among a selected multiple of the population
- Per capita amount of health-related costs per individual in the target population

Cost-Benefit and Net Present Value

One of the most sophisticated forms of economic evaluation applicable to health management programming is the use of cost-benefit (C/B) derivations and net present value (NPV) calculations. Indirect cost and direct costs for the program intervention are compared with the indirect benefit and direct benefit associated with the program intervention. If life-cycle effects, discounting, subsidiary assumptions, and scenario modifications are used, they can create very comprehensive C/B evaluation scenarios. C/B derivations attempt to determine the ratio of cost or investment to the production of economic savings. This method measures the "potency" of an intervention without determining the relative wealth created for the organization by a specific intervention. NPV calculations, on the other hand, meet the need for this key analytic process by projecting or confirming the net economic value of the specific health management intervention to the organization. NPV therefore is a more refined economic measure and allows a more discriminating analysis.

Common Form of Metrics

- Cost-benefit ratio for an identified time period (C/B ratio)
- Negative or positive number of dollars associated with the introduction of the proposed intervention (NPV)

CONCLUSIONS AND FUTURE TRENDS

Health promotion and disease prevention efforts in managed care are likely to have a positive future. The newer emerging prevention methods and technology and the growing societal need for prevention and health improvement are likely to be continuing factors in their widespread growth in the decades ahead (19, 23–25). The following major trends are likely to affect health promotion and disease prevention activities in managed care settings in the years ahead:

1. Increased focus on health promotion and disease prevention interventions with short-term yield (i.e., 1 to 3 years)

2. Increased movement to proactive forms of programming

3. Greater integration of disease prevention into clinical practice

4. More use of complementary healing arts

5. Expanded use of technology in prevention programming

6. Increased balance and integration among primary, secondary, and tertiary prevention concerns

7. Greater *customization* of preventive interventions

These trends will continue to change the face of prevention in American medicine and may ultimately lead to the capability of our health care system to successfully minimize the individual and collective burden of morbidity and premature mortality. Economic pressures will likely be the major force that moves prevention from the periphery of the U.S. health care system to its center in the years ahead.

REFERENCES

1. Chapman L. Worksite health promotion in the managed care era. The Art of Health Promotion (newsletter) 1998;1(6):6.

2. Harris J, Gordon R, White K, et al. Prevention and managed care: opportunities for managed care organizations, purchasers of health care, and public health agencies. MMWR 1995;44:1–12.

3. Ellwood P. Health maintenance strategy. Medical Care 1971;9: 291–297.

4. Chapman L. Affordable employee health care: a model benefit program. New York: AMACOM Publications, 1992:355.

5. Chapman L. Integrated prevention: applications for managed care settings. Seattle: Summex Corporation, 1996:146.

6. Brook R. Does free care improve adults' health? N Engl J Med 1983;319:342–346.

7. Chapman L. The challenge of managing the demand for health care: an imperative for future health care reform. J Amer Compensation Assoc 1994;3:2–13.

8. Chapman L. Worksite health promotion in the managed care era. The Art of Health Promotion Newsletter 1998;1:1–8.

9. Bernton C. What is the future for health promotion in HMOs? Amer J Health Prom 1987;1:24–27.

10. Chapman L, Nelson L, Sloan B, et al. Secondary and tertiary prevention capabilities of selected HMOs: findings of an employer survey. Amer J Health Prom 1997;12: 98–107.

11. Gemson D. Health promotion and disease prevention in HMOs: a survey of newly established IPAs in New York City. Amer J Preven Med 1995;6:333–338.

12. Fries J, Koop CE, Beadle C, et al. Reducing health care costs by reducing the need and demand for medical services. N Engl J Med 1993;329:321–325.

13. Gustafson D, Bosworth K, Chewning B, Hawkins R. Computer-based health promotion: combining technological advances with problem-solving techniques to effect successful health behavior changes. Ann Rev Public Health 1987;8:387–415.

14. Harber P, Czisny K, Hsu P, et al. An expert system-based preventive medicine examination adviser. J Occup Environ Med 1995;37: 563–570.

15. Kellie S, Griffith H. Emerging trends in assessing performance and managing in health care: expectations for implementing preventive services. Amer J Preven Med 1995;11:388–392.

16. Loeppke R. Prevention and managed care: the next generation. J Occup Environ Med 1995;37:558–562.

17. Chapman L. Health management: optimal approaches for managing the health of defined populations. Seattle: Summex Corporation, 1997:175.

18. Thompson R, McAfee T, Stuart M. A review of clinical prevention services at Group Health Cooperative of Puget Sound. Amer J Preven Med 1995;11:409–416.

19. Friede A, O'Carroll P, Nicola R, et al, eds. CDC prevention guidelines: a guide to action. Baltimore: Williams & Wilkins, 1997:1556.

20. National Committee on Quality Assurance. Health plan employer data information set (HEDIS), Version 3.0. Washington, DC: 1997.

21. Prochaska J. Stages of change and decisional balance for 12 problem behaviors. Health Psych 1994;13: 39–45.

22. Cardinal B. Development and evaluation of stage-matched written materials about lifestyle and structured physical activity. Percept Motor Skills 1995;80:543–546.

23. Thompson R, Taplin S, McAfee T, et al. Primary and secondary prevention services in clinical practice: twenty years experience in development, implementation, and evaluation. JAMA 1995;273: 1130–1135.

24. U.S. Preventive Services Task Force. Guide to clinical preventive services. 2nd ed. Baltimore: Williams & Wilkins, 1996:953.

25. Woolf S, ed. Health promotion and disease prevention in clinical practice. Baltimore: Williams & Wilkins, 1996:618.

Chapter 79

The Impact on Health of Workplace Health Promotion Programs and the Methodologic Quality of the Research Literature

Michael P. O'Donnell

A comprehensive review of the published literature on the health impact of workplace health promotion programs was conducted to determine the impact of these programs and the quality of the research methodology of the published literature.

METHODOLOGY

A literature search was conducted using all of the major computer databases, to identify all of the published literature on the health effects of workplace health promotion programs. The computer databases searched are shown in table 79-1, and topics searched are shown in table 79-2. Additionally, a manual search of the health promotion literature was conducted. Finally, the references cited in all the articles identified through the computer and manual search were gathered. Literature was included that was published between 1968 and 1994 (the central search was conducted in 1994), and empirical results of health promotion interventions in workplace settings were reported. This search identified 325 studies.

Reports of these studies were distributed to 11 sets of subject-matter experts who completed their own additional search using the same inclusion and exclusion criteria. The subject matter experts are named in table 79-3. These experts identified 58 additional studies, many of which were published in 1995, after the central literature search was conducted, for a total of 383 studies. A tally of the articles by intervention focus and program strategy is shown in table 79-4. The number of studies listed under "search" were found through the central literature search. The number listed under "review" represent the total number critiqued, including those

found through the central search and those found through the manual searches of each author. Some of the studies found in the initial search were not included in the final review because they have two-star ratings. Most (92%) of the studies focused on educating the employee, 6.5% reported on efforts to change policy, and only a handful reported on efforts to train managers or educate families.

Each set of authors critiqued the literature in their subject area and wrote a literature review. This chapter summarizes the results reported in those 11 reviews. The complete reviews have been published in the *American Journal of Health Promotion* (2–10).

The methodology for the body of literature for each intervention area was rated as conclusive, acceptable, indicative, suggestive, or weak using the criteria in table 79-5. The methodology of each individual study was rated on a one- to five-star scale, using the criteria shown at the bottom of table 79-6. In most cases, only five-, four-, or three-star studies were included in the final review. Two-star studies were included if they offered some unique findings or if there were very few higher-rated studies for the specific intervention area.

RESULTS

Ratings for the body of literature in each of the 11 intervention areas and a count of the number of studies at each of the research rating levels are shown in table 79-6. Brief comments about the conclusions that can be drawn from the studies in each area and the focus required for future research are discussed in this section. The ratings for the individual

Table 79-1 Computer Databases Searched

Medline
Aidsline
Psychological Abstracts
Combined Health Information Database
Employee Benefits Infosource
National Prevention Evaluation Research Collection
National Resource Center for Worksite Health Promotion
National Technical Information Service
Substance Abuse Information Database

Table 79-2 Topics Included in Search

Alcohol abuse
Back injury
Cancer
Cardiovascular disease
Drug abuse
Exercise
Health risk appraisal
HIV/AIDS
Hypertension
Hypercholesterolemia
Multicomponent programs
Nutrition
Seat belt use
Smoking
Stress management
Weight control

Table 79-3 Interventions and Authors

Alcohol: Paul M. Roman, Terry C. Blum
Exercise: Roy J. Shephard
Health risk appraisal: David R. Anderson, Michael J. Staufacker
Nutrition and cholesterol: Karen Glanz, Glorian Sorensen, Anna Farmer
Weight control: Deborah Hennrikus, Robert W. Jeffery
Hypertension: Andrea A. Foote
HIV/AIDS: Mark G. Wilson, Cynthia Jorgensen, Galin Cole
Multicomponent programs: Catherine Heaney, Ronald Goetzel
Seat belts: James M. Eddy, Eugene C. Fitzhugh, G. Greg Wojowicz, Min Qi Wang
Smoking: Michael P. Ericksen
Stress management: Lawrence R. Murphy

studies and more detailed results of the findings are reported in the published review for each subject area (2–10).

Hypertension

The highest quality research has been in hypertension control programs, with an overall research rating of "conclusive." There have been 32 studies published in this area; almost one-half were rated as five-star studies and almost two-thirds were rated as four- or five-star studies.

Program participation rates are high, with an average of 79% of eligible employees participating, and success rates in controlling hypertension are high, ranging from 60% to 85% while programs are in place. Educational programs by themselves, without medical treatment, have not yet been successful in controlling hypertension.

Future research can make the greatest contribution to the literature if hypertension control programs are investigated within the context of comprehensive programs. Research is also needed to identify the characteristics of the most effective programs.

Stress Management

The research in stress management has also been high-quality, with 64 published studies, over one-half with five-star ratings and over three-quarters with four- or five-star ratings. The research rating is indicative for the literature as a whole and acceptable for programs that use a combination of strategies.

Programs have been shown to have a positive effect on anxiety and muscle tension; minimal effect on blood pressure and job satisfaction; and the effect on depression, irritability, and somatic complaints has been unclear.

There is sufficient evidence to draw conclusions about the most effective methods for a variety of outcomes. Biofeedback has not been very effective as an intervention on any of the outcomes measured. Muscle relaxation has been most effective for physiologic improvements. Cognitive-behavioral training has been most effective for psychological outcomes and effective for job satisfaction. Custom programs designed for the specific needs of the organization have been most effective for organizational outcomes. Meditation has been an effective intervention for all the different outcomes measured, and the most successful programs used a combination of techniques.

The greatest progress in stress management can be made if research is directed toward programs that include both individual and organizational strategies. Also, the most powerful sources of stress in the work environment must be identified, and given the personal nature of the interventions, employees need to be involved in program design and evaluation. Many of the programs were developed on the basis of the individual strengths and biases of the program developers, and few were guided by theory. Developing programs guided by theory will facilitate transferring programs from one site to another and will help in standardizing evaluation efforts and in establishing causal relationships between programs and outcomes.

Weight Control

The quality of research has been fairly good for weight control programs, with 46 published studies, a quarter of which were five-star ratings and almost one-half of which had four- or five-star ratings. The overall rating for the literature was indicative.

Programs show short-term weight losses averaging 1 to 2 pounds per week, but there is little evidence of long-term weight loss, and the characteristics of the most successful strategies are not clear.

	Table 79-4 Studies Reviewed									
	NUMBER OF STUDIES									
	POLICY		**EMPLOYEE EDUCATION**		**FAMILY EDUCATION**		**MANAGER TRAINING**		**TOTAL STUDIES**	
INTERVENTION	**SEARCHED**	**REVIEWED**	**SEARCHED**	**REVIEWED**	**SEARCHED**	**REVIEWED**	**SEARCHED**	**REVIEWED**	**SEARCHED**	**REVIEWED**
Alcohol	2	0	24	19			5	5	31	24
Exercise			32	52					32	52
Health risk appraisal			3	11					3	11
Nutrition and cholesterol			27	24					27	24
Weight control			30	44					30	44
Hypertension			37	31					37	31
HIV and AIDS			7	12					7	12
Multicomponent	0	7	48	22	2	1			50	30
Seabelts			14	14					14	14
Smoking	17	19	42	49					59	68
Stress management			22	64					22	64
Total Studies	19	26	286	340	2	1	5	5	325	383

NOTE: The computer search found 325 articles. The review included 383 because additional studies were found through a manual search.

The quality of research in this area will be enhanced by more randomized designs, with replication of studies at multiple sites. Multiple outcomes beyond weight loss need to be examined, such as recruitment strategies and participation rates. The effect of organizational factors such as organization norms on weight loss and the impact of intervention programs on organizational factors should be examined. Very little is know about the most effective techniques: This must be studied. Finally, more consistent documentation of study results is required to facilitate replication of studies.

Smoking Control

Smoking control programs take two basic forms: smoking cessation and smoking policy. Given the significant difference between these two strategies, they were reviewed separately in this effort.

Thirty-nine studies of smoking cessation were published, 12 of which were five-star studies. The literature in this area was rated as acceptable for specific methods of cessation, indicative for competitions, and suggestive for minimal treatments and interventions. Quit rates for programs varied greatly, ranging from 20% to 60%. Accounting for the quality of methodology, a quit rate of 25% is most likely accurate. Programs with minimal treatment had lower quit rates, ranging from 1% to 20%. Group programs have higher quit rates than minimal interventions, but minimal interventions are often able to reach more people. Few studies have long-term follow-up. Incentives and contests are successful in increasing participation rates but do not seem to increase quit rates.

Twenty-seven studies were published for smoking cessation programs, 24 of which were three-star studies. The literature was only suggestive for reduction of smoking at work and weak for smoking cessation and overall cigarette consumption. Policies do seem be successful in reducing exposure to environmental tobacco smoke, and reduce cigarette consumption at work by about three cigarettes per day. The impact on total consumption or cessation is not clear.

To improve the quality of future research, studies should measure the impact of interventions designed for each of stages of readiness to change, use the worksite as unit of analysis, measure impact of worksite policies on self-reported smoking and exposure to environmental tobacco smoke, and measure the prevalance of policy coverage among worksites.

Nutrition and Cholesterol Programs

The total number of studies examining the impact of nutrition and cholesterol programs has been small at 26, but the quality has been fairly good, with one-half of the nutrition studies and almost one-third of the cholesterol studies rating five stars. The body of literature was rated "suggestive" to "indicative" for both areas.

The conclusions we can draw about the impact of nutrition programs are limited. Group education, combined with counseling, produces short-term changes, but the impact on long-term changes is not clear. Cafeteria programs show promise in changing cafeteria purchases. More intensive strategies have greater impact than less intensive strategies.

The conclusions we can draw about the impact of cholesterol reduction programs are also limited. Counseling combined with follow-up meetings or distribution of educational materials produces short-term changes. Group education also produces short-term changes. More intensive strategies have greater impact, but less intensive strategies may be able to reach more people and should thus sometimes be utilized.

The improvements needed in research on nutrition and cholesterol programs include using standard measures, using the worksite as the unit of analysis, using more rigorous research designs, and giving more attention to determining what strategies are most effective. Fortunately, six large-scale controlled trials are in progress that should address most of the deficiencies in the research (11–15).

Table 79-5 Research Ratings For Body of Literature
Conclusive • Cause and effect relationship between intervention and outcome supported by substantial number of well-designed studies with randomized control groups • Nearly universal agreement by experts in the field regarding impact
Acceptable • Cause and effect relationship supported by well-designed studies with randomized control groups • Agreement by majority of experts in the field regarding impact
Indicative • Relationships supported by substantial number of well-designed studies but few or no studies with randomized control groups • Majority of experts in the field believe that relationship is causal, based on existing body of evidence, but view it as tentative because of lack of randomized studies and potential alternative explanations
Suggestive • Multiple studies with consistent relationships, but no well-designed studies with randomized control groups • Majority of experts in the field believe causal impact is consistent with knowledge in related areas, but see support as limited and acknowledge plausible explanations
Weak • Research supporting relationship is fragmentary, nonexperimental, or poorly done • Majority of experts in the field believe causal impact is plausible, but no more plausible than alternative explanations

Exercise

Despite the long-standing presence of exercise programs in the workplace, and the relatively large number of studies conducted, the quality of the literature in this is only suggestive, with only 5 of the 52 studies earning five-star ratings and 14 earning four-star ratings.

We can conclude that workplace exercise programs do reduce body fat and body mass and improve aerobic power, muscle strength, and flexibility while people remain in the programs. The impact on long-term changes is not clear, and the impact on reduction in smoking and improvement in mood state is not clear.

To improve the quality of future research, we need larger scale studies with controlled designs, and we need to focus on measures beyond physical fitness, in areas such as blood pressure levels, emotional factors, and smoking behavior. Many fitness programs are now offered within the context of comprehensive health promotion programs, so it will be difficult to isolate the impact of the fitness program.

Safety Belt Programs

The number of studies examining the effect of safety belt programs has been limited, with only 14 reported in the literature, but more than two-thirds of these studies earned four-star ratings, and the body of literature as whole is rated "suggestive."

Seat belt programs increase seat belt use in the short term, and long-term relapse rates remain above baseline. Incentives, awareness programs, and goal-setting strategies are common, but it is not clear which strategies are most effective. Many programs were implemented during a national media blitz or when state seat belt laws changed, so it is difficult to determine the impact of the program independent of those influences.

The greatest improvements in research on seat belt programs can come from conducting controlled trials, identifying the intervention strategies that are the most effective, and determining how to reduce relapse. However, given the passage of laws requiring seat belt use, most employers are not implementing seat belt programs, and further funding for research in this area is not likely.

Health Risk Appraisals

Despite the widespread use of health risk appraisals (HRA) in workplace health promotion programs, only 11 studies have been published on their effects, and only 2 of those have been five-star level studies. The research rating for this body of literature was "weak" for stand-alone HRAs and "suggestive" for HRA use within comprehensive programs.

There is no evidence that HRAs change health conditions, but there is some evidence to show that they can increase seat belt use and physical activity. There has been very little research to measure changes at the precontemplation, contemplation, and preparation stages, which are the stages of change most appropriate to expect from HRAs.

The research most important for HRAs is a concentration on changes at the precontemplation,, contemplation, and preparation stages; identifying the characteristics of effective HRAs; and determining the characteristics of effective implementation.

Alcohol

There have been 25 studies on the impact of alcohol prevention programs. Most have been at the two-star level; the overall body of literature is rated "weak" to "suggestive"; and we can conclude very little from this literature.

We can conclude that alcohol programs within the context of employee assistance programs (EAP) are effective in reaching employees in crisis, and that educational programs are effective in changing attitudes toward alcohol, but the effect of programs on rates of drinking and the characteristics of successful programs are not clear.

Most of work site alcohol prevention programs have been implemented by recovering alcoholics and social workers who are often very effective in counseling alcoholics but have very little research training. Before effective research can be conducted in alcohol prevention programs, it will be necessary to build basic research infrastructures into intervention communities.

Table 79-6 Research Ratings for Individual Studies and for Bodies of Literature

	5-STAR #	5-STAR %	4-STAR #	4-STAR %	3-STAR #	3-STAR %	2-STAR #	2-STAR %	TOTAL #	RATING
Hypertension	14	44%	5	16%	12	38%	1	3%	32	Conclusive
Stress management	34	53%	15	23%	14	22%	1	2%	64	Indicative to acceptable (for combined programs)
Multicomponent programs	9	25%	16	44%	11	31%	—	—	36	Indicative to acceptable
Weight control	13	28%	9	20%	24	52%	—	—	46	Indicative
Smoking control	12	18%	14	21%	40	59%	—	—	68	
Nutrition	8	50%	1	6%	7	44%	—	—	16	Suggestive to indicative
Cholesterol	3	30%	1	10%	6	60%	—	—	10	Suggestive to indicative
Exercise	5	10%	14	27%	33	63%	—	—	52	Suggestive
Safety belt	—	—	10	71%	4	29%	—	—	14	Suggestive
Health risk appraisal	2	18%	4	36%	5	45%	—	—	11	Weak for stand-alone HRA; suggestive within comprehensive program
Alcohol	2	8%	4	16%	3	12%	16	64%	25	Weak to suggestive
HIV and AIDS	1	9%	2	18%	7	64%	1	9%	11	Weak
Total per rating	103	27%	95	25%	166	43%	19	5%	383	

Rating system:
Five-star, properly conducted study with randomized control group; four-star, properly conducted study with comparison group, but not randomized control group; three-star, evaluation without comparison or control group; two-star, no intervention, but might include long-term or dramatic results from dissemination of information or a medical agent into a population; one-star, descriptive, anecdotal, or authoritative.

HIV and AIDS

Research on the impact of HIV and AIDS programs is very limited, with only 11 published studies, most of which are at the two-star level. This body of literature is rated as "weak."

Very little can be concluded about the impact of HIV and AIDS programs. Most programs are educational and directed to populations in clinical settings who are at risk for exposure to HIV while caring for AIDS patients. None of the studies measured the impact on behaviors, but 10 of 12 studies showed improvements in knowledge or attitudes.

In comparison to alcohol prevention programs, the need for research in HIV and AIDS programs is more clearly recognized, but the research infrastructure is comparably undeveloped. Research in this area should focus on refinement of efficient and effective strategies to change knowledge, attitudes, and behaviors; attention to policy, manager training, family education, and community outreach strategies; development of valid and reliable measures of knowledge, attitudes, and behavior; measurement of individual, organizational, and community outcomes; and rigorous research designs.

Multicomponent Programs

Programs that included a number of interventions, such as exercise, nutrition, and stress management, or any combination of the intervention areas considered in this review, were considered multicomponent programs. The number of studies within this area was moderately large, with 36 published studies, and two-thirds of these studies were rated with four or

five stars. The body of literature for multicomponent programs was rated "indicative" to "acceptable."

Reviewing the impact of multicomponent programs is more complicated than assessing single-intervention studies, but also more revealing. Many of these programs used multiple strategies such as awareness, skill building, and organizational level change. Also, these multicomponent programs affect multiple intervention areas (e.g., fitness, nutrition, and stress management), and can affect knowledge, attitudes, behavior, and health conditions in each of these areas. To simplify reporting these results in aggregate, we classified program outcomes as those that are "mostly positive outcomes," "some positive outcomes," and "few positive outcomes." As shown in table 79-7, programs that included individual counseling had mostly positive outcomes almost twice as often (80%) as programs that did not (47%). This provides compelling evidence that programs will be more successful if they include an individual counseling component. Also, table 79-7 shows that programs that included a combination of information, skill building, and organizational enhancements were slightly more likely to have "mostly positive outcomes" than programs that did not include all three of these approaches. The difference in effectiveness was too modest for us to draw any conclusion.

The research in multicomponent programs can be improved by including measures of employee satisfaction as outcome and moderator variables, randomly assigning participants to different strategies, measuring the impact on each program subobjective, including a qualitative evaluation component, and reporting more detail on program content and objectives.

DISCUSSION

This review is the first comprehensive review of the literature on the health impact of workplace health promotion programs. A total of 365 studies published between 1968 and 1995 that reported empiric results of the effects of workplace health promotion programs were critiqued. The review aids understanding of both the quality of the research methods and the health effects of workplace health promotion programs.

Health Impact

This review shows us that health promotion programs *usually* produce short-term changes in knowledge, *often* produce changes in behavior, and *sometimes* produce changes in health, but there is little evidence that these changes last after programs end. From one perspective, this is discouraging. Our initial hope, when we started implementing programs more than 2 decades ago, was that we could educate people on the benefits of a healthy lifestyle and teach them some skills to improve their lifestyle and that this would produce a life-changing metamorphosis. Voila! They would become (like us) good health converts who maintain these practices for the rest of their lives. From another perspective, the impact we see from programs is encouraging,. In recent years, we have begun to realize that our original expectation was not realistic. Where else in our lives do we see such major changes through so little effort? Medical interventions often require weeks and months and sometimes years of intensive and expensive intervention to produce changes that revert when the treatment is withdrawn. Psychotherapy often takes 1 or 2 hours per week for 3 to 5 years to produce a change in a person's approach to one aspect of life. Educating ourselves to function in society and perform a job takes 30 to 50 hours per week for 13 to 20 years. Is it realistic to think we can forever change lives with health promotion budgets that average $10 to $20 and 4 to 5 hours of contact per person per year in basic programs and $200 per person per year in the most extensive programs? Of course not, but it is realistic to expect to make short-term changes and maintain these changes as long as people participate in programs. A more realistic strategy is probably to realize that we need to continue to engage people in programs to maintain the health habits we have helped them adopt.

Research Methodology

For the literature as a whole, 103 (27%) were properly conducted studies with randomized control groups (five-star), and 95 (21%) were properly conducted studies with nonrandomized comparison groups (four-star); thus 198 studies, over 50% of the total, had four- or five-star ratings. As a whole, the literature can be rated as "indicative" to "acceptable," which is very encouraging. As a body, this literature is comparable or superior to the body of literature supporting the outcomes of medical interventions. Despite this overall rating, the ratings in many of the individual areas, notably HIV and AIDS, alcohol use, HRAs, seat belt use, and exercise programs, were "weak" or only "suggestive."

This assessment of the literature compares favorably to a comprehensive review of the literature conducted by Warner et al of literature published through 1986 (16). Although their scoring key was different, their overall assessment of the impact of programs on behavior changes was comparable to the rating or "weak" on our scale. Compared to that review, research quality has improved two rungs on the scale, which is quite impressive progress in less than 1 decade.

In summary, we have made good progress in improving the methodologic quality of research on the health impact of workplace health promotion programs. In fact, the methodology and the health effects of our programs are probably of sufficient quality to satisfy all but the most conservative business decision makers. Nevertheless, we need to get better. Our short-term goal should be to raise the overall rating one additional rung on the scale to "acceptable" to "conclusive" and to raise the ratings in each area at least to the "indicative" to "acceptable" level. For the individual researcher, this means that studies lacking at least a comparison group (quasi experimental design) will not make a contribution to the literature accept as exploratory studies of new approaches, and our primary focus should be limited to experimental designs with randomized control groups. The focus of our research should be large-scale studies, utilizing randomized control groups, with more attention on what works best and on long-term results.

If we are able to raise our standard of research to this level, and we are able to demonstrate health improvements, health promotion is likely to become a standard business practice, a standard strategy in medical practice, and a funded priority in state and federal health policy.

THE EFFECT OF RESEARCH DESIGN ON REPORTED RESULTS

It is often difficult for practitioners to understand the importance of rigorous research methodology in health promotion research or in the evaluations of their programs. The need for comparison groups (quasi experimental design), especially randomly assigned control groups (experimental design), is often dismissed as a sophisticated research protocol that scientists love but that has no practical value. The importance of research design in showing the true impact of a program is illustrated by a closer look at the results of multicomponent

Table 79-7 Impact of Strategies on Program Outcomes

	PREDOMINANCE OF POSITIVE OUTCOMES		
PROGRAM STRATEGY	MOSTLY	SOME	FEW
Information only	62.5%	25%	12.5%
Information and skill building	57%	29%	14%
Information, skill building, and organizational enhancements	67%	25%	8%
Individual counseling	80%	13%	7%
No individual counseling	47%	37%	16%

Table 79-8 Impact of Research Design on Outcome Conclusions			
	OUTCOME CONCLUSIONS		
RESEARCH DESIGN	**MOSTLY POSITIVE**	**SOME POSITIVE**	**FEW POSITIVE**
Experimental	25%	50%	25%
Quasi experimental	56%	31%	12%
Nonexperimental	100%	0%	0%

change were comparable. These programs had to show some improvements in most of the outcome measures; those improvements needed to be statistically more significant than the improvements seen in a control group; and the control group members were just as motivated and able to make changes as the intervention group.

Practitioners not trained in statistics typically do not understand the importance of a quasi experimental or an experimental design. They often think it is an academic complication that makes program evaluation more difficult. As a result, they often use a nonexperimental design and conclude that their programs are successful, when in fact changes that occurred after the program may have resulted from other changes that occurred in the workplace or the individual motivation of the participants and may further have occurred without the program. Does this mean that practitioners should stop evaluating their programs if they can only afford to measure before and after changes without a comparison or control group? No, before and after changes are valuable for internal use within the program, especially to show trends over time. However, additional effort should be invested to include at least a comparison group (quasi experimental design) in the initial assessments of a program. Although it takes additional effort, it is usually not difficult to find people within the organization who have decided not to enroll in a program who can be used as a comparison group. Program managers should also explore the possibility of joint ventures with managers at other companies, program vendors, and local universities to conduct controlled trials with randomized designs.

programs as shown in table 79-8. The designs of the studies reviewed were divided into experimental (five-star), quasi experimental (four-star) and nonexperimental (two- and three-star) designs. As in table 79-7, the outcomes of these programs were classified as "mostly positive outcomes," "some positive outcomes," and "few positive outcomes." As the table shows, all of the nonexperimental studies, just over one-half of the quasi experimental studies, and only one-quarter of the experimental studies showed "mostly positive outcomes." This is the pattern a research methodologist would expect. All the nonexperimental studies showed mostly positive outcomes because, to achieve this level of success, the programs merely had to show some statistically significant improvement in most of the outcome measures. The success rate is smaller for the quasi experimental studies because the programs not only had to show some improvements in most of the outcome measures, but those improvements had to be statistically more significant than the improvements seen in a comparison group. The success rate was lowest for the experimental studies because people were randomly assigned to the intervention group and the control group, so their motivation, education, and other factors that might influence successful

This study was funded by the Office of the Associate Director for HIV/AIDS, at the Centers for Disease Control and Prevention as part of an effort to identify strategies that can be used for worksite AIDS prevention programs. This search was coordinated by Mark Wilson (1).

REFERENCES

1. Wilson M, Hollman P, Hammock A. A comprehensive review of the effects of worksite health promotion on health-related outcomes. Amer J Health Prom 1996;11: 429–435.

2. Anderson D, Staufacker M. The impact of worksite-based health risk appraisal on health related outcomes: a review of the literature. Amer J Health Prom 1996; 10:499–508.

3. Eddy J, Fitzhugh E, Wojowicz G, Wang M. The impact of worksite-based safety belt programs: a review of the literature. Amer J Health Prom 1997;11:281–290.

4. Glanz K, Sorensen G, Farmer A. The health impact of worksite nutrition and cholesterol interven-tion programs. Amer J Health Prom 1996;10:453–470.

5. Heaney C, Goetzel R. A review of health-related outcomes of multi-component workplace health promotion programs. Amer J Health Prom 1997;11:290–307.

6. Hennrikus D, Jeffrey R. Worksite intervention for weight control: a review of the literature. Amer J Health Prom 1996;10:471–498.

7. Murphy L. Stress management in work settings: a critical review of the health effects. Amer J Health Prom 1996;11:112–135.

8. Roman P, Blum T. Alcohol: a review of the impact of worksite interventions on health and behav-ioral outcomes. Amer J Health Prom 1996;11:136–149.

9. Shephard R. Workplace fitness and exercise programs: a review of methodology and health impact. Amer J Health Prom 1996;10: 436–452.

10. Wilson M, Jorgenson C, Cole G. The health effects of worksite HIV/AIDS interventions: a review of the research literature. Amer J Health Prom 1996;11:150–157.

11. Abrams D, Boutwell WB, Grizzle J, et al. Cancer control at the work-place: the working well trial. Preven Med 1994;23:15–27.

12. Sorensen G, Thompson B, Glanz K. Working well: results from a worksite-based cancer prevention trial. Amer J Public Health 1996.

13. Glasgow RE, Terborg JR, Hollis JF. Modifying dietary and tobacco use

patterns in the worksite: the Take Heart Project. Health Ed Q 1994; 21:69–82.

14. Tilley B, Vernon S, Myers R. Planning the next step: a screening promotion and nutrition intervention trial in the worksite.

Ann N Y Acad Sci 1995;768:292–295.

15. Havas S, Heimendinger J, Reynolds K. A day for better health: a new research initiative. J Amer Dietetic Assoc 1994;94:32–36.

16. Warner K, Wickizer R, Wolfe J, et al. Economic implications of workplace health promotion programs: a review of the literature. J Occup Med 1988;30:105–112.

Chapter 80

The Financial Impact of Worksite Health Promotion and Methodologic Quality of the Evidence

Steven G. Aldana

Many employers have tried to increase the quality of life of their employees by developing and funding health promotion programs designed to reduce employee health risk factors while reducing employee-related expenses. The *modus operandi* of these programs has been to facilitate lifestyle change through a combination of efforts to enhance awareness, change behavior, and create environments that support good health practices and prevent disease (1). Originally, these programs were an extension of the benefits offered to employees and were limited to companies that had strong support for employees and sufficient financial strength to afford such programs. A natural evolution of most programs has been to move from an employee "perk" to an increasingly comprehensive program. These expanded programs were designed to lower employee-related expenses by improving employee health and enhance quality of life by preventing disease. Today, some programs are initiated for the sole purpose of reducing employee-related expenses.

This evolution was not possible without additional corporate funding and support, which placed worksite health promotion programs under closer financial scrutiny. This financial examination forced health promotion professionals to be critical of their own programs, to question what was done and justify every expense, and to keep programs that could show a positive return on investment and terminate programs that cannot. In hindsight, having a corporate birthplace has been a blessing in disguise for the health promotion profession, because the profession was forced, while in its infancy, to carefully evaluate and demonstrate program effectiveness, both in terms of disease prevention and financial return on investment.

To accurately review the literature, a search was con-

ducted to identify all of the studies published between 1975 and 1997 in the English language that examined the financial impact of workplace health promotion programs. To be included, studies had to 1) be published in peer-reviewed journals, 2) report the results of a worksite–based program, 3) provide a health promotion intervention, and 4) report financial, absenteeism, or health care cost outcomes. Studies reported only in abstract form or presented at professional conferences and not published were excluded. Computer searches were conducted on the following databases: Medline, E.R.I.C, A.B.I. Inform, EDGAR, CARL UnCover, and Lexis–Nexis, using the following keywords: work site, health, promotion, cost, benefit, effectiveness, health care costs, medical, and absenteeism. This computer search was followed by a manual search of 16 journals that previously had published worksite health promotion findings. The final list of articles was sent to four established health promotion researchers to determine if they knew of any published findings not included in the list.

HEALTH PROMOTION ECONOMICS

The typical health promotion program consists of strategies and interventions designed to reduce health risks and prevent the onset of certain diseases. Tobacco control, physical activity, stress management, blood pressure, and weight control are a few examples of health risk areas affected by health promotion programs. More comprehensive programs include additional interventions targeted at cancer prevention, seat belt use, nutrition, substance abuse prevention, muscle strength and flexibility, and injury prevention. Programs that are successful at reducing employee health risks and improving worker satisfaction can affect a variety of employee-related expenses, including health care costs and utilization, disability, employee absenteeism, productivity, employee turnover and morale, workers' compensation, and smoking-related costs. In addition to these, the presence of a health promotion program can potentially alter the public image of the company and indirectly boost revenues.

The causal relationship between health promotion and reduced employee expenses is thought to take several paths, depending on the expense to be reduced. Employee health care costs for example, are caused by a variety of factors, including employee health risk. The ability of health promotion programs to reduce employee health risks has been well documented. In Chapter 79, Michael O'Donnell discusses the health impact of health promotion. In his review, he shows that many health promotion programs have been able to significantly reduce the health risks of participants. It is generally believed that reduced health risks should lead to a reduced incidence of disease and that reduced disease should translate into fewer medical claims.

It does seem logical that, if morbidity is reduced, the cost of treating that morbidity should be reduced. At the present, there is no causal evidence to support this hypothesis; however, there is some limited correlational research that demonstrates a significant positive association between the number of health risks an individual may have and the amount of money spent on medical care. Yen et al and Henritze et al revealed an increase in medical care costs as the number of health risks increase (2,3). The trend underlying the data suggests that as the number of health risks increase, there is a similar increase in medical care costs and that medical care costs could potentially be reduced by lowering health risks. Research that has been conducted on the financial benefit of health promotion programs has only evaluated health care cost outcomes as they relate to program participation, not as they relate to reduced health risk.

Another way to reduce the amount and severity of morbidity is with early disease detection. Regular medical screening is a common component of health promotion programs that may result in reduced medical expenses. Mammography screening, for example, has been shown to reduce overall medical expenses because less treatment is required to deal with cancers found in early stages (4). Thus, screening has the potential to reduce medical expenses and loss of productivity by reducing the quantity of treatment required.

The most common type of injury reported by employees is cumulative trauma disorders (CTDs). Back injury, one type of CTD, occurs in 75% of workers, and though the duration of back injuries is relatively short, the medical and workers' compensation costs can be substantial (5). Many health promotion programs are designed to reduce the incidence of CTDs through pre-work stretching routines, awareness campaigns, flexibility programs, ergonomic aids, and physical fitness programs. Programs that are able to reduce the incidence of CTDs should be able to realize savings in medical care costs, workers' compensation, and absenteeism.

Another common component of health promotion programs that are aimed at reducing injuries is seat belt interventions. Not only do seat belts save lives, but they also reduce injuries and fewer injuries may translate into fewer medical care expenses and less loss of productivity because of missed work (6). Several successful seat belt programs, which have demonstrated significant increases in seat belt use among program participants, have been developed (6). However, the relationship between medical care costs and seat belt use is undocumented.

Health promotion program participants may have improved work satisfaction, which can have a direct impact on employee productivity, job turnover, workers' compensation, and absenteeism. Of these four program outcomes, absenteeism is the only one that has been evaluated in a variety of health promotion settings. Although the methodologic quality of the absenteeism literature has some research design problems, the available findings suggest that participants in health promotion programs can lower rates of absenteeism by lowering their health risks or improving their job satisfaction (44).

The newest health promotion strategy for reducing employee health care costs is demand management, which is a cost-reducing scheme that uses 1) informed patient decision making programs, 2) acute and chronic disease management interventions, and 3) health care consumer education designed to increase appropriate and decrease inappropriate utilization of medical services. A typical demand management strategy might be to provide all program participants with a medical self-care book designed to assist them in determining if medical care is needed or if home remedies could be applied to a current illness or injury. Reductions in health care costs occur if participants who use the book are able to reduce inappropriate medical visits. Use of demand management strategies has been shown to be an effective technique in reducing employee health care expenses over the short term (7). At the present, there is considerable debate whether or not demand management approaches are part of traditional health promotion. Research that has evaluated demand management interventions is not included in this review, but readers who have additional interest in this subject should refer to the article by Lynch et al (8).

Research on the economic impact of health promotion has centered on employee medical expenses, including workers' compensation and disability, and employee absenteeism. These two financial outcome measures are used most often as outcome measures because they are relatively easy to measure and are objective. Only studies that evaluated health care costs savings and changes in absenteeism are considered in this review.

METHODOLOGIC QUALITY OF THE LITERATURE

The current body of literature on the cost-benefit of health promotion programs typifies the methodologic difficulties found in social science research. In order to evaluate an existing program and maintain ecologic validity, internal validity is often sacrificed. It is difficult to maintain both internal and external validity when most research conducted on health promotion programs is conducted in real world settings. Scientific criticisms ensue when health promotion research is too applied (high in ecologic validity) and lacks internal validity. This dilemma is played out each time research is conducted on a health promotion program. The underlying issue

Table 80-1 Summary of the Impact of Health Promotion Programs on Medical Expenses

STUDY (REFERENCE)	PURPOSE	SAMPLE SIZE	CONTROL GROUP	EVALUATION PERIOD
Canada & North America Life (11)	Assess medical care expense after initiation of a fitness intervention	Experimental: 534 Control: 113	Yes	1 year
Prudential (12)	Evaluate impact of fitness program on fitness, medical costs, and disability	Disability group: 184 Medical cost group: 121	No	Disability: 5 year Medical cost: 1 year
Blue Cross/Blue Shield of California (13)	Assess impact of health education program on outpatient visits	5191 employees	Yes	15 months
Los Angeles Fire Department (14)	Effect of health and fitness program on fitness and workers' compensation	4221 employees	No	10 years
Blue Cross/Blue Shield of Indiana (15)	Compare health care costs of health promotion participants and nonparticipants	Participants: 667 Nonparticipants: 892	No	5 years
Johnson & Johnson (16)	Evaluate the relationship between exposure to a comprehensive work site health promotion program and health care costs	Participants: 5192; 3259 Controls: 2955	Yes	5 years
Tenneco (17)	Compare medical utilization between exercisers and nonexercisers	Exercisers: 221 Nonexercisers: 296	No	1 year
Northern Telecom (18)	Evaluate impact of health promotion on lifestyle-related costs	NA	No	1 year
Control Data (19)	Evaluate impact of health promotion on medical costs and utilization	50,000 employees	No	6 years
Tenneco (20)	Determine the relationship between exercise and injury prevalence	6104 employees	No	2 years
Blue Cross/Blue Shield (21)	Assess impact of health promotion on health care utilization and health risk	Treatment group: 3466 from three sites	No for most groups	1–5 years
General Mills (22)	Compare health risks and medical costs for health promotion participants and nonparticipants	Controls varied with sites Treatment: 685 Control: 341	Yes	2 years
General Motors (23)	Compare medical care costs for treated employees, controls and normotensives	Three treatment sites with average subject size (n = 275) Control group: 169	Yes	4 years
Textile Plant (24)	Evaluate the effect of health promotion on medical costs	Treatment group consisted of employees from 38 plants	No	1 year
Travelers Insurance (25)	Impact of health promotion on risk age, medical care costs, absenteeism	Treatment group: 36,000	No	4 years with projections for 10 additional years
Bank of America (26)	Determine the cost-benefit of using assessment and printed media in a health promotion program for retirees	Two treatment groups: 3779 Control group: 1907	Yes	2 years
City of Mesa, Arizona (27)	Evaluate the effect of participation in a worksite health promotion program on health care costs	Participants: 340 Nonparticipants: 340	No	4 years
Bank of America (28)	Evaluate a randomized trial of health promotion using risk assessment and written materials targeted toward retirees	Two treatment groups: 3102 Control group: 1610	Yes	1 year
City of Birmingham (29)	Initiate and evaluate a city wide comprehensive health promotion program	4000 city employees	No	5 years
Blue Cross/Blue Shield of Indiana (30)	Determine if health promotion program participation is associated with reduced medical care expenses	Participants: 430 Controls: 313	No	7 years
Utility Company (31)	Determine health and cost outcomes of a worksite health promotion program on medical costs	Participants: 1188	Yes	1 year
California PERS (32)	Evaluate the impact of a mail-delivered intervention targeted at retirees	Participants: 54,902 Controls: 2366	Yes	1 year
First Bank of Chicago (33)	Evaluate the impact of a comprehensive worksite health promotion program on medical and disability costs	Sample represented claims, not participants	No	4 years
Manufacturing Company (34)	Investigate the relationship between changes in health risk and medical claims cost	796 employees	No	6 years

NA, not applicable.

SOURCE: Reprinted by permission of the American Journal of Health Promotion from: The art and science of health promotion, March/April 1998.

Outcome Measures	Evaluation Design	Design Rating*	Cost-Benefit Ratio	Findings
Health insurance claims, program participation, fitness scores	Before and after with participants compared to nonparticipants	***	NA	Participants had fewer medical claims and hospital days
Disability days, medical costs, fitness	Before and after one-group design	***	1.00 : 2.93	Medical costs reduced by 50%, disability cut by 20%
Self-reported physician visits	Before and after staggered time series, quasi experimental	****	NA	Program participants had significantly fewer visits
Fitness measures, workers' compensation costs	Before and after staggered time series	***	NA	Lower workers' compensation costs, improved fitness
Medical costs per person per year	7-month before and after measures, every 6 months	***	1.0 : 2.5	Participants had lower medical care expenses than nonparticipants (subsequent re-analysis of this data showed no significant differences) (10)
Inpatient costs, admissions, hospital days, outpatient costs	Two treatment groups of varying exposure and a control group	*****	NA	Exposed groups had lower hospital days, admissions, and inpatient costs: no difference in total medical costs
Medical costs, rate of claims increase, fitness	Self-selected before and after participants vs. nonparticipants	***	NA	Participants had lower nonhospital costs, but had higher rates of utilization
Medical costs and various health risks	Before and after	***	NA	Medical costs remained constant or declined over a 1-year period
Medical costs and utilization and health risk	6-year longitudinal	***	NA	Lower medical claims related to lower risk, reported savings of $1.8 million from lower medical costs and reduced absenteeism
Injury prevalence, fitness measures	Longitudinal, correlational with injury and fitness categories	***	NA	Exercisers and nonexercisers had equal number of injuries, exercisers over 50 had fewer medical costs and fitness levels increased
Health risk factors and medical utilization	Quasi experimental with self-selected participants	***	NA	Participants demonstrated fewer number of claims and lower total medical costs
Health risks, medical care costs, absenteeism	Before and after comparison of participants to nonparticipants	****	1.0 : 3.5	No difference between participants and nonparticipants, benefit due to reduced absenteeism
Medical claims	Quasi experimental, 3 treatment groups and 1 control group	****	1.0 : 2.3	Medical care costs for hypertensive workers at treatment sites were lower than control sites; costs for matched subjects did not differ
Medical utilization	Longitudinal correlation (regression)	***	NA	Age, sex, plant product, and medical access explained 23% of claim variance; health promotion and plant product explained 54% of variance
Health risk age, medical costs, absenteeism, life insurance costs	Quasi experimental, longitudinal, multiple-year comparisons	***	1.0 : 3.4	Participants had 1.2 fewer days absence, projected; program cost $57 million over 15 years and resulted in savings of $146 million
Self-reported health risk change, medical care utilization, medical care costs, days confined to home	Randomized, controlled trial	*****	NA	Treatment groups had lower medical visits, sick days, hospital days, and medical care costs
Medical care costs, utilization	Quasi experimental design with participants age- and sex-matched with nonparticipating control subjects	****	1.0 : 3.6	Both groups had lower health care costs, but participants had twice the decrease: no difference in substance abuse or emergency care costs
Health risk scores, self-reported medical utilization, medical care costs	Randomized, controlled trial	*****	1.0 : 5.9	Health risk scores improved by 12%, self-reported utilization decreased 20% among treatment groups, 48% lower claims for treatment group
Program cost, average per capita medical cost, hospital admissions	Quasi experimental, longitudinal design	***	1.0 : 2.7	Days of hospitalization per participant dropped 71.1% and hospital admissions dropped 62.5% from 1985 to 1990
Medical costs per year, program participation data	Quasi experimental before and after with 2 intervention groups and 2 control groups	****	NA	There was no significant difference in medical care cost between treatment and control groups
Medical costs, hospital days	Before and after intervention	****	NA	Four different levels of intervention showed reduced medical cost and hospital days as program intensity increased; benefit ranged from $145 for the least intense group to $421 for the most intense group
Risk factor scores, change in health risk, annual medical care costs increases, self-reported utilization	Before and after randomized, quasi experimental	*****	NA	Improved risk scores, reduced self-reported utilization, reduced medical costs compared to controls, reduced increase in annual medical costs
Number of depression diagnoses, days per depressive event	Quasi experimental, longitudinal	***	NA	Costs associated with depressive events were reduced after introduction of the program
Changes in health risk and medical care costs	Before and after intervention	***	NA	Changes in health risk were associated with changes in health care costs; as risks increased, costs increased

* Design ratings were as follows: ***, no comparison or control group;
****, properly conducted study with comparison group but not randomized; *****, properly conducted study with a randomized comparison or control group.
NA, not applicable.

Table 80-2 Summary of the Impact of Health Promotion Programs on Worker Absenteeism

Study (Reference)	Purpose	Sample Size	Control Group	Evaluation Period
Tenneco (17)	Determine the effect of a work site fitness program on absenteeism and health care costs	Participants: 221 Nonparticipants: 296	Yes	1 year
Dallas School District (35)	Evaluate the impact of a multi–work site wellness program	Participants: 3846 Control group: 8290	Yes	1 year
Control Data (19)	Evaluate the impact of the company's Staywell program on health risk, medical costs, utilization, and absenteeism	Longitudinal data on 50,000 employees	No	6 years
Coors (36)	Evaluate the health and cost benefit of a cardiac rehabilitation program	180 postcoronary patients	No	6 years
General Mills (22)	To compare rates of absenteeism and health care costs between health promotion participants and nonparticipants	Participants: 685 Nonparticipants: 341	Yes	2 years
Johnson and Johnson (37)	Evaluate the effect of health promotion program on rates of absenteeism in two groups of employees	Participants: 1406 Controls: 487	Yes	3 years
Travelers (38)	Determine the effect of a work site fitness program on absenteeism	Participants: 2232 Controls: 5218	No	2 years
Dupont (39)	Evaluate the effect of a comprehensive, multisite health promotion program on absenteeism	4 experimental sites: 29,315 employees; 19 control sites: 14,573 employees	Yes	2 years
Blue Cross Plans (21)	Evaluate the impact of traditional health promotion on absenteeism	Three experimental groups; 3466 total participants; one control group: 177	Yes	11 years
Travelers (25)	Evaluation of the effect of a comprehensive work site health promotion program on absenteeism	Participants: 36,000	No	4 years projected for 10
Canada Life Assurance Co. (40)	12-year follow-up of an employee fitness program	Participants: 486 Nonparticipants: 142	No	12 years
Bank of America (26)	Randomized evaluation of a health promotion program for retirees	Participants: 3779 Nonparticipants: 1907	Yes	2 years
32 Worksites (41)	Impact of a smoking cessation and weight control program on absenteeism	32 sites of 200 employees each: 6400	No	1 year
Utility Company (42)	Impact of health promotion program on medical care cost and absenteeism	Nine company divisions	No	1 year
Dupont (43)	Assess impact of a 5-phase health promotion program on selected health risks and absenteeism	Participants: 7178 Controls: 7101	Yes	2 years
Duke University (44)	Effects of the "Live for Life" health promotion program	15,500 participants	Yes	3 years
Work Sites in the Netherlands (49)	Assess effect of employee fitness programs on absenteeism	Experimental: 469 Control: 415	Yes	1 year

NA, not applicable.

SOURCE: Reprinted by permission of the American Journal of Health Promotion from: The art and science of health promotion, March/April 1998.

in this problem is the randomization or lack of randomization of subjects.

Randomization of program participants is not always possible, and sometimes is not recommended. Most health promotion programs are made available to the members or employees of a specific organization. When individuals are randomly selected to participate in a health promotion program, those same participants will be working alongside nonparticipating controls: there is considerable chance for social interaction and the sharing of common professional and personal experiences, including their participation in the health promotion program. When subjects of the treatment group share some of the treatment with subjects of the control group, contamination occurs and any measurable differences between the groups become diluted. One solution to this problem is to randomly select different geographic health promotion sites and provide the health promotion program to one treatment site and provide nothing to the control site. Under this design, contamination of the treatment is of less concern, but larger problems arise when socioeconomic, racial, religious, and other differences, which introduce a selection bias, are found between the treatment and control sites. Whether researchers randomize by subject or sites, there are still substantial threats to the outcome of the study.

Outcome Measures	Evaluation Design	Design Rating*	Cost-Benefit Ratio	Findings
Absenteeism in hours, level of exercise, medical claims data	Before and after randomized design	****	NA	Male and female exercisers had 20% and 46.8% lower rates of absenteeism than nonexercising controls; medical costs were lower for participants
Average annual absenteeism, exercise participation, health risk measures	Before and after randomized design	*****	NA	Program participants demonstrated 20% less absenteeism than controls; absenteeism for controls increased 5%, 1.25 days per person per year less for participants
Participation and adherence, health risk, absenteeism, medical costs	Longitudinal cross-sectional design of health risk, medical, and absenteeism data	***	NA	Reduced rates of absenteeism for employees with lower health risk scores, savings from absenteeism estimated at $1.8 million
Disability costs, absenteeism, fitness	Longitudinal cross-sectional design	***	1.0 : 10.1	Absenteeism was reduced 68.2% for program participants
Health risk scores, absenteeism rates per year	Randomized before and after design	****	1.0 : 3.5	36.3% lower mean days of absenteeism for participants vs. nonparticipants; 36% lower sick leave costs for participants
Self-reported sick leave, company-reported absenteeism	Before and after test, experimental and control group	****	NA	Adjusted mean levels of absenteeism were lower in the final year for wage earners, but no difference for salaried workers
Number of days of absenteeism per year, number of visits to the fitness center	Before and after test self-selected participant compared to nonparticipants	****	NA	After control for age and gender, participants had 13.8% less absenteeism; decrease related to level of participation
Disability days and absenteeism rates per employee, total program costs	Randomized experimental and control sites	****	1.0 : 2.5	Intervention sites had a 14% decline in disability days vs. 5.8% for controls; difference of 4 disability days per participant
Absence due to illness measured in hours per year	Quasi experimental, longitudinal	****	NA	Costs associated with absenteeism were 33.6% lower for participants
Health risk age, absenteeism costs, medical costs, program costs	Cross-sectional, longitudinal	***	1.0 : 3.4	Cost benefit believed to be caused by reduced absenteeism and medical care costs; absenteeism reduced 19%
Program participation rates, fitness measures, absenteeism, productivity	Quasi experimental, longitudinal	***	1.0 : 4.85	Statistical results not available, calculated benefits greater than program costs
Average annual absenteeism	Cross sectional analysis of 32 random worksites	****	NA	Absenteeism increased 4.5% by intervention; smoking was associated with sick days but participation in weight loss program was not
Medical visits, hospitalizations, and injuries; average absenteeism days per year	Longitudinal before and after	***	NA	Group with the most intense intervention had declines in medical visits, hospitalization, and injuries; as intensity increased, absenteeism decreased
Self-reported health risks before and after intervention, medical cost and utilization	Randomized controlled trial	*****	NA	Improvements in health risk scores, 12.1% lower sick days, 6.6% lower physician visits, and 32% lower medical costs
Seven behavior health risks and self-reported absenteeism	Quasi experimental before and after intervention, with comparison	****	NA	Portion of subjects with 3+ risk factors decreased, absenteeism decreased by 12%, six of seven risks were decreased
Free program with HRA screening, fitness and biometric data, and absenteeism	Cross-sectional, longitudinal two-group design	***	NA	Absenteeism increased for both participants and controls, but more for controls; participants had 4.6 fewer hours
Company gathered sick leave data	Before and after test experimental and control groups	****	NA	Only high participation in fitness programs was associated with a significant reduction in absenteeism

* For explanation, see note to Table 80-1 on page 931.

More often than not, health promotion researchers choose not to randomize groups. Once the decision not to randomize is made, a Pandora's box of methodologic woes opens wide and a whole host of threats to the validity of the study appear.

In addition to problems of internal validity, there are significant questions about the statistical analyses used in the research that has evaluated outcomes involving health care expenditures. Most employees generate no claims or very small claims, while a small number of employees have incurred very large medical costs. When the distribution of health care expenditures is graphed, the distribution is always highly, negatively skewed. Costs associated with premature childbirth, organ transplants, and some cancer treatments can be especially costly. When these high costs are included within the total cost base, the medical care expense of the average person is greatly inflated. This increases the potential for inaccurate findings, because if high-cost cases are more prevalent in the treatment group, the mean health care expenditure per program participant is inflated and the treatment group appears to have higher medical costs. If there are more high-cost cases in the control group, the average medical cost for program participants is lower, and it is easy to conclude that health promotion program participants have lower health care costs, when in reality participation may not have had any effect on medical costs.

Worse, skewed health care cost data dramatically violates the assumptions required for the use of parametric statistics, which are the type of statistics used in 90% of studies evaluating health care costs. A good example of this problem was brought to light when Gibbs et al completed a health care cost evaluation of the employees who participated in the health promotion program of Blue Cross and Blue Shield of Indiana (15). Using parametric statistics to analyze the highly skewed health care cost data, the researchers concluded that the program participants had significantly lower health care costs than nonparticipants. Seven years later, Sciacca et al completed a re-evaluation using the same data, only this time the skewed health care cost data was analyzed using nonparametric statistics, which eliminates the problems inherent in skewed data (10). In the second evaluation, the authors reported that program participation was not associated with reduced health care costs and concluded, "It would be prudent to remain guarded about the health cost savings effects of worksite health promotion programs" (10). Such diametric results highlight the need to use correct statistical analyses when the outcome data is medical cost reported in dollars and to cast shadow of concern over the existing body of literature, which fails to address this problem.

Lack of randomized groups and failure to use appropriate methods of analysis are the two most prominent limitations of the literature. But other limitations that exist in the literature include short intervention periods, subject drop out, and lack of information on the extent of participation, which could provide data on a possible dose response. Scientifically rigorous studies could control for all of these limitations. However, well-controlled studies are typically expensive and few worksite programs have the resources to conduct such studies. Joint research between companies, foundations, and government funding entities has a greater likelihood of completing good experimental studies.

Despite the apparently low methodologic quality of the existing literature, several points must be considered to objectively evaluate the financial impact of the literature. First, evaluation must be conducted on existing programs that provide high ecologic validity and somewhat reduced internal validity. Second, researchers are forced to work within the framework of existing programs and must make the best of a difficult research situation. This forces researchers to use backup methods to maintain validity when randomization is not possible. This is not an excuse to get the profession to accept less than stellar research, it is merely confirmation that controlled, randomized trials are extremely difficult to conduct in complex, real world settings. Lastly, regardless of the differences in the scientific rigor of the available literature, almost all published findings tend to support the hypothesis that participation in health promotion programs can reduce employee-related health care costs and absenteeism.

DOCUMENTED IMPACT

The cost impact of health promotion programs can be measured in terms of cost-effectiveness and cost-benefit ratios. Cost-effectiveness is a ratio of the cost of a program divided by the documented change in a health risk outcome. For example, a blood pressure control program might cost $20

Table 80-3 Summary of Health Promotion Cost-Effectiveness Studies

Study (Reference)	Purpose	Sample Size	Control Group	Evaluation Period
Coors (47)	Implement a voluntary program focused on multiple risk factor reduction for cardiovascular disease	692 "Lifecheck" program participants, 8 week program	No	1 year
Georgia Pacific Corp. (45)	Determine the cost effectiveness of different models of delivering a total cholesterol program	Participants: 3202	Yes	1–3 months
Minneapolis/St. Paul Metropolitan Area (41)	Measure impact of work site weight control and smoking cessation programs	10,000 total subjects, 16 control and 16 intervention sites	Yes	2 years
Metropolitan Toronto (48)	Improve hypertension detection in blue collar workers	7856 hypertensives	No	40 days and 1 year
AHCPR Recommendations (50)	Determine the cost-effectiveness of clinical recommendations in AHCPR's guideline	The guidelines' 15 recommendations	NA	NA

AHCPR, Agency for Health Care Policy and Research;
NA, not applicable.
SOURCE: Reprinted by permission of the American Journal of Health Promotion from: The art and science of health promotion, March/April 1998.

per participant per year and result in an average 5 mm/Hg reduction in systolic blood pressure per participant. The cost per 5 mm/Hg reduction would therefore be $20, or $4 per 1 mm reduction.

Cost-benefit analyses follow more of the "bottom-line" approach to evaluating a program's economic impact. Rather than comparing program cost to health outcome, cost-benefit analyses compare program costs with the financial savings associated with the health outcome or program participation. Applying the blood pressure control example above to a cost-benefit analysis, the cost portion of the ratio remains the same, i.e., $20. The benefit is the calculated financial gain associated with participating in the program, including reduced medical care costs, decreased absenteeism, decreased job turnover, higher productivity and morale, and any other financial savings caused by participation in the program. Assuming each participant saved an average of $40, the cost-benefit ratio for the program would be 20:40, or 1:2, meaning that for every dollar spent on the program, two dollars were saved. This bottom-line approach is appealing to managers and administrations accustomed to justifying expenses and is an accepted method of demonstrating financial benefit. It may also permit accurate comparison between programs, provided the methods used to calculate the cost and benefit are similar.

Most of the research on the economic impact of health promotion can be classified into two major categories on the basis of the outcome used to calculate cost savings: 1) medical expenses, including disability and workers' compensation, and 2) absenteeism. To locate all published studies on this topic, a data-based literature search was followed up by personal communication with several prominant researchers in the health promotion field. To date, there are 50 studies that measured medical costs or absenteeism and four additional studies that reported cost-effectiveness findings. Table 80-1 is a summary of the 24 health promotion program evaluations that have evaluated medical costs. Table 80-2 is a summary of the 16 evaluations that have included employee absenteeism as an outcome measure, and Table 80-3 highlights the four studies that conducted cost-effectiveness evaluations. Each table contains the following information: 1) name of the evaluation site, 2) purpose of the evaluation, 3) number of subjects in each study group, 4) use of a control group, 5) length of the evaluation period, 6) outcome measures, 7) evaluation design, 8) a design rating, 9) cost-benefit ratio, and 10) a brief summary of the findings. The design rating is a qualitative estimate of the methodologic rigor of each evaluation. The ratings range from three stars to five stars, wherein five stars represent a properly conducted study with a randomized comparison or control group; four reflect a properly conducted study with a comparison group that was not randomized; and three represent an evaluation without a comparison or control group.

The reductions reported in medical care cost and absenteeism are significant in most cases. The average cost-benefit ratio for the eight studies that measured health care costs and calculated cost-benefit ratios was 1.00:3.35. The five absenteeism studies produced an average cost-benefit ratio of 1.00:4.87 (Table 80-4). When taken collectively, the 13 studies that produced cost-benefit ratios tend to support the hypothesis that health promotion programs are cost-beneficial, based entirely on savings in reduced medical care expenditures and absenteeism. Benefits resulting from savings in reduced turnover, increased productivity, and improved

Outcome Measures	Evaluation Design	Design Rating*	Findings
Blood pressure, total, cholesterol, weight, physical activity, risk of ischemia within 8 years	Before and after design with participants acting as controls	***	The program cost $32 per participant; documented reductions in systolic blood pressure, cholesterol, weight, and risk of ischemia
Program costs, total cholesterol	Randomized case control group design with 4 groups, each receiving a different model and one control group	****	Interventions costs ranged from $6.33 to $31.71 per participant depending on intervention group; educational programs with incentives appeared most effective
Weight loss and smoking cessation	Randomized treatment and control sites, before and after designs	*****	Average weight loss was 4.8 lbs, and 2% quit rate for smokers; $1500 cost for 24 people who quit smoking
Employees randomly assigned to either physician care or scheduled for another screening	Two-group before and after design	***	Blood pressure declined (8.5 mm/Hg) for both groups; one stage screening is preferred and appears more cost-effective
Smoking intervention costs and cost per life year or quality-life-year	Computer modeling	***	Smoking cessation interventions would cost $6.3 billion to implement and result in 1.7 million quitters and add 2 years of life to each quitter

* For explanation, see note to Table 80-1 on page 931.

Table 80-4 Average Cost-Benefit Ratios for Absenteeism and Health Care Costs		
STUDY (REFERENCE)	HEALTH CARE	ABSENTEEISM
Prudential (12)	1:2.9	—
Blue Cross/Blue Shield of Indiana (15)	1:2.5	—
General Mills (22)	1:3.5	1:3.5
General Motors (23)	1:2.3	—
Travelers Insurance (24)	1:3.4	1:3.4
Bank of America (28)	1:5.9	—
City of Mesa, Arizona (27)	1:3.6	—
City of Birmingham (29)	1:27	—
Coors (36)	—	1:10.1
Dupont (39)	—	1:2.5
Canada Life Assurance Co. (40)	—	1:4.85
AVERAGE RATIOS	1:3.35	1:4.87

SOURCE: Reprinted by permission of the American Journal of Health Promotion from: The art and science of health promotion, March/April 1998.

company image are very difficult to quantify as evidenced by the dearth of literature that measured these variable as

outcomes. It is hypothesized that changes in turnover, productivity, and image would only add to the program benefits.

How long these benefits may last is unknown. The average length for all studies that had a control group was 2.8 years. The real payoff in risk reduction may not be realized until many years after the risk has been reduced. The average age of subjects in these studies is around 39 years. The leading cause of death, coronary heart disease, does not affect most victims until the 5th and 6th decades of life. And with a national job turnover rate of 11% per year, real financial benefits of health promotion programs are likely to be scattered and therefore realized by businesses that hire employees who have reduced their health risks at the expense of previous employers.

We will likely never know the actual economic impact of health promotion programs. The financial benefits are eventually realized by the entire society as Medicare costs are reduced, national productivity increases, costs of goods and services are reduced, and both the quality and quantity of life are extended.

This chapter was previously published under the same title in the March/April 1998 issue of the Art and Science of Health Promotion and is reprinted with permission of the American Journal of Health Promotion, Inc.

REFERENCES

1. O'Donnell MP, Harris JS, ed. Health promotion in the workplace. 2nd ed. Albany, NY: Delmar Publishers, 1994:1–18.

2. Yen DE, Witting P. Associations between health risk appraisal scores and employee medical claims cost in a manufacturing company. Am J Health Promo 1991;6:46–54.

3. Henritze J, Brammell H, McGloin J. LIFECHECK: a successful, low touch, low tech, in-plant cardiovascular disease risk identification and modification program. Am J Health Promo 1992;6:129–136.

4. Newhouse JP. Free for all: lessons from the Rand health insurance experiment. Cambridge, MA: Harvard University, 1993:9–16.

5. U.S Department of Labor, Bureau of Labor Statistics Newsletter. 1992; Nov 18:1–11.

6. Eddy JM, Fitzhugh EC, Wojtowics GG, Wang MQ. The impact of worksite-based safety belt programs: a review of the literature. Am J Health Promo 1997;11: 281–289.

7. Terry P. Health promotion, demand management, and social justice: three ships passing or a powerful flotilla? Worksite Health 1996;3: 8–15.

8. Lynch W, Vickery D. The potential impact of health promotion on health-care utilization: an introduction to demand management. Amer J Health Prom 1993;8:87–92.

9. Reed R, Mulvaney D, Billingham R, Skinner T. Health promotion service evaluation and impact study. Indianapolis, IN: Benchmark, 1986:1–25.

10. Sciacca H, Seehafer R, Reed R, Mulvaney D. The impact of participation in health promotion on medical costs: a reconsideration of the Blue Cross and Blue Shield of Indiana study. Am J Health Promo 1993;7:374–383.

11. Shephard R, et al. The influence of an employee fitness and lifestyle modification program upon medical care costs. Can J Pub Health 1982;73:259–263.

12. Bowne D, et al. Reduced disability and health care costs in an industrial fitness program. J Occup Med 1984;26:809–816.

13. Lorig K, Kraines R, Brown B, Richardson N. A workplace health education program that reduces outpatient visits. Medical Care 1985;23:1044.

14. Cady L, et al. Program for increasing health and physical fitness of fire fighters. J Occup Med 1985; 27:110–114.

15. Gibbs J, et al. Work-site health promotion: five year trend in employee health care costs. J Occup Med 1985;27:826–830.

16. Bly J, et al. Impact of worksite health promotion on health care costs and utilization: evaluation of Johnson and Johnson's live for life program. JAMA 1986;256:3236–3240.

17. Baun W, et al. A preliminary investigation: effect of a corporate fitness program on absenteeism and health care cost. J Occup Med 1986;28:18–22.

18. Harris J. Northern Telecom: a million dollar medically based program in a rapidly changing high tech environment. Am J Health Promo 1986;1:50–59.

19. Jose W, Anderson D, Haight S. The StayWell strategy for health care cost containment. In: Opatz J, ed. Health promotion evaluation: measuring the organizational impact. Stevens Point, WI: National Wellness Institute, 1987:15–34.

20. Tsai S, Bernacki E, Baun W. Injury prevalence and associated costs among participants of an employee fitness program. Preven Med 1988;17:475–482.

21. Conrad K, Riedel J, Gibbs J. Health promotion: a new direction in health care. Evaluation of four Blue Cross and Blue Shield plans' worksite health promotion programs. Executive Summary. Health Services Foundation, Indianapolis, IN, June 1988.

22. Wood E, et al. An evaluation of lifestyle risk factors and absenteeism after two years in a worksite health promotion program. Amer J Health Promo 1989;4:128–133.

23. Foote E, Erfurt J. The benefit-to-cost ratio of worksite blood pressure control programs. JAMA 1991;265:1283–1286.

24. Wheat JR, Graney MJ, Schachtman RH, et al. Does workplace health promotion decrease medical claims? Am J Prev Med 1992;8:110–114.

25. Golaszewski T, et al. A benefit-to-cost analysis of a worksite health promotion program. J Occup Med 1992;34:1164–1172.

26. Leigh JP, et al. Randomized controlled study of a retiree health promotion program: the Bank of America study. Arch Inter Med 1992;152:1201–1206.

27. Aldana S, et al. Influence of a mobile worksite health promotion program on health care costs. Am J Prev Med 1993;9:378–383.

28. Fries J, et al. Two-year results of a randomized controlled trial of a health promotion program in a retiree population: the Bank of America study. Am J Med 1993; 94:455–462.

29. Harvey M, et al. The impact of a comprehensive medical benefits cost management program for the city of Birmingham: results at five years. Am J Health Promo 1993;7:296–303.

30. Sciacca J, et al. The impact of participation in health promotion on medical costs: a reconsideration of the Blue Cross and Blue Shield of Indiana study. Am J Health Promo 1993;7:374–395.

31. Shi L. Worksite health promotion and changes in medical care use and sick days. J Health Behav Educ Promot 1993;17:9–17.

32. Fries J, et al. Randomized controlled trial of cost reductions from a health education program: the California public employees' retirement system (PERS) study. Am J Health Promo 1994;8:216–223.

33. Conti DJ, Burton WN. The economic impact of depression in a workplace. J Occup Med 1994;36:981–983.

34. Edington DW, Yen LT, Witting P. The financial impact of changes in personal health practices. J Occup Envir Med 1997;39:1037–1047.

35. Blair S, et al. Health promotion for educators: impact on absenteeism. Prev Med 1986;15:166–175.

36. Henritze J, Brammell HL. Phase II cardiac wellness at the Adolph Coors Company. Am J Health Promo 1989;4:25–31.

37. Jones R, et al. A study of a worksite health promotion program and absenteeism. J Occup Med 1990; 32:95–99.

38. Lynch W, et al. Impact of a facility-based corporate fitness program on the number of absentees from work due to illness. J Occup Med 1990;32:9–12.

39. Bertera R. The effects of workplace health promotion on absenteeism and employment costs in a large industrial population. Am J Pub Health 1990;80:1101–1105.

40. Shephard R. Twelve years' experience of a fitness program for the salaried employees of a Toronto life assurance company. Am J Health Promo 1992;6:292–301.

41. Jeffery R, et al. Effects of worksite health promotion on illness-related absenteeism. J Occup Med 1993;35:1142–1146.

42. Shi L. A cost-benefit analysis of a California county's back injury prevention program. Publ Health Rep 1993;108:204–211.

43. Bertera R. Behavioral risk factor and illness day changes with workplace health promotion: two-year results. Am J Health Promo 1993; 7:365–372.

44. Knight K, et al. An evaluation of Duke University's LIVE FOR LIFE health promotion program on changes in worker absenteeism. J Occup Med 1994;36:533–534.

45. Wilson M, Edmunson J, DeJoy D. Cost-effectiveness of work-site cholesterol screening and intervention programs. J Occup Med 1992;34:642–649.

46. Jeffery R, Forster J, French S, et al. The healthy worker project: a work-site intervention for weight control and smoking cessation. Am J Pub Health 1993;83:395–401.

47. Henritze J, Brammell H, McGloin J. LIFECHECK: a successful, low touch, low tech, in-plant cardiovascular disease risk identification and modification program. Am J Health Promo 1992;6:129–136.

48. Edward E, Koblin W, Irvine JM, et al. Small blue collar work site hypertension screening: a cost

effective study. J Occup Med 1994;36:346–355.

49. Lechner L, Vries H de, Adriaansen S, Drabbels L. Effects of an employee fitness program on reduced absenteesim. J Occup Med 1997;39:827–831.

50. Cromwell J, Bartosh W, Fiore M, et al. Cost-effectiveness of the clinical practice recommendations in the AHCPR Guideline for Smoking Cessation. JAMA 1997;278:759–766.

Chapter 81

The Future of Health Promotion

Jonathan E. Fielding

This chapter provides a perspective on how health promotion may evolve in the early twenty-first century. Starting with an inquiry into who will "own" health promotion and how it will be defined, I suggest how an increasing focus on population may alter its domain. The effects of free markets and the accompanying acceleration of technologic advances on development and delivery of health promotion products are explored, as is possible changes in notions of consumer protection. Also discussed is the growing importance of the systematic assessment of evidence on 1) intervention effectiveness and 2) cost-effectiveness analysis. Further likely changes in managed care, their effects on health promotion, and enhanced access to a wide range of relevant data are discussed. The implications of increasing attention to interventions to improve health at the beginning of life are considered. Finally, the potential for certification of health promotion professionals is explored.

WILL HEALTH PROMOTION BE HOMELESS?

In the future, where will health promotion live and who will have responsibility for it? Those of us who have nurtured the concept would be dismayed—nay, saddened—to see it homeless. Yet the risk exists, for several reasons. Health promotion is neither discipline- nor profession-specific. Instead, many disciplines are involved, from psychology and health education to kinesiology and nutrition. It blends elements of medicine and of public health. It is not localized to a specific site. It occurs where people live, study, work, or congregate for a variety of other purposes. A commonly accepted definition is elusive,

despite excellent attempts to capture its essence. Just as the WHO definition of health, "a state of complete physical, mental and social well-being and not merely the absence of disease or infirmity" (1) strikes many as overly broad, so do common definitions of health promotion. Determining who may lay claim to doing health promotion and how notions of it will be refined requires movement toward a consensus definition that does not have as many interpretations as interpreters.

DEFINITIONAL CONFUSION

Most of us concerned with finding a secure home for heath promotion agree that it is broader than health education or behavior change. Changes in institutions and environments that improve health are usually considered part of health promotion efforts. Yet Healthy People 2000 (2) makes distinctions between activities that fall under health promotion, health protection, and disease prevention. On the surface, it is easy to classify interventions based on this schema. Immunizations are disease prevention; fences around swimming pools or restaurant inspection are health protection; and exercise programs, education about menopause, and self-help groups for the bereaved are health promotion. Yet the distinctions quickly blur. Is education to erect fences around swimming pools health promotion or health protection? Are community fairs that feature immunization as one of many activities health promotion or disease prevention? Is a condom availability program for high school youth health protection or disease prevention?

DEFINITION AS THE FIRST DERIVATIVE OF MISSION

Because of the difficulties in drawing definitional boundaries, it may be easier to seek common ground by considering the *mission* of health promotion. I consider the mission of health promotion closely linked with that of public health. In the Institute of Medicine's 1988 study, The Future of Public Health, the public health mission was defined as "fulfilling society's interest in assuring conditions in which people can be healthy." Might health promotion's mission be to change conditions in a way that can positively influence the health of individuals and populations? If so, then Larry Green's operational definition comfortably follows: "any combination of educational, organizational, economic, and environmental supports for behavior and conditions of living conducive to health" (3).

HEALTH DETERMINANTS

Confidence in an expansive view of the mission and definition of health promotion is enhanced by our growing understanding of the determinants of health. Historical inquiry reveals that the health status of a population, and disparities among subgroups, does not depend solely on specific interventions to control a disease or efforts to change health behavior. Rather, it depends more on changes in social environment, particularly in levels of prosperity overall and its distribution (4). In the United States we have a high average per capita income, but health status, particularly of economically disadvantaged groups, is lower than what some might predict given our economic achievement. In fact, countries with the longest life expectancy are not the wealthiest measured by gross domestic product per capita. Rather, the healthiest among developed countries are those with the smallest income spreads among the population and the smallest percentage in poverty (5). In the United States, we have about 15% of our population (a higher percentage for children) living below the federal poverty line (6). This group is at much greater risk of many health problems—physical, mental, and social—than those better off economically.

Other aspects of the social environment are important determinants of population health. For example, being raised in a two-parent household reduces the likelihood of serious risk-taking behavior among adolescents (7). Family strife increases drug abuse (8). Exposure to excessive violence on television, movie, and video screens increases the risk of violent behavior in children and young adults (9). Advertising for tobacco products that associates smoking with being sexy, grown up, sophisticated, and rebellious increases youth smoking (10). Lack of social connections within families and communities increases the rate of many serious diseases and all-cause mortality (11). And social cohesion, the degree to which people feel a part of their neighborhood and community, appears to be an important determinant of health (12).

The physical environment also exerts enormous influence. From homelessness to ozone depletion and from lead to environmental tobacco smoke, the physical environment affects health in both obvious and subtle ways. For example, the introduction of thousands of new chemicals into the environment over the past decades may help account for the large increase in asthma incidence. More exposure to the sun, accelerated by ozone depletion, is a probable contributor to a large increase in skin cancers (13). Positive effects of small changes in the physical environment are exemplified by the dramatic effect of fluoridation on dental caries and of bicycle helmets on the rate of serious head injuries to riders.

To fulfill its mission to positively change conditions that can influence health of individuals and populations, health promotion must include intensive efforts to influence these broad determinants of the health of populations. In this quest, health promotion is adopting many professionals who might not have considered themselves in the business of health promotion. Yet the lawyers working to increase tobacco taxes through public referenda are health promotion practitioners. So are the politicians who work to reduce poverty, and the community organizers who seek to reduce the attractiveness of gang life to youth and those who fight for high-quality child care that promotes social and mental development. Of course, the formal education and skill set of health promotion practitioners who regulate food ingredients or use the law to get lead abated in housing may differ from those teaching breastfeeding to new mothers or conducting exercise classes at a worksite. But one of the jobs of those with an expansive perspective of health promotion is to elucidate the complementary nature of the work of these disparate and currently unconnected groups and to impress on each that improved health status and quality of life for the overall population will be advanced by their close collaboration.

In the future, therefore, the touchstone for health promotion may not be with those who have taken health promotion courses or who consider it their career. Rather, the touchstone may be the combinations of organizations and individuals who are concerned with population health and its determinants and who develop and monitor interventions to improve these—from the World Bank to public health agencies, and from those developing bioengineered seed for greater crop yields to "green" political parties and other environmental groups. In short, we many need to broaden the range of organizations who consider themselves engaged in health promotion to avoid it being considered too narrow—or worse, irrelevant—to major global health problems.

OVERCOMING BARRIERS

Inderpendent of definitions or organizations that speak for health promotion, the future will see a greater understanding of the synergy of those concerned with health-promoting products and services, those expert in marketing and in health applications of economic incentives, and those interested in strengthening community institutions. Take the example of exercise. Despite enormous efforts to increase public awareness of the value of regular exercise (14) and dramatic growth in the numbers of exercise physiologists, age-specific rates of sufficient exercise have barely moved, with the majority of adults in the deficient column (15). What will change this? A doubling in the number of exercise physiologists? More doctors giving exercise prescriptions? More work site health promotion programming? From available evidence, these measures could be helpful but, even collectively, they are unlikely to yield a large difference in the percentage of regular exercisers.

What other interventions offer hope of making a big difference in exercise rates? Economic barriers are substantial. Employer subsidies for gym memberships—contingent on regular use—might have a large impact and reduce the exercise gradient by income. Significant reductions in health benefit premiums, both under private insurance and under Medicare, for those exercising on a regular basis could also make a large difference. What about broader social interventions? If every local religious organization aggressively sponsored walking clubs, how many sedentary adults might join up?

TECHNOLOGIC ADVANCES

We need to harness the creative power of engineering and communications to combat the health problems that progress in these disciplines has exacerbated. The development of the cathode ray tube led to ubiquitous screens—televisions, computers, and video monitors—before which we spend too many immobile hours a week. We substitute watching physical activity for performing it.

In the future, we could we ask harder questions about how advances in engineering and communications technology can support health promotion. For example, might exercising be increased by an inexpensive exercise bicycle with a built-in television that required constant pedaling to remain on? A nonprofit organization, perhaps the American Heart Association, might develop and rent exercise bicycles to anyone with heart disease or serious risk factors, with the payment amount inversely proportional to the number of calories burned that month. They might require no payment if more than 2000 calories were consumed in exercise during the past 7 days.

What about an office chair with pedals that must be used to activate the telephone? Or a computer terminal with similar pedals? Pushing back the boundaries of what is usually considered health promotion to build everyday opportunities and incentives may be necessary to have the benefits of regular exercise visited upon the entire population.

What are the other likely advances and challenges for the beginning of the new millennium? A certain one is the fruits of investment in genetic and pharmacologic research. While predictions are perilous, it would not be surprising to see more effective pharmacologic therapy for weight control within the next 10 years. Such a development could have a major impact on population health, as the effects of obesity—higher rates of hypertension, hypercholesterolemia, type II diabetes, and acquired cardiovascular disease—are enormous. Also likely are effective genetic treatments for serious genetically influenced diseases, such as Alzheimers and many cancers. In short, drugs will be more important health promotion tools in the future than the past.

MARKET SEGMENTATION

The future will see increasing attention to market segmentation. What gets a 22-year-old single female who recently graduated from college and played soccer throughout her

schooling to continue to exercise regularly is different than what motivates a 22-year-old single mother of two living in a high-crime area who is trying to get off welfare and working the night shift in a garment factory. Consumer marketing firms that sell detergent, soap, or beer have different brands for different market segments and different marketing strategies for selling a brand to different segments. Health promoters need to make full use of these techniques.

MARKET FORCES

The world, with only a few exceptions, has accepted capitalism as the best economic structure to fuel growth. In this environment, we naturally think of how free markets can also serve social goals. For some aspects of health promotion, market forces are powerful allies. There are good markets for nicotine replacement products that significantly increase smoking cessation rates. For those who find it easier to exercise with others or who want or need specialized exercise equipment, a proliferation of sports clubs and gyms has broad appeal. And there is substantial demand for many safety devices, from child car seats to bicycle helmets.

However, the market does not always suffice. Particularly for those with limited economic resources, money to join a gym or buy a bicycle helmet for each child is an unaffordable luxury. Many families lack finances to purchase sufficient food for the family. Yet these segments of the population are also those at highest risk for poor development and preventable diseases and injuries. At an organizational level, most large employers can afford to invest in health promotion programming for their employees. Many smaller employers, especially those in businesses with a low profit margin, cannot. In the future, we will decide if it is in our collective interest to subsidize access to these health-promoting products and services. Subsidies or tax-supported payments for smoking cessation counseling and pharmacologic therapy for those with low incomes are likely to be among the first. Funds for smoking cessation and prevention will come, in part, from taxes on tobacco products or payments by manufacturers. For example, the Minnesota Tobacco Settlement allocates $102 million for cessation services (16).

CONSUMER PROTECTION

In the future, health promotion could unite behind a set of marketing principles that moves closer to the safety and efficacy principles of FDA-approved drugs. Currently, regulation of safety and efficacy only applies when health promotion uses or comes in the form of a drug or device. The Phen-Fen diet, for example, as most diets, was oversold to the growing throngs of obese people who wanted a painless way to reduce, until the FDA intervened when reports of serious heart damage surfaced. The FDA had not intervened previously, even though these drugs were being grossly oversold and used for indications and populations that had not been approved. The second form of regulation is regarding claims for health products and services, although the impact of such regulation is unclear. The question for the future is whether the government role will be extended beyond prohibiting unsubstantiated claims to letting the public know what are the probabilities of success. As an example, for most individuals, no diet program will ever work unless it is coupled with regular exercise. Perhaps in the future, ads for diet products and services will be required to include a Surgeon General's warning that diets rarely work except for a short period, that they can cause harm, and that long-term effectiveness requires coupling changes in eating habits with regular exercise.

EVIDENCE-BASED DECISIONS

One of the almost certain trends in the near future will be increased emphasis on evidence-based decision making. The U.S. Guide to Clinical Preventive Services (17) broke new ground in evaluating the effectiveness of all clinical preventive services on the basis of standardized rules of evidence and a reproducible approach to translating evidence into recommendations. An important parallel effort is under way to assess evidence underlying preventive interventions at the local, regional, and state levels (18). The U.S. Guide to Community Preventive Services (18) includes topics that range as widely as child safety seats, fluoridation, improving immunization rates, and decreasing teenage pregnancies. The results of this process are valuable in at least three ways. First they increase pressure for interventions that have been shown to be effective but are not currently in place. Second, they identify interventions in use that have been shown to be ineffective. Third, they highlight interventions for which there is no evidence or inconclusive evidence, yielding a rich and prioritized research agenda.

COST-EFFECTIVENESS

The Guide to Community Preventive Services summarizes evidence on cost-effectiveness. Marrying effectiveness to cost information is crucial to give a sense of relative value for investment. For example, available evidence currently suggests that for most populations, community-wide immunization campaigns that try to get children immunized through community care management outreach programs may be less cost-effective than efforts to improve the immunization reminder and recall systems of providers (19,20). Increasingly, we will find several different effective interventions with varying levels of effectiveness in reducing the preventable fraction of a health problem and with varying levels of health return on investment. Allocation of investment will increasingly make use of this type of information.

As both policy makers and purchasers of health promotion products and services increase in sophistication, they will want to go a step farther and understand the marginal cost-effectiveness of alternative measures to improve health, i.e., "Given where we are today, which investment yields the greater return in terms of health?" Immunizations have been shown not only to have high levels of health return on investment, but also to save money, on average. However, if 95% of children reaching age 2 are already fully immunized, further investment to get the last 5% immunized might cost more per year of life saved than other investments in health, such as providing bicycle helmets or breastfeeding education.

The immunization example illustrates a related problem that will receive more attention: how compliance issues change with use rates. To return to our exercise example, the cost to get one sedentary individual to exercise for 6 months may be X dollars when the percentage of regular exercisers is 20%, but 2X when it is 45%. This is because the at-risk population changes as those most likely to change do so, leaving a population with an average diminished propensity to change.

MANAGED CARE

One of the more interesting prognostications is what the impact of managed care will be on health promotion. Many managed care organizations (MCOs) have committed substantial resources to health promotion. Some have hired well-respected experts in health promotion, public health, and preventive medicine. It can be argued that MCOs have a strong financial incentive to keep their enrollee population healthy and therefore that the organization's interest aligns well with that of their enrollees and communities. However, this easy truth does not cover all situations. High rates of disenrollment still characterize some geographical regions and particular MCOs. Further, many of the benefits may accrue to the individual or to society, but may not result in lower costs to the plan. For example, the health benefits of smoking cessation are substantial in terms of individual health, but they accrue over a long period of time, while the costs of cessation are borne today by the plan.

Even assuming that all individuals stayed in same plan throughout their life, the plan will not get net dollar savings from smoking cessation but rather a good health return on investment. For an investor-owned company, this translates into higher costs and reduced profits, unless there are some other business benefits. An example of such a benefit is an employer willing to pay more for premiums to health plans whose programs increase worker productivity by decreasing absenteeism.

PERFORMANCE MEASURES

This is where performance measures come into play. The Nation Committee on Quality Assurance (NCQA), the Foundation for Accountability (FACCT), and the Joint Commission on Accreditation of Health Care Organizations offer voluntary programs for MCOs to measure their performance on an increasing number of measures, many of them prevention-oriented. There is strong pressure from private purchasers of health benefits, and a requirement from the Health Care Financing Administration (HCFA), for plans with Medicaid enrollees, that they report on Health Plan Employer Data Information Set (HEDIS) measures, such as mammography and cervical cancer screening rates, but also on physician advice for smoking cessation (21). Increasingly, these measures are incorporated into plan "report cards" that are being given to employees at the time of enrollment or re-enrollment. As most large employers provide employees the choice of several MCOs, how well each fares on these prevention measures can influence employee decisions. This is the other business benefit from investment in prevention. Competition among

MCOs will increasingly be based on results. There will be a strong emphasis on what percentage of the at-risk population has reduced their risk from, for example, high blood pressure, high cholesterol, or sedentary activity. To the degree that better health promotion translates into enhanced market share and higher revenues, the return on the health promotion investment will be not only in terms of health but also healthy returns to MCO shareholders.

CHILD HEALTH AND DEVELOPMENT

The first century of the new millennium will see more attention to health promotion applied at the beginning of life. We have made major advances in our understanding of the development of the human brain. Research has deepened our understanding of the trajectory of development. Small problems not addressed early in childhood can lead to serious problems in older children and adults that affect their social functions and their educational attainment. Yet we have done relatively little to assure that all children are benefiting from this knowledge in terms of parental roles and responsibilities or the services provided by child care providers. Providing a nurturing, safe, stimulating environment for our youngest children is likely to turn out to be our best health promotion investment, with effects reaching into many sectors—such as reduced juvenile crime, and improved educational attainment, mental health, social functioning, physical health, and parenting in the next generation.

INTERNET-ACCESSIBLE TOOLS AND DATABASES

Health promotion planning and evaluation will benefit from better, more accessible tools to easily understand the available databases of interventions and their context. The Internet is a great leveler. A moderately sophisticated web user can efficiently amass a tremendous amount of culled information on a particular health promotion topic in less than an hour. In addition, data from national, state, and local surveys on health will be easier to combine to provide actionable information along with databases on what interventions are effective and how to evaluate them. A program planner or manager will be able to rapidly develop a community diagnosis and determine the best alternative interventions to share with community partners. Further, health promotion professionals will increasingly use the Internet to share ideas and experiences and to provide consultation.

PROFESSIONAL CERTIFICATION

In the future, we are likely to see the evolution of certification processes available for health promotion professionals, focused on a core set of generic skills. We are also likely to see a clearer division between health promotion professionals who help individuals and those whose skills are population-based. The former could be a clinical nutritionist, a smoking cessation counselor, or a one-on-one fitness trainer, while the latter could be the health promotion corrdinator of an MCO or medical group. For both groups, however, what the public considers health promotion is likely to be enlarged. For example, developing a breastfeeding program at a corporation, designing a program to help parents find child care for children with episodic childhood illnesses, or devising a strategy to cost-effectively counsel those at high risk for a variety of genetic problems are all likely to be considered health promotion. An infant stimulation program also may be considered as part of health promotion, as may a home visiting program for the frail elderly.

The concept of health promotion, however construed, was born, nurtured, and developed rapidly during the last third of the twentieth century. The twenty-first century will see it take many new forms, avail itself of more powerful technologies, and strengthen its position as an important part of public efforts to improve health. Health promotion will have multiple homes and likely will still have many operational definitions. Such continuing confusion over what health promotion is won't detract from its increasing impact on population health.

REFERENCES

1. World Health Organization. Basic documents. 40th ed. Geneva: World Health Organization, 1994.

2. U.S. Department of Health and Human Services. Healthy people 2000: national health promotion and disease prevention objectives. Washington, DC: Government Printing Office, 1991.

3. Green LW. Prevention and health education. In: Last JM, Wallace RB, eds. Public health and preventive medicine. 13th ed. East Norwalk, CT: Appleton & Lange, 1992.

4. Hertzman C, Frank J, Evans RG. Heterogeneities in health status and the determinants of population health. In: Evans RG, Barer ML, Marmor TR, eds. Why are some people healthy and others not? Hawthorne, NY: Aldine de Gruyter, 1994.

5. Wilkinson RD. The epidemiological transition: from material scarcity to social disadvantage. Daedalus 1994;123:61–78.

6. U.S. Bureau of the Census. Statistical abstract of the U.S.: 1997. 117th ed. Washington, DC: Government Printing Office, 1997: 475–476.

7. Garfinkel I, McLanahan SS. Single mothers and their children. Washington, DC: The Urban Institute, 1986.

8. Newcomb MD, Maddahian E, Bentler PM. Risk factors for drug use among adolescents: concurrent and longitudinal analyses. Am J Public Health 1986;76:525–531.

9. Surgeon General's Scientific Advisory Committee on Television and Social Behavior. Television and growing up: the impact of televised violence. Washington, DC: Government Printing Office, 1972.

10. Pierce JP, Choi WS, Gilpin EA, et al. Tobacco industry promotion of cigarettes and adolescent smoking. JAMA 1998;279:511–515.

11. Syme SL. Social determinants of disease. In: Last JM, Wallace RB, eds. Public health and preventive medicine. 13th ed. East Norwalk: Appleton & Lange, 1992:687–700.

12. Syme SL. Social determinants of disease. In: Last JM, Wallace RB, eds. Public health and preventive medicine. 13th ed. East Norwalk: Appleton & Lange, 1992:687–700.

13. Ferrini RL, Perlman M, Hill L. Skin protection from ultraviolet light exposure: American College of Preventive Medicine practice policy statement. Am J Preven Med 1998;14:83–86.

14. U.S. Department of Health and Human Services. Physical activity and health: a report of the Surgeon General. National Center for Chronic Disease Prevention and Health Promotion. Atlanta, GA: Centers for Disease Control and Prevention, 1996.

15. U.S. Department of Health and Human Services. Physical activity and health: a report of the Surgeon General. National Center for Chronic Disease Prevention and Health Promotion. Atlanta, GA: Centers for Disease Control and Prevention, 1996.

16. Minnesota Attorney General's Office. Historic 6.1 billion dollar settlement of tobacco lawsuit. Available at http://www.ag.state.mn.us/settlement/settlementagreement.html.

17. U.S. Department of Health and Human Services. Guide to clinical preventive services. 1st ed. Report of the U.S. Preventive Services Task Force. Baltimore, MD: Williams & Wilkins, 1989.

18. U.S. Department of Health and Human Services. Guide to community preventive services. Atlanta: USDHSS, 1997.

19. Wood D, Halfon N, Donald-Sherbourne C, et al. Increasing immunization rates among inner-city, African American children. JAMA 1998;279:29–34.

20. Vaccine-preventable diseases. Draft chapter on infectious diseases. Presented at the Quarterly Meeting of the Task Force on Community Preventive Services, U.S. Department of Health and Human Services. Atlanta, GA, April 14, 1998.

21. Task Force on Community Preventive Services. HEDIS 3.0. Washington, DC: National Committee for Quality Assurance, 1997.

Part XV.

EXERCISE AND SPORT PSYCHOLOGY

Edited by
David R. Brown

Introduction to Exercise and Sport Psychology

David R. Brown

The field of exercise and sport psychology may be viewed as the counterpart to exercise physiology: they are two separate scientific disciplines devoted to the study of different aspects of the same behavior, physical activity. The fact that two fields have emerged to study one behavior, broadly defined as physical activity (including exercise and sport activity), is strong testament to the dualistic nature of this behavior, which has led researchers in exercise and sport psychology, such as William Morgan and Dan Landers, to advocate for viewing physical activity behavior from a psychophysiologic perspective, rather than from a psychological or physiologic perspective only. The author of the first chapter in this section, Steven Petruzzello, highlights evidence for the increasingly popular belief and "renewed" interest among the lay and scientific communities that mind and body are intricately related to behavior and health. His review is based on findings that have emerged from other fields in addition to exercise science and reinforces the importance of viewing behavior and health from a multidisciplinary perspective. The remaining chapters in this section capture what is often viewed as the more traditional "psychology" component of physical activity, but these chapters in their own right also reinforce the view that physical activity behavior involves both mind and body interactions and health outcomes. The two are inescapably interconnected, and this fact should guide physical activity research efforts and public health interventions to promote physical activity among the general population.

Lise Gauvin, John Spence, and Sandra Anderson review the research related to exercise and psychological well-being in the adult population. They point out that, depending on the psychological construct, there is scientific support for the view that physical activity is weakly to moderately associated with psychological well-being. The causal mechanisms mediating the association remain unclear, however, and the authors discuss what impact this has on framing public health messages to promote the psychological benefits of physical activity. Gauvin et al further emphasize the need for additional research to focus on intrapersonal factors that may influence or confound the exercise and psychological well-being association.

Karen Calfas extends the exploration of the psychological benefits associated with physical activity to youth, representative of both general and special populations. Her review suggests modest support for the view that psychological benefits are associated with physical activity in this population. Though the literature yields promising results, methodologic weaknesses in much of the research reviewed, and equivocal findings, do not allow Calfas to draw firm or strong conclusions. Calfas discusses future research directions that are required to increase confidence in findings related to the literature in this area.

James Krause discusses a series of studies that explore the relationship between physical activity and psychological well-being among persons with spinal cord injuries. His work expands our knowledge beyond what we know about persons without disabilities. His findings indicate that researchers in exercise science may benefit from thinking about activity in broader terms than leisure time activity (e.g., to include such factors as employment) and that researchers in the area of disabilities should consider giving greater attention to the benefits of leisure time activity.

Malani Trine reviewed the research related to physical activity and quality of life and found that the literature in this area is equivocal. Trine points out that this is a result of a lack of an agreed-on definition of quality of life, a lack of valid and reliable quality of life measures, and physical activity and quality of life studies that possess methodologic weaknesses. Her chapter is an excellent overview of the methodologic issues and difficulties that face researchers in the area of exercise and sport psychology, who are faced with achieving valid and reliable measurements of quality of life, life satisfaction, and well-being.

Although the benefits of physical activity are numerous, involvement in physical activity is not risk free. John Raglin and Lori Moger review the literature that shows that physical activity may be contraindicated for some individuals who take physical activity to the extreme. This includes recreational exercisers as well as competitive endurance athletes. For a small number of inactive persons who initiate a physical activity or exercise program, the risks of "too much" activity may become a reality that necessitates therapeutic interventions.

Although it is often thought that physical activity is related to eating disorders in some persons, especially girls and young women, these hypothesized relationships appear to be based more on opinion than the weight of scientific evidence. Pat O'Connor and J. Carson Smith point out that the prevalence of eating disorders is low, but disturbingly on the increase, and that the morbidity and mortality rates associated with the disorders are very concerning. However, after reviewing some known correlates of eating disorders, O'Connor and Smith conclude that there is no compelling evidence supporting a hypothesis that involvement in sports, or being physically active, *causes* eating disorders.

After reviews about the positive and potentially negative aspects of physical activity, Janet Buckworth and Rod Dishman tackle the difficult question about how to increase the number of persons who initiate and maintain physically active lifestyles. They review the state of the art with respect to determinants of physical activity. Despite early measurement problems and limitations with physical activity determinants research, progress has been made during the past 10 to 15 years. When possible, Buckworth and Dishman discuss the potential application of the knowledge gained from determinants research to physical activity and health promotion efforts. They also provide direction for future research that can fill current gaps in our knowledge.

Chapter 82

Recent Advances in Mind-Body Understandings

Steven J. Petruzzello

Mens sana en corpore sano—a sound mind in a sound body: this Latin phrase has been a mantra for the fledgling discipline of exercise psychology. At its essence, it seems to suggest that mind and body are intimately related to one another. Careful consideration of the available literature, however, could lead to the conclusion that mind and body are distinct entities, with the latter serving only as a place within which the former resides. The goal of this chapter is to examine advances in mind-body understandings. It would seem prudent to begin with an explanation of the term "mind-body." What exactly does this imply? Many have pointed to the thinking and writings of Rene Descartes for the origins of the dualistic distinction between mind and body (1–4). Since the early seventeenth century science has operated on the notion that mind and body can be separated. As Melnechuk put it,

> Back then, dualism made the body, as a ghost-free machine of mere meat, a permissible object of empirical investigation at a time when the Inquisition was dangerous to scientists, as shown by the contemporaneous trial of Galileo. In modern times it reinforced the biomedical avoidance of studying emotions as factors in health and disease (3).

This dualistic thinking still permeates much of science, although it is difficult to defend the position that mind and body are separate. What results from the continued distinction are physiologists studying physiologic processes as distinct entities (with no influence from the mind) and psychologists (or other "mind scientists") studying psychological processes as though they were distinct from physiologic sources. Consider the following: "All social cognitive approaches are based on a constructionist metatheory, where cognitively based variables such as intentions, attitudes, and self-efficacy are nonmaterial psychological constructions and not observable in the physical world" (5). Such thinking allows one to operate at a single level of organization (e.g., psychological) without concern for how such phenomena might extend to other, adjacent levels (e.g., physiological, social). Cacioppo et al (6,7) have stated,

> Traditionally, investigators have emphasized single levels of analysis of social psychological phenomena with survey and self-report measures being the most common methods used to investigate the mechanisms underlying these phenomena. The predictable yield from isolated research on discrete determinants of multiply determined social psychological phenomena is a portfolio of fact lists and disparate microtheories. These microtheories each provide a limited account for the phenomenon of interest and are at best pieces of a larger conceptual puzzle. Even determinants of a phenomenon that account for a modicum of variance are noteworthy if the goal is to achieve a comprehensive theory of the psychological phenomenon rather than a microtheory of the determinant. In addition, knowledge of the body and brain can usefully constrain and inspire concepts and theories of psychological function, because there are any number of ways in which a particular outcome might be achieved. Knowledge about the functional organization of ordered and disordered mental or social activities, however, can also usefully guide the study of the underlying brain processes because the nature of the particular physiological mechanisms and events could be suggested by the observed mentation, behavior, or interaction. Although there are neurophysiological processes that are affected,

for instance, by human association and which underlie the associated psychological and social phenomena, these phenomena shape physiological events in ways that may not be evident from studies of the physiology isolated from the social context in which they manifest (6).

The problem cuts both ways. The physiologist, often viewed as reductionistic, typically ignores the influence of psychological and social factors. To once again quote Cacioppo et al:

> . . . it [reductionism] undermines multilevel, integrative analyses, alienates scientists working at "unchosen" levels of organization who might otherwise contribute relevant data and theory, and renders it acceptable to ignore relevant theory and data on a phenomenon of interest simply because they were not born from one's preferred level of analysis (6).

While such approaches to viewing the world and answering questions about it are certainly valuable in their own right, the obvious point is that a much greater understanding of phenomena can be gained by examining across levels of analysis (i.e., psychological, physiologic). One conceptual approach to examining mind-body issues across analytic levels is the psychophysiologic approach. An aspect of this approach that aids in cross-level investigation is the *monistic identity thesis* (1), a central tenet of psychophysiology. At its essence, the monistic identity thesis holds that there is a counterpart in the physical domain for every psychological event. This leads to the realization that events taking place at any level in the individual occur simultaneously at all levels (8). As such, intentions, attitudes, and self-efficacy are *not* nonmaterial constructs and *can be* observed in the material world. The monistic identity thesis holds that events of the body are simultaneously events of the mind. Thus, "A mental perception or idea and the initial physical event (brain cells firing, neurotransmitter molecules moving) are not two separate things, but two different ways of describing the same event. An initial mental change must entail corresponding physical change" (8). If one espouses such a philosophy, then examining mind-body issues becomes potentially more fruitful. It becomes the challenge of science to find these corresponding physical changes.

Interest in the so-called interactions of mind and body continues to grow, particularly in the health domain. Goleman et al (9) discuss mind-body medicine, referring to it as a framework wherein the mind (i.e., emotions, thoughts) is viewed as having a significant influence on the body's health. There has also been a growing effort to uncover the physical events that correspond with psychological phenomena. As a way of illustrating the interconnectedness of mind-body, the remainder of this chapter examines findings from different areas of research that clearly show the linkages between mind and body or between body and mind. Intriguing findings have come from scientists who are focusing on cognitions and emotions using a mind-body perspective.

"WINDOWS INTO THE THINKING MIND"

Cognitions and cognitive function have historically held a place of prominence in psychophysiology. Cognitive processes such as attention, information processing, and even attitudes have been extensively studied using psychophysiologic paradigms and techniques. For example, researchers in motor behavior have long been interested in reaction time, or how long it takes an individual to respond to an environmental stimulus. Behaviorally, this is assessed by measuring the amount of time that elapses from the time a stimulus is presented until the subject makes some overt response (e.g., button press). This reveals little about how the response comes about, however. More information is gained if the motor system is examined using electromyographic (EMG) recordings. This still reflects a delay from the time the stimulus is processed by the nervous system to when a response is initiated.

Measures of brain activity (e.g., event-related potentials, or ERPs) have been used as "windows into the mind (i.e., cognition)" (10). Working with such techniques, investigators have been able to demonstrate partial information transmission, preparation of the motor system for action of some kind, and processes involved in the inhibition of responses (10). ERPs have been reported in the exercise literature as an effective method for indexing cognitive function. For example, Dustman et al (11) compared electroencephalographic (EEG) and ERP measures in younger and older individuals who were classified, based on their lifestyles (i.e., physical activity habits), as either being in poor-fair or excellent-superior condition. They found that more fit subjects had earlier visual evoked potential latencies (i.e., they perceived visual stimuli more quickly) and faster P300 latencies (i.e., they processed information more rapidly) than did less fit subjects. In addition, the older fit individuals were similar to the younger subjects in terms of P300 latency, suggesting that maintenance of aerobic fitness may offer some immunity against the functional loss that is often seen with "normal" aging. Similar findings have also been reported by Bashore (12).

Dustman et al also examined the central inhibition capacity of these subjects using a measure termed *cortical coupling*. The ability of the central nervous system (CNS) to inhibit unwanted or undesirable responses deteriorates with advancing age. A lessening of inhibitory strength is thus expected to adversely affect physical and cognitive functioning (13). EEG waveforms have been shown to be more homogeneous across electrode sites in older than in younger adults (14). Such loss of inhibition is reflected in cortical coupling, with greater cortical coupling values seen in diseased states (e.g., Down syndrome, dementia) and with advancing age. Because cortical coupling reflects the degree to which distinct cortical regions function similarly, an increase in cortical coupling with age would "suggest that aging is associated with a loss of functional autonomy of brain areas such that the older brain responds in a more homogeneous or global manner" (13). However, physically fit older subjects have been shown to be similar to young adults on measures of such functional autonomy (i.e., cortical coupling values), suggesting that endurance exercise can modulate excitation or inhibition relationships. A more contemporary measure of regional functioning is EEG coherence, which measures the similarity between two EEG signals at different brain regions. Like cortical coupling, it is thought to reflect structural and functional coupling of those brain regions (15). Higher coherence values reflect increasing similarity of response between different brain regions. Recent data from our laboratory has shown that older, active subjects had lower mean coherence values than older, sedentary individuals (16). How such differences might be manifested at the psychological level (i.e., cognitive function) requires further elaboration. At present, however, it appears that "body" manipulations (e.g., regular exercise) can have important effects as reflected in these "windows into the mind."

"Windows into the mind" are not exclusive to the brain. Numerous other psychophysiologic measures have been used to infer various psychological processes. As Kutas et al (7) point out, autonomic measures can be particularly useful for gaining insight into cognitive processes that individuals might have difficulty describing (17). Attitudes, or the direction and intensity of a feeling toward an object or concept, have been the subject of extensive investigation in the psychophysiologic domain. Cacioppo et al have performed numerous studies to investigate the relation between mind and body with respect to attitudes. For example, Cacioppo et al (18) showed that arm (but not leg) flexion and extension had differential effects on attitude formation, suggesting that motor processes (i.e., flexion, extension) influence evaluative judgments (i.e., how individuals think about things). These authors clearly demonstrated that motor processes can influence an individual's attitude. Attitudes can also be reflected in the CNS, again utilizing ERP measures. Using the late positive potential (LPP), Cacioppo et al (19) have shown that attitude stimuli that are evaluatively inconsistent (e.g., presenting a very negative trait in a sequence of predominantly very positive traits) result in a graded LPP response, with larger evoked responses to very negative traits. Cacioppo and colleagues have shown that the LPP is not linked invariantly to affective processes but could instead be considered a marker of specific evaluative categorizations (1).

"WINDOWS INTO THE FEELING MIND"

Probably more than any other class of behavior, emotion often involves frank biological changes that are frequently perceptible to the person in whom the emotion arises as well as to an observer (20).

Numerous individuals have suggested that understanding emotions is a necessary task for understanding human behavior. A strong case can be made for the importance of the brain in furthering our knowledge about human emotion and emotional function. It is clear that how we feel has direct effects on our central and peripheral physiology; changes in our physiology also influence how we feel. As LeDoux (21) has noted, "understanding emotions in the human brain is clearly an important quest, as most mental disorders are emotional disorders." Much of what is known about emotion is often based on self-reports of emotions or feeling states as a function of manipulations hypothesized to change how we feel. Davidson et al (22) note, however, that "inferences about emotion can be made on the basis of changes in behavior and physiology, and need not rely upon conscious introspective report." Indeed, as noted by Nisbett et al (17) many years ago, this is not a new idea. Psychophysiologic investigations of emotion have pro-

vided much greater understanding than could have ever been achieved from an exclusively self-report perspective.

Psychophysiologists have tried for some time to uncover the physiologic patterns of basic emotions. There has been a good deal of debate as to whether specific autonomic patterns accompany specific emotions. Although current opinion seems to hold that support for emotion-specific autonomic activity is inconclusive (23), a number of interesting findings have emerged in this area. Lang et al (24), using pictures that varied along dimensions of valence (pleasant-unpleasant) and arousal (excited-calm), showed that facial EMG (corrugator, zygomatic sites) readings were significantly related to self-rated valence of the pictures. Skin conductance response, however, was more strongly linked with arousal but not valence. This work highlights the *pattern* of physiologic responding, with different patterns depending on whether individuals were more expressive (via facial somatic system) or internalized (i.e., primarily sympathetic responders). Focusing exclusively on facial EMG patterns in response to manipulations designed to produce certain emotional states has been a more typical tactic in the autonomic specificity research. For example, it has been shown that smiles reflecting the experience of enjoyment have concomitantly different muscle activation patterns than smiles elicited in response to other stimuli (e.g., trying to appear pleasant while concealing negative emotion). Specifically, smiles referred to as "Duchenne smiles" (reflecting frank joy) include activity of both the zygomatic and orbicularis oculi muscles, whereas "other" smiles (e.g., reflecting fake joy) involve only zygomatic muscle activity (25).

Another perspective has also been entertained for the changes in muscle activity that appear to occur along with different kinds of emotions. It has been speculated that facial actions can change brain physiology. Zajonc and colleagues (26–28), in presenting the vascular theory of emotional efference, have suggested that changes in the facial musculature result in alterations in the volume of air inhaled through the nose. This altered air volume affects the temperature of blood in the brain (via the direct effect such changes have on hypothalamic temperature), which in turn has affective consequences. Negative facial expressions (achieved by having subjects vocalize phonemes) have been shown to result in less air movement through the nose, resulting in higher forehead temperatures (i.e., index of hypothalamic temperature) and more negative affect. Conversely, more positive facial expressions result in greater air movement through the nasal passages, lower forehead temperatures, and more positive affective responses. Some hypotheses (e.g., thermogenic hypothesis) (29) in exercise psychology have implicated temperature change as a potential mechanism for explaining exercise-related changes in affect. Investigations of such temperature change, however, have shown a general failure of manipulations in core body temperature during exercise to have any appreciable effect on exercise-related affect (30,31). Unfortunately, none of these studies have examined indices of brain temperature. Growing evidence indicates that brain temperature and body temperature may be independently regulated (32–34). Thus, while current data may allow the elimination of core body temperature as a factor in explaining exercise-related affective change, brain temperature remains a viable and theoretically appealing alternative.

Davidson has been instrumental in advancing what he has referred to as "affective neuroscience" (22). Evidence from numerous fronts has led to the proposal that the anterior regions of the cerebral cortex are particularly important in emotional behavior and experience. Davidson has proposed that the right and left anterior regions of the brain are specialized for withdrawal or aversive and approach or appetitive processes, respectively (20). Individuals who have damage to the left hemisphere have been characterized as having a deficit in approach behavior, often experiencing apathy, loss of interest or pleasure in people and things, and difficulty in initiating action. Robinson and Downhill (35) have noted that damage (i.e., lesion due to stroke) to the left hemisphere, specifically in the left dorsolateral frontal and the left basal ganglia area, is most often associated with depressive symptoms.

The basic approach-withdrawal distinction has been supported through a growing body of research on normal, neurologically intact individuals. Derived in large part through noninvasive measures of brain activity (i.e., EEG), although more recent work has also utilized advanced neuroimaging techniques (e.g., positron emission tomography, or PET; functional magnetic resonance imaging, or fMRI), it has been shown that greater relative activation of the left anterior brain region coincides with approach-related processes and emotions (i.e., positive affect), deficient activation of this region is associated with approach-related deficits (e.g., sadness, depression), and greater relative activation of the right anterior brain region is seen with withdrawal-related processes and emotions (i.e., fear, disgust, anxiety).

As noted by Kutas and Fedemeier (7), autonomic measures like EMG can be used in combination with CNS measures (e.g., EEG), thus providing examination of the nervous system at multiple levels (e.g., somatic, CNS). In addition to being able to distinguish among Duchenne smiles and other smiles using facial muscle activity patterns, Ekman and Davidson et al demonstrated such smiles (and, by inference, the accompanying emotion) could be distinguished by patterns of regional brain activation. Consistent with the approach-withdrawal distinction, Davidson et al (36) found that film clips designed to evoke either positive or negative emotions resulted in facial behavior classified as either happiness or disgust, respectively. EEG recorded from the scalp at the same time revealed that during the negative emotion–eliciting film clips, greater right-sided anterior activation was present, whereas during the positive emotion–eliciting film clips, greater left-sided anterior activation was present. In addition to the somatic activation patterns of the face that accompany positive and negative emotions, differential activation patterns emerge in the CNS. The work of Ekman et al (37) further showed that voluntarily produced Duchenne smiles (reflecting enjoyment) were distinguishable from other voluntary smiles as indicated by a left-sided anterior activation pattern. Other voluntary smiles did not produce this electrocortical pattern.

Patterns of regional brain activation at rest have also been shown to be related to dispositional affect (38) and to be predictive of emotional response (39). Davidson (20) has discussed this within the context of a diathesis-stress formulation whereby the asymmetrical activation of the anterior brain regions serves as a diathesis that predisposes an individual to respond, given an appropriate emotion elicitor, with a characteristic emotional response. For example, Wheeler et al (39) showed that individuals with greater resting left anterior brain activation (as assessed via scalp-recorded EEG), relative to the right anterior region, reported more intense positive affect and less intense negative affect in response to positive and negative film clips, respectively. Conversely, those individuals with greater resting right anterior brain activation, relative to the left anterior region, reported less intense positive affect and more intense negative affect in response to the same positive and negative film clips. Thus, in response to an emotion eliciting stimulus (i.e., positive or negative film clip), the individual's emotional response can be predicted by their resting cortical physiology.

Exercise has been suspected as an emotion-eliciting stimulus for some time, often resulting in reduced negative and enhanced positive affect. The perspective espoused here is that the physical changes that occur with exercise are intimately linked with these affective changes. Consider the following, as expressed by noted philosopher and psychologist William James:

> Everyone knows the effect of physical exercise on the mood: how much more cheerful and courageous one feels when the body has been toned up, than when it is "run down." . . . our moods are determined by the feelings which come up from our body. Those feelings are sometimes of worry, breathlessness, anxiety; sometimes of peace and repose. It is certain that physical exercise will tend to train the body toward the latter feelings. The latter feelings are certainly an essential ingredient in all perfect human character (40).

In a series of studies, we have shown that regional brain activation can predict affective responses to exercise (41–43), but is also associated with concurrent affective states after exercise (42,43). As Davidson does, we have shown that individuals with greater left anterior activation at rest report less anxiety and greater positive affect after acute, moderately intense, aerobic exercise. Our most recent work suggests that the relationship between resting brain activation and the affective response to exercise is mediated by level of aerobic fitness (41). Our data further supports the diathesis-stress hypothesis in that light-to-moderate aerobic exercise ($\leq$55% of maximum oxygen consumption, or Vo_2max) is not a sufficient enough stimulus to elicit an emotional response and can therefore not be predicted by resting brain activity (44). We also have some preliminary data that suggests that brain activation patterns during exercise reflect concomitant self-reported affect (45). It is from findings such as these that we are fairly comfortable in asserting that aerobic exercise is indeed an emotion-eliciting event. Furthermore, it is apparent that patterns of resting physiology of the CNS can reflect not only individual differences in dispositional affect but it can also be predictive of affective responses to rather robust psychophysiologic changes occurring as a result of moderately intense-to-heavy exercise loads ($\geq$70% Vo_2max).

Another noninvasive methodology that has potential promise in the exercise paradigm is the affect-modulated startle response, which is reflected in the eyeblink response to acoustic probes. There is a growing body of evidence showing that negative affect serves to potentiate the eyeblink response whereas positive or neutral affect inhibits the response (46). Beyond being simply another methodology, the startle response is a noninvasive index of activation of the amygdala, considered to be the center of emotional integration (47,48). This highlights the fact that a psychological event (i.e., affect) is simultaneously reflected in activity of the CNS as indexed by autonomic nervous system measures (i.e., EMG). In other words, psychological constructs can be observed in the physical world. To date, only one attempt has been made in the exercise literature to utilize the startle probe method (49). In this study, startle eyeblink responses were unrelated to changes in anxiety, but relying on anxiety to index affective change in nonanxious subjects is potentially problematic. Thinking of affect in terms of both activation and valence dimensions would perhaps be a more productive approach to examining the role of exercise intensity, and the startle method is ideally suited to examine such dimensions. Yet again, the point is that "mind" issues (i.e., affect or emotion) are intimately rooted in, and inseparable from, "body" issues.

"LOOKING THROUGH 'STRAINED'-GLASS WINDOWS"

From the perspective of Davidson, diathesis-stress is used as a formulation for examining emotional responsivity to environmental stimuli based on resting activation asymmetries. An individual with greater relative right anterior activation at rest would be likely to express more intense negative affect in response to a stressful event. Different approaches for examining stress occur in other domains. A particularly interesting field of research, which offers the promise of much greater understanding of how stress affects the body, is psychoneuroimmunology (PNI). PNI is a descriptor for research that examines the interplay among a variety of mind-body systems, particularly the nervous and immune systems. Furthermore, special attention is given to psychological and social-environmental factors and the effects these have on mind-body function. To follow up on the work of Davidson, he and his colleagues (50) have shown that individuals characterized by extreme right anterior brain activation, as opposed to extreme left anterior activation, had significantly lower levels of natural killer (NK) cell activity (a measure of immune function). No differences were found, however, for other immune measures (e.g., T-cell subsets, lymphocyte proliferation). These findings are consistent with the framework that greater relative right anterior brain activation is reflective of vulnerability to negative affective responsivity and dispositional negative affect. Kang et al speculated that such a pattern of neural activity and immune function could affect an individual's illness vulnerability. Gruzelier et al (51) carried such a proposition further by examining brain function (via EEG and neuropsychological assessment) and immune status in men infected with HIV. It was shown that greater left hemisphere activation upon entry to the study was associated with better immune function 30 months later. In both cases, it could be proposed that certain patterns of resting brain activation may serve as a biologic marker of the predisposition to respond to potential stressors, at least in terms of the immune response.

An influential model in the development of our understanding of the stress response involves two related yet distinct neuroendocrine axes: the sympathetic-adrenal-medullary (SAM) axis and the hypothalamic-pituitary-adrenocortical (HPA) axis. The SAM axis response to a stressor results in sympathetic outflow to the adrenal medulla, releasing norepinephrine into the bloodstream. The HPA axis response involves stimulation of the adrenal cortex from the hypothalamus, resulting in the release of glucocorticoids, namely cortisol, into the bloodstream. An important link in the HPA axis response involves the amygdala. As noted by Sothmann et al (21,52), threatening stimuli access a more direct pathway to the hypothalamus via the amygdala. If sufficiently aversive, cortical pathways are bypassed altogether, providing for a quicker initiation of the response. Both axes are involved in the stress response, with the SAM axis responding more rapidly and the HPA axis requiring longer recovery time.

Wittling (53) has suggested that the SAM axis reflects a "defense response" characterized by the active involvement of the individual in dealing with or trying to escape from the challenge. Based on evidence from presentations of either evocative or neutral film clips to either the left or right hemisphere, Wittling suggests that such defensive (i.e., active) coping is more strongly associated with activation of the left hemisphere. This is consistent with Davidson's work inasmuch as the defensive coping is similar to an approach orientation, which it would be, if approach is viewed as an active type of response. Wittling further suggests that an HPA axis response is a "conservation-withdrawal" response, enjoined by a passive response by the individual and the concomitant experience of loss of control. In contrast to the defense response, the withdrawal response is proposed as more strongly associated with right hemisphere activation. Using salivary cortisol (reflective of coping ability, i.e., less cortisol in response to challenge is postulated to be adaptive and more cortisol to be maladaptive) (54), Wittling et al (55) demonstrated that an emotionally aversive film projected to the right hemisphere resulted in the release of significantly more cortisol than when the film was projected to the left hemisphere.

Substantial evidence exists demonstrating decreased immunocompetence in response to numerous stressors (56). Kiecolt-Glaser et al (57), for example, point out the effects of exam stress on medical students. Such stress affects a wide range of immune functions: NK cell activity, which fights tumors and viral infections, declines; gamma interferon, which stimulates the growth and activity of NK cells, decreases; and the response of T-cells to stimulation is compromised. Dantzer (58) notes that positive, familiar social relationships can serve to buffer the stress response. In adults experiencing troubles in their marriages and in spouses caring for a mate with Alzheimer's disease, NK cell activity is diminished, cellular immune control is decreased, and lymphoproliferative responses are reduced. It is apparent that, in our dealings with others, things over which we have little perceived control can have profound effects on our mind/body.

It has become apparent, however, that a stressor in and of itself does not necessarily produce a stress reaction in a given individual. One important factor is the degree of control the individual has over the situation. A number of models have been examined in this regard (e.g., Dienstbier's (54) physiologic toughening model, Bandura's (59) social cognitive framework). Dealing with a stressor without distress, i.e., viewing the stressor as a challenge rather than a threat, has been shown to be associated with an increase in catecholamines coupled with relatively low levels of cortisol (i.e., relatively small HPA axis responses). The same stressor viewed as a threat is likewise accompanied by an increase in catecholamines; however, there is also an increase in cortisol production. Bandura et al (60) examined plasma catecholamine secretion as a function of perceived coping ability, which they refer to as "perceived coping efficacy." Phobics with varying levels of perceived coping efficacy were presented with coping tasks they had determined to be in their low, moderate, or high self-efficacy range. Blood samples were simultaneously taken via an indwelling catheter. Levels of plasma epinephrine and norepinephrine were relatively low during coping with tasks high in the self-efficacy range. Moderate self-efficacy tasks led to increased self-doubt, which was coupled with a sharp increase in plasma catecholamines. Interestingly, low self-efficacy tasks showed a sharp decline in catecholamine levels, and the phobics declined to perform the tasks. Bandura et al further showed that when perceived coping efficacy was enhanced through guided mastery, the stress-producing tasks did not elicit a catecholamine response. Catecholamine reactivity before efficacy enhancement was attributed to a mismatch between the demands of the task and the individual's ability to cope.

In another study with snake phobics (ophidiophobics), Wiedenfeld et al (61) measured immunologic changes during coping. It is known that the degree of control over stressors can have an important influence on immune system function. Wiedenfeld et al assessed immunocompetence (i.e., lymphocyte, T-cell, helper/suppressor cell, interleukin-2 levels), autonomic (i.e., heart rate), and neuroendocrine (i.e., salivary cortisol level) function at baseline and in response to a manipulation designed to enhance self-efficacy over controlling stressors. It was found that the development of a strong sense of self-efficacy had immunoenhancing effects. Specifically, slow development of perceived self-efficacy, high cortisol activation, and heart rate acceleration were related to poorer immune status. Conversely, subjects who developed a strong sense of efficacy quickly showed little decline in immunocompetence. Subjects also showed an overall decline in cortisol activation as perceived efficacy developed, indicating their increasing familiarity with the stressor.

For some individuals, coping with stress is a constant task. In cases of chronic, prolonged stress, the impact on health can be quite dramatic. Simply examining HPA axis activation, for example, may not be informative enough with respect to how the individual is coping with the stress. Appels (62) presents an interesting discussion of distinguishing between conditions associated with either increased or decreased activation of the HPA axis. As an example, melancholic depression is associated with increased HPA axis activation. In seasonal depression (accompanied by feelings of lethargy, hypersomnia, enhanced affective responses to environmental stimuli, fatigue), HPA axis activation is decreased. These individuals are more susceptible to inflammatory diseases, which includes atherosclerosis. Appels makes the case that these "exhausted" individuals are at greater risk for myocardial infarctions as a result of their divergent pattern of HPA axis activation.

It has been a popularly held belief that exercise can act as a buffer against the stress response (54). O'Connor et al (63) demonstrated a relationship between elevated salivary cortisol levels and increased depression in a sample of female swimmers during a period of heavy training (i.e., increased stress). With reduced stress, depression and cortisol level both returned to baseline levels. Rudolph and McAuley (64) examined relationships between self-efficacy and cortisol responses to acute exercise in adults who were classified as either very physically active or less active. The more active group evidenced a faster dissipation of cortisol after the exercise bout, and self-efficacy was found to be inversely related to the cortisol response (i.e., greater levels of efficacy were associated with smaller cortisol increases). Rudolph and McAuley (65) conducted another study examining how exercise history impacted the cortisol and affective response to acute aerobic exercise. Although there were no differences in the cortisol response to treadmill running at 60% of Vo_2max between cross-country runners and nonrunners, nonrunners did have higher perceptions of effort during the run. Cortisol level after running was significantly related to perceived effort, highlighting a link between in-task cognitions and neuroendocrine function. Cortisol levels 30 minutes after the run were also inversely related to affect, supporting the link between lower levels of cortisol and positive affect.

The impact of "body" interventions (i.e., exercise) has also been examined as a way of buffering the effects of stressors. An intriguing study by LaPerriere et al (66) showed that exercise training in an AIDS risk group of men served to attenuate the effects of notification of HIV-1 status. Specifically, asymptomatic men who exercised aerobically for 5 weeks had little change in psychometric and immunologic measures after they had been notified of positive results on HIV testing. Control subjects who did not exercise had significant changes reflective of decreased immunocompetence (i.e., decreased NK cell activity) accompanied by significant increases in anxiety and depression.

In conjunction with personal factors, social and environmental factors can also have an important effect on immune function. Kaplan et al (67) present a review of work detailing how psychosocial factors can influence coronary atherosclerosis. More specifically, their work has focused on how the expression of anger or hostility can lead to atherosclerosis and coronary heart disease. They argue that psychosocial factors, particularly those reflecting dominant social status and social group instability, can lead to the development of disease. Using an animal model, they have found that monkeys housed in unstable social environments (i.e., social groups were constantly changing) developed twice the amount of coronary atherosclerosis if they were dominant monkeys (i.e., high in social rank). This finding was interpreted as evidence that the behavioral demands of having to continually re-establish dominance in ever-changing social environments increases the likelihood of atherosclerotic development. The behavioral demands are reflected in continuing, excessive sympathetic activation with the concomitant increases in heart rate, blood pressure, and catecholamine release.

Cacioppo (68) presents an excellent review of studies that have shown that a variety of "socioemotional" factors can have a significant influence on the functioning of the body. For example, in work examining the social relationships in caregivers for individuals with Alzheimer's disease, evidence is available showing that interpersonal relations (e.g., closeness of relationship to spouse before illness, level of affection) are important in cardiovascular regulation. Specifically, caregiver spouses who spent a good deal of time and engaged in numerous activities with the spouse with Alzheimer's before the illness (i.e., had greater disruption in social lives after diagnosis) had higher resting blood pressure (both systolic and diastolic), whereas degree of positive emotional bond before illness was related to lower resting diastolic blood pressure and less heart rate reactivity (68). Furthermore, Cacioppo notes that cardiac reactivity can have important consequences with respect to stress responses. Specifically, individuals characterized by high sympathetic cardiac reactivity, as compared to those characterized by vagal (i.e., parasympathetic) cardiac reactivity, had greater stress-induced cortisol responses. Work of this type is exciting because it is beginning to uncover intricate relationships not only between mind and body, but also between environmental factors and mind-body relationships.

CLEANING OUR WINDOWS AND LOOKING FOR THE PATTERNS

One of the most striking aspects of examining mind-body research is that there is certainly great potential to increase understanding of how humans function. If investigators can be convinced to begin examining such functioning from multiple levels, as I argued in the beginning of this chapter, this will certainly be a step in the right direction. However, the functioning of human beings is not going to be easily understood. One need go back no further than the work of Cacioppo. In examining neuroendocrine responses to a stressor, he and his colleagues could have easily stopped with the finding that a psychological stressor activates the SAM axis (i.e., increased norepinephrine and epinephrine levels), but not the HPA axis (i.e., no change in cortisol level). However, when these responses were examined in individuals who were high or low heart rate responders, a different picture emerged. High heart rate responders had higher levels of cortisol in addition to the elevated catecholamine response; low heart rate responders did not. As Cacioppo (68) also points out, classifying an individual as a high or low heart rate responder ignores the origin of this reactivity. For example, high heart rate reactivity could be caused by elevated sympathetic reactivity, vagal withdrawal, or reciprocal activation of both sympathetic and vagal input to the heart. The point is, simply including measures from different levels of analysis isn't sufficient. Patterns or profiles of response must be sought, as opposed to expecting simple relationships to be discovered between mind and body measures.

Cacioppo et al (1) make a cogent case for how to examine these multiple measures from the physiologic and psychological domains and put them together in a manner that allows us to make sense out of the confusion. They argue that it is probably not realistic to expect to find simple one-to-one relationships between a psychological event and a physiologic event (e.g., to expect that heart rate will give us a

physiologic measure of anxiety). Such an assumption will lead to frustration because rarely will there be consistent correspondence between such measures. Cacioppo et al argue instead for examination of patterns or profiles of response. As an illustrative example, they present how two autonomic measures, skin conductance and heart rate, can be used to infer different psychological processes. The orienting, defense, and startle responses all share a relationship with skin conductance and heart rate, which would normally preclude the ability to infer the psychological processes from the physiologic signals. Such inferences can be made, however, when the patterns particular to each response are examined. The orienting response is associated with a phasic skin conductance response accompanied by a deceleration in heart rate. Both the startle and defense responses can be inferred from a phasic skin conductance response and an acceleration in heart rate but are differentiated by the fact that the startle response involves an abrupt acceleration in heart rate while the defense response involves a lingering acceleration in heart rate. The point is, it is only through the examination of patterns of responding, or response profiles, that we can uncover the complicated relationships between "body" measures and "mind" constructs. The cost of such an approach is not cheap, but the payoff is infinitely great.

CLOSING THE WINDOW

Although certainly not exhaustive, the evidence presented in this paper clearly shows that "mind" and "body" are intimately linked and inseparable from each other. Much more information is gained by examining human functioning from a mind-body perspective at multiple levels (i.e., psychophysiologic, social-environmental) simultaneously than could ever be obtained by looking at mind and body as separate entities or from single levels of analysis. It is my hope that such information will stimulate readers to examine their research questions more thoughtfully and to begin to explore phenomena of human functioning from a multilevel perspective. It is no longer enough to assume that the only reality that matters is that which individuals construct for themselves. Such perspectives are important but incomplete. The corporeal basis for such realities will aid in how we come to understand human behavior. The following quote from Miller sums it up well:

> The body is the medium of experience and the instrument of action. Through its actions we shape and organize our experiences and distinguish our perceptions of the outside world from sensations that arise within the body itself (69).

The author would like to gratefully acknowledge Panteleimon Ekkekakis, Eric E. Hall, and Lisa M. Van Landuyt for their helpful comments on an earlier draft of this manuscript. Preparation of this chapter and some of the author's own research reviewed within it were supported in part by grant RO3 MH55513-01 from the National Institute of Mental Health.

REFERENCES

1. Cacioppo JT, Tassinary LG. Psychophysiology and psychophysiological inference. In: Cacioppo JT, Tassinary LG, eds. Principles of psychophysiology: physical, social, and inferential elements. New York: Cambridge, 1990:3–33.

2. Kabat-Zinn J. Meditation. In: Moyers BD, ed. Healing and the mind. New York: Doubleday, 1993:115–143.

3. Melnechuk T. Emotions, brain, immunity, and health: a review. In: Clynes M, Panksepp J, ed. Emotions and psychopathology. New York: Plenum, 1988:181–247.

4. Pert C. The chemical communicators. In: Moyers BD, ed. Healing and the mind. New York: Doubleday, 1993:177–193.

5. Dzewaltowski DA. Physical activity determinants: a social cognitive approach. Med Sci Sports Exerc 1994;26:1395–1399.

6. Cacioppo JT, Berntson GG, Crites SL. Social neuroscience: principles of psychophysiological arousal and response. In: Higgins ET, Kruglanski AW, eds. Social psychology: handbook of basic principles. New York: Guilford, 1996:72–101.

7. Kutas M, Federmeier KD. Minding the body. Psychophysiol 1998;35:135–150.

8. Cunningham AJ. Pies, levels, and languages: why the contribution of mind to health and disease has been underestimated. Advances 1995;11:4–11.

9. Goleman D, Gurin J, eds. Mind/body medicine: how to use your mind for better health. Yonkers, NY: Consumer Reports Books, 1993:1–482.

10. Coles MGH. Modern mind-brain reading: psychophysiology, physiology, and cognition. Psychophysiol 1989;26:251–269.

11. Dustman RE, Emmerson RY, Ruhling RO, et al. Age and fitness effects on EEG, ERPs, visual sensitivity, and cognition. Neurobiol Aging 1990;11:193–200.

12. Bashore TR. Age, physical fitness, and mental processing speed. In: Lawton MP, ed. Annual review of gerontology. New York: Springer, 1989:120–144.

13. Dustman RE, Emmerson RY, Shearer DE. Physical activity, age, and cognitive neuropsychological function. J Aging Phys Activity 1994;2:143–181.

14. Dustman RE, LaMarche JA, Cohn NB, et al. Power spectral analysis and cortical coupling of EEG for young and old normal adults. Neurobiol Aging 1985;6:193–198.

15. Hugdahl K. Psychophysiology: the mind-body perspective. Cambridge, MA: Harvard University, 1995:1–429.

16. Hall EE, Petruzzello SJ. Frontal asymmetry, dispositional affect, and physical activity in older adults. J Aging Phys Activity 1999;7:76–90.

17. Nisbett RE, Wilson TD. Telling more than we can know: verbal reports on mental processes. Psychol Rev 1977;84:231–259.

18. Cacioppo JT, Priester JR, Berntson GG. Rudimentary determinants of attitudes. Part II: Arm flexion and extension have differential effects on attitudes. J Pers Soc Psychol 1993;65:5–17.

19. Cacioppo JT, Crites SL, Gardner WL, Berntson GG. Bioelectrical echoes from evaluative categorizations: Part I. A late positive brain potential that varies as a function of trait negativity and extremity. J Pers Soc Psychol 1994;67:115–125.

20. Davidson RJ. Cerebral asymmetry, emotion, and affective style. In: Davidson RJ, Hugdahl K, eds. Brain asymmetry. Cambridge, MA: MIT Press, 1995:361–387.

21. LeDoux J. The emotional brain: the mysterious underpinnings of emotional life. New York: Simon & Schuster, 1996:1–384.

22. Davidson RJ, Sutton SK. Affective neuroscience: the emergence of a discipline. Curr Opin Neurobiol 1995;5:217–224.

23. Cacioppo JT, Klein DJ, Berntson GG, Hatfield E. The psychophysiology of emotion. In: Lewis M, Haviland J, eds. Handbook of emotion. New York: Guilford, 1993:119–142.

24. Lang PJ, Greenwald MK, Bradley MM, Hamm AO. Looking at pictures: affective, visceral, and behavioral reactions. Psychophysiol 1993;30:261–273.

25. Ekman P, Davidson RJ, Friesen WV. The Duchenne smile: emotional expression and brain physiology. Part II. J Pers Soc Psychol 1990;58:342–353.

26. McIntosh DN, Zajonc RB, Vig PS, Emerick SW. Facial movement, breathing, temperature, and affect: implications of the vascular theory of emotional efference. Cogn Emotion 1997;11:171–195.

27. Zajonc RB, McIntosh DN. Emotions research: some promising questions and some questionable promises. Psychol Sci 1992;3:70–74.

28. Zajonc RB, Murphy ST, Ingelhart M. Feeling and facial efference: implications of the vascular theory of emotion. Psychol Rev 1989;96:395–416.

29. Morgan WP, O'Connor PJ. Exercise and mental health. In: Dishman RK, ed. Exercise adherence: its impact on public health. Champaign, IL: Human Kinetics, 1988:91–121.

30. Petruzzello SJ, Landers DM, Salazar W. Exercise and anxiety reduction: examination of temperature as an explanation for affective change. J Sport Exerc Psychol 1993;15:63–76.

31. Youngstedt S, Dishman RK, Cureton KJ, Peacock LJ. Does body temperature mediate anxiolytic effects of acute exercise? J Appl Physiol 1993;74:825–831.

32. Cabanac M, Caputa M. Natural selective cooling of the human brain: evidence of its occurrence and magnitude. J Physiol 1979;286:255–264.

33. White MD, Cabanac M. Physical dilatation of the nostrils lowers the thermal strain of exercising humans. Eur J Appl Physiol Occup Physiol 1995;70:200–206.

34. White MD, Cabanac M. Exercise hyperpnea and hyperthermia in humans. J Appl Physiol 1996;81:1249–1254.

35. Robinson RG, Downhill JE. Lateralization of psychopathology in response to focal brain injury. In: Davidson RJ, Hugdahl K, ed. Brain asymmetry. Cambridge, MA: MIT Press, 1995:693–711.

36. Davidson RJ, Ekman P, Saron CD, et al. Approach-withdrawal and cerebral asymmetry: emotional expression and brain physiology Part I. J Pers Soc Psychol 1990;58:330–341.

37. Ekman P, Davidson RJ. Voluntary smiling changes regional brain activity. Psychol Sci 1993;4:342–345.

38. Tomarken AJ, Davidson RJ, Wheeler RE, Doss RC. Individual differences in anterior brain asymmetry and fundamental dimensions of emotion. J Pers Soc Psychol 1992;62:676–687.

39. Wheeler RE, Davidson RJ, Tomarken AJ. Frontal brain asymmetry and emotional reactivity: a biological substrate of affective style. Psychophysiol 1993;30:82–89.

40. James W. Untitled. Am Phys Educ Rev 1899;4:220–221.

41. Hall EE, Ekkekakis P, Petruzzello SJ. Regional brain activation as a biological marker of affective responsivity to acute exercise: influence of fitness. Med Sci Sports Exerc 1988;30(suppl):S128.

42. Petruzzello SJ, Landers DM. State anxiety reduction and exercise: does hemispheric activation reflect such changes? Med Sci Sports Exerc 1994;26:1028–1035.

43. Petruzzello SJ, Tate AK. Brain activation, affect, and aerobic exercise: an examination of both state-independent and state-dependent relationships. Psychophysiol 1997;34:527–533.

44. Hall EE, Ekkekakis P, Van Landuyt LM, Petruzzello SJ. Inability of frontal asymmetry to predict affective changes to 10-min walk. J Sport Exerc Psychol 1999 (in press).

45. Petruzzello SJ, Tate AK. Brain activation and affect as a result of exercise. Med Sci Sports Exerc 1997;29(suppl):S31.

46. Lang PJ, Bradley MM, Cuthbert BN. Motivated attention: affect, activation, and action. In: Lang PJ, Simons RF, Balaban M, ed. Attention and orienting: sensory and motivational processes. Mahwah, NJ: Erlbaum, 1997:97–135.

47. LeDoux J. Emotion and the amygdala. In: Aggleton JP, ed. The amygdala: neurobiological aspects of emotion, memory, and mental dysfunction. New York: Wiley-Liss, 1992:339–351.

48. Irwin W, Davidson RJ, Lowe MJ, et al. Human amygdala activation detected with echo-planar functional magnetic resonance imaging. Neuroreport 1996;7:1765–1769.

49. Tieman JG, Dishman RK, Peacock LJ. The effects of acute exercise on state anxiety and the acoustic startle eyeblink response. Med Sci Sports Exerc 1991;23(suppl):S42.

50. Kang DH, Davidson RJ, Coe CL, et al. Frontal brain asymmetry and immune function. Behav Neurosci 1991;105:860–869.

51. Gruzelier J, Burgess A, Baldeweg T, et al. Prospective associations between lateralized brain function and immune status in HIV infection: analysis of EEG, cognition, and mood over 30 months. Intl J Psychophysiol 1996;23:215–224.

52. Sothmann MS, Buckworth J, Claytor RP, et al. Exercise training and the cross-stressor adaptation hypothesis. Exerc Sport Sci Rev 1996;24:267–287.

53. Wittling W. The right hemisphere and the human stress response. Acta Physiol Scand 1997;161(suppl):55–59.

54. Dienstbier RA. Arousal and physiological toughness: implications for mental and physical health. Psychol Rev 1989;96:84–100.

55. Wittling W, Pfluger M. Neuroendocrine hemisphere asymmetries: salivary cortisol secretion during lateralized viewing of emotion-related and neutral films. Brain Cogn 1990;14:243–265.

56. Kiecolt-Glaser JK, Glaser R. Psychoneuroimmunology: can psychological interventions modulate immunity? J Consult Clin Psychol 1992;60:569–575.

57. Kiecolt-Glaser JK, Glaser R. Mind and immunity. In: Goleman D, Gurin J, eds. Mind/body medicine: how to use your mind for better health. Yonkers, NY: Consumer Reports Books, 1993:39–61.

58. Dantzer R. Stress and immunity: what have we learned from psychoneuroimmunology? Acta Physiol Scand 1997;161(suppl):43–46.

59. Bandura A. Social foundations of thought and action: a social cognitive theory. Englewood Cliffs, NJ: Prentice-Hall, 1986:1–617.

60. Bandura A, Taylor CB, Williams SL, et al. Catecholamine secretion as a function of perceived coping self-efficacy. J Consult Clin Psychol 1985;53:406–414.

61. Wiedenfeld SA, O'Leary A, Bandura A, et al. Impact of perceived self-efficacy in coping with stressors on components of the immune system. J Pers Soc Psychol 1990;59:1082–1094.

62. Appels A. Exhausted subjects, exhausted systems. Acta Physiol Scand 1997;161(suppl):153–154.

63. O'Connor PJ, Morgan WP, Raglin JS, et al. Mood state and salivary cortisol levels following overtraining in female swimmers. Psychoneuroendocrinol 1989;14:303–310.

64. Rudolph DL, McAuley E. Self-efficacy and salivary cortisol responses to acute exercise in physically active and less active adults. J Sport Exerc Psychol 1995;17:206–213.

65. Rudolph DL, McAuley E. Cortisol and affective responses to exercise. J Sports Sci 1998;16:121–128.

66. LaPerriere AR, Antoni MH, Schneiderman N, et al. Exercise intervention attenuates emotional distress and natural killer cell decrements following notification of positive serologic status for HIV-1. Biofeedback Self-Regulation 1990;15:229–242.

67. Kaplan JR, Manuck SB. Using ethological principles to study psychosocial influences on coronary atherosclerosis in monkeys. Acta Physiol Scand 161(suppl):1997;96–99.

68. Cacioppo JT. Social neuroscience: autonomic, neuroendocrine, and immune responses to stress. Psychophysiol 1994;31:113–128.

69. Miller J. The body in question, New York: Random House, 1978:1–352.

Chapter 83

Exercise and Psychological Well-Being in the Adult Population: Reality or Wishful Thinking?

Lise Gauvin
John C. Spence
Sandra Anderson

There is general agreement that one component of the promotion of physical activity in the adult population consists of informing apparently healthy but sedentary persons of the health risks of remaining sedentary and the health benefits of achieving a more active lifestyle (1,2). As health promotion researchers have observed (3,4), this task is immensely complex because one is faced simultaneously with the responsibility of determining what the available evidence shows, what information will be most meaningful to recipients, whom to target with different sources of information, and how to deliver the information in an accurate and unbiased fashion.

Above and beyond these concerns, the dissemination of information on the relationship between physical activity and psychological well-being comprises an additional challenge—there are limitations on the quantity and quality of information available to substantiate any generalized claims. That is, current consensus statements (5,6) and the breadth of chapters in this textbook support the notion that a wealth of data is available on selected health benefits of physical activity (e.g., cardiorespiratory fitness). In comparison, however, there is a dearth of *high-quality* data on the link between physical activity and mental well-being (7,8). Furthermore, and perhaps more critically, the idea that physical activity can contribute to mental health, is met at once with enthusiasm and indifference. For example, in a previous review (7), we noted that a variety of national surveys and academic reviews show that the general population, physicians, and mental health practitioners believe that physical exercise is a useful means for improving and maintaining psychological well-being. Yet despite this overwhelming positive aura, there have been few efforts to systematically integrate knowledge dissemination about the mental health benefits of physical activity into public health practice or clinical practice, although there have been notable exceptions (9).

The purpose of this chapter is therefore twofold. First, we provide a concise overview of what is known about the benefits of physical activity for psychological well-being and highlight the quality of the evidence. Second, we offer guidelines intended for public health practitioners and clinicians regarding how to most effectively disseminate information on the link between physical activity and psychological well-being. Our efforts at formulating guidelines are guided by principles of health promotion rather than effectiveness trials (a test of whether a technology, treatment, procedure, intervention, or program does more good than harm when delivered under real-world conditions) (10), because effectiveness trials in this area have, to our knowledge, not been conducted. We conclude our discussion by pointing to promising areas of ongoing and future research. For ease of consultation, we use a question and answer format.

WHAT IS PSYCHOLOGICAL WELL-BEING?

Psychological well-being has been defined in a variety of ways by different social psychological theorists (11). The most widely accepted definition holds that psychological well-being refers to the extent to which people experience a preponderance of positive over negative emotions in their daily lives and the extent to which they feel satisfied with their past, present, and future life circumstances. On the one hand, people with high levels of psychological well-being typically have more positive (e.g., enjoyment, satisfaction, tranquillity) than negative feelings (e.g., anxiety, depression, anger) in their daily pursuits and report that they are satisfied with their life. On the other hand, people who report frequent episodes of negative emotions, few positive feelings, and low levels of satisfaction with life would be designated as persons with a low level of psychological well-being. Only a handful of investigations have examined the role of physical activity on global indicators of psychological well-being (7,8). Rather, researchers have concentrated their efforts on examining how acute bouts of exercise (i.e., single sessions) and chronic involvement in physical activity (i.e., repeated bouts of exercise over an extended period of time) could influence underlying measures of psychological well-being, such as levels of anxiety, depression, self-esteem, and satisfaction with life. Methodologies have been quite diverse, ranging from epidemiologic surveys to laboratory investigations. In the following paragraphs, we draw a general portrait of the knowledge base by stating what is known and describing the methodologies employed to yield findings.

WHAT IS KNOWN ABOUT THE RELATIONSHIP BETWEEN WELL-BEING AND ACTIVITY?

Amount of Data Available

Over 100 reviews have been conducted on the topic of physical activity and psychological well-being (7), and a cursory search of several computer databases (MEDLINE, Sport Discus, PsychLit) reveals at least 500 published studies on the topic. However, based on the reference lists in several meta-analyses (12–14), the number of unpublished studies on physical activity and psychological well-being may actually approach those in the published literature. Thus, there is a large quantity of data available. Unfortunately, as discussed further, the quality of the database is wanting: study design, measurement, and sampling procedures do not frequently meet high research standards (15).

Anxiety

Epidemiologic data suggest that physically fit or active people experience less anxiety than people who are not fit (16,17), thus supporting the notion that chronic involvement in physical activity is associated with higher psychological well-being (in this case caused by the possible anxiolytic effect of exercise). Because much of these data are cross-sectional, however, it is impossible to rule out the possibility that the relationship between physical activity and psychological well-being exists not because exercise is a causal factor, but because those persons with high psychological well-being are more likely to engage in physically active pursuits.

However, meta-analyses of the nonepidemiologic literature support the idea that chronic exercise interventions result in small decreases in anxiety (Table 83-1). In many of these studies, researchers have adequately manipulated level of exercise involvement. Whether it be state anxiety (i.e., transitory emotional state characterized by feelings of apprehension and tension and physiologic activation) or trait anxiety (i.e., tendency to experience a wide variety of situations as threatening and to react by experiencing state anxiety), studies show an effect size of approximately −0.33 SD. This can be interpreted as meaning that the anxiety of a person involved in chronic exercise would be, on average, one-third of a standard deviation below that of a nonexercising control individual. Hence, chronic involvement in exercise results in reductions in anxiety, but these reductions are small in magnitude. Bahrke and Morgan (18) and Petruzzello et al (14) found that exercise was as effective in reducing anxiety as more traditional therapeutic modalities (e.g., meditation, relaxation, quiet rest).

While useful in gauging the influence of chronic exercise, population data and chronic training studies provide very little in the way of evidence regarding the effects of acute bouts of exercise. Indeed, the study of transient mood changes as a function of single bouts of activity requires a

Table 83-1 Physical Activity, Anxiety, and Stress: Findings from Meta-Analyses

EXERCISE PARADIGM	STUDY	SPECIAL CHARACTERISTICS	OUTCOME	K	EFFECT SIZE (d)
Chronic					
	Crew et al (83)		Stress reactivity	67	−0.59
	Kugler et al (84)	Coronary patients	Anxiety	13	−0.31
	Landers et al (12)	Includes unpublished data	Trait anxiety	51	−0.40
			State anxiety	30	−0.38
	Long et al (60)		Trait anxiety	29	−0.38
			State anxiety	21	−0.34
	McDonald et al (26)	Aerobic exercise studies only	Trait anxiety	20	−0.25
			State anxiety	13	−0.28
	Petruzzello et al (14)	Includes unpublished data	Trait anxiety	62	−0.34
			State anxiety	88	−0.25
			Physiologic	53	−0.40
	Schlicht (85)	1980–1990	Anxiety	22	−0.30
Acute					
	Crew et al (83)		Stress reactivity	25	−0.11
	Landers et al (12)	Includes unpublished data	State anxiety	25	−0.53
	Petruzzello et al (14)	Includes unpublished data	State anxiety	119	−0.23

K = number of effect sizes. Note that the effect size for Schlicht (85) is from both chronic and acute studies.

more fine-grained analysis of changes in emotional states from before to after exercise. In this regard, the data on acute exercise show that an exercise bout is again associated with about a one-third of a standard deviation reduction in anxiety (see Table 83-1). It is, however, unclear how long this anxiolytic effect may persist, but findings from one study indicate that the duration may be 2 to 3 hours (19). In summary, exercise is related to reduced anxiety, but the reduction is small in magnitude.

Depression

Depression refers to an emotional state characterized by sadness, lethargy, withdrawal, and possibly even suicidal ideation (20). Persistent feelings of depression and lethargy are obviously characteristics of lower levels of positive well-being. Thus, the interest in studying depression relates to reducing episodes of ill-being in the general population and searching for an effective adjunct to treatment for depression.

To date, epidemiologic evidence suggests that physically active individuals are characterized by lower levels of depression in comparison to sedentary individuals (17,21–25). Odds ratios for depression in sedentary adults in comparison to more active adults range from 1.3 (22) to 1.8 (21). As in the case of anxiety, before and after training measures of depression have shown that chronic exercise results in decreases in depression (Table 83-2). However, these decreases are moderate-to-large, as opposed to the small decreases observed for anxiety. Across meta-analyses, effect sizes range from −0.46 SD to −0.97 SD. For example, North et al (13) found that exercise decreases depression more in individuals recruited from medical or psychological facilities than in individuals recruited from other locations (e.g., college students or faculty, community citizens). This finding is further supported by another meta-analysis (26) that found the antidepressant effect associated with exercise was 40% greater in depressed persons compared with healthy persons. Furthermore, in treating depressed patients, exercise has been found to be as effective as psychotherapy in reducing depression (13,27). However, to get optimal results, it is suggested that treatments be performed concurrently (13,28). Most modes of physical activity seem to be effective in reducing depression, with weight training and aerobic activities having the greatest effect (13).

Positive Affect and Other Mood Indicators

Oddly enough, positive affect (i.e., sentiments of enjoyment, happiness, and fun) has not been studied frequently in relation to exercise involvement. This seems surprising because physical activity is perceived very favorably by a large segment of the population. Nevertheless, some large-scale population surveys (17,24) suggest that greater involvement in physical activity is associated with more frequent reports of well-being (as assessed by the Bradburn affect balance scale) (29). Other correlational studies have shown that acute bouts of activity are related to greater positive affect (30–32). Unfortunately, the volume of research on this outcome is limited in comparison to the data available on outcomes such as reduction of anxiety and depression, suggesting that, although an association is apparent, further data are required before making generalized claims.

One dimension of positive affect that has shown more consistent associations with exercise involvement is perceived vigor or heightened perceptions of one's energy level. Other labels have been used to designate this phenomenon, including vitality (33–35). Perceptions of activation or arousal are identified as a central component of affective experience (36–38), hence the interest in understanding its link to physical activity. In this regard, Thayer (38) has argued that exercise can significantly heighten feelings of energy or vigor in the period following a bout of activity. The data, although limited in quantity, seem to support this claim. After a bout of vigorous exercise of at least 10 minutes, persons report heightened feelings of energy (39,40), suggesting that physical activity may have a powerful influence. Overall, the association of greater physical activity levels with higher levels of well-being holds true for positive affect and perceived vigor or energy.

Self-Concept

Apart from indicators of general well-being (17), little population-based evidence is available to indicate that physically active people have a more positive self-concept than sedentary people. However, the idea that our perceptions of self are affected by changes in physical fitness is both intuitively appealing and supported by narrative reviews on the topic. In fact, Folkins and Sime (41) identified self-concept as the psychological construct most likely to be enhanced with

Table 83-2 Physical Activity and Depression: Findings from Meta-Analyses

Exercise Paradigm	Study	Special Characteristics	K	Effect Size (d)
Chronic				
	Craft*	Clinical population	119	−0.72
	Kugler et al (84)	Coronary patients	15	−0.46
	McDonald et al (26)	Aerobic exercise studies only	17	−0.97
	North et al (13)	Includes unpublished data	226	−0.59
Acute				
	North et al (13)	Includes unpublished data	26	−0.31

K = number of effect sizes.
* Craft LL. The effect of exercise on clinical depression resulting from mental illness: a meta-analysis. Unpublished master's thesis, Arizona State University, 1997.

exercise. Findings from meta-analyses support the idea that physical activity participation enhances self-concept (Table 83-3), since a small-to-moderate effect is reported. One likely reason for the difference in findings among the meta-analyses is that one group of reviewers (42) treated self-concept as a multidimensional measure, providing effect sizes for global self-concept and physical self-concept, whereas another group (26) aggregated all self-concept measures under one global outcome. A case has been made for viewing self-concept as a multidimensional construct (43). In this regard, it is likely more reasonable to expect the beneficial effects of physical activity to manifest in the physical perceptions of self as opposed to at a global level (44,45). Thus, the benefits for physical activity in regard to global self-concept may be overstated in the physical activity literature.

Satisfaction with Life

Satisfaction with life refers to a person's judgment of the quality of their accomplishments and their current life circumstances. Although it is viewed as a central concept in conceptualization of psychological well-being, its relationship to physical activity has not been extensively studied and few consistent relationships have emerged that suggest that the two variables are related. A reasonable explanation for the absence of this relationship is that physical activity is only one activity among the person's numerous daily pursuits. Hence, to imagine that physical activity might significantly impact perceptions of life accomplishments or current life situation is probably oversimplistic. In other words, if physical activity is not a critical feature in daily activities, then such a relationship may be absent. However, to the extent that physical prowess or physical functioning is critical to the accomplishment of daily pursuits, one might expect a relationship between life satisfaction and increased physical activity. In this respect, in populations with chronic disabilities, physical activity may significantly influence satisfaction with life by allowing the person to engage in valued social and occupational activities (the interested reader is referred to 8). Evaluating the relationship between physical activity and satisfaction with life (such as quality of life) (see Chapter 86) is complicated by different definitions and the valid and reliable measurement of the construct.

Negative Impact of Physical Activity on Psychological Well-Being

Exercise has typically been associated with positive outcomes in relation to psychological well-being. However, there are at least two situations wherein the relationship may be reversed, namely in cases of excessive exercise (see Chapter 87) and in cases of patients with eating disorders (see Chapter 88). With respect to the idea of excessive exercise, several authors have attempted to conceptually and clinically define the concept of exercise addiction or obsessive exercise (46–48). The central feature of this idea is that certain persons chronically exercise beyond recommended guidelines, despite clear evidence that this behavior is harmful to their physical well-being or to their social functioning. Persons highly committed to exercise and who exercise excessively often report feelings of anxiety, irritation, depression, or physical symptoms when prevented from exercising in their habitual routine. In common parlance, this has been referred to as exercise addiction. Although the idea is appealing and selected authors have documented clinical cases of obligatory exercise (46,47), very little is known about the psychological well-being of persons who may be dealing with such problems. More data are needed on this real, but probably rare, behavior before any generalizations can be formulated.

Patients with eating disorders offer another case in point of the potential lack of generalizability of findings on the link between physical activity and psychological well-being. Excessive exercise is identified as a symptom of eating disorders (more particularly, anorexia nervosa) (20). However, patients with eating disorders also experience a great deal of negative affect (49), which indicates that the relationship may be reversed or that exercise is not serving as a buffer to negative affect in this subgroup of the population. Furthermore, very little data are available to explore the psychological outcomes of acute bouts of activity in these populations. More research is needed to explore the links between psychological well-being and special cases of excessive exercise, but according to O'Connor and Smith (see Chapter 88) the available evidence indicates that a causal link between physical activity and eating disorders has not been established.

WHAT IS KNOWN ABOUT DOSE-RESPONSE RELATIONSHIPS?

From the standpoints of exercise prescription and public health efforts to promote physical activity, one of the most central research issues has been to understand what amounts of physical activity (i.e., frequency, intensity, duration, type) result in any health benefits. Whereas researchers in the biologic sciences have documented dose-response relationships (50) that have provided a knowledge base from which to formulate public health pronouncements (51), the parallel in the psychological sciences has not come to fruition. There are at least three reasons for this gap.

First, as mentioned by Rejeski (52), the concept of dose-response relationships requires a broader conceptualization in the social sciences than in the biologic sciences. That is, while it is interesting and relevant to examine how different doses of physical activity (objective dose, or amounts, of activity

Table 83-3 Chronic Physical Activity and Self-Concept: Findings from Meta-Analyses

Study	Special Characteristics	K	Effect Size (d)
McDonald et al (26)	Aerobic exercise studies only	41	0.56
Spence et al (42)	Includes unpublished data	61	0.23

K = number of effect sizes.

determined by type, frequency, intensity, and duration) relate to different psychological outcomes, there is a need to also understand how people's subjective perceptions of the dose of physical activity (subjective dose) influence psychological outcomes. A vast array of research on social cognition (53), affect (36), and rate of perceived exertion (54) supports the notion that a person's perception, rather than the objective characteristics of the event or situation, determines their reactions to the event or situation. As an example in the realm of physical activity, Rejeski et al (39) studied the reactions of moderately fit women to different durations of physical activity (i.e., control, 10, 25, and 40 minutes). Only one indicator of psychological well-being was influenced by the duration of physical activity, although substantial portions of the variance in three of the four indicators of psychological well-being were explained by how good or bad the exerciser felt in the last minute of their exercise episode. In other words, those women who reported felling good or very good in the last minute of their exercise bout experienced greater improvements in psychological well-being than women who reported feeling neutral, bad, or very bad in the last minute of exercise, regardless of duration of activity. These findings were reproduced in another study of dose-response relationships reported by Gauvin et al (55) in which the intensity of the exercise bout was manipulated. Similarly, any changes in self-concept resulting from physical activity may be more related to perceived changes in physical fitness and skills as opposed to real absolute indicators (56).

Second, from a methodologic standpoint, it is very difficult to manipulate solely the objective dose of physical activity while controlling for other potential sources of influence on psychological well-being (57). For example, researchers have shown that different indicators of positive and negative affect can be influenced by diurnal variations, intrapersonal biologic events (e.g., physical symptoms may depress mood), the quality of interpersonal interactions, and the physical environment (38,58). For instance, in the area of exercise, Turner et al (59) found that a fitness instructor's behavior could influence psychological outcomes: participants interacting with an enthusiastic and positive instructor experienced more positive changes than those interacting with a neutral yet professional instructor. Thus, to demonstrate that physical activity influences psychological well-being, it is necessary to show that any changes are not confounded by any other social psychological or biologic factors. The available evidence has largely failed to control for such confounding variables and has prevented researchers from constructing such a demonstration.

Third, few data support the existence of strong dose-response relationships as a function of objective doses of activity (52). For example, Gauvin et al (55) showed that, in comparison to light- and moderate-intensity physical activity, vigorous physical activity made sedentary participants feel more fatigued but did not substantially influence any other indicators of psychological well-being. Dose-response relationships in the psychological domain may be intertwined with interpersonal influence processes or intraindividual differences (e.g., level of fitness) in addition to features of the exercise episode per se. The viability of this assertion obviously awaits further empiric data.

Unfortunately, the amount of data on dose-relationships is limited. Petruzzello et al (14) found that exercise lasting 20 minutes or more in duration results in larger decreases in state anxiety than shorter bouts of exercise. Furthermore, trait anxiety will be reduced much more if the length of the training program spans at least 6 to 8 weeks (60) and preferably more than 10 weeks (12). However, there is no clearly established exercise intensity that has consistently shown anxiolytic effects (12). Therefore, caution must be taken before accepting these findings as definitive, especially since the impact of the different components of dose of exercise (i.e., type, frequency, intensity, and duration) are poorly understood at this time.

As for depression, when the exercise program spans over a longer period of time and therefore includes more sessions completed overall, the effect is greater (13). However, weekly frequency per se and duration of activity per session seem to have no effect. Little information is available on intensity. However, there is some consensus that the dose of exercise required to achieve gains in psychological well-being is probably quite close to the standard exercise prescriptions for heart health (61).

DO THESE EFFECTS GENERALIZE ACROSS GENDER, AGE, AND HEALTH AND ACTIVITY STATUS?

A relevant concern for researchers and practitioners is to grasp whether or not any relationships between physical activity and psychological well-being generalize across gender, age groups, health status categories, and activity status. This type of information is important not only for knowledge development but also for knowledge dissemination—it should not be said that physical activity has positive mood outcomes to a population subgroup that has not consistently been shown to be influenced by exercise in a given way. The challenge in the area of physical activity and psychological well-being is that any systematic differences across gender, age, and health status be consistently reproduced. For example, although it has been shown that physical activity is associated with lower depression and anxiety in both men and women, the effect sizes reported in some meta-analyses are greater for men for depression and perhaps for anxiety (13,26,60). However, these findings are equivocal (28) and do not hold up for all indicators of psychological well-being. A more consistent finding is that persons with lower levels of psychological well-being at the outset of a training regimen or a single bout of activity (as evidenced by health status, diagnosed psychological problems, or depressed baseline levels of functioning), experience greater improvements in psychological well-being after acute or chronic exercise in comparison to persons with higher levels of well-being (13,39,55,62). Few, if any, differences on the basis of age have been documented in this area: most population segments show similar patterns of relationships. Identifying strong and consistent patterns of differences across gender, age, and health status are critical first steps to targeting physical activity messages and promotion efforts at different segments of the population.

As we have mentioned elsewhere (7,63), the three components of psychological well-being (i.e., positive affect, negative affect, satisfaction with life) have been shown to be systematically related to gender, age, and health status. For instance, women report higher affect intensity, as do people who are younger (64). A person's health status influences their satisfaction with life, in that people with lower subjective and objective health status report lower life satisfaction. Diener and colleagues (65–67) have shown cross-national differences in psychological well-being and have documented that socioeconomic status is systematically related to psychological well-being. In sum, social psychological research indicates that gender, age, health status, and socioeconomic status differences affect health behaviors and outcomes, and these variables need to be controlled for and understood in studies evaluating the relationships between physical activity and psychological well-being.

With respect to activity status, the formulation of generalizations is hampered by lack of data. Just as public health practitioners and clinicians struggle to increase levels of physical activity in the population and in their patients, researchers are faced with the challenge of inciting participants to volunteer for a study that requires them to engage in and maintain an activity that they do not normally choose to do. Furthermore, persons who do volunteer for physical activity studies are often favorably predisposed to activity at the outset of a study. Thus, they may expect and subsequently report positive outcomes. Methodologically, it is thus challenging to avoid creating confounds.

Nevertheless, there are some data to suggest that activity status may moderate the relationship between activity and well-being; sedentary persons may not reap the benefits reported by more active persons. For example, Lennox et al (62) found that a sample of sedentary hospital employees experienced no benefits in mood after a 13-week exercise program. Gauvin et al (55) also showed that persons recruited into an exercise study, specifically because of their sedentary status, experienced no systematic mood benefits after physical activity. While limited, some of the data points to the fact that those persons who are currently active may experience mood benefits as a result of activity, but those who are inactive may not reap such benefits. These generalizations also await further empiric support.

IS ACTIVITY A CAUSE OR A CONSEQUENCE OF WELL-BEING?

Given the relatively recent focus of scientific research on psychological outcomes of physical activity, much existing data speak to descriptive questions (i.e., how does physical activity relate to psychological well-being?) rather than explanatory questions (i.e., why is physical activity related to psychological well-being and under what circumstances?). Indeed, researchers (17) are emphatic in stating that the association between activity and well-being could exist because exercise causes improvements in psychological well-being or because psychological well-being provokes differing levels of activity. As a result, there are a plethora of hypotheses, none of which have unequivocal empirical support.

What Causal Mechanisms for Activity Mediate Changes in Well-Being?

The hypothesized processes underlying a link between psychological well-being and exercise can be subsumed under both biologic and psychosocial hypotheses. Among the biologic hypotheses, researchers have suggested that mood alterations could, among other things, be related to released beta-endorphins, changes in catecholamine levels, changes in core body temperatures, and changes in EEG patterns or muscle tension (14,68). The popular media has overstated the beta-endorphin hypothesis to the extent that many persons and health professionals believe this hypothesis to be the only tenable explanation. At the present time, the data do not heavily outweigh one explanation over the others.

In terms of psychosocial hypotheses, several ideas have dominated conceptualizations (68). Specifically, some authors have suggested that psychological benefits might result from the distraction provided by an acute bout of physical activity (18). Similarly, others have proposed that physical activity results in feelings of mastery, which in turn result in heightened mood or affect (14). More recently, some authors (59,69) have shown that the social environment could serve to enhance the benefits of acute physical activity on mood. Moreover, at least one group of authors (70) found the psychological outcomes of exercise may be nothing more than a placebo effect. While all are plausible, the data do not support one hypothesis over the others. Hence, more information is needed.

What Causal Mechanisms for Well-Being Mediate Changes in Activity?

In support for the position that selected patterns of psychological functioning elicit differential patterns of behavior, Hamid (71) studied 186 exercise program participants. Positive and negative affect were measured before and after the study. Results indicated that participants with greater positive affect reported greater participation in physical activity, while individuals with greater negative affect showed a reverse pattern, namely lower persistence. To our knowledge, no data shed light on whether any psychological outcomes of acute exercise serve to increase the likelihood of persistence in an exercise regimen, although more positive attitudes toward performing vigorous physical activity are linked to greater involvement in physical activity (72). Thus, positive moods could result in greater exercise involvement, as shown by Hamid (71).

However, research in the social psychology literature suggests that while positive moods elicit mood-congruent behaviors (i.e., behavioral activity, altruistic behaviors, search for opportunities for affiliation, competence, and achievement), negative moods can elicit either mood-congruent or mood-incongruent behaviors (73,74). For negative affect, mood congruent effects could be observed when no active self-regulation is elicited: Persons with a low level of psychological well-being would tend to remain sedentary. Mood-incongruent effects could occur when the person attempts to self-regulate their mood through involvement in activities designed to change their mood. Persons with a low level of psychological well-being might therefore become more physically active if they perceive exercise to be instrumental to regulation of well-being. Consistent with this latter possibility, Thayer et al (75) demonstrated that exercise was viewed and preferentially chosen as a self-regulation strategy for alleviation of depression and increasing energetic arousal by college students, community residents, and psychotherapists. These data suggest that selected moods (i.e., sadness and low energy) may lead persons to engage and persist in exercise to regulate these undesired moods. Thus, the presence of a negative mood state coupled with efforts towards self-regulation could predict exercise involvement. In sum, neither the view that exercise causes psychological changes nor that selected psychologic states enhance the likelihood of greater exercise adherence has unequivocal support, although each view is tenable.

GUIDELINES FOR PUBLIC HEALTH PRACTITIONERS AND CLINICIANS

The previous discussion serves to highlight several issues. First, higher levels of physical activity have been associated with higher levels of psychological well-being (mainly decreased anxiety and depression, but also heightened positive affect, self-concept, and feelings of vigor), but there is insufficient evidence to support the preponderance of one causal path over the other. Second, while associations do exist, they are of small-to-large magnitude for negative affect (e.g., anxiety, depression), moderate to large for positive affect and feelings of vigor, and small to nonexistent for self-concept and satisfaction with life. Third, while the effects seem generalizable across age in adults, there may be differences in magnitude related to gender and baseline health status. Fourth, it is unclear why these relationships exist, and more particularly, whether they are related to features in which exercise typically unfolds or whether they are linked to exercise per se.

With this information and these caveats in mind, we propose that the message to be delivered to the population at large should be that positive *associations* between physical activity and psychological well-being exist but that the direction of the relationships is unclear at this time and the associations are generally small to moderate in size. The rationale for this message is threefold. First, this message appears to accurately reflect the database. Second, as mentioned in the beginning of the chapter, many persons in the population believe that exercise is *strongly* (rather than weakly or moderately) related to psychological well-being. It is our belief that expectations may require some readjustments downward. Third, although research with clinical populations indicates that exercise is an effective treatment modality for some forms of depression and anxiety, it remains unclear whether these positive outcomes are due to exercise per se, or other factors related to the exercise experience (e.g., socialization, attention from therapist or exercise leader).

Despite these cautions about framing a public health message pertaining to physical activity and psychological well-being, we feel that it is prudent to promote the above message. The potential to society of reducing the serious nature of problems such as depression and anxiety and enhancing positive aspects related to psychological well-being by promoting physical activity far outweighs the alternative of not recommending physical activity as a means for improving psychological well-being until stronger evidence is available or causal mechanisms mediating the association are identified.

In terms of actual dissemination of information, it is our belief that these messages can and should be delivered through media campaigns designed to promote involvement in physical activity at the societal (e.g., organizations, institutions, policies) level and through interpersonal approaches to physical activity counselling (76). That is, with respect to media campaigns, messages designed for the general public that would encapsulate information about the physical benefits of physical activity alongside information about the psychological benefits of activity constitute a viable route of dissemination. In this regard, careful attention should be devoted to considerations elaborated by Rothman et al (4); these authors convincingly argue that the effectiveness of a message in motivating healthy behavior depends on proper decisions being made regarding 1) whether information should be presented in terms of gains (e.g., increases in psychological well-being) or losses (e.g., avoiding decrements in psychological well-being), and 2) whether the message should encourage persons to take action (e.g., increase involvement in physical activity) or to avoid pitfalls (e.g., avoid being sedentary) (77). In addition, as discussed by several authors (1,2,78), the groups most receptive to physical activity messages are those with neutral to moderately positive attitudes to physical activity. More research is required before formulating strong generalizations about framing messages and making associated decisions.

With reference to interpersonal approaches to physical activity counselling, we anticipate that information on the psychological well-being correlates of physical activity could be appropriately disseminated through application of decision balance sheet procedures. As discussed by several authors (1,79–81), decision balance sheets are a technique for exercise adoption that consists essentially of having the participant list the positive and negative outcomes of involvement in physical activity for self and significant others. "Feeling better" or in other words "increasing psychological well-being," is a coveted outcome for many exercisers (1,82). In the context of completing this exercise, the physical activity counselor or health care professional can reinforce accurate perceptions of the psychological well-being benefits as listed by participants or, alternatively, provide information to debunk myths about psychological benefits entertained by beginning exercisers. This, too, constitutes a viable route of application. For further discussion of additional strategies and interventions to promote physical activity, see Chapter 89.

WHERE DO WE GO FROM HERE?

Coming full circle with the introduction to this chapter, the previous discussion has highlighted the fact that the scientific knowledge base supports the existence of a relationship between psychological well-being and physical activity with higher activity levels being linked to more positive well-being outcomes. While this generalization seems warranted, many issues require further investigation. Notably, the direction of any causal link between activity and well-being remains unclear, as do dose-response relationships and the moderating or mediating role of a host of intrapersonal variables, such as gender and activity status. Similarly, the actual impact of disseminating information on the psychological well-being correlates of physical activity has not been examined through efficacy or effectiveness trials. We believe that these issues constitute fruitful directions for future research and application.

REFERENCES

1. Brawley LR, Rodgers WR. Social psychological aspects of fitness promotion. In: Seraganian P, ed. Exercise psychology: influence of physical exercise on psychological processes. New York: Wiley & Sons, 1993:254–298.

2. Donavan RJ, Owen N. Social marketing and population interventions. In: Dishman RK, ed. Advances in exercise adherence. Champaign, IL: Human Kinetics, 1994:249–290.

3. Green LW, Kreuter M. Health promotion planning: an educational and environmental approach. Mountain View, CA: Mayfield, 1991:1–506.

4. Rothman AJ, Salovey P. Shaping perceptions to motivate healthy behavior: the role of message framing. Psychol Bull 1997;121: 3–19.

5. Bouchard C, Shephard RJ, Stephens T, ed. Physical activity, fitness, and health: international proceedings and consensus statement. Champaign, IL: Human Kinetics, 1994:1–1055.

6. U.S. Department of Health and Human Services. Physical activity and health: a report of the Surgeon General. Atlanta: U.S. Department of Health and Human Services, Centers for Disease Control and Prevention, National Center for Chronic Disease Prevention and Health Promotion, 1996: 1–277.

7. Gauvin L, Spence JC. Physical activity and psychological well-being: knowledge base, current issues, and caveats. Nutr Rev 1996;54(suppl):S53–S65.

8. Rejeski WJ, Brawley LR, Shumaker SA. Physical activity and health-related quality of life. Exerc Sport Sci Rev 1996;24:71–108.

9. Martinsen EW. Physical fitness, anxiety, and depression. Br J Hosp Med 1990;43:194–199.

10. Flay BR. Efficacy and effectiveness trials (and other phases of research) in the development of health promotion research programmes. Prev Med 1986;15: 451–474.

11. Diener E. Subjective well-being. Psychol Bull 1984;95:542–575.

12. Landers DM, Petruzzello SJ. Physical activity, fitness, and anxiety. In: Bouchard C, Shephard RJ, Stephens T, eds. Physical activity, fitness, and health: international proceedings and consensus statements. Champaign, IL: Human Kinetics, 1994:868–882.

13. North TC, McCullagh P, Tran ZV. Effect of exercise on depression. Exerc Sport Sci Rev 1990;18: 379–415.

14. Petruzzello SJ, Landers DM, Hatfield BD, et al. A meta-analysis on the anxiety-reducing effects of acute and chronic exercise: outcomes and mechanisms. Sports Med 1991;11:143–182.

15. Campbell DT, Stanley JC. Experimental and quasi-experimental design for research. Chicago, IL: Rand McNally, 1966:1–84.

16. Ross CE, Hayes D. Exercise and psychologic well-being in the community. Am J Epidemiol 1988; 127:762–771.

17. Stephens T. Physical activity and mental health in the United States and Canada: evidence from four population surveys. Prev Med 1988;17:35–47.

18. Bahrke MS, Morgan WP. Anxiety reduction following exercise and meditation. Cog Ther Res 1978;2: 323–333.

19. Raglin JS, Morgan WP. Influence of exercise and quiet rest on state anxiety and blood pressure. Med Sci Sports Exerc 1987;19:456–463.

20. American Psychiatric Association. Diagnostic and Statistical Manual of Mental Disorders. 4th ed. Washington, DC: American Psychiatric Association, 1994:1–886.

21. Camacho TC, Roberts RE, Lazarus NB, et al. Physical activity and depression: evidence from the Alameda County study. Am J Epidemiol 1991;134:220–231.

22. Farmer ME, Locke BZ, Moscicki EK, et al. Physical activity and depressive symptoms: the NHANES I epidemiologic follow-up study. Am J Epidemiol 1988;128: 1340–1351.

23. Mobily KE, Rubenstein LM, Lemke JH, et al. Walking and depression in a cohort of older adults: the Iowa 65+ rural health study. J Aging Phys Activity 1996;4: 119–135.

24. Stephens T, Craig CL. The well-being of Canadians: highlights of the Campbell's survey. Ottawa: Canadian Fitness and Lifestyle Research Institute, 1990:1–123.

25. Weyerer S. Physical inactivity and depression in the community: evidence from the Upper Bavarian field study. Int J Sports Med 1992;13:492–496.

26. McDonald DG, Hodgdon JA. Psychological effects of aerobic fitness training. New York: Springer, 1991:1–224.

27. Greist JH, Klein MH, Eischens RR, Faris J, Gurman AS, Morgan WP. Running as a treatment for depression. Compr Psychiatry 1979;20: 41–54.

28. Morgan WP. Physical activity, fitness, and depression. In: Bouchard C, Shephard RJ, Stephens T, eds. Physical activity, fitness, and health: international proceedings and consensus statement. Champaign, IL: Human Kinetics Publishers, 1994:851–867.

29. Bradburn NM. The structure of psychological well-being. Chicago, IL: Aldine, 1969:1–318.

30. Clark LA, Watson D. Mood and the mundane: relations between daily life events and self-reported mood. J Pers Soc Psychol 1988;54:296–308.

31. Gauvin L, Rejeski WJ. The exercise-induced feeling inventory: development and initial validation. J Sport Exerc Psychol 1993;15: 413–423.

32. McAuley E, Courneya KS. The Subjective Exercise Experiences

Scale (SEES): development and preliminary validation. J Sport Exerc Psychol 1994;16:163–177.

33. Ryan RM, Frederick C. On energy, personality, and health: subjective vitality as a dynamic reflection of well-being. J Pers 1997;65:539–565.

34. Wood C, Magnello ME. Diurnal changes in perceptions of energy and mood. J R Soc Med 1992;85:191–194.

35. Wood C, Magnello ME, Jewell T. Measuring vitality. J R Soc Med 1990;83:486–489.

36. Ekman P, Davidson RJ, eds. The nature of emotion: fundamental questions. New York: Oxford, 1994:1–496.

37. Larsen RJ, Diener E. Problems and promises with the circumplex model of affect. Rev Pers Soc Psychol 1992;13:25–59.

38. Thayer RE. The biopsychology of mood and arousal. New York: Oxford, 1989:1–234.

39. Rejeski WJ, Gauvin L, Hobson ML, Norris J. Effects of baseline responses, in-task feelings, and duration of physical activity on exercise-induced feeling states in women. Health Psychol 1995;14:350–359.

40. Thayer RE. Energy, tiredness, and tension effects of a sugar snack versus moderate exercise. J Pers Soc Psychol 1987;52:119–125.

41. Folkins CH, Sime WE. Physical fitness training and mental health. Am Psychol 1981;36:373–389.

42. Spence JC, Poon P, Dyck P. The effect of physical activity on self-concept: a meta-analysis. J Sport Exerc Psychol 1997;19(suppl):S109.

43. Shavelson RJ, Hubner JJ, Stanton GC. Self-concept: validation of construct interpretations. Rev Educ Res 1976;46:407–411.

44. Fox KR, ed. The physical self: from motivation to well-being. Champaign, IL: Human Kinetics, 1997:1–329.

45. Sonstroem RJ, Morgan WP. Exercise and self-esteem: rationale and model. Med Sci Sports Exerc 1989;21:329–337.

46. Morgan WP. Negative addiction in runners. Phys Sportsmed 1979;7:56–63; 67–70.

47. Pierce EF. Exercise dependence syndrome in runners. Sports Med 1994;18:149–155.

48. DeCoverly Veale DMW. Exercise dependence. Br J Addict 1987;82:735–740.

49. Brownell KD, Fairburn CG, eds. Eating disorders and obesity: a comprehensible handbook. New York: Guilford, 1998:1–538.

50. Haskell WL. Health consequences of physical activity: understanding and challenges regarding dose-response. Med Sci Sports Exerc 1994;26:649–660.

51. Pate RR, Pratt M, Blair SN, et al. Physical activity and public health: a recommendation from the Centers for Disease Control and Prevention and the American College of Sports Medicine. JAMA 1995;273:402–407.

52. Rejeski WJ. Dose-response issues from a psychosocial perspective. In: Bouchard C, Shephard RJ, Stephens T, eds. Physical activity, fitness, and health: international proceedings and consensus statement. Champaign, IL: Human Kinetics, 1994:1040–1055.

53. Ross M, Fletcher GJO. Attribution and social perception. In: Lindzey G, Aronson E, eds. The handbook of social psychology. Vol 2. New York: Random House, 1985:73–122.

54. Dishman RK. Prescribing exercise intensity for healthy adults using perceived exertion. Med Sci Sports Exerc 1994;26:1087–1094.

55. Gauvin L, Rejeski WJ, Norris JL, Lutes L. The curse of inactivity: failure of acute exercise to enhance feeling states in a community sample of sedentary adults. J Health Psychol 1997;2:509–523.

56. Heaps RA. Relating physical and psychological fitness: a psychological point of view. J Sports Med Phys Fit 1978;18:399–408.

57. Ojanen M. Can the true effects of exercise on psychological variables be separated from placebo effects? Int J Sport Psychol 1994;25:63–80.

58. Etnier JL, Hardy CJ. The effects of environmental color. J Sport Behav 1997;20:299–312.

59. Turner EE, Rejeski WJ, Brawley LR. Psychological benefits of physical activity are influenced by the social environment. J Sport Exerc Psychol 1997;19:119–130.

60. Long BC, van Stavel R. Effects of exercise training on anxiety: a meta-analysis. J Appl Sport Psychol 1995;7:167–189.

61. American College of Sports Medicine. ACSM's guidelines for graded exercise testing and exercise prescription. Philadelphia: Williams & Wilkins, 1995:1–372.

62. Lennox SS, Bedell JR, Stone AR. The effects of exercise on normal mood. J Psychosom Res 1990;34:629–636.

63. Gauvin L, Spence JC. Challenges and issues in the measurement of exercise-induced changes in feeling states, affect, mood, and emotion. In: Duda JL, ed. Advances in sport and exercise psychology measurement. Morgantown, WV: Fitness Information Technology, 1998:325–336.

64. Larsen RJ, Diener E. Affect intensity as an individual difference characteristics: A review. J Pers 1987;21:1–39.

65. Diener E, Diener C. The wealth of nations revisited: income and quality of life. Soc Indic Res 1995;36:275–286.

66. Diener E, Sandivik E, Pavot W. Response artifacts in the measurement of subjective well-being. Soc Indic Res 1984;24:35.

67. Diener E, Suh EM, Shao L. National differences in reported subjective well-being: why do they occur? Soc Indic Res 1995;34:7–32.

68. Morgan WP, ed. Physical activity and mental health. Washington, DC: Taylor & Francis, 1997:1–288.

69. Iso-Ahola SE, Park CJ. Leisure-related social support and self-determination as buffers of stress-illness relationship. J Leisure Res 1996;28:169–187.

70. Desharnais R, Jobin J, Cote C, et al. Aerobic exercise and the placebo effect: a controlled study. Psychosom Med 1993;55:149–154.

71. Hamid NP. Positive and negative affectivity and maintenance of exercise programmes. Percept Mot Skills 1990;70:478.

72. Godin G. Social-cognitive models. In: Dishman RK, ed. Advances in exercise adherence. Champaign, IL: Human Kinetics, 1994:113–136.

73. Morris WM. Mood: the frame of mind. New York: Springer-Verlag, 1989:1–261.

74. Schaller M, Cialdini RB. Happiness, sadness, and helping: a motivational integration. In: Higgins T, Sorentino R, eds. Handbook of motivation and cognition. New York: Guilford, 1990:265–296.

75. Thayer RE, Newman JR, McClain TM. Self-regulation of mood: strategies for changing a bad mood, raising energy, and reducing tension. J Pers Soc Psychol 1994; 67:910–925.

76. King AC. Community intervention for promotion of physical activity and fitness. Exerc Sport Sci Rev 1991;19:211–260.

77. Epstein LH, Saelens BE, Myers MD, Vito D. Effects of decreasing sedentary behaviors on activity choice in obese children. Health Psychol 1997;16:107–113.

78. Olson JM, Zanna MP. Understanding and promoting exercise: a social psychological perspective. Can J Pub Health 1987;78:1–7.

79. Hoyt MF, Janis IL. Increasing adherence to a stressful decision via the balance sheet procedure: a field experiment on attendance at an exercise class. J Pers Soc Psychol 1975;31:833–839.

80. Pender NJ, Sallis JF, Long BJ, Calfas KJ. Health-care provider counseling to promote physical activity. In: Dishman RK, ed. Advances in exercise adherence. Champaign, IL: Human Kinetics, 1994:213–235.

81. Wankel LM. Enhancing motivation for involvement in voluntary exercise programs. In: Maehr ML, Kleiber DA, eds. Recent advances in motivation and achievement: enhancing motivation. Greenwich, CT: JAI, 1987:239–286.

82. Rodgers WM, Gauvin L. Heterogeneity of self-efficacy and incentives for physical activity in highly active and moderately active exercisers. J Appl Soc Psychol 1998; 28:1016–1029.

83. Crews D, Landers DM. A meta-analytic review of aerobic fitness and reactivity to psychosocial stressors. Med Sci Sports Exerc 1987;19(suppl):S114–S120.

84. Kugler J, Seelbach H, Kruskemper GM. Effects of rehabilitation exercise programmes on anxiety and depression in coronary patients: a meta-analysis. Br J Clin Psychol 1994;33:401–410.

85. Schlicht W. Does physical exercise reduce anxious emotions? a meta-analysis. Anxiety Stress Coping 1994;6:275–288.

Chapter 84

The Relationship Between Physical Activity and the Psychological Well-Being of Youth

Karen J. Calfas

While the majority (64%) of American youth participate in vigorous physical activity, the percentage declines with age, even during the childhood years (1,2). The same is true of participation in physical education classes and organized sports during adolescence (1). This decline causes concern because American children are becoming more obese (3). Increases in physical activity will reduce this trend, and recommendations to this end have been made (4).

Physical activity is associated with many physical benefits, including reduced risk of cardiovascular disease, diabetes, and some forms of cancer (1). Mental health benefits are also documented in the literature (5–7). The notion of a relationship between physical fitness and mental health dates back to ancient times and consideration of the mind-body connection. Currently there exists strong clinical lore that exercise or other forms of "hard work" lead to improvements in self-esteem and overall psychological well-being. There is cross-sectional data to support this relationship (8–10).

Additional studies have been conducted which examine treatment effects of physical activity interventions on mental health variables. However, much of the research in this area has focused on adult populations (11–14). Among adults, physical activity is associated with decreased symptoms of depression (12,14) and anxiety (11,15) and overall improvements in general mood (7) (see Chapter 83). These relationships evaluated among adults are not generalizable to children, and a smaller but separate literature on the mental health benefits of physical activity among youth is emerging.

Children and adolescents (birth to age 18) constitute approximately 29% of the U.S. population (16), and by a conservative estimate, 12% have one or more mental disorders (17). In 1985, the cost of treating mental disorders among youth less than age 14 was $1.5 billion per year, and other estimates indicate that only one-third of youth needing treatment for mental health disorders received it (17). Childhood disorders, particularly depression and anxiety, tend to persist into adulthood, so early identification and treatment are necessary. In addition to clinical mental disorders, increasingly complex and stressful lifestyles contribute to reduced quality of life.

Physical activity is frequently reported to increase feelings of well-being. While it is not a substitute for formal treatment, many support its use as an adjunct to treatment for various mental disorders. Still others hold that physical activity can improve overall well-being and self-esteem, even among nonclinical populations. Research to date among adults generally shows a stronger treatment effect of physical activity among clinical populations (or those with poorer scores on mood indicators at baseline) (18–19). These relationships are less clear among children and adolescents, partly because there are fewer well-designed experimental studies.

Psychological development during childhood and adolescence is important because it creates a foundation for psychological functioning as an adult. Self-concept, self-esteem, and symptoms of depression or anxiety are important markers of psychological development. Certainly primary and secondary education are devoted to both academic and emotional development of students, and there is evidence that increasing time spent in school physical education can have an overall positive effect on academic performance (20). The ultimate contribution of physical activity to this goal is less clear but of great interest among educators, parents, and youth.

The purpose of this chapter is to review the empiric evidence of mental health benefits of physical activity among children and adolescents (less than age 18). Interventions are likely to have different effects on different populations, so research conducted with both a general population of youth as well as special populations (e.g., psychiatric inpatients, learning disabled) is included. The potential psychological impact of physical activity is broad, so the variables of interest in the present chapter include symptoms of clinical mental disorders (e.g., depression, anxiety) as well as measures of positive affect and general well-being, such as self-concept and self-esteem.

METHODS OF INQUIRY FOR REVIEW

Index Medicus and social science databases that accumulated over the past 30 years were searched for studies or review articles on physical activity or exercise and for terms that describe mental health variables, such as self-esteem, self-concept, self-worth, anxiety, depression, and hostility, for children and adolescents. While other relevant outcomes have been examined (e.g., risk-taking behavior, academic achievement), they are beyond the scope of this chapter and were not included in the search. Review articles and experimental studies were examined and additional relevant references were retrieved and included, if appropriate.

Studies were included in this review if they met the following criteria:

1. Participants (or the vast majority of them) were under age 18.

2. Design included a physical activity intervention.

3. Because of greater confidence in the results of controlled studies, the design was required to include a before and after assessment tool and at least one control-comparison group and one intervention group.

4. At least one measure of a mental health variable in both intervention and control-comparison groups before and after testing was required.

5. The study had been published.

6. The study had been reported in English.

All potentially relevant studies were reviewed, and information was abstracted if the study met the eligibility criteria. Participant characteristics were summarized as total sample size at baseline and follow-up (if applicable), mean age in years (or grade level), percent female, ethnicity, and socioeconomic description. For the general population of children and adolescents, all studies reviewed included a control or comparison group. However, the method of group assignment varied and was reported under "design." For special populations, the specific design was indicated. To the extent possible, specific information about the physical activity intervention and control-comparison group intervention was extracted, including the total duration of the intervention, setting (e.g., school physical education or other), level of supervision, use of behavioral theory in the intervention, and frequency, intensity, type, and duration of physical activity.

Measurement techniques used to quantify physical activity-fitness and mental health variables were summarized. While several studies evaluated other dependent variables, only mental health effects were summarized in this review, including self-concept, self-esteem, self-efficacy, body image, depression, hostility, stress, and anxiety. The effects of the intervention on physical activity or physical fitness were reported, if available.

Changes in physical activity or fitness from before to after intervention were noted in the results column when reported in the original article. Since most studies did not report post-test means adjusted for baseline, unadjusted differences between groups at follow-up or the before-to-after change within groups were reported for psychological variables along with associated p values, where possible. A p value of less than 0.05 was considered statistically significant. For studies with more than one follow-up, differences between baseline and the longest-term follow-up were reported.

Studies including apparently healthy children and adolescents were of particular interest (Table 84-1). However, reviews of studies including youth with developmental or psychological problems or other special needs were included separately as "special populations" (Table 84-2). Since less research was available for participants of specific special populations, the design criteria requiring a control or comparison group was relaxed to include single-group prospective observational studies of special populations.

RESULTS OF THE DATA SEARCH
Summary of Studies of the General Population

Twelve studies of the general population were identified, including seven of children (ages 3 to 12), three of adolescents (ages 13 to 17), and one with participants from each age group. Age was not reported in one study. Notably, gender of subjects was not reported in five studies; two assessed boys only; two girls only; and the remainder mixed genders. Ethnicity and socioeconomic status went largely unreported. Ten studies were conducted in the United States; one in Canada; and one in England.

Five of the studies used random assignment of participants to condition, while the rest were either non-random assignment or random assignment of classes to condition. The majority of studies had one post-test assessment, one intervention, and one control group (exceptions are noted in Table 84-1). The number of participants ranged from 24 to 344.

All interventions were conducted in an educational setting, usually as part of a school or a summer program, and ranged in total duration from 1 session to 2 to 18 weeks of sessions. The physical activity intervention included an aerobic component in almost all of the studies; only one evaluated strength training alone. Generally, the interventions for older children were more likely to include aerobics classes and running, while interventions for younger children focused on motor and sport skill development. The intensity of physical activity was not reported in half of the studies, but usually included a vigorous-intensity component in those that did report intensity. The number of minutes per bout of exercise ranged from 15 to 60 minutes.

Seven of the studies reported significant improvements in fitness (21–23), strength (24), or motor skills (25–27). The

Table 84-1 Studies of General Population Children and Adolescents

REFERENCE	PARTICIPANTS	DESIGN	INTERVENTION SETTING DESCRIPTION OF PA	MEASUREMENT	RESULTS

Boyd et al, 1997 (39)	• N = 181, FU
	  n = NR
	• 9–16 yrs;
	  grades 4–5,
	  7–8, 9–10;
	  pre-, early,
	  and
	  midadolescent
	• 100% girls
	• Canada
	• Ethnicity NR
	• SES NR
		Nonrandom
		assignment of
		classes
		G1: intervention
		  (n = NR)
		G2: control
		  (regular PE)
		  (n = NR)
			• School-based (PE
			  classes)
			• Physical activity,
			  education, self-
			  monitoring,
			  tailored to age
			  specific
			  psychological and
			  developmental
			  tasks
			F = 9 sessions
			  (preadolescents);
			  12 sessions
			  (adolescent);
			  both for 6 wks
			I = NR
			T = aerobic,
			  strength,
			  flexibility, agility
			T = 40-min sessions
				• PA: not collected
				• Self-concept:
				  Self-Description
				  Questionnaire
				  (total, physical
				  abilities, and
				  physical
				  appearance)
					• Self-concept,
					  physical
					  appearance:
					  Tx > C, $p < .01$
					• Physical ability:
					  Preadolescents
					  > early/mid
					  adolescents,
					  $p < .01$
					  (no means
					  reported)

Norris et al, 1991 (22)	• N = 80, FU
	  n = 60
	• M = 16.5 yr,
	  Rng = 13–
	  17 yr
	• 50% girls
	• England
	• Ethnicity NR
	• Middle- to
	  upper-class
		Nonrandom
		assignment of
		groups based
		on free lesson
		periods with
		matched
		controls
		G1: high
		  intensity
		  (n = 22)
		G2: moderate
		  intensity
		  (n = 19)
		G3: flexibility
		  (n = 19)
		G4: no PA
		  control
		  (n = 20)
			• School-based
			  (special class
			  during school hrs
			• Aerobic training
			  program
			F = 2 × wk, 10 wks
			I = G1: vigorous
			  G2: moderate
			  G3: flexibility
			T = G1–G2: aerobic
			  G3: flexibility
			T = 25–30 min
			  sessions
				• Fitness: 2 min
				  step test,
				  recovery heart
				  rate
				• Anxiety,
				  depression and
				  hostility: Multiple
				  Adjective Check
				  List
				• Stress: Perceived
				  Stress Scale
					• Fitness
					  improved sig
					  for G1 vs G2,
					  $p < .001$
					• Anxiety, G1 vs
					  G2 △: Tx
					  = –1.00 C =
					  +0.94, $p < .05$
					• Stress, G1 vs
					  G4 △: Tx =
					  –2.86 C =
					  –0.38, $p < .01$
					Depression,
					hostility: NS

Alpert et al, 1990 (21)	• N = 24, FU
	  n = NR
	• M = 3.7 yr
	  Rng = 3–5 yr
	• % girls NR
	• US
	• Multiethnic,
	  % NR
	• Middle class
		Random
		assignment of
		children
		G1: intervention
		  (n = 12)
		G2: control,
		  play-ground
		  freeplay
		  (n = 12)
			• Pre-school
			• Aerobics Exercise
			  Period
			F = 5 × wk, 8 wks
			I = vigorous
			T = aerobic
			T = 20 min sessions
				• Fitness: graded
				  submax bicycle
				  ergometer test,
				  agility, observed
				  gross motor
				  activity, resting
				  heart rate
				• Self concept:
				  Thomas Self-
				  Concept Values
				  Test
					• Fitness, agility,
					  gross motor
					  activity, Tx > C,
					  all p's < .05
					• General self-
					  concept △: Tx
					  = +3.0 C =
					  –1.1, $p < .01$

Holloway et al, 1988 (24)	• N = 59, FU
	  N = 27
	• M = 16 yr
	• 100% girls
	• US
	• Ethnicity NR
	• Middle class
		Non-random
		assignment of
		participants
		G1: intervention
		  (n = 13)
		G2: mild
		  activity
		  (n = 23)
		G3: no PA
		  control (n =
		  18)
			• School-based
			  (after school hrs)
			• Weight training
			  program
			F = 3 × wk, 12 wks
			I = moderate
			T = strength
			T = 60 min sessions
				• Strength: 1 rep
				  maximum (wt
				  group only)
				• Physical Self-
				  Efficacy Scale
				• Ineffectiveness
				  scale on Eating
				  Disorder
				  Inventory
					• Strength: Tx >
					  C, $p < .03$
					*Post median
					scores:*
					• Total self-
					  efficacy Tx =
					  995, G2 =
					  640, G3 =
					  720 $p < .004$
					• Phys self-
					  efficacy
					  G1 = 103.5,

Table 84-1 continues

Table 84-1 (*Continued*)

REFERENCE	PARTICIPANTS	DESIGN	INTERVENTION SETTING DESCRIPTION OF PA	MEASUREMENT	RESULTS
					• G2 = 79.0, G3 = 84.0, $p < .02$ • Ineffectiveness G1 = 0.5, G2 = 3.5, G4 = 4.0, $p < .05$
Bahrke et al, 1985 (54)	• N = 65, post n = 65, 10 min FU n = 65 • M = 10.6 yr (SD = .8), • 54% girls • US • Ethnicity NR • Middle class	Random assignment of children G1: intervention (n = 22) G2: rest period (n = 22) G3: control, crafts (n = 21)	• School-based • Run/walk, 1/4 mile course F = 1 session I = moderate T = aerobic T = 15-min session	• Fitness: exercise heart rate using Insta-Pulse monitor directly and 10 min post exercise. • State Trait Anxiety Inventory for Children	• Only acute effects assessed • Anxiety △ for G1 vs G3: Tx = −0.7 C = −2.3, NS
Lydon et al, 1984 (25)	• N = 310, FU n = 285 • Grades 1–5 • % girls NR • US • 27% white • SES NR (urban inner city)	Non-random assignment of matched schools G1: intervention (n = 206)* G2: control, no PE (n = 104) *Note: the original study compared two teaching styles in G1	• School-based (PE class) • Physical Education Program-outdoor movement exploration, physical fitness, gymnastics F = 5 × wk, 1 semester I = NR T = aerobic, strength, flexibility T = 45-min sessions	• Motor skill development: Schilling Body Coordination Test • Global self-concept: Martinek-Zaichkowsky Self-Concept Scale	• Motor skills: Tx > C, P < .01 • Self-concept at post: Tx = 22.85 C = 22.40, NS
Schempp et al, 1983 (26)	• N = 208, FU n = 174 • Grades 1–5 • % girls NR • US • Ethnicity NR • SES NR	Random assignment of children G1: intervention (n = 148)* G2: control (NR) (n = 60) *Note: the original study compared two teaching styles in G1	• School-based (classroom setting) • Physical education instruction: movement, motor skills, gymnastics F = 1 × wk, 8 wk I = NR T = aerobic, flexibility T = 45-min sessions	• Motor skills: Johnson Fundamental Skills Test • Global self-concept: Martinek-Zaichkowsky Self-Concept Scale	• Motor skills: Tx > C, $p < .05$ • Self-concept: NS (no means reported)
Percy et al, 1981 (59)	• N = 30, FU n = NR • Grades 5–6 • % girls NR • US • Ethnicity NR • SES NR	Children randomly selected and assigned G1: intervention (n = 15) G2: control (NR) (n = 15)	• School-based (non-class) • Running program: students chose when and where they ran the required 1 mile F = ≥ 3 × wk, 7 wk I = moderate/vigorous T = aerobic T = NR	• PA: Teacher log for attendance and distance run. • Self-esteem: Coopersmith Self-Esteem Inventory	• PA compliance NR • Self-Esteem △: Tx = +13.4 C = −2.7, $p < .002$
Martinek et al, 1978 (27)	• N = 344, FU n = 344 • Grades 1–5 • % girls NR • US • Caucasian,	Randomly selected children, non-randomly assigned G1: intervention	• University-based PE center (class) • Physical activity program, perceptual motor, gymnastic activity	• Motor development: Korper Coordination Test • Self-concept:	• Motor skills: Tx > C, $p < .05$ • Self-concept post scores adjusted for baseline:

Table 84-1 (*Continued*)

REFERENCE	PARTICIPANTS	DESIGN	INTERVENTION SETTING DESCRIPTION OF PA	MEASUREMENT	RESULTS
	• SES NR	PE) (n = 114)	T = aerobic, flexibility, motor skills T = 45-min sessions	Self-Concept Scale	$p < .01$
Bruya, 1977 (60)	• N = 72, FU n = NR • 9–11 yr • 50% female in each grp • US • Ethnicity NR • SES NR	Classes randomly assigned G1: intervention (n = 36) G2: control (no skills training) (n = 36)	• School-based (class) • Basketball Movement Program F = 2 × wk, 4 wk I = NR T = sports skills T = 30-min sessions	• PA: no measures • Self-concept: Piers-Harris Children's Self-Concept Scale	• Self-concept △: Tx = +2.9 C = +4.3, NS
McGowen et al, 1974 (23)	• N = 37, FU N = NR • Grade 7 • 0% female • US • Ethnicity NR • SES NR	Random assignment of students G1: intervention (n = NR) G2: no PA control (n = NR)	• School-based (PE Class) • Running Training Program F = 3–4 × wk, 18 wk I = vigorous T = aerobic T = NR	• Fitness: Cooper 12-min run • Self-concept: Tennessee Self-Concept Scale	• Fitness: Tx > C, $p < .005$ • Self-concept: Tx > C, $p < .05$ (no means reported)
Koocher, 1971 (61)	• N = 65, FU n = 65 • 7–15 yr M = 10.3 • 0% female • US • Ethnicity NR • Middle class	Assignment based on results of swimming test G1: intervention, learned to swim (n = 19) G2: did not learn to swim (n = 16) G3: passed initial swim test, control (n = 30)	• Resident summer camp • Swim Program F = 12 consecutive days I = Vigorous T = aerobic T = NR	• Swimming test: 25 yards unassisted • Self-concept, discrepancy between self-concept and ideal self: index of adjustment and values	• Groups defined by change in swimming skills • Change in difference between perceived and ideal self: G1 = −4.89 G2 = +1.87 G3 = −1.53, NS

FU, follow-up; NR, not reported; Rng, range; Tx, treatment; C, control; PE, physical education; PA, physical activity; FITT, frequency, intensity, type, and time (duration) of physical activity; SES, socioeconomic status.

other studies did not assess physical activity as an outcome. A wide range of psychological variables were assessed and the assessment techniques were generally age-appropriate. Overall, the utility of physical activity interventions to improve psychological outcomes was mixed for the general population of children and adolescents. Table 84-3 summarizes the findings by specific psychological outcome and study population.

Summary of Studies of Special Populations
Nine studies of special populations were identified, representing eight different populations (i.e., incarcerated youth, delinquent youth, learning disabled, mentally retarded, physically disabled, obese, pregnant teens, and psychiatric inpatients). Participants ranged in age from 4 to 20 years, and the majority of studies were of adolescents aged 13 to 18. Studies evaluated girls only (one study), boys only (four studies), or both (four studies). Ethnicity and socioeconomic status were largely unreported. Two studies were conducted in Canada and seven in the United States.

Two studies did not include a control or comparison

group. Four of the studies used a no-activity control group and three used standard physical education or a light physical activity intervention as the comparison group. Participants were randomly assigned to condition in four of the studies. The interventions were delivered in school, camp, or residential facilities and lasted from 3 to 20 weeks. Many of the interventions included multiple types of physical activity (e.g., aerobic and strength exercises) and intensity was often not measured. Sports programs, physical education classes, motor skill training, and ski camp are examples of the interventions tested. Participants attended physical activity classes 1 to 5 times per week for 25 to 120 minutes per session. Two of the studies also included additional time for counseling (28,29), and the effects of these interventions cannot be separated from that of the physical activity intervention alone.

Eight studies showed significant improvement in fitness (28–32), motor skills and coordination (33,34), or sport skills (35). Koniak et al (36) did not assess physical activity outcomes. Again, a wide variety of psychological outcomes were assessed, and 11 of 17 showed significant improvement. A list

Table 84-2 Review of Studies Including Special Populations

REFERENCE	PARTICIPANTS	DESIGN	INTERVENTION SETTING DESCRIPTION OF PA	MEASUREMENT	RESULTS
Koniak et al, 1994 (36)	• Pregnant teens • N = 58, FU n = 58 • *M* = 16.6 yr, Rng = 14–20 yr • 100% girls • US • 34% Hispanic, 28% African-Amer, 24% white, 12% mixed, 2% other • SES NR	Non-random assignment of volunteers into self-selected groups* G1: intervention (n = 35) G2: control (n = 23) *Note: comparison group chose not to exercise	• Residential maternity home • Aerobic exercise class F = 2 × wk, 6 wk I = vigorous T = aerobic, strength T = 65-min sessions	• PA not assessed • CES-D (Center for Epidemiological Studies Depression Scale) • Coopersmith Self-Esteem Inventory	• Depression △: Tx = −5.44 C = −0.48, NS • Self-esteem, total △: Tx = +3.52 C = +3.81, NS • Self-esteem, general △: Tx = +0.59 C = +0.13, NS
Brown et al, 1992 (30)	• Psychiatric inpatients with dysthymia or conduct disorder • N = 27, post FU n = 16, 4 wk FU n = 11 • *M* = 16.5 yr Rng = NR • 41% female • US • Ethnicity NR • Working class to affluent	Random assignment of classes G1: intervention (n = 17) G2: control (regular PE) (n = 10)	• Private psychiatric institution • Running/ aerobic exercise program, in addition to regular PE F = 3 × wk, 9 wk I = vigorous T = aerobic T = NR	• Fitness (resting, exercise and recovery heart rate, time to complete 1 mile run, BMI) • Beck Depression Inventory • Profile Of Mood States (baseline differences in BDI and POMS not controlled in analyses, very low n's at 4 wk FU)	• Recovery heart rate, Tx > C, $p < .05$ • Depression △: boys: Tx = 0.0, C = 0.0, NS girls: Tx = −15.75, C = −0.66, NS • Anxiety △: boys: Tx = −1.0, C = −2.0, NS girls: Tx = −21.75, C = +5.0, NS • Hostility △: boys: Tx = +17.0, C = −10.0, NS girls: Tx = −18.69, C = +8.67, NS • Total self-efficacy △: Tx = +6.33, C = −0.4, NS
MacMahon et al, 1988 (31)	• Incarcerated youth • N = 98, FU n = 69 • *M* = 16.3 yr, Rng = 14–18 yr • 0% female • US • 51% white, 42% Hispanic, 6% black, 1% Asian • SES NR	Random assignment of adolescents G1: intervention (n = 45) G2: control, less strenuous sports (n = 53)	• Incarceration facility (PE class) • Exercise program, addition to PE curriculum F = 3 × wk, 12 wk I = vigorous T = aerobic T = 40-min sessions	• Submax cycle ergometer • Piers-Harris Children's Self-Concept Scale • Beck Depression Inventory	• Tx > C on change in fitness; Tx: 73.05 vs 21.55, $p < .001$ • Self-concept △, NS • Depression △: Tx = −4.78 C = −1.35, $p < .02$
MacMahon et al, 1987 (32)	• Learning disability with average to above average intelligence • N = 54, FU n = 54 • *M* = 9.7 yr, Rng = 7–13 yr • 0% female • US	Random assignment of children G1: intervention (n = 27) G2: control, structured games and less vigorous physical activity	• Private school for learning disabled with average or above average IQ • Aerobic Exercise Program F = 5 × wk, 20 wk I = vigorous	• Fitness: submaximal text on cycle ergometer • Self-concept (Piers-Harris Children's Self-Concept Scale; read aloud)	• Fitness, Tx > C, $p < .05$ • Self concept △: Tx = +6.7 C = +0.5, $p < .05$

Table 84-2 (*Continued*)

REFERENCE	PARTICIPANTS	DESIGN	INTERVENTION SETTING DESCRIPTION OF PA	MEASUREMENT	RESULTS
	• Ethnicity NR • Middle class	(n = 27)	T = aerobic T = 25-min sessions		
Roswal et al, 1984 (33)	• Educable mentally retarded • N = 32, FU n = 32 • M = 10.2 yr Rng = 5–13 yr • 37% female • US • Ethnicity NR • SES NR	Non-random assignment of children G1: intervention (n = 16) G2: no PA control, (n = 16)	• University • Children's developmental play program F = 1 × wk, 9 wk I = NR T = aerobic, motor skills T = 120-min sessions	• Motoric functioning Bruininks-Oseretsky Test of Motor Proficiency • Martinek-Zaichkowksy Self Concept Scale (global score) (analyses combined PA and mental health effects)	• Exp group showed greater increase in both motor proficiency and self concept, $p < .001$
Hilyer et al, 1982 (28)	• High security risk delinquents • N = 60, FU n = 43 • Mean NR, Rng = 15–18 yr • 0% female • US • 55% African-Amer. 45% Caucasian • SES NR	Random assignment of boys G1: intervention (n = 30) G2: control, regular PE program (n = 30)	• State industrial school for youth offenders • Physical fitness training Program, physical activity and counseling F = 3 × wk, 20 wk I = NR T = aerobic, strength, flexibility T = 90-min sessions (10–15 min was counseling)	• Cooper 1.5 mile run, submax VO$_2$, sit and reach, grip strength, bench press, situps, pullups, skinfolds • Coopersmith Self-Esteem Inventory • Profile of Mood States • Beck Depression Inventory • State-Trait Anxiety Inventory for Children	• Tx improved on multiple measures; C did not improve. • Total self-esteem △: Tx = +11.2, C = −11.53, p NR • General self-esteem △: Tx = +2.49, C = −2.94, $p < .001$ • Depression, BDI △: Tx = −8.17, C = +6.77, p NR • Depression, POMS △: Tx = −5.66, C = +5.33, NS • Anger, POMS △: Tx = −.12, C = +6.13, $p < .001$ • State anxiety △: Tx = −3.20, C = +1.77, $p < .03$ • Trait anxiety △: Tx = −6.46, C = +5.83, p NR • Tension, POMS △: Tx = −0.9, C

Table 84-2 continues

Table 84-2 (*Continued*)

Reference	Participants	Design	Intervention Setting Description of PA	Measurement	Results
					= +6.97, $p < .002$
Simpson et al, 1979 (35)	• Trainable mentally retarded, IQ = 40–60 • N = 20, FU n = 19 • Mean NR Rng = 14–20 yr • boys & girls (% NR) • Canada • Ethnicity NR • SES NR	Non-random assignment of adolescents, NS differences at baseline for age and IQ G1: intervention (n = 14) G2: control, regular school curriculum (n = 6)	• School-based (group class outside school, during school hours) • Snow ski program, 0.5 hrs instruction and 1 hr skiing F = 1 × wk, 5 wk I = moderate/vigorous T = aerobic T = 60-min session	• Videotaped ski skills each week, rated improvement, GI only • Self-concept scale for children (modified for mentally retarded children)	• PA: documented improvement in skiing skills • Self-concept △: Tx = +11.7 C = −1.7, $p < .05$
Mauser et al, 1977 (34)	• Children with perceptual motor and social interaction problems • N = 12, n at FU NR • M = 8.4 yr, Rng 4–12 yr • 20% girls • Canada • Ethnicity NR • SES NR	Single group design, results compared to published norms for non-disabled children G1: intervention (n = 12)	• Setting NR • Developmental Physical Activity Program F = NR, 8 wk I = NR T = NR T = NR	• Documented improvement in body coordination, $p < .01$ • Martinek-Zaichkowski Self-Concept Scale △: Tx = +0.75, NS pre to post, baseline NS different from normative data.	• Sig improved body coordination 62.8 (14.9) pre, 69.0 (15.0) post, $p < .01$ • Self-concept NS
Collingwood et al, 1971 (29)	• Obese adolescents • N = 5, n at FU NR • Mean NR, Rng = 13–16 yr • 0% female • US • Ethnicity NR • SES NR	Single group design G1: intervention (n = 5)	• YMCA (structured sessions) • Physical training program 1 hr in gym, 1 hr in pool (jogging, strength training, swimming) plus 3 total hr of group counseling F = 5 × wk, 3 wk I = moderate/vigorous T = aerobic T = 120-min sessions	• Fitness (body weight, waist circumference, resting heart rate, lung capacity, Kraus Webber fitness series; balance, chalk jump, pushups; situps) • Body attitude scale (evaluative; potency; activity) • Self-concept, self acceptance, ideal self.	• Fitness: significant improvements in weight, resting heart rate, Kraus Webber fitness, balance, chalk jump, pushups and situps) all $p < .05$ • Body attitude, evaluative: improved, $p < .05$ • Self-concept: improved, $p < .05$ • Discrepancy between self-concept and ideal self: reduced, $p < .05$ (no means reported)

FU, follow-up; NR, not reported; Rng, range; Tx, treatment; C, control; PE, physical education; PA, physical activity; FITT, frequency, intensity, type and time (duration) of physical activity intervention; BMI, body mass index; SES, socioeconomic status.

Table 84-3 Summary of Findings by Psychological Outcome for General and Special Populations

PSYCHOLOGICAL OUTCOME	SIGNIFICANT IMPROVEMENTS		NS FINDINGS	
	GENERAL POPULATION	SPECIAL POPULATION	GENERAL POPULATION	SPECIAL POPULATION
Positive Affect				
• Self-Concept	Y Alpert (21) Y Martinek (27) O McGowen (23) Y Boyd (39)	O Collingwood (29) Y MacMahon, 1987 (32) Y Roswal (33) O Simpson (35)	Y Lydon (25) Y Schempp (26) Y Bruya (60) O Boyd (39) Y Koocher (61)	Y Mauser (34) O MacMahon, 1988 (31)
• Self-Esteem	NR Percy (59)	O Hilyer (28)		O Koniak (36)
• Self-Efficacy	O Holloway (24)			O Brown (30)
• Body Attitude		O Collingwood (29)		
Negative Affect				
• Depression		O MacMahon, 1988 (31)	O Norris (22)	O Koniak (36) O Brown (30) O Hilyer (28)
• Hostility, Anger		O Hilyer (28)	O Norris (22)	O Brown (30)
• Perceived Stress	O Norris (22)			
• Anxiety	O Norris (22)	O Hilyer (28)	Y Bahrke (54)	O Brown (30)
• Ineffectiveness (EDI)	O Holloway (24)			

EDI, subscale of Eating Disorder Inventory; Y, younger sample (~5–12 years old); O = older sample (~13–18 years old); NR = not reported; NS = nonsignificant.

of special population studies and their specific psychological outcomes is included in Table 84-3.

DISCUSSION AND RECOMMENDATIONS BASED ON THE REVIEW

The results of this literature review are discussed in terms of treatment effects on psychological outcomes, treatment effects on physical activity outcomes, potential mediators, limitations of the current review, and implications for further research.

Treatment Effects of Psychological Variables

Approximately half of the effects were significant improvements on psychological variables (51%). There did not appear to be differences between general and special populations in that the findings from the literature in both areas were mixed. Older children from special populations were evaluated more frequently than younger children, and the reverse was true for the general population. Among younger and older children regardless of population, physical activity improved psychological outcomes about half the time. Self-concept was the most frequently evaluated outcome, and significant improvements were detected in 8 of 14 studies. There was moderate support for improvements in self-esteem, and this is consistent with other reports in the literature (19,37,38). Results for self-efficacy were mixed. Reductions in depression and hostility received little support, since three-quarters of the findings were nonsignificant. Results for stress and anxiety were also mixed. However, all of the interventions, regardless of statistical significance, produced changes in the expected direction, except Brown et al (30), in which hostility increased nonsignificantly in treated boys. This study had a small total study

population (N = 2) at follow-up and significant differences between groups at baseline on several variables, so the direction of this result is probably spurious.

Surprisingly, none of the studies interpreted the clinical significance of the psychological improvements. Improvements in self-concept were not interpreted in light of normative data, except in one study where disabled children were found to have self-concept scores no lower than normative data (34). In a study of incarcerated boys, a physical activity intervention produced a reduction in depression scores that was both statistically and clinically significant. While Beck Depression Inventory (BDI) scores increased for the control condition ($M = 20$ to 26) from pre- to post-test, it decreased for the intervention group ($M = 23$ to 14). BDI scores from 19 to 29 indicate moderate to severe depression, and boys in this study not only reduced depressive symptoms, but their symptoms were reduced to the mild range (28). Future researchers need to interpret the clinical significance of changes in psychological outcomes.

Differences in design of the studies and methodologic flaws made interpretation of results difficult. Two of the problems with study design included nonrandom assignment of participants to conditions (53% of studies with two or more groups) and use of various comparison conditions (i.e., alternate forms of physical activity) that were not adequately described. Twelve studies did not report adequate information about their findings (i.e., all means and standard deviations): this is a weakness of the literature. Additionally, several studies (24,30) reported differences between conditions on psychological variables at baseline, which were not controlled in subsequent analyses.

The nature of the physical activity interventions varied. For younger children the interventions focused more on movement, coordination, and play; those for older children tended to be planned "exercise" sessions (more like adult exercise classes). For example, Boyd et al (39) tailored the physical activity intervention to the developmental interests of pre-adolescent and adolescent girls. Younger girls received a skill-related intervention to foster coordination, speed, and agility; older girls participated in strength and aerobic training to maintain or lose weight. While ratings of satisfaction with physical appearance increased for both younger and older adolescents in this study, planners of physical activity interventions need to take care not to remove all aspects of play from physical activity interventions and replace them with an emphasis on energy expenditure and physical appearance. In a recent controlled study, a 3-month physical activity intervention produced increased body dissatisfaction among women (40). Physical activity interventions have the capacity of over-sensitizing participants to body image-satisfaction issues. This may be particularly true for older adolescent girls, and we should develop interventions that emphasize health-related physical activity and body acceptance.

In addition to the interventions being quite differen from one another, the intervention components were not well described in most of the studies. Some utilized a behavioral approach to motivate participants to continue taking part in the intervention. The majority of interventions included some type of adult contact, but it varied greatly from an adult "coach" who supervised appropriate use of exercise equipment to counseling about physical activity or other issues. In fact, two studies, both of special populations, included a counseling component in the intervention, and the effects of the physical activity intervention independent of the counseling cannot be determined. One study, of obese adolescent boys, included "counseling-discussion" for a total of 3 hours over the course of the 3-week intervention at a summer camp (29). The content of the counseling is not described at all, but participants improved their self-assessment of body attitudes and self-concept.

The second study, of incarcerated adolescent boys, included a counseling component, described in much greater detail (29). As part of the 90-minute physical activity intervention, 10 to 15 minutes/week for 20 weeks were spent with a counselor who used behavioral techniques to reinforce fitness gains. Praise and goal setting were used to support incremental successes. Generalizations of success from self-discipline gained in the exercise intervention were drawn to other parts of the subjects' lives, including delinquent behavior and substance abuse. It is not surprising that this is the study that showed significant clinical reductions in depression because affect was addressed in the counseling component of the intervention. Future research should consider the utility of combined physical activity and psychological interventions and possible synergistic effects they may have.

Potential Negative Psychological Effects of Exercise

All of the studies showed either an improvement or no significant difference in psychological outcomes. No study showed a significant negative intervention effect. However, participation in physical activity is not without risks, both physical and psychological. Excessive training can lead to

overuse injuries (1) or disrupted sleep (41), and there is some evidence of increased mood disturbances among athletes who overtrain (18,42,43) (see Chapter 87). Compulsive and excessive exercising is a characteristic of eating disorders (44) and has been reported in almost one-third of patients with a diagnosis of an eating disorder (45). However, there is no evidence to suggest that exercise causes eating disorders (46,47) (see Chapter 88). Rather, eating disorders are likely brought about by a complex interplay of interpersonal and environmental factors (48). Literature on overtraining indicates that negative psychological outcomes are usually seen among athletes or those performing considerable amounts of physical activity and may be prevented or ameliorated by reducing physical activity, so this should not be a significant barrier for the majority of children and adolescents.

Intervention Effects on Physical Activity Outcomes

In the current literature, eight studies evaluated and reported increases in estimates of cardiorespiratory fitness (e.g., submaximal bicycle ergometer tests); seven studies assessed some other physical activity outcome (e.g., coordination, sport skills, motor skills, or strength); and the other six studies did not assess physical activity variables. All of the studies measuring a physical activity outcome documented an improvement. Changes in psychological outcomes may be associated with increases in physical activity or physical fitness. Among adults, changes in psychological outcomes were independent of changes in fitness (49). In the current studies under review, there does not appear to be a differential effect on psychological outcomes based on increases in fitness versus physical activity, because about half of the studies with changes in fitness and about half of the studies with changes in other physical activity measures showed significant improvements in psychological variables.

Potential Mediators of the Effect on Psychological Variables

Several potential mediating factors have been hypothesized in the literature (50–52), but none has been widely accepted in the literature on children and adolescents. One proposed mechanism is an increase in the level of endogenous endorphins (e.g., beta-endorphin) after high-intensity exercise, which has been related to improved mood. Second, alpha brain waves, known to be associated with relaxed states, increase during exercise and persist for a period of time afterward. Third, neurotransmitters with known relationships to affect are altered by physical activity. For example, norepinephrine and serotonin are related to depression, and exercise has been shown to increase the level of these neurotransmitters, providing a plausible explanation for decreased symptoms of depression after regular physical activity (53). Finally, the relationship could be mediated by simple distraction from worries and stressful cues in the environment. There is little evidence to support one mechanism over another, especially among children and adolescents, because few studies address this important issue. In fact, none of the studies reviewed in this chapter measured or reported suspected mediators of the psychological benefits. This area deserves further empiric consideration.

Potential Limitations

There are several factors that may limit the conclusions drawn from this review. First, there are very few controlled studies in this age group, and this is especially true for individual special populations. Second, methodologic flaws in many of the studies make it difficult to interpret their results. Participants from ethnic minority groups were underrepresented in most of the studies, and all of these factors jeopardize the external validity of the results. This review was limited to published papers, and studies with significant findings may be more likely to be published, so these studies may overestimate the true effect.

Finally, this is a descriptive review. Quantitative analysis of the results is necessary to make better estimations of the strength of the effect of the literature as a whole. Also, descriptive reviews give equal weight to results from studies with good and poor implementation (e.g., high attrition rates). Therefore, the reader is urged to interpret these conclusions with appropriate caution. However, it should be remembered that regardless of whether a qualitative or quantitative review is used, many studies in this area possess methodologic weaknesses that make it difficult to form strong conclusions.

Implications for Future Research

More well-designed empiric studies with diverse populations are needed to draw firm conclusions about the effect of physical activity on psychological outcomes among children and adolescents. Future research should carefully document the nature of the physical activity intervention including the frequency, intensity, type, and duration as well as compliance with the physical activity intervention.

Little is known about the dose of physical activity required to produce psychological changes. Several studies comparing more vigorous physical activity to a less active comparison group showed significant improvement in psychological outcomes (21,31,32). Norris and colleagues (22) found greater reductions in anxiety in a high-intensity group compared to a moderate-intensity physical activity group. Other aspects of the dose-response relationship, such as frequency and total duration of physical activity necessary to bring about changes in psychological outcomes, are unknown in this population and deserve further study.

Future research should carefully consider what psychological outcomes are important for specific populations. Studies of special populations should tailor the outcome measures to clinical needs and symptoms of the population. However, it is not terribly interesting to assess depression and anxiety among "normal" children or adoles-

cents who do not have clinical symptoms of depression or anxiety disorders, though two (22,54) of the studies in this review did. A floor effect and difficulty detecting significant differences is one reason for this; however, a more important reason is that there is no psychopathology to treat. A psychiatrist does not prescribe antidepressants to someone without depressive symptoms and expect their mood to improve. So, even if physical activity interventions produce reductions in negative affect, but all in the clinically "normal" range, that finding is not very useful. Rather, studies of non-clinical populations should focus on developmental issues relevant to *all* children and adolescents, such as self-esteem building, social-peer interactions, "quality of life," and stress management.

Another general psychological issue relevant to all children and adolescents is body image. Physical activity is positively associated with body image (55,56), and increases in body mass are related to decreases in self-concept and body image (57). This issue is particularly important to adolescent girls, and physical activity interventions should emphasize health benefits of exercise and body acceptance. Eleven studies in this review documented changes in these general psychological areas, and results from these and future studies like them will be highly relevant to general populations of children and adolescents.

SUMMARY

In summary, the psychological effects of physical activity interventions were reviewed in 21 studies of general and special population children and adolescents under age 18. Intervention characteristics and study designs varied greatly. There was only modest support for psychological benefits of physical activity programs and significant improvements were seen in about half of the studies. This is consistent with other literature showing modest intervention effects on psychological outcomes (13,58). However, this is still a very promising area (37), and it deserves further evaluation with well-designed and well-implemented studies. Although there are inconsistent findings about the psychological benefits associated with physical activity among youth, health care professionals, and others interested in the health and well-being of this population, should promote physical activity for its known physical health benefits and potential, if not yet consistently confirmed, psychological benefits.

REFERENCES

1. US Department of Health and Human Services. Physical activity and health: a report of the Surgeon General. Atlanta: Centers for Disease Control and Prevention, 1996:175–207.

2. Sallis JF. Epidemiology of physical activity and fitness in children and adolescents. Crit Rev Food Sci Nutr 1993;33:403–408.

3. Gortmaker SL, Dietz WH, Sobol AN, et al. Increasing pediatric obesity in the U.S. Am J Diseas Childr 1987;14:535–540.

4. Sallis JF, Patrick K. Physical activity guidelines for adolescents: consensus statement. Pediatr Exerc Sci 1994;6:302–314.

5. Gleser J, Mendelberg H. Exercise and sport in mental health: a review of the literature. Isr J Psychiatr Relat Sci 1990;27:99–112.

6. Kugler J, Seelbach H, Kruskemper GM. Effects of rehabilitation exercise programmes on anxiety and depression in coronary patients: a meta-analysis. Brit J Clin Psychol 1994;33:401–410.

7. Gauvin L, Spence JC. Physical activity and psychological well-

being: knowledge base, current issues, and caveats. Nutr Rev 1996;54(suppl):S53–S65.

8. Weyerer S. Physical inactivity and depression in the community: evidence from the Upper Bavarian field study. Int J Sports Med 1992;13:492–496.

9. Stephens T. Physical activity and mental health in the United States and Canada; evidence from four population surveys. Prev Med 1988;17:35–47.

10. Ross CD, Hayes D. Exercise and psychologic well-being in the community. Am J Epidemiol 1988; 127:762–771.

11. Petruzzello SL, Landers DM, Hatfield BD, et al. A meta-analysis on the anxiety-reducing effects of acute and chronic exercise: outcomes and mechanisms. Sports Med 1991;11:143–182.

12. North TC, McCullagh P, Tran ZV. Effect of exercise on depression. Exerc Sport Sci Rev 1990;18:379–415.

13. Spence JC, Poon P, Dyck P. The effect of physical activity participation on self-concept: a meta-analysis. J Sport Exer Psychol 1997;19(suppl):S109.

14. Martinsen EW. Benefits of exercise for the treatment of depression. Sports Med 1990;9:380–389.

15. Long BC, van Stavel R. Effects of exercise training on anxiety: a meta-analysis. J Appl Sport Psychol 1995;7:167–189.

16. U.S. Department of Health and Human Services. Child health USA '96–'97. Washington, DC: Health Resources and Services Administration, Maternal & Child Health Bureau, 1997:1–73.

17. U.S. Department of Health and Human Services. Research on children and adolescents with mental, behavioral and developmental disorders. Rockville, MD: United States Department Health Human Services, National Institute of Mental Health, 1990.

18. Raglin JS. Exercise and mental health: beneficial and detrimental effects. Sports Med 1990;9:323–329.

19. Gruber, JJ. Physical activity and self-esteem development in children: a meta-analysis. In: Stull GA, Eckert HM, eds. Effects of physical activity on children (the American Academy of Physical Education papers, No. 19.) Champaign, IL: Human Kinetics, 1986:30–48.

20. Shephard RJ, Wolle M, Lavallee H, et al. Required physical activity and academic grades: a controlled study. In: Ilmarinen J, Valimake I, eds. Children and sport: pediatric work physiology. Berlin: Springer-Verlag, 1984:58–63.

21. Alpert B, Field T, Goldstein S, et al. Aerobics enhances cardiovascular fitness and agility in preschoolers. Health Psychol 1990;9:48–56.

22. Norris R, Carrol D, Cochrane R. The effects of physical activity and exercise training on psychological stress and well-being in adolescent population. J Clin Psychol 1991; 36:55–65.

23. McGowan R, Jarman B, Pederson D. Effects of a competitive endurance training program on self-concept and peer approval. J Psychol 1974;86:57–60.

24. Holloway J, Beuter A, Duda J. Self-efficacy and training for strength in adolescent girls. J Appl Soc Psych 1988;18:699–719.

25. Lydon M, Cheffers J. Decision-making in elementary school-age children: effects upon motor learning and self-concept development. Res Q Exer Sport 1984;55:135–140.

26. Schempp P, Cheffers J, Zaichkowsky D. Influence of decision-making on attitudes, creativity, motor skills, and self-concept in elementary children. Res Q Exer Sport 1983;54:183–189.

27. Martinek J, Cheffers J. Physical activity, motor development, and self-concept: race and age differences. Percept Motor Skills 1978;46:147–154.

28. Hilyer JC, et al. Physical fitness training and counseling as treatment for youth offenders. J Couns Psychol 1982;29:292–303.

29. Collingwood T, Willet L. The effects of physical training upon self-control and body attitude. J Clin Psychol 1971;27:411–412.

30. Brown SW, et al. Aerobic exercise in the psychological treatment of adolescents. Percept Motor Skills 1992;74:555–560.

31. MacMahon J, Gross RT. Physical and psychological effects of aerobic exercise in delinquent adolescent males. Sports Med 1988; 142:1361–1366.

32. MacMahon J, Gross RT. Physical and psychological effects of aerobic exercise in boys with learning disabilities. Dev Behav Pediatr 1987;8:274–277.

33. Roswal G, Frith G, Dunleavy AO. The effect of a developmental play program on the self-concept, risk-taking behaviors, and motoric proficiency of mildly handicapped children. Physical Ed 1984;41:43–50.

34. Mauser H, Reynolds R. Effects of a development physical activity program on children's body coordination and self-concept. Percept Motor Skills 1977;44:1057–1058.

35. Simpson HM, Meaney C. Effects of learning to ski on the self-concept of mentally retarded children. Am J Mental Defic 1979;84:25–29.

36. Koniak-Griffin D. Aerobic exercise, psychological well-being, and physical discomforts during adolescent pregnancy. Res Nursing Health 1994;17:253–263.

37. Folkins CH, Sime WE. Physical fitness training and mental health. Am Psych 1981;9:380–389.

38. Sonstrom RJ. Exercise and self-esteem. Exerc Sport Sci Rev 1984;12:123–155.

39. Boyd K, Hrycaiko D. The effect of a physical activity intervention package on the self-esteem of pre-adolescent and adolescent females. Adolescence 1997;32:693–708.

40. Zabinski MF, Calfas KJ, Sallis JF. Effects of a physical activity inter-

vention on body image in university seniors: project GRAD. Ann Behav Med 1998;20:B148.

41. Montgomery I, Trinder J, Paxton S, et al. Sleep disruption following a marathon. J Sports Med 1985;25:69–74.

42. Morgan WP, Brown DR, Raglin JS, et al. Psychological monitoring of overtraining and staleness. Br J Sports Med 1987;21:107–114.

43. Morgan WP, Costill DL, Flynn MG, et al. Mood disturbance following increased training in swimmers. Med Sci Sports Exerc 1988;20:408–414.

44. American Psychiatric Association. Diagnostic and Statistical Manual of Mental Disorders. 4th ed. Washington, DC: American Psychiatric Association, 1994:539–550.

45. Brewerton TD, Stellefson EJ, Hibbs N, et al. Comparison of eating disorder patients with and without compulsive exercising. Intern J Eating Dis 1995;17:413–416.

46. Dishman RK. Exercise and sport psychology in youth 6–18 years of age. In: Gisolfi CV, Lamb DR, eds. Perspectives in exercise science and sports medicine. Vol 2. Youth

exercise and sport. Indianapolis: Benchmark, 1989:47–97.

47. Yates A, Leehy K, Shisslak CM. Running: an analogue to anorexia? N Eng J Med 1983;308:251–255.

48. Thompson KJ, ed. Body image, eating disorders, and obesity. Washington, DC: American Psychological Association, 1996:173–362.

49. Thirlaway K, Benton D. Participation in physical activity and cardiovascular fitness have different effects on mental health and mood. J Psychosom Res 1992;36:657–665.

50. Morgan WP. Affective beneficence of vigorous physical activity. Med Sci Sports Exerc 1985;17:94–100.

51. Petruzzello SJ, Landers DM. State anxiety reduction and exercise: does hemispheric activation reflect such changes? Med Sci Sport Exerc 1994;26:1028–1035.

52. Rowland TW. Exercise and children's health. Champaign, IL: Human Kinetics, 1990:161–180.

53. Morgan WP, O'Connor PJ. Exercise and mental health. In: Dishman RK, ed. Exercise adherence. Champaign, IL: Human Kinetics, 1988:91–124.

54. Bahrke M, Smith R. Alterations in anxiety of children after exercise and rest. Am Correct Ther J 1985;39:90–94.

55. Ameika CL, Calfas KJ, Sallis JF. Physical activity and body image in college men and women. Ann Behav Med 1998;20(suppl):S188.

56. McAuley E, Bane S. Exercise and body image in college females. Med Sci Sports Exerc 1996;28(suppl):S138.

57. Kolody B, Sallis JF. A prospective study of ponderosity, body image, self-concept, and psychological variables in children. Dev Behav Pediatr 1995;16:1–5.

58. Calfas K, Taylor W. Effects of physical activity on psychological variables in adolescents. Pediatr Exerc Sci 1994;6:406–423.

59. Percy L. Analysis of effects of distance running on self-concepts of elementary students. Percept Motor Skills 1981;52:42.

60. Bruya L. Effect of selected movement skills on positive self-concept. Percept Motor Skills 1977;45:252–254.

61. Koocher GP. Swimming, competence, and personality change. J Personality Soc Psych 1971;18:275–278.

Chapter 85

Physical Activity and Well-Being Among Persons with Spinal Cord Injuries

J. Stuart Krause

Traumatic spinal cord injury (SCI) occurs instantly and unexpectedly to nearly 10,000 people each year in the United States. It generally results in permanent loss of sensory and motor functioning, the extent of which depends on the level of injury (where the spinal cord is damaged) and the neurologic completeness of injury (the extent to which there is intact sensory or motor functioning below the level of the lesion). In complete injuries, there is no sensory or motor functioning below the level of the lesion (about 48% of all cases) (1). Historically, individuals with SCI did not live long after injury. However, life expectancy has increased dramatically over the past few decades (2–4), with estimates of life expectancy varying as a function of age, severity of injury, and a number of factors related to quality of life (5–8).

Maintaining an active lifestyle is challenging after SCI, particularly among individuals with more severe limitations. Not only may normal activity patterns be disrupted (e.g., employment), but ability to do planned exercise may be severely compromised, if not totally absent. Loss of ability to perform even the most basic types of exercise raises questions as to the potential impact of inactivity on health and general well-being.

Despite the potential importance of maintaining an active lifestyle after SCI, there has been rather limited investigation of the relationship between physical activities and outcomes after SCI. Research that attempts to identify relationships among activities and multiple aspects of well-being, including both objective (health) and subjective (psychological or emotional) outcomes, is generally lacking. The limitations in research relate to both general activities, such as maintaining gainful employment or an overall

active lifestyle, and to specific health-related behaviors (e.g., planned exercise).

The purpose of this chapter is to provide a general overview of the 20-year Minnesota Longitudinal Study (MLS), an ongoing line of research that has generated data on activities and well-being after SCI, and to analyze data from this study to further ascertain the relationships between activities and well-being after SCI. Because this study was not developed with the specific intention of solely investigating the relationships between activities and well-being, the variables used in the study are only a subset of those of interest. Nevertheless, there is a large amount of data that, when analyzed, can provide insights into the relationships between activities and well-being after SCI.

SUMMARY OF REPORTED DATA

Types of Activities

There are two classes of activities that may be investigated in relation to SCI outcomes. The first class is comprised of general activities or behaviors that are not necessarily intended to promote heath or wellness. Examples of activities fitting this category include employment, interpersonal relationships, participation in organizations, leaving the home on outings, and time spent out of bed. Performing these types of activities may be associated with a global favorable effect on many SCI outcomes.

In contrast to these general activities, the second set of variables are more directly linked to specific health outcomes. There are two subsets of specific behaviors: 1) those that are intended to produce a positive outcome, and 2) those that

980

may have an unintended negative outcome. Behaviors intended to produce specific positive outcomes include planned exercise, attention to nutrition, and SCI–specific health maintenance behaviors (e.g., weight shifts intended to prevent pressure ulcers). Behaviors that may have an unintended negative effect on well-being include tobacco, alcohol, and drug misuse. These two types of activities may be assessed independently along separate dimensions and may be associated with a specific pattern of health outcomes (9). They may be associated with a differential pattern of subjective well-being (SWB), particularly if they indeed lead to different health outcomes, which may in turn be related to differing levels of SWB.

The majority of data from the MLS fits the former category (general activities). As a result, there is very little data in the current study regarding specific types of health-related behaviors. However, the research on general activities has helped lay the foundation for new research (in progress) that is addressing the relationships between specific health behaviors and multiple aspects of well-being after SCI. These topics are discussed further, after review, analysis, and summary of existing data.

Minnesota Longitudinal Study

In 1974, researchers at the University of Minnesota initiated a study of life after SCI. Although not initially intended as a longitudinal study, subsequent follow-up has occurred in 1985, 1989, and 1994. Over the past two decades, this study has generated data on multiple aspects of quality of life (QOL), including both activities and SWB. The majority of this research has focused on general activity patterns, including employment and educational pursuits, social activities, and time spent out of bed (sitting tolerance). However, during later stages of the study there was an increase in the number of activity variables. The expanded number of variables paid more attention to the types of social activities in which individuals participated, sedentary activities, exercise, and self-reported fitness (a proxy for healthy behaviors and a healthy lifestyle). Particular activities were correlated with several outcomes in previous publications.

Assessment of Outcomes

The Life Situation Questionnaire (LSQ) has been used to measure outcomes throughout the study. This instrument was developed to measure a wide range of outcomes related to QOL after SCI, including both activity patterns and subjective evaluations of various areas of life. The LSQ has been revised on several occasions, with content expanded on each occasion. Earlier versions of this instrument, as well as the Multi-Dimensional Personality Questionnaire (10), are described in the following paragraphs, as they are pertinent to the review of earlier studies; whereas, a complete description of the current version of the LSQ is described later in this chapter along with the methods to analyze the data.

The preliminary version of the LSQ (11) contained three psychosocial adjustment scales, two related to satisfaction and a third related to adjustment. The adjustment scale include two 10-point items, each of which asked individuals to rate their overall adjustment on a scale from 1 to 10. They rated their current adjustment, as well as predicted what their adjustment would be in 5 years. The two satisfaction scales were derived from factor analysis of six satisfaction self-rating items. The first scale (interpersonal satisfaction) measured items related to social life, sex life, and general health; the second scale measured employment and finances (economic satisfaction).

A later revision to the LSQ expanded the number of satisfaction items to 11 and added a new set of 20 self-rated problems items, each of which also used five-point scales. The adjustment scale remained unchanged. However, factor analysis was performed on the life satisfaction and problems items set (independent analyses). There remained two satisfaction scales, with the second scale again comprised of the same two items. The interpersonal satisfaction scale was replaced by an eight-item general satisfaction scale that included a broader range of items (e.g., control over life, life opportunities, recreational opportunities). Three problems scales were derived from analysis of the 20 problems items (12). These scales included emotional distress (e.g., depression, loneliness, sadness); dependency (e.g., lack of transportation, lack of control over life, dependency); and poor health (pain, health problems).

The Multi-Dimensional Personality Questionnaire (MPQ) was developed to generate conceptually informative scales that are clear and replicable using an iterative process of data collection and scale modification (10). Eleven primary dimensions, three higher-order dimensions, and six validity scales are included in the MPQ. The higher-order dimensions include positive affectivity, negative affectivity, and constraint. Higher scores on positive affectivity tap feelings of joy, excitement, and vigor, while lower scores are indicative of fatigue and loss of interests (well-being, social potency, achievement). The negative affectivity scale is marked by feelings of anxiety and anger for high scores, and calm and relaxed feelings for low scores (stress reaction, alienation, aggression). Finally, higher scores on constraint indicate cautiousness, while lower scores are indicative of self-indulgence or impulsivity (control, harm avoidance, traditionalism). The 11 primary dimensions are subscales that are reflective of the three higher-order dimensions. The MPQ scales have been found to be internally consistent (0.83 to 0.89 alpha coefficients for individual scales), and stable over a 30-day period (0.82 to 0.92 for the primary dimensions) (10).

Studies of Employment and Well-Being

Clear relationships have been established between gainful employment, avocational productive activities, and multiple aspects of SWB. In the first report of these data (11), several aspects of general activities, recent medical history, life satisfaction, problems, and self-rated adjustment were compared among three groups of participants: 1) those who were gainfully employed, 2) those who were unemployed, but doing avocational, productive activities (e.g., attending school, doing volunteer work, homemaking), and 3) those who were neither employed nor doing other types of productive activities. The results indicated that participants who were employed reported the best outcomes, followed by those who were doing unpaid productive activities. Activities, such as sitting tolerance and outings, were highly correlated with being employed or doing other types of productive activities. In sum, this study suggested that: 1) individuals who score high on one type of activity are active in other areas of life as well; 2) being active is central to life satisfaction and the individuals' perception of the degree to which they have adapted to injury; and 3) being active relates to fewer physician visits and fewer hospitalizations.

In a second report (12), participants were reclassified as either: 1) currently employed; 2) currently unemployed, but employed at some time since injury; and 3) not employed at any time since injury. This study found that the positive impact of employment was maintained only while the individual was actively employed. In other words, the individuals needed to maintain their level of activity to experience associated gains in well-being.

A third analysis of data from this study (13) utilized data from both 1974 and 1985 (the first two stages of the study) to determine the temporal relationships underlying the observed correlations between employment activities and well-being. Two competing hypotheses were tested: 1) enhanced well-being predates being actively employed (those who are better adapted are more likely to become employed), or 2) the pattern of employment activities is present before enhanced well-being (employment activities may actually facilitate well-being). Employment status was cross-tabulated between 1974 and 1985, forming four groups of participants: 1) employed on both occasions; 2) employed in 1974 but unemployed in 1985, 3) unemployed in 1974 but employed in 1985, and 4) unemployed on both occasions. Measures of activities, recent medical history, and well-being were compared among groups in both 1974 and 1985. The results supported the second hypothesis: those who were employed in 1974 but unemployed by 1985 reported well-being scores in 1974 that were similar to those who remained employed on both occasions. However, in 1985, they no longer reported superior well-being scores. Conversely, those who were unemployed in 1974 but employed by 1985 were found to have the opposite pattern (i.e., their well-being scores improved in 1985). In fact, some aspects of their well-being in 1985 exceeded that of those who were actively employed in both 1974 and 1985.

Prospective Studies of Mortality

A series of prospective studies were conducted to investigate the relationships among the full range of activity, health, and well-being variables and mortality among study participants. Prospective data collections had been conducted at routine intervals (1974, 1985, 1989, and 1994), with mortality status ascertained at the time of each new data collection. At each stage of the study, data obtained during the previous data collection were used to compare and contrast the life adjustment of participants who had survived until the next data collection (survivors) with those who had died over the interval between studies (deceased). For example, all participants who first participated in 1974 were classified into survivor and deceased groups in 1985. The 1974 data on life adjustment was then used to identify prospective predictors of mortality after SCI. Similarly, the new data collected in 1985 was used to identify prospective differences in life adjustment between people who survived until 1989 and those who had died by 1989. A more complete description of each study is presented in the following paragraphs.

In 1985, Krause and Crewe (5) ascertained the survival status of the 256 participants from 1974. One hundred seventy-nine former participants were found to be alive (70%), 46 were deceased (18%), and the status of the remaining 31 could not be determined (12%). The deceased sample averaged 16.9 years since injury at the time of death. After statistically controlling any age differences, the authors compared the survivor and deceased groups on three sets of adjustment measures: 1) psychological ratings of psychosocial, vocational, and medical adjustment; 2) indices of social activity, medical stability, and life satisfaction; and 3) seventeen single adjustment items.

Participants surviving until the 1984 follow-up were found to have superior ratings of vocational and psychosocial adjustment but not of medical adjustment. Participants in the survivor group were more active socially, had a greater sitting tolerance, and were more likely to be working or attending school than participants who had died since 1974. Somewhat surprising, none of the indicators of recent medical history (e.g., doctor visits, hospitalizations) differentiated between the survivor and deceased groups.

A replication of this study was carried out during the 1988 follow-up, 15 years after the preliminary data collection. Survival status was again ascertained for all previous participants, including a new sample (N = 193) that was added during the 1985 data collection. Separate analyses were carried out as a function of the year of data collection (1974 or 1985), but not as a function of participant sample. Therefore, survivor and deceased groups were compared on all 1974 variables (6) and then again on all 1985 data (7). Because there were two participant samples, only one of which participated during the 1974 data collection, the number of cases available from each time of measurement differs. There were 102 individuals with 1974 data only, 154 with data from both 1974 and 1985, and 193 cases from 1985 only.

In the first report, Krause (6) identified the survival status of all the original 1974 participants. By 1989, 161 of the original 256 participants were known to be alive, 60 were deceased, and the remaining 35 could not be located. A two-by-two analysis of covariance (ANACOVA) was used to compare the deceased and survival groups on three sets of adjustment variables. Injury severity (quadriplegia versus paraplegia) was cross-matched with survival status to statistically control for the disproportionate percentage of quadriplegics in the survivor group. Age was used as a covariate. The three sets of variables included: 1) the same three ratings of psychosocial, vocational, and medical adjustment as were used in the 11-year report (5); 2) a different set of five adjustment scales; and 3) the same 17 individual adjustment items. The five scales included the same medical scale, a revised activity scale, self-rated adjustment, and two satisfaction scales (broken down from the previous full scale).

Survivors again showed superior adjustment on both psychosocial and vocational ratings. Somewhat less impressive, but statistically significant, differences were noted on medical adjustment. Survivors also showed superior scores on each of the five adjustment scales, with the most significant relationship for activity and the least significant for medical instability. Consistent differences were found on most psychosocial variables including five of the six life satisfaction items (none of which were significant in the 11-year follow-up). In general, these results are consistent with the findings of the previous

11-year study; survivors showed superior prospective adjustment. However, many more significant differences were obtained over the 15-year period, particularly those related to life satisfaction. The most parsimonious explanation of these differences is the added statistical control for differences in injury severity. Paraplegics tended to be somewhat better adjusted than quadriplegics in this study, yet quadriplegics were disproportionately found in the survivor group. These findings suggest that the failure to control for injury severity in the preliminary study (5) may have led to a conservative estimate of the true differences between the survivor and deceased groups.

Krause and Kjorsvig (7) also analyzed the 4-year prospective data from 1985. In 1989, investigators found that 309 of the 347 participants with 1989 data were known to be alive, 22 were deceased, and 16 could not be located. The same data analytic procedures (two-by-two ANACOVA) were carried out, using an expanded number of variables that were not available in the original study. Five more life satisfaction items and a new set of 15 problems items were included in the 1985 LSQ. One of the satisfaction scales changed as a result of factor analysis of the larger item set. Similarly, three problems scales were available, all derived via factor analysis.

The results over this 4-year period again supported the major study findings: survivors were more active, rated their adjustment to be better, and were more satisfied with many areas of life than deceased participants. Recent medical history was again only marginally related (at best) to survival status. The most interesting findings were obtained with the newly added problems items: psychologically loaded problems scales (emotional distress and dependency) were more highly negatively correlated with survival status than were measures of life satisfaction. On specific items, deceased participants had reported significantly more boredom, loneliness, and depression. They also reported more problems related to environmental resources, including a lack of adequate transportation, conflicts with attendants, and negative attitudes towards persons with disabilities. Lastly, the deceased group had reported greater problems with alcohol and drug abuse.

A generally similar methodology was used during the most recent follow-up (8), although the statistical analysis was changed rather dramatically. A prospective design was used, because data on life adjustment was taken at one time (1985) and subsequent survival status ascertained 11 years later (1996). Logistic regression was used to identify the relative risk of mortality, given the level of adjustment on a number of predictor variables. A total of 345 participants with SCI completed study materials in 1985, 330 of whom could be definitively classified into survivor and deceased groups in 1996. Of these 330 participants, 84% were known to be alive in 1996 (n = 278) and the other 16% were deceased (n = 52). The LSQ was used to measure nine primary predictors related to life adjustment after SCI, including employment status and eight predictor scales: activity, medical instability, adjustment, general satisfaction, economic satisfaction, emotional distress, dependency, and poor health. The LSQ was also used to generate data on 34 individual items that were used in exploratory predictive analyses. Activities were significantly predictive of survival status, as one SD difference on the activity scale was associated with a 1.59 greater chance of surviving the 11-year period. The odds of surviving were also 1.72 higher per SD for frequency of outings and 1.64, for daily sitting tolerance. Individuals who were employed in 1985 were 2.38 times more likely to have survived until 1996.

Summary

Taken together, these studies suggest that leading an overall active lifestyle is associated with a pattern of health, emotional well-being, and longevity. The activity indicators were general in nature, such as employment, sitting tolerance, or number of outings. Ideally, more information would be available regarding the role of more specific activities and behaviors in relation to a broad range of well-being outcomes. The remainder of this chapter will focus on analyzing and describing the most recent data from the MLS in an attempt to identify associations between multiple activity indicators and measures of SWB, adjustment, needs for medical services, and the incidence of pressure ulcers. All available activities variables, exclusive of those already used and reported in the literature (i.e., employment, hobbies, homemaking, and volunteering), were investigated in relation to multiple aspects of well-being and are discussed next.

ANALYSIS OF EXISTING DATA

Participants

There were three inclusion criteria to be eligible for the study: 1) traumatic onset of SCI, 2) a minimum of 2 years since injury, and 3) at least age 18. Two participant samples were selected: The first consisted of 435 participants that were identified from outpatient files of the University of Minnesota hospital and the Sister Kenny Institute (both in Minneapolis, Minnesota); the second sample (n = 597) was identified from outpatient files of the Shepherd Center (in Atlanta, Georgia). There was a total of 1,032 participants.

Overall, 69% of the participants were male and 75% were Caucasian. The average age of the participants was 29 years at the time of injury and 42 years at the time of the study; an average of 13 years had passed since injury. The breakdown by injury severity was complete quadriplegia (28%), incomplete quadriplegia (28%), complete paraplegia (26%), and incomplete paraplegia (19%). The sample averaged 13.5 years of education. Thirty-six percent of the participants were employed at the time of the study.

Procedures

All prospective participants were sent cover letters to describe the study, to obtain their written informed consent, and to alert them that study materials were forthcoming, followed by a copy of the revised version of the Life Situation Questionnaire (LSQ-R), which was sent 4 to 6 weeks later. A LSQ-R was sent to all nonrespondents. Follow-up phone calls were made to all individuals who did not respond to either mailing. Participants were offered a $20 stipend and copies of the general study results as inducements to participate.

Instruments

The LSQ-R includes several sets of items that are appropriate for investigating the relationships between activities and well-being. These item sets included basic demographic and injury-related variables, including: gender, race or ethnicity, geographic region, current age, years since injury, and injury severity (classified into quadriplegia and paraplegia for the purpose of the current report). The other two important item sets included items related to activities (or proxies for activities) and outcome variables.

There were nine activity variables, which fall into three general categories: 1) specific types of behaviors, 2) general activity indicators, and 3) self-ratings of fitness, which serve as proxy variables for a healthy lifestyle. The first two activity variables were hours spent per week watching TV and frequency of exercising. Both items were presented in multiple-choice format, with the options representing grouped frequencies (e.g., exercise: rarely, once per month, two to three times per month, one to two times per week, three to four times per week, five or more times per week). The two general activity variables were the frequency of leaving home on social outings and daily sitting tolerance. The outings items were presented as grouped frequencies (using the same categories as frequency of exercise), whereas sitting tolerance was an open-ended item. Lastly, the five fitness variables, which served as proxies for a healthy lifestyle, asked participants to rate five aspects of fitness (i.e., overall fitness, coordination, flexibility, strength, and endurance) on a five-point scale (1 = poor; 5 = excellent).

There were two types of relevant well-being outcomes—those related to SWB and those related to health. The LSQ-R includes seven factor-analysis derived SWB scales, an adjustment scale, and several individual items related to health status (14). The seven SWB scales were developed from factor analysis of two item sets of the LSQ-R. The first item set includes 20 satisfaction items; the second was comprised of 30 problems items. The homogeneous item domains were used to develop the following SWB scales: 1) engagement, 2) negative affect, 3) health problems, 4) finances, 5) career opportunities, 6) living circumstances, and 7) interpersonal relations. Higher scores indicate more favorable SWB for all scales except negative emotions and health problems, where lower scores are more favorable. The adjustment scale was developed by summing two 10-point items that asked participants to rate their overall adjustment (i.e., current adjustment and predicted adjustment in 5 years). Alpha coefficients ranged from 0.79 to 0.92, with a mean of 0.86 for the seven-factor scale.

The five health outcomes all requested participants to identify events over the 2 years before the study. They included: 1) number of pressure ulcers, 2) days adversely affected by pressure ulcers, 3) number of nonroutine physician visits, 4) number of hospitalizations, and 5) days hospitalized. Days adversely impacted by pressure ulcers and days hospitalized were presented as grouped frequencies (e.g., none, less than 1 week, 1 to 2 weeks).

Analyses

Stepwise multiple regression was used to identify the optimal predictors of several aspects of well-being after SCI. The predictors fell into two groups: 1) biographic or injury-related and 2) activity-related. The biographic or injury-related predictors included: 1) geographic region, 2) gender, 3) race or ethnicity, 4) age at injury, 5) years since injury, and 6) severity of injury (quadriplegia or paraplegia). These variables were

essentially used as control variables, as the activity variables were of primary importance. Nine activity variables were used as predictors. They included: 1) hours spent watching TV, 2) frequency of exercising, 3) weekly outings, 4) sitting tolerance, and 5) five fitness variables that served as proxies for a healthy lifestyle (i.e., overall fitness, coordination, flexibility, strength, and endurance).

Thirteen regression analyses were implemented, one for each outcome. There were eight psychosocial and five health outcomes. The psychosocial outcomes included an adjustment scale and seven factor-analysis derived SWB scales.

RESULTS

Correlations

Table 85-1 summarizes the intercorrelations between the predictors, both biographic and activity-related and Table 85-2 summarizes the correlations between the predictors and the well-being outcomes.

An inspection of the correlation matrix reveals several trends with regard to co-linearity among the predictors. First, the subset of five fitness rating scales are highly intercorrelated (ranging from +0.58 to +0.71). This indicates that these variables share a great deal of common variance and are likely to be measuring a similar, single underlying construct. Second, there is only a moderately strong correlation (−0.34) between the two aging variables (age at injury onset and years since injury). However, age at injury onset is more highly correlated with the other predictors, because it was significantly correlated with each of the other predictors ($p < .001$). However, "years since injury" was only significantly correlated with one other predictor. This suggests that, given equally strong relationships with the outcomes, "years since injury" explains a greater percentage of unique variance than "age at injury onset." Third, the remaining predictors fall into two general categories, with hours spent watching TV and frequency of exercising minimally correlated with the other predictors, and frequency of outings and sitting tolerance moderately correlated with other predictors. Given equal correlations with the outcomes, the former two predictors would account for a greater amount of unique variance in comparison with the latter predictors.

Multiple Regression

Table 85-3 summarizes the multiple correlations (R) and squared multiple correlations (SMC) for the 13 outcomes, as well as the number of predictor variables that significantly enhanced the prediction.

Several observations are readily apparent from this table. First, the multiple correlations ranged from 0.23 (number of pressure sores and number of nonroutine physician visits) to 0.59 (engagement). The SMCs ranged from 0.05 to 0.35. Second, the predictors accounted for more variance in SWB outcomes than in health outcomes. In fact, the multiple correlation that was lowest for any SWB scale (0.29 for home life) was essentially the same as that obtained from the highest multiple correlation with a health outcome (0.28 for number of days hospitalized). Third, the SMCs for several outcomes (n = 6) failed to reach 0.10.

Table 85-1 Intercorrelations Among Predictor Variables

	Hours Watching TV	Exercise	Outings	Sitting Tolerance	Fitness	Coordination	Flexibility	Strength	Endurance	Age at Onset	Time Since Injury
Hours watching TV	—	—	—	—	—	—	—	—	—	—	—
Exercise	−.02	—	—	—	—	—	—	—	—	—	—
Outings	−.10	.09	—	—	—	—	—	—	—	—	—
Sitting tolerance	−.13*	−.08	.33*	—	—	—	—	—	—	—	—
Fitness	−.13*	.14*	.31*	.21*	—	—	—	—	—	—	—
Coordination	−.17*	.02	.34*	.30*	.61	—	—	—	—	—	—
Flexibility	−.14*	.08	.31*	.26*	.59*	.65*	—	—	—	—	—
Strength	−.15*	.11*	.33*	.27	.61*	.66*	.62*	—	—	—	—
Endurance	−.15*	.05	.31*	.28*	.63*	.61*	.58*	.71*	—	—	—
Age at onset	.11*	.21*	−.26*	−.32*	−.12*	−.23*	−.18*	−.20*	−.23	—	—
Time since injury	−.06	−.12*	.05	.09	.06	.05	−.02	.00	.09	−.34*	—

* $p < .001$.

Table 85-2 Correlations Among Predictor and Outcome Variables

Outcome Variables	Age at Onset	Time Since Injury	Hours Watching TV	Exercise	Outings	Sitting Tolerance	Fitness	Coordination	Flexibility	Strength	Endurance
Engagement	−.11*	.10	−.22*	.16*	.43*	.26*	.43*	.38*	.34*	.38*	.43*
Negative emotion	.01	−.09	.12*	−.16*	−.29*	−.16*	−.33*	−.25*	−.25*	−.28*	−.30*
Health	.12*	−.04	.16*	−.12*	−.33*	−.29*	−.44*	−.35*	−.33*	−.38*	−.37*
Finances	.10	.10*	−.09	.08	.21*	.16*	.18*	.13*	.11*	.13*	.14*
Employment	−.02	.19*	−.23*	.05	.28*	.27*	.28*	.27*	.22*	.22*	.27*
Home life	.06	.04	−.01	.12*	.19*	.12*	.20*	.15*	.16*	.13*	.18*
Interpersonal relationships	−.03	.04	−.10*	.12*	.24*	.10	.22*	.16*	.19*	.16*	.21*
Self-rated adjustment	−.27*	.09	−.13*	.06	.35*	.24*	.40*	.43*	.38*	.38*	.42*
Number of pressure sores	−.03	.00	.10*	−.06	−.12*	−.12*	−.12*	−.11*	−.09	−.12*	−.09
Days impacted by pressure sores	−.04	.02	.08	−.08	−.12*	−.22*	−.14*	−.06	−.09	−.11*	−.10
Treatment	.06	−.06	.05	−.05	−.07	−.14*	−.18*	−.11*	−.12*	−.17*	−.15*
Hospitalized	.09	−.08	.10*	−.02	−.16*	−.19*	−.15*	−.14*	−.09	−.17*	−.16*
Days in hospital	.10	−.07	.14*	.00	−.17*	−.20*	−.16*	−.14*	−.10	−.15*	−.12*

* $p < .001$.

Subjective Well-Being Outcomes

Findings for each of the individual SWB scales are highlighted first, followed by the health items (data are available in tabular form from the author upon request). Because there was such a large sample (N = 1032), several predictors were significantly related to the outcome variable, without accounting for a great deal of variance. Therefore, only the most important predictors are noted for each outcome.

Table 85-3 Efficacy of Predictors for Each Outcome Variable

Outcome Variable	No. of Predictors	R	SMC	F*
Engagement	9	.59	.35	$F_{9,882} = 52.57$
Negative emotions	7	.44	.19	$F_{7,916} = 30.56$
Health	5	.53	.28	$F_{5,914} = 72.14$
Finances	6	.37	.14	$F_{6,924} = 24.15$
Employment	9	.51	.26	$F_{9,799} = 31.04$
Home life	5	.29	.08	$F_{5,919} = 16.91$
Interpersonal relations	4	.33	.11	$F_{4,886} = 27.50$
Self-rated adjustment	6	.51	.26	$F_{6,920} = 54.61$
No. of pressure sores	6	.23	.05	$F_{6,927} = 8.83$
No. of days impacted by pressure sores	2	.26	.07	$F_{3,889} = 21.90$
No. of visits to the doctor	3	.23	.05	$F_{3,927} = 16.77$
No. of visits to the hospital	4	.26	.07	$F_{4,935} = 16.85$
No. of days in hospital	4	.28	.08	$F_{5,928} = 15.94$

R, multiple correlations; SMC, squared multiple, correlations; F, variance ratio test.
* All F values are significant at $p < .001$.

The most general measure of global well-being was the engagement factor scale. The predictors accounted for a total of 35% of the variance in engagement scores. Higher scores on this scale were most strongly predicted by a greater frequency of leaving home on social outings (accounting for 19% of the variance in engagement) and by self-reported endurance (accounting for another 9% of variance). Although not accounting for a great deal of variance (no other predictors accounted for more than 2% of additional variance), higher overall ratings of fitness, spending less time watching TV, and exercising more frequently were also associated with higher engagement scores.

The predictors accounted for only 19% of the variance in negative affect, which was most strongly associated with lower overall reports of fitness (11% of the variance) and leaving the home less frequently on social outings (4% of the variance). Although not accounting for much further variance, negative affect was associated with less exercise and endurance, a younger age at injury onset, and a greater amount of time spent watching TV.

Activities accounted for a moderate amount of variance (28%) in self-reported health problems. Health problems were negatively correlated with self-rated overall fitness (20% of the variance). Frequency of leaving home on outings and sitting tolerance were also negatively correlated with health problems. Individuals with cervical injuries reported more health problems.

None of the predictors for finances accounted individually for more than 5% of the variance and, in total, they accounted for only 14%. The leading predictor of finances was the number of weekly outings followed by three demographic variables (i.e., race, age at onset, time since injury). Individuals with greater well-being related to finances left their homes more frequently on social outings and were more likely to be Caucasian, to be older at injury onset, and to have lived more years with SCI.

Several predictors were significantly related to career opportunities and accounted for 25% of the total variance.

The primary predictor was endurance, which accounted for 8% of the variance, followed by race. Only five other predictors accounted for approximately 2% of the variance. Higher career opportunity scores were related to greater self-reported endurance, being Caucasian, spending fewer hours watching TV, leaving home more frequently on social outings, being older at injury onset, having lived more years with SCI, and having a greater sitting tolerance.

There were fewer predictors that were significantly related to living circumstances. In total, five predictors accounted for only 8% of the variance in living circumstances. Only two variables accounted for at least 2% of the variance (rounded): self-reported fitness and number of outings. Individuals who reported greater well-being also reported higher levels of fitness and more frequent outings. Although not accounting for a large portion of variance, individuals who were older, Caucasian, and who had higher self-reported endurance also reported higher well-being scores related to living circumstances.

On the final well-being factor scale, four variables significantly contributed to the prediction of interpersonal relations scores and accounted for a total of 11% of the variance. Participants who reported greater well-being resulting from interpersonal relations were those who left their homes more frequently on outings, were female, had higher self-reported endurance, and exercised more frequently.

Adjustment

Six variables significantly added to the prediction of self-rated adjustment and accounted for a total of 26% of the variance. However, only three of these variables accounted for at least 2% of the variance; one variable (coordination) accounted for 16% of the variance. Individuals who left their homes more frequently on outings and who had higher self-reported endurance also reported higher overall adjustment scores (as did those who had higher self-reported level of coordination).

Health-Related Outcomes

In terms of more health-related variables, the prediction tended not to be as strong. On the first health variable, number of pressure ulcers within the past 2 years, six variables significantly added to the prediction, although they only accounted altogether for 5% of the variance. Only two accounted for as much as 1.5% of the variance. The number of sores reported within the past 2 years was greater among individuals with cervical injuries and those with lower self-reported fitness levels.

For "days adversely impacted by pressure ulcers" over the past 2 years, the predictors accounted for a slightly greater percentage of the variance (7%). However, only three variables significantly added to the prediction: individuals who reported lower sitting tolerance, a younger age at injury, and lower fitness level were more likely to report being adversely affected by pressure ulcers within the last year.

Only three variables added to the prediction of number of nonroutine doctor visits within the 2 years before this study. These variables accounted for only 5% of the variance and included self-reported fitness, sitting tolerance, and gender. The number of nonroutine doctor visits was greater among males, individuals with lower self-reported fitness, and those with a lower sitting tolerance.

The predictors also failed to account for a great deal of variance (7%) in the hospital visits in the 2 years before the study. Only two variables (sitting tolerance and self-reported strength) accounted for at least 2% of the variance. The number of hospitalizations was negatively correlated with sitting tolerance, self-reported strength, and the number of weekly outings but was positively correlated with the amount of time spent watching TV.

The number of days hospitalized was predicted by five variables which, as with the other health variables, accounted for only a small percent of the variance in participants responding (8%). Of the predictors, only two accounted for a minimum of 2% of the variance (rounded). "Days hospitalized" was negatively correlated with sitting tolerance and self-reported fitness. Of the less important variables, the amount of time watching television was positively correlated with the number of days hospitalized, whereas the number of outings and being in the Midwestern sample were negatively correlated with days hospitalized.

DISCUSSION

The purpose of this chapter was to summarize the existing literature on activities and well-being after SCI and to present new analyses relating to the relationship between activities and well-being. Data were generated by an ongoing longitudinal study. Most of the study variables that were used as predictors in this study reflect a general, rather than specific, health relevant behavior. The primary variables of interest included sitting tolerance, frequency of leaving home on outings, several proxy variables for a healthy lifestyle (self-rated fitness), and frequency of exercising. Several biographic and injury-related variables were also studied in relation to general well-being.

The most basic conclusion to be drawn from the data is that general activity level is predictive of well-being after SCI. However, the nature of the predictors that are most efficacious in predicting the outcome varied depending on the outcome under study. In general, self-reported fitness (either global fitness, strength, or endurance) and frequency of leaving the home on social outings were the best predictors of the majority of well-being outcomes. It must be kept in mind that other important general activity variables, particularly employment and educational activities, were not studied in the current analyses because they have been the focus of a great deal of previous research (at least relative to the total body of research available).

General SWB outcomes, such as engagement and the adjustment scale, were those that were best predicted by the general activity, proxy, and biographic variables. More specific aspects of SWB were not well predicted by these variables. These outcomes included interpersonal relations, living circumstances, and finances. In contrast with the modest to moderate relationships between the predictors and SWB outcomes, there were a very limited number of relationships detected between specific health outcomes and the predictors. For example, the number of variables accounted for in the five specific health outcomes ranged between 5% and 8% of the variance. Clearly, the general activity variables, although statistically significant, did not help a great deal in predicting these outcomes.

There are several implications of these findings. First, leading an overall active life appears to be predictive of several positive outcomes, mostly related to general well-being. This may reflect the fact that people who are more active in terms of working, attending school, or simply leaving their homes are less likely to be doing sedentary types of activities or smoking or drinking. These findings must be considered only hypothetical at this point, because there is no concrete evidence in this study to verify them. It is also likely that there are some direct positive effects from simply having a more active lifestyle.

The current project also suggests that more research is needed on specific behaviors or activities that may be related to health outcomes. First and foremost, researchers should turn their attention to behaviors that have been previously identified as related to health in the more general population. These may be either protective behaviors or risk behaviors. Protective behaviors buffer an individual from adverse outcomes (e.g., proper nutrition, exercise); risk behaviors lead directly to an increased risk of adverse outcomes. Tobacco and alcohol misuse are prime examples of risk behaviors that should be studied in relation to outcomes among people with SCI. Future research should be either theory-based or guided by empiric models that help to account for the relationships between protective and risk behaviors with well-being outcomes.

A new study is currently under way that is investigating the relationship between both risk and protective behaviors and multiple outcomes after SCI. The outcomes cut across a wide range of areas, including SWB, secondary conditions, and mortality. This study is being guided by a behavioral model that accounts for independent dimensions for protective and risk behaviors (9). The data collection for this study is nearly complete, with just under 1400 individuals with SCI already having participated. The intention of this study is to draw upon previous research with general activity variables but with an emphasis on more specific activities in behaviors, in an attempt to identify information that sets the stage for both prevention and treatment strategies among individuals with SCI. It is only through diligent research effort that we will progress and enhance our understanding of these relationships and reach our ultimate goal of prevention.

This research was supported by two grants from the National Institute for Disability and Rehabilitation Research (NIDRR) of the United States Department of Education, a field initiated grant (#H133G20200-93) and the SCI Model Systems grant (#H133N00023-95), and a grant from the Shepherd Center, Atlanta, Georgia.

REFERENCES

1. National Spinal Cord Injury Statistical Center. Annual report for the model spinal cord injury care systems. Birmingham, AL: National Spinal Cord Injury Statistical Center, 1997.

2. Devivo MJ, Black KJ, Stover SL. Causes of death during the first 12 years after spinal cord injury. Arch Phys Med Rehab 1993;74:248–254.

3. DeVivo MJ, Kartus PL, Stover SL, et al. Causes of death for patients with spinal cord injuries. Arch Int Med 1989;149:1761–1766.

4. Devivo MJ, Stover SL. Long term survival and causes of death. In: SL Stover, JA DeLisa, GG Whiteneck, eds. Spinal cord injury: clinical outcomes from the model systems. Gaithersberg MD: Aspen, 1955:289–316.

5. Krause JS, Crewe NM. Prediction of long-term survival of persons with spinal cord injury: an 11-year prospective study. Rehab Psych 1987;32:205–213.

6. Krause JS. Survival following spinal cord injury: a fifteen-year prospective study. Rehab Psych 1991;36:89–98.

7. Krause JS, Kjorsvig JM. Mortality after spinal cord injury: a four-year prospective study. Arch Phys Med Rehabil 1992;73:558–564.

8. Krause JS, Sternberg M, Maides J, Lottes S. Mortality after spinal cord injury: an 11-year prospective study. Arch Phys Med Rehabil 1997;78:815–821.

9. Krause JS. Secondary conditions and spinal cord injury: a model for prediction and prevention. Top SCI Rehabil 1996;2:58–70.

10. Tellegen A. Brief manual for the differential personality questionnaire. Minneapolis: University of Minnesota, 1982.

11. Krause JS, Crewe NM. Chronologic age, time since injury, and time of measurement: effect on adjustment after spinal cord injury. Arch Phys Med Rehab 1991;72:91–100.

12. Krause JS. The relationship between productivity and adjustment following spinal cord injury. Rehabil Coun Bull 1990;33:188–199.

13. Krause JS. Employment after spinal cord injury. Arch Phys Med Rehabil 1992;73:163–169.

14. Krause JS. Employment after spinal cord injury: transition and life adjustment. Rehabil Coun Bull 1996;39:244–255.

Chapter 86

Physical Activity and Quality of Life

Malani R. Trine

There has been a great deal of interest in the psychological construct known as "quality of life" in recent years, and there are a number of reasons for this development. The early work involving quality of life developed out of an interest in quantifying the status of society, and this work has been known as social indicators research. The principal approach focused on the development of questionnaires and the administration of large-scale surveys to national samples (1–4). There has also been increased interest in quality of life in the medical field, especially as life expectancy has increased, and investigators have become interested in the quality of those extra years lived. This development has led to an explosion of research in this area, and in 1992, the first journal specifically focusing on the topic of quality of life was published, *Quality of Life Research*. This research has included the development of over 300 quality-of-life scales (5), some of which are intended for individuals with specific diseases (e.g., coronary heart disease, cancer, AIDS) and others that are for the general population or for specific age groups within the general population. In addition, a series of published articles has been compiled that focus on the use of health-related quality-of-life measures, and the most recent publication in this series is the 1994 update, which lists over 200 articles published in the latter half of 1993 and throughout 1994 (6).

Another area in which there has been increased interest in quality of life is the study of physical activity. There are a number of health benefits of physical activity, and investigators are interested in learning whether or not increased quality of life can be considered one of those benefits.

In all of these areas of interest, similar questions can be raised about the psychological construct known as quality of life. What is meant by quality of life? What are the compo-nents included in quality of life? How is quality of life measured? What factors influence quality of life? There are many different views on all of these issues, and this review explores these issues in relation to the definition and measurement of quality of life in physical activity research.

DEFINITION AND MEASUREMENT OF QUALITY OF LIFE

Many different terms have been used in discussions of quality of life, but the "quality of life" rubric is used throughout this chapter. Terms used to describe concepts related to the subjective assessment of life quality include quality of life, health-related quality of life, life satisfaction, happiness, psychological well-being, and subjective well-being. All of these terms have been defined in slightly different ways. Quality of life has been defined as "individuals' perception of their position in life in the context of the culture and value systems in which they live and in relation to their goals, expectations, standards and concerns" (7). Health-related quality of life has been defined as "the impact of health conditions on function" (8). Life satisfaction has been defined as "the perceived discrepancy between aspiration and achievement, ranging from the perception of fulfillment to that of deprivation" (3). Happiness has been viewed as a preponderance of positive affect over negative affect (2). Psychological well-being includes self-acceptance, positive relations with others, autonomy, environmental mastery, purpose in life, and personal growth (9). Subjective well-being has been defined as including both the affective and cognitive satisfaction components of well-being (10).

As illustrated by the variety of definitions, there is no consensus about the meaning of quality of life, but there are some common themes that do appear across multiple definitions. One theme is the idea that quality of life is subjective and influenced by individuals' perceptions. A second theme is the idea that the assessment of quality of life involves some kind of comparison process (e.g., to objective criteria, to others, to one's own past, to one's own expectations). A third theme that appears in some definitions is the idea that quality of life is multidimensional. Although many investigators agree that quality of life is multidimensional, there is some disagreement about what components should be included in quality of life and how they should be selected. Some investigators have focused on assessments of an individual's life-as-a-whole, whereas others have focused on assessments of multiple life domains (e.g., work, family, money, housing) or multiple facets of health (e.g., physical, psychological, social, spiritual).

This issue is very important and it is directly related to the measurement of quality of life. If particular elements are selected by the investigators, whether through theoretical, empirical, or intuitive means, it is possible that some elements may not be important to particular individuals in terms of assessing their own quality of life. Most quality-of-life scales do not allow individuals to choose their own elements of importance, but one exception to this generalization is the approach of Flanagan (4).

Flanagan employed the critical incident technique to survey about 3000 individuals of varying ages, and subsequently used this empiric basis for selecting 15 areas of needs:

1) material comforts;

2) health;

3) relationships with relatives;

4) having and raising children;

5) close relationship with a spouse;

6) close friends;

7) helping and encouraging others;

8) participation in local and national government;

9) learning;

10) understanding yourself;

11) work;

12) creative expression;

13) socializing;

14) passive recreation; and

15) active recreation.

Flanagan then developed a questionnaire and administered it to three age cohorts: 30-year-olds, 50-year-olds, and 70-year-olds. The questionnaire consisted of two parts: First, respondents were asked how important each of the 15 factors was to them in terms of their overall quality of life; and second, respondents were asked to indicate how well their needs were being met in each area. This novel approach allows for individuality in terms of assessing quality of life, although it does present some interesting scoring challenges. Flanagan scored responses to each of the two questions sepa-

rately, but a worthwhile endeavor would be to develop a method to combine the two response sets.

Another example of an instrument that allows individuals to select their own components of importance is the Satisfaction with Life Scale (SWLS), developed by Diener et al (11). This instrument does not contain items about particular life domains or particular facets of health; rather it includes five items, rated on a scale of one to seven, which are all general enough to allow each respondent to decide what components or elements are important in making a judgment about his or her life-as-a-whole. In addition, the SWLS is an improvement over earlier one-item instruments in terms of reliability. Examples of items on the SWLS include, "I am satisfied with my life," and "The conditions of my life are excellent." The SWLS and Flanagan's questionnaire are unique among quality-of-life measurement instruments because they allow individuals to choose their own criteria for assessing their quality of life.

Limitations of Existing Measures of Quality of Life

As noted previously, over 300 scales have been employed to measure quality of life (5), and reviews of some of these instruments have been published (12,13). A major problem with many of the existing measures of quality of life is a lack of construct validity. One of the requirements for construct validity is discriminant evidence, and this means that a measure should not be unduly related to measures of other distinct constructs. This requirement seems to be lacking for a number of quality-of-life measures, and instruments such as the Minnesota Multiphasic Personality Inventory (MMPI) (14), the State-Trait Anxiety Inventory (STAI) (15), and the Profile of Mood States (POMS) (16) have been used as "quality of life" measures, when in fact, they are psychometrically sound measures of other distinct constructs. If the intent is to measure depression, for example, then a validated measure of depression should be used. It is unreasonable to employ a measure that consists of a number of questions related to depression, and then refer to it as a quality-of-life measure. Of course, this would apply to many other variables as well (e.g., anxiety, cognitive function, physical health, bodily symptoms). Conversely, if the intent is to measure "quality of life," then a validated measure of quality of life should be employed.

Another requirement for construct validity is convergent evidence; that is, a measure should be substantially related to other measures of the same construct and also related to other variables that it relates to on theoretical grounds. This requirement appears to be fulfilled more often for quality-of-life measures, but sometimes one measure is correlated with another invalid measure in an attempt to fulfill this requirement. An alternative view of the validation process is the one put forth by Landy (17), who suggested that rather than discussing validity as including specific types, such as content, criterion, and construct validity, the validation process should be viewed as hypothesis testing about the inferences that may be drawn from test scores. This view appears to have been largely ignored in the development of quality-of-life measures.

Although many investigators have created specific definitions and developed instruments for their own conceptualization of quality of life, there is certainly no consensus regarding the definition or measurement of this psychological construct. In order for quality of life to be a distinct construct, it must be conceptualized as something different from other constructs, and an emphasis on construct validity is necessary to advance our understanding of quality of life. Fava (18) has noted that there is a tendency to regard any psychosocial measurement as an indicator of quality of life, and Andrews et al (1) have commented that "the notion of measuring the quality of life could include the measurement of practically anything of interest to anybody." These comments seem to accurately summarize the problems related to the definition and measurement of this construct, and there is a great need for further clarification and consensus about the definition of quality of life.

DEFINITION AND MEASUREMENT OF PHYSICAL ACTIVITY

The psychological construct known as quality of life has been increasingly used as an outcome variable in the study of physical activity. Physical activity has been most commonly defined as "bodily movement produced by skeletal muscles that results in energy expenditure," while exercise is defined as a "subset of physical activity that is planned, structured, and repetitive and has as a final or an intermediate objective the improvement or maintenance of physical fitness" (19). Although there seems to be some consensus about the definition of physical activity, the assessment and measurement of physical activity are problematic. Some investigators have compiled a set of various self-report questionnaires (20), but there is certainly no consensus about which assessment tool is best.

RELATED REVIEW ARTICLES

There has been quite a bit of research dealing with the health benefits of physical activity, including both physiologic and psychological benefits (21). In terms of psychological benefits specifically, the research literature has typically focused on depression (22), anxiety (23), and self-esteem (24) (see Chapters 83 and 84). In contrast, the intent of this review is to explore the relationship between physical activity and the psychological construct known as quality of life. There have been a number of review articles published that have focused on related issues, such as: 1) exercise and quality of life in individuals with specific diseases or conditions (e.g., spinal cord injury) (25) (see Chapter 85); 2) exercise and quality of life in the general population (26); 3) physical activity and quality of life in the frail elderly (27); 4) physical activity and quality-of-life outcomes in older adults (28); 5) physical activity and psychological well-being in the elderly (29); and 6) physical activity and health-related quality of life (30).

PURPOSE OF REVIEW

The purpose of this review is to examine the relationship between physical activity and quality of life in healthy adults. To avoid the confounding of a particular disease with quality of life, studies of individuals with specific diseases are not included. An additional requirement for inclusion in this review is that the quality-of-life measure must include an assessment of life in general and must be a measure of something distinct from other constructs (e.g., anxiety, depression, self-esteem). The articles reviewed in this chapter are summarized in Table 86-1.

CROSS-SECTIONAL STUDIES

Three small-scale survey studies produced somewhat different results. In the first study, 54 men and 68 women (aged 18 to 77) were recruited from fitness, language, and art classes at a YMCA in a large Canadian city, and these individuals were categorized into four groups: 1) autonomous exercisers (N = 51); 2) fitness program enrollees (N = 24); 3) fitness program dropouts (N = 17); and 4) nonexercisers (N = 29) (31). The individuals who were more physically active did not differ from less active individuals on quality of life, as measured by the SWLS (11).

In contrast to these findings, in a study of 286 first-year medical students, significantly more of the individuals who reported being very satisfied with life reported participating in regular physical activity than those who reported being less satisfied with life (32). Quality of life and physical activity were each assessed with one item on the Health Risk Appraisal (HRA) (33).

In a third study, it was found that the exercise or sport component of a leisure activity questionnaire was related to quality of life, as measured by a six-item modification of the Life Satisfaction Index (LSI) (34). This sample consisted of 136 men and 264 women (age 40 or older), and although the relationship was significant for all of the age groups combined, there were no significant relationships in any of the four specific age groups (35).

There are a number of potential explanations for the lack of congruence in the findings of these three studies, one of which relates to sample size. Positive findings were reported in the two studies with larger sample sizes, and in the third study, positive findings were reported for the entire sample, but none of the specific age groups. Correlation coefficients are directly influenced by sample size: this is apparent here.

Two studies of masters athletes reported that these athletes had higher quality of life than comparison groups of sedentary individuals. The first study, conducted with 10 women masters athletes over age 40 (36), showed that these national-caliber long-distance runners scored significantly higher than other adults and college students on Pflaum's Life Quality Inventory (37). Similarly, in a survey of an international sample of 551 male and 199 female masters athletes (ages 40 to 81) participating in the first World Masters Games, it was found that 67% of these athletes rated their overall quality of life as much higher than that of their sedentary peers, as measured by a five-point self-report scale (38). Athletes in general may have lives of high quality, and this characteristic may be independent of physical activity levels. Perhaps the high quality of these individuals' lives has allowed them to excel at something they enjoy. This hypothesis was tested in a follow-up study of 313 college athletes and nonathletes (39). Analyses revealed that 20 years after entering the university, former athletes were no different than nonathletes on quality of life, as measured by Flanagan's quality of life questionnaire (4), but when current physical activity patterns

Table 86-1 Summary of Reviewed Articles

Investigators	No. and Description of Participants	Measures Used	Design	Results
Gauvin, 1989 (31)	54 men & 68 women, age 18–77 yr ($\bar{x}$ = 32.7)	SWLS Classified participants into 4 categories of physical activity	Cross-sectional	–
Parkerson, et al, 1990 (32)	185 men & 101 women, $\bar{x}$ = 22.3 yr	Life satisfaction—1 item on HRA Physical activity—1 item on HRA	Cross-sectional	+
Kelly, et al, 1987 (35)	136 men & 264 women, age ≥40 yr	LSI—6 items Physical activity questionnaire	Cross-sectional	+
Morris, et al, 1982 (36)	10 female athletes, age >40 yr ($\bar{x}$ = 43.8)	Pflaum's Life Quality Inventory Mileage: 46/wk.	Cross-sectional	+
Shephard, et al, 1995 (38)	551 male & 199 female master's athletes, age 40–81 yr ($\bar{x}$ = 58)	Self-reported quality of life (5-point scale)	Cross-sectional	+
Morgan, 1985 (39)	313 men, $\bar{x}$ = 38 yr	Flanagan's quality of life questionnaire Physical activity questionnaire	Cross-sectional	+
Kaplan, et al, 1991 (40)	1,787 men & 2,238 women age 20–94 yr	Self-reported life satisfaction (4 items) Physical activity index (4 items)	Cross-sectional	+
Paffenbarger, et al, 1994 (42)	8,018 men, age 45–84 yr ($\bar{x}$ = 58.2)	2 questions implying satisfaction with life Paffenbarger physical activity questionnaire	Cross-sectional	+
Brown, et al, 1993 (44)	685 Canadian adults 18–70+ yrs.	LSI Canada Fitness Survey (adapted)	Cross-sectional	+ for overall sample & some age groups
Ruuskanen, et al, 1995 (46)	1224 Finnish adults, age 65–84 yr	Self-reported meaningfulness of life Self-reported physical activity (extent and intensity)	Cross-sectional	+
Ho, et al, 1995 (47)	843 Chinese men & 714 women, age 70+ yr	Self-reported life satisfaction Self-reported daily physical activity	Cross-sectional	+
Young, 1979 (48)	16 men & 16 women, age 23–62 yr	Life satisfaction—Cantril's ladder	10 wk Calisthenics & walk/jog	–
Sidney, et al, 1976 (50)	14 men & 28 women, age 60+ yr	LSI	14 wk Endurance training	–
Morris, et al, 1978 (51)	36 men & 15 women, age $\bar{x}$ ≈ 20 yr	Pflaum's Life Quality Inventory	15 wk Conditioning class Sport history class	+
McMurdo, et al, 1992 (52)	37 men & 40 women, age 60–81 yr ($\bar{x}$ ≈ 65)	LSI	32 wk Aerobic Health education	+
Norris, et al, 1990 (53)	77 policemen, age 20–50 yr	LSS	10 wk Aerobic training Anaerobic training control	+
Blumenthal, et al, 1989 (55)	50 men & 51 women, age 60–83 yrs. ($\bar{x}$ = 67)	LSI	16 wk Aerobic Yoga & flexibility Wait-list control	–
Brown, et al, 1995 (56)	66 men & 69 women, age 40–69 yrs. ($\bar{x}$ ≈ 53)	LSES	16 wk 4 physical activity groups Control—paid	+ for all 5 group, including control group

$\bar{x}$, average age; +, positive relationship between physical activity and quality of life; –, no relationship between physical activity and quality of life. SWLS, Satisfaction with Life Scale; HRA, health risk appraisal; LSI, Life Satisfaction Index; LSS, Life Situation Survey; LSES, Life Satisfaction in the Elderly Scale.

were assessed with a physical activity questionnaire, currently active men scored significantly higher than sedentary men on quality of life. These findings suggest that the association between physical activity and quality of life depends on current physical activity patterns, rather than former activity patterns, or athletic status. It is possible, however, that changes in physical activity level are also important in the relationship between physical activity and quality of life, but this hypothesis was not tested in this study, because physical activity levels were not assessed while the students were in college.

Two studies were located in which changes in physical activity over time were studied. In a 9-year follow-up of 4025 men and women (ages 16 to 94) in Alameda County (40), it was reported that increases in physical activity were associated with high quality of life, as measured by items about satisfaction with life in general and satisfaction with particular aspects of life, such as marriage, children, and work (41). Physical activity was measured with a four-item leisure-time physical activity index. In the Harvard Alumni Study (42), 8018 men (ages 45 to 84) completed the Paffenbarger Physical Activity Questionnaire (43) in 1962 or 1966 and again in 1977, and they completed a questionnaire about quality of life in 1988. Men who expended at least 1500 or more kcal per week in physical activity in 1977 were significantly different than less active men on questions that implied satisfaction with life in 1988. For example, 94% of those who expended at least 1500 kcal per week in physical activity reported that they "feel fine and enjoy life" compared with 92% of less active men, and 87% of the more active men reported that they "feel younger than their years" compared with 82% of the less active men. In terms of changes in physical activity, it was found that men who increased their physical activity levels to 1500 kcal per week from 1962 or 1966 to 1977 differed from less active men in a similar fashion. The sample size in this study was fairly large (N = 8018), and although these differences in proportions were statistically significant, these small differences may not be of practical significance. These two studies, in conjunction with the reports of previously mentioned studies, provide some evidence that not only are current physical activity levels related to quality of life, but changes in physical activity may be related to quality of life as well.

Many of the studies reviewed thus far dealt with individuals residing in the United States, but there is also some cross-cultural evidence of the relationship between physical activity and quality of life. Three fairly large-scale epidemiologic studies reported results from three countries other than the United States: 1) Canada; 2) Finland; and 3) China; all three studies reported an association between physical activity and quality of life. In a survey of 685 Canadians (44), it was found that physical activity, as measured by questions adapted from the Canada Fitness Survey (45), was significantly related to quality of life, as measured by the LSI (34), for the overall sample as well as for the age groups of 25 to 34 years, 35 to 44 years, 55 to 64 years, and 70+ years. However, this relationship was not significant for the age groups of 18 to 24, 45 to 54, and 65 to 69. All of the correlations were relatively small, ranging from R = 0.10 to R = −0.31. In a study of 1224 elderly residents of Jyväskylä, Finland (ages 65 to 84), it was found that a greater proportion of those individuals who engaged in regular physical activity rated their life as meaningful on a five-point self-report scale than those who performed mild or no physical activity (46). In addition, for the women, there was a significant correlation between physical activity and meaningfulness of life (R = .20), whereas this relationship was not significant for the men. In a cross-sectional survey study of 1557 Chinese men and women (older than 70 years), it was found that a quality-of-life score of more than 6 was associated with daily physical activity (47), when quality of life was assessed with a 0-to-10 point scale (0 = very dissatisfied with life, 10 = very satisfied with life), and daily physical activity was assessed with a questionnaire.

Of the 11 cross-sectional studies reviewed here, eight reported positive results regarding the association between quality of life and physical activity, one reported negative results, and two reported positive results for some age groups and negative results for other age groups. Different age groups and different countries were represented in these studies, making comparisons between studies difficult. In addition, these 11 studies employed 10 different measures of quality of life and eleven different measures of physical activity. The presence of many methodologic problems, which are discussed later in this chapter, makes it difficult to draw firm conclusions about the nature of the cross-sectional relationship between physical activity and quality of life.

INTERVENTION STUDIES

Two of the intervention studies that were located employed a single-group design to examine quality-of-life changes over the course of a chronic physical activity program. Young (48) found no change in quality of life, as measured by Cantril's ladder (49), following a 10-week physical activity program for 16 men and 16 women (ages 23 to 62). The physical activity program consisted of one hour of group calisthenics and walking-jogging at 70% of maximal working capacity for 3 days a week. Similar results were reported by Sidney and Shephard (50), who found that quality of life, as measured by the LSI (34), did not change over a 14-week physical activity training program in 14 men and 28 women (age 60 or older). The intervention consisted of 1 hour, 4 days per week of fast walking, jogging, and other forms of endurance work. These two studies suggest that perhaps chronic physical activity programs do not result in changes in quality of life.

Two studies were located that included a physical activity group and a control group, and both reported positive results for the physical activity group and no change for the control group. Morris and Husman (51) studied college-aged men (N = 36) and women (N = 15) in two intact groups, one from a conditioning class (2 hours, twice per week for 15 weeks, long-distance running), and the other from a history of sport class (the individuals did not participate in any formal physical activity program). Both groups completed the Pflaum Life Quality Inventory (37) on the first day of class and at the end of the class, and it was found that the conditioning class had a significant increase in quality of life (mean score improved from 145.5 to 155.7), whereas the history of sport class had no change (mean score decreased from 155.0 to 154.2). Although the authors do note that the baseline scores of the two groups are within one SD of Pflaum's reported mean, they do not report whether a 9.5 unit difference between the groups was significant. Calculation of the effect size for the initial mean difference reveals an effect size of 0.64, and it is possible that the group with lower scores at the outset had more room for improvement in quality of life. McMurdo and Burnett (52) randomly assigned 37 men and 40 women, aged 60 to 81, to an aerobic class or a health education class for a 32-week study. The physical activity group performed exercise to music for 45 minutes three times per week, while the health education group attended six lectures over the 32-week study about the aging process, the benefits of exercise, the importance of diet, the dangers of smoking tobacco and how to stop, osteoporosis, and stress management. The group that performed physical activity increased significantly on quality-of-life rating, whereas the control group did not change, as measured by the LSI (34). Although both of these studies included a control group, the first study lacked random assignment to groups; however, participants in the second study were randomly assigned to groups. In addition, neither of these studies employed a placebo group, so the changes found for the experimental groups could have resulted from the expectations of the participants.

Three studies were located that included an aerobic physical activity intervention, a control condition, and in addition, employed an alternative physical activity intervention that could be viewed as an alternative or minimal treatment (e.g., weight training, yoga, tai chi). In the first study, Norris et al (53) studied men, ages 20 to 50, on the police force over a 10-week period. They were assigned to one of three groups: 1) aerobic physical activity (30 to 40 minutes of running, 2 to 3 days/week); 2) anaerobic physical activity (30 to 40 minutes of weight training, 2 to 3 days/week); or 3) control (unaware of other two groups). The two physical activity groups had a significant improvement in quality of life, as measured by the Life Situation Survey (LSS) (54), and the control group had significantly worse scores on the LSS after 10 weeks. In the second study, Blumenthal et al (55) randomly assigned 101 adults (ages 60 to 83) for a 16-week intervention period to one of three groups: 1) aerobic physical activity (leg ergometer, jogging, and arm ergometer at 70% of heart rate reserve [HRR]), 2) yoga, or 3) wait-list control. The physical activity group completed 3 sessions a week of 60 minutes of bicycle ergometry, walking-jogging, and arm ergometry at 70% maximum HRR, and the yoga group performed 2 sessions a week of 60 minutes of yoga exercises. There were no changes in quality of life, as measured by the LSI (34), in any of the groups.

In the third study, Brown et al (56) randomly assigned 135 men and women (ages 40 to 69) to one of five groups: 1) moderate-intensity walking, 2) low-intensity walking, 3) low-intensity walking plus the relaxation response, 4) mindful exercise, or 5) control. The four physical activity groups completed a 16-week intervention program in which they walked 2.0 to 2.5 miles or performed tai chi for 30 to 50 minutes three times a week. Quality of life was assessed with the Life Satisfaction in the Elderly Scale (LSES) (57), which consists of 40 items, 5 items each in the subscale areas of daily activities, meaning, goals, mood, self-concept, health, finances, and social contacts. The authors reported that total life satisfaction increased significantly after the program and that none of the groups differed, meaning that total life satisfaction increased for the four physical activity groups as well as the control group. It is interesting to note that although total life satisfaction scores increased for both men and women, there were some gender differences on some of the subscales. For example, only the subscales of satisfaction with daily activities and satisfaction with physical health changed significantly for the women; however, the subscales related to meaning of life, life goals, mood, self-concept, and health changed significantly for the men. Inspection of the items on these scales reveals that the subscales related to meaning of life and life goals are probably the ones most related to an assessment of life-as-a-whole, whereas the others are more specific to particular domains (e.g., finances, physical health, mental health, social contacts, daily activities).

Of these three studies, the first one reported positive changes for aerobic and anaerobic physical activity groups and negative changes for the control group, the second one reported no change for the physical activity groups or the control group, and the third one reported positive changes for the physical activity groups and the control group. The first study lacked random assignment whereas the second and third studies did employ random assignment in the creation of the groups. The results of these three studies may result from the expectations of the participants, and it is also possible that different measures of quality of life may be more sensitive to change than others.

Of the seven intervention studies reviewed here, three reported positive changes in quality of life associated with physical activity, three studies reported no change in quality of life, and one study reported positive changes for the groups performing physical activity but also for the control group. There may be a number of reasons for these equivocal findings. The length of time of the interventions ranged from 10 weeks to 32 weeks, and observation of changes in a variable such as quality of life may require a longer intervention. The three studies that reported positive results employed the LSS, Pflaum's Life Quality Inventory, and the LSI; one of the three studies that reported negative results employed Cantril's ladder, and the two others employed the LSI. An instrument such as the LSI may not be sensitive to change over a time period of 14 to 16 weeks, for example, but a 32-week intervention may be more likely to be accompanied by changes in LSI scores. The LSI appears to consist of questions about life in general, and the questions often ask the respondent to evaluate his or her life as he or she looks back on it, so it is possible that the interaction between quality-of-life instruments and the length of the physical activity intervention may explain some of the lack of congruence in these findings.

Another plausible explanation is the observation that personality structure is associated with quality of life. Costa and McCrae (58) have reported that extroversion accounts for about 8% of the variance in well-being scores, and neuroticism accounts for as much as 27%. In addition, it has been reported that personality in the early years is effective in predicting quality of life in the middle years. Morgan (39) has found that personality at age 18 is effective in predicting quality of life 20 years later, with an average prediction accuracy of 73%. Since personality has been found to be relatively stable over the years (58), and since personality has been shown to be associated with quality of life, these observations suggest that for an intervention to be effective in changing quality of life, it should be initiated early in life.

METHODOLOGIC ISSUES

There are numerous methodologic problems with much of the research in the area of physical activity and quality of life, just as there are in the area of physical activity and mental health in general (59). The primary problem is the lack of psychometrically sound measures of quality of life and physical activity. For example, some of the measures employed in these studies consisted of a single item, many were unpublished scales, and others may have been used inappropriately (e.g., for a different population or inappropriate time frame). In addition, some studies lacked random assignment; that is, intact groups were selected as comparison groups (e.g., particular classes), or participants were assigned to groups in a nonrandom fashion (e.g., the first 50 persons assigned to the first group). Other studies lacked a control group, and instead focused on changes in a single group performing physical activity, and in the cases where a control group was employed, there were often no controls for the Hawthorne effect.

The Hawthorne effect describes the case where individuals have improvements simply resulting from special attention, so a placebo group is needed to control for these effects. In addition, demand characteristics were rarely controlled for in these studies. Particularly in physical activity research, participants often have expectations about how the intervention may affect them, and it is also possible that the investigator may knowingly or unknowingly communicate his or her own expectations to the participants. There is some empiric research showing that when participants were led to believe they would have improvements in psychological well-being, these individuals had significant increases in self-esteem after a 10-week physical activity program, but participants who were not given explicit expectations did not change on self-esteem scores (60).

Demand characteristics were seldom considered in the studies reviewed in this chapter, but an exception to this generalization is the study by Brown et al (56). These investigators conducted a survey at the end of their study, which consisted of questions related to the participants' expectations, and performed statistical analyses to quantify the effects of expectations. These analyses revealed that the control group expected significantly less improvement in their physical fitness and overall health compared with the groups performing physical activity, but all groups expected similar changes in psychological well-being, and these expectations were accompanied by improvements in overall life satisfaction in all five groups. It is difficult to explain why the control group expected to have changes in psychological well-being, although a potential explanation is that these individuals received special attention,

knowledge about their physical fitness level, and payment for maintaining their usual lifestyle behaviors. Pretest sensitization is always a potential problem in before and after test designs, and this design was employed in all of the intervention studies. In addition, sample size may also have affected some of the results reported in these studies, particularly where small effects were observed for very large samples. Because of the numerous methodologic problems present in most of these studies, it is not possible to draw firm conclusions about the relationship between physical activity and quality of life.

POTENTIAL MECHANISMS

A number of physiologic explanations have been advanced for the relationship between acute physical activity and mood states, such as the serotonin hypothesis (61), the norepinephrine hypothesis (62), the endorphin hypothesis (63), and the thermogenic hypothesis (64), and some of these hypotheses could also be proposed as explanations for any relationship between physical activity and quality of life. However, none of these hypotheses have been tested in relation to quality of life, so there is a need for further research in this area.

SUMMARY

On the basis of the studies of physical activity and quality of life reviewed in this chapter, the current research evidence can be regarded as equivocal. Many studies are plagued with methodologic problems, and a principal problem is the lack of agreement about the definition and measurement of quality of life. If quality of life is a distinct construct, then its definition and measurement should reflect something different than other constructs (e.g., anxiety, depression, and self-esteem).

Different quality-of-life scales were developed for different purposes, and it is recommended that investigators evaluate the adequacy of existing scales for answering their particular research questions before undertaking the development of a new questionnaire. If existing scales are found to be inadequate for answering a specific research question, then the development of a new scale is recommended, and measures such as Flanagan's (4) and Diener's (11) that allow persons to self-select what quality-of-life components are important to them personally serve as good models for future scale development. The development and use of psychometrically sound instruments will enable investigators to gain further knowledge about the nature of the relationship between physical activity and quality of life.

REFERENCES

1. Andrews FM, Withey SB. Social indicators of well-being: Americans' perceptions of life quality. New York: Plenum Press, 1976.

2. Bradburn NM. The structure of psychological well-being. Chicago: Aldine, 1969.

3. Campbell A, Converse PE, Rodgers WL. The quality of American life. New York: Russell Sage Foundation, 1976.

4. Flanagan JC. A research approach to improving our quality of life. Am Psychol 1978;33:138–147.

5. Spilker B, Molinek FR, Johnston KA, et al. Quality of life bibliography and indexes. Med Care 1990; 28(suppl):DS1–DS77.

6. Berzon RA, Donnelly MA, Simpson RL, et al. Quality of life bibliography and indexes: 1994 update. Qual Life Res 1995;4:547–569.

7. The WHOQOL Group. The World Health Organization Quality of Life Assessment (WHOQOL): position paper from the World Health Organization. Soc Sci Med 1995;41:1403–1409.

8. Kaplan RM, Anderson JP, Wu AW, et al. The Quality of Well-Being Scale. Med Care 1989;27(suppl):S27–S43.

9. Ryff CD. Happiness is everything, or is it? Explorations on the meaning of psychological well-being. J Pers Soc Psychol 1989;57:1069–1081.

10. Diener E. Subjective well-being. Psychol Bull 1984;95:542–575.

11. Diener E, Emmons RA, Larsen RJ, et al. The Satisfaction with Life Scale. J Pers Assess 1985;49:71–75.

12. Bowling A. Measuring health: a review of quality of life measurement scales. Philadelphia: Open University, 1991.

13. Hollandsworth JG. Evaluating the impact of medical treatment on the quality of life: a 5-year update. Soc Sci Med 1988;26:425–434.

14. Hathaway SR, McKinley JC. Minnesota Multiphasic Personality Inventory. Minneapolis: University of Minnesota, 1967.

15. Spielberger CD. Manual for the State-Trait Anxiety Inventory (form Y). Palo Alto, CA: Consulting Psychologists Press, 1983.

16. McNair DM, Lorr M, Droppleman LF. Profile or Mood States Manual. San Diego, CA: Educational and Testing Service, 1992.

17. Landy FJ. Stamp collecting versus science: validation as hypothesis testing. Am Psychol 1986;41:1183–1192.

18. Fava GA. Methodologic and conceptual issues in research on quality of life. Psychother Psychosom 1990;54:70–76.

19. Caspersen CJ, Powell KE, Christenson GM. Physical activity, exercise, and physical fitness: definitions and distinctions for health-related research. Public Health Rep 1985;100:126–130.

20. Kriska AM, Caspersen CJ, eds. A collection of physical activity questionnaires for health-related research. Med Sci Sports Exerc 1997;29(suppl):S1–S205.

21. Bouchard C, Shephard RJ, Stephens T, eds. Physical activity, fitness, and health. Champaign, IL: Human Kinetics, 1994.

22. Martinsen EW, Morgan WP. Antidepressant effects of physical activity. In: Morgan WP, ed. Physical activity and mental health. Washington, DC: Taylor & Francis, 1997:93–106.

23. Raglin JS. Anxiolytic effects of physical activity. In: Morgan WP, ed. Physical activity and mental health. Washington, DC: Taylor & Francis, 1997:107–126.

24. Sonstroem RJ. Physical activity and self-esteem. In: Morgan WP, ed. Physical activity and mental health. Washington, DC: Taylor & Francis, 1997:127–143.

25. Noreau L, Shephard RJ. Spinal cord injury, exercise, and quality of life. Sports Med 1995;20:226–250.

26. Berger BG, McInman A. Exercise and the quality of life. In: Singer RN, Murphy M, Tennant LK, eds. Handbook of research in sport psychology. New York: Macmillan, 1993:729–760.

27. Spirduso WW, Gilliam-MacRae P. Physical activity and quality of life in the frail elderly. In: Birren JE, Lubben JE, Rowe JC, Deutchman DE, eds. The concept and measurement of quality of life in the frail elderly. San Diego, CA: Academic Press, 1991:226–255.

28. Stewart AL, King AC. Evaluating the efficacy of physical activity for influencing quality-of-life outcomes in older adults. Ann Behav Med 1991;13:108–116.

29. Brown DR. Physical activity, aging, and psychological well-being: an overview of the research. Can J Sport Sci 1992;17:185–193.

30. Rejeski WJ, Brawley LR, Shumaker SA. Physical activity and health-related quality of life. Exerc Sport Sci Rev 1996;24:71–108.

31. Gauvin L. The relationship between regular physical activity and subjective well-being. J Sport Behav 1989;11:107–114.

32. Parkerson GR, Broadhead WE, Tse CJ. The health status and life satisfaction of first-year medical students. Acad Med 1990;65:586–588.

33. Lasco R, Moriarity D, Nelson CF. CDC Health Risk Appraisal user manual. Atlanta, GA: Centers for Disease Control, 1982.

34. Neugarten BL, Havighurst RJ, Tobin SS. The measurement of life satisfaction. J Gerontol 1961;16:134–143.

35. Kelly JR, Steinkamp MW, Kelly JR. Later-life satisfaction: does leisure contribute? Leisure Sci 1987;9:189–200.

36. Morris AF, Lussier L, Vaccaro P, et al. Life quality characteristics of national class women masters long distance runners. Ann Sports Med 1982;1:23–26.

37. Pflaum JH. Development of a life quality inventory. Ph.D. dissertation, University of Maryland, 1973.

38. Shephard RJ, Kavanagh T, Mertens DJ, et al. Personal health benefits of masters athletics competition. Br J Sports Med 1995;29:35–40.

39. Morgan WP. Athletes and nonathletes in the middle years of life. In: McPherson BD, ed. Sport and aging. Champaign, IL: Human Kinetics, 1985:167–186.

40. Kaplan GA, Lazarus NB, Cohen RD, et al. Psychosocial factors in the natural history of physical activity. Am J Prev Med 1991;7:12–17.

41. Berkman LF, Breslow L. Health and ways of living: the Alameda County study. New York: Oxford University Press, 1983.

42. Paffenbarger RS, Kampert JB, Lee I-M, et al. Changes in physical activity and other lifeway patterns influencing longevity. Med Sci Sports Exerc 1994;26:857–865.

43. Paffenbarger RS, Wing AL, Hyde RT. Physical activity as an index of heart attack risk in college alumni. Am J Epidemiol 1978;180:161–175.

44. Brown BA, Frankel BG. Activity through the years: leisure, leisure satisfaction, and life satisfaction. Soc Sport J 1993;10:1–17.

45. Fitness Canada: fitness and aging—Canada Fitness Survey. Ottawa: Fitness and Amateur Sport, 1982.

46. Ruuskanen JM, Ruoppila I. Physical activity and psychological well-being among people aged 65 to 84 years. Age Aging 1995;24:292–296.

47. Ho SC, Woo J, Lau J, et al. Life satisfaction and associated factors in older Hong Kong Chinese. J Am Geriatr Soc 1995;43:252–255.

48. Young RJ. The effect of regular exercise on cognitive functioning and personality. Br J Sports Med 1979;13:110–117.

49. Kilpatrick FP, Cantril H. Self-anchoring ladder scaling. J Indiv Psychol 1960;16:158–173.

50. Sidney KH, Shephard RJ. Attitudes towards health and physical activity in the elderly: effects of a training program. Med Sci Sports 1976;8:246–252.

51. Morris AF, Husman BF. Life quality changes following an endurance conditioning program. Am Corrective Ther J 1978;32:3–6.

52. McMurdo MET, Burnett L. Randomised controlled trial of exercise in the elderly. Gerontology 1992;38:292–298.

53. Norris R, Carroll D, Cochrane R. The effects of aerobic and anaerobic training on fitness, blood pressure, and psychological stress and well-being. J Psychosom Res 1990;34:367–375.

54. Chubon RA. Development of a quality-of-life rating scale for use in health care evaluation. Eval Health Prof 1987;10:186–200.

55. Blumenthal JA, Emery CF, Madden DJ, et al. Cardiovascular and behavioral effects of aerobic exercise training in healthy older men and women. J Gerontol 1989;44:M147–M157.

56. Brown DR, Wang Y, Ward A, et al. Chronic psychological effects of exercise and exercise plus cognitive strategies. Med Sci Sports Exerc 1995;27:765–775.

57. Salamon MJ, Conte VA. Manual for the Salamon-Conte Life Satisfaction in the Elderly Scale. Odessa, FL: Psychological Assessment Resources, 1984:1–23.

58. Costa PT, McCrae RR. Personality as a lifelong determinant of well-being. In: Izard CZ, ed. Emotion in adult development. Beverly Hills, CA: Sage, 1984:141–157.

59. Morgan WP. Methodological considerations. In: Morgan WP, ed. Physical activity and mental health. Washington, DC: Taylor & Francis, 1997:3–32.

60. Desharnais R, Jobin J, Côté C, et al. Aerobic exercise and the placebo effect: a controlled study. Psychosom Med 1993;55:149–154.

61. Chaouloff F. The serotonin hypothesis. In: Morgan WP, ed. Physical activity and mental health. Washington, DC: Taylor & Francis, 1997:179–198.

62. Dishman RK. The norepinephrine hypothesis. In: Morgan WP, ed. Physical activity and mental health. Washington, DC: Taylor & Francis, 1997:199–212.

63. Hoffmann P. The endorphin hypothesis. In: Morgan WP, ed. Physical activity and mental health. Washington, DC: Taylor & Francis, 1997:163–177.

64. Koltyn KF. The thermogenic hypothesis. In: Morgan WP, ed. Physical activity and mental health. Washington, DC: Taylor & Francis, 1997:213–226.

Chapter 87

Adverse Consequences of Physical Activity: When More is Too Much

John S. Raglin
Lori Moger

The physical benefits of exercise have long been acknowledged. Regular participation in exercise, even at relatively mild levels, can forestall many of the major health disorders of modern life, such as heart disease and hypertension (1). Exercise is an important aspect of treatment for these and other physical diseases. Physical activity can also have a significant impact on mental health (2). Single sessions of exercise are typically associated with reduced anxiety, enhanced mood, and attenuated stress responsiveness (3). These benefits, however, are transitory and dissipate within 2 to 4 hours after the cessation of activity. Long-term participation in physical activity programs can result in more persistent changes in mental health. Reduced depression and trait anxiety have been commonly noted after long-term exercise, although changes are often quite modest or even absent in healthy individuals. In contrast, psychological benefits are generally more pronounced in persons with emotional disorders of mild to moderate severity (4). Available research indicates the efficacy of exercise compares well with standardized forms of psychotherapy (5).

In spite of these benefits and the fact they are widely recognized by the public at large, the most liberal estimates indicate that only about 45% of the adult population of the United States is currently physically active (6). Barely over one in five adults exercises three times a week or more at an intensity sufficient to improve cardiovascular capacity. Even more sobering, approximately 50% of individuals who begin an exercise program will quit, with the majority dropping out within the initial weeks (6).

Based on this information, it may seem that there would be virtually no incidence of overexercise in the population, yet some individuals exercise to an extent where physical and psychological health are adversely affected. This chapter describes salient examples of excessive physical activity. Exercise abuse is a debilitating condition largely found in recreational exercisers. Serious competitive athletes face the strain of overtraining and the risk of developing the staleness syndrome. The major symptoms of these conditions are presented along with hypothesized contributing factors. In instances where information is available, potential means of prevention or treatment are provided.

EXERCISE ABUSE

Accounts of detrimental psychological consequences of excessive exercise have long been noted (7). However, an article published in 1979 by the psychologist William Morgan (8) has been recognized as the first to bring this problem to the attention of sport scientists (9). The article presented a series of case studies of recreational and competitive athletes who developed adverse psychological and physical symptoms as a consequence of their running programs. Morgan labeled this condition "running addiction," but it has since been referred to by others as obligatory exercise, exercise dependency syndrome, activity anorexia, and compulsive exercise (10). The term "addiction" was initially intended to refer to dependencies on physical substances; because of this and concerns whether habitual behaviors, such as exercise, can truly qualify as addictions, Morgan now prefers the term exercise abuse (11).

A number of psychometric scales have been developed in efforts to identify persons who abuse exercise (9), but the relative efficacy of these measures has not been established.

Moreover, there is a strong potential for affected individuals to falsify their answers to these questionnaires (i.e., response distortion), particularly in a manner that conforms to a perceived desirable stereotype in which symptoms are not acknowledged. Unfortunately, none of the extant scales include items or "lie scales" designed specifically to identify forged responses. As a consequence, exercise abuse is probably best identified by its symptoms. The following sections present the symptoms and signs most often associated with the disorder.

Excessive Reliance on Physical Activity

Perhaps the most commonly cited sign of exercise abuse is excessive reliance on physical activity, usually daily, as a means of coping (8,9,12). Although physical exercise has long been advocated as a way to deal with the stresses of daily life, for the exercise abuser it becomes the primary or even the sole means of coping. In turn, this overreliance spurs efforts to continually increase the level of exercise. More often this involves exercising more frequently and for longer periods instead of the same duration at a higher intensity level. Thus, the emphasis is more often on quantity rather than the quality of activity. This need for ever greater "doses" of exercise should be distinguished from the more healthy incentive that the dedicated exerciser may have to increase her or his workload (9,12). In the latter case, a training plateau is eventually reached, and the exerciser becomes content with maintaining this level of activity.

The excessive reliance on exercise often leads to a reprioritization of values whereby work, social, and family obligations take on secondary importance. Cases in which affected persons have lost jobs or gone through divorces because of a consuming devotion to exercise have been reported (8,9,12). Unfortunately, no single cutoff has been found that can be used to define the level of activity at which exercise takes on abusive properties. Some researchers have proposed that persons who exercise at least 6 days a week for an hour or more qualify as excessive exercisers (13). However, in other studies, persons at this level of activity were classified simply as habitual exercisers(14). This range contrasts with the much higher training volumes seen in high-level endurance athletes—sometimes exceeding 6 hours a day—who generally do not display signs of exercise abuse (15).

Defining exercise abuse by means of questionnaires is also problematic. In one study (16), 54% of members of an exercise club were classified as obligatory exercisers as defined by a widely used scale (17). An even higher percentage (82%) of marathon runners in a survey study acknowledged some degree of addiction to their sport (18). These inordinately high numbers suggest that some individuals perceive excessive exercise behavior as desirable, which is not inconceivable given the way physical activity is sometimes promoted in the fitness industry. This may result in a form of response distortion (referred to as simulation) to questions on exercise behavior, whereby individuals overprescribe to symptoms, including those not actually experienced. Yet, the potential for simulation has rarely been considered in questionnaire research on exercise behavior. Variation in exercise capacity, age, years of training, and other factors make it unlikely that exercise abuse can be reliably identified solely by the activity level of a given individual. Questionnaire data are also unlikely to be effective in many instances because of the lack of validity of exercise abuse scales and problems such as response distortion (either simulation or dissimulation).

Exercise During Injury

The constant and high levels of activity maintained by the exercise abuser raise the specter of serious injury. Reports consistently indicate that exercise abusers generally refuse to stop training when injured and will make as few adjustments or reductions as possible (8,9,12). Unfortunately, physician recommendations to stop or amend training are often ignored, even though the proper course is to make appropriate adjustments (e.g., cross-training or reducing training) or cease exercise until the injury heals. Paradoxically, cases have been reported in which some injured individuals continue exercising until a permanent disability occurs, making further activity essentially impossible (8).

The reason why some individuals refuse to alter their exercise patterns after an injury that threatens to become debilitating is not well understood. A variety of explanations have been proposed, including: 1) absence of alternative means of coping, 2) fear of experiencing withdrawal symptoms (12), 3) lack of strong self-identity (19), 4) fear of a loss in self-esteem associated with exercise (20), or 5) fear of potential weight gain or loss of fitness (21). Exercise abuse has also been proposed to be a manifestation of compulsive behavior (9). Each of these potential issues complicates treatment.

Withdrawal Symptoms

The third defining feature of exercise abuse is the experience of withdrawal symptoms when the individual must stop exercising for a period of time. Commonly reported symptoms of exercise withdrawal are similar to those seen in withdrawal from substance abuse and include sleep disturbances, changes in appetite, difficulty concentrating, and negative shifts in mood, particularly depression (8,12). Physical symptoms such as muscle pain and soreness have also been noted. As stated by an affected triathlete: "I began to experience a distorted self-image, leg cramps, stiffness, and altered sleep patterns" (22). These symptoms should be distinguished from feelings or sensations experienced by the committed, but healthy, recreational exerciser who must stop exercising for a period of time or who misses a planned exercise session. In the latter case, feelings of frustration, anger, or anxiety are not uncommon. Hence, some degree of discomfort may be anticipated when a committed exerciser misses a session, but it is usually minor and can be tolerated. However, in the case of the abusive exerciser, mood disturbances and other unpleasant symptoms experienced are far more pernicious.

The onset of some symptoms after the withdrawal from exercise can be quite rapid. In a study of exercise deprivation, Mondin et al (14) examined the psychological responses of highly physically active individuals who were paid to voluntarily stop exercising for a 3-day period. To qualify for the study, participants regularly exercised at least 5 days a week for sessions lasting an hour or more. After 2 days without exercise, significant elevations in mood disturbance and state anxiety resulted. Mood tended to improve somewhat on the final day without exercise but did not return to levels observed at baseline. This partial abatement may have occurred because the subjects began to habituate to being without exercise, but more likely resulted from the anticipation of the end of the deprivation period. In fact, three subjects exercised within 2 hours after the cessation of the study, and the remaining participants had all resumed their training regimens within the next 24 hours. Other research (23) has found negative shifts in mood to occur following 1 day of exercise deprivation.

The study by Mondin et al (14) is notable because the majority of studies on exercise deprivation effects have involved individuals who were only moderately active (24) or were forced to stop exercising because of injury (25). Hence, mood changes observed in some investigations may be confounded by disturbances resulting directly from the effects of the injury rather than the lack of exercise. The subjects in the Mondin et al (14) study voluntarily stopped exercising. The true exercise abuser may be unwilling to cease exercising, even for a brief period. Hence, it might be hypothesized that the elevation in mood disturbance would be even greater for the exercise abuser, given no choice but to stop.

Persons who abuse exercise often exhibit disordered eating, particularly anorexia nervosa (9,21,26). Traditionally, hyperactivity and excessive exercise were regarded simply as clinical symptoms of anorexia, in which some affected individuals adopt physical activity as an additional means of reducing body weight. However, an initial preoccupation with exercise may contribute to the development of an eating disorder in some cases (26). The percentage of individuals who develop anorexia in association with exercise is not known, nor is it clear what factors may predispose certain individuals to become excessively dependent on physical activity and to develop an eating disorder. Early explanations proposed that an exercise-induced release of endorphin, an endogenous opioid associated with mood change and analgesia, was responsible. This hypothesis continues to be a popular explanation for both mood changes associated with exercise and its potentially addictive qualities (9). However, research has not consistently supported an endorphin link with mood change after exercise (27), nor is there compelling evidence linking endorphin or other endogenous opioids to a dependence on physical activity. Psychological factors associated with excessive exercise and eating disorders, particularly body dissatisfaction (9,26) and obsessive-compulsiveness (28), have been implicated as contributing risk factors. It is likely that contributing factors differ across cases and that several may be involved. Moreover, the social environment present in many fitness settings often encourages and rewards pathologic exercise behavior (29).

The finding that excessive exercise is often associated with eating disorders such as anorexia might imply that exercise abuse is more prevalent in women, but little information exists on this issue. Additionally, in a review of this literature, O'Connor et al (see Chapter 88) conclude that a cause-and-effect relationship between physical exercise and eating disorders has not been established. There is also no research to examine whether some exercise modes are more likely to lead to problems with abuse. Exercise abuse probably occurs with many types of physical activity and may simply be most common in the most popular or accessible activities. If true, this may also imply that men and women are more apt to abuse different forms of exercise (30).

Treatment

Unfortunately, there is no information concerning effective means of prevention or treatment for exercise abuse. Some exercise facilities have adopted policies in attempts to promote healthy exercise habits and minimize compulsive behavior. For example, participants in organized fitness classes at Indiana University who wish to increase their exercise regimen are encouraged to consider cross-training (e.g., aerobic and strength training) instead of attending two successive exercise classes in the same activity. Options for shorter length classes are offered, and participants are limited to 30-minute sessions on exercise apparatus.

Exercise abusers should, of course, be encouraged to reduce their training load. Affected individuals should be approached with care since many may be apt to deny they have a problem. If the exercise abuser is unwilling to exercise less, then cross-training may at least provide some reduction to the risk of overuse injury. Training logs have been proposed as a means of alerting the exercise abuser into realizing just how much activity he or she is engaged in (31), but critics contend that such logs may simply strengthen compulsiveness about exercise (9). Because of the severity of dysfunctional behavior associated with exercise abuse, as well as the liability for physical complications and associated problems such as eating disorders, psychological and medical interventions are often necessary (9).

OVERTRAINING

The analog of exercise abuse for athletes might well be overtraining. In endurance sports as well as many nonendurance activities, a high degree of physical conditioning is required if athletes are to achieve their potential. As a result, competitive athletes undergo extended periods of extreme training—often referred to as overtraining—toward the goal of optimizing their performance. This "overload principle" of athletic conditioning has led to dramatic increases in both the volume and intensity of training in many sports. In the case of swimming, athletes may train up to 6 hours or more a day at distances of 15,000 m, and distances of more than 35,000 m a day have been reported (15). When followed by a sufficient period of reduced training (i.e., taper) or rest, overtraining generally results in small (e.g., 1% to 3%) but potentially significant improvements in performance.

The physical stress inherent in overtraining is not without consequences. Studies on competitive swimming and other endurance sports (32) have demonstrated that intense training is consistently associated with detrimental shifts in mood states in the majority of athletes who otherwise exhibit positive mental health (33). The results of overtraining research indicate that physical training exerts a predictable effect on emotional health. Increases in training load (volume or intensity) result in elevations in mood disturbance, with both training load and mood disturbance peaking concomitantly. The shift in mood can be extensive, and elevations in mood disturbance of one to two SDs on standardized psychological measures are not uncommon (34). When training is gradually tapered or reduced outright, mood disturbance also abates, so that by the end of a training season most individuals regain the positive emotional health profiles they possessed at the onset of training. An example of the association between training and mood state is presented in Figure 87-1.

Similar dose-response relationships between training load and mood state have been observed in athletes across a variety of endurance sports and may occur with nonendurance training, if the stimulus is sufficiently intense (15). While most training regimens slowly progress in intensity over a period of weeks or months, the effects of overtraining can develop quite quickly. Immediate and severe increases in training load can result in elevations in mood disturbances that become evident within as few as 2 days (35).

The Staleness Syndrome

Not all athletes benefit from the stress of overtraining. Perhaps between 10% and 20% of athletes who overtrain develop a chronic state of worsened performance, referred to as "staleness," or the overtraining syndrome (32). Along with a loss of performance, other common responses include endocrine hormone disturbances, increased susceptibility to infection, mood disturbances, changes in appetite, and soreness associated with actual muscle damage (15,36,37). Perceptual symptoms such as elevated perception of effort and sensations of heaviness are also common in stale athletes (36,38). A wide variety of other physical symptoms and biologic changes have been reported in the literature (e.g., increased resting or exercise heart rate), but few of these have been found to be consistently associated with staleness (36).

Of all the symptoms associated with staleness, psychological changes are among the most reliable (37). Research has found that stale athletes exhibit significant mood disturbances that are more severe than those experienced by athletes who overtrain but do not experience staleness. More important, approximately 80% of stale athletes exhibit depression of clinical magnitude (32). In contrast, athletes who do not develop staleness usually exhibit only small elevations in depression during heavy training (34,39).

Treatment and Prevention

At present, the primary accepted treatment for the staleness syndrome is to refrain from training. A minimal rest period of

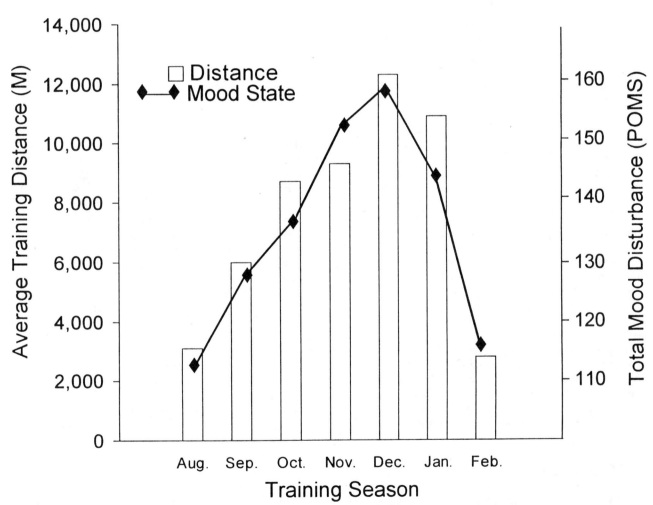

Figure 87-1 Mood state responses during a training season in a sample of collegiate swimmers (POMS = Profile of Mood States). (Adapted with permission from: Raglin JS. Overtraining and staleness: psychometric monitoring of endurance athletes. In: Singer RN, Murphey M, Tennant LK, eds. Handbook of research in sport psychology. New York: Macmillan, 1993: 846.)

2 weeks is commonly cited, but severe cases may require far longer layoffs, sometimes up to several months. Appropriate medical attention is also important for infectious disorders and other physical complications that are often present in stale athletes. Psychological counseling should also be considered, given the severity of depression seen in many stale athletes, and antidepressant mediation may be needed in the most serious cases. Sport psychology performance enhancement techniques, such as mental imagery or goal setting, have been advocated as effective means of treatment or prevention (40), but empiric evidence for the effectiveness of such methods is lacking and their use is not recommended.

Given the complications associated with staleness and its chronic nature, along with the fact that serious athletes cannot avoid intensive training, there has been considerable interest in identifying means to prevent the occurrence of this disorder. Some research has been conducted on preventing staleness using nutritional supplements or antiviral agents (36), but the bulk of effort has been directed toward identifying early warning signs or markers of staleness. The intent is to be able to identify affected individuals early enough for brief rests or training reductions to be effective in preventing staleness from developing fully.

Unfortunately, most physiologic markers of staleness have been found to be either insufficiently sensitive or too costly to be of practical use (15,36,37). Invasiveness is an additional concern with many physiologic measures. In contrast, psychological measures of mood state have been found to be reliably associated with staleness when properly administered and interpreted by trained psychologists. Moreover, this information can be more quickly obtained than hormonal or biochemical markers.

Only limited research exists involving the use of mood-state monitoring as an intervention strategy for athletes undergoing overtraining, but the extant findings suggest this approach may be efficacious (15). For example, in a study of elite race canoeists who were training for Olympic competition, Berglund and Säfström (41) employed a mood-state monitoring paradigm in the effort to prevent staleness. Mood state was assessed bimonthly during training in the canoeists by means of the Profile of Mood States (POMS) (42), the most commonly used psychological instrument in overtraining research. Athletes who exhibited excessively high mood-state scores had their training load reduced until the disturbance abated. The intervention operated in both directions, and workloads were increased in athletes who had a notable absence of mood disturbance. No instances of staleness occurred, although, based on previous experiences, the authors anticipated that at least 10% of the team would become stale by the end of the training season.

While the previous findings are promising, additional work is necessary to confirm the efficacy of this approach with other samples. Moreover, it is likely that the utility of mood-state monitoring will be enhanced by the addition of selected physiologic and perceptual measures (33). In the meantime, athletes and coaches can do much to reduce the occurrence of staleness by informal monitoring of mood, fatigue, and other common symptoms. Prophylactic measures, such as adequate nutrition and adequate sleep, are also important to help minimize risk.

CONCLUSIONS

For the majority of physically active people, exercise is associated with beneficial outcomes. However, some individuals exercise to excess, either out of compulsion or, in the case of the competitive athlete, by necessity. In each instance, physical activity results in detrimental physical and psychological changes.

Recreational exercisers may abuse physical activity and become overly dependent on it as a means of coping and as a source of self-esteem. The continual quest to increase the level of exercise often leads to injuries, which can become exacerbated by the unwillingness of the exerciser to rest or properly rehabilitate. Severe withdrawal symptoms have been noted in affected individuals who are forced to stop exercising because of illness, injury, or other circumstances.

Serious competitive athletes who overtrain in an effort to maximize performance typically experience mood disturbances that rise and fall in concert with the training load. Most athletes are capable of tolerating the stresses of intense training, but between 10% and 20% do not adapt and experience the staleness syndrome. Athletes who have become stale suffer from a chronic loss of performance, severe mood disturbances and depression, an increased risk of infectious disorders, and other symptoms.

The previous examples stand in direct contrast to research indicating that proper physical activity alleviates mood disturbances and improves mental health (2) (see Chapters 83 and 84). Together these results indicate that physical activity should be considered a complex stressor that can result in either beneficial (i.e., eustress) or detrimental (i.e., distress) outcomes (10). To a large degree, the response is dependent on the amount of exercise. Yet, a single demarcation between beneficial and detrimental training does not exist, in large part because of the considerable variation in the responses of recreational exercisers and competitive athletes to physical activity. Hence, acquired or inherent characteristics can mediate the psychological and physiologic responses to physical activity. A greater understanding of the factors that contribute to this heterogeneity would undoubtedly aid in preventing adverse responses to physical activity.

REFERENCES

1. Blair SN, Kohl H, Paffenbarger R. Physical fitness and all-cause mortality: a prospective study of healthy men and women. JAMA 1989;262:2395–2401.

2. Morgan WP. Physical activity and mental health. Washington, DC: Taylor & Francis, 1997.

3. Raglin JS. Anxiolytic effects of exercise. In: Morgan WP, ed. Physical activity and mental health. Washington, DC: Taylor and Francis, 1997:107–126.

4. Martinsen EH. Therapeutic implications of exercise for clinically anxious and depressed patients. Int J Sport Psychol 1993;24:185–199.

5. Greist JM. Exercise intervention with depressed patients. In: Morgan WP, ed. Exercise and mental health. Washington DC: Hemisphere, 1988:117–121.

6. Dishman RK. Advances in exercise adherence. Champaign, IL: Human Kinetics, 1994.

7. Parmenter DC. Some medical aspects of the training of college athletes. Boston Med Surgical J 1923;189:45–50.

8. Morgan WP. Negative addiction in runners. Phys Sportsmed 1979;7:57–70.

9. Polivy J. Physical activity, fitness, and compulsive behaviors. In: Bouchard C, Shephard RJ, Stephens T, eds. Physical activity, fitness, and health: international proceedings and consensus statement. Champaign, IL: Human Kinetics, 1994:883–897.

10. Raglin JS. Exercise and mental health: beneficial and detrimental effects. Sports Med 1990;9:323–329.

11. Morgan WP, O'Connor PJ. Exercise and mental health. In: Dishman R, ed. Exercise adherence: its impact on public health. Champaign, IL: Human Kinetics, 1989:91–121.

12. Veale DMW. Psychological aspects of staleness and dependence on exercise. Int J Sports Med 1991;12(suppl):s19–s22.

13. Nudelman S, Rosen JC, Leitenberg N. Dissimilarities in eating attitudes, body image distortion, depression, and self-esteem between high school runners and women with bulimia nervosa. Int J Eating Dis 1988;7:625–634.

14. Mondin GW, Morgan WP, Piering PN, et al. Psychological consequences of exercise deprivation in habitual exercisers. Med Sci Sports Exerc 1996;28:1199–1203.

15. Raglin JS, Wilson G. Overtraining and staleness in athletes. In: Hanin YL, ed. Emotion and sport. Champaign, IL: Human Kinetics, 1999 (in press).

16. Stuppy LA. Group differences on obligatory exercise behaviors and level of body size. Master's thesis, 1997, Boise State University.

17. Pasman L, Thompson JK. Body image and eating disturbance in obligatory runners, obligatory weightlifters, and sedentary individuals. Int J Eating Dis 1988;7:759–769.

18. Summers JJ, Machin VJ, Sargent GI. Psychosocial factors related to marathon running. J Sport Psychol 1983;5:314–331.

19. Dishman RK. Medical psychology in exercise and sport. Med Clin North Am 1985;69:123–143.

20. Little JC. The athlete's neurosis—a deprivation crisis. Acta Psychiatr Scand 1969;45:187–197.

21. Davis C, Fox J. Excessive exercise and weight preoccupation in women. Addictive Behav 1993;18:201–211.

22. Israel D. Reflections on depression. Inside Triathlon 1995;Sept, 30:30.

23. Thaxton L. Physiological and psychological effects of short-term exercise addiction on habitual runners. J Sport Psychol 1982;4:73–82.

24. Morris MH, Steinberg H, Sykes EA, et al. Effects of temporary withdrawal from regular running. J Psychosom Res 1990;34:493–500.

25. Chan CS, Grossman HY. Psychological effects of running loss on consistent runners. Percept Mot Skills 1988;66:875–883.

26. Davis C, Kennedy SH, Ravelski E, et al. The role of physical activity in the development and maintenance of eating disorders. Psychol Med 1994;24:957–967.

27. Hoffmann P. Endorphin hypothesis. In: Morgan WP, ed. Physical activity and mental health. Washington, DC: Taylor & Francis, 1997:163–177.

28. Leon GR, Fulkerson JA, Perry CL, et al. Personality and behavioral vulnerabilities associated with risk status for eating disorders in adolescent girls. J Abnorm Psychol 1993;102:438–444.

29. Raglin JS. The endless workout. IDEA Today 1996;14:55–61.

30. Wroblewska AM. Androgenic-anabolic steroids and body dysmorphia in young men. J Psychosom Res 1997;42:225–234.

31. Beamount PJ, Arthur B, Russell JD et al. Excessive physical activity in dieting disorder patients: proposals for a supervised exercise program. Int J Eating Dis 1994;15:21–36.

32. Morgan WP, Brown DL, Raglin JS, et al. Psychological monitoring of overtraining and staleness. Brit J Sports Med 1987;21:107–114.

33. Morgan WP. Selected psychological factors limiting performance: a mental health model. In: Clarke DH, Eckert HM, eds. Limits of human performance. Champaign, IL: Human Kinetics, 1985:70–80.

34. Raglin JS. Overtraining and staleness: psychometric monitoring of endurance athletes. In: Singer RN, Murphey M, Tennant LK, eds. Handbook of research in sport psychology. New York: Macmillan, 1993:840–850.

35. O'Connor PJ, Morgan WP, Raglin JS. Psychobiologic effects of three days of increased training in female and male swimmers. Med Sci Sports Exerc 1991;23:1055–1061.

36. Kreider RB, Fry AC, O'Toole ML. Overtraining in sport. Champaign, IL: Human Kinetics, 1988.

37. O'Connor PJ. Overtraining and staleness. In: Morgan WP, ed. Physical activity and mental health. New York: Hemisphere, 1997:145–160.

38. Morgan WP, Costill DL, Flynn MG, et al. Mood disturbance following increased training in swimmers. Med Sci Sports Exerc 1988;20:408–414.

39. O'Connor PJ, Morgan WP, Raglin JS, et al. Mood state and salivary

cortisol changes following overtraining in female swimmers. Psychoneuroendocrinol 1989;14:303–310.

40. Henschen KP. Athletic staleness and burnout: diagnosis, prevention and treatment. In: William JM, ed. Applied sport psychology: personal growth to peak performance. 3rd ed. Mayfield View, CA: Mayfield, 1997:398–408.

41. Berglund B, Säfström H. Psychological monitoring and modulating of training load of world class canoeists. Med Sci Sports Exerc 1994;26:1036–1040.

42. McNair DM, Lorr M, Dropplemann LF. Profile of mood states manual. San Diego: Educational and Industrial Testing Services, 1992.

Chapter 88

Physical Activity and Eating Disorders

Patrick J. O'Connor
J. Carson Smith

The aims of this chapter are twofold: first, to provide an overview of eating disorders, and second, to examine the strength of the scientific evidence linking participation in physical activity, athletics, and sports with eating disturbances. A number of related, previously published books and review articles are available to the interested reader (1–8).

WHAT ARE EATING DISORDERS?

Mental disorders that are characterized by severe disturbances in eating behavior are known as eating disorders. A mental disorder can be defined as "a clinically significant behavioral or psychological syndrome or pattern that occurs in an individual and that is associated with present distress (e.g., a painful symptom) or disability (i.e., impairment in one or more important areas of functioning) or with a significantly increased risk of suffering death, pain, disability, or an important loss of freedom" (9). Currently, there are two eating disorders that have garnered significant attention from both clinicians and researchers: anorexia nervosa and bulimia nervosa.

One of the most important developments in the last 25 years has been the use of standardized criteria for diagnosis of eating disorders (10). This development has resulted in greater consistency in diagnosis and treatment and an improvement in our understanding of the two major eating disorders. The diagnostic criteria for anorexia nervosa are presented in Table 88-1. The essence of anorexia nervosa is a refusal to maintain a normal body weight. The diagnostic criteria for bulimia nervosa are provided in Table 88-2. The primary criteria for bulimia nervosa involve eating binges followed by inappropriate compensatory methods to prevent weight gain. Binge eating, without accompanying methods to prevent weight gain, has been suggested as a separate, third major eating disorder. Although experts determined that there was inadequate scientific evidence to include binge eating disorder in the fourth edition of the *Diagnostic and Statistical Manual of the American Psychiatric Association (DSM-IV)*, provisional criteria for the condition were established (9). The provisional criteria are presented in Table 88-3.

Because clinical cases present in diverse ways, diagnostic nomenclature rarely covers every possible presentation of an eating disorder. Accordingly, *DSM-IV* includes a category labeled "eating disorders not otherwise specified (NOS)" to identify cases that present with symptoms that do not meet the criteria for a primary disorder. Examples of such instances are presented in Table 88-4.

Questionnaires such as the Eating Disorders Inventory (EDI) or the Eating Attitudes Test (EAT) have been frequently employed to obtain a standardized assessment of the severity of symptoms relevant to eating disorders. These psychometric tools are supported by published evidence as to their reliability and validity. An individual with an elevated score on the drive for thinness subscale of the EDI, for example, cannot be considered to have psychopathology, but the person is highly weight-preoccupied and is at increased risk for meeting the diagnostic criteria for an eating disorder. Some authors have suggested that individuals not meeting the criteria for a primary eating disorder but who exhibit eating disturbances and possess elevated scores on relevant psychometric instruments can be classified as having a "subclinical eating disorder" (1).

HOW SERIOUS ARE EATING DISORDERS?

The prevalence of anorexia nervosa is about 1%—estimates have ranged from 0.2% to 1.3% (9,11). Estimates of the prevalence of bulimia range from 1% to 4% (9,11,12). Unfortunately, prevalence rates for eating disorders have increased during the past two decades, especially among women aged 15 to 25 (13).

It is generally agreed that subclinical eating disturbances are more prevalent than anorexia or bulimia; however, consensus or accurate estimates are presently unavailable, in part because of a lack of agreement about what defines subclinical eating disorders.

The severity of anorexia nervosa can also be illustrated by the high all-cause mortality rate for individuals with the disorder. Several studies indicate mortality rates in young women with the disorder of between 3% to 20% over 6 to 20 years (14–17). Other adverse health consequences of anorexia include dry skin, hypotension, cardiac rhythm disturbances, osteoporosis, cerebral atrophy, anemia, and abnormalities in the hypothalamic-pituitary-adrenal, -gonadal, and -thyroidal axes. Adverse health consequences of bulimia include tooth decay, cardiac rhythm disturbances, gastrointestinal damage, hypokalemia, hypochloremia, metabolic acidosis, cerebral atrophy, amenorrhea, and osteoporosis. Without question, eating disorders are associated with significant negative health outcomes.

WHAT ARE EFFECTIVE TREATMENTS FOR EATING DISORDERS?

Anorexia

Treatment for anorexia is extremely difficult. The course and outcome are quite variable. Often, the first step is inpatient hospitalization in which the initial focus is on weight restoration. Cognitive-behavioral or family therapy occurs in conjunction with or after weight restoration. Treatment is often multifaceted, involving family members as well as a variety of professionals, including physicians, psychologists, and nutritionists. A common component of a behavioral program is to make the patient's access to pleasurable activities contingent on weight gain.

Bulimia

Two primary types of treatment have been employed; namely, pharmacologic and cognitive-behavioral therapy. Cognitive-behavioral therapists consider the main problem of bulimia to be a morbid fear of becoming fat. Thus, treatment focuses on altering attitudes and behaviors relevant to body shape, weight, and image. In more than 30 clinical trials, cognitive-behavioral therapy has been found to be effective compared to wait-list control (18). Antidepressant medications, such as fluoxetine, also have been found to be effective in controlling the symptoms of bulimia (19). While drug treatment is one option, several large-scale clinical trials found that cognitive-behavioral therapy resulted in superior outcomes in comparison to pharmacotherapy (20–21).

Table 88-1 Diagnostic Criteria for Anorexia Nervosa

A. Refusal to maintain body weight at a level normal for age and height (weight loss to less than 85% of expected normal level)
B. Intense fear of becoming fat or gaining weight despite being underweight
C. Body image disturbance, undue influence of weight or shape on self-evaluation, or denial of seriousness of current low weight
D. Amenorrhea in postmenarcheal females

Types of anorexia nervosa:
Binge eating or purging: during current episode the person regularly engaged in binge eating or purging behavior
Restricting: during current episode the person has not regularly engaged in binge eating or purging behavior

Source: American Psychiatric Association. Diagnostic and statistical manual of mental disorders. 4th ed. Washington, DC: American Psychiatric Association, 1994: 544–545.

Table 88-2 Diagnostic Criteria for Bulimia Nervosa

A. Recurrent episodes of binge eating
   1. Rapid consumption of a large amount of food in a short time
   2. A sense of lack of control of eating during the episode
B. Recurrent compensatory behavior to prevent weight gain, such as the use of laxatives, diuretics, fasting, or excessive exercise
C. Episodes occur at least twice per week for 3 months
D. Self-evaluation unduly influenced by body shape or weight
E. Does not occur exclusively during periods of anorexia nervosa

Types of bulimia nervosa:
Purging: during current episode the person regularly purges via laxatives, diuretics, enemas, or self-induced vomiting
Nonpurging: during current episode the person does not purge but engages in other inappropriate compensatory behaviors such as fasting or excessive exercise

Source: American Psychiatric Association. Diagnostic and statistical manual of mental disorders. 4th ed. Washington, DC: American Psychiatric Association, 1994:549–550.

Table 88-3 Provisional Diagnostic Criteria for Binge Eating Disorder

A. Recurrent episodes of binge eating
   1. Rapid consumption of a large amount of food in a short time
   2. A sense of lack of control of eating during the episode
B. Episodes are associated with three or more of the following
   1. Eating faster than usual
   2. Eating until feeling uncomfortably full
   3. Eating large amounts when not hungry
   4. Eating alone because of embarrassment about how much one is eating
   5. Guilt, depression, or disgust following overeating
C. Marked distress about binge eating
D. Episodes occur on average 2 days per week for 6 months
E. Binges are not associated with the regular use of inappropriate compensatory behaviors

SOURCE: American Psychiatric Association. Diagnostic and statistical manual of mental disorders. 4th ed. Washington, DC: American Psychiatric Association, 1994:731.

Table 88-4 Examples of an Eating Disorder Labeled as "Not Otherwise Specified"

1. All criteria for anorexia nervosa are met except that regular menses occurs
2. All criteria for anorexia nervosa are met except that current weight is in the normal range
3. All criteria for bulimia nervosa are met except that episodes are less frequent than twice per week or of a duration of less than 3 months
4. Repeatedly chewing and spitting out large amounts of food, but not swallowing

SOURCE: American Psychiatric Association. Diagnostic and statistical manual of mental disorders. 4th ed. Washington, DC: American Psychiatric Association, 1994:550.

Binge Eating Disorder

Short-term group cognitive-behavioral therapy is commonly employed; however, at the present time there is a lack of scientific evidence on what type of treatment to recommend. Opioid antagonism (infused naloxone hydrochloride) has been associated with a reduction in the consumption of fat-rich snacks, including chocolate candy and cookies, and a reduced hedonic preference for mixtures of milk, cream, and sugar in binge eaters (22). Thus, it is conceivable that opioid receptor blockade ultimately may prove to be a useful treatment for binge eating disorder.

Exercise-Related Treatment Issues

Strenuous exercise is contraindicated for some patients. For example, electrolyte imbalances associated with anorexia and bulimia can increase a patient's risk for an adverse cardiac event during strenuous exercise. From a more practical standpoint, if exercise during refeeding prevents weight gain in anorexics, then patients' hospitalization is longer and more costly. However, one study has found that the addition of a formal exercise program to standard behavioral therapy did not compromise weight gain during recovery from anorexia (23). Also, a single bout of exercise has been found to reduce anxiety and depression scores in females with bulimia (24). This idea is of importance because mood and anxiety disorders are commonly co-morbid conditions (25). There are also case studies suggesting that running can be combined with psychotherapy to effectively treat anorexia (26). These findings, combined with the evidence that

central nervous system adaptations such as alterations in serotonin neurotransmission and endogenous opioid systems do occur in response to exercise (27–28), suggest that physical activity could prove to be an effective adjunct in the treatment of eating disorders. Exercise counseling is an important, but often neglected, aspect in comprehensively treating patients with eating disorders (23,29). Treating athletes with eating disorders presents additional challenges because of their unique physical activity patterns and nutritional needs. In short, the decision to recommend exercise for patients with eating disorders is complex. Exercise by these patients should be conducted under the care of a physician who may wish to consult with a multidisciplinary medical team, including an individual with training in exercise science (30,31).

WHAT ARE THE MAJOR RISK FACTORS FOR THESE EATING DISORDERS?

It is axiomatic that prevention of a disorder is better than treating a medical condition after the illness is manifested. Thus, the incidence and prevalence of eating disorders could be reduced through large-scale educational programs. To date, school-based educational interventions aimed at preventing eating disorders by reducing the prevalence of dieting have uniformly failed (32–34). Indeed, there is recent evidence that these programs may do more harm than good (35). Given the lack of success, an alternative approach is to identify those individuals at increased risk for eating disorders and focus interventions on those people.

The etiology of eating disorders is multifactorial and includes a complex interaction among cultural, social, behavioral, psychological, and biologic factors. Comprehensive investigations using ideal methodology (e.g., large samples selected to be representative of the population at large) to examine risk factors for eating disorders have yet to be conducted. Despite limitations in the available data, some facts have emerged.

Cultural Factors

Eating disorders are significantly more prevalent in industrialized countries, such as Australia, Canada, England, France, and the United States, in comparison to less industrialized nations. Also, in recent years, it has been found that minority groups are vulnerable to the development of eating disorders, although in the past, it had been suggested that minorities were relatively immune to these disorders (e.g., 36).

Social Factors

One of the most well-designed investigations to date that has examined potential risk factors for eating disorders has been conducted by Fairburn et al (37). The case-control technique was employed to examine risk factors for bulimia nervosa. Females with bulimia nervosa (n = 102) were recruited from a British community, and in an interview, they were asked to recall information about their personal lives before the development of their eating disorder. Similar interviews were conducted with age-matched and social class-matched healthy controls (n = 102) and with a group of patients with other psychiatric problems (n = 102). Those who developed bulimia reported significantly worse social relationships compared to the healthy controls. The major social factors that increased the risk for the development of bulimia were: 1) being sexually or physically abused, 2) the presence of a parental psychiatric disorder (e.g., depression, alcoholism, or substance abuse), or 3) other problems with parents, such as minimal affection, frequent teasing, criticism, low levels of maternal care, or overprotection. Other important risk factors were the presence of a premorbid psychiatric condition, such as depression or drug abuse, during adolescence and parental or childhood obesity. When those with bulimia nervosa were compared with general psychiatric controls fewer differences between the groups emerged, and the risk factors that best discriminated between these two groups were: 1) being sexually or physically abused, 2) parental alcoholism or substance abuse, and 3) childhood obesity. In addition, menarche occurred earlier in the bulimia nervosa group (31% between ages 9 to 11) compared to both the healthy controls (11%) and the general psychiatric controls (13%).

Exposure to mass media images that emphasize current societal preferences is thought to be a factor that contributes to the development of eating disorders. Although the focus used to be simply on being thin, more recent evidence shows that women consider a thin physique with a muscular, athletic-looking upper body as ideal, regardless of whether they are personally involved in athletics (38). A recent study showed that reading popular magazines (e.g., *Shape, Cosmo-*

politan) known to contain numerous articles about diet and exercise was the most consistent predictor of disordered eating symptoms when compared with other forms of mass media exposure (39). With regard to television, a recent investigation showed that the total time exposed to watching TV was less relevant than the type of program watched. Soap operas were positively related to symptoms of eating disorders, while time spent watching sporting events was negatively correlated to eating disorder symptoms (40).

Behavioral Factors

Dieting is common in industrialized societies. One study of 11,467 students found that more than 40% of high school females surveyed were attempting to lose weight (41). Hsu (42) reviewed the literature on the role of dieting in the development of eating disorders. The results of five independent longitudinal investigations pointed ". . . unanimously to the role of dieting behaviour in the pathogenesis of an eating disorder. Obviously, not all dieters proceed to develop an eating disorder; and therefore, other risk factors must also be involved if a dieter is to develop an eating disorder" (42).

Psychological Factors

Several psychological factors, including depression, neuroticism, low self-esteem, and body image disturbances, have been implicated in the development of eating disorders. One of the most consistent of these appears to be body image disturbances. There is evidence that body image disturbances predict the severity of problematic eating patterns. Several independent, prospective investigations with large numbers of adolescents (e.g., N = 800 boys and 800 girls) as well as structural modeling studies have found that body image disturbances are predictive of eating disorders (43–46). The largest differences between patients and controls have been reported using measures of cognitive-evaluative body image dissatisfaction, such as the body dissatisfaction scale of the EDI (47), which asks respondents to indicate the frequency with which they are dissatisfied with certain body parts (e.g., "I think my thighs are too large," "I think my hips are too big").

Biologic Factors

In addition to the biologic risk factors mentioned earlier (i.e., propensity toward obesity and early onset of menarche) eating disorders are strongly gender-linked. For instance, for every 10 female cases of anorexia and bulimia there is 1 male case (9). Age also is a risk factor for the development of an eating disorder. Eating disorders occur most commonly in females between the ages of 12 and 20.

There is clearly evidence that eating disorders aggregate within families. However, two major investigations have provided only a limited amount of evidence for genetic influences on bulimia (48) and no evidence for anorexia nervosa (49). This, combined with the fact that eating disorders are essentially nonexistent in some cultures, argues strongly that biologic risk factors are significantly less powerful than cultural and psychosocial factors.

In summary, although most people do not have an eating disorder, there is evidence that selected cultural, social, behavioral, psychological, and biologic factors interact to put certain individuals at increased risk for an eating disorder.

WHAT EVIDENCE LINKS PHYSICAL ACTIVITY WITH EATING DISTURBANCES?

The purpose of this section is to summarize the evidence linking participation in physical activity, athletics, and certain types of sports with eating disturbances.

Expert Opinions

Some experts feel strongly that physical activity and eating disorders are related. For example, Striegel-Moore et al (50) in reviewing the literature on bulimia wrote: "Although the possible health benefits are very real, the current emphasis on fitness may itself be contributing to the increased incidence of bulimia."

Based on clinical cases, Yeager et al (51) outlined a syndrome they labeled as the "female athlete triad." The authors argued that while any young woman could be negatively affected by adopting a pattern of disordered eating, emerging evidence suggested that women athletes, especially those participating in certain sports, were at increased risk not only for developing disordered eating behaviors but also amenorrhea and premature bone loss. Subsequent research shows that this syndrome can occur in a range of individuals from physically active girls who are not involved in competitive athletics to elite female athletes. The prevalence of this syndrome is presently unknown, and the implication that participation in exercise or sport plays a key role in the development of these health problems has been challenged (52). Nevertheless, it has been hypothesized that participation in 1) subjectively scored sports (e.g., figure skating), 2) sports requiring body-contour–revealing clothing for competition (e.g., swimming), 3) endurance sports emphasizing a low body weight (distance running), 4) sports using weight categories for participation (e.g., martial arts), and 5) sports in which possessing a low level of body fat is a competitive advantage for performance (e.g., gymnastics, figure skating) can all increase an individual's risk for disordered eating patterns and the female athlete triad (5). The veracity of these hypotheses awaits future research.

Superficial Similarities

Endurance athletes are thin; anorexics are thin. This superficial similarity apparently led some authors to suggest that endurance athletes, therefore, are anorexic (53). Subsequent investigations have revealed the error of this simplistic syllogism (54,55).

Case Studies

Cases in which serious long-distance running apparently triggered the emergence of anorexia have been reported (56). Also, there have been several documented cases of elite or near-elite athletes suffering from an eating disorder. Perhaps the most well-known is the case of former elite U.S. gymnast Christy Henrich, who died from complications of anorexia. It is possible that the worldwide publicity generated by the death of this single athlete has led people to believe that eating disorders are more prevalent among athletes in general and in participants in sports that emphasize leanness, gymnasts in particular, than the population at large.

Empiric Evidence Regarding Physical Activity and Eating Disturbances

Despite a lack of compelling empirical evidence, a current misconception is that excessive exercise leads to the development of anorexia nervosa. Beyond the case studies, this notion has been supported by animal studies of "activity-based anorexia" (57,58) and cross-sectional studies in which anorexic patients have retrospectively reported being more physically active than control subjects before the onset of their eating disorder (e.g., 59).

Activity-Based Anorexia in the Rat

The model of activity-based anorexia in rats proposed by Epling et al has been considered analogous to human anorexia nervosa; indeed, these researchers contend that ". . . most cases of anorexia nervosa are in fact instances of activity anorexia" (57). "Activity anorexia" has been functionally defined as occurring when a decline in food consumption leads to increases in physical activity; furthermore, these two factors have been proposed to mutually reinforce each other. It has been shown that when previously sedentary adolescent (2-month-old) Sprague-Dawley rats were placed on a restricted diet (one 60- to 90-minute meal per day) and were given ad libitum access to an activity wheel during nonmeal times, they steadily reduced their daily food consumption (to nearly zero) and increased their distance run on the activity wheel (up to 15 km/day) (57). Control rats provided with the same diet but with no access to an activity wheel adapted to the diet and remained healthy while the experimental rats lost weight and became emaciated or died.

While it may seem surprising to some (58,60) that rats would run excessively in the face of caloric restriction, it is important to recognize that foraging is a natural behavior for rats. Indeed, some Sprague-Dawley rats provided with ad libitum access to food, water, and an activity wheel exercise spontaneously for distances up to 18 km/day (61).

Increased physical activity in the rat can be accompanied by an increase, decrease, or no change in caloric intake. Furthermore, multiple factors may influence the response, including the amount of time between cessation of activity and measurement of food intake (62); the mode, intensity, duration, and frequency of the activity; and perhaps, gender. In rats, short-term, high-intensity exercise has been shown to decrease the caloric intake and weight of males but to increase the caloric intake of females (63).

While it has been shown that rats will run when food-deprived, others have shown that this effect occurs in response to other factors that energize behavior, such as water deprivation (64). Rieg et al compared weight loss in three groups: 1) rats that were maintained on a restricted water schedule (with free access to food and access to running wheels, except during 10 minutes per day when water was provided); 2) rats that were water deprived only; and 3) a weight-matched control group (by limiting food access) with no access to activity wheels. The weight-matched control group and the experimental group lost the same amount of weight over the last 10 days of the experiment (approximately 25% from baseline), and both groups lost significantly more weight compared to sedentary water-deprived control rats (about 8% from baseline). These results have important implications that challenge whether activity-based anorexia in the rat approximates the human condition: first, excessive activity-wheel running in the rat is not contingent solely upon caloric restriction, since water deprivation and caloric restriction also served to energize the rat's natural foraging behavior; second, the fact that an equal amount of weight was lost for the experimental group and the weight-matched control group (the former via exercise, the latter via caloric restriction) suggests that weight loss in the rat is not contingent upon excessive activity-wheel running; and third, despite their differences in weight loss, the two water-deprived groups consumed similar amounts of food and water, showing that excessive activity-wheel running per se did not affect the appetite of the experimental rats. These data suggest that while caloric restriction may be a sufficient condition, it is not a necessary condition to induce high levels of physical activity in the rat, and further, that a high level of physical activity in the rat does not necessarily lead to reduced food consumption. This also brings into question whether excessive activity-wheel running and caloric restriction should be characterized as mutually reinforcing behaviors. Animal models of human disorders are useful, especially when generally accepted criteria are employed to assess the strength and generalizability of the model (65). Despite the utility of the activity-based anorexia model for exploring physiologic and pharmacologic manipulations not possible in humans, this animal model cannot be considered analogous to human anorexia nervosa.

Physical Activity and Anorexia Nervosa in Humans

Currently available studies conducted with humans do not indicate a causal relationship between hyperactivity and anorexia nervosa. Prospective human studies have not been conducted. Relevant published research has largely failed to use physical activity assessments with adequate supportive validity evidence. Also, rarely have key terms, such as "hyperactivity" or "excessive exercise," been operationally defined in a compelling way. Physical activity norms are needed both for patients with eating disorders and aged-matched healthy controls if the term "excessive" is to be used in a nonarbitrary fashion. Despite the lack of evidence to indicate a causal relationship between participation in physical activity and the development of anorexia nervosa, some still express this view. For example, Davis writes, ". . . the psychology and the biology of physical activity can play a *causal* [her emphasis] role in the development and maintenance of some eating disorders" (59).

Logic and empirical evidence dictate that excessive exercise cannot be a sole cause of anorexia nervosa. Up to about 12% of the adult population participate in regular vigorous physical activity (66); however, the overwhelming majority of these never develop anorexia nervosa. Increased physical activity with anorexia is paradoxical because starvation has been found to result in reduced physical activity and fatigue (67). Hyperactivity in anorexia nervosa has been associated with poor clinical prognosis, despite at least one report

of a positive correlation between the amount of physical activity performed and weight gain in anorectic patients during their first 2 weeks of hospitalization (68). Early reports (69) seemingly have prompted a clinical consensus that hyperactivity *may* be a primary feature of anorexia nervosa, but it is clearly not a feature in all cases.

Davis et al (59) conducted a retrospective study of the exercise habits of 45 female anorexia nervosa patients (mean age, 21.3 ± 2.4 yr). These patients completed: 1) a questionnaire regarding their current amount of physical activity and their past activity habits at age 8, age 13, and age 18; 2) a semi-structured interview in which the interviewer encouraged detailed responses regarding ". . . her participation in, and commitment to, sport and physical activity from childhood onwards, whether or not she was involved in competitive athletics, the chronology of her dieting and exercise behaviours, and her perceptions concerning any causal associations between the two behaviours"; and 3) a seven-item checklist of eating disorders symptoms.

Although the patients reported being significantly more physically active at ages 13, 18, and at the time they were interviewed, these data should be viewed with caution since validity data for the instrument employed to quantify physical activity have not been reported, despite the fact that validity data, albeit imperfect, are available for several other physical activity instruments (70). During the interview, 70% of the patients reported being more physically active than their peers during childhood, 60% reported participation in competitive athletics, and 78% reported exercising beyond what, in their opinion, would be considered normal for women their age. Also, 93% considered their exercise routine as compulsive and ritualized, 75% reported that their physical activity increased as weight and food intake decreased, and 60% reported that sport or exercise participation preceded regular dieting, while 13% reported that these events began simultaneously. Interview and symptom checklist data were not obtained from the controls, so it is not clear whether the patients differed from healthy individuals on these items. In a subsequent study, Davis (60) found that 82% of a small group of adolescent female anorexic patients reported excessive exercise at the time of admission, but only 51% of adult anorexic patients reported excessive exercise at the time of admission.

Bouten et al (71) have reported data suggesting that hyperactivity in anorexics is related to body size and mass. In a study of 11 nonhospitalized females with anorexia and 13 normal-weight controls, daily physical activity was measured by a movement counter, daily metabolic rate was measured via doubly-labeled water, and sleeping metabolic rate was measured in a metabolic chamber. On average, daily physical activity did not differ between the anorexics and the controls, and this is consistent with other investigations (72) in which the controls were found to be inactive (73). However, anorexic women with a very low body mass index (BMI) ($<17 \text{ kg/m}^2$) tended to be less active than the controls, but anorexic women with a higher BMI ($\geq 17 \text{ kg/m}^2$) tended to be more or equally active compared with the controls (71). This study is the only one that we are aware of in which normal daily physical activity was assessed in nonhospitalized anorexics. Studies with larger samples of anorexics and specially selected matched controls are needed to more conclusively determine the physical activity patterns of anorexics.

Beyond eating disorders per se, several investigations have examined relationships between physical activity and symptoms of eating disorders. In one study of 1494 adolescents a small positive correlation (R, about 0.20) was found between the preference for healthy foods and participation in leisure sports, such as biking, skiing, and tennis (74). Nevertheless, in this study physical activity was found to be a consistent predictor of eating disorder symptoms in a series of regression analyses. The percent of variance in eating disorder symptoms accounted for by physical activity, however, was quite small (1.7%) compared to body mass index (10%). Sands et al (75) studied elementary school children (26 girls and 35 boys) and found that a child version of the EDI's drive for thinness scale was *negatively* related to "time per week participating in sport" for the girls but not for the boys. Furnham et al (76) reported that EAT scores did not differ between an active group of women (i.e., those enrolled in an aerobics class) and sedentary controls. Moreover, both these groups possessed EAT scores that were lower than women participating in a Weight Watchers program. Female aerobics instructors, however, have been found to possess elevated scores on the drive for thinness and body dissatisfaction scales of the EDI (77).

There is a limited amount of research suggesting that exercise may moderate food preferences. Female varsity athletes and women who reported exercising for more than 3 hours per week displayed reduced preferences for high-sugar and high-fat dairy solutions compared to women who were sedentary or less physically active (78). In a separate study, women who reported exercising for more than 3 hours per week displayed increased preferences for samples of popcorn (79). The authors speculated that people who engage in regular exercise are similar to those who engage in dietary restraint—they have a more positive view of a "safe" food, such as popcorn, and more negative views of "unsafe" foods known to be high in fat or sugar.

In summary, the weight of the available evidence with human subjects does not support the hypothesis that physical activity causes eating disorders. Indeed, there is little good evidence describing the physical activity patterns of women with either eating disorders per se or those who may be at increased risk for an eating disorder. Thus, participation in physical activity does not appear to be contraindicated for females at increased risk for an eating disorder and may be a useful adjunct in the treatment of eating disorders.

Empiric Evidence Comparing Athletes and Nonathletes

No scientifically compelling study of the prevalence of eating disorders in female athletes has yet been conducted. Consequently, the incidence and prevalence of eating disorders in athletes is unknown. The available data are mixed. One study of students at a large public university in the U.S. (80) found a low percentage (0.8%) of female athletes (n = 126) who met the *Diagnostic and Statistical Manual of Mental Disorders*, third

edition (*DSM-III*) criteria for bulimia compared with the total group studied (n = 716; 2.7%), or a subgroup of dance majors (n = 50, 4.0%), or students visiting a primary care clinic (n = 143; 4.2%), or a subgroup of sorority members (n = 200; 3.0%). In contrast, Sundgot-Borgen (7) obtained a total of 522 returns on a battery of questionnaires sent to the total population (n = 603) of elite (defined as members of a national sport team) female athletes in Norway (7). Twenty-two percent of those responding exhibited elevated scores on the drive for thinness and body dissatisfaction subscales of the Swedish version of the EDI. Those with elevated scores were classified as "at risk" for the development of an eating disorder, and 103 of these individuals were subsequently interviewed. The interviews revealed that 1.3% (7 of 522) of athletes met the *DSM-III* diagnostic criteria for anorexia while 8.0% (42 of 522) met the criteria for bulimia. These data suggest that bulimia is at least twice as prevalent among elite Norwegian female athletes as among the general U.S. population; however, it is unclear whether acceptable methods were employed. For example, the time frame (e.g., point, six-month, or lifetime) of the prevalence data obtained was not specified. In addition, these investigations, unlike that of Kurtzman et al (80), appear to have been completed without collaboration with a clinical psychologist or a psychiatrist.

Several investigations have compared athletes to nonathletes on eating disorder symptoms. Ashley et al (81) found that 145 NCAA Division I female athletes in various sports did not exhibit EDI-2 scores that were elevated in comparison to the published norms or a control group of university female students enrolled in an advanced program of academic study. EDI scores were also not elevated in a sample of 21-year-old women participating in the 1994 Canadian Indoor National Field Hockey Championship. Indeed, only 4 of 111 participants had elevated scores (>15) on the drive for thinness scale (82). In a study of 650 female high school students, the athletes (n = 302) did not differ on EAT scores compared with nonathletes (n = 259), and the results for both groups were generally consistent with normative values for high school girls (83). This study illustrates the importance of using control groups. A seemingly high number of athletes (19.5%) scored above a cutoff that has been used to identify disturbed eating patterns; however, an even greater percentage of the control group (23.6%) had scores above the cutoff. The need to use a control group for scientifically defensible conclusions to be drawn seems obvious, but control groups have not been employed in several studies that, unfortunately and inappropriately, have been widely cited as evidence that disordered eating is more prevalent among athletes (84,85).

Several studies have reported that small samples of amenorrheic athletes exhibit higher mean scores on psychometric questionnaires designed to assess eating disorder symptoms than eumenorrheic athletes and sedentary control groups (86,87). This is potentially important for several reasons. Elevated scores on the drive for thinness scale of the EDI have been linked to reduced bone mineral density in athletes (88) and have been found to distinguish clinical eating disorder patients from healthy individuals (89). It is clear that exercise training combined with dietary restriction can lead to neuroendocrine abnormalities, such as a reduction in gonadotropin-releasing hormone and luteinizing hormone pulse-generator activity. This reduced hormonal activity is more marked in amenorrheic athletes and likely accounts for the lack of menstrual periods in these women (90). Whether psychological factors play a causal role in relationships among dietary restriction, neuroendocrine abnormalities, and amenorrhea remains to be discovered.

Empiric Evidence from Athletes in Sports That Emphasize Leanness

Athletes possessing a low percentage of body fat (and consequently a greater strength-body mass ratio) enjoy a competitive advantage in performing certain sports—typically those requiring the athlete to lift his or her body against gravity (e.g., gymnastics, distance running, diving, figure skating), but also in sports such as martial arts, weight lifting, and wrestling, which require athletes to compete against others of roughly the same body weight. In addition, thinness appears to be a competitive advantage for aesthetic reasons in some sports, such as rhythmic gymnastics. Researchers have labeled all of these as sports that emphasize leanness.

There are no scientifically compelling large-scale studies of the prevalence of eating disorders per se among participants in sports that emphasize leanness. However, Sundgot-Borgen has reported that 16.7% (2 of 12) of the Norwegian modern rhythmic gymnastics team were found to meet the criteria for anorexia nervosa (91).

Several investigations have found that participants in sports that emphasize leanness exhibit greater symptoms of disordered eating. The percentage of elite female Norwegian athletes meeting the criteria for anorexia, bulimia, or anorexia athletica (a "subclinical" eating disturbance) was highest among those who participated in weight-dependent (27%) and aesthetic (34%) sports (7). Also, EDI drive for thinness scores have been found to be higher for groups of athletes participating in sports that emphasize leanness than for control groups (92,93). This has been observed for female weight lifters and body builders (94), female gymnasts (95), and in reports in which lean sport groups were combined to form a single group (96). Moreover, this has been observed when comparisons were made with age-, height-, and weight-matched controls and after deleting those subjects suspected of providing false answers on the EDI (88). In interpreting these findings, it is important to consider that it is not only reasonable, but indeed necessary, for competitive athletes in sports that emphasize leanness to be concerned about their body composition. Consequently, when a competitive female gymnast, for example, indicates that she is usually or always "preoccupied with being thinner" when responding to the EDI, it may represent a rationale response given her desire to perform well, especially in light of the time she has devoted to her sport. In other words, elevated scores on the EDI drive for thinness scale may represent appropriate dedication rather than psychopathology. In further support of this are reports that: 1) the average elevation in EDI scores for participants in sports that emphasize leanness has always been reported to be lower than average scores for groups of women with anorexia or bulimia, 2) athletes tend to possess more positive mental health on average than nonathletes (97), and 3) eating disorder symptoms abate after retirement from participation in competitive sports (98).

SUMMARY

This review has provided an overview of eating disorders and examined the strength of the scientific evidence linking participation in physical activity, athletics, and sports with eating disturbances. The current diagnostic criteria, based on clinical experience, imply links between excessive exercise and bulimia (see Table 88-2). However, there is a lack of scientific evidence documenting the frequency with which individuals with bulimia compensate their binging behavior by engaging in exercise. Moreover, there is no consensus as to what constitutes exercise that is excessive. Additional research is needed to clarify the usefulness of including excessive exercise as part of the criteria for bulimia nervosa. The weight of the available scientific evidence does permit the conclusion that selected cultural, social, behavioral, psychological, and biologic factors place individuals at increased risk for an eating disorder. Physical activity per se, even when performed to an extreme level, does not result in an eating disorder. Indeed, there is no compelling evidence in humans to suggest that women or men should refrain from participating in sports or exercise because it would contribute in a meaningful way to the risk of an eating disorder. There is evidence that females who participate in sports that emphasize leanness report greater symptoms of disordered eating; however, it is not yet clear whether this represents a first step toward psychopathology or the rationale response of a dedicated athlete who wants to do everything in her power to perform optimally. It is recommended that, among those athletes who participate in sports that emphasize leanness, increased preventive efforts be aimed at those athletes possessing multiple risk factors for an eating disorder.

This review has focused on females because most people with eating disorders are female and because the majority of available research has used females as test subjects. However, males are not immune to eating disorders and related concerns about the management of body weight. For example, three previously healthy college wresters died from dehydration- and hypothermia-related events associated with rapid weight loss during a 1-month period in late 1997 (99). In each case, the wrestler sought to lose 3.5 to 9.0 pounds over a 3- to 9-hour period by restricting their food and water intake and exercising vigorously in a hot environment while wearing a vapor-impermeable suit. Moreover, in the 10 to 13 weeks before the acute rapid weight loss, all three athletes had lost from 21 to 23 pounds from their September preseason body weight. These cases highlight the seriousness of weight concerns in male athletes and underscore the importance of preventing unsafe weight-loss practices. The education of coaches and athletes about proper diet and weight management techniques is a critical step toward this goal.

Preparation of this manuscript was supported by a grant from the Office of Research on Women's Health in conjunction with the National Institute on Child Health and Human Development (1 RO1 HD 35592-01).

REFERENCES

1. Beals KA, Manore MM. The prevalence and consequences of subclinical eating disorders in female athletes. Int J Sport Nutr 1994;4:175–195.

2. Benson JE, Engelbert-Fenton KA, Eisenman PA. Nutritional aspects of amenorrhea in the female athlete triad. Int J Sport Nutr 1996;6:134–145.

3. Brownell KD, Rodin J, Wilmore JH. Eating, body weight, and performance in athletes. Malvern, PA: Lea & Febiger, 1992:1–374.

4. O'Connor PJ, Lewis RD, Boyd A. Health concerns of female gymnasts. Sports Med 1996;21:321–325.

5. Otis CL, Drinkwater B, Johnson M, et al. The female athlete triad. Med Sci Sports Exerc 1997;29:i–ix.

6. Smith AD. The female athlete triad: causes, diagnosis, and treatment. Phys Sportsmed 1996;24:67–76.

7. Sundgot-Borgen J. Risk and trigger factors for the development of eating disorders in female elite athletes. Med Sci Sports Exerc 1994;26:414–419.

8. Wilmore JH. Eating and weight disorders in the female athlete. Int J Sport Nutr 1991;1:104–117.

9. American Psychiatric Association. Diagnostic and statistical manual of mental disorders. 4th ed. Washington, DC: American Psychiatric Association 1994:1–750.

10. Stunkard A. Eating disorders: the last 25 years. Appetite 1997;29:181–190.

11. Hoek HW. The distribution of eating disorders. In: Brownell KD, Fairburn CG, eds. Eating disorders and obesity: a comprehensive handbook. New York: Guilford, 1995:207–211.

12. Warheit GJ, Langer LM, Zimmerman RS, Biafora FA. Prevalence of bulimic behaviors and bulimia among a sample in the general population. Am J Epidemiol 1993;137:569–577.

13. Ash JB, Piazza E. Changing symptomatology in eating disorders. Int J Eating Dis 1995;18:27–38.

14. Crisp AH, Callender JS, Halek C, Hsu LKG. Long-term mortality in anorexia nervosa: a 20-year follow-up of the St. George's and Aberdeen cohorts. Br J Psychiatr 1992;161:104–107.

15. Eckert ED, Halmi KA, Marchi P, et al. Ten-year follow-up of anorexia nervosa: clinical course and outcome. Psychol Med 1995;25:143–156.

16. Noring CE, Sohlberg SS. Outcome, recovery, relapse, and mortality across six years in patients with clinical eating disorders. Acta Psychiatr Scandia 1993;87:437–444.

17. Ratnasuriya RH, Eisler I, Szmukler GI, Russell GF. Anorexia nervosa: outcomes and prognostic factors after 20 years. Br J Psychiatr 1991;158:495–502.

18. Fairburn CG. The prevention of eating disorders. In: Brownell KD, Fairburn CG, eds. Eating disorders and obesity: a comprehensive handbook. New York: Guilford, 1995:289–293.

19. Pope HG, Hudson JI. Treatment of bulimia with antidepressants. Psychopharmacol 1982;78:176–179.

20. Agras WS, Rossiter EM, Arnow B, et al. Pharmacological and cognitive-behavioral treatment for bulimia nervosa: a controlled comparison. Am J Psychiatr 1992;149:82–87.

21. Mitchell JE, Pyle RL, Eckert ED, et al. A comparison study of antidepressants and structured intensive group psychotherapy in the treatment of bulimia nervosa. Arch Gen Psychiatr 1990;47:149–155.

22. Drewnowski A, Krahn DD, Demitrack MA, et al. Naloxone, an opiate blocker, reduces the consumption of sweet high-fat foods in obese and lean female binge eaters. Am J Clin Nutr 1995;61:1206–1212.

23. Touyz SW, Lennerts W, Arthur B, Beumont PJV. Anaerobic exercise as an adjunct to refeeding patients with anorexia nervosa: does it compromise weight gain? Eur Eat Dis Rev 1993;1:177–182.

24. Glazer AR, O'Connor PJ. Mood improvements following exercise and quiet rest in bulimic women. Scand J Med Sci Sports 1992;3:73–79.

25. Cooper PJ. Eating disorders and their relationship to mood and anxiety disorders. In: Brownell KD, Fairburn CG, eds. Eating disorders and obesity: a comprehensive handbook. New York: Guilford, 1995:159–164.

26. Kostrubala T. The joy of running. New York: JB Lippincott, 1976:1–158.

27. Chaouloff F. The serotonin hypothesis. In: Morgan WP, ed. Physical activity and mental health. Washington DC: Taylor & Francis, 1997:179–198.

28. Hoffmann P. The endorphin hypothesis. In: Morgan WP, ed. Physical activity and mental health. Washington DC: Taylor & Francis, 1997:163–178.

29. Beumont PJV, Arthur B, Russell JD, Touyz SW. Excessive physical activity in dieting disorder patients—proposals for a supervised exercise program. Int J Eating Dis 1994;15:21–36.

30. Joy E, Clark N, Ireland ML, et al. Team management of the female athlete triad. Part 1: What to look for, what to ask. Phys Sportsmed 1997;25:95–110.

31. Joy E, Clark N, Ireland ML, et al. Team management of the female athlete triad. Part 2: Optimal treatment and prevention tactics. Phys Sportsmed 1997;25:55–69.

32. Killen JD, Taylor CB, Hammer LD, et al. An attempt to modify unhealthful eating attitudes and weight regulation practices of young adolescent girls. Int J Eating Dis 1993;13:369–384.

33. Moreno AB, Thelen MH. A preliminary prevention program for eating disorders in a junior high school population. J Youth Adolesc 1993;22:109–124.

34. Shisslak CM, Crago M, Neal ME. Prevention of eating disorders among adolescents. Am J Health Prom 1990;5:100–106.

35. Carter JC, Stewart DA, Dunn VJ, Fairburn CG. Primary prevention of eating disorders: might it do more harm than good? Int J Eating Dis 1997;22:167–172.

36. Wilfley DE, Schreiber GB, Pike KM, et al. Eating disturbance and body image: a comparison of a community sample of adult black and white women. Int J Eat Dis 1996;20:377–387.

37. Fairburn CG, Welch SL, Doll HA, et al. Risk factors for bulimia nervosa: a community-based case-control study. Arch Gen Psychiatr 1997;54:509–517.

38. Lenart EB, Goldberg JP, Bailey SM, et al. Current and ideal physique choices in exercising and nonexercising college women from a pilot athletic image scale. Percept Motor Skills 1995;81:831–848.

39. Harrison K, Cantor J. The relationship between media consumption and eating disorders. J Commun 1997;47:40–67.

40. Tiggemann J, Pickering AS. Role of television in adolescent women's body dissatisfaction and drive for thinness. Int J Eat Dis 1996;20:199–203.

41. Serdula MK, Collins ME, Williamson DF, et al. Weight control practices of United States adolescents and adults. Ann Intern Med 1993;119:667–671.

42. Hsu LKG. Can dieting cause an eating disorder? Psychol Med 1997;27:509–513.

43. Attie I, Brooks-Gunn J. Development of eating problems in adolescent girls. Develop Psychol 1989;25:70–79.

44. Leon GR, Fulkerson JA, Perry CL, Cudeck R. Personality and behavioral vulnerabilities associated with risk status for eating disorders in adolescent girls. J Abnorm Psychol 1993;102:438–444.

45. Striegel-Moore RH, Silberstein LR, Frensch P, Rodin J. A prospective study of disordered eating among college students. Int J Eat Dis 1989;8:499–509.

46. Thompson JK, Coovert MD, Richards KJ, et al. Development of body image, eating disturbance, and general psychological functioning in female adolescents: covariance structure modeling and longitidinal investigations. Int J Eat Dis 1995;18:221–236.

47. Cash TF, Deagle EA. The nature and extent of body-image disturbances in anorexia nervosa and bulimia nervosa. Int J Eat Dis 1997;22:107–125.

48. Kendler KS, Maclean C, Neale M, et al. The genetic epidemiology of bulimia nervosa. Am J Psychiatr 1991;148:1627–1637.

49. Walters E, Kendler KS. Anorexia nervosa and anorexic-like syndromes in a population-based female twin sample. Am J Psychiatr 1995;152:64–71.

50. Striegel-Moore RH, Silberstein LR, Rodin J. Toward an understanding of risk factors for bulimia. Am J Psychiatr 1986;152:246–263.

51. Yeager KK, Agostini R, Nattiv A, Drinkwater B. The female athlete triad. Med Sci Sports Exerc 1993;25:775–777.

52. DiPietro L, Stachenfeld NS. The female athlete triad. Med Sci Sports Exerc 1997;29:1669–1671.

53. Yates A, Leehey K, Shisslak CM. Running—an analogue of anorexia nervosa? N Engl J Med 1983;398:251–255.

54. Blumenthal JA, O'Toole LC, Chang JL. Is running an analogue of anorexia? An empirical study of obligatory running and anorexia nervosa. JAMA 1984;252:520–523.

55. McSherry JA. The diagnostic challenge of anorexia nervosa. Am Fam Phys 1984;29:141–145.

56. Katz JL. Long distance running, anorexia nervosa, and bulimia: a report of two cases. Compr Psychiatr 1986;27:74–82.

57. Epling WF, Pierce WD. Activity-based anorexia: a biobehavioral perspective. Int J Eating Dis 1988;7:475–485.

58. Pierce WD, Epling WF. Activity anorexia: an interplay between basic and applied behavior analysis. Behavior Analyst 1994;17:7–23.

59. Davis C, Kennedy H, Ravelski E, Dionne M. The role of physical activity in the development and maintenance of eating disorders. Psychol Med 1994;24:957–967.

60. Davis C. Eating disorders and hyperactivity: a psychobiological perspective. Can J Psychiatr 1997;42:168–175.

61. Gisiger V, Belisle M, Gardiner PF. Acetylcholinesterase adaptation to voluntary wheel running is proportional to the volume of activity in fast, but not slow, rat hindlimb muscles. Eur J Neurosci 1994;6:673–680.

62. Tokuyama K, Saito M, Okuda H. Effects of wheel running on food intake and weight gain of female rats. Physiol Behav 1982;23:899–903.

63. Oscai LB. The role of exercise in weight control. Exerc Sport Sci Rev 1973;1:103–123.

64. Rieg TS, Doerries LE, O'Shea JG, Aravich PF. Water deprivation produces an exercise-induced weight loss phenomenon in the rat. Physiol Behav 1993;53:607–610.

65. Suomi SJ. Relevance of animal models for clinical psychology. In: Kendall PC, Butcher JN, eds. Handbook of research methods in clinical psychology. New York: Wiley, 1982:249–270.

66. Dishman RK. Introduction: concensus, problems, and prospects. In: Dishman RK, ed. Advances in exercise adherence. Champaign, IL: Human Kinetics, 1994:1–27.

67. Keys A, Brozek J, Henschel A, et al. The biology of human starvation. Minneapolis: University of Minnesota Press, 1950:714–721.

68. Falk JR, Halmi KA, Tryon WW. Activity measures in anorexia

nervosa. Arch Gen Psychiatr 1985; 42:811–814.

69. Kron L, Katz JL, Gorzynski G, Weiner H. Hyperactivity in anorexia nervosa: a fundamental clinical feature. Comprehen Psychiatr 1978;19:433–440.

70. Krista AM, Caspersen CJ. A collection of physical activity questionnaires for health-related research. Med Sci Sport Exer 1997;29 (suppl):S1–S205.

71. Bouten CV, Van Marken Lichtenbelt WD, Westerderp KR. Body mass index and daily physical activity in anorexia nervosa. Med Sci Sports Exerc 1996;28:967–973.

72. Platte P, Pirke KM, Trimborn P, et al. Resting metabolic rate and total energy expenditure in acute and weight-recovered patients with anorexia nervosa and in healthy young women. Int J Eating Dis 1994;16:42–47.

73. Casper RC, Schoeller DA, Kushner R, et al. Total daily energy expenditure and activity level in anorexia nervosa. Am J Clin Nutr 1991; 53:1143–1150.

74. French SA, Perry CL, Leon GR, Fulkerson JA. Food preferences, eating patterns, and physical activity among adolescents: correlates of eating disorders symptoms. J Adolesc Health 1994;15:286–294.

75. Sands R, Tricker J, Sherman C, et al. Disordered eating patterns, body image, self-esteem, and physical activity in preadolescent school children. Int J Eating Dis 1997;21:159–166.

76. Furnham A, Boughton J. Eating behaviour and body dissatisfaction among dieters, aerobic exercisers, and a control group. Eur Eat Dis Rev 1995;3:35–45.

77. Olson MS, Williford HN, Richards LA, et al. Self-report on the eating disorder inventory by female aerobic instructors. Percept Motor Skills 1996;82:1015–1058.

78. Crystal S, Frye CA, Kanarek RB. Taste preferences and sensory perceptions in female varsity swimmers. Appetite 1995;24:25–36.

79. Kanarek RB, Ryu M, Przpek J. Preferences for foods with varying levels of salt and fat differ as a function of dietary restraint and exercise but not menstrual cycle. Physiol Behav 1995;57:821–826.

80. Kurtzman FD, Yager J, Landsverk J, et al. Eating disorders among selected female student populations at UCLA. J Am Diet Assoc 1989;89:45–53.

81. Ashley CD, Smith JF, Robinson JB, Richardson MT. Disordered eating in female collegiate athletes and collegiate females in an advanced program of study: a preliminary investigation. Int J Sport Nutr 1996;6:391–401.

82. Marshall JD, Harber VJ. Body dissatisfaction and drive for thinness in high performance field hockey athletes. Int J Sports Med 1996; 17:541–544.

83. Taub DE, Blinde EM. Disordered eating and weight control among adolescent female athletes and performance squad members. J Adolesc Res 1994;9:483–497.

84. Rosen LW, McKeag DB, Hough DO. Pathogenic weight-control behavior in female athletes. Phys Sportsmed 1986;14:79–86.

85. Rosen LW, Hough DO. Pathogenic weight-control behaviors of female college gymnasts. Phys Sportsmed 1988;16:141–144.

86. Perry AC, Crane LS, Applegate B, et al. Nutrient intake and psychological and physiological assessment in eumenorrheic and amenorrheic female athletes: a preliminary study. Int J Sports Nutr 1996;6:3–13.

87. Myerson M, Gutin B, Warren MP, et al. Resting metabolic rate and energy balance in amenorrheic and eumenorrheic runners. Med Sci Sports Exerc 1991;23:15–22.

88. O'Connor PJ, Lewis RD, Kirchner EM. Eating disorder symptoms in female college gymnasts. Med Sci Sports Exerc 1995; 27:550–555.

89. Garner DM, Olmsted MP, Polivy J. Development and validation of a multidimensional eating disorder inventory for anorexia nervosa and bulimia nervosa. Int J Eat Dis 1983;2:15–34.

90. Laughlin GA, Yen SSC. Nutritional and endocrine-metabolic aberrations in amenorrheic athletes. J Clin Endo Metab 1996;81:4301–4309.

91. Sundgot-Borgen J. Eating disorders, energy intake, training volume, and menstrual function in high-level modern rhythmic gymnasts. Int J Sport Nutr 1996;6:100–109.

92. Borgen JS, Corbin CB. Eating disorders among female athletes. Phys Sportsmed 1987;15:89–95.

93. Davis C, Cowles M. A comparison of weight and diet concerns and personality factors among athletes and non-athletes. J Psychosom Res 1989;33:527–536.

94. Walberg JL, Johnston CS. Menstrual function and eating behavior in female recreational weight lifters and competitive body builders. Med Sci Sports Exerc 1991;23:30–36.

95. Warren BJ, Stanton AL, Blessing DL. Disordered eating patterns in competitive female athletes. Int J Eating Dis 1990;9:565–569.

96. Petrie TA. Differences beween male and female college lean sport athletes, nonlean sport athletes, and nonathletes on behavioral and psychological indices of eating disorders. J Appl Sport Psychol 1996;8:218–230.

97. Morgan WP. Selected psychological factors limiting performance: a mental health model. In: Clarke DH, Eckert HM, eds. Limits of human performance. Champaign, IL: Human Kinetics, 1985:70–80.

98. O'Connor PJ, Lewis RD, Kirchner EM, Cook DB. Eating disorder symptoms in former female college gymnasts: relations with body composition. Am J Clin Nutr 1996;64:840–843.

99. Remick D, Chancellor K, Pederson J, et al. Hyperthermia and dehydration-related deaths associated with intentional rapid weight loss in three collegiate wrestlers. MMWR 1998;47:105–107.

Chapter 89

Determinants of Physical Activity: Research to Application

Janet Buckworth
Rod K. Dishman

For centuries, philosophers and scientists have attempted to describe and predict human behavior with varying degrees of success. Understanding physical activity behavior has practical implications for researchers and practitioners today, considering the continued evidence for health benefits of an active lifestyle (1,2). However, few controlled studies have been conducted to experimentally manipulate variables presumed to operate as determinants of physical activity behavior, and no population trials have been completed (3). The term "determinant" is thus frequently misused in the literature to imply a causal relationship. In this chapter, "determinant" will be used to denote a reproducible association or predictive relationship and not to imply cause and effect.

Physical activity and exercise are terms that also warrant clarification. Both are associated with health benefits and physical fitness (1,4), but exercise is planned, structured, and repetitive bodily movement with the purpose of improving or maintaining physical fitness components, and physical activity is any bodily movement via skeletal muscles that results in increased energy expenditure (5). Physical inactivity is a level of activity less than that needed to maintain good health (6).

Defining determinants of physical activity is important for several reasons. First, expanding our knowledge of the dynamics of physical activity behavior facilitates the design and application of more appropriate theoretical models of behavior change. Second, identification of inactive segments of the population can guide allocation of resources earmarked to increase exercise adoption and adherence. Third, determining malleable variables that influence behavior change can direct interventions to target those variables. In addition, expanding our knowledge of characteristics that influence physical activity in specific populations fosters personalized interventions more

likely to meet the needs of the target group, and thus, increase maintenance of behavior change.

The objectives of this chapter are to review the evidence related to the determinants of physical activity and to describe how this research can be used to help people initiate and maintain an active lifestyle. We begin by presenting the current consensus on determinants of physical activity based, in part, on several earlier, more detailed reviews (7–9). Next, we describe the contextual dynamics of interventions to increase adoption and maintenance of physical activity and provide examples of specific strategies. Finally, we summarize some of the issues in research that have limited our understanding of exercise behavior.

DETERMINANTS OF PHYSICAL ACTIVITY

Although most studies of determinants have been correlational or predictive, there are reliable associations between certain variables and physical activity. The known determinants of physical activity can be classified as characteristics of the person, the environment, and the physical activity itself. Identifying determinants that reside in the individual specifies population segments that may be more responsive to different types of interventions. Personal attributes such as smoking, education, income, and ethnicity can be markers of underlying stereotypical habits or circumstances that reinforce sedentary living (3). Identifying environmental factors in exercise behavior can guide policy and facility planning at the national and community levels and can help direct program development in school, church, health care, and recreational settings (7,10,11). Identifying specific aspects of physical activity that enhance adoption and adherence is especially important to practitioners prescribing exercise in a variety of settings (3).

The significance of specific determinants must also be considered in the context of other personal, environmental, and behavioral factors. Determinants of physical activity are not isolated variables, but interact dynamically to influence behavior over time. For example, someone who has just started exercising might be motivated to walk when the weather is nice, regardless of whether he or she is alone, but will only walk when it is cold if family or friends come along. After physical activity is an established behavior, external support becomes less important and walking does not depend on the company of others. In addition, it is believed that determinants may differ somewhat for supervised versus free-living settings and for type of physical activity (9).

Table 89-1 presents a summary of physical activity determinants and their association with supervised and unsupervised exercise programs.

Table 89-1 Summary of Physical Activity Determinants Literature for Studies Conducted in Supervised Settings and with Free-Living Samples During Two Time Periods

Determinant	Supervised		Free-Living	
	Pre-1988 Results	1988–1991 Results	Pre-1988 Results	1988–1991 Results
Personal attributes:				
Demographics				
Age	00	-	-	—
Blue-collar occupation	—	-	-	
Childless				+
Education	+		++	++
Gender (male)			++	++
High risk for heart disease	-	-	-	
Income/socioeconomic status			++	++
Injury history				+
Overweight/obesity	-	0	-	00
Race (nonwhite)			-	—
Cognitive Variables				
Attitudes	0	+	0	
Barriers to exercise		-		—
Control over exercise				0
Enjoyment of exercise	+		+	0
Expect health and other benefits	0	+	+	+
Health locus of control	+	0		
Intention to exercise	0		+	++
Knowledge of health and exercise	0		0	0
Lack of time	—		-	-
Mood disturbance	-		-	—
Normative beliefs	0			0
Perceived health or fitness	++		-	++
Self-efficacy for exercise	+	+	+	++
Self-motivation	+	++	++	+
Self-schemata for activity			+	+
Stress				0
Susceptibility to illness				0
Value exercise outcomes	0		0	
Behaviors				
Alcohol				0
Contemporary program activity			0	
Diet	00		+	0
Past free-living activity during childhood			0	0
Past free-living activity during adulthood	+		+	++
Past program participation	++	+	+	
School sports	0		0	00
Smoking	—	1 -	0	0

Table 89-1 continues

Table 89-1 (*Continued*)				
	SUPERVISED		**FREE-LIVING**	
DETERMINANT	**PRE-1988 RESULTS**	**1988–1991 RESULTS**	**PRE-1988 RESULTS**	**1988–1991 RESULTS**
Sports media use				0
Environmental Factors:				
Social Environment				
Class size		+		
Exercise models				0
Group cohesion		+		
Physician influence			+	
Social isolation				-
Past family influences			+	0
Social support; friends/peers			+	++
Social support; spouse/family	++		+	++
Social support; staff/instructor	+	0		
Physical Environment				
Climate/season	-		-	0
Cost	0		0	
Disruptions in routine	-			
Access to facilities: actual	+			+
Access to facilities: perceived	+		0	0
Home equipment				0
Physical Activity Characteristics				
Intensity	-		-	
Perceived effort	—		-	-

++, repeatedly documented positive association with physical activity; +, weak or mixed evidence of positive association with physical activity; 00, repeatedly documented lack of association with physical activity; 0, weak or mixed evidence of no association with physical activity; —, repeatedly documented negative association with physical activity; -, weak or mixed evidence of negative association with physical activity. Blank spaces indicate no data available.

Reprinted by permission from Dishman RK, Sallis JF. Determinants and interventions for physical activity and exercise. In: Bouchard C, Shephard RJ, Stephens T, eds. Physical activity, fitness, and health: international proceedings and consensus statement. Champaign, IL: Human Kinetics, 1994:223–224.

Characteristics of the Person

Characteristics of the person include demographic variables, biomedical status, past and present behaviors, and psychological traits and states, such as knowledge, attitudes, and beliefs that are related to physical activity.

Demographic Variables

Demographics such as sex, age, ethnicity, education, and income are consistent correlates of physical activity. Females are more likely to be inactive than males (12,13). According to data summarized in the *1996 Surgeon General's Report on Physical Activity and Health from the Behavioral Risk Factor Surveillance System (BRFSS)*, 30.7% of females and 26.5% of males aged 18 and over reported no leisure-time physical activity over the past month (12). Sex differences are consistent for different racial or ethnic groups and across age groups. For example, Kelley (14) examined gender differences in physical activity for 127 African-American college freshmen using the Lipid Research Clinic's Physical Activity Questionnaire. Significantly more males (19%) than females (6%) were in the high-active group, and more females (71%) than males (45%) were in the very

low- or low-active groups. Results from the 1995 College Health Risk Behavior Survey (N = 4609) indicate no gender difference in participation in moderate intensity activity, but significantly more males (43.7%) than females (33.0%) reported vigorous physical activity (13). Female high school students are also less active than males; 52.1% of the girls compared to 74.4% of the boys sampled in the 1995 Youth Risk Behavior Survey (YRBS) reported participation in vigorous activity over the past week surveyed (15).

Participation in physical activity decreases with age (12,15–17). According to the YRBS, vigorous activity decreases from grade nine to grade twelve. In the ninth grade, 79.9% of males and 61.6% of females reported vigorous activity compared to 67.2% of males and 42.1% of females in the twelfth grade (15). This decrease in activity is especially noticeable in African-American females, only 9% of whom reported vigorous activity in the twelfth grade (17). Participation in moderate activity is also different as a function of race or ethnicity in youth. African-American and Hispanic youth are more likely to participate in moderate physical activity than Caucasian youth. Generally, non–Hispanic whites appear to be more active than other ethnic groups regardless of age, but in this case, it is difficult or impossible to disentangle the effects of ethnicity and socioeconomic status.

Generally, income and education are positively associated with physical activity (7,8) and have been associated with increased activity in prospective studies (18–20). For example, Anderson (18) found that Danish adolescents with similar aerobic capacities in high school had significantly lower aerobic capacities 8 years later if they were in blue-collar jobs or unemployed than if they were civil servants, white-collar workers, or students. However, because there are associations between low income, fewer years of education, and low activity, these variables may not be a cause per se, but may be selection bias.

Biomedical Variables

Significant genetic contributions to aerobic fitness are approximately 25% (21). There is also some evidence for a genetic influence on physical activity. Pérusse et al (22) examined pairs of biologic and cultural relatives (N = 1610) to quantify genetic and nongenetic sources of variation in physical activity. There was no genetic influence on exercise participation, but 29% of the variability in level of habitual physical activity was accounted for by genetic factors. The investigators speculate that the intrinsic drive to engage in spontaneous physical activity could be influenced by genotype, but exercise participation is entirely cultural (22).

Other physiologic characteristics of individuals can play a critical role in behavior and may interact significantly with psychosocial constructs (23). For example, body mass index, obesity, and physical discomfort have been negatively correlated with self-report of physical activity (7) and those who perceive their health as poor are unlikely to adopt and adhere to an exercise program (9).

Even though symptoms may prompt an individual to act on a physician's advice to begin an exercise program, cardiovascular disease and low metabolic tolerance for physical activity are not reliable predictors of adherence to clinical exercise programs (9). When physical activity is defined by observation, those who do not adopt or adhere to supervised rehabilitative and work site exercise programs typically have high CHD risk profiles.

Past and Present Behaviors

Associations between physical activity and other health behaviors in high school were explored by Pate et al (24). They divided 11,631 high school students in the 1990 YRBS into subsets of 2652 high-active (22.8% of total) and 1641 low-active (14.1% of total) groups. Low levels of physical activity were associated with cigarette smoking, marijuana use, lower amount of fruit and vegetable consumption, greater amount of TV watching, failure to wear a seat belt, one or more sexual partners in the past 3 months, and a low perception of academic performance (24). Smoking has also been negatively associated with physical activity in adult males (25).

Longitudinal population studies that evaluate concurrent changes in physical activity and changes in purported determinants can provide stronger evidence for the role of specific variables in exercise adoption and adherence. Declines in physical activity in adults over time have been associated with social isolation, lower levels of education and income, a blue-collar occupation, unmarried status, depression, low levels of life satisfaction, and less than excellent perceived health (26).

Being active in the recent past predicts present and future participation, but playing sports when young does not influence future physical activity (27). No prospective study has shown a relationship between interscholastic or intercollegiate athletics and free-living physical activity in adults, and there is little evidence that activity patterns in childhood are predictive of later physical activity (9). There is evidence of a relationship between exercise history and sports media use; being active in sports as a child predicted frequent use of sports media rather than physical activity as an adult (25).

Psychological States and Traits

Psychological constructs can account for variability in behavior within population segments that are demographically homogeneous and across settings that differ in place and time. Because they can also reflect past behavior history but exist in the present, they offer promise for more precise predictions of physical activity than the determinants considered up to this point. Psychological traits are relatively stable, but they can be changed. However, they are resistant to change over the narrow ranges of time, exposure, and settings characteristic of medical and public health interventions.

Personality theorists suggest that certain enduring characteristics of a person's drive behavior can account for a variety of behaviors and the relationships among them, but it is questionable whether any single determinant explains more than a small part of the variance in exercise behavior (28). Enduring personality traits, such as achievement motivation, stress tolerance, and independence, as well as attitudes, beliefs, and values, show weak or no association with physical activity in children (29). However, knowledge of how to become physically active may be a significant influence on behavior in this population (29).

The cognitive variable with the most support as a determinant is self-efficacy, which is the belief in one's capability to perform exercise behavior and one's perception of anticipated benefits (30–34). For example, in a community analysis, Sallis et al (25) found that the strongest correlates with self-report of vigorous activity were self-efficacy and perceived barriers to exercise, in addition to weaker correlations with modeling, dietary habits, and age. However, we are not sure how much of the relationship between physical activity and self-efficacy is a selection bias, i.e., active individuals reporting a high self-efficacy because of past success. This is because studies looking at psychosocial variables have been cross-sectional or prospective, not experimental, and have not done a good job of measuring past habits and the causes of past habits. Thus, the correlation between current or future physical activity and self-efficacy may have been inflated, because it is old habits that are predicting current physical activity, perhaps operating through increased self-efficacy associated with success, but other factors that led to the original habit were the actual cause.

Other cognitive variables positively associated with physical activity are self-schemata (seeing oneself as an exerciser), expectations of benefits, self-motivation, perceived barriers, and behavioral intentions (25,35,36). Knowledge is not enough to change behavior, but clear, relevant information about the benefits of physical activity and how to become more active can influence attitudes and beliefs. Mood disorders are negatively associated with physical activity. There has been little research on anxiety traits and states and exercise adherence.

Those who believe exercise has little value for health and fitness, do not expect health outcomes from physical activity, and believe health outcomes are out of their personal control have been found to exercise less frequently and to drop out sooner in fitness-related programs than peers holding opposite views. However, because most entrants into supervised programs share similarly positive attitudes and beliefs about expected outcomes from exercise, their self-perceptions of exercise ability, feelings of health responsibility, and attitude toward exercise have not reliably predicted who will adhere to the program (3,31,37).

Characteristics of the Environment

Environmental factors include access to facilities, time, and social support. They can act as determinants of physical activity by facilitating or hindering exercise adoption or maintenance.

Access to Facilities

Access to facilities is perceived as an important participation influence (12). Access can be considered in terms of geography, economics, safety, and perceptions. When access to facilities has been measured by objective methods (e.g., distance), access typically has been related to both the adoption and maintenance of physical activity. When perceived access has been measured by self-report, it typically has not been related to the adoption and maintenance of physical activity (38).

Time

A perceived lack of time is the principal and most prevalent reason given both for dropping out of supervised clinical and community exercise programs and for inactive lifestyles. For many, however, this may reflect a lack of interest or commitment to physical activity. Population surveys indicate that regular exercisers are more likely than sedentary persons to view time as an activity barrier. It is not yet clear whether time represents a true environmental determinant, a perceived determinant, poor behavioral skills (such as time management), or a rationalization for a lack of motivation to be active.

Social Support

Social influences in the form of modeling, social support, and prompting appear to be strong correlates of physical activity. When social influences on physical activity are studied, they are usually found to be correlated with physical activity. Social support from family and friends is consistently related to physical activity in cross-sectional and prospective studies (39–42). Spousal influences on exercise appear to be reliable correlates of participation. Group factors may be important in adherence to exercise programs as well.

Social interactions and social influences appear to be more important in physical activity participation for women (39,42) than for men. For example, adherence to a structured exercise program was predicted by perceptions of females that they received adequate levels of guidance and reassurance of worth, while social provisions did not predict adherence in males (39).

Characteristics of the Behavior

The current guidelines for physical activity promoted by the U.S. Public Health Service and the American College of Sports Medicine (43) are to accumulate 30 minutes or more of moderate-intensity exercise most days of the week. The available studies strongly indicate that moderate and vigorous physical activities are controlled by different factors, but few studies have examined differences in activity patterns, determinants of moderate and vigorous physical activity, or components of an exercise prescription. Jakicic et al (44) tested the effects of prescribing exercise in short bouts versus one long bout on exercise adherence, cardiorespiratory fitness, and weight loss. Fifty-six sedentary, overweight women were randomized to a short bout (three or four 10-minute bouts per day) or continuous (one 30- to 40-minute bout per day) of brisk walking for 5 days per week. After 20 weeks of exercise and dietary restrictions, the short bout group had significantly better adherence and trends toward greater exercise duration and weight loss (44). However, because only self-report of physical activity was increased, with no change in aerobic capacity or motion sensor readings, the self-reports may have been biased.

The strong decline in total and vigorous activity with age is not seen with moderate-intensity activities. Studies reporting separate analyses for moderate-intensity activities have consistently noted increased levels with age. Walking is the most commonly reported form of moderate-intensity activity and its frequency increases for older adults (12). Walking and other forms of moderate activity appear to have important health benefits, and they may be more acceptable to older adults and to women.

Factors controlling adoption and maintenance of different types and intensities of exercise have not been explored, and specific determinants of adopting, maintaining, or resuming exercise after dropping out have not been identified (8). We have evidence that exercise self-efficacy increases as one moves from an established sedentary lifestyle to long-term maintenance of regular exercise (45,46), but there is little information about what causes someone to make these behavioral transitions or to drop out of a structured exercise program (8).

Auweele et al (47) attempted to identity the attitudes and beliefs associated with adoption of exercise in 268 sedentary middle-aged adults in Belgium. Reasons for not exercising were related to self-concept, negative feelings, and perceptions of cost-benefit. Subjects would have been willing to exercise if they believed exercise would decrease a health risk or improve a health problem, or if they believed there were few barriers to participation and exercise would meet personal needs (47). In addition, the longer someone had been inactive, the more irrelevant exercise was for them.

INTERVENTIONS

There are gaps in our knowledge about exercise determinants, in part because physical activity participation is a dynamic process. Factors that support an active lifestyle may not be the same over time, across populations, in different settings, or for different exercise programs. In addition, there is no consensus of guidelines for interventions to increase and maintain physical activity. Traditional interventions have not addressed the cyclical or dynamic nature of exercise behavior, and the drop-out rate from structured exercise programs has remained at 50% for the past 20 years (23). Participating in regular physical activity is a complicated behavioral process, and designing and implementing strategies to help people become more active and stay that way is a challenge.

To determine the efficacy of interventions and factors that moderate their success, we conducted a quantitative meta-analysis of 127 studies and 14 dissertations on interventions to increase physical activity published between 1965 and 1975 (9). Overall, we found a moderately large effect for increasing exercise adherence. Weighted by sample size, we found no difference as a function of age, sex, or race. The most successful interventions applied behavioral modification strategies to healthy subjects in a group setting. Effects were greater in studies using mediated approaches (e.g., print mailings, telephone) than in those using face-to-face or face-to-face and mediated approaches and in studies promoting low-intensity leisure activities. However, because of limited numbers of studies with various moderator variables, we were unable to analyze interactions among factors such as setting and intervention type.

Interventions to change exercise behavior are described in the context of the target group, the setting in which the intervention is implemented, and the level at which it is directed. Characteristics of the target group, such as age, living situation, and education, influence intervention selection. The setting can range from a high school physical education class to a factory and presents a variety of resources and limitations. Interventions can be applied on an individual, group, or community level, which can affect the choice of specific strategies. A wide range of strategies has been used to influence physical activity, and examples are used to illustrate the more effective approaches.

Target Group

It is becoming increasingly evident that the application of one theory or type of intervention in general without considering the unique demands of the population has limited impact. Certain characteristics of the target group must be taken into account to select the best strategy, setting, and level of intervention. Demographic variables, such as age, sex, ethnicity, and education, can provide important information about structuring an intervention to be more appealing to participants.

Exercise stage refers to a classification based on the transtheoretical (stages of change) model, which presents behavior change as a dynamic process that occurs through a series of stages characterized by exercise history and motivational readiness (48,49). Empiric analysis of the model established five distinct stages that are stable but open to change. This model has been applied to exercise to place people in stages according to their past and present exercise behavior and their intentions. People in the *precontemplation* stage are inactive and have no plans to start exercising. People in the *contemplation* stage are also inactive, but they are considering starting an exercise program. During the *preparation* stage, a

plan has been made but not implemented. People in the *action* stage have started regular exercise within the past 6 months but are at greater risk of not adhering than those individuals in the *maintenance* stage, who have been active for more than 6 months and for whom exercise behavior is more established.

Most interventions are for people who are prepared to take action (49). However, studies that have measured stages of change typically have reported that 10% to 20% of their subjects had no plans to change their behavior, 20% to 35% were thinking about changing, and only 25% were actually ready to change (45,48,50–53). According to this model, traditional participant recruitment strategies have little effect on people who are not ready to change. Other strategies must be used to persuade disinterested people to consider change and then motivate them to take action. In addition, strategies to increase exercise adoption in motivated individuals use different cognitive and behavioral techniques than interventions designed to help newly active individuals maintain adherence to exercise. Programs that have matched interventions to stage of change have been effective in increasing exercise adoption and adherence in community (34,54) and medical settings (51,55).

Intervention Setting

Interventions to increase physical activity can be applied in the home, schools, work sites, and community. Settings in which the intervention is implemented have real and perceived barriers, as well as supports for physical activity, depending on the target group. Home-based programs may offer accessibility and convenience, but should provide initial instruction in self-management strategies and appropriate exercise prescriptions. This would be particularly important for those just beginning to exercise. Project PACE (Physician-Based Assessment and Counseling for Exercise) has been used successfully in health care settings to increase exercise adoption and adherence (51,55). Patients are triaged based on the stages of change model and are given customized information packets and counseling by their physician and supported by nurses and staff.

Several interventions have been implemented in the schools and at work sites. Schools are a critical setting for the development of health behaviors, but most physical education classes do not teach the skills necessary to increase activity out of class or maintain physical activity after graduation. Several comprehensive health promotion programs have been implemented in the schools, such as CATCH (56), SPARK (57), and "Know Your Body" (58). There is some evidence for moderate effects of these school-based programs, but there is a disturbing national trend toward reduction in required physical education classes as grade level increases. According to the 1995 YRBS, although 80.7% of ninth graders were enrolled in physical education classes, this proportion decreased to 42.2% by the twelfth grade (15). Since physical activity significantly declines in adolescents, more community opportunities for recreational activities and sports should be considered.

In 1992, 42% of work sites offered physical activity and fitness programs, up from 22% in 1985 (12). These programs vary widely in available facilities, activities offered, target audiences, costs to employees, and incentives. Work site fitness programs have had equivocal success, and onsite facilities may be a barrier to individuals who are dependent on others for transportation home. A recent meta-analysis of 25 studies published between 1972 and 1997 found a small (0.25 SD) effect size for work site interventions (59). The generally poor scientific quality of the literature on this topic precludes the judgment that interventions at work sites cannot increase physical activity or fitness. Work site programs may provide information and encouragement to get employees to begin exercising, but additional studies using valid research designs and measures are needed.

Community interventions can be provided by churches, private and nonprofit fitness centers, and city or county recreational departments. The type of intervention can range from exercise classes to mass media campaigns. Programs in churches can provide social support, encouragement, positive role models, peer-led exercise classes, and information about exercise through church channels (60). For-profit and nonprofit fitness centers, such as the YMCA, are natural sites for interventions. Comprehensive facilities, flexible hours of operation, promotion of classes for beginners, and low-cost or complimentary child care are features that can address some barriers to exercise participation. Many city or county recreational departments have neighborhood recreational centers. The effectiveness of their physical activity programs depends on safety, privacy, hours of operation, transportation, child care, and their ability to identify and address special needs of a specific community.

Within each setting, interventions can be implemented at different levels. Strategies can be applied on an individual level, such as with the PACE program; on an interpersonal level, such as in an aerobics class; or on a community level, such as the Minnesota Heart Health Project (61). Community-based fun runs or walks supporting a local charity may stimulate individuals who primarily want to help the organization to promote exercise for its own sake. However, interventions at the level of the community or society must also provide an environment that supports an active lifestyle. Proposing legislation and environmental engineering to ensure safe, accessible facilities for exercise, which include well-equipped buildings and safe neighborhoods in which to walk, jog, and bicycle, can be implemented on a community-wide and state-wide level to address barriers to participation (11).

Barriers to physical activity can also be defined on different levels. Barriers can be personal, such as low levels of exercise self-efficacy or perceived lack of time. Past injuries and chronic diseases can be physical barriers to adopting an active lifestyle. Barriers can also be interpersonal. Peer pressure to engage in sedentary behaviors or discouraging comments about attempts to be more active can hinder adoption and maintenance. Environmental barriers to exercise include inclement weather or lack of transportation to an exercise facility. Sociocultural factors, such as associating thinness with fitness, can influence motivation to exercise. Life transitions, such as graduation, marriage, childbirth, or divorce, can disrupt an established exercise routine.

Strategies to Increase Physical Activity

The goals of an intervention such as a *media campaign* vary according to the individual's stage of readiness. The primary goal of a media campaign may be to capture the individual's attention and motivate him or her to contemplate becoming more active. For those who are already considering participation in an activity program, the desired outcome is to motivate them toward action by increasing the relevance of the behavior change or decreasing the barriers they perceive. Mass media campaigns and marketing strategies, such as health fairs, can be useful to individuals in the precontemplation and contemplation stages by increasing awareness and providing concrete information about exercise classes and programs. *Health screenings* and *health risk appraisals* (HRAs) can relate health information to individual circumstances and enhance motivation to become more active. For individuals in an action phase, the utility of the media campaign is diminished, but continued support and reinforcement should be provided to encourage continuation or maintenance of activity and the development of strategies to resume activity after relapse.

By itself, an *exercise prescription* has not been effective in increasing exercise adherence. In 1993, the American College of Sports Medicine (ACSM) and the U.S. Centers for Disease Control and Prevention (CDC) began promoting an active lifestyle program (43). Rather than prescribe 15 to 60 minutes of a specific percentage of someone's exercise capacity 3 to 5 days per week, this recommendation is to accumulate 30 or more minutes of moderate intensity exercise in multiple bouts of at least 10 minutes most days of the week. This alternative approach may reduce perceived barriers to participation, such as time and effort, and make regular physical activity more psychologically accessible. For example, a sedentary postmenopausal woman might not have considered regular exercise when the previous prescriptions were promoted, but would consider the current recommendation, especially if she is already walking at some level. However, few studies have tested the effects of the active lifestyle recommendations on health outcomes and adherence. These training studies that have compared short multiple bouts of activity to one longer continuous bout have focused primarily on cardiovascular fitness benefits (44,62,63).

Other strategies have been used to change exercise behavior and may be useful in conjunction with a lifestyle approach. *Behavioral management approaches* are based on behavioral modification theory and generally target the antecedents and consequences of exercise behavior. *Stimulus control* involves manipulating antecedent conditions, or cues, which can prompt behavior; this method is frequently used with individuals and small groups but can be applied on a community level. A classic study by Brownell et al (64), which was replicated by Blamey et al (65) in 1995, successfully used a point of decision cue in the form of a poster placed near the escalator and stairs encouraging people to take the stairs (64,65).

Motivation to exercise depends on anticipated future benefits and more immediate intrinsic and extrinsic rewards (42,66). *Reinforcement management* is crucial when someone begins to exercise, because the longer someone has been inactive, the longer it takes for exercise itself to become reinforcing. Immediate feedback from exercise can be pain and fatigue, so external, immediate, positive rewards are especially necessary for beginners.

Self-monitoring has been used as a cognitive-behavior modification strategy to help identify cues and barriers to exercise and scheduling changes that must be made to fit in an exercise routine. Effective *goal-setting* is also critical (7,67,68). Flexible goals that are consistent with capabilities, values, resources, and needs are more effective than general, nonspecific goals. Since self-efficacy can be increased with mastery experiences, initial goals should be challenging but realistic to foster confidence.

Increasing physical activity in our society entails a fundamental challenge to the established and powerful social and technologic inducements to be sedentary, such as TV and labor-saving technologies. Recently, *community-based interventions* have applied psychological behavioral theories for behavior change on a broad basis (10). These approaches go beyond the traditional practice of individual counseling to include organizational (e.g., community recreation centers, churches, diffusion strategies through schools), environmental (e.g., facility planning), and social (e.g., family interventions) macrochanges. They have also used cost-effective or pragmatically convenient avenues (e.g., mailings, telephone campaigns) for reaching large numbers of individuals who might not be accessible or amenable to traditional clinically based interventions.

Examples of environmental strategies that are being implemented in communities include restricting downtown centers to foot or bicycle traffic to encourage walking or bicycling to work. Other policy approaches suggest changing building codes to make stairs more accessible and safe and passing legislation to fund more parks and recreation centers. Many states are now considering legislation to offer companies incentives for employer-sponsored fitness programs.

In summary, interventions must be applied based on characteristics of the target group, limitations of the setting, and consideration of potential barriers to participation. Multilevel, multicomponent programs are more likely to be effective in fostering long-term behavior change and creating environments that prompt increased activity, offer accessible facilities, reward physical activity, and remove real and perceived barriers.

RESEARCH ISSUES

Research on determinants as a whole is characterized by an absence of uniform standards for defining and assessing physical activity and its determinants, differences in sample characteristics, and limited application of theoretical models. The diversity of the variables, population segments, time periods, and settings sampled in published studies makes it difficult to interpret and compare results. We also know little about determinants in different populations. There are too few studies of children, elderly and physically challenged persons, and ethnic or minority groups and too few comparisons between men and women to permit conclusions about how determinants in these cases differ from general observations (7,8,10,29,69–71).

Measurement of Physical Activity

One of the major research issues in identifying determinants of physical activity is accurate and reliable assessment of the behavior in question. Physical activity has been quantified using self-report data gathered through questionnaires, interviews, and activity diaries and with more objective methods, such as motion sensors and observation. Considering that there are more than 30 different methods to measure physical activity in children and youth alone (29), the difficulty in comparing results across studies without uniform assessment methods is obvious. Recently, a collection of the latest versions of popular physical activity questionnaires, along with descriptions of their use and information about reliability and validity, was published as a supplement to *Medicine and Science in Sports and Exercise* (72). Hopefully, this publication will support more appropriate and consistent measurement of physical activity and forestall new research with unvalidated questionnaires.

Specific methods of physical activity assessment have their own limitations. Self-reports of physical activity are dependent on recall accuracy, which can be influenced by the time between the activity and the recall, the salience of the behavior, the social desirability of the response, demographics, and the structure of the instrument (73). Surveys with longer time frames are subject to recall bias and are difficult to validate. Self-reports of physical activity are also less accurate for the sporadically active.

Motion sensors can give us information about total activity for a specified period, but do not tell us type or intensity and may not be able to measure activities such as cycling or swimming. In addition, physical activity has several definitions as an outcome variable, such as number of days active per week or total energy expenditure, which make it difficult to compare studies.

Moderate- and low-intensity exercise programs have better adherence rates than high-intensity exercise (8), but activities at moderate and low intensities are easily forgotten and difficult to measure (74), making it difficult to discover if different factors control their adoption and adherence. We also know little about determinants of different types of physical activity, which include sports and leisure-time activities, as well as endurance exercise and strength training.

Measurement of Determinants

Research on determinants as a whole is characterized by limitations of measurement methods (e.g., lack of standardized psychological variables), the limited number of studies that have used the same variables or instruments, and differences in sample characteristics. There is a plethora of instruments to measure purported psychosocial determinants, many of which do not have established reliability and validity. In addition, there may be several different instruments reported in the literature that measure the same construct. For example, two recent studies of the influence of enjoyment on the maintenance of physical activity reported opposite results but used different measures of enjoyment (33,75)

In recent years, investigators have begun to develop psychometrically sound instruments to measure potential determinants of physical activity. These include physical self-concept (76), physical activity enjoyment (75), exercise motivation (77,78), expected outcomes and barriers for physical activity (80), social support (79), and self-efficacy (45,81).

Lack of experimental studies and good measures of past habits and the causes of past habits has also limited our ability to clarify the issue of selection bias. Without knowing exercise history, we do not know if people are more active because they have higher self-efficacy, or they have higher self-efficacy because of past success with exercise and their experience is the true determinant of their current behavior. Not knowing exercise history can also affect our ability to identify differences, if any, in factors influencing adoption, drop out, maintenance, and resumption of exercise after a period of inactivity.

Some progress has been made recently regarding research on adoption of physical activity. Sedentary students who perceived themselves as exercisers (self-schemata) were likely to adopt exercise in the near future (82). Adoption of vigorous exercise by a community sample of sedentary men during a 2-year period was predicted by self-efficacy, age, and neighborhood environment. Adoption by women was predicted by education, self-efficacy, and friend and family support for exercise (83). In the same study, maintenance of vigorous exercise was predicted by some of the same variables. While some variables predicted both adoption and maintenance, the model was more successful in predicting adoption.

An ongoing shortcoming of the determinants research is that studies have poorly distinguished between adoption and maintenance (adherence) and have not examined determinants of periodicity of exercise (i.e., resumption after dropout). The biggest gap in the physical activity behavior literature in the past 10 years is that studies have not explained why people drop out of regular exercise. Although the stages of change model offers potential for designing interventions to help people begin an exercise program, it does a poor job accounting for why people in the maintenance stage drop out.

Theory

Most social psychology models of the determinants of behavior recognize that ability moderates the impact that social and psychological variables have on behavior, or these models posit an assumption of equal ability among persons. Because physical activity is biologically based behavior, the role of genetic (22) and biologic influences on physical activity must be understood, since these factors may interact with, or modify, social and psychological determinants. Applications of social-cognitive variables to understanding physical activity typically have not included measures of biologic influences on physical activity. Hence, nearly all of the exercise adherence literature has failed to recognize that social determinants of physical activity occur in a biocultural context. It seems unlikely that psychological models that exclude or minimize considerations about biologic aspects of physical activity are sufficient to explain and predict physical activity.

SUMMARY

Gains have been made over the past 15 years in understanding the determinants of physical activity and interventions targeted to the initiation, maintenance, and resumption of exercise behavior. Determinants that reside or originate in the individual are practically important because they can identify population segments that may be responsive or resistive to physical activity interventions. Smoking behavior, occupation, ethnicity, education, income, and obesity are examples of personal attributes that can present barriers to physical activity or be sentinel markers of underlying habits or circumstances that reinforce sedentary living. Too few studies are available on children, elderly and physically challenged persons, and ethnic and minority groups and there are too few direct comparisons of men and women to permit conclusions about determinants and successful interventions in these subgroups.

Reconstructing past activity history is important for interpreting past and present determinants, designing and evaluating plausible interventions, and for predicting future activity. However, currently there is no standardized method for assessing lifetime activity history or stage of behavior change. Attitudes, beliefs and expectations, values, and intentions are amenable to change, but they alone do not predict behavior with sufficient accuracy for practical purposes. Similarly, personality traits do not predict exercise behavior with sufficient accuracy for practical purposes, but they may help explain why cognitive and attitudinal theories offer incomplete predictions of exercise activity (35). Exercise programs with strong social support or reinforcement conducted in settings requiring low-frequency, low-intensity activity may offset differences in personality that might otherwise predispose a person to inactivity. Physical environment variables, such as access to facilities and legislative initiatives, have not been widely studied but have potential for being equally as practical as altering knowledge and attitudes.

REFERENCES

1. Fletcher GF, Blair SN, Blumenthal J, et al. Statement on exercise: benefits and recommendations for physical activity programs for all Americans. Circulation 1992;86:340–344.

2. Physical activity and cardiovascular health. NIH Consensus Statement. 1995;13:1–33.

3. Dishman RK, Buckworth J. Adherence to physical activity. In:

Morgan WP, ed. Physical activity and mental health. Washington, DC: Taylor & Francis, 1996:63–80.

4. Blair SN, Kampert JB, Kohl HW, et al. Influences of cardiorespiratory fitness and other precursors on cardiovascular disease and all-cause mortality in men and women. JAMA 1996;276:205–210.

5. Caspersen CJ, Powell KE, Christenson GM. Physical activity, exercise, and physical fitness: definitions and distinctions for health-related research. Pub Health Rep 1985;100:126–131.

6. NIH Consensus Conference. Physical activity and cardiovascular health. JAMA 1996;276:241–246.

7. Dishman RK, Sallis JF. Determinants and interventions for

physical activity and exercise. In: Bouchard C, Shephard RJ, eds. Physical activity, fitness and health: international proceedings and consensus statement. Champaign, IL: Human Kinetics, 1994: 214–238.

8. Sallis JF, Hovell MF. Determinants of exercise behavior. Exerc Sport Sci Rev 1990;11:307–330.

9. Dishman RK, Buckworth J. Increasing physical activity: a quantitative synthesis. Med Sci Sports Exerc 1996;28:706–719.

10. King AC, Blair SN, Bild D, et al. Determinants of physical activity and interventions in adults. Med Sci Sports Exerc 1992;24(suppl): S221–S236.

11. Blair SN, Booth M, Gyarfas I, et al. Development of public policy and physical activity initiatives internationally. Sports Med 1996; 21:157–163.

12. U.S. Department of Health and Human Services. Physical activity and health: a report of the Surgeon General. Atlanta, GA: U.S. Department of Health and Human Services, Centers for Disease Control and Prevention, National Center for Chronic Disease Prevention and Health Promotion, 1996.

13. Douglas KA, Collins JL, Warren CW, et al. Results from the 1995 national college health risk behavior survey. J Am College Health 1997;46:55–66.

14. Kelley GA. Gender differences in the physical activity levels of young African-American adults. J Natl Med Assoc 1995;87:545–548.

15. Kann L, Warren CW, Harris WA, et al. Youth risk behavior surveillance—United States, 1995. MMWR 1996;45(SS-4):1–83.

16. Booth ML, Macaskill P, Owen N, et al. Population prevalence and correlates of stages of change in physical activity. Health Ed Q 1993;20:431–440.

17. Dietz WH. The role of lifestyle in health: the epidemiology and consequences of inactivity.

Proc Nutr Soc 1996;55:829–840.

18. Anderson LB. Tracking of risk factors for coronary heart disease from adolescence to young adulthood with special emphasis on physical activity and fitness: a longitudinal study. Ph.D. dissertation, Danish State Institute of Education, 1996.

19. Kaplan GA, Strawbridge WJ, Cohen RD, et al. Natural history of leisure-time physical activity and its correlates: associations with mortality from all causes and cardiovascular disease over 28 years. Am J Epidemiol 1996;144:793–797.

20. Schmitz K, French SA, Jeffery RW. Correlates of changes in leisure time physical activity over 2 years: the healthy worker project. Prev Med 1997;26:570–579.

21. Bouchard C, Pérusse L. Heredity, activity level, fitness, and health. In: Bouchard C, Shephard RJ, eds. Physical activity, fitness, and health: international proceedings and consensus statement. 2nd ed. Champaign, IL: Human Kinetics, 1994:106–118.

22. Pérusse L, Tremblay A, LeBlanc C, et al. Genetic and environmental influences on level of habitual physical activity and exercise participation. Am J Epidemiol 1989; 129:1012–1022.

23. Dishman RK. Predicting and changing exercise and physical activity: what's practical and what's not. In: Quinn HA, Gauvin L, Wall AET, eds. Toward active living: proceedings of the International Conference on Physical Activity, Fitness, and Health. Champaign, IL: Human Kinetics, 1994:97–106.

24. Pate RR, Heath GW, Dowda M, et al. Associations between physical activity and other health behaviors in a representative sample of US adolescents. Am J Pub Health 1996;86:1577–1581.

25. Sallis JF, Hovell MF, Hofstetter CR, et al. A multivariate study of determinants of vigorous activity in a community sample. Prev Med 1989;18:20–34.

26. Kaplan GA, Cohen RD, Lazarus NB, et al. Psychosocial factors in the natural history of physical activity. Am J Prev Med 1991;7: 12–17.

27. Dishman RK. Supervised and free-living physical activity: no differences in former athletes and nonathletes. Am J Prev Med 1988; 4:153–160.

28. Young DR, Steinhardt MA. An analysis of the psychobiological model in a supervised exercise setting. Health Values 1991;15: 42–48.

29. Sallis JF, Simons-Morton BG, Stone EJ, et al. Determinants of physical activity and interventions in youth. Med Sci Sports Exerc 1992;24:S248–S257.

30. Armstrong CA, Sallis JF, Hovell MF, et al. Stages of change, self-efficacy, and the adoption of vigorous exercise: a prospective analysis. J Sport Exerc Psychol 1993;15:390–402.

31. McAuley E, Jacobson L. Self-efficacy and exercise participation in sedentary adult females. Am J Health Prom 1991;5:185–191.

32. Wilcox S, Storandt M. Relations among age, exercise, and psychological variables in a community sample of women. Health Psychol 1996;15:110–113.

33. Garcia AW, King AC. Predicting long-term adherence to aerobic exercise: a comparison of two models. J Sport Exerc Psychol 1991;13:394–410.

34. Morgan WP, O'Connor PJ. Exercise and mental health. In: Dishman RK, ed. Exercise adherence: its impact on public health. Champaign, IL: Human Kinetics, 1988: 91–92.

35. Dzewaltowski DA. Physical activity determinants: a social cognitive approach. Med Sci Sports Exerc 1994;26:1395–1399.

36. Klonoff EA, Annechild A, Landrine H. Predicting exercise adherence in women: the role of psychological and physiological factors. Prev Med 1994;23:257–262.

37. Dishman RK, Ickes W. Self-motivation and adherence to therapeutic exercise. J Behav Med 1981;4:421–437.

38. Sallis JF, Hovell MF, Hofstetter CR, et al. Distance between homes and exercise facilities related to frequency of exercise among San Diego residents. Public Health Rep 1990;105:179–185.

39. Duncan TE, Duncan SC, McAuley E. The role of domain and gender-specific provisions of social relations in adherence to a prescribed exercise regimen. J Sport Exerc Psychol 1993;15:220–231.

40. MacDougall C, Cooke R, Owen N, et al. Relating physical activity to health status, social connections, and community facilities. Aust New Zealand J Pub Health 1997; 21:557–558.

41. Treiber FA, Baranowski T, Braden DS, et al. Social support for exercise: relationship to physical activity in young adults. Prev Med 1991;20:737–750.

42. Wankel LM. The importance of enjoyment to adherence and psychological benefits from physical activity. Int J Sport Psychol 1993; 24:151–169.

43. Pate RR, Pratt M, Blair SN, et al. Physical activity and public health: a recommendation from the Centers for Disease Control and Prevention and the American College of Sports Medicine. JAMA 1995;273:402–407.

44. Jakicic JM, Wing RR, Butler BA, et al. Prescribing exercise in multiple short bouts versus one continuous bout: effects on adherence, cardiorespiratory fitness, and weight loss in overweight women. Int J Obes Metab Disord 1995; 19:893–901.

45. Marcus BH, Selby VC, Niaura RS, et al. Self-efficacy and the stages of exercise behavior change. Res Q Exerc Sport 1992;63:60–66.

46. Marcus BH, Banspach SW, Lefebvre RC, et al. Using the stage of change model to increase the adoption of physical activity among community participants. Am J Health Promo 1992;6: 424–429.

47. Auweele YA, Rzewnicki R, Van Mele V. Reasons for not exercising and exercise intentions: a study of middle-aged sedentary adults. J Sports Sci 1997;15:151–165.

48. Marcus BH, Simkin LR. The stages of exercise behavior. J Sport Med Phys Fitness 1993;33:83–88.

49. Prochaska JO, Marcus BH. The transtheoretical model: applications to exercise. In: Dishman RK, ed. Advances in exercise adherence. Champaign, IL: Human Kinetics, 1994:161–180.

50. Marcus BH, Rossi JS, Selby VC, et al. The stages and processes of exercise adoption and maintenance in a worksite sample. Health Psychol 1992;11:386–395.

51. Calfas KJ, Long BJ, Sallis JF, et al. A controlled trial of physician counseling to promote the adoption of physical activity. Prev Med 1996;25:225–233.

52. Prochaska JO, Velicer WF, Rossi JS, et al. Stages of change and decisional balance for 12 problem behaviors. Health Psychol 1994; 13:39–46.

53. Godin G. The theories of reasoned action and planned behavior: overview of findings, emerging research problems, and usefulness for exercise promotion. J Appl Sport Psychol 1993;5:141–157.

54. Dunn AL, Marcus BH, Kampert JB, et al. Reduction in cardiovascular disease risk factors: six-month results from Project Active. Prev Med 1997;26:883–892.

55. Patrick K, Sallis JF, Long B, et al. A new tool for encouraging activity: Project PACE. Phys Sportsmed 1994;22:45–55.

56. Luepker RV, Perry CL, McKinlay SM, et al. Outcome of a field trial to improve children's dietary patterns and physical activity: the child and adolescent trial for cardiovascular health. JAMA 1996; 275:768–776.

57. Sallis JF, McKenzie TL, Alcaraz JE, et al. Effects of a two-year health-related physical education program on physical activity and fitness in elementary students: SPARK. 1996(in press).

58. Bush PJ, Zuckerman AE, Theiss PK, et al. Cardiovascular risk prevention in black schoolchildren: two-year results of the know your body program. Am J Epidemiol 1989;129:466–482.

59. Dishman RK, Oldenburg B, O'Neal H, et al. Worksite physical activity interventions. Am J Prev Med 1998;15:344–361.

60. Hatch JW, Cunningham AC, Woods WW, et al. The fitness through churches project: description of a community-based cardiovascular health promotion intervention. Hygiene 1986;5:9–12.

61. Blake SM, Jeffery RW, Finnegan JR, et al. Process evaluation of a community-based physical activity campaign: the Minnesota Heart Health program experience. Health Ed Res 1987;2:115–121.

62. DeBusk RF, Stenestrand U, Haskell WL. Training effects of long versus short bouts of exercise in healthy subjects. Am J Cardiol 1990;65:1010–1013.

63. Edisu T. Splitting the distance of endurance training on cardiovascular endurance and blood lipids. Jap J Phys Ed 1985;30:37.

64. Brownell K, Stunkard AJ, Albaum J. Evaluation and modification of exercise patterns in the natural environment. Am J Psychiatr 1980;136:1540–1545.

65. Blamey A, Mutrie N, Aitchison T. Health promotion by encouraged use of stairs. Br Med J 1995;311: 289–290.

66. Rutherford WJ, Corbin CB, Chase LA. Factors influencing intrinsic motivation towards physical activity. Health Values 1992;16:19–24.

67. Buckworth J. Behavior modification. In: Howley ET, Franks DB, eds. Health fitness instructor's handbook. 3rd ed. Champaign, IL: Human Kinetics, 1997:389–403.

68. O'Connor MJ. Exercise promotion in physical education: application of the transtheoretical model. J Teach Phys Ed 1994;1:2–12.

69. Gregg EW, Narayan KMV, Kriska AM, et al. Relationship of locus of

control to physical activity among people with and without diabetes. Diabetes Care 1996;19:1118–1121.

70. Douthitt VL. Psychological determinants of adolescent exercise adherence. Adolescence 1994;29:711–722.

71. Shephard RJ. Determinants of exercise in people aged 65 years and older. In: Dishman RK, ed. Advances in exercise adherence. Champaign, IL: Human Kinetics, 1994:343–360.

72. Kriska AM, Caspersen CJ. A collection of physical activity questionnaires for health-related research. Med Sci Sports Exerc 1997;29 (suppl):S5–S9.

73. Durante R, Ainsworth BE. The recall of physical activity: using a cognitive model of the question-answering process. Med Sci Sports Exerc 1996;28:1282–1291.

74. Kriska AM, Casperson C. Introduction to a collection of physical activity questionnaires. Med Sci Sports Exerc 1997;29(suppl):S5–S9.

75. Kendzierski D, DeCarlo KJ. Physical activity enjoyment scale: two validation studies. J Sport Exerc Psychol 1991;13:50–64.

76. Marsh HW, Richards GE, Johnson S, et al. Physical self-description questionnaire: psychometric properties and a multitrait-multimethod analysis of relations to existing instruments. J Sport Exerc Psychol 1994;16:270–305.

77. Markland D, Hardy L. The exercise motivation inventory: preliminary development and validity of a measure of individuals' reasons for participation in regular physical exercise. Person Individ Diff 1993;15:289–296.

78. Marcus BH, Rakowski W, Rossi JS. Assessing motivational readiness and decision making for exercise. Health Psychol 1992;11:257–261.

79. Sallis JF, Grossman RM, Pinski RB, et al. The development of scales to measure social support for diet and exercise behaviors. Prev Med 1987;16:825–836.

80. Steinhardt M, Dishman RK. Reliability and validity of expected outcomes and barriers for habitual physical activity. J Occup Med 1989;31:536–546.

81. Sallis JF, Pinski RB, Grossman RM, et al. The development of self-efficacy scales for health-related diet and exercise behaviors. Health Ed Res 1988;3:283–292.

82. Kendzierski D. Exercise self-schemata: cognitive and behavioral correlates. Health Psychol 1990;9:69–82.

83. Sallis JF, Hovell MF, Hofstetter CR. Predictors of adoption and maintenance of vigorous physical activity in men and women. Prev Med 1992;21:237–251.

Part XVI.

OBESITY AND WEIGHT MANAGEMENT

Edited by
John P. Foreyt
Walker S. Carlos Poston

Introduction to Obesity and Weight Management

John P. Foreyt
Walker S. Carlos Poston

Obesity is one of the most pressing public health problems facing the United States and many other industrialized nations (1). Obesity is defined as a body mass index (BMI) 30 or greater and current standards define three severity levels: class I (BMI 30 to 34.9), class II (BMI 35 to 39.9), and class III (BMI ≥ 40) (2). The age-adjusted prevalence rates of class I, class II, and class III obesity in U.S. adults are estimated to be 14.4%, 5.2%, and 2.9%, respectively, which represent substantial increases over the last several decades (2). Although the prevalence of obesity has been increasing at alarming rates, cures have remained elusive. Given the multifactorial nature of obesity, most experts have come to recognize it as a chronic disease that requires long-term, multidisciplinary management (2).

The successful management of obese patients involves multiple treatment strategies, most of which focus on modifying aspects of the patient's lifestyle (i.e., changing dietary and physical activity habits). Behavior modification, although not an intervention in and of itself, is a method for systematically modifying eating, exercise, or other behaviors that are thought to contribute to or maintain obesity. Thus, the first chapters in this section provide comprehensive reviews of the literature on the exercise and dietary management of the obese patient.

In the first chapter, Tamara and David Lombard examine the importance of energy expenditure in weight loss and maintenance and how energy expenditure is affected by exercise and lifestyle activity. They then turn their attention to the potential mechanisms by which exercise and lifestyle activity may contribute to weight loss (i.e., exercise-related changes in resting metabolic rate and caloric intake). They conclude by reviewing important barriers to modifying physical activity and the behavioral strategies that have been found most helpful in promoting long-term adherence.

In the second chapter, Sachiko St. Jeor, Judith Ashley, and Jon Schrage address the role of dietary change in the successful management of obese patients. In this chapter they present a review of the use of low-calorie diets and very-low-calorie diets in obesity management. In addition, they present a stepped-care model for matching patients to the different dietary interventions and provide guidelines on how to ensure that the various diets provide adequate nutrition. They discuss methods for developing dietary prescriptions that incorporate an obese patient's current weight, goals for weight loss, and activity level. Finally, they provide information on methods for promoting adherence to dietary change, the role of dietary supplements and fat and sugar substitutes, and the future of dietary treatments.

Even though physical activity and dietary change are crucial to long-term obesity management, results of lifestyle programs are modest due to poor long-term adherence and limited applicability for the severely obese (i.e., BMI ≥ 40). For example, in most studies with extended follow-up, patients gradually return to baseline within several years after treatment termination unless some form of maintenance program with sustained contact is implemented. Given that obesity is a chronic disease, the importance of adjunctive pharmacotherapy cannot be overlooked. In the third chapter, Nikhil Dhurandhar and Richard Atkinson review current obesity pharmacotherapies and their primary mechanisms (i.e., reducing food intake, nutrient partitioning, or increasing energy expenditure). They provide an overview of drugs currently approved by the Food and Drug Administration (FDA) and describe several experimental drugs that may be on the market in the future. They provide current guidelines for selecting appropriate patients for adjunctive drug treatments and review the literature on drug efficacy and safety.

Some patients suffer from such severe obesity that nothing short of surgical intervention is appropriate. In the fourth chapter, Harvey Sugerman, Eric DeMaria, John Kellum, and Michael Schweitzer review the research evaluating surgical procedures for severely obese patients. They discuss selection criteria, the effectiveness of the various procedures, common adverse effects, and the role of the surgeon in the long-term follow-up of obese patients who have undergone surgical treatment.

In the final chapter, Risa Stein, C. Keith Haddock, W. S. Carlos Poston, and John Foreyt discuss the future of obesity research. In this chapter they examine the value of broadening obesity management outcomes assessment to include factors such as improved psychological and metabolic health (e.g., body acceptance, fitness, etc.) and the importance of viewing treatment as a life-long process. In addition, they discuss future trends in lifestyle management and pharmacotherapy, including the application of psychosocial therapies to address interpersonal problems that many obese patients experience and the development of new drugs that may improve long-term outcomes, particularly neuropeptide agonists/antagonists and gene products. Finally, they discuss the importance of viewing obesity from a public health perspective and describe population-based measures that may help to address the growing epidemic.

REFERENCES

1. World Health Organization (WHO). Obesity: Preventing and managing the global epidemic. Report of a WHO consultation on obesity. Geneva: World Health Organization, 1998.

2. National Institutes of Health (NIH), National Heart, Lung, and Blood Institute (NHLBI). Clinical guidelines on the identification, evaluation, and treatment of overweight and obesity: The evidence report. Washington D.C.: U.S. Government Printing Office, 1998.

Chapter 90

Exercise Management of the Obese Patient

Tamara Neubauer Lombard
David Neubauer Lombard

Even given decades of research, weight management is still a matter of creating a deficit between caloric intake and energy expenditure. Is decreasing caloric intake the most appropriate goal for weight reduction programs? Population studies would suggest not. In both the United States and Europe population surveys indicated that over the past several decades the average daily caloric intake has been decreasing, yet the average weight and rates of obesity have been increasing (1). This has led to the conclusion that energy expenditure, not caloric intake, should be the focus for successful weight loss efforts.

Past research indicates physical activity is the single most important behavior for long-term weight management in obese people (2,3). Many controlled trials demonstrate that individuals who are physically active lose more weight than nonactive individuals. Moreover, individuals who maintain weight loss typically report exercising regularly versus those who do not maintain their weight loss (4,5). Physical activity produces behavioral, psychological, and physiologic effects that facilitate weight loss and the ultimate maintenance of weight loss (6,7). This chapter briefly examines the physiologic effects of physical activity that promote weight loss and weight maintenance and then discusses the difficulty in initiating and maintaining a physical activity program. A brief review of strategies shown to be helpful in maintaining physical activity also is presented.

ENERGY EXPENDITURE

Physical activity is the most easily controllable way to increase energy expenditure. Daily bouts of physical exercise increase the energy expenditure by the number of calories needed to perform the chosen activity. Simple, but is there an optimal amount or intensity of exercise? The American College of Sports Medicine (ACSM) has set guidelines for recommended physical activity of 30 minutes, 3 times per week, at 70% capacity (8). But, remember the ACSM guidelines are for aerobic fitness, not weight loss. For weight loss, there is the need to create a calorie deficit each day, not just 3 days per week. The greater the deficit, the greater the weight loss. Brownell (9) and others have recommended daily bouts of physical activity of up to 60 minutes to create continuous weight loss through daily deficits between energy intake and energy expenditure.

ENERGY EXPENDITURE DURING PHYSICAL ACTIVITY

If daily bouts of physical exercise are optimal, then at what level of intensity should the activity be done? Should exercise be performed at a low intensity over a long duration to burn numerous calories without much stress on the body (8)? Or, should exercise be performed at a high intensity for a short duration (10)? Research indicates the higher-intensity exercise shows a greater decrease in subcutaneous skinfolds compared to low-intensity exercise even when total energy expenditure is controlled (11).

What are the factors that influence energy expenditure during exercise and why would higher-intensity exercise be more successful in decreasing weight? Several factors influence energy expenditure during physical activity. The first is the total amount of work performed. For example, running 5 miles requires five times the work to run 1 mile if the running pace is the same. Energy expenditure is a fairly linear relationship as long as the task performed is at the same intensity. Second, the efficiency of work can greatly influence energy expenditure. As intensity of the activity performed increases, there appears to be a decrease in the efficiency of the human body to perform the activity. This reduction in efficiency has been shown in cycling (12–14), walking (15), and weight training (16–18). For example, 22% more energy is required to bike at high intensity versus low intensity for the same distance (14). Also, 200% more energy is required for one bench press at 80% of maximum versus four bench presses at 20% of maximum (16).

Why do we see this relationship between increased intensity of activity causing decreases in work efficiency and thus greater energy expenditure? There are numerous theories. First, as intensity increases, there is an increased dependence on the inefficient fast twitch muscle fibers (19), an increase in recruitment of the heart and respiratory muscles (16), and an increased recruitment of stabilizing muscles (16). Second, as intensity increases, there is increased energy expenditure required to remove excess lactate. The third theory targets the changes in the myosis of ATPase activity to cross-bridge sweep ratio and sympathetic nervous activity (10). Regardless of which factors most impact this change in energy expenditure, at higher volumes of high-intensity exercise there will be the greatest effect in increasing energy expenditure during physical activity. Unfortunately, high-intensity, high-volume exercise is very fatiguing, has increased risk for injury, and has a low patient compliance rate. Therefore, we recommend the use of interval training: a mixture of high- and moderate-intensity time periods within the workout session.

RESTING ENERGY EXPENDITURE

Increased energy expenditure during activity is only one target for weight management. A second target is to increase resting energy expenditure. For decades people have attempted to increase their resting energy expenditure with the use of stimulants and other very questionable supplements. Recent research has suggested that increasing the frequency of intense exercise bouts may be the optimal natural process for increasing resting energy expenditure.

What impact does an individual exercise session have on resting energy expenditure? There is a 5% to 15% increase in resting energy expenditure for 1 to 2 days after aerobic exercise of at least 70% of Vo_2max, but not for lower levels of physical activity (14,20–22). Athletes have approximately 5% to 20% higher resting energy expenditure compared to sedentary controls (22a) even after controlling for total body fat. These studies suggest high-intensity exercise will not only increase energy expenditure during the exercise bout, but will also continue creating a calorie deficit for up to 2 days by increasing the energy the body uses when at rest.

Why is there this observed increase in resting energy expenditure? One theory is that the increase in muscle mass is the cause, but there is little increase in muscle mass for each acute episode of exercise. Therefore, this theory is unlikely to be true. Another theory is driven by the fact there are

increases in serum norepinephrine levels following high-intensity aerobic exercise (20) for up to 24 hours. This increase in norepinephrine and the increase in sympathetic tone may be partially responsible for the observed exercise-induced increase in resting energy expenditure. Whatever the reason, high-intensity exercise can increase the body's resting energy expenditure up to 200 kcal/day for 48 hours (10).

So far the research covered only examined aerobic exercise, not weight training. Increasing muscle mass or fat-free mass requires high-intensity training. Weight training is generally done as a high-intensity exercise over a short duration to increase fat-free muscle mass and to increase energy expenditure. But we also see subsequent increases in resting energy expenditure. Professional bodybuilders have resting energy expenditures up to 30% higher than controls (10). Even amateur weight trainers compared to controls have a 5% to 15% higher resting energy expenditure (23–26). These findings are independent of the increase in resting energy expenditure for 1 to 2 days after each acute episode of exercise (10,27).

Given all the correlated findings above, what can we actually say about physical activity as well as the intensity of the activity and its relationship with realized weight loss? Several studies have shown high-intensity exercise is inversely related to rates of obesity (28–30) and lower waist to hip ratios (31). Furthermore, high intensity exercise is independently and negatively related to weight gain on 2-year follow-up after initial weight loss (29). But the problem remains that a large number of people do not like engaging in high-intensity exercise, in some cases because of low baseline fitness levels (32). Perhaps the best recommendation is for a combination of daily moderate-intensity exercise to increase daily expenditure of energy with semidaily episodes of higher-intensity exercise to increase optimal energy expenditure.

AEROBIC EXERCISE IMPACT ON CALORIC INTAKE

Given the recommendations for increased energy expenditure through physical activity, should there be the concern of possible increased calorie consumption secondary to the increased activity levels? A recent review by Perri et al (33) suggested low to moderate levels of exercise are not associated with increases in appetite. Further, Wood et al (34) found moderate exercise may limit preference for dietary fat. But what about higher-intensity exercise?

One theory suggests there is the potential existence of exercise-induced suppression of energy intake/hunger (35–37). Kissileff et al (38) had two groups each of obese and nonobese subjects exercise at either a strenuous or moderate level. After each acute bout of exercise, the subjects were offered food to eat. The researchers found no difference in amount of food eaten for the obese subjects. But, in the nonobese groups, those who engaged in high-intensity exercise ate less than those in the moderate level of exercise. Kissileff et al's results suggested that obese subjects' desire for food may have a psychological nature that overrides the exercise-induced suppression of appetite.

Although this study found changes in food consumed, most others have only found decreases in reported hunger after high-intensity exercise, but not for actual caloric intake (39). Still others (35–37,40,41) report suppression of hunger immediately following bouts of intense exercise. Why do we see this decrease? Theories include elevations in body temperature (42), increases in levels of lactic acid (43), and increases in tumor necrosing factor (44). Regardless of why this difference occurs, the suppression of appetite is short-acting and may not actually decrease overall daily caloric intake.

Does how long one waits to eat after an exercise session impact caloric consumption? Verger et al (45) assessed the impact of offering immediate or delayed meals to subjects after 2 hours of physical activity. Food was offered immediately, 1 hour, or 2 hours after the exercise session. Their results indicated a 2-hour delay was related to decreased hunger and caloric intake. Other results confirm the lack of decrease in caloric consumption if one eats too close to the bout of exercise (39,46).

LIFESTYLE ACTIVITY AND CALORIC CONSUMPTION

What impact does lifestyle activity have on caloric consumption? Mayer et al's classic study (47) of mill workers first found sedentary workers ate as much as the highly active workers, resulting in increased weight. On the other hand, some cross-sectional studies have found highly active individuals have high intake compared to sedentary individuals, but the active individuals tended to be leaner, suggesting a better intake to expenditure ratio (48–50). Hardman (51) also found that highly active subjects had a relatively higher carbohydrate intake. However, others have not found such nutrient-specific selection (48,52).

Numerous longitudinal studies have examined the question of increased activity's impact on caloric intake. Most studies have revealed no increase in energy intake in response to intervention to increase physical activity (53–56). Dempsey (54) had both obese and nonobese subjects engage in three different physical activity programs with varying intensities. Dempsey found no difference in energy consumption due to increased intensity of exercise. Leon et al (55) found no impact on caloric consumption for a 16-week high-intensity walking program. McGowan et al (56) compared the impact of three different intensities of running and found no impact on total caloric intake.

Population, cross-sectional, and longitudinal studies have all suggested that having people increase their physical activity level, even to a high-intensity level, will not create a significant increase in caloric intake. Since food preference may be mostly psychologically and environmentally controlled, dietary choices may be relatively immune to the energy requirements of acute exercise bouts (35–37,57).

DIFFICULTIES IN INITIATING AND MAINTAINING PHYSICAL ACTIVITY

Given the information presented above, it is clear that physical activity is essential in the management of the obese patient. Fortunately most individuals in weight loss programs are successful in initiating exercise programs (7). Unfortunately, just like the nonobese population, individuals who initiate physical activity fail to maintain it over time (8). In addition, although we know exercising at a greater intensity increases the likelihood of weight loss and the corresponding increases in self-efficacy, we also know initiating an exercise program at a high intensity for a sedentary population is almost doomed to fail (58). Further, methods for maintaining physical activity among the population have shown limited effectiveness (58). Similarly, effective methods for maintaining physical activity in obese individuals are not yet known (7).

Methods showing the most promise in the general population for increasing and maintaining physical activity can be examined for application to the obese population. Fortunately, as noted above, health benefits and weight loss and/or maintenance are associated with moderate-intensity, frequent physical activity (i.e., walking, lawn mowing, swimming, housework). This type of activity corresponds well with obese individuals who are likely to be sedentary, who may have issues associated with exercising at a high intensity or in public, and who may never have participated in physical activity in their lifetime.

STRATEGIES FOR IMPROVING INITIATION AND MAINTENANCE OF PHYSICAL ACTIVITY

A brief review of the literature reveals behavior change strategies that have been somewhat effective in increasing physical activity. These strategies are: prompting, goal setting, feedback, problem solving, and self-monitoring. However, although these strategies have been used to increase initiation of physical activity, they have not shown much effect, if any, on maintenance of physical activity. It is hypothesized that these strategies show potential for maintenance of physical activity when program development combines initiation strategies with those designed for maintenance of behavior change.

Prompting

Kazdin (59) defined prompting as behavior initiation through antecedent events. A prompt is delivered immediately before the opportunity for the behavior. Brownell et al (60) used posted prompts at escalator/stair choice points in a variety of community settings and showed an increase in the use of stairs. After removal of the prompts, the increase in stair use maintained at 1 month, but fell after 3 months. Thus, use of posted prompts showed good effects for initiation if present, but poor continued behavior when removed.

Other researchers have used telephone prompts to increase exercise. Telephone prompts increased attendance and maintenance at a health club (61) and adherence to a home-based program (62). King et al (63) found the addition of weekly phone calls to a home-based intervention had good effects for adoption of physical activity and for fitness levels.

These authors used stimulus control and prompting strategies appropriately for initiation but not for maintenance. Kazdin (59), stated that, ideally, a program would continue to use the initial cues and then develop other cues to prompt the behavior (e.g., gradually moving toward using environmental or social cues as prompts for the behavior). Importantly, the prompt needs to be specific and within close temporal and spatial proximity to the target behavior. For instance, rather than someone associated with a program calling the exerciser, a friend or spouse could prompt physical activity. A posted cartoon could be used. For example, a cartoon posted on the back of the remote control, on the television dial, on the refrigerator, or on the dashboard of the car could prompt physical activity at an active-sedentary choice point. Thus, prompting could potentially be effective for maintenance of physical activity.

Goal Setting

Kazdin (59) defined goal setting as specification of a behavior or set of behaviors to be performed at a specified period of time. Bandura (64) stated goal setting is most effective when individuals set challenging but achievable goals.

Through several studies, Martin et al (65) assessed the differential effects of individual goal setting. One study examined the effect of distance goals (i.e., distance to walk) versus time goals (i.e., time to walk). Adherence required class attendance plus a third-day run outside of class. Results show greater adherence for time goals (76.4%) than for distance goals (67.3%). At 3-month follow-up, time goals and distance goals showed similar maintenance (23% versus 29%).

The next study examined distance goals (because they were more convenient to administer) within a fixed-goal (i.e., consistent goal over time) or a flexible-goal condition (i.e., changing goal over time). Flexible goal setting showed a greater effect (83.7%) than fixed goal setting (67.8%). In addition, the flexible goal-setting condition showed the lowest dropout rate (0%).

The next study examined the effect of distal (mileage goals set at the beginning and middle of program) versus proximal (new mileage goals set each week) goal setting with a flexible-distance goal. Results indicated greater adherence for the distal goal-setting condition (83%) than for the proximal goal-setting condition (71%). The investigators found a more pronounced effect at follow-up: distal (67%) and proximal (33%). This result is interesting because behavior modification techniques for initiation stress continual reinforcement and proximal goal setting for continued success. However, this study showed greater short-term and long-term effects for a distal goal. Perhaps initiation with distal goals generalized better for longer-term adherence than initiation with proximal goals.

Several conclusions were drawn from the goal-setting studies reviewed. First, when individuals set their goals, effects were stronger. Second, although time goals were effective initially, results did not hold for maintenance. Third, distance goals were more convenient to administer and thus, more practical, while showing only slightly smaller adherence rates than time goals. Fourth, flexible, distal goals showed greater initiation and maintenance rates than fixed or proximal goals. Thus, the use of goal-setting strategies can increase initiation and maintenance rate, but these studies only examined maintenance for 3 months and longer study is necessary for confident conclusions about maintenance.

Feedback

Kazdin (59) defined feedback as information about performance. Feedback is more potent when given for an explicitly defined performance criterion (e.g., physical activity goal). Research shows feedback to be less effective when applied alone than in combination with other reinforcers (59).

Juneau et al (66) provided a portable heart rate monitor that emitted a tone when the exerciser's heart rate increased or decreased from prescribed levels. This home-based program involved self-monitoring of activity levels. Individuals were prescribed exercise 5 days per week. Results showed a fitness increase measured by an increase in Vo_2max for both men and women by 12 weeks and continued fitness for 24 weeks. Adherence rates for men were 90% and adherence for women was 75%. In addition, the investigators found greater fitness gains corresponded with greater adherence to the program. Another study involving portable heart rate monitors (67) showed Vo_2max increases of 14% in men and 10% in women (95% achieved during the first 12 weeks) with high adherence to the heart rate prescription compared to controls.

These programs involved an explicit performance goal (heart rate prescription) and immediate feedback (when heart rate increased or decreased outside the prescription). This exemplifies an ideal application of feedback. Adherence levels were higher than most studies e.g., 90% versus 50%). Unfortunately, the studies provided no follow-up information about maintenance effects.

Martin et al (65) systematically assessed group versus individual feedback in their series of studies. They encouraged individuals to participate in pairs or small groups. Investigators defined group feedback as information about performance given at the end of a group session and individual feedback as praise twice per exercise session. Individual feedback showed a greater effect on adherence than did group feedback (77.2% versus 65.8%). At 3-month follow-up both individual and group feedback showed decreased adherence, yet the individual feedback condition decreased significantly less than the group feedback condition (54% and 17%, respectively).

Weber et al (68) compared three conditions: 1) standard treatment (fitness exam, encouragement, and assessment), 2) self-monitoring plus goal setting, and 3) self-monitoring and goal setting plus individual positive feedback. Approximately 78% of participants completed at least 4 weeks of the program in both the self-monitoring and the self-monitoring plus feedback group, with 42% completing at least 10 weeks. Unexpectedly, self-monitoring alone had a greater effect on attendance than self-monitoring plus additional feedback (possibly because additional feedback had no added value on the effect of self-monitoring).

In sum, when feedback was explicit and immediate, adherence was high. Individual feedback showed better initiation and 3-month maintenance effects compared with group feedback. Thus, feedback, when appropriately used and applied with a specific performance criterion (e.g., goal setting), can be effective in increasing and maintaining exercise.

Problem-Solving Techniques
Cost-Benefit Analysis

Cost-benefit analysis can be defined as any procedure designed to examine the positive aspects and the negative aspects associated with behavior change. Besides the many benefits of exercise (e.g., reduced risk of coronary heart disease, cancer, and obesity), there are many costs to an activity program designed to increase exercise (e.g., sore muscles, time commitment). Often, the costs are much more salient to the individual than the benefits, especially since the costs tend to be encountered immediately, with the benefits far away. Programs typically do not attempt to increase the benefits or decrease the costs associated with physical activity increases. If a program does not fit into an individual's lifestyle, he or she probably will have difficulty adopting the change and even more difficulty maintaining the change. In addition, Prochaska et al (69) have found that when individuals assess their pros as greater than the cons (i.e., benefits greater than costs), they move from contemplation to preparation (i.e., from thinking about performing a behavior to preparing to perform). Some programs have attempted to assess the costs and benefits by use of a decision-balance sheet (70,71).

Decision-Balance Sheets

The decision-balance sheet categorizes anticipated gains (benefits) and anticipated losses (costs) into four major types of consequences: 1) utilitarian gains or losses to self, 2) utilitarian gains or losses for significant others, 3) approval or disapproval from significant others, and 4) self-approval or disapproval (70). This process involves having individuals consider all information relative to making a decision (e.g., positive consequences, negative consequences), and then on a balance-sheet grid (with the four headings listed above describing the four major types of decisional consequences) filling in the pros and cons for selected decisions (e.g., time commitment to exercise).

Two of the studies reviewed used decision-balance sheets (70,71). Both studies found a significant increase in program adherence when the decision-balance sheet was used. The method required little specialized training and only about 20 minutes per participant. Wankel (72) has found the decision-balance sheet effective in a variety of other settings (university-based fitness classes, commercial fitness center classes, and community-based fitness classes).

Despite the efficacy of decision-balance sheet interventions, some limitations should be noted. First, both studies were less than 2 months in duration and did not allow assessment of effects beyond initial attendance. Thus, while the balance sheet procedure showed initial effects, long-term usage and maintenance effects are unknown. Second, the magnitude of the positive effects was not large, perhaps reflecting methodologic factors (e.g., definition of adherence, intensity of intervention). Thus, while the decision-balance sheet method appeared to have some success, more research is needed to draw definite conclusions.

Other studies attempted to assess costs and benefits by the use of problem-solving strategies (73) and identification of costs and benefits (74). Studies using these techniques showed modest increases in physical activity and modest gains in maintenance. The use of problem-solving procedures in one study focused these strategies on maintenance (73). This study showed no significant results. Daltroy (74) applied identification of benefits and drawbacks to increase adoption and maintenance and found significant increases in attendance (controlling variables related to the exposure of the intervention). But, investigators showed a 50% dropout rate by week 12, suggesting this method may not have adequately addressed maintenance issues.

Thus, when investigators implemented cost-benefit procedures, they showed mixed results. Some showed greater initial adoption with poor maintenance, and others showed little effect. Two issues may explain these inconsistencies. First, cost-benefit analyses performed at the start of a program may be different from analyses performed midway through or after a program. For instance, items or events identified initially as costly may be resolved with new unexpected costs occurring after program initiation (i.e., walking shoes are initially costly, and sore muscles and injuries occur later). Second, focusing on the initial benefits of exercise may initiate program entry, but once realized, these benefits lose their reinforcing quality. For instance, identifying quick weight loss after initiating regular, high-intensity activity may be experienced for a few weeks as a wonderful benefit and a reason to continue exercising. But, after a few weeks the weight losses slow and may no longer be an identifiable benefit and no longer reinforcing.

Given its flaws, cost-benefit analysis can still effect increases in physical activity. However, assessment should occur throughout the program to allow for shifts in costs and benefits and to allow for programmed planning to increase the benefits and reduce the costs. Further assessment should continue throughout a program to address maintenance costs and benefits of physical activity.

Self-Monitoring

Most exercise researchers have used some form of self-monitoring strategies to increase exercise adherence. As stated previously, Weber et al (68) combined self-monitoring with goal setting and feedback and found 78% of participants in a gym setting completed at least 4 weeks of the program. They also found self-monitoring alone had a greater effect on attendance than self-monitoring plus additional feedback.

Other researchers have found combining self-monitoring with other behavior change strategies increased physical activity in a variety of settings including worksites (75), physician's offices (76), home-based programs (63), and cardiac rehabilitation programs (77). Thus, self-monitoring is shown to be a simple and effective strategy to increase physical activity. However, no effects for maintenance of activity are noted.

Maintenance

Initiation and adoption of physical activity through behavioral or cognitive behavioral strategies have shown good results (65,70,76,78,78a). However, maintenance of this behavior change has shown poor results (65,73,79). When physical activity promotion programs are examined, it is apparent they are designed to increase rather than maintain activity. The strategies used are designed for initiation, not maintenance (e.g., frequent reinforcement, continual feedback). Kazdin (59) suggested *response maintenance* and *transfer of training* as appropriate strategies for maintenance. He defined response maintenance as the extension of behavior change over time and transfer of training as the extension of behavior change to new situations and new settings. Unfortunately, response maintenance and transfer of training are not often used in physical activity promotion programs.

One strategy to promote maintenance is gradually removing or fading the contingencies. Ideally, withdrawing reinforcers gradually leads to complete elimination of the initial reinforcer without a return of behavior change to baseline (59). (for example, an individual who is vacuuming for exercise and receiving an encouraging phone call each week initially, then biweekly, once a month, bimonthly, once a year, and then no phone calls, but continues to exercise). This procedure prepares participants for normal conditions (i.e., conditions under which they must normally perform the behavior).

Self-control and cognitively based procedures are also potential maintenance strategies. Kazdin (59) stated that self-control training involves teaching individuals to control their own behavior through the use of self-reinforcement, self-monitoring, and self-evaluation (alone or together). This training aids in the transition from externally managed programs to environmentally managed programs. Kazdin (59) defined cognitively based procedures as self-instructional training and problem-solving skills training, which are specialized forms of self-control strategies. Developing self-control strategies allows individuals to develop skills that can be applied across settings and situations. For example, walking program participants can be taught to self-monitor their walking, reward themselves frequently initially, and then fade their reinforcement over time based on self-evaluation (e.g., goal setting and feedback). In addition, participants can be taught to generate problem situations (e.g., walking while on vacation or while the children are sick), plan a solution, and then practice carrying out the plan (e.g., walk while on vacation). These strategies have been found effective in maintaining both a walking program (80) and a lifestyle physical activity program (81).

LIFESTYLE PHYSICAL ACTIVITY

One of the most important decisions in conducting physical activity research is what type of physical activity to promote. As stated before, some of the barriers to performing physical activity are the perceived discomfort of the activity, the time allowed for activity, and access to facilities (82). Individuals should be allowed to choose the activity they

Table 90-1 Maintenance Strategies and Applications to Physical Activity	
MAINTENANCE STRATEGY	**APPLICATION**
Bring Behavior Under the Control of Natural Contingencies	Walker initially receives praise and support from staff and following program a friend continues to praise.
Programming Naturally Occurring Reinforcers	Walking friends receive praise and support from staff and are instructed to give praise and support to each other when goals are met outside of program.
Gradually Removing or Fading Contingencies	Individual walker receives a supportive phone call each week initially, then biweekly, then once a month, bimonthly, once a year, and then no phone calls.
Expanding Stimulus Control over Behavior	Walkers meet weekly for informational meeting and then walk after the meeting. Gradually, different staff members walk with group; participants are encouraged to walk with different partners and to vary their route. They are encouraged to develop partners for walking outside of class.
Training Individual to Respond to the General Case	Walkers identify how walking can occur across different situations: times during the week, at different locations, and under different circumstances, and these situations and their solutions are discussed and taught.
Altering Schedules of Reinforcement Increasing the Delay of Reinforcement	Walkers are rewarded daily at beginning of a program and after walking is consistent, they are rewarded weekly and then biweekly on a random schedule with reinforcement gradually withdrawn.
Using Peer Facilitators	Walkers are encouraged to bring a walking partner or choose a partner from the group. The partner is involved with administering rewards for goals achieved.
Using Self-Control Procedures	Walkers are taught to self-monitor their walking, reward themselves frequently initially, fading rewards over time based on self-evaluation.
Using Cognitively Based Procedures	Walkers are taught to generate problem situations, plan solutions, and practice carrying out their plan.

feel "fits best" with their lifestyle. Recent studies suggest the activity need not be what individuals typically think constitutes exercise (e.g., jogging, aerobics classes, stairmasters). Rather, lifestyle activities such as gardening, vacuuming, walking, and choosing stairs over the elevator can result in health-related improvements if performed consistently over time. In fact, it may prove easier to maintain an activity that "fits" into one's lifestyle, rather than activity which requires an individual to "make time." Thus, individuals should choose the activity that they believe they can perform (i.e., self-efficacy) over time, that they will enjoy, and that can produce health benefits if performed consistently over time.

The Centers for Disease Control recently published a report emphasizing the importance and the health benefits achieved by lifestyle activity (8). In addition, Rippe et al (83) reviewed the physical and psychological benefits of low- to moderate-intensity exercise. They found physical activity at this level had several health benefits including decrease in cholesterol level (84), control of hypertension through lower blood pressure (85), increases in Vo_2max (86), control of weight loss through decreased appetite (87), and increases in overall mood state (88). Furthermore, Rippe et al (83) indicated that walking is an ideal target behavior for people with varying medical conditions, including diabetes (89) and pregnancy (90), and for people in cardiac rehabilitation (87).

Lifestyle activity has several other benefits for increased maintenance of activity. There can be no cost associated with the individual's choice (e.g., choosing to take the stairs over the elevator, walking, gardening). There is no need for expensive facilities, membership fees, or equipment. In addition, individuals can choose to look for opportunities to engage in lifestyle activity within their day, and thus may continue to engage in activity when away from home, away on business,

or on vacation. Thus, they have the ability to *maintain* their exercise program even when their schedule or location varies. Further, lifestyle activity allows the individual choice and variety in his or her activity program, which may alleviate some of the boredom of routine programs that correlates with exercise dropout (90).

SUMMARY

Research on the effects of physical activity on obesity has repeatedly shown its benefits. Yet, the percentage of the U.S. population who exercise regularly is very low, approximately 10% to 20%. A review of the literature indicates the obese population may respond best with a physical activity program that increases in intensity, recognizes the barriers associated with physical activity and obesity, and "fits" within the individual's lifestyle. A review of the determinants of exercise literature suggested the use of behavior change techniques was important for long-term adherence to physical activity and therefore associated with greater weight loss maintenance. Furthermore, a review of the behavioral strategies used in the exercise area indicated several conclusions: 1) telephone prompting can be effective; 2) individual feedback can also be effective; 3) goal setting, specifically individualized, flexible, and distal goals, can increase adherence; 4) self-monitoring can both increase adherence and offer outcome data; and 5) lifestyle activity may relate to long-term maintenance while providing health benefits. Thus, a physical activity program incorporating these self-control and prompting strategies with lifestyle activity should be more effective than a program without them. Table 90-1 illustrates how a walking program could be designed using strategies designed to maintain behavior change.

REFERENCES

1. Heine AF, Weinsier RL. Divergent trends in obesity and fat intake patterns: the American paradox. Am J Med 1997;102:259–267.

2. Foreyt JP, Goodrick K. Do's and don'ts for weight management: exercise is always good, but are some foods bad? Obes Res 1994; 2:378–379.

3. Pronk NP, Wing RR. Physical activity and long-term maintenance of weight loss. Obes Res 1994;2:587–599.

4. Jeffrey RW, Bjornson-Benson WM, Rosenthal BS, et al. Correlates of weight loss and its maintenance over two years of follow-up among middle-aged men. Prev Med 1984;13:155–168.

5. Kayman S, Bruvold W, Stern JS. Maintenance and relapse after weight loss in women: behavioral aspects. Am J Clin Nutr 1990; 52:800–807.

6. Bouchard C, Despres JP, Tremblay A. Exercise and obesity. Obes Res 1993;1:133–147.

7. Grilo CM, Brownell KD, Stunkard AJ. The metabolic and psychological importance of exercise in weight control. In: Stunkard AJ, Wadden TA, eds. Obesity: Theory and therapy. New York: Raven Press 1993:253–273.

8. Pate RR, Pratt M, Blair SN, et al. Physical activity and public health: a recommendation from the Centers for Disease Control and Prevention and the American College of Sports Medicine. JAMA 1995;273:402–407.

9. Brownell KD. The LEARN program for weight control. Dallas: American Health, 1998.

10. Hunter GR, Weinsier RL, Bamman MM, et al. A role for high intensity exercise on energy balance and weight control. Int J Obes 1998;22:489–493.

11. Tremblay A, Simoneau JA, Bouchard C. Impact of exercise intensity on body fatness and skeletal muscle metabolism. Metabolism 1994;43:814–818.

12. Gaeser GA, Brooks GA. Muscular efficiency during steady-rate exercise: effects of speed and work rate. J Appl Physiol 1975;38: 1132–1139.

13. Gladden LB, Welch HC. Efficiency of anaerobic work. J Appl Physiol 1978;44:564–570.

14. Treuth MS, Hunter GR, Williams MJ. Effects of exercise intensity on 24-h energy expenditure/substrate oxidation. Med Sci Sports Exerc 1996;2:1138–1143.

15. Donovan CM, Brooks GA. Effects of walking speed and work rate. J Appl Physiol 1977;43:431–439.

16. Hunter GR, Belcher LA, Dunnan L, Fleming G. Bench press metabolic rate as a function of exercise intensity. J Appl Sports Sci Res 1988;2:1-6.

17. Hunter GR, Kekes-Szabo T, Schnitzler A. Metabolic cost/vertical work relationship during knee extension and knee flexion weight training exercise. J Appl Sports Sci Res 1992;6:42–48.

18. Kalb J, Hunter GR. Weight training economy as a function of intensity of the squat and overhead press exercise. J Sports Med Physical Fitness 1991;31:154–160.

19. Coyle EF, Sidossis LS, Horowitz JF, Beltz JD. Cycling efficiency is related to the percentage of type I muscle fibers. Med Sci Sports Exerc 1992;24:782–788.

20. Poehlman EG, Danforth E. Endurance training increases metabolic rate and norepinephrine appearance rate in older individuals. Am J Physiol 1991; 261:E233–E239.

21. Poehlman EG, Horton ES. The impact of food intake and exercise on energy expenditure. Nutr Rev 1989;47:129–137.

22. Poehlman ET, McAuliffe T, Danforth E. Effects of age and level of physical activity on plasma epinephrine kinetics. Am J Physiol 1990;258:E256–E262.

22a. Burke CM, Bullough RC, Melby CL. Resting metabolic rate and postprandial thermogenesis by level of aerobic fitness in young women. Eur J Clin Nutr 1993;47:585.

23. Treuth MS, Hunter GR, Weinsier RL, Kell SH. Energy expenditure and substrate utilization in older women after strength training: 24-h Calorimetry results. J Appl Physiol 1995;78:2140–2146.

24. Bosselaers I, Buemann B, Victor OJ, et al. Twenty-four hour energy expenditure and substrate utilization in body builders. Am J Clin Nutr 1994;59:10–12.

25. Poehlman ET. A review: exercise and its influence on resting energy metabolism in man. Med Sci Sports Exerc 1989;21:515–525.

26. Poehlman ET, Garner AW, Ades PA, et al. Resting energy metabolism and cardiovascular disease risk in resistance and aerobically trained males. Metabolism 1992; 41:1351–1360.

27. Campbell WW, Crim MC, Young VR, Evans UW. Increased energy requirements and changes in body composition with resistance training in older adults. Am J Clin Nutr 1994;60:167–175.

28. DiPietro L, Williamson DF, Caspersen CJ, et al. The descriptive epidemiology of selected physical activities and body weight among adults trying to lose weight: the Behavioral Risk Factor Surveillance System Survey. Int J Obes 1989;17:69–76.

29. French SA, Jeffery RW, Forster JL, et al. Predictors of weight change over two years among a population of working adults: the Healthy Worker Project. Int J Obes 1994;18:145–154.

30. Khalidk MEM. The association between strenuous physical activity and obesity in high and low altitude populations in southern Saudi Arabia. Int J Obes 1995; 19:776–778.

31. Tremblay A, Despres JP, Leblanc C, et al. Effects of intensity of physical activity on body fatness and fat distribution. Am J Clin Nutr 1990;51:153–157.

32. Mattsson E, Larsson UE, Rossner S. Is walking for exercise too exhausting for obese women? Int J Obes 1997;21:380–386.

33. Perri MG, Martin D, Leermakers EA, et al. Effects of group- versus home-based exercise in the treatment of obesity. J Consult Clin Psychol 1997;65(2):278–285.

34. Wood PD, Terry RB, Haskell WL. Metabolism of substrates: diet, lipoprotein metabolism and exercise. Federal Proc 1985;44:358–363.

35. King NA, Burley VJ, Blundell JE. Exercise-induced suppression of appetite: effects on food intake and implications for energy balance. Eur J Clin Nutr 1994;48:715–724.

36. King NA, Blundell JE. High-fat foods overcome the energy expenditure due to exercise after cycling and running. Eur J Clin Nutr 1995;49:114–123.

37. King NA, Blundell JE. Effects of exercise and macronutrient availability on appetite: is there a difference between men and women? Int J Obes 1995;19 (suppl 4):91.

38. Kissileff HR, Pi-Sunyer XF, Egal K, et al. Acute effects of exercise on food intake in obese and non-obese women. Am J Clin Nutr 1990;52:240–245.

39. Thompson DA, Wolfe LA, Eikelboom R. Acute effects of exercise intensity on appetite in young men. Med Sci Sports Exerc 1988;20:222–227.

40. Maxwell BD. Serum free fatty acid concentration during post-exercise recovery. PhD thesis. Tucson, AZ: University of Arizona.

41. Reger WE, Alison TG. Exercise and appetite. Med Sci Sports Exerc 1987;19:S38.

42. Andersson B, Larson B. Influence of local temperature changes in the preoptic area and rostral hypothalamus in the regulation of food and water intake. Acta Physiol Scand 1961;52:75–89.

43. Baile CA, Zinn WN, Mayer J. Effects of lactate and other metabolites on food intake of monkeys. Am J Physiol 1970;219:1606–1613.

44. Grunfield C, Finegold KR. The metabolic effects of tumor necrosis factor and other cytokines. Biotherapy 1991;3:143–158.

45. Verger PM, Lanteaume T, Louis-Sylvestre J. Human intake and choice of foods at intervals after exercise. Appetite 1992;1:1–7.

46. Schoeller DA. Measurement of energy expenditure in free living human by using doubly labeled water. J Nutr 1988;11:1278–1289.

47. Mayer J, Roy P, Mitra KP. Relation between caloric intake, body weight and physical work: studies in an industrial male population in West Bengal. Am J Clin Nutr 1956;4:169–175.

48. Blair SN, Ellsworth NW, Haskell WL, et al. Comparison of nutrient intake in middle-aged men and women runners and controls. Med Sci Sports Exerc 1981;13:310–315.

49. Maughan RJ, Robertson JD, Bruce AC. Dietary energy and carbohydrate intakes of runners in relation to training load. Proc Nutr Soc 1989;48:170A.

50. Richard D. Exercise and the neurobiological control of food intake and energy expenditure. Int J Obes 1995;19:S73–S79.

51. Hardman AE. Exercise and health. CHO Int Dialogue 1991; 2:1–3.

52. Woo R, Pi-Sunyer FX. Effect of increased physical activity on voluntary intake in lean women. Metabolism 1985;34: 836–841.

53. Andersson B, Xu M, Rebuffee-Scrive K, et al. The effects of exercise training on body composition and metabolism in men and women. Int J Obes 1991; 15:75–81.

54. Dempsey JA. Anthropometrical measurements on obese and nonobese young men undergoing a program of vigorous physical exercise. Res Q 1964;35:275–287.

55. Leon AS, Conrad J, Hunninghake DB, Serfass R. Effects of a vigorous walking program on body composition and lipid metabolism of obese young men. Am J Clin Nutr 1979;33:1776–1787.

56. McGowan CR, Epstein LH, Kupfer DJ, et al. The effects of exercise on non-restricted caloric intake in male joggers. Appetite 1986;7: 97–105.

57. Reger WE, Allison RA, Kurucz RL. Exercise, post-exercise metabolic rate and appetite. Sports Health Nutr 1986;2:117–123.

58. Dishman RK. Exercise adherence: its impact on public health. Champaign, IL: Kinetics Books, 1988.

59. Kazdin AE. Behavior modification in applied settings. Pacific Grove, CA: Brooks/Cole, 1993.

60. Brownell KD, Stunkard AJ, Albaum JM. Evaluation and modification of exercise patterns in the natural environment. Am J Psychiatry 1980;137(12):1540–1545.

61. Wankel LM, Thompson CE. Motivating people to be physically active: self-persuasion vs. balanced decision-making. J Appl Soc Psychol 1977;7:332–340.

62. Acquista VW, Wachtel TJ, Gomes CI, et al. Home-based health risk appraisal and screening program. J Community Health 1988;13(1): 43–52.

63. King AC, Taylor CB, Haskell WL, DeBusk RF. Strategies for increasing early adherence to and long-term maintenance of home-based exercise training in healthy middle-aged men and women. Am J Cardiol 1988;61:628–632.

64. Bandura A. Social foundations of thought and action: a social cognitive theory. Englewood Cliffs, NJ: Prentice Hall, 1986.

65. Martin JE, Dubbert PM, Katell AD, et al. Behavioral control of exercise in sedentary adults: studies 1–6. J Consult Clin Psychol 1984;52(5):795–811.

66. Juneau M, Rogers F, DeSantos V, et al. Effectiveness of self-monitored, home-based, moderate intensity exercise training in middle-aged men and women. Am J Cardiol 1987;60:66–70.

67. Rogers F, Juneau M, Taylor CB, et al. Assessment by a microprocessor of adherence to home-based moderate-intensity exercise training in healthy, sedentary middle-aged men and women. Am J Cardiol 1987;60: 71–75.

68. Weber J, Wertheim EH. Relationships of self-monitoring, special attention, body fat percent, and self-motivation to attendance at a community gymnasium. J Sport Exerc Psychol 1989;11:105–111.

69. Prochaska JO, Velicer WF, Rossi JS, et al. Stages of change and decisional balance for 12 problem behaviors. Health Psychol 1994;13(1):39–46.

70. Hoyt MF, Janis IL. Increasing adherence to a stressful decision via a motivational balance-sheet procedure: a field experiment. J Pers Soc Psychol 1975;31(5): 833–839.

71. Wankel LM, Yardley JK, Graham J. The effects of motivational interventions upon the exercise adherence of high and low self-motivated adults. Can J Sports Sci 1985;10(3):147–156.

72. Wankel LM. Decision-making and social support strategies for increasing exercise involvement. J Card Rehabil 1984;4:124–135.

73. Meyer AJ, Nash JD, McAlister AL, et al. Skills training in a cardio-vascular health education campaign. J Consult Clin Psychol 1980;48(2):129–142.

74. Daltroy LH. Improving cardiac patient adherence to exercise regimens: a clinical trial of health education. J Card Rehabil 1985;5:40–49.

75. Durbeck DC, Heinzelman F, Schacter J, et al. The National Aeronautics and Space Administration—U.S. Public Health Service Evaluation and Enhancement program: Summary of results. Am J Cardiol 1972;30: 784–790.

76. Epstein LH, Wing RR. Aerobic exercise and weight. Addict Behav 1980;5:371–378.

77. Oldridge NB, Jones NL. Improving patient compliance in cardiac exercise rehabilitation: effects of written agreement and self-monitoring. J Card Rehabil 1983;3:257–262.

78. Gettman LR, Ward P, Hagan RD. A comparison of combined

running and weight training with circuit weight training. Med Sci Sports Exerc 1982;14(3):229–234.

78a. King AC, Frederickson LW. Low-cost strategies for increasing exercise behavior. Behav Modif 1984;18:3–21.

79. Reid EL, Morgan RW. Exercise prescription: a clinical trial. Am J Public Health 1979;69(6):591–595.

80. Lombard DN, Lombard TN, Winett RA. Walking to meet health guidelines: the effects of prompting frequency and prompting structure. Health Psychol 1995;14(2):164–170.

81. Lombard TN, Lombard DN, Winett RA. Improving physical activity adherence: the effects of self-control strategies and telephone prompting using lifestyle physical activity. Unpublished manuscript.

82. Dishman RK. Compliance/adherence in health-related exercise. Health Psychol 1982;1:237–267.

83. Rippe JM, Ward A, Porcari JP, Freedson PS. Walking for health and fitness. JAMA 1988;259:2720–2724.

84. Goldberg L, Elliot DL. The effects of exercise on lipid metabolism in men and women. Sports Medicine 1987;4:307–321.

85. Blackburn H. Physical activity and hypertension. J Clin Hypertens 1986;2:154–162.

86. Dehn MM, Bruce RA. Longitudinal variations in maximal oxygen intake with age and activity. J Appl Physiol 1972;33:805–807.

87. Rippe JM, Maher PM, Ockene J. Care and rehabilitation of the patient following myocardial infarction. In: Rippe JM, Irwin RS, Alpert JS, eds. Intensive care medicine. Boston: Little, Brown, 1985:366–376.

88. Porcari JP, Ward A, Morgan W. Effect of walking on state anxiety and blood pressure. Med Sci Sports Exerc 1988;20:85.

89. Laws A, Reaven GM. Physical activity, glucose tolerance, and diabetes in older adults. Ann Behav Med 1991;13(3):125–132.

90. Kashiwa A, Rippe J. Fitness walking for women. New York: Putnam, 1987.

Chapter 91

Dietary Management of the Obese Patient

Sachiko St. Jeor

Judith M. Ashley

Jon P. Schrage

New challenges have developed in the dietary management for obese patients (body mass index (BMI) ≥ 30 kg/m²) as well as for overweight adults (BMI of 25 to 29.9 kg/m²), currently estimated to be 55 percent of the American population (1). The growing global epidemic of obesity calls attention to its serious nature and treatment limitations as a worldwide public health threat (2). Importantly, newer treatment recommendations now recognize obesity as a disease that is rarely, if ever, cured (3,4). Longer-term weight management strategies and shorter-term weight reduction efforts, accepting smaller weight losses of 5% to 10% of initial body weight as successful outcome measures, are being emphasized (1–5). Additionally, lifestyle changes of diet and activity remain essential to the treatment and prevention of obesity, but combined therapies, including pharmacotherapy (for adults with a BMI ≥ 30 or ≥ 27 kg/m² with two or more risk factors) and surgery (BMI ≥ 40 or BMI ≥ 35 with coexisting morbidities), may also be appropriate for treatment-resistant individuals (1,4). Nonetheless, diet remains essential to all management strategies, but environmental factors that promote overeating, such as convenient, relatively inexpensive, highly palatable, energy-dense foods in large portion sizes, make successful dietary interventions extremely difficult (6).

New treatment guidelines (1) recommend a reasonable time line of 6 months for a 10% reduction in body weight at a rate of 1 to 2 pounds per week, 30 minutes or more of physical activity per day, and lifestyle therapy for at least 6 months before embarking on pharmacotherapy. Surgical interventions for the severely obese also offer renewed interest with balanced perspectives on long-term outcomes. Further, emphasis is placed on weight maintenance for the prevention of weight gain at any point and the assessment of BMI in normal weight individuals every 2 years (1).

There remains no doubt that weight management and maintenance of overall health are both related to the quantity as well as the quality of what we eat. Thus, the role of the diet in producing successful outcomes for the treatment and prevention obesity is to 1) provide essential nutrients to achieve and maintain an optimal nutrition status, 2) produce an energy deficit to yield a reasonable weight loss or to provide sufficient energy to prevent further weight gain, and 3) to provide enjoyment of eating while supporting healthy eating patterns. Dietary management is essential for any treatment for obesity to succeed.

TRADITIONAL DIETS: DEFINITIONS

The major classification of diets for weight management has been based on the total level of energy (in kilocalories per day) provided. Although there will always be some controversy, the types of traditional diets and their descriptions are outlined below (1–3).

Low-calorie diets (LCDs) are those which provide a caloric deficit and usually average 1000 to 1500 kcal/day. The anticipated weight loss is approximately 0.25 kg/week or 1 lb/week for every 500-kcal/day deficit (3). These diets focus on the use of regular foods but also include formulated, fortified, and/or prepackaged and portioned products. Diets less than 1000 kcal/day may require vitamin and mineral supplementation (3). Reported weight losses approximate 0.5 to 1.5 kg/week (8.5 kg over 20 weeks) or approximately 2 lb/week (3) and produce an average loss of 8–10% of body weight over a period of 3 to 12 months (1). *Balanced deficit diets* (BDDs) have been defined as LCDs generally above 1200 kcal/day and are nutritionally adequate; they provide the essential nutrients by using a variety of well-chosen foods (3).

Very-Low-Calorie Diets (VLCDs) are those that usually provide approximately 400 to 500 kcal/day (no more than 800 kcal/day) and are considered to induce a modified fast (7). Regular foods are usually replaced with special formulated foods and/or drinks and supplements. Emphasis is placed on provision of 40 to 100 g (or 0.8 to 1.5 g/kg of ideal body weight) of protein of high biological value (HBV) to meet minimum protein requirements. Up to 100 g of carbohydrates, a minimum of fat as essential fatty acids, and recommended allowances of vitamins, minerals, and electrolytes are also usually provided. Weight loss averages 20 kg over 12 weeks or approximately 3 lb/wk (3). Although initial weight loss is greater on VLCDs, overall long-term weight loss (>1 year) is not different from LCDs.

Although LCDs and VLCDs are effective on the shorter term, weight regain generally occurs 3 to 5 years after treatment intervention ends (5,6). Thus, the dietary management of obesity is one of the greatest challenges today, and newer strategies that will have longer-term benefits are needed. Individualized behavioral approaches, designed to target major lifestyle changes in increasing physi-

cal activity and exercise, as well making healthier modifications in diet, are still the hallmark of any treatment for obesity (8–10).

DIETARY TREATMENT MODEL: SPECTRUM OF CARE

A treatment model adapted from the Blackburn Model (3) for obesity is summarized in Figure 91-1 and emphasizes dietary involvement (assessment, management, and/or treatment as well as follow-up) at every stage. It is always advisable to recommend medical advice and to conduct baseline nutrition assessment before embarking on any weight reduction regimen so that individualized intervention strategies can be developed. However, at any point at which weight loss is desired, a balanced deficit diet of greater than 1200 kcal/day may be initiated and is generally safe. Other LCDs less than 1200 kcal/day should be used with caution since they may not provide the essential nutrients needed. It should be recognized that the majority of dieting individuals will embark on weight reduction regimens without professional advice and will engage in self-help forms of treatment, including books and/or organized commercial groups. Generally, these are safe for individuals without medical complications over

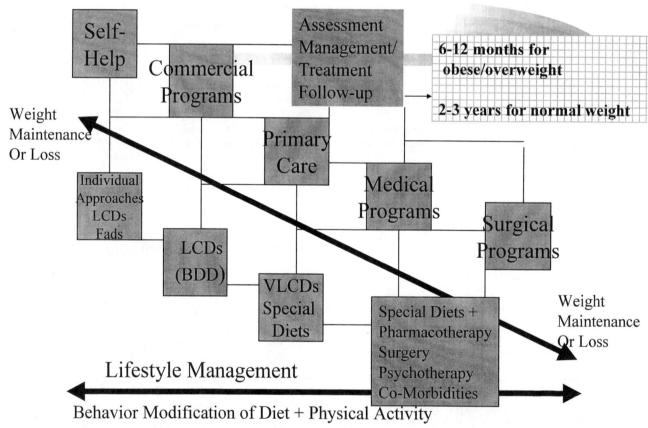

Figure 91-1 Spectrum of Care for the Treatment of Obesity (Adapted from the Blackburn model from Committee to Develop Criteria for Evaluating the Outcomes of Approaches to Prevent and Treat Obesity. Food and Nutrition Board, Institute of Medicine. Thomas PR, ed. Weighing the options: Criteria for evaluating weight management programs. Washington, D.C.: National Academy Press, 1995:99.)

the short term and involve LCDs using a variety of individual approaches and diet fads currently in vogue.

LCDs and VLCDs are used in medical settings (primary care, medical, and/or surgical programs) because they may pose some unexpected burden on or consequence to the body. Monitoring by a nutritionist (registered dietitian) is recommended for LCDs and VLCDs, and physician monitoring and evaluation should accompany VLCDs and other special dietary interventions. Dietary management is important to the success of pharmacotherapy as well as pre- and postsurgical interventions. Thus, the spectrum of care progresses in medical management as the severity of diet and combined therapies increase. However, the longer-term basic approaches for preventing weight gain or regain, in addition to shorter-term approaches for weight reduction, include lifestyle management of diet and physical activity, which is essential and supportive to all. Current trends also promote the effectiveness of the primary care setting for earlier, less intensive interventions with support from the physician in conjunction with trained office staff (11,12).

In the new treatment paradigm, prevention of adult weight gain or regain is critically important. The saying that "if you can't lose, don't gain" applies to both the prevention of obesity in normal-weight individuals and exacerbation of the obese state in already obese or overweight individuals. Weight maintenance has been defined as less than ±5 lb over any two points in time (13). This concept of weight maintenance (or overall energy balance) should be applied for serious evaluation in 6-month intervals for already overweight or obese individuals and no less than 2-year intervals for normal-weight individuals (1,2). It is also important to consider that weight maintainers tend to have healthier profiles overall (14) and that weight maintenance requires less intervention than weight loss and can concentrate on smaller, additive changes in behaviors, which may be more feasible to maintain.

NUTRIENT ADEQUACY AND BASIC 1200-KCAL BALANCED DEFICIT DIET

The focus of any diet is to provide adequate nutrition. The obese patient poses multiple and complex dietary challenges. The total energy (kilocalorie) intake is of central importance, however, in weight management, and reductions in intake are too often accompanied by consequential compromises in essential nutrients and the overall quality of the diet. A major outcome of dietary treatment should be a notable improvement in diet, as evidenced by adherence to the Food Guide Pyramid the majority of the time (or at least 4 days of the week) (3). A basic 1200-kcal (3) diet adapted from the Food Guide Pyramid (15) can serve as an excellent starting point and is outlined in Table 91-1. The dietary pattern is based on the minimum number of servings recommended, with the addition of 1 teaspoon (4 g) of added sugar and 5 g of added fat for flexibility, the meat group limited to 4 oz of lean, and use of skim milk products. Increased calcium recommendations, however, emphasize the need for either an additional serving of the skim milk products (+80 to 100 kcal), which may need further accommodation or wise choices of calcium-rich and fortified foods.

Table 91-1 Modification of the Food Guide Pyramid for a 1200-kcal Diet	
FOOD GROUP	NUMBER OF SERVINGS FOR A 1200-KCAL DIET*,a
Bread Group	6[b]
Vegetable Group	3
Fruit Group	2
Milk Group	2[c]
Meat Group (ounces)	4[d]

* Not recommended for pregnant or lactating women, children (depending on age), or those who have special dietary needs. At or below this low level of kilocalorie intake, it may not be possible to obtain recommended amounts of all nutrients from foods; therefore, it is important to make careful food choices, and the need for dietary supplements should be evaluated.
[a] This plan allows up to 1 teaspoon (4 g) of added sugar and 5 g of added fat.
[b] For maximum nutritional value, make whole-grain, high-fiber choices.
[c] Choose skim milk products. The discretionary 5 g of added fat can be used here to select low- or reduced-fat dairy products. With the increase in recommendations for calcium intake, if three servings from this group are encouraged, the 80 to 100 kcal additional to be provided should be accommodated.
[d] Select lean meat and use cooking methods that do not require added fat.
Adapted from U.S. Department of Agriculture. USDA's Food Guide Pyramid. Home and Garden Bulletin No. 252. Washington, D.C.: USDA Human Nutrition Information Service, 1992; and from Committee to Develop Criteria for Evaluating the Outcomes of Approaches to Prevent and Treat Obesity. Food and Nutrition Board. Institute of Medicine. Thomas, PR, ed. Weighing the options: criteria for evaluating weight management programs. Washington, D.C.: National Academy Press, 1995:109.

The adequacy of low-calorie diets that are not carefully selected poses particular concern for intakes of calcium, folic acid, and vitamin B_{12}.

Calcium

The recent Dietary Reference Intakes (DRIs) have outlined increased levels for calcium and outline recommendations that are higher than the 1989 Recommended Dietary Allowances (RDAs) (16–18). The current Adequate Intakes (AIs) for both males and females are 1000 mg/day for ages 19 to 50 years and 1200 mg/day for ages 50 + years (15,17). Practically speaking, it is difficult to achieve this level of calcium intake without consuming two to three servings of milk (approximately 250 to 300 mg per 8-oz serving) or dairy products (300 to 450 mg of calcium per 3 oz of cheese), dark green leafy vegetables (approximately 50 to 100 mg per half cup), nuts and seeds (25 to 75 mg per 1-oz serving), and calcium-fortified foods (200 to 300 mg per 8-oz serving, such as orange juice or soy milk) (19,20). All LCDs should especially encourage maximal intake of these foods emphasizing low-fat, lower-calorie items. Related to increasing the bioavailability of calcium in the body is its dependence on vitamin D for absorption. It is important to consider the new AI level established for vitamin D, which increases with age (5, 10, and 15 μg/day for the two decades following 30, 50, and 70 years, respectively) as cholecalciferol (where 1 μg cholecalciferol = 40 IU vitamin D) (16,18). Thus, the level of vitamin D formerly recommended by the 1989 RDAs (10 μg/day to age 24 years and 5 μg/day thereafter) (17) has been significantly reversed with increasing needs for vitamin D recommended with increasing age. This stresses the need for adequate exposure to sunlight, which could be practically encouraged with recommendations to increase physical activity (such as walking) outdoors.

Folic Acid

The recent DRI consisting of a new RDA of 400 μg/day of folate is more than double that recommended by the 1989 RDA (16,17,20). Dieting individuals are at particular risk for reduced intake of foods high in folate coming from "foliage," particularly fruits and vegetables. Thus, because of the evidence linking low folate intake with neural tube defects in the developing fetus, synthetic folic acid from fortified foods and/or supplements is recommended in addition to the food folate from a well-chosen, varied diet in women of childbearing age (16).

AIs of naturally occurring folate in foods or synthetic folic acid supplementation in all adults is also viewed as particularly important in preventing hyperhomocysteinemia associated with increased arteriosclerotic plaque formation and increased cardiovascular disease (21–24). Foods high in folate include leafy green vegetables, orange juice, and grain products (23). However, because of the inadequate intake of folate in general, the fortification of folic acid in cereals and grains starting January 1998 was introduced as a significant public health strategy to help ensure better health for all Americans. Grain products were targeted for fortification with folic acid (140 μg per 100 g of flour) since they are consumed by 90% of the target population. The effect of consuming six servings of folic-acid-enriched grain products has been calculated at 80% of the current RDA (four servings of bread = 160 μg, + one serving of cereal = 100 μg, + one serving of pasta = 60 μg = total of 320/400 μg = 80% RDI) (23).

An upper tolerable limit of synthetic folic acid has been set at 1000 μg/day for adults 19 years and older to prevent masking of the neurologic symptoms of vitamin B₁₂ deficiency or pernicious anemia (21). The current level of folic acid in over-the-counter vitamin supplements is limited to 400 μg/tablet (25). Thus, it is important to target the five servings of fruits and vegetables as sources of folate in foods along with the six servings of folic-acid-enriched grain products to meet the current recommendations for folate. The upper tolerable level of intake, thus, still will not be exceeded with the consumption of 12 servings of fortified grain products, but vitamin supplements should then be used with caution. The new ADIs that replace the old 1989 RDAs consider dietary folate equivalent (DFE) as 1 DFE = 1 μg of food folate = 0.6 μg of folic acid (from fortified food or supplement) consumed with food = 0.5 μg synthetic (supplemental) folic acid taken on an empty stomach (16,21). Thus, the best way to ensure adequate intakes of folate/folic acid DFEs, particularly when consuming LCDs, is by consuming a Balanced Deficit Diet (BDD) meeting the minimum requirements of the Food Guide

Pyramid as outlined in Table 91-1 and making sure the diet is rich in the best sources of folate-containing foods and folic-acid-fortified grain products.

Vitamin B₁₂

The new DRIs include RDAs for vitamin B₁₂ of 2.4 μg/day for both adult men and women over 14 years of age (16). These recommendations are higher than those suggested in 1989 (17). Because approximately 10% to 30% of older people may malabsorb vitamin B₁₂, current recommendations encourage persons 50 years or older to consume foods fortified with vitamin B₁₂ or take supplements (16,21). Clinical signs and symptoms of vitamin B₁₂ deficiency are not clearly exhibited in the elderly; many have undiagnosed deficiencies, and it has been recommended that suspected individuals not receive folic acid supplementation before their vitamin B₁₂ status is evaluated (26). Since vitamin B₁₂ is found in animal foods, consideration for protein adequacy is related, especially in older dieting Americans. Thus, LCDs should consist practically of no less than 50 g of protein, mainly from high biologically available and complete sources of essential amino acids, as provided by such foods as milk products, meat, poultry, fish, and eggs, which are all animal sources. Skim milk products are the best low-fat, high-protein choices because of their quality of protein, high calcium content, and provision of other nutrients, including vitamin B₁₂.

THE DIETARY PRESCRIPTION: ENERGY BALANCE AND DEFICITS

When energy *intake* (food) equals energy *expenditure* [basal metabolic rate (BMR) + activity + thermogenesis], weight maintenance is achieved. Resting energy expenditure (REE) is currently measured today in lieu of BMR using a variety of methods for indirect calorimetry. REE has been approximated to be 10% above BMR, accounting for 65% to 70% of total energy expenditure, or 24-hour TEE (27). The thermic effect of food (TEF) and physical activity (PA) account for the remaining 10% to 15% and 20% to 30% respectively, of 24-hour TEE. Since the 10% of kilocalories from thermogenesis (TEF), or metabolic response to food, is offset by the increase of 10% in REE above BMR, it is not figured into most formulas using REE.

Thus, the following formula is recommended for estimating total energy needs or 24-hour TEE:

$$24\text{-hour TEE} = \text{REE} \times \text{AF} + \text{PA}$$

or

24 - hour total energy expenditure (24 - hour TEE) = resting energy expenditure (REE) × activity factor (AF) + physical activity (PA)

The REE can be calculated or measured by indirect calorimetry using a gas exchange system and special metabolic apparatus, such as the Metabolic Measurement Cart Horizons Systems (Sensor Medics, Anaheim, California). Because indirect calorimetry is expensive and usually unavailable in general office settings, the following formula for calculating REE for healthy normal-weight and obese adults (BMI

18 to 36) is recommended (Mifflin–St. Jeor equation, or MSJE) and is based on sex, height, weight, and age (27):

$$\text{REE (men)} = 10 \times \text{weight (kg)} + 6.25 \times \text{height (cm)} - 5 \times \text{age (years)} + 5$$

$$\text{REE (women)} = 10 \times \text{weight (kg)} + 6.25 \times \text{height (cm)} - 5 \times \text{age (years)} - 161$$

However, because BMI, or weight(kg)/height(m)^2 is currently being used in the assessment of overweight and obesity, work to convert REE to BMI units is underway. Table 91-2 outlines REE conversions to BMI by age in two separate calculations according to sex using the following equations derived from the same population as the MSJE for REE above (28):

$$\text{REE (men)} = (\text{BMI} \times 28.15) - (\text{age} \times 6.41) + 1290$$

$$\text{REE (women)} = (\text{BMI} \times 28.15) - (\text{age} \times 6.44) + 905$$

Interpretations of regression coefficients indicated the following influences on REE: a 28-kcal increase per BMI unit, a −6.5-kcal decrement per year of age, and a +385-kcal increase for men relative to women (28). Although work is in progress to establish an international REE registry to expand these charts, they can be usefully applied to project REE from BMI in healthy, normal to overweight/obese (BMI 18 to 36) individuals ages 18 through 70+ years, as was the population from which these charts are based (29).

The AF consists of two components: a multiplication of the REE by an AF and an average estimated contribution of daily PA. We believe the AF of 1.3 × REE projects the best estimate of energy expenditure for both men and women of sedentary activity, which includes the majority of Americans (30,31). This activity factor of 1.3 × REE has also been recognized as the minimum value reflecting approximately 14 hours of very light activity and 10 hours at rest (17,32). Past recommendations have generally focused on recommendations of 1.5 to 1.6 × REE for light activity and 1.6 to 1.7 × REE for moderate activity, as set forth by the World Health Organization in 1985 (17,32), but these have been relatively high when used in our population (31). Thus, we have chosen to add an additional estimated amount of energy (kilocalories per day) contributed by a personalized assessment of physical activity, which is reflected by PA in the formula above. The PA can be calculated by those general activities and/or exercise patterns that can be estimated on a daily or weekly basis and approximates less than 4 to more than 7 kcal/min or 100 to 200 kcal per 30 minutes, depending on the intensity of effort as outlined from Table 91-3 (32) and recommended for practical application by the most recent U.S. Dietary Guidelines for Americans to encourage 30 minutes of moderate activity on most days (5). For example, to expend 200 kcal, one must walk 2 miles at moderate intensity (3 to 4 mph), which should then take about 20 to 30 minutes (32). Thus, the approximate amount of PA (kilocalories per 24 hours) expended can be added into the formula above either daily or averaged over the week and reflects a more personalized adjustment of the highly variable activity levels from day to day and from person to person. Two examples of these calculations follow:

1. A 50-year-old female office worker who walks 1 mile on her lunch hour every day of the week: height = 64 inches; weight = 145 lb; BMI = 25.

Table 91-2 Predicted Resting Energy Expenditure (REE) from Body Mass Index (BMI)

BMI	AGE RANGE					
	18–29	30–39	40–49	50–59	60–69	70
Women: Predicted REE (kcal per 24 hours) = (BMI × 28.15) − (Age × 6.44) + 905						
18	1260	1190	1125	1061	996	932
19	1289	1218	1153	1089	1024	960
20	1317	1246	1181	1117	1053	988
21	1345	1274	1210	1145	1081	1016
22	1373	1302	1238	1173	1109	1045
23	1401	1330	1266	1201	1137	1073
24	1429	1358	1294	1230	1165	1101
25	1457	1387	1322	1258	1193	1129
26	1486	1415	1350	1286	1222	1157
27	1514	1443	1378	1314	1250	1185
28	1542	1471	1407	1342	1278	1213
29	1570	1499	1435	1370	1306	1242
30	1598	1527	1463	1399	1334	1270
31	1626	1555	1491	1427	1362	1298
32	1654	1584	1519	1455	1390	1326
33	1683	1612	1547	1483	1419	1354
34	1711	1640	1576	1511	1447	1382
35	1739	1668	1604	1539	1475	1410
36	1767	1696	1632	1567	1503	1439
Men: Predicted REE (kcal per 24 hours) = (BMI × 28.15) − (Age × 6.41) + 1290						
18	1645	1575	1510	1446	1381	1317
19	1674	1603	1538	1474	1409	1345
20	1702	1631	1566	1502	1438	1373
21	1730	1659	1595	1530	1466	1401
22	1758	1687	1623	1558	1494	1430
23	1786	1715	1651	1586	1522	1458
24	1814	1743	1679	1615	1550	1486
25	1842	1772	1707	1643	1578	1514
26	1871	1800	1735	1671	1607	1542
27	1899	1828	1763	1699	1635	1570
28	1927	1856	1792	1727	1663	1598
29	1955	1884	1820	1755	1691	1627
30	1983	1912	1848	1784	1719	1655
31	2011	1940	1876	1812	1747	1683
32	2039	1969	1904	1840	1775	1711
33	2068	1997	1932	1868	1804	1739
34	2096	2025	1961	1896	1832	1767
35	2124	2053	1989	1924	1860	1795
36	2152	2081	2017	1952	1888	1824

Reproduced by permission from Harrington, ME, St Jeor ST, Silverstein LJ. Predicting resting energy expenditure from body mass index: Practical applications and limitations. Obes Res 1997;5:17s. Abstract.

$$\text{REE (from chart in Table 91-2)} = 1258 \times \text{AF of } 1.3$$
$$= 1635 \text{ kcal/day}$$

$$1635 + \text{PA of } 100 \text{ (1-mile walk/day)} = 1735 \text{ kcal/day}$$

2. A 32-year-old male business executive who travels a lot, but works out two times a week for 1 hour of vigorous activity (conditioning, exercise) at the health

Table 91-3 Examples of Common Physical Activities for Healthy US Adults by Intensity of Effort Required in MET Scores and Kilocalories per Minute

Light (<3.0 METs or <4 kcal/min)	Moderate (3.0–8.0 METs or 4–7 kcal/min)	Hard/Vigorous (>6.0 METs or >7 kcal/min)
Walking, slowly (strolling) (1–2 mph)	Walking, briskly (3–4 mph)	Walking, briskly uphill or with a load
Cycling, stationary (<50 W)	Cycling for pleasure or transportation (≤10 mph)	Cycling, fast or racing (>10 mph)
Swimming, slow treading	Swimming, moderate effort	Swimming, fast treading or crawl
Conditioning exercise, light stretching	Conditioning exercise, general calisthenics	Conditioning exercise, stair ergometer, ski machine
...	Racket sports, table tennis	Racket sports, singles tennis, racketball
Golf, power cart	Golf, pulling cart or carrying clubs	...
Bowling	...	...
Fishing, sitting	Fishing, standing/casting	Fishing in stream
Boating, power	Canoeing, leisurely (2.0–3.9 mph)	Canoeing, rapidly (≥4 mph)
Home care, carpet sweeping	Home care, general cleaning	Moving furniture
Mowing lawn, riding mower	Mowing lawn, power mower	Mowing lawn, hand mower
Home repair, carpentry	Home repair, painting	...

The METs (work metabolic rate/resting metabolic rate) are multiples of the resting rate of oxygen consumption during physical activity. One MET represents the approximate rate of oxygen consumption of a seated adult at rest, or about 3.5 mL/min·kg. The equivalent energy cost of 1 MET in kilocalories/min is about 1.2 for a 70-kg person, or approximately 1 kcal/hr·kg.
SOURCE: Pate RR, Pratt M, Blair SN, et al. Physical activity and public health: a recommendation from the Centers for Disease Control and Prevention and the American College of Sports Medicine. JAMA 1995;273:402–407.

club and jogs two times per week for 1 hour (5 miles): height = 70 inches; weight = 192 lb; BMI = 27.

REE (from chart in Table 91-2) = 1828 × AF of 1.3
= 2376 kcal/day

2376 + PA of 120 (60 minutes × 2) = 120 ×
7 kcal/min = 840 kcal/week/7 = 120 kcal/day +
105 (10 miles @ 100 kcal/mile = 1000 kcal/week/7
= 143 kcal/day

2376 + PAs of 120 + 143 = 2639

Note that PA can be figured either by the day or by the week. Intake can then be adjusted accordingly.

Another way of monitoring daily physical activity is with the use of an activity monitor, such as the Digi-Walker digital step counter. The goal is to increase readouts in steps gradually by increasing physical activity. However, it is important to also generally quantitate the type of activity being done. Thus, the overall goal of such activity monitors is to provide a baseline reading and motivate individuals to do more by providing them with direct feedback. Such increases in activity can then be more simply traced and recorded on monitoring forms.

ESTIMATING DIETARY INTAKE AND PROMOTING CHANGE

One of the most difficult tasks in weight management is to estimate dietary intake. Most obese individuals underestimate their intake and fail to adequately describe their intake on a recall basis. Thus, a 7-day prospective food record is recommended to be kept by all potential patients in as much detail as possible. This record should reflect the patients' "usual" diet prior to intervention and should also be sensitive to the pattern of eating (time, place, and occasion), portion size, and method of preparation. Patients should be instructed in detail how to keep the food record and counseled with regard to why it is important to establish a true baseline before any interventions.

The 7-day food record should then reflect a good pattern on which to base any dietary interventions or recommendations for change (29). A general calculation for caloric intake can be done by categorizing foods into food groups, estimating portion sizes according to the Food Guide Pyramid, and separating out fats, sweets, and alcoholic and other caloric drinks for added caloric value. The dietary intervention should begin with this usual pattern in mind. The first goal is either to achieve caloric balance to maintain weight or to achieve a caloric deficit to reflect a desired weight loss. An intervention plan can then be made using the Food Guide Pyramid, as outlined for the 1200-kcal BDD in Table 91-1 or by examples of the 1600-, 2200- and 2800-kcal diets outlined to guide healthy changes (14). Foods eaten that are not listed conveniently in the Food Guide Pyramid are then targeted for evaluation jointly with the patient. It is important to be realistic about what can be achieved and what weight loss can be expected. Thus, the usual food pattern derived from the 7-day food record can be used to begin recommendations for change (increasing or decreasing food groups, assessing food portion sizes, changing or substituting foods especially of high caloric and/or high fat value, and changing eating patterns where feasible).

Our monthly monitoring chart is presented in Figure 91-2. This is an example of how self-monitoring can be used to reinforce behavioral changes and to encourage adherence to prescribed dietary and activity changes. By simply asking patients to log daily or weekly weights or weight changes and using a simpler system of /, +, or − to indicate usual and

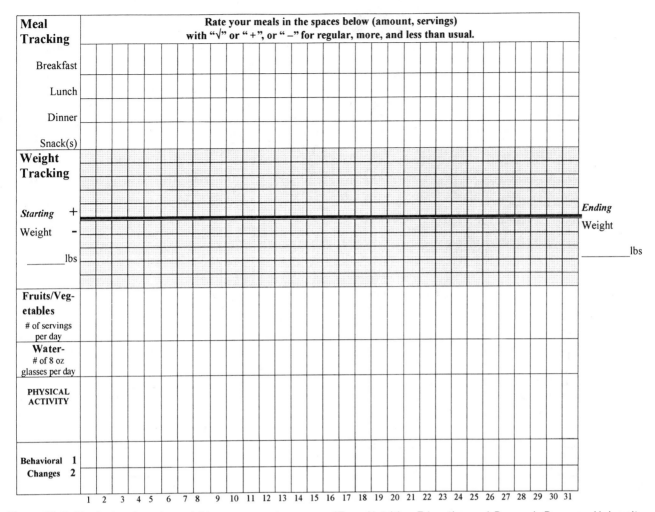

Meal Tracking	Rate your meals in the spaces below (amount, servings) with "√" or " + ", or " – " for regular, more, and less than usual.																														
Breakfast																															
Lunch																															
Dinner																															
Snack(s)																															

Figure 91-2 Monitoring form for weight management program. (From Nutrition Education and Research Program, University of Nevada School of Medicine, Reno, NV 89557.)

more or less than usual, simple changes can be encouraged, monitored, and assessed. The goal is to encourage small, incremental changes in behaviors toward the prescribed BDD diet, with increases in PA monitored by a simple activity monitor (Digi-Walker) and awareness of weight changes. This chart has been useful not only in our weight reduction programs but also in weight maintenance protocols.

DIET COMPOSITION

The ideal composition of the diet for weight loss and weight maintenance has not been established. During weight reduction, it appears that the greatest impact of diet is from its total energy deficit, and the diet composition has little effect on the rate or magnitude of weight loss over the short term (33–35). On the other hand, over the long term or conditions of weight maintenance, the total energy requirement may be affected by many factors and diet composition, mainly high fat intake, may make a contribution to weight gain (36).

Although consensus was seemingly being established around the efficacy of diets low in fat, the increasing incidence of obesity despite lower fat intakes in the United States

has raised many questions regarding associated trends in higher total caloric intakes (37). Concomitant higher carbohydrate intakes are now also being questioned with regard to their relative efficacy compared to diets higher in monounsaturated fats and low in carbohydrates that have been demonstrating more favorable overall effects on HDL cholesterol, triglycerides, insulin, and glucose (38). Simultaneously, popularized high-protein diets continue to be suggested as an alternative, but the role of alcohol in weight management is largely ignored. Thus, many new theories are emerging regarding the type and amount of fats in the diet, the role of carbohydrates beyond substitution for fat calories, the efficacy of high-protein diets for weight loss, the contributions of alcohol beyond its caloric load, the importance of water, and the impact of energy density on the selection of foods.

The effects of diet composition on total energy balance through increased intake and/or increases in energy expenditure through the thermic effect of food need further study. Further, the role of fat intake on fat stores through selective oxidative processes and the genetic predisposition to gain weight and deposit fat centrally are important issues still to be addressed (39). Behavioral, psychological, and environmental factors also affect eating patterns and food intake, thus ultimately affecting diet composition. Additionally, physiologic stimulators as well as genetic factors may predispose the selection of foods higher in carbohydrates and/or fat. Thus, dietary patterns are highly individual and highly variable, resulting in unpredictable outcomes. Importantly, long-term compliance to dietary interventions is affected by how well the diet composition meets the most important of these established needs.

A low-calorie step I diet has been outlined by the recent guidelines for the treatment of obesity (1) and is recommended to guide the formulation of diets to be used for weight reduction while providing adequate nutrition. It incorporates guidelines outlined by other organizations, particularly those of the American Heart Association, and represents a balanced perspective that should be initiated in most cases (40,41). New additions are included for calories, protein, calcium, and fiber with the recommendation that alcohol be minimized because it displaces more nutritious foods. These guidelines are outlined in Table 91-4 (1) and should serve to guide the nutrient composition of LCDs used for weight reduction.

BEYOND DIET

Fat and sugar substitutes have a role in the dietary management of overweight and obese individuals primarily because they can potentially lower fat and caloric intake overall. However, it is important that they are used in the context of a regular diet, used in moderation and balance with other foods, are appreciated for total energy and nutrient value, and do not replace other nutritious foods (42,43). Likewise, *meal replacements*, which are formulated products, have value because they provide a regulated amount of calories per serving, are usually fortified with essential nutrients and fiber, and are economical, safe, and convenient to use. They also provide a departure from normal eating patterns and can serve as a venue for reeducation about and/or reformulation of what foods can be substituted or reintroduced. Finally, *dietary supplements* should be considered when eating patterns are compromised, erratic, limited in choices, or less than 1200 kcal/day (3). Approximately 50% of the U.S. population uses such supplements (44). The most common supplements are a multivitamin tablet, a calcium-containing supplement, and/or a vitamin C tablet. Vitamin and mineral supplements should never be used in lieu of a healthy diet, and their use should be evaluated on a case-by-case basis. As previously discussed, special attention should be placed on folate/folic acid, vitamin B_{12}, and calcium for dieting men as well as women. *Meal patterns and food portion sizes* are also deemed important in regulating dietary intake overall and should be evaluated as part of the dietary history and 7-day food records. Interventions should be focused on the total diet, eating patterns rather than specific foods, and obtaining nutrient adequacy through

Table 91-4 Low-Calorie Step I Diet	
NUTRIENT	**RECOMMENDED INTAKE**
Calories[a]	Approximately 500 or 1000 kcal/day reduction from usual intake
Total Fat[b]	30% or less of total calories
Saturated Fatty Acids[c]	8% to 10% of total calories
Monounsaturated Fatty Acids	Up to 15% of total calories
Polyunsaturated Fatty Acids	Up to 10% of total calories
Cholesterol[c]	<300 mg/day
Protein[d]	Approximately 15% of total calories
Carbohydrate[e]	55% or more of total calories
Sodium Chloride	No more than 100 mmol per day (approximately 2.4 g of sodium or approximately 6 g of sodium chloride)
Calcium[f]	1000 to 1500 mg
Fiber[e]	20 to 30 g

[a] Alcohol provides unneeded calories and displaces more nutritious foods; it should be minimized.

[b] Fat-modified foods may provide a helpful strategy for lowering total fat intake but will only be effective if they are also low in calories and if there is no compensation of calories from carbohydrate or protein.

[c] Patients with high blood cholesterol levels may need to use the step II diet to achieve further reductions in LDL cholesterol levels; in the step II diet, saturated fatty acids are reduced to less than 7 percent of total calories, and cholesterol levels to less than 200 mg/day. All of the other nutrients are the same as in step 1.

[d] Protein should be derived from plant sources and lean sources of animal protein.

[e] Complex carbohydrates from different vegetables, fruits, and whole grains are good sources of vitamins, minerals, and fiber. A diet rich in soluble fiber, including oat bran, legumes, barley, and most fruits and vegetables may be effective in reducing risk factors. A high-fiber diet may also aid in weight management by promoting satiety at lower levels of calorie and fat intake. Some authorities recommend 20 to 30 g daily with 6 g from soluble fiber.

[f] Moderate weight loss may be associated with a loss of bone and thus may increase the risk of fracture. Many patients on weight loss diets consume less than the recommended amount of calcium and most mineral supplements do not supply adequate calcium supplementation, with 1000 mg calcium the rate of bone turnover during weight loss in premenopausal women. Dieters should maintain recommended calcium and vitamin D intakes during caloric restriction.

From Expert Panel on the Identification, Evaluation and Treatment of Overweight and Obesity in Adults, National Heart, Lung, and Blood Institute Education Initiative, National Institutes of Health. Clinical guidelines on the identification, evaluation and treatment of overweight and obesity in adults, Bethesda, MD: National Institutes of Health, 1998.

a variety of foods. Finally, the enjoyment of eating should not be overlooked, and flexibility in a meal plan must be included to maximize the potential for long-term adherence rather than short-term compliance.

THE FUTURE OF DIETARY TREATMENT

Diet fads come and go, and there will always be a popular diet or dietary strategy that will seemingly monopolize the current marketplace. Education of consumers toward realistic goals, maintenance of diets that comply with the dietary guidelines, and the rationale that there is no one food, nutrient, or strategy that will be uniquely successful will always be a major challenge. Fad diets usually emphasize 1) large weight losses in short amounts of time; 2) the best or ideal macronutrient composition of the diet (fat, carbohydrate, or protein); 3) special attributes of a special ingredient, food, or substance; 4) a rationale for a specific mechanism of a food or food combination that is preferred; 5) featured and/or structured meal plans and recipes; 6) foods or food combinations with special actions; and/or 7) a focus on why other diets don't work. Diet recommendations should be seriously evaluated with regard to efficacy, safety, and long-term effects. Although there can usually be some "half-truth" imbedded in any claims, the best way to evaluate a diet fad is by asking the following questions (all of which should be answered affirmatively) (45).

1. Is the diet well-balanced and does it include a variety of foods? Are all the major food groups included?

2. Does the diet impose a consistent caloric deficit or balance? Are the weight loss expectations reasonable? Is a safe weight loss (0.5 to 3 lb per week) consistent?

3. Is a minimum of 50 g protein provided daily?

4. Is a minimum of 100 g of carbohydrate provided daily?

5. Are the meal plans practical, flexible, and individualized? Does the plan allow for special foods and preferences?

6. Is increased energy expenditure or physical activity emphasized without compensation by foods?

7. Are total kilocalories emphasized along with other aspects of the diet (fat, carbohydrate, protein, alcohol) in a totally integrated lifestyle change approach?

8. Are reasonable dietary goals established?

9. Is nutrition education provided?

10. Is positive behavior change for both diet and activity incorporated into the program?

It is important to recognize that the majority of the weight loss industry flourishes without medical involvement. Approximately 62% of men and 71% of women are dieting, and these dieters include normal-weight as well as underweight and obese individuals (46). An additional problem is the recognition that binge eating disorder (BED) occurs in 30% of obese people in treatment (47). All of these underlying issues makes the dietary management of obesity extremely complex.

Practical approaches that emphasize normalized eating patterns and a variety of foods as part of a long-term, inte-grated lifestyle should form the foundation of a solid dietary approach. Special efforts to maximize individual treatment considerations should be given when the dietary management includes attention to adjunctive therapies, such as pharmacotherapy or pre- or postsurgical interventions for weight loss and/or special dietary needs for the management of obesity-related conditions, such as diabetes, hypertension, and cardiovascular diseases. Caution should be taken to ensure adequate intake because some patients may compromise their intake because of increased motivation to new treatments, such as pharmacotherapy, and lose weight more rapidly than anticipated. Additionally, special requirements for the treatment of obesity-related comorbidities should be carefully addressed and included in the total dietary plan.

Importantly, losses of 5% to 10% of body weight are significant. Thus, interventions that encourage small, incremental weight losses over time that can be maintained are proving to be more successful. A 200-kcal deficit per day (100 kcal in expenditure by 30 minutes of walking plus 100 kcal in intake by omitting 2 teaspoons of high-fat sources) can result in 1400 kcal/week, equal to approximately a half pound or approximately 26 lb over 1 year.

The dietary management of obesity is key to the treatment and management of obesity and prevention of further weight gain. The greatest challenge for health professionals in this area is to develop innovative methods to help patients continue to enjoy eating while successfully controlling their weight. Further, as reimbursement for professional services are extremely limited, the patients must also assume responsibility in their own long-term care. Proactive consumer organizations, such as the American Obesity Association, support patients to help educate the public about obesity, to help professionals to provide the best possible care, to encourage the prevention of obesity, especially in children, and to encourage insurance companies and third-party payers to provide adequate coverage for obesity treatment and prevention (48).

The future of dietary treatment for obesity includes innovation to meet these new challenges. Because we have not been successful in the long term, new treatment strategies must include the consideration of obesity as a disease. A seven-step process is recommended before initiating any dietary treatment for obesity: 1) Establish and assess BMI and related risks (waist measurements for men ≥ 40 in. and women ≥ 35 in.); 2) assess weight-related comorbidities (diabetes, hypertension, cardiovascular diseases), readiness to diet, and any contraindication to a low-calorie diet (pregnancy, cancerous cachexia, and other debilitating diseases); 3) calculate and evaluate REE from BMI; 4) estimate level of activity and usual activity; 5) estimate dietary intake and/or establish a dietary intake pattern; 6) project energy balance and prescribe a level of energy deficit and other dietary parameters; and 7) develop long-term, practical dietary strategies and individual goals with individuals.

Thus, as we begin to better assess the needs and future directions for the dietary management of the obese, as well as overweight individuals, we can project important successful outcomes that take time and effort. Short-lived, unhealthy diet fads should be avoided, and emphasis should be placed on practical interventions that support health and the enjoyment of eating.

REFERENCES

1. Expert Panel on the Identification, Evaluation and Treatment of Overweight and Obesity in Adults. National Heart, Lung, and Blood Institute Education Initiative, National Institutes of Health. Clinical guidelines on the identification, evaluation and treatment of overweight and obesity in adults. Bethesda, MD: National Institutes of Health, 1998.

2. World Health Organization. Obesity. Preventing and managing the global epidemic. Report of a WHO consultation on obesity. Geneva: World Health Organization, 1998.

3. Committee to Develop Criteria for Evaluating the Outcomes of Approaches to Prevent and Treat Obesity. Food and Nutrition Board, Institute of Medicine. Thomas PR, ed. Weighing the options: Criteria for evaluating weight-management programs. Washington, D.C.: National Academy Press, 1995.

4. Shape Up America and American Obesity Association, Guidance for the treatment of adult obesity. Bethesda, MD: Shape Up America, 1996.

5. U.S. Department of Agriculture and U.S. Department of Health and Human Services. Dietary guidelines for Americans. 4th ed. Home and Garden Bulletin No. 232. Washington, D.C.: U.S. Government Printing Office, 1995.

6. Hill JO, Peter JC. Environmental contributions to the obesity epidemic. Science 1998;280:1371–1373.

7. National Task Force on the Prevention and Treatment of Obesity, National Institutes of Health. Very low-calorie diets. JAMA 1993;270: 967–974.

8. Wadden TA. The treatment of obesity: an overview. In: Stunkard AJ, Wadden TA, eds. Obesity theory and therapy. New York: Raven Press, 1993:197–217.

9. Foreyt JP, Goodrick GK. Impact of behavior therapy on weight loss. Am J Health Promotion 1994;8: 466–468.

10. Stunkard AJ. Diet, exercise and behavior therapy: a cautionary tale. Obes Res 1996;4(3):293–294.

11. Wadden TA, Berkowitz RI, Vogt RA, et al. Lifestyle modification in the pharmacologic treatment of obesity: a pilot investigation of a potential primary care approach. Obes Res 1997;5:218–226.

12. Simkin-Silverman LR, Wing RR. Management of obesity in primary care. Obes Res 1997;5:603–612.

13. St. Jeor ST, Brunner RL, Harrington ME, et al. A classification system to evaluate weight maintainers, gainers, and losers. J Am Diet Assoc 1997;97:481–488.

14. St. Jeor ST, Brunner RL, Harrington ME, et al. Who are the maintainers? Obes Res 1995;3:249s–259s.

15. U.S. Department of Agriculture. USDA's Food Guide Pyramid. Home and Garden Bulletin No. 252. Washington, D.C.: USDA Human Nutrition Information Service, 1992.

16. Yates AA, Schlicker SA, Suitor CW. Dietary reference intakes: the new basis for recommendations for calcium and related nutrients, B vitamins, and choline. J Am Diet Assoc 1998;98:699–706.

17. Institute of Medicine, Food and Nutrition Board. Recommended dietary allowances. 10th ed. Washington, D.C.: National Academy Press, 1989.

18. Institute of Medicine, Food and Nutrition Board. Dietary reference intakes for calcium, phosphorus, magnesium, vitamin D, and fluoride. Washington, D.C.: National Academy Press, 1997.

19. National Institutes of Health. Optimal calcium intake. NIH Consensus Statement 1994;12:1–31.

20. Mullins VA, Houtkooper L. Calcium supplement guidelines. Tucson: Cooperative Extension, The University of Arizona, College of Agriculture, 1998.

21. Institute of Medicine, Food and Nutrition Board. Dietary reference intakes for thiamin, riboflavin, niacin, vitamin B-6, folate, vitamin B-12, pantothenic acid, biotin, and choline. Washington, D.C.: National Academy Press, 1998.

22. Bailey LB. Evaluation of a new recommended dietary allowance for folate. J Am Diet Assoc 1992; 92:463–468.

23. Hine J. What practitioners need to know about folic acid. J Am Diet Assoc 1996;96:451–452.

24. Rimm EB, Willett WC, Hu FB, et al. Folate and vitamin B6 from diet and supplements in relation to risk of coronary heart disease among women. JAMA 1998;279: 359–364.

25. U.S. Department of Health and Human Services. Part 3. Federal Register 1996;61:8750–8806.

26. Stabler SP, Lindenbaum J, Allen RH. Vitamin B-12 deficiency in the elderly: current dilemmas. Am J Clin Nutr 1997;66:741–749.

27. Mifflin MD, St. Jeor ST, Hill LA, et al. A new predictive equation for resting energy expenditure in healthy individuals. Am J Clin Nutr 1990;51:241–247.

28. Harrington ME, St. Jeor ST, Silverstein LJ. Predicting resting energy expenditure from body mass index: practical applications and limitations. Obes Res 1997;5:17s. Abstract.

29. St. Jeor ST, ed. Obesity assessment: tools, methods, interpretations. A reference case: the RENO Diet-Heart Study. New York: Chapman and Hall, 1997.

30. St. Jeor ST, Stumbo PJ. Energy needs and weight maintenance in controlled feeding studies. In: Dennis B, Ershow A, Obarzanek E, Clevidence B, eds. Well controlled diet studies in humans. A practical guide to design and management. Chicago: American Dietetic Association, 1998.

31. World Health Organization. Energy and protein requirements. Report of a Joint WHO/UNU expert consultation. Technical Report Series

724. Geneva: World Health Organization, 1985.

32. Pate RR, Pratt M, Blair SN, et al. Physical activity and public health: a recommendation from the Centers for Disease Control and Prevention and the American College of Sports Medicine. JAMA 1995;273:402–407.

33. Hill JO, Drougas H, Peters JC. Obesity treatment: can diet composition play a role? Ann Intern Med 1993;119:694–697.

34. Golay A, Allaz AF, Morel Y, et al. Similar weight loss with low- or high-carbohydrate diets. Am J Clin Nutr 1996;63:174–178.

35. Hill JO, Peters JC, Reed GW, et al. Nutrient balance in humans: effects of diet composition. Am J Clin Nutr 1991;54:10–17.

36. Lichenstein A, Kennedy E, Bauer P, et al. Dietary fat consumption and health. Nutr Rev 1998;56: S3–S28.

37. Connor WE, Connor SL. Should a low-fat, high carbohydrate diet be recommended for everyone? New Engl J Med 1997;337:562–563.

38. Katan MB, Grundy SM, Willett W. Beyond low fat diets. New Engl J Med 1997;337:563–566.

39. Swinburn B, Ravussin E. Energy balance or fat balance? Am J Clin Nutr 1993;57:766S–771S.

40. National Cholesterol Education Program. Second Report of the Expert Panel on Detection, Evaluation and Treatment of High Blood Cholesterol in Adults (Adult Treatment Panel II). Circulation 1994;89:1333.

41. National High Blood Pressure Education Program, NHLBI, NIH. The Sixth Report of the Joint National Committee on Prevention, Detection, Evaluation and Treatment of High Blood Pressure. NIH Publication No. 98-4080. Washington, D.C.: National Institutes of Health, 1997.

42. American Dietetic Association. Position of the American Dietetic Association: fat replacements. J Am Diet Assoc 1991;91:1285–1288.

43. American Dietetic Association. Position of the American Dietetic Association: use of nutritive and non-nutritive sweeteners. J Am Diet Assoc 1993;93:816–821.

44. Report of the Commission on Dietary Supplement Labels. Washington, D.C.: Department of Health and Human Services, 1997.

45. St. Jeor ST, Dwyer JT. The optimal diet: does it exist? Weight Control Digest 1991;11(7):105.

46. Levy AS, Heaton AW. Weight control practices of US adults trying to lose weight. Ann Intern Med 1993;119:661–666.

47. American Psychiatric Association. Diagnostic and statistical manual of mental disorders, 4th ed. Washington, D.C.: American Psychiatric Association, 1994.

48. Atkinson RL. Let's give obesity the attention it deserves! AOA Rep 1996;1:1–2.

Chapter 92

Pharmacologic Management of the Obese Patient

Nikhil V. Dhurandhar
Richard L. Atkinson

Obesity is the most common disease in the United States and in much of the world. The National Health and Nutrition Examination Survey (NHANES) carried out by the U.S. government demonstrated that by the end of 1994, 22.5% of the population was obese [body mass index (BMI) > 30] and 55% of the total population was overweight (BMI > 25) (33,34). This is an increase in the prevalence of obesity of more than 50% since 1980. Obesity produces numerous comorbidities such as diabetes mellitus, hypertension, dyslipidemia, sleep apnea, cancer, and gall bladder disease, all of which contribute to the increase in mortality with obesity, particularly in younger individuals (7,26,45,52). It has been estimated that more than 300,000 people die each year from obesity-related diseases (40,54).

Historically, the clinical treatment of obesity has been limited to a low-calorie, low-fat, high-fiber diet, an exercise regimen, and lifestyle behavior modification. It is estimated that many people who lose weight will regain most of the weight lost after 5 years. The reasons for this regain are not completely clear. Although the lifestyle modification of the diet and exercise are extremely important for long-term weight maintenance and overall health, some obese patients may need additional help.

Physicians have often been reluctant to prescribe medication for the treatment of obesity. This reluctance has been primarily due to the addictive potential of early obesity drugs such as dexamphetamine and methamphetamine. However, the new generation of obesity drugs offers physicians new treatment strategies for their patients. Recent research has begun to change the perception of obesity drugs. In 1992, Weintraub (58) reported that obesity drugs produced reductions of body weight and complications of obesity for up 3.5

years. Coupled with discoveries of the genetic basis for several animal models of obesity (10,12,28,43,61), these studies altered the perception of pharmacologic treatment of obesity and led to a rapid expansion of research on obesity drugs and to a dramatic increase in the long-term use of drugs to treat obesity.

In this chapter, we discuss the pharmacologic treatment of obesity, including a discussion of recently approved drugs, those still available, and others that may soon become available. It should be pointed out that the obesity drugs should be regarded as a *supplement* and not a *substitute* to the patients' effort at weight reduction with lifestyle changes to improve the diet and physical activity.

MECHANISMS OF ACTION OF OBESITY DRUGS

Obesity is a disease of storage in the body of excess energy as fat. In order to reduce body fat, there must be a period of negative energy balance. This must be accomplished either by a reduction of food intake or an increase in energy expenditure. Pharmacologic agents act by different mechanisms on the energy balance equation (Table 92-1).

Reduction of Energy Intake

Reduction of energy intake may occur in several ways. Most obesity drugs are thought to reduce appetite or hunger, so food-seeking behavior is reduced (27,36,51). However, there also is evidence for increased satiety, resulting in reduced amounts of energy being consumed in a meal. There is limited evidence that obesity drugs may alter dietary preference. Studies by Wurtman et al (60) suggested that serotonin

Table 92-1 Obesity Drugs: Mechanisms of Action

1. Reduce Energy Intake
   a. Decrease hunger and/or appetite
   b. Increase satiety
   c. Decrease fat and/or carbohydrate preference
   d. Reduce nutrient absorption
2. Increase Energy Expenditure
   a. Stimulate physical activity
      1) Tremor
      2) Spontaneous physical activity
   b. Increase metabolic rate
      1) Increase resting metabolic rate
      2) Increase thermogenesis with eating, cold, exercise

agonists may reduce cravings for carbohydrate, and Blundell et al (5) reported that dexfenfluramine may reduce preference for dietary fat. If the total quantity of food remains unchanged, reduction of the proportion of calories as fat will reduce energy intake.

Energy intake could also be reduced by reduction of absorption of nutrients from the gastointestinal (GI) tract, in effect producing malabsorption. As described below, two drugs are available that block absorption from the GI tract by binding or inactivating enzymes that digest fat or carbohydrate (4,18,19).

Increase in Energy Expenditure

Obesity drugs may increase energy expenditure by stimulating an increase in activity levels or by increasing metabolic rate directly. Some patients complain of tremor, particularly during the initial phase of treatment with certain pharmacologic agents (14,55). Tremor is muscle contraction and requires energy expenditure. Anecdotally, patients report an increase in willingness to exercise and an increase in comfort when active, but there have been no studies that have clearly documented this. Most studies include behavioral therapy that focuses on increasing activity, so the independent contribution of medications is difficult to determine.

Numerous studies have evaluated the effects of obesity drugs on metabolism. This literature is controversial, but some animal and human studies suggest that some obesity drugs may increase energy expenditure by increasing resting metabolic rate (RMR) and others report increased dietary-induced thermogenesis (DIT) (36,56). Levitsky et al (36) reported that rats given fenfluramine had a normal RMR, but an exaggerated rise in energy expenditure after a meal, when compared with untreated control animals. Troiano et al (56) demonstrated a similar phenomenon in humans. However, other investigators have found no increase in either RMR or in DIT with fenfluramine or dexfenfluramine (48).

The combination of ephedrine and caffeine has been shown to increase energy expenditure, probably by stimulating beta-adrenergic receptors (37,53). Liu et al (37) and Stock (53) demonstrated that beta$_1$ and beta$_2$ receptors were initially stimulated, but tachyphylaxis occurred rapidly. However, the

chronic increase in metabolic rate suggested a continued stimulation of beta$_3$ receptors.

Theory of Altered Defense of Body Weight

Some authors advance the theory that obesity drugs may reduce the level at which body weight is defended. Keesey et al (31) have argued that animals and people have a "set point" around which weight is defended. Other authors suggest this is a "settling point" caused by the confluence of numerous factors that affect body weight (20). There is no doubt that with weight loss induced by dieting, both animals and humans lower metabolic rate (31). It appears that treatment with obesity drugs reduces body weight, and this reduction is maintained at the lower level. Levitsky et al (36) showed that animals initially decreased food intake and lost weight with fenfluramine or dexamphetamine, but that food intake returned to baseline without a regain in body weight. This phenomenon also is seen in animals or patients after intestinal bypass or ileal transposition surgeries (2).

CATEGORIES OF OBESITY DRUGS

Maintenance of energy balance is so critical to survival that there are many redundant mechanisms that influence food intake and energy expenditure (8). Numerous areas of the brain have been shown to participate in the regulation of energy balance, and they respond to different neurotransmitters. Many of the drugs approved for the treatment of obesity in the United States act on two of the more important neurotransmitters systems to regulate energy balance: the centrally active adrenergic and serotonergic systems.

Centrally Active Serotonergic Agents

Sibutramine is the only currently approved obesity drug that prevents the reuptake of serotonin in the neural clefts. Fluoxetine and sertraline are antidepressant agents that are not approved for obesity, but have been shown to produce weight loss in humans or animals, and have been used by clinicians for obesity. They are thought to act exclusively as serotonin reuptake inhibitors. Weight loss with fluoxetine reaches maximum at about 6 months; then there is a gradual regain so that 1-year loss is not significantly different from placebo (22).

There are a variety of centrally active adrenergic agents that are approved by the Food and Drug Administration (FDA) and available in the United States for the treatment of obesity (Table 92-2). These adrenergic agents either stimulate secretion of norepinephrine from central nervous system (CNS) nerve terminals or inhibit its uptake, thus leading to actions on food intake and energy expenditure.

Sibutramine is a norepinephrine as well as a serotonin reuptake inhibitor. Unlike phentermine and fenfluramine, sibutramine does not cause the release of norepinephrine or serotonin. In animals and humans, sibutramine was shown to decrease food intake by prolonging the appetite-regulating neurotransmitters to enhance feelings of satiety. In animals, sibutramine has produced a sustained increase in metabolic rate (with 30% greater oxygen consumption) for more than 6 hours after the drug was given.

The drugs shown in Table 92-2 in Drug Enforcement Agency (DEA) schedule II are not routinely used or are used

Table 92-2 Current Pharmacologic Agents Used for Obesity and Their DEA Schedule Category

GENERIC NAME	TRADE NAME	DEA SCHEDULE
Catecholaminergic Drugs		
Amphetamine	Dexedrine	II
Methamphetamine	Desoxyn	II
Phenmetrazine	Bontril	II
Benzphetamine	Didrex	III
Chlorphentermine		III
Choltermine		III
Phendimetrazine	Plegine, Prelu-2	III
Diethylpropion	Tenuate	IV
Mazindol	Sanorex, Mazinor	IV
Phentermine	Ionamin, Fastin, Adipex	IV
Phenylpropanolamine	Dexatrim, Accutrim	OTC
Ephedrine and caffeine	Numerous names	NA
Serotonergic Drugs		
Fluoxetine	Prozac	NA
Sibutramine	Meridia	IV?
Enzyme Inhibitors		
Orlistat	Xenical	

* OTC = over-the-counter; NA = not currently approved by the FDA for the treatment of obesity.

only in extremely rare circumstances by responsible physicians. These include dexamphetamine, methamphetamine, and phenmetrazine. These drugs have significant abuse potential and do not produce significantly greater weight loss than do less addictive agents (51). Schedule III drugs include benzphetamine, chlorphentermine, chlortermine, and phendimetrazine and are thought to have less abuse potential, but are not used by most physicians for treating obesity.

Adrenergic drugs in DEA schedule IV include phentermine, diethylpropion, and mazindol, and are the adrenergic drugs most used by physicians in the United States to treat obesity. All three of these drugs have minimal addiction or abuse potential (25), and the popularity of phentermine over the other two is due primarily to the publicity of the Weintraub regimen (58). Griffiths et al (25) demonstrated in non-human primates that diethylpropion had somewhat higher reinforcement potential than did phentermine. Phentermine and diethylpropion stimulate norepinephrine from CNS nerve terminals and mazindol acts predominantly as a reuptake inhibitor. Silverstone (51) concluded that all of the drugs in this category produce approximately the same weight loss.

Enzyme Inhibitors

Orlistat (Xenical) reduces absorption of fat by binding to lipase in the intestine and inhibiting its action (18,19). Clinical trials have recently been concluded in the United States and the drug has received approval from the FDA, but there are few data published in the literature on orlistat. Orlistat has an advantage over the centrally active adrenergic and serotonergic agents listed above because it acts peripherally and is not

expected to have any adverse effects on cardiovascular function. Orlistat produces about 8% to 10% weight loss of initial body weight. Side effects include intestinal gas, cramping, and diarrhea, which may make it unacceptable to some patients. Also, patients treated with orlistat had lower levels of beta-carotene and vitamin D. A vitamin supplement is recommended for patients taking this drug. During its review by the FDA, questions arose because, compared to the placebo group, the incidence of breast cancer was greater in the group treated with orlistat (120 mg three times a day). The increased incidence of breast cancer was not noted in the group receiving orlistat 60 mg three times a day. A careful reanalysis of the data has shown that it seems very unlikely that orlistat causes breast cancer. Nevertheless, most experts recommend that women should be followed more carefully than usual to detect any early breast cancer.

Experimental Drugs or Drugs Not Currently Approved by the FDA

Acarbose is an alpha-glucosidase inhibitor that reduces digestion of complex carbohydrates, allowing them to pass unabsorbed into the large intestine (4). The appearance of undigested complex carbohydrates in the colon is associated with increased intestinal gas, flatulence, abdominal pain, and diarrhea. Acarbose is approved in the United States for treatment of diabetes, but its effects in studies for the treatment of obesity were disappointing. It is not an adequate weight loss agent.

There have been a few studies of the combination of ephedrine with caffeine and/or aspirin for obesity (14,55). It appears that this combination results in chronic stimulation of the beta$_3$-adrenergic system, with an attendant increase in lean body mass and decrease in fat mass (14,37,53,55). Ephedrine stimulates norepinephrine secretion, whereas caffeine appears to delay the degradation of norepinephrine and inhibits phosphodiesterase in the postsynaptic neurons, thereby potentiating the effect of ephedrine. Aspirin inhibits the activity of prostaglandins that degrade norepinephrine in the neural cleft. Thus, the end result of treatment with these three agents is a prolonged increase in norepinephrine activity. During the initial phase of treatment with these agents, norepinephrine stimulation of beta$_1$ and beta$_2$ receptors produces increases in heart rate and blood pressure, and elevates serum insulin levels, occasionally worsening glucose intolerance or diabetic control. Some patients report a tremor. However, tachyphylaxis occurs fairly rapidly and over about 1 month, and these symptoms resolve (37,53).

Ephedrine may be extracted from the Chinese plant ma huang, caffeine from coffee beans, and acetosalicylic acid (aspirin) from willow bark. Since such extracts may be marketed as "supplements" in the United States and are subject to minimal FDA oversight, sales of varieties of this combination are currently booming. The FDA and Federal Trade Commission (FTC) have become concerned and issued warnings because a number of people have had cardiac events or even died while taking these compounds, but a direct cause and effect relationship has not been established.

Gene Products

The discovery of the gene defect responsible for obesity in ob/ob mice and the subsequent identification of the ob gene protein generated intense publicity (10,28,43,61). This was rapidly followed by discovery of a defective receptor for ob gene protein, causing the defect identified as the db/db mice and the Zucker obese rat. The ob gene product was named leptin, and there is hope that leptin will be useful for the treatment of obesity (61). The optimism about the role of leptin in the treatment of human obesity was dampened by the findings that most obese humans have elevated levels of leptin (13), and some investigators have speculated that leptin will not be effective in reducing body weight in obese humans.

However, the findings that rodents made obese by feeding them a high-fat diet have high leptin levels, yet respond to leptin injections, suggests that there may be leptin resistance similar to insulin resistance in type II diabetes. Since much human obesity is exacerbated by high-calorie, high-fat diets, there is hope that with sufficient doses of leptin, humans will achieve weight loss. Clinical trials to assess the effect of leptin administration in humans are in progress.

DRUG TREATMENT OF OBESITY: SELECTION OF PATIENTS, DRUGS, AND REGIMEN

Who Should Be Treated with Obesity Drugs?

Several sets of guidelines have been advanced to guide clinicians in selecting appropriate patients for treatment (41,44,50,54). The National Institutes of Health (NIH) National Task Force on the Prevention and Treatment of Obesity recommends against long-term use of obesity drugs by general physicians until additional research has been performed (41). The FDA released guidances for the pharmaceutical industry for the types of studies necessary to obtain approval for new obesity drugs. These guidances suggested that obesity drugs may be used in individuals with a BMI of 30 without comorbidities and a BMI of 27 with comorbidities.

The North American Association for the Study of Obesity (NAASO) convened a broad-based group consisting of academicians, clinicians, industry representatives, and representatives from several government agencies, including the NIH, FDA, Federal Trade Commission, and the U.S. Health Care Financing Administration (HCFA) developed guidelines for the use of obesity drugs (44). These guidelines recommended that drugs might be considered for individuals with a BMI of 27 if no comorbidities were present. Drugs may be considered for individuals with a BMI below 27 in the presence of comorbidities after careful consideration of the risks and benefits of drug use.

Shape Up America! and the American Obesity Association (AOA) developed a comprehensive set of guidances for physician treatment of obesity that includes recommendations for obesity drugs (50). These guidances follow the FDA model of a BMI of 30 without comorbidities and a BMI of 27 for individuals with comorbidities, but allow a greater leeway for physicians to assess individual patients and come to a rational decision based on the individual risk factors and risk-benefit ratio.

The Shape Up America!-AOA document (50) suggested that obesity drugs be restricted to adults aged 18 and above, and listed conditions that are contraindications or cautions to their use (Table 92-3). Because of the limited research on

---

Table 92-3 Contraindications or Cautions to the Use of Obesity Drugs

1. Pregnancy or lactation
2. Unstable cardiac disease
3. Uncontrolled hypertension
4. Unstable severe systemic illness
5. Unstable psychiatric disorder or anorexia
6. Other drug therapy, if incompatible (e.g., MAO inhibitors, migraine drugs)
7. Closed-angle glaucoma (caution)
8. General anesthesia (absolute contraindication, except emergencies)

---

long-term use of obesity drugs, it was recommended that these agents not be used in patients with unstable medical or psychological conditions. Closed-angle glaucoma may be exacerbated by both adrenergic and serotonergic agents, so this condition requires careful follow-up if obesity drugs are used. Age above 65 years is a caution (3). Obesity drugs generally do not interact negatively with other drugs, with some notable exceptions. Antidepressant agents, including tricyclic and selective serotonin reuptake inhibitor drugs should be used only with caution, and monamine oxidase inhibitors are absolutely contraindicated because of the possibility of excess serotonin activity in the CNS.

The National Heart, Lung, and Blood Institute (NHLBI) issued clinical guidelines on the identification, evaluation, and treatment of overweight and obesity in adults (42). According to these guidelines, individuals with a BMI of 25 to 29.9 are considered overweight, and individuals with a BMI of 30 or greater are considered obese. Treatment of overweight is recommended only when two or more risk factors are present. The initial goal for weight loss should be 10% weight loss from baseline, and upon reaching the goal further weight loss may be attempted after further assessment. The rate of this weight loss should be about 1 to 2 lb per week. The guidelines further state that weight loss and maintenance therapy should use the combination of low-calorie diet, increased physical activity, and behavior therapy. As an adjunct to this strategy, weight loss drugs approved by the FDA may be used for patients with a BMI of 30 or greater with no concomitant obesity-related risk factors and for patients with a BMI of 27 or greater with concomitant obesity-related risk factors. The NHLBI guidelines also stress the need for a weight maintenance therapy and recommend that a weight maintenance program should be a priority after the initial 6 months of weight loss therapy.

How Should Obesity Drugs Be Used?

There is growing sentiment among clinicians and scientists who prescribe obesity drugs that, in individuals who have significantly severe obesity to warrant the use of drugs, long-term, including life-long, use may be necessary (50). The NHLBI guidelines (42) recommend that an obesity drug may be continued if it helps patients to lose and/or maintain weight loss and if there are no serious side effects. The guidelines emphasize that obesity drug safety and efficacy beyond 1 year of total treatment have not been established and a continued assessment for drug efficacy and safety is necessary. Because the initial period of treatment with obesity drugs is associated with a high number of side effects, a stepped-dose approach has been recommended (50,54). Table 92-4 lists initial and maximum doses for the most commonly used obesity drugs.

RESULTS OF TREATMENT

Studies with Single Drugs

The vast majority of clinical trials with obesity drugs have involved the use of single agents for short periods of time. Scoville (49) reviewed the results of over 200 studies of single agents and concluded that all of the agents available at that time produced essentially comparable results. The average additional weight loss above the placebo-treated control groups was about a half pound per week (49). Silverstone (51) reached similar conclusions when comparing short-term results from different agents.

Unfortunately, there are very few long-term studies that have evaluated any obesity drug for longer than a year. Goldstein et al (23) surveyed the literature and found only nine studies that had followed subjects for a year or more (Table 92-5). As seen in Table 92-5, with the exception of fluoxetine, longer-term weight loss ranged from about 5 to about 14 kg and most of the drugs produced better weight loss than placebo. Placebo weight losses in several studies were very good, demonstrating that the studies were not simple tests of drug versus placebo, but both groups underwent standard obesity therapy with diet, exercise, and behavioral therapy. Mazindol produced the largest weight losses (14.2 kg) seen with a single agent in the review by Goldstein et al (23), but the large loss in the placebo group (10.2 kg) suggests that the behavioral component was quite strong in this study.

Fluoxetine produces excellent weight loss over the first 6 months of treatment (15,22,39), although weight regain occurs thereafter and 1 year weight was not different between the placebo and experimental groups in 8 of 10 studies reported in a summary paper by Goldstein et al (23). Two studies, Marcus et al (39) and Darga et al (15), included a strong behavioral program and were able to obtain significant weight loss at 1 year.

Sibutramine, the obesity drug recently approved by the FDA, produced weight losses of about 7 to 10 kg in a dose-dependent manner (6,47). Weight loss was very rapid in the first 12 weeks of treatment but continued after 24 weeks of treatment. Although the weight loss was accompanied with significant reductions in serum cholesterol, triglycerides, and LDL cholesterol, the drug produced less decrease in blood pressure of hypertensive patients than does placebo with a comparable degree of weight loss (47). Blood pressure may rise slightly in normotensive patients, as does pulse rate (47). These side effects have raised concern and led to recommendations that patients should be very carefully followed early in the course of treatment and medications stopped if weight loss is not satisfactory or if blood pressure rises.

Studies with Drug Combinations

Three main combinations of drugs have been reported: phenylpropanolamine-benzocaine, ephedrine-methylxanthines-aspirin, and fenfluramine-phentermine (3,14,24,55,57,58). Phenylpropanolamine (PPA) is an adrenergic agent that is sold over the counter in the United States and has no reinforcement potential in animals (25). It produces modest weight loss when used alone (24). Benzocaine is a local anesthetic agent contained in some over-the-counter weight reduction aids. The rationale for its use is to anesthetize the taste buds and thus reduce food intake. In the only publication using this combination, Greenway (24) found weight loss in an 8-week trial was similar in the drug and placebo groups.

The combination of ephedrine and caffeine, with or without aspirin, produces results that are among the best of any drug regimen reported (14,55). Toubro et al (55) compared placebo, ephedrine alone, caffeine alone, and the combination of ephedrine and caffeine over a period of 24 weeks in 180 patients. The combination of ephedrine and caffeine

Table 92-4 Obesity Drugs: Dosage Regimens

	Initial (mg/day)	Maximum (mg/day)
Dexfenfluramine	15	30
Fenfluramine	10–20	60
Diethylpropion (CR)	75	75
Mazindol	1	3
Phentermine HCl	8–19	37.5
Phentermine resin	15	30
PPA	75	75
Sibutramine	15	39

Table 92-5 Long-Term Clinical Trials with Obesity Drugs

Obesity Drug	1-Year Weight Loss (kg)	
	Placebo	Active Agent
Diethylpropion	−10.5	−8.9
Mazindol	−10.2	−14.2
	—	−12.0
Fenfluramine	−4.5	−8.7
Dexfenfluramine	−7.2	−9.8
	−2.7	−5.7
	−4.6	−5.2
Fluoxetine	+0.6	−13.9
	−4.5	−8.2
	−1.5	−2.3
Sibutramine	−1.8	−6.0

Sibutramine data from Bray GA, Ryan DH, Gordon D, et al. A double-blind randomized placebo-controlled trial of sibutramine. Obes Res 1996;4:263–270; and Ryan DH, Kaiser P, Bray GA. Sibutramine: A novel new agent for obesity treatment. Obes Res 1995; 3(suppl 4):5535–5595. Table adapted from Goldstein DJ, Potvin JH. Long-term weight loss: The effect of pharmacologic agents. Am J Clin Nutr 1994;60: 647–657.

produced weight loss of about 16 kg at 24 weeks. Of the initial 180 patients, 99 were followed for another 26 weeks in an open label study. Weight loss persisted for as long as the drugs were given. Daly et al (14) treated six patients in an open label study for periods of up to 26 months and noted a persistent, modest weight loss.

Dhurandhar et al (17) reported that the combination of fluoxetine (20–60 mg/day) and phentermine HCl (18.75–37.5 mg/day) produced significant weight losses that were similar to those produced by the combination of fenfluramine (20–60 mg/day) and phentermine HCl (18.75–37.5 mg/day). This study extended only to 6 months, so it is not possible to determine if the weight regain reported with fluoxetine after 6 months (22) will be prevented by the addition of phentermine.

The combination of fenfluramine, a serotonin agonist, and phentermine, an adrenergic agonist, was first reported in 1984 by Weintraub et al (57). Weintraub (58) then performed a 4-year follow-up study that generated an enormous amount of publicity and changed the perception of the use of drugs for obesity. A total of 121 patients started treatment with the combination or placebo in a double-blind, randomized trial for an initial period of 34 weeks. All patients received diet, exercise, and behavior modification throughout the study. Weight loss reached a plateau at about 25 weeks into the initial 34-week period. All patients were then treated with the combination in an open label fashion, and at 60 weeks, a 15.8-kg weight loss persisted. When all medications were terminated at about 3.5 years and all patients were followed for 6 months off drugs, virtually all regained back to or near their baseline weights. Side effects included dry mouth, fatigue, sweating, insomnia, and other sleep disturbances. In general, the side effects were tolerable, and few patients discontinued drugs for this reason.

Atkinson et al (3) treated over 1300 patients with phentermine and fenfluramine for periods of up to 2 years. They noted weight losses of about 16 kg that persisted for 2 years in subjects who continued on drugs. Fenfluramine-phentermine was the best studied of the combinations. However, fenfluramine and dexfenfluramine have been withdrawn from the market and are not available for treatment. The reasons leading to the withdrawal of fenfluramine and dexfenfluramine are discussed separately.

Withdrawal of Fenfluramine and Dexfenfluramine from the Market

Although fenfluramine and dexfenfluramine produced promising results, they were withdrawn from the market in September 1997 when they were found to be associated with increased incidence of fibrosis of mitral and/or aortic heart valves, resulting in regurgitation. An increased level of circulating serotonin was initially proposed as the mechanism responsible for this observation. However, fenfluramine does not increase the circulating serotonin, and the exact mechanism responsible for the heart valve problems associated with the use of these drugs is unclear. No cases of heart valve problems due to phentermine alone have been reported and phentermine has not been withdrawn from the market.

Recently, three separate articles and an editorial published in an issue of the *New England Journal of Medicine* dealt with the issue of valvular heart disease and the obesity drugs (16,30,32,59). In the study by Khan et al (32) the prevalence of cardiac valve abnormalities that met the FDA definition was 1.3% among the obese controls who had not taken the appetite suppressants, whereas, out of those who had taken the appetite suppressants when they were available, 13% of those receiving fenfluramine, 23% of those receiving dexfenfluramine, and 25% of those receiving fenfluramine and phentermine had cardiac valve abnormalities. Jick et al (30) followed a large number of patients divided in four different groups for clinically detected valvular heart disease and found that during the 4 years of follow-up, the incidence was 0.14 per 1000 patient-years in the two groups who had taken fenfluramine or dexfenfluramine for less than 4 months and 0.7 per 1000 patient-years for those who had taken fenfluramine or dexfenfluramine for more than 4 months. No such cases were detected in the group receiving phentermine or in the group that had not taken appetite suppressants. In another retrospective study, Weissman et al (59) found a 4.5% prevalence of cardiac valve abnormality that met the FDA definition in the dexfenfluramine-treated patients versus 6.9% prevalence in the placebo-treated group. Although results of the three studies differ in magnitude from one another, they clearly show an association of fenfluramine and/or dexfenfluramine use and heart valve regurgitation.

CONCERNS ABOUT DRUG TREATMENT OF OBESITY

Some scientists in the field have expressed strong reservations about some of the obesity drugs for potentially major adverse events such as cardiac valve problems and primary pulmonary hypertension. A case report suggested that the fenfluramine-associated valvular regurgitation disappeared or reduced after discontinuation of the drug(s) (11). This suggests that the physicians should use caution in recommending valve replacement surgery unless absolutely necessary. Careful follow-up is important for those who have taken fenfluramine or dexfenfluramine in the past. An echocardiogram is indicated if a heart murmur or symptoms such as dyspnea on exertion, easy fatigue, fainting, or chest pain are present. Many physicians believe that if there are no symptoms or physical findings, an echocardiogram is not necessary. Others feel that all those who have taken fenfluramine or dexfenfluramine need an echocardiogram. Although, fenfluramine and dexfenfluramine are serotonergic agents, similar associations with cardiac valve regurgitation in other serotonergic agents used for the treatment of obesity, such as fluoxetine or sibutramine, have not been reported.

Primary pulmonary hypertension (PPH) is a rare disorder characterized by hyperplasia of the vascular endothelium of pulmonary blood vessels (9). In the 1960s, aminorex fumarate, a drug used for weight control in Europe, was reported to increase the risk of PPH (9). From a case-control study, Brenot et al (9) suggested that d-fenfluramine and other obesity drugs increase the risk of PPH. A larger case-control study, reported by Abenhaim et al (1), found 95 cases of PPH after screening 306 medical centers in Europe. The authors noted that dexfenfluramine and many other antiobesity drugs are associatd with an increase in the prevalence of PPH that may be as high as 1 in 20,000. This study has been attacked because of potential problems of patient selection bias and differential recall of use of obesity drugs between cases of PPH and the controls (38). However, patients taking obesity drugs should be monitored for signs of pulmonary disease, such as sudden and unexplained reduction in exercise tolerance, edema of legs and feet, chest pain, or syncope.

A COMPREHENSIVE OBESITY TREATMENT PROGRAM

Obesity drugs should be only a part of a comprehensive program that includes diet, exercise, increased activity, and alteration of behavior to attain a healthy lifestyle (50). Few patients treated with drugs reach their goal weight and almost none reach "ideal" weight (3). The focus of the treatment should be on improving the physical and the mental health of the patient and not on achieving an unrealistic dream weight (21). Patients need to understand that obesity is a chronic disease and that they will have to be persistent in their efforts at managing their weight. Medical treatment currently offered for obesity is far from being ideal. Weight reduction and maintenance regimens require a strong commitment and may not be easy for everyone. In appropriately selected individuals obesity drugs can supplement the efforts and the commitment

necessary for the management of the body weight. Currently available obesity drugs help in producing a mean weight loss of about 10%, although the range of weight loss can vary enormously.

Because obesity is a chronic disease, education of patients is critical. Education requires a significant commitment of time, and physicians rarely have sufficient time to accomplish the necessary degree of education. Several guidelines suggest that obesity treatment be conducted by a healthcare team that includes a physician and one or more allied health professionals, such as a dietitian, nurse, exercise physiologist, psychologist, or counselor (44,46,50,54).

SUMMARY

Obesity is a chronic disease that requires lifelong treatment. Experience with long-term use of obesity drugs is limited, but early data suggest drugs improve the outcome of standard therapy. There are insufficient data to assume that treatment with these drugs for the long term is safe or efficacious. Weight loss usually is modest with obesity drugs, but there are significant improvements in comorbidities of obesity. Obesity drugs must be used with caution and only in patients with medically significant obesity. Careful follow-up and continuous assessment for efficacy and appearance of side effects are mandatory.

REFERENCES

1. Abenhaim L, Moride Y, Brenot F, et al. Appetite-suppressant drugs and the risk of primary pulmonary hypertension. N Engl J Med 1996; 335:609–616.

2. Atkinson RL. Mechanisms of weight loss with obesity surgery. In: Angel A, Bouchard C, eds. Progress in obesity research: VII. London: John Libbey, 1996.

3. Atkinson RL, Blank RC, Schumacher D, et al. Long term drug treatment of obesity in a private practice setting. Obes Res 1997; 5:578–586.

4. Berger M. Pharmacological treatment of obesity: digestion and absorption inhibitors—clinical perspective. Am J Clin Nutr 1992; 55:318S–319S.

5. Blundell JE, Lawton CL, Halford JCG. Serotonin, eating behavior, and fat intake. Obes Res 1995;3 (suppl 3):471S–476S.

6. Bray GA, Ryan DH, Gordon D, et al. A double-blind randomized placebo-controlled trial of sibu-

tramine. Obes Res 1996;4:263–270.

7. Bray GA. The risks and disadvantages of obesity. In: The obese patient. Philadelphia: WB Saunders, 1976:215–251.

8. Bray GA. Peptides affect the intake of specific nutrients in the sympathetic nervous system. Am J Clin Nutr 1992;55:265S–271S.

9. Brenot F, Herve P, Petitpretz P, et al. Primary pulmonary hypertension and fenfluramine use. Br Heart J 1993;70:537–541.

10. Campfield LA, Smith FJ, Guisez Y, et al. Recombinant mouse OB protein: evidence for a peripheral signal linking adiposity and central neural networks. Science 1995; 269:546–549.

11. Cannistra LB, Cannistra AJ. Regression of multivalvular regurgitation after the cessation of fenfluramine and phentermine treatment. N Engl J Med 1998; 339:771.

12. Coleman DL. Genetics of obesity in rodents. In: Bray GA, ed. Recent advances in obesity research: II. London: Newman Publishing, 1978:142–152.

13. Considine RV, Sinha MK, Heiman ML, et al. Serum immunoreactive-leptin concentrations in normal-weight and obese humans. N Engl J Med 1996;334: 292–295.

14. Daly PA, Krieger DR, Dulloo AG, et al. Ephedrine, caffeine and aspirin: safety and efficacy for treatment of human obesity. Int J Obes 1993;17(suppl 1):S73–S78.

15. Darga LL, Carroll-Michals L, Botsford SJ, Lucas CP. Fluoxetine's effect on weight loss in obese subjects. Am J Clin Nutr 1991;54: 321–325.

16. Devereux RB. Appetite suppressants and valvular heart disease. N Engl J Med 1998;339:765–767. Editorial.

17. Dhurandhar NV, Atkinson RL. Comparison of serotonin agonists in combination with phentermine

for treatment of obesity. FASEB J 1996;10:A561.

18. Drent ML, van der Veen EA. Lipase inhibition: a novel concept in the treatment of obesity. Int J Obes 1993;17(4):241–244.

19. Drent ML, van der Veen EA. First clinical studies with orlistat: a short review. Obes Res 1995;3 (suppl 4):623S–625S.

20. Flatt JP. Effect of carbohydrate and fat intake on postprandial substrate oxidation and storage. Top Clin Nutr 1987;2:15–27.

21. Foster GD, Wadden TA, Vogt RA, Brewer G. What is a reasonable weight loss? patient's expectations and evaluations of obesity treatment outcomes. J Consult Clin Psychol 1997;65(1):79–85.

22. Goldstein DJ, Rampey AH Jr, Dornseif BE, et al. Fluoxetine: a randomized clinical trial in the maintenance of weight loss. Obes Res 1993;1:92–98.

23. Goldstein DJ, Potvin JH. Long-term weight loss: the effect of pharmacologic agents. Am J Clin Nutr 1994;60:647–657.

24. Greenway FL. Clinical studies with phenylpropanolamine: a meta-analysis. Am J Clin Nutr 1992;55 (suppl 1):203S–205S.

25. Griffiths RR, Brady JV, Bradford LD. Predicting the abuse liability of drugs with animal drug self-administration procedures: psychomotor stimulants and hallucinogens. Adv Behav Pharmacol 1979;2:163–208.

26. Grundy SM, Barnett JP. Metabolic and health complications of obesity. Dis Mon 1990;36(12):641–731.

27. Guy-Grand B, Apfelbaum M, Crepaldi G, et al. International trial of long-term dexfenfluramine in obesity. Lancet 1989;2:1142–1145.

28. Halaas JL, Gajiwala KS, Maffei M, et al. Weight-reducing effects of the plasma protein encoded by the obese gene. Science 1995;269:543–546.

29. Hartley GG, Nicol S, Halstenson C, et al. Phentermine, fenfluramine, diet, behavior modification, and exercise for treatment of obesity. Obes Res 1995;3(suppl 3):340S.

30. Jick H, et al. A population based study of appetite-supressant drugs and the risk of cardiac-valve regurgitation. N Engl J Med 1998;339:719–724.

31. Keesey RE, Powley TL. The regulation of body weight. Ann Rev Psychol 1986;37:109–133.

32. Khan MA, et al. The prevalence of cardiac valvular insufficiency assessed by transthoracic ecocardiography in obese patients treated with appetite-suppressant drugs. N Engl J Med 1998;339:713–718.

33. Kuczmarski RJ, Flegal KM, Campbell SM, Johnson CL. Increasing prevalence of overweight among US adults. JAMA 1994;272:205–211.

34. Kuczmarski RJ, Carrol MD, Flegal KM, Troiano RP. Varying body mass index cutoff points to describe overweight prevalence among US adults: NHANES III (1988 to 1994). Obes Res 1997;5:542.

35. Leibowitz SF. Brain peptides and obesity: pharmacologic treatment. Obes Res 1995;3:(suppl 4)573S–589S.

36. Levitsky DA, Troiano R. Metabolic consequences of fenfluramine for the control of body weight. Am J Clin Nutr 1992;55:167S–172S.

37. Liu YL, Toubro S, Astrup A, Stock MJ. Contribution of β_3-adrenoceptor activation to ephedrine-induced thermogenesis in humans. Int J Obes 1995;19:678–685.

38. Manson JE, Faich GA. Pharmacotherapy for obesity—do the benefits outweigh the risks? N Engl J Med 1996;335:659–660.

39. Marcus MD, Wing RR, Ewing L, et al. A double-blind, placebo-controlled trial of fluoxetine plus behavior modification in the treatment of obese binge-eaters and non-binge-eaters. Am J Psychiatry 1990;147:876–881.

40. McGinnis JM, Foege WH. Actual causes of death in the United States. JAMA 1993;270:2207–2212.

41. National Task Force on the Prevention and Treatment of Obesity. Long term pharmacotherapy in the management of obesity. JAMA 1996;276:1907–1915.

42. National Heart, Lung, and Blood Institute, National Institutes of Health. Clinical guidelines on the identification, evaluation and treatment of overweight and obesity in adults: the evidence report. Obes Res 1998;6(suppl 2):51S–209S.

43. Pelleymounter MA, Cullen MJ, Baker MB, et al. Effects of the obese gene product on body weight regulation in ob/ob mice. Science 1995;269:540–543.

44. Pi-Sunyer X. Guidelines for the approval and use of obesity drugs. Obes Res 1995;3:473–478.

45. Pi-Sunyer FX. Medical hazards of obesity. Ann Intern Med 1993;119:655–660.

46. Ricaurte GA, Molliver ME, Martello MB, et al. Dexfenfluramine neurotoxicity in brains of non-human primates. Lancet 1991;338:1487–1488.

47. Ryan DH, Kaiser P, Bray GA. Sibutramine: a novel new agent for obesity treatment. Obes Res 1995;3(suppl 4):553S–559S.

48. Schutz Y, Munger R, Deriaz O, Jequier E. Effect of dexfenfluramine on energy expenditure in man. Int J Obes 1992;16(suppl 3):S61–S66.

49. Scoville BA. Review of amphetamine-like drugs by the Food and Drug Administration. In: Bray GA, ed. Obesity in perspective. Fogarty International Center for Advanced Studies in the Health Sciences, series on preventive medicine, Vol. II. Washington, D.C.: U.S. Government Printing Office, 1976:441–443.

50. Shape Up America! and American Obesity Association. Guidance for treatment of adult obesity. Bethesda, MD: Shape Up America!, 1996.

51. Silverstone T. Appetite suppressants: a review. Drugs 1992;43:820–836.

52. Simopoulos AP, Van Itallie TB. Body weight, health and longevity. Ann Intern Med 1984;100:285–295.

53. Stock MJ. Potential for β_3-adrenoceptor agonists in the treatment of obesity. Int J Obes 1996;20(suppl 4):4–5.

54. Thomas PR, ed. Weighing the options. Criteria for evaluating weight-management programs. Washington D.C.: National Academy Press, 1995.

55. Toubro S, Astrup AV, Breum L, Quaade F. Safety and efficacy of long-term treatment with ephedrine, caffeine, and an ephedrine/-caffeine mixture. Int J Obes 1993;17(suppl 1):S69–S72.

56. Troiano RP, Levitsky DA, Kalkwarf HJ. Effect of dl-fenfluramine on thermic effect of food in humans. Int J Obes 1990;14:647–655.

57. Weintraub M, Hasday JD, Mushlin AI, Lockwood DH. A double blind clinical trial in weight control: use of fenfluramine and phentermine alone and in combination. Arch Intern Med 1984;144:1143–1148.

58. Weintraub M. Long-term weight control: the National Heart, Lung, and Blood Institute funded multi-modal intervention study. Clin Pharmacol Ther 1992;51:581–646.

59. Weissman NJ, et al. An assessment of heart-valve abnormalities in obese patients taking dexfenfluramine, sustained release dexfenfluramine, or placebo. N Engl J Med 1998;339:725–732.

60. Wurtman JJ, Wurtman RJ, Reynolds S, et al. Fenfluramine suppresses snack intake among carbohydrate cravers but not among non-carbohydrate cravers. Int J Eat Dis 1987;6:687–699.

61. Zhang Y, Proenca R, Maffei M, et al. Positional cloning of the mouse obese gene and its human homologue. Nature 1994;372:425–431.

Chapter 93

Surgery for Morbid Obesity

Harvey J. Sugerman
Eric J. DeMaria
John M. Kellum
Michael Schweitzer

Severely obese patients suffer from a multitude of medical problems, some of which may be life-threatening and others of which may severely limit their ability to lead productive lives, giving rise to the term *morbid obesity* (Table 93-1). Premature death is much more common in severely obese individuals. Comorbid conditions that can be associated with an earlier mortality include an increased incidence of coronary artery disease, hypertension, impaired cardiac function, adult-onset diabetes mellitus, obesity hypoventilation and/or sleep apnea syndromes (known collectively as the *Pickwickian syndrome*), venous stasis disease and hypercoagulability leading to an increased risk of pulmonary embolus, and necrotizing panniculitis.

Of special importance to surgeons is the increased difficulty in recognizing peritonitis in a morbidly obese patient. Severe obesity is also associated with an increased risk of uterine, breast, and colon carcinoma. A number of obesity-related problems are not threatening to life but can cause significant physical or psychological disability, including degenerative osteoarthritis, pseudotumor cerebri, cholecystitis, skin infections, chronic venous stasis ulcers, stress and/or urge overflow urinary incontinence, gastroesophageal reflux, sex hormone imbalance with dysmenorrhea, hirsutism, infertility, and an increased incidence of all types of hernias: incisional, inguinal, and umbilical. Many of these individuals suffer from severe psychological and social disability, including marked prejudice regarding employment.

CENTRAL OBESITY: SYNDROME X VERSUS INCREASED INTRA-ABDOMINAL PRESSURE

There are data documenting that central, or android, obesity is much more dangerous than peripheral, or gynoid, obesity. This is thought to be secondary to increased visceral fat metabolism leading to hyperglycemia, diabetes, and insulin-induced sodium reabsorption, leading to hypertension. This combination of metabolic problems is known as *syndrome X* (1,2). We have found that central obesity also is associated with a marked increase in intra-abdominal pressure (Figure 93-1), as estimated from urinary bladder pressure (3). Bladder pressures in patients with central obesity, as measured by sagittal abdominal diameter, are often as high, or higher, than those in patients with an acute abdominal compartment syndrome in which it is recommended that they undergo abdominal decompression. Increased intra-abdominal pressure may lead to venous stasis ulcers, obesity hypoventilation syndrome, gastroesophageal reflux, increased intracranial pressure associated with pseudotumor cerebri, systemic hypertension, and incisional hernias. Studies have shown that increased intra-abdominal pressure will push the diaphragm superiorly, decrease lung volume, and raise intrapleural pressure, which will increase central venous pressure and decrease venous return from the brain and raise intracranial pressure. The presumed pathophysiology of systemic hypertension and microalbuminuria in morbid obesity is secondary to increased renal venous pressure, leading to a glomerulopathy and increased renin and angiotensin secretion that also occurs secondary to increased pleural pressure and decreased venous return to the heart with a decreased cardiac output, leading to activation of the renin-angiotensin system; finally, direct renal compression may also lead to activation of the renin-angiotensin system. The urinary bladder pressure was found to be significantly higher in patients with three or more comorbidity problems per patient than in those with two or less (Figure 93-2).

SURGERY FOR OBESITY

Although many individuals can lose weight successfully through dietary manipulation, the incidence of recidivism in the morbidly obese approaches 95% (4). In 1991, a National Institutes of Health (NIH) Consensus Conference stated that patients with a body mass index (BMI) of $40\,kg/m^2$ or greater could be considered eligible for gastric surgery for obesity in the absence of comorbidity or a BMI of $35\,kg/m^2$ or greater with obesity-related comorbidity (5). Another NIH Health Consensus Conference in 1992 concluded that dietary weight reduction with, or without, behavioral modification or drug therapy has an unacceptably high incidence of weight regain in the morbidly obese within 2 years after maximal weight loss (6).

Intestinal Bypass

The initial operation for severe obesity was the jejunoileal (J–I) bypasss, connecting a small amount of jejunum (usually 8 in.) to a short segment of ileum (about 4 in.) either as an end-to-side anastomosis or as an end-to-end procedure with the bypassed intestine connected to the colon. Although effective for weight loss, this procedure is associated with a number of complications that can be divided into metabolic, nutritional, and electrolyte abnormalities or problems secondary to bacterial overgrowth in the bypassed, "blind-limb," intestine (7). This operation is a model of iatrogenic bacterial translocation with hepatic, renal, and joint abnormalities associated with the absorption of endotoxin or bacteria from the bypassed intestine. Many of these patients respond to metronidazole therapy. Cirrhosis may develop insidiously after J–I bypass in the absence of abnormal liver function tests (7). Randomized studies found the gastric bypass procedure to have an equivalent weight loss with a significantly lower incidence of complications (8). Since patients who have the J-I bypass dismantled will invariably regain their lost weight, they should be offered conversion to a gastric procedure for obesity, unless they have advanced cirrhosis with portal hypertension (9).

Gastric Surgery for Obesity

The two procedures that were supported by the 1991 NIH Consensus Conference on Surgery for Obesity are the gastric bypass (GBP) (10) (Figure 93-3) and the vertical banded gastroplasty (VBGP) (11) (Figure 93-4) or silastic ring gastroplasty. In a randomized, prospective trial, it was found that GBP had a significantly greater weight loss than VBGP (Figure 93-5), which was especially true for patients who were addicted to sweets (10). This has been supported by three other randomized, prospective trials (12–14) and two retrospective studies (15,16). It was found that "sweets eaters" did very poorly after VBGP but well after GBP, presumably because of the development of dumping syndrome symptoms following the ingestion of foods rich in sugar following GBP (Table 93-2) (10). Even when patients were selectively assigned to GBP (sweets eaters) or VBGP ("non–sweets eaters"), there was still a

---

Table 93-1 Morbidity of Severe Obesity

Central Obesity
- Metabolic complications (syndrome X)
  - Non-insulin-dependent diabetes (adult onset/type II)
  - Hypertension
  - Dyslipidemia: elevated triglycerides, cholesterol
  - Cholelithiasis, cholecystitis
- Increased intra-abdominal pressure
  - Stress overflow urinary incontinence
  - Gastroesophageal reflux
  - Venous disease: thrombophlebitis, venous stasis ulcers
  - Pulmonary embolism
  - Obesity hypoventilation syndrome
  - Nephrotic syndrome
  - Hernias (incisional, inguinal)
  - Pre-eclampsia

Respiratory Insufficiency of Obesity (Pickwickian Syndrome)
- Obesity hypoventilation syndrome
- Obstructive sleep apnea syndrome

Cardiovascular Dysfunction
- Coronary artery disease
- Increased complications after coronary bypass surgery
- Heart failure subsequent to:
  - Left ventricular concentric hypertrophy—hypertension
  - Left ventricular eccentric hypertrophy—obesity
  - Right ventricular hypertrophy—pulmonary failure
- Prolonged Q-T interval with sudden death

Sexual Hormone Dysfunction
- Amenorrhea, hypermenorrhea
- Stein-Leventhal syndrome: hirsutism, ovarian cysts
- Infertility
- Endometrial carcinoma
- Breast carcinoma

Other Carcinomas: Colon, Renal Cell, Prostate

Infectious Complications
- Difficulty recognizing peritonitis
- Necrotizing pancreatitis
- Necrotizing subcutaneous infections
- Wound infections, dehiscence

Pseudotumor cerebri (idiopathic intracranial hypertension)

Degenerative Osteoarthritis:
- feet, ankles, knees, hips, back, shoulders

Psychosocial Impairment

Decreased Employability, Work Discrimination

Table 93-2 Percentage Decrease in Excess Weight in Sweets Eaters versus Non–Sweets Eaters with GBP versus VBGP

PROCEDURE		SWEETS EATERS	NON–SWEETS EATERS
GBP	(1)	69 ± 17 <12>	67 ± 17 <7>
	(2)	62 ± 19 <11>	75 ± 19 <7>
	(3)	59 ± 17 <11>	71 ± 21 <7>
		$p < .001$	NS
VBGP	(1)	36 ± 13 <12>	57 ± 18 <6>
	(2)	35 ± 14 <11>	53 ± 22 <6>
	(3)	32 ± 18 <11>	50 ± 21 <5>
		$p < .05$	

Reprinted by permission from Sugerman HJ, Starkey JV, Birkenhauer R. A randomized prospective trial of gastric bypass versus vertical banded gastroplasty for morbid obesity and their effects on sweets versus non-sweets eaters. Ann Surg 1987;205: 613–624.

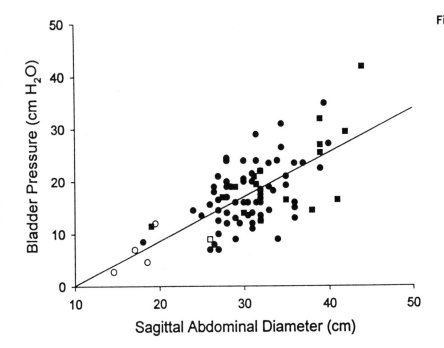

Figure 93-1 Correlation between urinary bladder pressure and sagittal abdominal diameter in 84 morbidly obese patients (women ●, men ■) and 5 "control" nonobese patients (women ○, men □) with ulcerative colitis, r = +.67, $p < .0001$. (Reprinted by permission from Sugerman H, Windsor A, Bessos M, Wolfe L. Intra-abdominal pressure, sagittal abdominal diameter and obesity co-morbidity. J Intern Med 1997;241:71–79.)

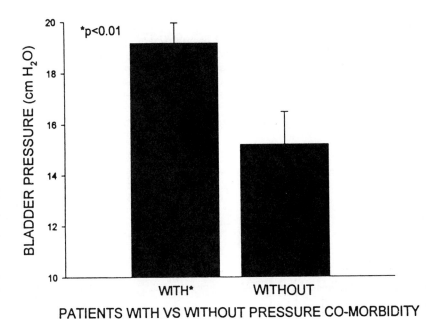

Figure 93-2 Increased urinary bladder pressure in patients with three or more than those with two, one, or no probable or possible pressure related comorbidity problems. (Reprinted by permission from Sugerman H, Windsor A, Bessos M, Wolfe L. Intra-abdominal pressure, sagittal abdominal diameter and obesity co-morbidity. J Intern Med 1997;241:71–79.)

significantly better weight loss with GBP and no loss of efficacy with all sweets eaters now assigned to GBP (Figure 93-6), and many of the VBGP patients failed to lose enough weight to correct their obesity-related comorbidity (17). The GBP was found to be associated with significantly higher levels of enteroglucagon than the VBGP and a lower area under the curve for both insulin and glucose following 100 g of oral glucose (18).

The GBP may be associated with iron, vitamin B_{12}, and calcium deficiencies, which usually respond to oral supplementation (10,17). Rapid weight loss following surgery for obesity is associated with a 32% risk of gallstone formation, which can be decreased to 2% with 300 mg of prophylactic

ursodiol taken twice daily for 6 months (19). Stomal stenosis or marginal ulcer may occur in approximately 12% of patients each, but usually respond to endoscopic balloon dilation or antacid therapy, respectively (20). There are three potential spaces for internal herniation, which may have a normal upper gastrointestinal radiographic barium series and be very difficult to diagnose. Recurrent, cramping periumbilical pain should lead to consideration for abdominal exploration.

Three studies have shown that weight loss following GBP is long-lasting in the vast majority of patients, with the average weight loss at 2 years 66% of excess weight, 60% at 5 years, and in the mid-50s at 5 to 10 years following surgery,

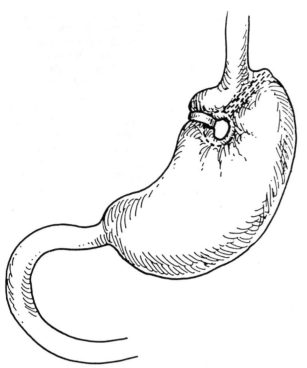

Figure 93-3 Vertical banded gastroplasty. (Reprinted by permission from Sugerman HJ, Starkey JV, Birkenhauer R. A randomized prospective trial of gastric bypass versus vertical banded gastroplasty for morbid obesity and their effects on sweets versus non-sweets eaters. Ann Surg 1987;205:613–624.)

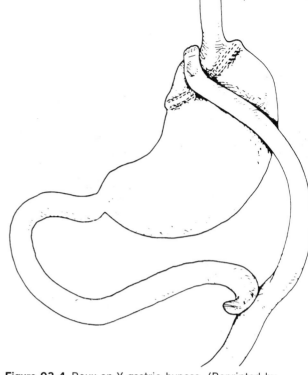

Figure 93-4 Roux-en-Y gastric bypass. (Reprinted by permission from Sugerman HJ, Starkey JV, Birkenhauer R. A randomized prospective trial of gastric bypass versus vertical banded gastroplasty for morbid obesity and their effects on sweets versus non-sweets eaters. Ann Surg 1987;205:613–624.)

Figure 93-5 Percentage of excess weight ± SD (n) over 3 years after Roux-en-Y gastric bypass (RYGBP) compared to vertical banded gastroplasty (VBGP). (Reprinted by permission from Sugerman HJ, Starkey JV, Birkenhauer R. A randomized prospective trial of gastric bypass versus vertical banded gastroplasty for morbid obesity and their effects on sweets versus non-sweets eaters. Ann Surg 1987;205: 613–624.)

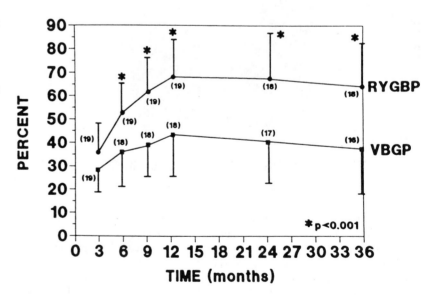

an acceptable risk of complications, and a mortality rate of 0.5% or less (15,21,22). Ten to fifteen percent of patients will fail the operation as defined by the loss of 40% or less of excess weight. Vertical banded gastroplasty may be associated with a high incidence of outlet stenosis, gastroesophageal reflux disease (GERD) (23), or failed weight loss caused by maladaptive eating behavior (many patients are unable to tolerate normal, nutritious foods and become sweets or junk food eaters). Conversion to gastric bypass has had a low risk of morbidity and weight loss results equivalent to primary

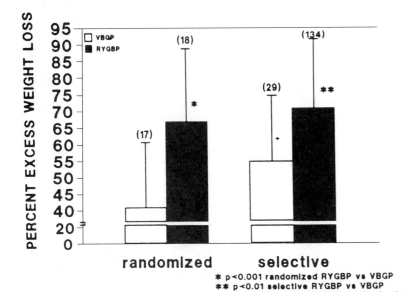

Figure 93-6 Percentage excess weight loss at 2 years following selective assignment of sweets eaters to GBP and non–sweets eaters to VBGP as compared to random assignment. (Reprinted by permission from Sugerman HJ, Londrey GL, Kellum JM, et al. Weight loss with vertical banded gastroplasty and Roux-Y gastric bypass for morbid obesity with selective versus random assignment. Am J Surg 1989;157:93–100.)

* p<0.001 randomized RYGBP vs VBGP
** p<0.01 selective RYGBP vs VBGP
\+ p<0.05 selective VBGP vs randomized VBGP

gastric bypass with correction of GERD symptoms (24). Patients who are superobese (BMI ≥ 50 kg/m^2) only lose one half of their excess weight at 2 years (17,25); lengthening the Roux-en-Y limb from 45 to 150 cm (long-limb GBP) was found to increase their weight loss to two thirds of excess weight, without any apparent increased nutritional deficiencies (25).

All forms of horizontal gastroplasty have been found to have an unacceptable incidence of weight loss failure, as well as a high complication rate related to gastric leaks or splenic injury (26). There are several types of gastric banding procedures. Swedish studies found that gastric banding has an extremely variable and often inadequate weight loss as well as frequent mechanical problems associated with outlet obstruction. A more recent modification using a laparoscopic adjustable silicone gastric band may have more favorable results (27) but awaits convincing data from prospective studies and is currently under evaluation in the United States at seven medical centers before approval for generalized use can be provided by the Food and Drug Administration (FDA). Concerns with the procedure include risk of band erosion into the stomach, band slippage with outlet obstruction, and inadequate weight loss. Laparoscopic gastric bypass is a surgical tour de force and is currently being evaluated for safety and efficacy. Because of the increased intra-abdominal pressure there is a high incidence (20%) of incisional hernia following a midline laparotomy incision (28); laparoscopic approaches should markedly reduce the risk of this complication.

Partial Biliopancreatic Bypass and Duodenal Switch Operations

A more radical procedure proposed for the treatment of severely obese patients is the *partial biliopancreatic diversion*, which involves a subtotal gastrectomy leaving a 400-cc gastric pouch for the average obese patient and a 200-cc gastric pouch for the superobese patient (29). The distal small bowel is transected 250 cm proximal to the ileocecal valve, and the proximal, bypassed bowel is anastomosed to the ileum 50 cm proximal to the ileocecal valve. This leaves a 200-cm "alimentary tract," a 300- to 400-cm "biliary tract" of bypassed intestine, and a 50-cm "common absorptive alimentary tract," where the ingested food mixes with bile and pancreatic juices for digestion and absorption. Thus, this is both a gastric restrictive and intestinal malabsorptive procedure. The biliopancreatic diversion has had excellent weight loss results and does not appear to be associated with the high incidence of bacterial overgrowth and translocation problems of the J-I bypass, since bile and pancreatic juices wash out the bypassed small intestine. However, the biliopancreatic diversion may be associated with severe protein-calorie malnutrition, necessitating hospitalization and total parenteral nutrition; frequent, foul-smelling steatorrheic stools that float leading to fat-soluble vitamin deficiencies; and calcium loss secondary to chelation with fat, leading to severe osteoporosis. Patients in Italy, where the operation was developed, seem to have fewer nutritional problems since their diet is high in complex carbohydrates (e.g., pasta) as compared to American patients whose diet is much higher in fat (e.g., fried foods, potato or corn chips). A randomized, prospective trial using a much smaller stomach (50 cc) without gastric resection and a longer common absorptive intestinal tract (150 cm) in superobese patients, called a distal GBP, was associated with a much greater weight loss than a standard GBP, but had a 25% incidence of severe malnutrition necessitating conversion to the standard GBP (30). We currently reserve this type of distal GBP for superobese patients who fail a standard GBP and have severe obesity-related comorbidity (e.g., diabetes, Picwickian syndrome), recognizing that there will be a need for fat-soluble vitamin supplementation as well as a risk of severe malnutrition (30).

A modified malabsorptive procedure, known as the *duodenal switch operation* (31), has been developed with the hope that there will be less protein and fat-soluble vitamin malabsorption. This procedure involves wedge resection of the greater curvature of the stomach and division of the

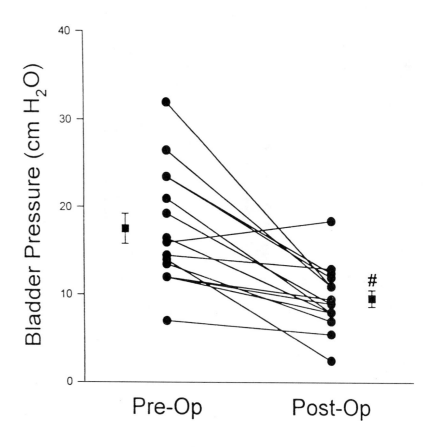

Figure 93-7 Urinary bladder pressure before and 1 year following gastric bypass–induced loss of 69 ± 4% excess weight. (Reprinted by permission from Sugerman H, Windsor A, Bessos M, et al. Effects of surgically induced weight loss on urinary bladder pressure, sagittal abdominal diameter and obesity co-morbidity. Int J Obes Relat Metab Disord 1998;22:230–235.)

duodenum in the distal bulb and the ileum 250 cm proximal to the ileocecal valve with anastomosis of the proximal duodenal segment to the distal ileal segment; the distal end of the transected duodenum is oversewn as a duodenal stump. The proximal segment, which carries the biliary and pancreatic secretions, is anastomosed end to side for an enteroenterostomy 50 to 100 cm proximal to the ileocecal valve. It is not clear yet if this operation will prevent the protein malnutrition, calcium, and fat-soluble vitamin deficiencies associated with a malabsorptive procedure.

SUMMARY

In conclusion, the gastric bypass has significantly better weight loss than the vertical banded or silastic ring gastroplasty, but may be associated with iron, vitamin B_{12}, and calcium deficiencies, which usually can be overcome with oral prophylaxis, as well as stomal stenosis or marginal ulcer that also usually respond to medical treatment. Horizontal gastroplasties have a very high failure and complication rate and should no longer be performed. Gastric banding appears to have results similar to gastroplasty in addition to problems with outlet obstruction. The laparoscopic adjustable gastric band is currently under evaluation for the FDA. The long-limb GBP appears to be the procedure of choice for superobese patients. Biliopancreatic diversion, distal gastric bypass, and, possibly, the duodenal switch operation have a high incidence of protein-calorie malnutrition, fat-soluble vitamin deficiencies, and osteoporosis, especially in American patients.

Significant, long-lasting weight loss follows gastric surgery for obesity, and this loss of weight is associated with amelioration, or complete resolution, of the morbidity associated with severe obesity, including obstructive sleep apnea syndrome (32,33), obesity hypoventilation (32), gastroesophageal reflux (34), pseudotumor cerebri (35), systemic hypertension (36,37), hypercholesterolemia (38), cardiac dysfunction of obesity (39), type II diabetes (22,40), female sexual hormone dysfunction (41), chronic lower extremity joint and back pains (42), venous stasis ulcers (43), stress incontinence (44), and improved self-image and employability (45). The increased intra-abdominal pressure associated with an increased sagittal abdominal diameter in central obesity decreases significantly with surgically induced weight loss which is associated with improvement or resolution of intra-abdominal-pressure-related and nonrelated comorbidity (46) (Figure 93-7). It is not often that a surgeon can perform one operation and cure four or five diseases. Although insurance coverage for bariatric surgery can be a problem with some state Medicaid programs, as well as health maintenance organizations (HMOs), inappropriate procedures in the morbidly obese would most likely be supported, such as ventriculoperitoneal shunts for pseudotumor cerebri, skin grafts (which usually won't take) for venous stasis ulcers, Nissen fundoplication for gastroesophageal reflux, and bladder suspension for stress and/or urge overflow urinary incontinence. It is tragic that patients with these severe comorbidities are prevented from having access to a procedure that may not only be life-saving but may also markedly improve the quality of their lives. These HMOs seem to be more concerned with this year's financial "bottom line" than the ultimate cost of care over 5 to 10 years.

Gastric surgery for obesity mandates surgeons dedicated to the treatment of the morbidly obese and long-term follow-up with the assistance of dieticians to maximize dietary compliance and weight loss, as well as to prevent micronutrient deficiencies. The potential complications are significant; however, the surgeon who is aware of these problems can minimize the risks and be rewarded with a very grateful group of patients.

REFERENCES

1. Kissebah A, Vydelingum N, Murray R, et al. Relation of body fat distribution to metabolic complications of obesity. J Clin Endocrinol Metab 1982;54:254–257.

2. Kvist A, Chowdhury B, Grangard U, et al. Total and visceral adipose tissue volumes derived from measurements with computed tomography in adult men and women: predictive equations. Am J Clin Nutr 1988;49:1351–1361.

3. Sugerman H, Windsor A, Bessos M, et al. Abdominal pressure, sagittal abdominal diameter and obesity co-morbidity. J Intern Med 1997;241:71–79.

4. Johnson D, Drennick EJ. Therapeutic fasting in morbid obesity. Arch Intern Med 1977;137:1381–1383.

5. NIH Conference. Gastrointestinal surgery for severe obesity: Consensus Development Conference Panel. Ann Intern Med 1991;115:956–961.

6. NIH Conference: Methods for voluntary weight loss and control. NIH Technology Assessment Conference Panel. Ann Intern Med 1992;116:942–949.

7. Hocking MP, Duerson MC, O'Leary PJ, et al. Jejunoileal bypass for morbid obesity: late follow-up in 100 cases. N Engl J Med 1983;308:995.

8. Griffen WO, Young VL, Stevenson CC. A prospective comparison of gastric and jejunoileal bypass for morbid obesity. Ann Surg 1977;186:500–508.

9. Halverson JD, Gentry K, Wise L, et al. Reanastomosis after jejunoileal bypass. Surgery 1978;84:241–249.

10. Sugerman HJ, Starkey JV, Birkenhauer R. A randomized prospective trial of gastric bypass versus vertical banded gastroplasty for morbid obesity and their effects on sweets versus non-sweets eaters. Ann Surg 1987;205:613–624.

11. Mason EE. VBG: Effective treatment of uncontrolled obesity. Bull Am Coll Surg 1991;76:18–22.

12. MacLean LD, Rhode BM, Sampalis J, et al. Results of the surgical treatment of obesity. Am J Surg 1993;165:155–160.

13. Howard L, Malone M, Michalek A, et al. Gastric bypass and vertical banded gastroplasty—a prospective randomized comparison and 5-year follow-up. Obes Surg 1995;5:55-60.

14. Capella JF, Capella RF. The weight reduction operation of choice: vertical banded gastroplasty or gastric bypass? Am J Surg 1996;171:74–79.

15. Yale CE. Gastric surgery for morbid obesity: complications and long-term weight control. Arch Surg 1989;124:941–946.

16. Kenler HA, Brolin RE, Cody RO. Changes in eating behavior after horizontal gastroplasty and Roux-en-Y gastric bypass. Am J Clin Nutr 1990;52:87–91.

17. Sugerman HJ, Londrey GL, Kellum JM, et al. Weight loss with vertical banded gastroplasty and Roux-Y gastric bypass for morbid obesity with selective versus random assignment. Am J Surg 1989;157:93–100.

18. Kellum J, Kuemmerle J, O'Dorisio T, et al. Gastrointestinal hormone responses to meals before and after gastric bypass and vertical banded gastroplasty. Ann Surg 1990;211:763–771.

19. Sugerman HJ, Brewer WH, Shiffman ML, et al. A multicenter, placebo-controlled, randomized, double-blind, prospective trial of prophylactic ursodiol for the prevention of gallstone formation following gastric-bypass-induced rapid weight loss. Am J Surg 1995;169:91–97.

20. Sanyal AJ, Sugerman HJ, Kellum JM, et al. Stomal complications of gastric bypass surgery: incidence and natural history. Am J Gastroenterol 1992;87:1165–1168.

21. Sugerman HJ, Kellum JM, Engle KM, et al. Gastric bypass for treating severe obesity. Am J Clin Nutr 1992;55:560S–566S.

22. Pories WJ, MacDonald KG, Morgan EJ, et al. Surgical treatment of obesity and its effects on diabetes: 10-y follow-up. Am J Clin Nutr 1992;55:582S–585S.

23. Kim CH, Sarr MG. Severe reflux esophagitis after vertical banded gastroplasty for treatment of morbid obesity. Mayo Clin Proc 1992;67:33–35.

24. Sugerman HJ, Kellum JM, DeMaria EJ, et al. Conversion of failed or complicated vertical banded gastroplasty to gastric bypass in morbid obesity. Am J Surg 1996;171:263–269.

25. Brolin RE, Kenler HA, Gorman JH, et al. Long-limb gastric bypass in the superobese. A prospective randomized study. Ann Surg 1992;215:387–392.

26. Sugerman HJ, Wolper JL. Failed gastroplasty for morbid obesity: revised gastroplasty versus Roux-en-Y gastric bypass. Am J Surg 1984;148:331–336.

27. Belachew M, Legrand M, Vincent V, et al. Laparoscopic placement of adjustable silicone gastric band in the treatment of morbid obesity: how to do it. Obes Surg 1995;5:66–70.

28. Sugerman HJ, Kellum JM, Reines HD, et al. Greater risk of incisional hernia with morbidly obese than steroid dependent patients and low recurrence with prefascial poly-

propylene mesh. Am J Surg 1996;
171:80–84.

29. Scopinaro N, Gianetta D, Adami G, et al. Biliopancreatic diversion for obesity at eighteen years. Surgery 1996;119:261–268.

30. Sugerman HJ, Kellum JM, DeMaria EJ. Conversion of proximal to distal gastric bypass for failed gastric bypass for superobesity. J Gastrointest Surg 1997;1: 517–525.

31. Lagace M, Marceau P, Marceau S, et al. Biliopancreatic diversion with a new type of gastrectomy: some previous conclusions revisited. Obes Surg 1995;5:411–418.

32. Sugerman HJ, Fairman RP, Sood RK, et al. Long-term effects of gastric surgery for treating respiratory insufficiency of obesity. Am J Clin Nutr 1992;55:597S–601S.

33. Charuzi I, Ovnat A, Peiser J, et al. The effect of surgical weight reduction on sleep quality in obesity-related sleep apnea syndrome. Surgery 1985;97:535–538.

34. Deitel M, Khanna RK, Hagen J, Ilves R. Vertical banded gastroplasty as an antireflux procedure. Am J Surg 1988;155:512–514.

35. Sugerman HJ, Felton WL, Sismanis A, et al. Effects of surgically induced weight loss on pseudotumor cerebri in morbid obesity. Neurology 1995;45:1655–1659.

36. Foley EF, Benotti PN, Borlase BC, et al. Impact of gastric restrictive surgery on hypertension in the morbidly obese. Am J Surg 1992; 163:294–297.

37. Carson JL, Ruddy ME, Duff AE, et al. The effect of gastric bypass surgery on hypertension in morbidly obese patients. Ann Intern Med 1994;154:193–200.

38. Gleysteen JJ, Barboriak JJ, Sasse EA. Sustained coronary-risk-factor reduction after gastric bypass for morbid obesity. Am J Clin Nutr 1990;51:774–778.

39. Alpert MA, Lambert CR, Terry BE, et al. Effect of weight loss on left ventricular mass in nonhypertensive morbidly obese patients. Amer J Cardiol 1994;73:918–921.

40. Pories WJ, Swanson MS, MacDonald KG, et al. Who would have thought it? An operation proves to be the most effective therapy for adult-onset diabetes mellitus? Ann Surg 1995;222: 339–350.

41. Deitel M, Toan BT, Stone EM, et al. Sex hormone changes accompanying loss of massive excess weight. Gastroenterol Clin N Amer 1987;16:511–516.

42. Bostman OM. Body mass index and height in patients requiring surgery for lumbar intervertebral disc herniation. 1993;18:851–854.

43. Kellum JM, DeMaria EJ, Sugerman HJ. Surgery for morbid obesity. Curr Probl Surg 1998;35:791–858.

44. Bump RC, Sugerman HJ, Fantl JA, et al. Obesity and lower urinary tract function in women: effects of surgically induced weight loss. Am J Obstet Gynecol 1992;167:392–397.

45. Stunkard AJ, Wadden TA. Pschological aspects of severe obesity. Am J Clin Nutr 1991;55:532S–534S.

46. Sugerman HJ, Windsor A, Bessos M, et al. Effects of surgically induced weight loss on urinary bladder pressure, sagittal abdominal diameter and obesity co-morbidity. Int J Obes Relat Metab Disord 1998;22:230–235.

Chapter 94

Obesity Research in the New Millenium

Risa J. Stein
C. Keith Haddock
Walker S. Carlos Poston
John P. Foreyt

For the past 30 years, obesity research has been characterized by many changes in treatment design and delivery (11). The number of treatments that have been tested for obesity is impressive; researchers have been quite creative in their attempt to discover a therapy that produces sustained weight loss. However, if success in obesity treatment research is defined as significant weight loss that is maintained indefinitely, our vast array of therapies have produced disappointing results. Foreyt (25), in reviewing the obesity literature, concluded that "obesity appears to be very difficult to treat and there are no prospects of a long-term solution or cure on the near horizon." Foreyt's comments suggest the need for researchers to think in terms of different treatment paradigms (6). In this chapter we outline several trends we predict will characterize obesity research of the future. Some of these trends have a long history whereas others require changing our paradigms about obesity treatment.

CHANGING THE GOALS OF OBESITY TREATMENTS

Given that traditional obesity treatment programs do not produce sustained reductions in weight, researchers are reconsidering the reasons for using pounds lost as the benchmark criteria for success in obesity treatment as well as whether a different indicator of success may be more meaningful and effectable. Perhaps more important indicators of "success" in obesity treatment would include medical, psychological, and behavioral measures (3).

Historically, obesity researchers have justified their craft by pointing to the improvement in health parameters following weight loss rather than by the questionable goal of helping patients reach a subjective aesthetic standard. Therefore, it seems reasonable that weight loss would evolve to be, at best, a secondary outcome in obesity treatment research. As more obesity specialists advocate treatment programs that improve health-related indices rather than focus on body weight, sheer measurement of pounds lost (usually with the accompanying goal of reaching a societally influenced ideal weight) will continue to fall into disrepute. Future research will attempt to develop treatments that are designed to improve health parameters rather than to promote weight loss per se (25).

PROMOTING BODY ACCEPTANCE

It will be difficult to socially market obesity programs focused on health rather than pounds lost if the primary reason patients pursue treatment is to improve their appearance. Therefore, future research should be directed toward developing treatments that reduce the level of weight obsession and the seemingly desperate attempt to control weight seen in many patients (25). There is a growing realization that body weight is not readily malleable, even on a short-term basis. For instance, a 1990 study by Stunkard et al (46) of 93 monozygotic twins reared apart found that 77% of the variance in body weight could be accounted for by genetics. Moreover, the amount of weight gain while on a fixed-calorie diet and body fat distribution patterns are both influenced considerably by genetics (8,9). Thus, the control an obese individual can exert over his or her weight may be significantly limited. Patients who harbor unrealistic expectations eventually run up against their biologic limits and inevitably suffer a blow to their self-esteem.

Given that most patients will not be able to reach and maintain their ideal body weight, a more relaxed and realistic approach to treatment that focuses on health seems reasonable, at least to professionals. However, a large body of evidence suggests that patients primarily join obesity treatment programs to improve their appearance through large weight losses. For instance, Foster et al (27) asked 60 obese women involved in a treatment program to define their goal weight losses. These women defined their goal weight loss as a 32% reduction in body weight, an objective quite different from the 5% to 10% reduction usually suggested by health professionals. These researchers also asked their patients about factors that influenced the selection of their goal weights. The principal reasons given for the selection of weight loss goals were appearance and physical comfort. Finally, although these women lost weight at a rate which would be considered quite reasonable in the obesity literature (i.e., 16 kg in 48 weeks), most patients reported dissatisfaction with their weight loss following treatment. Thus, developing successful obesity programs that encourage patients to focus on health rather than weight loss is likely to be a difficult, albeit important, undertaking.

FOCUS ON EXERCISE AND FITNESS

Physical activity has been linked to a large number of medical and psychological benefits, including the promotion of healthy body composition (40). In terms of obesity, studies have demonstrated that exercise alone may be the preferred treatment for obesity (31,44). Regular exercise offers several important benefits for obese patients, including facilitation of energy release from adipose tissue (7), reduction of hypertension (40), reducing preference for dietary fats (50), and increased adherence to healthy eating habits (12). Furthermore, regular physical activity may mitigate many of the health concerns associated with obesity in those who remain overweight (4).

Additional research efforts are necessary to determine how best to involve the obese in physical activity and how to help them maintain exercise as a new habit. Obese patients who are working to develop a healthy exercise habit need to master several new skills (35). They need to become comfortable with sensations of perspiration and increased heart rate and breathing rate, as well as the ability to change their schedules to accommodate exercise. One suggestion King et al (35) present is to provide ample social support at early stages of exercise incorporation because benefits are slight and discomfort is often high.

Exercise should be presented to patients as a method to promote health, energy, and fitness rather than weight loss. Patients should learn that moderate exercise that can be maintained, rather than extreme exercise goals, results in improved health and weight control as well as decreased attrition and injuries (26). Monitoring changes in health parameters (e.g., blood lipids, hypertension) and mood (e.g., depression) rather than body weight during an exercise program may provide incentives for overweight patients to continue physical activities despite slow or no changes in weight.

One very promising model for increasing exercise par-ticipation involves home-based programs (33,34,42). Home-based exercise programs are based on the presumption that exercising at home facilitates the long-term adherence to exercise goals because the new skills are gained in and incorporated into the patient's natural environment. Added to the fact that most individuals prefer to exercise on their own rather than in a group format (51), home-based exercise programs provide an exciting line of obesity research. Perri et al (42) directly compared a traditional group exercise program with a home-based treatment in a group of obese women. At follow-up, patients in the home-based program demonstrated more exercise participation, greater treatment adherence, and significantly greater weight losses than those in the traditional, group exercise program. Future obesity treatments should exploit the benefits of home-based programs and determine which specific factors are related to the success of these programs (e.g., supportive family environment, location and time of exercise).

TREATMENT AS A LIFELONG PROCESS

"Cure" is perhaps an outdated notion with regard to obesity treatment. Brownell (11) states that if cure is defined as weight loss to ideal body weight and maintenance of that weight status for 5 years, then "the cure rate for most forms of cancer is greater than that for obesity." Instead of the outdated notion of curing obesity with a specific time-limited treatment, new approaches will likely stress a "chronic" or "continuous care" model of obesity similar to that applied to the management of diabetes (26,41). Such a model would de-emphasize the promotion of long-term results based on a single treatment attempt and would instead espouse directing patients on how to rebound after episodes of overeating and gaining weight, thus continuing weight management across the lifespan.

Fairburn et al (22) point out two significant barriers to the ongoing maintenance of weight loss. First, many treatment programs do not teach weight maintenance behaviors or do not monitor the implementation of maintenance strategies. This barrier to weight maintenance could be overcome by replacing short-term treatments with a continuous care model similar to that used for diabetes or hypertension (41). In fact, we suggest that a continuous care plan implemented and rigorously monitored following initial treatment be adopted as a new standard of care for obesity treatment. Second, because most patients do not reach their ideal weight following treatment, many are unmotivated to maintain a weight loss they consider inconsequential. This barrier may be overcome with strategies designed to increase body shape acceptance. That is, if patients are able enjoy the increased energy and fitness resulting from treatment and accept that they will not reach the cultural ideal of body shape, weight maintenance becomes more likely.

IDENTIFYING AND ADDRESSING PSYCHOSOCIAL PROBLEMS

Although a large body of research suggests that the obese do not have a higher prevalence of psychopathology compared to nonobese individuals (28,36), psychiatric comorbidities such as depression, low self-esteem, or eating disorders will likely moderate the effectiveness of obesity treatment. Also, one unique group of obese patients who have a relatively high prevalence of psychopathology are binge eaters (26). Future obesity treatment programs should screen for problems with binge eating since surveys have shown that 25% to 45% of individuals who present for obesity treatment report binge eating, depending on the criteria used. Thus, the psychological presentation of the patient should play a role in the individualized development of obesity treatment strategies.

Both cognitive-behavioral therapy (CBT) and interpersonal therapy (IPT) have demonstrated promise as effective treatments for psychiatric problems that may present comorbidly with obesity. CBT assumes that both styles of thinking and coping skills need to change in order to effect lasting changes in emotions and behaviors (48). IPT, while sharing several core features with CBT, suggests that negative affect and problematic behaviors are primarily the result of dissatisfaction with relationships and social impairment (1). Both of these therapies have demonstrated clinical and cost-effectiveness for psychiatric disorders such as depression, binge eating, and bulimic behaviors (2,23,49). Future obesity treatments will likely further integrate strategies to alter cognitive style and interpersonal functioning into current treatment modalities.

CONTINUED SEARCH FOR EFFECTIVE AND SAFE PHARMACOTHERAPIES

Drug therapies for obesity have long suffered from a negative public image, and the recent withdrawal prompted by the Food and Drug Administration (FDA) of two popular drugs, fenfluramine and dexfenfluramine (Fen-Phen), will likely only further tarnish the view of pharmacotherapies (47). However, the development and prescription of drug treatments for obesity will likely continue. Several new pharmacotherapies are under study or have recently been granted FDA approval and will likely figure prominently in future treatment research. The new pharmacotherapies can be categorized as those that reduce energy intake, reduce nutrient absorption (nutrient partitioning), or increase energy expenditure.

Pharmacotherapies That Reduce Energy Intake

Sibutramine was recently approved by the FDA while leptin and brain and gut peptides are under development as obesity therapies. Sibutramine, a norepinephrine and serotonin reuptake inhibitor, has both satiating and thermogenic effects and produces weight losses of 4.7 to 7.6 kg in treatment trials lasting from 12 to 52 weeks (45). Leptin is a protein that may inhibit neuropeptide Y (NPY) gene expression and appears to increase satiety and energy expenditure. Leptin appears to control body weight through a feedback system that regulates fat storage. It has been suggested that low levels of leptin may increase the risk for developing obesity. Unfortunately, several recent human studies demonstrated that obese individuals produce significant amounts of leptin and that leptin levels are highly correlated with body weight (15,39). It is also possible that obese individuals are insensitive to endogenous leptin

production, although there are currently no known defects in the leptin-effector system (15). It is also possible that premorbidly low levels of leptin predisposed some individuals to develop obesity (43).

Brain and Gut Peptides

Research has found elevated levels of beta-endorphin in obese individuals when compared to lean patients, findings that persist after weight loss (21). Elevated beta-endorphin levels have also been found in binge eaters, regardless of their weight status (19,21). As a result, opiate peptide antagonists are now under investigation for applications to obesity and binge eating. For instance, naloxone, an opiate blocker, has shown promise in decreasing the desire for and consumption of sweet, high-fat foods in binge-eating women (20).

Pharmacotherapies That Reduce Nutrient Absorption

Orlistat, a lipase inhibitor, produces significant (i.e., 4.74 + 0.38 kg at a dosage of 360 mg/day after 12 weeks), dosage-dependent weight losses (16–18,30). However, some patients report mild and transient gastrointestinal side effects during treatment. Orlistat has received final FDA approval for the treatment of obesity.

Pharmacotherapies That Increase Energy Expenditure

β_3 agonists are under investigation for their ability to increase energy expenditure and produce weight loss. However, initial studies of the effectiveness of β_3 agonists for obesity have produced disappointing outcomes (13,14,52). β_3 agonists are currently not approved by the FDA for the treatment of obesity.

Adherence and Attrition Rates of Pharmacotherapies

Although pharmacotherapies will continue to be an important clinical tool for the treatment of obesity, future research will need to address the poor adherence and attrition characteristic of these therapies. Attrition rates for clinical trials of obesity medications, even in specialty treatment centers, are substantial. For instance, Bray et al (10) reported 85% attrition in a 96-week trial of sibutramine. If attrition is high in tightly controlled trials in which considerable resources are often directed at reducing attrition and increasing compliance, it is likely to be a greater problem in other settings. Therefore, it is imperative that behavioral interventions specifically designed to increase compliance to obesity medications be developed. It may be that behavioral interventions designed to increase the patient's focus on health parameters, accept realistic weight loss, and increase acceptance of body shape would increase compliance with pharmacologic interventions.

INCREASED RELIANCE ON PUBLIC HEALTH APPROACHES

Obesity is one of the most prominent public health problems in the United States. The prevalence of obesity has increased approximately 25% in the past 15 years (29). Currently, approximately 25% of men and 34.7% of women are obese (37). The increase in obesity among ethnic minority groups has been even more dramatic, with nearly 46% of African-American and Mexican-American women meeting the NHANES III definition of overweight (37). Given that over a third of the population is obese, it is unlikely that current treatments will reach the majority of overweight individuals. As a consequence, several researchers have suggested that future obesity research focus on public health approaches (5,32).

Public health approaches to obesity require the researcher to take a different perspective on the causes of obesity. Most current obesity treatments are based on the view that particular characteristics of individuals, such as genetics or a lack of control over eating, cause obesity. However, several factors strongly argue against the assumption that answers to the riddle of obesity are primarily found within the skin of our patients. The dramatic rise in the prevalence of obesity over the past decade cannot be explained by changes in the gene pool, with the presumption that successive generations have dramatically lower levels of self-control, or with the suggestion that people have recently learned to crave dietary fats and detest exercise. Also, treatments based on an individual approach have failed to stem the tide of obesity.

In contrast to the "within the skin" explanations of the rising tide of obesity, many researchers have argued that a paradigm shift is needed that looks to the environment for the causes of obesity (5,25,32). Many investigators have pointed to the "toxic environment" that has developed in industrialized countries as the principal reason for the high prevalence of obesity. For instance, Battle and Brownell (5, p. 761) suggest that "the environment provides access to and encourages consumption of a diet that is high in fat, high in calories, delicious, widely available, and low in cost" and that "with energy-saving devices and less physically demanding work, the number of individuals who maintain physical activity in day-to-day activities is diminishing."

How do we alter our toxic environment in order to increase the likelihood that the public will consume a healthy diet and remain physically active? Several regressive approaches have been suggested, such as controlling food advertising and increasing taxation on high-fat foods (5,25,32). However, it is questionable whether public support would exist for such efforts because they may be viewed as infringements on one's right to determine one's own diet and activity level without intrusion by the federal government. For example, during congressional hearings (16 July 1997) Robert A. Levy of the Cato Institute (38) stated: "Proposals from supposedly intelligent people in positions of responsibility include grading goods for their fat content, taxing them accordingly, and using the revenues for public bike paths and exercise trails. When decisions about the products we choose to consume are entrusted to an unelected and unaccountable bureaucracy, the loss of personal freedom is inescapable."

Public health interventions based on a nonregressive, incentive-based approach may be more acceptable to the public (5,25,32). Healthy foods (i.e., fruits and vegetables) could be subsidized to encourage increased consumption, insurance companies could provide premium reductions to those who regularly exercise, and cities could receive grants to provide easily accessable and safe opportunities for physical activity (e.g., bike paths, well-maintained sidewalks, fitness centers). Also, private firms could be encouraged to provide fitness facilities and showers for their employees and allow workers to transfer sick leave to vacation time. Public health programs based on an incentive-based approach should receive increased attention in future obesity research.

SUMMARY

The past 3 decades have seen great changes in treatments for obesity. However, despite extensive research in the area, few findings have significantly advanced the treatment of this condition. This chapter has presented several courses of exploration that may redirect the area of obesity research toward novel, and hopefully more productive, avenues. Central to the current state-of-the-art treatment of obesity is a cognitive shift on behalf of providers as well patients away from number of pounds lost and achievement of an aesthetic ideal to improved health and increased energy across the lifespan. Consistent with an emphasis on health, obesity researchers must continue to explore ways of involving the obese in regular, moderate, or vigorous exercise programs. New areas of exploration will almost certainly involve pharmacologic approaches to obesity management. However, public health approaches aimed at prevention and treatment of obesity through external agencies such as insurance premium reductions and exercise facilities provided by employers are likely to receive the most attention.

An integration of the new themes in obesity research suggests that an obese patient may experience the following when seeking treatment in the new millenium. First, the patient will be told that today's treatment programs take an individualized approach to care, which is likely to differ from the group programs the patient previously attended. This message will serve to emphasize that the practitioner is concerned about each individual and his or her health. Second, the chronic care approach will be outlined for the patient in a detailed fashion. Ideally, the patient will understand that weight management will be approached as a lifelong process. Because treatment is framed as a continuous process across the lifespan, the patient will likely feel less stigmatized about returning for treatment following inevitable relapses and slips. As part of continued care, progress toward improved health, as well as the pros and cons of continued attempts at weight loss, will be routinely discussed with the patient's healthcare providers.

One of the most prominent features of treatment will be the continual reinforcement of a cognitive shift toward self-esteem independent of body weight. The program leaders will offer the patient both social skills training and counseling on healthful methods of achieving nurturance and recognition. Instead of rapid weight loss goals achieved through severely restricted diet and acute strenuous exercise, a more gradual approach to increased health will be espoused. Gradual increases in exercise that is both pleasurable and vigorous will be coupled with a personally tailored diet that is modified in terms of composition but is not severely restrictive. After several weeks of treatment, the patient will most likely experience a 10% reduction in weight. However, during later treatment sessions the clinicians will primarily reinforce the decrease in blood pressure and the increase in physical fitness and energy the patient has experienced.

Once the initial treatment program is completed, the emphasis will be placed on maintenance of health and fitness gains. The patient will enroll in a comprehensive health maintenance program that is regularly monitored by area clinicians but is conducted at a local community center by volunteers. Periodically, the patient will return to the treatment program for medical check-ups and "booster" sessions. Also, weight maintenance will be enhanced by a number of programs sponsored by local employers and the city government. For example, on warm days the patient will ride his or her bike to work on the newly constructed path through town. Fortunately, the patient's employer installed a shower in the office area for individuals who either bike to work or who exercise at lunch.

Maintaining the healthy diet the patient began during treatment is also easier since the company cafeteria instituted its healthy lunch program. High-fat and high-calorie foods are hard to find at the cafeteria, whereas inexpensive fruits and vegetables (subsidized by the company owner) are plentiful. Finally, a number of initiatives in the patient's community and in the national media are sending the message that body weight and beauty are not necessarily linked. The patient is becoming convinced that he or she is attractive at current weight. Healthy and fit models with a variety of body shapes grace the covers of popular magazines and television commercials.

Some may suggest that increasing patient acceptance of modest weight losses, incorporating public health approaches to weight management, and promoting positive changes in public attitudes toward varying body shapes could only occur within the fantasies of obesity researchers. However, in the course of 3 decades cigarette smoking has evolved from a socially prized behavior that was sanctioned by sectors of the medical community to a deadly addiction that is viewed negatively by the public. The change in attitudes toward smoking was driven by dedicated public health and grass roots organizations that fought against prevailing public attitudes and an entrenched tobacco lobby. We are convinced that the obesity research community can accomplish similar goals.

The development of this chapter was supported by a Faculty Research Grant from the University of Missouri–Kansas City and a Minority Scientist Development Award from the American Heart Association and its Puerto Rican affiliate.

REFERENCES

1. Agras WS. Nonpharmacological treatments of bulimia nervosa. J Clin Psychiatry 1991;52(suppl): 29–33.

2. Agras WS. Short-term psychological treatments for binge eating. In: Fairburn CG, Wilson GT, eds. Binge eating: nature, assessment, and treatment. New York: Guilford Press, 1993:270–286.

3. Atkinson RL. Proposed standards for judging the success of the treatment of obesity. Ann Intern Med 1993;119:677–680.

4. Barlow CE, Kohl HW, Gibbons LW, Blair SN. Physical fitness, mortality, and obesity. Int J Obes Relat Metab Disord 1995;19(suppl 4): S41–S44.

5. Battle EK, Brownell KD. Confronting a rising tide of eating disorders and obesity: treatment vs. prevention and policy. Addict Behav 1996;21:755–765.

6. Beliard D, Kirschenbaum DS, Fitzgibbon ML. Evaluation of an intensive weight control program using a priori criteria to determine outcome. Int J Obes 1992;16: 505–517.

7. Bielenski R, Schutz Y, Jequier E. Energy expenditure and postprandial thermogenesis in obese women before and after weight loss. Am J Clin Nutr 1985;42:69–82.

8. Bouchard C, Perusse L, Leblanc C, et al. Inheritance of the amount and distribution of body fat. Int J Obes 1988;12:205–215.

9. Bouchard C, Tremblay A, Despres JP, et al. The response to long-term overfeeding in identical twins. N Engl J Med 1990;322: 1477–1482.

10. Bray GA, Ryan DH, Gordon D, et al. A double-blind placebo-controlled trial of sibutramine. Obes Res 1996;4:263–271.

11. Brownell KD. Obesity: understanding and treating a serious, prevalent, and refractory disorder. J Consult Clin Psychol 1982;50: 820–840.

12. Brownell KD. Exercise in the treatment of obesity. In: Brownell KD, Fairburn CG, eds. Eating disorders and obesity: A comprehensive handbook. New York: Guilford Press, 1995:473–478.

13. Connacher AA, Bennet WM, Jung RT. Clinical studies with beta-adrenoreceptor agonist BRL 26830A. Am J Clin Nutr 1992; 55(suppl 1):S258–S261.

14. Connacher AA, Jung RT, Mitchell PE. Weight loss in obese subjects on a restricted diet given BRL 26830A, a new atypical beta adrenoreceptor agonist. BMJ 1988;296:1217–1220.

15. Considine RV, Sinha MK, Heiman ML, et al. Serum immunoreactive-leptin concentration in normal-weight and obese humans. N Engl J Med 1996;334:292–325.

16. Drent ML, Larsson I, William-Olsson T, et al. Orlistat (RO 18-0647), a lipase inhibitor, in the treatment of human obesity: a multiple dose study. Int J Obe Relat Metab Disord 1995;19: 221–226.

17. Drent ML, van der Veen EA. Lipase inhibition: a novel concept in the treatment of obesity. Int J Obes Relat Metab Disord 1993;17:241–244.

18. Drent ML, van der Veen EA. First clinical studies with Orlistat: a

short review. Obes Res 1995;3 (suppl 4):S623–S625.

19. Drewnowski A. Metabolic determinants of binge eating. Addict Behav 1995;20:733–745.

20. Drewnowski A, Krahn DD, Demitrack MA, et al. Naloxone, an opiate blocker, reduces the consumption of sweet high-fat foods in obese and lean female binge eaters. Am J Clin Nutr 1995;61:1206–1212.

21. Ericsson M, Poston WSC, Foreyt JP. Common biological pathways in eating disorders and obesity. Addict Behav 1996;21:733–743.

22. Fairburn CG, Cooper Z. New perspectives on dietary and behavioural treatments for obesity. Int J Obes 1996;20(suppl 1):S9–S13.

23. Fairburn CG, Norman PA, Welch SL, et al. A prospective study of outcome in bulimia nervosa and the long-term effects of three psychological treatments. Arch Gen Psychol 1995;52:304–312.

24. Foreyt JP. Issues in the assessment and treatment of obesity. J Consult Clin Psychol 1987;55:677–684.

25. Foreyt JP, Poston WSC, Goodrick GK. Future directions in obesity and eating disorders. Addict Behav 1996;21:767–778.

26. Foster GD, Kendall PC. The realistic treatment of obesity: changing the scales of success. Clin Psychol Rev 1994;14:701–736.

27. Foster GD, Wadden TA, Vogt RA, Brewer G. What is reasonable weight loss? patient's expectations and evaluations of obesity treatment outcomes. J Consult Clin Psychol 1997;65:79–85.

28. Friedman MA, Brownell KD. Psychological correlates of obesity: moving to the next research generation. Psychol Bull 1995;117:3–20.

29. Garfinkel PE. Forward. In: Brownell KD, Fairburn CG, eds. Eating disorders and obesity: a comprehensive handbook. New York: Guilford Press, 1995:vii–viii.

30. Guerciolini R. Mode of action of Orlistat. Int J Obes Relat Metab Disord 1997;21(suppl 3):S12–S23.

31. Gwinup G. Effect of exercise alone on the weight of obese women. Arch Intern Med 1975;135:676–680.

32. Jeffery RW. Public health approaches to the management of obesity. In: Brownell KD, Fairburn CG, eds. Eating disorders and obesity: a comprehensive handbook. New York: Guilford Press, 1995:558–563.

33. King AC, Haskell WL, Taylor CB, et al. Group- vs. home-based exercise training in healthy older men and women. JAMA 1991;266:1535–1542.

34. King AC, Haskell WL, Young DR, et al. Long-term effects of varying intensities and formats of physical activity on participation rates, fitness, and lipoproteins in men and women aged 50 to 65 years. Circulation 1995;91:2596–2604.

35. King AC, Taylor CB, Haskell WL, DeBusk RF. Strategies for increasing early adherence to and long-term maintenance of home-based exercise training in healthy middle-aged men and women. Am J Cardiol 1988;61:628–632.

36. Klesges RC, Haddock CK, Stein RJ, et al. Relationship between psychosocial functioning and body fat in preschool children: a longitudinal investigation. J Consult Clin Psychol 1992;60:793–796.

37. National Institutes of Health (NIH), National Heart, Lung, and Blood Institute (NHLBI). Clinical guidelines on the identification, evaluation, and treatment of overweight and obesity: the evidence report. Washington, DC: US Government Printing Office, 1998.

38. Levy RA. Global Tobacco Settlement. Statement of Robert A. Levy, Ph.D., J.D., Senior Fellow in Constitutional Studies, Cato Institute, Washington, D.C., before the Committee on the Judiciary, United States Senate, July 16, 1997. Washington, D.C.: Cato Institute, 1997.

39. Maffei M, Halaas J, Ravussin E, et al. Leptin levels in human and rodent: measurement of plasma leptin and ob RNA in obese and weight-related subjects. Nature Med 1995;1:1155–1161.

40. Pate RR, Pratt M, Blair SN, et al. Physical activity and public health: a recommendation from the Centers for Disease and Prevention and the American College of Sports Medicine. Physical Activ Public Health 1995;273:402–407.

41. Perri MG, Fuller PR. Success and failure in the treatment of obesity: where do we go from here? Med Exerc Nutr Health 1995;4:255–272.

42. Perri MG, Martin D, Leermakers EA, et al. Effects of group- versus home-based exercise in the treatment of obesity. J Consul Clin Psychol 1997;65:278–285.

43. Ravussin E, Pratley RE, Maffei M, et al. Relatively low plasma leptin concentrations precede weight gain in Pima Indians. Nature Med 1997;3:238–240.

44. Skender ML, Goodrick GK, del Junco DJ, et al. Comparison of 2-year weight loss trends in behavioral treatment of obesity: diet, exercise, and combination interventions. J Am Diet Assoc 1996;96:342–346.

45. Stock MJ. Sibutramine—a review of clinical efficacy. Int J Obes Relat Metab Disord 1997;21(suppl 1):S30–S36.

46. Stunkard AJ, Harris JR, Pedersen NL, McClearn GE. The body-mass index of twins who have been reared apart. N Engl J Med 1990;322:1483–1487.

47. U.S. Food and Drug Adminstration. FDA announces withdrawal of fenfluramine and dexfenfluramine. FDA announcement, 15 September 1997.

48. Wessler RL. Conceptualizing cognitions in the cognitive-behavioral therapies. In: Dryden W, Golden WL, eds. Cognitive-behavioral approaches to psychotherapy. New York: Hemisphere, 1987:1–30.

49. Wilfley DE, Agras WS, Telch CF, et al. Group cognitive behavioral therapy and group interpersonal

psychotherapy for non-purging bulimics: a controlled comparison. J Consult Clin Psychol 1993;61: 296–305.

50. Wood PD, Terry RB, Haskell WL. Metabolism of substrates: diet, lipoprotein metabolism and exercise. Fed Proc 1985;44;358–363.

51. King AC, Taylor CB, Haskell WL, DeBusk RF. Identifying strategies for increasing employee physical activity levels: findings from the Stanford/Lockheed Exercise Survey. Health Educ Q 1990;17: 269–285.

52. Chapman BJ, Farquahar DL, Galloway SM, et al. The effects of a new beta-adrenoreceptor agonist BRL26830A in refractory obesity. Int J Obes Relat Metab Disord 1998;12:119–123.

Part XVII.

FITNESS AND EXERCISE

Edited by
James S. Skinner

Introduction to Fitness and Exercise

James S. Skinner

There is now a broad consensus that regular physical activity makes positive contributions to health and well-being. However, there has been a shift in emphasis regarding exercise and fitness over the past few decades. While fitness and performance were the main reasons given for regular physical activity during the 1970s and 1980s, there has been much more emphasis on the health-related aspects of exercise in the 1990s. At this time, public health officials and scientists recommend that people do 30 minutes of moderate-intensity physical activity on most days of the week (1–4).

This change has been reflected in the position stands of the American College of Sports Medicine during this same time period. Starting in 1978, they discussed the recommended quality and quantity of exercise for developing and maintaining fitness in healthy adults (5). In 1983, there was a position stand on proper and improper weight loss programs (6). In 1990, they added muscular fitness to the position and flexibility was added in 1998 (7,8). The section in this book on exercise and fitness also reflects and is consistent with the latest trends.

Kaminsky and Whaley discuss how to evaluate aspects of health-related fitness such as body composition, cardiovascular-respiratory endurance, and muscular strength and endurance. They give examples of common protocols for measuring these aspects, as well as some factors to consider when interpreting the results.

In his chapter, Going provides a detailed discussion of the changes in body composition that come as a result of exercise training. As he points out to the reader, this is a complex area because body composition and the changes induced by regular exercise can be influenced by such important factors as age, gender, initial body composition, genetics, quality and quantity of nutrients and energy ingested, and the characteristics of the exercise program itself.

Whaley and Kaminsky discuss some of the health benefits of and adaptations to regular physical activity and endurance training. They point out that the epidemiologic evidence strongly suggests that increased physical activity is associated with a reduced risk of such chronic diseases as coronary heart disease, stroke, some types of cancer, and non–insulin dependent diabetes mellitus. To help understand why this occurs, they then discuss the adaptations that occur in the body that might contribute to a decreased rate of morbidity and mortality for various chronic diseases.

Finally, Skinner discusses how exercise should be prescribed for the general population and those with special health states. The reader is reminded that the same principles apply to everyone but may have to be modified depending on the person's age, how long he or she has been inactive, the severity of the disease(s) the person has, and the limitations imposed by the disease(s). Giving examples of these general principles and how and why the exercise prescription may have to be modified, the emphasis is more on exercise and health than on exercise and fitness, per se. The reader should realize that there are many ways that one can increase physical activity and obtain similar results for health. Because of this, patients should select those activities that they enjoy, so that activity will become part of their lifestyle. If they become regularly active, then the types of changes outlined in this section should occur.

REFERENCES

1. Physical activity and health: a report of the Surgeon General. Atlanta: U.S. Department of Health and Human Services, Centers for Disease Control and Prevention, National Center for Chronic Disease Prevention and Health Promotion, 1996.

2. NIH consensus development panel on physical activity and cardiovascular health. JAMA 1996;276:241–246.

3. Pate RR, Pratt M, Blair SN, et al. Physical activity and public health: a recommendation from the Centers for Disease Control and Prevention and the American College of Sports Medicine. JAMA 1995;273:402–407.

4. Fletcher GF, Balady G, Blair SN, et al. Statement on exercise: benefits and recommendations for physical activity programs for all Americans: a statement for health professionals by the Committee on Exercise and Cardiac Rehabilitation of the Council of Clinical Cardiology, American Heart Association. Circulation 1996;94:857–862.

5. American College of Sports Medicine. Position stand on the recommended quantity and quality of exercise for developing and maintaining fitness in healthy adults. Med Sci Sports Exerc 1978;10:vii–x.

6. American College of Sports Medicine. Position stand on proper and improper weight loss programs. Med Sci Sports Exerc 1983;15:ix–xii.

7. American College of Sports Medicine. Position stand on the recommended quantity and quality of exercise for developing and maintaining cardiorespiratory and muscular fitness in healthy adults. Med Sci Sports Exerc 1990;22:265–274.

8. American College of Sports Medicine. Position stand on the recommended quantity and quality of exercise for developing and maintaining cardiorespiratory and muscular fitness, and flexibility in healthy adults. Med Sci Sports Exerc 1998;29:975–991.

Chapter 95

Physical Fitness Evaluation

Leonard A. Kaminsky
Mitchell H. Whaley

Physical fitness has been defined in a variety of ways (1). For the purposes of this chapter, physical fitness will be defined as: *a set of attributes that people have or achieve that relates to the ability to perform physical activity* (2). The specific attributes or components of physical fitness covered are: 1) body composition, 2) cardiorespiratory endurance, 3) flexibility, 4) muscular endurance, and 5) muscular strength.

Since physical fitness evaluations are often performed on individuals before beginning an exercise program, a health or medical screening may be recommended before initiating the evaluation process. Specific guidelines for performing a health or medical screening have been established by the American College of Sports Medicine (ACSM) (3) and should be followed.

BODY COMPOSITION

Body composition evaluations can range from the simple height and weight measurements to sophisticated assessments of the relative amounts of many different types of body tissues (e.g., muscle, bone, fat). In most settings, measurement of body composition as part of a physical fitness evaluation uses a two-component model of assessing the relative amounts of fat and fat-free tissue. The rationale for this approach is that excess body fat is associated with a number of chronic diseases and conditions (4).

Height and Weight Indices

The most basic approach for body composition assessment is to compare an individual's body weight to values established as normal for height. This method is commonly employed by physicians and other clinicians and is probably the most understood by the lay population. Many different height-weight tables have been produced. Some tables break down weight categories by frame size within each height, some require nude weights, others require shoes to be off, and most break down weights into categories by gender. The most common and useful version of these is one that was adapted (to eliminate constants used for weight of clothing and height of shoes) from standards for "desirable" weight developed in 1959 by the Metropolitan Life Insurance Company (Table 95-1). For each height, a range of body weight is given that represents a variance of approximately ±10% of the midpoint value. The advantages of this table are that it is widely recognized, and since the values were generated based on data on mortality, they do reflect a gross measure of health. The disadvantages are all related to limitations of the sample population used for the data set, such as an age range of only 25 to 59 years, underrepresentation of certain racial and socioeconomic groups, and measures of height and weight that were self-reported in 20% of cases (5).

For those who do not have ready access to a reference table, a "rule of thumb" method for determining an acceptable weight per height can be substituted. A well-recognized approach is to use the "Hamwi formula" (6), which states:

> 5 foot tall men = 106 lbs
> 5 foot tall women = 100 lbs
> add 5 lbs for each inch above 5 feet

Once a reference weight or weight range is determined, it is often helpful to express an individual's weight status as a relative weight (i.e., relative to the "reference" weight for height). Note the midpoint of the range of weights for height

Table 95-1 Height-Weight Classifications

HEIGHT (IN)*	WEIGHT (LB)*	
	MEN	WOMEN
58		92–121
59		95–124
60		98–127
61	105–134	101–130
62	108–137	104–134
63	111–141	107–138
64	114–145	110–142
65	117–149	114–146
66	121–154	118–150
67	125–159	122–154
68	129–163	126–159
69	133–167	130–164
70	137–172	134–169
71	141–177	
72	145–182	
73	149–187	
74	153–192	
75	157–197	

* Height without shoes; weight without clothing.
SOURCE: Neiman DC. Fitness and sports medicine. Palo Alto: Bull, 1995:114.

Table 95-2 Classifications of Weight Status

Desirable weight	20.0–24.9 kg/m^2
Grade I Obesity	25.0–29.9 kg/m^2
Grade II Obesity	30.0–40.0 kg/m^2
Grade III Obesity	>40.0 kg/m^2

from Table 95-1 is used as the reference weight for relative weight calculations. For example, the midpoint weight for a 66-inch-tall man and woman would be 137 and 134 lbs., respectively.

$$\text{Relative weight} = [(\text{Actual Weight}/\text{Reference Weight}) \cdot 100]$$

Given the reference weight equals 100%, the overweight percentage can be computed by subtracting 100 from the relative weight percentage. It is generally accepted that obesity is defined as 20% or more above the reference weight.

A third height-to-weight method is that of calculating the body mass index (BMI).

$$\text{BMI} = \text{kg} / \text{m}^2$$
(body weight in kg and height in meters^2)

The BMI is used extensively in research studies, particularly with large sample sizes. Nomograms are available to ease the calculations, although in many laboratories or offices the formula can be programmed into a computer. At an international symposium on diet and health, the Panel on Energy, Obesity, and Body Weight Standards adopted classifications of weight status based on the BMI (Table 95-2) (7).

These classifications have been recommended for use as a reference by the ACSM (3), because a consensus of research literature has demonstrated an increase in health risks begins with BMIs in the range of 25 to 30 kg/m^2.

The advantages of the height-to-weight methods are that measurements are easily understood by both clinicians and patients, simple to make (usually with a high degree of accuracy), inexpensive, and require little time. The primary disadvantage of the height-to-weight methods is that for the subset of the population that are regular exercisers, some may

be classified as overweight or obese as a result of excess body weight, even though the excess weight is composed of fat-free mass. This is especially true of athletes who compete in sports that require powerful movements, such as football. The fact that these measures can be derived from self-reported values of height and weight can be both an advantage and a disadvantage, depending on the knowledge or honesty of the patient.

Measurement Recommendations

Although measures of height and weight are considered routine, a few measurement considerations should be mentioned. Related to height, the measurements should be made with the patient not wearing shoes. This is a simple requirement that should not pose any trouble to a patient and adds only a minimal amount of time. Ideally, this should be performed with a stadiometer (a vertical ruler attached to a wall with a movable horizontal headboard) on a floor without carpeting. Patients should stand with their heels together, against the wall, and look straight ahead away from the wall. The measurement is obtained by lowering the headboard to the highest point on the head with enough pressure to compress any hair. Measurements with balance-beam scale height bars, although commonly performed, may produce widely variant results.

Measurement of weight should be performed on a professional-quality balance-beam scale. These scales should be placed on a level, uncarpeted surface. Before each measurement, the zero point should be checked and, if necessary, adjusted to assure the scale is in balance. Many electronic scales are being marketed with features of high resolution and interfaces with computers. If an electronic scale is used, the accuracy should be established by regular comparison to balance-beam scale measurements.

In summary, height-to-weight measures provide a simple and easy-to-understand first step in body composition evaluation. If the rationale for performing the body composition evaluation is simply to determine if an individual may have excess weight (fat) that could be detrimental to their health or ability to perform activities, then height-to-weight measures may provide all the information that is necessary. However, if there is a concern that a classification of obesity may be erroneous for a patient based on visual observation or the patient's reported exercise habits, more sophisticated body composition measurements are indicated.

Body Fat Distribution

One additional measurement that is simple to make and can be helpful in identifying health risks of obesity is that of waist circumference. Evidence is mounting that most of the deleterious effects of obesity are associated with an accumulation of excess body fat in the upper half of the body (8). Among the terms used to describe this condition are upper-body obesity, android obesity, "apple-shaped" body type, or central obesity.

Much of the early work on this topic actually compared the ratio of the waist circumference to that of the hip circumference (i.e., the waist-hip ratio). Although no universally accepted standard was established, the ACSM (3) used values of 0.95 or more for men and 0.86 or more for women as thresholds that identified increased health risks.

More recently, it has been reported that the use of waist circumference alone can be used to identify increased health risks. A study in 1994 reported that a waist circumference of more than 100 cm (40 inches) was associated with excess visceral abdominal fat, which would be predictive of the metabolic syndrome (hyperinsulinemia, hypertension, hypertriglyceridemia, low high-density lipoprotein levels) (9). This study was delimited to adults less than age 40. A subsequent report suggested that the waist circumference threshold may be even lower in older adults (ages 40 to 60) and recommended a value of less than 90 cm (36 inches) be used as the risk threshold (10).

Measurement Recommendations

Measurement of circumferences should be made with a nonelastic measuring tape with metric unit markings and a tension gauge to allow for consistent pressure. A popular brand that offers these features is the Gulick II (Country Technology, Inc., Gays Mills, Wisconsin). The actual measurement of the waist circumference should be made on bare skin (i.e., not over clothing) using the following description of the site location: *the narrowest part of the torso (above the umbilicus and below the xiphoid process)* (11).

Body Fat Estimation

The most important factor to consider in making measurements of body fat percentage is that all available in vivo measurements are indirect. As with any predicted variable, the measure should be interpreted with consideration of the measurement error range.

Even though all in vivo measurements of body fat are made by indirect methods, there are a number of methods that would be considered *reference*, or *criterion*, methods. Among them are hydrostatic weighing, measurement of total body water, measurement of dual energy radiography, and air displacement plethysmography. The total body water and dual energy radiography methods are not widely used in nonresearch applications and thus are not discussed here. Interested readers are referred to Lohman's monograph for more information on these methods (12).

Hydrostatic Weighing

Undoubtedly, the most widely used criterion method for body fat estimation in fitness evaluations is hydrostatic weighing. A thorough explanation of this procedure is beyond the scope of this chapter (13); however, a brief overview is provided. The outcome measurement from the hydrostatic weighing procedure is body density. Body density is defined as body mass (weight) divided by body volume (loss of weight in water, with specific correction factors applied). The body density value is

then used in an equation (14) that predicts body fat percentage using a two-compartment model of the human body (fat versus fat-free mass). The actual density values assigned to fat and fat-free tissue are based on a small number of studies on cadavers with samples limited in size and characteristics (mostly middle-aged white males). The two-compartment model assumes that the density of both fat and fat-free tissue is stable both within and among individuals. Although it appears that the density of fat tissue is relatively stable, it is known that the density of fat-free tissue is not. A nice review of the issues related to variability in density of fat-free tissue is provided by Lohman (12). The measurement error for body fat estimates derived from body density measures is ±2.77% (12).

For those desiring to perform hydrostatic weighing, a number of measurement issues should be considered. A facility with adequate space and access to plumbing and good ventilation is required. The effort and ability required of the individuals being measured are considerable: the procedure requires the individual to exhale completely to residual volume and then remain as motionless as possible under the water until a stable weight can be obtained. This requires multiple trials, and for subjects who are not comfortable in the water, it can be very difficult. A third issue relates to the requirement to correct for gases trapped in the body. Gastrointestinal gas is usually assumed to be of minor consequence, although some (15) suggest the use of a constant of 100 mL to correct for such gas. Accounting for residual lung volume should be done by measuring it, which requires additional time and instrumentation. Pollock and Wilmore (13) have noted that estimating residual lung volume can result in errors of up to ±5% body fat.

Air Displacement Plethysmography

Recently, a new instrument (the BOD POD) has been developed to provide measures of body volume using a long-accepted technique (air displacement plethysmography) (16). Although only a few studies have been published on this method, the findings suggest that it may be useful as a criterion method for body fat estimation in fitness evaluations (17,18).

The principle of the measurement is based on applying Boyle's law:

$$P_1V_1 = P_2V_2$$

A volume measurement is first made of the empty chamber and then repeated with an individual sitting in the chamber. Essentially, body volume is determined by subtraction (i.e., empty chamber volume minus chamber volume with body). Two correction factors are required for this measurement. The first is related to the influence that temperature changes have on pressure and volume. There is a difference in temperature in the air on the skin's surface and in the lung compared with the air in the chamber. Thus, a correction factor is made for what is called *surface area artifact*. Additionally, a correction must be made for the lung volume component of body volume. A measurement of average thoracic gas volume is made and applied as a correction factor in the determination of body volume. The thoracic gas volume measurement is made in the plethysmograph through a special port and thus does not require any additional instrumentation. The one study published to date found excellent agreement with hydrostatically determined body fat percentage, with an r^2 of 0.93 and a standard error of the estimate (SEE) of ±1.81% (17).

Just as in hydrostatic weighing, there are some measurement-related issues that should be considered. First, the location in the facility that houses the **BOD POD** must be free of environmental disturbances that may cause changes in pressure and temperature. Because of the sensitivity of the plethysmograph, small changes in the room environment (e.g., an air vent blowing in the room or a door shutting) can affect the body volume measurement. Because of the need to correct for surface area artifact, individuals being measured should wear only a tight-fitting swimsuit made of a spandex synthetic fiber (Lycra). Additional clothing traps air at a different temperature from that of the chamber and thus would affect the body volume calculation.

Skinfold Measurements

Since criterion reference methods are not available to all and may not be feasible because of time and expense constraints, other methods have been developed. The most common and widely used of these methods is the measurement of skinfold fat. The basic premises of this technique are that: a majority of the body fat is located in subcutaneous fat deposits, the distribution of subcutaneous fat to visceral fat is similar between individuals, and selected skinfold sites are representative of the fat distribution in the entire body.

There is a wealth of research on skinfold measurements as a method of estimating body fat percentage. The reader is referred to the *Anthropometric Standardization Manual* (11) for a thorough review of methodologic issues related to skinfold measurement. Provided here is a brief overview of methods required for obtaining estimates of body fat from skinfold measures. The majority of research on using skinfold measures to estimate body fat was done in comparison to hydrostatic weighing, thus leading some to refer to this as a *double*

indirect method. There are literally hundreds of prediction equations that have been developed to derive body fat percentage from skinfold measurements. Many of these equations were developed for specific populations (e.g., college-aged women basketball players) and thus would be ideal for use with individuals with the same characteristics. However, if the individuals to be evaluated have a wide range of characteristics, equations developed for a more generalized population should be used. The most widely used equations for fitness evaluations are those developed by Jackson and Pollock (19). These equations and the skinfold site descriptions are presented in Table 95-3. Note that the equations give a value for body density; the estimate of body fat requires use of a further equation, such as that developed by Siri (14).

$$\text{Body fat \%} = (495 \, / \text{body density}) - 450$$

Although these investigators developed equations using different numbers and combinations of skinfold sites, only one equation for men and one for women are presented—both using only three sites. The advantage of improved technical accuracy outweighs any benefit from using more sites or different equations. Two of the largest sources of error in skinfold measurements are variability in site location and variability among the measurers' technique. Concentration on technician training and practice on three specific standardized sites results in less variability in skinfold measurements and consequently reduces measurement error. Specific measurement technique guidelines are presented in Table 95-4. A high-quality caliper should be used to make the measurement. The caliper should come with a certificate verifying that it is calibrated, and the arms should apply a constant pressure of $10 \, \text{g/mm}^2$. The distance measure should be periodically checked with a certified calibration block.

Since the skinfold measures are considered a double indirect method, it is logical to assume that the measurement error will be greater than the criterion reference methods. Generally, measurement errors in body fat percentage have ranged from approximately 3.5% to 5.0% for skinfold methods. The error

---

Table 95-3 Description of Skinfold Sites and Generalized Body Fat Equations

SKINFOLD SITE	DESCRIPTION
Abdominal	Vertical fold; 2 cm to the right side of the umbilicus
Triceps	Vertical fold; on the posterior midline of the upper arm, halfway between the acromion and olecranon processes, with the arm held freely to the side of the body
Suprailiac	Diagonal fold; in line with the natural angle of the iliac crest taken in the anterior axillary line immediately superior to the iliac crest

BODY FAT EQUATIONS
Men Body Fat (%) = 0.39287·(sum of abdomen, suprailiac, triceps) − 0.00105·(sum of abdomen, suprailiac, triceps) + 0.15772·(Age) − 5.18845
Women Body Fat (%) = 0.41563·(sum of triceps, abdomen, suprailiac) − 0.00112·(sum of triceps, abdomen, suprailiac) + 0.03661·(Age) + 4.03653

SOURCE: American College of Sports Medicine. Guidelines for exercise testing and prescription. 5th ed. Baltimore: Williams & Wilkins, 1995:56–57.

Table 95-4 Technique Tips for Skinfold Measurement

1. The skinfold should be grasped firmly by the thumb and index finger of the left hand and pulled away from the body. Do not grasp underlying muscle. If you are unsure that you have a fat fold, have the subject contract the underlying muscle.
2. The caliper should be held perpendicular to the skinfold by the right hand, with the caliper dial facing upward. The caliper should be 1 cm away from thumb and finger so that the pressure of the caliper is not affected. Gradually release the pressure on the caliper arms so that full tension is exerted.
3. The caliper should not be placed too far in nor too far away from the tip of the skinfold. Try to visualize where a true double fold of skin thickness is and place the caliper heads there.
4. The dial should be read approximately 1 to 2 seconds after the grip has been released. (Note: The needle should be stabilized by this time). Read dial to the nearest 0.5 mm.
5. A minimum of two measures should be taken at each site with at least 15 seconds allowed between measures. Additional measures should be taken if the first two vary by more than 1 mm, or 10%, whichever is greater, until there is consistency. A mean of the measures is reported. (Note: An outlier value should not be included in the calculation of the mean.)

ranges for the two equations provided in Table 95-3 are ±3.4% for men and ±3.9% for women.

Body Fat Interpretation

Unfortunately, no national standards or universally accepted categorization exists for body fat percentage measurements. We use values of 15% for men and 22% for women to represent an "acceptable" body fat percentage standard for participants in the Ball State University adult physical fitness program. With age, body fat percentage increases. However, it is debatable how much of this increase in body fat percentage is a normal consequence of aging versus a result of lifestyle changes. For those who desire a more "average" value, we recommend that the 15% and 22% figure be increased by 2% for each decade of life beginning at age 30.

Summary

Before making body composition evaluations, the rationale for the measurement must be determined. In most fitness settings, the rationale is the relationship of body composition status to risk factors for a number of chronic diseases and conditions. For most individuals, this data may be obtained from simple measures of body height, weight, and waist circumference. In cases where an estimate of body fat is desired, interpretation must be made with consideration of the relatively large measurement errors of these methods.

CARDIORESPIRATORY ENDURANCE

Cardiorespiratory endurance, also called *functional capacity* or *aerobic fitness*, is often considered the most important health-related component of physical fitness. The reason for this can be gleaned by thinking about the determinants of the criterion measurement of cardiorespiratory endurance, namely maximal oxygen uptake (VO_2max).

$$VO_2max = \text{cardiac output} \cdot \text{arteriovenous oxygen content difference}$$

Since cardiorespiratory endurance is affected by the capabilities of the cardiovascular system, respiratory system, and the skeletal musculature, it provides a global measure of function of much of the body.

The criterion measurement of cardiorespiratory endurance, VO_2max, is obtained via the actual measurement of ventilation and inspired and expired oxygen and carbon dioxide concentrations during a maximal exercise effort. These tests can be done on a variety of different ergometers (e.g., treadmill, cycle, arm, wheelchair, step, swim). Treadmill testing is most common in the United States. Maximal exercise tests with measurement of VO_2max can be expensive (both in necessary equipment and personnel costs) and time consuming and require additional monitoring with electrocardiography and blood pressure cuff (in most populations) and a high level of cooperation and effort from the individual being tested. Specific protocols and procedures for maximal exercise testing are reviewed elsewhere in this text. Due to the limitations in being able conduct maximal exercise tests with measurement of VO_2max, other methods have been developed to estimate the measurement.

Estimation of Cardiorespiratory Endurance Without Exercise

Methods to provide predictions of VO_2max based on demographic characteristics of individuals have been available for many years. Most of these formulas are based on two characteristics, age and gender, that are known to have a significant relationship to VO_2max (20). As with other prediction equations, these are of limited use for predicting the VO_2max of an individual because of the relatively large SEE.

In the 1990s, a number of studies were reported that examined the role of additional demographic variables that have been shown to be related to VO_2max (21–23). The goal of these studies was to determine if adding additional variables to a prediction equation could significantly lower the SEE to improve the ability to provide estimates for individuals. Among the different variables studied and shown to have a significant relationship to VO_2max were body composition (both BMI and percentage of body fat), physical activity habits, resting heart rate, and smoking status. The study by Jackson et al (21) demonstrated that indeed the addition of these other variables to the regression equation resulted in a statistical improvement in the prediction. However, the SEE for their generalized equations ranged from 5.35 to 5.7 mL/kg/min. Heil et al (22) also studied this topic with a different, albeit smaller, sample (n = 229 women, n = 210 men) than that of Jackson et al (n = 195 women, n = 1814 men) (21). Interestingly, they found a slightly lower SEE (4.9 mL/kg/min) for their generalized equation. However, when they attempted to cross-validate the equations by Jackson et al with their study sample, they observed a much higher SEE (ranging from 5.54 to 8.59 mL/kg/min). Whaley et al (23) also investigated this topic with a large sample size of both women (n = 935) and men (n = 1415). Table 95-5 presents the multiple regression equations for three models, two of which included all variables that were significant (one used percentage of body fat and one used BMI as the body composition measurement) and one reduced model with only four vari-

Table 95-5 Multiple Regression Equations for Predicting Relative V_{O_2} peak (mL/kg/min)

Variable	Full Model	Full Model	Reduced Model
Intercept	61.66	64.62	50.55
Age (yr)	−0.328	−0.339	−0.324
Sex (female, 0; male, 1)	5.45	9.006	5.664
Physical Activity Status	1.832	2.069	2.157
Percent Body Fat	−0.436		−0.460
BMI (kg/m)		−0.601	
Resting HR (bpm)	−0.143	−0.143	
Cigarette Smoking Status	−0.446	−0.409	
R	0.852*	0.838*	0.837*
R^2	0.726	0.703	0.701
SEE	5.38	5.60	5.61

NOTE: Values represent regression equation coefficients. Two full model equations are presented. The first uses % body fat and results in a slightly smaller SEE. The second full model equation can be used with BMI in situations where % body fat data is not available. The reduced model equation can be used when information on smoking status and resting HR is not available.
* $p < 0.001$
BMI, body mass index; HR, heart rate; R, correlation coefficient; R^2, multiple correlation coefficient; SEE, standard error of the estimate
Cigarette smoking codes: 1 = non-smoker; 2 = former smoker (quit > 1 year ago); 3 = cigar smoker; 4 = cigarette smoker (<0.5 pack/day); 5 = 0.5–0.9 pack/day; 6 = 1.0–1.4 pack/day; 7 = 1.5–2.0 pack/day; 8 = >2.0 pack/day.
Physical activity habits codes: 1 = sedentary lifestyle; 2 = sedentary occupation with moderate recreational activity; 3 = moderate occupational and recreational activity; 4 = heavy occupational with moderate recreational activity; 5 = participates regularly in endurance exercise (e.g., 3 times/week of walking, running, swimming, cycling, aerobic dancing); 6 = highly trained (e.g., >20 miles/week of running, cycling, swimming).
SOURCE: Reproduced by permission from Whaley MH, et al. Failure of predicted V_{O_2} peak to discriminate physical fitness in epidemiological studies. Med Sci Sports Exerc 1995;27:89.

ables included. The SEE for the three models (ranging from 5.38 to 5.61 mL/kg/min) is similar to that of the other two studies. The conclusion was that, although these equations may be useful as a normative reference for a group, they lack the accuracy needed for deriving values for individuals. To demonstrate this point, Figure 95-1 shows the 95% confidence intervals for a hypothetical man and woman. This figure shows that the error range overlaps the "low" and "high" fitness categories from the widely recognized norms developed at the Cooper Institute for Aerobic Research.

Measurement Recommendations

Most or all of the information needed for these types of prediction equations is available from patient records, with the exception of physical activity status. This may require completion of a short questionnaire or patient responses to a few questions. The code scheme used for participants in Ball State University's adult physical fitness program is presented in Table 95-5. If a body composition variable is used, height and weight data from a patient file would allow the calculation of BMI. Obviously, the equations that require body fat percentage would require one of the methods discussed above to provide that measure.

Estimation of Cardiorespiratory Endurance from Submaximal Exercise Tests

Another common method to provide predictions of V_{O_2}max uses data collected during submaximal exercise tests, usually performed on a cycle ergometer. The physiologic basis for most of these tests is the known linear relationship between heart rate and oxygen consumption. Thus, if both are measured at submaximal levels, and if maximal heart rate is predicted, an extrapolation can be made to estimate V_{O_2}max.

Two common versions of submaximal exercise tests are the Åstrand test (24) and the YMCA test (3). The Åstrand test actually recommends that both heart rate and oxygen consumption be measured, whereas the YMCA protocol uses estimates for oxygen consumption based on power output values on the cycle ergometer. Both of these methods require a number of assumptions to allow for a reasonable prediction of V_{O_2}max: 1) the linear relationship between heart rate and oxygen consumption holds through maximal levels, 2) the decline in maximal heart rate is uniform with age, 3) the mechanical efficiency is the same for all individuals, 4) submaximal heart rates are reliable at fixed workloads, and 5) maximal oxygen uptake can be predicted from maximal power output values on the cycle ergometer (24–26). However, the reality is that individuals' responses do not always meet these assumptions, resulting in prediction error. Astrand and Rodahl noted the SE on the Astrand test was ±10% for well-trained individuals and ±15% for moderately trained subjects (24). These values are about the midpoint of the SE range (7% to 27%) from other studies of submaximal exercise tests (25).

Measurement Recommendations

The measurement error from predicting V_{O_2}max from submaximal exercise tests is not much lower than that of nonexercise prediction equations. Thus, there is some question about the usefulness of these tests. In fact, Åstrand and Rodahl provided the following answer: "can the maximal oxygen uptake be predicted accurately from data recorded during a submaximal exercise test? . . . definitely no." However, these methods may be useful in some situations, such as those in which serial testing of the same subject is used to demonstrate relative changes. When this method is used, the cycle ergometer must be properly calibrated and the measures of heart rate must be accurate.

Estimation of Cardiorespiratory Endurance from Maximal Exercise Tests

Another method to obtain predictions of VO_2max uses data collected during maximal exercise testing in situations where metabolic measurements are not made. Maximal exercise tests involve varying levels of risk for different populations. The ACSM has issued guidelines on exercise testing and has reviewed issues related to indications and contraindications for exercise testing, test personnel, measurement recommendations, and test termination criteria (3). Thus, those whose primary interest is in obtaining a measure of cardiorespiratory endurance should make sure they are following appropriate procedures for conducting maximal exercise tests.

In many environments, maximal exercise tests are performed for clinical evaluations. These test data can be used to obtain a prediction of VO_2max. If standardized protocols are used, equations are available to predict VO_2max from treadmill exercise test time. Table 95-6 provides a summary of different equations that have been published from the Balke, Bruce, and the BSU/Bruce ramp protocols. Although the SEEs are markedly lower than those obtained from nonexercise models or submaximal exercise tests, significant variability is observed for some individuals.

Measurement Recommendations

In predicting VO_2max from maximal exercise test data, a number of factors are important, but the first and foremost is the effort level of the patient during the test. All of the published equations used subjects who were encouraged to give a true maximal effort, and an age-predicted heart rate attainment was not used for termination of the test. A second factor, which is equally important, is that patients not use handrail support during these tests. Handrail support lowers metabolic requirements and thus would invalidate the equations.

One other issue should be mentioned related to predicting VO_2max from maximal exercise tests—the practice of attempting to estimate VO_2max from maximal speed and grade. The equations used to provide these estimates are only validated for submaximal, steady-state exercise efforts. Thus, use with maximal data results in increased error that varies widely among individuals.

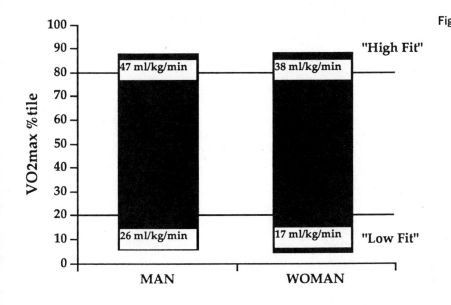

Figure 95-1 The 95% confidence interval for predicted VO_2peak expressed as a percentile score for a hypothetical man and woman. Reproduced by permission from Whaley MH et al. Failure of predicted VO_2peak to discriminate physical fitness in epidemiological studies. Med Sci Sports Exer 1985;27:89.

Table 95-6 Estimation of VO_2max (mL/kg/min) from Treadmill Exercise Test Time

PROTOCOL	REGRESSION EQUATION	STUDY POPULATION AND SAMPLE SIZE
Balke (29)	$9.42 + 1.25 \cdot (min)$	181 women, 55 ± 1 yr
Bruce (30)	$6.7 - 2.82 \cdot (sex^*) +$	157 women, 41 ± 11 yr
	$0.056 \cdot (sec)$	138 men, 49 ± 11 yr
BSU/Bruce Ramp	$3.9 \cdot (min) - 7.0 \pm 3.4$	318 women, 43 ± 11 yr
(31)		380 men, 46 ± 12 yr

*Sex code for Bruce equation is men = 1, women = 2.

Summary

Since cardiorespiratory endurance is considered the most important health-related component of physical fitness, its measurement is desirable. Obtaining metabolic measurements during maximal exercise tests is obviously the method of choice. However, since it is not practical in all situations, other procedures are available. The error ranges of the tests must be considered relative to the indication for the measurement to be most helpful for each situation.

FLEXIBILITY, MUSCULAR ENDURANCE, MUSCULAR STRENGTH

Certainly, body composition and cardiorespiratory endurance have been studied and evaluated more than any of the three other health-related components of physical fitness. The reason for this is that they represent measures of function of the entire body. The major issue or problem with measurement of flexibility, muscular endurance, and muscular strength is that there is not a single test that can be performed that represents the overall capacity of the body for any of these three components. That is, flexibility varies from one joint to another. Similarly, endurance and strength vary among muscle groups.

Since no one single test or, for that matter, group of tests exists to quantify an overall capacity for these three components of physical fitness, they are less commonly performed. We will briefly review some methods that can be used for each of these three components. The rationale for obtaining measurements of flexibility, muscular endurance, and muscular strength is the determination of whether the functional ability to perform certain tasks that require specific joints and muscle groups is present.

Flexibility

Basically, flexibility can be thought of as the ability to perform a complete range of motion around a joint. Although research is lacking on the health-related risks of poor flexibility, inadequate flexibility is believed to predispose an individual to injury. For example, one of the more significant health problems associated with poor hamstring flexibility is low back pain.

A variety of tests can be performed to evaluate flexibility: a recent review of these tests is provided by Protas (27). These evaluations range from the simple visual observation by a health care provider of a patient performing a range of motion about a joint to the use of electronic inclinometers to measure complex movements.

Probably the most widely used fitness measure of flexibility is the sit and reach test. This test gained popularity resulting from the following factors: 1) the perceived relationship of poor lumbar flexibility with the incidence of low back pain, 2) the simplicity of the measurement, and 3) the fact that some norms exist for adult populations (28). Some measurement-related concerns for this test include: 1) the lack of correction for individuals with different limb lengths (legs and arms), 2) whether a standardized warm-up should be performed before the test, and 3) whether the measurement point should be required to be held for a fixed time period. Other

somewhat common tests of flexibility that are relatively simple to perform are the back-extension test, the total body rotation test, and the shoulder flexibility test.

Obviously, more investigation is needed to develop an acceptable test battery for flexibility assessment. Despite these limitations, many clinicians remain interested in obtaining some type of flexibility evaluation on individual patients. One recommendation would be to use a universal goniometer, which can provide a reasonable assessment of range of motion for a variety of joints in the body. Even though there are not any established norms to use in interpreting test data, these measures can be useful in measuring change in flexibility resulting from a flexibility training program.

Muscular Endurance and Muscular Strength

Muscular endurance is the ability of a muscle group to perform repeated contractions or to sustain an isometric contraction for a period of time. Although muscular endurance is related to muscular strength, it is a separate component of physical fitness. Muscular strength is the capacity of a muscle group to develop force. The basic rationale for assessing muscular endurance and strength is that both are logically assumed to be related to an individual's ability to perform physical tasks. Although lacking in depth, research data is evolving to demonstrate many health-related aspects of muscular strength and endurance (4). The health benefits cited for muscular endurance and strength include: 1) increased bone density, 2) less risk of fracture from falling, 3) increased resting metabolic rate, and 4) improved insulin sensitivity.

Again, because of the principle of specificity, there are no global measures of total body muscular endurance or strength. The two most widely used fitness measurements of muscular endurance are the sit-up and push-up tests. Unfortunately, there are many variations of both of these tests (i.e., bent-knee sit-ups, kneeling push-ups, timed versus total number to exhaustion), which makes interpretation of the tests, in comparison to a set norm, difficult. Another commonly used procedure to evaluate muscular endurance is assessing the maximal number of repetitions of a set weight. The amount of weight may be set as a percentage of the one-repetition maximum or a percentage of the body weight. A slightly more sophisticated measurement can be obtained with an electronic dynamometer, which can assess force production over time. Similar to flexibility assessment, although lacking in normative comparison interpretation, muscular endurance and strength assessments can be useful for performing serial measurements over time for individuals.

Strength measures can be obtained from a variety of types of equipment, such as dynamometers, tensiometers, strain-gauges, free weights, and electromechanical instruments. A relatively popular measure of strength in fitness settings is the grip strength test. Although norms for this test are available, the usefulness of this measure is questionable. Although many research and clinical settings utilize sophisticated electromechanical instruments for assessing strength, the practicality of obtaining these measurements is a major issue. Potentially the most useful measure of strength is the assessment of a one-repetition maximum. This can be done relatively easily for a variety of muscle groups and contraction types. The major limiting factor for this measurement is that there is a learning effect, which results in an increased time period for the assessment.

Summary

The principle of specificity complicates the assessment of flexibility, muscular strength, and muscular endurance. Since no single test, or battery of tests, exists to assess any of these components of physical fitness, it is difficult to classify an individual's ability in these components. Despite these limitations, promoting fitness in these three areas is important. At the present time, the assessment and interpretation of results should focus on individualized measures for given patients and evaluation of how the measures change over time.

REFERENCES

1. Miller AJ, Grais IM, Winslow E, et al. The definition of physical fitness. J Sports Med Phys Fit 1991;31:639–640.

2. Caspersen CJ, Powell KE, Christenson GM. Physical activity, exercise and physical fitness: definitions and distinctions for health-related research. Pub Health Rep 1985;100:126–130.

3. American College of Sports Medicine. Guidelines for exercise testing and prescription. 5th ed. Baltimore: Williams & Wilkins, 1995:1–373.

4. U.S. Department of Health and Human Services. Physical activity and health. Washington, DC: United States Department of Health and Human Services, Centers for Disease Control and Prevention, National Center for Chronic Disease Prevention and Health Promotion, 1996:1–278.

5. Robinett-Weiss N, Hixson ML, Keir B, et al. The Metropolitan height-weight tables: perspectives for use. J Am Diet Assoc 1984;84:1480–1481.

6. Hamwi G. Changing dietary concepts. In: Dankowski TS, ed. Diabetes mellitus and treatment. New York: American Diabetes Association, 1964.

7. Jéquier E. Energy, obesity, and body weight standards. Am J Clin Nutr 1987;45:1035–1036.

8. Després JP: Visceral obesity, insulin resistance, and dyslipidemia: contribution of endurance training to the treatment of the plurimetabolic syndrome. In: Holloszy JO, ed. Exercise and sport science reviews. Baltimore: Williams & Wilkins, 1997:271–300.

9. Pouliot MC, Després JP, Moorjani S, et al. Waist circumference and abdominal sagittal diameter: best simple anthropometric indexes of abdominal visceral adipose tissue accumulation and related cardiovascular risk in men and women. Am J Cardiol 1994;73:460–468.

10. Lemieux S, Prudhomme D, Nadeau A, et al. A single threshold value of waist girth to identify non-obese and overweight subjects with excess visceral adipose tissue. Am J Clin Nutr 1996;64:685–693.

11. Lohman TG, Roche AF, Martorell R. Anthropometric standardization reference manual. Champaign, IL: Human Kinetics, 1988:1–177.

12. Lohman TG. Advances in body composition assessment. Champaign, IL: Human Kinetics, 1992:1–150.

13. Pollock ML, Wilmore JH. Exercise in health and disease: evaluation and prescription for prevention and rehabilitation. 2nd ed. Philadelphia: W.B. Saunders, 1990:1-741.

14. Siri NE. Body composition from fluid spaces and density. In: Brozek J, Henschel A, eds. Techniques for measuring body composition. Washington, DC: National Academy of Science, 1961:223–224.

15. Buskirk ER. Underwater weighing and body density: a review of procedures. In: Brosek J, Henschel A, eds. Techniques for measuring body composition. Washington, DC: National Academy of Sciences, 1961:90–105.

16. Dempster P, Aitkens S. A new air displacement method for the determination of human body composition. Med Sci Sports Exerc 1995;27:1692–1697.

17. McCrory MA, Gomez TD, Bernauer EM, et al. Evaluation of a new air displacement plethysmograph for measuring human body composition. Med Sci Sports Exerc 1995;27:1686–1691.

18. McCrory MA, Mole PA, Gomez TD, et al. Body composition by air-displacement plethysmography by using predicted and measured thoracic gas volumes. J Appl Physiol 1998;84:1475–1479.

19. Jackson AS, Pollock ML. Practical assessment of body composition. Phys Sports Med 1985;13:76–90.

20. Myers JN. Essentials of cardiopulmonary exercise testing. Champaign, IL: Human Kinetics, 1996:1–177.

21. Jackson AS, Blair SN, Maha MT, et al. Prediction of functional aerobic capacity without exercise testing. Med Sci Sports Exerc 1990;22:863–870.

22. Heil DP, Freedson PS, Ahlquist LE, et al. Nonexercise regression models to estimate peak oxygen consumption. Med Sci Sports Exerc 1995;27:599–606.

23. Whaley MH, Kaminsky LA, Dwyer GB, et al. Failure of predicted Vo_2peak to discriminate physical fitness in epidemiological studies. Med Sci Sports Exerc 1995;27:85–91.

24. Åstrand PO, Rodahl K. Textbook of work physiology. 3rd ed. New York: McGraw-Hill, 1986.

25. Greiwe JS, Kaminsky LA, Whaley MH, et al. Evaluation of the ACSM submaximal cycling ergometer test for estimating Vo_2max. Med Sci Sports Exerc 1995;27:1315–1320.

26. Whaley MH, Kaminsky LA, Dwyer GB, et al. Predictors of over- and underachievement of age-predicted maximal heart rate in adult men and women. Med Sci Sports Exerc 1992;24:1173–1179.

27. Protas E. Flexibility and range of motion. In: Roitman JL, ed. ACSM's resource manual for guidelines for exercise testing and prescription. Baltimore: Williams & Wilkins, 1998;368–377.

28. Golding LA, Myers CR, Sinning WE. Y's way to physical fitness: the complete guide to fitness testing and instruction. 3rd ed. Champaign IL: Human Kinetics, 1989.

29. Martin AD, Notelovitz M, Fields C, et al. Predicting maximal oxygen uptake from treadmill testing in trained and untrained women. Am J Obstet Gynecol 1989;161:1127–1132.

30. Bruce RA, Hosmer F, Kusumi F. Maximal oxygen intake and nomographic assessment of functional aerobic impairment in cardiovascular disease. Am Heart J 1973;85:546–562.

31. Kaminsky LA, Whaley MH. Evaluation of a new standardized ramp protocol: the BSU/Bruce ramp protocol. J Cardiopul Rehab 1998 (in press).

Chapter 96

Body Composition Alterations with Exercise

Scott Going

Body composition refers to the absolute and relative amounts of body constituents assessed on atomic, chemical, cellular, tissue-system, and whole body levels (1). The components on the various levels are interrelated, and changes in elements or compartments on one level are necessarily reflected on the other levels. The aim of this chapter is to describe exercise-induced changes in body composition. While an understanding of changes on all levels is important, this chapter focuses on changes on the chemical (e.g., bone, mineral, fat, and fat-free mass [FFM]) and tissue-system (e.g., muscle, bone, and adipose tissue) levels, since changes on these levels have practical significance and are most often assessed.

As Ballor has noted, the description of exercise-induced changes in body composition is not an easy task (2). The adaptations to exercise depend on many factors, including age, gender, and initial composition and distribution of components. Genetic makeup; nutrient and energy intake; mode, intensity, and duration of exercise; and total exercise energy expenditure are other significant factors. Too few studies have adequately described or controlled these and other influential factors, making it difficult to compare studies and draw generalizations. Another major limiting factor has been the short duration (i.e., a few weeks to a few months) of most studies. Using short-term exercise studies to predict how long-term exercise affects body composition is fraught with problems, since the changes are likely to plateau (2). Extrapolating from cross-sectional comparisons of habitual exercisers versus their inactive peers is also problematic, because cross-sectional studies suffer from self-selection bias. Thus, this chapter emphasizes the findings from studies of exercise training. Because of biologic heterogeneity and methodologic differences, the effects of exercise on body composition are discussed relative to other variables that may mitigate the results.

EXERCISE AND BODY WEIGHT

In previously inactive individuals, exercise has been shown to have modest effects on body weight (2). Although some individuals may achieve more dramatic results, weight changes generally average about 1 to 2 kg with exercise, unless some type of dietary modification is also pursued (3). Whether weight is lost or gained depends on the type of exercise and energy balance. Aerobic activities that result in a daily caloric deficit are accompanied by weight loss; resistance exercise results in an approximately equal weight gain. A focus on weight changes without consideration of compositional changes can be misleading, because meaningful changes in different components in opposite directions result in minimal weight change.

Epstein and Wing (4), Thomson et al (5), Wilmore (6), and Ballor et al (3) have published comprehensive reviews of the effects of exercise on body weight. These authors' results generally are in agreement, showing that initial body mass and composition, energy expenditure, and exercise frequency are the most robust predictors of weight loss with aerobic exercise. In general, heavier and fatter individuals, and individuals with greater exercise frequency and weekly energy expenditure, lose the greatest amounts of weight. The optimal exercise energy expenditure to maximize weight loss is not clear because, at some level of expenditure, appetite and caloric intake are expected to increase and counter the effect.

In animal studies, a sex-specific response has consistently been found: females conserve weight and males lose weight in response to exercise training (7). There is evidence that these gender-specific responses are related to differences in gonadal steroids (8). Also, it has been suggested that exercise may stimulate appetite more in females than in males (9). While the results of Ballor and Keesey (3) support a sex-specific response, the effect is only a modest one, and the influence of potential confounders, such as differences in initial mass and composition and exercise energy expenditure, cannot be discounted.

Recent studies have clearly demonstrated the large individual differences in the effects of exercise on body weight and composition (10,11). While initial weight and composition and energy expenditure are consistent predictors of the response, together they account for only 50% to 70% of the change in body mass. Further research is required to identify other factors that moderate the response of body weight and composition to different types of exercise.

EXERCISE AND FAT FREE BODY MASS

The FFM is a heterogeneous compartment that includes all nonfat body components. Many traditional body composition assessment methods are designed to measure the FFM (12). Since FFM is generally easier to measure than its components, changes in FFM are often reported in intervention studies. An increase or decrease in FFM represents the composite of changes in muscle, bone, connective tissue, vital organs, and body water; it is impossible to determine the relative contributions of changes in various compartments without applying multiple methods. Nevertheless, a change in FFM is generally interpreted as a change in muscle or body cell mass, since these are the major compartments of FFM and seem to respond most rapidly to exercise.

Ballor and Keesey (3) have reviewed the short-term effects of exercise on FFM. Both aerobic and resistance exercise result in modest increases in FFM in males and females, about 0.5 to 1.0 kg (aerobic) and about 2.0 kg (resistance). Observations of individuals involved in long-term resistance exercise, such as body builders and football players, suggest much larger increases are possible, although the time course of these changes is not well studied and the effects of nutritional interventions and performance-enhancing drugs must be considered. In contrast, with aerobic exercise, there appears to be a ceiling effect. In a recent analysis, Ballor reported a weak and negative association between duration of aerobic training and change in FFM in males (2). Moreover, higher levels of weekly aerobic exercise energy expenditure were not associated with greater increases in FFM.

Whether age and gender differentially affect exercise-induced changes in FFM remains to be determined. Studies of master athletes (13) and comparisons between young and old men and women who were habitually active or inactive suggest similar responses in males and females at young and old ages (14). These studies are cross-sectional, however, and susceptible to sampling bias. Studies of exercise training also support the notion of similar exercise-induced responses in young and old men and women (15–17), although the overall effect on FFM may be less in older men and women who have lost significant numbers of muscle cells with aging (18).

EXERCISE AND MUSCLE MASS

The muscle-building effects of resistance exercise are well known (19). Ballor et al reported an average increase in FFM of 2.2 kg as a result of weight lifting for an average of 9.6 weeks (3). Although, as noted, FFM and muscle mass are not equivalent, the majority of the change in FFM with resistance exercise is likely the result of an increase in muscle mass. The largest increases in FFM are slightly greater than 3 kg in about 10 weeks of training. This is equivalent to an increase in FFM of about 0.66 kg/week. Muscle cell hypertrophy (20) and an increase in FFM (3) have also been reported as a result of aerobic exercise, although the increases in FFM are more modest than with weight training. Aerobic exercises with higher resistance components, such as cycling and rowing, are likely to elicit greater increases in muscle and FFM than low-resistance exercise, such as walking or running (3).

Increased muscle size with exercise is attributed to hypertrophy of existing muscle cells (19). Muscle cell hypertrophy is thought to occur through remodeling of protein within the cell and increased size and number of myofibrils. In addition, increases in the number of contractile myofilaments and sarcomeres contribute to increased muscle-cell size and ultimately to increases in muscle mass. The contractile proteins and fluid in muscle turn over every 7 to 15 days (21). Resistance exercise affects this process by influencing the type of protein and the quantity of proteins that are produced (19). Changes in the types of proteins produced have been observed very early after the start of training (22), whereas a longer duration of training (>8 sessions) is required to demonstrate significant muscle-cell enlargement. The degree of hypertrophy depends on the duration and intensity of training. Muscle fiber composition also influences the increase in muscle mass with training (19). All cells hypertrophy, but not to the same extent. Ultimately, the degree of hypertrophy is dependent on the upper genetic limits for cell size.

Whether similar degrees of hypertrophy are possible in males and females at different ages remains unclear. Before puberty, boys and girls respond similarly, with increases in muscle strength and little or no increase in muscle mass (24,25), whereas adolescent, young adult, and middle-aged males (25–27) achieve significant hypertrophy with resistance training. Adolescent girls and women are also capable of significant muscle hypertrophy (28–32). Whether one concludes that hypertrophy in females is similar to that in males is influenced by the approach used for gender comparisons, since muscle strength and mass before training are greater in men. Similar *relative* increases in muscle mass would indicate greater absolute increases in men than women; similar *absolute* increases would indicate greater relative increases in women (33). Assuming muscle dimensions increase in a geometrically proportional manner, similar relative increases would represent similar "trainability" (28,34). Using this criteria, studies to date suggest similar training adaptations in men and women.

An additional way to address the relative trainability of men and women would be to assess the change in the ratio of women's to men's muscle mass during training. An increase in this ratio would suggest greater trainability of women and a decrease would suggest greater trainability in men (33). Most studies show no change in this ratio with training. Thus, analyzing the results in this way also supports similar trainability of men and women.

In a series of studies, Frontera et al (24) and Fiatarone et al (17) have examined the muscular adaptation to resistance exercise in old and very old men and women. In contrast to the notion that trainability is impaired in old age, significant increases in muscle strength and mass were demonstrated in men and women in the ninth and tenth decades of life. The results suggest that inactivity is a major correlate of muscle atrophy and weakness in old men and women. These studies also showed that older men and women are capable of resistance exercise at relative loads (>75% of maximum voluntary contraction) similar to those employed with younger subjects. Other investigators have also studied the effects of strength training in older men and women with similar results (15, 35–37). Although few gender comparisons have been made, those that have been done suggest trainability is similar in older men and women (38,39).

Although controversial, it has been suggested that resistance exercise may also elicit an increase in the number of muscle cells (hyperplasia) that would contribute to the increase in muscle size as a result of training (19). Hyperplasia after resistance exercise has not been demonstrated in humans because of methodologic difficulties, but it has been shown in animals and birds (40,41). Findings of hyperplasia have been questioned on the basis of methodologic limitations and the possibility of damage to the samples and degeneration that would account for any observed hyperplasia, although in studies that attempted to control these factors, increases in muscle cell number continued to be observed (41). Thus, although there is no clear evidence supporting hyperplasia in humans, it remains a possibility. Kraemer et al (19) speculate that hyperplasia may represent an adaptation that occurs when some fibers reach an upper limit in cell size. If hyperplasia does occur, it probably accounts for only a small (>10%) portion of the increase in muscle size.

The effect of exercise on muscle mass has also been studied in regard to its influence on muscle composition, i.e., the predominant type of cells within the muscle. Muscle cells are classified along a continuum. While it is doubtful that exercise transforms cells from one major type to another (e.g., from type I to type II), there is evidence of movement along the continuum. Muscle plasticity exists in part as a result of the complex yet adaptable group of myosin contractile and regulatory proteins. There is evidence that when a type IIB muscle cell is stimulated, it begins a process of transformation toward the type IIA profile by changing the quality of proteins and expressing different types and amounts of adenosine triphosphatase (ATPase) (42,43). Thus, very few type IIB cells remain after resistance training. These alterations in muscle cell types are supported by myosin heavy chain (MHC) analyses with the replacement of MHC IIB chains with MHC IIA chains. Muscle cell conversions may occur very early in training, although they do not appear to be related to the rate of change in the cross-sectional area of the cell. Systematic com-

parisons of the effects different types of training on transformations have not been done, although when resistance training and aerobic training are done simultaneously, the adaptive response seems different than when either mode of exercise is done alone (23).

EXERCISE AND BONE MASS

Bone loss with aging is universal. The onset and rate of loss vary at different skeletal sites, averaging about 0.1% to 0.3% per year in males (44). The rate of loss is generally similar in females, except at menopause, when the rate is accelerated for 7 to 10 years. As a result, females may lose as much as 30% of bone mass by age 80 to 90, whereas the loss in males is generally less than 10%.

Osteoporosis—excessive bone loss leading to increased risk of bone fractures with minimal trauma—is a major public health concern, accounting for 1.3 million fractures per year with the estimated cost increasing to $45 billion over the next 10 years (45). Many more women are affected than men. Traditional therapeutic regimens for osteoporosis have focused primarily on diet modification with calcium and vitamin D, fluoride, and hormone therapy, often with only limited success. Hormone replacement therapy (HRT), more than other strategies, has proved effective for retarding bone loss and maintaining bone mass, yet many women are unwilling or unable to initiate and comply with HRT (46,47). Consequently, considerable research has been done to develop safe, acceptable alternative regimens for osteoporosis prevention and treatment.

Adequate mechanical stimuli are clearly needed for optimal bone growth and maintenance of bone mass. Initial enthusiasm for exercise as an effective intervention was based on indirect evidence from comparisons of habitually active individuals versus their inactive peers, as well as athletes versus nonathletes (48,49). While these studies almost universally showed that athletes and active individuals have greater bone mass and density than the general population, the exercise effect was most certainly overestimated as a result of self-selection bias (48,50,51). More valid evidence of an effect of chronic exercise on bone comes from comparisons of bone mass and density in the dominant arms versus nondominant arms of tennis players, which show hypertrophy of bone that exceeds the usual bilateral differences in the general population (52).

The optimal exercise regimen for increasing bone mass and density is not known. The results of animal studies suggest that bone adapts in response to the magnitude of strain placed on it. Rubin et al (53), for example, found that the change in the cross-sectional area of turkey ulnae was closely correlated with magnitude of strain imposed upon it and not the total amount of strain. These results suggest that weight-bearing exercises would cause greater increases in bone mineral density (BMD) than non–weight-bearing exercises. In addition, resistance exercise may induce greater site-specific increases than other forms of training, because the localized stresses on bone during resistance exercise are commonly five times greater than those for aerobic exercises, such as walking, running, and cycling (54). The results from the few well-designed prospective studies that have tested these ideas suggest that weight-bearing exercise may be effective for slowing bone loss and maintaining bone mass, while resistance exercise elicits significant, though small (1% to 2%), increases in BMD (16,55–59). Whether further increases are possible with long-term training is not known, since most studies have lasted only 6 to 12 months and cover only a few bone remodeling cycles (60).

Perhaps the strongest evidence to date for an exercise effect comes from a study by Kerr et al (55), who examined the effects of resistance exercise on regional BMD of one side of the body, using the opposite side as the control. Effects of high-intensity versus low-intensity exercise on BMD were also compared. Exercise intensity and exercised side of body were randomly assigned. The results clearly showed that high-intensity exercise resulted in a greater exercise response, although the magnitude was similar to what was observed in other studies (16,58,61). Other recent studies have demonstrated that moderate-to-high impact exercise also stimulates significant increases in BMD (62–64). While feasible for younger women and women who have little bone loss, impact exercise is contraindicated in women with significant bone loss (65).

A number of factors may modify the bone response to exercise, including calcium intake, endocrine status, initial BMD, age, and gender. Of these factors, the permissive effect of estrogen in women may have the most potent effect, since BMD has been shown to decline in young exercising women with amenorrhea (48,66). Also, available data suggest estrogen replacement plus exercise in postmenopausal women may have additive or at least synergistic effects (67,68). Although adequate calcium intake is necessary to support increases in BMD, when exercise is discontinued BMD is lost despite continued calcium supplementation (69). The effects of different types of exercise in males and females at different ages has not been systematically investigated, although it appears that similar responses are possible in young and old males and females (44). While it is plausible that individuals with lower initial BMD would achieve the greatest increases in BMD (58), there is little data to support this point of view.

The peak bone mass, the highest BMD achieved before the onset of decline, is an important predictor of future osteoporosis and fracture risk. Interventions aimed at maximizing peak bone mass may prove important for osteoporosis prevention. Studies of general activity in children and adolescents suggest that active boys and girls have greater BMD than their less active peers, although these studies are inconclusive as a result of their cross-sectional design (44). There are few controlled prospective studies of the effects of resistance exercise on BMD in children and adolescents, and these have yielded mixed results (44). Recent studies with college-aged gymnasts, however, demonstrate significant increases in BMD over a competitive season, suggesting that it may be possible to alter peak BMD with high impact exercise (63,70).

EXERCISE AND BODY FAT

The results of volunteer-based studies have repeatedly shown that athletes and active individuals have considerably less body fat than their less active peers (6). While it is tempting to conclude that the exercise involved in sport participation is responsible for the lower level of body fat, the two groups are likely to differ in many ways besides athletic and weight status. Randomized controlled trials are the best way to assess the effects of exercise on body fat, provided the sample adequately represents the population and is large enough to offer adequate statistical power to detect group differences. The designs should specify the type of exercise, frequency, intensity, and duration of exercise, as well as the subjects' compliance with the protocol, all of which may affect the results.

In one of the more comprehensive reviews of exercise intervention studies, Ballor et al (3) evaluated over 500 studies of exercise and body composition. Using meta-analytical techniques, they examined the effects of exercise type, frequency, intensity, and duration on changes in body weight, fat weight, and fat as a percentage of weight in adult males and females in 53 studies that met their inclusion criteria of at least five previously sedentary subjects of a single gender per group. Other inclusion criteria included adequate reports of pre- and post-exercise body mass and composition, exercise energy expenditure, and exercise type (with no mixing of exercise types). Studies that involved exercise sessions longer than 60 minutes or programs of more than 36 weeks were excluded from the analysis.

The results of Baylor et al (3) showed that all exercise was associated with a reduction in fat mass. Cycling exercise and weight lifting in males were associated with an increase in FFM such that the actual loss of body fat was greater than total weight loss. No studies of weight lifting in females were included in the analysis. The rates of change in fat mass (−0.11 to −0.12 kg/week) and percent fat (−0.12% to −0.16%/week) were remarkably similar for walking, jogging, cycling, and resistance training in males. In females, fat was lost more rapidly as a result of walking or jogging (−0.10 kg/week) compared with cycling exercise (−0.05 kg/week), although the changes in percent fat were similar (−0.10% to −0.11%/week). The energy expended during exercise and initial fat levels or body mass accounted for most of the variance in the changes in composition; in females, weeks of training and duration of exercise per session were also significant predictors.

The role of initial weight and composition on the change in composition with exercise is important to emphasize. Based on a model of two energy reservoirs, Forbes (71) has examined the relationship between FFM and fat and shown that the former is a curvilinear function of the latter. Thus, in persons losing or gaining weight as a result of restricted or excess energy intake, the change in FFM is inversely related to body fat content. A similar relationship exists in exercising persons (72). Based on a variety of data from the literature, Forbes estimates that individuals with small or modest amounts of body fat tend to lose or gain about 0.5 kg of FFM for every kilogram of change in body weight with exercise. Persons who maintain their weight tend to gain 0.67 kg of FFM while losing an equal amount of fat. If these same persons lose more than 1.5 kg of weight, they tend to lose FFM, despite engaging in an exercise program, although there is evidence that resistance training may preserve the FFM even when there is a substantial energy deficit (73,74). These estimates of compositional change represent average values and individuals may deviate substantially from these average figures.

In contrast, having larger fat stores serves to protect the individual from loss of FFM as weight is lost and hence favors the loss of body fat during exercise. Individuals with larger fat stores lose or gain only about 0.25 kg of FFM for every kilogram of body weight change, and those whose weight is maintained during exercise gain almost twice as much FFM as do leaner individuals and so lose more fat (75).

The distribution of body fat along with total fat may influence the change in body weight and body fat with exercise. The two largest adipose tissue regions in humans are the subcutaneous and intra-abdominal (visceral) fat depots. There is considerable evidence that the regulation of intra-abdominal and subcutaneous fat depots differs, as does regulation among subcutaneous fat depots. Subcutaneous abdominal adipocytes have been shown to be four to five times more responsive to norepinephrine than are gluteal adipocytes (76). Catecholamines have also been shown to be more lipolytic in omental than in subcutaneous adipocytes (77,78), and omental fat is less responsive to the antilipolytic effect of insulin than subcutaneous fat (79). In addition to different lipolytic responses, adipose tissue lipoprotein lipase (LPL) activity has been shown to be higher in abdominal subcutaneous tissue than gluteal adipose tissue in men. The opposite was true in women (80), for whom reproductive hormone status has been shown to relate to the activity of both femoral and subcutaneous abdominal adipose tissue LPL, and also the lipolytic responsiveness of these depots to catecholamines and insulin (81,82).

Insomuch as the android pattern of fat distribution is characterized by higher central or truncal (visceral) fat, while the gynoid pattern is characterized by peripheral or extremity fat, fat distribution may contribute to gender differences in alterations in body fat as a result of exercise. Aerobic exercise training has been shown to decrease trunk fat more than extremity fat in men (83). Moreover, aerobic exercise decreases intra-abdominal fat as well as abdominal subcutaneous fat in younger and older men (84), and in obese premenopausal women, greater loss of intra-abdominal fat compared with thigh fat has been observed (85). It has been suggested that women with an android distribution of fat may benefit more from exercise for weight and fat reduction than do women who deposit fat in the more resistant gluteal and thigh areas, possibly because of preferential lipolysis of intra-abdominal fat with stimulation of the sympathetic nervous system during exercise (86). It follows that obese men may benefit more from exercise training than women (87), which may explain why changes in fatness with 20 weeks of aerobic exercise were correlated with initial fatness in men but not in women (88). Further investigations of men and women at different ages with upper and lower body fat patterns are needed to better explain the role of gender, initial fat, and fat distribution in the success or failure of exercise to induce fat loss.

Adipocyte number and morphology may also contribute to variability in exercise-induced loss of body fat. Lipoprotein lipase activity, which facilitates fat storage, increases when adipocyte volume is reduced (89), whereas enlarged adipocytes become insulin-resistant and their capacity to store fat is reduced (90). Thus, the regulation of adipocyte volume may impose limits on body fat loss with exercise. Individuals who are already near the lower limits of adipocyte volume would be expected to lose less fat than individuals with larger adipocytes. Moreover, losses of body fat with exercise would be proportional to exercise energy expenditure until adipocyte volume was reduced to a critical level, after which dietary intake would increase to stabilize weight. Since the number of adipocytes varies among individuals, stabilization can occur at a variety of body weights and levels of body fat.

If a relationship does exist between fat cell volume and exercise adaptations, obese individuals with enlarged adipocytes would be expected to lose body fat in response to training more readily than obese individuals with larger numbers of average-size cells (91). This notion is supported by studies showing greater fat loss in men with larger initial adipocyte volume (4.6 kg of fat loss over 20 weeks) in comparison to men with smaller adipocytes (0.7 kg of fat loss) (88). In contrast, females did not significantly reduce their body fat and there were no differences between women with large or small initial adipocyte volumes. Boileau et al (1971) also showed greater fat loss (5.9 kg) in obese men compared with loss (2.1 kg) in lean men who expended 3000 kcal per week for 9 weeks. Thus, the same total energy expenditure does not necessarily elicit the same reduction in fat mass.

Postmenopausal women are more likely to be overfat and to deposit fat in beta-mediated adipocytes in which the fat is more labile, especially in the abdominal region. Thus, older women may lose more body fat with exercise than younger premenopausal women. Data from Kohrt et al (93) showing greater differences in body fat between trained and untrained old women compared to trained and untrained young women support this idea. A similar finding was made in men. Additional evidence comes from a second study by Kohrt et al (93) in which the effects of a 9- to 12-month aerobic training program on fat mass and adipose tissue distribution were studied in men and women aged 60 to 70. Both men and women lost body fat (on average, 3.1 kg and 1.6 kg, respectively), and in both sexes, the greatest loss occurred in the truncal area, suggesting preferential loss of fat from this region.

Diet composition may play a role in the cause of obesity (74,87,94). Reports of significant positive correlations between percent body fat and intake of total, saturated, and monounsaturated fats (95,96) and negative correlations between percent fat and carbohydrates and plant protein (95) would seem to support this point. The macronutrient content of the diet may also influence the effect of exercise on body composition. This notion has not been systematically tested, although results from the Stanford Weight Control Project (87) and from Walberg et al (74) suggest the composition of weight-reducing diets may influence the effects of exercise on body fat (87) and FFM (74).

SUMMARY

Optimal body weight and composition, although difficult to define because of individual variation, are important determinants of good health, functional capacity, and physical performance. There is a large body of evidence showing that exercise can modify composition of body fat, muscle, and bone in males and females at all ages. The direction and magnitude of the change depends on many factors, including the mode and duration of exercise, energy expenditure, the age and sex of the participant, initial body composition and the distribution of components, energy intake, and the composition of dietary intake. The relative importance of each of these factors depends on the component under investigation. Energy expenditure, for example, seems to be more important than intensity and mode for modifying body fat, whereas intensity and mode are significant determinants of the changes in muscle and bone. Adolescent and adult males and females at all ages seem to respond similarly to training, especially when matched for initial differences in weight and whole body and regional composition. Generally, the average changes with exercise are modest in magnitude, although there is considerable individual variation: some individuals undergo impressive changes. Undoubtedly, genetic factors place a "ceiling" on the response to exercise. Persons who are furthest away from their individual optimal composition will likely experience the greatest response. More research is needed to determine the relative contribution of various factors that predict a person's optimal body composition and that determine the response to exercise.

REFERENCES

1. Wang ZM, Pierson RN, Heymsfield SB. The five level model: a new approach to organizing body composition research. Amer J Clin Nutr 1992;56:19–28.

2. Ballor DL. Exercise training and body composition changes. In: Roche AF, Heymsfield SB, Lohman TG, eds. Human body composition. Champaign, IL: Human Kinetics, 1996:287–304.

3. Ballor DL, Keesey RE. A meta-analysis of the factors affecting exercise-induced changes in body mass, fat mass, and fat-free mass in males and females. Int J Obesity 1991;15:717–726.

4. Epstein LH, Wing RR. Aerobic exercise and weight. Addict Behav 1980;5:371–388.

5. Thompson JK, Jarvie GJ, Lahey BB. Exercise and obesity: etiology, physiology, and intervention. Psych Bull 1982;91:55–79.

6. Wilmore JH. Body composition in sport and exercise: directions for future research. Med Sci Sports Exerc 1983;15:21–31.

7. Oscai LB. The role of exercise in weight control. Exerc Sci Sports Rev 1973;1:103–123.

8. Nance DM, Bromley B, Barnard RJ, et al. Sexually dimorphic effects of forced exercise on food intake and body weight in the rat. Physiol Behav 1977;19:155–158.

9. Anderson B, Xu X, Rebuffe-Scrive M, et al. The effects of exercise training on body composition and metabolism in men and women. Int J Obesity 1991;15:75–81.

10. Bouchard C, Tremblay A, Després JP, et al. The response to long-term overfeeding in identical twins. N Engl J Med 1990;322:1477–1482.

11. Bouchard C, Tremblay A, Després JP, et al. The response to exercise with constant energy intake in identical twins. Obesity Res 1994;2:400–410.

12. Roche AF, Heymsfield SB, Lohman TG, eds. Human body composition. Champaign, IL: Human Kinetics, 1996:3–190.

13. Marti B, Howald H. Long-term effects of physical training on aerobic capacity: controlled study of former elite athletes. J Appl Physiol 1990;69:1451–1459.

14. Kohrt W, Malley MT, Dalsky GP, et al. Body composition of healthy sedentary and trained, young and older men and women. Med Sci Sports Exerc 1992;24:832–837.

15. Charette SL, McEvoy L, Pyka G, et al. Muscle hypertrophy response to resistance training in older women. J Appl Physiol 1991;70:1912–1916.

16. Nelson ME, Fiatarone MA, Morganti CM, et al. Effects of high-intensity strength training on multiple risk factors for osteoporotic fractures: a controlled clinical trial. JAMA 1994;272:1909–1914.

17. Fiatarone MA, Marks EC, Ryan ND, et al. High-intensity strength training in nonagenarians: effect on skeletal muscle. JAMA 1990;263:3029–3034.

18. Lexell J, Taylor CC, Sjöström M. What is the cause of the aging atrophy? Total number, size, and proportion of different fiber types studied in whole vastus lateralis muscle from 15- to 83-year-old men. J Neurol Sci 1988;84:275–294.

19. Kraemer WJ, Volek JS, Fleck SJ. Chronic musculoskeletal adaptations to resistance training. In: Roitmann JL, ed. ACSM's resource manual for guidelines for exercise testing and prescription. 3rd ed. Baltimore: Williams & Wilkins, 1998:174–181.

20. Costill DL. Inside running: basics of sports physiology. Indianapolis, IN: Benchmark, 1986:9.

21. Goldspink C. Cellular and molecular aspects of adaptation in skeletal muscle, In: Komi P, ed. Strength and power in sports: the encyclopedia of sports medicine. Oxford, England: Blackwell Scientific, 1992:211–229.

22. Staron RS, Karapondo DL, Kraemer WJ, et al. Skeletal muscle adaptations during the early phase of heavy-resistance training in men and women. J Appl Physiol 1994;76:1247–1255.

23. Kraemer WJ, Patton J, Gordon SE, et al. Compatibility of high intensity strength and endurance training on hormonal and skeletal muscle adaptations. J Appl Physiol 1995;78:976–989.

24. Ramsay JA, Blimkie CJR, Smith K, et al. Strength training effects in prepubescent boys. Med Sci Sports Exerc 1990;22:605–614.

25. Sale DG. Strength training in children. In: Gisolfi CV, Lamb DR, eds. Perspectives in exercise science and sports medicine. Vol. 2. Youth, exercise, and sport. Indianapolis: Benchmark, 1989:165–222.

26. Frontera WR, Meredith CN, O'Reilly HG, et al. Strength conditioning in older men: skeletal muscle hypertrophy and improved function. J Appl Physiol 1988; 64:1038–1044.

27. Tesch PA. Skeletal muscle adaptations consequent to long-term heavy resistance exercise. Med Sci Sports Exerc 1988;20(suppl): S132–S134.

28. Cureton KJ, Collins MA, Hill DW, et al. Muscle hypertrophy in men and women. Med Sci Sports Exer 1988;20:338–344.

29. Krotkiewski M, Aniansson A, Grimby G, et al. The effect of unilateral isokinetic strength training on local adipose and muscle tissue morphology, thickness, and enzymes. Eur J Appl Physiol 1979;42:271–281.

30. O'Hagan FT, Sale DG, MacDougall JD, et al. Response to resistance training in young women and men. Int J Sports Med 1995;16:314–321.

31. Staron RS, Malicky ES, Leonardi MJ, et al. Muscle hypertrophy and fast fiber type conversions in heavy resistance-trained women. Eur J Appl Physiol 1989;60:71–79.

32. Wang N, Hikida RS, Staron RS, et al. Muscle fiber types of women after resistance training: quantitative ultrastructure and enzyme activity. Pflüg Arch Eur J Physiol 1993;424:494–502.

33. Sale DG, Spriet LL. Skeletal muscle function and energy metabolism. In: Bar-Or O, Lamb DR, Clarkson PM, eds. Perspectives in exercise science and sports medicine. Vol 9. Exercise and the female: a life span approach. Carmel, IN: Cooper, 1996:289–359.

34. Holloway JB, Baechle TR. Strength training for female athletes: a review of selected aspects. Sports Med 1990;9:216–228.

35. Connelly DM, Vandervoort AA. Improvement in knee extensor strength of institutionalized elderly women after exercise with ankle weights. Physiother Can 1995;47: 15–23.

36. Nichols JF, Omizo DK, Peterson KK, et al. Efficacy of heavy resistance training for active women over sixty: muscular strength, body composition, and program adherence. J Amer Geriatr Soc 1993; 41:205–210.

37. Pyka G, Lindenberger E, Charette S, et al. Muscle strength and fiber adaptations to year-long resistance training program in elderly men and women. J Gerontol 1994;49: M22–M28.

38. McCartney N, Hicks AL, Martin J, et al. Long-term resistance training in the elderly: effects on dynamic strength, exercise capacity, muscle, and bone. J Gerontol Biol Sci 1995;50A:B97–B104.

39. Häkkinen K, Pakarinen A. Serum hormones and strength development during strength training in middle-aged and elderly males and females. Acta Physiol Scand 1994;150:211–219.

40. MacDougall JD. Hypertrophy or hyperplasia. In: Komi P, ed. Strength and power in sports: the encyclopedia of sports medicine. Oxford, England: Blackwell Scientific, 1992:230–238.

41. Antonio J, Gonyea WJ. Muscle fiber splitting in stretch-enlarged avian muscle. Med Sci Sport Exerc 1994;26:973–977.

42. Fry AC, Allemeier CA, Staron RS. Correlation between percentage fiber type area and myosin heavy chain content in human skeletal muscle. Eur J Appl Physiol 1994; 68:246–251.

43. Staron RS. Correlation between myofibrillar ATPase activity and myosin heavy chain composition in single human muscle fibers. Histochem 1991;96:21–24.

44. Blimkie CJR, Chilibeck PD, Davison KS. Bone mineralization patterns: reproductive endocrine, calcium, and physical activity influences during the life span. In: Bar-Or O, Lamb DR, Clarkson PM, eds. Perspectives in exercise science and sports medicine. Vol 9. Carmel, IN: Cooper Publishing Group, 1996:73–142.

45. Chrischilles C, Sherman T, Wallace R. Cost and health effects of osteoporotic fractures. Bone 1994;15: 377–386.

46. Ryan PJ, Harrison R, Black GM, et al. Compliance with hormone replacement therapy after screening for postmenopausal osteoporosis. Br J Obstet Gynaecol 1992; 99:325–328.

47. Brett KM, Madans JH. Use of postmenopausal hormone replacement therapy: estimates from nationally representative cohort study. Am J Epidemiol 1997; 145:536–545.

48. Drinkwater BL. Does physical activity play a role in preventing osteoporosis? Res Q Exerc Sport 1994;65:197–206.

49. Drinkwater BL. Physical activity, fitness, and osteoporosis. In: Bouchard C, Shephard RJ, Stephens T, eds. Physical activity, fitness, and health. Champaign, IL: Human Kinetics, 1994:724–736.

50. Block JE, Smith R, Friedlander A, Genant HK. Preventing osteoporosis with exercise: a review with emphais on methodology. Med Hypoth 1989;30:9–19.

51. Forwood MR, Burr DB. Physical activity and bone mass: exercises in futility. Bone Min 1993;21: 89–112.

52. Huddleston AL, Rockwell D, Kuland D, et al. Bone mass in lifetime tennis athletes. JAMA 1980; 244:1107–1109.

53. Rubin CT, Lanyon CE. Regulation of bone mass by mechanical strain magnitude: the effect of peak strain magnitude. Calcif Tissue Int 1985;37:411–417.

54. Frost HM. Why do marathon runners have less bone than weight

lifters? A vital-biomechanical view and explanation. Bone 1997;20: 183–189.

55. Kerr DA, Morton A, Dick I, Prince R. Exercise effects on bone mass in postmenopausal women are site-specific and load dependent. J Bone Min Res 1996;11:218–225.

56. Kohrt WM, Ehsani AA, Birge Jr SJ. Effects of exercise involving predominantly either joint-reaction or ground-reaction forces on bone mineral density in older women. J Bone Min Res 1997;12:1253–1261.

57. Lohman TG, Going SB, Parmenter RW, et al. Effects of resistance training on bone mineral density in premenopausal women: a randomized, prospective trial. J Bone Min Res 1995;10:1015–1024.

58. Shaw JM, Witzke KA. Exercise for skeletal health and osteoporosis prevention. In: Roitman JL, ed. ACSM's resource manual for guidelines for exercise testing and prescription. 3rd ed. Philadelphia: Williams & Wilkins, 1998:288–293.

59. Snow-Harter C, Marcus R. Exercise, bone mineral density, and osteoporosis. Exer Sport Sci Rev 1991;19:351–358.

60. Block JE. Interpreting studies of exercise and osteoporosis: a call for rigor. Contr Clin Trials 1997; 18:54–57.

61. Chillibeck PD, Sale DG, Webber CE. Exercise and bone mineral density. Sports Med 1995;19: 103–122.

62. Heinonen A, Sievanen H, Oja P, et al. Randomized controlled trial of effect of high-impact exercise on selected risk factors for osteoporotic fractures. Lancet 1996; 348:1343–1347.

63. Taaffe DR, Robinson TL, Snow CM, et al. High-impact exercise promotes bone gain in well-trained female athletes. J Bone Min Res 1997;12:255–260.

64. Welsh L, Rutherford OM. Hip bone mineral density is improved by high-impact aerobic exercise in postmenopausal women and men over 50 years. Eur J Appl Physiol 1996;74:511–517.

65. American College of Sports Medicine. ACSM position stand on osteoporosis and exercise. Med Sci Sports Exerc 1995;27:i–vii.

66. Drinkwater BL, Milson K, Chestnut CH III. Bone mineral content of amenorrheic and eumenorrheic athletes. N Engl J Med 1984; 311:277–281.

67. Kohrt WM, Snead DB, Slatopolsky E, et al. Additive effects of weight-bearing exercise and estrogen on bone mineral density in older women. J Bone Min Res 1995; 10:1303–1311.

68. Notelovitz MD, Martin R, Tesar K, et al. Estrogen therapy and variable-resistance weight training increase bone mineral in surgically menopausal women. J Bone Min Res 1991;6:583–590.

69. Dalsky GP, Stocke KS, Ehsani AA, et al. Weight-bearing exercise training and lumbar bone mineral content on postmenopausal women. Ann Intern Med 1988; 108:824–828.

70. Nichols DL, Sanborn CF, Bonnick SL, et al. The effects of gymnastics training on bone mineral density. Med Sci Sports Exerc 1994;26:1220–1225.

71. Forbes GB. Lean body mass-body fat interrelationships in humans. Nutr Rev 1987;45:225–231.

72. Forbes GB. Exercise and lean weight: the influence of body weight. Nutr Rev 1992;50:157–161.

73. Ballor DL, Katch VL, Becque MD, et al. Resistance weight training during caloric restriction enhances lean body weight maintenance. Am J Clin Nutr 1988;47: 19–25.

74. Walberg JL. Aerobic exercise and resistance weight-training during weight reduction: implications for obese persons and athletes. Sports Med 1989;47:343–346.

75. Forbes GB. Exercise and body composition. J Appl Physiol 1991; 70:994–997.

76. Wahrenberg H, Bolinder J, Arner P. Adrenergic regulation of lipolysis in human fat cells during exercise. Eur J Clin Invest 1991;21:534–541.

77. Efendic S. Catecholamine and metabolism of human adipose tissue. Part 3. Comparison between the regulation of lipolysis in omental and subcutaneous adipose tissue. Acta Med Scand 1970;187:477–483.

78. Ostman J, Arner P, Engfeldt, et al. Regional differences in the control of lipolysis in human adipose tissue. Metab 1979;28:1198–1205.

79. Bolinder J, Kager L, Ostman J, et al. Differences at the receptor and post-receptor levels between human omental and subcutaneous adipose tissue in the action of insulin on lipolysis. Diabetes 1983;32:117–123.

80. Arner P, Lithell H, Wahrenberg H, et al. Expression of lipoprotein lipase in different human subcutaneous adipose tissue regions. J Lipid Res 1991;32: 423–429.

81. Rebuffe-Scrive M, Enk L, Crona N, et al. Fat cell metabolism in different regions in women: effect of menstrual cycle, pregnancy, and lactation. J Clin Invest 1985;75: 1973–1976.

82. Rebuffe-Scrive J, Lonnroth P, Marin P, et al. Regional adipose tissue metabolism in men and postmenopausal women. Int J Obesity 1987;11: 347–355.

83. Després JP, Bouchard C, Tremblay A, et al. Effects of aerobic training on fat distribution in male subjects. Med Sci Sports Exerc 1985; 17:113–118.

84. Schwartz RS, Shuman WP, Larson V, et al. The effect of intensive endurance exercise training on body fat distribution in young and older men. Metab 1991;40:545–551.

85. Després JP, Poulot MC, Moorjani S, et al. Loss of abdominal fat and metabolic response to exercise training in obese women. Am J Physiol 1991;261:E159–167.

86. Krotkiewski M, Björntorp P. Muscle tissue in obesity with different distribution of adipose tissue: effects of physical training. Int J Obesity 1986;10:331–341.

87. Stefanik ML. Exercise and weight control. In: Holloszy JO, ed. Exercise and sport sciences reviews. Vol 21. Baltimore: Williams & Wilkins, 1993:363–396.

88. Tremblay A, Després JP, LeBlanc C, et al. Sex dimorphism in fat loss in response to exercise-training. J Obes Weight Reg 1984; 3:193–203.

89. Kern PA, Ong JM, Saffari B, et al. The effects of weight loss on the activity and expression of adipose tissue lipoprotein lipase in very obese humans. N Engl J Med 1990;322:1053–1059.

90. Craig BW, Garthwaite SM, Holloszy JO. Adipocyte insulin resistance: effects of aging, obesity, exercise, and food restriction. J Appl Physiol 1987;62:95–100.

91. Björntorp P. Adipose tissue adaptation to exercise. In: Bouchard C, Shephard RJ, Stephens T, et al, eds. Exercise, fitness and health: a consensus of current knowledge. Champaign, IL: Human Kinetics 1990:315–323.

92. Boileau RA, Buskirk ER, Horstman DH, et al. Body composition changes in obese and lean men during physical conditioning. Med Sci Sports 1971;3:183–189.

93. Kohrt WM, Obert KA, Holloszy JO. Exercise training improves fat distribution patterns in 60- to 70-year-old men and women. J Gerontol Med Sci 1992;47:M99–M105.

94. Shah M, Jeffrey RW. Is obesity due to overeating and inactivity, or to a defective metabolic rate? a review. Ann Behav Med 1991;13:73–81.

95. Dreon DM, Frey-Hewitt B, Ellsworth N, et al. Dietary fat: carbohydrate ratio and obesity in middle-aged men. Am J Clin Nutr 1988;47:995–1000.

96. Miller WC, Lindeman AK, Wallace J, et al. Diet composition, energy intake, and exercise in relation to body fat in men and women. Am J Clin Nutr 1990;52:426–430.

Chapter 97

Health Benefits and Cardiovascular Adaptations to Physical Activity and Endurance Training

Mitchell H. Whaley
Leonard A. Kaminsky

Health benefits that have been associated with habitual physical activity include a lower incidence of all-cause and cause-specific mortality, lower morbidity from various chronic diseases, and maintenance or improvements in physical function across the life span. Many of the health benefits are related to chronic changes in the function of the cardiovascular system in response to regular endurance exercise training. This chapter focuses first on reductions in chronic disease risk associated with physical activity and then details various adaptations of the cardiovascular system that contribute to reductions in morbidity and mortality from selected chronic diseases.

CHRONIC DISEASE RISK

Reductions in risk for several chronic diseases have been associated with participation in a regular physical activity program. While evidence for such benefits has been accumulating for several decades, recent reports from prominent health organizations have brought much needed attention to the importance of a physically active lifestyle (10,34,40). The strength of the available evidence relates to a reduction in risk for all-cause and coronary heart disease mortality. However, reductions in risk for other chronic diseases, such as various site-specific cancers, non–insulin-dependent diabetes mellitus, stroke, and hypertension have also been shown in prospective studies.

Numerous observational studies have linked a sedentary lifestyle or low cardiorespiratory fitness (CRF) to greater risk for cardiovascular disease (CVD), or more specifically, coronary heart disease (CHD) morbidity and mortality. Reviews of

early research (5,36) concluded that the CHD risk for sedentary individuals is double that of more active individuals, and studies using better epidemiologic methods reported stronger inverse associations between physical activity or CRF and CHD. Although a consensus exists regarding the association between CVD and CHD risk and physical inactivity, more information is needed regarding: 1) the dose-response relationship between physical activity or CRF and premature morbidity or mortality from CHD, and 2) whether adoption of a more active lifestyle or improvements in CRF would confer the protection from CHD inferred by earlier studies.

Leisure-Time Physical Activity and Coronary Heart Disease

Several recent studies compared CVD and CHD rates among multiple ordinal categories of leisure-time physical activity (LTPA) (20,22,25,30,42,43) and provided information about the dose-response relationship between physical activity and CVD. Three of the reports (25,42,43) suggested that moderate amounts and intensities of physical activity are adequate for protection from CHD, while others reported more vigorous physical activity—designed to increase CRF—was necessary to reduce risk for CHD (20,30) or death due to any cause (22). Although the results of these studies appear to be sending a mixed signal regarding the appropriate dose of activity, the differences may not be as large as they first appear. Leon et al (26) reported that less than 5% of the men in the Multiple Risk Factor Intervention Trial (MRFIT) cohort participated in 1 hour or more of "vigorous" exercise per week. These authors concluded that their study lacked sufficient statistical power to assess whether more vigorous exercise would have further lowered the risk of mortality from CVD. In addition, when combined fatal and nonfatal myocardial infarction (MI) was used as the end point in the above analyses, three of the four studies reported a lower risk for only the most active men (20,26,30).

With these points in mind, the results from the available studies indicate that high-risk men who engage in mostly light- to moderate-intensity physical activities and accumulate an average of 1500 kcal per week of total energy expenditure in physical activity are likely to experience a 25% to 50% lower risk of CHD (25,26,33,42). However, those who engage in more intense activities, e.g., more than 6 metabolic equivalents (METs), on a regular basis may experience a 60% to 70% lower CHD risk (20,30) and greater longevity (22). Collectively, these studies support the notion of an inverse dose-response relationship between LTPA and the incidence of CHD, and recommendations for regular exercise training should reflect this relationship.

Cardiorespiratory Fitness and Coronary Heart Disease

Recently, various studies have assessed the association between CRF and CHD. These studies include a more objective measure of cardiovascular function as the exposure variable with the analyses. Each of the studies used a maximal exercise test to quantify CRF and reported an independent, inverse relationship between CRF and CHD/CVD (7,20,39). Using maximal test time during a treadmill test to quantify CRF, Blair et al (7) reported a seven- to ninefold greater risk for CVD mortality for the least compared to the most fit men or women in the Aerobics Center Longitudinal Study (ACLS) cohort. The other two studies were based on maximal exercise tests on a leg cycle ergometer. Sandvik et al (39) reported a 2.4-fold greater risk for CVD mortality when comparing the least to the most fit men, and Lakka et al (20) reported a 2.9-fold greater risk for combined fatal and nonfatal MI when comparing the least to the most fit men. These results, derived from studies that included strong, objective measures of CRF, strengthen the findings from earlier studies of CRF in men and extend the findings to women (7).

Both Blair et al (7) and Lakka et al (20) used measures of CRF that allowed identification of quantitative fitness thresholds within their data. Based on the treadmill time cutoff points for the low and high fitness categories from Blair et al, age-specific minimal and optimal levels of CRF for men and women are presented in Table 97-1. In addition, Lakka et al divided their cohort of men into tertiles (thirds), with the thresholds for maximal oxygen uptake for the middle and high tertiles at 28 mL/kg/min and 33.6 mL/kg/min, respectively. When adjusting for the 10% to 15% lower Vo_2max measured during maximal leg cycling compared with treadmill exercise, the CRF thresholds for the middle (9 METs) and upper (11 METs) tertiles from Lakka et al are consistent with those reported for similarly aged men by Blair et al (7).

Based on the available studies of CRF and CHD/CVD, it appears as though a fitness level below 8 to 9 METs represents a threshold for middle-aged men that is associated with significantly greater risk. Because Blair et al (7)

represents the only study where fitness data are available for women, the thresholds presented in Table 97-1 are reasonable until more data on women become available.

Changes in Leisure-Time Physical Activity and Coronary Heart Disease

As previously stated, most of the observational studies that assess the relationship between physical activity or fitness and CHD risk have been based on a single measure of either variable at study baseline. A stronger test of the association between either variable and CHD would come from a research design that assessed changes in LTPA or CRF using two or more measures across time. Several reports of this nature (6,32,33) strongly support the notion that maintaining or adopting a more physically active lifestyle—or increasing one's CRF level—leads to a significant reduction in CHD risk. Paffenbarger et al (32) reported that alumni who took up moderately vigorous physical activity (≥4.5 METs) during the follow-up period had a 41% lower risk of CHD mortality compared with those who never engaged in such activity. In a similar study design, Blair et al (6) assessed change in CRF in male members of the ACLS, and those considered to be fit at both exams had 67% and 78% lower risk of all-cause and CVD mortality, respectively, compared to those who were unfit at both exams. In addition, all-cause and CVD mortality risks for those who changed their level of fitness between exams (increase or decrease) were approximately 50% less than those who were unfit at both exams.

LEISURE-TIME PHYSICAL ACTIVITY, CARDIORESPIRATORY FITNESS, AND CANCER

Cancer is the second leading cause of death for adult men and women in the United States, trailing only heart disease. Some recent papers reviewing the available epidemiologic studies related to physical activity or fitness and risk of cancer (18,21,44) concluded that there was significant evidence to support an inverse association between physical activity and colon cancer, but studies had not shown consistent relation-

Table 97-1 Values (MET) for Low and High Cardiorespiratory Fitness in Adult Men and Women

Age Category (yr)	Men		Women	
	Low	High	Low	High
20–39	10.1	13.4	7.1	11.1
40–49	9.1	12.5	6.6	9.7
50–59	8.4	11.7	6.0	8.9
60+	7.0	10.5	5.4	8.0

NOTE: MET values based on fitness categories as described by Blair et al (7).
Reprinted with permission from Whaley MH Blair SN. Epidemiology of physical activity, physical fitness, and coronary heart disease. J Cardiovasc Risk 1995;2:289–295.

ships between physical activity and cancers of the rectum, lung, breast, pancreas, or other sites.

Results from four of five recent studies (4,12,23,41) support an inverse association between leisure-time physical activity and colon cancer risk, which confirms the findings from earlier reports reviewed elsewhere (18,21,44). Despite the dissimilar physical activity assessment instruments among these recent studies, the average relative risk for colon cancer among the most sedentary men was approximately double that of the most active men. However, based on the results from two of the studies (3,4), the association between physical activity and colon cancer is less clear in women.

Several recent prospective investigations have assessed the association between leisure time physical activity (LTPA) or fitness and risk of prostatic cancer in men (3,24,31,41). Three of the four studies reported an inverse association (3,24,31), while the other reported null results (41). Albanes et al reported a twofold greater risk for the least recreationally active men compared with the most active. Lee et al observed an 82% lower risk for men who reportedly expended more than 4000 kcal/wk during leisure time at both assessments (1962 to 66 and 1977). Lee et al also reported that older men (age 70 and older) who reportedly expended more than 4000 kcal/wk in leisure pursuits at either assessment had a 50% lower risk. The above two studies were consistent in finding that only the most active men within their cohorts had a reduced risk for prostatic cancer during the follow-up period, and thus, both appear to suggest a protective threshold at the upper end of the physical activity spectrum. In a subsequent report from the ACLS cohort, Oliveria et al (31) assessed the association between prostatic cancer and CRF. They reported a significant inverse trend ($p = 0.004$) for incidence of prostatic cancer across CRF categories with the least fit quartile having a fourfold risk compared with the most fit quartile.

The results from prospective studies assessing the association between other site-specific cancers and LTPA or fitness have been mixed. There appears to be little or no association between LTPA and cancers of the rectum (3,23,41), breast (3,9), lung (3,41), cervix, stomach, or urinary bladder (3,41).

In conclusion, the results from the recent studies of LTPA/CRF and cancer provide support for an inverse association for risk of cancers of the colon (in men, not women) and prostate. When combined with results from studies reviewed previously (21), more recent evidence would confirm no association between LTPA and rectal cancer. The associations between LTPA/CRF and other site-specific cancers remain unclear and should continue to be a focus of future prospective studies, particularly of women.

LEISURE-TIME PHYSICAL ACTIVITY, CARDIORESPIRATORY FITNESS, AND STROKE

Stroke is the third leading cause of death in the United States, trailing CHD and cancer. In a recent review of physical activity and stroke, Kohl and McKenzie (19) concluded that the available data were "equivocal concerning the role that physical activity and physical fitness may play in the risk of stroke." Five prospective epidemiologic studies have assessed the association between LTPA and incidence of stroke (1,14,17,27,45). Each of these studies included results from

multivariate analyses where other variables that might confound the relationship between physical activity and stroke, e.g., body mass index (BMI), traditional CHD risk factors, and alcohol use, were controlled. All of the studies included men (1,14,17,27,45); only one included women (17).

In a report on incident cases of stroke from a large cohort of Swedish men, Harmsen et al (14) found no association between their measure of physical activity and stroke. The investigators used a four-point scale to quantify LTPA habits within the study but chose to compare only the lowest physically active group to the upper three groups combined. The null findings may have resulted from the crude measure of physical activity used within the study. In a study from the Seventh Day Adventist cohort, Linsted et al (27) reported a 22% lower risk for men who reported being moderately active. Those who reported being more highly active did not appear to acquire this protection from fatal stroke during the follow-up period. In another report, based on data from the British Regional Heart Study, Wannamethee and Shaper (45) reported that moderate and moderately vigorous levels of activity were associated with a 50% lower risk of stroke, and the benefit from vigorous activity was even greater (about 80% lower risk). In a recent analysis from the Honolulu Heart Program, Abbott et al (1) reported a three- to fourfold greater risk of hemorrhagic stroke for the least active compared to most active men. However, this protective effect of physical activity was observed only for older men (age 55 to 68 years at baseline). The authors also reported a two- to threefold greater risk for thromboembolic stroke for less active, older men. However, the protective effect of physical activity was observed only in those men who were nonsmokers. For men who smoked, there was no protective effect associated with increased physical activity. Similar to the findings from Wannamethee et al, the benefit was greater for the most active group of men. Finally, in an analysis from the Framingham Heart Study, Kiely et al (17) reported lower risk for both the middle and most active tertiles of men compared to the least active tertile. However, similar to an earlier report (38), they did not observe any protective effect for LTPA for women after adjusting for other risk factors in multivariate analyses.

In summary, most of the available studies (17,45) reported a graded relationship with significantly lower stroke rates for the most active men, but the existing data are not conclusive regarding a relationship between physical activity and stroke in men or women. However, since hypertension is a major risk factor for stroke, exercise prescriptions designed to lower blood pressure should be emphasized for those with mild to moderate hypertension. Future studies should continue to assess the relationship between physical activity and stroke risk, as well as further defining the relationship within subtypes of stroke (e.g., hemorrhagic versus thromboembolic).

LEISURE-TIME PHYSICAL ACTIVITY, CARDIORESPIRATORY FITNESS, AND NON–INSULIN-DEPENDENT DIABETES MELLITUS

Non–insulin-dependent diabetes mellitus (NIDDM) affects some 12 million people in the United States and is a major risk factor for cardiovascular disease morbidity and mortality. Several prospective epidemiologic studies have assessed the relationship between LTPA or CRF and the risk of developing NIDDM (8,15,16,28,29). Four studies have provided results from multivariate analyses where other variables that might confound the relationship between activity or fitness and NIDDM (e.g., BMI, traditional CHD risk factors) were taken into consideration. Of these, all of the studies included men (8,15,16,28), and two included women (16,29). In addition, four studies used self-report of physical activity habits as the exposure variable (8,15,28,29), while one assessed the risk of NIDDM as a function of CRF (16).

In a study from the University of Pennsylvania alumni, Helmrich et al (15) focused on the amount of energy expended per week during leisure time and risk for NIDDM. They reported an inverse gradient across LTPA deciles with a 6% lower risk for every 500 kcal/wk increase in total energy expenditure and a 50% lower risk when comparing the least active group (<500 kcal/wk) to the most active group of men (>500 kcal/wk). Two other reports focused more on the quality of LTPA (e.g., intensity) and risk of NIDDM. In both the Nurses Health Study (29) and the Physicians Health Study (28), Manson et al reported that men or women who participated in vigorous exercise at least once per week were significantly less likely to develop NIDDM compared to those who reported no vigorous exercise. In this study, vigorous exercise was defined as activity such as brisk walking, jogging, or bicycling, performed long enough to work up a sweat. In a recent analysis from the Honolulu Heart Program cohort, Burchfiel et al (8) quantified physical activity by combining both the amount and intensity of physical activity. They reported an inverse gradient across five physical activity categories, with a 50% lower risk for the most active compared to the least active men. Finally, Jackson et al (16) assessed the relationship between physical fitness (as defined by maximal treadmill test time) and risk for NIDDM among men and women from the ACLS. The least fit men (lowest 20% of the ACLS fitness distribution for age) were 4 times as likely to develop NIDDM compared with the most fit men (highest 40%). Although a significant relationship was not observed for women within the ACLS, the number of incident cases of NIDDM was rather low (n = 22) during the follow-up period. Thus, the results may be inconclusive.

Although the available studies differed significantly in the way they quantified LTPA or physical fitness, collectively they support the finding of an inverse relationship between LTPA and risk for development of NIDDM for both men and women. The studies that included more elaborate measures of LTPA (8,15) or a measure of CRF (16) also reported stronger associations between inactivity or low fitness level and the risk for NIDDM. Because obesity is a major risk factor for NIDDM, exercise prescriptions designed to promote loss of excess body fat should be emphasized for individuals at risk for the development of NIDDM. Future studies should focus on further defining the relationship between the quantity and quality of physical activity and risk of NIDDM.

CARDIOVASCULAR ADAPTATIONS TO ENDURANCE TRAINING

In addition to the many health benefits associated with a physically active lifestyle, numerous adaptations in the cardio-vascular system occur after participation (e.g., 3 to 6 months) in regular endurance training (2,11,37,46). These cardiovascular adaptations contribute to many of the long-term health benefits associated with an active lifestyle. Cardiovascular adaptations to chronic endurance training generally follow a dose-response pattern: greater training intensity, frequency, and duration produce larger adaptations. The components of a cardiovascular endurance training program that result in clinically relevant cardiovascular adaptations are summarized in Table 97-2. Individuals who participate in light to moderate physical activity that does not reach the quality and quantity described in Table 97-2 may attain many of the health benefits described earlier in the chapter but will probably not accrue the cardiovascular adaptations described here. The exercise prescription information in Table 97-2 applies mainly to sedentary, apparently healthy adults. Specifics about exercise programs for those with various chronic diseases are covered elsewhere.

Following an endurance training program, cardio-respiratory fitness—defined as the maximal amount of oxygen (Vo_2max) one can utilize during exhaustive exercise (35)—typically increases between 10% and 30% in previously untrained adults (2). The improvement in Vo_2max after the training program is inversely related to the initial or baseline value; this means that after adjusting for other variables known to influence the training response (e.g., training intensity, duration), the less fit an individual is before the training program, the larger the improvement in fitness. Although older individuals have the ability to improve their Vo_2max to a similar relative degree as younger individuals, the rate of change in Vo_2max is slower, and so a longer training duration (months) would be necessary in older individuals.

Several key physiologic adaptations that contribute to the increase in Vo_2max are summarized in Table 97-3. Maximal oxygen uptake is the product of cardiac output (heart rate times stroke volume) and the amount of oxygen

Table 97-2 Components of an Exercise Training Program for Apparently Healthy adults

VARIABLE	RECOMMENDATIONS
Intensity*	55/65%–90% of HRmax or 40/50%–85% of Vo_2max or maximal HRR
Frequency	3–5 days/week
Duration	20–60 min of continuous activity
Mode	Aerobic activities

* the lower intensity ranges (55–64% of HRmax or 40–49% of Vo_2max or maximal HRR should be used initially for those who are quite unfit.
HRmax = maximal exercise heart rate; Vo_2max = measured maximal oxygen consumption; HRR = measured heart rate reserve (HRmax − HR rest).
SOURCE: American College of Sports Medicine. The recommended quantity and quality of exercise for developing and maintaining cardiorespiratory and muscular fitness, and flexibility in healthy adults. Med Sci Sports Exerc 1998;30: 975–991.

Table 97-3 Expected Physiologic Adaptations to Endurance Training in Previously Untrained Individuals

VARIABLE	UNIT OF MEASURE	TRAINING CHANGE	RANGE OF CHANGE
Maximal Exercise			
VO_2max	mL/kg/min	↑	≈10–30%
Cardiac Output	L/min	↑	≈10–20%
HRmax	beats/min	↔ or ↓	Very little change, if any
Stroke Volume	mL/beat	↑	Varies
$a–\bar{v}O_2$	mL O_2/100 mL blood	↑	Varies
Submaximal Exercise			
Heart Rate	beats/min	↓	20–40 beats/min
Stroke Volume	mL/beat	↑	Varies
Cardiac Output	L/min	↔ or ↓	Minimal
Systolic/Diastolic BP	mm Hg	↔ or ↓	Varies
Rate Pressure Product	HR·SBP	↓	Varies
$a–\bar{v}O_2$	mL O_2/100 mL blood	↑	8–10%
Resting			
Heart Rate	beats/min	↓	Varies (≈10 beats/min)
Stroke Volume	mL/beat	↑	Varies
Systolic/Diastolic BP	mm Hg	↔ or ↓	≈10 mm Hg
Cardiac Output	L/min	↔	

VO_2max, maximum oxygen consumption; ↑, increase; HR, heart rate; ↓, decrease; ↔, little if any change; $a–\bar{v}O_2$ = arteriovenous oxygen difference; BP, blood pressure; SBP, systolic blood pressure.

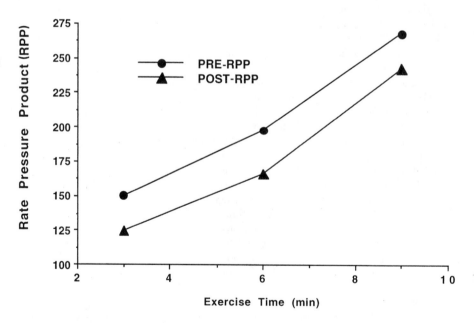

Figure 97-1 Changes in rate pressure product during the BSU/Bruce ramp treadmill protocol for 38-year-old male following 6 months of endurance exercise training. The plotted exercise intensities span 5 to 10 METs, which represents the submaximal training intensity range for this individual.

extracted from the circulation at peak exercise. Oxygen extraction is referred to as the arteriovenous oxygen difference $(a – \bar{v}O_2)$. Increases in both of these variables contribute to the overall improvement in VO_2max after a training program; however, they may not contribute equally in all cases or at the same rate. Physiologic changes that contribute to an increase in oxygen extraction by skeletal muscle (increase in $a – \bar{v}O_2$) may occur sooner during the training program than the adaptations that contribute to an increase in blood flow (not equal to cardiac output) (37). The increase in cardiac output is brought about primarily by an increase in stroke volume, which is the result of several factors (e.g., an increase in plasma volume and preload, a decrease in peripheral vascular resistance) (37). Maximal $a – \bar{v}O_2$ is brought about primarily by an increase in oxidative capacity and capillary density within the recruited skeletal muscle mass (37). Maximal heart rate does not appear to change much with chronic training, but some people might encounter a slight decline (3 to 4 beats/min).

Numerous adaptations contribute to a more efficient

cardiovascular response to submaximal exercise loads. These changes are usually compared as values at a given submaximal workload or oxygen consumption. These changes are summarized in Table 97-3. At a given or fixed oxygen consumption, both heart rate and systolic blood pressure are generally reduced following a training regimen. Therefore, the product of these variables—known as the rate pressure product (RPP) or double product—is also lower. This adaptation has clinical implications because RPP correlates well with the myocardial oxygen demand. Reductions in RPP indicate a reduction in myocardial stress during submaximal exercise after completing an endurance training program. Figure 97-1 illustrates the reduction in RPP at several submaximal intensities during an incremental exercise test for a 38-year-old man following 6 months of endurance exercise training. Left ventricular stroke volume is generally increased at a given sub-

maximal workload resulting primarily from the combination of an expanded plasma volume and reduced heart rate response (greater ventricular filling time). The increase in oxidative capacity and capillary density within the recruited skeletal muscle mass leads to an increase in the $a - \bar{v}O_2$ at a given submaximal workload, which can lead to a slight reduction in the cardiac output necessary to provide the oxygen requirements of the muscle.

After chronic endurance training, one can expect a reduction in resting heart rate coupled with an increase in left ventricular stroke volume. These changes result in a fairly stable resting cardiac output. Adaptations in resting blood pressure depend on the baseline or pre-training value with little or no change for normotensives, but clinically significant reductions in both systolic and diastolic pressure for those with mild to moderate hypertension (13).

REFERENCES

1. Abbott RD, Rodriquez BL, Burchfiel CM, Curb JD. Physical activity in older middle-aged men and reduced risk of stroke: the Honolulu Heart Program. Am J Epidemiol 1994;139:881–893.

2. American College of Sports Medicine. The recommended quantity and quality of exercise for developing and maintaining cardiorespiratory and muscular fitness, and flexibility in healthy adults. Med Sci Sports Exerc 1998;30:975–991.

3. Albanes D, Blair A, Taylor PR. Physical activity and risk of cancer in the NHANES I population. Am J Public Health 1989;79:744–750.

4. Ballard-Barbash B, Schatzkin A, Albanes D, et al. Physical activity and risk of large bowel cancer in the Framingham Study. Cancer Res 1990;50:3610–3613.

5. Berlin JA, Colditz A. A meta-analysis of physical activity in the prevention of coronary heart disease. Am J Epidemiol 1990; 132:612–627.

6. Blair SN, Kohl HW, Barlow CE, et al. Changes in physical fitness and all-cause mortality: a prospective study of healthy and unhealthy men. JAMA 1995;273:1093–1098.

7. Blair SN, Kohl HW, Paffenbarger RS, et al. Physical fitness and all-cause mortality: a prospective study of healthy men and women. JAMA 1989;262:2395–2401.

8. Burchfiel CM, Sharp DS, Curb JD, et al. Physical activity and incidence of diabetes: the Honolulu Heart Program. Am J Epidemiol 1995;141:360–368.

9. Dorgan JF, Brown C, Barrett M, et al. Physical activity and risk of breast cancer in the Framingham Heart Study. Am J Epidemiol 1994;139:662–669.

10. Fletcher GF, Balady G, Blair SN, et al. Statement on exercise: benefits and recommendations for physical activity programs for all Americans. Circulation 1996;94:857–862.

11. Franklin BA, Roitman JL. Cardiorespiratory adaptations to exercise. In: Roitman JL, ed. ACSM's resource manual for guidelines for exercise testing and prescription. Baltimore: Williams & Wilkins, 1998:156–163.

12. Giovannucci E, Ascherio A, Rimm EB, et al. Physical activity, obesity, and risk for colon cancer and adenoma in men. Ann Intern Med 1995;122:327–334.

13. Gordon NF. Hypertension. In: Durstine JL, ed. ACSM's exercise management for persons with chronic diseases. Champaign, IL: Human Kinetics, 1997:269.

14. Harmsen P, Rosengren A, Tsipogianni A, et al. Risk factors and stroke in middle-aged men in Göteborg, Sweden. Stroke 1990; 21:223–229.

15. Helmrich SP, Ragland DR, Leung RW. Physical activity and reduced occurrence of non–insulin-dependent diabetes mellitus. N Engl J Med 1991;325:147–152.

16. Jackson S, Barlow C, Brill P, Blair SN. The association between physical fitness and non–insulin-dependent diabetes in men and women. Med Sci Sports Exerc 1992;24(suppl):S61.

17. Kiely DK, Wolf PA, Cupples LA, et al. Physical activity and stroke risk: the Framingham Study. Am J Epidemiol 1994;140:608–620.

18. Kohl HW, LaPorte RE, Blair SN. Physical activity and cancer: an epidemiological perspective. Sports Med 1988;6:222–237.

19. Kohl HW, McKenzie JD. Physical activity, fitness and stroke. In: Bouchard C, Shephard RJ, Stephens T, eds. Physical activity, fitness, and health. Champaign, IL: Human Kinetics, 1994:609–621.

20. Lakka TA, Venalainen JM, Rauramaa R, et al. Relation of leisure-time physical activity and cardiorespiratory fitness to the risk of acute myocardial infarction. N Engl J Med 1994;330:1549–1554.

21. Lee I-M, Physical activity, fitness and cancer. In: Bouchard C, Shephard RJ, Stephens T, eds. Physical activity, fitness, and health. Champaign IL: Human Kinetics, 1994:814–831.

22. Lee I-M, Hsieh CC, Paffenbarger RS. Exercise intensity and longevity in men: the Harvard Alumni Health Study. JAMA 1995;273:1179–1184.

23. Lee I-M, Paffenbarger RS, Hsieh CC. Physical activity and risk of developing colorectal cancer among college alumni. J Natl Cancer Inst 1991;83:1324–1329.

24. Lee I-M, Paffenbarger RS, Hsieh CC. Physical activity and risk of prostatic cancer among college alumni. Am J Epidemiol 1992; 135:169–179.

25. Leon AS, Connett J. Physical activity and 10.5 year mortality in the Multiple Risk Factor Intervention Trial (MRFIT). Int J Epidemiol 1991;20:690–697.

26. Leon AS, Connett J, Jacobs DR, Rauramaa R. Leisure-time physical activity levels and risk of coronary heart disease and death: the Multiple Risk Factor Intervention Trial. JAMA 1987;258:2388–2395.

27. Lindsted KD, Tonstad S, Kuzma JW. Self-report of physical activity and patterns of mortality in Seventh-Day Adventist men. J Clin Epidemiol 1991;44:355–364.

28. Manson JE, Nathan DM, et al. A prospective study of exercise and incidence of diabetes among US male physicians. JAMA 1992;268: 63–67.

29. Manson JE, Rimm EB, et al. Physical activity and incidence of non–insulin-dependent diabetes mellitus in women. Lancet 1991;338: 774–778.

30. Morris JN, Clayton DG, et al. Exercise in leisure time: coronary attack and death rates. Br Heart J 1990;63:325–334.

31. Oliveria SA, Kohl HW. The association between cardiorespiratory fitness and prostate cancer. Med Sci Sports Exerc 1996;28:97–104.

32. Paffenbarger RS, Hyde RT, et al. The association of changes in physical-activity level and other lifestyle characteristics with mortality among men. N Engl J Med 1993;328:538–545.

33. Paffenbarger RS, Kampert JB, et al. Changes in physical activity and other lifeway patterns influencing longevity. Med Sci Sports Exerc 1994;26:857–865.

34. Pate RR, Pratt M, et al. Physical activity and public health: a recommendation from the Centers for Disease Control and Prevention and the American College of Sports Medicine. JAMA 1995; 273:402–407.

35. Pollock ML, Wilmore JH. Exercise in health and disease: evaluation and prescription for prevention and rehabilitation. 2nd ed. Philadelphia: W.B. Saunders, 1990:93.

36. Powell KE, Thompson PD, Caspersen CJ, Kendrick JS. Physical activity and the incidence of coronary heart disease. Ann Rev Public Health 1987;8:253–287.

37. Rowell LB. Human circulation regulation during physical stress. New York: Oxford University, 1986:416.

38. Salonen JT, Puska P, Tuomilehto J. Physical activity and risk of myocardial infarction, cerebral stroke, and death: a longitudinal study in Eastern Finland. Am J Epidemiol 1982;115:526–537.

39. Sandvik L, Erikssen J, et al. Physical fitness as a predictor of mortality among healthy, middle-aged Norwegian men. N Engl J Med 1993;328:533–537.

40. U.S. Department of Health and Human Services. Physical activity and health: a report of the Surgeon General. Atlanta: U.S. Department of Health and Human Services, Centers for Disease Control and Prevention, National Center for Chronic Disease Prevention and Health Promotion, 1996.

41. Severson RK, Nomura AMY, et al. A prospective analysis of physical activity and cancer. Am J Epidemiol 1989;130:522–529.

42. Shaper AG, Wannamethee G. Physical activity and ischaemic heart disease in middle-aged British men. Br Heart J 1991;66:384–394.

43. Shaper AG, Wannamethee G, Walker M. Physical activity, hypertension, and risk of heart attack in men without evidence of ischaemic heart disease. J Hum Hypertens 1994;8:3–10.

44. Shephard RJ, Exercise in the prevention and treatment of cancer: an update. Sports Med 1993;15: 258–280.

45. Wannamethee G, Shaper AG. Physical activity and stroke in British middle-aged men. Br Med J 1992; 304:597–601.

46. Wilmore JH, Costill DL. Physiology of sport and exercise. Champaign, IL: Human Kinetics, 1994:549.

Chapter 98

Exercise Prescription for Apparently Healthy Individuals and for Special Populations

James S. Skinner

According to the American College of Sports Medicine, "Exercise prescription is the process whereby a person's recommended regimen of physical activity is designed in a systematic and individualized manner" (1). This chapter discusses some of the information that should be obtained to prescribe exercise, the principles of training, and the components of a good training program. The reader is then shown how this can be applied to those who 1) exercise for their general health, 2) train for improved fitness or performance, or 3) have special problems or health states that need more guidance. This chapter gives only an overview and cannot go into detailed discussions of each topic. Many books and articles have been written about all of these topics and they should be consulted for more information (1–6).

Whether persons need an individualized exercise prescription depends on their present level of fitness, their health status, how much of a change in activity they are contemplating, and their ultimate goal. For example, a young healthy person who wishes to begin hiking probably does not need a medical examination or an exercise prescription. On the other hand, an older person who either has heart disease or has risk factors associated with the development of heart disease or an older person who wishes to train to run a marathon will need more testing and an individualized prescription.

There is a general public health and scientific consensus that regular physical activity makes positive contributions to health and well-being (7). The general recommendation for health is to obtain 30 minutes of moderate-intensity physical activity, such as brisk walking, on most days of the week. It is obvious that most people can do this without an exercise prescription.

Only two types of people need careful and precise prescriptions. Athletes are interested in increasing their fitness and their performance and, because of the principle of training specificity, require precise exercise prescriptions. Similarly, persons who have a disease that negatively affects their ability to exercise or for whom exercise may cause an increased health risk also need a more precise exercise prescription.

The same principles of training apply to everyone. Any modifications that are made are usually associated with 1) the presence or absence of medical restrictions, limitations, or contraindications; 2) types of activities to emphasize or to avoid; 3) initial fitness level; 4) desired fitness level; and 5) intensity of participation. The longer people have been sedentary and the more restrictions and limitations they have, the more modifications will be required in their exercise prescription.

To prescribe exercise correctly, one needs to consider age, health (any special problems), fitness level, and individual needs, goals, and interests. Because those who need exercise most are often the ones who do less, are less motivated to exercise, have more problems and limitations when they do exercise, need more guidance, and have been studied less, it is obvious that some information is required to prescribe safe, effective, and enjoyable exercise programs.

Is exercise testing needed? Again, if the exercise program is to be undertaken by young healthy individuals or by those who plan only minor increases in physical activity, exercise testing is useful but not required. As with exercise prescription, however, the older people are, the longer they have been sedentary, and the more risk factors they have, the greater the need for exercise testing.

Exercise tests should be standardized, reproducible tests with known quantities of work and with many submaximal stages so that more information can be gained. While the Bruce test is a good test for diagnosis of coronary heart disease, it is not a good test for exercise prescription in people who are older and are more likely to have limitations in their health and work capacity. For example, many patients may not be able to complete or go beyond the third stage; this gives an insufficient amount of information on only three different levels of work. On the other hand, a modified Balke test begins at 3 mph and 0% grade for 3 minutes, followed by increases of 2.5% grade every 2 to 3 minutes. This test, with its smaller increments in power output, allows persons being tested to complete many more stages before they reach the same power output at which they had to stop on the Bruce test. These extra stages allow the physician to have a better idea of the relationship between heart rate and power output, which will be used to prescribe exercise. In addition, with the smaller exercise increments, the physician or allied health professional has a better idea of when and under what conditions any medical problems or symptoms occur. All of these factors are useful in prescribing exercise.

To have standardized, reproducible treadmill tests, patients should not hold on to the rails. Many clinicians allow patients to hold the rails for balance and feelings of security. While this is appropriate for a test whose main purpose is to diagnose disease, it is not appropriate for a test designed to prescribe exercise, because the patient may hold more or less firmly onto the rail. As a result, it is not known exactly how much work they are doing. Because the work done may vary from one test to another, it is also less useful to evaluate any changes that might occur after training or if there is further progression of the disease being diagnosed or evaluated. The reader is referred to Chapter 95 and other references (1,3–5) for more information.

EXERCISE PRESCRIPTION FOR HEALTH

There are well-done epidemiologic and experimental research findings to suggest that regular aerobic physical activity is associated with lower morbidity and mortality rates from cardiovascular disease (i.e., coronary artery disease, stroke, hypertension), some forms of cancer, and overall death rates from all causes (7). The greatest health benefits appear to be associated with moving from a low to a moderate amount and intensity of activity or from a low to a moderate level of fitness, in comparison to going from moderate levels of activity or fitness to high levels. For people who are young, healthy, and moderately active, any gradual increase in physical activity to moderate levels generally does not require an exercise prescription.

There is no one program that is best for all persons. The best program is one that is safe and that people enjoy so that they continue to do it on a regular basis. It is this regularity of physical activity that seems to be the most protective in terms of health.

EXERCISE PRESCRIPTION FOR FITNESS AND PERFORMANCE

Exercise is a form of acute stress on the various body systems. The degree to which these body systems are taxed depends on the intensity, duration, and type of exercise. Training is the adaptation by the different body systems to the repeated stimulus of exercise. The body attempts to adapt to the habitual demands placed on it. If the body has no problem adjusting to these demands, then the adaptation is complete and there are no problems. On the other hand, if the demands placed on the body require more adaptation than is possible because these demands are applied at an intensity, frequency, or duration that is too great, then adaptation is incomplete, with the usual result of fatigue, soreness, pain, or injury.

There are four principles of training that are particularly applicable to training to improve fitness or performance. A more detailed discussion of these principles may be found in my book (4).

Theory of Overload

For adaptation to occur, the body and its various parts and systems must be stimulated to levels greater than those they habitually encounter. An adequate and effective program of training is one that progressively overloads the body and its various parts and that permits adequate amounts of time to adapt to each new level.

Theory of Specificity

The effects of training are specific to those parts and systems of the body that have been overloaded. For example, lifting weights produces muscular hypertrophy and strength, while long-distance running develops cardiorespiratory endurance but not muscle hypertrophy. Adaptation is also specific to the muscle groups, parts of the body, or systems of energy production that have been stimulated. This theory of specificity is probably most important for people who have very specific objectives (for example, to compete in a particular sport), but it is less important for those who are exercising for health or just to develop their general physical condition.

Theory of Reversibility

Because the body adapts to its habitual level of stimulation, it can adapt to training and to inactivity. A good example of this would be the muscle hypertrophy that comes with weight lifting and the muscle atrophy that results when the muscle is put in a cast.

Theory of Maintenance

It takes less time and effort to maintain a high level of physical fitness than it does to obtain it. If the body is not overloaded, then it does not require additional adaptation. Thus, when persons become satisfied with their current level of fitness or physical activity, they should be able to maintain it by doing the same amount of exercise each week or even with a slight reduction in exercise for brief periods. The higher the level of fitness, the more that needs to be done to maintain it.

BASIC COMPONENTS OF AN EXERCISE PROGRAM

The five basic components of an exercise program are frequency, duration, intensity, type of exercise, and progression. A more detailed discussion of these components is available (4).

Training is the product of frequency, duration, and intensity of exercise, i.e., the total quantity of stimulation or overload. The type of exercise is associated with the principle of specificity as well as with its duration and intensity: high-intensity exercise tends to be brief and anaerobic; low-intensity exercise tends to be prolonged and aerobic.

With all of the possible combinations of these first four components, it is obvious that training can be very general or very specific. The main point to remember about a good exercise program to improve fitness or performance is that people should select activities that they enjoy and will do with sufficient frequency, duration, and intensity to produce a training effect.

Frequency

The general recommendation in terms of exercising for health is that one should do some exercise most or preferably all days of the week. If one is trying to improve fitness or performance, then the exercise should be done at least 3 to 5 times per week. How long it takes people to get to this frequency depends on their health status, their fitness level, and their usual level of activity, as well as the intensity and duration of the exercise being done. To maintain a desired level of fitness or performance, one should continue to exercise at least 3 times per week. It is possible to maintain a good level of fitness by exercising twice a week for a while, but after 2 to 4 weeks the fitness level may drop. The higher the level of fitness or performance, the greater the frequency of exercise must be to maintain it. As an example, it is highly unlikely that an elite athlete can maintain a high level of performance by training only 3 to 4 times per week.

Duration

As mentioned previously, the duration of an activity is closely associated with its intensity: prolonged exercise tends to be of low intensity, while high-intensity exercise tends to be brief. If the goal of the exercise program is to improve cardiorespiratory fitness, then the exercise should be of long duration. On the other hand, if the desire is to improve strength and speed, then the exercise should be done in a more intermittent fashion with short periods of high-intensity activity. For cardiorespiratory fitness, exercise sessions should be 20 to 30 minutes at the beginning, gradually increasing to 40 to 60 minutes. The minimal duration for overloading the endurance system and for losing weight should be 20 minutes.

An optimal program has three phases: 1) warm-up (5 to 10 minutes), 2) overload (15 to 40 minutes), and 3) cool-down (5 to 10 minutes), for a total of 25 to 60 minutes. The warm-up phase includes walking, slow jogging, stretching, and moderate exercises for strength and endurance. The older and less fit the individual, the more important this phase is and the longer it should be. The cool-down phase involves slow movements similar to those done during the warm-up phase. Less fit and older persons require more time to recover from exercise. As well, more time will be required if the intensity of exercise was too high, was done for a very long time, or was done in a warm environment.

Intensity

While duration (minutes per session) and frequency (sessions per week) are absolute terms and can be the same for persons who differ greatly in fitness, intensity is a relative term. The intensity of an exercise is defined as the energy required to do that exercise relative to the maximal quantity of energy that can be delivered aerobically; this quantity of energy is expressed as a percentage of the person's maximal aerobic power ($\dot{V}o_2$max). Exercise intensity is the most difficult to adjust because a precise prescription assumes that the person's $\dot{V}o_2$max has been either determined or estimated from the results of an exercise test. Even if test results are not available, however, it is possible to give some general guidelines.

As mentioned before, the higher the intensity, the shorter the duration and the more anaerobic the activity. To improve cardiorespiratory fitness, the intensity should be 30% to 50% of $\dot{V}o_2$max during the warm-up and cool-down phases and 60% to 85% during the exercise phase. Sedentary people who have low fitness levels should begin at 40% to 60% of $\dot{V}o_2$max and increase gradually to 60% to 70% and then to 70% to 85%.

Current American College of Sports Medicine recommendations to improve fitness and performance in aerobic activities (2) include the use of endurance-type exercise at a frequency of 3 to 5 times a week, a duration of 20 to 60 minutes per session, and an intensity of 40% to 85% of $\dot{V}o_2$max.

Total Amount of Exercise

Training is the product of frequency, duration, and intensity, or the total amount of exercise done. After reviewing evidence on the inverse relationship between physical activity and death rates, Blair (8) concluded that the total energy expended appeared to be the "single most important component of a physical activity regimen" to promote health. If this is true, then both health and fitness benefits can be obtained by various combinations of frequency, duration, and intensity. What is not known is the minimal amount of exercise needed to improve health. On the other hand, there is more information on the minimal frequency, duration, and intensity required to improve fitness and performance; these have been mentioned previously.

Once certain minimal levels of frequency, duration, and intensity are obtained and the total amount of exercise done per week is similar, the effects of aerobic training are also similar. In other words, similar results can be obtained by many different types of programs. Thus, one may, and probably should, vary the types of exercises done, depending on such factors as the season of the year, the facilities available, or the interests or needs of the person exercising. Varying the program should help increase or maintain the adherence to and the regularity of exercise without negatively affecting fitness.

Type of Exercise

Following the principle of specificity, the type of exercise influences the type of adaptation required. For example, overloading the aerobic system is best done by prolonged, continuous, and moderate-intensity exercise involving rhythmic contractions of large muscle groups (e.g., running, jogging, swimming, cycling). Strength and speed tend to be more anaerobic and are best developed by brief, intermittent, and high-intensity activities. There is also a specificity related to the muscle groups involved (i.e., upper or lower extremities) and whether the exercise is static or dynamic. For general health and fitness, many types of activities can and should be done. To improve specific performances, the exercises should also be specific.

Exercise Progression

The older participants are, the more limitations they have, and the longer they have been sedentary, the slower the rate of progression in the total amount of exercise done per week should be. Once participants have adjusted to a regular program of activity, a general rule is to increase the total amount of exercise done by no more than 10% per week. Young, healthy, moderately active or moderately fit persons may be able to increase the total amount of work done by more than 10%. In general, the person should exercise at the same level for several weeks to make certain that the adaptation has been complete. If there are no problems, such as fatigue or soreness, then the total amount of exercise can be increased.

EXERCISE PRESCRIPTIONS FOR SPECIAL POPULATIONS

The general principles of exercise prescription for special populations are not much different from those used with healthy people, except that the exercise prescription may have to be modified because of restrictions caused by aging, the disease or health state, and the goals or objectives of the program.

To understand what modifications in exercise prescriptions are needed, one should have knowledge of the particular health state, how it affects the ability to exercise, and how exercise may affect the health state. Understanding these factors should help the reader clarify why certain exercises are to be emphasized or avoided.

It is not possible in this chapter to discuss the details of each health state and what exercise programs should be prescribed. Instead, examples will be given of certain common health states and how exercise programs can be modified. The reader is referred to other references that go into much more detail about specific topics, including my book *Exercise Testing and Exercise Prescription for Special Cases*, which discusses each special population named in this chapter (3–5).

Exercise Prescription for the Elderly

With increasing age, there is a decrease in the size and/or number of functional units in almost every system of the body, as well as a loss in function of those units that remain. As a result, aging can be defined as the decreased ability to adapt to and recover from stimuli. The greater the intensity of the stimulus and the greater the number of physiologic mechanisms needed to adjust to the stimulus, the greater will be the loss in function with age. As an example, the rate of increase in heart rate and oxygen intake during exercise is slower in older persons, and it takes longer for the older person to recover after exercise. For this reason, the older person should have longer warm-up and cool-down periods and should not have major fluctuations in exercise intensity.

Because exercise is a stimulus requiring many forms of regulation and interaction among many systems in the body, it is logical that there is decreased performance with age. Because training is a form of adaptation and aging has been defined as a decreased ability to adapt, it is logical that older people do not adapt as well to training and that it takes them longer to adapt to the repeated stimulus of exercise. This does not mean that older persons cannot adapt, just that it may take them longer to do it.

The goals of exercise programs for the elderly are to improve functional ability, functional independence, and quality of life. The most important factors associated with functional independence are muscular strength, cardiovascular endurance, and flexibility. Therefore, exercise programs should concentrate on these aspects, even though a well-rounded program also works to improve balance and body composition.

Many elderly people have been inactive for long periods of time or may have health problems associated with aging and various diseases, so they should begin at a low frequency, duration, and intensity of exercise and the rate of progression should be slower.

Although there is a decrease in $\dot{V}o_2$max with age, the energy required to do the same activity (e.g., walking at 3 mph) remains the same or increases slightly because of a reduced efficiency of movement. As a result, the same activity has a higher intensity (% of $\dot{V}o_2$max). There is little change in the ability to work at or below 50% of $\dot{V}o_2$max, but older people have difficulty maintaining activities at higher intensities. Therefore, it is best to let them select their own work rate and not to impose it on them. The risk of cardiovascular and musculoskeletal problems is much greater with intense exercise. Therefore, training programs should start at a low intensity and allow for a more gradual increase in activity than would be the case for younger people.

In general, the selection of activities for older persons depends on the number and types of limitations they have. For example, if an older person has a problem with balance, exercise can be performed while sitting, lying on the floor, standing while holding a chair, or in warm water. Because the older adult is generally less adaptable, more time should be spent at each level of exercise to allow for more complete adaptation before increasing the total amount of work done. Finally, exercise is also a social activity for many older persons. For this reason, exercise programs should be safe, effective, and most of all, enjoyable, so that elderly persons make regular activity a routine part of their lifestyle.

Exercise Prescription for the Obese

Multiple health problems (e.g., hypertension, cardiovascular disease, type 2 diabetes) and increased mortality are associated with obesity. Because obesity is influenced greatly by lifestyle, weight control may best be achieved by using behavioral therapies that include regular exercise and diet. Exercise programs to reduce body fat and body mass should include high levels of total energy expenditure daily. One of the easiest ways to do this is to transport the body mass. Walking a given distance requires a specific amount of energy per kilogram of body mass moved. Therefore, obese persons walking a mile expend the same amount of energy relevant to their body mass as normal weight persons but expend more absolute energy because they have more body mass to move.

The same number of kilocalories are needed to run 10 miles, whether a person runs the 10 miles in 1 day or runs 1 mile per day for 10 days. How fast one runs has little effect on the total energy expended per mile, i.e., the same amount of energy is required to transport the body mass each mile, even though the intensity or power output varies with the speed. The total amount of work done is more important for weight loss, while the intensity of the work is more important for improving fitness.

Perhaps the best way to start an effective exercise program is to encourage obese individuals to walk regularly, in addition to the normal walking done at the job or at home. They should be encouraged to walk as many miles as possible to increase the total amount of energy expended.

Because obese persons have problems with heat tolerance and increased sweating, as well as the associated problems of chafing of the arms and legs, swimming is another exercise that can be useful. Exercising in water can reduce strain on the joints. Adequate amounts of energy can be expended if the person has sufficient skills to swim for a long period of time. The disadvantages of swimming are that obese persons are often embarrassed to be seen in a bathing suit and their low body density makes it easier for them to float and may make it harder for them to reach sufficient exercise intensity.

A major challenge in treating obesity is not the initial weight loss but maintaining the lower body weight and fatness later on. Therefore, achievement of a relatively permanent lifestyle change must be emphasized, using multiple behavioral modification techniques that include diet and regular exercise.

Exercise Prescription for Diabetes Mellitus

When discussing exercise for patients with diabetes, one must distinguish between type 1 diabetes (which requires the administration of exogenous insulin) and type 2 diabetes (which is more related to reduced insulin sensitivity and increased glucose intolerance). This disease is very complex, as is its cause and treatment. Readers are requested to review other references for more complete information.

Patients with Type 1 Diabetes

In type 1 diabetes, the metabolic response to exercise is determined primarily by the adequacy of the diabetic control of insulin. If insulin levels are adequate, exercise can reduce blood glucose. With insulin deficiency, exercise can cause an increase in the levels of blood glucose, free fatty acids, and ketone bodies. For this reason, the person with type 1 diabetes should not exercise if there is ketoacidosis or a fasting blood glucose of more than 250 to 300 mg/dL.

One of the most important aspects of diabetic control is consistency in daily lifestyle. If patients with diabetes exercise at the same time of day and at similar intensities and durations of exercise, then they can adjust food intake and insulin for better control. This is especially important if the

amount of energy expended can be quantified and remain relatively constant.

At the onset of an exercise program, patients with type 1 diabetes should reduce their insulin dose by about 20% and then determine whether this control is adequate. If it is, then they should maintain the insulin dose and regulate food intake.

Patients with type 1 diabetes should not exercise at the time of the peak insulin effect. Instead, they should exercise when glycosuria occurs, because exercise produces a reduction in blood glucose levels. Similarly, they should not inject insulin into the exercising limbs, as this will increase the washout from those muscles during exercise. Instead, insulin should be injected into the abdominal fat tissue.

Patients with Type 2 Diabetes

Type 2 diabetes causes fewer complications than type 1 diabetes, but there is a higher incidence of coronary heart disease, hypertension, stroke, and other complications associated with obesity. The vast majority of persons with type 2 diabetes are classified as obese. If they are obese and insulin-resistant at the same time, then they should be treated with diet and exercise to achieve both weight control and to restore the sensitivity to insulin. Training and weight loss both increase cell sensitivity to insulin. However, because the acute effect of exercise on insulin sensitivity is lost after a few days of inactivity, exercise and diet should be part of the lifestyle of these patients.

The longer the diabetes is present, the older the person, and the longer he or she has been sedentary, the more important it is to begin an exercise program at a low intensity and low duration. The best type of exercise seems to be rhythmic, aerobic exercise with major muscle groups at moderate intensities for a prolonged duration of 45 minutes or more. This type of exercise program has been shown to produce maximal benefits for diabetic control, weight control, aerobic fitness, and reduction of risk factors for cardiovascular disease.

Patients with both types of diabetes should have a carbohydrate snack 15 to 30 minutes before exercise, so that they will begin exercising with a mild hyperglycemia. They should then take snacks every 15 minutes to maintain a slightly higher blood glucose level. Because high-intensity, brief exercise may increase blood glucose and insulin requirements and also increases blood pressure, this kind of exercise is to be de-emphasized in patients with diabetes.

Exercise Prescription for Hypertension

Mean blood pressure is directly related to blood flow (i.e., heart rate × stroke volume = cardiac output, or $\dot{Q}$) and the resistance to flow in the periphery (systemic vascular resistance, or SVR), i.e., an increase in either or both of these factors causes a rise in mean blood pressure.

The characteristic hemodynamic patterns of hypertension vary according to the stage and severity of the disease. In stage 1 (mild, borderline) hypertension, there is a high $\dot{Q}$ and a normal SVR. Stage 2 (moderate, fixed) hypertension is characterized by a normal $\dot{Q}$ and a high SVR. Stage 3 (severe, advanced) hypertension is characterized by a low $\dot{Q}$ and a very high SVR, as well as by organ damage.

In general, patients with hypertension should do dynamic, aerobic exercise with large muscle groups at a frequency of 3 to 4 sessions per week, a duration of 30 to 45 minutes per session, and at an intensity of 55% to 70% of $\dot{V}o_2$max or a rating of perceived exertion of 12 to 14 (somewhat hard to hard). Light weight training (30% to 50% of the maximal amount of weight that can be lifted once) can be done if there is not an excessive rise in blood pressure during the activity.

There appears to be an inverse relationship between activity or fitness and blood pressure (9). Research suggests that there is little response in blood pressure to static training, while the response to aerobic training depends on the initial blood pressure status. For example, persons with normal blood pressure had a drop of approximately 3 mm Hg in both systolic and diastolic pressures after aerobic training. Persons with borderline hypertension had a decrease of 6 to 7 mm Hg in both pressures, while those with stage 2 hypertension had a reduction of 8 to 10 mm Hg in both pressures. No data were available for persons with stage 3 hypertension, but it is unlikely that exercise has a major effect because these persons have significant organ damage.

It should be stated that exercise is only one part of the management of hypertension. The Clinical Practice Guidelines (10) recommend "a multifactorial education, counseling, behavioral, and pharmacological approach to manage hypertension." They state that "neither education, counseling, and behavioral interventions nor rehabilitative exercise training as sole interventions have been shown to control elevated blood pressure levels."

Exercise Prescription for Peripheral Vascular Occlusive Disease

Peripheral vascular occlusive disease (PVOD) is an atherosclerotic disease affecting the arteries of the lower extremities. Because of arterial narrowing or obstruction, there is the classic symptom of claudication pain when the demands for the increased blood flow during exercise exceed the ability of the narrowed arteries to supply it.

The types of exercise programs for patients with PVOD that have shown the greatest improvements have the following characteristics. These programs generally lasted more than 6 months and involved walking intermittently to near-maximal pain for more than 30 minutes per session and for 3 or more sessions per week. These exercise programs provoked the ischemic response and stimulated the need for adaptation over a prolonged period of time with regular physical activity.

In general, exercise training programs increase the functional tolerance and reduce the symptoms of claudication

in patients with PVOD. However, there is a high incidence of coronary artery disease in PVOD patients and these people are at high risk.

SUMMARY

There has not been an attempt in this chapter to intensively and thoroughly discuss all health states and diseases. As an example, so much has been written on exercise for coronary heart disease that it would be impossibly to treat this adequately in a few paragraphs. Instead, this chapter has discussed the general principles of exercise prescription and tried to show how they can be applied to the average person as well as to those who are older and have various medical problems.

Generally speaking, people of below-average health and fitness need more precise and controlled guidance on how to improve their functional capacity and possibly to reduce further degeneration. The amount and rate of improvement as a result of exercise programs is probably less in these people. They also need more precise exercise prescriptions to know the types of exercise to emphasize and to avoid. In addition, they may have to exercise under varying degrees of supervision. The need for supervision depends on the degree of risk associated with exercise for each individual person and on his or her limitations.

As stated before, the general principles are the same for everyone, but must be modified according to the restrictions and limitations imposed on each person. Increased exercise may not change the status or course of a problem or disease, but may improve the ability to adapt to any restrictions associated with that problem or disease.

As long as a given type of exercise does not create a higher risk for the person involved, the best activities during all phases of an exercise program are those that are safe, effective, and enjoyable. While specific types of activities may need to be avoided by certain people, there are so many different ways that one can exercise: benefits can be obtained from many different forms of exercise programs. There is no one single exercise program that is correct for everyone or even for the same person over time.

Unless there are specific exercises to be avoided for medical reasons or unless there are specific exercises to be emphasized to improve performance, there are many kinds of activities available, and precise exercise prescriptions are not needed. For most people, it is the process of being active that is more important than the product of being fit. We need to communicate to the public that regular, moderate physical activity leads to a healthier lifestyle and to a substantially reduced risk of death from cardiovascular diseases and other major diseases.

REFERENCES

1. American College of Sports Medicine. Guidelines for graded exercise testing and exercise prescription, 5th ed. Philadelphia; Lea & Febiger, 1995:1–372.

2. American College of Sports Medicine. Position stand on the recommended quantity and quality of exercise for developing and maintaining cardiorespiratory and muscular fitness and flexibility in healthy adults. Med Sci Sports Exerc 1998;29:975–991.

3. American College of Sports Medicine. Resource manual for guidelines for exercise testing and

prescription. Philadelphia: Lea & Febiger, 1988:1–436.

4. Skinner JS, ed. Exercise testing and exercise prescription for special cases. 2nd ed. Philadelphia: Lea & Febiger, 1993:1–395.

5. Pollock ML, Schmidt DH, ed. Heart disease and rehabilitation. 3rd ed. Champaign, IL: Human Kinetics, 1995:1–471.

6. Bouchard C, Shephard RJ, Stephens T, ed. Physical activity, fitness, and health. Champaign, IL: Human Kinetics, 1994:1–1055.

7. Pate RR, Pratt M, Blair SN, et al. Physical activity and public health: a recommendation from the Centers for Disease Control and Prevention and the American College of Sports Medicine. JAMA 1995;273:402–407.

8. Blair SN. Exercise prescription and health. Quest 1995;47:338–353.

9. American College of Sports Medicine. Position stand on physical activity, physical fitness, and hypertension. Med Sci Sports Exerc 1995;25:i–x.

10. U.S. Department of Health and Human Services. Cardiac rehabilitation: clinical practice guideline. Publication No. 96–0672 17. Washington, DC: Agency for Health Care Policy and Research 1995;1–202.

Part XVIII.

IMMUNOLOGY

Edited by
David C. Nieman

Introduction to Immunology

James M. Rippe

The relationship between physical activity and immune function represents an area of intense scientific investigation. Chapters in this section summarize current knowledge and point toward future directions of possible fruitful inquiry. The opening chapter by David Nieman explores the relationship between exercise and respiratory function. Since respiratory tract infections are extremely common, the implications of any relationship between physical activity and immunity function hold great interest not only for public health, but also for performance of individual athletes and sports-active children and adults. The author posits a J curve in which moderate exercise may decrease the likelihood of respiratory infection while heavy exertion may increase the likelihood of such infections. The existing literature supporting this argument is reviewed in detail.

The chapter by Jeffrey Woods reviews knowledge of the effects of acute bouts of exercise on immune function (with *acute* defined as a single bout of exercise) and explores how this interaction may be of practical consequences to the athlete.

Laurel Mackinnon follows up with the equally important issue of how chronic exercise interacts with the immune system. The author reviews the evidence supporting mild suppression of some immune parameters in athletes. The chapter emphasizes that athletes are not clinically immune-deficient and that upper respiratory tract infection appears to be the only illness to which they are more susceptible.

Since there is a clearly established relationship between exercise and immune function, an exploration of how this might impact on immunocompromised patients such as those with HIV carries enormous clinical significance. Bente Klarlund Pedersen reviews this topic in the chapter "HIV Infection—Exercise and Immune Function" and concludes that HIV-seropositive patients should be encouraged to perform moderate-level physical activity.

The part concludes with the chapter by Robert Mazzeo, "Exercise, Aging, and Immunity." Older patients are increasingly being urged to participate in regular exercise programs to achieve a variety of health benefits. Such increased levels of physical activity have been shown to lower the risk of coronary artery disease and other chronic conditions, as well as improving quality of life. Much less is known about the relationship between physical activity and the immune system in older patients. As the author points out, although much research remains to be done, recent studies have suggested positive relationships between physical activity and improved immune function in older patients, adding yet another reason to encourage them to participate in regular physical activity.

Chapter 99

Exercise and Respiratory Infection

David C. Nieman

Among elite athletes and their coaches, a common perception is that heavy exertion lowers resistance and is a predisposing factor to upper respiratory traction infections (1–6). In a 1996 survey by the Gatorade Sports Science Institute of 2700 high school and college coaches and athletic trainers, 89% checked "yes" to the question, "Do you believe overtraining can compromise the immune system and make athletes sick?" (personal communication, Gatorade Sports Science Institute, Barrington, IL). Many elite athletes including Sebastian Coe, Uta Pippig, Liz McColgan, Michelle Akers-Stahl, Alberto Salazar, and Steve Spence have reported significant bouts with infections that have interfered with their ability to compete and train (4). During the Winter and Summer Olympic Games, it has been regularly reported by clinicians that "upper respiratory infections abound" (5) and that "the most irksome troubles with the athletes were infections" (6).

On the other hand, there is also a common belief among many individuals that regular exercise confers resistance against infection. For example, a 1989 *Runner's World* subscriber survey revealed that 61% of 700 runners reported fewer colds since beginning to run, whereas only 4% felt they had experienced more (7). In a survey of 170 nonelite marathon runners (personal best time, average of 3 hours 25 minutes) who had been training for and participating in marathons for an average of 12 years, 90% reported that they definitely or mostly agreed with the statement that they "rarely get sick" (unpublished personal observations). A survey of 750 Masters athletes (ranging in age from 40 to 81 years) showed that 76% perceived themselves as less vulnerable to viral illnesses than their sedentary peers (8).

The U.S. Centers for Disease Control and Prevention has estimated that over 425 million upper respiratory tract infections (URTIs) occur annually in the United States, resulting in $2.5 billion in lost school and work days, and in medical costs (9). The National Center for Health Statistics reports that acute respiratory conditions (primarily the common cold and influenza) have an annual incidence rate of 90 per 100 persons (10). Understanding the relationship between exercise and infection has potential implications for public health, and for the athlete it may mean the difference between being able to compete or performing at a subpar level or missing an event altogether because of illness.

The relationship between exercise and URTI may be modeled in the form of a J curve (Figure 99-1). This model suggests that although the risk of URTI may decrease below that of a sedentary individual when one engages in moderate exercise training, risk may rise above average during periods of excessive amounts of high-intensity exercise (2). At present, there is more evidence, primarily epidemiologic in nature, exploring the relationship between heavy exertion and infection, and these data will be reviewed first followed by a brief section on moderate exercise training and infection (Table 99-1). Much more research using larger subject pools and improved research designs is necessary before this model can be wholly accepted or rejected.

The ten epidemiologic studies summarized in Table 99-1 all used self-reported URTI data (primarily retrospective, with two studies using 1-year daily logs). None have attempted to verify symptomatology using viral identification or verification by physicians. There is some concern that the symptoms reported by endurance athletes following competitive race events may reflect those associated with an inflammatory response rather than URTI (11–13). Nonetheless, the data are consistent in supporting the viewpoint that

Figure 99-1 J-Shaped model of relationship between varying amounts of exercise and risk of URTI. This model suggests that moderate exercise may lower risk of URTI whereas excessive amounts may increase the risk.

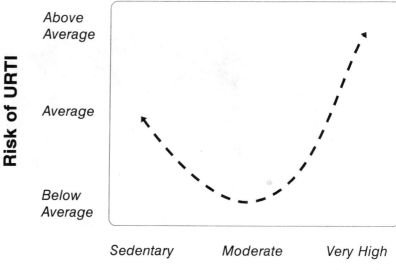

Table 99-1 Epidemiologic and Exercise Training Research on the Relationship Between Exercise and Upper Respiratory Tract Infection

INVESTIGATORS	SUBJECTS	METHOD OF DETERMINING URTI	MAJOR FINDING
Epidemiologic Studies			
Peters et al (16)	141 South African marathoners, 124 controls	2-week recall of URTI incidence and duration after 56-km race	URTI incidence twice as high in runners after 56-km race vs. controls (33.3% vs. 15.3%)
Linde (15)	44 Danish orienteers, 44 matched nonathletes	URTI symptoms self-recorded in daily log for 1 year	Orienteers vs. controls had 2.5 vs. 1.7 URTIs during year
Nieman et al (23)	294 California runners training for race	2-month recall of URTI incidence; 1-week recall, 5-, 10-, and 21-km races	Training 42 vs. 12 km/week associated with lower URTI; no effect of race on URTI
Peters (17)	108 South African marathoners, 108 controls	2-week recall of URTI incidence and duration after 56-km race	URTI incidence 28.7% in runners vs. 12.9% in controls after 56-km race
Nieman et al (14)	2311 Los Angeles Marathon runners	2-month recall of URTI incidence during training for marathon; 1-week recall after winter race	Runners training ≥97 vs. <32 km/week at higher URTI risk; odds ratio 5.9 for participants vs. nonparticipants 1 week after 42.2-km race
Heath et al (22)	530 runners in South Carolina	1-year daily log using self-reported, precoded symptoms	Increase in running distance positively related to increased URTI risk
Peters et al (18)	84 South African marathon runners, 73 nonrunner controls	2-week recall of URTI incidence and duration after 90-km race	URTI incidence 68% in runners vs. 45% in controls after 56-km race; 33% in runners using vitamin C vs. 53% in controls
Nieman (unpublished data, 1993)	170 North Carolina marathon runners	1-week recall of URTI incidence after summer marathon race	URTI reported by only 3% of marathoners during week after summer race
Peters et al (19)	178 South African runners, 162 controls	2-week recall of URTI incidence and duration after 90-km race	URTI incidence 40.4% in placebo runners vs. 15.9% using vitamin C (500 mg/day for 3 wks); vitamins A and E had no additional effect
Castell et al (21)	151 endurance athletes in the United Kingdom	1 week recall of URTI incidence after heavy exertion	URTI reported by 81% of athletes using placebo vs. 49% using a glutamine-based beverage
Exercise Training Studies			
Nieman et al (24)	36 mildly obese, inactive women in California	Daily logs using self-reported, precoded URTI symptoms for 15 weeks during winter season	Walking group reported fewer days with URTI symptoms than controls (5.1 vs. 10.8)
Nieman et al (25)	42 elderly women (30 inactive, 12 athletes) in North Carolina	Daily logs using self-reported, precoded URTI symptoms for 12 weeks during fall season	Incidence of URTI 8% in athletes; inactives randomized to 12 weeks walking vs. controls with 21% in walkers, 50% in sedentary controls
Nieman et al (26)	90 overweight and 30 normal-weight women	Daily logs using self-reported, precoded URTI symptoms for 12 weeks during winter season	Number of days with URTI symptoms, 9.4 ± 1.1, 5.6 ± 0.9, and 4.8 ± 0.9 in overweight walkers, overweight controls, and normal-weight controls

heavy exertion increases the risk of URTI, while moderate exercise training is associated with a decreased risk.

HEAVY EXERTION AND URTI: EPIDEMIOLOGIC EVIDENCE

Several epidemiologic reports suggest that athletes engaging in marathon-type events and/or very heavy training are at increased risk of URTI (see Table 99-1). Nieman et al (14) researched the incidence of URTI in a group of 2311 marathon runners who varied widely in running ability and training habits. Runners retrospectively self-reported demographic, training, and URTI episode and symptom data for the 2-month period (January, February) prior to and the 1-week period immediately following the 1987 Los Angeles Marathon race. During the week following the race, 12.9% of the marathoners reported an URTI compared to only 2.2% of control runners who did not participate (odds ratio, 5.9) (Figure 99-2). Forty percent of the runners reported at least

one URTI episode during the 2-month winter period prior to the marathon race. Controlling for various confounders, it was determined that runners training more than 96 km/week doubled their odds for sickness compared to those training less than 32 km/week.

Linde (15) studied URTI in a group of 44 elite orienteers and 44 nonathletes of the same age, sex, and occupational distribution during a 1-year period. Athletes and controls recorded symptoms of sickness using daily logs for 1 year. The orienteers experienced significantly more URTI episodes during the year in comparison to the control group (2.5 versus 1.7 episodes, respectively). Although one-third of the controls reported no URTI during the year-long study period, this applied to only 10% of the orienteers. The average duration of symptoms in the group of orienteers was 7.9 days compared to 6.4 days in the control group (NS). The control group had the expected seasonal variation with the peak incidence in winter and relatively few cases in summer, while the orienteers tended to show a more even distribution.

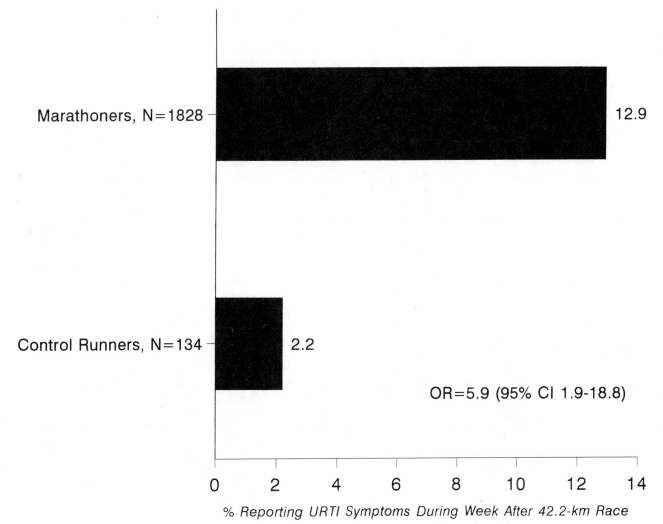

Figure 99-2 Self-reported URTI in 2300 Los Angeles marathon runners during the week following the 1987 Los Angeles Marathon. (Data from Nieman DC, Johanssen LM, Lee JW, et al. Infectious episodes in runners before and after the Los Angeles Marathon. J Sports Med Phys Fitness 1990;30:316–328.)

Peters et al (16) studied the incidence of URTI in 150 randomly selected runners who took part in a 56-km Cape Town race in comparison to live-in controls who did not run. Symptoms of URTI occurred in 33.3% of runners compared with 15.3% of controls during the 2-week period following the race, and were most common in those who achieved the faster race times. The most prevalent symptoms after the race were reported to be sore throats and nasal symptoms. Of the total number of symptoms reported by the runners, 80% lasted for longer than 3 days, suggesting an infective origin.

Several subsequent studies from this group of researchers have confirmed this finding (17–20). During the 2-week period following the 56-km Milo Korkie Ultramarathon in Pretoria, South Africa, 28.7% of the 108 subjects who completed the race reported non-allergy-derived URTI symptoms as compared to 12.9% of controls (17). In another study, 68% of runners reported the development of symptoms of URTI within 2 weeks after the 90-km Comrades Ultramarathon (18). Using a double-blind placebo research design, it was determined that only 33% of runners taking a 600-mg vitamin C supplement daily for 3 weeks prior to the race developed URTI symptoms. The incidence of URTI was greatest among the runners who trained the hardest coming into the race (85% versus 45% of the low- or medium-training-status runners).

In subsequent research, vitamin C, but not vitamin A and E, supplements have not been found to alter URTI rates following ultramarathon competitions (19,20). As depicted in Figure 99-3 and summarized in Table 99-1, 15.9% of runners using vitamin C supplements (500 mg/day) reported URTI during the 2-week period following the 1993 90-km Comrades Ultramarathon in comparison to 40.4% of runners using placebo, 20% to 26% of runners using vitamin C with vitamin E and beta-carotene, and 24.4% of controls on placebo. The authors suggested that because heavy exertion enhances the production of free oxygen radicals, vitamin C, which has antioxidant properties, may be required in increased quantities (18–20). One research team has reported reduced URTI rates following marathon race events in runners consuming beverages containing glutamine, an amino acid used by various cells of the immune system (11,21). However, further research is needed to confirm these findings.

Heath et al (22) followed a cohort of runners (N = 530) who self-reported URTI symptoms daily for 1 year. The average runner in the study was about 40 years of age, ran 32 km/week, and experienced a rate of 1.2 URTIs per year. Controlling for various confounding variables using logistic regression, the lowest odds ratio for URTI was found in those running less than 16 km/week. The odds ratio more than doubled for those running more than 27 km/week. This study demonstrated that total running distance for a year is a significant risk factor for URTI, with risk increasing as the running distance rises.

URTI risk following a race event may depend on the distance, with an increased incidence conspicuous only following marathon or ultramarathon events. For example, Nieman et al (23) were unable to establish any increase in prevalence of URTI in 273 runners during the week following 5-, 10-, and 21.2-km events as compared to the week before. URTI incidence was also measured during the 2-month winter period prior to the three races, and in this group of recre-ational runners, 25% of those running 25 or more km per week (average of 42 km/week) reported at least one URTI episode, as opposed to 34% training less than 25 km/week (average of 12 km/week) (p = .09). These findings suggest that, in recreational running, an average weekly distance of 42 versus 12 km is associated with either no change in or even a slight reduction of URTI incidence. Further, they suggest, that racing 5 to 21.1 km is not related to an increased risk of sickness during the ensuing week.

URTI rates after endurance races may also vary depending on the season. As summarized in Table 99-1, only 3% of marathon runners reported URTI symptoms during the week after the July 1993 Grandfather Mountain Marathon (Boone, NC).

Together, these epidemiologic studies imply that heavy acute or chronic exercise is associated with an increased risk of URTI. The risk appears to be especially high during the 1- or 2-week period following marathon-type race events. Among runners varying widely in training habits, the risk for URTI is slightly elevated for the highest distance runners, but only when several confounding factors are controlled.

MODERATE EXERTION AND URTI

A common belief among fitness enthusiasts is that regular physical activity is beneficial in decreasing URTI risk. Very few studies, however, have been conducted in this area, and more research is certainly warranted to investigate this interesting question.

At present, there are no published epidemiologic reports that have retrospectively or prospectively compared incidence of URTI in large groups of moderately active and sedentary individuals. Three randomized experimental trials have provided important preliminary data in support of the viewpoint that moderate physical activity may reduce URTI symptomatology (see Table 99-1). All three studies have been consistent in establishing that near-daily brisk walking when compared to inactivity reduces the number of sickness days in half over a 12- to 15-week period.

In one randomized, controlled study of 36 overweight women (mean age 35 years), exercise subjects walked briskly for 45 minutes, 5 days a week, and experienced one-half the days with URTI symptoms during the 15-week period compared to that of the sedentary control group (5.1 ± 1.2 versus 10.8 ± 2.3 days, p = .039) (24).

In a study of elderly women, the incidence of the common cold during a 12-week period in the fall was measured to be lowest in highly conditioned, lean subjects who exercised moderately each day for about 1.5 hours (8%) (25). Elderly subjects who walked 40 minutes, five times per week had an incidence of 21%, as compared to 50% for the sedentary control group (X = 6.36, p = .042). These data suggest that elderly women not engaging in cardiorespiratory exercise are more likely than those who do exercise regularly to experience an URTI during the fall season.

The effect of exercise training (five 45-minute walking sessions per week at 60% to 75% maximum heart rate) and/or moderate energy restriction (4.19 to 5.44 MJ or 1200 to 1300 kcal per day) on URTI was studied in nonobese, physically active women (N = 30) and obese women (N = 91, body

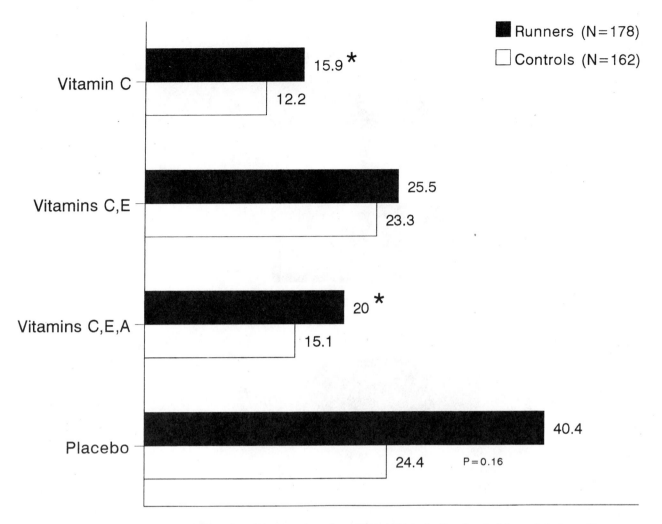

■ Runners (N=178)
□ Controls (N=162)

Vitamin C — 15.9 * / 12.2

Vitamins C,E — 25.5 / 23.3

Vitamins C,E,A — 20 * / 15.1

Placebo — 40.4 / 24.4   P=0.16

% URTI Incidence During Two-Week Period After 90-km Race

Figure 99-3 Vitamin C supplementation (500 mg/day for 3 weeks) significantly reduced URTI incidence in ultramarathon runners after a 90-km race, with no added benefit provided through vitamins A or E. *$p < .05$ relative to placebo runners. (Data from Peters EM, Goetzsche JM, Joseph LE, Noakes TD. Vitamin C as effective as combinations of antioxidant nutrients in reducing symptoms of upper respiratory tract infection in ultramarathon runners. S Afr J Sports Med 1996;11(3):23–27.)

mass index 33.1 ± 0.6 kg/m^2) randomized to one of four groups: control, exercise, diet, exercise and diet (26). All subjects self-reported symptoms of sickness in health logs using a precoded checklist. Energy restriction had no significant effect on URTI incidence, and subjects from the two exercise groups were contrasted with subjects from the two nonexercise groups. The number of days with symptoms of URTI for subjects in the exercise groups was reduced relative to the nonexercise groups (5.6 ± 0.9 and 9.4 ± 1.1 sickness days, respectively), similar to that of the nonobese controls (4.8 ± 0.9) (Figure 99-4).

POTENTIAL MECHANISMS

It naturally follows that if heavy and fatiguing exertion leads to an increased risk of URTI, various measures of immune function should be negatively affected. And conversely, if moderate exercise decreases URTI risk, there should be some aspect of immune function that is chronically or at least transiently improved. In other chapters of this text, the relationship between acute and chronic exercise and immunity is reviewed in more detail.

In general, studies comparing various measures of resting immunity in athletes and nonathletes have demonstrated few significant differences except for impaired neutrophil function (27–35). Pyne et al (35), for example, reported that elite swimmers undertaking intensive training have lower neutrophil oxidative activity at rest than do age- and sex-matched sedentary individuals, and that function is further suppressed during periods of strenuous training prior to national-level competition. Neutrophils are considered the body's best phagocyte; thus suppression of neutrophil function during periods of heavy training may have clinical

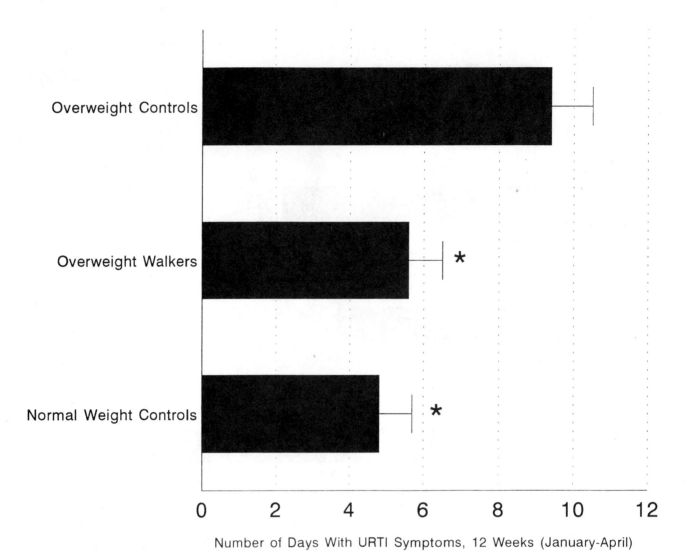

Figure 99-4 Number of days with URTI symptoms in obese nonexercising subjects (n = 48), obese exercising subjects (n = 43), and nonobese controls (n = 30). F(2,117) = 5.96, ≪0.001. *p < .05 compared to obese nonexercising subjects. (Data from Nieman DC, Nehlsen-Cannarella SL, Henson DA, et al. Immune response to exercise training and/or energy restriction in obese women. Med Sci Sports Exerc 1998;30:679–686.)

significance. Müns (36) has reported that neutrophils in the upper airway passages of athletes have a decreased phagocytic capacity when compared to nonathletes, and that following heavy exertion, a further suppression is experienced for 1 to 3 days afterward. Repeated cycles of heavy exertion may thus put the athletes at increased risk of URTI.

Several authors have posited that prolonged cardiorespiratory endurance exercise (defined in this chapter as ≥1.5 hours) leads to transient but significant perturbations in immunity and host defense (4,37,38). This has been described as the "open window theory," or the 3- to 24-hour immunosuppression period following heavy exertion that allows viruses to multiply and establish clinically detectable infection. Many components of the immune system exhibit change after heavy exertion, including the following (3,37,38):

- Neutrophilia and lymphopenia appear
- Increase in blood granulocyte and monocyte phagocytosis, but a decrease in nasal neutrophil phagocytosis

- Decrease in granulocyte oxidative burst activity
- Decrease in nasal mucociliary clearance
- Decrease in natural killer cell cytotoxic activity (NKCA)
- Decrease in mitogen-induced lymphocyte proliferation (a measure of T-cell function)
- Decrease in the delayed-type hypersensitivity response
- Increased pro- and anti-inflammatory cytokines (e.g., IL-6 and IL-1ra)
- Decrease in nasal and salivary IgA concentration

Most impressive are the data showing that immunity in the upper respiratory tract is diminished for an extended period following heavy exertion (36,39,40). The increase in phagocytosis and IL-6 suggests a strong proinflammatory response, whereas the rise in cortisol and IL-1ra shows that anti-inflammatory forces are also at work. Taken together, these data suggest that the immune system is suppressed and stressed, albeit transiently, following prolonged endurance exercise, supporting the viewpoint that host protection is compromised. This may be especially apparent when the athlete goes through repeated cycles of heavy exertion, has been exposed to novel pathogens, and has experienced other stressors to the immune system including lack of sleep, severe mental stress, malnutrition, or weight loss (2,3).

MANAGEMENT OF THE ATHLETE DURING INFECTION

Endurance athletes are often uncertain of whether they should exercise or rest during an infectious episode. There are few data available in humans to provide definitive answers. Most clinical authorities in this area recommend that if the athlete has symptoms of a common cold with no constitutional involvement, then regular training may be safely resumed a few days after the resolution of symptoms. Mild exercise during sickness with a common cold does not appear to be contraindicated. Weidner et al (41), for example, have shown that rhinovirus-caused upper respiratory illness does not impair short-duration submaximal or maximal exercise performance. In addition, moderate exercise training did not influence URTI symptomatology (42). However, it should be cautioned that rhinoviruses account for only 40% of URTI, and further research is needed with other pathogens to determine their relationship to exercise. Some clinicians feel that if there are symptoms or signs of systemic involvement (fever, extreme tiredness, muscle aches, swollen lymph glands, etc.), then at least 2 weeks should probably be allowed before resumption of intensive training (2,43).

Data from animal studies have been difficult to apply to the human condition but, in general, have supported the finding that one or two periods of exhaustive exercise following inoculation leads to a more frequent appearance of infection and a higher fatality rate (but results differ depending on the pathogen, with some more affected by exercise than others) (43,44). In humans, it is well established that various measures of physical performance capability are reduced during an infectious episode (43). Several case histories have been published demonstrating that sudden and unexplained deterioration in athletic performance can be traced to either recent URTI or subclinical viral infections that run a protracted course. In some athletes, a viral infection may lead to a debilitating state known as *postviral fatigue syndrome* (45,46). The symptoms include lethargy, easy fatigability, and myalgia, and can persist for several months.

Athletes must train hard to prepare for competition. Although this increases the risk for infection if the training becomes too intensive, there are several practical recommendations the athlete can follow to minimize the impact of other stressors on the immune system (2):

- Keep other life stresses to a minimum. Mental stress in and of itself has been linked to an increased risk of upper respiratory tract infection (47).
- Eat a well-balanced diet to keep vitamin and mineral pools in the body at optimal levels. Although there is insufficient evidence to recommend nutrient supplements, ultramarathon runners may benefit by taking vitamin C

supplements before ultramarathon races (600 mg/day for at least 1 week) (18–20). Vitamin C may help reduce oxidative damage to important immune cells.

- Avoid overtraining and chronic fatigue.
- Obtain adequate sleep on a regular schedule. Sleep disruption has been linked to suppressed immunity (48).
- Avoid rapid weight loss (which has also been linked to negative immune changes) (26).
- Avoid putting hands to the eyes and nose (which is a primary route of introducing viruses into the body) (49–51). Before important race events, avoid sick people and large crowds when possible.
- For athletes competing during the winter months, flu shots are recommended (2).
- Use carbohydrate beverages before, during, and after marathon-type race events or unusually heavy training bouts (52,53). This may lower the impact of stress hormones on the immune system.

Various attempts have been made to alter the negative changes in immunity following heavy exertion through nutritional or chemical means. Indomethacin, which inhibits prostaglandin production, has been administered to athletes prior to exercise, or used in vitro to determine whether the drop in NKCA can be countered. However, in one study of experienced marathon runners, indomethacin had no affect in countering the drop in NKCA following 2.5 hours of intensive running (54).

Only a few studies have been conducted investigating the role of nutritional supplementation on the immune response to intense and prolonged exercise, including zinc, vitamin C, glutamine, and carbohydrate. Most impressive have been the carbohydrate supplementation studies. A double-blind, placebo, randomized study was designed to investigate the effect of carbohydrate fluid (6% carbohydrate beverage, Gatorade) ingestion on the immune response to 2.5 hours of running in 30 experienced marathon runners (52,53,55). In prior research, carbohydrate versus water ingestion during prolonged endurance exercise had been associated with an attenuated cortisol and epinephrine response through its effect on the blood glucose concentration (56). Drinking the carbohydrate beverage before, during (1 liter/hour), and after 2.5 hours of running attenuated the rise in both cortisol and the neutrophil/lymphocyte ratio. The immediate postrun blood glucose level was significantly higher in the carbohydrate versus placebo group and was negatively correlated with cortisol ($r = -.67$, $p < .001$). Trafficking of most leukocyte and lymphocyte subsets was lessened in accordance with the lower cortisol levels in the carbohydrate subjects. Carbohydrate intake also blunted the rise in interleukin-6 and interleukin-1 receptor antagonist, cytokines involved in the inflammatory cascade in response to heavy exertion.

In another study of 10 triathletes, carbohydrate ingestion was studied for its effect on the immune response to 2.5 hours of running and cycling (57,58). Each triathlete ran or cycled for 2.5 hours at 75% Vo$_2$max, ingesting carbohydrate or placebo fluids (random order, double-blind conditions). Carbohydrate ingestion (but not activity mode) strongly influenced plasma glucose and hormonal responses to the intense exercise bouts, leading to diminished perturbations in blood immune cell and cytokine concentrations, natural killer cell activity, and granulocyte phagocytosis and oxidative burst activity. Together, these data suggest that carbohydrate ingestion before, during, and after prolonged endurance exercise may help to lessen the stress on the immune system, and attenuate cytokine levels in the inflammatory cascade.

SUMMARY

Epidemiologic and experimental data suggest that moderate exercise enhances host protection from URTI whereas heavy exertion places endurance athletes at increased risk. Following acute bouts of prolonged heavy endurance exercise, several components of the immune system demonstrate suppressed function for several hours. This has led to the concept of the "open window" theory, described as the 3- to 24-hour time period following prolonged endurance exercise when host defense is decreased and risk of URTI is elevated. Further research is needed to provide a better understanding of underlying mechanisms before definitive clinical applications can be drawn. Nonetheless, there is sufficient evidence to caution athletes to practice various hygienic measures to lower their risk of URTI and to avoid heavy exertion during systemic illness.

REFERENCES

1. Nieman DC. Physical activity, fitness and infection. In: Bouchard C, Shephard RJ, Stephens T, eds. Exercise, fitness, and health. Champaign, IL: Human Kinetics, 1994:796–813.

2. Nieman DC. Exercise immunology: practical applications. Int J Sports Med 1997;18(suppl 1):S91–S100.

3. Nieman DC. Immune response to heavy exertion. J Appl Physiol 1997;82:1385–1394.

4. Nieman DC. Exercise, infection, and immunity. Int J Sports Med 1994;15:S131–S141.

5. Hanley DF. Medical care of the US Olympic team. JAMA 1967; 12:236:147–148.

6. Jokl E. The immunological status of athletes. J Sports Med 1974; 14:165–167.

7. Anonymous. Up with people. Runner's World, April 1990.

8. Shephard RJ, Kavanagh T, Mertens DJ, et al. Personal health benefits of Masters athletics competition. Br J Sports Med 1995;29:35–40.

9. The Office of Disease Prevention and Health Promotion, U.S. Public Health Service, U.S. Department of Health and Human Services. Disease prevention/health promotion: The facts. Palo Alto, CA: Bull Publishing, 1988.

10. Adams PF, Benson V. Current estimates from the National Health Interview Survey. National Center for Health Statistics. Vital Health Stat 1991;10(181).

11. Castell LM, Poortmans JR, Leclercq R, et al. Some aspects of the acute phase response after a marathon race, and the effects of glutamine supplementation. Eur J Appl Physiol 1997;75:47–53.

12. Drenth JP, Van Uum SHM, Van Deuren M, et al. Endurance run increases circulating IL-6 and IL-1ra but down regulates ex vivo TNF-α and IL-1β production. J Appl Physiol 1995;79:1497–1503.

13. Nehlsen-Cannarella SL, Fagoaga OR, Nieman DC, et al. Carbohydrate and the cytokine response to 2.5 hours of running. J Appl Physiol 1997;82:1662–1667.

14. Nieman DC, Johanssen LM, Lee JW, et al. Infectious episodes in runners before and after the Los Angeles Marathon. J Sports Med Phys Fitness 1990;30:316–328.

15. Linde F. Running and upper respiratory tract infections. Scand J Sport Sci 1987;9:21–23.

16. Peters EM, Bateman ED. Respiratory tract infections: an epidemiological survey. S Afr Med J 1983; 64:582–584.

17. Peters EM. Altitude fails to increase susceptibility of ultramarathon runners to post-race upper respiratory tract infections. S Afr J Sports Med 1990;5:4–8.

18. Peters EM, Goetzsche JM, Grobbelaar B, et al. Vitamin C supplementation reduces the incidence of postrace symptoms of upper-respiratory-tract infection in ultramarathon runners. Am J Clin Nutr 1993;57:170–174.

19. Peters EM, Goetzsche JM, Joseph LE, Noakes TD. Vitamin C as effective as combinations of anti-oxidant nutrients in reducing symptoms of upper respiratory tract infection in ultramarathon runners. S Afr J Sports Med 1996;11(3):23–27.

20. Peters-Futre EM. Vitamin C, neutrophil function, and upper respiratory tract infection risk in distance runners: the missing link. Exerc Immunol Rev 1997;3:32–52.

21. Castell LM, Poortmans JR, Newsholme EA. Does glutamine have a role in reducing infections in athletes? Eur J Appl Physiol 1996;73:488–490.

22. Heath GW, Ford ES, Craven TE, et al. Exercise and the incidence of upper respiratory tract infections. Med Sci Sports Exerc 1991;23:152–157.

23. Nieman DC, Johanssen LM, Lee JW. Infectious episodes in runners before and after a roadrace. J Sports Med Phys Fitness 1989;29:289–296.

24. Nieman DC, Nehlsen-Cannarella SL, Markoff PA, et al. The effects of moderate exercise training on natural killer cells and acute upper respiratory tract infections. Int J Sports Med 1990;11:467–473.

25. Nieman DC, Henson DA, Gusewitch G, et al. Physical activity and immune function in elderly women. Med Sci Sports Exerc 1993;25:823–831.

26. Nieman DC, Nehlsen-Cannarella SL, Henson DA, et al. Immune response to exercise training and/or energy restriction in obese women. Med Sci Sports Exerc 1998;30:679–686.

27. Nieman DC, Brendle D, Henson DA, et al. Immune function in athletes versus nonathletes. Int J Sports Med 1995;16:329–333.

28. Nieman DC, Buckley KS, Henson DA, et al. Immune function in marathon runners versus sedentary controls. Med Sci Sports Exerc 1995;27:986–992.

29. Tvede N, Steensberg J, Baslund B, et al. Cellular immunity in highly-trained elite racing cyclists and controls during periods of training with high and low intensity. Scand J Sports Med 1991;1:163–166.

30. Baj Z, Kantorski J, Majewska E, et al. Immunological status of competitive cyclists before and after the training season. Int J Sports Med 1994;15:319–324.

31. Hack V, Strobel G, Rau J-P, et al. The effect of maximal exercise on the activity of neutrophil granulocytes in highly trained athletes in a moderate training period. Eur J Appl Physiol 1992;65:520–524.

32. Hack V, Strobel G, Weiss M, et al. PMN cell counts and phagocytic activity of highly trained athletes depend on training period. J Appl Physiol 1994;77:1731–1735.

33. Pyne DB. Regulation of neutrophil function during exercise. Sports Med 1994;17:245–258.

34. Smith JA, Telford RD, Mason IB, et al. Exercise, training and neutrophil microbicidal activity. Int J Sports Med 1990;11:179–187.

35. Pyne DB, Baker MS, Fricker PA, et al. Effects of an intensive 12-wk training program by elite swimmers on neutrophil oxidative activity. Med Sci Sports Exerc 1995;27:536–542.

36. Müns G. Effect of long-distance running on polymorphonuclear neutrophil phagocytic function of the upper airways. Int J Sports Med 1993;15:96–99.

37. Mackinnon LT, Hooper S. Mucosal (secretory) immune system responses to exercise of varying intensity and during overtraining. Int J Sports Med 1994;15:S179–S183.

38. Pedersen BK, Ullum H. NK cell response to physical activity: possible mechanisms of action. Med Sci Sports Exerc 1994;26:140–146.

39. Müns G, Liesen H, Riedel H, Bergmann KC. Einfluß von langstreckenlauf auf den IgA-gehalt in nasensekret und speichel. Deut Zeit Sportmed 1989;40:63–65.

40. Müns G, Singer P, Wolf F, Rubinstein I. Impaired nasal mucociliary clearance in long-distance runners. Int J Sports Med 1995;16:209–213.

41. Weidner TG, Anderson BN, Kaminsky LA, et al. Effect of a rhinovirus-caused upper respiratory illness on pulmonary function test and exercise responses. Med Sci Sports Exerc 1997;29:604–609.

42. Weidner T, Cranston T, Schurr T, Kaminsky L. The effect of exercise training on the severity and duration of a viral upper respiratory illness. Med Sci Sports Exerc 1998;30:1578–1583.

43. Friman G, Wesslen L, Karjalainen J, Rolf C. Infectious and lymphocytic myocarditis: epidemiology and factors relevant to sports medicine. Scand J Med Sci Sports 1995;5:269–278.

44. Ilbäck NG, Friman G, Crawford DJ, et al. Effects of training on metabolic responses and performance capacity in streptococcus pneumoniae infected rats. Med Sci Sports Exerc 1991;23:422–427.

45. Parker S, Brukner P, Rosier M. Chronic fatigue syndrome and the athlete. Sports Med Train Rehabil 1996;6:269–278.

46. Maffulli N, Testa V, Capasso G. Post-viral fatigue syndrome: a longitudinal assessment in varsity athletes. J Sports Med Phys Fitness 1993;33:392–399.

47. Cohen S, Tyrrell DA, Smith AP. Psychological stress and susceptibility to the common cold. N Engl J Med 1991;325:606–612.

48. Boyum A, Wiik P, Gustavsson E, et al. The effect of strenuous exercise, calorie deficiency and sleep deprivation on white blood cells, plasma immunoglobulins and cytokines. Scand J Immunol 1996;43:228–235.

49. Ansari SA, Springthorpe VS, Sattar SA, et al. Potential role of hands in the spread of respiratory viral infections: studies with human parainfluenza virus 3 and rhinovirus 14. J Clin Microbiol 1991;29:2115–2119.

50. Jackson GG, Dowling HG, Anderson TO, et al. Susceptibility and immunity to common upper respiratory viral infections—the common cold. Ann Intern Med 1960;53:719–738.

51. Jennings LC, Dick EC. Transmission and control of rhinovirus colds. Eur J Epidemiol 1987;3:327–335.

52. Nehlsen-Cannarella SL, Fagoaga OR, Nieman DC, et al. Carbohydrate and the cytokine response to 2.5h of running. J Appl Physiol 1997;82:1662–1667.

53. Nieman DC, Fagoaga OR, Butterworth DE, et al. Carbohydrate supplementation affects blood granulocyte and monocyte trafficking but not function after 2.5h of running. Am J Clin Nutr 1997;66:153–159.

54. Nieman DC, Ahle JC, Henson DA, et al. Indomethacin does not alter natural killer cell response to 2.5 hours of running. J Appl Physiol 1995;79:748–755.

55. Nieman DC, Henson DA, Garner EB, et al. Carbohydrate affects natural killer cell redistribution but not activity after running. Med Sci Sports Exerc 1997;29:1318–1324.

56. Murray R, Paul GL, Seifert GJ, Eddy DE. Responses to varying rates of carbohydrate ingestion

during exercise. Med Sci Sports Exerc 1991;23:713–718.

57. Nieman DC, Nehlsen-Cannarella SL, Fagoaga OR, et al. Influence of mode and carbohydrate on the cytokine response to heavy exertion. Med Sci Sports Exerc 1998;30:671–678.

58. Nieman DC, Nehlsen-Cannarella SL, Fagoaga OR, et al. Influence of mode and carbohydrate on the granulocyte and monocyte response to intensive, prolonged exercise. J Appl Physiol 1998; 84:1252–1259.

Chapter 100

Immune Responses to Acute Exercise: Practical Applications for Exercise Prescription

Jeffrey A. Woods

The immune response to acute exercise has received attention since the documentation of elevated incidence rates of upper respiratory tract infection (URTI) after stressful exercise in humans (1–3). Animal evidence also supports a role for acute bouts of exercise in experimental infectious disease depending on the model used (4–6). In addition to studies of clinical significance, acute bouts of exercise have been utilized as a model of the stress response in an attempt to identify factors involved in regulating immune responsiveness (7). This chapter is dedicated to the review of knowledge concerning the effects of acute exercise on immune function. Throughout this chapter acute exercise is defined as a single bout of exercise. The effects of chronically performed exercise (i.e., over periods of weeks to years) are discussed in Chapter 101. In acute exercise studies, immune responses are usually measured before, during, immediately after, and/or at several time points (up to 1 day or week) after a single bout of exercise. This chapter focuses on the immune responses during this time frame with respect to different intensities and durations of exercise bouts. Moderate exercise is defined as exercise between 40% to 65% of maximal oxygen uptake (Vo_2max), whereas intense exercise is defined as >65% Vo_2max. Acute exercise affects individuals differently depending on their fitness level; therefore, this chapter contrasts studies performed in athletes versus sedentary people when available. The majority of the studies cited will be human studies; however, where human data are lacking, animal studies will be cited.

LEUKOCYTE QUANTIFICATION IN RESPONSE TO ACUTE EXERCISE

Blood Leukocytes

Total Leukocytes

The most well-documented change in any immune measure with exercise is that of blood leukocytosis. Exercise-induced leukocytosis has been observed at least as far back as 1902 (8). Exercise results in an immediate (<5 minutes) substantial increase (50% to 100%) in the number of circulating leukocytes, the magnitude and kinetics of which are dependent on the intensity and duration of exercise (9,10). This exercise-induced leukocytosis reflects the combined influence of increases in polymorphonuclear neutrophils (PMNs), lymphocytes, and monocytes, with minor increases in eosinophils and basophils. In general, the neutrophilia persists into recovery, resulting in a sustained leukocytosis (up to 24 hours). In contrast, lymphocyte counts may fall below pre-exercise values in recovery. Figure 100-1 provides an indication of the relative percentage changes in blood leukocyte (Figure 100-1A) and lymphocyte subpopulations (Figure 100-1B) in response to prolonged intense exercise.

Neutrophils

PMNs are the most abundant leukocytes in the blood compartment and are potent phagocytic cells. In response to chemotactic signals, they are among the first cells to arrive at sites of tissue inflammation (11). They play an important role in ingesting and killing microbes and in the regulation of the inflammatory process. They also may cause tissue damage through the release of toxic granules. Exercise induces a neu-

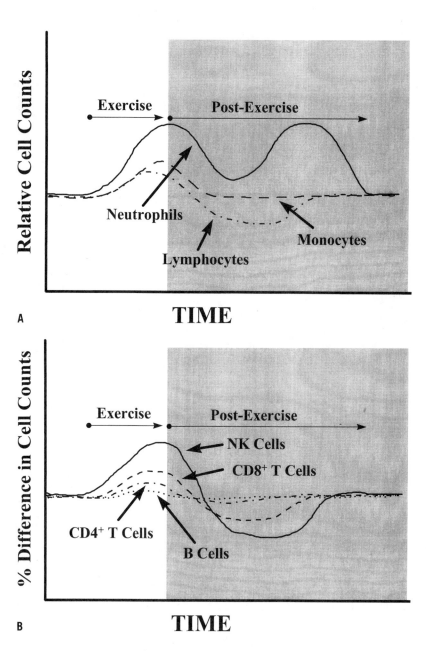

Figure 100-1 The effects of prolonged, intense exercise on blood leukocyte (A) and lymphocyte subsets (B).

trophilia of approximately 20% to 60% regardless of exercise intensity between the ranges of 40% to 100% Vo₂max (9,10). However, there is some evidence suggesting a dose-dependent increase such that at very low exercise intensities there is no increase in PMNs (12,13). Different exercise modes (i.e., running, cycling, weight lifting), at the same exercise intensity, all appear to result in similar responses. In general, intense long-duration exercise leads to very large (100% to 400%) increases in blood PMN numbers. PMN number may drop to pre-exercise values within 30 minutes postexercise, but often a rise occurs in the recovery period (9), leading to a characteristic biphasic response.

It has been hypothesized that the initial rise in PMN number is due to demargination of PMNs that were adhered to the vascular endothelium, especially in the lungs (9,14). This demargination is thought to occur due to exercise-induced increases in blood pressure, perfusion, and the pro-duction of catecholamines that tend to decrease leukocyte adhesion (9,15). The second more prolonged peak in PMNs in recovery is thought to be due to the delayed influence of cortisol and other inflammatory mediators (e.g., complement split products, cytokines) on bone marrow PMN production and may account for the large increases in PMNs seen immediately after long-duration exercise (9,10).

Lymphocytes

Lymphocytes are specialized leukocytes involved in the generation of specificity and immunologic memory. They are central to the recovery from infectious disease and the outbreak of neoplastic cells. They can be broadly categorized as either B or T lymphocytes. B lymphocytes are cells that produce soluble protein antibodies involved in humoral immunity, whereas T lymphocytes recognize antigen through unique T-cell receptors (TCRs) on their cell surface and are involved in cell-mediated immunity (CMI).

T Lymphocytes

T cells are characterized by the expression of CD3 (a molecule associated with the antigen-specific TCR) and exist as several distinct subsets, each having different physiologic roles. Helper T cells are defined as expressing CD4 (a molecule associated with the TCR that recognizes major histocompatibility complex (MHC) II on antigen-presenting cells) on their cell surface. These cells are important in recognizing antigen and secreting immune regulatory cytokines. Two main subclasses of CD4$^+$ cells have recently been identified. T$_{H1}$ CD4$^+$ cells act as proinflammatory cells and promote CMI by secreting the cytokines interleukin-2 (IL-2), which drives T-cell proliferation, and IL-12 and IFN-γ, which activate natural killer (NK) cells and macrophages (MΦ's). T$_{H2}$ CD4$^+$ cells promote humoral immunity by secreting IL-4, IL-5, IL-6, and IL-10, which cause the maturation of B lymphocytes into antibody-producing plasma cells. These responses are reciprocally regulated in that T$_{H1}$ cytokines can down-regulate T$_{H2}$ cytokine production and vice versa, thus polarizing the immune response toward either CMI or humoral immunity. CD8$^+$ T cells (CD8 recognizes MHC I) are either cytotoxic cells (high expressors of CD28) or suppressor cells (high expressors of CD11b). Cytotoxic T cells play an important role in combating intracellular pathogens such as viruses and play a role similar to the NK cell, except that they have a unique specificity. Suppressor cells provide feedback countering the actions of helper T cells.

Short-term exercise (<1 hour) of various intensities (moderate to severe) results in an immediate increase (up to 150%) in the total number of T cells in the circulation when measured during and immediately after exercise (10). During recovery from such exercise, the number of T cells quickly (<30 minutes) returns to baseline and, in some instances, falls below the pre-exercise values, especially if the exercise was intense. Following prolonged (>1 hour) intense exercise, T-lymphocyte counts are generally decreased, especially in recovery (16). During and immediately following short-term exercise, there is a small increase (0% to 40%) in the CD4$^+$ cell count with a correspondingly larger (50% to 150%) increase in the CD8$^+$ cell count that is especially sensitive to increasing exercise intensities. These effects lead to a decrease in the CD4$^+$/CD8$^+$ ratio (~20%) (17). Although a definitive role for epinephrine in exercise-induced increases in CD4$^+$ and CD8$^+$ T cells has yet to be substantiated, it is interesting to note that CD8$^+$ cells have an increased β_2-adrenergic receptor density when compared to CD4$^+$ cells (18).

In recovery, CD4$^+$ T cells decline somewhat below baseline, whereas CD8$^+$ T cells tend to decline more (10). It has been suggested that perhaps CD8$^+$ cells are either sequestered in secondary lymphoid organs or mobilized to damaged muscle tissue in the postexercise recovery period. Immediately after prolonged exercise CD4$^+$ and CD8$^+$ counts are depressed relative to pre-exercise values. There is little evidence concerning the effect of exercise on T$_{H1}$ and T$_{H2}$ cell subsets most probably because of a lack of definitive cell surface markers to be used in identification. Rhind et al (19) suggest, however, that exercise has the potential to shift the T-cell cytokine response toward a T$_{H2}$ phenotype because of the potential negative influence of glucocorticoids on T$_{H1}$ responses.

In addition to the variety of subsets, T cells (CD4$^+$ or CD8$^+$ cells) exist as either naive or memory cells. CD45 or leukocyte common antigen consists of a group of high molecular weight glycoproteins that are selectively expressed on the surface of leukocytes in different isoforms and act as accessory molecules in cellular activation, perhaps by interacting with ligands on other cells (20). In humans, naive cells are cells that have not yet come in contact with specific antigen and express CD45RA on their cell surfaces (21). In contrast, memory cells have been exposed to specific antigen and express CD45RO (21). Double positives (i.e., CD45RA$^+$RO$^+$) are thought to be in transition to a memory phenotype. Analysis of these subsets is important for it is thought that accumulation of memory cells may lead to immunosuppression and inability to respond to new challenges, as is the case in aged individuals (22). In addition, because memory and naive cells are typically stored in different anatomic sites and have distinct patterns of recirculation (23), study of these subsets may shed light on which tissues are being affected by exercise in terms of cell mobilization.

Unfortunately, to date, few studies have examined memory and naive lymphocyte numbers. Following brief high-intensity exercise, Gabriel et al (24) found that naive (CD45RO$^-$) CD8$^+$ cells increased most dramatically when compared to memory (CD45RO$^+$) CD8$^+$ cells or memory or naive CD4$^+$ cells. In another study by this same group (25), a prolonged bout (12 hours) of endurance exercise increased the number of CD4$^+$ and CD8$^+$ CD45RA$^+$RO$^+$, but not CD45RA$^-$RO$^+$, cells when measured at rest 8 days later. They concluded that the endurance exercise bout caused T-cell activation that would ultimately lead to an increased memory cell population. In contrast, Gannon et al (26) found that CD4$^+$ T cells mobilized to the blood during prolonged, intense exercise are predominantly (~80%) CD45RA$^-$RO$^+$, whereas equal percentages (CD45RA$^+$RO$^-$ and CD45RA$^-$RO$^+$) of CD8$^+$ cells were mobilized.

The increase in T lymphocytes that occurs during and immediately following exercise is thought to be mediated by mechanisms similar to those that induce neutrophilia (i.e., demargination). A role for exercise-induced increases in mean arterial pressure, perfusion, and catecholamines have all been suggested. Regarding epinephrine, it is interesting to note that CD8$^+$ T cells are more sensitive to exercise intensity than are CD4$^+$ cells, both in terms of the exercise-induced cell increases and postexercise decreases. This coupled with the fact that CD8$^+$ cells express higher levels of β_2-adrenergic receptors when compared to CD4$^+$ T cells suggests involvement of a mechanism whereby exercise-induced increases in epinephrine alter leukocyte-endothelial cell interactions. The mechanism behind the postexercise decrease in T lymphocytes is unclear.

B Lymphocytes

B lymphocytes are commonly characterized by the expression of CD19 and are involved in antigen recognition with subsequent antibody production and antigen presentation to T cells. When compared to other leukocyte types, CD19$^+$ B cells demonstrate the least amount of change in response to exercise (10). A number of reports have documented no change in peripheral blood B-cell count in response to various exercise modalities of different intensities and durations (27,28), whereas other studies (typically employing prolonged intense exercise) (16,29) have shown subtle (<50%) increases. Although B cells have a high density of β-adrenergic receptors, they fail to generate appreciable cyclic adenosine monophosphate (AMP) upon epinephrine exposure (30), which may explain the failure of exercise to mobilize this population of marginating cells.

Natural Killer Cells

Natural Killer (NK) cells consist of a subset of large granular lymphocytes that exhibit a high ratio of cytoplasm to nucleus and spontaneous (non-MHC-restricted) cytotoxic activity against a wide variety of virally infected and tumor cells (31). Upon stimulation with IL-2, IL-12, or IFN-γ they become even more potent lytic effector cells (32). Although controversy exists (33), NK cells express a characteristic set of cell surface markers (CD3$^-$, CD2$^+$, CD16$^+$, and CD56$^+$).

NK cells have been the most extensively studied cells in exercise immunologic literature. A threshold exercise intensity corresponding to 30% to 40% Vo$_2$max is required to significantly increase blood NK-cell numbers (34). Above this threshold, the increase in NK-cell numbers is correlated with increasing exercise intensity regardless of subject fitness level, such that at maximal exercise elevations in NK-cell numbers can be two- to fivefold higher than pre-exercise values, contributing substantially to the overall lymphocytosis (34,35). Resistance exercise also increases NK-cell numbers (36). NK cells have the highest density of β$_2$-adrenergic receptors (versus CD8$^+$ > CD4$^+$ T cells), which may explain why blood counts increase during high-intensity exercise when concentrations of epinephrine are high (18). Epinephrine, by decreasing the adhesive interactions between NK cells and endothelial cells, can induce recruitment of NK cells from the marginating to the circulating pool (37). Indeed, administration of epinephrine at doses similar to exercise-induced levels causes similar changes in NK-cell numbers (38), and β-blockade has been shown to reduce NK-cell mobilization in response to other stressors (39).

The post-exercise increase in NK cells is transient and within 30 minutes NK cells exit the circulation, probably under the influence of cortisol (40,41), with the lowest values occurring 30 minutes to 3 hours postexercise. This decrease in NK-cell numbers below pre-exercise values may persist up to 24 hours postexercise following prolonged intense exercise (16,42). Immediately following long-term (>90 minutes duration), high-intensity exercise, little increase in blood NK-cell counts is seen, most likely due to high plasma cortisol levels that counteract epinephrine-induced NK-cell recruitment (43). At present, the tissue destination of the NK cells that egress from the blood after exercise is unknown.

Monocytes

Monocytes (Mo's) are mononuclear leukocytes that are produced in the bone marrow, stored briefly, and released into the circulation in response to a variety of signals including colony-stimulating factors and IL-3 (44). In the blood they function as phagocytic cells, producers of cytokines, antigen presenters, and regulators of blood clotting. However, Mo's are actually immature cells that are in transit to tissues. When they reach these sites, they mature into larger more functionally capable MΦ's.

Exercise-induced monocytosis is more highly related to exercise intensity than neutrophilia, such that low-intensity exercise gives rise to a small (~30% to 50%) monocytosis, whereas intense exercise results in a substantial (~50% to 150%) monocytosis (10). Very prolonged exercise results in still higher counts (~75% to 200%). The rise in Mo's is quite transient, returning to baseline levels within 30 minutes if the exercise bout is not too intense or prolonged. Mo numbers may even fall below baseline in the ensuing hours of recovery (45). The mechanisms responsible for this exercise-induced monocytosis are unclear, but are likely similar to the ones outlined above for PMNs and lymphocytes (i.e., demargination and mobilization from extravascular sites). Indeed, Kappel et al (38) could mimic the exercise-induced increase in Mo number by infusing epinephrine. Interestingly, Gabriel et al (46) found a postexercise decrease in Mo's bearing high levels of the adhesion molecule LFA-1 (CD11a/CD18) when compared to low expressors. They speculated that exercise increased mature Mo (high expressors of adhesion molecules) trafficking into tissues like damaged muscle. Evidence to support this contention comes from studies showing increases in mononuclear phagocyte staining in cross sections of exercised damaged muscle (47,48). Comparisons of exercise-induced changes in Mo numbers among people of different fitness levels reveal no significant differences (10).

Eosinophils and Basophils

Both eosinophils and basophils constitute a small fraction of peripheral blood leukocytes. Eosinophils are large granular cells involved in phagocytosis. Brief exercise (<30 minutes) leads to increases (10% to 100%) in eosinophils regardless of exercise intensity, whereas prolonged exercise usually results in decreases (~–50%) when compared to pre-exercise values (10). Likewise, the decrease in eosinophils may persist into the recovery period. Basophils play a role in acute allergic and inflammatory reactions. Exercise either results in a small increase in circulating basophils or has no effect (10).

Mechanisms, Physiologic Significance, and Future Directions

Several questions arise when reviewing the literature surrounding acute exercise-induced leukocytosis and immune cell trafficking. First, *from what source are the leukocytes being mobilized into the blood and what are the mechanisms involved in their mobilization?* The possible sources include: 1) cells attached to the vascular endothelium of various organs (marginating cells), 2) cells housed in secondary lymphoid organs (i.e., spleen, lymph nodes) or lymphatic vessels, or 3) cells housed in primary lymphoid organs (i.e., bone marrow, thymus). Because of the rapid nature of the response and the fact that hormones such as epinephrine can decrease leukocyte-endothelial cell interactions, most evidence suggests that most cells are coming from the marginating pool. Baum et al (49) and others (9) found that exercise induced a similar leukocytosis in splenectomized patients when compared to controls, thus ruling out the spleen as a major contributor to exercise-induced leukocytosis. However, more studies need to be performed to elucidate which organ(s) are responsible for the release of leukocytes. Likewise, exercise studies using β-antagonists need to be performed to definitively determine the role of epinephrine in exercise-induced leukocytosis.

Second, *where are the mobilized cells going?* Are they being mobilized to exercise-induced areas of tissue damage? Some evidence suggests an infiltration of leukocytes into muscle tissue, especially following eccentric exercise (48). Or are the cells migrating back to the marginal pool? Future studies focusing on cellular adhesion molecules and histochemistry may be able to shed light on this area. A common finding in many of the studies is that in the postexercise period there is an apparent loss of some cell subsets from the circulation, particularly NK cells and CD8$^+$ T cells. Why are these cells being selectively depleted from the circulation?

Lastly, *what is the physiologic significance of acute exercise-induced leukocytosis and cell trafficking?* Do transient changes in blood leukocyte numbers play any role in host protection against disease reflecting a heightened state of readiness? Or are the changes due to the need to "clean up" debris resulting from exercise-induced tissue (muscle) damage. Clearly, changes in peripheral blood leukocyte numbers do not permit a direct assessment of integrated host defense. However, analysis of such a response may aid in the understanding of the role of stress hormones on immune cell trafficking. Perhaps a more relevant question pertains to whether or not chronic exercise increases subset specific leukocyte production from tissues such as bone marrow or removal via apoptosis.

Other Sites

Animal models have aided in garnering information concerning the effects of exercise on leukocyte numbers in tissues other than blood. Analysis of sites other than blood is vital to a comprehensive understanding of how exercise affects immunity because only a small fraction of leukocytes are present in blood at any given time. Indeed, it could be argued that tissues such as the thymus, spleen, and lymph nodes are actually more important to analyze than blood because of their role in leukocyte production and differentiation. Unfortunately, very few studies have focused on these tissues, perhaps because of their relative inaccessibility in humans.

Thymus

The thymus gland is the primary lymphoid organ responsible for the maturation of T lymphocytes. Upon entry into the thymus, T cells lack critical markers (TCR, CD3, CD4, CD8) that characterize mature T cells. Because they lack CD4 and CD8, these immature cells are called *double negative cells*. In the process of maturation, these cells acquire a double positive (CD4$^+$/CD8$^+$) phenotype and also express low levels of CD3 and the TCR. At this point, cells with a high affinity for self-molecules are deleted (i.e., negative selection). Another important positive selection occurs when T cells that can recognize self-MHC molecules with low to intermediate affinity are retained. These cells mature into single positive CD4 or CD8 T lymphocytes and emigrate from the thymus into the periphery (50).

In early studies, Hoffman-Goetz et al (51) found that an acute bout of exhaustive exercise in mice decreased total T-cell numbers in the thymus due to a reduction in T cytotoxic/suppressor (Lyt2$^+$), but not T helper (L3T4$^+$) cells. Two consecutive days of exhaustive exercise in 4-week trained rats was found to decrease total thymocyte numbers by 75% (52). This reduction was mainly due to decreases in the CD4$^+$CD8$^+$ population of cells, but reductions in double negative and single positive populations were also seen. The researchers also injected dexamethasone and found similar but greater effects, suggesting, perhaps, that exercise-induced increases in glucocorticoids were responsible for the observed changes. Glucocorticoids are known to cause programmed cell death or apoptosis, especially in rodent lymphocytes (53). In a follow-up study, Concordet et al (54) found that administration of the glucocorticoid antagonist RU-486 in rats could block the acute exercise-induced apoptosis of thymocytes. It is unknown if exercise results in a loss of thymocytes in humans.

Spleen and Lymph Nodes

The spleen is the largest lymphoid organ, containing about 25% of the body's lymphocytes. It consists of two regions. The red pulp functions as a filter, removing particulate matter and damaged erythrocytes from the circulation. The white pulp constitutes the major initiator of immune responses against blood-borne antigens and serves as a microenvironment for the development of immune responses. Lymph nodes are located at strategic locations throughout the body and, like the spleen, serve as a microenvironment for the development of specific immune responses.

Hoffman-Goetz et al (51,55) found no alteration in the absolute numbers or percentages of total T cells or T helper or T suppressor cells in the spleens or lymph nodes of exhaustively exercised mice. Lin et al (56) found no changes in total cell numbers or percentages of CD3$^+$, CD4$^+$, CD8$^+$, or B cells in spleens of moderately run rats. However, there was a small decrease in total cell numbers and CD8$^+$ and B-cell subsets after exhaustive running. Likewise, Bouix et al (57) found decreases in total splenocytes, splenic PMNs, and splenic CD4$^+$ cells in rats swum to exhaustion (~2.5 hours). Therefore, it appears that there can be a reduction in specific populations of splenocytes in response to exhaustive, but not moderate, exercise. Clearly, more studies need to be performed.

Sites of Inflammation

Unfortunately, few studies have analyzed the effects of exercise on the cellular response to inflammation or other immune challenges. Assessment of this response may be more physiologically relevant than assessment of exercise-induced changes in cell populations in the spleen or blood because they represent the host-pathogen interface. In response to an intraperitoneal (i.p.) injection of the sterile inflammatory agent thioglycolate, Woods et al (58) found no significant differences in mouse peritoneal exudate number or the percentage of MΦ's in response to moderate or exhaustive exercise over the 3-day inflammatory process. In contrast, this same group (59,60) documented a significant decrease in MΦ number and MHC II expression in response to i.p. injection of heat-killed

Propionibacterium acnes after exhaustive, but not moderate, exercise in mice. Along these same lines, daily moderate, but not exhaustive, exercise increased the number and activity of phagocytic cells (i.e., MΦ's) in tumors obtained from mice 14 days after inoculation (61). Taken together, these data suggest that exercise may affect cellular inflammation in an intensity- and inflammatory-stimulus–dependent fashion. Although untested, exhaustive exercise may act in an anti-inflammatory manner, perhaps because of the effects of glucocorticoids.

LEUKOCYTE FUNCTION IN RESPONSE TO ACUTE EXERCISE

Influence of Changes in Blood Leukocyte Numbers on Functional Assays

The effects of moderate and intense exercise on a wide range of leukocyte functions have been reported. Table 100-1 summarizes some of the salient findings. It should be noted, however, that the results of functional assays are dependent not only on the functional activity of each individual leukocyte in the assay but also on the number of leukocytes (or particular subsets) in the assay. Because exercise has a profound affect on leukocyte distribution, cell number needs to be accounted for in order to interpret data from functional assays. Some studies have expressed functional data on a per-cell basis; unfortunately, the majority of studies have not. In addition, the function of one cell type may be affected by the number or functional activity of other cell subsets in the assay sample. Therefore, in order to best interpret functional data, potential influencing cells should be quantified and their influences tested. This has not been done in most studies; in fact, all the regulatory influences on most immune function assays have yet to be identified.

Lymphocyte Function
Mitogenesis

Because cell division is central to the effectiveness of lymphocyte-mediated immunity, one of the most common ways to assess lymphocyte function is to measure the ability of lymphocytes to proliferate. This has been done predominantly in vitro using stimuli such as polyclonal mitogens [concanavalin A (Con A), phytohemagglutinin (PHA)]; however, at least one study has utilized in vivo delayed-type hypersensitivity responses to recall antigens (62) as a means of assessing CMI.

There is a large literature on the effects of acute (single bout) exercise on in vitro T-lymphocyte mitogenesis in response to Con A and PHA. Human isolated peripheral blood mononuclear cell (PBMC) or whole blood mitogenic responsiveness transiently decreases 30% to 60% following (up to 4 hours after) acute moderate or intense exercise (27,29,63–65). This suppressant effect does not vary greatly among individuals of different fitness levels and is greater following intense exercise when compared to moderate exercise (64). Some have shown no suppression due to moderate exercise (66). The exercise-induced changes in lymphocyte proliferation are thought to be largely due to exercise-induced decreases in the number of responsive cells (i.e., CD3+, CD4+, CD8+) in peripheral blood samples (65). However, intense exercise may also suppresses T-lymphocyte mitogenesis independently of cell number and although the mechanisms are unknown, it is believed that exercise-induced increases in immunosuppressive hormones like glucocorticoids or epinephrine may be responsible (27). Others argue that postexercise Mo production of prostaglandin E_2 (PGE_2) depresses T-cell responsiveness to mitogens (67). Whatever the mechanism, it is apparent that there is a decreased capacity for lymphocyte proliferation in blood following exercise.

Table 100-1 Effects of Acute Moderate and Exhaustive Exercise on Various Functional Measures of Immunity

IMMUNE MEASURE	MODERATE EXERCISE	EXHAUSTIVE EXERCISE
Lymphocyte Functions	↔ Proliferation	↓ Proliferation ↓ In vivo DTH response
Antibody Levels	↔ Serum antibodies	↔ Serum antibodies ↔ Antibody titre postvaccination ↓ salivary IgA
PMN Functions	↑ ROS production ↑ Chemotaxis ↑ Phagocytosis ↑ Microbial killing	↑ Phagocytosis (blood) ↓ ROS production ↓ Microbial killing ↓ Phagocytosis (airways)
NK Cell Function	↓ Tumor killing (during exercise)	↑ Tumor killing (during exercise) ↓ Tumor killing (postexercise)
Mo/Mφ Functions	↑ Chemotaxis ↑ Phagocytosis ↑ Tumor killing	↑ Chemotaxis ↑ Phagocytosis ↑ Tumor killing ↓ Antiviral activity (lung) ↓ MHC expression
Cytokine Levels	↔ Most cytokines	↑ Proinflammatory cytokines (IL-6, TNF-α, IL-1) ↓ Cytokine levels in response to stimulation

Because in vitro tests may not always provide accurate measures of host defense, Bruunsgaard et al (62) measured in vivo CMI (by way of delayed hypersensitivity skin tests to various antigens) in a group of triathletes following a 6.5-hour triathlon. They found that although the numbers of positive indurations were similar between those having competed in the triathlon and resting triathletes or sedentary controls, the exercisers demonstrated significantly reduced skin test scores (sum of diameters of indurations) especially for tuberculin and tetanus antigens. This lends evidence to the contention that prolonged intense exercise may result in immunosuppression.

Antibody Concentrations

The functional activity of B cells is usually assessed by their in vitro production of antibody or immunoglobulin (Ig) or by assessing serum or mucosal Ig levels. Few studies have examined the role of exercise in specific antibody production such as after a vaccination.

The effects of acute exercise on in vitro Ig synthesis are equivocal (68). Hedfors et al (69) and Tvede et al (70) have reported decreased production of IgA, IgM, and IgG in response to pokeweed mitogen and other factors after both moderate (69) and intense (70) exercise. Although the mechanisms for this decrease are unknown, Hedfors believed that the postexercise reduction in the percentage of $CD4^+$ helper cells reduced the ability of B cells to respond appropriately. Tvede et al documented that removal of Mo's or addition of indomethacin (which blocks PGE_2 production) could restore depressed antibody production, suggesting that Mo production of PGE_2 was responsible. In contrast, Mackinnon et al (71) failed to detect any reduction in antibody synthesis following a 2-hour bout of exercise performed at 70% to 80% Vo_2max. However, this latter study used trained athletes, whereas the previous two studies used untrained individuals. It may be that the suppression of antibody production is only seen after exercise in those who are unaccustomed to it.

Small or no differences in serum Ig concentrations have been reported after either moderate or intense exercise over a wide range of durations (68,72). For example, serum IgA, IgM, IgG, and IgE were all unchanged in men distance runners following a 12.8-km run at 70% to 80% Vo_2max (71). In some studies small (<20%) increases in some classes of Ig have been reported, and these differences have been attributed mainly to hemoconcentration brought about by a reduction in plasma volume following acute exercise (72). In some cases hemoconcentration cannot explain the modest increases in Ig seen postexercise; therefore other mechanisms such as systemic endotoxemia or influx of antibody from lymph or extravascular pools (72) have been put forth.

Gross levels of Ig in blood and tissue are likely not to give valuable information relative to the host's ability to mount an antigen-specific antibody response. Only two studies have examined the effect of acute exercise on the production of antibodies to defined antigens (62,73). It should be noted however, that acute exercise studies are confounded by the fact that antibody response takes time to develop, during which time further bouts of exercise may take place. Eskola et al (73) inoculated four runners with tetanus toxoid immediately after a marathon run, measured antitetanus antibody

titres 14 days later, and compared the response with nonexercising controls. They found no impairment in antibody titres and concluded that intense exercise had no effect on the development of humoral immunity. Likewise, Bruunsgaard et al (62) demonstrated that the antibody titres (measured 14 days postexercise) to diptheria, tetanus, and pneumococcal antigens were no different in athletes injected after a 6.5-hour triathlon when compared to inoculated nonexercising triathletes or sedentary controls. Therefore, unlike T-cell function and CMI, it appears that B-cell function is not impaired by acute bouts of exercise.

The secretory immune system is important in the protection of mucosal surfaces such as the eyes, nose, and respiratory tracts. In light of epidemiologic evidence that intense, prolonged exercise increases incidence of URTI and the fact that low levels of secretory IgA correlate with increased URTI incidence (68), analysis of this system is relevant. The humoral immune response of mucosal surfaces is mediated by antibodies of the IgA subclass. Secretory IgA inhibits attachment of viruses and bacteria to host cells and opsonizes microorganisms for rapid clearance.

Several studies have noted 25% to 65% decreases in salivary IgA when expressed micrograms per milligram or milliter of protein in response to nordic ski racing for 2 to 3 hours (74), running competitions of 20 minutes to 3 hours (75,76), controlled cycling for 2 hours (71), kayaking (77), or sprint interval training (75). In general studies that have failed to detect changes in salivary IgA in response to exercise have failed to adjust IgA concentrations for changes in salivary protein or albumin (68). Indeed, it is known that exercise, in a dose-dependent manner, will reduce saliva flow rates, which may lead to an artificial elevation in salivary IgA. In contrast, moderate exercise does not appear to alter IgA concentration or secretion rate (68). For example, McDowell et al (76) found no change in salivary IgA after 15 to 45 minutes of treadmill running at 60% Vo_2max. Taken together these studies indicate that salivary IgA concentration and secretion rates decline after intense and/or prolonged exercise and this effect may last for several hours.

Neutrophil Function

PMNs play an important role in the nonspecific killing of infectious agents, especially bacteria. PMN uptake of pathogens by phagocytosis triggers a series of non-oxygen- and oxygen-dependent processes, creating an extremely hostile environment that damages and ultimately destroys ingested microbes (78). However, PMNs have also been implicated in the pathology of various inflammatory diseases by release of their toxic products into the extracellular environment. PMNs are the first immune cells to be recruited to sites of infection or inflammation, exhibiting an orchestrated sequence of events including endothelial adherence, diapedesis, chemotaxis and migration, and phagocytosis. PMN functional assays involve isolations of these cells from a blood sample followed by assessment of a particular function in vitro. The PMNs are usually incubated in the absence or presence of a specific stimulus such as bacteria or their products, chemotactic peptides, or other nonphysiologic agents that activate biochemical cascades.

Contrasting responses in PMN function have been

reported after moderate exercise. The findings so far suggest that although some functional responses are enhanced, others are not affected significantly. Although some studies show that the capacity of PMNs to generate microbicidal reactive oxygen species (ROS) and kill ingested microbes is enhanced following exercise (79–81), others have reported a temporary suppression (82,83). In general, most studies have found that moderate exercise leads to increases in PMN chemotaxis and phagocytosis (84). Others have reported that the expression of certain cell surface molecules increases after exercise (81,85), although the functional significance of these changes is unknown, this provides further evidence that PMNs are affected by moderate exercise.

In contrast to moderate exercise, the reported responses to maximal exercise are more consistent. With the exception of phagocytosis and degranulation, which increase in response to both moderate and intense exercise, most PMN functions decrease significantly after a single bout of intense exercise. The capacity of PMNs to generate ROS in response to stimulation is suppressed immediately following intense exercise (80,86–88). Several groups have shown that progressive exercise to exhaustion increases phagocytic capacity (89,90). Since evidence of degranulation (i.e., elastase activity increase in plasma) has been found after maximal and prolonged exercise (91), and given that degranulation is indicative of PMN activation in vivo, it is possible that activated cells will not respond to secondary stimulation until a certain recovery time has elapsed. In other words, PMNs may be in a refractory state in the period following intense exercise because they were activated during exercise. Several studies have shown a suppression in the oxidative burst immediately following exercise (83,89,90). Since the magnitude of degranulation is proportional to run distance (92), it is likely that the majority of the PMN population is in an unresponsive state after maximal exercise. This postexercise refractory period may create a window of opportunity for opportunistic infections to become established.

In summary, although conflicting results have been found, blood PMN responses to a single episode of exercise are, in general, intensity-dependent. Although exercise at low to moderate intensity enhances some aspects of PMN function, maximal exercise is generally suppressive. Irrespective of these trends, the release of elastase and other degradative enzymes into the circulation in response to both moderate and intense exercise indicates that acute exercise has affected the PMN population.

One group has examined PMN function in the upper respiratory system in response to exercise. Muns (93) found that a 20-km race resulted in a 1.5- to 2-fold increase in the number of PMNs obtained by nasal lavage immediately and 1 day after the race. Interestingly, the phagocytic activity of these PMNs (including the percentage of phagocytizing cells and ingestion on a per-cell basis) was reduced approximately by half for up to 1 day after the run (93). It may be that exercise recruits hyporesponsive PMNs to the upper respiratory tract. In a subsequent study, they found that the in vitro chemotactic activity of PMNs obtained from nasal lavage was increased after a marathon run (94), which may explain the elevated numbers of PMNs in nasal secretions postexercise. These findings suggest that strenuous exercise impairs upper airway antimicrobial defense and may contribute to the higher incidence of URTI in the periods after strenuous exercise.

Natural Killer Cell Function

Much of the work on NK cells has focused on their ability to lyse target cells that have undergone malignant transformation (95). The "gold standard" measure for NK cell activity (NKCA) has been the chromium release assay, using cultured tumor cells (usually NK-sensitive K562 cells) labeled with ^{51}Cr as targets and peripheral blood mononuclear cells (PBMCs) isolated from blood as effectors. Cytokines, especially IFN-α, IFN-γ, IL-2, and IL-12 are efficient activators of NKCA.

Exercise affects unstimulated NK cell activity, and the magnitude and time course of these responses depend upon the intensity and duration of exercise (34). Acute moderate and exhaustive exercise appear to have a biphasic effect on human peripheral blood NK cell cytolytic activity, such that during and immediately after exercise there is a 50% to 100% increase in activity, followed later (1 to 6 hours) by a suppression when compared to pre-exercise values (27,96). The suppression after exhaustive exercise is greater than that manifested after moderate exercise. Immediately following long-duration, high-intensity exercise bouts, no increase in NKCA is seen, and the drop in NKCA during recovery is greater and more sustained than with bouts lasting less than 1 hour (40,42,97,98). Adjustment for changes in NK cell concentration completely eliminates this increase in NKCA during and immediately postexercise (40). Unresolved are issues involving destination sites for NK-cell trafficking activity, whether blood compartment NK cells reflect the NKCA capacity of other lymphoid sites, and overall effects on host protection (96).

Unfortunately, few exercise studies have examined the effects of exercise on the ability of cytokines to stimulate NK cells. Nielsen et al (99) found that maximal exercise (e.g., rowing) increased Lymphokine Activated Killer (LAK) cell activity twofold (when compared to pre-exercise), despite a threefold increase in NK cell number in competitive athletes. They believed that this reflected an exercise-induced recruitment of immature NK cells having low IFN or IL-2 responsiveness. Woods et al (100) demonstrated that, while INF-α augmented NKCA in both the pre– and post–maximal-exercise samples from young and old subjects, the percentage increase in NKCA in the postexercise samples was smaller than in the pre-exercise samples. They reasoned that this could have resulted from a "ceiling effect" at the high E:T ratios or high basal killing in the unstimulated samples, or exercise may have induced recruitment of NK cells that lacked IFN-α sensitivity, perhaps recruiting immature NK cells. Alternatively, exercise may have recruited NK cells that were already highly cytotoxic. Further study, perhaps using the CD56$^+$CD57$^-$ (immature NK cell) or CD56$^+$CD57$^+$ (mature NK cell) NK markers (101), is required to resolve this issue.

Although most researchers agree that the immediate postexercise increase in NKCA is due to the recruitment of NK cells into the circulation, they tend to disagree on the reasons for the transient NKCA decrease during recovery. Some researchers believe that the decrease is related to numerical shifts in NK cells (29,40,65), whereas others report that prostaglandins from activated monocytes and neutrophils (96) suppress the ability of NK cells to function appropriately. Both in vitro and in vivo studies have failed to demonstrate that epinephrine has an effect on NKCA beyond its effect on redistributing mononuclear cell subsets (38). Whatever the reason, the loss of NK cells from the circulation following exercise means that the blood compartment as a whole suffers a transient decrease in NKCA capacity.

Mo and Mϕ Function

Although it is clear that acute exercise can increase the number of Mo's in peripheral blood, much less information is available regarding exercise-induced changes in Mo function, perhaps because of their relatively small numbers in blood. In response to 30 minutes of graded exercise to exhaustion, blood Mo's exhibited increased glucose uptake and oxidative metabolism (102). In another study, acute maximal exercise had no effect on blood Mo adherence (103).

Much more information is available regarding the effects of acute exercise on Mϕ's from various tissue sources (i.e., peritoneal cavity, lung). Most of these studies have been performed in rodents with one exception (104). Both acute moderate and exhaustive exercise have been shown by several groups, and in several different species, to enhance a variety of Mo and Mϕ capacities including chemotaxis (104–106), adherence (107,108), oxidative metabolism (108), and phagocytic activity (104,105,107–110). Woods et al (58,61) have shown that both moderate and exhaustive treadmill running increases the antitumor cytotoxic activity of murine peritoneal Mϕ's. This effect was not due to altered numbers of Mϕ's in the assay system but was attributable in part to increased production of TNF-α and nitric oxide. In a similar study, Lotzerich et al (111) found that the cytostatic activity, but not antibody-dependent cytolytic activity, of murine peritoneal Mϕ's was enhanced after a single exhaustive running session. It is important to note that the results of the two studies are consistent despite the fact that different strains of mice, tumor targets, and exercise protocols were used. Moreover, these results indicated that this increase in Mϕ activity took place in the face of elevated corticosterone, a hormone known to suppress Mϕ functions (53). Therefore, in general, exercise is different from other stressors (i.e., psychological) that tend to suppress peritoneal Mϕ functions caused by stress-induced elevations in adrenal steroids (112). In contrast, Woods et al (60) demonstrated that peritoneal Mϕ MHC II expression in response to inflammation is reduced following exhaustive, but not moderate, treadmill running in mice. This raises the possibility that exercise affects different measures of Mϕ function differently.

Recent studies of Davis et al (5,113) have analyzed the role of exercise on the ability of alveolar Mϕ's to inhibit viral replication and tumor metastasis. Treadmill exercise to fatigue in mice resulted in greater morbidity and mortality due to herpes simplex virus 1 (HSV 1) infection when compared to sedentary or moderately exercised mice. This observation correlated with reduced in vitro alveolar Mϕ anti-HSV 1 resistance. In contrast, exhaustive exercise resulted in a reduction in the retention of B16 melanoma cells in the lungs of mice when compared to sedentary or moderately exercised mice. This correlated with an increased ability of alveolar Mϕ's to inhibit B16 growth in vitro (113). Taken together, these complex data suggest that exercise has intensity-related effects on various Mϕ functions depending on the function measured, the immune challenge introduced, and the tissue source of Mϕ's.

Cytokines

Cytokines are hormones produced by immune cells that regulate both local immune and systemic functions and are likely to provide a missing link between immunology and physiology. They are diverse in nature and act on a wide variety of cells and tissues, exerting positive or negative influences. In a broad sense, they can be classified into proinflammatory (i.e., IL-1, IL-6, TNF-α) or anti-inflammatory (i.e., IL-4, IL-10, TGF-β) categories. Assessment of the effects of acute exercise have included measurement of in vitro cytokine production from human PBMCs and plasma, urine, and tissue cytokine concentrations.

Interestingly, physical exercise has been shown to increase plasma and urine levels and in vitro PBMC production of a number of cytokines, the most consistent and quantifiably largest being IL-6 (114–123). IL-6 is a multifunctional cytokine produced in large amounts by Mo's and Mϕ's and to a lesser extent by T lymphocytes, fibroblasts, and vascular endothelial cells (124). IL-6 has been described as an "alarm hormone" whose productions is increased by events such as infection, inflammation, and tissue damage.

Initial studies revealed that plasma and PBMC supernatants from exercised subjects contained a factor that induced fever (endogenous pyrogen) in rats (114). This pyrogenic effect was later attributed to IL-1 by the use of column chromatography and the murine thymocyte bioassay (115). This same group detected an increase in plasma IL-1 bioactivity in humans in response to unaccustomed eccentric exercise (125). They suggested that elevated IL-1 may promote the apparent acute phase response seen following high-intensity and/or damaging exercise. However, unbeknownst to them at the time, it was later found that the murine thymocyte bioassay and fever induction could also be attributable to the presence of IL-6 in their samples. In fact, it was later suggested that IL-6 was actually the cytokine responsible for the fever and acute phase induction seen in the earlier studies (120). Using a very specific IL-6 bioassay, this latter group found that IL-6, but not IL-1 (thymocyte assay) or IL-1β [enzyme-linked immunosorbent assay (ELISA)] was elevated in plasma following a marathon run (120).

More recently, elevated plasma levels of IL-6, but not IL-1β or TNF-α, have been found in humans following a 20-km run (122). This group was, however, able to detect elevations in all three cytokines in urine by ELISA. Elevations in plasma TNF have also been detected after prolonged strenuous exercise (117). Unlike strenuous prolonged or eccentric exercise, moderate exercise does not appear to alter immunoreactive plasma IL-1β, TNF-α, or IL-6 (126). Other cytokines including IFN-γ, IL-10, IL-12, and IL-2 have not been detected consistently in plasma, urine, or tissue in response to acute exercise (122,127–129). Indirect evidence for elevated cytokine levels comes from the apparent acute phase response seen during and following strenuous exercise (130). Taken together, these data suggest that exercise, especially prolonged and intense exercise, results in an increase in proinflammatory cytokine concentrations.

Although it is evident that strenuous exercise can elevate blood cytokine levels, the source of exercise-induced increases and the mechanisms contributing this effect are unknown. Analysis of tissues other than plasma or urine may shed light on the mechanism of why exercise increases proinflammatory cytokines. Several attempts have been made to attribute increases to production by PBMCs. Haahr et al (119) found no immuno- or bioactive IL-1, IL-1β, or IL-6 in unstimulated PBMCs, but did find elevated lipopolysaccharide (LPS) induced production of these cytokines. In another study, the spontaneous release of IL-6 and TNF-α was slightly increased in response to a short-term maximal exercise test; however, serum TNF-α was undetectable and IL-6 was not measured (121). Natelson et al (131) failed to detect messenger ribonucleic acid (mRNA) for IL-1α, IL-1β, IL-2, IL-4, IL-6, IL-10, or IFN-γ in PBMCs via reverse transcriptase-polymerase chain reaction following an acute maximal exercise test. Ullum et al (123) recently found elevated levels of immunoreactive plasma IL-6, but not IL-1α, IL-1β, or TNF-α in response to 1 hour of cycling at 75% Vo_2max. However, they could not detect elevated IL-6 mRNA in PBMC and concluded that these circulating cells were not responsible for the increase in IL-6 seen in plasma.

Although there exists controversy as to the source of circulating cytokines, one potential explanation is that local production (perhaps from damaged muscle) in response to a variety of stimuli leads to "spillover" into blood. Indeed, excessive physical exercise can cause injury to skeletal muscle as evidenced by muscle soreness, increased activity of lysosomal enzymes, and elevated serum levels of intracellular enzymes from muscle (i.e., creatine kinase). Lengthening (eccentric) contractions appear to cause greater injury to skeletal muscle than shortening (concentric) contractions (47). Reports from the laboratories of Cannon, Evans, and Pedersen et al have shown that unaccustomed eccentric exercise is associated with elevated levels of immunoreactive IL-1β in muscle biopsies of humans (116,118) and increased plasma and muscle IL-6 levels (132,133). In addition, their work and the work of others supports the notion that eccentric and/or

strenuous, prolonged exercise induces inflammation in the affected muscles and results in inflammatory cell (neutrophils and Mφ's) infiltration (48). Other plausible, but as yet untested, mechanisms as to how exercise increases proinflammatory cytokine levels include systemic endotoxemia, hyperthermia, and epinephrine.

In addition, few studies have determined whether exercise can regulate induction of cytokines in response to infectious stimuli. Bagby et al (134) have recently demonstrated that prior exhaustive exercise dramatically decreases the ability of LPS to stimulate TNF production. In addition, Chao et al (135) found that daily swimming exercise reduced serum TNF in mice inoculated with *Toxoplasma gondii* Me49 when compared to nonexercising, infected controls. They believed that this reduction may have been responsible for a more rapid recovery seen in the exercised mice. Lastly, lower levels of serum IL-1 and IL-6 in exhaustively exercised mice have been correlated to reduced mortality following *P. acnes* and lipopolysaccharide injection when compared to sedentary controls (136). Therefore, intense exercise may attenuate proinflammatory cytokine production in response to infectious stimuli, perhaps through activation of the hypothalamic-pituitary-adrenal (HPA) axis and production of glucocorticoids. Because high levels of cytokines mediate many of the negative consequences of disease (i.e., endotoxic shock), exercise-induced cytokine reduction may be beneficial.

PRACTICAL CONSIDERATIONS FOR EXERCISE PRESCRIPTION

Epidemiologic and observational evidence have defined a relationship between acute exercise dose and susceptibility to URTI. Intense prolonged exercise has been shown to increase risk for URTI. More data regarding the beneficial effect of moderate exercise are needed before we can definitively say this type of exercise lowers infectious disease risk. At the present time, it is virtually impossible to establish a direct "cause-and-effect" link between changes in the incidence of

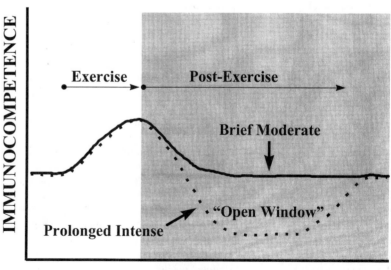

Figure 100-2 The "open-window" hypothesis. (Adapted from Pedersen BK, Ullum H. NK cell response to physical activity: Possible mechanisms of action. Med Sci Sports Exerc 1994; 26:140–146.)

infection and exercise-induced changes in immune function. However, the fact that many immune function measures are negatively affected after strenuous, but not moderate, exercise (Table 100-1) has led to the advancement of an "open-window" hypothesis (96) (Figure 100-2). According to this theory, exercise-induced immunosuppression in the postexercise period increases a person's risk for the development of infection. Therefore, based on the evidence at hand, it is prudent to recommend that athletes and those working stren-uously avoid exposing themselves to pathogens in the recovery from such exercise. Also, it is recommended that additional stressors such as lack of sleep, psychological stress, malnutrition, and dieting be minimized when strenuous exercise is anticipated. Clearly, the biggest challenge in this area of research is to link exercise-induced changes in immune function with altered susceptibility to disease. When this is done, more definitive public health recommendations regarding exercise, immune function, and disease will be available.

REFERENCES

1. Nieman DC, Johannsen LM, Lee JW, et al. Infectious episodes in runners before and after the Los Angeles Marathon. J Sports Med Phys Fitness 1990;30:316–328.

2. Peters EM, Bateman ED. Ultra-marathon running and upper respiratory tract infections. S Afr Med J 1983;64:582–584.

3. Peters EM, Goetzsche JM, Grobbelaar B, et al. Vitamin C supplementation reduces the incidence of postrace symptoms of upper respiratory tract infection in ultramarathon runners. Am J Clin Nutr 1993;57:170–174.

4. Chao CC, Strgar F, Tsang M, et al. Effects of swimming exercise on the pathogenesis of acute murine Toxoplasma gondii Me49 infection. Clin Immunol Immunopathol 1992;62:220–226.

5. Davis JM, Kohut ML, Colbert LH, et al. Exercise, alveolar macrophage function, and susceptibility to respiratory infection. J Appl Physiol 1997;83:1461–1466.

6. Gatmaitan BG, Chason JL, Lerner AM. Augmentation of the virulence of murine coxsackie virus B-3 myocardiopathy by exercise. J Exp Med 1970;131:1121–1136.

7. Hoffman-Goetz L, Pedersen BK. Exercise and the immune system: a model of the stress response? Immunol Today 1994;15:382–387.

8. Larrabee RC. Leukocytosis after violent exercise. J Med Res 1902;7:76–82.

9. McCarthy MM, Dale DA. The leukocytosis of exercise: a review and model. Sports Med 1988;6:333–363.

10. Shephard RJ. Physical activity, training and the immune response. Carmel, IN: Cooper Publishing, 1997.

11. Smith JA, Pyne DB. Exercise, training and neutrophil function. Exerc Immunol Rev 1997;3:96–116.

12. Barriga C, Pedrera MI, Maynar M, et al. Effect of submaximal physical exercise performed by sedentary men and women on some parameters of the immune system. Rev Esp Fisiol 1993;49:79–85.

13. Ferry A, Picard F, Duvallet A, et al. Changes in blood leukocyte populations induced by acute maximal and chronic submaximal exercise. Eur J Appl Physiol 1990;59:435–442.

14. McCarthy DA, MacDonald I, Grant M, et al. Studies on the immediate and delayed leucocytosis elicited by brief (30 min) strenuous exercise. Eur J Appl Physiol 1992;64:513–517.

15. Foster N, Martyn J, Robertson D, et al. Leukocytosis of exercise: role of cardiac output and catecholamines. J Appl Physiol 1986;61:2218–2223.

16. Haq A, al Hussein K, Lee J, et al. Changes in peripheral blood lymphocyte subsets associated with marathon running. Med Sci Sports Exerc 1993;25:186–190.

17. Shephard RJ, Shek PN. Exercise and CD4+/CD8+ cell counts: influence of various factors contributing in health and HIV infection. Exerc Immunol Rev 1996;2:65–83.

18. Khan MM, Sansoni P, Silverman ED, et al. Beta-adrenergic receptors on human suppressor, helper, and cytolytic lymphocytes. Biochem Pharmacol 1986;35:1137–1142.

19. Rhind SG, Shek PN, Shephard RJ. The impact of exercise on cytokines and receptor expression. Exerc Immunol Rev 1995;1:97–148.

20. Thomas ML. The leukocyte common antigen family. Annu Rev Immunol 1989;7:339–369.

21. Cossarizza A, Ortalani C, Paganelli R, et al. CD45 isoforms expression on CD4$^+$ and CD8$^+$ T cells throughout life, from newborns to centenarians: implications for T cell memory. Mech Ageing Dev 1996;86:173–195.

22. Ernst DN, Weigle O, Hobbs MV. Aging and lymphokine gene expression by T cell subsets. Nutr Rev 1995;53:S18–S26.

23. Mackey CR. Homing of naive, memory and effector lymphocytes. Curr Opin Immunol 1993;5:423–427.

24. Gabriel H, Schwarz L, Born P, et al. Differential mobilization of leucocyte and lymphocyte subpopulations into the circulation during endurance exercise. Eur J Appl Physiol 1992:65:529–534.

25. Gabriel H, Schmitt B, Urhausen A, et al. Increased CD45RA$^+$CD45RO$^+$ cell indicate activated T cells after endurance

exercise. Med Sci Sports Exerc 1993;25:1352–1357.

26. Gannon GA, Rhind SG, Shek PN, et al. The majority of CD4+, but not CD8hi, T-cells mobilized to the peripheral blood during exercise express a CD45RO+ memory phenotype. Data presented at the 3rd International Symposium: Exercise and Immunology, Paderborn, Germany, 1997.

27. Nieman DC, Miller AR, Henson DA, et al. Effect of high versus moderate intensity exercise on lymphocyte subpopulations and proliferative response. Int J Sports Med 1994;15:199–206.

28. Pizza FX, Mitchell JB, Davis BH, et al. Exercise-induced muscle damage: effect on circulating leukocyte and lymphocyte subsets. Med Sci Sports Exerc 1995;27:363–370.

29. Field CJ, Gougeon R, Marliss EB. Circulating mononuclear cell numbers and function during intense exercise and recovery. J Appl Physiol 1991;71:1089–1097.

30. Maisel AS, Knowlton KU, Fowler P, et al. Adrenergic control of circulating lymphocyte subpopulations: effects of congestive heart failure, dynamic exercise, and terbutaline treatment. J Clin Invest 1990;85:462–467.

31. Herberman RB. Natural killer cells. Annu Rev Med 1986;37:347–352.

32. Bloom ET. Natural killer cells, lymphokine-activated killer cells, and cytolytic T lymphocytes: compartmentalization of age-related changes in cytolytic T lymphocytes? J Gerontol 1994;49:B85–B92.

33. Robertson MJ, Ritz J. Biology and clinical relevance of human natural killer cells. Blood 1990;76:2421–2438.

34. Gannon GA, Shek PN, Shephard RJ. Natural killer cells: modulation by intensity and duration of exercise. Exerc Immunol Rev 1995;1:26–48.

35. Mackinnon LT. Exercise and natural killer cells: what is the relationship? Sports Med 1989;7:141–149.

36. Nieman DC, Henson DA, Sampson CS, et al. The acute immune response to exhaustive resistance exercise. Int J Sports Med 1995;16:322–328.

37. Benschop RJ, Oostveen FG, Heijnen CJ, et al. Beta 2-adrenergic stimulation causes detachment of natural killer cells from cultured endothelium. Eur J Immunol 1993;23:3242–3247.

38. Kappel M, Tvede N, Galbo H, et al. Evidence that the effect of physical exercise on NK cell activity is mediated by epinephrine. J Appl Physiol 1991;70:2530–2534.

39. Benschop RJ, Nieuwenhuis E, Tromp E, et al. Effects of β-adrenergic blockade on immunologic and cardiovascular changes induced by mental stress. Circulation 1994;89:762–769.

40. Nieman DC, Miller AR, Henson DA, et al. The effects of high-versus moderate-intensity exercise on natural killer cell cytotoxic activity. Med Sci Sports Exerc 1993;25:1126–1134.

41. Tonnesen E, Christensen NJ, Brinklov MM. Natural killer cell activity during cortisol and adrenaline infusion in healthy volunteers. Eur J Clin Invest 1987;17:497–503.

42. Berk LS, Nieman DC, Youngberg WS, et al. The effect of long endurance running on natural killer cells in marathoners. Med Sci Sports Exerc 1990;22:207–212.

43. Nieman DC, Ahle JC, Henson DA, et al. Indomethacin does not alter natural killer cell response to 2.5 h of running. J Appl Physiol 1995;79:748–755.

44. Woods JA, Davis JM. Exercise, macrophages, and cancer defense. Med Sci Sports Exerc 1994;26(2):147–157.

45. Gabriel H, Brechtel L, Urhausen A, et al. Recruitment and recirculation of leukocytes after an ultramarathon run: preferential homing of cells expressing high levels of the adhesion molecule LFA-1. Int J Sports Med 1994;15:S148–S153.

46. Gabriel H, Urhausen A, Brechtel L, et al. Alterations of regular and mature monocytes are distinct, and dependent of intensity and duration of exercise. Eur J Appl Physiol 1994;69:179–181.

47. Evans WJ, Cannon JG. The metabolic effects of exercise-induced muscle damage. Exerc Sports Sci Rev 1991;19:99–125.

48. Tidball JG. Inflammatory cell response to acute muscle injury. Med Sci Sports Exerc 1995;27:1022–1032.

49. Baum M, Geitner T, Leisen H. The role of the spleen in the leukocytosis of exercise: consequences for physiology and pathophysiology. Int J Sports Med 1996;17:604–607.

50. Sprent J. T lymphocytes and the thymus. In: Paul WE. Fundamental immunology. 3rd ed. New York: Raven Press, 1993:75–109.

51. Hoffman-Goetz L, Thorne L, Randall-Simpson JA, et al. Exercise stress alters murine lymphocyte subset distribution in spleen, lymph nodes and thymus. Clin Exp Immunol 1989;76:307–310.

52. Ferry A, Rieu P, Le Page C, et al. Effect of physical exhaustion and glucocorticoids (dexamethasone) on T-cells of trained rats. Eur J Appl Physiol 1993;66:455–460.

53. Munck A, Guyre PM. Glucocorticoids and immune function. In: Ader R, Felten DL, Cohen N, Psychoneuroimmunology. 2nd ed. San Diego: Academic Press, 1991:447–474.

54. Concordet JP, Ferry A. Physiological programmed cell death in thymocytes is induced by physical stress (exercise). Am J Physiol 1993;265:C626–C629.

55. Hoffman-Goetz L, Thorne RJ, Houston ME. Splenic immune responses following treadmill exercise in mice. Can J Physiol Pharmacol 1988;66:1415–1419.

56. Lin YS, Jan MS, Chen HI. The effect of chronic and acute exercise on immunity in rats. Int J Sports Med 1993;14:86–92.

57. Bouix O, El Mexouini M, Oresetti A. Effects of naloxone opiate blockade on the immunomodulation induced by exercise in rats. Int J Sports Med 1995;16:29–33.

58. Woods JA, Davis JM, Mayer EP, et al. Exercise increases inflammatory macrophage anti-tumor cytotoxicity. J Appl Physiol 1993;75:879–886.

59. Woods JA, Davis JM, Mayer EP, et al. Effects of exercise on macrophage activation for anti-tumor cytotoxicity. J Appl Physiol 1994;76:2177–2185.

60. Woods JA, Ceddia MA, Kozak C, et al. Effects of exercise on the macrophage MHC II response to inflammation. Int J Sports Med 1997;18:483–488.

61. Woods JA, Kohut ML, Davis JM, et al. The effects of exercise on the immune response to cancer. Med Sci Sports Exerc 1994;26(9):1109–1115.

62. Bruunsgaard H, Hartkopp A, Mohr T, et al. In vivo cell-mediated immunity and vaccination response following prolonged, intense exercise. Med Sci Sports Exerc 1997;29:1176–1181.

63. Ceddia MA, Price EA, Kohlmeier CK, et al. Effects of maximal exercise on the blood leukocyte response in the young and old. Med Sci Sports Exerc 1999 (in press).

64. MacNeil B, Hoffman-Goetz L, Kendall A, et al. Lymphocyte proliferation responses after exercise in men: fitness, intensity, and duration. J Appl Physiol 1991;70:179–185.

65. Shinkai S, Shore S, Shek PN, et al. Acute exercise and immune function: relationship between lymphocyte activity and changes in subset counts. Int J Sports Med 1992;13:452–461.

66. Nehlsen-Cannerella SL, Nieman DC, Jessen J, et al. The effects of acute moderate exercise on lymphocyte function and serum immunoglobulin levels. Int J Sports Med 1991;12:391–398.

67. Smith JD, Chi S, Salazar G, et al. Effect of moderate exercise on proliferative responses of peripheral blood mononuclear cells. J Sports Med Phys Fitness 1993;33:152–158.

68. Mackinnon LT. Immunoglobulin, antibody, and exercise. Exerc Immunol Rev 1996;2:1–34.

69. Hedfors E, Holm G, Ivansen M, et al. Physiological variation of blood lymphocyte reactivity: T-cell subsets, immunoglobulin production, and mixed lymphocyte reactivity. Clin Immunol Immunopathol 1983;27:9–14.

70. Tvede N, Heilman C, Halkjaer-Kristensen J, et al. Mechanisms of B-lymphocyte suppression induced by acute physical exercise. J Clin Lab Immunol 1989;30:169–173.

71. Mackinnon LT, Chick TW, van As A, et al. Decreased secretory immunoglobulins following intense endurance exercise. Sports Train Med Rehabil 1989;1:202–218.

72. Nieman DC, Nehlsen-Cannerella SL. The effects of acute and chronic exercise on immunoglobulins. Sports Med 1991;11:183–201.

73. Eskola J, Ruuskanen O, Soppi E, et al. Effect of sport stress on lymphocyte transformation and antibody formation. Clin Exp Immunol 1978;32:339–345.

74. Tomasi TB, Trudeau FB, Czerwinski D, et al. Immune parameters in athletes before and after strenuous exercise. J Clin Immunol 1982;2:173–178.

75. Mackinnon LT, Jenkins DG. Decreased salivary immunoglobulins after intense interval exercise before and after training. Med Sci Sports Exerc 1993;25:678–683.

76. McDowell SL, Chalos K, Housh TJ, et al. The effect of exercise intensity and duration on salivary immunoglobulin A. Eur J Appl Physiol 1991;63:108–111.

77. Mackinnon LT, Ginn EM, Seymour GJ. Decreased salivary immunoglobulin A secretion rate after intense interval exercise in elite kayakers. Eur J Appl Physiol 1993;67:180–184.

78. Smith JA. Neutrophils, host defense, and inflammation: a double-edged sword. J Leukoc Biol 1994;56:672–686.

79. Dziedziak W. The effect of incremental cycling on the physiological functions of peripheral blood granulocytes. Biol Sport 1990;7:239–247.

80. Smith JA, Telford RD, Mason IB, et al. Exercise, training and neutrophil microbicidal activity. Int J Sports Med 1990;11:179–187.

81. Smith JA, Gray AB, Pyne DB, et al. Submaximal exercise triggers both priming and activation of neutrophil microbicidal activity. Am J Physiol 1996;270:R838–R845.

82. Macha M, Shlafer M, Kluger MJ. Human neutrophil hydrogen peroxide generation following physical exercise. J Sports Med Phys Fitness 1990;30:412–419.

83. Pyne DB, Baker MS, Smith JA, et al. Exercise and the neutrophil oxidative burst: biological and experimental variability. Eur J Appl Physiol 1996;74:564–571.

84. Ortega E, Barriga C, De la Fuente M. Study of the phagocytic function of neutrophils from sedentary men after acute moderate exercise. Eur J Appl Physiol 1993;66:60–64.

85. Kurokawa Y, Shinkai S, Torii J, et al. Exercise-induced changes in the expression of surface adhesion molecules on circulating granulocytes and lymphocyte populations. Eur J Appl Physiol 1995;71:245–252.

86. Gabriel H, Muller HJ, Urhausen A, et al. Suppressed PMA-induced oxidative burst and unimpaired phagocytosis of circulating granulocytes one week after a long endurance exercise. Int J Sports Med 1994;15:441–445.

87. Gray AB, Telford RD, Collins M,

et al. Granulocyte activation induced by intense interval running. J Leukoc Biol 1993;53: 591–597.

88. Kokot K, Schaefer RM, Teschner M, et al. Activation of leukocytes during prolonged physical exercise. Adv Exp Biol Med 1988; 240:57–63.

89. Hack V, Stobel G, Raul JP, et al. The effect of maximal exercise on the activity of neutrophil granulocytes in highly-trained athletes in a moderate training period. Eur J Appl Physiol 1992;65:520–524.

90. Hack V, Stobel G, Weiss M, et al. PMN cell counts and phagocytic activity of highly-trained athletes depend on training period. J Appl Physiol 1994;77:1731–1735.

91. Dufaux B, Order U. Plasma elastase, α_1-antitrypsin, neopterin, tumor necrosis factor and soluble interleukin-2 receptor increase after prolonged exercise. Int J Sports Med 1989;10:434–438.

92. Hanson J-B, Wilsgard L, Osterud B. Biphasic changes in leucocytes induced by strenuous exercise. Eur J Appl Physiol 1991; 62:157–161.

93. Muns G. Effect of long-distance running on polymorphonuclear neutrophil phagocytic function of the upper airways. Int J Sports Med 1993;15:96–99.

94. Muns G, Rubinstein I, Singer P. Neutrophil chemotactic activity is increased in nasal secretions of long-distance runners. Int J Sports Med 1996;17:56–59.

95. Trinchieri G. Natural killer cells wear different hats: effector cells of innate resistance and regulatory cells of adaptive immunity and of hematopoiesis. Semin Immunol 1995;7:83–88.

96. Pedersen BK, Ullum H. NK cell response to physical activity: possible mechanisms of action. Med Sci Sports Exerc 1994;26: 140–146.

97. Pedersen BK, Tvede N, Klarlund K, et al. Indomethacin in vitro and in vivo abolishes postexercise suppression of natural killer cell activity in peripheral blood. Int J Sports Med 1990; 11:127–131.

98. Shek PN, Sabiston BH, Buguet A, et al. Strenuous exercise and immunological changes: a multiple-time-point analysis of leukocyte subsets, CD4/CD8 ratio, immunoglobulin production and NK cell response. Int J Sports Med 1995;16:466–474.

99. Nielsen HB, Secher NH, Kappel M, et al. Lymphocyte, NK and LAK cell responses to maximal exercise. Int J Sports Med 1994; 17:60–65.

100. Woods JA, Wolters BW, Ceddia MA, et al. Effects of maximal exercise on natural killer (NK) cell activity and responsiveness to interferon-α in young and old. J Gerontol Biol Sci 1998;53A: B430–437.

101. Krishnaraj R, Svanborg A. Preferential accumulation of mature NK cells during human immunosenescence. J Cell Biochem 1992;50:386–391.

102. Bieger WP, Weiss M, Michne G, et al. Exercise-induced monocytosis and modulations of monocyte function. Int J Sports Med 1980;1:30–36.

103. Lewicki R, Tchorzewski H, Denys A, et al. Effect of physical exercise on some parameters of immunity in conditioned sportsmen. Int J Sports Med 1987;8: 309–314.

104. Michna H. The human macrophage system: activity and functional morphology. Bibl Anat 1988;31:1–38.

105. Ortega E, Collazos ME, Barriga C, et al. Stimulation of the phagocytic function in guinea pig peritoneal macrophages by physical activity stress. Eur J Appl Physiol 1992;64:323–327.

106. Forner MA, Collazos ME, Bariga C, et al. Effect of age on adherence and chemotaxis capacities of peritoneal macrophages: influence of physical activity stress. Mech Ageing Dev 1994; 75:179–189.

107. De La Fuente M, Martin MI, Ortega E. Changes in the phagocytic function of peritoneal macrophages from old mice after strenuous physical exercise. Comp Immunol Microbiol Infect Dis 1990;13:189–198.

108. Ortega E, Forner MA, Barriga C, et al. Effect of age and of swimming-induced stress on the phagocytic capacity of peritoneal macrophages from mice. Mech Ageing Dev 1993;70:53–63.

109. Fehr HG, Lotzerich H, Michna H. Influence of physical exercise on peritoneal macrophage functions: histochemical and phagocytic studies. Int J Sports Med 1988; 9:77–81.

110. Fehr HG, Lotzerich H, Michna H. Human macrophage function and physical exercise: phagocytic and histochemical studies. Eur J Appl Physiol 1989;58:613–617.

111. Lotzerich H, Fehr HG, Appell H. Potentiation of cytostatic but not cytolytic activity of murine macrophages after running stress. Int J Sports Med 1990;11:61–65.

112. Pavlidis N, Chirigos M. Stress-induced impairment of macrophage tumoricidal function. Psychosom Med 1980;42:47–53.

113. Davis JM, Kohut ML, Jackson DA, et al. Exercise effects on lung tumor metastases and in vitro alveolar macrophage antitumor cytotoxicity. Am J Physiol 1998;5:R1454–1459.

114. Cannon JG, Kluger MJ. Endogenous pyrogen activity in human plasma after exercise. Science 1983;220:616–619.

115. Cannon JG, Evans WJ, Hughes VA, et al. Physiological mechanisms contributing to increased interleukin-1 secretion. J Appl Physiol 1986;61(5):1869–1874.

116. Cannon JG, Fielding RA, Fiatarone MA, et al. Increased interleukin-1β in human skeletal muscle after exercise. Am J Physiol 1989;257:R451–R455.

117. Dufaux B, Order U. Plasma elastase-α-1-antitrypsin, neopterin, tumor necrosis factor, and soluble interleukin-2 receptor after prolonged exercise. Int J Sports Med 1989;10:434–438.

118. Fielding RA, Manfredi TJ, Ding W, et al. Acute phase response in exercise III: neutrophil and IL-1β accumulation in skeletal muscle. Am J Physiol 1993;265: R166–R172.

119. Haahr PM, Pedersen BK, Fomsgaard A, et al. Effect of physical exercise on in vitro production of interleukin-1, interleukin-6, tumor necrosis factor-α, interleukin-2 and interferon-γ. Int J Sports Med 1991;12(2): 223–227.

120. Northoff H, Berg A. Immunologic mediators as parameters of the reaction to strenuous exercise. Int J Sports Med 1991;12(suppl 1):S9–S15.

121. Rivier A, Pene J, Chanez P, et al. Release of cytokines by blood monocytes during strenuous exercise. Int J Sports Med 1994;15(4):192–198.

122. Sprenger H, Jacobs C, Nain M, et al. Enhanced release of cytokines, interleukin-2 receptors, and neopterin after long-distance running. Clin Immunol Immunopathol 1992;63(2): 188–195.

123. Ullum H, Haahr PM, Diamant M, et al. Bicycle exercise enhances plasma IL-6 but does not change IL-1α, IL-1β, IL-6, or TNF-α pre-mRNA in BMNC. J Appl Physiol 1994;77(1):93–97.

124. Kishimoto T. The biology of inter-leukin-6. Blood 1989;74(1): 1–10.

125. Evans WJ, Meredith CN, Cannon JG, et al. Metabolic changes following eccentric exercise in trained and untrained men. J Appl Physiol 1986;61(5): 1864–1868.

126. Smith JA, Telford RD, Baker MS, et al. Cytokine immunoreactivity in plasma does not change after moderate endurance exercise. J Appl Physiol 1992;73(4): 1396–1401.

127. Espersen GT, Elbaek A, Ernst E, et al. Effect of physical exercise on cytokines and lymphocyte subpopulations in human peripheral blood. APMIS 1990;98: 395–400.

128. Gannon GA. Peripheral blood lymphocyte trafficking and natural killer cell cytolytic activity during prolonged exhaustive aerobic exercise: a focus on cell adhesion molecules and β-endorphin. Unpublished doctoral dissertation. University of Toronto, 1998.

129. Viti A, Muscettola M, Paulesu L, et al. Effect of exercise on plasma interferon levels. J Appl Physiol 1985;59:426–428.

130. Weight LM, Alexander D, Jacobs P. Strenuous exercise: analogous to the acute-phase response? Clin Sci 1991;81:677–683.

131. Natelson BH, Zhou X, Ottenweller JE, et al. Effect of acute exhausting exercise on cytokine gene expression in men. Int J Sports Med 1996;17:299–302.

132. Bruusgaard H, Galbo H, Halkjaer-Kristensen J, et al. Exercise-induced increase in serum IL-6 in humans is related to muscle damage. J Physiol 1997; 15:833–841.

133. Rohde T, MacLean DA, Richter EA, et al. Prolonged submaximal eccentric exercise is associated with increased levels of plasma IL-6. Am J Physiol 1997;273: E85–E91.

134. Bagby GJ, Sawaya DE, Crouch LD, et al. Prior exercise suppresses the plasma tumor necrosis factor response to bacterial lipopolysaccharide. J Appl Physiol 1994;77(3):1542–1547.

135. Chao CC, Strgar F, Tsang M, et al. Effects of swimming exercise on the pathogenesis of acute murine Toxoplasma gondii Me49 infection. Clin Immunol Immunopathol 1992;62: 220–226.

136. Ishizashi H, Yoshimoto T, Nakanishi K, et al. Effect of exercise on endotoxin shock with special reference to changes in concentrations of cytokines. Jpn J Physiol 1995;45:553–560.

Chapter 101

Chronic Exercise and Immunity: Practical Applications for Athletes

Laurel T. Mackinnon

As discussed in the two previous chapters, endurance athletes experience a high incidence of symptoms of upper respiratory tract infection (URTI) during periods of intense training and after competition. In contrast, the risk of URTI is not elevated in less competitive "recreational" athletes who train more moderately and, if they compete, generally do so at a much slower pace. Chapter 100 also discussed evidence showing that certain immune parameters may be suppressed for some time after a single bout of intense exercise. These data form the basis of the so-called J-curve hypothesis, which suggests that although intense exercise increases risk of illness, moderate exercise may have no effect or may actually decrease risk of illness (1). Although recent evidence suggests mild suppession of some immune parameters in athletes, it is important to note that athletes are not clinically immune-deficient; that is, they do not experience illnesses generally associated with immunodeficiency. URTI appears to be the only illness to which they are more susceptible. This chapter discusses evidence supporting the notion of mild immunosuppression during intense exercise training in high-performance athletes.

EXPERIMENTAL MODELS TO STUDY THE CHRONIC IMMUNE RESPONSE IN ATHLETES

There are three basic experimental models with which to study the chronic immune system response to exercise training. The simplest method is to compare immune parameters in athletes with clinical norms or to cross-sectionally compare these values with those obtained from age- and sex-matched nonathlete control subjects; it is preferable that the latter are exposed to similar environmental influences except for exercise (e.g., living in the same household). In the second model, athletes are followed over a training season, and immune parameters are measured at time points corresponding to low- and high-intensity training. Ideally, a nonathlete group is included to control for possible seasonal variability. This model provides useful information about the immune responses to exercise training in the athlete's "natural" training environment, that is, during a normal training season. However, potentially confounding influences such as competition, illness, travel, psychological stress, dietary changes, and alterations to training programs cannot be fully controlled. In the third model, training is intensified over a limited time period, usually up to 4 weeks; for ethical reasons, coaches and scientists are reluctant to intensify training for longer because of the risk of overtraining syndrome (2–6). Immune function is then compared within the same athletes from before to after the intensified training period. Although this model provides better control of training loads, not all athletes respond similarly to increased training loads. That is, some positively adapt whereas others experience symptoms of negative adaptation such as mood state changes, poor performance, and hormonal changes (3–5,7,8), which may significantly influence immune function. In addition, training load is often increased far in excess of what would be considered normal (e.g., doubling of training volume over 4 weeks). Although no single experimental approach is ideal, by combining data from each model it is possible to gain a comprehensive understanding of the immune system response to chronic exercise training in

Table 101-1 Summary of Immune System Changes During Intense Training in Athletes

Immune Parameter	In Athletes at Rest* (Representative Reference)	After Intense Exercise Training[a] (Representative Reference)
Leukocyte Number	Normal (10,12) or low (7)	No change (9,11) or decrease to clinically low levels (7)
Neutrophil Number	Normal (20)	No change or slight increase (20)
Neutrophil Activation	Lower in athletes (20,24)	Lower during intense versus moderate training (20,22)
Lymphocyte Number	Normal (8,9,12,13,28)	No change (8,9,19)
Lymphocyte Activation	Normal (9) or higher (30)	Increase (15,19)
Lymphocyte Proliferation	Normal (31,32)	Increase (6,31)
NK Cell Number	Normal (12,32,34) or higher (33)	Normal (31) or decreased (9,29,35)
NK Cell Cytotoxic Activity	Normal (13) or higher (32,34,36)	No change (33) or decrease (35)
Serum Immunoglobulin	Normal (27,39) or low IgG_1 and IgG_2 (9); normal specific antibody response (42)	No change (9)
Mucosal Immunoglobulin	Normal (39) or low (9,45,46)	No change (45) or decrease (9,47); decrease in athletes who later develop URTI (48)
Plasma Glutamine	Normal (5,49) or low (50,51)	Decrease (49) or increase or no change (5)

* At rest, in athletes compared with nonathletes or clinical norms.
[a] In athletes, after compared with before a period of intense training or compared with moderate training.

athletes. The chronic responses of various immune parameters to intense exercise training are summarized in Table 101-1.

EFFECTS OF EXERCISE TRAINING ON IMMUNE PARAMETERS IN ATHLETES

Immune Cells

Immune cells are involved in virtually all aspects of immune function. The immune response involves coordinated activity of specialized immune cells that may act directly to kill foreign organisms (e.g., phagocytes and natural killer cells) or indirectly by releasing soluble factors capable of activating other immune cells or inhibiting foreign agents (e.g., cytokines, antibody). As discussed below, cellular responses vary by exercise intensity, and not all immune cell subsets respond similarly to chronic exercise training.

Leukocyte Number

Resting peripheral blood leukocyte number is generally normal in well-trained athletes compared with clinical norms or values in nonathlete control subjects (9–14). Moreover, resting leukocyte number does not change over many months of normal training in high-performance athletes (9,10,15). In contrast, low resting leukocyte counts have been observed during periods of intense training in distance runners and road cyclists (3,7,16). Cell counts near the low end of the clinically normal range ($\sim 4 \times 10^9$/L) were reported in middle- and long-distance runners (3,7,17). These clinically low cell counts may reflect chronic suppression of circulating leukocyte number. Alternatively, low cell counts may also reflect the relatively larger expansion of plasma volume in proportion to

cell volume known to occur during endurance exercise training.

Peripheral blood leukocyte count does not change appreciably during short- and long-term normal training in elite athletes (9,10,14,18). Resting leukocyte counts may or may not be influenced by short-term intensified training (3,7,8,11). For example, leukocyte counts were unchanged after 4 weeks of intensified training in triathletes and cyclists (11). In another study, when training was intensified over 4 weeks in competitive swimmers, cell numbers increased significantly after 2 weeks, but returned to prestudy levels after 4 weeks; leukocyte numbers were well within the clinically normal range at all times (8). Moreover, in this study no differences were observed in cell counts between athletes showing symptoms of short-term overtraining ("overreaching") compared with those who positively adapted to the increased training. In contrast, leukocyte counts progressively declined toward the low end of the clinically normal range (mean 4.2×10^9/L) during 4 weeks of intensified training (doubled volume) in distance runners, all of whom showed symptoms of overreaching (Figure 101-1) (3,7). Taken together, these data suggest that leukocyte count remains relatively constant in athletes provided that training intensity progresses gradually throughout the normal training season; cell counts may decline to clinically low levels after sudden and excessive increases in training volume leading to symptoms of overtraining syndrome.

Neutrophil Number and Function

Resting circulating neutrophil number is generally within the clinically normal range in athletes and is relatively resistant to change during normal training cycles or during short periods of increased training (8,10,19,20). Despite the normal cell

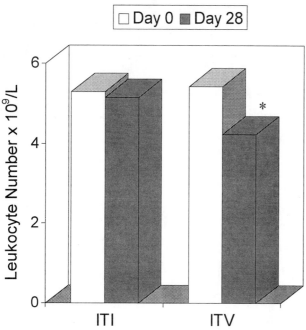

Figure 101-1 Leukocyte number before (day 0) and after (day 28) 4 weeks intense training in men distance runners. Training was intensified by either increasing training intensity (ITI) or training volume (ITV). *Significant decrease ($p < .05$) after 4 weeks training only in ITV. (Data from Lehmann M, Mann H, Gastmann U, et al. Unaccustomed high-mileage vs intensity training-related changes in performance and serum amino acid levels. Int J Sports Med 1996;17:187–192.)

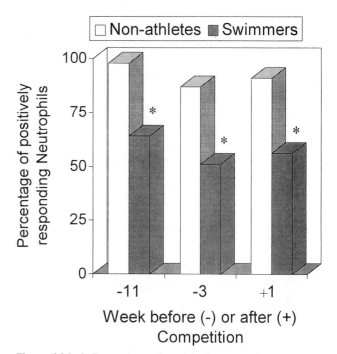

Figure 101-2 Percentage of positively responding neutrophils in elite swimmers and nonathlete control subjects during 12 weeks intense swim training before and recovery after major competition. *Significantly lower ($p < .05$) percentage of neutrophils stimulated to increase oxidative burst activity in an in vitro system in swimmers compared with nonathletes. (Data from Pyne DB, Baker MS, Fricker PA, et al. Effects of an intensive 12-wk training program by elite swimmers on neutrophil oxidative activity. Med Sci Sports Exerc 1995;27:536–542.)

counts, however, morphologic evidence showing an increase in the number of immature neutrophils (21) suggests an increased turnover of cells. In contrast, in distance runners, lower neutrophil counts were observed in samples obtained during intense compared with moderate training and with matched nonathletes; training was intensified over 3 months by increasing both volume and intensity (22). It appears, then, that circulating neutrophil count remains clinically normal in most training situations, declining only during prolonged periods of excessive training, a pattern similar to that observed for leukocyte number, as discussed above.

Despite clinically normal neutrophil counts, however, there is good evidence for downregulation of both resting and postexercise neutrophil function in trained athletes (20,22–24). Markedly lower neutrophil activation was noted both at rest and after moderate exercise in cyclists compared with nonathletes (24). Resting and postexercise neutrophil activation and phagocytic activity were lower in distance runners during intense compared with moderate training cycles and compared with nonathletes (22). Resting neutrophil activation and the number of cells capable of responding to in vitro stimulation were also lower in elite swimmers at the start of a

training season compared with matched nonathletes (Figure 101-2) (20). Moreover, in this study neutrophil activation and the number of responsive cells declined further during 12 weeks of intense training, partially recovering during the 2-week taper (reduced training) before major competition.

It has been suggested that downregulation of neutrophil function may reflect persistent activation of neutrophils after a single exercise bout resulting in depletion of granule content within neutrophils, leaving these cells refractory to further stimulation for some time (20,24). Daily intense exercise performed by competitive athletes may thus contribute to a persistently refractory (inactive) neutrophil in the circulation. It has also been proposed that, since these cells migrate to damaged skeletal muscle, where they release toxic factors and mediate inflammation, downregulation of neutrophil function may be protective by limiting their inflammatory activities (25,26). It is unclear whether such downregulation contributes to increased susceptibility to infection in athletes, since no correlation was found between lower neutrophil function and incidence of URTI over 12 weeks of intense training in elite swimmers (20).

Lymphocyte Number, Activation, and Proliferation

As with other immune cells, resting lymphocyte count is usually normal in athletes from various endurance and power sports (8,9,12,13,15,19,27,28). Periods of intense training up to several months in duration generally do not influence lymphocyte number (8–11,18,19,22), nor are the relative proportions of lymphocyte subsets (B cells, T cells, and T-cell subsets) altered by exercise training (9,10,19).

Lymphocytes may be activated both acutely after a single exercise session and chronically as a result of exercise training, depending on the activation markers studied. In athletes, enhanced expression of cell surface activation markers, such as the low- and high-affinity IL-2 receptor subunits (CD25 and CD122, respectively) and HLA-DR antigen, has been reported (15,29,30), although other studies have failed to note such differences (9,12). For example, the number of resting lymphocytes expressing HLA-DR antigen did not differ between distance runners and matched nonathletes (12), nor between elite swimmers and nonathletes followed over 7 months (9). In contrast, expression of the high-affinity IL-2 receptor (CD122) was greater in resting T and NK cells obtained from distance runners compared with nonathletes (30). Significant increases in expression of the low-affinity IL-2 receptor (CD25) were observed after 10 days of intense interval training in endurance athletes (29), and after a competitive season in track athletes (15). Taken together, these data suggest that lymphocyte activation may occur in response to prolonged periods of intense training despite no changes in circulating lymphocyte number.

Lymphocyte activation and function may be indirectly assessed by studying the ability of lymphocytes to respond to in vitro mitogenic challenge. In cells obtained at rest, lymphocyte proliferation is normal in athletes during moderate training (31,32), and may be stimulated during periods of intense training (6,31). For example, although T cell proliferation was initially similar in cyclists and matched nonathletes, proliferation increased after 6 months of intense training in cyclists, while remaining unchanged in control subjects (31). This increase could not be attributed to changes in T cell number, and may reflect the enhanced activation during intense training, as discussed above.

Natural Killer Cells

Natural Killer (NK) cells are a distinct lymphocyte subset capable of cytotoxic activity against certain types of virally infected and tumor cells. NK cells are involved in early host defense against viral infection and some types of tumors. Circulating NK cell number may be normal, low, or high in athletes compared with nonathletes, depending on the training phase at which samples are obtained from athletes. Normal NK cell number has been recorded in various groups of endurance and power athletes (12,31–33). However, higher resting NK cell number has been reported in runners, cyclists, and swimmers during low- to moderate-intensity training compared with nonathletes (9,30,33,34). In contrast, resting NK cell number may decline during prolonged periods of intense exercise training (9,29,35). For example, decreases in NK cell number were observed in competitive swimmers during a 7-month training season (9) and after 4 weeks of

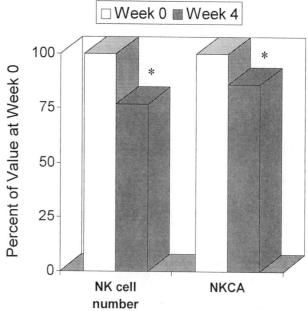

Figure 101-3 Changes in NK cell number and NK cell cytotoxic activity (NKCA) from before (week 0) to after (week 4) 4 weeks intensified training in competitive swimmers. Training was intensified by 40% increasing swimming volume (distance) over the 4 weeks. *Significant decrease in cell number ($p < .05$) and NKCA ($p < .01$) week 4 compared with week 0. (Data from Gedge VL, Mackinnon LT, Hooper SL. Effects of 4 wk intensified training on natural killer (NK) cells in competitive swimmers. Med Sci Sports Exerc 1997;29:S158. Abstract.)

intensified training (Figure 101-3) (35), and in runners after 10 days intense interval training (29). In these studies, numbers of other lymphocyte subsets remained unchanged by exercise training, suggesting a specific effect on NK cell number.

NK cell cytotoxic activity (NKCA) may also be normal or elevated in athletes. Two studies have reported significantly higher resting NKCA in endurance athletes compared with matched nonathletes (32,34,36). The higher NKCA could not be attributed to higher NK cell number, suggesting enhanced cytotoxic activity of each NK cell (32). However, a subsequent study from the same laboratory did not show higher NKCA in another group of distance runners compared with nonathletes (12). Differences may relate to the small sample sizes in some studies, or to the training phase at which blood samples were obtained from athletes. There are few studies focusing on the effects of intense exercise training on NKCA. A recent study published in abstract form (35) reported significant decreases in NKCA after 4 weeks of intensified training in swimmers (see Figure 101-3). Thus, while moderate exercise training may enhance NKCA in previously sedentary individuals (37) or in athletes (32,33,36,38), prolonged periods of intense exercise training appear to suppress NK cell number and cytotoxic activity (9,29,35).

Soluble Factors

In addition to cellular activity, an effective immune response also requires many soluble factors such as immunoglobulin (Ig) produced by B cells, cytokines produced by many types of cells, and substrates such as glutamine required for energy production by lymphocytes.

Immunoglobulin

In athletes, serum Ig levels may be clinically normal (27,39,40) or low (9,41,42). Significantly lower serum IgA, IgG, and IgM concentrations were recorded throughout a 7-month training season in elite swimmers compared with matched nonathletes; although within the clinically normal range, these values were within the lowest 10th percentile for their population. Clinically low serum IgG_2 and IgG_3 concentrations were also reported in these swimmers (9,42). Lower serum Ig concentrations could not be explained by differences in the numbers of B or T cells or activated lymphocytes, suggesting possible impairment of Ig production. Serum Ig levels do not appear to change during moderate exercise training (43), whereas declining concentrations of total Ig, IgM, IgG, and subclasses IgG_1 and IgG_2 were observed after 3 months of intense exercise training in athletes (41). However, although serum Ig levels may be low, athletes appear capable of mounting a clinically appropriate antibody response to antigenic challenge even during intense training (42). Thus, the clinical significance, if any, of low serum Ig levels is unclear at present.

The secretory or mucosal immune system is a major effector of host resistance to organisms colonizing the body's external surfaces, and in particular, those causing viral URTI. Because of the apparently high incidence of URTI among athletes, several research groups have studied the response of secretory (usually salivary) IgA, the major Ig in mucosal secretions, to acute and chronic exercise [reviewed by Mackinnon (44)]. Resting salivary IgA concentration has been reported to be either normal (39,45) or low (9,46) in competitive athletes compared with nonathletes or clinical norms. Although clinically normal, significantly lower IgA concentration was found throughout a 6-month training season in swimmers diagnosed as overtrained compared with those considered well-trained (45). Both resting and postexercise IgA concentrations declined progressively over 4- to 7-month training seasons in swimmers (9,47). One study has shown a temporal relationship between acute exercise-induced decreases in IgA concentration and subsequent appearance of URTI (48), suggesting that low IgA levels may predispose athletes to URTI. In contrast to intense exercise training, more moderate training is not associated with suppression of secretory IgA concentration [reviewed by Mackinnon (44)].

Plasma Glutamine

Glutamine is an essential requirement as an energy source and for nucleotide synthesis in proliferating lymphocytes. Plasma glutamine concentration declines acutely after prolonged exercise, during intense exercise training, and in overtrained athletes. It has been suggested that low plasma glutamine levels may compromise lymphocyte function, and thus immunity to infection (49–52). A recent brief report sug-

gests the possibility that glutamine supplementation may prevent URTI after endurance competition (distance running) (53). However, although low plasma glutamine concentration was observed in overtrained compared with non-overtrained athletes, lymphocytes from overtrained athletes exhibited normal in vitro proliferation in response to mitogenic challenge (50). Moreover, despite marked declines in plasma glutamine concentration, lymphocyte activation markers and IL-2 production were enhanced after 10 days of intense interval training (29). In another recent study, despite significantly lower plasma glutamine concentration in overtrained compared with well-trained swimmers, glutamine levels did not differ between athletes who developed URTI and those who did not during 4 weeks of intensified training (5). Thus, the significance, if any, of low plasma glutamine concentration in overtrained athletes and during intense exercise training is unclear at present.

MECHANISMS UNDERLYING APPARENT SUPPRESSION OF IMMUNITY DURING INTENSE EXERCISE TRAINING

It is unlikely that a single mechanism is responsible for the variety of changes in immune parameters reported in athletes during periods of intense training. As shown in the previous chapter, a single bout of intense exercise is sufficient to suppress a number of immune parameters, including lymphocyte proliferative response to mitogenic challenge, specific serum antibody response to immunization, mucosal immunoglobulin concentration, neutrophil activation, and a delayed suppression of NK cell cytotoxic activity. Many of these effects persist for several hours, and possibly days, after a single session of intense exercise. The "open-window" model suggests that the athlete may be susceptible to infection during the extended period of immune suppression after each exercise session (54). Competitive athletes train intensely on a daily or more frequent basis over many weeks. It has been suggested that chronic suppression of immune function may result if the athlete begins a training session before full recovery from the previous session (i.e., during the open window) (25,44). Thus, it is possible that immune function is somewhat compromised by the additive and interactive effects of small changes in several parameters central to host defense during recovery after intense exercise.

The observation that clinically normal cell counts are maintained in athletes except during excessively rigorous exercise training suggests that the processes involved in cell turnover remain in balance. Declining leukocyte counts during very high volume training (7) may indicate increased turnover of cells, possibly similar to that observed in red blood cells (55). Although it is unlikely that a single mechanism is responsible for the apparent suppression of immune cell function during intense training, many of the observed changes may be related to neuroendocrine factors.

Regulation of neutrophil function is complex, and there is no simple explanation for the apparent downregulation of neutrophil activity during intense exercise training. Several hormones and cytokines can modulate neutrophil function, including catecholamines, corticosteroids, opioid peptides, IL-1, and TNFα; intense exercise training has been shown to alter at least catecholamines and possibly corticosteroids and some cytokines (56). As discussed above, it is possible that downregulation of neutrophil function reflects a beneficial adaptation that limits chronic inflammation and tissue damage in response to intense exercise training.

Mechanisms responsible for low secretory and serum Ig concentrations are also likely to be complex and to possibly involve neuroendocrine factors. Ig-producing B lymphocytes exhibit β-adrenergic receptors, and both serum and mucosal Ig synthesis are influenced by catecholamines or sympathetic activity. Depletion of catecholamines and/or downregulation of receptors may occur during intense exercise training (3,7,56), possibly influencing Ig synthesis. Despite lower levels of serum Ig, however, the antibody response to specific antigenic challenges appears to be normal in athletes (42), suggesting maintenance of this function despite neuroendocrine changes.

Intense exercise training is also associated with psychological stress, leading to alterations in mood state and anxiety levels. It is known that psychological stress may modulate a wide variety of immune parameters. It is likely that, in athletes, mild immune suppression during prolonged periods of intense exercise training reflects the combined effects of physical and psychological stress.

PRACTICAL CONSIDERATIONS FOR THE ATHLETE

There are, at present, no clear guidelines as to how athletes may avoid immunosuppression and illness during intense training and competition, nor is it clear what level of exercise an athlete may undertake during illness. Although intense exercise on a daily or more frequent basis has been associated with chronic suppression of certain immune parameters, it is impractical to suggest that high-performance athletes avoid such exercise. Overtraining syndrome is also associated with increased illness rates, and practical suggestions to help athletes avoid this syndrome, such as periodization of training with programmed rest days, regular monitoring of indicators of well-being and stress, and sufficient recovery between sessions and competitive seasons (57), may help prevent immunosuppression and illness. However, this has yet to be tested experimentally.

There is some evidence that URTI may be prevented by supplementation with vitamin C (58) or glutamine (53) after endurance competition (e.g., a marathon). It is unclear at present, however, whether supplementation can prevent URTI during periods of intense training or in athletes other than distance runners. There is also evidence that, during endurance exercise, carbohydrate supplementation (e.g., sports drinks) may attenuate some of the acute exercise effects on immune parameters (59). Although it is premature to recommend supplements to all athletes, it is important to ensure their diets contain sufficient intake of total energy, carbohydrate, vitamins, minerals, and fluids to optimize immune function, training responses, and maintenance of body mass.

Simple, localized viral illness such as the common cold without systemic involvement may require only slight modification of training intensity and relief of symptoms (e.g., nasal congestion) for a few days until illness is resolved (60,61). In contrast, systemic infections such as influenza or other bacterial or viral infections may require at least 2, and possibly 4, weeks of recovery (1,60), and even longer (2 to 6 months) may be needed for full recovery from more serious illnesses such as infectious mononucleosis (60). Systemic viral illness is associated with impaired physical capacity, including decreased muscular strength and endurance exercise capacity. Thus, the athlete may find it difficult to maintain training loads during systemic illness, and attempts to do so may lead to musculoskeletal injury or persistent fatigue, and eventually to overtraining syndrome. It is significant that many athletes experiencing chronic fatigue syndrome (CFS) cite continued training during a previous systemic viral illness as a main contributing factor to subsequent development of symptoms of CFS; symptoms of CFS may last months to years and may effectively end an athlete's career (62). Furthermore, structural and biochemical changes in skeletal and cardiac muscle during systemic viral infection may limit physiologic training adaptations in these tissues, and may exacerbate illness and possibly lead to further complications (e.g., rare instances of viral myocarditis). The general recommendation is that a simple head cold (i.e., nasal symptoms with no systemic involvement, the so-called *above-the-neck* rule) requires little modification of training. However, more extensive illness, especially involving fatigue, fever, enlarged lymph nodes, or gastrointestinal symptoms, requires cessation of training until assessed by a physician who can recommend the proper treatment and need for alteration of training.

SUMMARY

Athletes are not clinically immune-deficient; that is, they do not generally experience serious illnesses associated with immune deficiency, and URTI appears to be the only illness to which athletes are more susceptible. However, evidence published over the past few years suggests that long periods of intense exercise training (e.g., weeks to months) are associated with changes in a number of immune parameters including low resting leukocyte counts, decreasing NK cell number and cytotoxic activity, low serum and secretory Ig concentrations, suppression of neutrophil activation and antimicrobial activity, and low plasma glutamine concentration. Although many of these alterations are relatively small, it is possible that, in athletes, immune function is compromised by the additive and interactive effects of small changes in several parameters important to host defense. Exercise capacity may be limited during infection, and athletes may experience difficulty in maintaining training loads during illness. Simple, localized viral illness such as the common cold without systemic involvement ("above the neck" rule) may require only slight modification of training intensity, whereas systemic infections such as influenza or other bacterial or viral infections may require 2 to 4 weeks of rest or reduced training. Although moderate exercise training is not associated with suppression of immune parameters (suggesting that immune suppression can be avoided by training only moderately), periods of intense exercise training are necessary for most high-performance athletes. Attention to other details such as regularly monitoring athletes' adaptation to training, periodized and individualized training that permits athletes to recover adequately between sessions, and ensuring optimal nutrition and fluid replacement may help athletes avoid overtraining and associated illness.

REFERENCES

1. Nieman DC, Nehlsen-Cannarella SL. Exercise and infection. In: Watson RR, Eisinger M, eds. Exercise and disease. Boca Raton, FL: CRC Press, 1992: 122–148.

2. Flynn MG, Pizza FX, Boone JB Jr, et al. Indices of training stress during competitive running and swimming seasons. Int J Sports Med 1994;15:21–16.

3. Lehmann M, Baumgartl P, Wiesenack C, et al. Training-overtraining: influence of a defined increase in training volume vs training intensity on performance, catecholamines and some metabolic parameters in experienced middle- and long-distance runners. Eur J Appl Physiol 1992;64:169–117.

4. Lehmann M, Foster C, Keul J. Overtraining in endurance athletes: a brief review. Med Sci Sports Exerc 1993;25:854–862.

5. Mackinnon LT, Hooper SL. Plasma glutamine concentration and upper respiratory tract infection during overtraining in elite swimmers. Med Sci Sports Exerc 1996;28: 285–290.

6. Verde TJ, Thomas SG, Shephard RJ. Potential markers of heavy training in highly trained distance runners. Br J Sports Med 1992; 26:167–175.

7. Lehmann M, Mann H, Gastmann U, et al. Unaccustomed high-mileage vs intensity training—related changes in performance and serum amino acid levels. Int J Sports Med 1996;17:187–192.

8. Mackinnon LT, Hooper SL, Jones S, et al. Hormonal, immunological and hematological responses to intensified training in elite swimmers. Med Sci Sports Exerc 1997;29:1637–1645.

9. Gleeson M, McDonald WA, Cripps AW, et al. The effect on immunity of long term intensive training in elite swimmers. Clin Exp Immunol 1995;102:210–216.

10. Hooper S, Mackinnon LT, Howard A, et al. Markers for monitoring overtraining and recovery in elite swimmers. Med Sci Sports Exerc 1995;27:106–112.

11. Ndon JA, Snyder AC, Foster C, Wehrenberg WB. Effects of chronic intensive exercise training on the leukocyte response to acute exercise. Int J Sports Med 1992;13: 176–182.

12. Nieman DC, Brendle D, Henson DA, et al. Immune function in athletes versus nonathletes. Int J Sports Med 1995;16: 329–333.

13. Nieman DC, Simandle S, Henson DA, et al. Lymphocyte proliferative response to 2.5 hours of running. Int J Sports Med 1995;16:404–408.

14. Tvede N, Pedersen BK, Hansen FR, et al. Effect of physical exercise on blood mononuclear cell subpopulations and in vitro proliferative responses. Scand J Immunol 1989;29:383–389.

15. Baum M, Liesen H, Enneper J. Leucocytes, lymphocytes, activation parameters and cell adhesion molecules in middle-distance runners under different training conditions. Int J Sports Med 1994;15:S122–S126.

16. Blannin AK, Chatwin LJ, Cave R, Gleeson M. Effects of submaximal cycling and long-term endurance training on neutrophil phagocytic activity in middle aged men. Br J Sports Med 1996;30:125–129.

17. Green RL, Kaplan SS, Rabin BS, et al. Immune function in marathon runners. Ann Allergy 1981;47:73–75.

18. Mujika I, Chatard J-C, Geyssant A. Effects of training and taper on blood leucocyte populations in competitive swimmers: relationships with cortisol and performance. Int J Sports Med 1996; 17:213–217.

19. Fry RW, Morton AR, Garcia-Webb P, et al. Biological responses to overload training in endurance sports. Eur J Appl Physiol 1992; 64:335–344.

20. Pyne DB, Baker MS, Fricker PA, et al. Effects of an intensive 12-wk training program by elite swimmers on neutrophil oxidative activity. Med Sci Sports Exerc 1995;27: 536–542.

21. Keen P, McCarthy DA, Passfield L, et al. Leucocyte and erythrocyte counts during a multistage cycling race ("The Milk Race"). Br J Sports Med 1995;29:61–65.

22. Hack B, Strobel G, Weiss M, Weicker H. PMN cell counts and phagocytic activity of highly trained athletes depend on training period. J Appl Physiol 1994;77: 1731–1735.

23. Espersen GT, Toft E, Ernst E, et al. Changes of polymorphonuclear granulocyte migration and lymphocyte proliferative responses in elite runners undergoing intense exercise. Scand J Med Sci Sports 1991;1:158–162.

24. Smith JA, Telford RD, Mason IB, Weidemann MJ. Exercise, training and neutrophil microbicidal activity. Int J Sports Med 1990;11: 179–187.

25. Mackinnon LT. Future directions in exercise and immunology: regulation and integration. Int J Sports Med 1998;19(suppl 3):S205–S208.

26. Smith JA. Neutrophils, host defense, and inflammation: a

double-edged sword. J Leukoc Biol 1994;56:672–686.

27. Nieman DC, Tan SA, Lee JW, Berk LS. Complement and immunoglobulin levels in athletes and sedentary controls. Int J Sports Med 1989;10:124–128.

28. Nieman DC, Henson DA, Sampson CS, et al. The acute immune response to exhaustive resistance exercise. Int J Sports Med 1995;16:322–328.

29. Fry RW, Grove JR, Morton AR, et al. Psychological and immunological correlates of acute overtraining. Br J Sports Med 1994;28:241–246.

30. Rhind SG, Shek PN, Shinkai S, Shephard RJ. Differential expression of interleukin-2 receptor alpha and beta chains in relation to natural killer cell subsets and aerobic fitness. Int J Sports Med 1994;15:911–918.

31. Baj Z, Kantorski J, Majewska E, et al. Immunological status of competitive cyclists before and after the training season. Int J Sports Med 1994;15:319–324.

32. Nieman DC, Buckley KS, Henson DA, et al. Immune function in marathon runners versus sedentary controls. Med Sci Sport Exerc 1995;27:986–992.

33. Tvede N, Steensberg J, Baslund J, et al. Cellular immunity in highly trained elite racing cyclists during periods of training with high and low intensity. Scand J Sci Med Sport 1991;3:163–166.

34. Pedersen BK, Tvede N, Christensen LD, et al. Natural killer cell activity in peripheral blood of highly trained and untrained persons. Int J Sports Med 1989;10:129–131.

35. Gedge V, Mackinnon LT, Hooper SL. Effects of 4 wk intensified training on natural killer (NK) cells in competitive swimmers. Med Sci Sports Exerc 1997;29:S158. Abstract.

36. Nieman DC, Ahle JC, Henson DA, et al. Indomethacin does not alter natural killer cell response to 2.5 h of running. J Appl Physiol 1995;79:748–755.

37. Nieman DC, Nehlsen-Cannarella SL, Markoff PA, et al. The effects of moderate exercise training on natural killer cells and acute upper respiratory tract infections. Int J Sports Med 1990;11:467–473.

38. Nieman DC, Henson DA, Gusewitch G, et al. Physical activity and immune function in elderly women. Med Sci Sports Exerc 1993;25:823–831.

39. Mackinnon LT, Chick TW, van As A, Tomasi TB. Decreased secretory immunoglobulins following intense prolonged exercise. Sports Med Train Rehabil 1989;1:1–10.

40. Mackinnon LT. Exercise, immunoglobulin and antibody. Exerc Immunol Rev 1996;2:1–32.

41. Garagiola U, Buzzetti M, Cardella E, et al. Immunological patterns during regular intensive training in athletes: quantification and evaluation of a preventive pharmacological approach. J Int Med Res 1995;23:85–95.

42. Gleeson M, Pyne DB, McDonald WA, et al. Pneumococcal antibody response in elite swimmers. Clin Exp Immunol 1996;105:238–244.

43. Nehlsen-Cannarella S, Nieman DC, Jessen J, et al. The effects of acute moderate exercise on lymphocyte function and serum immunoglobulin levels. Int J Sports Med 1991;12:391–398.

44. Mackinnon LT. Advances in Exercise Immunology. Champaign, IL: Human Kinetics, 1999.

45. Mackinnon LT, Hooper SL. Mucosal (secretory) immune system responses to exercise of varying intensity and during overtraining. Int J Sports Med 1994;15:S179–S183.

46. Tomasi TB, Trudeau FB, Czerwinski D, Erredge S. Immune parameters in athletes before and after strenuous exercise. J Clin Immunol 1982;2:173–178.

47. Tharp GD, Barnes MW. Reduction of saliva immunoglobulin levels by swim training. Eur J Appl Physiol 1990;60:61–64.

48. Mackinnon LT, Ginn E, Seymour GJ. Temporal relationship between exercise-induced decreases in salivary IgA and subsequent appearance of upper respiratory tract infection in elite athletes. Aust J Sci Med Sport 1993;25:94–99.

49. Keast D, Arstein D, Harper W, et al. Depression of plasma glutamine concentration after exercise stress and its possible influence on the immune system. Med J Aust 1995;162:15–18.

50. Parry-Billings M, Budgett R, Koutedakis Y, et al. Plasma amino acid concentrations in the overtraining syndrome: possible effects on the immune system. Med Sci Sports Exerc 1992;24:1353–1358.

51. Rowbottom DG, Keast D, Goodman C, Morton AR. The haematological, biochemical and immunological profile of athletes suffering from the overtraining syndrome. Eur J Appl Physiol 1995;70:502–509.

52. Rowbottom DG, Keast D, Morton AR. The emerging role of glutamine as an indicator of exercise stress and overtraining. Sports Med 1996;21:80–97.

53. Castell LM, Newsholme EA, Poortmans JR. Does glutamine have a role in reducing infections in athletes? Eur J Appl Physiol 1996;73:488–490.

54. Pedersen BK, Ullum H. NK cell response to physical activity: possible mechanisms of action. Med Sci Sports Exerc 1994;26:140–146.

55. Smith JA. Exercise, training and red blood cell turnover. Sports Med 1995;19:9–31.

56. Urhausen A, Gabriel H, Kindermann W. Blood hormones as markers of training stress and overtraining. Sports Med 1995;20:251–276.

57. Hooper SL, Mackinnon LT. Monitoring overtraining in athletes: recommendations. Sports Med 1995;20:321–327.

58. Peters EM, Goetzsche JM, Grobbelaar B, Noakes TD. Vitamin C supplementation reduces the incidence of postrace symptoms of upper respiratory tract infection in ultramarathon runners. Am J Clin Nutr 1993;57:170–174.

59. Nieman DC, Henson DA, Garner EB, et al. Carbohydrate affects natural killer cell redistribution but not activity after running. Med Sci Sports Exerc 1997;29:1318–1324.

60. Roberts JA. Viral illnesses and sports performance. Sports Med 1986;3:296–303.

61. Simon HB. Exercise and infection. Phys Sportsmed 1987;15:135–141.

62. Parker S, Brukner PD, Rosier M. Chronic fatigue syndrome and the athlete. Sports Med Train Rehabil 1996;6:269–278.

Chapter 102

HIV Infection: Exercise and Immune Function

Bente Klarlund Pedersen

Several studies have shown that exercise modulates the immune system (1–3). In essence lymphocytes are mobilized to the circulation during moderate as well as intense exercise; however, in the recovery period of strenuous exercise the immune system is impaired. For several hours subsequent to heavy exertion, the number of lymphocytes declines, natural immunity is impaired, and the mucosal immunity (saliva secretory IgA) is suppressed. At the same time, pro- and anti-inflammatory cytokines increase. The postexercise temporary immunosuppression and concomitant inflammatory response may provide a physiologic rationale for increased frequency of infections in athletes performing strenuous exercise (4).

Given the fact that exercise modulates the immune system and potentially alters resistance to infections, it is obviously important to determine how exercise influences the immune system in immunocompromised individuals such as patients infected with the human immunodeficiency virus (HIV). This chapter describes the HIV-associated immune deficiency and defines immune parameters of prognostic importance for progression of HIV disease. Thereafter, the effects of acute and chronic exercise on these immunologic prognostic markers are described in healthy subjects as well as in HIV-seropositive individuals.

IMMUNOLOGIC MARKERS OF HIV DISEASE PROGRESSION

The natural course of the HIV infection is dominated by a progressive immunosuppression leading to development of AIDS with the occurrence of severe opportunistic infections and malignant diseases in the majority of infected individuals (5–7). The primary immunologic defect in individuals infected with HIV is a depletion of the CD4$^+$ T-cell subset (5,6), and the number and percentage of CD4$^+$ cells have been established as strong and reliable predictors for progression to AIDS and death (8,9). However, the immune defect in HIV is not thoroughly described by a CD4$^+$ cell count, and several immunologic parameters are associated with advanced disease and possess prognostic value (Table 102-1).

Within the CD4$^+$ T-cell population an early loss of memory CD45RO$^+$ cells is followed by an increased loss of naive CD45RA$^+$ cells, which in advanced infection is highly predictive to death (10). In the population of CD8$^+$ T cells early increases in numbers (11) and expression of activation markers (12) have been related to a poorer outcome.

The functional capacity of lymphocytes has been evaluated by the lymphocyte proliferation, either spontaneous or stimulated by mitogens or antigens. A defective proliferative response has been detected early in HIV infection and has been related to a poorer prognosis (13).

The specific antibody response following tetanus and pneumococcal vaccination, an in vivo estimate of B-cell function, has been shown to be impaired in HIV-seropositive patients with advanced disease (14,15). The delayed-type hypersensitivity skin test response to recall antigens, a functional measure of in vivo cellular immunity, has been shown to be an independent predictor of progression to AIDS in persons with HIV infection (16).

The function of natural killer (NK) cells and lymphokine-activated killer (LAK) cells is suppressed early in the disease (17) and high levels of HIV RNA are associated with low levels of non-MHC class I restricted cytotoxic activity (18). Recently, it has been shown in a cohort of 347 HIV-

Table 102-1 Prognostic Immunological Markers of HIV Progression

Low lymphocyte count
Low concentration of CD4 count
Low percentage of CD4 count
Early increases in concentration of CD8[+] cells
Low proliferative response to mitogens
Impaired specific antibody response to recall antigens
Decreased delayed-type hypersensitivity response (skin test)
Decreased natural killer cell activity
Decreased lymphokine-activated killer cell activity
Increased concentration of β_2-microglobulin and neopterin
Elevated plasma concentrations of TNF-α
Elevated plasma concentrations of TNF receptors
Decreased production of TNF-α and interleukin-1β
Decreased production of interferon-γ
Decreased production of MIP-1β

TNF-α = tumour necrosis factor-α.
MIP-1β = macrophage inflammatory protein-1β.

Table 102-2 The Effect of Intense Exercise of Long Duration on Various Immune Parameters

PARAMETER	DURING STRENUOUS EXERCISE	FOLLOWING STRENUOUS EXERCISE
Lymphocyte count	↑	↓
CD4[+] cell count	↑	↓
Percentage of CD4[+] cells	(↓)	—
CD8[+] cell count	↑	↓
Proliferative response to mitogens	↓	-(↓)
Antibody response in vitro	↓	↓
Antibody response in vivo	n.d.	—
Delayed-type hypersensitivity response (skin test)	n.d.	↓
Natural killer cell activity	↑	↓
Lymphokine-activated killer cell activity	↑	↓
Neopterin	n.d.	↑
Plasma concentrations of TNF-α, IL-1β	—	(↑)
Plasma concentrations of IL-6, IL-1 receptor antagonist	—	↑↑
Plasma concentrations of TNF receptors	n.d.	↑
Plasma concentrations of MIP-1β and IL-8	—	↑
Production of interferon-γ, IL-2, TNF-α, IL-1β, IL-6	—	↓

TNF = α tumor necrosis factor -α; IL = interleukin; MIP-1β = macrophage inflammatory protein; ↑ = increase; ↓ = decrease; ( ) = slight; — = no change; n.d. = not done.

seropositive subjects that the LAK cell activity is an age-, CD4[+]-, and HIV RNA–independent prognostic marker of HIV disease progression to AIDS and death (19).

Altered production of plasma concentrations have been described for several cytokines (20–24). The inflammatory cytokines' tumour necrosis factor (TNF)-α and interleukin (IL)-1β stimulate the replication of HIV (25). The possible detrimental effects of TNF-α or IL-1β have led to the hypothesis that these cytokines are important in the pathogenesis of HIV infection (20). However, conflicting results have been obtained regarding the production of TNF-α (20,24). Whereas some studies report increased plasma concentration of TNF-α (20), the production of TNF-α from lipopolysaccharide whole blood cultures was decreased in both AIDS and non-AIDS patients, whereas the production of IL-1β was decreased in AIDS patients only (24). Increased circulating levels of IL-6 have been described in patients with HIV disease (21). Recent findings show that low production of interferon-γ (22) and the β-chemokine macrophage inflammatory protein (MIP)-1β (23) are associated with HIV disease progression to AIDS and death. The serum levels of neopterin and β_2-microglobulin (indicators of activation of monocytes and lymphocytes, respectively) each had nearly as much predictive power as the CD4 count (9). Furthermore, serum levels of TNF receptors increase with disease progression (26).

ACUTE EXERCISE AND THE IMMUNE SYSTEM IN HEALTHY SUBJECTS

Exercise can be employed as a model for temporary immunosuppression that occurs after physical stress (27). There are several consistent patterns that emerge regarding exercise effects on various immune parameters in the blood (Tables 102-2 and 102-3). During acute exercise the lymphocyte concentration increases during exercise and falls below prevalues following intense long-duration exercise (28). The monocyte concentration is unchanged during exercise but increases following exercise. The neutrophil concentration increases during exercise and continues to increase after intense exercise (27).

Several reports describe exercise-induced changes in subpopulations of blood mononuclear cells (BMNC) [reviewed by Pedersen (1)]. The increased lymphocyte concentration is due to recruitment of all lymphocyte subpopulations to the blood. Thus, both CD3[+]CD4[+] T cells, CD4[+]CD45RA[+] naive T cells, CD4[+]CD45RO[+] memory T cells, CD3[+]CD8[+] T cells, CD19[+] B cells, CD3[−]CD16[+] NK cells, and CD3[−]CD56[+] NK cells increase during exercise. Simultaneously, the CD4/CD8 ratio decreases, because the CD8 count increases more than the CD4 count. The percentage CD4[+] cells declines mainly because the number of NK increases more than any other lymphocyte subpopulation. The NK cells are more sensitive to exercise stress and other physical stressors than any other lymphocyte subpopulation. The mechanisms underlying the acute exercise effects on lymphocyte subpopulations are most related to effects mediated by catecholamines, and in particular adrenaline (1,27,29).

Table 102-3 The Effect of Moderate Exercise on Various Immune Parameters

Parameter	During Moderate Exercise	Following Moderate Exercise
Lymphocyte count	↑	—
CD4$^+$ cell count	↑	—
Percentage of CD4$^+$ cells	(↓)	—
CD8$^+$ cell count	↑	—
Proliferative response to mitogens	(↓)	—
Antibody response in vitro	—	—
Antibody response in vivo		↑
Delayed-type hypersensitivity response (skin test)		n.d.
Natural killer cell activity	↑	—
Lymphokine-activated killer cell activity	↑	—
Neopterin	—	—
Plasma concentrations of TNF-α, IL-1β	—	—
Plasma concentrations of IL-6, IL-1 receptor antagonist	—	(↑)

TNF = α tumor necrosis factor -α; IL = interleukin; MIP-1β = macrophage inflammatory protein; ↑ = increase; ↓ = decrease; ( ) = slight; — = no change; n.d. = not done.

NK cells are thought to play an important role in the first line of defense against acute and chronic virus infections and tumor spread (30). Studies in various stress models, in humans and animals, show that high numbers of NK cells are recruited to the circulation within a few minutes after the onset of the stress and that NK cells are more sensitive to stress stimuli than any other subpopulations (31). Results from the area of stress immunology indicate that the rapid increased NK cell response in relation to infections probably also includes immediate recruitment of NK cells to the circulation and the site of infection.

Exercise of various types, duration, and intensity causes recruitment to the blood of cells expressing characteristic NK cell markers, such as CD16 and CD56. The NK cells have been studied in various models, including laboratory and field studies, studies on running, cycling and rowing, studies on concentric, eccentric, or combined concentric and eccentric models, and exercise lasting from few minutes to several hours [reviewed in Pedersen et al (32) and Pedersen (1)].

In general the NK and LAK cell activities (the ability of NK/LAK cells to kill tumor target cells or virus-infected cells) are increased when measured immediately after or during both moderate and intense exercise of a few minutes. The intensity more than the duration of exercise is responsible for the degree of increment in the number of NK cells. If the exercise has lasted for very long and has been very intense (e.g., a triathlon race), only a modest increase in NK cells is found postexercise (33). The NK cell count and the NK cell activity are suppressed only following intense exercise of a certain duration; 1 hour seems to be a critical duration of exercise in terms of postexercise immunosuppression. Initial fitness level or sex do not influence the magnitude of exercise-induced changes in NK cells (34).

The assessment of lymphocyte function in relation to exercise has involved the analysis of induced lymphocyte proliferation as a central issue. It is difficult to study the proliferation of normal lymphocytes in response to specific antigens, because only a minor proportion of cells will be stimulated to divide, and most studies on lymphocyte proliferation have used so called polyclonal mitogens, which induce many or all lymphocytes of a given type to proliferate. Although the polyclonal mitogens probably do not act directly on the antigen-specific receptors of lymphocytes, they seem to trigger the same growth response mechanisms as antigens. Highly variable results on lymphocyte proliferation in humans have been found. However, most studies in humans show that the mitogen response declines during exercise, and this has been a consistent finding in animal studies also [reviewed in Pedersen (1) and Nielsen et al (35)].

Suppressed levels of salivary immunoglobulin A (IgA) have been described after cross-country skiing (36), cycling (37), swimming (38), marathon running, and incremental treadmill running to exhaustion (39). Although the percentage of B cells does not change in relation to exercise, the ability of B cells to produce IgG, IgA, and IgM was suppressed, indicating that the suppressed antibody production was due to a functional inhibition. Altogether it was concluded that the exercise-induced suppression of the plaque-forming cell response was mediated by monocytes (40).

Several studies have investigated the immune system in relation to exercise, employing in vitro immunologic methods. Only a few studies have monitored the immune system in relation to exercise using in vivo immunologic methods. A recent study (41) investigated if an in vivo impairment of cell-mediated immunity and specific antibody production could be demonstrated after intense exercise of long duration (a triathlon race). The cellular immune system was evaluated as the skin test response to seven recall antigens, and the humoral immune system was evaluated as the antibody response to pneumococcal polysaccharide vaccine, which is generally considered to be T-cell-independent, and two toxoids (tetanus and diphtheria) that are dependent on T cells. The skin test response was significantly suppressed in the group who performed a triathlon race compared to triathlete controls and untrained controls, who did not perform the race. No differences in specific antibody titers were found between the groups, which is in accordance with the findings by others (42,43).

Thus, in vivo cell-mediated immunity was impaired in the first days after prolonged, high-intensity exercise, whereas there was no impairment of the in vivo antibody production measured 2 weeks after vaccination. The explanation of this may be that mainly unspecific immunity is influenced by exercise, whereas the specificity of the immune system is not altered. Alternatively, the time factor may be taken into consideration; thus, during the 2 weeks intermission the immune system may have had time to regenerate.

Moderate exercise training may influence the antibody response to vaccination differently than following intensive exercise. Thus, 8 weeks of moderate exercise resulted in 40% greater specific antibody response to tetanus toxoid (44).

Studies from the 1980s indicated that exercise induced elevated levels of IL-1 (45–47). Later studies reported on increased plasma levels of IL-6 after exercise (48–54). Several studies have failed to detect TNF-α after exercise (49,55–57), although some studies reported on increased levels (58,59). In relation to The Copenhagen Marathon 1996, we found a twofold increase in the concentrations of TNF-α, whereas the concentrations of IL-6 increased roughly fiftyfold, followed by a marked increase in the concentration of IL-1ra (Ostrowski et al, unpublished data). These results have recently been confirmed in a study performed in relation to The Copenhagen Marathon 1997 (Ostrowski et al, unpublished data). Recent studies in our laboratory have shown that strenuous exercise is followed by increased plasma concentrations of cytokine inhibitors (TNF receptors and IL-ra) and by increased concentration of the antiinflammatory cytokine IL-10. The findings that plasma levels of neopterin were increased after strenuous exercise (50,60) further support the idea of exercise-induced immune activation. The stimulated release of TNF-α, IL-1β, IL-6, IFN-γ, and IL-2 were suppressed after intense exercise (53).

Chemokines are small polypeptides that function mainly as chemoattractants for monocytes, neutrophils, and lymphocytes. Recent results from our laboratory found increased levels of the beta-chemokines IL-8 and MIP-1β after strenuous exercise (Ostrowski, Pedersen, unpublished data).

CHRONIC EXERCISE AND THE IMMUNE SYSTEM IN HEALTHY SUBJECTS

In contrast to the large number of studies on the immune response to acute exercise, much less is known concerning the effect of physical conditioning or training on immune function (Table 102-4). This is largely due to the difficulties in separating fitness effects from the actual physical exercise.

Table 102-4 Effect of Chronic Exercise Training on Resting Levels of the Immune System

PARAMETER	EFFECT
Lymphocyte count	—
Concentration of CD4+ cells	—
Percentage of CD4+ cells	—
Concentration of CD8+ cells	—
Proliferative response to mitogens	—
Antibody response	(↑)
Delayed-type hypersensitivity response	n.d.
Natural killer cell activity	↑
Lymphokine-activated killer cell activity	↑
Circulating levels and production of cytokines and their receptors	n.d.

— = no change; ↑ = increase; ( ) = slight; n.d. = not done.

Thus, the changes induced by intense physical exercise may last at least 24 hours, and even moderate acute exercise induces significant immune changes for several hours. Since it is not easy to persuade athletes to abstain from their normal training program even for just 1 day, it may be difficult to obtain results on really "resting levels." A good indicator of chronic exercise as a lifestyle factor is to compare resting levels of the immune system in untrained controls and in athletes who have been competing for several years. The effects of chronic exercise have also been studied in longitudinal designs, which have the advantage that the studies can be conducted using randomization, thus in principle excluding other confounding factors. The disadvantage is that most studies investigate at most 16 weeks of training, whereas the cross-sectional studies reflect many years of training.

Chronic exercise or training has been described in most studies to have no effect on lymphocyte proliferation in healthy HIV-seronegative individuals (61–65), although decreased (66) and increased (67,68) resting levels have been reported in trained individuals. One study showed that chronic exercise enhanced resting levels of the CD4 count (69), but most studies found no effect on concentrations or percentages of CD4+ cells in HIV-seronegative subjects (61–64,68,70–72). However, most cross-sectional studies show that the NK cell activity is increased in trained HIV-seronegative athletes compared to untrained subjects (27,70,72,73). In randomized, longitudinal studies chronic training has not shown a consistent effect on NK cell activity (68,70,72,74), whereas animal studies report an increased natural immunity in response to training (75–78).

EFFECTS OF ACUTE EXERCISE ON THE IMMUNE SYSTEM IN HIV-SEROPOSITIVE INDIVIDUALS

Given the fact that acute exercise causes alterations in the concentrations of lymphocyte subpopulations, proliferative responses, and NK and LAK cell functions in normal healthy individuals (27), and given the fact that HIV induces impairment in these immune parameters and that these changes are of clinical importance, it is obviously important to determine if exercise influences the immune system differentially in HIV-seropositive and HIV-seronegative subjects (1).

A study (57) on acute exercise was designed to determine to what extent HIV-infected individuals were able to mobilize immunocompetent cells to the blood in response to physical exercise. The study included eight asymptomatic men infected with HIV and eight HIV-seronegative controls who cycled for 1 hour at 75% of Vo₂max. The HIV-seropositive subjects were without AIDS or AIDS-related complex and had a CD4 count of 200 to 500 cells/μL. The percentages of CD4+, CD4+45RA+, and CD4+45RO+ cells did not change in response to exercise, whereas the concentration of CD4+ cells increased twofold during exercise.

The level of CD4+ cells in the circulation has prognostic value for predicting the development of acquired immunodeficiency syndrome (AIDS) (79–81) in HIV-infected patients and for predicting mortality resulting from complications of HIV infection in AIDS (82,83). However, increases in the concentration of CD4+ cells (the CD4 count) and in the CD4 percentage in response to treatment may not always reflect a better prognosis (84,85).

It has been debated which of the immunological markers to use: the absolute number or the percentage of CD4$^+$ cells. A study (86) showed that the percentage of CD4$^+$ lymphocytes had slightly greater prognostic significance and showed slightly less variability on repeated measurement. The finding that the CD4 count, but not the percentage of CD4$^+$ cells, changed in response to acute exercise offers one explanation of the variability in the absolute numbers of CD4$^+$ cells. Furthermore, it also strengthens the idea, that the percentage of CD4$^+$ cells is preferable to the number of CD4$^+$ cells in monitoring patients seropositive for HIV.

Interestingly, HIV-seropositive subjects were shown to possess an impaired ability to mobilize neutrophils and cells mediating NK cell activity. Furthermore, only control persons showed increased LAK cell activity in the blood in response to exercise, whereas HIV-seropositive subjects did not (57). Because exercise is accepted as a model of physical stress, the study on acute exercise suggests that HIV-seropositive subjects, although only moderately immunosuppressed, possess an impaired ability to generate unspecific immunity toward microbial agents in response to various physical stimuli.

In another study (87) the effects of acute exercise on mitogen-induced lymphocyte proliferation were studied. The HIV-seropositive subjects were without clinical symptoms, and the baseline CD4$^+$ count was 200 to 500 cells/μL). The lymphocytes from HIV-infected subjects had an overall lower mitogen-stimulated proliferative response than the lymphocytes from the HIV-seronegative subjects. The mitogen-induced proliferative response was lower in the HIV-seropositive subjects compared with HIV-seronegative subjects at all time points. The proliferative response was lower during the last 5 minutes of exercise in both the HIV-seropositive and HIV-seronegative groups.

The mechanisms behind the defective recruitment of cells to the blood are not fully understood, but may include 1) an impaired stress hormone response (e.g., the increase in catecholamines and growth hormone during physical exercise may be lower in HIV-seropositive subjects), 2) low expression of β-receptors on the surface of NK cells, or 3) alternatively, HIV-seropositive persons may simply have a smaller reservoir of cells available for recruitment (88).

EFFECT OF CHRONIC EXERCISE ON THE IMMUNE SYSTEM OF HIV-SEROPOSITIVE INDIVIDUALS

There are only few controlled studies on the effect of chronic exercise on the immune system in HIV-seropositive subjects. A controlled, randomized study was performed (89), including 19 HIV-seropositive subjects [groups II, III and IV according to Centers for Disease Control (CDC)] who performed bicycle exercise training for 12 weeks. Eighteen HIV-seropositive individuals, who did not exercise, were included as controls. Immune monitoring included flow cytometry analysis of lymphocyte subpopulations. Although training induced significant increases in neuromuscular strength and cardiorespiratory

fitness, there were no significant effects on the CD4 count or other lymphocyte subpopulations.

A similar randomized, controlled training study was performed (90). The study included 10 HIV-seropositive subjects who performed bicycle exercise training for 45 minutes three times a week for 10 weeks. The study also included HIV-seropositive control subjects, who did not train. The CD4 count, the CD56 count, and the NK cell activity measured per CD56$^+$ cell in whole blood were initially reported not to change as a result of training. However, a later review article by LaPerriere et al (91) reported increases in the CD4 count and in the number of CD4$^+$CD45RA$^+$ cells, using the same exercise protocol and number of subjects (90). One study (92) included five HIV-seropositive subjects in a 1-year training study, and another study (93) reported on six HIV-seropositive subjects, CDC stage IV, who performed 24 weeks of training. Training had no effect on the CD4 count in either of the studies (92,93).

Unfortunately, one study did not report the number of dropouts (90). However, other studies reported 1 of 5 (29%) (92), 4 of 23 (17%) (89), and 19 of 25 (76%) (93) dropouts. Clinical deterioration in some patients may be a major cause of the high dropout rates reported in training studies including seropositive patients. Thus, although one study (89) did not find differences between the training group and the control group regarding the number of subjects who dropped out or died, it can not be excluded that HIV-seropositive subjects dropped out because exercise training worsened their disease. These dropouts therefore constitute a clinically very important group. If training induces an immunologic and clinical deterioration in some patients, who then dropped out of the training program, this would be a major source of error.

Some of the studies have shown an insignificant increase in CD4 count in patients that train. Based on these results it has been concluded that training increases the CD4 count in HIV-seropositive patients (91). This is a very important conclusion since it could lead to the acceptance of physical training as a treatment of HIV infection. However, no study has to our knowledge been able to show any significant effect of training on the CD4 count in HIV-infected patients. If patients with declining CD4 counts drop out of the exercise regimen due to declining health, this could lead to a false impression of an increasing CD4 count caused by physical training.

THE OPEN-WINDOW HYPOTHESIS IN HIV DISEASE

In essence the immune system is enhanced during moderate and severe exercise, and only intense long-duration exercise is followed by suppressed concentration of lymphocytes, suppressed NK and LAK cell activities, and decreased secretory IgA in mucosa. Thus, following intense long-duration exercise the immune system is temporarily suppressed. This period of postexercise temporary immunosuppression has also been called the "open window" in the immune system (32). During the open window, microbacterial agents, especially viruses, may invade the host and infections may be established. One reason for the increased susceptibility to infections seen in elite athletes could be that this window of opportunism for pathogens is longer and the degree of immunosuppression more pronounced. We have previously suggested that severe immunodepression may occur if athletes do not allow the immune system to recover, but initiate a new bout of exercise while still immunodepressed. It has recently been suggested that neutrophils serve as a last line of defense (94). During the open window immune suppression of lymphoid cells, neutrophils are being mobilized to plug these gaps. The removal of this backup system following extreme activity would be compatible with the increased frequency of upper respiratory tract infections in athletes (94).

Regarding HIV-seropositive subjects, it was shown that these subjects have an impaired ability to mobilize neutrophils to the blood during exercise. Thus HIV-seropositive subjects have an impaired immune system when measured at rest, and furthermore an impaired ability to mobilize neutrophils to the blood during exercise stress. Therefore, HIV-seropositive subjects may in theory be more prone to enter the so-called open window in the immune system, and may more easily acquire infections during the time of postexercise immunosuppression. Moderate exercise boosts the immune system without inducing postexercise immunosuppression. Although there is no systemic research available regarding the effects of moderate exercise on the immune system of HIV-seropositive subjects, there is no reason to think that moderate exercise is detrimental to the immune system of HIV-infected individuals. Strenuous exercise such as a marathon induces immune activation, including most aspects of a classical acute phase response. It remains to be shown whether exercise-induced systemic inflammation is harmful to patients with HIV infection.

SUMMARY

There are no consistent findings regarding an effect of chronic training on resting levels of the immune system in HIV-seropositive patients. It is therefore not possible to conclude whether an endurance training program may alter HIV-associated immune impairment. The major reason for this uncertainty is related to the scarcity of data addressing the issue of exercise training and immune function in HIV infection. Thus, the available amount of data does not allow the drawing of any strong conclusions regarding possible beneficial or detrimental effects of training on the immune system in HIV-seropositive subjects. It has, however, been proven that exercise has positive effects in HIV-seropositive patients. Thus, improved muscle strength, retarded weight loss, and increased oxygen uptake as well as psychological relief have been demonstrated in patients that are able to participate in a training program (89,95).

New treatment strategies including the use of effective HIV-specific protease inhibitors such as ritonavir or indinavir have swept the scientific community with hope caused by dramatic reductions of viral load and similar increases of CD^+ cell counts (96,97). Similarly, the use of protease inhibitors and triple therapy in clinical practice has been associated to a marked lowering of HIV-related morbidity (25). It is not possible to tell to what extent the new treatment strategies will influence the survival of patients with HIV infection, but complete suppression of HIV replication without development of resistance has been shown in some patients for up to 3 years. Thus, in principle HIV replication can be continually suppressed, leading to partial or total immune reconstitution in the patients. Therefore, patients with HIV disease living in the Western world today with access to triple or quadruple antiretroviral treatment may, in principle, not have reduced longevity. It is obviously important to support the patients to be compliant with their antiretroviral treatment. Helping the patients to cope with their medication must have a higher priority than instructing the patients in the potential beneficial (but not proven) effects of moderate training in boosting their immune system. On the other hand, since HIV-seropositive patients will probably have increased longevity in the future compared to those patients who acquired the disease and died before the new treatment strategies, it is important that they (and everybody else) embrace healthy lifestyles. Thus, it may be equally important for patients with chronic infections such as HIV disease to perform regular moderate exercise in order to obtain the many positive effects of regular exercise, including lowering blood pressure, decreased risk of atherosclerosis, improved lipid profile, enhanced mood, decreased sensitivity to pain, and decreased risk of some cancers (98–105).

Recently, the ability to measure HIV-RNA in plasma has contributed to our understanding of the pathogenesis of HIV infection. Recent date demonstrate that a continuous high replication of HIV leads to an exhaustion of the vast proliferative capacity of the immune system; in other words, the destruction of the $CD4^+$ T cells eventually exceeds their replenishment (96,97). The use of both CD4 counts and plasma HIV-RNA measurements in the monitoring of HIV-infected patients has added greatly to the prognostic value of the isolated use of the CD4 count for predicting progression of the HIV infection. Furthermore, the concomitant measurements of neopterin and β_2-microglobulin are useful prognostic markers for predicting disease progression (9). Thus, in order to accept exercise as a treatment of HIV infection, exercise must be shown not only to increase CD4 counts but also to reduce the viral load and the immunologic activation as expressed by plasma HIV-RNA, neopterin, and serum β_2-microglobulin. Furthermore, since HIV infection is known to inhibit the function of the cellular immune response, a true positive clinical effect of any treatment of HIV infection would also lead to increases in the functional capacity of the cellular immune system. However, there are a lack of studies on the effect of training on viral load and immune activation as measured by plasma HIV-RNA, neopterin, β_2-microglobulin, and cytokines, including chemokines. Furthermore, there are no data showing a beneficial effect of chronic exercise or training on resting levels of lymphocyte proliferation and cytotoxic functions in HIV-seropositive patients.

Thus, encouragement for HIV-seropositive patients to perform physical activity relies on 1) the before-mentioned general positive effects of regular exercise, 2) the positive effects obtained in HIV patients in particular, including effect on muscle strength, cardiorespiratory fitness, and psychological relief, and 3) the fact that there is no evidence for a risk of transmission of HIV when infected persons, without bleeding wounds or skin lesions, engage in sports.

REFERENCES

1. Pedersen BK, ed. Exercise immunology. Austin, TX: R. G. Landes, 1997:1–206.

2. Nieman DC. Immune response to heavy exertion. J Appl Physiol 1997;82:1385–1394.

3. Mackinnon LT. Immunity in athletes. Int J Sports Med 1997; 18:S62–S68.

4. Nieman DC. Exercise, upper respiratory tract infection, and the immune system. Med Sci Sports Exerc 1994;26:128–139.

5. Fauci AS. Immunologic abnormalities in the acquired immunodeficiency syndrome (AIDS). Clin Res 1984;32:491–499.

6. Fauci AS. The human immunodeficiency virus: infectivity and mechanisms of pathogenesis. Science 1988;239:617–622.

7. Rosenberg ZF, Fauci AS. Immunopathogenic mechanisms of HIV infection: cytokine induction of HIV expression. Immunol Today 1990;11.

8. Phillips AN, Pezzoti P, Cozzi Lepri A, Rezza G. CD4 lymphocyte count as a determinant of the time from seroconversion to AIDS and death. Evidence from the Italian Seroconversion Study. AIDS 1994;7:975–982.

9. Fahey JL, Taylor JM, Detels R, et al. The prognostic value of cellular and serologic markers in infection with human immunodeficiency virus type 1. N Engl J Med 1990;322:166–172.

10. Ullum H, Lepri AC, Victor J, et al. Increased losses of CD4$^+$CD45RA$^+$cells in late stage of HIV infection is related to increased risk of death: evidence from a cohort of 347 HIV-infected individuals. AIDS 1997; 11:1479–1485.

11. Phillips AN, Sabin CA, Elford J, et al. CD8 lymphocyte counts and serum immunoglobulin A levels early in HIV infection as predictors of CD4 lymphocyte depletion during 8 years of follow-up. AIDS 1993;7:975–980.

12. Bruunsgaard H, Pedersen C, Scheibel E, Pedersen BK. Increase in percentage CD45RO$^+$CD8$^+$cells is associated with previous severe primary HIV infection. J AIDS 1995;10:107–114.

13. Hoffmann B, Jakobsen KD, Odum N, et al. HIV-induced immunodeficiency: relatively preserved phytohemagglutinin as opposed to decreased pokeweed mitogen responses may be due to possibly preserved responses via CD2/phytohemagglutinin pathway. J Immunol 1989;142:1874–1880.

14. Opravil M, Fierz W, Matter L, et al. Poor antibody response after tetanus and pneumococcal vaccination in immunocompromised HIV-infected patients. Clin Exp Immunol 1991;84:185–189.

15. Loeliger AE, Rijkers GT, Aerts P, et al. Deficient antipneumococcal polysaccharide responses in HIV-seropositive patients. FEMS Immunol Med Microbiol 1995; 12:33–41.

16. Blatt SP, Hendrix CW, Butzin CA, et al. Delayed-type hypersensitivity skin testing predicts progression to AIDS in HIV-infected patients. Ann Intern Med 1993; 119;177–184.

17. Ullum H, Gotzsche PC, Victor J, et al. Defective natural immunity: an early manifestation of human immunodeficiency virus infection. J Exp Med 1995;182:789–799.

18. Ullum H, Katzenstein T, Gerstoft J, et al. Increased plasma HIV-1 RNA levels are associated with low levels of non MHC class I restricted cytotoxicity. J AIDS 1996;13:255–256.

19. Ullum H, Lepri A, Katzenstein T, et al. Lymphokine activated killer cell activity—a new prognostic marker for disease progression in human immunodeficiency virus infection. AIDS 1999(in press).

20. Matsuyama T, Kobayashi N, Yamamoto N. Cytokines and HIV infection: is AIDS a tumour necrosis factor disease? AIDS 1991;5:1405–1417.

21. Ullum H, Diamant M, Victor J, et al. Increased circulating levels of interleukin-6 in HIV seropositive subjects. AIDS 1996;13:93–99.

22. Ullum H, Gotzsche P, Victor J, et al. Production of interferon-gamma is increased in early HIV infection but decreased in AIDS patients. AIDS Res Hum Retroviruses 1997;13:1039–1046.

23. Ullum H, Lepri AC, Victor J, et al. Production of beta-chemokines in HIV infection: evidence that high levels of MIP- 1 beta are associated with a decreased risk of HIV disease progression. J Infect Dis 1998; 177:331–336.

24. Ullum H, Victor J, Katzenstein T, et al. Decreased short term production of tumour necrosis factor-alfa and interleukin- 1 beta in HIV seropositive subjects. J Infect Dis 1997;175:1507–1510.

25. Osborn L, Kunkel S, Nabel GJ. Tumor necrosis factor-alpha and interleukin-1 stimulate the human immunodeficiency virus enhancer by activation of the nuclear factor kbeta. Proc Natl Acad Sci U S A 1989;86:2336–2340.

26. Aukrust P, Liabakk NB, Muller F, et al. Serum levels of tumor necrosis factor-alpha (TNF-alpha) and soluble TNF receptors in human immunodeficiency virus type 1 infection—Correlations to clinical, immunologic, and virologic parameters. J Infect Dis 1994;169:420–424.

27. Hoffman-Goetz L, Pedersen BK. Exercise and the immune system: a model of the stress response? Immunol Today 1994;15:382–387.

28. McCarthy DA, Dale MM. The leucocytosis of exercise: a review

and model. Sports Med 1988;6: 333–363.

29. Pedersen BK, Bruunsgaard H, Klokker M, et al. Exercise-induced immunomodulation—Possible roles of neuroendocrine factors and metabolic factors. Int J Sports Med 1997;18:S2–S7.

30. Whiteside TL, Herberman RB. The role of natural killer cells in human disease. Clin Immunol Immunopathol 1989;53:1–23.

31. Pedersen BK, Kappel M, Klokker M, et al. The immune system during exposure to extreme physiologic conditions. Int J Sports Med 1994;15:S116–S121.

32. Pedersen BK, Ullum H. NK cell response to physical activity: possible mechanisms of action. Med Sci Sports Exerc 1994;26:140–146.

33. Rohde T, MacLean DA, Hartkopp A, Pedersen BK. The relationship between plasma glutamine level and cellular immune responses in relation to triathlon race. Eur J Appl Physiol 1996;74:428–434.

34. Brahmi Z, Thomas JE, Park M, Dowdeswell IR. The effect of acute exercise on natural killer-cell activity of trained and sedentary human subjects. J Clin Immunol 1985;5:321–328.

35. Nielsen HB, Pedersen BK. Lymphocyte proliferation in response to exercise. Eur J Appl Physiol 1997;75:375–379.

36. Tomasi TB, Trudeau FB, Czerwinski D, Erredge S. Immune parameters in athletes before and after strenuous exercise. J Clin Immunol 1982;2:173–178.

37. Mackinnon LT, Chick TW, van As A, Tomasi TB. The effect of exercise on secretory and natural immunity. Adv Exp Med Biol 1987;216A:869–876.

38. Tharp GD, Barnes MW. Reduction of saliva immunoglobulin levels by swim training. Eur J Appl Physiol 1990;60:61–64.

39. McDowell SL, Hughes RA, Hughes RJ, et al. The effect of exhaustive exercise on salivary immunoglobulin A. J Sports Med Phys Fitness 1992;32:412–415.

40. Tvede N, Heilmann C, Halkjaer Kristensen J, Pedersen BK. Mechanisms of B-lymphocyte suppression induced by acute physical exercise. J Clin Lab Immunol 1989;30:169–173.

41. Bruunsgaard H, Hartkopp A, Mohr T, et al. In vivo cell mediated immunity and vaccination response following prolonged, intense exercise. Med Sci Sports Exerc 1997;29:1176–1181.

42. Eskola J, Ruuskanen O, Soppi E, et al. Effect of sport stress on lymphocyte transformation and antibody formation. Clin Exp Immunol 1978;32:339–345.

43. Gleeson M, Pyne DB, McDonald WA, et al. Pneumococcal antibody responses in elite swimmers. Clin Exp Immunol 1996; 105:238–244.

44. Kapasi ZF, Catlin PA, Geis C, et al. Effects of moderate exercise training on anti-tetanus antibody responses in young sedentary individuals. Int J Sports Med 1997;18(suppl 1):S45.

45. Cannon JG, Kluger MJ. Endogenous pyrogen activity in human plasma after exercise. Science 1983;220:617–619.

46. Cannon JG, Evans WJ, Hughes VA, et al. Physiological mechanisms contributing to increased interleukin-1 secretion. J Appl Physiol 1986;61:1869–1874.

47. Evans WJ, Meredith CN, Cannon JG, et al. Metabolic changes following eccentric exercise in trained and untrained men. J Appl Physiol 1986;61:1864–1868.

48. Northoff H, Berg A. Immunologic mediators as parameters of the reaction to strenuous exercise. Int J Sports Med 1991;12:S9–S15.

49. Ullum H, Haahr PM, Diamant M, et al. Bicycle exercise enhances plasma IL-6 but does not change IL-1α, IL-1β, IL-6, or TNFα pre-mRNA in BMNC. J Appl Physiol 1994;77:93–97.

50. Sprenger H, Jacobs C, Nain M, et al. Enhanced release of cytokines, interleukin-2 recep-

tors, and neopterin after long-distance running. Clin Immunol Immunopathol 1992;63:188–195.

51. Castell LM, Poortmans JR, Leclercq R, et al. Some aspects of the acute phase response after a marathon race, and the effects of glutamine supplementation. Eur J Appl Physiol 1997;75:47–53.

52. Bruunsgaard H, Galbo H, Halkjaer-Kristensen J, et al. Exercise-induced increase in interleukin-6 is related to muscle damage. J Physiol Lond 1997;499:833–841.

53. Weinstock C, Konig D, Harnischermacher R, et al. Effect of exhaustive exercise stress on the cytokine response. Med Sci Sports Exerc 1997;29:345–354.

54. Rohde T, MacLean DA, Richter EA, et al. Prolonged submaximal eccentric exercise is associated with increased levels of plasma IL-6. Am J Physiol 1997;273: E85–E91.

55. Rivier A, Pene J, Chanez P, et al. Release of cytokines by blood monocytes during strenuous exercise. Int J Sports Med 1994;15: 192–198.

56. Smith JA, Gray AB, Pyne DB, et al. Moderate exercise triggers both priming and activation of neutrophil subpopulations. Am J Physiol 1996;270:R838–R845.

57. Ullum H, Palmo J, Halkjaer Kristensen J, et al. The effect of acute exercise on lymphocyte subsets, natural killer cells, proliferative responses, and cytokines in HIV-seropositive persons. J Acquir Immune Defic Syndr 1994;7:1122–1133.

58. Dufaux B, Order U. Plasma elastase-alpha 1-antitrypsin, neopterin, tumor necrosis factor, and soluble interleukin-2 receptor after prolonged exercise. Int J Sports Med 1989;10:434–438.

59. Espersen GT, Elbaek A, Ernst E, et al. Effect of physical exercise on cytokines and lymphocyte subpopulations in human peripheral blood. APMIS 1990;98: 395–400.

60. Tilz GP, Domej W, Diez Ruiz A, et al. Increased immune activation during and after physical exercise. Immunobiol 1993;188:194–202.

61. Pedersen BK, Tvede N, Christensen LD, et al. Natural killer cell activity in peripheral blood of highly trained and untrained persons. Int J Sports Med 1989;10:129–131.

62. Tvede N, Steensberg J, Baslund B, et al. Cellular immunity in highly trained elite racing cyclists during periods of training with high and low intensity. Scand J Med Sci Sports 1991;1:163–166.

63. Nieman DC, Brendle D, Henson DA, et al. Immune function in athletes versus nonathletes. Int J Sports Med 1995;16:329–333.

64. Nieman DC, Buckley KS, Henson DA, et al. Immune function in marathon runners versus sedentary controls. Med Sci Sports Exerc 1995;27:986–992.

65. Oshida Y, Yamanouchi K, Hayamizu S, Sato Y. Effect of acute physical exercise on lymphocyte subpopulations in trained and untrained subjects. Int J Sports Med 1988;9:137–140.

66. Papa S, Vitale M, Mazzotti G, et al. Impaired lymphocyte stimulation induced by long-term training. Immunol Lett 1989;22:29–33.

67. Baj Z, Kantorski J, Majewska E, et al. Immunological status of competitive cyclists before and after the training season. Int J Sports Med 1994;15:319–324.

68. Nieman DC, Henson DA, Gusewitch G, et al. Physical activity and immune function in elderly women. Med Sci Sports Exerc 1993;25:823–831.

69. LaPerriere A, Antoni MH, Ironson G, et al. Effects of aerobic exercise training on lymphocyte subpopulations. Int J Sports Med 1994;15(suppl 3):S127–S130.

70. Nieman DC, Nehlsen Cannarella SL, Markoff PA, et al. The effects of moderate exercise training on natural killer cells and acute upper respiratory tract infections. Int J Sports Med 1990;11:467–473.

71. Barnes CA, Forster MJ, Fleshner M, et al. Exercise does not modify spatial memory, brain autoimmunity, or antibody response in aged F-344 rats. Neurobiol Aging 1991;12:47–53.

72. Crist DM, Mackinnon LT, Thompson RF, et al. Physical exercise increases natural cellular-mediated tumor cytotoxity in elderly women. Gerontology 1989;35:66–71.

73. Nieman DC. Prolonged aerobic exercise, immune response, and risk of infection. In: Hoffman-Goetz L, ed. Exercise and immune function. Boca Raton, FL: CRC Press, 1996:143–162.

74. Baslund B, Lyngberg K, Andersen V, et al. Effect of 8 wk of bicycle training on the immune system of patients with rheumatoid arthritis. J Appl Physiol 1993;75:1691–1695.

75. MacNeil B, Hoffman-Goetz L. Chronic exercise enhances in vivo and in vitro cytotoxic mechanisms of natural immunity in mice. J Appl Physiol 1993;74:388–395.

76. MacNeil B, Hoffman-Goetz L. Effect of exercise on natural cytotoxicity and pulmonary tumor metastases in mice. Med Sci Sports Exerc 1993;25:922–928.

77. MacNeil B, Hoffman-Goetz L. Exercise training and tumor metastasis in mice: influence of time of exercise onset. Anticancer Res 1993;13:2085–2088.

78. Hoffman-Goetz L, MacNeil B, Arumugam Y, Randall Simpson J. Differential effects of exercise and housing condition on murine natural killer cell activity and tumor growth. Int J Sports Med 1992;13:167–171.

79. Detels R, Visscher BR, Fahey JL, et al. Predictors of clinical AIDS in young homosexual men in a high-risk area. Int J Epidemiol 1987;16:271–276.

80. Moss AR, Bacchetti P, Osmond D, et al. Seropositivity for HIV and the development of AIDS or AIDS related condition: three year follow up of the San Francisco General Hospital cohort. Br Med J Clin Res Ed 1988;296:745–750.

81. Polk BF, Fox R, Brookmeyer R, et al. Predictors of the acquired immunodeficiency syndrome developing in a cohort of seropositive homosexual men. N Engl J Med 1987;316:61–66.

82. Safai B, Johnson KG, Myskowski PL, et al. The natural history of Kaposi's sarcoma in the acquired immunodeficiency syndrome. Ann Intern Med 1985;103:744–750.

83. Taylor J, Afrasiabi R, Fahey JL, et al. Prognostically significant classification of immune changes in AIDS with Kaposi's sarcoma. Blood 1986;67:666–671.

84. Anonymous. Concorde: MRC/ANRS randomised double-blind controlled trial of immediate and deferred zidovudine in symptom-free HIV infection. Concorde Coordinating Committee. Lancet 1994;343:871–881.

85. Kovacs JA, Baseler M, Dewar RJ, et al. Increases in CD4 T lymphocytes with intermittent courses of interleukin-2 in patients with human immunodeficiency virus infection: a preliminary study. N Engl J Med 1995;332:567–575.

86. Taylor JM, Fahey JL, Detels R, Giorgi JV. CD4 percentage, CD4 number, and CD4:CD8 ratio in HIV infection: which to choose and how to use. J Acquir Immune Defic Syndr 1989;2:114–124.

87. Rohde T, Ullum H, Palmo J, et al. Effects of glutamine on the immune system—influence of muscular exercise and HIV infection. J Appl Physiol 1995;79:146–150.

88. Doweiko JP. Hematologic aspects of HIV infection. AIDS 1993;7:753–757.

89. Rigsby LW, Dishman RK, Jackson AW, et al. Effects of exercise training on men seropositive for the human immunodeficiency

virus-1. Med Sci Sports Exerc 1992;24:6–12.

90. LaPerriere A, Antoni MH, Schneiderman N, et al. Exercise intervention attenuates emotional distress and killer cell decrements following notification of positive serologic status for HIV-1. Biofeedback Self Regul 1990; 15:229–242.

91. LaPerriere A, Fletcher MA, Antoni MH, et al. Aerobic exercise training in an AIDS risk group. Int J Sports Med 1991;12:S53–S57.

92. Birk TJ, MacArthur RD. Chronic exercise training maintains previously attained cardiopulmonary fitness in patients seropositive for human immunodeficiency virus type 1. Sports Med Train Rehabil 1994;5:1–6.

93. MacArthur RD, Levine SD, Birk TJ. Supervised exercise training improves cardiopulmonary fitness in HIV-infected persons. Med Sci Sports Exerc 1993;25:684–688.

94. Brines R, Hoffman-Goetz L, Pedersen BK. Can you exercise to make your immune system fitter? Immunol Today 1996;17:252–254.

95. LaPerriere A, Ironson G, Antoni MH, et al. Exercise and psychoneuroimmunology. Med Sci Sports Exerc 1994;26:182–190.

96. Ho DD, Neumann AU, Perelson AS, et al. Rapid turnover of plasma virions and CD4 lymphocytes in HIV-1 infection. Nature 1995;373:123–126. Comments.

97. Wei X, Ghosh SK, Taylor ME, et al. Viral dynamics in human immunodeficiency virus type 1 infection. Nature 1995;373: 117–122. Comments.

98. Paffenbarger RS, Kampert JB, Lee IM, et al. Changes in physical activity and other lifeway patterns influencing longevity. Med Sci Sports Exerc 1994;26: 857–865.

99. Lakka TA, Vwnalainen JM, Rauramaa R, et al. Relation of leisure-time physical activity and cardiorespiratory fitness to the risk of acute myocardial infarction in men. New Engl J Med 1994;330:1549–1554.

100. Williams PT. High-density lipoprotein cholesterol and other risk factors for coronary heart disease in female runners. N Engl J Med 1996;334:1298–1303.

101. Thune I, Brenn T, Lund E, Gaard M. Physical activity and the risk of breast cancer. N Engl J Med 1997;336:1269–1275.

102. Petruzzello SJ, Landers DM, Hatfield BD, et al. A meta-analysis on the anxiety-reducing effects of acute and chronic exercise: outcomes and recommendations. Sports Med 1991;11:143–182.

103. Thoren P, Floras JS, Hoffmann P, Seals DR. Endorphins and exercise: Physiological mechanisms and clinical implications. Med Sci Sports Exerc 1990;22:417–428.

104. Hoffman-Goetz L, Husted J. Exercise and cancer: do the biology and epidemiology correspond? Exerc Immunol Rev 1995;1:81–96.

105. Pedersen BK, Clemmensen IH. Exercise and cancer. In: Pedersen BK, ed. Exercise immunology. Austin, TX: R. G. Landes, 1997:171–201.

Chapter 103

Exercise, Aging, and Immunity

Robert S. Mazzeo

Participation by older individuals in regular exercise programs is being highly promoted by healthcare professionals including the National Institute on Aging. Among the documented benefits associated with regular exercise include increased cardiovascular fitness, retention of muscle mass and strength, improved balance and flexibility (thus, reducing the risk of falling), increase/retention of bone density (reducing the risk of osteoporosis), and an enhancement in psychosocial variables (e.g., depression). Additionally, involvement in exercise results in the reduction in risk factors associated with various life-threatening diseases (coronary heart disease, diabetes, certain cancers, etc.). Taken together, these benefits from regular exercise contribute to an improved quality of life in this age group.

The extent to which regular exercise affects the immune system in older populations is less understood. Although it is well documented that immune function deteriorates with advancing age, the influence of exercise intervention remains unclear. The major questions that need to be addressed are: 1) Does participation in regular exercise alter immune function? 2) Does this translate into a reduced risk for infectious diseases, cancer, and autoimmune disorders? and 3) How do acute bouts of exercise affect immune function in this population? This chapter examines what the research, to date, has revealed regarding these issues. Although there have been few studies addressing the effect of exercise and age on immune function, recent evidence is encouraging.

THE AGING IMMUNE SYSTEM

Declines in immunoresponsiveness and function are known consequences associated with the aging process (1–3). As a result of this immunosenescence, older individuals are more susceptible and are at greater risk for infectious diseases, tumorigenesis, and autoimmune disorders. The clinical significance is apparent since the age-related decline in immune function can contribute to increased mortality from various causes (4). In individuals over 60 years of age, those who exhibit an age-related dysfunction in their immune system have significantly greater mortality rates compared to age-matched individuals with normal immune function (5). It is noteworthy, however, that not all components of the immune system demonstrate this age-related dysfunction to the same extent or degree.

Innate Immunity

Natural Killer Cells

The evidence examining influence of age on natural killer (NK) cell number and function must be addressed with caution. When looking at NK-cell number and activity in the spleen from both mice and rats, there is a clear and consistent decline in NK-cell number and activity (6–9). However, when examining peripheral blood NK-cell activity in humans, it is frequently reported that no age-related change is found (10–12), and in some cases an increase in NK-cell number and activity has been observed (13–15). Although this may be related to species differences, it is also likely that the immune compartments examined play a major role. In this regard, whereas murine splenic NK-cell activity is well documented to decline with advancing age, NK-cell activity measured in murine peripheral blood does not decline. Thus, when peripheral blood is used, a similar response is observed in mice and humans. To date, we know of no studies examining human

1159

splenic NK-cell activity to see if the age-related decline found in animal models also exists in humans. The functional significance of these differences between blood, spleen, and potentially other immune compartments remains to be determined.

Macrophages

Because macrophages play an essential role in the recognition and presentation on antigens for both cell-mediated and humoral immunity, any age-related alterations in macrophage function would have significant adverse effects on both T- and B-cell responses. It is generally found that macrophage number, phagocytotic activity, and ability to process antigens is unaffected by age (16–18). Further, splenic macrophage ability to interact with T and B cells, necessary to initiate and regulate both effective antibody and lymphocyte responses, was also found to be unchanged with age (16,19). However, it has been reported that the ability to produce interleukin-1 is reduced with age in peritoneal macrophages (20).

Cell-Mediated Immunity

It is clear that cell-mediated immunity is the branch of the immune system affected most adversely by advancing age. This can be directly attributed to the well-documented involution of the thymus associated with aging (21–23). Responsibilities of the thymus include those of an endocrine gland as well as being a major site for lymphocyte differentiation. Immature lymphocytes originating from bone marrow migrate to the thymus gland for cellular differentiation and maturation. The thymus gland also produces a number of polypeptide hormones that help to regulate the differentiation of pre- and post-thymic lymphocytes. Thus, the dramatic thymic involution (Figure 103-1) that occurs with advancing age

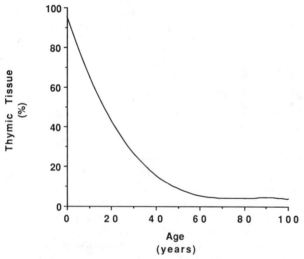

Functional Thymic Tissue

Figure 103-1 Change in functional thymic tissue as a result of human aging. (Modified from George AJT, Ritter MA. Thymic involution with ageing: Obsolescence or good housekeeping? Immunol Today 1996;17: 267–272.)

severely alters the ability of T-lymphocyte function. Consequently, total T-cell numbers, subset distributions, and responsiveness are compromised with aging. Reduction in numbers of T cytotoxic/suppressor subset (CD8$^+$) and CD4$^+$CD45RA$^+$naive T cells is most prominent. Diminished responsiveness to mitogen-induced [phytohemagglutinin (PHA), concanavalin A Con A] proliferation of T lymphocytes is commonly observed with advancing age. Further evidence of age-related declines in T-cell-dependent functions is provided by the delayed-hypersensitivity reaction skin test as well as mixed lymphocyte reaction analysis (24,25).

Age-related defects in a number of other components related to cell-mediated immunity have also been reported including cytokine production, receptor number, and expression; mechanisms of signal transduction; and cell differentiation (26–30). A consistent observation across species studied is an age-related decline in both the ability for IL-2 production and the number of cells synthesizing IL-2 mRNA. As IL-2 plays an integral role in humoral and cell-mediated immunity, loss of IL-2 activity will have a negative effect on overall immune function. This is supported by the observation that exogenous administration of IL-2 can partially restore immune function in older individuals (28).

Other techniques, including thymic and bone marrow cell grafts (31,32), administration of thymic hormones, and the addition of calcium ionophores, have also been shown to improve immune function (28,29,33–36). These results further support the importance of the loss of functional thymic tissue and hormones as contributors to cell-mediated immunosenescence.

Caloric restriction is another technique or intervention that has been consistently shown to prevent or delay dysfunctions of the immune system (37–40). This preserved immune function is reflected by increased mitogen-induced proliferation, interleukin-2 (IL-2) induction and synthesis, cytotoxic T-cell function, and a greater percentage of T cells in spleen. Caloric restriction also results in a lower cancer rate and tumor development associated with advancing age, improved immune responsiveness after inoculation with an infectious agent, and a reduction in autoimmune disorders (41–43). The increased longevity and life span associated with caloric restriction has, in part, been attributed to the improvement in immune function. As caloric restriction slows or retards the aging of many biological systems (cardiovascular, endocrine, reproductive, skeletal, etc.), its contribution to longevity, as well as the precise mechanisms involved, remains to be elucidated.

Humoral Immunity

It is generally reported that B-cell function is only marginally affected by the aging process (44,45). As T-cell function and activity are adversely affected with age, regulation of B-cell function by dysfunctional T-cell mechanisms likely contribute to this observation. Thus, alterations in B-cell function with age may be indirectly related to the documented impairment in T-cell function. Calcium mobilization, cyclic nucleotides fluxes, and membrane transmission through surface receptors are diminished, thereby affecting responsiveness. The decline in B-cell function can also be attributed to the decline in cytokine secretion associated with age-related T-cell function. It has been reported that antibody production to human gammaglobulin (HGG) in aged CBA/CaJ (24 to 27 months) and C57BL/6JNNia (24 to 25 months) mice decreases significantly when compared to young mice (6 to 8 weeks) of respective strains (46). Although CBA/CaJ mice have better antibody responses to HGG than C57BL/6JNNia mice at each age, both groups showed large decreases in antibody production with age. However, for the most part, B-cell function appears to be well preserved with advancing age.

ACUTE EXERCISE AND IMMUNE FUNCTION IN OLDER INDIVIDUALS

A lack of knowledge exists regarding the influence that a single bout of acute exercise has on immune function in this population. This has both physiological as well as clinical implications when one considers that an acute bout of exercise is known to be immunosuppressive and the elderly are at greater risk from infectious diseases.

Depending upon the intensity and duration, it is generally agreed that an acute bout of exercise is immunosuppressive (47,48). However, these studies are based upon data collected from young populations only, with very little information available regarding the response in older individuals. The immunoresponsiveness to an acute bout of exercise is important from both a mechanistic as well as clinical perspective.

Although few studies have been performed to date, recent evidence suggests that the ability of the immune system in older individuals to respond to the stress imposed from a single bout of exercise is maintained with age (49–51). Fiatarone et al (52) investigated the influence of a single bout of cycling in young (30 ± 1 years) and old (71 ± 1 years) untrained women. No differences were observed between age groups in baseline NK-cell numbers and function in peripheral blood lymphocytes. In response to exercise, NK-cell activity increased significantly in both groups; however, no difference was observed between age groups. Thus, NK-cell activity was enhanced immediately postexercise, as is generally reported in young populations, and the effect was similar in both age groups.

The NK-cell activity in elderly women following acute exercise was also examined by Crist et al (53). This investigation also compared individuals after participation in 16 weeks of aerobic training with age-matched sedentary controls (72 ± 1 years). Following the training program, women demonstrated a 33% increase in baseline NK tumor cytotoxicity in peripheral blood lymphocytes when compared with age-matched sedentary controls. An acute bout of progressive treadmill exercise produced an increase in NK activity in both groups; however, the trained women achieved significantly greater values of NK activity compared to controls (50.3% versus 31.1%, respectively). Unfortunately, no comparisons were made with younger women of either training status.

Using acute maximal exercise as the stimulus, it has been recently reported that similar increases in NK-cell number and cytotoxicity are found in both young (23 ± 2 years) and older (64 ± 4 years) subjects, supporting results from the above studies (51). The information from the above studies is limited in that they only examined NK activity,

which is generally not altered with age when compared to components of cell-mediated immunity.

Recent experiments from our laboratory on human subjects have yielded novel findings regarding the influence of an acute bout of exercise on immune function (49). Peripheral blood lymphocyte numbers and percentages as well as responsiveness to PHA were studied in young (n = 6, 23 ± 2 years) and old (n = 7, 68 ± 3 years) male subjects both prior to and immediately after 20 minutes of supine bicycle ergometry at approximately 60% of maximal work capacity. The baseline proliferative responsiveness was significantly lower (22%) in the old compared to the young subjects. In response to submaximal exercise, proliferative responsiveness to PHA increased significantly (55%) in the young subjects; however, for the old subjects this response did not differ significantly from resting values increasing by 18%. No age-related differences in the percentage of $CD3^+$, $CD4^+$, and $CD19^+$ peripheral blood lymphocytes were observed; however, the percentage of $CD8^+$ cells was significantly reduced in the old subjects. As total number of lymphocytes declined with age, this resulted in a lower number of cells expressing $CD3^+$, $CD4^+$, and $CD8^+$ with age. These findings are consistent with the majority of literature examining T-cell subsets as a function of age. Total lymphocyte numbers as well as individual T-cell subsets measured increased in response to the 20-minute bout of submaximal exercise. This lymphocytosis, which is associated with an acute bout of exercise (47,48), occurred to the same extent in both age groups, suggesting that the mechanisms responsible are unaffected by age. Thus, a consistent finding, as indicated in Figure 103-2, was that exercise-induced increases in T-cell subset populations were similar across age groups. It was concluded that, although having lower initial T-cell numbers and PHA responsiveness, immunoresponsiveness during a single bout of exercise is, in general, maintained in old when compared to young individuals.

These findings have also been observed in response to an acute bout of maximal exercise in young (23 ± 2 years) and older (65 ± 4 years) subjects (50). The mitogenic response (Con A) to maximal exercise was similar in both young and older subjects. Further, the exercise-induced alterations in leukocyte subsets did not differ as a function of age.

Although results from animal studies can be more extensive, again there are very few studies available. Studies using young and old BALB/c mice that were required to swim until exhaustion (194 ± 28 minutes) found that spleen, thymus, and axillary node lymphocyte responsiveness to PHA was suppressed in both groups (54). However, it is noteworthy that although baseline responsiveness to mitogen was significantly lower in old versus young mice, the acute bout of exhaustive exercise had a greater immunosuppressive effect in the young (62% decrease for splenocytes) when compared to the old (26% decrease for splenocytes) mice.

The responsiveness to several neuroendocrine regulators is significantly altered with advancing age, and this may contribute to the attenuated immune responses observed during acute exercise in the older individuals. The neuroendocrine system plays a critical role in modulating immune function in response to both an acute bout as well as chronic endurance exercise in young populations. As the aging process is associated with functional declines in many facets of the neuroen-

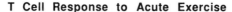

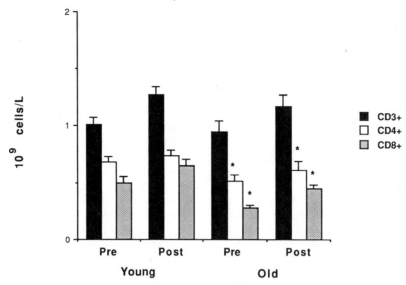

Figure 103-2 Alterations in T-cell numbers in response to 20 minutes of submaximal cycling exercise. Six young (26 ± 3 years) and nine older (69 ± 5 years) healthy, nonsmoking male subjects participated in the study. Peripheral blood lymphocytes were collected before and immediately after exercise. Although initial baseline values were lower for old subjects, the response to exercise was similar across age groups. *Significantly different from young subjects for similar time period. (Modified from Mazzeo RS, Rajkumar C, Rolland J, et al. Immune response to a single bout of exercise in young and elderly subjects. Mech Ageing Dev 1998;100:121–132.)

docrine system, this could potentially influence the immune response to both acute and chronic stressors (e.g., exercise) in this population. Included among this diminished neuroendocrine responsiveness are a reduction in innervation of spleen, alterations in receptor number, density, and affinity, diminished receptor responsiveness and various components of signal transduction, as well as a reduction in the ability to synthesize and release hormones and neurotransmitters. For example, Bellinger et al (55) have proposed a causal relationship between the diminished sympathetic innervation of the spleen and the decline of T-lymphocyte immune functions with advancing age. As a result of these neuroendocrine changes, older individuals are likely to respond differently to both acute and chronic exercise stimulation. Specifically, age-related changes exist in overall catecholamine metabolism and receptor responsiveness, tissue-specific sympathetic nerve activity, stress-induced corticosteroid production and effectiveness, and sensitivity to prostaglandin E$_2$, including T lymphocytes (56). All of these variables are documented to alter immune function, particularly during exercise.

EXERCISE TRAINING AND IMMUNE FUNCTION IN OLDER INDIVIDUALS

A limited number of studies have addressed the effect of endurance training adaptations on immune function in older individuals. As cited above, Crist et al (53) examined the influence of 16 weeks of aerobic training (3 days per week at 50% heart rate reserve) in older women. Compared to age-matched sedentary controls, trained women demonstrated a 33% increase in basal NK cytotoxic activity. Additionally, a

progressive treadmill exercise test resulted in a 32% increase in NK-cell activity in the control group, whereas a significantly greater increase was found for the trained women (50%). Thus, it was concluded that long-term aerobic training enhances NK-mediated cytotoxicity in elderly women.

In contrast, Nieman et al (57) have shown that 12 weeks of moderate aerobic training (5 days per week at 60% heart rate reserve) had no effect on basal NK-cell activity and T-cell function (PHA responsiveness) in previously sedentary women (73 ± 1 years). However, in a group of highly conditioned female endurance competitors (n = 12, 73 ± 2 years), it was found that T-cell function was significantly greater when compared to age-matched sedentary controls. Differences in the training intensity, duration, and frequency may be responsible for the changes in immune function between the moderately trained and highly conditioned women. Alternatively, the age at which exercise training is initiated may be a factor since the highly conditioned women had begun an exercise program earlier in life. This is supported by a recent cross-sectional study (58) that found that older male runners (63.8 ± 3.3 years) who had been active for the previous 17.2 ± 6.1 years had significantly greater circulating T-cell function and related cytokine production than age-matched sedentary controls (Figure 103-3).

In the only study examining the effect of strength training on healthy elderly subjects (70 ± 5 years), lymphocyte subpopulations, cytokine production, proliferative response to PHA and Con A, and delayed-type hypersensitivity skin response were determined before and after 12 weeks of progressive resistance strength training (59). It was concluded that this type of exercise training had no affect on immune func-

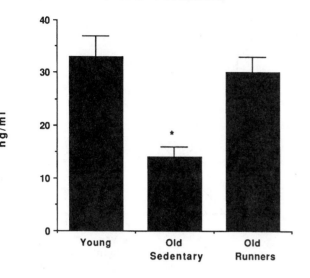

IL-2 Production

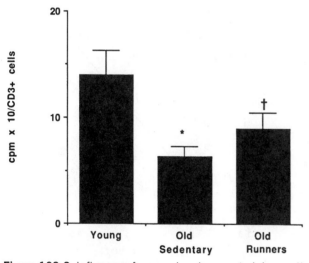

PHA-Induced Proliferation

Figure 103-3 Influence of age and endurance training on IL-2 production and mitogen (PHA)-induced proliferation in young (24 ± 2 years), old sedentary (66 ± 4 years), and old runners (64 ± 3 years). The old runners had been exercising regularly for an average of 17 ± 6 years. All subjects were healthy male volunteers. Participation in regular exercise significantly reduced the normal age-related decline in IL-2 production and proliferation responses. *Significantly different from young subjects. †Significantly different from both young and old sedentary subjects. (Modified from Shinkai S, Kohno H, Kimura K, et al. Physical activity and immune senescence in men. Med Sci Sports Exerc 1995;27:1516–1526.)

tion in this population. Additionally, subjects with rheumatoid arthritis, an autoimmune disorder, did not demonstrate any improvement in immune function as a result of the same training regimen.

Finally, in a study with frail elderly men (75 ± 5 years) who participated in 3 months of a combination of strength, balance, and aerobic exercise, it was suggested that exercise had an adverse effect on NK-cell cytotoxicity (60). A significant decrease in NK activity was observed in these frail subjects that led the authors to speculate that, in this population, the added stress of training on an already weakened immune system contributed to this decline.

Although animal studies allow for a more thorough analysis of immune function (spleen, thymus, and axillary nodes), there still is a lack of data related to exercise training, aging, and immune function.

Pahlavani et al (61) investigated the role of exercise training on immunosenescence in male Fischer 344 rats. Rats of four different age groups (1, 6, 12, and 18 months of age, initially) were examined after a 6-month training program (swimming for 60 minutes, twice daily, 5 days per week). Mitogen-induced proliferation of isolated splenocytes in both trained (41%) and untrained (52%) rats declined significantly with increasing age. Con-A–stimulated proliferation was actually reduced with training in the 7- and 12-month-old rats (32% and 23%, respectively) when compared to age-matched control groups. However, in the older animals, no differences were observed between groups. An age-related decline in IL-2 synthesis was observed in both the trained and the untrained rats, which was unaltered by training (except for a decrease in the young group). These authors concluded that exercise training did not prevent the age-related decline in lymphocyte proliferation as well as IL-2 production. Further, training had an adverse effect on mitogen-induced proliferation and IL-2 production in the younger animals.

In a separate study, markers of immune function were measured in endurance-trained (15 weeks at 75% maximal running capacity) male Fischer 344 rats across age groups (7). Mitogen-induced (Con A) lymphocyte proliferation, IL-2 production, and NK cytotoxicity were determined in splenocytes from 8-, 17-, and 27-month-old rats. The proliferative response and IL-2 production were significantly reduced with age in both trained and untrained animals. Although exercise training significantly reduced both proliferation and IL-2 production in 8- and 17-month-old animals, these variables were increased in the 27-month-old trained group compared to age-matched controls. Training did not effect NK-cell activity across any age group, which was found to significantly decline with age.

Spleen-weight-adjusted total T-cell numbers were lower for old animals regardless of training status. As found for mitogen-induced proliferation, training lowered T-cell numbers for young and middle-aged animals but increased numbers in the old animals. CD4+ and CD8+ T cells followed a similar pattern to that of total T cells, such that percentages and numbers declined with age. Again, although a reduction in CD4+ and CD8+ T-cell numbers was observed with training for young (25%) and middle-aged (47%) animals, a training-induced increase was found for the old animals (53%). Thus, splenocyte subpopulations as well as mitogen-induced splenocyte proliferation and IL-2 production are altered with age and training. A significant interaction was observed such that these immunological markers decreased with training in the younger groups but increased in the older trained animals.

The training-induced reduction in spleen weight observed may contribute to the diminished T-cell numbers reported. Further, the repeated stress of forced treadmill running may confound data interpretation and contribute to the training-induced reductions in immune function and spleen weight reported for the younger animals.

Immune function has been measured in vivo by administration of keyhole-limpet hemocyanin (KLH, a T-cell-dependent antigen) in young and old Fischer 344 rats (62). KLH antibody production, determined 10 and 17 days after administration, was found to be significantly lower in old compared to young animals (77%). Ten weeks of endurance training by treadmill running did not improve this response in old animals.

The effect of endurance training and aging on the immune response to acute exercise has been examined, to date, in only one study. De la Fuente et al (54) measured the PHA-induced proliferative response in spleen, thymus, and axillary nodes from young (15 ± 2 weeks) and old (60 ± 5 weeks) BALB/c mice, both at rest and after an exhaustive bout of swimming. When compared to control mice that did not exercise, exhaustive exercise significantly suppressed the proliferative response in both young and old untrained mice. The suppressive effect of exercise was abolished in mice from both age groups that had been swim-trained (90 minutes a day for 20 days). Thus, the acute bout of exercise was not found to be immunosuppressive in the swim-trained group; however, this protective effect of training was found to be greater in the young compared to the old animals.

CLINICAL IMPLICATIONS

Infectious disease remains a significant cause of death in the elderly, which has been suggested to be a direct result of the age-related decline in immune function (63). Infectious diseases such as pneumonia and urinary tract infections are leading causes of death in individuals over the age of 60 years, suggesting that an impaired immune system reduces these individuals' capacity to fight common types of infections. Other evidence has been provided indicating that both animals and humans who demonstrate reduced immune function with age demonstrate significantly greater mortality rates compared with individuals whose immune function is within the normal range (5,64). Thus, any intervention that can slow or prevent the age-related decline in immune function would have significant health implications.

A program of regular cardiovascular exercise has been shown to have many benefits including a reduction in risk factors associated with various life-threatening diseases (coronary heart disease, diabetes, certain cancers, etc.). Preliminary evidence suggests that participation in a regular exercise program can have a beneficial effect on the aging immune system. This is particularly true when the exercise program is begun earlier in life. Nieman et al (57) have found a significant correlation between cardiovascular fitness levels (maximal oxygen consumption) with those of NK cell cytotoxic activity as well as PHA-induced lymphocyte proliferation (Figure 103-4). In that study, highly conditioned women (mean age = 73 years) who had been physically active for a

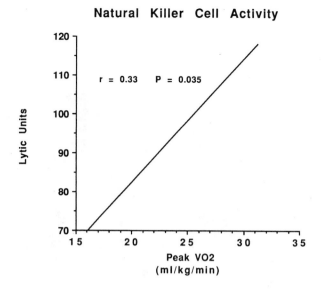

Natural Killer Cell Activity

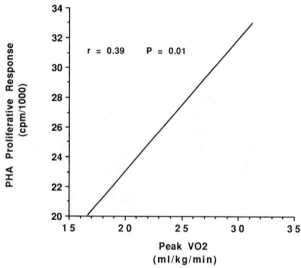

Proliferation Response

Figure 103-4 Relationship between cardiovascular fitness and makers of immune function in 42 elderly women (73 ± 1 years). Within this age group, both natural killer cell activity and PHA-induced proliferation increased as a function of fitness and was significantly correlated with peak V_{O_2}. (Modified from Nieman DC, Henson DA, Gusewitch G, et al. Physical activity and immune function in elderly women. Med Sci Sports Exerc 1993;25: 823–831.)

number of years demonstrated significantly superior immune function when compared to age-matched controls. Further, women (mean age = 73 years) who participated in a 12-week moderate exercise program did not show any improvement in immune function. The differences between these two groups of women may be related to the intensity and duration of the exercise program or the age of initiation of exercise training. What is of interest is the finding that the highly conditioned women (with the greater baseline immune function) had significantly fewer incidences of upper respiratory tract infections when compared to two other groups of age-matched women (Figure 103-5).

Similar findings were found in a group of Japanese men (mean age = 64 years) who had been running approximately 4 to 5 days per week on average for 17 years. Compared to aged-matched sedentary controls, the elderly runners exhibited significantly greater mitogen-induced proliferative responses as well as higher rates of IL-2, IL-4, and IFN-γ production (58). It was concluded that endurance training was associated with a lesser age-related decline in T-cell function and related cytokine production.

Thus, given the known susceptibility and potential adverse consequences of contracting infectious diseases in elderly populations, any improvement in baseline immune function could significantly impact health and reduce morbidity and mortality. Clearly, more research in this important area of gerontology remains to be conducted. Future research should be targeted at: 1) determining mechanisms whereby regular endurance training may improve immune function in older individuals; 2) the extent to which such adaptations translate into less susceptibility to infectious diseases and improvements in overall health; and 3) examining if an interaction exists between exercise training, improved immune function, and lessening the risk of cancer development as one ages.

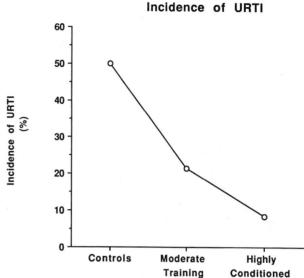

Incidence of URTI

Figure 103-5 Incidence of upper respiratory tract infections (URTIs) over a 12-week period in 42 elderly women (73 ± 1 years). Highly conditioned elderly women (5 years of regular aerobic exercise) demonstrated a significantly lower incidence of URTI compared to age-matched sedentary and moderately trained (12 weeks of walking) women. (Modified from Nieman DC, Henson DA, Gusewitch G, et al. Physical activity and immune function in elderly women. Med Sci Sports Exerc 1993;25:823–831.)

REFERENCES

1. Hausman PB, Weksler ME. Changes in the immune response with age. In: Finch CE, Schneider EL, eds. Handbook of biology of aging. New York: Van Nostrand Reinhold, 1985:414–432.

2. Makinodan T, Kay MMB. Age influence on the immune system. Adv Immunol 1980;29:287–330.

3. Miller RA. The cell biology of aging: immunological models. J Gerontol 1989;44:B4–B8.

4. Ohstu S. Morphology and causes of death in extremely elderly people. The 3rd Symposium in Tokyo Metropolitan Institute of Gerontology, Tokyo, 1979.

5. Roberts-Thomson IC, Whittingham S, Youngchaiyud U, et al. Ageing, immune response and mortality. Lancet 1974;2:368–370.

6. Bash JA, Vogel D. Cellular immunosenescence on F344 rats: decreased natural killer activity involves changes in regulatory interactions between NK cells, interferon, prostaglandins and macrophages. Mech Ageing Dev 1984;24:49.

7. Nasrullah I, Mazzeo RS. Age-related immunosenescence in Fischer 344 rats: influence of exercise training. J Appl Physiol 1992;73:1932–1938.

8. Saxena RK, Saxena QB, Alder WH. Interleukin-2-induced activation of natural killer activity in spleen cells from old and young mice. Immunology 1984;51:719–726.

9. Weindruch R, Devens BH, Raff HV. Influence of dietary restriction and ageing on natural killer cell activity in mice. J Immunol 1983;130:993–996.

10. Ferguson FG, Wikby V, Maxson P, et al. Immune parameters in a longitudinal study of a very old population of Swedish people: a comparison between survivors and nonsurvivors. J Gerontol 1995;50A:B378–B382.

11. Ligthart GJ, Schuit HRE, Hijmans W. Natural killer cell function is not diminished in the healthy aged and is proportional to the number of NK cells in the peripheral blood. Immunology 1989;68:396–402.

12. Murasko DM, Nelson BJ, Silver R, et al. Immunologic response in an elderly population with a mean age of 85. Am J Med 1986;81:612–618.

13. Batory G, Benczur M, Varga M, et al. Increased killer cell activity in aged humans. Immunobiol 1981;158:393.

14. Krishnaraj R, Blandford G. Age-associated alterations in human natural killer cells. Clin Immunol Immunopathol 1987;45:268–285.

15. Sansoni P, Cossarizza A, Brianti V, et al. Lymphocyte subsets and natural killer cell activity in healthy old people and centenarians. Blood 1993;82:2767–2773.

16. Callard RE. Immune function in aged mice III. Eur J Immunol 1978;8:697–705.

17. Perkins EH. Phagocyte activity of aged mice. J Reticuloendothel Soc 1971;9:642–643.

18. Shelton E, Davis S, Hemmer R. Quantitation of strain Balb/c mouse peritoneal cells. Science 1970;168:1232–1234.

19. Heidrick ML, Markinodan T. Presence of impairment of humoral immunity in non-adherent spleen cells of old mice. J Immunol 1973;111:1502–1506.

20. Inamizu T, Chang MP, Makinodan T. Influence of age on the production and regulation of interleukin-1 in mice. Immunology 1985;55:447–455.

21. Hirokawa K, Makinodan T. Thymic involution: effect on T cell differentiation. J Immunol 1975;114:1659–1664.

22. Hirokawa K, Utsuyama M, Kasai M. Role of the thymus in aging of the immune system. In: Goldstein AL, ed. Biomedical advances in aging. New York: Plenum Publishing, 1990:375–384.

23. Utsuyama M, Kasai M, Kurashima C, et al. Age influence on the thymic capacity to promote differentiation of T cells: induction of different composition of T cell subsets by aging thymus. Mech Ageing Dev 1991;58:267–277.

24. Canonica GW, Ciprandi G, Caria M, et al. Defect of autologous mixed lymphocyte reaction and interleukin-2 in aged individuals. Mech Ageing Dev 1985;32:205–212.

25. Gilhar A, Aizen E, Pillar T, et al. Response of aged versus young skin to intradermal administration of interferon gamma. J Am Acad Dermatol 1992;27:710–716.

26. Nordin AA, Proust JJ. Signal transduction mechanisms in the immune system: Potential implication in immunosenescence. Endocrinol Metab Clin North Am 1987;16:919–945.

27. Proust JJ, Filburn CR, Harrison SA, et al. Age-related defect in signal transduction during lectin activation of murine T lymphocytes. J Immunol 1987;139:1472–1478.

28. Thoman M, Weigle WO. Reconstitution of in vivo cell-mediated lympholysis responses in aged mice with interleukin 2. J Immunol 1985;134:949–952.

29. Thoman ML, Weigle WO. Partial restoration of Con A-induced proliferation, IL-2 receptor expression, and IL-2 synthesis in aged murine lymphocytes by phorbol myristate acetate and ionomycin. Cell Immunol 1988;114:1–11.

30. Vie H, Miller RA. Decline, with age, in the proportion of mouse T cells that express IL-2 receptors after mitogen stimulation. Mech Ageing Dev 1986;33:313–322.

31. Hirokawa K, Sato K, Makinodan T. Influence of age of thymic grafts on the differentiation of T cells in nude mce. Clin Immunol Immunopathol 1982;24:251–262.

32. Hirokawa K, Utsuyama M. Combined grafting of bone marrow and thymus, and sequential multiple thymus graftings in various strains of mice: the effect on immune functions and life span. Mech Ageing Dev 1989;49:49–60.

33. Fagiolo U, Amador A, Borghesan F, et al. Immune dysfunction in the elderly: effect of thymic hormone administration on several in vivo and in vitro immune function parameters. Aging 1990;2:347–355.

34. Frasca D, Adorini L, Mancini C, et al. Reconstruction of T-cell functions in aging mice by thymosin alpha one. Immunopharmacol 1986;11:155–163.

35. Miller RA. Immunodeficiency of aging: restorative effects of phorbol ester combined with calcium ionophore. J Immunol 1986;137:805–808.

36. Miller RA, Jacobson B, Weil G, et al. Diminished calcium influx in lectin-stimulated T cells from old mice. J Cell Physiol 1987;132:337–342.

37. Richardson A, Cheung HT. The relationship between age-related changes in gene expression, protein turnover, and the responsiveness of an organism to stimuli. Life Sci 1984;31:605–613.

38. Umezawa M, Hanada K, Naiki H, et al. Effects of dietary restriction on age-related immune dysfunction in the senescence accelerated mouse (SAM). J Nutr 1990;120:1393–1400.

39. Weindruch R, Kristie JA, Naeim F, et al. Influence of weaning-initiated dietary restriction on response to T cell mitogens and on splenic T cell levels in a long-lived mouse hybrid. Exp Gerontol 1982;17:49–64.

40. Weindruch R, Gottesman SRS, Walford RL. Modification of age-related immune decline in mice dietarily restricted from or after midadulthood. Proc Natl Acad Sci 1982;79:898–902.

41. Effros RB, Walford RL, Weindruch R, et al. Influence of dietary restriction on immunity to influenza in aged mice. J Gerontol 1991;46:B142–B147.

42. Gilman-Sachs A, Kim YB, Pollard M, et al. Influence of aging, environmental antigens, and dietary restriction on expression of lymphocyte subsets in germ-free and conventional Lobound-Wistar rats. J Gerontol 1991;46:B101–B106.

43. Kubo C, Day NK, Good RA. Influence of early or late dietary restriction on life span and immunological parameters in MRL/Mp-lpr/lpr mice. Proc Natl Acad Sci 1984;81:5831–5835.

44. Ben-Yehuda A, Weksler ME. Immune senescence: mechanisms and clinical implications. Cancer Invest 1992;10:525–531.

45. Ennist DL, Jones KH, St. Pierre RL, et al. Functional analysis of the immunosenescence of the human B cell system: Dissociation of normal activation and proliferation from impaired terminal differentiation into IgM immunoglobulin-secreting cells. J Immunol 1986;136:99–105.

46. Gahring LC, Weigle WO. The effect of aging on the induction of humoral and cellular immunity and tolerance in two long-lived mouse strains. Cell Immunol 1990;128: 142–151.

47. Keast D, Cameron K, Morton AR. Exercise and the immune response. Sports Med 1988;5: 248–267.

48. Nieman DC, Nehlsen-Cannarella SL. The immune response to exercise. Semin Hematol 1994;31: 166–179.

49. Mazzeo RS, Rajkumar C, Rolland J, et al. Immune response to a single bout of exercise in young and elderly subjects. Mech Ageing Dev 1998;100:121–132.

50. Ceddia MA, Wolters BW, Price EA, et al. Effects of acute maximal exercise on leukocytosis, leukocyte subsets, and mitogenesis in the elderly. Med Sci Sports Exerc 1997;29:S298.

51. Woods JA, Wolters BW, Ceddia MA, et al. Effects of maximal exercise on natural killer (NK) cell activity and responsiveness to interferon-α in young and old. Med Sci Sports Exerc 1997;29: S159.

52. Fiatarone MA, Morley JE, Bloom ET, et al. The effect of exercise on natural killer cell activity in young and old subjects. J Gerontol 1989;44:M37–M45.

53. Crist DM, Mackinnon LT, Thompson RF, et al. Physical exercise increases natural cellular-mediated tumor cytotoxicity in elderly women. Gerontology 1989;35: 66–71.

54. De la Fuente M, Ferrandez MD, Miquel J, et al. Changes with aging and physical activity in ascorbic acid content and proliferative response of murine lymphocytes. Mech Ageing Develop 1992;65:177–186.

55. Bellinger DL, Felten SY, Collier TJ, et al. Noradrenergic sympathetic innervation of the spleen: IV. Morphometric analysis in adult and aged F344 rats. J Neurosci Res 1987;18:55–63.

56. Sonntag WE. Hormone secretion and action in aging animals and man. Rev Biol Res Aging 1987; 3:299–335.

57. Nieman DC, Henson DA, Gusewitch G, et al. Physical activity and immune function in elderly women. Med Sci Sports Exerc 1993;25:823–831.

58. Shinkai S, Kohno H, Kimura K, et al. Physical activity and immune senescence in men. Med Sci Sports Exerc 1995;27:1516–1526.

59. Rall LC, Roubenoff R, Cannon JG, et al. Effects of progressive resistance training on immune response in aging and chronic inflammation. Med Sci Sports Exerc 1996;28:1356–1365.

60. Rincon HG, Solomon GF, Benton D, et al. Exercise in frail elderly men decreases natural killer cell activity. Aging Clin Exp Res 1996;8:109–112.

61. Pahlavani MA, Cheung TH, Cheskey JA, et al. Influence of exercise on the immune function of rats at various ages. J Appl Physiol 1988;64:1997–2001.

62. Barnes CA, Forster MJ, Fleshner M, et al. Exercise does not modify spatial memory, brain autoimmunity, or antibody response in aged F-344 rats. Neurobiol Aging 1991;12:47–53.

63. Hirokawa K. Understanding the mechanism of the age-related decline in immune function. Nutr Rev 1992;50:361–366.

64. Hirokawa K, Utsuyama M, Goto H, et al. Differential rate of age-related decline in immune functions in genetically defined mice with different tumor incidence and life span. Gerontology 1984;30: 223.

Part XIX.

ENVIRONMENTAL STRESS

Edited by
Scott J. Montain

Introduction to Environmental Stress

Scott J. Montain

Physical activity, consumption of the proper mix of carbohydrate, fat, and protein and five or more servings of fruits and vegetables each day are behavioral strategies that can reduce morbidity and premature mortality. The environment in which we live and work can also impact on our health and well-being. In our fast-paced modern society we now travel more, travel farther, and have fast access to geographical regions that heretofore were not accessible. As a consequence, we can travel to areas with vastly different ambient weather conditions and dramatically different altitudes—each of which can impact on our exercise tolerance and can compromise health. In this section, C. Bruce Wenger, Nigel Taylor et al, and James Anholm discuss the impact of working in hot, cold, and high-altitude environments, respectively. The authors discuss the physiologic responses to acute exposure and the adaptions that occur with chronic exposure. The medical risks of working in these environmental extremes are presented, as are methods to reduce risk.

Technologic advances have also altered our work and leisure environments. Pollutants in the air we breathe can impact on our health and physical comfort. Lack of sleep or sleep disturbances brought on by personal behaviors, work stress, or long-distance travel can compromise both our physical and cognitive abilities, and increase susceptibility to illness and injury. William Linn and Henry Gong discuss the impact of various airborne pollutants on health and physical comfort. They also present practical solutions to minimize exposure. Gila Lindsley and Lou Stephenson complete the section by discussing the role of sleep in health, how sleep disturbances can impact on physical and cognitive abilities, and methods to diagnose and treat individuals suspected of having chronic sleep disorders.

Chapter 104

Physiologic and Pathologic Responses to Heat Stress

C. Bruce Wenger

Temperatures low enough to freeze tissue, and temperatures higher than about 45°C (113°F) (1), can directly injure living tissue. Even within these limits, temperature changes alter biological function both through configurational changes that affect the function of protein molecules, such as enzymes, receptors, and membrane channels, and through a general effect on chemical reaction rates. Most reaction rates vary approximately as an exponential function of temperature within the physiologic range, and raising temperature by 10°C increases the reaction rate two- to threefold. A familiar clinical example of the effect of body temperature on metabolic processes is the rule that each 1°C of fever increases a patient's fluid and calorie needs 13% (2). Homeotherms, through their thermoregulatory processes, keep their internal or body *core* temperatures within a fairly narrow range near 37°C (98.6°F), and thus provide a more stable physicochemical environment for their biological processes. (Temperatures of the skin and superficial tissues, of course, vary more widely.)

The level of normal body temperature is conventionally given as 37°C (98.6°F), and this figure may create a misleading impression of the constancy of body temperature. Core temperature at rest undergoes a daily or circadian rhythm, with an amplitude of about 1°C, and is lowest in the early morning and highest in the late afternoon (3–5). In women of childbearing age, this circadian rhythm is superimposed on another rhythm, with a somewhat smaller amplitude, associated with the menstrual cycle (6–8). These rhythms are produced by underlying rhythms in the control of the thermoregulatory responses, in what we may think of as the setting of the body's "thermostat." These rhythms, plus other factors such as individual variation and acclimatization to

heat, account for a range of core temperatures of healthy subjects at rest (Figure 104-1). In addition core temperature may increase several degrees with heavy exercise or fever; still higher temperatures may result from extreme conditions of exercise, neurologic disease, or heat stress that overwhelm the capacity of the thermoregulatory system.

Adverse effects of heat stress include impairment of physical and mental performance (9,10), heat-related illnesses, and syndromes (11–13), aggravation of other preexisting illnesses, and direct injury caused by high tissue temperatures. Direct thermal injury includes burns (which, however, are not the subject of this chapter) and perhaps some injury associated with heat stroke. In healthy people, however, the thermoregulatory responses are ordinarily so powerful and effective that tissue temperatures rarely reach harmful levels during heat stress, and most adverse effects of heat stress owe much more to secondary consequences of thermoregulatory and other homeostatic responses than they do to direct thermal injury to tissue. This chapter discusses normal physiologic responses to heat and to combined exercise-heat stress, events that lead to deterioration of performance in the heat or frank heat illness, factors that affect heat tolerance and susceptibility to heat-related illnesses, and preventive measures. In addition, clinical aspects of heat illness are briefly summarized.

REGULATION OF BODY TEMPERATURE
Physiologic and Behavioral Temperature Regulation
Two distinct control systems, physiologic and behavioral, operate in parallel to regulate body temperature. Physiologic

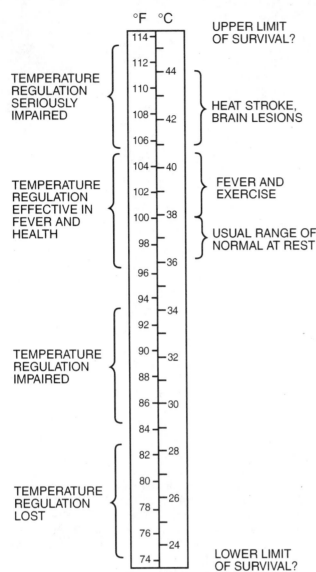

TEMPERATURE REGULATION SERIOUSLY IMPAIRED

TEMPERATURE REGULATION EFFECTIVE IN FEVER AND HEALTH

TEMPERATURE REGULATION IMPAIRED

TEMPERATURE REGULATION LOST

UPPER LIMIT OF SURVIVAL?

HEAT STROKE, BRAIN LESIONS

FEVER AND EXERCISE

USUAL RANGE OF NORMAL AT REST

LOWER LIMIT OF SURVIVAL?

Figure 104-1 Ranges of rectal temperature found in healthy persons, patients with fever, and in persons with impairment or failure of thermoregulation. (Modified with permission of the publisher from DuBois EF. Fever and the regulation of body temperature. Spring field IL: Charles C Thomas, 1948.)

thermoregulation employs involuntary responses. In humans the most important physiologic responses for thermoregulation in the heat are 1) vasomotor responses, which control blood flow from the interior of the body to the skin, and 2) sweating. (In addition, hyperthermic humans often pant, but panting is not a major avenue of heat loss in humans.) The physiologic control system is capable of fine adjustments in these responses, and enables homeotherms to achieve fairly precise regulation of their core temperatures. These responses will be discussed further below. Behavioral thermoregulation involves the conscious, willed use of whatever means are available, and operates primarily to reduce the level of thermal discomfort. Since thermal discomfort is closely related to the underlying

physiologic strain (14), behavioral thermoregulation reduces the demand on the physiologic thermoregulatory responses. Familiar behavioral responses to heat stress include shedding excess clothing, reducing physical activity to decrease heat production, seeking a more comfortable environment, and drinking cool fluids. Behavioral thermoregulation is strongly influenced by learned responses, and may be compromised or overridden when there is enough motivation to persist in a situation that produces a high degree of thermal stress, as during intense physical training or athletic competition, or in the performance of certain jobs. In healthy young individuals, heat illness is frequently the result of failure to make the necessary behavioral responses to heat strain, owing either to excessive motivation or to improper supervision.

Balance Between Heat Production and Heat Loss

Although the body exchanges some energy with the environment in the form of mechanical work, most is exchanged as heat by conduction, convection, and radiation and as latent heat through evaporation or (rarely) condensation of water (Figure 104-2). If the sum of energy production and energy gain from the environment does not equal energy loss, the extra heat is "stored" in, or lost from, the body. This is summarized in the heat balance equation

$$M = E + R + C + K + W + S \qquad (104\text{-}1)$$

where M is the metabolic rate; E is the rate of heat loss by evaporation; R and C are rates of heat loss by radiation and convection, respectively; K is the rate of heat loss by conduction (only to solid objects in practice, as explained later); W is the rate of energy loss as mechanical work; and S is the rate of heat storage in the body (15,16), which is positive when body temperature is increasing.

Metabolic Rate and Sites of Heat Production

At thermal steady state, the rate of heat production in the body is equal to the rate of heat loss to the environment, and can be measured precisely by direct calorimetry, a rather cumbersome technique in which all heat and water vapor leaving the body are captured and measured using special apparatus. More usually, metabolic rate is estimated by *indirect calorimetry* (17) from measurements of O_2 consumption, since virtually all energy available to the body depends ultimately on oxygen-consuming chemical reactions. The heat production associated with consumption of 1 liter of O_2 varies somewhat with the fuel—carbohydrate, fat, or protein—that is oxidized. An average value of $20.2\,kJ$ ($4.83\,kcal$) per liter of O_2 is often used for metabolism of a mixed diet. Since the ratio of CO_2 produced to O_2 consumed varies according to the fuel, indirect calorimetry can be made more accurate by also measuring CO_2 production and calculating the amount of protein oxidized from urinary nitrogen excretion.

Metabolic rate at rest is approximately proportional to body surface area. In a fasting young man it is about 45 W/m^2 ($81\,W$ or $70\,kcal/hr$ for $1.8\,m^2$ of body surface area, corresponding to an O_2 consumption of about $240\,mL/min$). At rest the trunk viscera and brain account for about 70% of energy production, even though they comprise only about 36% of the body mass (Table 104-1). During exercise, however, the muscles are the chief site of energy production,

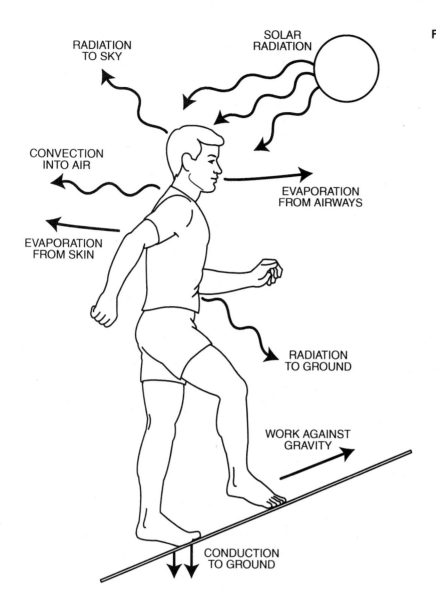

Figure 104-2 Exchange of energy with the environment. This hiker gains heat from the sun by radiation, and loses heat by conduction to the ground through the soles of his feet, by convection into the air, by radiation to the ground and sky, and by evaporation of water from his skin and respiratory passages. In addition, some of the energy released by his metabolic processes is converted into mechanical work, rather than heat, since he is walking uphill. (Redrawn from Wenger CB: The regulation of body temperature. In: Rhoades RA, Tanner GA, eds. Medical physiology. Boston: Little, Brown, 1995:587–613, with permission of the publisher.)

and may account for 90% during heavy exercise (Table 104-1). A healthy but sedentary young man performing moderate exercise may reach a metabolic rate of 600 W, and a trained athlete performing intense exercise may reach 1400 W or more. The overall mechanical efficiency of exercise varies enormously, depending on the activity; at best, no more than one quarter of the metabolic energy is converted into mechanical work outside the body, and the remaining three quarters or more is converted into heat within the body (18). Since exercising muscles produce so much heat, they may be nearly 1°C warmer than the core. They warm the blood that perfuses them, and this blood, returning to the core, warms the rest of the body.

Biophysics of Heat Exchange with the Environment

Radiation, convection, and evaporation are the dominant means of heat exchange with the environment. In humans, respiration usually accounts for only a minor fraction of total

Table 104-1 Relative Masses and Rates of Metabolic Heat Production of Various Body Compartments During Rest and Severe Exercise

	Body Mass (%)	Heat Production (%) Rest	Heat Production (%) Exercise
Brain	2	16	1
Trunk Viscera	34	56	8
Muscle and Skin	56	18	90
Other	8	10	1

Modified from Wenger CB, Hardy JD. Temperature regulation and exposure to heat and cold. In: Lehmann JF, ed. Therapeutic heat and cold. 4th ed. Baltimore: Williams & Wilkins, 1990:150–178.

heat exchange and is not predominantly under thermoregulatory control, although hyperthermic subjects may hyperventilate. Therefore, humans exchange the most heat with the environment through the skin, and the rate of heat exchange between the body and the environment depends on the surface area of the skin.

Every surface emits energy as electromagnetic radiation with a power output that depends on its area, reflectivity, and temperature. Every surface absorbs electromagnetic radiation from its environment at a rate that depends on its area and reflectivity, and on the radiant temperature of the environment (T_r). Radiative heat exchange (R) between the skin and the environment is proportional to the difference between the fourth powers of the surfaces' respective absolute temperatures; however, if the difference between skin temperature (T_{sk}) and T_r is much smaller than the absolute temperature of the skin, R is approximately proportional to ($T_{sk} - T_r$). At ordinary tissue and environmental temperatures, virtually all radiant energy is in the far infrared range, where nearly all surfaces except polished metals have low reflectivities. However, bodies like the sun that are hot enough to glow emit large amounts of radiation in the near infrared and visible range, in which light-colored surfaces have higher reflectivities than dark ones. The practical importance of this is that skin and clothing color have little effect on heat exchange except in sunlight or intense artificial light.

Convection is the transfer of heat via a moving fluid, either liquid or gas. In thermal physiology the fluid is usually air or water in the environment, or blood inside the body, as discussed later in the chapter. Fluids conduct heat in the same way as solids do, and a perfectly still fluid transfers heat only by conduction. Since air and water are not good conductors of heat, perfectly still air or water is not very effective in heat transfer. Fluids, however, are rarely perfectly still, and even nearly imperceptible movement produces enough convection to have a large effect on heat transfer. Thus, although conduction plays a role in heat transfer by a fluid, convection so dominates the overall heat transfer that we refer to the entire process as convection. Therefore, the conduction term (K) in Equation (104-1) is in practice restricted to heat flow between the body and other solid objects, and usually represents only a small part of the total heat exchange with the environment. Convective heat exchange between the skin and the ambient air is proportional to the skin surface area and the difference between skin and air temperatures. Convective heat exchange depends also on geometrical factors that affect heat exchange with moving air, and on the degree of air movement. It is approximately proportional to the square root of air speed, except when air movement is very slight.

A gram of water that is converted into vapor at 30°C absorbs 2425 J (0.58 kcal) in the process. In subjects who are not sweating, evaporative water loss is typically about 13 to 15 g/(m²·hr), corresponding to a heat loss of 16 to 18 W for a surface area of 1.8 m². About half of this amount is lost through breathing and half as *insensible perspiration* (19,20) (i.e., evaporation of water that diffuses through the skin). Insensible perspiration is unrelated to the sweat glands and is not under thermoregulatory control. These modes of water loss, however, are quite small compared to sweating. Evaporation of sweat from the skin is proportional to the skin surface area that is wet with sweat, and depends also on air movement,

since water vapor is carried away by moving air, and on the temperature of the skin and the moisture content of the air. The most familiar way of expressing the moisture content of the air is the relative humidity, which is the ratio between the actual moisture content of the air and the maximum moisture content that is possible at the temperature of the air. However, relative humidity is not the most useful measure of the evaporative cooling power of the environment for thermal physiology, and may be misleading. A more useful index is the wet-bulb temperature, which is the temperature of a completely wet ventilated surface that is not artificially heated or cooled, and may be measured with a psychrometer. The temperature inside a closed vehicle or poorly ventilated building in direct sunlight may easily reach 50°C (122°F); if there are sources of moisture inside, the relative humidity may reach 37%—which may not sound particularly high. However the wet-bulb temperature in such an environment is 35°C (95°F), the same as in a 35°C environment at 100% relative humidity.

Tissue Blood Flow and Heat Transport in the Body

Heat travels within the body by two parallel means: *conduction* through the tissues and *convection* by the blood, the process by which flowing blood carries heat from warmer to cooler tissues. Heat flow by conduction is proportional to the change of temperature with distance in the direction of heat flow, and to the thermal conductivity of the tissues. Heat flow by convection depends on the rate of blood flow through the tissue and the temperature difference between the tissue and the blood supplying it. The power of the body to transport heat through a layer of tissue by conduction and convection combined is expressed as a quantity called *conductance, C,* defined as $C = HF/(\Delta T)$, where HF is the rate of heat flow through the tissue layer, and ΔT is the temperature difference across the tissue layer.

The most important conductance for thermal physiology is that involved in heat transfer from body core to skin. The skin and other superficial and peripheral tissues are, in general, cooler than the core. These cooler tissues, lying between the core and the skin surface, comprise the shell. (The shell is defined functionally rather than anatomically, and is thinnest when the body is warm and skin blood flow is high.) Since all heat leaving the body via the skin passes through the shell, the shell insulates the core from the environment. In a cold subject, vasoconstriction reduces skin blood flow so much that the conductance of the shell, and thus core-to-skin heat transfer, is dominated by conduction. A representative value for shell conductance of a lean man under these conditions is 8.9 W/(m²·°C), or about 16 W/°C for a whole body with a typical surface area of 1.8 m². The subcutaneous fat layer adds to the insulation value of the shell of a vasoconstricted subject, because it increases the thickness of the shell and has a conductivity only about 0.4 times that of dermis or muscle. In a warm subject, however, the shell is relatively thin and provides little insulation. Furthermore a warm subject's skin blood flow is high, so that heat flow from the core to the skin is dominated by convection. In these circumstances the subcutaneous fat layer—which affects conduction but not convection—has little effect on heat flow. (Obese individuals do tend to be less heat-tolerant than thinner individuals. However, the major reasons for this difference are first, that the obese are at a relative disadvantage for dissipating heat because they have less skin surface area in proportion to their weight than do their thinner counterparts, and second, obese individuals tend to be less physically fit and thus, as discussed later, to have less well-developed thermoregulatory responses.)

Let us return to our vasoconstricted man with a shell conductance of 16 W/°C. Under these conditions a temperature difference between core and skin of 5°C allows a typical resting metabolic heat production of 80 W to be conducted to the skin surface. In a cool environment, T_{sk} may be low enough for this to occur easily. However in a warm environment or, especially, during exercise, shell conductance must increase substantially to allow all the heat produced to be conducted to the skin without at the same time causing core temperature to rise to dangerous or lethal levels. [For example without an increase in shell conductance, T_c (core temperature) would have to be 30°C higher than T_{sk} to allow a heat production of 480 W during moderate exercise to be carried to the skin.] Fortunately, under such circumstances increases in skin blood flow occur that can raise shell conductance tenfold or more. Thus, a crucial thermoregulatory function of skin blood flow is to control the conductance of the shell and the ease with which heat travels from core to skin. A closely related function is to control T_{sk}; in a person who is not sweating, an increase in skin blood flow tends to bring T_{sk} toward T_c, and a decrease allows T_{sk} to approach ambient temperature. Since convective and radiative heat exchange $(R + C)$ depend directly on skin temperature, the body can control heat exchange with the environment by adjusting skin blood flow. If the heat stress is so great that increasing R + C through increasing skin blood flow is not enough to maintain heat balance, the body secretes sweat to increase evaporative heat loss. Once sweating begins, skin blood flow continues to increase as the person becomes warmer, but now the tendency of an increase in skin blood flow to warm the skin is approximately balanced by the tendency of an increase in sweating to cool the skin. Therefore, after sweating has begun, further increases in skin blood flow usually cause little change in skin temperature or dry heat exchange. Nevertheless, the increases in skin blood flow that accompany sweating are important to thermoregulation, since they deliver to the skin the heat that is being removed by evaporation of sweat, and facilitate evaporation by keeping the skin warm. Skin blood flow and sweating thus work in tandem to dissipate heat that is produced in the body.

Physiologic Heat-Dissipating Responses

Responses of Skin Vascular Beds, and Pooling of Blood

Blood vessels in human skin are under dual vasomotor control, involving separate nervous signals for vasoconstriction and for vasodilation (21–23). Reflex vasoconstriction, occurring in response to cold and also as part of certain nonthermal reflexes such as baroreflexes, is mediated primarily through adrenergic sympathetic fibers distributed widely over most of the skin (24). Reducing the flow of impulses in these nerve fibers allows the blood vessels to dilate. In the so-called acral regions—lips, ears, nose, palms of the hands, and soles of the feet (23,24)—and in the superficial veins (23), vasoconstrictor fibers are the predominant vasomotor innervation, and the vasodilation occurring during heat exposure is largely a result of withdrawal of vaso-

constrictor activity (25). Reflex control of skin blood flow in these regions, unlike that in the rest of the skin (25), is sensitive to small temperature changes in the thermoneutral range (i.e., the range of thermal conditions in which the body is neither chilled nor sweating) and may "fine tune" heat loss to maintain heat balance in this range.

In most of the skin the vasodilation occurring during heat exposure depends on sympathetic nervous signals that cause the blood vessels to dilate, and is prevented or reversed by regional nerve block (26). Since it depends on the action of nervous signals, such vasodilation is sometimes referred to as *active* vasodilation. Active vasodilation occurs in almost all the skin outside the acral regions (25). In skin areas where active vasodilation occurs, vasoconstrictor activity is minimal in the thermoneutral range; as the body is warmed, active vasodilation does not begin until near the onset of sweating (23,27). The neurotransmitter or other vasoactive substance(s) responsible for active vasodilation in human skin is not known (24). However, since sweating and vasodilation operate in tandem in the heat, there has been considerable interest in the notion that the mechanism for active vasodilation is somehow linked to the action of sweat glands (23,28). Active vasodilation does not occur in the skin of patients with anhidrotic ectodermal dysplasia (29), even though their vasoconstrictor responses are intact, implying that active vasodilation either is linked to an action of sweat glands, or is mediated through nerves that are absent or nonfunctional in anhidrotic ectodermal dysplasia.

The superficial venous beds, which receive blood from the skin, are fully dilated at mild levels of heat stress. Therefore, in regions below the level of the heart, these veins readily become engorged with blood, especially when skin blood flow is high, and the resulting peripheral pooling of blood impairs venous return, reduces central blood volume, compromises diastolic filling of the heart, and limits cardiac output, especially during exercise. The most important physiologic compensatory mechanism is constriction of the renal and splanchnic vascular beds. Reduction of blood flow through these beds increases the fraction of cardiac output that is available to perfuse exercising muscle. In addition, the splanchnic vascular bed is very compliant, so that a reduction in splanchnic blood flow reduces the volume of blood contained in the splanchnic vascular bed, allowing a partial restoration of central blood volume and cardiac diastolic filling. The effect of pooling of blood in the skin on central blood volume, and the compensatory effect of splanchnic vasoconstriction are shown schematically in Figure 104-3. The degree of splanchnic vasoconstriction is graded according to the levels of heat stress and exercise intensity. During strenuous exercise in the heat, renal and splanchnic blood flows may fall to 20% of their values in a cool resting subject (23,30). Such intense splanchnic vasoconstriction may help to explain the intestinal symptoms that some athletes experience after endurance events (31).

Sweating and Loss of Fluid and Electrolytes

Humans can dissipate large amounts of heat by secretion and evaporation of sweat, and when the environment is warmer than the skin—usually when the environment is warmer than about 35°C—evaporation is the only way to lose heat. Human sweat glands are controlled through postganglionic sympathetic nerves that release acetylcholine (32) rather than

Figure 104-3 Schematic diagram of the effects of skin vasodilation on peripheral pooling of blood and the thoracic reservoirs from which the ventricles are filled, and also the effects of compensatory vasomotor adjustments in the splanchnic circulation. The valves drawn at the right sides of liver/splanchnic, muscle, and skin vascular beds represent the resistance vessels that control blood flow through those beds. Arrows show the direction of the changes during heat stress. (Redrawn from Rowell LB. Cardiovascular adjustments to thermal stress. In: Shepherd JT, Abboud FM, eds. Handbook of physiology. The cardiovascular system. Peripheral circulation and organ blood flow. Bethesda, MD: American Physiological Society, 1983:sect. 2, vol. 3, 967–1023; and Rowell LB. Cardiovascular aspects of human thermoregulation. Circ Res 1983;52:367–379.)

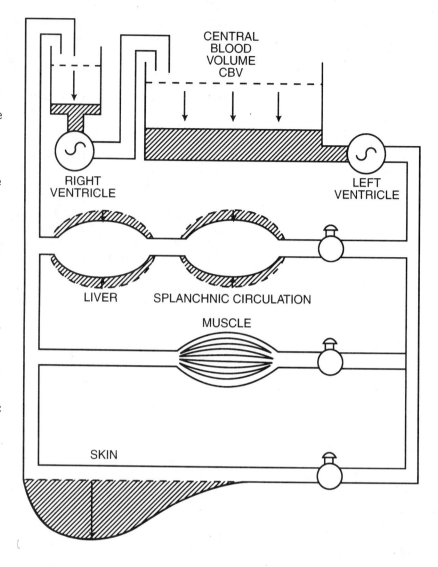

norepinephrine like most other sympathetic nerves. Human skin contains 2 to 3 million functional eccrine sweat glands (32), the histologic type most important in thermoregulation. Their secretory capacity can be increased by aerobic exercise training and heat acclimatization; a fit man well acclimatized to heat can achieve a peak sweating rate greater than 2.5 liters per hour (33,34). Such rates cannot long be maintained, however, and the maximum daily sweat output is probably about 15 liters (35).

Eccrine sweat is formed from a precursor fluid in the secretory coil of the gland. This fluid is initially isotonic with plasma; however, as it moves along the duct, Na^+ is reabsorbed from the fluid by active transport. When it emerges from the duct as sweat, it is the most dilute body fluid, with $[Na^+]$ ranging from less than 5 to 60 mEq/L (36). As the rate of sweat secretion increases, the precursor fluid moves through the duct more quickly, so that a smaller fraction of its initial sodium content is reabsorbed, and $[Na^+]$ in the resulting sweat is higher. Thus salt losses through sweating increase disproportionately as sweat production rises.

At high sweating rates, large volumes of water can be lost in a few hours, and the consequent reduction in plasma volume may compromise cardiovascular homeostasis and cardiac output. In addition, since sweat is hypotonic to plasma, loss of sweat progressively increases the osmolality of the bodily fluids if the water is not replaced. Both the reduction in plasma volume and the increase in osmolality will compromise thermoregulation by shifting the thresholds for sweating and vasodilation in the skin toward higher core temperature. If large amounts of salt are lost, and only the water but not the salt is replaced, plasma volume will not return to normal because the loss of salt reduces the total number of osmoles in the extracellular fluid, so that the water that is replaced goes preferentially into the intracellular space.

During prolonged (several hours) heat exposure with high sweat output, sweat rates gradually diminish and the sweat glands' response to locally applied cholinergic drugs is reduced also. The reduction of sweat-gland responsiveness is sometimes called sweat-gland "fatigue." One mechanism involved is hydration of the stratum corneum, which swells and mechanically obstructs the sweat duct, causing a reduction in sweat secretion, an effect called *hidromeiosis* (37). The glands' responsiveness can be at least partly restored if the skin is allowed to dry [e.g., by increasing air movement (38)], but prolonged sweating also causes histologic changes in the sweat glands (39).

Control of Thermoregulatory Responses

Integration of Thermal Information

Temperature receptors in the body core and the skin transmit information about their temperatures through afferent nerves to the brain stem, and especially the hypothalamus, where much of the integration of temperature information takes place. Although temperature receptors in other core sites, including the spinal cord and medulla, participate in the control of thermoregulatory responses (40); the core temperature receptors involved in thermoregulatory control are concentrated especially in the hypothalamus (40); temperature changes of only a few tenths of 1°C in the anterior preoptic area of the hypothalamus elicit changes in the thermoregulatory effector responses of experimental mammals.

Most physiologic control systems produce a response that is graded according to the disturbance in the regulated variable. In many of these systems, including those that control the heat-dissipating responses, changes in the effector responses are proportional to displacements of the regulated variable from some threshold value (19); such control systems are called *proportional control* systems. Changes in the heat-dissipating

responses are proportional to displacements of core temperature from some threshold value (Figure 104-4). Each response in Figure 104-4 has a core-temperature threshold, a temperature at which the response starts to increase; these thresholds depend on mean skin temperature. Thus, at any given skin temperature, the change in each response is proportional to the change in core temperature; increasing the skin temperature lowers the threshold level of core temperature and increases the response at any given core temperature. (Control of the heat-dissipating responses is more complicated than a basic proportional-control system, since these responses are controlled according to both core and skin temperature.) The sensitivity of the thermoregulatory system to core temperature allows it to adjust heat loss so as to resist disturbances in core temperature, and the system's sensitivity to skin temperature allows it to respond appropriately to moderate changes in the environment with little or no change in body core temperature. For example, the skin temperature of someone who enters a hot environment rises and may elicit sweating even if there is no change in core temperature. On the other hand, an increase in heat production due to exercise elicits the appropriate heat-dissipating responses through a rise in core temperature.

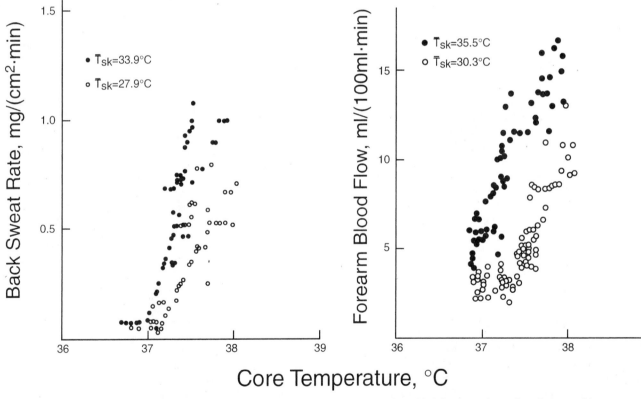

Figure 104-4 The relationships of back sweat rate (left) and forearm blood flow (right) to esophageal and mean skin temperatures (T_{es} and T_{sk}). Sweating data are from four subjects performing cycle exercise at an O_2 consumption rate of 1.6 L/min. Blood flow data are from one subject. During measurements of blood flow, forearm temperature was kept at 36.8°C to eliminate a difference in local temperature between experiments. Local temperature was not controlled independently during measurements of sweating, so that the difference between conditions includes a small effect of local skin temperature, appearing as a difference in slope. (Left panel drawn from data of Sawka MN, Gonzalez RR, Drolet LL, Pandolf KB. Heat exchange during upper- and lower-body exercise. J Appl Physiol 1984;57:1050–1054; right panel modified from Wenger CB, Roberts MF, Stolwijk JAJ, Nadel ER. Forearm blood flow during body temperature transients produced by leg exercise. J Appl Physiol 1975;38:58–63.)

Both sweating and skin blood flow participate in other reflexes besides thermoregulatory responses. For the purposes of this chapter, the most important nonthermoregulatory reflexes are those that involve the blood vessels of the skin in responses that help to maintain cardiac output, blood pressure, and tissue O_2 delivery. During heat stress, thermoregulatory requirements usually dominate the control of these responses, but in conditions of high cardiovascular strain thermoregulatory requirements for skin blood flow may be overridden to support circulatory function. An important and dramatic example is the reduction in skin blood flow that accounts for the cool, ashen skin characteristic of heat exhaustion, discussed below.

Thermoregulatory Responses During Exercise

At the start of exercise, metabolic heat production increases rapidly; however, there is little change in heat loss initially, so heat is stored in the body and core temperature rises. The increase in core temperature, in turn, elicits heat-loss responses, but core temperature continues to rise until heat loss has increased enough to match heat production, so that heat balance is restored and core temperature and the heat-loss responses reach new steady-state levels. The rise in core temperature that elicits heat-dissipating responses sufficient to re-establish thermal balance during exercise is an example of a *load error* (19), which occurs when any proportional control system resists the effect of some imposed disturbance or "load." The load error is proportional to the load, so that the elevation in core temperature during exercise is proportional to the rate of heat production. Although the elevated core temperature during exercise superficially resembles that during fever due to resetting of the body's thermostat, there are some crucial differences. First, although heat production may increase substantially (through shivering) at the beginning of a fever, it does not need to stay high to maintain the fever, but in fact returns nearly to prefebrile levels once the fever is established; during exercise, however, an increase in heat production not only causes the elevation in core temperature, but is necessary to sustain it. Second, the rate of heat loss while core temperature is rising during a fever, is, if anything, lower than before the fever began, but the rate of heat loss during exercise starts to increase as soon as core temperature starts to rise and continues to increase as long as core temperature is rising.

FACTORS AFFECTING HEAT TOLERANCE

Acclimatization and Physical Fitness

Prolonged or repeated heat stress, especially when combined with exercise sufficient to elicit profuse sweating, produces *acclimatization* to heat (41), a set of physiologic changes that reduces the physiologic strain associated with exercise-heat stress. The classic signs of heat acclimatization are reductions in the levels of core and skin temperatures and heart rate, and increases in sweat production during a given level of exercise in the heat. These changes begin to appear during the first few days and approach their full development within a week. Figure 104-5 illustrates some of these effects in three young men who were acclimatized by daily treadmill walks in dry heat for 10 days (42). On the first day in the heat, heart rate

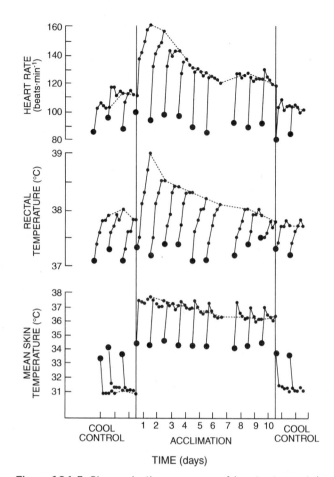

Figure 104-5 Change in the responses of heart rate, rectal temperature, and mean skin temperature during exercise in a 10-day program of acclimatization to dry heat (50.5°C, 15% relative humidity), together with responses during exercise in a cool environment before and after acclimatization. (The "cool control" condition was 25.5°C, 39% relative humidity.) Each day's exercise consisted of five 10-minute treadmill walks at 2.5 mph (1.12 m/s) up a 2.5% grade. Successive walks were separated by 2-minute rest periods. Large circles show values before the start of the first exercise period each day, small circles show values at the ends of successive exercise periods, and dotted lines connect final values each day. (Redrawn from Eichna LW, Park CR, Nelson N, et al. Thermal regulation during acclimatization in a hot, dry (desert type) environment. Am J Physiol 1950;163:585–597.)

and rectal temperature during exercise reached much higher levels than in cool control (25°C) conditions; however, on the tenth day in the heat, final heart rate and rectal temperature during exercise were 40 beats/min and 1°C, respectively, lower than on the first day. In addition, sweat production increased 10%, skin temperature was about 1.5°C lower, and the metabolic cost of treadmill walking decreased 4%. The mechanisms that produce these changes are not fully understood, but include a modest (~0.4°C) reduction in the setting of the body's thermostat (thus reducing the thresholds for sweating and cutaneous vasodilation), increased sensitivity of the sweat glands to cholinergic stimulation (43,44), a decrease in the sweat glands' susceptibility to hidromeiosis and fatigue, and retention of salt and water and expansion of plasma volume to compensate for peripheral pooling of blood in dilated blood vessels in the skin. Heat acclimatization produces other changes (41) also, including an improved ability to sustain high rates of sweat production; an aldosterone-mediated reduction of sweat sodium concentration (to levels as low as 5 mEq/L at low sweat rates), which minimizes salt depletion; an increase in the fraction of sweat secreted on the limbs; and perhaps other changes that help protect against heat illness. The effect of heat acclimatization on performance can be quite dramatic, so that acclimatized subjects can easily complete exercise in the heat that previously was difficult or impossible (see Reference 45). The benefits of acclimatization are lessened or reversed by sleep loss, infection, alcohol abuse, dehydration, and salt depletion (41). Heat acclimatization disappears in a few weeks if not maintained by repeated heat exposure.

Some of the changes that occur with heat acclimatization are mediated by "training" the heat-dissipating responses, particularly sweating, through repeated use (41). Repeated aerobic exercise of sufficient intensity and duration to improve maximal O_2 consumption also trains the heat-dissipating responses and expands plasma volume, and produces an improvement in heat tolerance similar to that associated with heat acclimatization (41). This effect probably explains the association of physical fitness with heat tolerance.

Gender, Age, Obesity, Drugs, and Skin Disorders

Although women as a group are less tolerant to exercise-heat stress than men, the difference appears to be explained by differences in size, acclimatization, and maximal O_2 consumption; when subjects are matched according to these variables, gender differences largely disappear (46). Curiously, the exertional form of heat stroke is quite rare in women (13), but it is unknown whether the explanation for its rarity is biological or behavioral. The effect of phase of the menstrual cycle has not been well studied. However Pivarnik et al (47), studying women's responses during cycle exercise at 22°C, found that after 60 minutes of exercise heart rate was 10 beats/min higher in the luteal than in the follicular phase; rectal temperature increased 1.2°C in the luteal phase and was still rising, whereas it increased 0.9°C in the follicular phase and was near steady state. Although they examined only one set of experimental conditions, using a temperate rather than a warm environment, their data suggest a decline in tolerance to exercise-heat stress during the luteal phase.

The effectiveness of the thermoregulatory system is reduced with increasing age, but it is not clear how much of the decrease is a direct effect of aging itself, and how much owes to changes that tend to accompany increased age, such as reduced physical fitness (46). Obesity also is associated with reduced heat tolerance, and Kenney (46) reviews mechanisms that may explain this association. Thermoregulation is also impaired by salt and water depletion, and by a number of drugs, including diuretics, which may cause loss of fluid and electrolytes, and various drugs that suppress sweating, including anticholinergics, antiparkinsonians, antihistamines, and phenothiazines (11). In addition some drugs, including tricyclic antidepressants, butyrophenones, and amphetamines, increase the risk of heat illness through other mechanisms (11).

Several congenital and acquired skin disorders impair sweating, and may greatly reduce heat tolerance. Anhidrotic ectodermal dysplasia is especially interesting in this regard, since not only sweating, but also active vasodilation in the skin, is impaired or absent. Thus artificially wetting the skin only partially corrects the thermoregulatory deficit during exercise, when large amounts of body heat need to be carried to the skin. Artificial wetting is probably most effective in a dry environment, in which evaporation can produce a cool skin.

ADVERSE EFFECTS OF HEAT AND EXERCISE

Although hyperthermia is often associated with heat disorders, and may be involved in the pathogenesis, the relation between body temperature and clinical manifestations is complex (48), and levels of core temperatures that are typically associated with heat stroke have been observed in athletes who apparently suffered no ill effects (49,50). For convenience the heat disorders may be divided into two groups: those whose manifestations are primarily local, and those having more general manifestations. This division is not absolute, however, since miliaria rubra may impair thermoregulation.

For more detailed discussion of pathogenesis and clinical management the reader is referred elsewhere (11,13).

Heat Disorders
Disorders with Primarily Local Manifestations

Heat edema, a dependent edema of the hands, legs, and feet, typically occurs within the first week of adaptation to tropical heat, and is worsened by prolonged standing. Heat edema is probably due to the retention of salt and water that is a normal part of acclimatization to heat, and peripheral vasodilation probably has a contributory role. Heat edema is a benign and self-limited condition. Treatment with diuretics is not indicated and will impair development of acclimatization by interfering with retention of salt and water.

Miliaria rubra (commonly called heat rash or prickly heat) is characterized by blockage of the sweat ducts with plugs of keratin debris, and typically occurs following repeated or prolonged exposure to heat. The resulting rash is irritating, but the most serious effect is marked impairment of sweating in the affected skin, which may precede the appearance of the rash by up to a week and may persist for some time after the rash clears (51). Some patients may be unable to sweat below the neck. The impairment of sweating, if extensive, substantially limits the ability to tolerate exercise in the heat.

Heat Syncope

Heat syncope is a temporary circulatory failure due to pooling of blood in the peripheral veins and a consequent decrease in diastolic filling of the heart. The primary cause of the peripheral pooling is the large increase in skin blood flow that occurs as part of the thermoregulatory response to heat exposure, but an inadequate baroreflex response may be an important contributing factor. It usually occurs in individuals who are standing with little activity. Symptoms may range from lightheadedness to loss of consciousness. Core temperature typically is no more than slightly elevated except when an attack follows exercise, and the skin is wet and cool. Recovery is rapid once the patient sits or lies down, although complete recovery of blood pressure and heart rate often takes an hour or two. Heat syncope affects mostly those who are not acclimatized to heat, presumably because the expansion of plasma volume that occurs with acclimatization compensates for the peripheral pooling of blood. Patients being treated for hypertension with diuretics or medications that impair the baroreflexes are at particular risk, and should exercise care when standing in crowds or lines in hot surroundings.

The Continuum of Heat Cramps, Heat Exhaustion, and Heat Stroke

Traditionally heat cramps, heat exhaustion, and heat stroke were considered to be three distinct clinical entities. However these disorders have overlapping features, and the concept that they are syndromes representing different parts of a continuum (52,53) has gained favor. In keeping with this concept, some recent literature describes a syndrome called *exertional heat injury*, intermediate in severity between heat exhaustion and heat stroke. However, there does not seem to be a consensus on diagnostic criteria for distinguishing exertional heat injury from heat exhaustion on one hand or heat stroke on the other (compare, for example, References 54 and 55).

Water loss from the sweat glands can exceed 1 liter per hour during exercise in the heat. The amount of salt lost in the sweat is quite variable, and persons who are well acclimatized to heat can often secrete very dilute sweat. However, those who are less well acclimatized may lose large amounts of salt in their sweat and become substantially salt-depleted.

Heat Cramps

Heat cramps is an acute disorder consisting of brief, recurrent, and often agonizing cramps in skeletal muscles of the limbs and trunk. The cramp produces a hard lump in the affected muscle, which typically has recently participated in intense exercise. Although the cramps are brief, generally lasting only a few minutes, they may recur for many hours in severe, untreated cases. Patients are characteristically physically fit men, well acclimatized to heat, who have been drinking adequate amounts of water but not replacing salt lost in the sweat. They are usually hyponatremic, and the hyponatremia is thought to be involved in the pathogenesis of the cramps, although the mechanism is obscure. Hyponatremia is rather common, however, whereas heat cramps are an unusual accompaniment. Intravenous infusion of 0.5 to 1 liter of normal saline, or alternatively, somewhat smaller amounts of hypertonic saline, is the treatment of choice in severe cases. However, administration by mouth of 0.1% salt in water is also effective (11), somewhat unexpectedly given the usual association of heat cramps with hyponatremia. The immediate goal of treatment is relief of the cramps, not restoration

of salt balance, which takes longer and is best achieved by giving salted food or fluids by mouth.

Heat Exhaustion

Heat exhaustion is characterized by circulatory collapse occurring after prolonged or repeated exercise-heat stress. Most patients have lost both salt and water, but heat exhaustion may be associated either predominantly with salt depletion or predominantly with water depletion. Salt-depleted patients are hypovolemic out of proportion to the degree of dehydration (and are hypovolemic even if not greatly dehydrated), since their body water is distributed preferentially to the intracellular space in order to maintain osmotic balance between the intra- and extracellular spaces. They tend either to be unacclimatized to heat or to be consuming small amounts of salt in their diet, and they have replaced at least some of their water loss. Heat exhaustion caused primarily by water depletion tends to develop more rapidly than that caused by salt depletion, and is characterized by greater thirst. In addition, hypovolemia occurring during water-depletion heat exhaustion is associated with less hemoconcentration, since water is lost from both the red cells and the plasma.

Heat exhaustion spans a clinical spectrum from fairly mild disorders that respond well to rest in a cool environment and fluid replacement by mouth to severe forms with collapse, confusion, and hyperpyrexia. Loss of consciousness is uncommon, but there may be vertigo, ataxia, headache, weakness, nausea, vomiting, pallor, tachycardia, and low blood pressure. The patient usually is sweating profusely. Muscle cramps indistinguishable from heat cramps may occur, especially if salt depletion is part of the pathogenesis. Treatment consists primarily of laying the patient down away from the heat and replacing fluid and salt, as needed. In severe cases, intravenous administration of normal saline may be required. Active cooling measures may be called for if the patient's core temperature is 40.6°C (105°F) or higher, since water-depletion heat exhaustion may lead to heat stroke.

Restoration of Fluid Loss

As [Na$^+$] in the extracellular fluid is reduced, fluid moves from the extracellular fluid into the intracellular fluid to maintain osmotic balance, causing the cells to swell. Since the brain occupies most of the space within a rigid case, even a modest degree of cerebral edema can increase intracranial pressure, leading to encephalopathy and brain stem herniation in extreme cases. By removal of interstitial fluid and by loss of solutes from within the cells, the brain can protect itself from osmotic swelling if plasma [Na$^+$] changes slowly enough (56). Although osmotic swelling of the brain is usually associated with hyponatremia, its occurrence is related to the rate of change of plasma [Na$^+$] rather than the level of [Na$^+$]. For this reason care should be taken to avoid reducing plasma [Na$^+$] too rapidly when replacing water in water-depleted patients (11). In addition, a few individuals who are drinking large amounts of fluid during sustained exercise in the heat may become hyponatremic if they lose excessive amounts of salt in their sweat or drink and retain more fluid than is required to replace their losses (57–59). Although this condition is far less common than water-depletion heat exhaustion, it may be difficult to distinguish the two conditions from each other in the early stages without laboratory tests. Patients with water-depletion heat exhaustion respond rather quickly to fluid replacement, whereas hyponatremia is aggravated by administering hypotonic fluids, and may progress to life-threatening cerebral edema. Therefore, in a patient who was presumed to have heat exhaustion but does not improve quickly in response to administration of hypotonic fluids, such treatment should not be continued without further medical evaluation. (A rule suggested for field use is that a patient with presumed heat exhaustion should be given 2 quarts of water to drink over the course of an hour, and needs medical evaluation if noticeable improvement has not occurred by the end of the hour.)

Heat Stroke

Heat stroke is the most severe heat disorder and is characterized by rapid development of hyperthermia and severe neurologic disturbances, frequently including convulsions. Although these disturbances typically are characteristic of a nonfocal encephalopathy, some patients may show abnormalities of cerebellar function, which may be transient or may persist. Heat stroke may be complicated by liver damage, electrolyte abnormalities, and especially in the exertional form, by rhabdomyolysis, disseminated intravascular coagulation, or renal failure.

Loss of consciousness may occur suddenly, or may be preceded by up to an hour of prodromata, including headache, dizziness, drowsiness, restlessness, ataxia, confusion, and irrational or aggressive behavior. The physiologic pathology is not well understood, and there is some indication that factors other than hyperthermia contribute to the development of heat stroke. Heat stroke may be divided into two forms depending on the pathogenesis. In the classic form, the primary pathogenic factor is environmental heat stress that overwhelms an impaired thermoregulatory system, whereas in exertional heat stroke the primary factor is metabolic heat production. (See Reference 11 for a more extensive discussion.) Consequently, victims of the exertional form tend to be younger and physically fitter (typically soldiers, athletes, and laborers) than victims of the classic form. The traditional diagnostic criteria of heat stroke—coma, hot dry skin, and temperature above 41.3°C (106°F)—reflect experience primarily with the classic form. Adherence to these criteria will lead to underdiagnosis, since cessation of sweating may be a late event, especially in exertional heat stroke. Moreover, patients may come to medical attention either in the prodromal phase or after they have had a chance to cool somewhat and regain consciousness, especially if they still are sweating.

Measurements of rectal temperature or other deep body temperature are essential for clinical evaluation of hyperthermic patients and following response to treatment. A diagnosis of heat stroke must not be excluded on the basis either of oral temperature, or of temperature measured at the external auditory meatus or tympanic membrane. Because of hyperventilation, oral temperature may be 2 to 3°C lower than rectal temperature in heat stroke; the temperature of the external auditory meatus or tympanum may be as much as 5°C lower than rectal temperature in collapsed hyperthermic athletes (60). (Low values of the temperature of the tympanum may owe in part to cooling of its blood supply, which comes mostly from branches of the external carotid artery and thus follows a superficial course.) It is sometimes asserted that since the tympanum is so close to the cranium, tympanic temperature represents intracranial temperature—and thus the temperature of the brain—more accurately than any other noninvasive temperature measurement. Thus tympanic temperature measurements that are appreciably lower than measurements of trunk core (e.g., rectal or esophageal) temperature in hyperthermic human subjects are sometimes adduced to argue for the existence of physiologic heat-exchange mechanisms that protect the human brain during hyperthermia by cooling it below the temperature of the central blood. However, there is little empirical support either for the claims made for tympanic temperature or for the existence of special mechanisms to cool the human brain. (See References 28 and 61 for further discussion.)

Heat stroke is an extreme medical emergency, and prompt appropriate treatment is critically important in reducing morbidity and mortality. Cooling the patient to lower core temperature is the cornerstone of early treatment, and should begin as soon as possible. The patient should be removed from hot surroundings without delay, excess clothing and any equipment that obstructs free flow of air should be removed, the patient's skin should be wet if water is available, and the patient should be fanned to promote evaporative cooling. Although helpful, these measures are no substitute for more vigorous cooling once appropriate means are available, and cooling is accomplished most effectively by immersion in cold water. Costrini et al (62) lowered the rectal temperatures of their heat stroke patients at a mean rate of 0.18°C/min by immersing them in ice water. There is some disagreement as to the optimal water temperature, since lowering the temperature not only increases the core-to-skin thermal gradient for heat flow, but also reduces skin blood flow. Observations on heat-stroked dogs suggest that while 15 to 16°C (59 to 61°F) water is more effective than warmer water, little further advantage is gained with lower water temperatures (63). However there is no empirical support for the superiority of cooling methods, such as tepid baths or evaporation of sprayed water, that achieve only modest skin cooling. Some arguments in favor of such cooling methods are based on studies comparing different cooling methods in mildly hyperthermic normal subjects, whose peripheral vascular and other thermal responses may, however, be substantially different from those of heat stroke patients. The pitfalls in relying on such studies may be seen by comparing the following two reports: In tests on hot but normal young subjects, an evaporative cooling method was reported to be more effective than other cooling methods, causing tympanic temperature to fall at a rate of 0.31°C/min (64). However in a series of heat stroke patients the same authors found that the same cooling method lowered rectal temperature at a rate of only 0.06°C/min (65), one fifth the rate that they had reported in healthy individuals (64), and one third the rate that Costrini et al (62) achieved.

There is evidence for a systemic inflammatory component in heat stroke (53), and elevated levels of several inflammatory cytokines have been reported in patients presenting with heat stroke (66–68). Leakage of gram-negative endotoxin from the gut, perhaps facilitated by splanchnic ischemia, may be a trigger for secretion of these cytokines, since treatments aimed at preventing leakage of (69,70) or neutralizing (71) endotoxin partially protect experimental animals against heat stroke during subsequent heating. Gaffin et al (72) have discussed the implications of these concepts for prevention and treatment of heat stroke, but the efficacy of their proposed measures has not been sufficiently tested to allow their recommendation.

Heat stroke is to be distinguished from malignant hyperpyrexia, a rare process provoked in genetically susceptible individuals by inhalational anesthetics or neuromuscular blocking agents (73). Reuptake of calcium ion by the sarcoplasmic reticulum is severely impaired so that concentrations in the cytoplasm rise, leading to an uncontrolled hypermetabolic process that produces a rapid rise in core temperature. Dantrolene sodium, which reduces release of calcium ion from the sarcoplasmic reticulum, is an effective treatment and has dramatically reduced the mortality rate of this disorder.

Aggravation of Other Diseases

Besides causing the more or less characteristic disorders discussed above, heat stress can worsen the clinical state of patients with a number of other diseases. For example, patients with congestive heart failure have substantially impaired sweating and circulatory responses to environmental heat stress, and exposure to moderately hot environments worsens the signs and symptoms of congestive heart failure (74). Conversely, air conditioning improves the clinical progress of patients hospitalized in the summer with a variety of cardiorespiratory and other chronic diseases (74). The harmful effects of heat stress on those suffering from other diseases are also shown by analysis of the effects of unusually hot weather on total mortality and causes of death. Ellis (75), in a study of U.S. Public Health Service vital statistics reports for the years 1952 to 1967, examined monthly mortality statistics for 5 "heat wave" years, defined as those having more than 500 deaths reported as caused by "excessive heat and insolation." June and July of the heat wave years had excess mortality (i.e., above that expected for the month) from diabetes; cerebrovascular accidents; arteriosclerotic, degenerative, and hypertensive heart disease; and diseases of the blood-forming organs. He estimated the total number of excess deaths was more than 10 times as great as the number of deaths actually reported as due to heat.

Epidemiologic studies of individual heat waves demonstrate the effects of heat stress even more strikingly. For example Bridger et al (76) analyzed the July 1966 heat wave in eastern Missouri and central Illinois and related the death rates of various age groups to the reported daily temperatures. Using 1965 as a "normal" period for comparison of death rates, the authors computed 3-week moving averages as shown in Figure 104-6. Of the population at risk, people 65 years old and older suffered the greatest increase in mortality, attributed chiefly to diseases of the cardiovascular system, particularly cerebrovascular disease and arteriosclerosis. Since this heat wave began suddenly and was the first truly hot spell of the year, it may have struck an essentially unacclimatized population and thus have had an especially severe effect (76).

Prevention

Prevention of heat illness depends on careful attention to risk factors. Candidates for occupations or other activities that

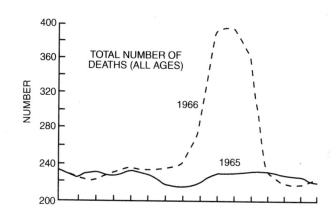

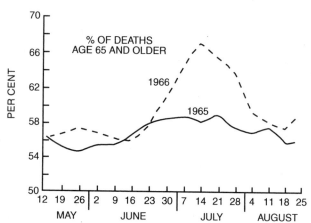

Figure 104-6 Three-week moving average of number of deaths per week in St. Louis, Mo, during the summers of 1965 and 1966 (top), and deaths occurring in those age 65 years and over expressed as a percentage of all deaths (bottom). There was a heat wave in July 1966, while the summer of 1965 was taken to represent normal weather. (Redrawn from Bridger CA, Helfand LA. Mortality from heat during July in Illinois. Int J Biometeorol 1968;12:51–70.)

subject them to prolonged or severe exercise-heat stress should be screened for individual risk factors, including use of therapeutic or recreational drugs that would increase their risk of heat illness. Unacclimatized personnel—especially those who are physically unfit—should be allowed to acclimatize gradually. Consideration should be given to excusing personnel with mild infections from activities that involve prolonged or severe exercise-heat stress. Provision should be made for adequate sleep, and alcohol abuse should be guarded against. Perhaps the most important preventive measure is ample provision of cool palatable water or other beverages, with frequent opportunity to drink. It should be stressed that although acclimatization reduces loss of salt, it does not reduce water requirements—indeed, the biophysics of heat exchange largely precludes any such effect. The persistent myth that withholding water during exercise-heat stress produces toughening is unsupported by evidence, unless rigor mortis is taken as evidence of toughness.

Persons undergoing prolonged exercise-heat stress should be encouraged to drink frequently and not to wait until they feel thirsty. Thirst is not a reliable guide to water requirements under such conditions, and complete water replacement during prolonged heat stress is difficult even if ample water is available. Soldiers on a long march, for example, gradually become progressively dehydrated if they drink only according to their feelings of thirst (77). Provision of flavored beverages may enhance consumption, but beverages should not be carbonated or caffeinated, since the former may cause a sense of fullness and the latter may promote fluid loss by diuresis. Consideration should be given to beverages containing electrolytes during intense sustained exercise-heat stress or in settings where food intake is reduced.

The views, opinions, and findings in this chapter are those of the author and should not be construed as an official Department of the Army position, policy, or decision unless so designated by other official documentation. Approved for public release, distribution is unlimited.

REFERENCES

1. Moritz AR, Henriques FC Jr. Studies of thermal injury II: the relative importance of time and surface temperature in the causation of cutaneous burns. Am J Pathol 1947;23:695–720.

2. Du Bois EF. Fever and the regulation of body temperature. Springfield, IL: C. C. Thomas, 1948.

3. Gisolfi CV, Wenger CB. Temperature regulation during exercise: old concepts, new ideas. Exerc Sport Sci Rev 1984;12:339–372.

4. Mackowiak PA, Wasserman SS, Levine MM. A critical appraisal of 98.6°F, the upper limit of the normal body temperature, and other legacies of Carl Reinhold August Wunderlich. JAMA 1992; 268:1578–1580.

5. Aschoff J. Circadian rhythm of activity and of body temperature. In: Hardy JD, Gagge AP, Stolwijk JAJ, eds. Physiological and behavioral temperature regulation. Springfield, IL: C. C. Thomas, 1970:905–919.

6. Hessemer V, Brück K. Influence of menstrual cycle on shivering, skin blood flow, and sweating responses measured at night. J Appl Physiol 1985;59:1902–1910.

7. Kolka MA. Temperature regulation in women. Med Exerc Nutr Health 1992;1:201–207.

8. Stephenson LA, Kolka MA. Menstrual cycle phase and time of day alter reference signal controlling arm blood flow and sweating. Am J Physiol 1985;249:R186–R191.

9. Sawka MN, Pandolf KB. Physical exercise in hot climates: physiology, performance and biomedical issues. In: Burr RE, Pandolf KB, eds. Medical aspects of deployment to harsh environments. Washington, D.C.: Office of the Surgeon General, Department of the Army, 1999 (in press).

10. Johnson RF, Kobrick JL. Psychological aspects of military performance in hot environments. In: Burr RE, Pandolf KB, eds. Medical aspects of deployment to harsh environments. Washington, D.C.: Office of the Surgeon General, Department of the Army, 1999 (in press).

11. Knochel JP, Reed G. Disorders of heat regulation. In: Maxwell MH, Kleeman CR, Narins RG, eds. Clinical disorders of fluid and electrolyte metabolism. New York: McGraw-Hill, 1987:1197–1232.

12. Leithead CS, Lind AR. Heat stress and heat disorders. Philadelphia, PA: FA Davis, 1964.

13. Knochel JP. Heat stroke and related heat stress disorders. Dis Mon 1989;35:301–377.

14. Cabanac M. Physiological role of pleasure. Science 1971;173: 1103–1107.

15. Bligh J, Johnson KG. Glossary of terms for thermal physiology. J Appl Physiol 1973;35:941–961.

16. Gagge AP, Hardy JD, Rapp GM. Proposed standard system of symbols for thermal physiology. J Appl Physiol 1969;27:439–446.

17. Ferrannini E. Equations and assumptions of indirect calorimetry: some special problems. In: Kinney JM, Tucker HN, eds. Energy metabolism: Tissue determinants and cellular corollaries. New York: Raven Press, 1992: 1–17.

18. Åstrand P-O, Rodahl K. Temperature regulation. In: Åstrand P-O, Rodahl K, eds. Textbook of work physiology. New York: Mc-Graw-Hill, 1977:523–576.

19. Hardy JD. Physiology of temperature regulation. Physiol Rev 1961; 41:521–606.

20. Kuno Y. Human perspiration. Springfield, IL: C. C. Thomas, 1956:3–41.

21. Fox RH, Edholm OG. Nervous control of the cutaneous circulation. Br Med Bull 1963;19:110–114.

22. Sawka MN, Wenger CB. Physiological responses to acute exercise-heat stress. In: Pandolf KB, Sawka MN, Gonzalez RR, eds. Human performance physiology and environmental medicine at terrestrial extremes. Indianapolis, In: Benchmark Press, 1988:97–151.

23. Rowell LB. Cardiovascular adjustments to thermal stress. In: Shepherd JT, Abboud FM, eds. Handbook of physiology, section 2: The cardiovascular system, vol. 3. Peripheral circulation and organ blood flow. Bethesda, MD: American Physiological Society, 1983: 967–1023.

24. Johnson JM, Proppe DW. Cardiovascular adjustments to heat stress. In: Fregly MJ, Blatteis CM, eds. Handbook of physiology, section 4. Environmental physiology. New York: Oxford University Press for the American Physiological Society, 1996:215–243.

25. Roddie IC. Circulation to skin and adipose tissue. In: Shepherd JT, Abboud FM, eds. Handbook of physiology, section 2: The cardiovascular system, vol. 3. Peripheral circulation and organ blood flow. Bethesda, MD: American Physiological Society, 1983:285–317.

26. Rowell LB. Active neurogenic vasodilatation in man. In: Vanhoutte PM, Leusen I, eds. Vasodilatation. New York: Raven Press, 1981:1–17.

27. Love AHG, Shanks RG. The relationship between the onset of sweating and vasodilatation in the forearm during body heating. J Physiol (Lond) 1962;162:121–128.

28. Sawka MN, Wenger CB, Pandolf KB. Thermoregulatory responses to acute exercise-heat stress and heat acclimation. In: Fregly MJ, Blatteis CM, eds. Handbook of physiology, section 4. Environmental physiology. New York: Oxford University Press for the American Physiological Society, 1996:157–185.

29. Brengelmann GL, Freund PR, Rowell LB, et al. Absence of active cutaneous vasodilation associated with congenital absence of sweat glands in humans. Am J Physiol 1981;240:H571–H575.

30. Rowell LB. Human cardiovascular adjustments to exercise and thermal stress. Physiol Rev 1974;54:75–159.

31. Fogoros RN. "Runner's trots:" gastrointestinal disturbances in runners. JAMA 1980;243:1743–1744.

32. Kuno Y. Human perspiration. Springfield, IL: C. C. Thomas, 1956:42–97.

33. Eichna LW, Ashe WF, Bean WB, Shelley WB. The upper limits of environmental heat and humidity tolerated by acclimatized men working in hot environments. J Indust Hyg Toxicol 1945;27:59–84.

34. Ladell WSS. Thermal sweating. Br Med Bull 1945;3:175–179.

35. Kuno Y. Human perspiration. Springfield, IL: C. C. Thomas, 1956:251–276.

36. Robinson S, Robinson AH. Chemical composition of sweat. Physiol Rev 1954;34:202–220.

37. Brown WK, Sargent F II. Hidromeiosis. Arch Environ Health 1965;11:442–453.

38. Nadel ER, Stolwijk JAJ. Effect of skin wettedness on sweat gland response. J Appl Physiol 1973;35:689–694.

39. Dobson RL, Formisano V, Lobitz WC Jr, Brophy D. Some histochemical observations on the human eccrine sweat glands: III: the effect of profuse sweating. J Invest Dermatol 1958;31:147–159.

40. Jessen C. Interaction of body temperatures in control of thermoregulatory effector mechanisms. In: Fregly MJ, Blatteis CM, eds. Handbook of physiology, section 4. Environmental physiology. New York: Oxford University Press for the American Physiological Society, 1996:127–138.

41. Wenger CB. Human heat acclimatization. In: Pandolf KB, Sawka MN, Gonzalez RR, eds. Human performance physiology and environmental medicine at terrestrial extremes. Indianapolis, In: Benchmark Press, 1988:153–197.

42. Eichna LW, Park CR, Nelson N, et al. Thermal regulation during acclimatization in a hot, dry (desert type) environment. Am J Physiol 1950;163:585–597.

43. Collins KJ, Crockford GW, Weiner JS. The local training effect of secretory activity on the response of eccrine sweat glands. J Physiol (Lond) 1966;184:203–214.

44. Kraning KK, Lehman PA, Gano RG, Weller TS. A non-invasive dose-response assay of sweat gland function and its application in studies of gender comparison, heat acclimation and anticholinergic potency. In: Mercer JB, ed. Thermal physiology 1989. Amsterdam: Elsevier, 1989:301–307.

45. Pandolf KB, Young AJ. Environmental extremes and endurance performance. In: Shephard RJ, Åstrand PO, eds. Endurance in sport. Oxford: Blackwell Scientific, 1992:270–282.

46. Kenney WL. Physiological correlates of heat intolerance. Sports Med 1985;2:279–286.

47. Pivarnik JM, Marichal CJ, Spillman T, Morrow JR Jr. Menstrual cycle phase affects temperature regulation during endurance exercise. J Appl Physiol 1992;72:543–548.

48. Kark JA, Gardner JW, Hetzel DP, et al. Fever in classification of exertional heat injury. Clin Res 1991;39:143A.

49. Maron MB, Wagner JA, Horvath SM. Thermoregulatory responses during competitive marathon running. J Appl Physiol 1997;42:909–914.

50. Pugh LGCE, Corbett JL, Johnson RH. Rectal temperatures, weight losses, and sweat rates in marathon running. J Appl Physiol 1967;23:347–352.

51. Pandolf KB, Griffin TB, Munro EH, Goldman RF. Persistence of impaired heat tolerance from artificially induced miliaria rubra. Am J Physiol 1980;239:R226–R232.

52. Lind AR. Pathophysiology of heat exhaustion and heat stroke. In: Khogali M, Hales JRS, eds. Heat stroke and temperature regulation. Sydney: Academic Press, 1983:179–188.

53. Hales JRS, Hubbard RW, Gaffin SL. Limitation of heat tolerance. In: Fregly MJ, Blatteis CM, eds. Handbook of physiology, section 4. Environmental physiology. New York: Oxford University Press for the American Physiological Society, 1996:285–355.

54. Petersdorf RG. Hypothermia and hyperthermia. In: Wilson JD, Braunwald E, Isselbacher KJ, et al, eds. Harrison's principles of internal medicine. New York: McGraw-Hill, 1991:2194–2220.

55. Kark JA, Ward FT. Exercise and hemoglobin S. Semin Hematol 1994;31:181–225.

56. Berl T. Treating hyponatremia: damned if we do and damned if we don't. Kidney Int 1990;37:1006–1018.

57. Armstrong LE, Curtis WC, Hubbard RW, et al. Symptomatic hyponatremia during prolonged exercise in heat. Med Sci Sports Exerc 1993;25:543–549.

58. Frizzell RT, Lang GH, Lowance DC, Lathan SR. Hyponatremia and ultramarathon running. JAMA 1986;255:772–774.

59. Noakes TD, Goodwin N, Rayner BL, et al. Water intoxication: a possible complication during endurance exercise. Med Sci Sports Exerc 1985;17:370–375.

60. Roberts WO. Assessing core temperature in collapsed athletes: what's the best method? Physician Sportsmed. 1994;22:49–55.

61. Brengelmann GL. Dilemma of body temperature measurement. In: Shiraki K, Yousef MK, eds. Man in stressful environments: Thermal and work physiology. Springfield, IL: C. C. Thomas, 1987:5–22.

62. Costrini AM, Pitt HA, Gustafson AB, Uddin DE. Cardiovascular and metabolic manifestations of heat stroke and severe heat exhaustion. Am J Med 1979;66: 296–302.

63. Magazanik A, Epstein Y, Udassin R, et al. Tap water, an efficient method for cooling heatstroke victims—a model in dogs. Aviat Space Environ Med 1980;51:864–867.

64. Weiner JS, Khogali M. A physiological body-cooling unit for treatment of heat stroke. Lancet 1980;1:507–509.

65. Khogali M, Weiner JS. Heat stroke, report on 18 cases. Lancet 1980; 2:276–278.

66. Bouchama A, Parhar RS, El-Yazigi A, et al. Endotoxemia and release of tumor necrosis factor and interleukin 1α in acute heatstroke. J Appl Physiol 1991;70:2640–2644.

67. Bouchama A, Al-Sedairy S, Siddiqui S, et al. Elevated pyrogenic cytokines in heatstroke. Chest 1993;104:1498–1502.

68. Chang DM. The role of cytokines in heat stroke. Immunol Invest 1993;22:553–561.

69. Butkow N, Mitchell D, Laburn H, Kenedi E. Heat stroke and endotoxaemia in rabbits. In: Hales JRS, ed. Thermal physiology. New York: Raven, 1984:511–514.

70. Bynum G, Brown J, DuBose D, et al. Increased survival in experimental dog heatstroke after reduction of gut flora. Aviat Space Environ Med 1978;50:816–819.

71. Gathiram P, Wells MT, Brock-Utne JG, Gaffin SL. Antilipopolysaccharide improves survival in primates subjected to heat stroke. Circ Shock 1987;23:157–164.

72. Gaffin SL, Hubbard RW. Experimental approaches to therapy and prophylaxis for heat stress and heatstroke. Wildern Environ Med 1996;4:312–334.

73. Gronert GA. Malignant hyperthermia. Anesthesiology 1980;53: 395–423.

74. Burch GE, DePasquale NP. Hot climates, man and his heart. Springfield, IL: C. C. Thomas, 1962.

75. Ellis FP. Mortality from heat illness and heat-aggravated illness in the United States. Environ Res 1972; 5:1–58.

76. Bridger CA, Helfand LA. Mortality from heat during July in Illinois. Int J Biometeorol 1968;12:51–70.

77. Rothstein A, Adolph EF, Wills JH. Voluntary dehydration. In: Visscher MB, Bronk DW, Landis EM, Ivy AC, eds. Physiology of man in the desert. New York: Interscience, 1947:254–270.

Chapter 105

Physiologic Responses to Acute and Chronic Cold Stress

Nigel A.S. Taylor

Jodie M. Stocks

Karen D. Mittleman

DYSTHERMIA

Dysthermia results when the regulation of body-core temperature (T_{core}) is disturbed, either transiently or permanently. Normally, the body's T_{core} remains relatively unchanged during heat gains from, or losses to, most thermal environments, and varies around 36.7°C (98.1°F) [standard deviation = 0.3°C (1)]. From a clinical perspective, if T_{core} varies more than 2°C to either side of 37°C, then dysthermia exists and is classified as either *hypothermia* (<35°C), or *hyperthermia* (>39°C). Although man can tolerate a vast range of thermal environments (2,3), utilizing both physiologic and behavioral strategies, T_{core} must be maintained within a very narrow range. The focus of this chapter is the acute and chronic physiologic changes (*strain*) accompanying human exposure to cold gases and liquids (*stress*), and the factors that modify these responses.

Heat Balance

One of the most significant scientific generalizations is the *law of conservation of energy*, which, in terms of thermal physics, becomes the *First Law of Thermodynamics*. This law tells us that, within a closed system, energy is neither created nor destroyed. Instead, the total amount of energy is conserved, but not necessarily the forms or location of that energy. We may consider our solar system as a closed system, in which thermal energy is continuously transferred from one site (heat source) to another (heat sink), due to temperature differences between those sites. When an inadequately protected person is exposed to a cold environment, the body becomes the primary heat source, and the surrounding environment the heat sink. Examples of heat sinks include surrounding air, water, and solids to which heat is transferred via convection,

conduction, or radiation. For every 3.47 kJ/kg of heat lost to the environment, the average tissue temperature will decline by 1°C (*specific heat*: 0.83 kcal/kg/°C). In this chapter, we are concerned with the thermal energy exchanges between man and cold environments, as well as energy conservation. These interrelationships are best summarized by the *heat balance equation*:

$$S = M - (\pm W) \pm E \pm R \pm C \pm K$$

in watts per square meter, where S = heat storage (+ for storage; − for loss) (W/m²), M = metabolic heat production (W/m²), W = work performed (+ for energy leaving system) or received (− for energy entering system) (W/m²), E = heat exchange via evaporation (−) or condensation (+) (W/m²), R = heat exchange via radiant exchange (− for loss; + for gain) (W/m²), C = heat exchange via convective heat flow (− for loss; + for gain) (W/m²), and K = heat exchange via conductance (− for loss; + for gain;) (W/m²).

Thermoreceptors

Thermosensitive sites exist in the skin, viscera, spinal cord, midbrain, medulla oblongata, and hypothalamus (4,5). However, the first perception of a thermal stimulus is obtained via cutaneous thermoreceptors, found close to the skin surface, and within deeper cutaneous (shell) tissues (6). Assuming the uniform T_{core} did not extend to within about 2.5 cm of the skin surface, Burton (7) calculated that over 50% of the body mass was within these shell tissues. Thus, a considerable fraction of the body is capable of providing immediate input concerning our thermal environment. Cutaneous thermoafferents from the limbs and trunk enter the spinal cord through the spinal ganglion and dorsal root, synapsing in the dorsal horn with second-order afferents and ascend via the lateral spinothalamic tract (8,9). It is believed that the subcoeruleus region [pontine reticular formation (10)], and the raphe system [pons and midbrain (11)] relay these messages to the hypothalamus for integration. Facial cutaneous afferents pass to the hypothalamus via the trigeminal ganglion, synapsing with second-order neurons in the trigeminal nucleus caudalis (9).

During any cold exposure, a sequence of three events occurs. First, there is a reduction in skin temperature (T_{skin}). This elicits neural feedback to the hypothalamus, and also induces localized venoconstriction and, depending upon the intensity of the stimulus, centrally mediated vasoconstriction. The net result is a further reduction in T_{skin}, which, during cold-water immersion, will eventually approximate water temperature. Second, as a direct result of reduced skin blood flow, heat loss is briefly diminished. Prior to cold exposure, thermal equilibrium (zero heat storage) existed, so this rapid reduction in cutaneous heat loss transiently disturbs heat balance, producing a paradoxical elevation in T_{core}, which may last more than 30 minutes in some conditions. Third, T_{core} starts to decrease. The spinal cord, brain stem, and preoptic anterior hypothalamus receive and integrate both central and peripheral thermal signals (12,13), enabling the generation of a thermal load error signal, to which the hypothalamus produces its autonomic responses: cutaneous vasoconstriction and thermogenesis.

AUTONOMIC RESPONSES

Although the temperatures of solids, liquids, and gases may be identical, it is incorrect to assume that all environments at the same absolute temperature elicit equivalent thermal strain, since several physical properties, in addition to temperature, dictate heat flow to and from the body. Consider a person moving from one sealed tank to another (each at 10°C), with each tank containing one of five substances: 1) air at 1 atm, 2) air at 5 atm absolute, 3) water, 4) snow, 5) and helium. In each case, the person will lose heat. The increase in air density experienced on moving from tank 1 to 2 (such as encountered in hyperbaric facilities) will elevate convective and conductive heat losses, but will have minimal effect upon thermal conductivity (ability of heat to flow through a substance), so the quantity of heat transferred will probably be the same, but it will occur faster. Moving into tank 3 will have a dual effect. First, the thermal conductivity of water is about 23 times that of air. Second, the specific heat of water is about four times greater, and since specific heat is a function of mass and water is more than 1000 times denser than air, it will take over 4000 times the amount of heat to equilibrate an equal volume of water than air. In tank 4, the thermal conductivity is about 5.5 times greater than air (due to air surrounding solid particles) and the specific heat is about twofold greater. In the final tank we have helium, which is used to replace nitrogen in diving gas mixtures. This gas is less dense, but its thermal conductivity is six times greater, while its specific heat is close to five times that of air. Therefore, although each heat sink is at 10°C, the rate of heat loss and the total heat energy lost are unequal. If we consider the thermoneutral

state to occur under conditions in which T_{core} remains stable and is regulated only through changes in vascular tone (14), then the resting thermoneutral temperature for our person will vary between each of the tanks: air (23 to 26°C), water (34 to 36°C), and helium (31 to 32°C). Since exercise adds to the total heat content, but also enhances convective losses, these temperatures are reduced according to the exercise intensity.

Altered Cutaneous Blood Flow

Constriction of cutaneous veins and arteries is a primary autonomic cold response. Such stress stimulates sympathetic nervous activity, leading first to venoconstriction and then vasoconstriction, via activation of α-adrenergic receptors and through an elevation in plasma norepinephrine (15). The result of cutaneous vasoconstriction is reduced heat loss, by increasing the thickness of the insulating layer to reduce conductive heat transfer and by minimizing exposure of warm blood to the cold environment to restrict mass transfer. This constriction response reflects the integration of both static and dynamic thermoreceptor influences from the core and periphery (16). Furthermore, local T_{skin} reductions elicit local and generalized vasoconstriction, because of thermoreceptor and local effects. However, the magnitude of this local response is, in part, T_{core}-dependent. Thus, when T_{core} has been reduced, a given T_{skin} reduction augments vasoconstriction beyond that observed for the same T_{skin} change at a higher T_{core}. These direct local effects are believed to play a role in cold-induced vasodilation, along with abolishing the constrictive effect of catecholamines at very low temperatures (4).

Although the above trends are universally observed, the cutaneous blood flow response varies at the extremities (hands, feet, ears, nose, lips), trunk and proximal limbs, and the head (4). This is largely due to local variations in the role of vasoconstrictor control. The extremities, for example, are under strong sympathetic influence, whereas the head has minimal constrictor response to cold stress. The extremities also contain specialized networks of arteriovenous anastomoses, which, when activated, help control blood flow and reduce heat loss from deeper tissues.

Thermogenesis

When homeotherms experience heat loss, heat production (shivering thermogenesis) will be activated via autonomic thermoregulation to maintain a stable T_{core} (17). Shivering intensity is dependent upon several factors. First, the initial increase is driven by enhanced peripheral sensory activity, as T_{skin} declines. Second, if heat loss exceeds thermogenesis, T_{core} will decline, stimulating core thermoreceptors, which will induce greater thermogenesis. In this state, heat production is proportional to the magnitude of the T_{core} change. Third, there is an interaction between T_{skin} and T_{core} in determining thermogenic intensity during cold exposure (18). For example, when T_{core} is elevated prior to skin cooling, thermogenesis will be smaller for a given T_{skin} stimulus. On the other hand, a lower initial T_{core} will enhance thermogenesis. Finally, in addition to the importance of absolute temperature (i.e., static influence), the rates of T_{skin} and T_{core} change also affect thermogenesis [i.e., dynamic influence (4,19,20)]. Each of these factors are reflected in an elevation in oxygen consumption, which, during intense shivering, can undergo a fivefold increase.

In extreme environments, or when thermogenesis is impaired (e.g., age, drug influences), heat production fails to prevent T_{core} decline, and hypothermia ensues. For example, since shivering is mainly fueled by glucose, reduced muscle glycogen content may limit shivering (21–23). Hypoglycemia itself may be considered an index of imminent hypothermia (24), because of its impact upon both autonomic nervous system and cognitive functions, and the resultant shivering cessation (25).

Body-Fluid and Hormonal Responses

Acute cold-air exposure generally decreases intravascular volume, reducing plasma volume by 7% to 15% (26,27) and increasing plasma osmolality and sodium concentration. Hemoconcentration was attributed to a greater diuresis, whereby vasoconstriction increases central blood volume, stimulates baroreceptors, inhibits vasopressin secretion, and ultimately reduces plasma volume (28,29). Cold-induced diuresis can be considerable, increasing fluid losses almost twofold (30). However, hemoconcentration has also since been suggested to result from a fluid and ion redistribution from the intravascular to the interstitial space due to altered capillary exchange, evoked by peripheral vasoconstriction, which elevates total peripheral resistance and blood pressure (31). Although this is plausible, the fluid shift remains speculative, and there is a lack of information pertaining to the distribution and regulation of body fluids during acute cold-air exposure.

Information concerning body-fluid regulation during cold-water immersion is also sparse, with the primary focus again upon plasma volume changes. However, an important consideration is the hydrostatically induced redistribution of blood into the thorax (32,33), which perturbs the Starling forces and modifies intravascular fluid flux. Plasma volume is typically reduced 15% to 20% during cold-water immersion, despite differences in thermal stress (27,34). Notwithstanding these response similarities, determination of the mechanisms responsible for plasma volume change has remained difficult. Rochelle et al (35) suggested that plasma was lost to the urine. The plasma volume decrease has been correlated with body fat, and the magnitude of the plasma volume shift could be related to the degree of body cooling. However, Young et al (27) found no correlation between decreased plasma volume and shivering, diuresis, or T_{core} or T_{skin} responses. No doubt, there are both hydrostatic and thermal factors involved in fluid regulation during immersion.

Cold exposure elicits a number of hormonal responses that, in some cases, depend more upon the severity of the ensuing hypothermic strain than they do upon the type of stress. For instance, thyroid hormone increases within 15 to 30 minutes of cold exposure in animals, possibly increasing heat production via sodium pump stimulation. However, this outcome is less certain in man (36). Cold air and immersion induce thoraco-abdominal hypervolemia, elevate blood pressure, and induce cardiovascular distension, eliciting several hormonal changes. Atrial natriuretic peptide is released from the left atrium in response to atrial stretching and enhances both sodium and water excretion (sodium diuresis). There is also a transient reduction in vasopressin (antidiuretic hormone) secretion (posterior pituitary), which controls water permeability at the nephron. Finally, circulating aldosterone

(sodium-retaining hormone), and its regulating hormone renin (released from the juxtaglomerular cells) are reduced. Although some changes result from thermal stress and may occur to varying extents during air and immersion exposures, others are associated with hydrostatic changes accompanying immersion. For instance, Jansky et al (37) observed a 50% decrease in plasma renin activity during a 14°C immersion. Since similar results were observed during thermoneutral immersion, this was interpreted as a hydrostatic rather than a thermal effect. In contrast, plasma aldosterone was unchanged across these trials and, since aldosterone secretion is suppressed during thermoneutral immersion, it was possible that cold stress countered this hydrostatic effect. In addition, we have recently shown that atrial natriuretic peptide secretion, during cold-water immersion, is primarily mediated by thermal rather than hydrostatic influences (38).

Thermal Responses in Some Cold-Adapted Ethnic Groups

Adaptations are physiologic and morphologic changes modifying physiologic strain. When such a transformation occurs within the lifetime of an organism, it is classified as a phenotypic adaptation (genotypic adaptation accompanies genetic selection). Two forms of thermal, phenotypic adaptations are recognized: adaptation to naturally occurring exposures (acclimatization) and adaptation to experimentally induced stress (acclimation).

Several human populations exhibit acclimatization to air and water exposure (39,40). Acclimatization to cold air is classically described within the Australian Aborigines, and studies on this once-isolated people were among the earliest on human thermoregulation. Hicks studied central Australian Aborigines during the 1930s, when they were nomadic and wore little clothing (41). When Aborigines and nonadapted Europeans slept in the cold, the metabolic rate of the former remained virtually unchanged (blunted thermogenesis), while skin temperature continued to decrease (41). Subsequent research confirmed these observations, finding that the T_{core} in Aboriginals also decreased further (42,43). This adaptation was described as an insulative-hypothermic response, since T_{skin} and T_{core} were allowed to drop. In this circumstance, it is possible that the body tolerates mild hypothermia, reserving more powerful physiologic responses for even more threatening cold stress (44). Circumpolar inhabitants (e.g., Norwegian Lapps, Canadian Eskimos) also show cold-induced adaptation, with perhaps the most frequently reported observation being a blunted (habituated) shivering thermogenesis, combined with the maintenance of warmer T_{skin}, when compared to nonadapted people (45–47).

Cold-water acclimatization has also been identified. For example, the Korean breath-hold divers (Ama) dive daily in water temperatures from 10 to 25°C (winter-summer), experiencing year round T_{core} reductions to 35°C (48). The Ama show: 1) reversible increases in basal metabolic rate during winter [metabolic adaptation (40)]; 2) significantly lower critical water temperature for shivering onset (49); 3) lower limb heat loss during immersion, for a given blood flow, indicating more efficient countercurrent heat exchange (50); and 4) the maintenance of higher limb muscle temperature [vascular adaptation (51)]. Thus, whereas the Aborigines and Lapps demonstrated an habituated metabolic response, the Ama revealed heightened thermogenic and insulative adaptations.

FACTORS AFFECTING COLD-STRESS RESPONSES

Body Composition and Physique

Heat lost from an unclothed body is dependent, in part, on the insulation provided by subcutaneous adipose (52), which has a thermal conductivity approximately 50% that of muscle (53). The regional distribution of these deposits may also affect heat loss (54). For instance, individuals who have a relatively greater limb adiposity may have a thermal advantage during cold-water swimming, since they insulate a major heat source (active muscle). However, cold-adapted, relatively lean swimmers have been shown to adequately tolerate cold stress (55). This was achieved through cold habituation. Moreover, adipose is not the only insulating tissue. Veicsteinas et al (56) demonstrated that inactive, unperfused muscle provides effective insulation during cold-water immersion. Toner et al (57) similarly found that when larger and smaller men, matched for adiposity, were exposed to cold (rest), the larger men increased overall tissue insulation to a greater extent. This difference was associated with differences in muscle mass.

In addition to body composition, anthropometric characteristics also influence heat loss. For example, the surface area–to-mass ratio (58) and the relative linearity [(height/mass^3) (59)] affect cooling rates. Thus, small children and people tending towards ectomorphy lose heat more rapidly. In the former, rapid heat loss, and its impact upon metabolism, is a critical determinant of survival following protracted submersion.

Core temperature cooling is ultimately determined by the balance between heat loss and production. Although the latter is influenced by disease states and various chemical agents, it is uncertain to what extent it is affected by body composition. For instance, although some have found an inverse relation between subcutaneous adiposity and heat production during cold-water immersion (60,61), others have not observed this pattern (62). More recently, Mittleman (63) found that morphology did not influence the thermosensitivity of heat production in men with similar peripheral and central thermal drives. Strong et al (64) proposed that thermal mass, rather than adiposity per se, was related to shivering thermogenesis during cold-water immersion.

Gender

Two fundamental gender differences are readily apparent: 1) T_{core} is a function of menstrual phase, being about 0.5°C higher during the luteal phase; and 2) during cold-air exposures, the T_{skin} of women is typically lower than that observed in men (65,66). The combination of these factors means that women tend to lose less heat via tissue conductance since, in the cold, they maintain a lower cutaneous blood flow, which is even noticeable while resting in the heat (67). Thus, the skin-to-air temperature gradient is smaller, as is cutaneous heat flow. Although some gender-related contrasts are a function of body composition and anthropometric differences (68), others are intricately related to endocrine functions, in particular the hormonal changes associated with the menstrual cycle (69). These effects express themselves through a number of physiologic functions related to, as well as the outcomes from, thermoregulation.

The menstrual cycle interacts with regulatory hormones that affect both body-fluid balance and electrolyte regulation (70). It has also been shown to alter the thresholds for both thermal comfort (71) and thermogenesis (72), and to modify resting muscle glycogen levels (73), a factor which impacts upon long-term cold tolerance, through its role in shivering. Moreover, there is even evidence to indicate that estrogen may affect the thermosensitivity of the hypothalamus (74). At this time, our knowledge of cold tolerance in women is limited; however, we are unaware of evidence to indicate that women are more prone to cold injury.

Aging

In the years 1979 to 1990, more than 9300 people died in the United States from hypothermia (75). Similar epidemiologic studies reveal that people at either end of the age spectrum are susceptible to environmental extremes (76–78). Laboratory-based research has shown the aged may experience impaired autonomic function (79), an altered skin blood flow sensitivity to thermal stimuli (80–82), a reduced sweating response (83), and more variable T_{core} regulation (84). Furthermore, aging is generally accompanied by reduced subcutaneous adipose. Such changes predispose the elderly to thermal instability caused by a reduced ability to generate, conserve, and dissipate heat. Keatinge et al (85) further found that prolonged skin cooling increased erythrocyte counts, blood viscosity, and arterial blood pressure in young adults, and postulated this as a mechanism to account for the increased winter-related incidence of coronary and cerebral thromboses in the elderly. In addition, we must recognize the affects of various prescription drugs, which alter heat production, heat loss, or mood state.

Although several physiologic factors contribute to age-related dysthermia, it is uncertain whether this is a consequence of autonomic dysfunction, or combined with a failure to detect thermal changes and initiate behavioral responses. Research shows that, equivalently clothed, older subjects maintain room temperature as well as the young, but the young made more frequent temperature changes, keeping air temperature within a narrower range (86). Field studies have shown the aged maintain home temperatures below the recommended minimal winter levels (87,88). Although the cost of heating is undoubtedly a factor for some, the possibility exists that inappropriate behavioral responses may have prevented adequate temperature control. Consequently, we investigated age-related differences in air temperature control, thermal perception, and affect state in two groups (aged 23 and 67 years) during rest (89). After equilibration at 24°C, temperature controllers were set into cooling mode. Subjects adjusted air temperature using a dual position switch when it moved outside their preferred range. Switch operation resulted in maximal cooling or heating, without a steady state. Subjective ratings of thermal sensation, discomfort, and affect were provided at each activation. Although both groups controlled temperature equivalently, T_{skin} (calf, thigh, chest, hand) was significantly lower in the elderly at the cold-induced change points, yet they reported being more comfortable than the young subjects. Assuming thermal discomforture drives behavior, these observations were interpreted to indicate that the elderly may require a more intense thermal stimulus to elicit appropriate behavioral responses.

Physical Fitness

It has long been known that endurance training enhances heat tolerance. It is also known that endurance training affects a number of physiologic variables that may impact upon cold tolerance: suppressing basal T_{core}, increasing the vascular bed in limb muscles, elevating metabolic efficiency, and reducing adiposity. Certainly, peak shivering thermogenesis may be related to endurance fitness, with a strong relationship between aerobic power and peak shivering intensity (90). Nevertheless, while some have found elevated fitness improves cold tolerance (43,91), research evidence is far from unequivocal (92). There is even evidence to show covariation between endurance and body composition, such that leaner, trained subjects displayed an elevated shivering thermogenesis, whereas fatter subjects showed no change in heat production (93,94). Consequently, this question remains unresolved.

Cold Adaptation

The second form of phenotypic adaptation is acclimation, achieved through artificial cold exposure (94,95). However, despite a number of studies, the adaptive mechanisms have not been clearly identified, and no single picture of human cold adaptation has been consistently characterised. Three different, but not necessarily exclusive, patterns of cold adaptation exist (96): 1) metabolic adaptation [altered thermogenesis, associated with both nonshivering thermogenesis in animals and blunted shivering thermogenesis in man (42,95,97)]; 2) hypothermic adaptation [T_{core} decline with reduced thermogenesis (95,98)]; and 3) an insulative adaptation [lowered skin temperature while T_{core} and thermogenesis remain stable; (99,100)]. Unlike heat adaptation, cold acclimation is associated with a blunting (habituation) of thermoeffector responses (101,102), in which there is an apparent desensitization to cold stress.

Although cold-enhanced thermogenesis occurs in animals (103), in man, one typically observes thermogenic blunting or habituation (95,97). This habituated shivering response is accompanied by greater T_{core} reductions following acclimation [hypothermic adaptation (37,95,104)]. Blunting is believed to be centrally controlled, negative conditioning (105), but the nature of the thermogenic blunting is somewhat unclear. However, Young et al (95) reported a delay in shivering onset, which may be attributed to a reduced thermogenic threshold (94,98). Prior to adaptation, shivering is activated via peripheral thermoreceptors and then controlled by central and peripheral thermoreceptors. Following adaptation, the importance of the peripheral thermoreceptors is believed to be diminished, with shivering evolving only after T_{core} decreases (94). Confirmation of such changes has been obtained in cold-adapted rats (106); nonetheless evidence for central thermoreceptor modification in humans remains speculative. Taken in conjunction with a stable sweating threshold, following cold-air acclimation (107), data suggest a decreased sensitivity of the thermoregulatory system to cold stress, and a widening of the interthreshold zone (97).

Evidence for an insulative adaptation is primarily found in response to repeated cold-water immersions (94,95), rather than cold-air exposures, and is possibly caused by differences in the magnitude of the thermal stimuli. Young et al (95) reported lower T_{skin} following cold-water acclimation (cutaneous vasoconstriction), resulting in a larger core-to-skin temperature gradient, increasing heat transfer to the muscles, with the lower T_{skin} impeding heat loss to the environment.

Although humans experience common thermoregulatory reactions to cold, with three general acclimation trends being identified, cold adaptation may be widely variable (94,98,102). Furthermore, the characteristics that dictate the form of adaptation have not been clearly identified. It has been suggested that acclimation is a phasic response, with the maintenance of a constant T_{core}, with minimal shivering thermogenesis, being the final stage of adaptation (108).

POPULATIONS AT RISK OF DYSTHERMIA

Neonates and the Elderly

The Royal College of Physicians estimated that 0.68% of hospital admissions during winter were associated with hypothermia (109). Recently, Taylor et al (78) used the morbidity (1979 to 1986) and mortality files (1977 to 1986) of the National Health Statistics Centre (New Zealand) to identify 1815 hypothermia hospitalizations (6.9 per 100,000 per year) and 176 deaths from hypothermia. The incidence of hypothermia-related hospitalizations was highest among neonates, but this group rarely died from hypothermia. However, the hospitalization incidence was 12.7 times the fatality incidence, with 88% being of domestic origin (urban hypothermia) with neonates and the elderly accounting for majority of such cases. Hypothermia-related deaths represented 0.07% of deaths from all causes (0.537 per 100,000 people per year), lower than reported for the United Kingdom. Of these fatalities, 72% occurred within a domestic environment. For the domestic fatalities, 87% occurred in people over 65 years, with a male-female ratio of approximately 1:2. Although it has previously been assumed that hypothermia was largely confined to people in the age extremes, 69% of all New Zealand deaths were among the elderly. Thus, in this western population, the risk of death from hypothermia among the aged was no greater than that associated with any other cause. However, the aged case-fatality ratio, for this largely preventable disorder, was three times greater, highlighting the need for improving both prevention and management strategies for this age group.

Recreational and Military Groups

Hypothermia outside urban zones accounts for about 30% of hypothermia-related fatalities in New Zealand (78). Of these deaths, 76% occurred in people aged 13 to 65 years (95% men), and about one third were associated with water immersion. Clearly, younger active men are another risk group, as are military personnel exposed to severe thermal stress. In fact, hypothermia can even occur in situations that are not excessively cold (110). While better education would certainly reduce the incidence, little can be done to remove the prime cause: exposure to extreme and often isolated conditions. Furthermore, it is almost impossible to determine whether immersion fatalities are due to hypothermia [either overt or symptomless (110)], or to the cold-shock response accompanying unexpected immersion (111).

Atypical States

Numerous atypical states predispose to dysthermia through effects upon heat production, heat loss, and thermal awareness. For instance, in one epidemiologic investigation, alcohol consumption was estimated to be a contributory factor in almost 80% of the urban hypothermia cases (112). This causal relationship was possibly due to hypoglycemia accompanying intoxication, fatigue, and hunger, which inhibits shivering and induces cutaneous vasodilation and sweat secretion (25,113). Therefore, the ensuing hypothermia may be ascribed more to the consequences of hypoglycemia upon heat loss than to the effects of alcohol upon heat production. Similarly, various medications act to suppress the central nervous system, inhibiting hypothalamic control of thermogenesis and also the neural control of shivering (e.g., phenothiazines, barbiturates).

Although hypothermia per se may occur without other disorders or diseases, this may not be the case for urban hypothermia, which includes almost 90% of hypothermia-related hospitalizations and deaths (78). For instance, Woodhouse et al (114) reported in their urban hypothermia cases (occurring indoors) that all elderly patients had at least one serious disease, with 70% suffering cardiopulmonary dysfunction. Thus, the primary cause of hypothermia was collapse, or incapacitation, caused by the primary disease, with the ensuing cold exposure a secondary consequence. Incapacitation, which may also be due to falls, can leave people inadequately clothed and malnourished, with the latter suppressing heat production (115). Moreover, Kramer et al (116) found sepsis was the most common accompanying disorder, occurring in about 80% of their 54 elderly hypothermia cases. Acute ischemic tissue damage, accompanying various thromboses, will also impair shivering thermogenesis, as does tissue hypoxia (117), which may result from a wide range of cardiopulmonary diseases. Thus, in many instances, hypothermia may really be a secondary disorder.

Endocrine dysfunction, such as hypothyroidism, lowers basal metabolism and impairs cold-induced heat production, whereas insulin-dependent diabetics are at risk through inadvertent hypoglycemia (118). There is even a report to the effect that iron-deficiency anemia impaired temperature regulation, with iron supplementation correcting both anemia and cold tolerance, possibly via an interaction with thyroid function (119). Other metabolic disorders associated with hypothermia include hypopituitarism, hypoadrenalism, and anorexia nervosa (120).

PREVENTION OF DYSTHERMIA

Clothing

Although man can employ a wide range of behavioral cold responses, the most versatile involves clothing. With modern clothing, man can enter previously lethal environments with no threat to T_{core} stability. Perhaps the most significant milestones in the development of cold-weather clothing were World Wars I and II. Instead of wars being waged during favorable seasons, the world wars crossed many seasons,

taking place in many inhospitable climates. However, while we are able to insulate ourselves from the cold, the limiting factors that determine survival for most people include access to clothing (cost), portability (mass and volume), and the need for different protection levels during rest and exercise (clothing layers).

Although various textiles and ensembles may be selected, the key determinant of success is its impact upon the microclimate at the skin, between the skin and clothing, and between clothing layers. If clothing becomes even moderately wet, the thermal protection it affords will be greatly diminished due to both the replacement of air with water (greater conductivity) and the compression of clothing layers (reduced thickness). These effects are most pronounced during immersion, where Allan et al (121) found an insulation reduction of 30% for a 500-g water influx. A similar effect can occur if prolonged exercise in protective clothing increases heat storage, stimulating sweat secretion. During heavy exercise, sweating can approach 2 to 3 liters per hour, with a consequent reduction in thermal protection, which is most noticeable when the previously exercising person rests, escalating the possibility of nonfreezing cold injury. Furthermore, sweating also reduces comfort and adds to the physiologic strain by elevating hydration requirements. While respiratory water losses are negligible, the combined sweat and cold-induced urine losses result in a progressive dehydration. These effects may be offset by implementing appropriate water replacement procedures, and by using layered clothing ensembles. Such ensembles are best arranged using multiple layers of lightweight clothing, rather than fewer layers of heavy clothing, thus providing the wearer with finer control over garment insulation to optimize comfort and reduce heat storage. Furthermore, the use of undergarments that encourage water movement away from the skin surface (wicking) is advantageous, while a waterproof outer layer reduces the chance of environmental wetting. However, since these materials may also prevent removal of sweat, the inclusion of appropriate ventilation openings is frequently employed to minimize water accumulation. Users of nonventing garments should modify air flow by opening zippers and changing the area of clothing surface coverage.

Nutrition

Daily diet must serve both basal and work-related energy requirements. In the cold, there are two additional sources of energy expenditure: shivering thermogenesis and the added metabolic cost associated with wearing protective clothing. In the latter instance, it has long been known that the use of multiple clothing layers increases the energy cost of exercise by up to 20% (122), and this is further exacerbated when exercise is performed in water, snow, and over rough terrain. Thus, there is both an additional metabolic cost, necessitating dietary adjustments, and a possibly greater heat storage, requiring clothing modification and increased water consumption. Since thirst may be suppressed in the cold (123), additional attention must be directed toward fluid replacement to prevent dehydration, which will reduce the capacity to perform physical work. Much water is replaced via food intake; however, cold-weather drinking can be encouraged through the provision of warm drinks, preferably with a minimal caffeine content, which has a strong diuretic affect.

A major fuel for shivering thermogenesis is muscle glycogen. Since carbohydrate loading prior to endurance competition has long been known to improve physical performance (124), it has been postulated that a similar dietary manipulation, prior to exposure, may enhance cold tolerance (125). In trials conducted on eight individuals, this group found that although such a diet improved the ability of these individuals to perform intermittent work in cool water (25°C), it had only a marginal effect upon thermal tolerance. During immersion in cooler water (18°C), carbohydrate loading did not influence thermal tolerance at rest (22). It is possible the benefits of such a manipulation may become evident when more extreme cold exposure is combined with prolonged exercise.

Improved Physical Fitness

Adams et al (126) first reported endurance training–induced physiologic changes that were not unlike those elicited by cold adaptation, that is, metabolic habituation resulting in hypothermic adaptation. Thus, when an endurance-trained person is exposed to cold, the threshold for shivering thermogenesis appears to be lower than in untrained counterparts (127). This would appear to make the trained person more efficient during the early stages of cold exposure, and, like some ethnic groups, better able to conserve energy for more stressful stages of an exposure. However, there is very little research evidence pertaining to more extreme conditions. That is, although these responses are observable with mild hypothermia, we know very little about how improved physical fitness, or even prolonged acclimatization, affects cold tolerance when individuals are taken to the point of thermoregulatory failure. Nevertheless, it can be stated with some certainty that, for a given workload, an endurance-trained person will fatigue more slowly than an untrained person in whom shivering thermogenesis is more easily impaired. This is even further compounded by sleep deprivation. Thus, since there is a strong interaction between fatigue, hypoglycemia, and hypothermia, it is not unreasonable to conclude that endurance training has potentially beneficial outcomes for the cold-exposed person.

TREATMENT OF DYSTHERMIA

Rewarming from hypothermia may be traced back to biblical times (128), so a detailed coverage of treatment and rewarming is beyond this chapter. Ideally, primary treatment of hypothermia commences in the field, aimed at halting heat loss and stabilizing and then elevating T_{core}: 1) remove the patient from the problem (water, ice, snow, or wind); 2) follow standard first-aid procedures to stabilize injuries or conditions (e.g. bleeding); 3) if possible, replace wet clothing with warm dry clothing, and insulate from the heat sink (e.g., heated blankets, reflective films); 4) attempt to heat the patient (e.g., body heat from another person); and 5) if possible, administer intravenous infusion (500 mL of 5% dextrose solution). It is vital that an accurate diagnosis (esophageal not rectal temperature) be obtained as rapidly as possible, and that first-aid and emergency-ward personnel be encouraged to routinely screen for hypothermia in unconscious patients. Furthermore, attempts to resuscitate suspected

hypothermia patients should be continued for as long as possible, since effective resuscitation, sometimes hours after both breathing and cardiac contractions cease, have been reported (129).

Rewarming may commence in the field but, with profound hypothermia (<25°C), it is most effective in clinical settings. Rewarming may be classified as either passive (i.e., shivering thermogenesis provides heat), which is adequate for conscious patients with mild hypothermia (T_{core} >33°C), or active techniques (externally or internally applied heat source), in which T_{core} is <32°C and the patient may be unconscious. This dichotomy is largely determined by the patient's ability to shiver, which is lost below 32°C (3). Examples of the active techniques include warm bathing, airway rewarming (130), blood infusions (131), tissue irrigation (132), and extracorporeal heating [T_{core} <21°C (131,133)]. Active rewarming is not without risk. For instance, with an inadequate local blood flow, tissues have a reduced means for dissipating heat, and excessive local heat storage and thermal damage may accompany rewarming. Furthermore, since surface heating elicits cutaneous vasodilation, the patient may be exposed to undue cardiac stress, since the blood volume has been reduced (diuresis) and blood pressure may be low.

Supplementary clinical treatment of moderate and profound hypothermia has been adequately covered elsewhere (134–136), with the following summary provided. Arterial and venous catheters should be positioned for glucose, fluid, and electrolyte management (central lines may precipitate cardiac abnormalities). Identify alcohol and drug use possibilities, since these may impact upon treatment. Frequently monitor blood chemistry: 1) Blood glucose and muscle glycogen levels will be low following extended shivering, and hypoglycemia must be treated; 2) since insulin secretion is suppressed, hyperglycemia can accompany vigorous glucose replacement prior to central rewarming; 3) hyperkalaemia may be present, but can turn to hypokalaemia with very rapid rewarming and an insulin response to infusions; and 4) intravascular coagulation is common with hypothermia. Infuse heated dextrose (5%) or saline solutions, but the volume and flow should be monitored to avoid tissue edema. Regularly screen for infections. The recognition and prompt treatment of hypothermia largely determines the prognosis, particularly in the elderly, in whom the case-fatality ratio may be three times greater than in young adults (78).

SUMMARY

In cold environments, dysthermia occurs when T_{core} regulation is disturbed, typically resulting in hypothermia (<35°C), in which heat loss to the environment exceeds heat production. Thermosensitive sites in the skin and deep tissues relay thermal information to the hypothalamus, which initiates thermoefferent responses: thermogenesis and constriction of cutaneous veins and arteries. Some cold-adapted ethnic groups show evidence of phenotypic adaptation, which may also be seen following repeated exposure to experimentally induced cold stress (acclimation). This most frequently takes the form of a blunted metabolic response, which may also occur in endurance-trained individuals. During acute cold exposure, thermal tolerance is influenced by body composition and physique, gender, age, previous exposure history, and possibly physical fitness. Groups at greatest risk of thermal strain during cold stress are those with compromised cardiovascular and endocrine function, neonates and the aged, and recreational and military groups exposed to severe thermal environments. Although unprotected man has a limited capacity to tolerate cold, dysthermia is largely preventable through behavioral responses (e.g., protective clothing), with its principal treatment being tissue rewarming.

REFERENCES

1. Ivy AC. What is normal or normality? Q Bull Northwestern Univ Med Sch 1944;18:22–32.

2. Hales JRS, Hubbard RW, Gaffin SL. Limitation of heat tolerance. In: Fregly MJ, Blatteis CM, eds. Environmental physiology: vol. 1. Handbook of physiology. New York: Oxford University Press, 1996:285–355.

3. Pozos RS, Iaizzo PA, Danzl DF, et al. Limits of tolerance to hypothermia. In: Fregly MJ, Blatteis CM, eds. Environmental physiology: vol. 1. Handbook of physiology. New York: Oxford University Press, 1996:557–575.

4. Hensel H. Thermoreception and temperature regulation. London: Academic Press, 1981.

5. Hellon R. Thermoreceptors. In: Shepherd JT, Abboud FM, eds. Handbook of physiology. The cardiovascular system: vol. III. Peripheral circulation and organ blood flow: part 2. Bethesda, MD: American Physiological Society, 1983:659–673.

6. Ivanov KP. The location and function of different skin thermoreceptors. In: Bligh J, Voigt K, eds. Thermoreception and temperature regulation. Berlin: Springer-Verlag, 1990:37–43.

7. Burton AC. Human calorimetry: II: the average temperature of the tissues of the body. J Nutr 1935; 9:261–280.

8. Willis WD, Trevino DL, Coulter JD, et al. Responses of primate spinothalamic tract neurons to natural stimulation of hindlimb. J Neurophysiol 1974;37:358–372.

9. Brück K, Hinkel P. Thermoafferent networks and their adaptive modifications. In: Schönbaum E, Lomax P, eds. Thermoregulation: physiology and biochemistry. New York: Pergamon Press, 1990: 129–153.

10. Hinkel P, Schröder-Rosenstock K. Responses of pontine units to skin-temperature changes in the guinea-pig. J Physiol 1981; 314:189–194.

11. Dickenson AH. Neurons in the raphè nuclei of the rat responding to skin temperature. J Physiol 1976;256:110P.

12. Boulant JA. Hypothalamic mechanisms in thermoregulation. Fed Proc 1981;40:2843–2850.

13. Simon E, Pierau F-K, Taylor DCM. Central and peripheral thermal control of effectors in homeothermic temperature regulation. Physiol Rev 1986;66: 235–300.

14. Commission for Thermal Physiology. Glossary for thermal physiology. 2nd ed. Pflugers Arch 1987;410:567–587.

15. Rowell LB. Human circulation: Regulation during physical stress. New York: Oxford University Press, 1986.

16. Bligh J. Regulation of body temperature in man and other mammals. In: Shitzer A, Eberhart RC, eds. Heat transfer in medicine and biology. Analysis and applications: vol. I. New York: Plenum Press, 1985:15–51.

17. Jacobs I, Martineau L, Vallerand AL. Thermoregulatory thermogenesis in humans during cold stress. Exerc Sport Sci Rev 1994;22:221–250.

18. Benzinger TH. Peripheral cold reception and central warm reception, sensory mechanisms of behavioral and autonomic thermostasis. In: Hardy JD, Gagge AP, Stolwijk JAJ, eds. Physiological and behavioral temperature regulation. Springfield, IL: C. C. Thomas, 1970:831–855.

19. Brown AC, Brengelmann GL. The interaction of peripheral and central inputs in the temperature regulation system. In: Hardy JD, Gagge AP, Stolwijk JAJ, eds. Physiological and behavioral temperature regulation. Springfield, IL: C. C. Thomas, 1970:684–702.

20. Mittleman KD, Mekjavic IB. Contribution of core cooling rate to shivering thermogenesis during cold water immersion. Aviat Space Environ Med 1992;62: 842–848.

21. Haight JSJ, Keatinge RW. Failure of thermoregulation in the cold during hypoglycaemia induced by exercise and ethanol. J Physiol 1973;229:87–97.

22. Martineau L, Jacobs I. Muscle glycogen utilization during shivering thermogenesis in humans. J Appl Physiol 1988;65:2046–2050.

23. Passias TC, Meneilly GS, Mekjavic IB. Effect of hypoglycemia on thermoregulatory responses. J Appl Physiol 1996;80:1021–1032.

24. Thompson RL, Hayward JS. Wet-cold exposure and hypothermia: thermal and metabolic responses to prolonged exercise in rain. J Appl Physiol 1996;81: 1128–1137.

25. Gale EAM, Bennett T, Green JH, et al. Hypoglycaemia, hypothermia and shivering in man. Clin Sci 1981;61:463–469.

26. Bass DE, Henschel A. Responses of body fluid compartments to heat and cold. Physiol Rev 1956; 36:128–144.

27. Young AJ, Muza SR, Sawka MN, et al. Human vascular fluid

responses to cold stress are not altered by cold acclimation. Undersea Biomed Res 1987;14: 215–228.

28. Raven P, Niki I, Dahms T, et al. Compensatory cardio-vascular responses during an environmental cold stress (5°C). J Appl Physiol 1970;29:417–421.

29. LeBlanc J. Factors affecting cold acclimation and thermogenesis in man. Med Sci Sports Exerc 1988;20:193–196.

30. Lennquist S, Grandberg PO, Wedin B. Fluid balance and physical work capacity in humans exposed to cold. Arch Environ Health 1974;29:241–249.

31. Vogelaere P, Savourey G, Deklunder G, et al. Reversal of cold induced haemoconcentration. Eur J Appl Physiol 1992;64:244-249.

32. Arborelius M, Balldin UI, Lilja B, et al. Hemodynamic changes in man during immersion with the head above water. Aerospace Med 1972;43:592–598.

33. Epstein M. Renal effects of head-out water immersion in man: implications for an understanding of volume homeostasis. Physiol Rev 1978;58: 529–581.

34. Deuster PA, Smith DJ, Smoak BL, et al. Prolonged whole-body cold water immersion: fluid and ion shifts. J Appl Physiol 1989;66:34–41.

35. Rochelle RD, Horvath SM. Thermoregulation in surfers and nonsurfers immersed in cold water. Undersea Biomed Res 1978;5:377–390.

36. Fregly MJ. Activity of the hypothalamic-pituitary axis during cold exposure. In: Schönbaum E, Lomax P, eds. Thermoregulation: physiology and biochemistry. New York: Pergamon Press, 1990: 437–494.

37. Jansky L, Janakova H, Ulicny B, et al. Changes in thermal homeostasis in humans due to repeated cold water immersions. Pflugers Arch 1996;432:368–372.

38. Regan JM. Human physiological responses to cold-water immersion: effects of acute and repeated exposures. Doctoral dissertation. University of Wollongong, Australia, 1998.

39. Scholander PF, Hammel HT, Andersen KL, et al. Metabolic acclimation to cold in man. J Appl Physiol 1958;12:1–8.

40. Kang BS, Song SH, Suh CS, et al. Changes in body temperature and basal metabolic rate of the Ama. J Appl Physiol 1963; 18:483–488.

41. Hicks CS. Terrestrial animals in cold: exploratory studies of primitive man: In: Dill DB, Adolph EF, Wilber CG, eds. Handbook of physiology, Adaptation to the environment. Washington, D.C.: American Physiological Society, 1964:405–412.

42. Scholander PF, Hammel HT, Hart JS, et al. Cold adaptation in Australian Aborigines. J Appl Physiol 1958;13:211–218.

43. Hammel HT, Elsner RW, LeMessurier DH, et al. Thermal and metabolic responses of the Australian aborigine exposed to moderate cold in summer. J Appl Physiol 1959;14:605–615.

44. Bittel JHM, Nonotte-Varly C, Livecchi-Gonnot GH, et al. Physical fitness and thermoregulatory reactions in a cold environment in men. J Appl Physiol 1988;65: 1984–1989.

45. Andersen KL, Loyning Y, Nelms JD, et al. Metabolic and thermal response to a moderate cold exposure in nomadic Lapps. J Appl Physiol 1960;15:649–653.

46. Andersen KL, Hart JS, Hammel HT, et al. Metabolic and thermal response of Eskimos during muscular exertion in the cold. J Appl Physiol 1963;18:613–618.

47. Hildes JA. Comparison of coastal Eskimos and Kalahari Bushmen. Fed Proc 1963;22:843–845.

48. Hong SK, Rennie DW, Park YS. Cold acclimatization and deacclimatization of Korean women divers. Exerc Sport Sci Rev 1986;14:231–268.

49. Hong SK. Comparison of diving and nondiving women of Korea. Fed Proc 1963;28:831–833.

50. Hong SK, Lee CK, Kim JK, et al. Peripheral blood flow and heat flux of Korean women divers. Fed Proc 1969;28:1143–1148.

51. Paik KS, Kang BS, Han DS, et al. Vascular responses of Korean ama to hand immersion in cold water. J Appl Physiol 1972;32: 446–450.

52. Nunneley SA, Wissler EH, Allan JR. Immersion cooling: effect of clothing and skinfold thickness. Aviat Space Environ Med 1985; 56:1177–1182.

53. Hatfield HS, Pugh LGC. Thermal conductivity of human fat and muscle. Nature 1951;168:918–919.

54. Wade CE, Dacanay S, Smith RM. Regional heat loss in resting man during immersion in 25.2°C water. Aviat Space Environ Med 1979;50:590–593.

55. Golden FStC, Hampton IFG, Smith DJ. Lean long distance swimmers. J Royal Naval Med Service 1980;66:262.

56. Veicsteinas A, Ferretti G, Rennie DW. Superficial shell insulation in resting and exercising men in cold water. J Appl Physiol 1982; 52:1557–1564.

57. Toner MM, Sawka MN, Foley ME, et al. Effects of body mass and morphology on thermal responses in water. J Appl Physiol 1986; 60:521–525.

58. McArdle WD, Magel JR, Gergley TG, et al. Thermal adjustment to cold-water exposure in resting men and women. J Appl Physiol 1984;56:1565–1571.

59. Morrison JB, Conn ML, Hayward JS. Accidental hypothermia: the effect of initial body temperatures and physique on the rate of rewarming. Aviat Space Environ Med 1980;51:1095–1099.

60. Keatinge WR. The effects of subcutaneous fat and previous exposure to cold on the body temperature, peripheral blood flow and metabolic rate of men

in cold water. J Physiol 1960;
153:166–178.

61. Mekjavic IB, Mittleman KD, Kakitsuba N. The role of shivering thermogenesis and total body insulation in core cooling rate. Ann Physiol Anthropol 1987;6: 61–68.

62. Hayward MG, Keatinge WR. Roles of subcutaneous fat and thermoregulatory reflexes in determining ability to stabilize body temperature in water. J Physiol 1981;320:229–251.

63. Mittleman KD. Role of morphology on central thermosensitivity of heat production (HP) during cold water immersion. FASEB J 1990;4:A278.

64. Strong LH, Gee GK, Goldman RF. Metabolic and vasomotor insulative responses occurring on immersion in cold water. J Appl Physiol 1985;58:964–977.

65. Hardy JD, DuBois EF. Differences between men and women in their response to heat and cold. Proc Nat Acad Sci 1940;26:389–398.

66. Graham TE. Thermal, metabolic and cardiovascular changes in men and women during cold stress. Med Sci Sports Exerc 1988;20:S185–S192.

67. Fox RH, Löfstedt BE, Woodward PM, et al. Comparison of thermoregulatory function in men and women. J Appl Physiol 1969;26:444–453.

68. Nunneley SA. Physiological responses of women to thermal stress: a review. Med Sci Sports Exerc 1978;10:250–255.

69. Stephenson LA, Kolka MA. Thermoregulation in women. Exerc Sport Sci Rev 1993;21:231–262.

70. De Souza MJ, Maresh CM, Maguire MS, et al. Menstrual status and plasma vasopressin, renin activity, and aldosterone exercise response. J Appl Physiol 1989;67:736–743.

71. Cunningham DJ, Cabanac M. Evidence from behavioral thermoregulatory responses of a shift in setpoint temperature related to

the menstrual cycle. J Physiol (Paris) 1971;63:236–238.

72. Hessemer V, Brück K. Influence of menstrual cycle on shivering, skin blood flow, and sweating responses measured at night. J Appl Physiol 1985;59:1902–1910.

73. Hackney AC. Effects of the menstrual cycle on resting muscle glycogen content. Horm Metab Res 1990;22:644.

74. Silva NL, Boulant JA. Effects of testosterone, estradiol, and temperature on neurons in preoptic tissue slices. Am J Physiol 1986;250:R625–R632.

75. MMWR. Morbidity and Mortality Weekly Report. Hypothermia-related deaths: Cook County, Illinois, November 1992–March 1993. MMWR Morb Mortal Wkly Rep 1993;42:558–560.

76. Bull GM, Morton J. Environment, temperature and death rates. Age Ageing 1978;7:210–224.

77. Keatinge WR. Seasonal mortality among elderly people with unrestricted home heating. Br Med J 1986;293:732–733.

78. Taylor NAS, Cotter JD, Griffiths RF. Epidemiology of hypothermia: fatalities and hospitalisations in New Zealand. Aust N Z J Med 1994;24:705–710.

79. Collins KJ, Exton-Smith AN, James MH, et al. Functional changes in autonomic nervous responses with ageing. Age Ageing 1980;9:17–24.

80. Collins KJ, Easton JC, Belfield-Smith H, et al. Effects of age on body temperature and blood pressure in cold environments. Clin Sci 1985;69:465–470.

81. Wagner JA, Horvath SM. Cardiovascular reactions to cold exposures differ with age and gender. J Appl Physiol 1985;58:187–192.

82. Richardson D, Shepherd S. The cutaneous microcirculation of the forearm in young and old subjects. Microvasc Res 1991;41:84–91.

83. Kenney WL, Fowler SR. Methylcholine-activated eccrine sweat gland density and output as a function of age. J Appl Physiol 1988;65:1082–1086.

84. Marion GS, McGann KP, Camp DL. Core temperature in the elderly and factors which influence its measurement. Gerontology 1989;37:225–232.

85. Keatinge WR, Coleshaw SRK, Cotter F, et al. Increases in platelet and red cell counts, blood viscosity and arterial pressure during mild surface cooling: factors in mortality from coronary and cerebral thrombosis in winter. Br Med J 1984;289: 1405–1408.

86. Collins KJ, Exton-Smith AN, Dore C. Urban hypothermia: preferred temperature and thermal perception in old age. Br Med J 1981; 282:175–177.

87. Salvosa CB, Payne PR, Wheeler EF. Environmental conditions and body temperatures of elderly women living alone or in local authority home. Br Med J 1971; 4:656–659.

88. Fox RH, Woodward PM, Exton-Smith AN, et al. Body temperatures in the elderly: a national study of physiological, social, and environmental conditions. Br Med J 1973;1:200–206.

89. Taylor NAS, Allsopp NK, Parkes DG. Preferred room temperature of young versus aged males: the influence of thermal sensation, thermal comfort and affect. J Gerontol 1995;50:M216–M221.

90. Golden FStC, Hampton IFG, Hervey GR, et al. Shivering intensity in humans during immersion in cold water. J Physiol 1979;290:48P.

91. Jacobs I, Romet T, Frim J, et al. Effects of endurance fitness on responses to cold water immersion. Aviat Space Environ Med 1984;55:715–720.

92. Horvath SM. Exercise in a cold environment. Exerc Sport Sci Rev 1981;9:221–263.

93. Kollias J, Boileau R, Buskirk ER. Effects of physical conditioning

in man on thermal responses to cold air. Int J Biometeorol 1972; 16:389–402.

94. Bittel JHM. Heat debt as an index for cold adaptation in men. J Appl Physiol 1987;62:1627–1634.

95. Young AJ, Muza SR, Sawka MN, et al. Human thermoregulatory responses to cold air are altered by repeated cold water immersion. J Appl Physiol 1986;60:1542–1548.

96. Hammel HT. Summary of comparative thermal patterns in man. Fed Proc 1963;22:846–847.

97. Golden FStC, Tipton MJ. Human adaptation to repeated cold immersions. J Physiol 1988;396:349–363.

98. Brück K, Baum E, Schwennicki HP. Cold-adaptive modifications in man induced by repeated short-term cold exposures and during a 10-day and -night cold exposure. Pflugers Arch 1976; 363:125–133.

99. Hong SK. Pattern of cold adaptation in women divers of Korea (Ama). Fed Proc 1973;32:1614–1622.

100. Park YS, Rennie DW, Lee IS, et al. Time course of deacclimatization to cold water immersion in Korean women divers. J Appl Physiol 1983;54:1708–1716.

101. LeBlanc J, Pouliot M. Importance of noradrenaline in cold adaptation. Am J Physiol 1964;207:853–856.

102. Radomski MW, Boutelier C. Hormone response of normal and intermittent cold-preadapted humans to continuous cold. J Appl Physiol 1982;53:610–616.

103. LeBlanc J. Mechanisms of adaptation to cold. Int J Sports Med 1992;13:S169–S172.

104. Keatinge WR. The effect of repeated daily exposure to cold and of improved physical fitness on the metabolic and vascular responses to cold air. J Physiol 1961;157:209–220.

105. Glaser EM, Griffin JP. Influence of the cerebral cortex on habituation. J Physiol 1962;160:420–445.

106. Werner J, Schingnitz G, Hensel H. Influence of cold adaptation on the activity of thermoresponsive neurones in thalamus and midbrain of the rat. Pflugers Arch 1981;391:327–330.

107. Brück K, Zeisberger E. Significance and possible central mechanisms of thermoregulatory threshold deviations in thermal adaptation. In: Wang LCH, Hudson JW, eds. Strategies in cold. New York: Academic Press, 1978:655–694.

108. Skreslet S, Aarefjord F. Acclimatization to cold in man induced by frequent scuba diving in cold water. J Appl Physiol 1968;24:177–181.

109. Prescott LF, Peard MC, Wallace IR. Accidental hypothermia: a common condition. Br Med J 1962;2:1367–1370.

110. Hayward MG, Keatinge WR. Progressive symptomless hypothermia in water: possible cause of diving accidents. Br Med J 1979;183:1182–1183.

111. Tiption MJ. The initial responses to cold-water immersion in man. Clin Sci 1989;77:581–588.

112. Fitzgerald FT. Hypoglycaemia and accidental hypothermia in an alcoholic population. West J Med 1980;133:105–107.

113. Madison LL. Ethanol-induced hypoglycaemia. Adv Metab Disord 1968;3:85–109.

114. Woodhouse P, Keatinge WR, Coleshaw SRK. Factors associated with hypothermia in patients admitted to a group of inner city hospitals. Lancet 1989;18:1201–1205.

115. Fellows IW, MacDonald IA, Bennett T, et al. The effect of undernutrition on thermoregulation in the elderly. Clin Sci 1985;69:525–532.

116. Kramer MR, Vandijk J, Rosin AJ. Mortality in elderly patients with thermoregulatory failure. Arch Intern Med 1989;149:1521–1523.

117. Gautier H, Bonora M, Schultz SA, et al. Hypoxia-induced changes in shivering and body temperature. J Appl Physiol 1987;62:2477–2484.

118. Kedes LH, Field JB. Hypothermia: a clue to hypoglycaemia. N Engl J Med 1964;271:785–787.

119. Beard JL, Borel MJ, Derr J. Impaired thermoregulation and thyroid function in iron-deficiency anemia. Am J Clin Nutr 1990; 52:813–819.

120. Wongsurawat N, Davis BB, Morley JE. Thermoregulatory failure in the elderly. St Louis University geriatric grand rounds. J Am Geriatr Soc 1990;38:899–906.

121. Allan JR, Higenbottam C, Redman PJ. The effect of leakage on the insulation provided by immersion protection clothing. Aviat Space Environ Med 1985;56:1107–1109.

122. Teitlebaum A, Goldman RF. Increased energy cost with multiple clothing layers. J Appl Physiol 1972;32:743–744.

123. Rogers TA, Setliff JA, Klopping JC. Energy cost, fluid and electrolyte balance in subarctic survival situations. J Appl Physiol 1964;19:1–8.

124. Karlsson J, Saltin B. Diet, muscle glycogen, and endurance performance. J Appl Physiol 1971;31:203–206.

125. Thorp JW, Mittleman KD, Haberman KJ, et al. Work enhancement and thermal changes during intermittent work in cold water after carbohydrate loading. NMRI Report 90–14. Bethesda, MD: Naval Medical Research Institute, 1990.

126. Adams T, Heberling EJ. Human physiological responses to a standardized cold stress are modified by physical fitness. J Appl Physiol 1958;13:226–230.

127. Dressendorfer RM, Smith RM, Baker DG, et al. Cold tolerance

of long-distance runners and swimmers in Hawaii. Int J Biometeorol 1977;21:51–58.

128. Wislicki L. A biblical case of hypothermia-resuscitation by rewarming (Elisha's method). Clio Med 1974;9:213–214.

129. Southwick FS, Dalglish PH. Recovery after prolonged asystolic cardiac arrest and profound hypothermia. JAMA 1980;243: 1250–1253.

130. Lloyd EL. Equipment for airway warming in the treatment of accidental hypothermia. J Wilderness Med 1991;2:330–350.

131. Iserson KV, Huestis DW. Blood warming: current applications and techniques. Transfusion 1991;31:558–571.

132. Levitt MA, Kane V, Henderson J, et al. A comparative rewarming trial of gastric versus peritoneal lavage in a hypothermic model. Am J Emerg Med 1990;8:282–288.

133. Walpoth BH, Locher T, Leupi F, et al. Accidental deep hypothermia with cardiopulmonary arrest: Extracorporeal blood warming in 11 patients. Eur J Cardiothorac Surg 1990;4:390–393.

134. Keatinge WR. Survival in cold water: the physiology and treatment of immersion hypothermia and drowning. Oxford: Blackwell Scientific, 1969.

135. Hamlet MP. Human cold injuries. In: Pandolf KB, Sawka MN, Gonzalez RR, eds. Human performance physiology and environmental medicine at terrestrial extremes. Indianapolis, IN: Benchmark Press, 1988:435–466.

136. Lee-Chiong TI, Stitt JT. Accidental hypothermia: when thermoregulation is overwhelmed. Postgrad Med 1996;99:77–88.

Chapter 106

High-Altitude Acclimatization and Illness

High mountains have inspired and tantalized man for hundreds of years. By the end of the nineteenth century most of the peaks in the Alps along with a few high mountains elsewhere had been climbed. Many early climbers described their euphoria on attaining the summit and a few mentioned the symptoms we now describe as mountain sickness. By the turn of the century it was known that the major cause of these symptoms was hypoxia, but even nearly 100 years later, despite intensive study, many unanswered questions remain.

Despite the obvious dangers inherent in climbing and the altitude-related illness experienced by nearly all who spend much time in the mountains, people still seek the remoteness and pleasures of high places. Not everyone seeks to climb the highest peaks in the world; many travel to altitude for skiing or other recreation or for work. These individuals frequently experience acute illness soon after ascent. With longer stay at altitude, these symptoms improve in a process known as acclimatization.

This chapter describes the altitude environment, the acclimatization process during stay at altitude, and the various medical problems that occur following ascent. Several recent reviews provide a more comprehensive description of altitude illness and acclimatization (1,2).

THE ALTITUDE ENVIRONMENT

As one ascends to altitude, the most important change from a physiologic standpoint is the drop in partial pressure of oxygen. At sea level oxygen comprises about 20.9% of the atmosphere with a barometric pressure of 760 mm Hg. At higher elevations, the fraction of oxygen in the atmosphere remains unchanged as the barometric pressure progressively decreases to only 253 mm Hg on the summit of Mt. Everest (29,028 ft, 8848 m).

Barometric pressure does not decrease linearly with altitude, but follows a complex curvilinear relationship affected by temperature and other factors. Various equations describing these relationships have been proposed over the years. With the advent of aviation, the need for standardization became apparent, leading to the development of a "standard atmosphere" that could be used by all aviators to calibrate their altimeters. The U.S. Standard Atmosphere is nearly the same as that adopted by the International Civil Aviation Organization (ICAO) (3) and is given by:

$$P_B - P_{B_0}((288 - 0.0065z) / 288)^{5.256}$$

where z is the altitude in meters above sea level, P_{B_0} is the sea level barometric pressure (760 mm Hg), and 0.0065 represents the "lapse rate" or the decrease in temperature in degrees centigrade for every kilometer of increase in altitude (4).

The standard atmosphere was meant for calibration of barometers, not for predicting barometric pressure. Figure 106-1 shows the altitude – barometric pressure relationship and the discrepancy at high altitudes. Using the standard atmosphere, one would predict the barometric pressure on the summit of Mt. Everest to be only 236 mm Hg, whereas the actual measured barometric pressure is 253 mm Hg (5). This difference has important physiologic significance since a climber on the summit is very close to the limit of human tolerance of hypoxia, even disregarding the exertion necessary for climbing.

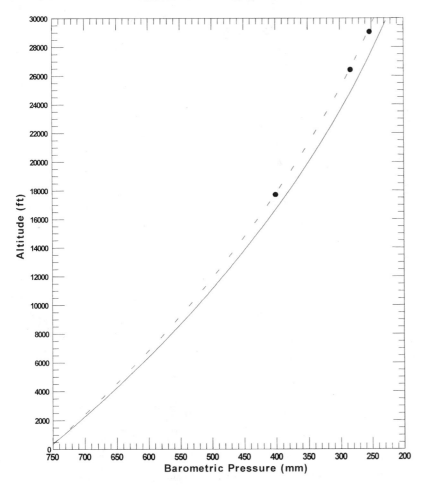

Altitude vs. Barometric Pressure

Figure 106-1 The relationship between altitude and barometric pressure. The solid line shows the U.S. Standard Atmosphere (or ICAO) altitude/pressure curve (from International Civil Aviation Organization. Manual of the ICAO Standard Atmosphere, Montreal: ICAO, 1964; Smithsonian Institution. Smithsonian meteorological tables, Washington, D.C.: Smithsonian Institution, 1949; and National Oceanic and Atmospheric Administration. US standard atmosphere, 1976. Washington, D.C.: NOAA, 1976) while the dashed line, that of West (from West JB. Prediction of barometric pressures at high altitude with the use of model atmospheres. J Appl Physiol 1996;81:1850–1854). The filled circles are reported barometric pressures on the summit and two lower camps on Mt. Everest (from West JB, Lahiri S, Maret KH, et al. Barometric pressures at extreme altitudes on Mt. Everest: physiological significance. J Appl Physiol 1983; 54:1188–1194).

ACCLIMATIZATION TO ALTITUDE

With ascent to altitude, numerous changes occur in the body. Some of these changes begin immediately, whereas others are delayed, and some are complete only after months or years of living at altitude. Rapid ascent to the summit of Mt. Everest would render sea-level dwellers unconscious almost immediately, but by taking several weeks to accomplish the ascent, it is quite possible to survive without supplemental oxygen at this altitude. The process by which the body makes changes allowing it to accomplish this is termed *acclimatization*. The acclimatization changes occurring at the cellular level are probably the most important, but are the least understood.

Houston (6) divided the changes during acclimatization into early (or struggle) responses and later (or adaptive) changes. The early (struggle) responses include increases in pulmonary ventilation, cardiac output, and hemoglobin concentration; changes in the affinity of hemoglobin for oxygen; increased alkalinity of the blood; and alterations in the distribution of blood flow. The later (adaptive) changes include alterations in glucose and substrate utilization; changes in hormone secretion; alterations in metabolic pathways, and in the number of mitochondria in the cells; changes in neurotransmitters; and at least a partial restoration of the blood acid-base balance. Although these processes do not describe all of the myriad alterations in the body, they do provide a convenient framework for describing many of the changes occurring after ascent.

In describing the changes that occur at altitude, it is useful to refer to different altitudes: Moderate or intermediate altitude is between about 5000 and 8000 ft (1500 to 2400 m). High altitude refers to elevations between 8000 and 14,000 ft (2400 to 4300 m), and very high altitude refers to elevations between 14,000 and 18,000 ft (4300 to 5500 m). Extreme altitude is used to describe the area from 18,000 ft (5500 m) up to the summit of Mt. Everest at 29,028 ft (8848 m) (1,pp 4–5).

Cardiovascular Changes During Acclimatization

The normal response of the cardiovascular system to acute exposure to altitude is an increase in the resting heart rate, an increase in resting cardiac output, and an increase in blood pressure. These responses are minimized in both high-altitude natives and in sea-level dwellers who have acclimatized to altitude. The cardiovascular changes are produced by increased sympathetic activity brought about by the hypoxic stimulation of the carotid bodies (7–9).

During physical activity at altitude, heart rate is higher than at sea level (10). During maximal exercise, however, the heart rate is lower than at sea level; the amount of decrease in maximal heart rate is proportional to the

Figure 106-2 The effect of increasing cardiac output (during cycle ergometer exercise) and hypoxia on mean pulmonary artery pressure. Data are from simulated altitude in a hypobaric chamber during Operation Everest II. (Redrawn from Groves BM, Reeves JT, Sutton JR, et al. Operation Everest II: Elevated high-altitude pulmonary resistance unresponsive to oxygen. J Appl Physiol 1987;63:521–530.) There was no further increase in pulmonary artery pressure above 25,000 ft (7620 m); in fact, at the highest altitude, equivalent to the summit of Mt. Everest, pulmonary artery pressure was lower than at 25,000 ft.

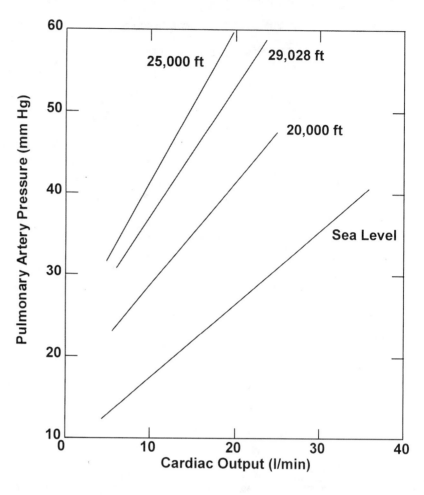

barometric pressure. For example, during Operation Everest II (a hypobaric chamber study) maximal heart rate at sea level was 177 beats per minute, but at 29,028 ft (8848 m) the maximal heart rate had decreased to 124 beats per minute (11).

Changes in cardiac output generally mirror those of heart rate responses as cardiac output is increased both at rest and during submaximal exercise (11–13). Furthermore, cardiac output is lower during maximal effort exercise than it is at sea level. Interestingly, after only 5 to 10 days of acclimatization, cardiac output at rest and during submaximal exercise trends back toward the sea-level values (9,12,14).

Numerous studies of cardiac function at altitude have been performed. These include measurements of systolic time intervals, echocardiograms, and left ventricular diastolic pressure. In general, all of these studies indicate that most indices of left ventricular function in healthy persons remain within normal limits at altitude both at rest and during exercise (8,11,15–17).

Pulmonary Circulation and Acclimatization

An important change following ascent to altitude is the rise in pulmonary artery pressure. The increase in pressure is caused by hypoxic pulmonary vasoconstriction resulting from alveolar hypoxia. Although the precise mechanism for hypoxic pulmonary vasoconstriction is unknown, it is dependent on calcium influx into the pulmonary artery smooth muscle fibers. The main site of vasoconstriction is in the precapillary

arterioles (18). As discussed below, an excessive rise in pulmonary artery pressure contributes to the development of high-altitude pulmonary edema.

Pulmonary artery wedge pressure, an estimate of left ventricular filling pressure, remains normal following acute exposure to altitude. In 1985, the Operation Everest II study provided a unique opportunity to study the pulmonary circulation and other aspects of acclimatization in individuals during a simulated ascent of Mt. Everest. In this study, eight individuals lived continuously for 40 days in a decompression chamber, during which time the barometric pressure was gradually decreased. Cardiac output, pulmonary artery pressure, pulmonary capillary wedge pressure, and pulmonary vascular resistance were measured at rest and during exercise at sea level prior to decompression and at barometric pressures simulating 20,000 ft (6100 m), 25,000 ft (7620 m), and 29,028 ft (8848 m). Figure 106-2 shows some of these results, including the rise in pulmonary artery pressure with altitude and with exercise.

With ascent from 25,000 ft (7620 m) to 29,028 ft (8848 m), there was no increase in either pulmonary artery pressure or pulmonary vascular resistance. The cause of this is unknown, although it is possibly due to a plateau in cardiac output above 25,000 ft (7620 m). Additionally, when individuals breathed supplemental oxygen, there was a prompt reduction in pulmonary artery pressure but not in pulmonary vascular resistance. The pulmonary artery pressure, however, did not return to sea-level values (19).

Long-term altitude residents develop medial hypertrophy of their pulmonary arteries that slowly regresses at sea level (20). The individuals in Operation Everest II may also have developed medial hypertrophy during the several weeks of acclimatization in the hypobaric chamber.

An important finding in Operation Everest II and other high-altitude studies is the large interindividual variation in pulmonary artery pressure with acute altitude exposure (21,22), possibly relating to the thickness of the pulmonary arteriolar medial wall (23). The clinical importance of the marked individual variation is demonstrated by the fact that those persons with a history of high-altitude pulmonary edema (HAPE) or who are susceptible to HAPE show a greater increase in pulmonary artery pressure at altitude than do those without a history of HAPE (24).

Persons born and raised at altitude have *higher* pulmonary artery pressures than do newcomers to altitude, as was first suggested by Hurtado (25) in 1932. Among high-altitude natives, pulmonary artery pressures vary considerably both within and between geographic regions. Tibetans, for example, show *lower* pulmonary artery pressures than do high-altitude natives from South America (26,27). These lower pulmonary artery pressures may account, in part, for the reason why fewer cases of chronic mountain sickness and other high-altitude problems are reported in this population. Similar circulatory changes also contribute to the legendary performance of Sherpas at extreme altitude.

Ventilatory Changes at High Altitude

Following ascent to altitude, ventilation increases largely due to hypoxic stimulation of the peripheral chemoreceptors (28). The extent of the increase in ventilation is related to the altitude and thus to the alveolar P_{O_2}, as described by Rahn et al (28). With stay at altitude, there is a further increase in ventilation over the next several days to weeks. The increase in alveolar ventilation causes a rise in Pa_{O_2} along with a fall in Pa_{CO_2}. This decrease in Pa_{CO_2} acts on the central chemoreceptors in the brain stem to blunt the increased ventilation (29–31).

The changes in alveolar ventilation with ascent to altitude represent one of the most important acclimatization responses. Without this hypoxia-driven increase in ventilation, ascent to extreme altitude would not be possible (32). The strength of the hypoxic ventilatory response varies greatly among individuals (33) and accounts for some of the differences in susceptibility to altitude illness (34–40).

The hypoxic ventilatory response (HVR) is altered by many factors. For example, men have lower HVRs than women, older persons have lower HVRs than young adults, and persons who have lived at high altitude for many years have blunted HVRs compared with sea-level natives acutely exposed to hypoxia. Various ethnic differences in HVR also exist, with those from South America having more blunted responses than do Sherpas from Nepal (33,41–43).

Hematologic Changes

An increase in erythropoietin occurs rapidly following altitude exposure. This results in production of red blood cells and increased hemoglobin and hematocrit. The hematologic changes begin soon after ascent but take many months to be complete (44). High-altitude natives generally show a hemoglobin concentration proportional to the altitude of residence (45).

An increased hemoglobin results in increased oxygen-carrying capacity, which allows increased oxygen delivery to the working tissues without an increase in cardiac output. A side effect of the increased hemoglobin, however, is an increase in blood viscosity. These counteracting responses suggest that the polycythemia at altitude is probably a relatively minor factor in acclimatization for most people (46–48).

Many years ago, Monge (49) described chronic mountain sickness in high-altitude natives who appeared to have lost the benefits of acclimatization and whose hemoglobin increased more than in healthy lifelong high-altitude residents. These patients with chronic mountain sickness, in addition to having increased hemoglobin, showed right ventricular strain, cor pulmonale, and a beneficial response to phlebotomy (50–52).

HIGH-ALTITUDE ILLNESS

A wide spectrum of medical problems occurs at altitude, some of which are benign, whereas others are potentially life-threatening. There is no universally accepted nomenclature, and considerable overlap occurs among these syndromes (2, pp 367–368; 53, p 9). Even so, it is useful to discuss the following illnesses: acute mountain sickness (AMS), high-altitude pulmonary edema (HAPE), and high-altitude cerebral edema (HACE).

Acute Mountain Sickness

Case Report: A 21-year-old healthy student living near sea level drove to 8000 ft (2438 m) in the Sierra Nevada mountains to go skiing. After spending one restless night at altitude, he awoke the next morning with a headache. During the day, he felt more tired than his friends and did not have much appetite, but skied anyway.

Nearly everyone, if they ascend too rapidly, will experience at least some of the symptoms of AMS. For many these symptoms are only a minor annoyance; for others, they are nearly incapacitating. The symptoms have been known for many years and were colorfully described by a Dr. Jacottet on Mont Blanc in 1881: "I was unable to sleep and passed so bad a night that I would not wish it on my worst enemy."

Another early description from South America also graphically describes AMS:

I got up and tried once more to go on but I was only able to advance one or two steps at a time, and then I had to stop, panting for breath, my struggles alternating with violent fits of nausea. At times I would fall down, and each time had greater difficulty rising; black specks swam across my sight; I was like one walking in a dream, so dizzy and sick that the whole mountain seemed whirling about me . . . As I got lower . . . I improved.

The symptoms of AMS are common and easily recognized by anyone, but the exact cause of AMS is still unknown, although cerebral edema probably plays a role.

At a 1991 conference on mountain medicine at Lake Louise, Canada, definitions of the various types of altitude illness were proposed. AMS was defined as follows (54): "In the setting of a recent gain in altitude, the presence of headache and at least one of the following symptoms: gastrointestinal (anorexia, nausea or vomiting), fatigue or weakness, dizziness or lightheadedness, difficulty sleeping."

Incidence

The incidence and severity of AMS depends on many factors, such as the rate of ascent, the altitude attained (especially the altitude of sleep), duration of altitude exposure, and how much exercise is undertaken at altitude. Probably the most important variable is the underlying physiologic susceptibility of the individual. Very few experience significant symptoms below 7000 to 8000 ft (2130 to 2440 m), whereas most unacclimatized persons going to 10,000 ft (3050 m) or higher will experience symptoms.

In one large study of tourists visiting the Colorado Rocky Mountains, 71% had at least some symptoms of AMS after arrival at altitudes between 6900 and 9700 ft (2100 to 2960 m) (55). Other studies at various altitudes generally confirm the conclusion that AMS is related to the rate of ascent and the altitude which is reached (56–61). Individuals with a history of altitude illness may tolerate ascent better if the rate of ascent is slowed or if they spend a day or two acclimatizing at an intermediate altitude (60,62,63). In some studies, women had more symptoms than did the men (55,64).

Treatment and Prevention

The best method of preventing AMS is slow, gradual ascent with adequate time for acclimatization as one ascends. The rate of ascent will necessarily vary based on the susceptibility to AMS. With the onset of symptoms of AMS, additional time for acclimatization before going higher is usually the only treatment needed for mild AMS.

If symptoms of AMS worsen despite additional time to acclimatize, descent to lower altitude (especially sleeping altitude) is indicated. Normally a descent of 1000 to 3000 ft (300 to 900 m) is adequate. Supplemental oxygen, although rarely available, also very effectively relieves symptoms of AMS.

Numerous studies over the last 30 years have established the effectiveness of acetazolamide (Diamox) both for the prevention and treatment of AMS. Forwand et al (65) demonstrated that 250 mg of acetazolamide every 8 hours dramatically reduced symptoms of AMS compared to subjects taking a placebo during a sojourn to the 12,800-ft (3900-m) summit of Mt. Evans, Colorado. Other studies confirmed these findings (62,66–68). In addition, Sutton et al showed that acetazolamide decreased hypoxemia during sleep by reducing the amount of periodic breathing (69).

Acetazolamide is a carbonic anhydrase inhibitor that causes a bicarbonate diuresis resulting in a metabolic acidosis. Acetazolamide also decreases production of cerebrospinal fluid. Exactly why it is effective for AMS is unclear. Current recommendations are 250–500 mg per day, in either single or divided doses, starting 1 or 2 days before ascent (or waiting until symptoms develop) and continuing for a couple days at altitude or even for the duration of stay at altitude (70).

Recently the steroid dexamethasone, 2–4 mg every 6 hours, has been shown to be effective in both preventing and treating AMS (71–76). The mechanism of action of dexamethasone on AMS symptoms is unknown, and its relative effectiveness compared to acetazolamide has not been established.

Portable hyperbaric bags (Gamow bags) simulate descent to a lower altitude and are effective for treating AMS as well as high-altitude pulmonary edema (see below) (77–79).

Prediction

It is impossible to accurately predict who will suffer from AMS, although a previous history of AMS makes it much more likely that it will recur. Those with a lower vital capacity (80,81) and lower HVR (34,36,38,40) are more likely to experience altitude illness.

Etiology

The precise cause of AMS is still unknown, although a relative hypoventilation probably is important, and fluid retention may or may not play a role (82–84). Secretion of antidiuretic hormone and atrial natriuretic factor is altered in those with AMS, suggesting that CNS changes that cause secretion of hormones that promote fluid retention may be important (85,86). Sutton et al proposed the theory that hypoxia stimulates increased cerebral blood flow that results in vasogenic cerebral edema (87). Many factors seem to be important in the pathophysiology of AMS, as proposed by Hackett et al (53) (Figure 106-3).

Sleep at High Altitude

Most newcomers to altitude, even those without other serious altitude symptoms, report difficulty sleeping at night. Many factors, besides altitude, contribute to sleep disruption and loss at altitude, including the cold windy environment and often crowded sleeping conditions. During sleep, periodic breathing causes further disruption of sleep continuity. At extreme altitude, loss of sleep is nearly complete, further compromising the already exhausted climbers.

Sleep disturbances, including frequent nighttime awakenings, disrupt high-altitude sleep (88–90). The Operation Everest II decompression chamber study provided an opportunity to monitor changes in sleep across various altitudes up to an altitude equivalent to the South Col of Mt. Everest (~8040 m; Pв 282 mm Hg). These studies confirmed earlier findings and additionally found severe sleep fragmentation and periodic breathing (with central sleep apneas) at the highest altitudes. Brief, 2- to 5-second arousals from sleep (not full awakenings) increased from an average of 22 ± 6 times per hour at sea level to 161 ± 66 times per hour at 25,000 ft (7620 m; Pв 282 mm Hg) (91). Even those with the fewest arousals had more than one arousal from sleep every minute, whereas the more severely affected had three to four arousals each minute. Frequent arousals cause fragmentation of sleep resulting in impairment of daytime performance even without concomitant hypoxia (92,93). These arousals usually are not remembered the next morning, yet act similarly to hypoxia itself to alter judgment and performance, without the realization of the affected person.

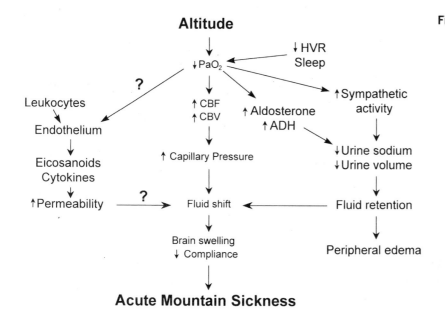

Altitude

Acute Mountain Sickness

Figure 106-3 Pathophysiology of acute mountain sickness. (Redrawn from Hackett PH, Roach RC. High-altitude medicine. In: Auerbach PS, ed. Wilderness medicine: Management of wilderness and environmental emergencies. 3rd ed. St. Louis: Mosby, 1995:1–37.).

Another unique aspect of sleep at high altitude is the breathing pattern. Many years ago, Mosso described this periodic breathing pattern, which consists of a series of three to five breaths followed by a short apnea (94). This breathing pattern is nearly universal in sojourners to high altitude (Figure 106-4), but far less common in highland Sherpas who have a blunted hypoxic ventilatory response (95). The amount of the night spent with periodic breathing is related in part to ventilatory drive; those with the strongest hypoxic ventilatory response have the most periodic breathing (96). Periodic breathing occurs in all sleep stages, including REM sleep, although at very high altitude the time spent in slow wave and REM sleep is quite limited (91).

Periodic breathing results from a destabilization of the respiratory control system (97–99). This is brought about because of changes in sleep state, hypocapnia, and hypoxic stimulation of the peripheral chemoreceptors. In a model of periodic breathing developed by Khoo et al an increase in chemoreceptor gain (such as occurs in those with a strong hypoxic ventilatory response) leads to destabilization of the respiratory system and periodic breathing (100). This model also predicts a decrease in cycle length (time from one apnea to the next) as altitude increases. Studies performed at high altitude on Mt. Everest confirm this prediction, although cycle time decreased less than predicted by the model (101).

Much of the sleep disruption at high altitude has been attributed to periodic breathing. Brief arousals from sleep have been noted at the onset of the hyperpneic phase of the periodic breathing (90,102). Data from the Operation Everest II study, however, found that nearly one half of the apneic episodes were not associated with EEG arousals (103). Alteration in sleep state may also serve to destabilize respiratory control. Thus there is a complex interplay between sleep state and breathing pattern.

Because of the fall in arterial oxygen saturation during sleep at high altitude, nighttime represents the most profound hypoxic insult during high-altitude sojourn. At 25,000 ft

(7620 m) during Operation Everest II, mean arterial oxygen saturation at night was only $52 \pm 2\%$ whereas daytime Sao_2 was $71 \pm 7\%$ (91). The lower Sao_2 at nighttime compared with daytime may, in part, result from periodic breathing (101). Periodic breathing does appear to be a risk factor for high-altitude illness (104,105). Carbonic anhydrase inhibitors (such as acetazolamide) decrease nocturnal periodic breathing, improve Sao_2, and decrease daytime symptoms of AMS (69,106,107).

High-Altitude Pulmonary Edema

Case Report: A 25-year-old student drove from sea level to approximately 7800 ft (2380 m) in the Sierra Nevada mountains of California, and then hiked with friends to 9000 ft (2740 m), where they spent their first night. The next day they hiked and skied to 11,000 ft (3350 m). The day after that, they continued to 12,400 ft (3780 m), where they dug a snow cave and spent the third night at altitude. That night the student developed a slight cough, but otherwise was asymptomatic. The next morning, about 60 hours after leaving sea level, the group departed camp for a day of ice climbing. Initially all went well, except that the student noted fatigue and shortness of breath, and he was unable to keep up with his climbing partners. In the early afternoon, they abandoned the climb and began the descent. By this time, the student was extremely fatigued but had only a slight headache. His cough increased, and soon he began coughing up thin straw-colored fluid. He was able to descend slowly, and after midnight, some 12 hours or more after starting the descent, the party arrived at their car. A chest radiograph obtained some 18 hours after descent is shown in Figure 106-5. Three days later, a follow-up chest film was much improved.

HAPE is one of the most serious and potentially dangerous manifestations of altitude illness. Descriptions of HAPE in the medical literature can be traced back to at

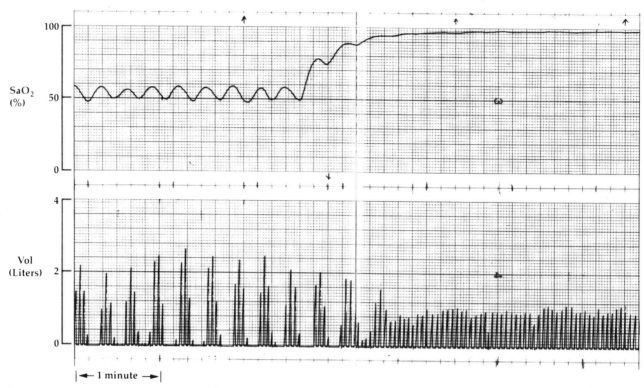

Figure 106-4 Nocturnal periodic breathing in subject no. 8 at 20,000 ft (6100 m) from Operation Everest II. Note that the administration of oxygen rapidly eliminates the apneas even though slight periodicity in tidal volume is still present.

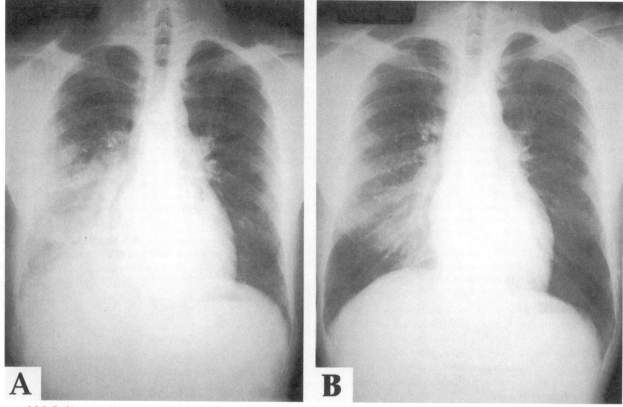

Figure 106-5 Chest radiograph in subject with high-altitude pulmonary edema. The radiograph on the left (A) was taken soon after return to sea level from high altitude; the film on the right (B), three days later, shows nearly complete resolution of the earlier findings.

least Mosso, who in 1898 described a fatal case on Mont Blanc (94). In 1913, Ravenhill published a report describing the different types of mountain sicknesses, including HAPE, in the Andes (108). These reports suggested that HAPE was of cardiac origin and were largely ignored. When Houston's pivotal paper described the first case of HAPE in the United States and suggested that cardiac failure was not the cause, the medical community finally began to take notice (109). Subsequent reports have further clarified this unusual form of pulmonary edema, but many uncertainties remain.

Signs and Symptoms

Twenty-four to 72 hours after arrival at altitude, the first symptoms of HAPE may appear. Frequently in adults, these symptoms occur after exercise and consist of cough, shortness of breath, chest tightness, and fatigue. About half of the time, these symptoms are combined with symptoms of AMS. Initially the cough is nonproductive, but later, a thin, clear, yellowish-colored sputum is produced. In some cases, the sputum is tinged with blood. Fatigue is an early symptom that may occur before dyspnea develops. Often the afflicted individual is unable to keep up with others and stops frequently to rest. Physical findings in HAPE include cyanosis, fever to 101°F (if higher, then this creates suspicion of pneumonia), flat neck veins, and crackles over the posterior and mid-chest. Heart and respiratory rates are increased.

Diagnosis

The diagnostic criteria for HAPE are (54):

In the setting of a recent gain in altitude, the presence of the following:
Symptoms: At least two of: dyspnea at rest, cough, weakness or decreased exercise performance, chest tightness or congestion.
Signs: At least two of: rales or wheezing in at least one lung field, central cyanosis, tachypnea, tachycardia.

In areas with medical facilities, a chest radiograph and measurement of arterial oxygen saturation may contribute to making the diagnosis and excluding other disorders. An important finding in HAPE is marked hypoxemia. Shown in Table 106-1 are arterial blood gas and saturation data in persons with and without HAPE:

Radiographic Features

Chest radiographs in patients with HAPE are useful to confirm the diagnosis and may show abnormalities even 24 to 48 hours after descent to sea level. The radiographic picture of HAPE is that of homogeneous or patchy opacities in the mid-lung areas involving one or both sides of the chest. Opacities are more likely to be present in the right than the left lung. Unilateral involvement of only the left lung is rare and should alert one to the possibility of congenital absence or hypoplasia of the right pulmonary artery (110,111). The heart size is normal, but the pulmonary arteries are frequently enlarged (112–115). Early reports did not describe the presence of Kerley lines (113); however, in a recent study of 60 cases of HAPE, Vock et al indicate that Kerley lines were present in some cases (114).

Incidence

Many factors affect the incidence of HAPE, such as rate of ascent, age, gender, physical exertion, and perhaps most importantly, individual susceptibility. In a large survey of skiers traveling to 8200 ft (2500 m) in Colorado, 0.1% developed HAPE (116). Trekkers in Nepal had an incidence of 4.5% at 14,000 ft (4270 m) (57). On Mt. McKinley, the incidence is about 2% to 3% (117).

Subclinical HAPE occurs much more frequently than full-blown cases (57), and children, not infants, appear to be more susceptible than adults. Men are more likely to develop HAPE than are women, but the reasons for this are unknown (116,118).

An intriguing aspect of HAPE is what is known as "reascent" HAPE or "re-entry" HAPE. Acclimatized individuals who descend to lower altitude and then reascend have an increased likelihood of developing HAPE. These individuals were found to have spent 3 to 5 days (119) or as much as 10 to 14 days (112) at low altitude before returning to higher elevations.

Pathophysiology

Establishing the precise etiology and mechanism for the development of HAPE is hampered by the lack of a good animal model of HAPE. Any hypothesis needs to take into account several factors: 1) elevated pulmonary artery pressures with normal wedge and left atrial pressures; 2) no evidence of left ventricular failure; 3) capillary and arterial thromboses in many fatal cases of HAPE; and 4) the fact that intense

Table 106-1 Arterial Blood Gases in Subjects with HAPE				
	Data from 12,400 ft (3779 m)*		Data from 14,953 ft (4558 m)[a]	
	HAPE Subjects	Normal Values at 3779 m	HAPE Subjects	Subjects Without HAPE or AMS
Po$_2$	40	53	31.7+5.5	45.8±6.9
Pco2	28.5	32.5±2.5	24.6±2.6	23.5±2.3
pH	7.45	~7.4	—	—

* From Hultgren HN, Wilson R. Blood gas abnormalities and optimum therapy in high altitude pulmonary edema. Clin Res 1981;29:99A. Abstract.
[a] From Bärtsch P, Vock P, Maggiorini M, et al. Respiratory symptoms, radiographic and physiologic correlations at high altitude. In: Sutton JR, Coates G, Remmers JE, eds. Hypoxia: The adaptations. Philadelphia: B.C. Decker, 1990:241–245.

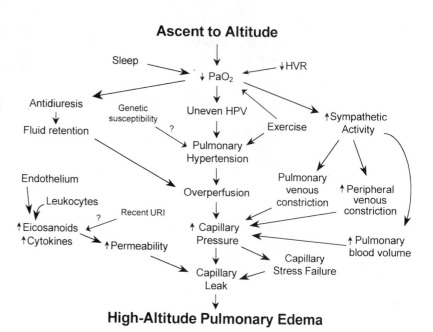

Figure 106-6 Pathophysiology of high-altitude pulmonary edema. (Adapted from Hackett PH, Roach RC. High-altitude medicine. In: Auerbach PS, ed. Wilderness medicine: Management of wilderness and environmental emergencies. 3rd ed. St. Louis: Mosby, 1995:1–37; and from Hackett PH, Roach RC. High altitude pulmonary edema. J Wilderness Med 1990;1:3–26.)

exercise makes HAPE more likely, whereas bed rest is beneficial. Additionally, at least in children, a recent viral upper respiratory tract infection precedes many cases of HAPE (120). Shown in Figure 106-6 is a summary of the pathogenesis of HAPE.

Pulmonary artery hypertension plays an important role in the development of HAPE. Hypoxic pulmonary vasoconstriction occurs to some extent in everyone after ascent to altitude; however, the amount of vasoconstriction varies widely (53). Individuals with HAPE have more severe pulmonary hypertension than average at altitude, but not everyone with this degree of pulmonary hypertension develops HAPE (24). Some HAPE-susceptible individuals appear to have an immunogenetic susceptibility by virtue of the higher prevalence of human leukocyte antigens HLA-DR6 and HLA-DQ4 (121).

Hultgren proposed what is now known as the "overperfusion" concept as the cause of HAPE (122,123). This overperfusion mechanism for HAPE postulates uneven hypoxic pulmonary vasoconstriction resulting in some lung areas with decreased blood flow and other areas with excessive flow. These overperfused lung areas are where the proposed leakage of edema fluid occurs.

Studies using bronchoalveolar lavage show that the edema fluid in HAPE has a high protein concentration. The edema fluid also contains various inflammatory markers, such as complement C5a and leukotriene B_4 (124,125).

Recently West et al have suggested that HAPE results from damage (i.e., rupture) of pulmonary capillaries subjected to high wall stresses from the high pressure in the vessels. The nonhomogeneous vasoconstriction proposed by Hultgren results in high pressures being transmitted to pulmonary capillaries (126,127).

Treatment and Prevention

The overperfusion and stress failure mechanisms for HAPE both imply that reduction of the excessive hypoxic pulmonary

vasoconstriction is important in the treatment of HAPE. Rapid descent to lower altitude results in dramatic improvement. Often a descent of only 1000 to 3000 ft (300 to 900 m) is necessary. Descent is thus the most important therapeutic maneuver. Early descent, before HAPE becomes severe, can potentially save more lives than any other treatment (1).

Use of supplemental oxygen will reduce pulmonary artery pressure and is useful; however, rarely are sufficient quantities of oxygen available to be able to rely on oxygen alone.

Nifedipine and other vasodilators are useful in treating HAPE. Subjects with HAPE treated by Oelz et al with 10 mg nifedipine followed by 20 mg every 6 hours of slow-release nifedipine showed improvement in oxygenation and overall condition, even without descent to lower altitude (128). Subsequently, Hackett et al found that several other vasodilators decrease pulmonary artery pressure and thus are useful in treating HAPE (129). Reliance on any of these medications should not cause one to forget the cardinal rule of treatment: descent.

Recently portable hyperbaric bags (e.g., Gamow bags) have become available. These fabric hyperbaric chambers increase the pressure approximately 2 psi (103 mm Hg), simulating descent. Several trials indicate these hyperbaric bags are effective in treating HAPE (77,79,130).

The best method of prevention for HAPE is gradual ascent, allowing adequate time for acclimatization, along with early recognition of HAPE symptoms and prompt descent. A recent study by Bärtsch et al found that in susceptible individuals, nifedipine taken prophylactically before ascent reduced the risk of developing HAPE (131).

High-Altitude Cerebral Edema

HACE is an extreme form of mountain sickness. The Lake Louise definition (54) states that HACE "can be considered 'end stage' or severe AMS. In the setting of a recent gain in altitude, [HACE is] the presence of a change in mental status and/or ataxia in a person with AMS, or the presence of both mental status change and ataxia in a person without AMS." Progression of the neurologic findings and death are likely without prompt treatment by descent, oxygen, or hyperbaric bag.

Most cases of HACE also have HAPE. It is difficult to determine the incidence of HACE, although it is considerably less common than HAPE. Singh et al (84) reported an incidence of HACE of 1.25%, whereas Hackett reported a 1.8% incidence in trekkers in Nepal (57). More cases of HACE in men have been reported, but due to the small numbers, it is unclear whether men are more likely than women to develop HACE (1, p 332).

Early signs and symptoms of HACE may progress rapidly (within 12 hours) to coma, but usually the progression occurs more slowly. Frequently, symptoms of HACE begin at night, sometimes resulting in loss of consciousness during sleep (132). In most cases, individuals have been at altitude for several days prior to the onset of HACE.

The pathophysiology of HACE shares many similarities to the pathophysiology of AMS. It is unclear why a few persons with AMS go on to develop HACE. MRI scans in patients with HACE show edema of the white matter, especially in the corpus callosum (133). Hansen et al proposed that cytotoxic cellular edema of the brain from hypoxia caused many of the signs and symptoms of both AMS and HACE (134). A few years later, however, Lassen et al suggested a vasogenic etiology whereby increased cerebral blood flow caused leakage of fluid into areas of the brain (135). Severinghaus has recently proposed roles for angiogenesis, osmotic swelling, and ischemia in the pathogenesis of HACE (136).

Treatment

Mild cases of AMS do not require descent to lower altitude. At the same time, early recognition of HACE is crucial. Any change in level of consciousness or the onset of ataxia makes descent mandatory. Patients with HACE should also receive supplemental oxygen, if available, and dexamethasone, 4–8 mg initially and 4 mg every 6 hours thereafter. Diuretics such as furosemide and mannitol are not recommended, as they may result in orthostatic hypotension from decreased intravascular volume, making descent difficult or impossible. Early use of a hyperbaric bag (Gamow bag) may relieve symptoms and make descent easier, but should not be considered a substitute for descent, especially since recovery often requires 10 or more days, even with treatment at low altitude (132,137).

In summary, the keys to the prevention and treatment of HACE, HAPE, and severe AMS are 1) learn to recognize early symptoms, 2) never ascend to a higher sleeping altitude with new symptoms, 3) descend to lower altitude if symptoms worsen, and 4) never leave someone with altitude illness alone.

SPECIAL POPULATIONS AT ALTITUDE

Given the large numbers of individuals going to altitude, it is not surprising that some will have special medical problems. Even though most of the problems of acclimatization and illness at altitude are similar to those in healthy individuals, persons with underlying cardiac disease, pulmonary disease, and sickle cell anemia deserve special mention (1,138).

Coronary Artery Disease

Ascent to altitude in an unacclimatized person with coronary artery disease may result in increased anginal symptoms caused by an increase in cardiac work as well as by possible vasoconstriction of the coronary arteries (139). Cardiac arrhythmias including atrial fibrillation or flutter may worsen after rapid ascent to altitude even without underlying coronary artery disease. During exercise testing at 10,150 ft (3100 m), cardiac patients developed angina or ST segment depression at the same double product (heart rate times systolic blood pressure) as they did at 5280 ft (1600 m) (140). Thus mild hypoxia to altitudes near 10,000 ft (3050 m) has little direct effect on myocardial ischemia but acts by increasing heart rate and blood pressure during submaximal exercise.

Despite the increase in cardiac symptoms following rapid ascent to altitude, the increased risk for cardiac death is probably small. In a large survey of trekkers in Nepal, trauma was the most common cause of death. No deaths from cardiac disease were reported although several individuals were evacuated for cardiac problems (141). Other studies done at moderate altitudes in unacclimatized individuals suggest a relatively low risk of cardiac events, both in elderly individuals and in those with known coronary artery disease (142–144). Recently Hultgren reviewed the effects of altitude on patients with cardiovascular disease and has suggested an approach (including when to perform a preascent exercise test) for evaluation of the patient with heart disease prior to trekking at high altitude (145).

With proper time for acclimatization, patients with coronary heart disease are likely to experience decreased symptoms because of a lower blood pressure (146). With long-term exposure to altitude, coronary artery disease mortality is actually lower than at sea level (147).

Pulmonary Disease
Chronic Obstructive Pulmonary Disease

One of the hallmarks of ascent to altitude is the shortness of breath experienced by everyone, including those with no heart or lung disease. Patients with chronic obstructive pulmonary disease (COPD) frequently are limited, even at sea level, by impaired lung mechanics and by dyspnea. Because of the increased ventilatory requirements of exercise at altitude, COPD patients may have worsening of their symptoms during exposure to altitude. COPD patients without evidence of cor pulmonale were exposed to 6300 ft (1920 m) altitude by Graham et al. These patients developed few altitude-related symptoms except fatigue (and headache in one subject) despite a decrease in resting arterial Po_2 from 66 to 52 mm Hg (148). The authors attributed the lack of symptoms of acute mountain sickness to partial acclimatization caused by hypoxemia in these COPD patients. They concluded that patients with mild or moderate COPD, without cor pulmonale, tolerate altitude exposure quite well.

Patients with COPD who live at altitude for longer periods of time, as opposed to sojourners, develop cor pulmonale and have an increased mortality when compared with similar patients living at low altitude. The mechanism by which altitude residence causes this increased mortality is unknown, but it is presumably related to the higher pulmonary artery pressure in those living at altitude (149,150).

Pulmonary Hypertension

Hypoxic pulmonary vasoconstriction increases pulmonary artery pressure in sojourners to high altitude. In the presence of primary pulmonary hypertension ascent to altitude is likely to raise pulmonary pressure even higher. These patients are likely to experience more symptoms such as fatigue, dyspnea, or even syncope. An increase in supplemental oxygen or in pulmonary vasodilators may be useful to ameliorate altitude symptoms. Prior to traveling to altitude, persons with primary pulmonary hypertension should consult a physician familiar with altitude problems who can evaluate the potential risks. Primary pulmonary hypertension may be more common among persons living at altitude, and those with pulmonary hypertension should be encouraged to consider moving to lower altitude (151,152).

Asthma

Many young, active people suffer from asthma so it is likely that a significant number of altitude sojourners will have asthma or reactive airways. The dry, cold air likely to be encountered at altitude may cause bronchoconstriction; however, this climate also contains fewer allergens. As a result, many asthmatics report doing as well or even better at altitude than at lower elevations. The reduced barometric pressure results in decreased air density. Thus, even though the ventilatory demands of activity at altitude are greater, the reduced air density at least partially compensates. Asthmatic patients wishing to travel to altitude should be encouraged to do so, being sure to take along an adequate supply of their medications and paying attention to their respiratory symptoms.

Air Travel

As global travel becomes more readily available and affordable, an increasing number individuals with preexisting cardiac and pulmonary problems are using this mode of transportation. Pressurized cabins on modern airliners increase the barometric pressure by about 385 to 445 mm Hg above the outside ambient pressure (153,154). Since commercial aircraft fly at altitudes ranging from about 10,000 ft (3048 m) to 60,000 ft (18,288 m), passengers are acutely exposed to altitude (155). Cottrell measured the cabin altitude in over 200 commercial flights. The median altitude was 6214 ft (1894 m) with an average cabin altitude of 5673 ft (1724 m) and standard deviation of 2019 ft (615 m) (153). The maximum altitude observed in this study was 8915 ft (2717 m). Newer aircraft models had significantly higher cabin altitudes than that of older planes.

Normal individuals adapt without difficulty to these altitudes, but those already hypoxic at sea level may require supplemental oxygen during their flight. Studies of patients with COPD suggest that significant arterial oxygen desaturation occurs. In one study (154), the arterial Po_2 decreased from 68 ± 8 mm Hg to 51 ± 9 mm Hg, whereas in another (156) the Pao_2 decreased from about 72 to 47 mm Hg. These oxygen levels indicate the need for oxygen supplementation for these patients. An altitude simulation test, measuring arterial blood gases while breathing a hypoxic gas mixture, may be useful in order to estimate the oxygen requirements for aircraft travel (157).

Sickle Cell Disease

Many variations of the hemoglobin molecule occur throughout the world. A few of these, such as hemoglobin with a high oxygen affinity, may be beneficial for altitude acclimatization and function (158). Others such as sickle cell disease make ascent to altitude inadvisable.

Sickle cell disease refers to several types of abnormal hemoglobins including hemoglobin AS and hemoglobin SS. Under conditions of hypoxia, the red blood cells in these individuals become deformed and take on a "sickle" shape. The change in cell shape and function causes blood viscosity to increase, the cells to clump together more readily, and the microcirculation to become blocked. The major determinate of sickling is the concentration of hemoglobin S in the circulation. Bone pain and splenic infarction may occur. Approximately 6% to 8% of African-Americans in the United States carry at lease one abnormal hemoglobin gene. Most of these have sickle cell trait and are largely asymptomatic, whereas a few have the far more severe sickle cell anemia. Patients with sickle cell anemia are likely to already know about their disease, whereas those with only sickle cell trait may be unaware of the problem and therefore are more likely to go to altitude and experience problems (159).

Patients with sickle cell anemia are likely to have had episodes of sickle cell crises. Given the susceptibility of their red cells to hypoxia, these individuals should not attempt to go to high altitude. Airline travel for those with sickle cell anemia may even precipitate symptoms. Consideration should be given to providing supplemental oxygen to those with sickle cell anemia during aircraft flights (160). Travel by commercial airline is generally safe for patients with sickle cell trait; however, rarely they may experience symptoms during plane flights (161,162). Most individuals with sickle cell trait can safely go to altitudes of 8000 to 10,000 ft (2440 to 3048 m), although a few may have difficulties (159). Although most persons with sickle cell disease are of African-American ancestry, sickle cell trait and even sickle cell crisis are known to occur in Caucasians (163).

REFERENCES

1. Hultgren HN. High altitude medicine. Stanford, CA: Hultgren Publications, 1997.

2. Ward MP, Milledge JS, West JB. High altitude medicine and physiology. London: Chapman & Hall, 1995.

3. International Civil Aviation Organization. Manual of the ICAO standard atmosphere. Montreal: International Civil Aviation Organization, 1964.

4. Smithsonian Institution. Smithsonian meteorological tables. Washington, DC.: Smithsonian Institution, 1949.

5. West JB, Lahiri S, Maret KH, et al. Barometric pressures at extreme altitudes on Mt. Everest: physiological significance. J Appl Physiol 1983;54:1188–1194.

6. Houston CS. Acclimatization. In: Sutton JR, Jones NL, Houston CS, eds. Hypoxia: Man at altitude. New York: Thieme-Stratton, 1982:158–160.

7. Hartley H. Effects of high-altitude environment on the cardiovascular system of man. JAMA 1971;215:241–244.

8. Hultgren H, Grover RF. Circulatory adaptation to high altitude. Annu Rev Med 1968;19:119–152.

9. Wolfel EE, Selland MA, Mazzeo RS, et al. Systemic hypertension at 4300 m is related to sympathoadrenal activity. J Appl Physiol 1994;76:1643–1650.

10. Kellogg RH. Altitude acclimatization, a historical introduction emphasizing the regulation of breathing. Physiologist 1968;11:37–57.

11. Reeves JT, Groves BM, Sutton JR, et al. Operation Everest II: preservation of cardiac function at extreme altitude. J Appl Physiol 1987;63:531–539.

12. Alexander JK, Hartley LH, Modelski M, et al. Reduction of stroke volume during exercise in man following ascent to 3100 m altitude. J Appl Physiol 1967;23:849–858.

13. Reeves JT, Groves BM, Sutton JR, et al. Oxygen transport during exercise at extreme altitude: Operation Everest II. Ann Emerg Med 1987;16:993–998.

14. Pugh LGCE. Cardiac output in muscular exercise at 5800 m (19,000 ft). J Appl Physiol 1964;19:441–447.

15. Fowles RE, Hultgren HN. Left ventricular function at high altitude examined by systolic time intervals and M-mode echocardiography. Am J Cardiol 1983;52:862–866.

16. Hirata K, Ban T, Jinnouchi Y, et al. Echocardiographic assessment of left ventricular function and wall motion at high altitude in normal subjects. Am J Cardiol 1991;68:1692–1697.

17. Suarez J, Alexander JK, Houston CS. Enhanced left ventricular systolic performance at high altitude during Operation Everest II. Am J Cardiol 1987;60:137–142.

18. Voelkel NF, McDonnell T, Chang S, et al. Mechanisms of hypoxic vasoconstriction. In: Ueda G, Kusama S, Voelkel NF, eds. High-altitude medical science. Matsumoto, Japan: Shinshu University, 1988:13–28.

19. Groves BM, Reeves JT, Sutton JR, et al. Operation Everest II: elevated high-altitude pulmonary resistance unresponsive to oxygen. J Appl Physiol 1987;63:521–530.

20. Sime F, Penaloza D, Ruiz L. Bradycardia, increased cardiac output, and reversal of pulmonary hypertension in altitude natives living at sea level. Br Heart J 1971;33:647–657.

21. Doyle JT, Wilson JS, Warren JV. The pulmonary vascular responses to short-term hypoxia in human subjects. Circulation 1952;5:263–271.

22. Viswanathan R, Jain SK, Subramanian S, et al. Pulmonary edema of high altitude II: clinical, aerohemodynamic, and biochemical studies in a group with history of pulmonary edema of high altitude. Am Rev Respir Dis 1969;100:334–341.

23. Wagenvoort CA, Wagenvoort N. Hypoxic pulmonary vascular lesions in man at high altitude and in patients with chronic respiratory disease. Pathol Microbiol 1973;39:276–282.

24. Hultgren HN, Grover RF, Hartley LH. Abnormal circulatory responses to high altitude in subjects with a previous history of high-altitude pulmonary edema. Circulation 1971;44:759–770.

25. Hurtado A. Respiratory adaptation in the Indian natives of the Peruvian Andes: studies at high altitude. Am J Phys Anthropol 1932;17:137–165.

26. Groves BM, Droma T, Sutton JR, et al. Minimal hypoxic pulmonary hypertension in normal Tibetans at 3658 m. J Appl Physiol 1993;74:312–318.

27. Moore LG, Curran-Everett L, Droma TS, et al. Are Tibetans better adapted? Int J Sports Med 1992;13:S86–S88.

28. Rahn H, Otis AB. Man's respiratory response during and after acclimatization to high altitude. Am J Physiol 1949;157:445–462.

29. Dempsey JA, Forster HV. Mediation of ventilatory adaptations. Physiol Rev 1982;62:262–346.

30. Eger EI, Kellogg RH, Mines AH, et al. Influence of CO_2 on ventilatory acclimatization to altitude. J Appl Physiol 1968;24:607–615.

31. Huang SY, Alexander JK, Grover RF, et al. Hypocapnia and sustained hypoxia blunt ventilation on arrival at high altitude. J Appl Physiol 1984;56:602–606.

32. West JB, Hackett PH, Maret KH, et al. Pulmonary gas exchange on the summit of Mount Everest. J Appl Physiol 1983;55:678–687.

33. Weil JV, Byrne-Quinn E, Sodal IE, et al. Hypoxic ventilatory drive in normal man. J Clin Invest 1970; 49:1061–1072.

34. King AB, Robinson SM. Ventilation response to hypoxia and acute mountain sickness. Aerospace Med 1972;43:419–421.

35. Mathew L, Gopinathan PM, Purkayastha SS, et al. Chemoreceptor sensitivity and maladaptation to high altitude in man. Eur J Appl Physiol 1983;51:137–144.

36. Moore LG, Harrison GL, McCullough RE, et al. Low acute hypoxic ventilatory response and hypoxic depression in acute altitude sickness. J Appl Physiol 1986;60:1407–1412.

37. Richalet JP, Keromes A, Dersch B, et al. Physiological characteristics of high altitude climbers. Sci Sports (Paris) 1988;3:89–108.

38. Schoene RB. Control of ventilation in climbers to extreme altitude. J Appl Physiol 1982; 53:886–890.

39. Schoene RB, Lahiri S, Hackett PH, et al. Relationship of hypoxic ventilatory response to exercise performance on Mount Everest. J Appl Physiol 1984;56:1478–1483.

40. Sutton JR, Bryan AC, Gray GW, et al. Pulmonary gas exchange in acute mountain sickness. Aviat Space Environ Med 1976;47: 1032–1037.

41. Byrne-Quinn E, Sodal IE, Weil JV. Hypoxic and hypercapnic ventilatory drives in children native to high altitude. J Appl Physiol 1972;32:44–46.

42. Milledge JS, Lahiri S. Respiratory control in lowlanders and Sherpa highlanders at altitude. Respir Physiol 1967;2:310–322.

43. Severinghaus JW, Bainton CR, Carcelen A. Respiratory insensitivity to hypoxia in chronically hypoxic man. Respir Physiol 1966;1:308–334.

44. Faura J, Ramos J, Reynafarje C, et al. Effect of altitude on erythropoiesis. Blood 1969;33: 668–676.

45. Beall CM, Strohl KP, Brittenham GM. Reappraisal of Andean high altitude erythrocytosis from a Himalayan perspective. Semin Respir Med 1983;5:195–201.

46. Lenfant C, Sullivan K. Adaptation to high altitude. N Engl J Med 1971;284:1298–1309.

47. Sarnquist FH, Schoene RB, Hackett PH, et al. Hemodilution of polycythemic mountaineers: effects on exercise and mental function. Aviat Space Environ Med 1986;57:313–317.

48. Winslow RM, Samaja M, West JB. Red cell function at extreme altitude on Mount Everest. J Appl Physiol 1984;56:109–116.

49. Monge C. Chronic mountain sickness. Physiol Rev 1943;23:166–184.

50. Cruz JC, Diaz C, Marticorena E, et al. Phlebotomy improves pulmonary gas exchange in chronic mountain polycythemia. Respiration 1979;38:305–313.

51. Penaloza D, Sime F. Chronic cor pulmonale due to loss of altitude acclimatization (chronic mountain sickness). Am J Med 1971;50:728–743.

52. Winslow RM, Monge CC, Brown EG, et al. Effects of hemodilution on O_2 transport in high-altitude polycythemia. J Appl Physiol 1985;59:1495–1502.

53. Hackett PH, Roach RC. High-altitude medicine. In: Auerbach PS, ed. Wilderness medicine: Management of wilderness and environmental emergencies. 3rd ed. St. Louis: Mosby, 1995:1–37.

54. Anonymous. The Lake Louise Consensus on the definition and quantification of altitude illness. In: Sutton JR, Coates G, Houston CS, eds. Hypoxia and mountain medicine. Burlington, VT: Queen City Printers, 1992:327–330.

55. Honigman B, Theis MK, Koziol-McClain J, et al. Acute mountain sickness in a general tourist population at moderate altitudes.

Ann Intern Med 1993;118:587–592.

56. Carson RP, Evans WO, Shields JL, et al. Symptomatology, pathophysiology and treatment of acute mountain sickness. Fed Proc 1969;28:1085–1091.

57. Hackett PH, Rennie D, Levine HD. The incidence, importance, and prophylaxis of acute mountain sickness. Lancet 1976;2: 1149–1155.

58. Hall WH, Barila TG, Metzger E, et al. A clinical study of acute mountain sickness. Arch Environ Health 1965;10:747–753.

59. Kamat SR, Banerji BC. Study of cardiopulmonary function on exposure to high altitude: I. acute acclimatization to an altitude of 3500 to 4000 meters in relation to altitude sickness and cardiopulmonary function. Am Rev Respir Dis 1972;106:404–413.

60. Kayser B. Acute mountain sickness in western tourists around the Thorong pass (5400 m) in Nepal. J Wilderness Med 1991; 2:110–117.

61. Maggiorini M, Bühler B, Walter M, et al. Prevalence of acute mountain sickness in the Swiss Alps. BMJ 1990;301:853–855.

62. Evans WO, Robinson SM, Hortsman DH, et al. Amelioration of the symptoms of acute mountain sickness by staging and acetazolamide. Aviat Space Environ Med 1976;47:512–516.

63. Hansen JE, Harris CW, Evans WO. Influence of elevation of origin, rate of ascent and a physical conditioning program on symptoms of acute mountain sickness. Military Med 1967; 132:585–593.

64. Harris CW, Shields JL, Hannon JP. Acute altitude sickness in females. Aerospace Med 1966; 37:1163–1167.

65. Forward SA, Landowne M, Follansbee JN, et al. Effect of acetazolamide on acute mountain sickness. N Engl J Med 1968; 279:839–845.

66. Gray GW, Bryan AC, Frayser R, et al. Control of acute mountain sickness. Aerospace Med 1971; 42:81–84.

67. Greene MK, Kerr AM, McIntosh IB, et al. Acetazolamide in prevention of acute mountain sickness: a double-blind controlled cross-over study. BMJ 1981;283:811–813.

68. Larson EB, Roach RC, Schoene RB, et al. Acute mountain sickness and acetazolamide. JAMA 1982;248:328–332.

69. Sutton JR, Houston CS, Mansell AL, et al. Effect of acetazolamide on hypoxemia during sleep at high altitude. N Engl J Med 1979;301:1329–1331.

70. Birmingham Medical Research Expeditionary Society Mountain Sickness Study Group. Acetazolamide in control of acute mountain sickness. Lancet 1981;1: 180–183.

71. Ellsworth AJ, Meyer EF, Larson EB. Acetazolamide or dexamethasone use versus placebo to prevent acute mountain sickness on Mount Rainier. West J Med 1991;154:289–293.

72. Hackett PH, Roach RC, Wood RA, et al. Dexamethasone for prevention and treatment of acute mountain sickness. Aviat Space Environ Med 1988;59:950–954.

73. Johnson TS, Rock PB, Fulco CS, et al. Prevention of acute mountain sickness by dexamethasone. N Engl J Med 1984;310:683–686.

74. Montgomery AB, Luce JM, Michael P, et al. Effects of dexamethasone on the incidence of acute mountain sickness at two intermediate altitudes. JAMA 1989;261:734–736.

75. Rock PB, Johnson TS, Cymerman A, et al. Effect of dexamethasone on symptoms of acute mountain sickness at Pikes Peak, Colorado (4300 m). Aviat Space Environ Med 1987;58:668–672.

76. Rock PB, Johnson TS, Larsen RF, et al. Dexamethasone as prophylaxis for acute mountain sick-

ness: effect of dose level. Chest 1989;95:568–573.

77. King SJ, Greenlee RR. Successful use of the Gamow hyperbaric bag in the treatment of altitude illness at Mount Everest. J Wilderness Med 1990;1:193–202.

78. Robertson JA, Shlim DR. Treatment of moderate acute mountain sickness with pressurization in a portable hyperbaric (Gamow) bag. J Wilderness Med 1991;2: 268–273.

79. Taber RL. Protocols for the use of a portable hyperbaric chamber for the treatment of high altitude disorders. J Wilderness Med 1990;1:181–192.

80. Anholm JD, Houston CS, Hyers TM. The relationship between acute mountain sickness and pulmonary ventilation at 2835 meters (9300 feet). Chest 1979;75:33–36.

81. Hackett PH, Rennie D, Hofmeister SE, et al. Fluid retention and relative hypoventilation in acute mountain sickness. Respiration 1982;43:321–329.

82. Aoki VS, Robinson SM. Body hydration and the incidence and severity of acute mountain sickness. J Appl Physiol 1971;31: 363–367.

83. Hackett PH, Rennie D. Rales, peripheral edema, retinal hemorrhage and acute mountain sickness. Am J Med 1979;67:214–218.

84. Singh I, Khanna PK, Srivastava MC, et al. Acute mountain sickness. N Engl J Med 1969;280: 175–183.

85. Bärtsch P, Maggiorini M, Schobersberger W, et al. Enhanced exercise-induced rise of aldosterone and vasopressin preceding mountain sickness. J Appl Physiol 1991;71:136–143.

86. Bärtsch P, Shaw S, Franciolli M, et al. Atrial natriuretic peptide in acute mountain sickness. J Appl Physiol 1988;65:1929–1937.

87. Sutton JR, Lassen N. Pathophysiology of acute mountain sickness

and high altitude pulmonary oedema: an hypothesis. Bull Physiopathol Respir (Nancy) 1979;15:1045–1052.

88. Miller JC, Horvath SM. Sleep at altitude. Aviat Space Environ Med 1977;48:615–620.

89. Powles ACP. Sleep at altitude. In: Sutton JR, Jones NL, Houston CS, eds. Hypoxia: Man at altitude. New York: Thieme-Stratton, 1982:182–185.

90. Reite M, Jackson D, Cahoon RL, et al. Sleep physiology at high altitude. Electroencephalogr Clin Neurophysiol 1975;38:463–471.

91. Anholm JD, Powles ACP, Downey R III, et al. Operation Everest II: arterial oxygen saturation and sleep at extreme simulated altitude. Am Rev Respir Dis 1992;145:817–826.

92. Bonnet MH. Effect of sleep disruption on sleep, performance, and mood. Sleep 1985;8:11–19.

93. Downey R, Bonnet MH. Performance during frequent sleep disruption. Sleep 1987;10:354–363.

94. Mosso A. Life of man on the high Alps. London: T. Fisher Unwin, 1898.

95. Lahiri S, Maret KH, Sherpa MG, et al. Sleep and periodic breathing at high altitude: Sherpa natives versus sojourners. In: West JB, Lahiri S, eds. High altitude and man. Bethesda, MD: American Physiological Society, 1984:73–90.

96. Lahiri S, Maret K, Sherpa MG. Dependence of high altitude sleep apnea on ventilatory sensitivity to hypoxia. Respir Physiol 1983;52:281–301.

97. Berssenbrugge A, Dempsey J, Iber C, et al. Mechanisms of hypoxia-induced periodic breathing during sleep in humans. J Physiol (Lond) 1983;343:507–524.

98. Douglas CG, Haldane JS. The causes of periodic or Cheyne-Stokes breathing. J Physiol (Lond) 1909;38:401–419.

99. Khoo MCK, Gottschalk A, Pack AI. Sleep-induced periodic breathing and apnea: a theoretical study. J Appl Physiol 1991; 70:2014–2024.

100. Khoo MCK, Kronauer RE, Strohl KP, et al. Factors inducing periodic breathing in humans: a general model. J Appl Physiol 1982;53:644–659.

101. West JB, Peters RM, Aksnes G, et al. Nocturnal periodic breathing at altitudes of 6300 and 8050m. J Appl Physiol 1986; 61:280–287.

102. Weil JV. Sleep at high altitude. In: Kryger MH, Roth T, Dement WC, eds. Principles and practice of sleep medicine. Philadelphia: W. B. Saunders, 1989:269–275.

103. Khoo MC, Anholm JD, Ko SW, et al. Dynamics of periodic breathing and arousal during sleep at extreme altitude. Respir Physiol 1996;103:33–43.

104. Eichenberger U, Weiss E, Riemann D, et al. Nocturnal periodic breathing and the development of acute high altitude illness. Am J Respir Crit Care Med 1996;154:1748–1754.

105. Powles AP, Sutton JR, Gray GW, et al. Sleep hypoxemia at altitude: Its relationship to acute mountain sickness and ventilatory responsiveness to hypoxia and hypercapnia. In: Folinsbee LJ, Wagner JA, Borgia JF, et al, eds. Environmental stress: Individual human adaptations. New York: Academic Press, 1978:221–229.

106. Sutton JR, Gray GW, Houston CS, et al. Effects of duration at altitude and acetazolamide on ventilation and oxygenation during sleep. Sleep 1980;3:455–464.

107. Swenson ER, Leatham KL, Roach RC, et al. Renal carbonic anhydrase inhibition reduces high altitude sleep periodic breathing. Respir Physiol 1991;86:333–343.

108. Ravenhill TH. Some experiences of mountain sickness in the Andes. J Trop Med Hyg 1913; 16:313–320.

109. Houston CS. Acute pulmonary edema of high altitude. N Engl J Med 1960;263:478–480.

110. Fiorenzano G, Rastelli V, Greco V, et al. Unilateral high-altitude pulmonary edema in a subject with right pulmonary artery hypoplasia. Respiration 1994;61:51–54.

111. Hackett PH, Creagh CE, Grover RF, et al. High-altitude pulmonary edema in persons without the right pulmonary artery. N Engl J Med 1980;302:1070–1073.

112. Hultgren HN, Spickard H, Houston CS. High altitude pulmonary edema. Medicine 1961; 40:289–313.

113. Maldonado D. High altitude pulmonary edema. Radiol Clin North Am 1978;16:537–549.

114. Vock P, Brutsche MH, Nanzer A, et al. Variable radiomorphologic data of high altitude pulmonary edema. Chest 1991;100:1306–1311.

115. Vock P, Fretz C, Franciolli M, et al. High-altitude pulmonary edema: Findings at high-altitude chest radiography and physical examination. Radiology 1989; 170:661–666.

116. Sophocles AM. High-altitude pulmonary edema in Vail, Colorado, 1975–1982. West J Med 1986; 144:569–573.

117. Hackett PH, Roach RC. High altitude pulmonary edema. J Wilderness Med 1990;1:3–26.

118. Hultgren HN, Honigman B, Theis K, et al. High-altitude pulmonary edema at a ski resort. West J Med 1996;164:222–227.

119. Scoggin CH, Hyers TM, Reeves JT, et al. High-altitude pulmonary edema in the children and young adults of Leadville, Colorado. N Engl J Med 1977;297:1269–1272.

120. Durmowicz AG, Noordeweir E, Nicholas R, et al. Inflammatory processes may predispose children to high-altitude pulmonary edema. J Pediatr 1997;130:838–840.

121. Hanaoka M, Kubo K, Yamazaki Y, et al. Association of high-altitude pulmonary edema with the major histocompatibility complex. Circulation 1998;97:1124–1128.

122. Hultgren HN. High altitude pulmonary edema. In: Hegnauer AH, ed. Biomedicine of high terrestrial elevations. Natick, MA: U. S. Army Research Institute of Environmental Medicine, 1969: 131–148.

123. Hultgren HN. High altitude pulmonary edema. In: Staub NC, ed. Lung water and solute exchange. New York: Marcel Dekker, 1978:437–464.

124. Schoene RB, Hackett PH, Henderson WR, et al. High-altitude pulmonary edema, characteristics of lung lavage fluid. JAMA 1986;256:63–69.

125. Schoene RB, Swenson ER, Pizzo CJ, et al. The lung at high altitude: bronchoalveolar lavage in acute mountain sickness and pulmonary edema. J Appl Physiol 1988;64:2605–2613.

126. West JB, Colice GL, Lee YJ, et al. Pathogenesis of high-altitude pulmonary oedema: direct evidence of stress failure of pulmonary capillaries. Eur Respir J 1995;8:523–529.

127. West JB, Tsukimoto K, Mathieu-Costello O, et al. Stress failure in pulmonary capillaries. J Appl Physiol 1991;70:1731–1742.

128. Oelz O, Maggiorini M, Ritter M, et al. Nifedipine for high altitude pulmonary oedema. Lancet 1989;2:1241–1244.

129. Hackett PH, Roach RC, Hartig GS, et al. The effect of vasodilators on pulmonary hemodynamics in high altitude pulmonary edema: a comparison. Int J Sports Med 1992;13(suppl 1):S68–S71.

130. Kasic JF, Yaron M, Nicholas RA, et al. Treatment of acute mountain sickness: hyperbaric versus oxygen therapy. Ann Emerg Med 1991;20:1109–1112.

131. Bärtsch P, Maggiorini M, Ritter M, et al. Prevention of high-

altitude pulmonary edema by nifedipine. N Engl J Med 1991; 325:1284–1289.

132. Dickinson JG. High altitude cerebral edema: cerebral acute mountain sickness. Semin Respir Med 1983;5:151–158.

133. Hackett PH, Yarnell P, Hill RP. MRI in high altitude cerebral edema: evidence for vasogenic edema. In: Sutton JR, Coates G, Remmers JE, eds. Hypoxia: The adaptations. Philadelphia: B. C. Decker, 1990:295. Abstract.

134. Hansen JE, Evans WO. A hypothesis regarding the pathophysiology of acute mountain sickness. Arch Environ Health 1970;21: 666–669.

135. Lassen NA, Harper AM. High altitude cerebral oedema. Lancet 1975;2:1154. Letter.

136. Severinghaus JW. Hypothetical roles of angiogenesis, osmotic swelling, and ischemia in high-altitude cerebral edema. J Appl Physiol 1995;79:375–379.

137. Houston CS, Dickinson J. Cerebral form of high-altitude illness. Lancet 1975;2:758–761.

138. Rennie D, Wilson R. Who should not go high. In: Sutton JR, Jones NL, Houston CS, eds. Hypoxia: Man at altitude. New York: Thieme-Stratton, 1982:186–190.

139. Grover RF, Tucker CE, McGroarty SR, et al. The coronary stress of skiing at high altitude. Arch Intern Med 1990;150:1205–1208.

140. Morgan BJ, Alexander JK, Nicoli SA, et al. The patient with coronary heart disease at altitude: observations during acute exposure to 3100 meters. J Wilderness Med 1990;1:147–153.

141. Shlim DR, Houston R. Helicopter rescues and deaths among trekkers in Nepal. JAMA 1989; 261:1017–1019.

142. Erdmann J, Sun KT, Masar P, et al. Effects of exposure to altitude on men with coronary artery disease and impaired left ventricular function. Am J Cardiol 1998;81:266–270.

143. Rennie D. Will mountain trekkers have heart attacks? JAMA 1989; 261:1045–1046.

144. Roach RC, Houston CS, Honigman B, et al. How well do older persons tolerate moderate altitude? West J Med 1995;162: 32–36.

145. Hultgren HN. Effects of altitude upon cardiovascular diseases. J Wilderness Med 1992;3:301–308.

146. Hultgren HN. Reduction of systemic arterial blood pressure at high altitude. Adv Cardiol 1979;5:49–55.

147. Mortimer EA, Monson RR, MacMahon B. Reduction in mortality from coronary heart disease in men residing at high altitude. N Engl J Med 1977;296:581–585.

148. Graham WGB, Houston CS. Short-term adaptation to moderate altitude: patients with chronic obstructive pulmonary disease. JAMA 1978;240:1491–1494.

149. Moore LG, Rohr AL, Maisenbach JK, et al. Emphysema mortality is increased in Colorado residents at high altitude. Am Rev Respir Dis 1982;126:225–228.

150. Renzetti AD Jr, McClement JH, Litt BD. The Veterans Administration cooperative study of pulmonary function: 3: Mortality in relation to respiratory function in chronic obstructive pulmonary disease. Am J Med 1966;41: 115–129.

151. Grover RF, Vogel JHK, Voigt GC, et al. Reversal of high altitude pulmonary hypertension. Am J Cardiol 1966;18:928–932.

152. Khoury GH, Hawes CR. Primary pulmonary hypertension in children living at high altitude. J Pediatr 1963;62:177–185.

153. Cottrell JJ. Altitude exposures during aircraft flight: flying higher. Chest 1988;93:81–84.

154. Schwartz JS, Bencowitz HZ, Moser KM. Air travel hypoxemia with chronic obstructive pulmonary disease. Ann Intern Med 1984;100:473–477.

155. Gong H Jr. Advising patients with pulmonary diseases on air travel. Ann Intern Med 1989;111:349–351.

156. Dillard TA, Berg BW, Rajagopal KR, et al. Hypoxemia during air travel in patients with chronic obstructive pulmonary disease. Ann Intern Med 1989;111:362–367.

157. Gong H Jr. Air travel and oxygen therapy in cardiopulmonary patients. Chest 1992;101:1104–1113.

158. Hebbel RP, Eaton JW, Kronenberg RS, et al. Human llamas: adaptation to altitude in subjects with high hemoglobin oxygen affinity. J Clin Invest 1978;62:593–600.

159. Winslow RM. Notes on sickle cell disease. In: Sutton JR, Jones NL, Houston CS, eds. Hypoxia: Man at altitude. New York: Thieme-Stratton, 1982: 179–181.

160. Claster S, Godwin MJ, Embury SH. Risk of altitude exposure in sickle cell disease. West J Med 1981;135:364–367.

161. Green RL, Huntsman RG, Serjeant GR. The sickle-cell and altitude. BMJ 1971;4:593–595.

162. Mahony BS, Githens JH. Sickling crises and altitude: occurrence in the Colorado patient population. Clin Pediatr (Phila) 1979;18: 431–438.

163. Lane PA, Githens JH. Splenic syndrome at mountain altitudes in sickle cell trait. Its occurrence in nonblack persons. JAMA 1985;253:2251–2254.

164. National Oceanic and Atmospheric Administration. US standard atmosphere, 1976. Washington, DC: NOAA, 1976.

165. West JB. Prediction of barometric pressures at high altitude with the use of model atmospheres.

J Appl Physiol 1996;81:1850–1854.

166. Hultgren HN, Wilson R. Blood gas abnormalities and optimum therapy in high altitude pulmonary edema. Clin Res 1981;29:99A. Abstract.

167. Bärtsch P, Vock P, Maggiorini M, et al. Respiratory symptoms, radiographic and physiologic correlations at high altitude. In: Sutton JR, Coates G, Remmers JE, eds. Hypoxia: The adaptations. Philadelphia: B.C. Decker, 1990:241–245.

Chapter 107

Air Pollution, Exercise, Nutrition, and Health

William S. Linn
Henry Gong, Jr.

This chapter reviews scientific evidence concerning the effects of common air pollutants on human health and the modifying influences of exercise, nutrition, and other personally controllable factors. Both indoor and outdoor pollutants are discussed. Although outdoor pollution receives more public attention, indoor pollution may be a greater threat to individuals who spend the large majority of their time indoors. This chapter aims to provide general advice to promote healthy lifestyles; it may also provide guidance in advising individual patients whose illnesses may be exacerbated by their pollution exposures. As in some other areas of medicine, the scientific evidence concerning specific air pollution effects is often limited, ambiguous, or unclear in its clinical implications. Thus, cautious interpretation, judgment, and careful application are essential.

Climate and topography, as well as human activities, determine the variety and distribution of air pollution possible in a given locality. Weather changes may affect pollution levels not only outdoors, but also indoors, as windows are opened or closed and heaters or air conditioners start or stop. It is important, though often difficult, to distinguish weather effects from pollution effects when evaluating health problems either in a single patient or in a large population.

CHARACTERISTICS AND KNOWN EFFECTS OF COMMON AIR POLLUTANTS

Sources of Further Information

The relevant scientific literature is voluminous, and only a small sample can be cited here. Recent review articles and monographs provide more detailed surveys of specific air

pollutant effects (1–10), effects of bioaerosols (airborne allergens of biologic origin) (11), and the broader applications of toxicologic science to environmental problems (12). The United States Environmental Protection Agency (EPA) periodically publishes criteria documents concerning the outdoor pollutants it regulates, with comprehensive reviews of recent health studies and other scientific evidence relevant to regulatory policy. The National Library of Medicine's MEDLINE database allows efficient on-line searches for literature on specific pollutants or effects, provided that search terms are chosen judiciously (13). Relevant Medical Subject Heading (MeSH) terms include "air-pollution," "air-pollutants," "air-pollutants-environmental," "air-pollution-indoor," and "air-pollutants-occupational." These are best used in combination with more specific search terms to define the pollutant or effect of interest.

Outdoor Pollutants Subject to Federal Air Quality Regulations

Introduction

Table 107-1 summarizes current health-based air quality standards established by EPA. These standards relate to "criteria" pollutants (i.e., pollutants with many sources and widespread exposures), which can be controlled but not eliminated. Another important category, "air-toxics" or "hazardous pollutants," includes substances (mostly organic compounds) with relatively few sources and more geographically restricted exposures (1,2). Table 107-2 lists acute symptoms which typically result from short-term exposures (8 hours or less) to specific criteria pollutants, within or modestly above the ambient concentration range, as judged from relevant

Table 107-1 Primary National Ambient Air Quality Standards (NAAQS), Established by U.S. Environmental Protection Agency for the Protection of Public Health

POLLUTANT	AVERAGING TIME	CONCENTRATION*
Ozone (O_3)	1 hour	0.12 ppm (235 μg/m^3)
	8 hours[a]	0.08 ppm (157 μg/m^3)[a]
Particulate matter <10 μm diameter (PM$_{10}$)	24 hours	150 μg/m^3
	1 year	50 μg/m^3
Particulate matter <2.5 μm diameter (PM$_{2.5}$)	24 hours[a]	65 μg/m^{3a}
	1 year[a]	15 μg/m^{3a}
Sulfur dioxide (SO_2)	3 hours	0.50 ppm (1300 μg/m^3)
	24 hours	0.14 ppm (365 μg/m^3)
	1 year	0.03 ppm (80 μg/m^3)
Nitrogen dioxide (NO_2)	1 year	0.053 ppm (100 μg/m^3)
Carbon monoxide (CO)	1 hour	35 ppm (40 mg/m^3)
	8 hours	9 ppm (10 mg/m^3)
Lead (Pb)	3 months	1.5 μg/m^3

* News media may report pollution in terms of the Pollutant Standard Index (PSI) rather than concentration. A PSI of 100 represents 100% of the NAAQS concentration.
[a] New standard issued in 1997.

Table 107-2 Short-Term Symptomatic Responses to Common Air Pollutants

POLLUTANT	TYPICAL SYMPTOMS	OBSERVED BY
O_3	Substernal irritation, becoming more painful as exposure continues; dry cough	Lab exposures and field studies
SO_2	Postexercise wheeze and dyspnea in asthmatics	Lab exposures
CO	Faster onset of exercise angina in cardiac patients	Lab exposures (above ambient range)
PM	Uncertain (various cardiopulmonary conditions may be exacerbated)	Epidemiology
NO_2	Symptoms unlikely at ambient concentrations. Accidental high-level occupational exposures may cause only mild eye and respiratory irritation immediately, but life-threatening small-airway inflammation may ensue.	

laboratory or field studies. Any symptom reports associated with pollution exposure should be interpreted cautiously. A given exposure may induce different symptoms in different individuals; the pollutant dose necessary to induce symptoms may vary markedly in different people; and the intensity of symptoms may not be a good indication of the severity of health risk, either short-term or long-term.

Ozone

Ozone (O_3) is most prominent among "secondary photochemical oxidant" pollutants. Other secondary photochemical oxidants (e.g., organic peroxides) may resemble O_3 in their toxic properties, but usually occur at lower concentrations. *Secondary* means that O_3 is not emitted directly by common pollution sources; it forms in the atmosphere through chemical reactions among directly emitted (primary) pollutants. *Photochemical* means that these reactions require sunlight. Specifically, solar ultraviolet radiation acts on volatile organic compounds (VOCs) in the presence of nitrogen oxides (NO_x) to form O_3. Normal fuel burning in vehicles, industries, and

homes emits VOCs and No$_x$, along with other pollutants. Thus, calm sunny summer weather in urban areas with many combustion sources encourages O_3 pollution.[1] Ozone levels are usually highest in the afternoon and lowest at night or in early morning.

Oxidant refers to the O_3 molecule's strong tendency to revert to normal oxygen (O_2) by giving up an oxygen free radical. By that means, O_3 can destroy many important biologic molecules, especially those containing carbon-carbon double bonds or sulfhydryl (—SH) groups. Accordingly, inhaled O_3 has the potential to disrupt many physiologic processes. However, for O_3, as for most other common air pollutants, current knowledge is not sufficient to relate specific

---

[1] Los Angeles and Mexico City are the most prominent examples, but many other areas, in developing as well as industrialized nations, can experience medically significant O_3 pollution. Once formed, O_3 may travel hundreds of kilometers downwind, and thus may affect rural areas with few pollution sources.

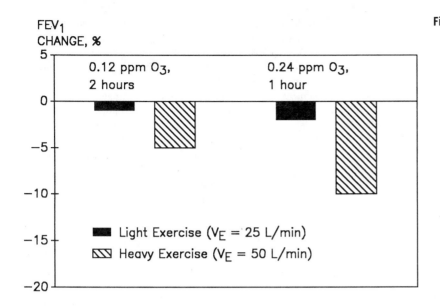

FEV$_1$
CHANGE, %

0.12 ppm O$_3$,
2 hours

0.24 ppm O$_3$,
1 hour

■ Light Exercise (V$_E$ = 25 L/min)
▧ Heavy Exercise (V$_E$ = 50 L/min)

Figure 107-1 Short-term losses in lung function expected in typical young adult men exposed to ozone at different concentrations, durations of exposure, and ventilation rates, as determined from prediction formulas in McDonnell WF, Stewart PW, Andreoni S, et al. Prediction of ozone-induced FEV$_1$ changes. Am J Respir Crit Care Med 1997; 156:715–722.

chemical reactions with specific toxic responses at cell, tissue, or organ levels.

Ozone is not highly soluble in water or biological fluids. Thus, some inhaled O$_3$ is not "scrubbed" by the upper respiratory tract, but penetrates to distal bronchioles and proximal alveoli. This "small-airway" region is the site of most prominent pathologic changes in laboratory animals exposed to O$_3$, although upper-airway injury may be detectable also. In humans, breathing route (oral versus nasal) has little effect on the acute lower-respiratory response to O$_3$ as measured by symptoms and decrements in common tests of lung function. Inflammatory injury from experimental O$_3$ inhalation has been documented not only in animals, but also in human volunteers studied by postexposure nasal or bronchoalveolar lavage. Lavage fluid typically shows increases in biochemical mediators and inflammatory cells, as well as increased protein levels, which indicate increased permeability of the alveolar-capillary membranes. A person who exercises heavily (e.g., with ventilation rates above 40 liters/min) outdoors for several hours may inhale enough O$_3$ to elicit inflammatory responses, even when air quality meets the current National Ambient Air Quality Standard (NAAQS) for O$_3$.

Physiologically, O$_3$ inhalation impairs performance on conventional lung function tests, temporarily reducing vital capacity (primarily inspiratory capacity) and forced expiratory flow rates. Ozone also increases airway responsiveness to inhaled histamine or cholinergic drug aerosols (i.e., it causes normal airways to behave more like asthmatic airways). Interestingly, volunteers with diagnosed asthma exposed to O$_3$ generally show a range of lung function losses similar to healthy volunteers. Nevertheless, similar function losses may result in more severe symptoms or exercise limitations in asthmatics, who may have diminished respiratory reserve. The typical symptomatic response to O$_3$ begins with slight substernal pain and dry cough on deep inspiration. The effects are seen in controlled laboratory O$_3$ exposures in otherwise clean air, and in field studies of people exercising outdoors. Physiologic and symptomatic responses usually reverse within a few hours at rest in cleaner air, but inflammatory responses peak somewhat later—roughly 18 hours after

exposure. The O$_3$ concentration, the ventilation rate during exposure, and the duration of exposure influence the severity of response, with concentration being most important (Figure 107-1). One or two hours of intermittent heavy exercise at 0.2 to 0.3 ppm (concentrations attainable in Los Angeles or Mexico City) or several hours of heavy exercise at 0.12 ppm (the 1-hour NAAQS level, attainable in many areas) may evoke symptoms and appreciable lung function losses.

If O$_3$ exposures are repeated on several successive days, function losses and symptoms diminish, but many inflammatory responses seem to persist. In single exposures, lung function changes do not appear to correlate with inflammatory response intensity, although function changes and inflammatory responses show reasonably similar dose-response relationships when averaged over groups of exposed volunteers. Thus, assuming that inflammation represents the greater threat of eventual chronic lung damage, a marked symptom or lung function response may have a useful protective effect (i.e., it may inhibit further exercise and thus limit the inhaled O$_3$ dose). Individual characteristics that govern any of these responses are not well known, but seem to be reasonably stable over periods of weeks or months. Middle-aged and older adults appear less responsive than younger adults, in terms of lung function and symptoms. Although relevant evidence is limited and not entirely consistent, O$_3$ exposure appears to enhance airway reactivity to subsequent allergen inhalation in patients with allergic asthma or rhinitis.

In a number of metropolitan areas, including some with relatively mild air pollution, daily O$_3$ levels have shown statistical associations with daily hospital admissions for respiratory illnesses (1,4). As in most air pollution epidemiology, the interpretation is complicated because other pollutants, especially particulates, and weather stresses may covary with O$_3$. *Acid summer haze* is a general term to describe the combination of O$_3$ with particulate pollutants (usually including sulfuric acid and sulfate salts) associated with excess respiratory illness in the northeastern United States and in Canada. In metropolitan Los Angeles, daily rates of death from cardiovascular illness or from all nontrauma causes have shown a relationship to daily O_3 levels, and this association appears to be independent of particulate pollution (14).

Long-term effects of repeated O_3 exposures have been difficult to investigate directly in humans. However, the aging-associated reductions in lung function have been suggested to be faster in residents of highly O_3-polluted regions; long-term animal studies have demonstrated the development of chronic lung lesions, primarily in terminal and respiratory bronchioles, at exposure levels not much higher than occur in outdoor air pollution (1).

Particulate Matter

Under EPA regulations, any substance that forms airborne solid and/or liquid particles 10 micrometers (μm) or less in diameter[2] is a component of particulate pollution. Thus, particulate pollutants' physical, chemical, and biologic properties may differ greatly in different locations, or in different seasons at the same location. Particles 2.5 to 10 μm in diameter (*coarse* particles) consist mostly of minerals from the earth's crust, and are mildly alkaline and not very water-soluble. Particles less than 2.5 μm in diameter (*fine* particles) consist mostly of combustion products. Fine particles often contain water-soluble strong acids, or salts formed by these acids' reaction with atmospheric ammonia, along with insoluble elemental carbon and organic compounds of relatively high molecular weight. The acids and salts typically are secondary pollutants, formed by atmospheric reactions of primary pollutant gases—oxides of nitrogen and sulfur. The carbon-containing substances may be primary or secondary. Fly ash—fragments of insoluble mineral constituents of coal or oil, often containing heavy metals—is another common primary constituent of fine particulate pollution.

Certain combustion processes yield large numbers of *ultrafine* particles, 0.1 μm or less in diameter, which later agglomerate into larger particles. Some animal studies indicate that fresh ultrafine particles may be much more toxic than larger particles, at much lower concentrations. The implications for ambient air pollution and human health are currently unknown.

The EPA has issued a new regulation specific to fine particles ($PM_{2.5}$), intended to concentrate pollution control efforts on combustion products rather than on windblown dust (coarse particles). Both chemical composition and aerodynamic properties suggest a greater health risk from fine particles. Inhaled coarse particles tend to deposit in larger conducting airways, from which they can be removed by mucociliary clearance within minutes, and then either expectorated or swallowed and eliminated through the gastrointestinal tract. Inhaled fine particles are more likely to deposit in peripheral airways or alveoli, where clearance is much slower. Insoluble particles there may be phagocytized by macrophages and carried to the mucociliary escalator or to regional lymph nodes. Fine particles constitute most of

the foreign material found at autopsy in the lung parenchyma of elderly nonsmokers (15).

With a few notable exceptions, animal toxicologic studies have shown little effect on lung function or symptoms from any component of particulate pollution, except at concentrations far above the present-day range in ambient air (1–4,9). Sulfuric acid aerosols appear to affect mucociliary clearance at concentrations close to the ambient range, increasing clearance rates in some circumstances and decreasing them in others (9). In one series of studies with guinea pigs, a species highly susceptible to respiratory insults, fresh combustion-derived ultrafine zinc oxide particles coated with sulfuric acid appeared to cause biologically significant and persistent lung lesions, at acid concentrations within the ambient range (as low as 20 μg/m^3). Ordinary aqueous aerosols of sulfuric acid showed no such effects (16). In another series of studies with rats, fresh ultrafine particles generated by heating polytetrafluoroethylene, a chemically inert substance, appeared to be lethal at concentrations below 60 μg/m^3 (17). A preliminary report has indicated that ordinary urban particulate pollution, if aerodynamically concentrated to several times its usual level, can be lethal to rats with preexisting pulmonary inflammation or chronic bronchitis (18). Another preliminary report has indicated subtle electrocardiographic abnormalities, suggestive of increased vulnerability to ventricular fibrillation, in dogs inhaling particulate matter from an oil-burning power plant (19). Thus, it may be that ill effects of particulate pollution depend on some combination of multiple toxic substances (perhaps only existing in fresh combustion products), small particle sizes, and highly susceptible hosts.

Controlled human exposure studies most often use sulfuric acid or a sulfate salt to model typical water-soluble secondary particles. Elemental carbon particles also have been studied in combination with H_2SO_4 (20). Most of these human studies have shown little short-term effect from any particulate exposure at a realistic concentration (1–4). However, changes in mucociliary clearance rates have been reported (9,21), as well as slight lung function reductions in adolescent asthmatics (22).

Despite the limited positive laboratory evidence, there is major concern about particulate health effects among health scientists, arising from numerous epidemiologic studies of urban populations that have shown that cardiopulmonary illness and death rates vary in relation to ambient particulate concentrations (1–8). These statistical associations have been observed in Europe, Asia, and the Americas, in summer and winter, in warm and cold climates, and across a broad range of socioeconomic circumstances. The only obvious common factor is a combustion source for the particulate pollution—whether motor vehicles, industries, or home heating and cooking. Associations of morbidity and mortality with particles are evident even in comparatively unpolluted cities where PM_{10} concentrations meet existing air quality standards. Increased ill health is usually evident within 1 or 2 days after a rise in pollution levels. Less serious acute effects—subtle changes in lung function, increased likelihood of lower-respiratory symptoms in healthy people, and increased frequency or severity of asthma attacks—also are associated with particulate pollution.

---

[2]For present purposes, particles are defined not by physical diameter, but by aerodynamic diameter, which depends on particle shape and density as well as size. Any particle that moves in air similarly to a spherical water droplet of 10 μm physical diameter has an aerodynamic diameter of 10 μm.

Pathophysiologic mechanisms to explain the epidemiologic observations are largely speculative at present. To what extent the particulate-health associations reflect cause and effect, and to what extent they are explained by confounding factors such as weather or other coexisting pollutants, are still matters of debate (23). Presumably, the people most at risk of serious acute effects (whatever the immediate cause) are the elderly with preexisting chronic cardiopulmonary diseases. Whether any of these chronic diseases can be caused or exacerbated by long-term particulate pollution exposure is another important question. Early studies showing shorter life expectancy in more highly polluted areas were criticized for inadequate control of confounding factors, smoking in particular. However, more recent studies of populations with documented smoking histories, or of nonsmoking populations, have found increased death rates from respiratory cancers and non-neoplastic cardiopulmonary diseases, as well as increased prevalence of chronic respiratory symptoms and subnormal lung function, in areas with elevated particulate pollution (1,2,5,24,25).

Airborne allergens of biologic origin may be an important component of particulate pollution. Although airborne pollen and fungus spores are usually considered part of the natural environment, some of them are airborne byproducts of human economic activity (either agriculture or ornamental landscaping), and may be considered pollutants in that sense. Exposures to these bioaerosols vary with location, season, and current weather, in patterns which may or may not track the variation of criteria (combustion-related) pollutants. The diversity of aeroallergens and the widely varying patterns of sensitivity within exposed populations make it difficult to investigate exposures and effects. In the few epidemiologic studies that examined aeroallergens as well as criteria pollutants, both appeared to be important influences on short-term respiratory health (26,27).

Numerous agricultural products release aeroallergens that may cause illness in exposed susceptible people. Allergens from one such product, bulk soybeans, have been implicated in asthma outbreaks in the population living near cargo-loading terminals (28).

Sulfur Dioxide

Most human exposure to atmospheric sulfur dioxide (SO_2) results from the burning of coal or oil containing sulfur. Other less common SO_2 sources are metal smelters and active volcanoes. Once in the atmosphere, SO_2 may be oxidized to form secondary particulate sulfuric acid and sulfate salts (see the previous section). Most SO_2 sources also emit primary particulates. Thus, atmospheric SO_2 and particulate levels usually correlate strongly, making it difficult to distinguish their health effects by epidemiologic investigation. In Britain, particulate controls appeared to decrease premature deaths even when SO_2 remained uncontrolled, suggesting that particulates were the more toxic constituent of the "SO_2-particulate complex." That conclusion is strengthened by newer findings of adverse health effects in areas with appreciable particulate pollution but little SO_2 (1,2). Nevertheless, unfavorable effects from present-day SO_2 levels cannot be ruled out.

Sulfur dioxide is highly soluble in water. Thus, unlike O_3, SO_2 can be "scrubbed" from the upper airway effectively, and nasal breathing mitigates its effects, relative to oral breathing. Laboratory studies of animals and healthy human volunteers generally have shown little effect at realistic exposure concentrations. However, asthmatics appear consistently more sensitive to SO_2 than people with no history of chronic respiratory problems (1–4,9,29). Some patients with upper-respiratory allergies but without diagnosed asthma also are responsive to SO_2. Asthmatics' typical response, as shown in controlled laboratory studies, is acute bronchoconstriction during or shortly after exercise. This may occur after only a few minutes' exposure to SO_2 at 0.25 to 0.5 ppm. Ambient concentrations in that range are uncommon in areas with modern pollution controls, but may be experienced occasionally near large SO_2 sources. The severity of response depends on dose rate (SO_2 concentration times ventilation rate) more than on total inhaled dose. In other words, prolonging the exposure does not appear to increase the intensity of bronchoconstriction.

Sulfur dioxide–induced bronchoconstriction resembles exercise-induced bronchoconstriction (EIB), in terms of its time course and its response to medications. The SO_2 response is often manifested as an exacerbation of EIB—a greater degree of constriction than would occur after similar exercise in clean air. [By contrast, O_3 exposure seems to have no effect on EIB (30).] However, at sufficiently high SO_2 exposure concentrations (possible in some occupational settings), bronchoconstriction can occur at rest. Bronchoconstriction after exercise at sub-ppm levels of SO_2 usually reverses after 10 to 30 minutes' rest, even if SO_2 exposure continues, and does not commonly lead to a full-blown asthmatic attack. Because cold, dry air also exerts a bronchoconstrictive effect, the effect of SO_2 may be exacerbated at low temperatures. Conventional beta-adrenergic bronchodilator drugs are effective in blocking or reversing SO_2-induced bronchoconstriction as well as EIB. Other asthma medications are less effective in preventing SO_2 effects, but may mitigate them by improving baseline lung function. Severity of asthma does not appear to predict the degree of bronchoconstriction evoked by a given SO_2 exposure. However, even relatively slight SO_2 responses may be clinically important in severe asthmatics.

Nitrogen Dioxide

Nitrogen and oxygen, the major constituents of air, combine chemically at high temperature to produce nitric oxide (NO) during all conventional fuel-burning processes. Atmospheric oxygen can oxidize NO further to nitrogen dioxide (NO_2), which is relatively persistent in the atmosphere, although it may be converted to nitric acid (still in the gas phase) and nitrate salts (secondary particulate matter). Except in the most heavily polluted urban areas (Los Angeles in particular), indoor exposures to NO_2 (discussed below in the section on indoor pollution) are likely to be more important than outdoor exposures.

Nitrogen dioxide, like O_3, is a relatively insoluble oxidizing gas that can penetrate to the deep lung. However, NO_2 is a less powerful oxidant than O_3. In laboratory animal studies, NO_2 appears to target the respiratory bronchioles, as does O_3; however, much higher concentrations of NO_2 (above the range in ambient pollution) are required to cause damage, and the details of pathologic change appear somewhat different (1,2,9).

Controlled human exposure studies with NO_2 have yielded a mixture of negative results and equivocally positive results (1–4,9). Respiratory symptoms or changes in conventional lung function tests generally are not found even with exercise at concentrations of several ppm. Some investigators have reported increased airway responsiveness to inhaled cholinergic drugs after NO_2 exposures at only 0.1 to 0.3 ppm; others have been unable to replicate these findings. More recently, NO_2 exposure has been reported to increase responsiveness to inhaled allergens in allergic asthmatics. Recent findings from bronchoalveolar lavage studies of healthy volunteers (31) indicate that lower-airway inflammation follows a single 4-hour exposure at 2 ppm NO_2. The clinical implications for common outdoor pollution exposures, at concentrations an order of magnitude lower, are uncertain.

Epidemiologic studies have sought to demonstrate health effects of NO_2 in outdoor exposures related to a large point source, and in indoor exposures related to gas stoves. The tendency of other pollutants to accompany NO_2 complicates the interpretation of all these studies. Results have been mixed, but some studies indicate an increased incidence of acute lower-respiratory illnesses in more highly exposed populations, particularly for infants and children. A recent large-scale, rigorous study of infants exposed indoors found no effect of NO_2 (32), although the range of exposures may have been lower for this population than for some others. Acute accidental high-level indoor NO_2 exposures can present appreciable health risk; see the section below on indoor pollution.

Carbon Monoxide

Carbon monoxide (CO) results from incomplete combustion of any carbon-containing fuel. Motor vehicle exhaust is the major outdoor source, although emissions and ambient CO concentrations have fallen considerably with widespread use of catalytic converters. Oxygenated organic compounds such as methyl tertiary-butyl ether (MTBE) are added to gasoline with the intent of reducing CO emissions further. Outdoor CO concentrations may vary considerably over short distances. Concentrations in or near heavy traffic may be much higher than "background" levels measured at monitoring stations.

The important physiologic property of CO is its tendency to bind to hemoglobin (1–4,9). In doing so it reduces blood oxygen transport, not only by direct displacement of oxygen molecules, but also by altering the shape of the hemoglobin molecule such that it less readily releases oxygen to tissues. Metabolic production of CO maintains a carboxyhemoglobin (COHb) concentration near 0.5% in otherwise unexposed healthy people. Steady exposure to atmospheric CO at X ppm will result in a COHb concentration of about 0.16X%, if the exposure continues long enough to allow equilibration between atmosphere and blood. Equilibration may take 8 hours or longer in a large adult at rest, but occurs faster with increased ventilation rate and smaller body size. Thus, if air quality just meets the NAAQS of 9 ppm over an 8-hour period, a blood COHb concentration around 1.4% can be expected. For comparison, typical cigarette smokers intermittently inhale 20,000 ppm of CO or more, and maintain COHb concentrations of 5% or higher.

Organs most vulnerable to CO effects are those most sensitive to hypoxia—the heart and brain. People most susceptible are those with preexisting impairments of oxygen delivery caused by chronic cardiopulmonary disease. Slightly more rapid onset of myocardial ischemia during exercise (documented both by angina and by ST-segment depression in the electrocardiogram) has been found in patients with coronary artery disease after controlled CO exposures that raised COHb above 2% (1,2,33). This is the lowest level at which any physiologic or clinical effect has been clearly documented. Increased incidence of ventricular arrhythmia has been reported at concentrations near 5%, although the evidence is mixed (1,2). Neurologic effects appear to require COHb concentrations of 5% or higher. Acute accidental high-level exposures to CO indoors may cause serious cardiovascular and neurologic effects, including death; see the section below on indoor pollution. Hospital admissions of Medicare beneficiaries for congestive heart failure have shown associations with ambient CO concentrations in several large U.S. metropolitan areas (34). Measured concentrations in most of these cities were usually well within the NAAQS; but, as mentioned before, this does not rule out higher exposures to people close to CO sources. It is not clear whether this effect is specific to CO.

Lead

Airborne lead occurs in various chemical forms as a component of particulate pollution. From the 1920s through the early 1980s, lead was a widespread and important air pollutant because of the routine addition of lead compounds to gasoline to improve its burning characteristics. Since the general adoption of catalytic converters and unleaded gasoline, airborne exposure to lead has become relatively unimportant in the United States, with the exception of a few areas near industrial or natural sources. Lead may still be found in soil previously exposed to leaded gasoline exhaust, as well as inside and outside older buildings with lead-based paint. Exposure may occur both by ingestion and by inhalation. Lead accumulates in the body, primarily in bone, and exerts a variety of chronic effects (1,2,9), the best documented of which are neurobehavioral dysfunction in children and increased blood pressure in adults. Blood lead concentrations above 10 μg/dL appear to increase the risk of these effects.

Indoor Pollution

This section addresses conventional homes and public indoor spaces, excluding occupational exposures in indoor workplaces. Sources of pollutants in indoor air may be entirely indoors (usually the case with environmental tobacco smoke, for example), entirely outdoors (usually the case with O_3 or SO_2), or both indoors and outdoors (often the case with NO_2 and CO).[3] Thus, the indoor/outdoor (I/O) concentration ratio differs importantly for different pollutants, depending on

---

[3]Certain appliances or air cleaning devices, including photocopiers, electrostatic precipitators, and odor-control devices, which generate O_3 to react with foul-smelling organic compounds, may be significant indoor sources of O_3 if they malfunction or are used improperly, especially in poorly ventilated rooms.

physical and chemical properties, sources of pollutants, and air exchange rates between indoors and outdoors.

For O_3, which has few indoor sources and which reacts readily with wall and furniture surfaces, the I/O ratio is usually well below 1. The ratio may approach zero in indoor areas with air conditioning, air filtration (especially with activated carbon), and no open windows. In other words, the indoor environment usually provides appreciable protection against O_3 exposure. That is also true to some extent for another reactive gas, SO_2.

At the other extreme is CO, which is unreactive with indoor surfaces and cannot be removed from air by common filter media. With no indoor sources, the I/O ratio for CO will remain close to 1 on average, and staying indoors will provide no protection against CO exposure.[‡] Indoor sources of CO, such as smoking and fuel-burning appliances, may increase the ratio well above 1. In the extreme, hundreds of deaths per year occur in the United States from CO poisoning caused by defective or misused appliances, usually space heaters.

Nitrogen dioxide, somewhat like CO, is difficult to filter out of incoming outside air, and may have indoor sources, particularly smoking and fuel-burning appliances. Thus, the I/O ratio for NO_2 is likely to be 1 or higher. Users of indoor ice rinks, where exhaust gases from fuel-burning ice resurfacers may accumulate, have experienced clinically significant toxic exposures to NO_2 on a number of occasions (35,36). These situations exemplify the risks from pollution sources in poorly ventilated indoor spaces, and from vigorous exercise during high-level pollution exposure.

Particulate matter is another form of pollution for which both indoor and outdoor sources may be important. Outdoor fine particles penetrate indoors efficiently, and coarse particles somewhat less efficiently; thus, I/O ratios are likely to be close to 1 without indoor sources, or higher than 1 with them. Particles can be removed from indoor air by suitable filters or electrostatic precipitators (see the section below on preventive measures), but few homes or other buildings are so equipped. Smoking markedly increases the indoor level of particulate pollution. Cooking and dust-creating hobby activities also may be important indoor sources. Conventional vacuum cleaning generates large quantities of airborne particles. Vacuum cleaners with high-efficiency particulate filters minimize this problem, but cost more than conventional models. Indoor sources of bioaerosols, including chronic dampness (a source of mold and mildew), carpets or bedding (dust mite habitats), furry pets, and insect pests (e.g., cockroaches) are significant risk factors for chronic respiratory health problems (11,37–40).

Various VOCs may reach medically significant concentrations in indoor air (9,39,40). One of the most important is formaldehyde (HCHO), a product of normal metabolism,

but also a potent eye/respiratory irritant and a suspected human carcinogen. Formaldehyde and other VOCs are released by smoking, and by indoor structures and furnishings (bonding agents of particle board and plywood, carpets, upholstery fabrics), especially when new.

Indoor air pollutants without short-term health effects, but with potential for catastrophic effects from long-term exposure, include asbestos fibers (particulate matter), as well as radon (a radioactive chemically inert gas) and radon daughter nuclei (found on particles). Most homes built before the mid-1970s contain asbestos in some building materials, which should present little hazard as long as it remains in place. When indoor asbestos release is suspected, qualified professional help should be sought to evaluate the problem and take appropriate action, which may involve either sealing the asbestos in place or removing it (39). Possible long-term effects of asbestos exposure include interstitial fibrosis, peribronchiolitis, pleural mesothelioma, and lung cancer (41). Such effects are rare apart from occupational exposures. Radon is emitted by natural rocks and soils, and enters buildings via gaps in their foundations. Occasionally, building materials or the water supply are important sources. Lung cancer is the principal hazard from radon (39). Control measures may involve sealing the routes of entry from soil, or increasing the indoor air exchange rate to reduce the concentrations of radioactive species.

Summary

Of common outdoor pollutants, ozone, a strong oxidizing agent with marked irritant and inflammatory effects, shows the most evidence of acute and chronic health risks in laboratory toxicologic studies. In epidemiologic studies, particulate matter shows the most evidence of acute and chronic health risks; the specific chemical and physical agents responsible, and the mechanisms of their effects, are unknown. Nitrogen dioxide somewhat resembles ozone in its effects, but appears less toxic at similar concentrations. Sulfur dioxide may acutely exacerbate asthma, and carbon monoxide may exacerbate cardiac ischemia, at worst-case outdoor ambient concentrations.

Ozone and sulfur dioxide exposures are usually higher outdoors than indoors. Nitrogen dioxide and carbon monoxide exposures may be higher indoors if there are indoor sources such as gas appliances, especially if they are not properly vented. Other common indoor pollutant health risks include volatile organic compounds and airborne allergens.

INFLUENCES OF EXERCISE AND RELEVANT PREVENTIVE MEASURES

Basic Strategies for Health Protection

Regular exercise is clearly important for good health. On the other hand, exercise, by increasing ventilation, increases the inhaled dose of pollutants and thus the risk of toxic effects. Thus, for people routinely exposed to air pollution, the basic strategy for health promotion is to choose exercise conditions that minimize pollution effects. This may mean significantly reducing the intensity and/or the duration of exercise during

---

[‡]However, since many buildings are designed for relatively slow exchange of air with the outdoors, at least partly under the occupants' control, it may be possible to keep the I/O ratio below 1 by admitting outdoor air faster at times of low CO pollution, and slower at times of high CO pollution (usually peak traffic hours).

pollution episodes, rescheduling exercise periods to times of day when pollution is low, relocating the exercise to a cleaner area, or using an air cleaning device when no better alternative exists.

Strategies to Minimize Specific Exposures

Ozone

As mentioned previously, O_3 tends to peak on warm, sunny summer afternoons. In urban areas, O_3 levels usually fall in late afternoon, as traffic peaks and exhaust gases consume O_3. In less populous downwind areas, peak O_3 levels may be lower, but elevated concentrations may persist until late evening. Early morning is probably the best time to exercise outdoors while minimizing the inhaled dose of O_3. When outdoor O_3 is high, exercising indoors may provide considerable protection, if indoor air exchanges with the outside relatively slowly, so that O_3 can react with indoor surfaces, and/or if air conditioning with filtration is in use.

Particulate Matter

Outdoor particulate pollution does not necessarily show a marked diurnal pattern. It is likely to be highest closest to sources (e.g., heavily traveled roads). As mentioned previously, staying indoors provides only slight protection against outdoor fine particles. Indoor exercise with avoidance of indoor sources, especially smoking, and filtration of indoor air (see the section below on protective equipment) may be the best alternative in localities with heavy particulate pollution.

Sulfur Dioxide

Sulfur dioxide effects are primarily important to asthmatics, as indicated previously. Pre-exercise prophylaxis with a common inhaled beta-adrenergic asthma medication (e.g., albuterol) usually will block bronchoconstrictive effects from SO_2 and from exercise itself. Exposure avoidance involves staying away from large SO_2 sources such as coal-burning power plants and smelters. Staying indoors may offer some protection when SO_2 is elevated outdoors.

Nitrogen Dioxide

Outdoor NO_2 tends to be highest at times and places of heavy motor vehicle traffic. Indoor sources of exposure seem more important than outdoor sources, except perhaps in high-pollution areas like Los Angeles. Indoor exposures can be minimized by properly venting gas appliances and avoiding their use during exercise periods.

Carbon Monoxide

Carbon monoxide exposures are high in the vicinity of motor vehicle exhaust, not only outdoors in heavily trafficked and poorly ventilated areas, but sometimes indoors, in buildings with attached garages and/or with air intakes near roads or driveways. Combustion appliances are the other major source of indoor CO pollution, which can be lethal in the event of serious malfunction or misuse, as mentioned previously. Deliberate use of an unvented cooking appliance (e.g., a charcoal grill) to heat a tightly closed room is a frequent cause of death or near-death from CO poisoning, but these incidents also can occur during normal operation of an appliance

with a blocked or damaged exhaust apparatus. Minimizing emissions and maximizing ventilation with cleaner air when emissions are unavoidable are the appropriate control measures for indoor CO, since filtering CO-polluted air is seldom feasible.

Air Exchange Rates and Indoor Exposures

Harmful indoor pollution exposures often result from inadequate ventilation of a building (12,39,40), which often results from energy-saving measures. The appropriate air exchange rate for a given indoor space depends on the level of unavoidable indoor pollutant emissions (including those from human bodies), the costs of conditioning outdoor air to acceptable indoor temperature and humidity levels, and the costs of cleaning pollutants (whether of indoor or of outdoor origin) from indoor air. If relatively clean and comfortable outdoor air is available, rapid air exchange rates are indicated. If outdoor air is polluted and/or at extreme temperature, slower air exchange and indoor air cleaning are indicated. Typical central air conditioning systems recirculate a high proportion of indoor air, and mix in only a small amount of outdoor "makeup" air (e.g., 10%). Thus, if indoor pollution sources are significant, air cleaning devices must operate on the entire air flow. If only outdoor pollution is significant, only the makeup air need be cleaned.

Protective Equipment

Various filter masks (also known as respirators) are available for personal protection against occupational exposures. Some of these may offer a degree of protection against ambient particulate pollution, including bioaerosols. Masks that contain activated carbon may also offer some protection against O_3 or SO_2, but not NO_2 or CO. To be effective, masks must be designed to remove the pollutants of concern, must fit properly so that all inhaled air passes through them, and must not unduly increase the work of breathing.

Many devices intended to recirculate and purify the air in a room are available commercially. To remove particulate pollution, electrostatic precipitators and high-efficiency particulate air filters (HEPA filters) have proven effective. (Filters commonly used in air conditioning systems are not very effective at removing the fine particles of health concern.) Activated carbon is the most common medium for removal of gaseous pollutants, including VOCs; aluminum oxide impregnated with potassium permanganate also may be effective. These "chemical filter" media are ineffective against CO and not very effective against NO_2. To be effective, a recirculating air purifier not only must use appropriate air cleaning technology, but also must deliver clean air at a flow rate appropriate to the volume of the room and its air exchange rate (39,40). Even the better household air purifiers can clean only one room, with doors and windows closed to minimize air exchange (often impractical in an exercise area).

Given the limitations of smaller-scale devices, the best way to minimize pollution exposure during indoor exercise is to equip central air conditioning systems with air cleaning accessories, such as electrostatic precipitators, HEPA filters, and chemical filter media. The cost to purchase and maintain such equipment is substantial, and energy costs also increase if more powerful blowers are required. Of course, for any size air cleaner, regular maintenance (cleaning of electrostatic precipitators, replacement of filters) is essential to adequate performance.

Summary

Exercise exacerbates effects of air pollutants by increasing the dose to the primary target organ system, the respiratory tract, while increasing the demands on that system. Therefore, exercise should be planned to minimize pollution exposure. This may involve changing the time or the location of exercise. In general, exposures are more easily controlled indoors than outdoors. Good indoor air quality requires control of indoor pollution sources, as well as adequate air exchange with the outside. Air cleaning devices may be needed to deal with pollutants that are otherwise unavoidable.

INFLUENCES OF NUTRITION AND RELEVANT PREVENTIVE MEASURES

In general, good nutrition promotes good health, which implies good defenses against external stresses, presumably including air pollution. (Part II of this book discusses nutrition in depth.) The extent to which specific nutrients can protect against specific air pollutant effects, or mitigate diseases (e.g., asthma) that increase susceptibility to air pollution, is not yet clear.

Some pollutants, O_3 and NO_2 in particular, exert toxic effects through oxidative mechanisms. Dietary antioxidants might strengthen antioxidant defenses in the lung, and thus prevent or mitigate those effects. Considerable evidence from animal studies shows that vitamins C and E protect against lung pathology caused by O_3 or NO_2 (42–45). Vitamin A also may protect against oxidant gases, as well as carcinogens (46,47). Relatively few human experimental studies have addressed protective effects of nutrients. Early work in the present authors' laboratory failed to detect any effect of vitamin E supplementation, at 800 or 1600 international units (IUs) per day, on lung dysfunction or symptoms in volunteers exposed to O_3 (48). Others' more recent work indicates that vitamin C supplementation (500 mg four times per day) may prevent airway hyperresponsiveness to bronchoconstrictor drugs after exposure to NO_2 above the ambient concentration range (49), and that a combination of vitamins E (400 IU/day) and C (500 mg/day) may have a similar effect in O_3 exposures at realistic levels (50). These findings indirectly suggest that vitamin supplementation can mitigate inflammatory response in the lung. Apparently, there have been no direct investigations of dietary supplements and inflammatory response in humans. Nitrogen dioxide exposure (above the ambient concentration range) has been reported to reduce the concentration of vitamin C in bronchoalveolar lavage fluid (51), implying that the vitamin plays a specific protective role that might be enhanced by supplementation.

From available evidence, it seems reasonable to assume that dietary antioxidants, vitamins C and E in particular, may mitigate inflammatory responses to oxidant pollutants, and thus protect to some degree against long-term chronic lung damage, even if they have little effect on short-term clinical effects of pollutant exposure. Further research will be needed to confirm this.

Asthma and perhaps other chronic respiratory diseases increase susceptibility to some pollutants, as mentioned previously. Any nutritional strategy that mitigates the disease might also mitigate the pollutant effects. There is no well-established nutritional therapy for asthma, except in the few cases exacerbated by specific food allergies; however, vitamin C and manganese appear to combat airway hyperresponsiveness (52,53). Also, in the general population increased dietary vitamin C intake is associated with better lung function (54). This relationship is evident in smokers as well as nonsmokers, suggesting that the vitamin mitigates effects of at least some pollutants found in tobacco smoke. Optimum protective levels of any of these nutrients, and unfavorable side effects (if any) from higher-than-optimum doses, remain to be determined.

REFERENCES

1. Bascom R, Bromberg PA, Costa DA, et al. Health effects of outdoor air pollution, part I. Am J Respir Crit Care Med 1996;153:3–50.

2. Bascom R, Bromberg PA, Costa DA, et al. Health effects of outdoor air pollution, part II. Am J Respir Crit Care Med 1996;153:477–498.

3. Gong H, Linn WS. Air pollution: Health effects. In: Encyclopedia of Energy Technology and the Environment. New York: Wiley, 1995:160–194.

4. Gong H, Linn WS. Health effects of criteria air pollutants. In: Tierney DF, ed. Current pulmonology, vol. 15. St. Louis: Mosby, 1995:341–397.

5. Lipfert FW, Wyzga RE. Air pollution and mortality: issues and uncertainties. J Air Waste Manage Assoc 1995;45:949–966.

6. Pope CA, Bates DV, Raizenne ME. Health effects of particulate air pollution: time for reassessment? Environ Health Perspect 1995;103:472–480.

7. Dockery DW, Pope CA. Acute respiratory effects of particulate air pollution. Annu Rev Public Health 1994;15:107–132.

8. Lipfert FW. Air pollution and community health: a critical review and data sourcebook. New York: Van Nostrand Reinhold, 1994.

9. Lippmann M, ed. Environmental toxicants: human exposures and their health effects. New York: Van Nostrand Reinhold, 1992.

10. McKee DJ, ed. Tropospheric ozone. Boca Raton, FL: Lewis/CRC Press, 1994.

11. Burge HA, ed. Bioaerosols. Boca Raton, FL: CRC Press, 1995.

12. Ottoboni MA. The dose makes the poison: A plain-language guide to

toxicology. 2nd ed. New York: Van Nostrand Reinhold, 1991.

13. Lowe HJ, Barnett GO. Understanding and using the medical subject headings (MeSH) vocabulary to perform literature searches. JAMA 1994;271:1103–1108.

14. Kinney PL, Ozkaynak H. Associations of daily mortality and air pollution in Los Angeles County. Environ Res 1991;54:99–120.

15. Churg A, Brauer M. Human lung parenchyma retains $PM_{2.5}$. Am J Respir Crit Care Med 1997;155: 2109–2111.

16. Amdur MO. Sulfuric acid: The animals tried to tell us. Appl Indust Hyg 1989;4:189–197.

17. Oberdorster G, Gelein RM, Ferin J, et al. Association of particulate pollution and acute mortality: involvement of ultrafine particles? Inhal Toxicol 1995;7:111–124.

18. Godleski JJ, Sioutas C, Katler M, et al. Death from inhalation of concentrated ambient air particles in animal models of pulmonary disease. Am J Respir Crit Care Med 1996;153:A15.

19. Nearing BR, Verrier RL, Skornik WA, et al. Inhaled fly ash results in alteration in cardiac electrophysiologic function. Am J Respir Crit Care Med 1996;153:A543.

20. Anderson KR, Avol EL, Edwards SA, et al. Controlled exposures of volunteers to respirable carbon and sulfuric acid aerosols. J Air Waste Manage Assoc 1992;42: 770–776.

21. Spektor DM, Yen BM, Lippmann M. Effect of concentration and cumulative exposure of inhaled sulfuric acid on tracheobronchial particle clearance in healthy humans. Environ Health Perspect 1989;79:167–172.

22. Koenig JQ, Pearson WE, Horike M. Effects of inhaled sulfuric acid on pulmonary function in adolescent asthmatics. Am Rev Respir Dis 1983;128:221–225.

23. Vedal S. Ambient particles and health: lines that divide. J Air Waste Manage Assoc 1997;47: 551–581.

24. Euler GL, Abbey DE, Magie AR, et al. Chronic obstructive pulmonary disease symptom effects of long-term cumulative exposure to ambient levels of total suspended particulates and sulfur dioxide in Southern California Seventh-Day Adventist residents. Arch Environ Health 1987;42:213–222.

25. Dockery DW, Pope CA, Xu X, et al. An association between air pollution and mortality in six U.S. cities. N Engl J Med 1993;329: 1753–1759.

26. Neas LM, Dockery DW, Burge H, et al. Fungus spores, air pollutants, and other determinants of peak expiratory flow rate in children. Am J Epidemiol 1996;143: 797–807.

27. Delfino RJ, Coate BD, Zeiger RS, et al. Daily asthma severity in relation to personal ozone exposure and outdoor fungal spores. Am J Respir Crit Care Med 1996;154: 633–641.

28. Anto JM, Sunyer J, Rodriguez-Roisin R, et al. Community outbreaks of asthma associated with inhalation of soybean dust. N Engl J Med 1989;320:1097–1102.

29. Sheppard D, Saisho A, Nadel JA, et al. Exercise increases sulfur-dioxide-induced bronchoconstriction in asthmatics. Am Rev Respir Dis 1983;123:486–491.

30. Weymer AR, Gong H, Lyness A, et al. Pre-exposure to ozone does not enhance or produce exercise-induced asthma. Am J Respir Crit Care Med 1994;149:1413–1419.

31. Blomberg A, Krishna MT, Bocchino V, et al. Inflammatory effects of 2 ppm NO_2 on the airways of healthy subjects. Am J Respir Crit Care Med 1997;156:418–424.

32. Samet JM, Lambert WE, Skipper BJ, et al. Nitrogen dioxide and respiratory illness in infants. Am Rev Respir Dis 1993;148:1258–1265.

33. Allred EN, Bleecker ER, Chaitman BR, et al. Short-term effects of carbon monoxide exposure on the exercise performance of subjects with coronary artery disease. N Engl J Med 1989;321:1426–1432.

34. Morris RD, Naumova EN, Munasinghe RL. Ambient air pollution and hospitalization for congestive heart failure among elderly people in seven large U.S. cities. Am J Pub Health 1995;85:1361–1365.

35. Brauer M, Spengler JD. Nitrogen dioxide exposures inside ice skating rinks. Am J Pub Health 1994;84:429–433.

36. Pribyl CR, Racca J. Toxic gas exposures in ice arenas. Clin J Sport Med 1996;6:232–236.

37. Brunekreef B, Dockery DW, Speizer FE, et al. Home dampness and respiratory morbidity in children. Am Rev Respir Dis 1989;140: 1363–1367.

38. Dales RE, Burnett R, Zwanenburg H. Adverse health effects among adults exposed to home dampness and molds. Am Rev Respir Dis 1991;143:505–509.

39. American Thoracic Society, Samet J, workshop chairman. Environmental controls and lung disease. Am Rev Respir Dis 1990;142: 915–939.

40. American Thoracic Society, Samet J, Spengler JD, workshop chairmen. Achieving healthy indoor air. Am J Respir Crit Care Med 1997; 156:S33–S64.

41. Bates DV. Respiratory function in disease. Philadelphia: WB Saunders, 1989.

42. Mustafa MG. Biochemical basis of ozone toxicity. Free Radic Biol Med 1990;9:245–265.

43. Pryor WA. Can vitamin E protect humans against the pathological effects of ozone in smog? Am J Clin Nutr 1991;53:702–722.

44. Menzel DB. Antioxidant vitamins and prevention of lung disease. Ann N Y Acad Sci 1992;669: 141–155.

45. Kelly FJ, Mudway I, Krishna MT, et al. The free radical basis of air pollution: focus on ozone. Respir Med 1995;89:647–656.

46. Paquette NC, Zhang LY, Ellis WA, et al. Vitamin A deficiency enhances ozone-induced lung

injury. Am J Physiol 1996;270: L475–L482.

47. Redlich CA, Grauer JN, Van-Bennekum AM, et al. Characterization of carotenoid, vitamin A, and alpha-tocopherol levels in human lung tissue and pulmonary macrophages. Am J Respir Crit Care Med 1996;154:1436–1443.

48. Hackney JD, Linn WS, Buckley RD, et al. Vitamin E supplementation and respiratory effects of ozone in humans. J Toxicol Environ Health 1981;7:383–390.

49. Mohsenin V. Effect of vitamin C on NO_2-induced airway hyperresponsiveness in normal subjects.

Am Rev Respir Dis 1987;136: 1408–1411.

50. Trenga CA, Williams P, Koenig JQ. Dietary antioxidants attenuate ozone-induced bronchial hyperresponsiveness in asthmatic adults. Am J Respir Crit Care Med 1997; 155:A732.

51. Kelly FJ, Blomberg A, Frew A, et al. Antioxidant kinetics in lung lavage fluid following exposure of humans to nitrogen dioxide. Am J Respir Crit Care Med 1996;154: 1700–1705.

52. Monteleone CA, Sherman AR. Nutrition and asthma. Arch Intern Med 1997;157:23–34.

53. Soutar A, Seaton A, Brown K. Bronchial reactivity and dietary antioxidants. Thorax 1997;52: 166–170.

54. Schwartz J, Weiss ST. Relationship between dietary vitamin C intake and pulmonary function in the First National Health and Nutrition Examination Survey (NHANES I). Am J Clin Nutr 1994;59:110–114.

55. McDonnell WF, Stewart PW, Andreoni S, et al. Prediction of ozone-induced FEV_1 changes. Am J Respir Crit Care Med 1997;156:715–722.

Chapter 108

Sleep, Health, and Well-Being

Gila Lindsley
Lou A. Stephenson

Coronary artery disease, chronic obstructive pulmonary disease, breast cancer, osteoporosis, and disease associated with smoking are serious medical problems already addressed in this volume. These are disorders for which Western medicine has developed a significant arsenal of treatments. In the context of these serious illnesses, spending the highly stressed medical dollar on preventing or correcting sleep loss would seem trivial.

Unfortunately, we are a nation of sleepless people, in a culture that supports working hard, forging onward despite tiredness. Products such as No-Doze and the ever-present availability of stimulants such as coffee—in as many flavors as one would like—allow a person at least temporarily to override the sleepiness and tiredness that comes from sleep loss. Few people would (or could) "sleep loss" themselves to death. However, many would "sleep loss" themselves to the point of biologic dysfunction without being aware of it.

The National Sleep Foundation has as one of its central missions to sensitize Americans to the risks of excessive sleepiness with respect to automobile accidents—one instantly recognizable life-threatening outcome of chronic sleep loss. Less obvious are the compromises to the host defense system and to general health and well-being that chronic sleep loss causes.

The purposes of this chapter are to bring to the attention of medical practitioners what the extreme impact of sleep loss is on physiologic systems and to outline approaches that can be applied in clinical practice.

SLEEP

What is sleep, then, besides the approximately one third of each day when activity ceases, when—if sleep is not too disturbed—one has some rest and a time-out. Although the absence of transaction with the external world and the relinquishment of the upright position behaviorally signal the state of sleep, these observable events are actually just the tip of the iceberg. Generated by signals traveling along fibers arising from several small nuclei in the brain stem and prolifically terminating in higher parts of the brain, the result is a global state change in the nervous system that affects all parts of the organism under its control. As is so well documented in the now classic text of Orem et al (1), the parameters of control for virtually every system in the body are distinctly different during the state of sleep than during the state of wakefulness.

The purpose of sleep has been hard to define, although most agree that sleep serves a restorative function. It is known that cerebral metabolism decreases during sleep and that there is a homeostatic propensity to sleep (Process S) that builds during wakefulness (2). A chemical mediator of sleep (Factor S) was shown to be present in the cerebral spinal fluid of sleep-deprived goats and could induce sleep in control animals (3). Research to find the chemical mediators of sleep continues although there is now good evidence that adenosine (4,5), prostaglandin D_2 (6), and interleukin-1 (7) are important mediators of sleep in the brain.

Sleep Architecture

Referred to as *sleep architecture*, the organization of a typical night of sleep is characterized by repeated cycles of what is called non-REM (NREM) sleep alternating with what is called REM (rapid eye movement) sleep. In normal sleep architecture, the length of the non-REM/REM cycle is between 90 and 110 minutes. During an 8-hour sleep period, therefore, there are usually four or five such cycles.

Normative Sleep

As depicted in Figure 108-1, in normal sleep the duration of the NREM portion of a cycle is longest in the first cycle, and then shows progressive decreases in length with successive cycles. Conversely, the REM portion of the cycle is shortest during the first cycle, and then increases in duration with successive cycles.

Non-REM Sleep

Non-REM sleep, in turn, is divided into stages 1, 2, and 3 to 4. These are defined by the joint appearance of several polysomnographic (*poly*–many; *somno*–sleep; *graphic*–visual denotation) variables including specific EEG waveforms, eye movements, and muscle tone.

Stage 1 NREM sleep is a period of transition, generally quite brief, between wakefulness and sleep onset. The electro-oculogram (EOG) marks the beginning of slow, rolling eye movements that are referred to as SEMs (slow eye movements). Notably, with the onset of stage 1 NREM sleep, core temperature falls. In the normal sleeper it will continue to fall until it reaches its low point, called the *temperature minimum*, about 2 hours before spontaneous awakening in the morning. During sleep there is increased heat dissipation via increased blood flow in peripheral cutaneous blood vessels, accomplished by peripheral vasodilation (8), especially of the distal extremities (Figure 108-2).

The "sleeper" is not actually aware of him or herself as sleeping during this transitional stage. In cases such as obstructive sleep apnea, wherein obstructed respirations may develop as a person enters sleep and cause an almost constant oscillation between wakefulness and stage 1 sleep for many hours, the person appears to be asleep. However, since "sleep" has been almost exclusively stage 1, there will have been no subjectively appreciable sleep—and the person may be more exhausted upon "awakening" than upon retiring for the night.

In the normal sleeper, after several minutes of stage 1 NREM there appear in the EEG two distinctive waveforms, referred to as sleep spindles and K complexes. Their appearance signals the beginning of stage 2 NREM sleep, usually referred to as stage 2 sleep.

Whereas the stage 1 sleeper if awakened may not have appreciated that he or she had been asleep, the individual awakened from stage 2 NREM sleep will. For this reason polysomnographers (the specialists who read and

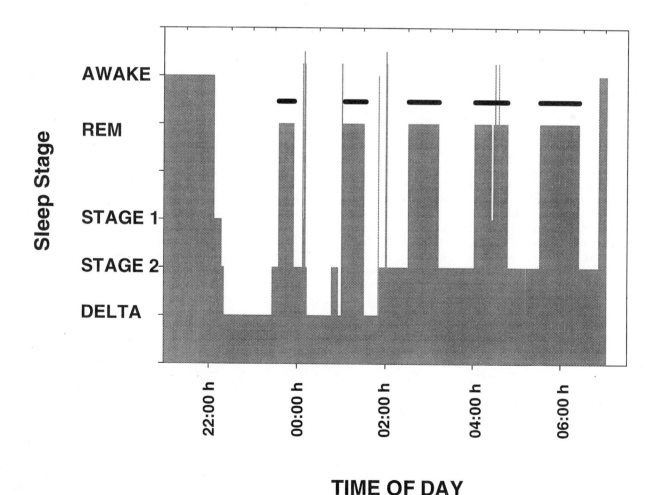

Figure 108-1 Sleep architecture during normal sleep.

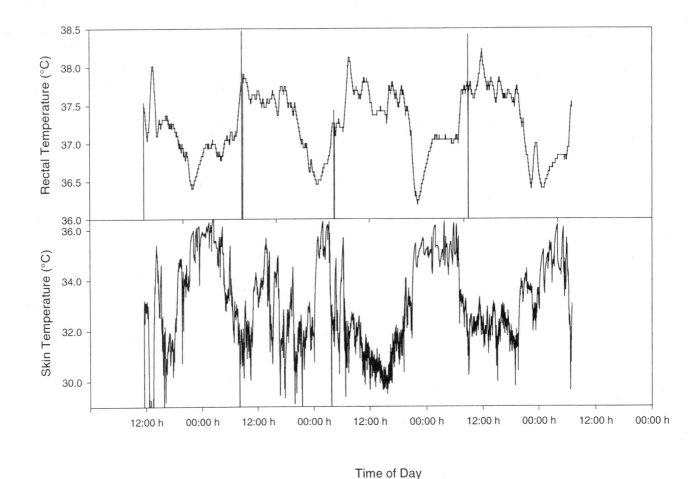

Figure 108-2 Core and a distal skin temperature plotted across 4 days.

interpret polysomnograms), following the criteria of Rechtschaffen et al (9), consider stage 2 to be the first stage of true sleep. It is nonetheless relatively easy to awaken a person from this sleep stage. When awakened, the individual will be relatively oriented with respect to time and place. This is not so for the next emerging NREM sleep stage in the progression, which is variously referred to as delta sleep, slow wave sleep (SWS), or stage 3–4. Large delta waves dominate the EEG. This is a stage of sleep from which it is far more difficult to awaken the individual. Awakenings from this stage leave the newly awakened person relatively disoriented with respect to time and place. It is the stage out of which sleep-walking and night terrors arise. Both sleepwalkers and those having a night terror not only will seem to be "in a fog" if talked to, but generally have no memory of the events when they awaken in the morning; such is the information process-ing state of the brain when it is dominated by delta wave activity.

Although cortical information processing is slow enough to create these changes in cognitive activity, endocrinologically this sleep state is quite dynamic. During delta sleep, human growth hormone (hGH) is secreted in a pulsatile fashion. The temporal association between NREM sleep and hGH release has suggested to many investigators that the function of SWS is physical restoration. Although this is a compelling hypothe-

sis that has a significant body of data to support it, it has yet to be validated (10).

REM Sleep

Toward the end of the NREM-REM cycle, the EEG slow waves will disappear, possibly to be replaced transiently by the polysomnographic events of stage 2 sleep. Strikingly, the electromyographic (EMG) activity recorded from the mental and submental musculature decreases dramatically in amplitude to the point of complete atonia, signaling a flaccid paralysis. Slow eye movements may briefly develop, often in association with erratic respirations (either hyperpneas or hypopneas) and generally in association with occasional twitches from various skeletal musculature. Heart rate variability is also likely to occur.

Finally, the events from which this stage (actually, state) of sleep takes its name will appear: rapid eye movements, or REMs. During REM sleep, active thermoregulation is suppressed. Mammals become essentially poikilothermic, so core body temperatures tend toward ambient temperature.

With respect to the EEG, it is sufficiently like the waking EEG for the stage at one time to have been referred to as paradoxical sleep (i.e., the person is profoundly asleep, yet the EEG resembles the waking EEG), and/or sufficiently like the stage 1 EEG for this sleep stage initially to have been referred to as re-emergent stage 1. Awakenings from this stage of sleep are accomplished easily, and the person awakened from the REM state is likely to have rich dream recall. This is interpreted to mean that dreaming has the highest probability of occurrence during REM. Long-term memory appears to be consolidated during REM sleep as well. Interference with REM sleep interferes with the consolidation of long-term memory and perceptual skills.

Of considerable clinical significance, not only does skeletal musculature tone decrease, but so does upper airway tone. When this decreases to a pathologic degree, the airway musculature becomes flaccid with snoring as the result—it is as if the inhaled air were playing the E string of a bass violin. Tonicity can decrease to the point that the airway closes entirely. This produces what is called an *obstructive apnea*—complete cessation of airflow caused by the collapse of the airway. Apneas can occur in all stages of sleep. However, REM sleep, because of the overall decrease in tonicity, is particularly vulnerable.

Variations in Sleep Architecture

There are age-related changes associated with sleep architecture. Although the percentage of REM sleep expected throughout the entire sleep period is remarkably constant throughout the majority of the life span, the percentage of total sleep time occupied by delta sleep changes. As a person ages, the percentage of delta sleep decreases. By mid-life or early old age, delta sleep may disappear entirely.

Enigmatic to the sleep disorders clinician and independent of a person's age, numerous variations on the theme described can be seen. Some examples of these variations are: 1) a period of delta sleep in the final cycle; 2) a temperature minimum that occurs close to sleep onset rather than toward the end of the sleep period; and 3) the occurrence of EEG waveforms expected in one state in the "wrong" place. For instance, the alpha EEG frequency is associated with relaxed awakening. However, it has also been observed to occur superimposed upon the delta waves of SWS. Termed the *alpha anomaly*, this has been associated with the clinical disorder termed *fibromyalgia syndrome* (11).

Summary

Normal sleep architecture, then, is composed of building blocks—NREM and REM sleep, and within NREM sleep, stages 1, 2, 3, and 4. In turn, each sleep stage is composed of physiologic events that tend to go together. The fact that permutations such as those described above can—and do—occur suggests that there is likely a hierarchical control system that when operative and healthy maintains the normative configuration described.

CIRCADIAN RHYTHM

Assuming a normal light/dark cycle and day-shift work schedule, there is a circadian pattern to the sleep/wake cycle. The term *circadian* refers to a period that approximates, but is not exactly equal to, the 24-hour day (12). There are predictable circadian rhythms in the output of homeostatic systems that synchronize regulatory systems and optimize function in humans. The sleep-wake cycle occurs in most people as an obvious circadian rhythm (process C) that is organized in the hypothalamus independently of Process S (2). Abnormalities either within a sleep stage, or within the organization of sleep stages with respect to each other, may derive from one or another abnormality in circadian timekeeping.

Figure 108-3 depicts the significant characteristics of a circadian rhythm waveform (13) using an idealized circadian core temperature curve. The oscillatory output is shown by the darkest curve. As can be seen in this figure, core temperature is normally at its lowest point or *nadir* about 2 hours before the end of the sleep period and at its highest level of temperature or *acrophase* in the late afternoon or early evening. The period or *tau* (τ) is the duration of an entire oscillatory output cycle, which is about 24 hours for circadian rhythms. *Amplitude* is defined as half the total predicted variation (e.g., in core temperature) during the circadian period.

Oscillatory outputs of different systems can be *phase advanced* or *phase delayed* relative to other rhythms. In the figure, a rhythm phase advanced relative to core temperature is depicted by the curve labeled ΦA. Both the nadir and the acrophase of the ΦA oscillatory output occur at an earlier circadian time than the corresponding points for core temperature. In a similar vein, the oscillatory output labeled ΦD is phase delayed relative to core temperature with both nadir and acrophase occurring later.

Identification of circadian oscillatory outputs in sleep and core temperature was the first step in the realization that temporal information must be propagated within the organism. As more oscillatory outputs were identified, it was clear that physiological and behavioral processes were controlled by a circadian timing system.

What Is the Circadian Timing System?

The circadian timing system (CTS) is an intrinsic regulatory system that provides temporal information to all homeostatic systems within an organism, specifying the dynamically changing set-point around which homeostatic control for the system is maintained. The endogenous CTS evolved as an adaptation to the geophysical world (14). In humans, τ appears to be genetically determined, with a value less than or greater than 24 hours in some individuals (15).

The CTS, by transmitting rhythmic circadian signals from the central nervous system to the periphery, orchestrates the tonic temporal organization and coordination of three communication systems: the autonomic nervous system, the immune system, and the endocrine-paracrine-autocrine systems. The highest-order endogenous circadian pacemaker is located in the suprachiasmatic nucleus (SCN) of the hypothalamus (16). It receives extrinsic information about the light-dark cycle from the retina. The lateral geniculate and dorsal raphe nuclei may also communicate extrinsic information to the SCN. The SCN also receives input from the numerous internal systems under its control, which provide the CTS with intrinsic information (17). Notably, the SCN has a reciprocal relationship (18) with the pineal gland, which secretes melatonin in a circadian output rhythm (19).

To determine what the *endogenous* period is, factors that modify it are eliminated. The paradigm used is referred to as *constant conditions*. In this paradigm, the geophysical light-dark cycle is eliminated. Ambient temperature is held constant.

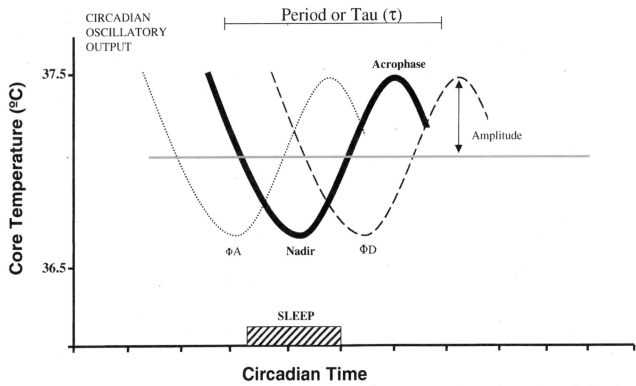

Figure 108-3 An idealized waveform depicting the circadian core temperature rhythm to show a phase advance (ΦA) and a phase delay (ΦD).

Although the CTS is internally stable because it is temperature compensated (14), ambient temperature extremes can affect the CTS as shown by phase shifts in monitored circadian output rhythms after exposure to high ambient temperature (20). Isocaloric food and water are consumed hourly. Sleep is prevented because of the masking effect of sleep on the temperature rhythm (21).

Implicit in the description of constant conditions is that the period of the endogenous circadian pacemaker can be modified so that its cycling is synchronized with the cycling of another event. This modification of the circadian pacemaker rhythm by another cyclic event is referred to as *entrainment*. The CTS is entrained by extrinsic stimuli, especially light, and some chemicals.

The extrinsic light-dark cycle entrains the CTS. Light stimulates the CTS, causing either a delay or an advance in its period, depending on the time in the circadian period when the light stimulation occurs. The effect of light stimulation on the CTS can be determined from the changes in the circadian output rhythm. Bright light treatment early in the subjective night would cause a ΦD in the circadian core temperature rhythm, whereas bright light treatment in the subjective night or early in the subjective day would cause a ΦA (22). This is the basis for using bright light therapy to treat circadian rhythm disorders, including seasonal affective disorder.

The CTS is also entrained by intrinsic signals such as cyclic melatonin secretion from the pineal gland. This is likely the mechanism by which extrinsic melatonin treatment causes phase shifts in the CTS (23,24).

The CTS provides circadian information to all homeostatic systems. In medicine, impairment of the CTS could have far-reaching effects on an individual's health (25,26). The impact of CTS dysregulation on the human organism can be appreciated by viewing a model of the basic elements of the mammalian CTS.

Figure 108-4 shows one model of the components of the CTS as originally diagrammed by Duncan (27). Entrainment to the external 24-hour light-dark cycle is accomplished by light entering through the eye and being transmitted to the primary endogenous pacemaker or SCN via the retinohypothalamic tract. Light entrains the SCN to an approximate 24-hour day although isolated SCN neurons show an intrinsic oscillatory firing rate (28) that approximates 24 hours. The SCN provides circadian oscillatory information to other brain regions that serve as secondary oscillators (depicted as S_1 to S_4), which in turn control oscillatory outputs (depicted as O_1 to O_4). The oscillatory output signals in turn provide feedback information back to the primary oscillator.

For a simple example, a primary oscillation generated in the SCN is sent through a circuitous route to a secondary oscillator (the pineal gland) ultimately via the superior cervical ganglion (19). Within the pineal gland the oscillatory signal modulates enzymatic control of serotonin *N*-acetyltransferase (29) to cause melatonin to be secreted in an oscillatory output rhythm.

Figure 108-5, reproduced from Cagnacci et al (30), shows the interrelationship of the circadian output rhythms of three secondary oscillators in normal women. Sleep, the core temperature nadir, and the melatonin acrophase all occur in a specific circadian relationship to each other. This figure shows how precisely the primary oscillator must direct circadian information to the secondary oscillators. If circadian informa-

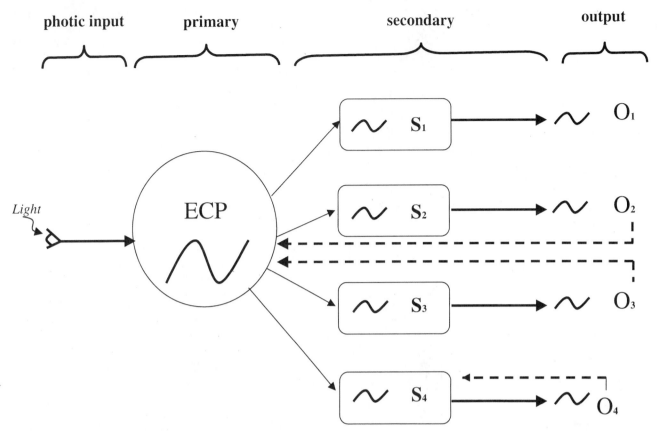

photic input   primary   secondary   output

Figure 108-4 A model of the critical elements of the circadian timing system. (Adapted with permission from Duncan WC. Circadian rhythms and the pharmacology of affective illness. Pharmacol Ther 1996;71:253–312, with permission from Elsevier Science.)

tion is slow arriving at one of the secondary oscillators, sleep quality is affected.

Figure 108-6 shows a more complex example of the CTS model, which is used to demonstrate how widespread the potential health problems might be if the CTS fails to convey entrainment information to even one of the many secondary oscillators. Control of the hypothalamic-pituitary-adrenal (HPA) axis, the immune system, and sleep interaction by the CTS is diagrammed. In this simplified scheme, the hypothalamus receives indirect input from the SCN (16), and in response secretes corticotropin releasing hormone (CRH) in a circadian rhythm. CRH in turn acts upon the anterior pituitary (31) to cause the release of corticotropin (ACTH) in a second circadian rhythm. The circadian ACTH output then triggers the release of cortisol from the adrenal cortex (32). Cortisol is also secreted in a circadian rhythm (32).

Corticosteroids provide negative feedback to the pituitary, but the sensitivity of this feedback depends on circadian time (33). If the HPA circadian coordination is disrupted, its synchronization with the immune system will be altered (34). Conversely, if the immune system is activated so that the circadian cytokine rhythm is affected, the HPA axis will be impacted.

There are circadian rhythms in circulating immune cells (35) and plasma cytokines produced from the immune cells (34,36). Cytokine oscillatory output might change in response to HPA perturbation, which in turn may affect the sleep-wake cycle. Once sleep disruption occurs, there is a domino effect that then affects the entrainment of the secondary oscillators. The circadian oscillatory outputs of the HPA axis also affect the metabolic aspect of cortisol and the circadian cytokine oscillations and therefore will have some effect on thermoregulation (37) (this axis is not diagrammed). The SCN likely transmits circadian signals to the preoptic area and anterior hypothalamus, where the circadian core temperature output rhythm is generated, because there are SCN efferents innervating the hypothalamus. Temperature regulation is of further importance to the CTS because neuronal temperature plays an integral part in the circadian oscillatory property of the SCN. Thermosensitive characteristics of some SCN neurons change across circadian time (38). This temperature sensitivity is either inherent to the SCN neuron or mediated by synaptic input (39). Other SCN temperature-insensitive neurons may provide temperature compensation in the SCN (39).

The oscillatory communications among the HPA axis, the immune system, sleep-wake system, and thermoregulation are primarily controlled by the SCN. Temporal signaling among just these homeostatic systems is very complex. A sustained physical or psychological stressor does impact on the HPA axis (40,41). If sleep is affected by the stress, then the CTS and several homeostatic systems could be affected and temporarily desynchronized. If the sleep disturbance persists, the individual may experience desynchronization symptoms similar to jet lag.

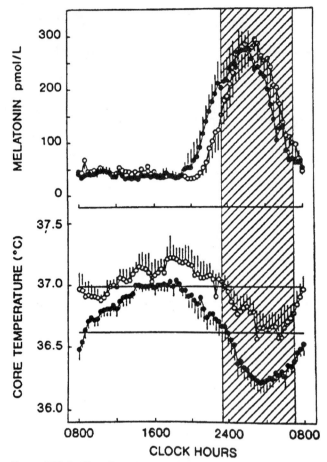

Figure 108-5 Circadian rhythms in core temperature and melatonin in relation to sleep in women. (From Cagnacci A, Soldani R, Laughlin GA, et al. Modification of circadian body temperature rhythm during the luteal menstrual cycle phase: Role of melatonin. J Appl Physiol 1996;80:25–29.)

In humans, it has been proposed that individual variation in circadian τ may be explained by genetic control (15). Genetic variation in the CTS in humans is probably as diverse as in other organisms (42–44). Genetically regulated oscillator mechanisms from different species appear to have common components (45,46), and these are predicted to be important in pacemaker control of circadian timing in humans (47).

Effects of Sleep Loss on the Circadian Timing System

Sleep disturbance may cause its greatest damage by its effect on the circadian timing system. Chronic sleep disturbance can eventually lead to establishment of an atypical circadian rhythm, and chronic disturbance of the circadian rhythm by external events such as a shift work schedule or the influence of a neonate awakening the mother at night, leading the mother to take compensatory naps during the daytime, can produce entrenched and long-lasting disturbances of sleep.

At the extreme, the numerous physiologic systems under circadian control may become desynchronized from each other, creating essentially the same situation for the biologic organism that defective timing in a car would cause for engine function. Jet lag is a commonly experienced example of CTS desynchronicity.

Internal desynchronization is common in an experimental paradigm referred to as a *free running* paradigm, wherein the research individual is deprived of cues such as the light-dark cycle, which would normally entrain the endogenous circadian rhythms to the geophysical day. There is evidence, however, that internal desynchronization may occur in some people under normal social conditions (15).

If the circadian synchronization of even one homeostatic system is disrupted by sleep loss, there is the potential for long-lasting dysfunction among several systems. Initial symptoms of sleep loss are impairments such as short-term memory loss and dysphoria, but persistence of the multisystem dysfunction could lead to other diseases, including sleep disorders and depression. The importance of circadian timing system dysfunction is not yet known for diseases of nonspecific origin, such as some allergies, premenstrual syndrome, and irritable bowel syndrome. Dysfunction within the CTS is a fertile area for etiologic investigation.

Drugs That Affect the Circadian Timing System

Disruption of the CTS in humans affects health and performance, as shown in shift workers (48). Drugs that act on the CTS as intrinsic synchronizers might also cause desynchronization with the external environment. Melatonin, caffeine, and benzodiazepines act to cause a phase shift in mammals when given at an appropriate time of the circadian cycle.

In humans, a short-acting benzodiazepine improved sleep in shift workers who slept during the day (49,50). Benzodiazepines sedate and also have a circadian impact. Depending upon the time of administration and delivery route, they can cause either a phase advance or a phase delay of the mammalian activity rhythm (51,52).

Circadian Timing System's Impact on Drug Action (Chronopharmacology)

Chronopharmacology, the circadian effects on pharmacology and homeostatic systems (53), is an important consideration for rhythmic changes in drug effectiveness (54). In humans, blood pressure varies in a circadian rhythm (55), as do plasma epinephrine and norepinephrine levels (56). Both systolic and diastolic blood pressure start to decrease before sleep onset, and then fall rapidly with sleep. Blood pressure begins to increase during the last two thirds of sleep and reaches maximum levels during the second half of the activity period. Plasma norepinephrine and epinephrine are at their nadirs during sleep and start to rise at its completion. The acrophases of both these catecholamines are in the morning. Norepinephrine peaks shortly after morning awakening and epinephrine reaches its acrophase in late morning.

In hypertensive patients the circadian rhythm in blood pressure is reported to be similar to normotensive controls (55), so the oscillatory nature of blood pressure regulation

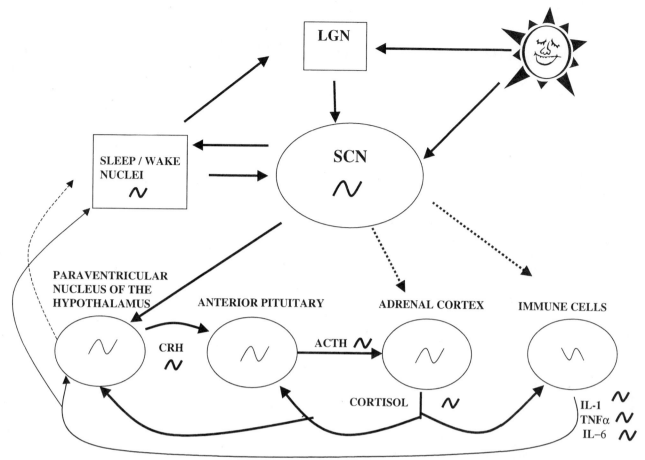

Figure 108-6 The complexity of the interaction between the CTS, the hypothalamic-anterior pituitary-adrenal gland axis, and the immune system is diagrammed. Abbreviations: LGN (lateral geniculate nucleus); SCN (suprachiasmatic nucleus of the hypothalamus); PVN (paraventricular nucleus); CRH (corticotropin releasing hormone); ACTH (corticotropin); IL-1 (interleukin-1); TNFα (tumor necrosis factor α); and IL-6 (interleukin-6). Sleep/wake nuclei include the LDT, PPT, ventromedial preoptic area of the hypothalamus, basal forebrain, and dorsal raphe.

must be considered when antihypertensive medications are prescribed. It is known that cardiovascular ischemic events occur most frequently in the morning (53), which might be partially explained by circadian endocrine and autonomic influences on the vasculature (57). The prominent circadian characteristics of increasing blood pressure and increased incidence of ischemic events in the morning underscore the importance that medications act *prior to awakening* in the hypertensive patient. Administration of antihypertensive medication at the appropriate circadian time is challenging because the individual's circadian phase rather than clock time is the factor that most influences medication efficacy. This can differ from individual to individual.

In normal, nondiabetic subjects, the rate of insulin secretion has a circadian rhythm with its acrophase between noon and 6:00 p.m. and its nadir between midnight and 6:00 a.m. (58). Importantly, plasma melatonin changes in the opposite direction, with the melatonin rhythm at an approximately 180° phase angle to the insulin secretion rate circadian curve.

There is also a circadian rhythm in the insulin requirement to maintain euglycemia in insulin-dependent diabetics.

The early morning requirement is double that of the daytime requirement (59). The increased demand (i.e., decreased insulin sensitivity) is related to increased early morning peaks of cortisol secretion. Plasma cortisol levels reach their acrophase at the end of the sleep period and their minimum at the beginning of the sleep period (60). The decreased insulin sensitivity and decreased glucose tolerance with increasing plasma levels of cortisol appear to be caused by circadian changes in hepatic glucose production (61).

The clinical implications of these associated rhythms in the carbohydrate metabolic pathways are important. There is a wide range of natural variation in the phase relationship of the circadian sleep-wake cycle to the day-night cycle. The sleep of "owls" is phase delayed relative to the day-night cycle, and the sleep of "larks" is phase advanced. Correspondingly, there will be an associated shift in the clock times for the acrophase and nadir of insulin sensitivity, plasma cortisol levels, and presumably also of hepatic glucose production for these two populations. The timing and dosage levels of exogenous insulin administration, therefore, must take the individual patient's circadian rhythm pattern into account.

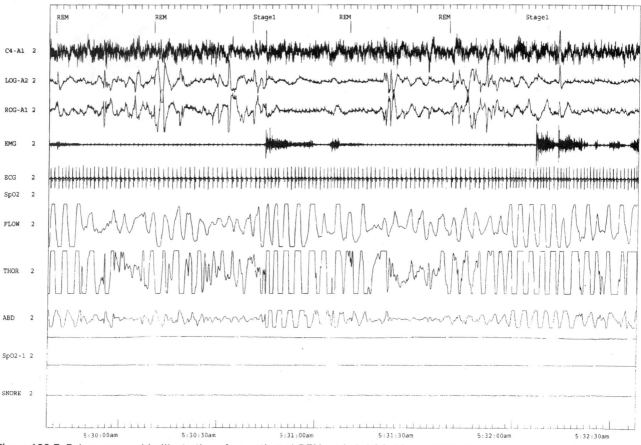

Figure 108-7 Polysomnographic illustration of an activated REM period. LOG-A2 and ROG-A1 are channels showing continuous rapid eye movements. The flow channel shows irregularities in oral and nasal air flow in association with dense REMs. Transitions to stage 1 following epochs of two arousals seen on the EMG channel illustrate the fragmentation of an activated REM period.

SLEEP LOSS AND CONCURRENT DISRUPTION OF THE CIRCADIAN RHYTHM

Effect of Alcohol and Benzodiazepines on Sleep Architecture

Sleep loss not only reduces the restorative function of sleep, but may also compromise the circadian timing system. With this in mind, we review some of the effects of sleep loss. The sleep period, with its several cycles of NREM sleep alternating with REM sleep, and with the changing proportions of NREM and REM sleep across the night, operates as a whole. That is, if one portion of sleep is disturbed, the entire architecture of sleep is disturbed. For instance, if REM sleep is disturbed during the first cycle, there will be an increase in what is called REM pressure during the second cycle. This, in turn, can affect the development of SWS in the second cycle.

Alcohol

In some people, selective deprivation of REM sleep can happen regularly. Alcohol is a powerful REM suppressor that causes selective REM sleep deprivation. A few drinks before bedtime leads to the suppression of REM sleep early in the sleep period, until the alcohol has been cleared by the liver. Once the alcohol is metabolized, the REM pressure

from the early part of the night leads to especially activated—and prolonged—REM periods in the second part of the night. The density of rapid eye movements becomes greater than normal. With increased REM density, there is an increase in other events of the phasic part of REM sleep, such as an increase in heart rate variability and an increase in respiratory irregularities (Figure 108-7). With prolonged repetitive trains of rapid eye movements, tachypnea (with respiratory rate increasing to as high as 32 breaths per minute) or central apneas develop. Significant atonicity of the upper airway may develop, leading to obstructive apneas. Bursts of EMG activity from any of the skeletal muscles are likely also to increase, as are runs of cardiac arrhythmias.

The immediate result of these kinds of events is that sleep becomes fragmented by brief awakenings. The subjective experience is of particularly vivid dreams, which at times incorporate the heart rate variability and respiratory disturbances into their content, producing nightmares. This series of events may be the basis of a morning hangover following too much alcohol the preceding night. Events that normally occur during REM sleep, such as the consolidation of the day's events into long-term memory, may fail to occur because REM sleep has not progressed normally.

Benzodiazepine Sedative-Hypnotics

Selective suppression of delta sleep can also happen in a normal social environment. The majority of benzodiazepine (BZD) sedative hypnotics, which act by potentiating GABA binding to the BZD receptors, suppress REM sleep to some degree, but suppress SWS sleep to a significant degree (62). This means that hGH secretion is also suppressed. The jury is still out regarding whether benzodiazepines completely suppress nocturnal hGH secretion—an issue which has tremendous bearing on whether benzodiazepines should be used postsurgically to help surgical patients sleep during recovery.

Sleep Forced in the Wrong Circadian Time

As mentioned earlier, Factor S mediates the propensity for sleep, which builds during wakefulness and likely indicates the magnitude of the homeostatic pressure for sleep (Process S) (2). Sleep occurs normally during the nighttime hours and is coupled to both the circadian core temperature rhythm and the circadian melatonin rhythm, but sleep onset can be delayed by using caffeine to cause arousal. A separate factor (Process C) originating from the CTS also affects the drive for sleep (2). Night shift work, delayed sleep phase syndrome, and jet lag have the common feature of an individual wanting to sleep when the CTS is not permitting sleep. Sleep is highly fragmented and unsatisfying in these conditions, probably because of circadian activation of arousal pathways in the brain when the individual is sleepy. As discussed earlier, there are specific treatments using entraining stimuli, such as bright light therapy or melatonin treatment, which help to synchronize the timing of sleep to the circadian time in which sleep is permitted.

Effect of Sleep Loss on Health

Sustained sleep loss in rats is associated with increased morbidity and mortality rates (63). This may be a product of a compromised immune system. Rechtschaffen et al made the initial finding that continuous sleep deprivation led, ultimately, to death. More recently, Everson (64) demonstrated a high rate of bacteremia in near-terminally sleep-deprived rats. There are obviously no research studies in humans comparable to the animal research studies in sustained sleep deprivation. A recent review of human studies indicated that sleep deprivation does affect the immune system, but the results are conflicting (65). It was suggested that study differences may be due to individual differences, difference in the stress magnitude as a consequence of the study, and the circadian timing of measurement of treatment effects. The experimental evidence to show that sleep deprivation impairs immunity in humans, despite the persistent anecdotal evidence, is still not available.

Sleep plays a probable role in host defense (66,67) as evidenced by the often-observed clinical finding that humans tend to sleep more while they are recuperating from an infectious illness, suggesting that sleep plays an important role in recuperation. Increased sleep during the course of an infectious illness is mediated by cytokines, including interleukin-1 (IL-1), a proinflammatory cytokine produced primarily by monocytes and macrophages, which mediates SWS (7).

IL-1 may actually be a normal component of SWS production. Recent research indicates that IL-1 has a spontaneous rhythm during a normal night of sleep, with the production of this cytokine significantly greater during the first 4 hours of sleep when SWS occurs than during the latter part of the sleep period. When host defense mechanisms are activated, as with an infectious illness, the increase in IL-1 production appears to increase the amount of SWS. A logical deduction, therefore, is that one function perhaps specifically of SWS is in host defense, such that compromise of SWS and the associated immunologic events might lead to a compromise of the immune system.

The clinical implication of these findings is that for the patient with chronic infections, an exploration of the patient's sleep habits, as well as direct treatment of the infections, is in order. With the powerful, broad-spectrum antibiotics now available, there is a great temptation to rely upon these medications rather than searching for the cause of recurrent infectious illness. The lore urging a sick person to get plenty of sleep is well established in our culture. Yet, the concept that sufficient sleep may prevent some health problems is not well rooted in the medical community. Instructing the sleep-deficient patient to get more sleep on a regular basis may improve the patient's health.

Sleep Loss and the Endocrine System

Sleep deprivation causes a marked elevation of plasma thyroid stimulating hormone (TSH) during the nighttime (68). Conditions of sustained operation in the field in a 5-day military training course with heavy physical exercise and an almost complete lack of food and sleep led to the extinction of a circadian rhythm in thyroid stimulating hormone (TSH), 17-α-hydroxyprogesterone, progesterone, androstenedione, and dihydroepiandrosterone (DHEA) (69). Simply depriving subjects of sleep during the second half of the night led to significant increases in TSH, which then remained significantly elevated throughout the remainder of the day. Under these same conditions, T_4 and T_3 also increased, whereas prolactin (PRL) levels decreased (70).

Sleep Loss and Performance, Mood, and Behavior

Sleep loss over the course of one night affects performance of tedious and repetitive tasks, believed to be due to increased sleepiness and lack of arousal. Sleep loss for two consecutive nights affects performance of tasks independently of task novelty and task stimulation. Reduced sleep time each night for a week will also increase sleepiness and decrease vigilance. In particular, sleep loss alters complex performance by affecting response variability, attention, latency of motor and cognitive reactions, accuracy, and working memory (71). The catecholaminergic waking-arousal pathways in the brain are likely affected by sleep loss as the use of caffeine (72) and other noradrenergic and dopaminergic stimulants improve performance during sleep deprivation (73).

CLINICAL APPLICATION

Commentary

The front cover of the February 1998 Life Magazine (74) featured an obviously wide-eyed sleepless man staring at the reader with the caption, "Why 70 million of us are sleepless in America." As a nation, we are inured to sleeplessness—

even our healthcare providers. According to a recent study of young doctors, a single night on call decreases cognitive function and mood considerably (75).

It is essential that screening be done because poor sleep quality can underlie many medical disorders. Understanding the fundamental principles of sleep and its partner in health, the circadian timing system, allows the clinician to utilize them. Although it may not be feasible in the current managed-care medical practice for every patient showing signs of sleep disturbance to be screened, the process takes little time. There are only a few questions that need to be asked. It is therefore strongly recommended that the simple questions about sleep described below (Diagnostic Issues) be incorporated into at least each patient's routine annual visit.

Signs and Symptoms of Sleep Loss

Curious as it may seem, a large percentage of patients with symptoms stemming from sleep loss are not aware of the source but rather search for other answers. Whereas the food-deprived person is typically well aware of impending starvation, the sleep-deprived person is often much less aware of being "starved for sleep." Table 108-1 lists the usual signs and symptoms in a form that can be used by the clinician as a checklist. See Lindsley (76) for a more complete description.

Tiredness and *sleepiness* obviously are symptoms. However, these might be described by the patient as, "I don't have any energy or motivation. Am I depressed? Am I sick?" *Memory disturbance* and other cognitive disturbances are another indication. Typical memory problems associated with sleep loss are difficulties retrieving the word for a familiar object (e.g., hat, with the circumlocution" uh, that thing you wear on your head" being what a person might replace that word with) or blocking on the name of a very familiar person (e.g., one's significant other, one's child, or one's parent).

Other memory problems revolve around long-term memory (e.g., problems consolidating into long-term memory the events of the previous day). REM sleep, as described above, is the time during sleep when such consolidation of long-term memory takes place. REM deprivation is associated with impairment of this function. One wonders how often dementia is suspected in older people with such memory disturbances when simple and correctable sleep loss might be at its root. Sleep loss can also activate a stress response that independently compromises memory (77).

Difficulty concentrating is another cognitive disturbance that routinely follows upon chronically insufficient or poor-quality sleep. Intrusion of extraneous thoughts and ideas; decreased span of attention; difficulty in interpreting the meaning of a single, simple sentence that the reader might read and reread; and inability to hold a single train of thought are all symptoms.

Hypersensitivity of many of the sensory systems is also symptomatic. The odd parasthesias some patients describe as a vague tingling or as migrating pins and needles or other odd tactile sensations can be the product of sleep loss. Increased sensitivity to light or to sound, so that the patient finds lights of normal luminescence to be too bright or sounds with a normal decibel level to be too loud, is also symptomatic of sustained sleep loss. The unrested brain loses the ability to modulate perceptual intensity.

Irritability in other areas of function is also symptomatic.

Table 108-1 Signs and Symptoms of Sleep Loss

1. Tiredness or fatigue, without true sleepiness
2. Irritability, generally unexplained emotional lability
3. Hypersensitivity to visual, auditory, and tactile stimuli
4. Development of paresthesias
5. Unexplained aching of the body, often diagnosed as fibrositis
6. Alterations in body temperature experience
7. Increasing preference for foods high in carbohydrates
8. Difficulty retrieving names of common objects or familiar persons
9. Disruption of ability to concentrate
10. Blurry eyes, burning eyes, and puffiness under the eyes

Reprinted with permission from Lindsley G. The insomnia syndrome: Befuddler of the psychotherapeutic enterprise. In: Ellison JM, Weinstein CS, Hodel-Malinofsky T, eds. The psychotherapist's guide to neuropsychiatry. Diagnostic and treatment issues. Washington, DC: American Psychiatric Press, 1994:279–302.

Lowered thresholds of frustration, easy triggering of irascibility, and outright anger for no real reason are common symptoms of sleep loss. One wonders how much of the increasing amount of domestic violence reported in this country might be attributable to economic and other stressors that lead to insufficient quality sleep.

Finally, *energy production systems in the body become defective*. Sustained sleep deprivation in laboratory rats (78) would indicate that eventually body temperature drops significantly, and although food is made available to the subjects ad lib, the rats cannot maintain their weight or their internal temperatures. The mechanisms mediating the effects of sleep loss on inability to maintain weight or body temperature are not known, but the finding is well validated. The comparable symptoms in people with insufficient sleep are frequently *feeling too cold* even when other people in the same environment feel fine and a significant *increase in craving for high-energy foods*, most often carbohydrates.

There are more specific symptoms one might identify, depending upon the part of sleep that is especially deficient (e.g., REM sleep in the case of patients who routinely use REM-suppressant agents such as alcohol or barbiturates) and depending upon the etiology of the sleep loss (voluntary versus induced by pathologic events arising during sleep, such as obstructive apneas). However, independent of these factors, the more generic symptoms of sleep loss described above will always be present.

Diagnostic Issues

The most important questions to ask your patient are summarized in Table 108-2. The first set (questions 1 to 6) are specific questions about sleep, and the second set (questions 7 to 11) are questions about daytime wakefulness. If the responses to these simple questions verify that there is a problem with sleep, extrinsic and intrinsic factors that might be pertinent can be pursued.

Table 108-2 Sleep Assessment Questions

Name of Patient _____	Medical Record Number _____
Date of Birth: _____	Primary Physician: _____
Address: _____	
_____	Today's Date: _____

For each question please make an X through the number that indicates how often you have each symptom. 1 = Rarely or none of the time. 5 = Always or almost all of the time.

1. I sleep well at night, wake up feeling good, and am alert during the day   1   2   3   4   5
2. I sleep poorly at night (have insomnia)   1   2   3   4   5
3. It takes me a long time to fall asleep   1   2   3   4   5
4. I wake up a lot from sleep   1   2   3   4   5
5. I wake up too early in the morning and can't get back to sleep   1   2   3   4   5
6. My sleep is not refreshing   1   2   3   4   5
7. During at least part of the night I doze instead of really sleep   1   2   3   4   5

8. I feel so sleepy during the day I wish I could take a nap   1   2   3   4   5
9. I feel so sleepy during the day I have trouble resisting a nap   1   2   3   4   5
10. I have fallen asleep (or almost fallen asleep) driving a car   1   2   3   4   5
11. I don't really get sleepy but I do feel fatigue during the day   1   2   3   4   5

12. I thrash in my sleep   1   2   3   4   5
13. I do unusual things (like putting milk in the cupboard) while apparently preoccupied   1   2   3   4   5
14. I block on the names of people I know well, or on the words for common, familiar objects   1   2   3   4   5
15. I have difficulty concentrating   1   2   3   4   5
16. I get odd sensations on my skin   1   2   3   4   5
17. I overinterpret shadows, thinking they are actual forms   1   2   3   4   5
18. I get irritable for no really good reason   1   2   3   4   5
19. If things get complicated, I tend to let them slide because I don't have the energy to deal with them   1   2   3   4   5
20. I am very sensitive even to soft noises or dim lights   1   2   3   4   5
21. My eyes burn or blur when I am awake   1   2   3   4   5

22. Some of the problems in items 2–21 interfere with my life. I would be better off if I could correct some or all. This is true (use numbers to show how often this is true)   1   2   3   4   5

Reprinted with permission from Lindsley G. The insomnia syndrome: befuddler of the psychotherapeutic enterprise. In: Ellison JM, Weinstein CS, Hodel-Malinofsky T, eds. The psychotherapist's guide to neuropsychiatry: diagnostic and treatment issues. Washington, DC: American Psychiatric Press, 1994:279–302.

Extrinsic Sources of Compromised Sleep

Extrinsic factors include a host of sleep-hygiene factors, medications, or a primary medical problem. Factors such as these account for a large proportion of sleep-wake complaints but are frequently overlooked by the patient.

Sleep Hygiene

The highest-quality sleep occurs when the behavioral sleep-wake schedule follows the endogenous circadian rhythm (see Figure 108-5). Violations of this are probably *the primary source* of difficulty. Examples of how compromises occur are: 1) waking up before the beginning of the biologic waking phase, and then drinking caffeine to "charge up the engine"; 2) trying to get to sleep before the beginning of the true biologic sleep phase, perhaps helping it along with a glass of wine or can of beer or either a prescription or over-the-counter sleep aid; or 3) staying awake for a late evening meeting, to do paperwork, to have personal time, or whatever, beyond the time when the body "wants" to fall

asleep. These are the things of which disturbed circadian rhythmicity is made.

It is not difficult to elicit a history to determine compatibility with this profile. Eliciting questions are "How many nights a week, on the average, do you stay up late even though you know you are tired, because of plans you have? Do you work second shift, or for some other reason have an extended day of obligation and responsibility? Do you wake up in the morning before you really feel ready, knowing that at times when you can sleep a little later (such as on weekends or holidays) that you feel much better? How many ounces of caffeinated beverages do you drink as a rule, on work or school days, versus when you are free of those responsibilities? How many ounces of alcohol do you drink a week on the average? How much physical exercise do you get, and how sedentary are you?" Hauri et al (79) provide an excellent chapter on sleep hygiene, which the practitioner and patient both will benefit from reading.

The practitioner is likely to discover that the patient acknowledges most or all of the above (as any of us might) and might add that he or she has been taking one or another psychotropic drug to help depression or anxiety (common consequences of insufficient quality sleep combined with the lifestyle that may have given rise to the problem in the first place). The question then is how to proceed, since the solution involves changing how the patient organizes life, rather than offering medication that might mask or exacerbate the problem.

Solutions are individual. The key element is that the person be motivated to make the lifestyle changes if current habits interfere with sleep. The best approach is to help the person understand that consistently good sleep eliminates the emotional "echo chamber" that makes challenging tasks overwhelming. In the absence of good-quality sleep, productivity is less efficient. Sufficient sleep will eliminate the perceived need to reinforce adherence to work schedules by using sleep or wake aids.

Once the patient is motivated, the practitioner might either work with him or her about how to reorganize time and activities; to *slowly* withdraw from caffeine in much the same way as one would taper any other long-lasting medication; to *slowly* reduce alcohol intake; and to *slowly* withdraw from sedative-hypnotics or from antidepressant medications. Rapid, or cold-turkey, withdrawal from any of these substances can produce serious side effects and may thereby deter the patient from making the necessary changes.

Alternatively, this might be the point at which the patient is referred to a specialist in either sleep disorders medicine or behavioral medicine who is qualified to help the patient work out the details. There are often many layers of the onion to be peeled back and teased apart before everything falls into place, so that consistent support and direction from a professional skilled in doing this is extremely helpful.

Medications

Both psychotropic drugs and medications intended for a wide range of medical disorders can be at the heart of the problem. It is therefore especially important to elicit from the patient the name (and dosage if available) of every pharmaceutical agent taken on more than a rare basis. This includes aspirin or aspirin substitutes, oral contraceptives, vitamins and minerals, herbal agents, over-the-counter sleep aids or stimulants, and all other prescribed medication as well as recreational drugs. This information will then put the practitioner (in collaboration with the patient) in the position of evaluating the potential role of pharmaceutical agents in the development of the problem. In this context, it is also important to determine the time of day when the substances are taken (see Chronopharmacology above).

Finally, tobacco products should not be ignored in this inquiry. The effects of nicotine and carbon monoxide, the irritation of nasal and buccal mucosa that can interfere with sleep, the waking up in the middle of the night in response to lowered blood nicotine levels are all relevant in solving sleep problems.

Intrinsic Sources of Compromised Sleep

It is possible that efforts to correct factors related to sleep hygiene fail to correct the problem or that there is no reason to suspect sleep hygiene or related extrinsic factors as etiologic. Rather, the presenting complaints may derive from what the International Classification of Sleep Disorders (80) refers to as intrinsic sleep disorders. Obstructive sleep apnea, most saliently characterized by loud, disruptive snoring with incremental hypertension the longer the condition has been present; periodic limb movements of sleep (in the past referred to as nocturnal myoclonus), and narcolepsy—a genetically transmitted disorder primarily affecting the organization and distribution of REM sleep—are examples of these.

The topic of sleep disorders medicine is a large one. Coverage is beyond the scope of this chapter. The interested reader is referred to the International Classification of Sleep Disorders (80) and also to the text *Principles and Practice of Sleep Disorders Medicine* (81).

The physician might also consider medical illnesses that might affect sleep or circadian rhythmicity. Thyroid imbalance, diabetes, and GI illnesses are among some of the diseases that might disrupt sleep.

Sleep Disorders Centers, Clinics, and Clinicians

If an intrinsic sleep disorder is suspected, the primary recommendation is that the patient be referred for evaluation to a sleep disorders center or sleep disorders clinician who is accredited by the American Sleep Disorders Association (ASDA). The organization, in Rochester, Minnesota, maintains a listing of accredited centers and Fellows of the American Board of Sleep Medicine and can provide that information to the practitioner. The national office can be reached at (507) 287–6006.

Each center or clinic will have its own procedure. Typically the referring physician can expect the patient first to have a diagnostic interview with the sleep disorders clinician, who will then apprise the referring physician of the impressions in a written report. It is likely that a sleep study, referred to as a polysomnogram (PSG), will be ordered. The ensuing PSG report will provide results in narrative and/or numeric form. It typically will also offer an interpretation to the findings and make recommendations to the referring physician regarding follow-up and treatment.

Depending upon the circumstances and the needs of the patient, the study may be carried out in a sleep laboratory, or it may be carried out with ambulatory recording devices in the patient's own home environment.

DIRECTIONS FOR THE FUTURE

The field of sleep disorders medicine evolved in 1979 out of the field of sleep research, and chronobiology has been a subdiscipline within the practice of sleep disorders. The burgeoning increase in the knowledge base of chronobiology should be soon incorporated into the clinical practice of sleep disorders medicine and general medical practice. The application of chronobiologic principles in clinical practice provides a very inexpensive method for maintaining sleep, health, and well-being in the individual. It follows that sleep disorders medicine, sleep physiology, and chronobiology should be a central theme in the curricula of medical schools, in the training of interns and residents, and in postgraduate medicine.

REFERENCES

1. Orem J, Barnes CD, eds. Physiology in sleep. New York: Academic Press, 1980.

2. Borbély AA, Tobler I. Endogenous sleep-promoting substances and sleep regulation. Physiol Rev 1989;69:605–670.

3. Pappenheimer JR, Miller TB, Goodrich CA. Sleep-promoting effects of cerebrospinal fluid from sleep-deprived goats. Proc Natl Acad Sci 1998;58:513–517.

4. Radulovacki M. Role of adenosine in sleep in rats. Rev Clin Basic Pharm 1985;5:327–339.

5. Porkka-Heskanen T, Strecker RE, Thakkar M, et al. Adenosine: a mediator of the sleep-inducing effects of prolonged wakefulness. Science 1997;276:1265–1268.

6. Hayaishi O. Molecular mechanisms of sleep-wake regulation: roles of prostaglandins D_2 and E_2. FASEB J 1991;5:2575–2581.

7. Krueger JM, Walter J, Dinarello CA, et al. Sleep-promoting effects of endogenous pyrogen (interleukin-1). Am J Physiol 1984;246:R994–R999.

8. Kräuchi K, Wirz-Justice A. Circadian rhythm of heat production, heart rate, and skin and core temperature under unmasking conditions in men. Am J Physiol 1994;267:R819–829.

9. Rechtschaffen A, Kales A, Berger RJ, et al. A manual of standardized terminology, techniques and scoring system for sleep stages of human subjects. U.S. Public Health Service Publication 204. Washington D.C.: U.S. Government Printing Office, 1968.

10. Horne J. Why we sleep. The functions of sleep in humans and other mammals. Oxford: Oxford University Press, 1989.

11. Pillemer SR, Bradley LA, Crofford LJ, et al. The neuroscience and endocrinology of fibromyalgia. Arthritis Rheum 1997;40:1928–1939.

12. Halberg F. Temporal coordination of physiologic function. Cold Spring Harb Symp Quant Biol 1960;25:289–308.

13. Halberg F, Barnwell F, Hrushesky W. Chronobiology: a science in tone with the rhythms of life. Minneapolis: Earl Bakken, 1986:1–20.

14. Pittendrigh CS. Circadian rhythms and the circadian organization of living systems. Cold Spring Harb Symp Quant Biol 1960;25:159–182.

15. Ashkenazi IE, Reinberg A, Bicakova-Rosher A, et al. The genetic background of individual variations of circadian-rhythm periods in healthy human adults. Am J Hum Genet 1993;52:1250–1259.

16. Buijs RM. The anatomical basis for the expression of circadian rhythms: The efferent projections of the suprachiasmatic nucleus. In: Buijs RM, Kalsbeek A, Romijn HJ, et al, eds. Hypothalamic integration of circadian rhythms. Amsterdam: Elsevier, 1996:229–240.

17. Pittendrigh CS. Temporal organization: Reflections of a Darwinian clock-watcher. Annu Rev Physiol 1993;55:17–54.

18. McArthur AJ, Gillette MU, Prosser RA. Melatonin directly resets the rat suprachiasmatic circadian clock in vitro. Brain Res 1991;565:158–161.

19. Axelrod J. The pineal gland: A neurochemical transducer. Science 1974;184:1341–1348.

20. Barrett RK, Takahashi JS. Temperature compensation and temperature entrainment of the chick pineal cell circadian clock. J Neurosci 1995;15:5681–5692.

21. Czeisler CA, Weitzman ED, Moore-Ede MC, et al. Human sleep: Its duration and organization depend on its circadian phase. Science 1980;210:1264–1267.

22. Czeisler CA, Allan JS, Strogatz SH, et al. Bright light resets the human circadian pacemaker independent of the timing of the sleep-wake cycle. Science 1986;233:667–671.

23. Deacon S, English J, Arendt J. Acute phase-shifting effects of melatonin associated with suppression of core body temperature in humans. Neurosci Lett 1994;178:32–34.

24. Arendt J. Melatonin and the mammalian pineal gland. London: Chapman & Hall, 1995.

25. Halberg F. Chronobiology. Ann Rev Physiol 1969;31:675–725.

26. Moore-Ede MC, Czeisler CA, Richardson GS. Circadian timekeeping in health and disease. Part 2. Clinical implications of circadian rhythmicity. N Engl J Med 1983;309:530–536.

27. Duncan WC. Circadian rhythms and the pharmacology of affective illness. Pharmacol Ther 1996;71:253–312.

28. Inouye SIT, Kawamura H. Persistence of circadian rhythmicity in mammalian hypothalamic island containing the suprachiasmatic nucleus. Proc Natl Acad Sci 1979;76:5961–5966.

29. Coon SL, Roseboom PH, Baler R, et al. Pineal serotonin N-acetyltransferase: Expression cloning and molecular analysis. Science 1995;270:1681–1683.

30. Cagnacci A, Soldani R, Laughlin GA, et al. Modification of circadian body temperature rhythm during the luteal menstrual cycle phase: Role of melatonin. J Appl Physiol 1996;80:25–29.

31. Krieger DT. Circadian pituitary adrenal rhythms. In: Hedlund LW Jr, Franz JM, Kenney AD, eds. Biological rhythms and endocrine function. New York: Plenum Press, 1975:169–189.

32. Weitzman ED. Circadian rhythms and episodic hormone secretion in man. Annu Rev Med 1976;27:225–243.

33. Akana SF, Cascio CS, Du J-Z, et al. Reset of feedback in the adrenocortical system: an apparent shift in sensitivity of adrenocorticotropin to inhibition by corticosterone between morning and evening. Endocrinology 1986;119:2325–2332.

34. Hohagen F, Timmer J, Weyerbrock A, et al. Cytokine production during sleep and wakefulness and its relationship to cortisol in healthy humans. Neuropsychobiology 1993;28:9–16.

35. Born J, Lange T, Hansen K, et al. Effects of sleep and circadian rhythm on human circulating immune cells. J Immunol 1997;158:4454–4464.

36. Crofford LJ, Kalogeras KT, Mastorakos G, et al. Circadian relationships between interleukin (IL)-6 and hypothalamic-pituitary-adrenal axis hormones: Failure of IL-6 to cause sustained hypercortisolism in patients with early untreated rheumatoid arthritis. J Clin Endocrinol Metab 1997;82:1279–1283.

37. Kluger M. Fever role of pyrogens and cryogens. Physiol Rev 1991;71:93–127.

38. Derambure PS, Boulant JA. Circadian thermosensitive characteristics of suprachiasmatic neurons in vitro. Am J Physiol 1994;266:R1876–R1884.

39. Burgoon PW. Temperature sensitivity and temperature compensation of neurons in the suprachiasmatic nucleus. Dissertation. Columbus: Ohio State University, 1997.

40. Kirschbaum C, Gonzalez Bono E, Rohleder N, et al. Effects of fasting and glucose load on free cortisol responses to stress and nicotine. J Clin Endocrinol Metab 1997;82:1101–1105.

41. Larsen PJ, Mikkelsen JD. Functional identification of central afferent projections conveying information of acute "stress" to the hypothalamic paraventricular nucleus. J Neurosci 1995;15:2609–2627.

42. Garceau Y, Liu Y, Loros JJ, et al. Alternative initiation of translation and time-specific phosphorylation yield multiple forms of the essential clock protein FREQUENCY. Cell 1997;89:469–476.

43. Sehgal A, Price AJL, Mann B, et al. Loss of circadian behavioral rhythms and per RNA oscillations in the Drosophilia mutant timeless. Science 1994;263:1603–1606.

44. Ralph MR, Menaker M. A mutation of the circadian system in golden hamsters. Science 1988;241:1225–1227.

45. Albrecht U, Sun ZS, Eichele G, et al. A differential response of two putative mammalian circadian regulators, mper1 and mper2, to light. Cell 1997;91:1055–1064.

46. Shigeyoshi Y, Taguchi K, Yamamoto S, et al. Light-induced resetting of a mammalian circadian clock is associated with rapid induction of the mPer1 transcript. Cell 1997;91:1043–1053.

47. Tei H, Okamura H, Shigeyoshi Y, et al. Circadian oscillation of a mammalian homologue of the Drosophila period gene. Nature 1997;389:512–516.

48. Moore-Ede MC. Jet lag, shift work, and maladaptation. News Physiol Sci 1986;1:156–160.

49. Seidel WF, Roth T, Roehrs T, et al. Treatment of a 12-hour shift of sleep schedule with benzodiazepines. Science 1984;224:1262–1264.

50. Walsh JK, Muehlbach MJ, Schweitzer PK. Acute administration of triazolam for the daytime sleep of rotating shift workers. Sleep 1984;7:223–229.

51. Turek FW, Losee-Olson S. A benzodiazepine used in the treatment of insomnia phase-shifts the mammalian circadian clock. Nature 1986;321:167–168.

52. Van Reeth O, Turek FW. Adaptation of circadian rhythmicity to shift in light-dark cycle accelerated by a benzodiazepine. Am J Physiol 1987;253:R204–R207.

53. Smolensky MH, D'Alonzo GE. Medical chronobiology: concepts and applications. Am Rev Respir Dis 1993;147:S2–S19.

54. Reinberg A, Smolensky MH, eds. Biological rhythms and medicine: cellular, metabolic, physiopathology, and pharmacologic aspects. New York: Springer-Verlag, 1983.

55. Millar-Craig MW, Bishop CN, Raftery EB. Circadian variation of blood-pressure. Lancet 1978;1:795–797.

56. Prinz PN, Halter J, Benedetti C, et al. Circadian variation of plasma catecholamines in young and old men: relation to rapid eye movement and slow wave sleep. J Clin Endocrin Metab 1979;49:300–304.

57. Panza JA, Epstein SE, Quyyumi AA. Circadian variation in vascular tone and its relation to α-sympathetic vasoconstrictor activity. N Engl J Med 1991;325:986–990.

58. Boden G, Ruiz J, Urbain JL, et al. Evidence for a circadian rhythm of insulin secretion. Am J Physiol 1996;271:E246–E252.

59. Trumper BG, Reschke K, Molling J. Circadian variation of insulin requirement in insulin dependent diabetes mellitus: the relationship between circadian change in insulin demand and diurnal patterns of growth hormone, cortisol and glucagon during euglycemia. Horm Metab Res 1995;27:141–147.

60. Krieger DT, Allen W, Rizzo F, et al. Characterization of the normal pattern of plasma corticosteroid levels. J Clin Endocrinol Metab 1971;32:266–284.

61. Boden G, Chen X, Urbain UL. Evidence for a circadian rhythm of insulin sensitivity in patients with NIDDM caused by cyclic changes in hepatic glucose production. Diabetes 1996;45:1044–1050.

62. Nitz D, Siegel J. GABA release in the dorsal raphe nucleus: role in the control of REM sleep. Am J Physiol 1997;273:R451–R455.

63. Kripke DF, Simons RN, Garfinkel L, et al. Short and long sleep and sleeping pills. Arch Gen Psychiatry 1979;36:103–116.

64. Everson CA. Sustained sleep deprivation impairs host defense. Am J Physiol 1993;265:R1148–R1154.

65. Dinges DF, Douglas SD, Hamarman S, et al. Sleep deprivation and human immune function. Adv Neuroimmunol 1995;5:97–110.

66. Pollmacher T, Mullington T, Korth C, et al. Influence of host defense activation on sleep in humans. Adv Neuroimmunol 1995;205:174–181.

67. Benca R, Quintans J. Sleep and host defenses: a review. Sleep 1997;20:1027–1037.

68. Sadamatsu M, Kato N, Iida H, et al. The 24-hour rhythms in plasma growth hormone, prolactin, and thyroid stimulating hormone: effect of sleep deprivation. J Neuroendocrinol 1995;7:599–606.

69. Opstad K. Circadian rhythm of hormones is extinguished during prolonged physical stress, sleep and energy deficiency in young men. Eur J Endocrinol 1994;131:56–66.

70. Baumgartner A, Dietzel M, Saletu B, et al. Influence of partial sleep deprivation on the secretion of thyrotropin, thyroid hormones, growth hormone, prolactin, luteinizing hormone, follicle stimulating hormone, and estradiol in healthy young women. Psych Res 1993;48:153–178.

71. Dinges DF, Pack F, Williams K, et al. Cumulative sleepiness, mood disturbance, and psychomotor vigilance performance decrements during a week of sleep restricted to 4–5 hours per night. Sleep 1997;20:267.

72. Penetar D, McCann U, Thorne D, et al. Caffeine reversal of sleep deprivation effects on alertness and mood. Psychopharmacology 1993;112:359–365.

73. McCann UD, Penetar DM, Shaham Y, et al. Sleep deprivation and impaired cognition. Possible role of brain catecholamines. Biol Psychol 1992;31:1082–1097.

74. Sullivan R. Discovery: Sleepless in America. Life 1998; February:56–66.

75. Lingenfelser T, Kaschel R, Weber A, et al. Young hospital doctors after night duty: their task-specific cognitive status and emotional condition. Med Ed 1994;28:566–572.

76. Lindsley G. The insomnia syndrome: Befuddler of the psychotherapeutic enterprise. In: Ellison JM, Weinstein CS, Hodel-Malinofsky T, eds. The psychotherapist's guide to neuropsychiatry: diagnostic and treatment issues. Washington, D.C.: American Psychiatric Press, 1994:279–302.

77. Lupien SJ, Gaudreau S, Tchiteya BM, et al. Stress-induced declarative memory impairment in healthy elderly subjects: relationship to cortisol reactivity. J Clin Endocrinol Metab 1997;82:2070–2075.

78. Rechtschaffen A, Bergmann BM, Everson CA, et al. Sleep deprivation in the rat: X, integration and discussion of the findings. Sleep 1989;12:68–87.

79. Hauri P, Linde S. No more sleepless nights. New York: Wiley, 1990.

80. Diagnostic Classification Steering Committee, Thorpy MJ, chairman. International Classification of Sleep Disorders. Rochester, MN: American Sleep Disorders Association, 1989.

81. Kryger MH, Roth T, Dement WC, eds. Principles and practice of sleep disorders medicine. Philadelphia: W. B. Saunders, 1989.

Part XX.

DERMATOLOGY

Edited by
Gary R. Kantor

Introduction to Dermatology

James M. Rippe

The skin, just like every other organ, reacts to lifestyle practices whether they be positive or negative. In this section, a distinguished group of authors focuses on aspects of lifestyle that impact the skin.

The first chapter by Ashraf Hassanein focuses on issues of nutritional balance and nutritional adequacy and skin health. The author discusses a wide variety of nutritional disorders, ranging from deficiencies to excesses, that may impact on the skin. He also reminds us that nutritional practices can exert an impact on DNA, and either lower the risk of the likelihood of skin cancer or increase it.

The chapter by Susan Bittenbender and Gary Kantor focuses on how aging relates to dermatologic issues. As the authors point out, life expectancy is increasing in the United States and other industrialized countries. Thus it becomes increasingly important for all physicians caring for older patients to recognize the difference between normal effects of aging on the skin and pathologic changes.

The chapter on sun and the skin by Chris Scholes presents a detailed summary of what is known about ultraviolet radiation and its effect on skin. The author begins with a basic description of the physics and physiology of the sun/skin interaction. He then proceeds to explore interactions not only between the sun and the skin but also drugs, sunscreen, clothing, and other factors that may positively or negatively alter the sun/skin interaction.

Gary Kantor, in his chapter on exercise and the skin, reminds us that physicians and other healthcare workers are increasingly seeing individuals who are engaging in athletic activity for cardiovascular fitness and stress reduction. Because of these positive reasons for exercise, individuals may inadvertently develop a whole host of disorders of the skin that are either caused or exacerbated by exercise. This comprehensive chapter describes both characteristics and treatment options for various exercise-induced skin problems.

In the concluding chapter of the section, Elen Donahue and Gary Kantor provide a general approach to skin care for the sports active individual. They categorize those modalities that have been shown to carry positive value and those which have not. This final chapter provides useful information for all individuals active in sports and the practitioners caring for them.

Chapter 109

Nutritional Diseases and the Skin

Ashraf M. Hassanein

Maintenance of adequate normal nutrition is essential for the prevention and management of disease. The skin appearance of a patient reflects his or her general health, race, and age. Moreover, cutaneous manifestations of abnormal nutrition can help identify the deficient nutrient and evaluate the adequacy of dietary replacement. Nutritional disorders may result from insufficient intake of dietary constituents, malabsorption, repeated vomiting, diarrhea, and fistulas. In this chapter, diseases of nutrition will be discussed, with special emphasis on their cutaneous manifestations.

PROTEIN-ENERGY MALNUTRITION

Protein-energy malnutrition (PEM), also termed protein-calorie malnutrition, results when inadequate protein and/or energy is available to satisfy the metabolic demands. Insufficient dietary intake, increased metabolic demands due to disease, and increased nutrient losses are the most common causes of PEM (1). Furthermore, PEM could be the outcome of multiple conditions that can produce protein-losing enteropathy. This category of disease is exemplified by Ménétrier's disease, characterized by gastric mucosal hypertrophy with protein loss, lymphatic obstruction, intestinal lymphangiectasia, and constrictive pericarditis.

The two most common forms of PEM are marasmus and kwashiorkor. Marasmus results from prolonged starvation, whereas kwashiorkor is the result of marked protein depletion with relative carbohydrate excess.

Marasmus

Marasmus is a severe emaciation resulting from starvation. It usually affects infants who are deprived of breast feeding without adequate substitution of other nutrients. However, severely ill hospitalized patients may show signs of marasmus. Marasmic patients frequently express manifestations of other nutritional deficiencies, e.g., zinc and vitamin deficiencies (1). The main clinical finding is marked weight loss. The skin appears wrinkled, loose, thin, inelastic, and dry with loss of subcutaneous fat. Marasmic adults may show prominent follicular hyperkeratosis. Their hair is sparse and thin and their nails are fissured. Skin ulcers may occur. Loss of buccal fat pad results in a characteristic "monkey facies." In contrast to kwashiorkor, marasmic patients have neither hepatomegaly nor edema. Fat metabolism is probably normal, as evidenced by normal serum lipid levels and absent hepatic fatty change.

Kwashiorkor

Kwashiorkor is a nutritional syndrome resulting from severe dietary protein deficiency with relative high carbohydrate supply. It usually affects children older than one year who are weaned and who are fed a starch-rich, protein-poor diet. Kwashiorkor is most commonly seen in the tropical and subtropical developing countries. However, it may be seen in older severely ill patients, terminal cancer patients, alcoholics, and patients with severe malabsorption (2).

Patients with kwashiorkor usually manifest with edema that can be mild pitting edema or anasarca, hepatomegaly, muscle wasting, and growth and behavioral abnormalities. Cutaneous changes of kwashiorkor are especially prominent in dark-skinned individuals (3). The typical skin changes are described as "flaky paint" or "enamel paint" and consist of waxy plaques of hypópigmentation with fine, bran-like desquamation that usually develop in edematous and circumoral areas (2,4). The skin of the tibial shins is usually dry, glossy, pigmented, and fissured. The "flag sign," which consists of alternating bands of normal and hypopigmented scalp hair related to intermittent periods of insufficient nutrition, is also seen.

Laboratory findings include hypoalbuminemia, anemia, hypoferremia, hypotransferrinemia, and hypozincemia. Frequently, these patients develop hypoglycemia, hypoaminoacidemia, and hypolipemia with elevated free fatty acids. Secretory IgA levels are reduced, while the humoral immunity is not generally altered. On the other hand, cell-mediated immunity is affected as evidenced by diminished absolute T-helper cell count and abnormal in vitro lymphocyte stimulation test (5). Finally, it has to be emphasized that kwashiorkor patients may have altered pharmacokinetics due to altered drug metabolism, clearance, and/or binding.

FAT-SOLUBLE VITAMINS

Vitamin A

Vitamin A is a cyclic fat-soluble polyene that is present in the diet as the vitamin itself or as a precursor in the form of beta carotene. The main dietary sources are liver, butter, eggs, carrots, fruits, and green leafy vegetables. The recommended daily allowance is 5000 IU, while the normal blood level is approximately 1.5 μmol/L. Vitamin A has three molecular forms: retinol, retinal, and retinoic acid. Retinyl esters are hydrolized to retinol before being uptaken by intestinal mucosa. In the intestinal villi, retinal is reduced into retinol, which forms complexes with cellular retinol-binding protein, type II (CRBP II), and is esterified to retinyl esters. The latter enter the blood in a bound form with chylomicrons (6). In the liver, retinyl esters are hydrolyzed into retinol, which can be bound to either transthyretin (prealbumen) or retinol-binding protein (RBP). Zinc deficiency can lead to vitamin A deficiency as the former acts on RBP. Moreover, zinc deficiency may lead to alteration of the oxidation-reduction interconversion of vitamin A secondary to alteration of alcohol dehydrogenase, which is a zinc metalloprotein. Furthermore, nyctalopia (night blindness) in alcoholics may be the result of the combined deficiency of zinc and vitamin A (7). Vitamin A is essential for the integrity of epithelia. In humans, high doses of vitamin A can produce retardation of keratinocyte maturation (8). A high dose of vitamin A or sterioisomers of retinoic acid has been successful in treating some skin disorders with abnormal keratinization such as ichthyosis, pityriasis, rubra pilaris, and Darier's disease (9).

Vitamin A Deficiency

Vitamin A deficiency is rarely seen today in the developed countries. However, it may be observed as a manifestation of malabsorption and frequently is associated with other fat-soluble vitamin deficiencies. On the other hand, in developing countries, it may be seen due to inadequate nutrition. Cutaneous manifestations include xerostomia, follicular hyperkeratosis, and generalized xerosis (dry skin). Follicular papules are characteristically distributed symmetrically on dorsal and lateral aspects of extremities and referred to as "phrynoderma" or "toad skin" (3,10). Other clinical signs of vitamin A deficiency include hemeralopia, nyctalopia, Bitot's spots, corneal ulceration, and keratomalacia. Ocular manifestations,

with the exception of corneal ulceration, respond to replacement therapy faster than cutaneous manifestations, which resolve within weeks to few months (3).

Hypervitaminosis A

Most chronic vitamin A toxicities are observed in children who are overdosed with concentrated vitamin A preparations. However, adult cases have also been reported (11). These patients develop anorexia, lethargy, and loss of weight. Cutaneous manifestations include diffuse alopecia and pruritic rough dry skin with follicular hyperkeratosis, patchy erythema, and purpura (12).

Carotenoderma

This describes an orange discoloration of the horny layer due to excess carotenes in the sweat secondary to a high intake of carrots. Children are more susceptible to this condition than adults. Infants can develop carotenoderma after two months on breast milk of a carotenic mother. Adults, typically a pregnant woman with pica syndrome, need to consume 1.8 kg of carrots weekly to develop appreciable skin pigmentation (13). Skin pigmentation usually develops in palms, soles, and in seborrheic areas. Subcutaneous fat may also be bright yellow. This harmless condition must be differentiated from jaundice by absence of scleral or mucous membrane pigmentation, itching, or change in urine or stool color. It must be noted that carotenemia is noted in some patients with hyperlipemia, such as those with myxedema and diabetes mellitus and those with metabolic carotenemia (14).

Vitamin D

Vitamin D is a fat-soluble vitamin that plays a role in calcium homeostasis. Vitamin D synthesis starts in the skin under the influence of ultraviolet light, where provitamin D3 (7-dehydrocholesterol) is isomerized to previtamin D3. The latter is spontaneously isomerized in the skin to vitamin D3, which enters the circulation via dermal capillaries. In the liver, it is hydrolyzed to 25-hydroxyvitamin D3 (25-hydroxycholecalciferol), and then to 1,25 dihydroxyvitamin D3 (calcitriol; 1,25 dihydroxycholecalciferol) in the kidney (3). Consequently, the skin is of unique importance in the synthesis, storage, and release of vitamin D into the circulation. Furthermore, chronic use of sunscreens may cause decreased circulating levels of 25-hydroxyvitamin D (15).

Deficiency of vitamin D causes rickets in children and osteomalacia in adults. However, no cutaneous lesions are specific for these diseases (16). On the other hand, vitamin D intoxication leads to hypercalcemia, hypercalciuria, nephrocalcinosis, and possibly widespread metastatic calcification. The latter manifests in the skin as deposits of small yellow hard nodules. Some constitutional symptoms may accompany hypercalcemia in the form of fatigue, depression, anorexia, constipation, nausea, and vomiting.

Vitamin K

Vitamin K is a natural fat-soluble vitamin present in green vegetables as vitamin K1 and as a product of intestinal bacteria as vitamin K2. Intestinal bacteria can metabolize both forms to menadione that is absorbed and then metabolized to its active form menaquinone. Vitamin K is essential for hepatic synthesis of coagulation factors. These include the coagulation factors II, VII, IX, and X as well as the anticoagulant proteins C and S (16). Vitamin K deficiency is caused by poor fat absorption, e.g., obstructive jaundice, and prolonged use of broad-spectrum antibiotics that alter intestinal flora. Hemorrhagic disease of newborns occurs partially because of a sterile gut and because of failure of the placenta to properly transmit lipids and fat-soluble vitamins.

Vitamin E

Alpha-tocopherol is the most potent vitamin E derivative. It is not clearly understood whether vitamin E is essential to humans or not. However, vitamin E has been claimed to be used as an effective treatment of some dermatologic disorders (17) and wound healing (18).

WATER-SOLUBLE VITAMINS

Thiamin

Thiamin (vitamin B1) is present in most foods and particularly abundant in the outer layers of cereal grains. Increased thiamin requirement occurs in pregnancy, thyrotoxicosis, dialysis, PEM, and alcoholism. Thiamin deficiency causes beri beri, which occurs in two forms. Wet beri beri is associated with peripheral vasodilatation, edema, and arteriovenous shunting, creating hyperdynamic circulation and heart failure. On the other hand, dry beri beri is associated with atrophy of muscles and skin changes secondary to peripheral neuropathy.

Consequently, cutaneous findings in thiamin deficiency are nonspecific and occur as a systemic manifestation of beri beri (16).

Riboflavin

Riboflavin (vitamin B2) is an essential component of the flavoprotein coenzymes, e.g., flavin mononucleotide (FMN) and flavin-adenine dinucleotide (FAD). Riboflavin is present in many plant and animal sources. Clinical deficiency manifests after several months of deprivation, which can be caused by malnutrition or chronic disease such as achlorhydria and alcoholic cirrhosis. Biochemical evidence of deficiency is noted with hypothyroidism, acute boric acid intoxication, neonatal phototherapy for hyperbilirubinemia, and chlorpromazine use (3). Clinical manifestations of deficiency include corneal vascularization and conjunctivitis with consequent photophobia. Cheilosis, sore lips, and angular stomatitis are frequently present. Glossitis is commonly present with smooth purple-red tongue (Figure 109-1). A scaly seborrheic dermatitis-like eruption may develop especially along the nasolabial fold, nose, forehead, cheeks, and postauricular areas. Scrotal dermatitis may develop with scaly erythematous eruption and lichenification that usually spares the median commissure (19). These manifestations are referred to as oro-oculogenital syndrome.

Niacin

Niacin (nicotinamide, nicotinic acid, vitamin B3) is a vitamin B complex component that has the unique characteristic of

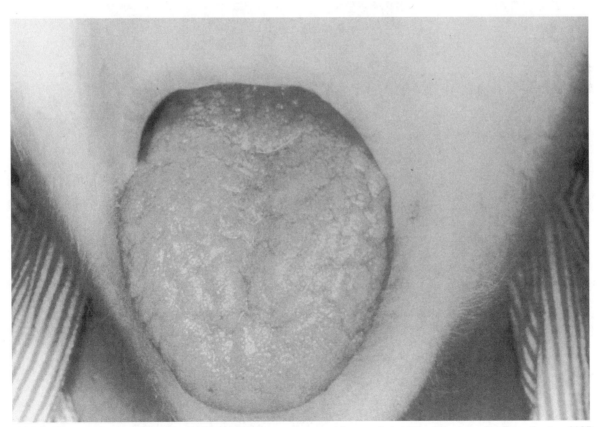

Figure 109-1 Tongue of a patient with riboflavin deficiency shows evidence of glossitis. (Courtesy Dr. Gary Kantor, MCP Hahnemann University, Philadelphia, PA.)

being synthesized in the body from the essential amino acid tryptophan. Niacin is a component of the ubiquitous coenzyme nicotinamide-adenine dinucleotide (NAD) and nicotinamide-adenine dinucleotide phosphate (NADP). Pellagra, the disease resulting from niacin deficiency, was first described by Casal in 1735 and was related to a maize diet (3). Pellagra is still seen in some areas of Asia where maize is the main diet. However, it may complicate some cases of malnutrition, as can occur in Crohn's disease, or following gastroenterostomy or subtotal gastrectomy. It may also complicate metabolic diseases that alter tryptophan metabolism, e.g., Hartnup disease and carcinoid syndrome.

Pellagra is classically characterized by the three Ds: diarrhea, dementia, and dermatitis. Erythema and superficial scaling appear on sun-exposed areas and at sites of trauma and friction. The eruption is symmetrically distributed on the dorsa of hands (Figure 109-2), forearms, legs (Figure 109-3), central chest, face, and neck.

Cutaneous manifestations begin as lesions resembling sunburn and resolve leaving dusky, brown-red coloration. A symmetric "butterfly" facial eruption occurs with marginated rash on the anterior aspect of the neck referred to as "Casal's necklace" (3).

Vitamin B6

Vitamin B6 is a pyridine derivative that has three interchangeable forms: pyridoxine, pyridoxamine, and pyridoxal. It is present in many foods including eggs, yeast, and various grains. Vitamin B6 deficiency is rare but can be seen in patients with chronic alcoholism, those treated with isonicotinic acid hydrazide (INH), and in some diseases associated with an increased demand for pyridoxine, e.g., homocystinuria and pyridoxine-responsive anemia (16). The most common cutaneous feature of pyridoxine deficiency is a seborrhea-like dermatitis of the face, neck, scalp, perineum, and buttocks. Other manifestations include glossitis, angular stomatitis, cheilosis, conjunctivitis, and intertrigo. Finally, pellagra-like dermatitis may rarely develop (3). In some instances, convulsions, anemia, and sensory neuritis with ascending paresthesias may develop (20).

Folic Acid

Folic acid is a glutamic acid derivative present in liver, meat, milk, and green leafy vegetables. In vivo, folic acid is converted to folinic acid with the aid of vitamin C. Folic acid deficiency is associated with greyish-brown discoloration on sun-exposed areas of the skin. Frequently, there is spotty pigmentation of palms and soles, with pigmented palmar creases (21), mucosal erosion, glossitis, and cheilitis.

Vitamin B12

Vitamin B12 (cyanocobalamine) is present mostly in animal sources and hence strict vegetarians are vulnerable to its deficiency. Pernicious anemia, the most common malabsorption disease, usually results from lack of the intrinsic factor. This is most commonly associated with atrophic gastritis and

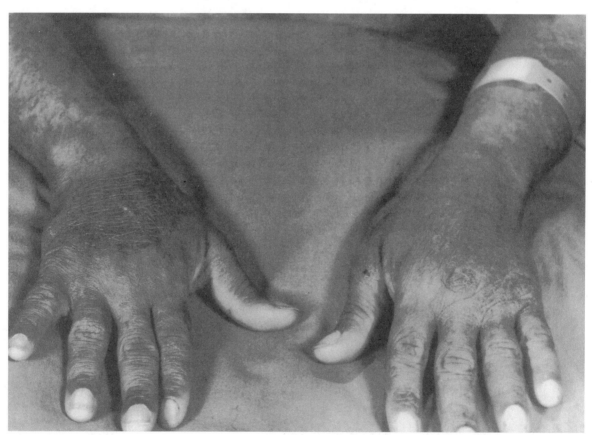

Figure 109-2 Dorsa of the hands of a pellagra patient show symmetrical hyperkeratosis and hyperpigmentation. (Courtesy Dr. Gary Kantor, MCP Hahnemann University, Philadelphia, PA.)

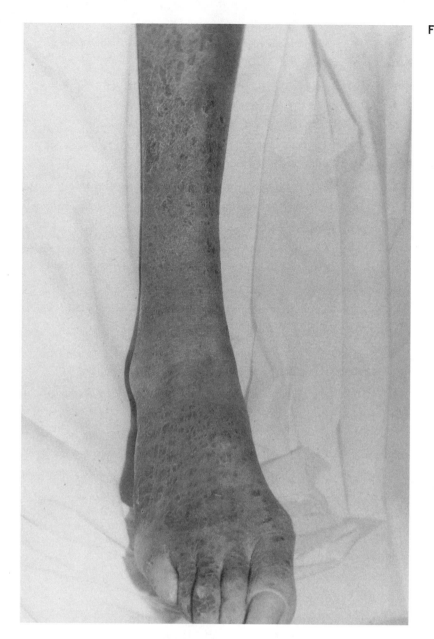

Figure 109-3 Hyperkeratotic, hyperpigmented plaques over the shin of the tibia and dorsum of the foot of this pellagra patient. (Courtesy Dr. Gary Kantor, MCP Hahnemann University, Philadelphia, PA.)

leads to megaloblastic anemia and neurologic manifestations secondary to subacute combined degeneration of the spinal cord. Vitamin B12 deficiency may also be caused by the fish tapeworm *Diphylobothrium latum*, which competes with the host's digestive system for vitamin B12 (16). Characteristically, vitamin B12 deficiency is associated with an enlarged, red tongue. Cutaneous hyperpigmentation can occur, especially in skin flexures, e.g., digits and palms.

Biotin

Biotin (vitamin H) is a water-soluble sulfur-containing coenzyme essential for carbohydrate and fat metabolism. Raw eggwhite contains avidin that binds biotin and prevents its absorption. Prolonged consumption of raw eggwhite has led to biotin deficiency. Other causes of biotin deficiency are parenteral nutrition and the autosomal recessive traits holocarboxylase and biotinidase deficiencies (22). Biotin-deficient patients may develop the "uncombable hair syndrome" char-

acterized by thin, slow-growing, straw-colored hairs with triangular cross section. These patients respond to oral biotin of 0.3 mg three times daily (23). Biotin deficiency manifests with dermatitis, eczema, alopecia, conjunctivitis, hyperesthesia, paraesthesia, muscle pains, and depression (24).

Vitamin C

Vitamin C (ascorbic acid) is abundant in fruits and vegetables. It plays an important role in collagen synthesis. Vitamin C deficiency (scurvy) occurs in elderly persons with an inadequate diet. Scurvy manifests with poor wound healing, bleeding gums, bone changes in the form of subperiosteal hemorrhages, and joint and bone aches. Follicular hyperkeratosis with perifollicular hemorrhages and "corkscrew" hairs are characteristic cutaneous features. Corkscrew hairs occur due to decreased number of reduced disulfide bonds necessary for keratin cross-linking and possibly also due to weak perifollicular connective tissue (3).

OTHER NUTRIENTS

Zinc

Zinc is an essential trace element. Approximately 20% to 30% of ingested zinc is absorbed mainly in the small intestine. Total body zinc can be estimated by measuring the neutrophil zinc levels. Zinc levels in the skin normally decrease with increasing depth in the skin. Therefore, it is highest in the epidermis (600 μg/g), lower in the papillary dermis (40 μg/g), and lowest in the reticular dermis (10 μg/g). Zinc deficiency occurs in premature infants, infants raised on a low-zinc formula, and in alcoholics. The latter occurs because alcohol increases urinary zinc excretion. Other causes of zinc deficiency include malabsorption syndromes, jejunoileal bypass, inflammatory bowel disease, chronic renal failure, burns, and cancer.

Acrodermatitis enteropathica is an autosomal recessive condition characterized by low zinc absorption (26). Clinical features of zinc deficiency involve many organ systems. Cutaneous manifestations include pustular and bullous dermatitis with acral and perioral distribution, pustular paronychia, angular stomatitis, glossitis, and alopecia (3). Deep transverse depressions ("Beau's lines") develop on fingernails due to temporary arrest of nail growth (27,28).

Essential Fatty Acids

Essential fatty acids (EFA) must be obtained in the diet since endogenous synthesis does not occur. EFA are the precursors of eicosanoids that include prostaglandins, hydroxyeicosatetraenoic acids, and leukotrienes. Major epidermal fatty acids include linoleic acid and arachidonic acid. Linoleic acid is necessary for proper lamellar granule formation, which is essential for providing the barrier function of the epidermis (29). EFA deficiency is seen in low-birthweight infants, infants with gastrointestinal anomalies, patients with inflammatory bowel disease, patients with intestinal surgery, and patients undergoing total parenteral nutrition (3). Cutaneous manifestations of EFA deficiency include alopecia, xerotic eczema, intertriginous erosions, and increased transepidermal water loss. Noncutaneous features include growth retardation, fatty change of the liver, anemia, thrombocytopenia, poor wound healing, and susceptibility to infection (3).

Copper

Copper deficiency is detected in infants with severe PEM, and those fed on low-copper milk. These infants develop anemia, neutropenia, and failure to thrive. Menke's hair (kinky hair) syndrome is an X-linked recessive disorder of copper metabolism. It is associated with low copper level in blood, liver, and hair. Children with Menke's syndrome have lethargy, drowsiness, hypotonia, seizures, and mental retardation. "Pili torti" describes a characteristic repetitive hair twisting (30). Trichorrhexis nodosa and monilethrix may occur. The former describes brushlike swellings of hair shafts that contain frayed cortical fibers, whereas the latter describes segmental hair shaft narrowings (3). Some patients have characteristic facies with pallor, pudgy cheeks, horizontal eyebrows, and an expressionless, lateral gaze (30).

SUMMARY

There is no doubt that the scope of nutritional disorders is broad, relating not only to deficiency of a variety of nutrients but also to an excess of some. Nutritional disorders arise secondary to primary dietary imbalance, or failure of utilization that could be familial, metabolic, or acquired. It is important to examine the skin when a patient presents with a gastrointestinal problem, since diseases of the skin and alimentary tract coexist more frequently than expected. On the other hand, nutrients and nutritional factors in the diet can protect DNA from being damaged and can delay or prevent cancer development even in people with an increased genetic risk for the disease (31).

REFERENCES

1. Mason JB, Rosenberg IH. Protein-energy malnutrition. In: Isselbacher AB, Martin JB, Braunwald E, et al, eds. Harrison's principles of internal medicine. 13th ed. New York: McGraw-Hill 1994:440.

2. Hennington VM, Carve E, Derbes V, et al. Kwashiorkor: a report of four cases from Louisiana. Arch Dermatol 1958;78:157–170.

3. Miller SJ. Nutritional deficiency and the skin. J Am Acad Dermatol 1989;21:1–30.

4. McLaren DS. Skin in protein energy malnutrition. Arch Dermatol 1987;123:1674a–1676a.

5. Chandra RK. T and B lymphocyte subpopulations and leukocyte terminal deoxynucleotidyltransferase in energy-protein undernutrition. Act Paediatr Scand 1979;68:841.

6. Org DE. Vitamin A-binding proteins. Nutr Rev 1985;43:225–232.

7. Solomons NW, Russell RM. The interaction of vitamin A and zinc: implications for human nutrition. Am J Clin Nutr 1980;33:2031.

8. Pinkus H, Hunter R. Biometric analysis of the effect of oral vitamin A on human epidermis. J Invest Dermatol 1964;42:131.

9. Thomas JR, Coke JP, Winkelman RK. High-dose vitamin A therapy for Darrier's disease. Arch Dermol 1982;118:891.

10. Logan WS. Vitamin A and keratinization. Arch Dermol 1972;105:748–753.

11. Raaschou-Nielsen W. Chronic intoxication with vitamin A in adults. Dermatologica 1961;123:293.

12. Soler-Bechara I, Socia JL. Chronic hypervitaminosis: report of a case in an adult. Arch Intern Med 1963;112:462.

13. McLaren DS. Cutaneous changes in nutritional disorders. In: Fitzpatrick T, Eisen A, Wolff K, et al, eds. Dermatology in general medicine. 4th ed. New York: McGraw-Hill, 1993:1821.

14. Monk BE. Metabolic carotenemia. Br J Dermol 1982;106:485–488.

15. Matsuoka LY, Wortsman J, Hanifan N, et al. Chronic sunscreen use decreases circulatory concentration of 25-hydroxyvitamin D: a preliminary study. Arch Dermol 1988; 124:1802–1804.

16. Hassanein AM, Atkinson BF. Nutritional pathology. In: Pathology review. Thousand Oaks, CA: Sage, 1998:121–126.

17. Ayers S, Mihan R. Vitamin E as a useful therapeutic agent. J Am Acad Dermol 1982;7:521.

18. Pollack SV. Wound healing: a review IV: systemic medications affecting wound healing. J Dermatol Surg Oncol 1983;8:667–672.

19. Hills OW, Liebert E, Steinberg A, et al. Clinical aspects of dietary depletion of riboflavin. Arch Intern Med 1951;87:682–693.

20. Viller RW, Mueller JF, Glazer HS, et al. The effect of vitamin B6 deficiency induced by desoxypyridoxine in human beings. J Lab Clin Med 1953;42:335–337.

21. Baumschlag N, Metz J. Pigmentation in megaloblastic anemia associated with pregnancy and lactation. BMJ 1969;II:737–739.

22. Champion RH, Burton JL, Ebling FJ. Metabolic and nutritional disorders. In: Champion RH, Burton JL, & Ebling FJ, eds. Rook/Wilkinson and Ebling Textbook of Dermatology. Oxford, England: Blackwell Scientific, 1992:2363.

23. Shelley WB, Shelley ED. Uncombable hair syndrome: observations on response to biotin and occurrence in siblings with ectodermal dysplasia. J Am Acad Dermatol 1985;13:97–102.

24. McClain CI, Baker H, Onstad GR. Biotin deficiency in an adult during parenteral nutrition. J Am Acad Dermatol 1982;247:3116.

25. Michaelsson G, Ljunghall K, Danielson BG. Zinc in epidermis and dermis in healthy subjects. Acta Derm Venereol (Stockh) 1980;60:295–299.

26. Danbolt N, Closs K. Acrodermatitis enteropathica. Acta Derm Venereol (Stockh) 1943;23:127–169.

27. Weismann K. Lines of Brau: possible markers of zinc deficiency. Acta Derm Venereol 1971;57:88.

28. Gonzalez JR, Botet MV, Sanchez JL. The histopathology of acrodermatitis enteropathica. Am J Dermatopath 1982;4:303–311.

29. Wertz PW, Swartzendruber DC, Abraham W, et al. Essential fatty acids and epidermal integrity. Arch Dermatol 1987;123:1381a–1384a.

30. Danks DM, Campbell PE, Stevens BJ, et al. Menke's kinky hair syndrome: an inherited defect in copper absorption with widespread defects. Pediatrics 1972;50:188–201.

31. The American Cancer Society, 1996 Advisory Committee on Diet, Nutrition, and Cancer Prevention. Guidelines on diet, nutrition, and cancer prevention: reducing the risk of cancer with healthy food choices and physical activity. CA Cancer J Clin 1996;46:325–341.

Chapter 110

Aging and the Skin

Susan Bittenbender
Gary R. Kantor

Life expectancy in the United States has been increasing over the last century with the most rapidly growing segment of the population in the over-65 age group. As a result, there will continue to be an increase in dermatologic disorders related to aging. It is important to know the effects of aging on the skin in order to differentiate between pathologic and normal age-related skin changes.

There are two types of cutaneous aging, intrinsic or chronologic aging, and extrinsic or photoaging. Intrinsic aging depends on physiologic and genetic factors, and the effects of disease and drugs. Race does not seem to play a role in cutaneous chronologic aging (1). Photoaging is the result of life-long cumulative exposure to ultraviolet radiation (UVR) from the sun. In habitually sun-exposed areas of the body, there are effects from both types of aging. However, most of the undesirable features associated with skin aging appear to be caused by photoaging (2).

Despite years of research, the precise mechanisms responsible for intrinsic aging are unknown, and controversy exists regarding some of the associated structural and functional changes that take place in the skin. Thus, continued research is needed to improve our understanding of normal skin aging. This chapter emphasizes alterations in the skin due to the intrinsic aging process.

EPIDERMIS

The skin is composed of three distinct layers that are affected by the aging process: the epidermis, dermis, and subcutaneous fat. The epidermis is the most superficial layer and is made up of rows of cells known as keratinocytes. The outermost epi-dermal layers contain flattened, terminally differentiated cells forming the stratum corneum, which is the main environmental barrier. The innermost row is made up of basal cells that form attachments with the underlying dermis and proliferate to form the other epidermal layers.

There are multiple age-related changes reported to occur in the epidermis (Table 110-1). The most consistent finding is flattening of the normally undulating dermal-epidermal junction (DEJ) resulting in a decreased area of contact between the two layers. This may explain why DEJ separation and subsequent blistering occurs more readily in the elderly due to minor trauma or edema (3). Other observations include a decrease in the epidermal turnover rate by 30% to 50% between the ages of 20 and 70, fewer basal cells per unit surface available to form the stratum corneum, and prolongation of stratum corneum replacement (1,3,6). These factors probably contribute to skin dryness associated with aging. In addition, there is a global decrease in lipid content of the stratum corneum with age, which may also contribute to a rougher, drier quality to the skin (4,5). Through their ability to bind water, stratum corneum lipids are thought to play a major role in skin hydration (5). There are also changes in epidermal drug permeability and cell cohesiveness in the stratum corneum (4,5). These abnormalities may result in a defective permeability barrier that is easier to disrupt and slower to repair (4). However, there is no consensus of opinion based on scientific investigation as to the effects of intrinsic aging on the epidermal barrier as a function of water content, transepidermal water loss, and percutaneous absorption. Finally, it has often been reported that there is an age-associated decrease in the thickness of the epidermis; however, this finding is disputed by other investigators (1,7).

Table 110-1 Changes in the Epidermis with Intrinsic Aging

- ↓ lipid content of stratum corneum
- ↓ cell cohesiveness in stratum corneum
- ↓ epidermal turnover rate
- altered epidermal drug permeability
- flattening of DEJ
- variable size, shape, and staining of keratinocytes
- ↓ number of melanocytes
- ↓ number of Langerhan's cells
- ↓ vitamin D synthesis

Morphologic alterations in keratinocytes such as variation in size, shape, and staining characteristics have been noted in aged epidermis (1,7). These cellular changes are more pronounced in photoaged skin. Other cells in the epidermis are also affected by the aging process, for example, melanocytes, which produce pigment in the skin, and Langerhans cells, which are immunologic cells involved in antigen recognition and presentation. The number of enzymatically active melanocytes decreases by 8% to 20% per decade after the age of 30 (1,7). Thus, there may be a decreased ability to tan resulting in a reduced protective mechanism against UVR. Langerhans cells decrease by 20% to 50% in the elderly, which may contribute to the age-associated decrease in immune responsiveness in the skin (3). An impairment in T-cell mediated immunity with a decline in delayed hypersensitivity reactions is noted (8). Antibody-mediated effector functions are also decreased, and there is an increase in autoantibody production with age (8). As a consequence of these changes, the elderly have an increased susceptibility to cutaneous infections and cancers.

Vitamin D synthesis is an important endocrine function of the epidermis that is also reported to decline with age. Provitamin D3 in keratinocytes is converted to previtamin D3 by ultraviolet B radiation and subsequently to vitamin D3, which is converted to its active form in the liver and kidney. The amount of the provitamin in the epidermis and previtamin production after exposure to UVR are both reduced in the aged (9). Deficiency of vitamin D can lead to osteomalacia and a predisposition to bone fractures.

DERMIS

The dermis is located just beneath the epidermis, to which it is attached by specialized connections. The dermis is mainly composed of a connective tissue matrix of collagen and ground substance made up of glycosaminoglycans and proteoglycans. Other components include elastic fibers, numerous cell types including fibroblasts and cells of the immune system, blood vessels, lymphatics, nerves, and adnexal structures (hair follicles, glands). There are two layers in the dermis: the papillary dermis, which is made up of finer, looser collagen fibrils, and the deeper reticular dermis where the collagen is more dense.

More striking alterations occur during the aging process in the dermis than in the epidermis (Table 110-2). There is a decrease in dermal thickness by as much as 20% in the elderly (3). It has been observed that the collagen content of the dermis decreases by 1% per year throughout adult life due to decreased synthesis by fibroblasts and increased proteolytic activity (1,7). The structural integrity of the collagen fibrils is also altered and their arrangement becomes disorganized (1). These abnormalities disturb the tensile strength of the dermis and may account for the thinned appearance of the skin often noted in the aged.

Hyaluronic acid is the major glycosaminoglycan (GAG) of the dermal extracellular matrix. GAGs are polysaccharide chains with water-attracting properties. They are necessary for water balance and the transport of substances in the skin, as well as for maintaining the structure and organization of the dermis (10–12). In addition, GAGs are believed to play a role in cell proliferation and migration (11). Studies have shown a decline in the content of hyaluronic acid in the skin with increasing age, which has been proposed to contribute to thinning of the dermis (10,11). Other investigators have found only an altered distribution of hyaluronic acid (12). These changes in GAGs probably also contribute to the clinical appearance of aging skin (10,11).

Elastic fibers are structural proteins in the dermis that give the skin its resilience and elasticity. There is a progressive disintegration of elastic tissue in the papillary dermis with intrinsic aging. The fibers have a decreased diameter and appear fragmented, especially in the area of the DEJ. In the reticular dermis there is an increased number of thickened haphazardly arranged fibers (1). These changes are speculated to result from changes in proteolytic and synthetic activity. The regression of the subepidermal elastic fiber network is considered to play a major role in the development of sagging and wrinkling of the skin (1,7).

Impairment of various steps in the process of wound healing has been reported in the elderly, including a decreased rate of epidermal repair and abnormal connective tissue remodelling (13). A decline in cell responsiveness to chemical signals in the epidermis and dermis and a progressive loss of dermal fibroblasts, mast cells, and macrophages with advancing

Table 110-2 Changes in the Dermis with Intrinsic Aging

- ↓ collagen
- disorganization of collagen fibers
- fragmented, disorganized elastic fibers
- ↓ GAGs
- ↓ fibroblasts
- ↓ mast cells
- ↓ papillary dermal blood vessels
- abnormal nerve endings
- ↓ eccrine and apocrine glands
- hyperplasia of sebaceous glands
- ↓ function of eccrine, apocrine, and sebaceous glands
- ↓ terminal hairs
- graying of hair
- ↓ growth rate of hair and nails
- abnormal nail plates

age has been reported and may affect wound healing (13,14). Other factors may also have an impact on wound healing, including infection, physical stress, disease, nutritional state, and drugs (14). Despite abnormalities in certain components of the process, wound healing in the elderly is essentially normal overall, provided that there are no complicating factors (13).

Blood vessels of the dermis provide the skin with oxygen and nutrients. A significant decline in the density of nutrient exchange vessels in the papillary dermis occurs during chronologic aging and may have significant physiologic consequences (15). Dermal mast cells, which stimulate angiogenesis, are reduced by 50% (7). Also, there is a progressive loss of structural support for the dermal vasculature that may contribute to increased bruising and dilated blood (telangiectasia) and lymphatic vessels (7). An age-related decrease in the dermal clearance of transepidermally absorbed substances has been observed and may be related to changes in the vascular bed as well as the extracellular matrix (3,15). In contrast, the effect of intrinsic aging on the function of the nervous system in the skin is still largely unknown. However, reported findings include a decrease in organized sensory nerve endings, diminished tactile sensation, and an increased pain threshold (1,3).

Three types of glands are found in the skin: 1) eccrine glands, which are distributed over nearly the entire body surface and produce sweat in response to increases in body temperature; 2) apocrine glands, which occur in the axilla and perineum and become functional around the time of puberty; and 3) sebaceous glands, which produce sebum and are associated with hair follicles. It is well known that the number and function of eccrine glands decreases with age, and structural changes have been noted (1,16). Apocrine glands also tend to decrease in size and limited studies show a declining function that is likely related to lower levels of circulating androgens (17). Sebum production in sebaceous glands peaks in late adolescence and then declines by about 23% and 32% per decade in men and women respectively (17). It has been proposed that decreasing androgen production is also responsible (1,17). Yet, a gradual increase in the size of some sebaceous glands, especially on the face, can occur and may explain the development of sebaceous hyperplasia, a lesion that appears commonly with age (1,17). Despite these alterations in sweat and sebum production, a significant association with the development of dry skin in the elderly is lacking (3).

Hair shows several changes with advancing age such as a decline in number, diameter, and growth rate (1). There are fewer terminal hairs and hair follicles on the body in both men and women, and more hairs are in the telogen or resting phase (7,15). Graying of the hair is a normal manifestation of aging in which heredity plays an important role (1). It reflects the progressive loss of functional melanocytes from the hair bulb, resulting in decreased melanin pigment in the hair shaft (1,3). There is also a slow decline in the rate of growth of the nails (1,3). Other common nail findings in the elderly include longitudinal ridging, brittleness with splitting of the distal nail, pigmentary changes, abnormal thinning or thickening, and dystrophy mainly of the toenails (1,3).

SUBCUTANEOUS TISSUE

The subcutaneous tissue is located beneath the dermis and is composed of fat cells, or adipocytes, in groups separated by fibrous septa. Primary functions include insulation and protection of internal structures from mechanical insults. In the elderly there is atrophy of the subcutaneous fat in certain locations, such as the face, backs of the hands, and the shins, leading to increased environmental vulnerability (1). In contrast, there is hypertrophy of the fat in other areas, especially the waist in men and the thighs in women (1).

NEOPLASIA

As humans age there is an increased incidence of benign and malignant tumors in many organ systems, particularly in the skin. One or more of the following benign growths is seen in nearly all adults over 65 years: acrochordon (skin tag), seborrheic keratosis (Fig. 110-1), cherry angioma, lentigo (liver spots or sun spots), and sebaceous hyperplasia (Fig. 110-2). Premalignant epithelial lesions, or actinic keratoses (Fig. 110-3), and malignant neoplasms, mainly basal cell and squamous cell carcinoma (Figs. 110-4 and 110-5), also occur with a higher frequency in the elderly. It is postulated that the factors governing tissue homeostasis become less well regulated with age (18). There is a decrease in local immune surveillance and DNA repair mechanisms are less efficient (18). These alter-

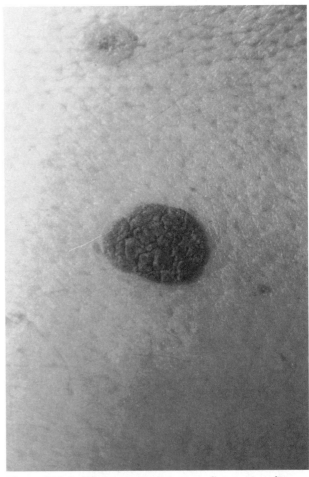

Figure 110-1 Seborrheic keratoses are flat, warty, often pigmented lesions that appear stuck onto the skin.

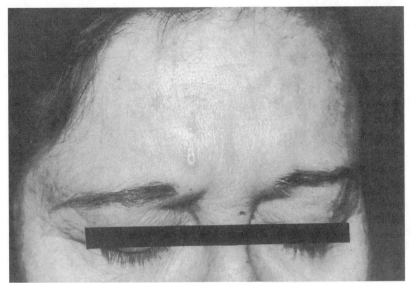

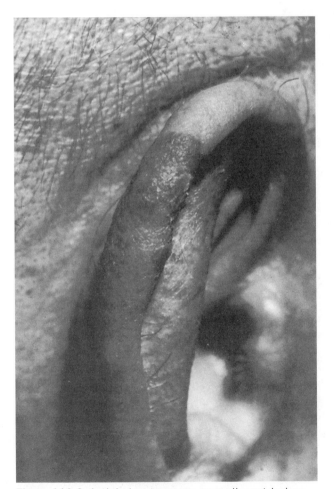

Figure 110-3 Actinic keratoses are premalignant lesions occurring in sun-exposed skin. They are scaly, erythematous, and rough to the touch.

ations are much more pronounced in sun-exposed skin and explain why skin cancers occur much more frequently in sun-damaged sites.

MECHANISMS OF AGING

Two major theories of aging focus on genetics and environmental insults (19). Alterations in gene expression occur in both intrinsic and extrinsic aging (20). Some of the proposed cellular and molecular mechanisms involved in the aging process include free radical formation leading to cellular and DNA damage, increased errors in DNA replication, decreased responsiveness of cells to growth stimuli and enhanced inhibitor sensitivity, and a finite cellular life span (19). More data is needed to discover the relevance of these mechanisms to dermatologic disorders in the elderly with regard to disease susceptibility and expression, and to determine optimal treatment. Many of the cellular manifestations of aging are more pronounced in photodamaged skin. Ultimately, the effects of extrinsic or photoaging lead to the more profound clinical changes associated with aging skin, such as deep wrinkling, laxity, roughness, nodularity, blotchiness, sallowness, and telangiectasias (Fig. 110-6).

SMOKING AND AGING

A link between cigarette smoking and premature wrinkling of facial skin has been recognized for many years (21). The mechanism by which smoking produces increased skin wrinkling is not known. Multiple hypotheses exist, such as alterations in elastic tissue, chronic ischemia and hypoxia of the dermis due to vasoconstriction, increased exposure to free radicals, lowering of estrogen levels in women, decreased stratum corneum moisture, and genetic factors (21). Smoking has also been found to impair the wound healing process (21).

Figure 110-4 Basal cell carcinoma showing rolled, semitranslucent border with telangiectasias and central crusted ulceration.

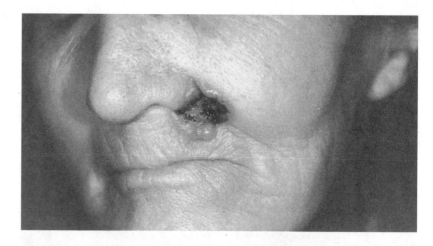

Figure 110-5 Erythematous, moist, and crusted lesion of squamous cell carcinoma on the posterior surface of the ear.

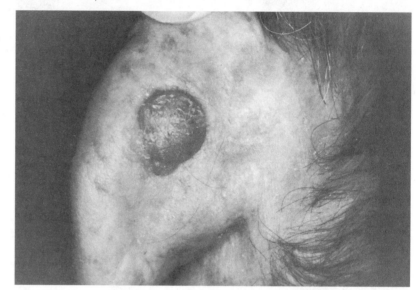

Figure 110-6 Photoaged skin with deep wrinkling, laxity, dryness, discoloration, and surface irregularities.

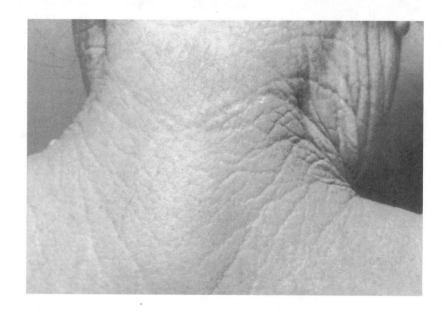

SUMMARY

In conclusion, there has been a great deal of interest in the effects of aging on the skin, reflected in the number of studies and reviews on this subject, but there is often a lack of agreement emerging from the research. Further knowledge of the histology of intrinsically aged skin as well as the molecular mechanisms at work will aid in understanding the structural and physiologic changes that take place in the skin with age. This knowledge will be essential for patient care as the elderly population continues to grow.

REFERENCES

1. Kurban RS, Bhawan J. Histologic changes in skin associated with aging. J Dermatol Surg Oncol 1990;16:908–914.

2. Leyden JJ. Clinical features of ageing skin. Br J Dermatol 1990; 122(suppl):1–3.

3. Gilchrest BA. Aging of skin. In: Fitzpatrick TB, Eisen AZ, Wolff K, et al, eds. Dermatology in general medicine. 4th ed. New York: McGraw-Hill, 1993:150–157.

4. Ghadially R, Brown BE, Sequeira-Martin SM, et al. The aged epidermal permeability barrier. J Clin Invest 1995;95:2281–2290.

5. Harvell JD, Maibach HI. Percutaneous absorption and inflammation in aged skin: a review. J Am Acad Dermatol 1994;31:1015–1021.

6. Cerimele D, Celleno L, Serri F. Physiological changes in ageing skin. Br J Dermatol 1990;122 (suppl):13–20.

7. West MD. The cellular and molecular biology of skin aging. Arch Dermatol 1994;130:87–95.

8. Thivolet J, Nicolas JF. Skin ageing and immune competence. Br J Dermatol 1990;122(suppl):77–81.

9. MacLaughlin J, Holick MF. Aging decreases the capacity of human skin to produce vitamin D3. J Clin Invest 1985;76:1536–1538.

10. Ghersetich I, Lotti T, Campanile G, et al. Hyaluronic acid in cutaneous intrinsic aging. Int J Dermatol 1994;33:119–122.

11. Manuskiatti W, Maibach HI. Hyaluronic acid and skin: wound healing and aging. Int J Dermatol 1996;35:539–544.

12. Meyer LJM, Stern R. Age-dependent changes of hyaluronan in human skin. J Invest Dermatol 1994;102:385–389.

13. Van de Kerkhof PCM, Van Bergen B, Spruijt K, Kuiper JP. Age-related changes in wound healing. Clin Exp Dermatol 1994;19: 369–374.

14. Ashcroft GS, Horan MA, Ferguson MW. The effects of ageing on cutaneous wound healing in mammals. J Anat 1995;187:1–26.

15. Kelly RI, Pearse R, Bull RH, et al. The effects of aging on the cutaneous microvasculature. J Am Acad Dermatol 1995;33:749–756.

16. Montagna W, Carlisle K. Structural changes in ageing skin. Br J Dermatol 1990;122(suppl):61–70.

17. Bolognia JL. Aging skin. Am J Med 1995;98(suppl):99S–103S.

18. Rogers GS, Gilchrest BA. The senile epidermis: environmental influences on skin ageing and cutaneous carcinogenesis. Br J Dermatol 1990;122(suppl):55–60.

19. Yaar M, Gilchrest BA. Cellular and molecular mechanisms of cutaneous aging. J Dermatol Surg Oncol 1990;16:915–922.

20. Gilchrest BA, Garmyn M, Yaar M. Aging and photoaging affect gene expression in cultured human keratinocytes. Arch Dermatol 1994; 130:82–86.

21. Smith JB, Fenske NA. Cutaneous manifestations and consequences of smoking. J Am Acad Dermatol 1996;34:717–732.

Chapter 111

Sun and the Skin

Chris Scholes

Ultraviolet radiation (UVR) is known to have several different effects on the skin, including the transformation of benign cells to a malignant phenotype. The single known beneficial effect of UVR on the skin is the production of vitamin D_3. As there are a great number of deleterious effects, it benefits the clinician to understand the interaction between sunlight and the skin. UVR is known to contribute to the development of skin cancers and to photoaging of the skin. These negative changes are largely both predictable and preventable with only simple interventions, but they require a modification in patient and physician behavior from the time of childhood. Prevention of actinic damage should become part of every physician's repertoire.

PHYSICS

The spectrum of electromagnetic radiation has been broken down in part into ultraviolet, visible light, and infrared radiation (Fig. 111-1). Although all of these may have effects on the skin, the most commonly encountered effects result from exposure of the skin to ultraviolet light. The amount of effective solar radiation at the earth's surface is affected by the distance through the atmosphere that the photons must travel, as well as by scattering of the photons by water and other particles in the atmosphere. A significant fraction (roughly 80%) of ultraviolet A (UVA) and ultraviolet B (UVB) is reflected by surfaces such as snow, sand, and water.

Ultraviolet C (UVC) radiation (200 to 290 nm), although composed of higher-energy photons than UVA or UVB, is for practical purposes entirely screened out by ozone in the earth's atmosphere. Laboratory work indicates that

UVC is capable of producing changes in DNA similar to those produced by UVB (formation of pyrimidine dimers), and also breakage of DNA strands.

Ultraviolet B radiation (290 to 320 nm) is a shortwave, high-energy radiation that has also been termed "sunburn" radiation, as it produces more erythema than does UVA. Fewer photons of UVB than UVA reach the earth's surface, but are sufficiently more erythemogenic than UVA to be largely responsible for sunburn as well as synthesis of vitamin D_3. The measurement of sun protection factor (SPF) on sunscreens is indicative of the degree of protection from ultraviolet B afforded by the sunscreen. A similar standard for measuring protection from UVA has not been developed.

Ultraviolet A radiation is subdivided into UVA1 (340 to 390 nm) and UVA2 (320 to 340 nm). Although greater in number, photons of UVA are less erythemogenic than those of UVB. UVA penetrates into the skin to a greater depth than does UVB. Ultraviolet A radiation is involved in photoallergic reactions, as well as an immediate pigment darkening (Meirowsky phenomenon).

PHYSIOLOGIC REACTION TO UV (ACTINIC DAMAGE)

UVR may produce both acute and chronic damage in the skin. The most common acute reaction is the inflammatory reaction known to all as a sunburn. Erythema develops with warmth, pain, and edema when the volume of blood present in the skin increases. Sunburn tends to be related to the total energy absorbed by the skin, rather than to specifics of time or fluence. In other words, two exposures, one with twice the

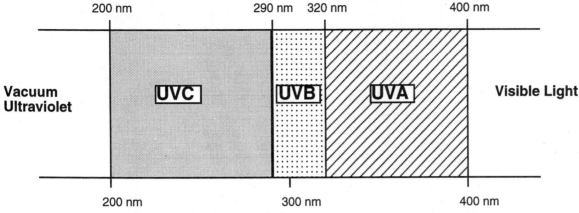

Figure 111-1 The spectrum of electromagnetic radiation.

Table 111-1 Fitzpatrick Skin Phototypes		
FITZPATRICK PHOTOTYPE	**DESCRIPTION**	**EXAMPLE**
I	Always burns, never tans	Albino, Celtic
II	Usually burns, sometimes tans	Fair-skinned, Northern European
III	Sometimes burns, usually tans	"Average" caucasoid
IV	Never burns, always tans	Mediterranean
V	Moderate constitutive pigmentation	Hispanic or Asian
VI	Marked constitutive pigmentation	Negroid

intensity and half the time of the other, would produce approximately the same magnitude of inflammatory response.

Risk of sunburn can be associated with several factors. The most important of these is skin coloration (Table 111-1). Darkly pigmented individuals may experience sunburn, albeit at a lower rate than that of persons with "Celtic" skin. Other factors such as altitude, with its attendant diminuition of atmospheric protection, play a role in the development of actinic damage.

Most of the sunburn reaction is caused by UVB, which has a delayed onset, beginning several hours after exposure and reaching maximum intensity after 12 to 24 hours. This erythema will fade over the next several days, sometimes with desquamation. Treatment with prostaglandin-inhibiting agents (aspirin or NSAIDS) or topical steroids immediately after exposure may attenuate discomfort. After the erythema has fully developed, further exposure should be avoided. Moisturizing creams may be soothing. However, the most effective treatment for sunburn is prevention. Use of high-SPF sunscreens and protective clothing should be stressed to all patients, especially those with fair skin. Sun exposures during the middle of the day (10 AM to 2 PM) should be avoided. Patients with severe sunburns may require hospitalization.

Exposure to ultraviolet radiation causes hyperpigmentation of two types, immediate and delayed. Immediate pigment darkening (IPD) is caused primarily by UVA. This darkening, most prominent in already pigmented skin, results from oxidation of existing melanin and a redistribution of melanin in the melanocytes. IPD provides no significant protection from further UV damage. This hyperpigmentation is most prominent immediately after ultraviolet exposure, and will fade over several days, sometimes overlapping with delayed hyperpigmentation.

Delayed hyperpigmentation, the more commonly recognized "suntan," results primarily from UVB exposure. This tanning becomes visible approximately 72 hours after UV exposure. The hyperpigmentation results from an increase in both the number and activity of melanocytes in the exposed areas, as well as some structural changes in the melanocytes. Depending on the skin type of the individual, this pigmentation may manifest as a smooth tan, or as discrete pigmented freckles in fair-skinned persons (Fitzpatrick type I skin). Even the darkest of tans provides minimal photoprotection and should not be considered a substitute for adequate sun protection.

Chronic exposure to ultraviolet radiation, seen commonly in outdoor laborers, farmers, and sailors, as well as those with outdoor avocations, results in distinct damage to the skin. This damage, referred to as "photoaging," "heliodermatitis," or "dermatoheliosis," appears clinically as dry, wrinkled, leathery skin, with loss of normal skin elasticity (Fig. 111-2). Photoaged skin may also show irregularities of pigmentation, with areas of both hypo- and hyperpigmentation. Epidermal atrophy may be apparent, as may dilated cutaneous capillaries or telangiectasias. These changes are most prominent on the face, posterior neck, dorsal hands, and upper chest (most commonly sun-exposed sites), with relative sparing of the area under the chin, the medial forearms, and the covered areas of the trunk. Comparison of the medial and lateral aspects of the

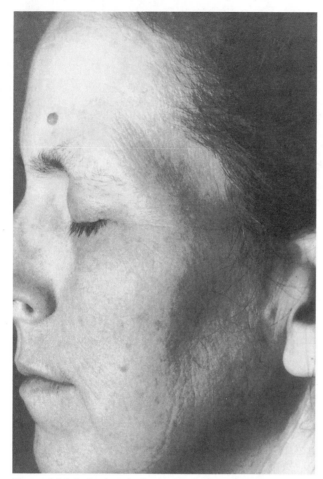

Figure 111-2 Dermatoheliosis. Note the fine wrinkling and leathery skin texture.

Table 111-2 Photosensitivity Disorders	
TYPES OF PHOTOSENSITIVITY DISORDERS	**EXAMPLES**
Idiopathic	Polymorphous light eruption
Secondary to exogenous agents	Phototoxicity Photoallergy
Secondary to endogenous agents	Porphyria cutanea tarda
Autoimmune diseases	Lupus erythematosus Dermatomyositis
Genodermatoses	Xeroderma pigmentosum
Infectious disease	Herpes simplex
Nutritional deficiencies	Pellagra
Primary dermatologic disease	Psoriasis

forearm in a chronically sun-exposed patient provides dramatic evidence of the effects of the sun.

Studies in both mice and humans have demonstrated a decrease in photoaging with the use of sunscreens (1–3). Tretinoin, a staple of acne therapy, has been found to speed repair of the photodamaged dermis, as well as to improve wrinkles and roughness clinically (4–5).

Histologically the most striking evidence of actinic damage is elastosis, production by fibroblasts of tangled, thickened fibers of elastin incapable of maintenance of normal skin elasticity.

It has been well documented tht ultraviolet radiation, even in suberythemogenic doses, causes suppression of the cutaneous immune system. Reactions to both exogenous (contact hypersensitivity) and endogenous (tumor) antigens have been found to be blunted (6–8). The precise role for this effect in photocarcinogenesis has not been completely elucidated. High SPF sunscreens are effective in blocking this immunosuppression (9).

PATHOLOGIC REACTIONS TO UV

In addition to the expected physiologic reactions to acute and chronic exposure to ultraviolet radiation, multiple states exist in which the body, sometimes through interaction with a foreign substance, reacts in an atypical way. Certain primary diseases of the skin may also be exacerbated by UV exposure (Table 111–2).

Examples of idiopathic photodermatoses include polymorphous light eruption, chronic actinic dermatitis, and solar urticaria. Polymorphous light eruption (PMLE) is an idiopathic eruption occurring primarily in young, fair-skinned females, usually after the initial exposure to significant UV. This generally occurs in the spring season, but may also appear after sun exposure on a vacation to warmer climes. PMLE is very common, affecting up to 21% of the population in some estimates (10,11). As the name indicates, PMLE has many different clinical appearances, including macules, papules, plaques, vesicles, and lesions resembling erythema multiforme. Treatment consists of limiting sun exposure through avoidance and the use of broad-spectrum (covering both UVA and UVB) sunscreens. A "hardening" effect with repeated UV exposures may be noted in some patients. This effect has been duplicated with psoralen and UVA (PUVA) therapy (12). Systemic therapies are rarely indicated.

Chronic actinic dermatitis, also known as persistent light reaction, is primarily a condition of light-skinned males over the age of 50. Clinically, these patients present with patchy or confluent eczematous plaques on the sun-exposed skin of the chest, face, or dorsal hands. The eruption tends to persist into or through the winter months, and not infrequently develops into erythroderma. Later stages of this process, known as actinic reticuloid, may resemble cutaneous lymphoma both clinically and histologically (13,14). In rare cases this condition may evolve into a true lymphoma (15). Treatment, which may be only partially effective, is strict avoidance of ultraviolet radiation and use of broad-spectrum sunscreens. In severe cases PUVA or immunosuppressives have been used (16–18).

Solar urticaria is a rare condition that appears clinically as wheals developing within a few minutes of exposure to UV or visible light. The wheals fade over 1 to 2 hours but will recur on re-exposure to light. Widespread involvement may lead to systemic symptoms of histamine release including headache, syncope, nausea, or bronchospasm. Treatment is avoidance of sunlight and photoprotection with broad-spectrum (UVA and UVB) sunblocks and clothing. Systemic

H1 blockers or antimalarials may be useful as adjuvant therapy.

INTERACTIONS BETWEEN DRUGS AND UV

Ultraviolet radiation may interact with various substances to produce changes in the skin. The interaction between the drug, the UVR, and the skin may be manifest in several ways, including phototoxicity, photoallergy, and photocontact dermatitis.

Phototoxicity is an exaggerated sunburn response after exposure to UVR. This reaction, which is mediated by histamine and prostaglandins (19,20), may occur after the initial medication dose, and will recur after sufficient UVR dose if the culpable medication is still present. In contrast to allergic reactions, phototoxicity is not idiosyncratic, and may be avoided with care in choice of medication. The action spectrum for most phototoxic reactions is in the UVA range. Most currently available sunscreens offer insignificant UVA protection. Prevention of a phototoxic reaction requires either broad-spectrum sunscreens or protective clothing.

Phototoxicity may occur with either systemic or topical exposure to the sensitizer. Tetracyclines are among the most commonly prescribed systemic photosensitizers. Doxycycline is a more potent photosensitizer than is its parent compound. Other common oral photosensitizing agents include non-steroidal anti-inflammatory drugs (NSAIDs), amiodarone, phenothiazines, quinolones, sulfa derivatives (including furosemide), systemic retinoids, sulfonamides, and griseofulvin. The photosensitizing properties of the psoralens have been harnessed to create a desired photosensitive state (e.g., PUVA). The most common topical photosensitizers are coal tar derivatives and furocoumarins, found in parsley, parsnip, limes, lemons, figs, and other plants (21). Linear phototoxicity on the extremities is most commonly from exposure to natural furocoumarins. "Bartender's dermatitis," localized photosensitivity of the hands, may result from contact with limes.

Photoallergic dermatitis is an immune-mediated delayed-type hypersensitivity reaction occurring when UVR converts a drug or drug-substrate complex into an immunologically active compound, which is then recognized by the cutaneous immune system. The precise mechanisms by which this happens are incompletely understood. Photoallergy occurs much less frequently than drug-induced phototoxicity. Topical photoallergy, also called photocontact dermatitis, is more common than systemic photoallergy. Common photocontactants include fragrance and musk ambrette. Systemic photoallergens include phenothiazines, sulfa derivatives, and NSAIDs (22,23). Clinically, photoallergic dermatitis appears as an eczematous eruption, usually pruritic, at sun-exposed sites. If the offending drug is topical, then the eruption appears at the sites of exposure to both allergen and ultraviolet light. Photoallergic dermatitis may rarely spread to involve covered sites not initially involved.

An excellent review of photosensitivity and photodermatoses was published by Gonzalez et al (24).

PHOTOEXACERBATED SKIN CONDITIONS

Several primary cutaneous diseases may be exacerbated by ultraviolet radiation. Examples include autoimmune diseases, such as dermatomyositis, lupus erythematosus, and pemphigus vulgaris, as well as some states of nutritional deficiency, such as pellagra. Several different genodermatoses fall into this category as well, such as the Rothmund-Thompson syndrome or xeroderma pigmentosum (25). The relevant action spectrum for photoexacerbation is generally in the UVA range. Broad-spectrum sunscreens and sun avoidance are mandatory for these patients. Significant sunburn may act as the inciting event for the isomorphic (Koebner) phenomenon, in which a pre-existing condition such as vitiligo or psoriasis may spread to involve the burned sites.

UVR AND MALIGNANCY

UVR is generally accepted to be the dominant environmental risk factor for the two most common forms of skin cancer, basal cell carcinoma and squamous cell carcinoma. Additionally, sunlight is thought to be a major etiologic factor in the development of melanoma. The mechanism (or mechanisms) for UV carcinogenesis is unknown, but may relate to alterations in DNA structure or cutaneous immunosuppression.

Basal cell carcinoma (BCC) is the single most common malignancy in the United States today, found primarily (though not exclusively) on sun-exposed sites of Caucasian patients (Fig. 111-3). The link between solar radiation and BCC is strong, since the incidence of BCC increases with decreasing latitude and tumors develop primarily on sun-damaged skin (26). Studies have demonstrated that light hair color, childhood sunburn, a family history of nonmelanoma skin cancer, and tendency to freckle rather than tan are predictors of later development of BCC (27). One study (28) suggests that recreational sunlight exposure in the first twenty years of life causes an increased lifetime risk of BCC development.

Squamous cell carcinoma (SCC) and its precursor lesion, actinic keratosis (AK), are increasing in frequency (29). Factors favoring the development of eventual SCC include light skin, light (red or blonde) hair, tendency to burn rather than tan, and tendency to freckle (30). Cumulative lifetime UVR dose (31) and occupational exposure over the previous 10 years (30) have also been implicated. The spectrum of UV-induced neoplasia begins with actinic keratoses, which are extremely common on the sun-exposed skin of photoaged persons (Fig. 111-4). Over time, AK may progress to squamous cell carcinoma in situ, and eventually to invasive squamous cell carcinoma. The rate of progression from AK to SCC is uncertain, but thought to be only a few percent. SCC that arises from actinic keratoses has a lower incidence of invasion and metastasis than does carcinoma on sun-protected skin. The combined immunosuppression of UV exposure and chronic lymphedema leading to formation of multiple sites of SCC has recently been described (Perkins et al, personal communication, 1997).

The relationship between UVR and melanoma is not as well defined as that for nonmelanoma skin cancers. Evidence suggests that fair skin and intense sun exposure during childhood are contributing factors. The incidence of melanoma is increasing faster than any other cancer (32), and this increase does not appear to be explainable solely by earlier diagnosis

Figure 111-3 Basal cell carcinoma on the forehead.

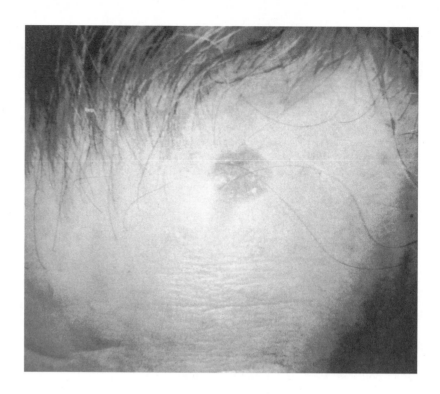

or by the aging of the population (33). Most melanomas are thought to be caused by sun exposure in the first 15 years of life (34,35). UV exposure may cause development of melanocytic nevi in susceptible persons, and it is known that approximately 20% of melanomas will arise in association with a pre-existing melanocytic nevus (36). This evidence suggests that broad-spectrum sunscreens should be used regularly, especially in childhood.

Conventional dermatologic wisdom suggests that basal cell and squamous cell carcinoma are related to chronic ultraviolet exposure of the type found in farmers, sailors, and other outdoor laborers. Development of melanoma, on the other hand, is related to acute, intermittent exposure (especially blistering burns in childhood), found in those persons with outdoor avocations such as golf or tennis (37).

Current recommendations for prevention of UV-induced neoplasia include avoidance of the sun during midday hours, use of protective clothing, and regular use of sunscreens. Sunscreens have been shown to decrease erythema and histologic changes in UV-exposed skin (38), as well as to decrease the incidence of actinic neoplasia (39).

SUNSCREENS

Sunscreens are topical preparations that have been recognized by the FDA since 1978 as drugs intended to protect the skin against actinic damage. They may act to absorb incident UVR (chemical sunscreens), or to reflect and scatter UV (physical blocking agents). Chemical sunscreens, which typically contain oxybenzone derivatives or cinnamates, must be applied 15 to 30 minutes prior to sun exposure. These cosmetically elegant preparations act as filters to prevent penetration of UVR into the skin. Most commercially available preparations act only to block UVB. The sun protection

factor (SPF) seen on the sunscreen container is an indication of the degree of protection offered by the sunscreen. An SPF of 15 means that on laboratory evaluation the sunscreen was found to prolong the duration of constant radiation required for development of erythema by a factor of 15. The actual protection experienced by the sunscreen wearer is likely to be lower, given inadequacy of application, washing or wiping off, or sweating.

PHOTOPROTECTION FROM CLOTHING

Clothing provides some degree of photoprotection, although this protection is limited. A typical T-shirt provides an SPF of 5 to 9 (40), with heavier fabrics providing more sun protection. The photoprotective ability of most fabrics diminishes when the fabric is wet. New fabrics have been developed over the past several years for people desiring greater photoprotection (41). These have a tested SPF of 30 or greater, and may be useful in persons unable to tolerate sunscreens.

TANNING PARLORS

The use of indoor tanning parlors is rising in the United States, and the tanning industry has become a $1 billion business (42). Indoor tanning entails the exposure of a person to UVR primarily in the UVA range, with lesser amounts of UVB and UVC. Despite the cultural fascination with a "healthy golden glow," there are no documented medical benefits to tanning. (43,44). The photoprotective effect from UVA is minimal, and mostly fades within minutes to hours of ultraviolet exposure (45).

Indoor tanning is responsible for the same type of deleterious effects caused by "natural" tanning. Acutely, users may

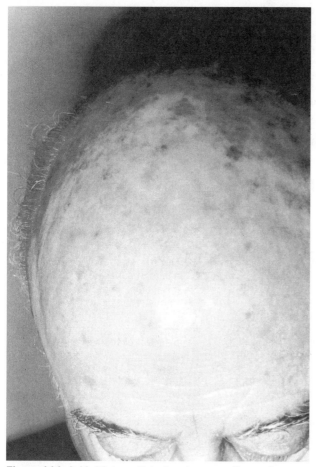

Figure 111-4 Multiple actinic keratoses on the scalp.

from indoor UVA include photoaging, carcinogenesis, and cataract formation. This last may be of special import, as the position of the body on a tanning bed denies the eyes the physical protection from UVR normally provided by the brows. Troubling also is the inconsistent use by tanning parlors of necessary eye protection (46).

Tanning beds have been implicated in carcinogenesis. As UVR given in many small doses has been shown to be more carcinogenic than an equal dose given in a few large doses (47), the method of UVR delivery in tanning parlors may be particularly harmful. Significant correlation with development of basal cell carcinoma (48) as well as cytologically atypical melanocytic lesions (49,50) have been reported. Studies have also linked tanning bed use with an increased risk of development of malignant melanoma (51,52). Given the lack of benefit from indoor tanning coupled with the well-documented health risks, the concensus conference statement from the National Institutes of Health rings particularly true: "UVR-induced tanning, whether from natural or artificial sources, is deleterious to the skin" (53).

SUMMARY

Sun exposure to some extent is unavoidable in everyday life. To minimize photodamage and photocarcinogenesis, it is recommended that a sunscreen with a rating of SPF 15 or higher be used daily. Application of the sunscreen should be repeated if extended sun exposure is expected. Additional protection with broad-brimmed hats and photoprotective clothing is beneficial, especially for persons with fair skin and hair (Fitzpatrick type I or II). Avoidance of excessive sun exposure, during the brightest hours of the day (10 AM to 2 PM) and avoidance of other sources of ultraviolet radiation (e.g., tanning parlors) will also help to prevent photodamage. Persons with photosensitivity disorders should be monitored closely in conjunction with a dermatologist.

experience pruritus, nausea, skin dryness, or erythema. Exacerbation of a previously existing skin disease, as detailed earlier, may also occur with tanning bed use. Chronic effects

REFERENCES

1. Gurish MF, Roberts LK, Krueger GG, et al. The effect of various sunscreen agents on skin damage and the induction of tumor susceptibility in mice subjected to ultraviolet irradiation. J Invest Dermatol 1981;78:246–251.

2. Kligman LH, Akin FJ, Kligman AM. Prevention of ultraviolet damage to the dermis of hairless mice by sunscreens. J Invest Dermatol 1982;78:181–189.

3. Boyd AS, Naylor M, Camergon GS, et al. The effects of chronic sunscreen use on the histologic changes of dermatoheliosis. J Am Acad Dermatol 1995;33:941–946.

4. Kligman LH, et al. Topical retinoic acid enhances the repair of ultraviolet damaged dermal connective tissue. Connect Tissue Res 1984; 12:139.

5. Schwartz E, et al. Topical all-trans retinoic acid stimulates collagen synthesis in vivo. J Invest Dermatol 1991;96:875.

6. Spellman CW, Daynes RA. Ultraviolet light induced murine suppressor lymphocytes dictate specificity of anti-ultraviolet tumor immune responses. Cell Immunol 1978;38:25–34.

7. Reeve VE, Bosnic M, Boehm-Wilcos C, Ley RD. Differential protection by two sunscreens from UV radiation-induced immunosuppression. J Invest Dermatol 1991;97:624–628.

8. Fisher MS, Kripke ML. Systemic alterations induced in mice by ultraviolet light irradiation and its relationship to UV carcinogenesis. Proc Natl Acad Sci USA 1977;74:1688–1692.

9. Whitmore SE, Morison WL. Prevention of UVB-induced immunosuppression in humans by a high sun protection factor sunscreen. Arch Dermatol 1995;131:1128–1133.

10. Morison WL, Stern RS. Polymorphous light eruption: a common reaction uncommonly recognized. Acta Derm Venereol 1982;62:237.

11. Ros A, Wennersten G. Current aspects of polymorphous light eruptions in Sweden. Photodermatology 1986;3:298.

12. Murphy GM, et al. Prophylactic PUVA and UVB therapy in polymorphic light eruption—a controlled trial. Br J Dermatol 1987;116:531.

13. Ive FA, Magnus IA, Warin RP. Actinic reticuloid: a chronic photodermatosis associated with severe photosensitivity and histological resemblance to lymphoma. Br J Dermatol 1969;81:469–485.

14. Toonstra J, Henquet CJM, van Weelden H. Actinic reticuloid. J Am Acad Dermatol 1989;21:205–214.

15. Leith IM, Hawk JLM. Treatment of chronic actinic dermatitis with azathioprine. Br J Dermatol 1984;131:209–214.

16. Murphy GM, et al. A double-blind controlled trial of azathioprine in chronic actinic dermatitis. Br J Dermatol 1987;117:16.

17. Norris PG, et al. Actinic reticuloid: response to cyclosporin A. J Am Acad Dermatol 1989;21:307.

18. Hindson C, et al. PUVA therapy of chronic actinic dermatitis. Br J Dermatol 1985;113:157.

19. Falk MS. Light sensitivity to demethychlortetracycline: report of four cases. JAMA 1960;172:156–158.

20. Lam SK, Tomlinson DR. Chlorpromazine-induced histamine release from guinea pig skin in vitro: a photosensitivity reaction. Arch Dermatol Res 1976;255:219–223.

21. Pathak MA, Daniels F, Fitzpatrick TB. The presently known distribution of furocoumarins (psoralens) in plants. J Invest Dermatol 1962;39:225–239.

22. Ikezawa Z, Kitamura K, Osawa J, et al. Photosensitivity to piroxicam is induced by sensitization to thimerisol and thiosalicylate. J Invest Dermatol 1992;98:918–992.

23. Maguire HC, Kaidbey K. Studies in experimental photoallergy. In: Parrish JA, ed. The effect of ultraviolet radiation on the immune system. Skillman, NJ: Johnson & Johnson, 1983:181–192.

24. Gonzales E, Gonzales SL. Drug photosensitivity, idiopathic photodermatoses, and sunscreens. J Am Acad Dermatol 1996;35:871–885.

25. Lim HW, Epstein J. Photosensitivity diseases. J Am Acad Dermatol 1997;36:84–90.

26. Scotto J, Fears TR, Fraumini JF Jr. Incidence of nonmelanomatous skin cancer in the United States. Washington, DC: US Dept of Health and Human Services, National Cancer Institute, 1983 Publication #83–2433.

27. Hogan DJ, To T, Gran L, et al. Risk factors for basal cell carcinoma. Int J Dermatol 1989;28:591–594.

28. Gallagher RP, Hill GB, Bajdik CD, et al. Sunlight exposure, pigmentary factors, and risk of nonmelanocytic skin cancer: I: basal cell carcinoma. Arch Dermatol 1995;131:157–163.

29. Glass AG, Hoover RN. The emerging epidemic of melanoma and squamous cell skin cancer. JAMA 1989;262:2097–2100.

30. Gallagher RP, Hill GB, Bajdik CD, et al. Sunlight exposure, pigmentary factors, and risk of nonmelanocytic skin cancer: II: squamous cell carcinoma. Arch Dermatol 1995;131:164–169.

31. Vitasa BC, et al. Association of nonmelanoma skin cancer and actinic keratosis with cumulative solar ultraviolet exposure in Maryland watermen. Cancer 1990;65:2811–2817.

32. Grin CS, Rigel DS, Friedman RJ. Worldwide incidence of malignant melanoma. In: Balch CM, et al, eds. Cutaneous melanoma. Philadelphia: JB Lippincott, 1992.

33. Rigel DS. Malignant melanoma: perspectives on incidence and its effects on awareness, diagnosis, and treatment. CA Cancer J Clin 1996;46:195–198.

34. Holman CDJ, Armstrong BK. Cutaneous malignant melanoma and indicators of total accumulated exposure to the sun: analysis by histogenetic types. J Natl Cancer Inst 1984;72:765–770.

35. Khlat M, Vail A, Parkin M, Green A. Mortality from melanoma in migrants to Australia: variation by age at arrival and duration of stay. Am J Epidemiol 1992;135:1103–1113.

36. Harley S, Walsh N: A new look at nevus-associated melanomas. Am J Dermatopath 1996;18:137–141.

37. Lew RA, et al. Sun exposure habits in patients with cutaneous melanoma: a case control study. J Dermatol Surg Oncol 1983;9:81.

38. Kaidbey KH. The photoprotective potential of the new superpotent sunscreens. J Am Acad Dermatol 1990;22:449–452.

39. Naylor MF, Boyd A, Smith DW, et al. High sun protection factor sunscreens in the suppression of actinic neoplasia. Arch Dermatol 1995;131:170–175.

40. Sayre RM, Hughes SNG. Sun protective apparel: advancements in sun protection. Skin Cancer J 1993;8:41–47.

41. Menter JM, Hollins TD, et al. Protection against UV photocarcinogenesis by fabric materials. J Am Acad Dermatol 1994;31:711–716.

42. The $1,000,000,000 industry. Looking Fit 1992;7:56–70.

43. Bickers DR, Epstein JH, Fitzpatrick TB, et al. Risks and benefits from high-intensity ultraviolet A sources used for cosmetic purposes. J Am Acad Dermatol 1985;12:380–381.

44. Council on Scientific Affairs. Harmful effects of ultraviolet radiation. JAMA 1989;262:380–384.

45. Black G, Matzinger E, Gange RW. Lack of photoprotection against UVB induced erythema by immediate pigmentation induced by 382 nm radiation. J Invest Dermatol 1985;85:448–449.

46. Bruyneel-Rapp F, Dorsey SB, Guin JD. The tanning salon: an area survey of equipment, procedures, and practices. J Am Acad Dermatol 1988;18:1030–1038.

47. Forbes PD, Davies RE, Urbach F. Experimental ultraviolet photocarcinogenesis: wavelength interactions and time-dose relationships. Natl Cancer Inst Monogr 1978;50:31–38.

48. Dinehart SM, Dodge R, Stanley WE, et al. Basal cell carcinoma treated with Mohs surgery. J Dermatol Surg Oncol 1992;18:560–566.

49. Roth DE, Hodge SJ, Callen JP. Possible ultraviolet-A-induced lentigenes: a side effect of chronic tanning salon usage. J Am Acad Dermatol 1989;20:950–954.

50. Jones SK, Moseley H, MacKie RM. UVA-induced melanocytic lesions. Br J Dermatol 1987;117:111–115.

51. Walter SD, Marrett LD, From L, et al. The association of cutaneous malignant melanoma with the use of sunbeds and sunlamps. Am J Epidemiol 1990;131:232–243.

52. Westerdahl J, Olsson H, Masback A, et al. Use of sunbeds or sunlamps and malignant melanoma in southern Sweden. Am J Epidemiol 1994;140:691–699.

53. National Institutes of Health Consensus Development Conference. Sunlight, ultraviolet radiation, and the skin. Bethesda, Md: National Institutes of Health, May 8–10, 1988.

Chapter 112

Exercise and the Skin

Gary R. Kantor

More and more people are engaging in athletic activities for fitness and stress reduction. As a result, patients are developing a host of disorders caused or exacerbated by their exercise program. For example, one of the many functions of the skin is the protection of underlying soft tissue and bone from injury. Various traumatic injuries can occur while engaging in exercise and exercise may also predispose the skin to infection or exacerbate a pre-existing skin condition. In addition, the use of certain types of equipment and athletic gear makes the participant susceptible to other skin disorders such as irritant or allergic contact dermatitis.

Sports dermatology is a growing subspecialty in dermatology and, with this growth, new and exotic exercise-related skin eruptions are being seen and described. This chapter reviews some common and some new skin diseases that are related to exercise participation.

TRAUMATIC INJURIES

Numerous traumatic injuries are related to exercise, and the skin of the feet is especially likely to be affected. Table 112-1 lists the traumatic injuries seen in sports participants.

Friction Blisters

Friction blisters develop on the feet in running sports such as track, basketball, baseball, and soccer; on the hands in stick and crew sports such as rowing and tennis; and on specific fingers in sports such as fencing and baseball (1). Shearing forces, primarily horizontal, are responsible and cause an intraepidermal split with the accumulation of serum and, occasionally, blood. Heat, humidity, and underlying bony abnormalities also contribute to blister development. The lesions are only slightly tender, but are much more symptomatic when they occur under calluses. Prevention is often difficult and most padding materials are ineffective. However, properly fitted shoes, wearing two pairs of powdered socks (preferably acrylic [2]), and the use of protective hand and foot gear are often helpful. Various padding materials based on organic polymers have also shown promise as preventive measures (3). Treatment consists of draining a tense blister with a sterile needle and covering with a topical antibiotic. An occlusive dressing such as an adhesive tape may also be used. A small patch of hydrocolloid dressing often decreases pain and accelerates healing.

Calluses

Calluses (Fig. 112-1) occur over bony prominences as a protective response to chronic, prolonged pressure and friction. Common sites for calluses include metacarpal and palmodigital aspects of the hand. Calluses are not always undesirable and may be advantageous in sports such as gymnastics, dancing, running, bowling, golfing, and tennis. When occurring in response to abnormal pressure or as a consequence of a structurally or functionally defective part, significant pain or tenderness may occur. Preventive measures help to evenly distribute applied pressure and include properly fitted shoes, shoe inserts, metatarsal bars, arch supports, or the use of properly designed padding (4). When needed, treatment consists of the paring or sanding of the callus with a scalpel or a pumice stone after hydration. Topical agents such as the nightly application of 5–10% salicylic acid in flexible collodion, 40% salicylic acid plaster, or 12% lactic acid cream help reduce the hyperkeratosis.

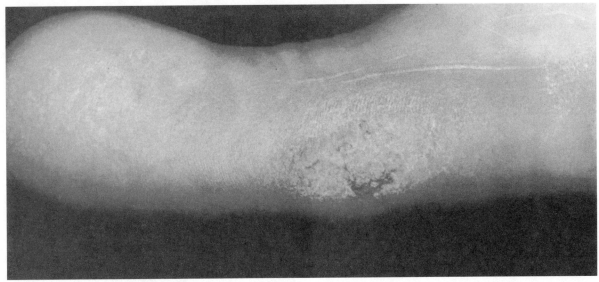

Figure 112-1 Callus on pressure bearing surface of foot.

Table 112-1 Traumatic Sports Injuries
Friction blisters
Calluses
Black heel
Striae distensae
Subungual hemorrhage
Tennis toe
Ingrown toenail
Athlete's nodules
Alopecia
Jogger's nipples
Bicyclist's nipples

Black Heel

Black heel (talon noir) arises from sudden, forceful halting and twisting movements of the foot, which produces a shearing stress on the delicate skin capillaries. As a result, extravasated red blood cells move upward throughout the epidermis into an intracorneal location to produce the clinical lesions. The posterior or lateral aspects of the heel are the most common sites, although lesions may be bilateral and multiple (5) and the palm may rarely be involved.

The lesions appear as painless aggregates of tiny black dots or streaks, often horizontally oriented. Because of the black color, patients will become alarmed and seek medical advice. Differential diagnosis should appropriately include malignant melanoma, benign melanocytic nevi, and verruca vulgaris. However, the sudden appearance, age of the patient, and characteristic location enables the correct diagnosis to be made. In addition, horizontal paring of black heel with the scalpel blade will reveal the intracorneal location of the lesion. No treatment is needed once it is recognized as a benign, trauma-induced condition. Use of a felt heel pad may reduce recurrence (5).

Striae Distensae

Striae distensae or "stretch marks" are commonly seen on the abdomen and thighs with pregnancy, obesity, Cushing's syndrome, or the prolonged use of potent fluorinated topical corticosteroids. However, athletes who utilize weight training such as body builders, gymnasts, or football players may develop striae of the chest, shoulder, upper-outer arm, thighs, and legs. When present in association with other high-androgen states such as acne or baldness, use of performance-enhancing anabolic steroids should be suspected.

Striae distensae appear as linear, pink or flesh-colored atrophic patches that are arranged perpendicular to the lines of skin tension (Fig. 112-2). Treatment is difficult, but one study showed significant improvement in 15 of 16 patients with topical 0.1% tretinoin cream (6). Patients should be counseled to avoid strenuous weight training and anabolic steroids.

Subungual Hemorrhage and Tennis Toe

Subungual hemorrhage results from repeated or sudden blunt trauma to the nail unit and is most common under the hallux or second toenail. When hemorrhage occurs in the nail matrix, it is incorporated into the nail plate while bleeding distal to the lunula is found in the nail bed (7). Subungual hemorrhage is particularly common in jogging and racket sports. It appears as a blue-black spot under the nail (Fig. 112-3) and must be distinguished from a subungual melanocytic nevus or melanoma. When acute or painful, incisional drainage or hot-wire puncture of the nail plate is indicated.

A particular form of subungual hemorrhage that occurs in tennis players has been referred to as "tennis toe" (8). It usually occurs on the longer of the first two toes. "Tennis toe" is believed to result from frequent trauma of the toe into the toebox and tip of the sneaker with the frequent abrupt stops made during tennis play (8). Hard surfaces and ill-fitting shoes are important aggravating factors. "Tennis toe" appears clini-

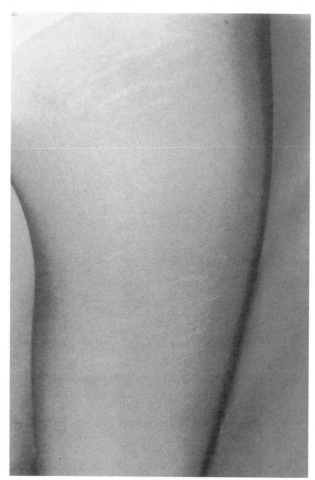

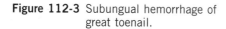
Figure 112-2 Striae distensae from strenuous biking.

cally as painful, vertically oriented lines of hemorrhage similar to splinter hemorrhages. The use of properly fitted shoes and padding of the distal toes may prevent hemorrhage from occurring. Tightly lacing the shoes and retying the laces when they become loosened are also helpful preventive measures.

Ingrown Toenail

Ingrown toenails are most common on the great toe, but any toe may be affected. Because of the associated pain and infection, ingrown toenails can have a profound effect on the ability to perform exercise.

Conservative treatment measures should be pursued first, including warm antiseptic soaks in Burow's solution 1 : 40, analgesics, rest, and elevating the corner of the nail with cotton. If conservative therapy fails, partial or complete nail avulsion to include the lateral nail bed is indicated.

Preventive measures include trimming of the nails straight across, rather than rounding them off, and allowing the nail to grow over the edge of the toe (9). Properly fitting footwear with a wide toebox is also recommended for prevention. If all of these measures fail, permanent removal of the nail with destruction of the nail matrix may be warranted.

Athlete's Nodules

Repeated local trauma and hemorrhage at specialized sites may induce fibrotic dermal or subcutaneous masses (10). One example is surfer's nodules, which are nontender nodular collections caused by kneeling on the surfboard. Common sites include the tibial prominences, mid-dorsa of the feet, and dorsal aspect of one or more metatarsophalangeal joints. Osseous changes may also be associated and ulceration may develop occasionally. Similar nodules develop also in boxers

Figure 112-3 Subungual hemorrhage of great toenail.

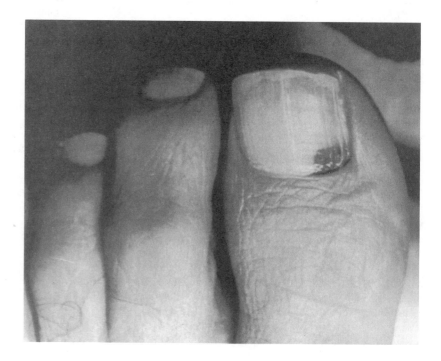

and football players and may occur on the feet from ill-fitting shoes ("Nike nodules") (11). Conservative treatment measures including intralesional corticosteroids should be tried first before surgical excision.

Alopecia

Traction alopecia resulting from wearing a tight-banded wide-stripped headphone while jogging has been reported (12). The use of a lighter headpiece halted the hair loss. Patchy alopecia in the occipitoparietal area was described in two male adolescents who practiced break dancing (12). Gymnasts who repeatedly practice headstands and rollovers on the balance beam may develop alopecia (13).

Jogger's and Bicyclist's Nipples

A frictional injury seen in joggers is abrasion of the nipple and areola resulting from frictional contact with the coarse fabric of a shirt during a long run. The condition has been called "jogger's nipples" (14) and manifests as painful, inflamed, fissured, and occasionally bleeding nipples. Wearing a brassiere made of soft fabric is curative in women. In men, the use of a garment made of a semisynthetic fabric or silk, taping the nipples, cutting out the fabric over the breasts, or applying petrolatum before running are helpful measures (15).

Bicyclist's nipples are primarily a thermal injury to the nipples that occurs during a cold-weather ride (16). Evaporation of sweat and the chill of the wind lower the temperature of the nipples to produce a painful injury that may continue for several days. Use of a cycling jacket, thermal undergarment, or some other protective material will prevent further recurrences.

ENVIRONMENTAL INJURIES

Cold Induced

Pernio

Pernio or chilblains results from repeated exposure to cold and dampness and commonly affects the hands, feet, nose, cheeks, and ears in children or people with poor circulation. Pernio is also associated with wearing waterproof boots with linings (17). This is because cold water accumulates in the inner lining of the boots and is prevented from evaporating, leaving the skin in contact with a cold, moist environment. Vasospasm occurs and produces the clinical lesions characterized by reddish-blue edematous plaques that itch and burn. A dermatitis with blisters may develop and lesions may become chronic.

Treatment consists of elimination of precipitating factors and rewarming of the affected part. Prevention by wearing wool socks that are changed as soon as dampness sets in, gentle massage of the affected area, and properly fitted boots are helpful measures.

Frostnip and Frostbite

Frostnip is a very superficial frostbite and affects exposed areas of the face, nose, cheeks, chin, and ears. It is common in skiers due to exposure in subfreezing temperatures with a significant wind-chill factor (17). Clinically, insensitive white patches of skin are present. Blistering may occur and numb-

ness may last for several days. Frostnip may be prevented by avoiding bathing and shaving the face until after the day's outing, thus minimizing removal of the skin's protective oils (17). The application of a petrolatum-based sunscreen cream or other emollient may also be a helpful preventive measure.

Frostbite is severe, deep cold injury affecting skin, subcutaneous tissue, muscle, and even bone. It occurs from prolonged exposure to temperatures of at least −2°C, at which point anoxia and vasoconstriction cause cellular metabolism to halt (17). Frostbite is unusual in downhill skiers, but may occur in cross-country skiers and winter hikers and climbers who become lost or trapped in a snowstorm. The anterior neck is most commonly affected and muscles, nerves, and blood vessels are damaged most rapidly. Depending on the time of presentation, a white, cold, and insensitive part with or without tissue necrosis is present. The preferred treatment is rapid rewarming in a warm-water bath regulated at 38°C to 44°C for 20 minutes (18). Analgesics, sedatives, whirlpool baths, and antibiotics are often needed (17). Proper apparel and safety precautions are the best measures to prevent frostbite.

Cold Urticaria

Cold urticaria is the most common form of acquired physical urticaria in participants in winter sports (19). The most frequent pathogenic mechanism is nonallergic, in which there is direct histamine liberation from mast cells. Clinically, symptomatic or asymptomatic, localized or generalized, urticarial wheals develop in response to cold exposure. Cold urticaria responds better than most other types of physical urticaria to antihistamines such as cyproheptadine, so athletes who are affected need not abandon training and exercise.

Raynaud's Disease

Raynaud's disease is an idiopathic cold hypersensitivity and results in vascular spasm with pallor, cyanosis, and, in severe cases, gangrene of the affected digits (17). Raynaud's phenomenon may occur secondary to systemic connective tissue disease such as scleroderma, lupus erythematosus, and cryoglobinemia (17). Patients with Raynaud's disease or phenomenon can find winter sports devastating and must be instructed to protect their hands and feet during these activities. Treatment with topical medications and corticosteroids has been generally unfavorable. However, treatment with nifedipine in low doses such as 10–20 mg once a day often produces significant improvement (20). Smoking must be prohibited and some patients have found battery-operated heated gloves and boots useful.

Heat Induced

Miliaria

Miliaria, commonly referred to as "prickly heat," results from occlusion of the sweat duct. It develops on body sites that are covered by clothing and occurs in participants in football, baseball, rugby, and skiing (21). Miliaria may occur in several different forms. The first type, miliaria crystallina, develops when duct occlusion occurs superficially within the epidermis. Asymptomatic, clear, noninflammatory blisters are present, which resolve within hours of cooling the area. Miliaria rubra is a second clinical type that develops when sweat duct occlusion occurs in the lower epidermis. Clinically, discrete reddish papules and blisters that itch are present. Treatment consists of exposing the area to cool air and applying a 1% hydrocortisone lotion. Loose clothing that is changed at regular intervals as sweat accumulates may help reduce recurrences. Two other types of miliaria, miliaria profunda and miliaria pustulosa, are rare in athletes and result from sweat duct occlusion deeper in the skin with associated inflammation.

Intertrigo

Intertrigo is an inflamed, itchy dermatitis that occurs in body folds, especially the groin, as a result of friction, maceration, and overheating. It is not a particular problem in lean, muscular athletes, but is common in football linemen and weightlifters who have been recruited for their large size and weight (1). Intertrigo appears clinically as reddish, macerated patches that may be secondarily colonized by bacteria or yeast. In the latter instance, it is referred to as candida intertrigo.

Treatment includes the application of compresses of Burow's solution 1:40 for 15 to 20 minutes three times daily followed by the application of 1% hydrocortisone cream with or without diiodohydroxyquin (4). Loose-fitting cotton underclothing, weight reduction, and gentle cleansing once daily with warm water and mild soap are helpful preventive measures.

Cholinergic Urticaria

Cholinergic urticaria is an acetylcholine-mediated disorder that is provoked by heat, emotion, and exertion (19). The etiology is unknown, but autoallergy to sweat and sweat metabolites is probably not causative as once proposed. Boxers, runners, swimmers, and weightlifters have been affected (19). Lesions consist of 1 to 2 mm urticarial wheals, surrounded by a large erythematous axonal reflex flare. Systemic symptoms such as generalized sweating, abdominal cramps, dizziness, wheezing, and bradycardia may also occur.

Treatment is not as effective as in cold urticaria. Antihistamines such as hydroxyzine and cyproheptadine may relieve symptoms, but do not cure the disorder. Some athletes may have to give up training and participation in their sport for an indefinite period (19).

Exercised-induced Urticaria

Exercise-induced urticaria differs from cholinergic urticaria by its failure to develop after exposure to heat without exercise (22). Cutaneous manifestations include giant urticaria, lesions indistinguishable from cholinergic urticaria, or angioedema (soft tissue swelling). The skin changes may be accompanied by systemic manifestations such as wheezing or hypotension, so that some cases may resemble exercise-induced anaphylaxis (23).

Treatment for exercise-induced urticaria has proven difficult. Antihistamines, anticholinergics, beta-agonists, or phosphodiesterase inhibitors given prophylactically have not been successful. Cromolyn sodium 20 mg three to four times daily, given by inhalation, not orally, has been reported to prevent attacks of exercise-induced urticaria and angioedema (24). When accompanied by systemic symptoms, the treatment of choice is subcutaneous epinephrine (23).

Sun Induced

Acute Sunburn

Everyone, not only athletes, should be concerned about an acute injury from the sun during outdoor activities. Individuals who participate in sports as diverse as swimming, sailing, golfing, fishing, mountain climbing, and skiing are all susceptible. Sunburns can be painful and disfiguring and may prevent subsequent participation in an athletic event. In addition, recent evidence has accumulated to incriminate acute sunburns at a young age with the later development of malignant melanoma. Exposed areas of the body are most affected, but reflection off sand, water, and snow may injure sites that are usually not exposed to the sun. Systemic symptoms such as fever, chills, nausea, and prostration may also occur (4). Treatment is similar to that for a burn, and oral corticosteroids may be necessary in severe cases.

Prevention is the key to dealing with sun-related disorders. Sunscreens are available in many forms and levels of sun protection factor (SPF) (25). The proper choice of a sunscreen and SPF will vary according to the patient's skin type and preference. I recommend at least an SPF 15 sunscreen applied to exposed skin 30 minutes before sun exposure. Application of a thin film of petrolatum around the eyes helps prevent stinging and irritation to the conjunctiva. Contact with water or excessive sweating usually necessitates additional application of the agent. The lips should also be protected with a suitable sunscreen stick. Wearing long sleeves and a cap, if feasible, will offer partial protection. If the sports participant takes these proper precautions, a number of uncomfortable days and spoiled vacations can be prevented.

Chronic Actinic Injury

Chronic sun exposure is associated with the development of wrinkling, aging, elastosis, and premalignant and malignant skin tumors. Light-complexioned, blue-eyed redheads and blonds are most susceptible. A variety of skin changes occur from chronic sun exposure. These include furrowing, wrinkling, and a yellow discoloration of the skin, comedones around the eyes, red scaly plaques, and frank skin cancer. The most commonly sun-damaged areas are the ones most exposed to the sun such as the face, scalp in bald men (Fig. 112-4), neck, arms, and hands.

Unfortunately, our society equates health with the presence of a golden tan. This is even more evident when considering the popularity of so-called "tanning salons." One can still enjoy the sun and outdoor activities by using sunscreens and appropriate clothing. These measures will prevent acute injury and reduce the aging and carcinogenic potential of the sun's rays.

Solar Urticaria

Solar urticaria is a rare type of physical urticaria and an uncommon cause of urticaria in sports participants (19). Pathogenically, solar urticaria is believed to result from nonallergic liberation of histamine by a direct effect of sunlight on mast cells. Clinically, urticarial wheals develop shortly after exposure to the causative wavelength of electromagnetic energy. Antihistamines may be helpful for acute episodes and anti-

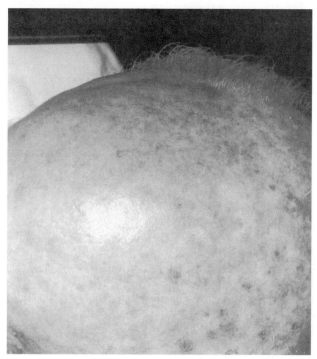

Figure 112-4 Chronic solar injury of scalp.

malarial drugs may be beneficial in some patients for prevention (19).

Photosensitivity Dermatitis

Photosensitivity dermatitis is classified into two types: phototoxic and photoallergic. Phototoxic dermatitis is a severe, exaggerated sunburn occurring after a small dose of ultraviolet light. Photoallergic dermatitis (Fig. 112-5) is a sun-induced eczema that is characterized by severe itching and blister formation. Outdoor sporting activities may expose a susceptible individual to sufficient ultraviolet light to precipitate a photosensitivity dermatitis.

Photosensitivity dermatitis has multiple causes including: systemic drugs (tetracycline, demeclocycline, sulfonamides, griseofulvin, hydrochlorothiazide, chlorpropamide, chlorpromazine); topical preparations (coal tar derivatives, antimicrobial soaps, sunscreens); plants and vegetables (fig, parsnip, parsley, dill, wild carrot, lime, celery, anise); and fragrances (colognes, perfumes, aftershave lotions). Often, the offending agent may be determined from the history, but photopatch testing may be needed to determine the cause. Treatment is symptomatic (topical corticosteroids and systemic antihistamines) and once the cause is found and discontinued, the athlete may resume normal sports participation.

INFECTIONS
Bacterial
Impetigo

Impetigo is a common superficial cutaneous infection caused by streptococcal and staphylococcal microorganisms. The infection may be acquired by contact with infected persons or

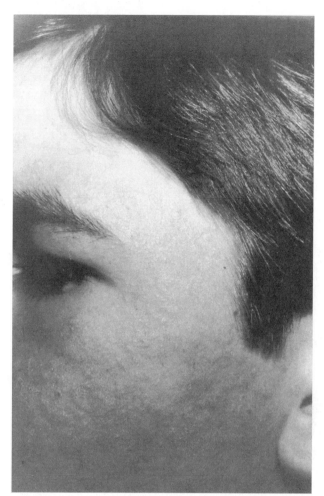

Figure 112-5 Photoallergic dermatitis of the face.

fomites, such as mats, equipment, or towels (26). Wrestlers, swimmers, and gymnasts are particularly susceptible to impetigo. Lesions appear as flaccid blisters (bullous type from *Staphylococcus aureus*) or erosions with golden-yellow crusting (contagiosa type from *Streptococcus*) (Fig. 112-6). Bacterial culture will confirm the clinical diagnosis. Because of the potential, though small, for associated glomerulonephritis, a urinalysis to examine for red blood cells and protein should also be obtained if streptococcal infection is found.

Treatment for bullous impetigo consists of a 7 to 10 day course of a systemic penicillinase-resistant penicillin or cephalosporin. The contagiosa type can be treated with topical mupirocin ointment (Bactroban) (27). Topical cleansing with mild soap and water is helpful for debridement. Impetigo is highly contagious, so the athlete must be restricted from activity until the infection has resolved.

Pitted Keratolysis

Pitted keratolysis is a superficial infection of the skin of the feet caused by a species of *Corynebacterium*. It is seen primarily in basketball and tennis players and is precipitated by occlusive footwear and hyperhidrosis (28). The patient presents with the complaint of malodorous feet and 1 to 3 mm pits with dirty-brown to black pigmentation involving the weight

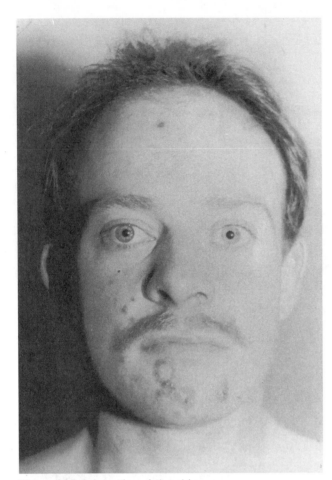

Figure 112-6 Impetigo of the chin.

bearing surfaces of the foot. The lesions clear rapidly when the occlusive moisture-contained environment is eliminated. When this fails, topical erythromycin, clindamycin, or 5% formalin are effective. Long-term treatment may be necessary. For resistant cases, oral erythromycin in therapeutic

doses can be used. Preventive measures include use of foot powder, absorbent socks, or a 20% aluminum chloride solution (Drysol) as a drying agent (28).

Pseudomonas Folliculitis

Outbreaks of a papulopustular skin eruption associated with the use of hot tubs, jacuzzis, whirlpools, and swimming pools have been described (29). The causative organism is *Pseudomonas aeruginosa*, which flourishes in the warm, turbulent, heavily-used, low-chlorinated water found in public hot tubs and whirlpools. The clinical lesions are reddish papules, pustules, or blisters that develop within two days after exposure, predominantly on the lateral trunk, axillae, proximal extremities, and buttocks. (Fig. 112-7) Pseudomonas folliculitis may also occur with use of a wet suit while diving (30).

The disease appears self-limited, lasting 7 to 10 days. Topical or systemic therapy does not appear to shorten the duration of the dermatitis. Since the disease was first recognized, measures such as frequent changing of water, automatic chlorination, frequent monitoring of disinfectant level, and maintenance of water at higher temperatures and at a pH of 7.2 to 7.8 have reduced the prevalence of pseudomonas folliculitis.

Otitis Externa

Acute otitis externa or "swimmer's ear" occurs uniquely in this specific group of athletes (31). It develops because prolonged exposure to water causes epidermal maceration and dissolution of cerumen in the ear canal, removing the protective seal for the skin. Trauma and anatomic anomalies also allow for invasion of bacteria, principally pseudomonas species. Pain, swelling, itching, fever, and diminished hearing are the most common symptoms. Treatment consists of cleansing the external auditory canal by gentle lavage and suctioning followed by the topical application of antibiotics or astringents. Prevention may be maintained by prophylactic installation of an acidic solution such as 2% acetic acid in propylene glycol (VoSol) and the use of wax or petrolatum-coated earplugs (32).

Figure 112-7 Pseudomonas folliculitis from hot tub.

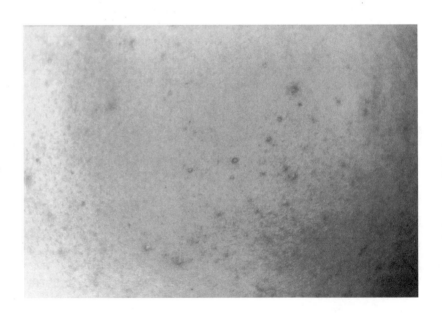

Viral

Herpes Simplex

Herpes simplex infections of the skin and mucous membranes are common problems in the general population. Participants in contact sports such as wrestling or rugby are particularly susceptible, and infection in these athletes has been termed herpes gladiatorum (33). Common sites of involvement are the head, neck, and upper extremities, although the trunk may be also be involved. The right side of the face and head is more frequently infected because the common "lock-up" position in wrestling in which the right cheeks of the opponents are repeatedly pressed together (34). (Fig. 112-8)

Typically, painful, grouped blisters on an inflamed base are present (Fig. 112-9); however, ulceration develops rapidly with secondary crusting. Because the fragile blisters are frequently traumatized, the characteristic eruption is not always present in the athlete and may be misdiagnosed as bacterial pyoderma or herpes zoster (28). Microscopic examination of the blister base for multinucleated giant cells and viral culture are helpful diagnostic aides. The infection heals in 10 to 14 days, but may recur in the same anatomic site. Factors or events such as trauma, sunlight, illness, surgery, stress, or menstruation may trigger a recurrence in an individual (4).

Cutaneous herpes infections are highly contagious and preclude the athlete from contact sports or swimming. Recommendations vary as to the length of time in which the athlete is prohibited from participation, but the most prudent approach is to prohibit competition until the lesions have fully healed (28).

Treatment of herpes gladiatorum is indicated to prevent complications such as herpes keratitis, meningitis, arthritis (35), or disseminated disease. Topical treatment with drying agents such as Burow's solution 1:40 or benzoyl peroxide gel 5% two to three times daily is helpful. Topical or systemic antibiotics for secondary bacterial colonization may be necessary. Systemic antiviral agents including acyclovir, famciclovir, and valciclovir accelerate healing and decrease viral shedding and pain. Frequent recurrences may mandate chronic suppressive oral antiviral therapy. Topical acyclovir is not effective alone and shows efficacy similar to drying agents. Prevention of herpes infection is possible with good personal hygiene, showering before and after events, and inspection of all participants before sport competition.

Molluscum Contagiosum

Molluscum contagiosum is a viral infection of the skin caused by a DNA pox virus. It is more contagious than common warts and is acquired by personal contact, or via contaminated swimming pools or gymnastic equipment. Minor epidemics have been reported in wrestlers and swimmers (36). Most commonly, the lesions are found on the trunk, axillae, face, perineum, and thighs and present as solitary or multiple pearly umbilicated papules on a noninflammatory base (Fig. 112-10). Occasionally, hyperkeratosis on frictional sites such as the elbows and knees may make the lesions difficult to recognize. Lesions may spread by direct inoculation through scratching.

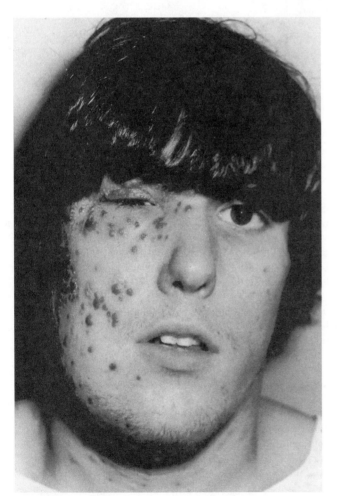

Figure 112-8 Herpes gladiatorum of the right side of the face.

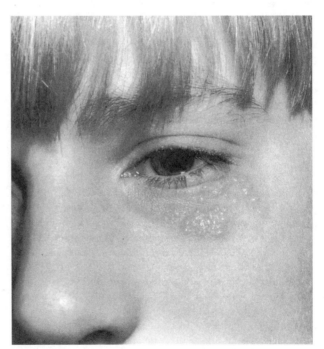

Figure 112-9 Cutaneous herpes simplex infection.

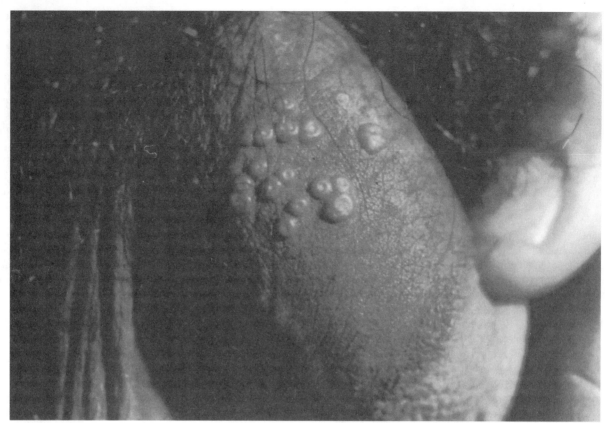

Figure 112-10 Molluscum contagiosum with characteristic central umbilication.

Treatment consists of curettage of each individual lesion followed by a chemical cauterizing agent. Liquid nitrogen cryotherapy and electrodesiccation are also effective. Topical agents such as tretinoin (Retin-A) or skin abrasion after bathing with a Buff-Puff pad, which is disposed after each treatment, have also been used.

Fungal

Superficial cutaneous fungal infections have been intimately associated with athletic participation as evidenced by the phrases "athlete's foot" and "jock itch." Factors implicated in predisposition to tinea infections include moisture (as created by constantly perspiring feet in athletic shoes), occlusion, increased carbon dioxide tension, and individual host factors (37). Showers and locker rooms provide a reservoir of dermatophyte infections and reinfection is common if proper precautions are not followed (9).

Tinea pedis or "athlete's foot" is the most common superficial fungal infection in athletes. It is most often caused by *Trichophyton rubrum* or *Trichophyton mentagrophytes*. Infection by the former generally causes an asymptomatic reddish plaque with peripheral scale and central clearing (Fig. 112-11), whereas infection by the latter may be associated with painful or itchy blisters. Many patients will self-treat and the clinical picture may be obscured. However, an important clue to diagnosis is involvement of the fourth toe web, which is nearly always affected (Fig. 112-12). Examination of potassium hydroxide scrapings from affected skin for the presence of septated fungal hyphae will confirm the diagnosis.

Treatment is helpful if measures are used to reduce dampness of the feet, such as frequent changes of absorbent socks and the use of a drying lotion or powder. Topical antifungals such as fungistatic imidazoles and fungicidal allylamines including naftifine and terbinafine are effective for most cases. For widespread or acute inflammatory lesions, oral griseofulvin, itraconazole, or terbinafine may be used. Prophylactic use of tolnaftate powder or topical antifungals can reduce the incidence of tinea pedis in high-risk groups (38). Wearing sandals in public showering facilities is also recommended. However, predisposed individuals may have a "localized" immune defect for certain fungal strains making eradication impossible and recurrences common.

Tinea cruris is a fungal infection of the groin and upper thighs and is often associated with tinea pedis. Most likely, the infection begins on the feet and spreads to the groin by clothing, towels, or other fomites. Lesions are itchy reddish plaques with peripheral scale and central clearing (Fig. 112-13). Examination of the feet and potassium hydroxide scrapings of peripheral scale should always be performed. Treatment is similar to that of tinea pedis with emphasis on loose, clean clothing for proper aeration and good hygiene (28). Other recommendations are for the athlete to wear socks before putting on underwear and to towel dry the feet last after a shower to reduce the chance of spreading infection from the feet (26).

Tinea corporis is a superficial fungal infection involving the body. The popular term "ringworm" is applied because the lesions appear as annular or circinate plaques with periph-

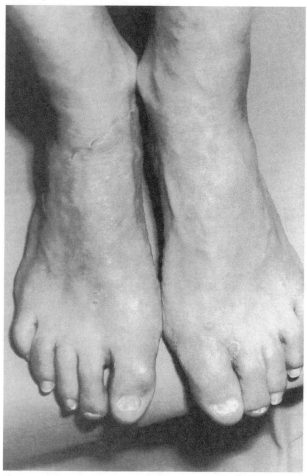

Figure 112-11 Tinea pedis of web spaces and medial feet.

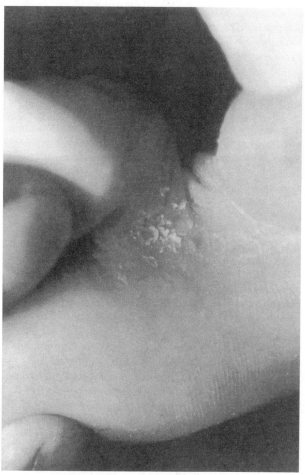

Figure 112-12 Scaling and maceration of toe web.

Figure 112-13 Tinea cruris showing annular ring on thigh.

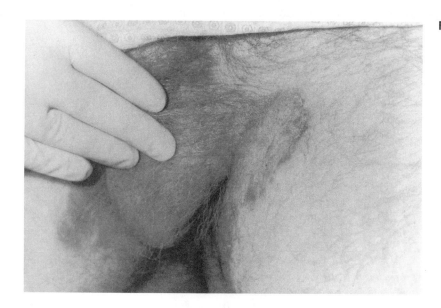

eral scaling and central clearing. Although not as common in athletes as tinea pedis and tinea cruris, epidemics among wrestlers have been reported (39). Treatment with topical or oral antifungals is effective.

CONTACT DERMATITIS

There are two types of contact dermatitis. Irritant contact dermatitis is nonallergic and results from exposure to a physical agent or irritating substance that produces dermatitis. Allergic contact dermatitis develops from acquired hypersensitivity to a specific allergen, such as poison ivy, applied to the skin.

Irritant contact dermatitis in athletes may occur by mechanical or chemical irritants. Some mechanical irritants include headbands or wristbands (runners), helmets (football players), gloves and fiberglass (hockey players), and adhesive tape (football and basketball players) (40). Irritant contact dermatitis due to chemicals may occur following application of antiseptics, medicaments, insect repellents, cosmetics, leakage of "cold pack" chemicals, or oily sunscreens (40).

The most common material causing allergic contact dermatitis in athletes is rubber-backed adhesive tape (21). Topical medications are also an important cause, and these include topical antibiotics (neomycin, nitrofurazone, penicillin) (Fig. 112-14), antihistamines (diphenhydramine, promethazine), anesthetics (benzocaine, dibucaine), and antiseptics (iodine) (40). Allergic contact dermatitis from tincture of benzoin, used to secure tape to the skin, is a common problem. Shoe dermatitis due to sensitivity to rubber, adhesives, dyes, or chemicals used in the tanning of leather may be seen in athletes, particularly runners (9). This characteristically presents on the dorsal aspects of the toes and feet (Fig. 112-15). The excessive moisture of the runner's foot makes it more susceptible to shoe dermatitis.

A thorough and complete history is essential to determine the underlying cause of allergic contact dermatitis. Cutaneous examination to determine the nature, configuration, and distribution of the eruption is also important. Typically in contact dermatitis, the clinical lesions are well demarcated and linear. Often, history and physical examination alone will identify the causative agent, but patch testing may be needed to determine the specific incriminating allergen.

Treatment for irritant and allergic contact dermatitis is similar, with elimination or avoidance of the precipitating cause being crucial. Medium-potency topical corticosteroid preparations are useful in limited disease, whereas severe cases may require systemic corticosteroids. Oral antihistamines for itching and oral antibiotics for secondary pyoderma may also be needed.

EXACERBATION OF PRE-EXISTING DERMATOSES

Exercise and its associated physiologic effects may worsen many skin diseases (Table 112-2). Patients with *atopic dermatitis* often have flares of their disease with sweating, friction, irritation, and increased bathing associated with strenuous exercise

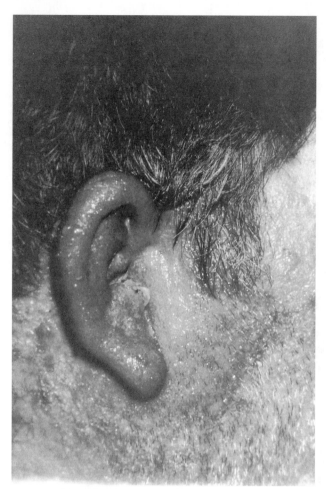

Figure 112-14 Allergic contact dermatitis from topical nitrofurazone antibiotic.

(40). Atopic individuals, especially swimmers (1), are very susceptible to dry skin and to secondary infections from staphylococcal organisms and herpes simplex. Certain protective skin measures are recommended including frequent use of emollients, avoidance of excessive cold or prolonged exposure, and reducing bathing to no more than once daily.

Athletes who are susceptible to *dry skin* need to follow similar measures as atopic patients. Dry skin is especially more prominent during the winter season when humidity is low. Swimmers, skiers, skaters, and hikers are particularly affected. Bathing with lukewarm water daily or every other day, use of a mild soap such as Dove, daily use of emollients, and humidifying the home air are often helpful preventive measures.

Dyshidrotic eczema occurs on the hands and feet as recurrent itchy blisters accompanied by redness, edema, and crusting. Stress is often associated with flares, although irritants and sweating may exacerbate the disorder. When the feet are affected, differentiation of dyshidrotic eczema from contact dermatitis or tinea pedis is a difficult problem. Tiny blisters on the lateral aspects of the toes favor a diagnosis of dyshidrosis since that symptom is rarely seen in contact dermatitis or tinea infections. In addition, potassium hydroxide examination

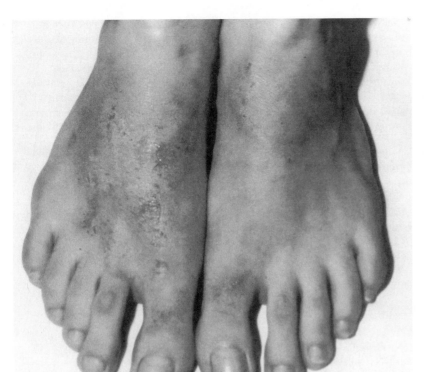

Figure 112-15 Shoe dermatitis.

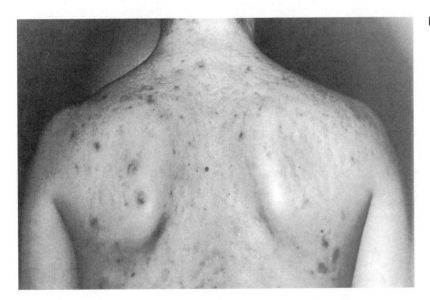

Figure 112-16 Severe acne on shoulders and back.

Table 112-2 Skin Diseases Exacerbated By Exercise
Atopic dermatitis
Dry skin
Dyshidrotic eczema
Psoriasis
Seborrheic dermatitis
Acne vulgaris

and patch testing give negative results in dyshidrotic eczema. Treatment includes measures to reduce moisture of the feet, such as application of an absorbent powder and frequent changing of white socks and shoes (21). Compresses with Burow's solution 1:40 and use of topical corticosteroid lotions or creams are also helpful.

Other common skin diseases such as *psoriasis* and *seborrheic dermatitis* are affected by athletic participation. Psoriasis often appears in areas that are susceptible to trauma such as the elbows, knees, and knuckles. Skin subjected to frictional or abrasional trauma may develop plaques of psoriasis, known as the Koebner phenomenon. For localized psoriasis, topical corticosteroids, calcipitrol (Donovex), and tar preparations are the mainstay of treatment. Seborrheic dermatitis presents as reddish plaques with greasy yellow scaling. The scalp, ears, eyebrows, and nasal crease are the most common sites although the axillae, mid-chest, umbilical area, and groin may also be affected. These latter sites would be most typically exacerbated in the athlete. Shampoos containing zinc pyrithione (Head and Shoulders), salicylic acid (Ionil), or tar (T Gel), mild corticosteroid creams (1% hydrocortisone) and topical ketoconazole cream (Nizoral) are effective for treatment.

Acne vulgaris may be worsened by gear or equipment used in exercise. This is particularly common in wrestlers and hockey and football players, and is associated with helmets with chin straps and shoulder pads (Fig. 112-16). Perspiration, heat, friction, and pressure are contributing factors. Treatment includes topical cleansing and antibacterial agents such as Lever 2000 and Dial during showers, topical antibiotics (erythromycin or clindamycin), benzoyl peroxide, and tretinoin (Retin A). Extensive or severe inflammatory cases may warrant systemic antibiotics such as tetracycline, doxycycline, minocycline, or erythromycin. Severe nodulocystic acne is treated with oral isotretinoin, but side effects including muscle and joint pain, lethargy, and decreased energy may inhibit performance in competitive events (41)

SUMMARY

The exercise enthusiast is susceptible to a whole spectrum of skin diseases that may or may not be unique to that particular sport or activity. Recognition and accurate diagnosis will lead to appropriate treatment and preventive measures and allow timely resumption of athletic participation or competition.

REFERENCES

1. Muller SA. Dermatologic disorders in athletes. J Ky Med Assoc 1976; 74:225–228.

2. Herring KM, Richie DM. Friction blisters and sock fiber composition: a double blind-controlled study. J Am Podiatr Med Assoc 1990;80:63–71.

3. Spence WR, Shields MN. New insole for prevention of athletic blisters. J Sports Med Phys Fitness 1968;8:177–180.

4. Stauffer LW. Skin disorders in athletes: identification and management. Physician Sports Med 1983;11:101–113, 117–121.

5. Bodine KG. Black heel. J Am Podiatry Assoc 1980;70:201.

6. Elston ML. Treatment of striae distensae with topical tretinoin. J Dermatol Surg Oncol 1990;16: 267–270.

7. Mortimer PS, Dawber RPR. Trauma to the nail unit including occupational skin injuries. Derm Clinics 1985;3:415–420.

8. Gibbs RC. Tennis toe. Arch Dermatol 1973;107:928.

9. Resnik SS, Lewis LA, Cohen BH. The athlete's foot. Cutis 1977; 20:351–353, 355.

10. Cohen PR, Eliezri YD, Silvers DN. Athlete's nodules: sports related connective tissue nevi of the collagen type (collagenomas). Cutis 1992;50:131–135.

11. Basler RSW, Jacobs SI. Athlete's nodules. J Am Acad Dermatol 1991;24:318.

12. Copperman SM. Two new causes of alopecia. JAMA 1984;252: 3367.

13. Ely PH. Balance beam alopecia. Arch Dermatol 1978;114:968.

14. Levit F. Jogger's nipples. N Eng J Med 1977;297:1127.

15. Brazin SA. Dermatologic hazards of long distance running. J Am Milit Dermatol 1979;5:8–9.

16. Powell B. Bicyclist's nipples. JAMA 1983;249:2457.

17. D'Ambrosia RD. Cold injuries encountered in a winter resort. Cutis 1977;20:351–353, 355.

18. Washburn B. Frostbite. N Engl J Med 1962;266:974–989.

19. Mikhailov P, Berova N, Andreev VC. Physical urticaria and sport. Cutis 1977;20:381–384, 389–390.

20. Rodeheffer RJ, Rommer JA, Wigley F, et al. Controlled double-blind trial of nifedipine in the treatment of Raynaud's phenomenon. N Engl J Med 1983;308:880–883.

21. Freeman MJ, Bergfeld WF. Skin diseases of football and wrestling participants. Cutis 1977;20: 333–339, 341.

22. Lewis J, Lieberman P, Treadwell G, et al. Exercise-induced urticaria, angioedema, and anaphylactoid episodes. J Allergy Clin Immunol 1981;68:432–437.

23. Sheffer AL, Austin KF. Exercise-induced anaphylaxis. J Allergy Clin Immunol 1984;73:699–703.

24. Hatty S, Mufti GJ, Hamblin TJ. Exercise-induced urticaria and angioedema with relief from cromoglycate insufflation. Postgrad Med J 1983;59:586–587.

25. Pathak MA. Sunscreens: topical and systemic approaches for protection of human skin against harmful effects of solar radiation. J Am Acad Dermatol 1982;7: 285–312.

26. Bart B. Skin problems in athletics. Minn Med 1983;66:239–241.

27. Leyden JJ. Mupirocin: a new topical antibiotic. J Am Acad Dermatol 1990;22:879–883.

28. Houston SD, Knox JM. Skin problems related to sports and recreational activities. Cutis 1977;19: 487–491.

29. Chandrasekar PH, Rolston KVI, Kannangara DW, et al. Hot tub-

associated dermatitis due to *Pseudomonas aeruginosa*. Arch Dermatol 1984;120:1337–1340.

30. Saltzer KR, Schutzer PJ, Weinberg JM, et al. Diving suit dermatitis: a manifestation of Pseudomonas folliculitis. Cutis 1997;59:245–246.

31. Hoadley AW, Knight DE. External otitis among swimmers and non-swimmers. Arch Environ Health 1975;30:445–448.

32. Garrity JD, Halliday TC. Prevention of swimmer's ear by simple prophylactic regimen. Curr Ther Res 1974;16:437–440.

33. Wheeler CE, Cabaniss WH. Epidemic cutaneous herpes simplex in wrestlers (herpes gladiatorum) JAMA 1965;194:145–149.

34. Becker TM. Herpes gladiatorum: a growing problem in sports medicine. Cutis 1992;50:150–152.

35. Shelly WB. Herpetic arthritis associated with disseminate herpes simplex in a wrestler. Br J Dermatol 1980;103:209–212.

36. Niizeki K, Kano O, Kondo Y. An epidemic study of molluscum contagiosum. Dermatologica 1984; 169:197–198.

37. Allen AM, King RD. Occlusion, carbon dioxide and fungal skin infections. Lancet 1978; 1:360–362.

38. Gentles JC, Jones GR, Roberts DT. Efficacy of miconazole in the topical treatment of tinea pedis in sportsmen. Br J Dermatol 1975; 93:79–84.

39. Beller M, Gessner BD. An outbreak of tinea corporis gladiatorum on a high school wrestling team. J Am Acad Dermatol 1994;31: 197–201.

40. Bergfeld WF, Taylor JS. Trauma, sports and the skin. Am J Indust Med 1985;8:403–413.

41. Basler RSW. Sports-related skin injuries. In: Callen JP, Dahl MV, Golitz LE, et al, eds. Advances in dermatology, vol 4. Chicago: Year Book, 1989:29–50.

Chapter 113

Skin Care

Elen Casso Donahue
Gary R. Kantor

MOISTURIZERS

A wide range of moisturizers are available to consumers as both over-the-counter and prescription formulations. The sheer number of products marketed and the various claims made by the manufacturers can cause confusion with regard to which products to use or recommend. In order to select the appropriate moisturizer for each individual, it is important to review the causes of dry skin and how the various ingredients in moisturizers function to treat this condition.

Causes of Dry Skin

Moisturizers can be used to maintain the condition of healthy skin as well as rehydrate dry skin (xerosis) (Fig. 113-1), which may be rough, scaly, and frequently pruritic. These signs and symptoms are primarily due to alterations in the barrier layer of the skin, the stratum corneum (1,2). A reduced water content in the stratum corneum can have a significant impact on the skin. In general, this occurs when excessive amounts of moisture are lost to the environment through evaporation. This causes the abnormal desquamation of corneocytes, which results in a rough, dry, and scaly texture (1–3). In order for the skin to appear normal and feel soft, the water content of the stratum corneum must be greater than 10% (4), and perhaps even as high as 20% to 35% (5).

Water loss alone, however, is not the only factor responsible for dry skin. Alterations in the intercellular lipid bilayer structure of the skin also contribute to the development of xerosis (1,3). A variety of different lipids are needed to retain moisture within the epidermis (6–8). Ceramide, which pos-

sesses long chain fatty acids and linoleic acid, is the major lipid found in the stratum corneum (3,9). In addition, sphingolipids, free sterols, free fatty acids (6), cholesterol sulfate, triglycerides, sterol wax/esters, squalene, and n-alkanes (10) all appear to play a role in maintaining barrier function. If they are depleted, then transepidermal water loss becomes significantly elevated (1) and cytokine actions, adhesion molecule expression, and growth factor production in the skin may be affected (11).

A third element that may be of importance in this process is pH (1). Some studies have shown that a pH range between 4.5 and 6.0 may be necessary for the formation of the lipid bilayers and the maintenance of corneocyte adhesion (12). Therefore, any factors that significantly alter the pH of the skin could potentially have detrimental effects on the barrier function.

Once this barrier layer has been altered in one or more of these ways, the skin becomes more susceptible to further damage. Certain external factors can cause xerosis or exacerbate the condition of previously damaged skin. The use of soaps, detergents, and household cleansers can result in dry skin by dissolving intercellular lipids and disrupting the lipid bilayers of the stratum corneum (2,13,14). For this reason, it is important that patients refrain from excessive washing and bathing. Another factor that commonly contributes to xerosis is the cycling phenomenon (1). This occurs in both the summer and winter seasons when patients are alternately exposed to cold dry and then warm humid conditions when traveling between indoor and outdoor environments. Furthermore, the application of water-based lotions to the skin immediately prior to exposure to a cold dry environment can worsen this situation by increasing the evaporation of mois-

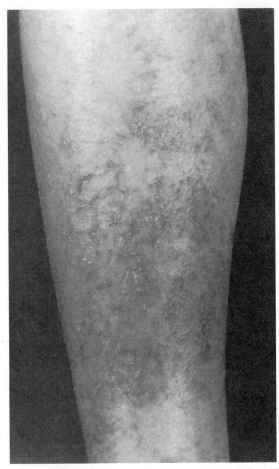

Figure 113-1 Scaling and fissuring of severe dry skin.

ture from the skin (1). Therefore, it is advisable to apply lotions at least 30 minutes prior to exposure to cold dry conditions in order to avoid this detrimental effect (1). Mechanical trauma or abrasion of the skin (1) and exposure to ultraviolet radiation or cold dry wind (2) can also damage the barrier function of the skin.

Methods of Rehydrating Dry Skin

Two basic treatment methods can be implemented to rehydrate dry skin: water delivery and occlusion. External water can be added to and retained in the stratum corneum by the use of humectants, and transepidermal water loss (TEWL) can be reduced by means of occlusive formulations (2).

Upon topical application, occlusives form a barrier over the skin's surface that reduces the amount of TEWL and allows the skin to retain more moisture (1,3). This barrier also serves as a protective agent against external environmental factors (1,3). However, studies have indicated that it is important for this artificial barrier to remain partially permeable in order for the skin to properly reestablish its own natural barrier function (10,15,16). When used alone, occlusives lack the ability to add water to the skin. Therefore, these formulations are best applied immediately after bathing when the skin is still damp. Unfortunately, patient compliance with the use of occlusives is often reduced because the formulations tend to feel sticky and greasy. Some commonly used occlusives

include: petrolatum, lanolin alcohols, fatty acids, phospholipids, cocoa butter, jojoba oil, paraffin, cholesterol, heavy mineral oil, heavy lipid mixtures, and propylene glycol.

Humectants are another class of chemicals that can rehydrate the skin. Glycerin, pyrrolidone carboxilic acid, sodium lactate, urea, propylene glycol, hyaluronic acid, vitamins, and sorbitol are some examples. In contrast to occlusives, humectants function by penetrating into the stratum corneum and increasing the amount of moisture that is associated with lipids and proteins (1). They slow the evaporative rate of water being delivered from the product, and increase the amount of water retained (2), thereby allowing the skin to feel smoother and softer (1). This is also accomplished by drawing water from the deeper epidermis and the dermis into the stratum corneum (1). It has also been proposed that water can be drawn into the stratum corneum directly from the environment if the humidity is greater than 70% (1). However, when used alone in low humidity conditions, humectants can actually draw moisture away from the skin by increasing TEWL (3). Therefore, effective moisturizers usually contain a combination of occlusive and humectant ingredients in order to maximize the beneficial properties of each (3).

Components of Moisturizers

In order for a moisturizer to be efficacious and marketable, it must fulfill at least three criteria. It must increase the water content of the skin, protect the cutaneous surface from harmful environmental factors, and make the skin feel soft and smooth (3). This last feature, referred to as emolliency, is necessary to make the formulations acceptable to the consumer (1,3). Ingredients such as silicone oils, cetyl alcohols, cholesterol, mineral oil, waxy esters, and quaternary compounds provide skincare products with the desired tactile and rub-in properties (1). They accomplish this immediate but temporary smoothing effect by filling the stratum corneum with oil droplets (1,3). Several categories of emollients exist, with each lending various characteristics to the final product (3). Protective emollients are fairly long lasting and feel smooth on application, whereas fatting emollients persist longer on the skin but feel greasy. Dry emollients are utilized to impart a dry feeling to the skin and astringent emollients are often added to minimize the oily feel of other emollients.

Most moisturizers are available in two basic formulations: water in oil (W/O) and oil in water (O/W). Water in oil emulsions are composed predominantly of oil, and therefore feel warm, glossy, and heavy after application. They function primarily as occlusives (2,15). Oil in water emulsions, on the other hand, contain water as their dominant ingredient. This affords them a cool, nonglossy, thinner, and more aesthetically pleasing feel when applied to the skin (17). They are usually available as creams and lotions, and function mostly by means of water delivery mechanisms (2).

Water is typically the main component of moisturizers, constituting 65% to 85% of the formulation. However, only minimal absorption of this water actually occurs after application of a moisturizer. Most of the water is lost to evaporation, leaving behind the lipid component to remoisturize the skin. The lipid phase of a moisturizer usually ranges from 5% to 20%, although some may contain up to 35%. The most commonly used lipids are mineral oil, petrolatum, and lanolin.

Also present may be fatty acids and alcohols, sphingolipids, and cholesterols. The lipids are thought to be the most effective components of moisturizers since they function to recondition the intercellular lipids in dry skin (18).

Another essential ingredient to moisturizers is an emulsifier that serves to bind the water and lipid components together in a stable form. Emulsifiers, such as stearic acid, triethanolamine, or various surfactants, are usually present in concentrations of 1% to 2% (18). For safety reasons, all moisturizers must contain preservatives. Chemicals such as parabens, formaldehyde donors, chelating agents, methylchoroisothiazolinone, methylisothiazolinone, and alcohols usually compose between 0.1% to 1% of the formulation (18). Fragrances are commonly added to moisturizers to mask the unpleasant odor of the lipid components. However, about 25% of moisturizers are now available as fragrance-free formulations (18). These are especially beneficial for patients with dry, sensitive skin or a history of hypersensitivity reactions (1).

Numerous other ingredients may be added to moisturizers. Alpha-hydroxy acids (AHAs) are commonly incorporated into both over-the-counter and physician-dispensed formulations. AHAs are a group of organic acids that include: glycolic, lactic, malic, tartaric, citric, mandelic, and ascorbic acids (2,3,19,20). These chemicals appear to have effects on the stratum corneum, epidermis, and dermis (2,3,19,20). Current theories suggest that AHAs cause a reduction in corneocyte cohesion that leads to desquamation (19–21) and a temporary thinning of the stratum corneum (19,21). In addition, sustained therapy in atrophic photoaged skin may result in an improved epidermal thickness and more orderly cellular differentiation (19,20,22,23). The potential dermal effects of AHAs may take 2 to 3 months to become apparent (22,24). An increase in dermal thickness may be related to an accumulation of dermal glycosaminoglycans (23,25) or an increase in collagen synthesis (19,20,26). The exact mechanisms by which AHAs produce these observed cutaneous changes are currently being investigated (19,20).

Many patients are interested in using AHAs because these products may aid in reducing some of the signs of photoaging. A number of studies have shown that an improvement in fine lines and wrinkles, dyspigmentation, dryness, and coarseness of the skin may be observed after sustained use of the higher concentrations of AHAs (3,20–23,27,28). AHA products most commonly contain glycolic acid in lotion, cream, or gel formulations (19). These products may have very different concentrations of AHAs and wide ranges of pH depending on their exact composition (19,20). In general, products intended to be applied to the face by the patient at home have a glycolic acid concentration between 4% and 15% and a pH in the range of 4.2 to 5.6 (20). In order to maximize the potential beneficial effects, these daily-use AHA moisturizers are often used in conjunction with periodic glycolic acid peels in the office that are more acidic and of higher concentrations (3,19,20). Topical tretinoin may also be added to this regimen because it may have additive effects with regard to the treatment of photoaging (3).

Lactic acid is another AHA that may also be incorporated into moisturizers. In addition to the previously stated actions of AHAs, lactic acid formulations appear to enhance the water uptake of the skin by increasing the water-binding capacity of the stratum corneum (3,28). This humectant property leads to an improved pliability of the skin (29). Moisturizers with lactic acid are commonly used to treat photoaging and severe xerosis.

Formulations for Different Skin Types

Moisturizer formulations are typically divided into categories based on the needs of various skin types. Products designed specifically for oily, dry, or normal skin differ in the types of oils they contain and in the water to oil ratios (2,3). Therefore, it is important that individual patients know how to select the proper formulation, especially with regards to facial moisturizers. Products for oily skin are usually oil-free and contain water and silicone derivatives that are noncomedogenic and nongreasy. Occasionally, small amounts of light oils like mineral oil may be used. Oil-absorbing substances, such as talc, clay, starch, or synthetic polymers may also be added to some products in order to further reduce the shiny look of oily skin (3). Dry skin responds best to W/O formulations that contain heavy oils like petrolatum, lanolin, propylene glycol, or mineral oil. These ingredients may improve the appearance of fine wrinkling and roughness that are due to dehydration (3). Products for normal or combination skin are usually O/W emulsions that contain light oils with small amounts of petrolatum or lanolin (3).

Products made for use on the body or hands follow the same basic principles. Body moisturizers are most commonly sold as O/W lotions because of their cosmetic acceptability. Typically, they contain 10% to 15% oil, 5% to 10% humectant, and 60% to 85% water (2,3). Hand lotions and creams are also most commonly of the O/W type. However, they tend to contain higher percentages of oils (15% to 40%) and smaller amounts of water (45% to 80%) (30). In addition, silicone derivatives are often added so that hand creams may better resist being washed off. Although the O/W products are the most frequently sold due to their acceptability to the consumer, it is important to inform patients that for severely dry or xerotic skin, the W/O formulations are much more effective.

Adverse reactions to moisturizers and their additives have been reported to occur in certain individuals. Preservatives and fragrances are most frequently implicated as the causative agents of allergic contact dermatitis (1,3,18). However, other ingredients may be responsible for eliciting allergic or irritant contact reactions (3,18). Additives such as propylene glycol, benzoic acid, cinnamic acid, lactic acid, glycolic acid, urea, emulsifiers, formaldehyde, and sorbic acid may cause burning or stinging sensations, especially if applied to damaged skin (3). If a patient develops signs or symptoms of an adverse reaction, it is recommended that a complete ingredient list be obtained in order to determine the most likely causative ingredient(s).

SKIN CLEANSERS

Numerous types of skin cleansers are available to the consumer. Their proper use is instrumental in maintaining the health and appearance of the skin. The majority of products can adequately perform the desired task of eliminating dirt, sebum, make-up, and dead corneocytes from the skin's surface

(2). However, it is important to recognize that these products do differ significantly in their propensity to induce adverse effects such as dryness and irritation. Numerous factors may contribute to the irritancy potential of a cleanser, including its specific chemical structure, pH, additives, and the amount of residue it deposits on the skin (31–33).

Cleansing products that strip the skin of essential lipids alter the barrier function of the stratum corneum (2). This results in increased transepidermal water loss (TEWL) and dryness as well as increased percutaneous absorption of substances that may induce irritant or allergic reactions (32,34). In addition, the irritant potential of a cleanser may be enhanced by the amount of detergent that persists on the skin after washing (17). This residue prolongs the contact time of the product with the skin, affording it a greater opportunity to interfere with the barrier function (32,34,35).

The importance of a cleanser's pH with regard to irritancy is controversial. It is known that the pH of normal skin is acidic and ranges between 4.0 and 6.5, with an average of about 5.5 (2,3,31,36–38). The use of a cleanser with an acidic to neutral pH causes minimal or no change in the cutaneous pH, whereas alkaline products, such as soaps, significantly elevate the normal pH (2,3,31,36). It has been suggested by some studies that this alteration in pH may cause irritation in some individuals (31,39) and may leave the skin feeling dry and tight (2,40). However, in healthy skin, the cutaneous buffering system restores the normal pH within several hours of washing (31,41). Therefore, many authors have concluded that the pH of a cleanser may actually have little influence on its irritancy potential (31,32). The pH may become important when the rinsability of a product is considered (32). In products that leave a residue, the alkaline pH may exert more of a lasting effect and therefore may result in more irritation.

Another way that the pH of a cleanser may affect the skin is its impact on the cutaneous microflora (2,36). The regular use of alkaline cleansers may result in elevated bacterial counts of *Propionibacterium acnes* (38), and, in certain patients, may cause increased numbers of acne lesions (Fig. 113-2) (42).

Allergic sensitization is an uncommon but not rare adverse effect of skin cleansers (31). Most products contain additives, such as preservatives and perfumes, that can precipitate allergic reactions (31). Even "unscented" cleansers contain fragrances that mask the unpleasant odor of the ingredients (31). Cutaneous reactions to dye additives (43) and to various photosensitizing ingredients (44) have also been reported.

Categories

Skin cleansers can be divided into four basic categories: soaps, synthetic detergents, cleansing creams, and astringents. True soaps are water-soluble products composed of long-chain fatty acid alkali salts that are created by the saponification of natural fats (3,31,33,45). Anionic surfactants, also called active surface agents, provide soaps with their effective detergent activity and good lathering ability (2). Some potential disadvantages of soaps are that they have an alkaline pH of between 9 and 10, and that they tend to strip the skin of essential lipids and cause increased TEWL and irritation (2,3,31). Therefore, true soaps should usually be avoided in patients with dry or sensitive skin.

Synthetic detergents (syndets) were developed to overcome some of the problems inherent in soaps. A few of the commonly used detergents in syndet bars are sodium cocoate, sodium tallowate, sodium cocoyl isethionate, sodium stearate, and sodium cocoglyceryl ether sulfonate. Liquid formulations often contain cocoamido propyl betaine, sodium laureth sulfate, and lauramide DEA (3). The pH of these products can be adjusted over a wide range (2,3,31,36), but most are formulated to have a slightly acidic pH between 5 and 7 (3,36,37). Depending on the particular formulation, clinical testing has shown that different syndets may vary from very mild to harsh (31). In general, however, most syndets cause less TEWL, and are less drying and irritating than are soaps.

In order to further improve the tolerability and versatility of cleansers, various other ingredients may be added to the formulations. Moisturizing agents such as free fatty acids are

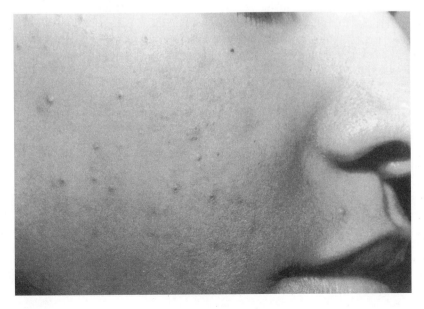

Figure 113-2 Comedones and pustules of acne vulgaris.

often incorporated into soaps and syndets to counteract the drying effects (2,3,31,33). Superfatted soaps are slightly less irritating than pure soaps but remain significantly more harsh than the syndets (33) Among the most mild products are the moisturizing syndets that are often labeled as "beauty bars" (3,33). Deodorant soaps are created by the incorporation of antibacterial agents. Triclocarban is effective at eradicating gram-positive organisms and triclosan can rid of both gram-positive and gram-negative bacteria (3). Unfortunately, most of the deodorant soaps tend to be harsh and irritating (3). Also available are medicated or acne soaps, which may contain ingredients such as benzoyl peroxide, sulfur, resorcinol, or salicylic acid (3).

Cleansing creams, which are composed of mineral oil, water, petrolatum, and natural waxes, are another category of skin cleansers (2,3,31). The solvent action of mineral oil removes heavy oil-based makeup and sebum more readily than does soap and water (2,31). Other benefits of these products are that they leave an emollient film on the skin's surface to help prevent delipidization, and they have a low potential for producing irritation (2,31). Older products, generally known as "cold creams," typically contained borax as an emulsifier (2,3,31). Newer formulations incorporate nonionic emulsifiers such as fatty acid esters, ethers, and alcohols that provide a lighter, less greasy texture and permit the pH to remain closer to that of normal skin (2,31). The addition of cationic conditioners can further reduce the oily feel and improve the emolliency (31). In general, cleansing creams are a good choice for patients with dry or sensitive skin (2,3,31). However, some products incorporate ingredients such as salicylic acid, resorcinol, or sulfur to make them more appealing to individuals with oily skin (31).

Astringents, or toners, are alcohol-based products intended for application to the face after washing with a cleanser in order to remove any residual oils, dirt, or soap residue (3,32). Use of these products may reduce the clinical safety of cleansing regimens and potentially worsen the cosmetic appearance of the skin by causing dryness, roughness, and erythema (32). This is particularly true for formulations that contain high concentrations of alcohol.

Guidelines for Selection

Many of the skin cleansers available are designed specifically for oily, dry, or sensitive skin types. In most cases, there is no perfect cleanser for any one individual. And, in fact, even products that claim to be in the same category of cleansers may have very different clinical effects (31). There are some general guidelines that can be given to patients regarding the category of cleanser that should be used. However, often personal preferences are also important in choosing a particular product.

In patients with oily skin, the purpose of cleansing is to remove dirt and excess sebum as well as control the process of regreasing and minimize the shiny appearance of the skin. In doing this, however, it is necessary to avoid extensive delipidization of the stratum corneum (2). Non-oily syndets or superfatted soaps followed by thorough but gentle rinsing are often recommended because they can accomplish both of these goals (2,46). Many patients with oily skin choose a deodorant or acne soap. Unfortunately, these harsh products can cause dryness and irritation, especially in patients who are being treated with concomitant acne medications that also may be irritants (2,46). In addition, they may even worsen the skin's oiliness because severe degreasing can actually intensify sebaceous secretion (2). With the purpose of controlling the recurrence rate of shininess after cleansing, oil-absorbing ingredients such as bentone and nylon powder may be added to formulations (2). However, these materials work only in cleansers that are not washed off, because the substances must remain on the skin in order to be effective. In addition, incorporating polyquaternary compounds into cleansers alters the distribution of sebum over the skin's surface, causing it to remain in furrows. This results in a reduction in the shiny appearance of oily skin (2).

Patients with dry or sensitive skin should be advised to use only products that will remove unwanted dirt, sebum, and makeup without stripping the skin of essential lipids necessary for the barrier function of the cutaneous surface. This is best accomplished with very mild formulations such as cleansing creams and moisturizing syndets (2,31). These cleansers have a low potential for irritation, are not likely to delipidize the skin, and leave a beneficial residual emollient film on the skin after cleansing (31). It is also important to advise these patients that harsh products such as true soaps and astringents as well as products with fragrances or other potentially irritating additives should be avoided.

In general, to maintain the health and appearance of any skin type, it is best to recommend the use of a mild cleanser. If a rinsable product is selected, warm but not hot water should be used to thoroughly but gently remove any detergent remaining on the skin. In addition, patients should be advised not to overuse any cleanser. Even the most mild product can cause irritation if utilized improperly (2,31,33,46).

INDOOR TANNING

The use of indoor tanning facilities for cosmetic purposes continues to grow despite convincing evidence of both acute and chronic adverse effects. The original tanning devices posed many potential health risks because they emitted mainly UVB radiation (290 to 320 nm) (47). UVB is the component of natural sunlight that is primarily responsible for the detrimental effects associated with excessive exposure to solar radiation. In an effort to improve safety, current tanning beds utilize primarily UVA radiation (320 to 400 nm). However, UVA is also biologically active, and actually penetrates more deeply into the skin than does UVB. In addition, between 0.5% and 4.6% of the total radiation emitted from these modern units is UVB (48). This percentage, although small, is potentially significant with regard to its possible biologic effects.

Acute Effects

The acute adverse effects of UVA exposure, which occur relatively frequently with the use of tanning beds, include the production of erythema, pruritus, dryness of the skin, and nausea (49,50). Although UVB is usually responsible for producing the erythema induced by excessive sunlight exposure, UVA alone can also induce erythema (51) if given at high enough doses (52). In one study of UVA sunbeds, 71% of the subjects experienced an immediate erythema that was thought to be due to UVA-induced inflammation (49). This immediate erythema produced by UVA often fades over a few hours but may be followed by a secondary phase of erythema (53,54). Tanning bed exposures can also result in acute cutaneous first-and second-degree burns, some necessitating emergency room visits (55).

Photosensitivity reactions are another type of acute adverse effect that can result from indoor tanning. The combination of UVA exposure and a variety of commonly prescribed medications, certain cosmetics, or even foods can cause serious photoallergic or phototoxic responses (48,56,57). Phototoxic reactions are nonimmunologic and can result in a sunburn-type response within hours after a UVA exposure (57). Systemic antibiotics, such as tetracyclines or sulfonamides, and foods containing psoralens, like celery or limes (58), are just a few of the chemicals that can provoke severe reactions (48,56,59–61). Photoallergic reactions can occur in individuals who have been previously sensitized to certain agents. A blistering dermatitis may develop 24 to 48 hours after exposure to UVA radiation. This reaction may be seen in sensitized patients taking certain diuretics, hypoglycemic agents, and phenothiazines among others.

Photosensitive diseases, such as systemic lupus erythematosus (Fig. 113-3), polymorphous light eruption, porphyria, melasma, and vitiligo can be exacerbated by exposure to tanning bed UV radiation (48,49,61,62). In addition, the induction of various diseases including polymorphous light eruption (Fig. 113-4) (48,49) pseudoporphyria (48,63,64), and mid-dermal elastolysis (48,65) have been reported following the use of sunbeds.

UVA tanning beds also pose a risk of causing ocular injuries. Corneal burns are one of the most frequent ocular complications (55). Fortunately, the corneal epithelium is highly regenerative and the damage is usually transient.

Repeated and prolonged exposure of the conjunctiva to UV radiation causes thickening and hypervascularity similar to the changes seen in actinically damaged skin (48,57). It also accelerates lens aging, dilates retinal vessels, alters the protein compounds in the eye, (59) and has been implicated in the formation of cataracts (48,55,57). Retinal damage is usually limited except in patients with aphakia or pseudoaphakia, in which there is no UV absorption by the lens (57). Based on the risk of serious injury to the eye, the FDA has mandated the use of protective goggles when tanning beds are used (66). However, despite these FDA guidelines, compliance with these recommendations appears to be poor among tanning salon patrons (50,67–70).

Delayed Effects

The potential delayed effects of UVA exposure in tanning beds include photoaging, immunologic alterations, and carcinogenesis. Photoaging refers to the skin changes that result from long-term exposure to UV radiation (71). Clinically apparent cutaneous alterations such as wrinkles, coarseness, dryness, mottled pigmentation, loss of elasticity, easy bruisability, telangiectasias, freckles, and lentigenes do not become evident until decades after exposure. The most striking histologic change of photodamage is elastosis in the dermis with thickened, tangled aggregates of degraded elastic fibers. UVA radiation has been shown to cause elastosis that extends more deeply into the dermis than that caused by UVB (71,72). The development of these clinical and histologic changes is determined not only by radiation exposure but by skin type as well. Individuals with light skin (skin types I and II) are at higher risk for developing more severe changes of photoaging than are dark-skinned persons (skin types V and VI) (71).

Cutaneous carcinogenesis represents the greatest potential risk of indoor tanning. Although UVB radiation is known to be three to four times more efficient at producing skin

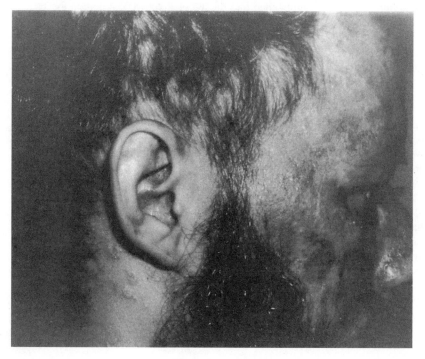

Figure 113-3 Scarring and hyperpigmented plaques on face, ear, and neck in a patient with lupus erythematosus.

Figure 113-4 Urticarial papules and plaques on sun-exposed areas of skin characteristic of polymorphous light eruption.

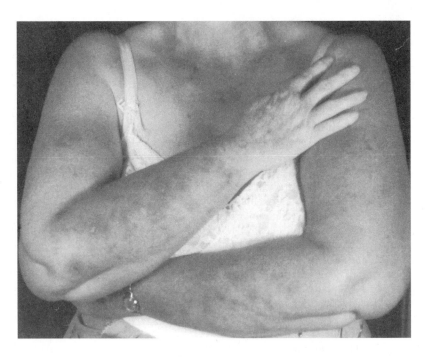

cancer than is UVA (51), experimental evidence indicates that UVA by itself can induce cutaneous carcinomas in laboratory animals (73,74). In addition, UVA tanning beds, when used in combination with sun exposure, may have additive and even augmentative effects with respect to carcinogenesis (48). Animal studies have illustrated that the pattern of exposure is also important in determining the long-term consequences of UV radiation. Many small doses are more carcinogenic for nonmelanoma skin cancer than the same amount of radiation given in a few large doses (75). This contradicts the notion that receiving many small doses of radiation from a tanning bed is a safe method of exposure.

The relevance of these findings as it relates to humans needs to be further clarified through large epidemiologic studies (48,76). Results of a few human studies offer some preliminary data. One study of relatively young people with basal cell carcinomas found a significant correlation with the use of tanning beds (77). The development of melanocytic lesions with lentiginous melanocytic proliferation has also been reported in association with tanning bed use (78,79). Several studies have even suggested a relationship between indoor tanning and melanoma (80–83). A number of mechanisms have been proposed to explain the process of UVA radiation-induced carcinogenesis. Direct DNA damage, pyrimidine dimer formation leading to DNA alteration, cell damage secondary to active oxygen species, and immunologic alterations may play a role in the pathogenesis (84–90).

Many patrons of tanning salons believe that obtaining a tan in this manner is protective against subsequent sun exposures. Indoor tanning with UVA can produce two types of tans referred to as immediate and delayed. Immediate tanning typically fades within minutes to hours and is not protective against burning (48,91). In certain individuals, delayed tanning may develop within 48 hours of exposure. Not all people exposed to UVA radiation are capable of delayed tanning. In those individuals who are, the various studies

examining the protective effects of a UVA-induced tan are conflicting (48). However, even if a mild protective effect is conferred against subsequent sun exposure, evidence indicates that a UVA-induced tan is produced at the expense of DNA damage (48).

Therefore, although some questions remain unanswered regarding the specific effects of UV radiation from indoor tanning, there is convincing evidence that both acute and chronic deleterious effects do occur. Based on the fact that the potential hazards outweigh any potential benefits, the Photobiology Task Force of the American Academy of Dermatology (56) and the British Photodermatology Group (92) have recommended that the use of indoor UV radiation for cosmetic purposes be discouraged.

TANNING WITHOUT THE SUN

Patients who desire the cosmetic appeal of a tan can be offered alternatives to sun exposure or tanning salons. A number of products are available that can impart the appearance of a tan without the potential risks of UV radiation. The two agents that are currently FDA approved in the United States are bronzing gels and self-tanning lotions (93,94). Bronzing gels are water-soluble dyes used to stain the skin (93,94). They impart a tanned appearance immediately but are easily removed by washing and can be messy to apply (93,94).

Self-tanning lotions contain dihydroxyacetone (DHA), a chemical that reacts with amino acids in the stratum corneum to create a brown-colored product that stains the skin within 1 to 3 hours of application (2,93,94). This product, referred to as a melanoidin, is incorporated into the amino acid structure of the cells and therefore resists being washed off (2,93). The staining process remains limited to the layers of the stratum corneum and appears to be nontoxic (2). However, infrequent cases of allergic contact dermatitis have been reported (95). The color fades gradually over 5 to 6 days as the stratum corneum naturally desquamates (2).

The self-tanning lotion formulations currently available, unlike the original products, produce a fairly even, natural-appearing, tan color, particularly in individuals with medium complexions (skin types II and III) (2,93,94). However, several factors can influence the staining characteristics. An alkaline pH can cause the color to appear an unnatural yellowish-orange. Therefore, any alkaline soap residue should be removed from the skin prior to application (2). In addition, the thickness of the stratum corneum and the anatomic location to which the lotion is applied can influence the intensity and duration of color. As a result, the hands stain more deeply and persistently than does the face (2,93). Finally, hyperkeratotic, mottled, or freckled skin may stain unevenly and cutaneous imperfections may be highlighted (2,3,93). In order to maximize the smoothness and duration of the color, it is best to gently exfoliate the skin prior to application (2,93).

It is important to inform patients that despite the tanned color produced on the skin, self-tanning lotions do not provide any significant protection against UV radiation (2,93). Additionally, the fact that some products advertise the incorporation of sunscreens into the formulations may further serve to falsely reassure consumers. Unfortunately, the duration of any sunscreen's effectiveness is significantly shorter than that of the tanned appearance produced (2,93). Therefore, sunscreens need to used as they routinely would, prior to each UV exposure.

Other types of tanning agents include tanning accelerators, promoters, and pills. None of these are currently approved for sale in the United States (93,94). Topical tan accelerators, which utilize tyrosine in conjunction with sun exposure to stimulate melanin production, have not proven to be very effective (93,96). The active ingredient in tanning promoters is 5-methoxypsoralen, which can cause phototoxicity and may be carcinogenic (94,97). Tanning pills induce a tanned appearance through the deposition of a carotenoid in the skin (98). Reported toxic effects of this canthaxanthin-containing drug include retinopathy (99,100), hepatitis (93), and aplastic anemia (101).

It can therefore be concluded that self-tanning lotions containing DHA, unlike some of the other preparations discussed, offer a cosmetically acceptable and apparently safe alternative means of obtaining a tanned appearance without the risks of UV radiation exposure. However, it must be emphasized to patients that the application of these agents does not eliminate the need for the use of sunscreens.

SUNSCREENS

The consistent use of sunscreens can be an important part of skin care for a number of reasons. Sun protection can reduce photoaging of the skin, may help to prevent skin carcinogenesis, and can decrease the risk of developing photosensitive reactions or exacerbating photosensitive diseases (3,102–104). Many manufacturers now incorporate various types of sunscreens into the formulations of facial foundations, moisturizers, and hair care products, among others.

Sunscreens can be divided into two broad categories: chemical and physical. Chemical sunscreens function by absorbing photons of UV radiation at the level of the stratum corneum (3,102). As a result of this absorption being wavelength specific, chemical sunscreens can be further subdivided into UVA and UVB types (3,102). UVB sunscreens absorb 90% to 95% of the radiation across the UVB spectrum from 290 to 320 nm (3,102). These products most commonly contain cinnamates, para-aminobenzoic acid (PABA) derivatives, and salicylates (3,102,103,105). Due to lower rates of skin sensitization and irritation, the PABA esters, such as padimate A and O, have essentially replaced pure PABA (3). UVA sunscreens have more limited absorption spectrums (102). Products containing benzophenones or anthranilates are effective for wavelengths of 300 to 350 nm whereas butylmethoxy-dibenzoylmethane (Parsol 1789) absorbs in the range of 340 to 350 nm (102,103,106).

Physical sunscreens are barriers that can reflect, scatter, or absorb UVA and UVB radiation as well as visible light and infrared wavelengths (3,102,103,107). Titanium dioxide and zinc oxide are the most common physical blockers (3,102,103). Combination sunscreens, which admix UVA and UVB chemical agents with a physical agent, offer the most complete protection (3,102,104). Combination sunscreens are especially valuable for individuals with fair skin (skin types I and II), a history of photosensitivity diseases, or for patients taking potentially photosensitizing medications (102,103).

Sunscreens are rated according to their sun protection factor (SPF), which indicates the ratio of UVB needed to produce a minimal erythema reaction in sunscreen-protected skin compared with unprotected skin (3,103). In use, an SPF of 6 will protect a person six times longer than if unprotected skin was exposed to the same amount of UVB radiation. Sunscreens with an SPF of 15 or greater are considered to be sunblocks, since more than 92% of the UVB is absorbed (103). Unfortunately, the SPF achieved in practice may be significantly less than that established through testing (103). This is usually due to a combination of factors including environmental conditions and the amount of sunscreen applied to the skin (3,103). If an insufficient amount is used, the SPF may be reduced by as much as half (108). Additionally, the SPF deteriorates over time and therefore the protective effects of the sunscreen will diminish if not reapplied frequently (103). Unfortunately, there exists no standard test to determine the photoprotective qualities of UVA sunscreens.

Another measure of the effectiveness of a sunscreen is substantivity, which is defined as the resistance of the product to being washed off or removed by perspiring (102,103). In order for a product to be called water resistant it must retain its SPF after 40 minutes of immersion in water (102,103). A waterproof sunscreen must retain its substantivity after 80 minutes of water exposure (102,103).

Sunscreens can cause adverse reactions in certain individuals. Chemical agents may induce irritant or allergic contact dermatitides as well as phototoxic or photoallergic reactions (3,102,109–117). In the past, PABA was a common sensitizer (103,118). However, the newer PABA esters have a lower sensitization potential (3,103,119). Benzophenones, cinnamates, and methoxydibenzoylmethane as well as added fragrances and preservatives may produce an allergic contact dermatitis (3,109,110,114,120–123). Salicylates and anthranilates are rare sensitizers and physical sunscreen agents are not sensitizers (3,102,115,124,125). If a reaction develops to a physical blocker, the most likely etiologic agent is a fragrance or preservative (3,102).

The American Academy of Dermatology Consensus Statement on Photoaging/Photodamage as a Public Health Concern recommends the use of a sunscreen with an SPF of 15 or higher (102,126). Combination sunscreens offer the most complete protection and are the most effective if used on a daily basis (102,103). This is particularly true since about two-thirds of an individual's lifetime sun exposure occurs on an incidental basis (103). In order to obtain the maximal effectiveness, sunscreens should be applied liberally and reapplied frequently (103).

REFERENCES

1. Spencer TS. Dry skin and skin moisturizers. Clin Dermatol 1988;6:24–28.

2. Baran R, Maibach HI, eds. Cosmetic dermatology. Baltimore: Williams & Wilkins, 1994.

3. Draelos ZD, ed. Cosmetics in dermatology. 2nd ed. New York: Churchill Livingstone, 1995.

4. Boisits EK. The evaluation of moisturizing products. Cosmet Toilet 1986;101:31–39.

5. Reiger MM. Skin, water and moisturization. Cosmet Toilet 1989;104:41–51.

6. Elias PM. Lipids and the epidermal permeability barrier. Arch Dermatol Res 1981;270:95–117.

7. Holleran WM, Man MQ, Wen NG, et al. Sphingolipids are required for mammalian epidermal barrier function. J Clin Invest 1991;88:1338–1345.

8. Downing DT. Lipids: their role in epidermal structure and function. Cosmet Toilet 1991;106:63–69.

9. Petersen RD. Ceramides key components for skin protection. Cosmet Toilet 1992;107:63.

10. Elias PM. Epidermal lipids, barrier function, and desquamation. J Invest Dermatol 1983; 80(suppl):44–49.

11. Nickoloff BJ, Naidu Y. Perturbation of epidermal barrier function correlates with initiation of cytokine cascade in human skin. J Am Acad Dermatol 1994;30: 535–554.

12. Osborne DW, Friberg SE. Role of stratum corneum lipids and moisture retaining agents. J Dispersion Sci Tech 1987;8:173–179.

13. Middleton JD. Mechanism of action of surfactants on water binding properties of isolated stratum corneum. J Soc Cosmet Chem 1969;20:399–412.

14. Elias PM, Bonar L, Grayson S, et al. X-ray diffraction analysis of stratum corneum membrane couplets. J Invest Dermatol 1983; 80:213–214.

15. Jass HE, Elias PM. The living stratum corneum: implications for cosmetic formulation. Cosmet Toilet 1991;106:47–53.

16. Holleran W, Feingold K, Man MO, et al. Regulation of epidermal sphingolipid synthesis by permeability barrier function. J Lipid Res 1991;32:1151–1158.

17. Frost P, Horwitz SN, eds. Principles of cosmetics for the dermatologist. St. Louis: CV Mosby, 1982.

18. Jackson EM. Moisturizers: what's in them? how do they work? Am J Contact Dermatitis 1992;3: 162–168.

19. Van Scott EJ, Ditre CM, Yu RJ. Alpha-hydoxyacids in the treatment of signs of photoaging. Clin Dermatol 1996;14:217–226.

20. Clark CP. Alpha hydroxy acids in skin care. Clin Plast Surg 1996; 23:49–56.

21. Van Scott EJ, Yu RJ. Hyperkeratinization, corneocyte cohesion, and alpha hydroxy acids. J Am Acad Dermatol 1984;11: 867–879.

22. Ditre CM, Griffin TD, Murphy GF, et al. Effects of α-hydroxy acids on photoaged skin: a pilot clinical, histologic, and ultrastructural study. J Am Acad Dermatol 1996;34:187–195.

23. Bernstein EF, Uitto J. Connective tissue alterations in photoaged skin and the effects of alpha hydroxy acids. J Geriatr Dermatol 1995;3(suppl):7A–18A.

24. Van Scott EJ, Yu RJ. Actions of alpha hydroxy acids on skin compartments. J Geriatr Dermatol 1995;3(suppl):19A–25A.

25. Lavker RM, Kaidbey K, Leyden JJ. Effects of topical ammonium lactate on cutaneous atrophy from a potent topical corticosteroid. J Am Acad Dermatol 1992;26:535–544.

26. Van Scott EJ, Yu RJ. Alpha hydroxy acids: therapeutic potentials. Can J Dermatol 1989;1: 108.

27. Van Scott EJ, Yu RJ. Alpha hydroxy acids: procedures for use in clinical practice. Cutis 1989; 43:222–228.

28. Ridge JM, Siegle RJ, Zuckerman J. Use of α-hydroxy acids in the therapy for photoaged skin. J Am Acad Dermatol 1990;23:932.

29. Idson B. Dry skin: moisturizing and emolliency. Cosmet Toilet 1992;107:69–77.

30. Williams DF, Schmitt WH, eds. Chemistry and technology of the cosmetics and toiletries industry. London: CV Mosby, 1992.

31. Oestreicher MI. Detergents, bath preparations, and other skin cleansers. Clin Dermatol 1988; 6:29–36.

32. Wortzman MS. Evaluation of mild skin cleansers. Dermatol Clin 1991;9:35–44.

33. Strube DD, Nicoll G. The irritancy of soaps and syndets. Cutis 1987;39:544–545.

34. Malten K. Thoughts on irritant contact dermatitis. Contact Dermatitis 1981;7:238–247.

35. White M, Jenkinson DM, Lloyd D. The effect of washing on the thickness of the stratum corneum in normal and atopic individuals. Br J Dermatol 1987;116:525–530.

36. Schmid MH, Korting HC. The concept of the acid mantle of the skin: its relevance for the choice of skin cleansers. Dermatology 1995;191:276–280.

37. Zlotogorski A. Distribution of skin surface pH on the forehead and cheek of adults. Arch Dermatol Res 1987;279:398–401.

38. Korting HC, Kober M, Muller M, et al. Influence of repeated washings with soap and synthetic detergents on pH and resident flora of the skin of forehead and forearm. Acta Derm Venereol (Stockh) 1987;67:41–47.

39. Jellinek JS. Formulation and function of cosmetics. New York: Wiley Interscience, 1970.

40. Prottey C, Ferguson T. Factors which determine the skin irritation potential of soap and detergents. J Soc Cosmet Chem 1975;26:29–46.

41. Wickett RR, Trobaugh CM. Personal care products. Cosmet Toilet 1990;105:41–46.

42. Korting HC, Ponce-Poschl E, Klovekorn W, et al. The influence of the regular use of a soap or an acidic syndet bar on pre-acne. Infection 1995;23:89–94.

43. Jordan WP. Contact dermatitis from D & C yellow 11 dye in a toilet bar soap. J Am Acad Dermatol 1981;4:613–614.

44. Fisher AA, ed. Contact dermatitis. Philadelphia: Lea & Febiger, 1986.

45. Wortzman MS, Scott RA, Wongg PS, et al. Soap and detergent bar rinsability. J Soc Cosmet Chem 1986;37:89–97.

46. Young D. Proper cleansing for the face. Cutis 1987;39:543.

47. American Cancer Society. Are tanning centers safe? Cancer News 1981;Spring/Summer:19.

48. Spencer JM, Amonette RA. Indoor tanning: risks, benefits, and future trends. J Am Acad Dermatol 1995;33:288–298.

49. Rivers JK, Norris PG, Murphy GM, et al. UVA sunbeds: tanning photoprotection, acute adverse effects and immunological changes. Br J Dermatol 1989;120:767–777.

50. Diffey BL. Use of UVA sunbeds for cosmetic tanning. Br J Dermatol 1986;115:67–76.

51. Parrish JA, Jaenicke KF. Erythema and melanogenesis action spectra in normal human skin. Photochem Photobiol 1982;36:187–190.

52. Kaidbey KH, Kligman AM. Acute effects of long wave ultraviolet irradiation on human skin. J Invest Dermatol 1979;72:253–256.

53. Parrish JA, Anderson RR, Ying CY, et al. Cutaneous effects of pulsed nitrogen gas laser irradiation. J Invest Dermatol 1976;67:603–608.

54. Hawk JLM, Black AK, Jaenicke KF, et al. Increased concentrations of arachidonic acid, prostaglandins E2, D2, and 6-oxo-fla, and histamine in human skin following UVA irradiation. J Invest Dermatol 1983;80:496–498.

55. Centers for Disease Control. Injuries associated with ultraviolet tanning devices—Wisconsin. JAMA 1989;261:3519–3520.

56. Bickers DR, Epstein JH, Fitzpatrick TB, et al. Risks and benefits from high-intensity ultraviolet A sources used for cosmetic purposes. J Am Acad Dermatol 1985;12:380–381.

57. Council on Scientific Affairs. Harmful effects of ultraviolet radiation. JAMA 1989;262:380–384.

58. Ljunggren B. Severe phototoxic burn following celery ingestion.

Arch Dermatol 1990;126:1334–1336.

59. Clore ER. Natural and artificial tanning. J Pediatr Health Care 1995;9:103–108.

60. Cohen JB, Bergstresser PR. Inadvertent phototoxicity from home tanning equipment. Arch Dermatol 1994;130:804–806.

61. Lichtenstein J, Sherertz EF. Harmful effects of indoor tanning. Am Family Practice 1985;32:142–146.

62. Stern RS, Docken W. An exacerbation of SLE after visiting a tanning salon. JAMA 1986;255:3120.

63. Farr PM, Marks JM, Diffey BL, et al. Skin fragility and blistering due to use of sunbeds. Br Med J 1988;296:1708–1709.

64. Murphy GM, Wright J, Nicholls DSH, et al. Sunbed-induced pseudoporphyria. Br J Dermatol 1989;120:555–562.

65. Snider RL, Lang PG, Maize JC. The clinical spectrum of mid-dermal elastolysis and the role of UV light in its pathogenesis. J Am Acad Dermatol 1993;28:938–942.

66. US Food and Drug Administration. The darker side of tanning: skin cancer, eye damage, skin aging, allergic reactions. Rockville, Md: US Public Health Service, 1987. HHS publication no. (FDA) 87-8270.

67. Fairchild AL, Gemson DH. Safety information provided to customers of New York City suntanning salons. Am J Prev Med 1992;8:381–383.

68. Fleischer AB, Lee WJ, Adams DP, et al. Tanning facility compliance with state and federal regulations in North Carolina: a poor performance. J Am Acad Dermatol 1993;28:212–217.

69. Bruyneel-Rapp F, Dorsey SB, Guin JD. The tanning salon: an area survey of equipment, procedures, and practices. J Am Acad Dermatol 1988;18:1030–1038.

70. Lillquist PP, Baptiste MS,

Witzigmann BS, et al. A population-based survey of sun lamp and tanning parlor use in New York State, 1990, J Am Acad Dermatol 1994;31:510–512.

71. Guercio-Hauer C, MacFarlane DF, DeLeo VA. Photodamage, photoaging, and photoprotection of the skin. Am Family Physician 1994;50:327–332.

72. Kligman LH, Akin FJ, Kligman AM. The contributions of UVA and UVB to connective tissue damage in hairless mice. J Invest Dermatol 1985;84:272–276.

73. Strickland PT. Photocarcinogenesis by near ultraviolet (UVA) radiation in Sencar mice. J Invest Dermatol 1986;87:272–275.

74. Sterenborg HJCM, van der Leun JC. Tumorigenesis by a long wavelength UVA source. Photochem Photobiol 1990;51:325–330.

75. Forbes PD, Davies RE, Urbach F. Experimental ultraviolet photocarcinogenesis: wavelength interactions and time-dose relationships. Natl Cancer Inst Monogr 1978;50:31–38.

76. Weinstock MA. Overview of ultraviolet radiation and cancer: what is the link? how are we doing? Environ Health Perspect 1995;103(suppl):251–254.

77. Dinehart SM, Dodge R, Stanley WE, et al. Basal cell carcinoma treated with mohs surgery. J Dermatol Surg Oncol 1992;18:560–566.

78. Roth DE, Hodge SJ, Callen JP. Possible ultraviolet A-induced lentigines: a side effect of chronic tanning salon usage. J Am Acad Dermatol 1989;20:950–954.

79. Jones SK, Moseley H, MacKie RM. UVA induced melanocytic lesions. Br J Dermatol 1987;117:111–115.

80. Retsas S. Sun beds and melanoma. Br Med J 1983;286:892.

81. Brodthagen H. Malignant melanoma caused by a UVA suntan bed? Acta Derm Venereol (Stockh) 1982;62:356–357.

82. Westerdahl J, Olsson H, Masback A, et al. Use of sunbeds or sunlamps and malignant melanoma in southern Sweden. Am J Epidemiol 1994;140:691–699.

83. Walter SD, Marrett LD, From L, et al. The association of cutaneous malignant melanoma with the use of sunbeds and sunlamps. Am J Epidemiol 1990;131:232–243.

84. Freeman SE, Gange RW, Sutherland JC, et al. Production of pyrimidine dimers in human skin exposed in situ to UVA irradiation. J Invest Dermatol 1987;88:430–433.

85. Peak MJ, Peak JG, Jones CA. Different (direct and indirect) mechanisms for the induction of DNA-protein crosslinks in human cells by far and near ultraviolet radiations (290 and 405 nm). Photochem Photobiol 1985;42:141–146.

86. Peak MJ, Peak JG, Carnes BA. Induction of direct and indirect single strand breaks in human cell DNA by far and near ultraviolet radiations: action spectrum and mechanisms. Photochem Photobiol 1987;45:381–387.

87. Willis I, Menter JM, Whyte HJ. The rapid induction of cancers in the hairless mouse utilizing the principle of photoaugmentation. J Invest Dermatol 1981;76:404–408.

88. Fisher MS, Kripke ML. Suppressor T lymphocytes control the development of primary skin cancers in ultraviolet irradiated mice. Science 1982;216:1133–1134.

89. Granstein RD. Photoimmunology. Semin Dermatol 1990;9:16–24.

90. Hersey P, MacDonald M, Henderson C, et al. Suppression of natural killer cell activity in humans by radiation from solarium lamps depleted of UVB. J Invest Dermatol 1988;90:305–310.

91. Black G, Matzinger E, Gange RW. Lack of photoprotection against UVB induced erythema by immediate pigmentation induced by 382 nm radiation. J Invest Dermatol 1985;85:448–449.

92. Diffey BL, Farr PM, Ferguson J, et al. Tanning with ultraviolet A sunbeds. BMJ 1990;301:773–774.

93. Levy SB. Dihydroxyacetone-containing sunless or self-tanning lotions. J Am Acad Dermatol 1992;27:989–993.

94. Jackson EM. Tanning without sun: accelerators, promoters, pills, bronzing gels, and self-tanning lotions. Am J Contact Dermatitis 1994;5:38–40.

95. Morren M, Dooms-Goossens A, Heidbuchel M, et al. Contact allergy to dihydroxyacetone. Contact Dermatitis 1991;25:326–327.

96. Jaworsky C, Ratz JL, Dijkstra JWE. Efficacy of tan accelerators. J Am Acad Dermatol 1987;16:769–771.

97. Cartwright LE, Walter JF. Psoralen-containing sunscreen is tumorigenic in hairless mice. J Am Acad Dermatol 1983;8:830–836.

98. Lober CW. Canthaxanthin—the "tanning" pill. J Am Acad Dermatol 1985;13:660.

99. Rousseau A. Canthaxanthin deposits in the eye. J Am Acad Dermatol 1983;8:123–124.

100. Barker FO. Canthaxanthin retinopathy. J Toxicol Cutaneous Ocular Toxicol 1988;7:223–236.

101. Bluhm R, Branch R, Johnston P, et al. Aplastic anemia associated with canthaxanthin ingested for "tanning" purposes. JAMA 1990;264:1141–1142.

102. Gonzalez E, Gonzalez S. Drug photosensitivity, idiopathic photodermatoses, and sunscreens. J Am Acad Dermatol 1996;35:871–885.

103. Sterling GB. Sunscreens: a review. Cutis 1992;50:221–224.

104. Roelandts R. Which components in broad-spectrum sunscreens are most necessary for adequate UVA protection? J Am Acad Dermatol 1991;25:999–1004.

105. Lowe NJ. Photoprotection. Semin Dermatol 1990;9:78–83.

106. Menter JM. Recent developments in UVA photoprotection. Int J Dermatol 1990;29:389–401.

107. Sayre RM, Kollias N, Roberts RL, et al. Physical sunscreens. J Soc Cosmet Chem 1990;41:103–109.

108. Lowe NJ, ed. Physician's guide to sunscreens. New York: Marcel Dekker, 1991.

109. Lowe NJ, Shaath NA, eds. Sunscreens: development, evaluation, and regulatory aspects. Cosmetic science and technology series, vol 10. New York: Marcel Dekker, 1990.

110. Foley F, Nickson R, Marks R, et al. The frequency of reactions to sunscreens: results of a longitudinal population-based study on the regular use of sunscreens in Australia. Br J Dermatol 1993; 128:512–518.

111. Pathak MA. Sunscreens: topical and systemic protection against solar radiation for human skin. Photochem Photophys 1987; 4(suppl):447–461.

112. Collins P, Ferguson J. Photoallergic contact dermatitis to oxybenzone. Br J Dermatol 1994;131: 124–129.

113. Szczurko C, Dompmartin A, Michel M, et al. Photocontact allergy to oxybenzone: ten years of experience. Photodermatol Photoimmunol Photomed 1994; 10:144–147.

114. DeLeo VA, Suarez SM, Maso MJ. Photoallergic contact dermatitis. Arch Dermatol 1992;128: 1513–1518.

115. Rietschel RL, Lewis CW. Contact dermatitis to homomenthyl salicylate. Arch Dermatol 1978;114: 442–443.

116. DeGroot AC, Weyland JW. Contact allergy to butyl methoxydibenzoylmethane. Contact Dermatitis 1987;16:278.

117. Motley RJ, Reynolds AJ. Photocontact dermatitis due to isopropyl and butyl methoxydibenzoylmethanes (Eusolex 8020 and Parsol 1789). Contact Dermatitis 1989;21: 109–110.

118. Mathias CGT, Maibach HI, Epstein J. Allergic contact photodermatitis to para-aminobenzoic acid. Arch Dermatol 1978; 114:1665–1666.

119. Fisher AA. Sunscreen dermatitis: para-aminobenzoic acid and its derivatives. Cutis 1992;50: 190–192.

120. Ramsay CA. Ultraviolet A protective sunscreens. Clin Dermatol 1989;7:163–166.

121. Thune P. Contact and photocontact allergy to sunscreens. Photodermatol 1984;1:5–9.

122. Knobler E, Almeida L, Ruzkowski AM, et al. Photoallergy to benzophenone. Arch Dermatol 1989; 125:801–804.

123. Ramsay DL, Cohen HJ, Baer RL. Allergic reaction to benzophenone. Arch Dermatol 1972;105:906–908.

124. Fisher AA. Sunscreen dermatitis: part IV—the salicylates, the anthranilates, and physical agents. Cutis 1992;50:397–398.

125. Menz J, Muller SA, Connolly SM. Photopatch testing: a six-year experience. J Am Acad Dermatol 1988;18:1044–1047.

126. American Academy of Dermatology. Consensus Conference on Photoaging/Photodamage as a Public Health Concern. Boston, 1988.

Part XXI.

PUBLIC POLICY

Edited by
Marjorie Speers

Introduction to Public Policy

James M. Rippe

Lifestyle issues in medicine increasingly involve public policy priorities and decisions. In this final section of the book, public policy approaches are examined in relation to the twin epidemics that plague modern America: inactivity and obesity. In the opening chapter, Dr. King provides a comprehensive approach to environmental and public policy approaches related to the promotion of physical activity. Dr. King includes not only an excellent historical perspective but also numerous analyses of outcomes and provides a road map for future public policy initiatives in physical activity.

The chapter by Howze, "Promoting Strategical Alliances to Increase Physical Activity," provides a practical strategy for how strategic alliances can assist in the national priority to increase physical activity across all population groups and all ages in modern America. The final chapter, by Rippe et al, explores public policy issues related to the modern obesity epidemic in the United States. In the decade between 1980 and 1990, the prevalence of obesity in the United States rose 40%. Clearly, if this epidemic is to be fought effectively, the actions not only of individual health care practitioners but also major efforts on the part of employers, healthcare systems, state, and the federal government will be required.

Chapter 114

Environmental and Policy Approaches to the Promotion of Physical Activity

Abby C. King

Over four decades' worth of epidemiologic, clinical, and laboratory research provide compelling evidence for the importance of physical activity to the health, functioning, and well-being of the American people (1). Regular physical activity can help to prevent and control a variety of chronic diseases and conditions, including cardiovascular disease, hypertension, non–insulin-dependent diabetes mellitus, obesity, and osteoporosis, that constitute the major threats to our nation's health (2,3). It also has been linked with lowered rates of at least some cancers (4). Further, physical activity is associated with greater longevity (5), and can help to promote enhanced functional independence, mental well-being, and improved quality of life for persons throughout the life span (6).

Despite the clear importance of regular physical activity to ongoing health and functioning, we remain a nation that is largely inactive. It has been estimated that only approximately 22% of American adults engage in regular, sustained physical activity during leisure time (defined as any type or intensity of activity occuring five times or more per week and 30 minutes or more per occasion) (1). Notably, 25% of U.S. adults do not engage in any leisure-time physical activity (1). Demographically, physical inactivity levels tend to be higher among women, minority populations, elderly persons, and those with less income or formal education (1).

The amount of underactivity among our nation's youth is equally alarming, with approximately 25% of children aged 6 through 17 years reporting no vigorous activity and another 25% reporting irregular levels of vigorous physical activity (1). Participation in all types of physical activity declines substantially with increases in age and grade in school (1). Levels of underactivity in youth likely play a major role in the increas-

ing prevalence rates of childhood and young adult obesity currently observed in this country (6).

The epidemic of underactivity observed in the U.S. and other industrialized nations is of relatively recent origin (i.e., one or two generations). It has been marked by dramatic declines over time in the amount of physical activity associated with work, home maintenance, and transportation. Much of this decrease can be attributed to technologic developments that have led to widespread availability of labor-saving devices throughout virtually all levels of society. These include motorized transportation (particularly the automobile), power machinery (which has eliminated the need for physical activity in virtually all jobs), and a host of devices at home, ranging from power lawn mowers to washing machines, electric garage door openers, and electric can openers. Such advances have greatly reduced the energy requirements of home maintenance. Some relatively new technologic developments, such as television, radio, recorded music devices, and interactive video games, may also have created a powerful inducement to spending leisure time in passive observation of events rather than active participation in them (7). A current trend toward a service-based, as opposed to a manufacturing-based, economy and a trend from an industrial toward an informational revolution may exacerbate inactivity rates even further.

In addition, despite the highly visible "fitness boom" occurring in the 1970s and 1980s, little actual progress has been observed during that time with respect to leisure-time physical activity participation rates. For instance, although intentional leisure-time physical activity has increased somewhat over the past several decades, this has occurred at a much lower rate than would be necessary to make up for the loss of more traditional sources of energy expenditure.

Related to this, recent indicators suggest that only 4 of the 11 physical activity objectives for the year 1990 contained in *Promoting Health, Preventing Disease: Objectives for the Nation* were accomplished (8). Given this failure to make progress in a number of the targeted areas related to physical activity participation, it is perhaps not surprising that physical activity is listed as the first of the 22 priority areas noted in *Healthy People 2000* (8). However, given current patterns of physical inactivity, the year 2000 goal of no more than 15% of the U.S. population aged 6 and older being completely sedentary will likely not be met until approximately 2024.

POPULATION-ATTRIBUTABLE MORTALITY AND ECONOMIC BURDEN CREATED BY A SEDENTARY LIFESTYLE

The substantial prevalence of physical inactivity across the American population has serious implications with respect to rates of cardiovascular disease morbidity and mortality as well as morbidity and mortality rates stemming from other chronic diseases and conditions. For example, as a consequence of the large prevalence of sedentariness and lack of fitness in their study population, Blair et al (9) found the population-attributable risks for both the unfit women and men in their longitudinal study to be comparable to or greater than that for the other major cardiovascular disease risk factors, including cigarette smoking, hypertension, and serum cholesterol level. Similarly, Paffenbarger et al have reported population-attributable risk data for inactivity in their studies of male Harvard alumni that were similar to the risks calculated for other cardiovascular risk factors (5).

From an economic perspective, the premature death and disability attributable to a sedentary lifestyle exact a tremendous toll with respect to health care expenditures. For example, it has been estimated that over $200 per worker-year of medical and related costs could be saved if persons participated regularly (i.e., weekly) in a recommended physical activity program, with the total fiscal benefit to a company from an employee fitness program estimated at $513 per worker-year (10).

Age-related decreases in physical activity likely exact a particularly large cost in light of the fact that a substantial proportion of chronic illness and disability strikes the older population (11). For instance, in 1987 persons with activity limitations or impaired functioning from chronic conditions represented 17% of the general population, but accounted for 47% of medical expenditures (12,13). It has been reported recently that 88% of elderly adults have at least one chronic condition; approximately 50% of middle-aged adults and 69% of elderly adults have more than one condition to manage (13).

In light of these statistics, efforts to prevent dependence and prolong the active life expectancy of elderly adults, ideally up to the time of death, have been increasingly espoused (14,15). Undertaking preventive efforts such as increased physical activity, even later in life, is likely to improve the quality of life of elderly adults while simultaneously increasing autonomy and reducing health care costs up to the terminal year (11,16).

WHY THE NEED FOR ENVIRONMENTAL AND POLICY-LEVEL INTERVENTIONS?

As the scope of the physical inactivity epidemic has become both increasingly pronounced and more explicitly recognized, an increased amount of energy has been spent in the dissemination of information to the general public concerning the desirability of increasing their levels of physical activity participation and fitness. As a result, public recognition of the issue is at a high level, and the majority of the population currently report a desire to increase their levels of activity. To date, however, such educational efforts have been ineffective in reversing the population trends of inactivity. The purpose of this chapter is to discuss the types of environmental and policy level intervention approaches that likely will be required, in combination with educational and other interpersonal level strategies, if we are to have a significant impact on the nation's physical activity levels. The chapter is divided into two general sections: 1) a brief discussion of some general issues that need to be considered in formulating environmental and policy-level intervention approaches; and 2) a description of the types of interventions at this level that have been or should be considered, in conjunction with some discussion of the population segments, modes of physical activity, and settings most likely to be suited to each strategy.

GENERAL ISSUES IN FORMULATING ENVIRONMENTAL AND POLICY-LEVEL INTERVENTIONS

Defining the Nature of the Physical Activity–Related Outcomes Being Sought

It is becoming increasingly clear that different types and amounts of physical activity may be necessary or optimal for obtaining different health benefits. For instance, while increases in overall levels of energy expenditure attained through daily increases in mild- to moderate-intensity activities may be sufficient for reducing risks of coronary heart disease or helping to control weight, regular participation in higher intensity physical activity may be necessary to obtain significant improvements in cardiorespiratory fitness or conditioning (1). Given this, clear determinations of the specific health-related goals to be achieved need to be decided upon before the development or initiation of specific interventions on any level of analysis (i.e., personal, organizational, environmental, societal).

In light of the large number of sedentary persons in the U.S. and the fact that energy expenditure levels appear to be an important determinant of risk for several of the more prevalent chronic diseases and conditions (1,3), a focus on moderate increases in energy expenditure throughout the week have in recent years been increasingly emphasized as a primary public health goal (6). The most recent U.S. Centers for Disease Control and Prevention (CDC) and American College of Sports Medicine (ACSM) recommendations state the goal of physical activity increases accumulating to at least 30 minutes or more of moderate-intensity activities such as walking, bicycling, or swimming on most days of the week, as well as increases in routine or lifestyle physical activities, such as stair climbing, that are more readily available and likely to be more easily undertaken by a large segment of the population throughout the week (17). The latter types of activities may be particularly amenable to environmental and policy-level intervention strategies.

Specifying the Intervention Goals or Objectives to Be Realized

Interventions of any type, whether implemented on a policy level or on a more personal level, typically are effective in meeting a specific type of behavioral goal and less effective for achieving other objectives. For example, interventions involving primarily mass media have been shown to be particularly effective in increasing awareness and in promoting other types of intervention programs but may be less effective in achieving actual changes in complex health behaviors such as physical activity, at least in some population segments (18,19). Other types of environmental or policy interventions may have similar limitations or special uses in terms of achieving awareness, increased knowledge or information dissemination, skill building or actual behavior change, or behavioral support and maintenance functions. This should be taken into account when interventions are being formulated for targeted subgroups. For instance, for the completely sedentary population subgroup who may not have begun even to contemplate or consider actions, no matter how small, for increasing daily activity levels, different objectives (e.g., awareness, knowledge) will likely require intervention first, before other objectives (e.g., intentional increases in physical activity) can be successfully targeted (20). Thus, environmental and policy intervention strategies should be matched to the behavioral needs of the population groups being targeted.

Developing Strategies for All Physical Activity Functions or Dimensions

Physical activity can be generally divided into activities required to accomplish work; those occurring to facilitate home life; those involved for transportation purposes; and those occurring during leisure time for sport or recreation. A large proportion of the effort that has gone into increasing physical activity levels in many communities has been focused primarily on programmed physical activity regimens that occur during leisure time. Leisure programming may be particularly useful for those who, by choice or force of circumstance, have increased free time (10). However, much of the U.S. population spends considerable amounts of time at work, in transportation activities, or in doing tasks in or around the home. These arenas present both challenges and opportunities with respect to physical activity intervention, and may be particularly appropriate for environmental and policy interventions. An increased focus on routine or task-oriented types of physical activity (e.g., taking stairs, walking) is especially germane in light of the shrinking amount of disposable income faced by much of the American public; diminished levels of disposable income have been linked in turn with reduced recreational spending in at least some population groups (10).

With respect to work, it seems unlikely that anyone would want to reverse the trends in mechanization of production in the workplace. However, many employers are increas-ingly interested in enhancing the fitness of their employees to improve efficiency and morale and to reduce health care expenses (10). As will be discussed in a later section, public policy intervention may be well-suited for increasing physical activity levels at the workplace, independent of the sedentary nature of most jobs. Policies and environmental initiatives to increase energy expenditure levels related to transportation and home activities in addition to leisure-time activities are also potentially important targets for intervention.

Applying Behavioral Science Principles to Facilitate the Success of Public Policy Interventions

An increasingly large body of evidence is being collected that shows that physical activity is amenable to certain principles of behavior modification that also govern the initiation and maintenance of other health behaviors (21,22). Although the development and applications of these principles have occurred largely on personal and interpersonal levels, it is likely that at least some of these principles can and should be applied in developing larger-scale interventions to influence physical activity levels (23).

Incorporating principles for physical activity promotion at the policy level in countries such as Australia has resulted in recommendations for policy intervention that have included:

1. Increasing the *appropriateness* and *convenience* of settings for targeted population subgroups (e.g., increasing access to facilities and physical activity venues where people go to school, work, or live)

2. Providing information and interventions appropriate for subgroups at different *stages of motivational readiness for behavior change* (e.g., precontemplation through maintenance phases) and at different stages of *diffusion* (e.g., early adopters, late adopters)

3. Focusing on the *immediate* as well as longer term benefits and barriers to promote change

4. Developing *realistic* behavioral targets, goals, and messages that are specific and subsume a variety of avenues and channels to promote behavior, including multiple levels (i.e., personal, interpersonal, environmental, organizational, institutional, societal, legislative)

5. Developing strategies and interventions that offer *choices* rather than directives

6. Promoting policies that focus on activities that provide *intrinsic value*, such as fun, skill development, variety, competition, feedback on ability, or positive social interactions

7. Increasing the *knowledge and instructional abilities* of appropriate messengers (e.g., physical education instructors, fitness leaders, teachers, physicians and other health professionals, journalists and reporters) to optimize the success of interventions and promote long-term maintenance of behavior change (23)

Considering Both Passive and Active Prevention Approaches to Physical Activity

For a number of health behaviors, populationwide risk reduction has often been accomplished through the implementation of public health policies that invoke passive prevention approaches to behavior change, i.e., strategies that do not require overt action on the part of the individual to be successful. Examples of such passive prevention approaches include modifying the filtering systems and the content of cigarettes to reduce toxic exposures; reducing the sodium, saturated fat, or cholesterol content of prepared or prepackaged foods; and adding air bags and other passive restraint systems to vehicles.

In contrast to these health areas, the nature of physical activity behavior makes it generally less amenable to such passive prevention approaches, and little effort has been expended on developing such strategies to date. Nonetheless, passive prevention approaches should be explored in this area, since they have a greater likelihood of achieving population-wide changes than do strategies that require individual action to attain effects. An example of such an approach is the designation of downtown centers as pedestrian malls that are open only to foot or bicycle traffic. Further examples might concern the placement of parking lots a suitable distance from buildings so that walking is encouraged or necessitated; designing buildings in which using stairways is equally or more convenient than using elevators or escalators; and developing alternative modes of transportation that significantly enhance physical activity (24). Increasing the availability of low-cost recreational facilities and programs is yet another form of passive intervention that can increase physical activity by reducing its response cost and enhancing its reinforcement value. Finally, as illustrated by cities such as Reston, Virginia, communities can be planned whereby businesses are built adjacent to residential areas and connected by a network of bicycling, hiking, or walking paths and public transportation interchanges.

Enhancing the Commitment to Evaluation

An integral part of the development of public policy interventions rests with an adequate evaluation of both the cost-benefit and the cost-effectiveness of the interventions being proposed. This is true perhaps now more than ever, in light of the constraints imposed by the current economic climate. Only through a concerted effort to evaluate programs introduced by work sites, schools, communities, states, or federal agencies can accurate and thoughtful decisions be made concerning which strategies to expand and develop further.

To date, the development of simple, low-cost evaluation strategies appropriate for the different types of environmental and policy-level physical activity interventions available or being proposed has lagged behind the implementation of many of these interventions. Given the scope of today's economic demands in the health arena, policy interventions must move ahead only in conjunction with the proper surveillance or evaluation strategies (25).

TYPES OF ENVIRONMENTAL AND POLICY-LEVEL INTERVENTIONS

The goal of this section is to highlight currently ongoing or potentially available environmental and policy-level interventions in the physical activity area. It is thus summative rather

than exhaustive in focus and is meant to provide examples of current initiatives and programs, as well as to highlight gaps.

Community Coalition Development and Advocacy

One of the major challenges to developing, prioritizing, and enacting policy approaches for increasing populationwide levels of physical activity is the creation of an organizational structure that can serve as an effective base of strategy and action. A systematic approach to policy development ideally evolves from broad consensus, cooperation, and coordination among diverse interest groups. There are many existing organizations, public and private, whose interests are relevant to the physical activity issue. For instance, conservation groups favor the enlargement of natural areas that are an attractive setting for physical activity. Recreation groups, including fish and wildlife, biking, running, camping, scouts, and 4H clubs, as well as recreation and parks departments, all promote forms of physical activity. Health conscious constituencies, including public health agencies, private health providers, mental health agencies, health and life insurance companies, and employers have direct and indirect interest in a more fit population. Additionally, transportation agencies and energy conservation groups are relevant to physical activity in so far as policy ideas may interact with their domains of interest and activity.

The development of broad-based coalitions to tackle health issues at a local or regional level has been found to be an effective means for heightening initial awareness of a health concern and providing a level of involvement and support across diverse segments of a community that will make the successful implementation of subsequent programs or strategies more likely. Such coalition building has been utilized successfully with a variety of other health, environmental, and sociopolitical issues but, to date, has been less formally used in the physical activity arena. A particularly useful model for community coalitions may be found in the effort to reduce tobacco consumption in this country. In this sphere, coalitions involving health interests, child protection interests, commercial interests, and nonsmokers' rights groups have successfully promoted a variety of policies, such as limiting access of children to tobacco (e.g., outlawing vending machines and promoting tighter enforcement of age restrictions on tobacco purchases) and increasing excise taxes on tobacco. Although physical activity is a more broad-based concept for which consensus on desirable courses of action would no doubt be more difficult to reach, similar approaches are worth exploring. Examples of potentially important physical activity coalition members are schools (representing primary, secondary, and college levels); parks and recreation departments; local public health departments; community service clubs; organizations representing senior citizens; sports organizations; local chapters of nonprofit agencies whose focus includes health or physical activity; religious organizations, which may be particularly effective in reaching underserved populations who may be able to reap the most benefits from increases in physical activity; representatives of the medical and health communities, including physician, nursing, exercise, public health, and psychological associations; hospital auxiliaries; clinics; and civic and business leaders, including community chambers of commerce and owners of exercise clubs and facilities. The inclusion of merchants or organizations who represent ethnic or racial subgroups and issues pertaining specifically to women is important if the coalition is to be effective in reaching all community members and, in particular, those at greatest risk for underactivity. Insurance groups, particularly those involved with life insurance, have in the past expressed interest in physical activity as a means for diminishing illness and should also be included in coalition-building efforts.

Other potential community partners include media services, tourism bureaus, mall organizations, homeowners' associations, realtors, neighborhood groups, sports associations, and foundations. As part of the identification process related to the development of community partnerships, it may be especially useful to outline approaches for making the most effective use of each partner's specific areas of expertise.

In light of the fact that communities typically have a number of health issues vying for attention, many of which will likely be viewed as more pressing than physical activity, it may be prudent for physical activity issues to be addressed by a task force nested within a larger health coalition. An initial first step in many communities may be to use this task force to "raise consciousness" among other coalition members and the community at large concerning the importance of making physical activity a priority. Another strategy might be to "piggyback" a physical activity task force onto an already established community or regional health coalition, such as a tobacco control coalition, because of potential commonalities of interests and goals. Given that fears related to weight gain and other symptoms after smoking cessation can interfere with quit attempts or impede maintenance of abstinence (26), physical activity issues become a natural complement to issues surrounding smoking cessation.

Examples of community-wide efforts to create a coalition around physical activity at the local level are contained in the intervention efforts of the four comprehensive, community-based cardiovascular disease risk reduction projects undertaken over the past decade: the Stanford Five-City Project, the Minnesota Heart Health Project, the Pawtucket Heart Health Project, and the Pennsylvania-based Community Health Improvement Project (27). The objectives of these federally funded initiatives were to bring about and evaluate change in several communities with respect to cardiovascular disease risk factors, including physical activity. As part of the interventions developed to effect change in the physical activity area, coalitions were developed with key community organizations. For instance, formal links were established between the Pawtucket Heart Health Project and the Pawtucket Parks and Recreation Department, among other organizations, as a means for institutionalizing program delivery within the target community (27). These coalitions were effective in heightening community awareness of health issues and attracting human and financial resources to support intervention activities.

At the national level, a number of major national health agencies and organizations have recently come together to form the National Coalition for Promoting Physical Activity (NCPPA). The goals of the NCPPA include the promotion of activities and initiatives aimed at enhancing physical activity levels across the U.S. population.

Other Issues Related to Coalitions

Successful policy implementation through the use of coalitions requires choosing goals whose time has come. Short-term goals are most successful if they are logical outgrowths of existing ideas and procedures (e.g., protecting children from unnecessary exposure to tobacco smoke is a more ideologically relevant or prominent issue in our current cultural climate than is the prohibition of sales and distribution to adults). In addition to the presence of a strong supporting coalition, successful policy implementation also involves the good fortune not to have good ideas blocked by disinterested gatekeepers or powerful counterforces. In the case of physical activity, there are few strong opponents. However, conflicts and competition among supporting groups may present challenges that have to be overcome if substantial gains are to be made in this area.

It has also become increasingly clear that, in addition to differences among communities in the types of organizational resources available for community coalition-building, socioeconomically disadvantaged communities may face particular barriers—both with respect to the number of organizations available and the feasibility of being able to activate those organizational resources that are present (28). Such issues should be addressed as directly in the physical activity area as in other health promotion activities.

ORGANIZATIONAL POLICY

Policies can be defined as statements or rules, either explicit or implicit, that provide a structure for the governance of organizations (29). Organizational policies for physical activity can be pursued at a variety of different levels. These include in organizations (e.g., worksites), in local communities, and at state, regional, and national levels. As a rule, the larger the unit involved, the less amenable it is to change. At a local level, all that may be needed is the enthusiastic support of one or two influential people in the community. In larger jurisdictional units, the politics are more complex and the number of competing priorities proportionately larger. Some policy initiatives are specific to a particular level of jurisdiction (e.g., funding for state parks or taxation to support physical activity programs). When this is not the case, however, it may be wise to focus on making changes at a low organizational level. If these are successful, they may serve as models for future applications on a larger scale.

The following sections highlight some of the community settings for which organizational policy change in the physical activity area may be particularly germane.

Worksites

In light of the sizeable sector of the American public that regularly works outside of the home, the worksite presents an important setting for the development of policies to foster increases in physical activity, both during the work day and outside of work. In addition to reaching the employee, worksite policies and programs also have the potential for reaching other family members and retirees, who are an important physical activity target group.

Physical activity programming in larger worksite settings has typically taken the form of on-site physical activity facilities or in-house physical activity classes. Such programs have been shown to be effective in increasing the fitness levels of regular users, who in general tend to be primarily white-collar employees (10), but often do not reach other large segments of the workforce. Programming efforts that have specifically targeted blue-collar employees have indicated the importance of involving employees early in the development of appropriate and appealing programs; offering a variety of programming options from which to choose; making available the means for providing ongoing feedback on performance; and using facilities that are convenient to where employees work (e.g., adjacent to the work location so that they can be easily reached at lunch time or after work) (30).

The relative importance of ongoing interpersonal support and education compared with the establishment of on-site exercise facilities to increase physical activity access and convenience was recently evaluated in a study undertaken by Heirich et al (31). Automotive plants were randomly assigned to four different types of worksite wellness programs. All sites had baseline and 3-year screenings. Results indicated that, after 3 years, almost one-half of employees at sites that offered either counseling or counseling combined with work-site organizational approaches reported exercising at least three times per week, compared to only about one-third of employees at either the control site, which consisted of health education classes only, or the site which had established a staffed and readily accessible fitness facility (31). These results suggest that personal conseling was more effective at increasing regular physical activity than ready access to fitness facilities. The costs of the programs were not substantially different among sites (31).

Over the past 15 years, large corporations, such as Johnson & Johnson, Control Data Corporation, Prudential Insurance Company, and Kimberly-Clark, have attempted to broaden the scope of their physical activity programming through offering programs to all employees (29). Johnson & Johnson provided a public health model for physical activity promotion across their worksites, which included an annual health assessment; a highly visible health education campaign using newsletters, contests, health fairs, and informational displays in hallways, cafeterias, and restrooms; and a series of health promotion seminars and physical activity classes (32). The program also included supportive policies, such as information regarding top management and supervisory support of the program and the availability of compensatory physical activity time and breaks to facilitate physical activity.

Physical activity participation and health outcomes in employees from four companies receiving this program were compared with those from employees in three comparison companies who received the annual health assessment only. During the first 24-month period, the amount of vigorous activity engaged in more than doubled in the intervention companies, compared with only a 33% increase among employees at the comparison companies (33). The changes in physical activity patterns were corroborated using estimates of maximal oxygen uptake obtained from a submaximal bicycle ergometer test. An added strength of this study was the high participation rates obtained for all sectors of the worksite. The relatively rigorous evaluation of this large-scale, comprehensive worksite effort is noteworthy, given that many

worksite physical activity programs, similar to programs initiated in other settings, have been inadequately evaluated or not evaluated at all.

Although these and similar efforts represent a model for a comprehensive package of policies and programs to promote physical activity at the worksite, few smaller companies (e.g., less than 100 employees), which employ the majority of American workers, are likely to have the resources to undertake all of the initiatives included in such large-scale efforts (34). In particular, convenient access to appropriate physical activity facilities and changing and showering areas may pose logistic problems for smaller companies that may require resolution through the development of consortia among such companies or with larger companies to facilitate the sharing of physical activity resources. Indeed, it has been argued that simply providing employees with shower and changing facilities may be the most effective means for promoting increased physical activity at smaller worksites (35), although, as demonstrated in the Heirich et al study (31), this may not work for all types of employees.

Alternatively, policies that encourage or facilitate increased participation in forms of physical activity, such as walking and stair climbing (36), in which facilities are not necessary, may provide the most effective means for increasing energy expenditure across a large segment of the workforce irrespective of company size (24). Policies that may be achievable by the majority of worksites, regardless of size, include explicit support by management for physical activity increases; the implementation of physical activity or walking breaks and compensatory time for physical activity; point of choice information related to the use of stairs rather than elevators or escalators in public venues (37,38); a system for formally recognizing employees who attempt or achieve physical activity changes; and worksite commuting policies and initiatives that encourage increases in foot or bicycle traffic (39,40). Such policies and environmental interventions should be explored further, particularly with respect to methods for evaluating their ease of implementation and their effectiveness in leading to increases in activity levels or energy expenditure (24). Ensuring that appropriate links are established with human resource personnel who manage employee orientation, training, and benefits packages will likely facilitate both program development and implementation efforts in this area. In addition, methods for extending physical activity policies and programs to include persons with disabilities, family members, and retirees require further exploration, particularly in light of the potentially significant health care and insurance costs incurred by these three groups for which the employer is often responsible.

With the advent of an increasing number of managed health care systems in this country, and their attendant emphasis on primary care, prevention, and reduced health care utilization patterns, worksites, working with health insurance organizations, have an additional incentive as well as opportunity to enact policies to promote health-enhancing behaviors such as physical activity. Methods for promoting physical activity in this context require further exploration.

The federal government, as a major employer, has become increasingly involved in promoting physical activity through the implementation of worksite programs. While several agencies, such as the Departments of the Interior,

Justice, and Defense, have initiated such programs, a comprehensive set of policies for federal worksites has yet to be established. Such a set of policies could serve as a model for business and other employers (29). A recent example of a successfully enacted federal worksite physical activity program has been the Centers for Disease Control and Prevention (CDC) 1996 Director's Physical Activity Challenge (41). The challenge, which targeted the entire CDC workforce, included a number of behavioral (e.g., self-monitoring, feedback), environmental (e.g., prompts, public displays), and organizational strategies (e.g., a team concept). Sixty-five percent of CDC employees joined the 50-day challenge, and 80% of those who joined reached the physical activity goals (organized on a point system) that they had initially set for themselves (41). Variants of this program are currently being initiated at several sites across the country.

Other Community Settings

The worksite policies and interventions being described potentially could be implemented in a variety of other settings, such as community or senior centers, clinics and other health care settings, and places of worship. Examples of churches that have initiated policies and programs to promote physical activity are the Health and Religion Project (HARP) of Rhode Island (42) and the Fitness Through Churches program, funded by the American Heart Association and sponsored by the University of North Carolina at Chapel Hill. This latter program is a demonstration project promoting aerobic activity along with education on other health behaviors among black residents of North Carolina (43). The program includes the use of media to increase awareness and knowledge with respect to physical activity, as well as the implementation of a common training program for the congregation-based organizers and physical activity instructors coming from ten participating inner-city churches. Enactment of such interventions at schools or similar settings could have the additional benefit of serving as a model for children and other site attendees with respect to the importance of and appropriate modes of physical activity and should be explored further (44).

In addition to other community settings, indoor shopping malls have become increasingly popular venues in recent years for walking groups and clubs. Encouraging the development of organizational policies for these and other settings that further legitimize and facilitate the use of such buildings as safe and appropriate places for physical activity for a broad segment of the population is indicated. As noted earlier, the use of simple, inexpensive informational signage in shopping malls and train stations, posted where people have to make the decision concerning using the escalator or the stairs, has been shown to significantly increase stair use in studies undertaken in both the U.S. (37) and Scotland (38).

Schools

Schools, from elementary through college levels, continue to represent an excellent means for promoting physical activity among our nation's youth. However, the actual amount of weekly energy expenditure derived from such programs and whether the activities and skills being taught adequately prepare individuals for a lifetime of physically active pursuits

have been increasingly questioned. School curricula in the physical education area remain focused largely on drills and competitive sports, which often do not adequately instill in students an appreciation of physical activity as a lifelong program to be engaged in by all. This may partially explain why, at present, most physical activity programs engaged in by youth occur outside of school (1,45). In addition, appropriate physical activity programs for persons with physical or mental disabilities are lacking in many locales.

Rather than modifying or replacing the traditional physical education curricula available in the schools, public health efforts to increase physical activity in youth through the school setting have been focused largely on complementing the physical education curriculum by targeting skills that may be better transferred to adulthood. These approaches have frequently utilized contests and other hands-on activities (e.g., logging of physical activity behavior; involvement of parents in home assignments) to encourage both interest and increased participation. Examples include the San Diego Family Heart Health Project (46), the Galveston Family Health Project (47), the Stanford Tenth Grader Project (48), and the multiple risk factor Know Your Body program (49). Most have reported a reasonable amount of success in obtaining short-term changes in reported physical activity levels. However, efforts to develop training programs to institutionalize such interventions as part of the ongoing school curriculum remain in their infancy. An example of one innovative program to incorporate walking into the ongoing curriculum of elementary schools in South Carolina is the Discover and Understand Carolina, Kids (DUCK) walking program (50). Objectives of this program include the promotion of walking as an enjoyable form of physical activity beginning at an early age, and the inclusion of teachers, parents, and students in the program. As part of this program, at least 20 minutes during one school day each week is devoted to aerobic walking, which is logged by each class. Teachers, parents, and students may choose a level of activity that best suits their needs.

Several programs have attempted to modify the actual structure and content of the physical education class itself to increase children's physical activity levels during the school day. One such program was the Go for Health project conducted in Texas (51). At baseline, observations of elementary school students attending physical education classes revealed that children moved continuously for an average of only about 2 minutes per class period (52). The program objectives included increasing the amount of physical education class time spent in moderate to vigorous physical activity to at least 50% of available class time, and increasing students' knowledge, confidence, and skills related to undertaking physical activity both in and outside of school. At the 2-year post-test, the intervention schools demonstrated a significant increase in the percentage of physical education class time devoted to moderate and vigorous physical activity relative to the control schools (53).

A more extensive effort to modify physical education curricula was undertaken as part of the Child and Adolescent Trial for Cardiovascular Health (CATCH)—a multicenter, randomized trial targeting 96 schools in four states (54). The intervention schools received a new physical education curriculum along with staff training and follow-up during a 2½-

year period. At the end of this period, observed participation in moderate-intensity and vigorous physical activity during physical education classes increased significantly in the intervention schools relative to control schools (54).

Clearly, given the restricted resources and competing educational demands placed on schools at all levels, the implementation of physical education curricula that provide the types of regular physical activities and skill training needed to meet the current national objectives will likely require legislative intervention at the state or federal levels, as well as changes in the philosophy, training, and certification of our nation's physical educators (24). Fostering creative ways of incorporating physical activity as part of other educational activities (e.g., through active field trips and homework assignments that involve movement) may provide a further means of promoting physical activity among the nation's youth (24).

Similar to primary and secondary schools, community colleges represent both an educational channel and environment that could potentially do much to promote physical activity for all adults in a community. The types of physical education courses offered through such colleges can be quite varied, increasing their appeal to a range of population segments, including women and obese and elderly adults. In addition to offering the more typical physical education class format, it is conceivable that community colleges could offer telephone and mail correspondence courses in the physical activity area, as well as other health education areas, that could be attractive to many persons who might not otherwise enroll in courses that require frequent on-site attendance at a physical activity facility (55,56). Exploring methods for continuing to link communities in their efforts to provide such innovative programming (i.e., information exchange) is indicated. Additionally, a majority of universities and colleges provide on-campus physical activity and fitness programs or facilities for community use.

Neighborhoods and Homes

As a setting, the home or neighborhood has received less systematic attention with respect to the promotion of physical activity than other community settings, such as the workplace or community center. Yet, this is the location where many Americans prefer to undertake their physical activity (56). The growth of "neighborhood watch" groups as a means of increasing safety and reducing crime in inner cities and suburban areas alike may provide an avenue for promoting increases in physical activity (e.g., group walks through the neighborhood). Such neighborhood walking groups may provide a safe, socially supportive means of increasing physical activity levels. Recently, the targeting of urban public housing settings as a focus for physical activity promotion also has been undertaken, with some success (57).

"Adopt a Highway" activities, or similar types of activities that have emerged in some locales for parks or beaches, may produce increases in energy expenditure levels (i.e., through clean-up activities that require walking) as well as civic benefits and should be explicitly encouraged (24). With respect to local parks and other recreation areas, regular clean-up and maintenance by such groups could have the additional benefit of maintaining the attractiveness of the park at a level that would make it more appealing to residents. Although it has been noted that municipal parks are often

significantly underused in at least some areas (10), local recreation and park services are generally perceived by the majority of the American public as having substantial benefit for the individual, household, as well as the community (58).

As noted earlier, at-home conveniences such as the electric can opener and riding lawn mower diminish the types of routine physical activities that are important to the maintenance of physical function, particularly as persons age. It would be worthwhile exploring the implementation of awareness and educational campaigns that inform the public about the full complement of trade-offs accompanying such "conveniences," as well as exploring the effects of value-added taxes or other economic disincentives that would discourage overdependence on such devices. In addition, the exploration of incentive-based policies (e.g., tax-based rebates or allowances) that would encourage the purchase of devices that promote greater levels of energy expenditure or physical effort is worth pursuing.

In the spirit of current efforts to build homes that are energy-efficient with respect to the environment, it may also be useful to evaluate policy methods (e.g., tax rebates) for encouraging the construction and purchase of homes that are "energy-producing" in terms of physical energy expenditure. For example, a two-story home may have the exact square footage as a single-story, but obviously would require extra caloric expenditure for stair climbing, and thus could be assessed and discounted appropriately. Similar strategies could be applied to reducing time-saving and electronic gadgetry built into homes, not only saving energy but necessitating increased physical exertion.

ENVIRONMENTAL SUPPORT

The integral relationship between people's health and their physical and social environments has been understood in some form for years and recently has been reemphasized in the context of the chronic diseases that are currently plaguing Western societies (59). The environment plays a prominent role both in providing a safe and disease-free setting in which to live and in promoting the kinds of healthful activities, including physical activity, that are integral to long-term health and functioning.

Environmental support can take the form of facilities that house or promote physical activities and of mass media programs that increase awareness concerning physical activity, provide information to set the stage for increases in physical activity, or promote specific programs in the community. Social environment also plays a role in improving physical activity adherence and overall levels of physical activity. Given this, peer and spouse involvement should be considered in programming efforts at all levels of intervention.

Access to Facilities

Facilities to promote physical activity generally consist of those made available for participation in primarily leisure time (e.g., public swimming pools or ice rinks, municipal or county parks, public tracks or par courses, community centers or health clubs) and those that encourage or require increases in physical activity or more routine forms of physical activity (24). Although lack of access to appropriate facilities or equipment is often cited by people as a barrier to becoming more active (21), the current scientific data on this issue are mixed. For instance, one cross-sectional study (60) found a reasonably weak relationship (correlation coefficients ranged from 0.20 to 0.25) between the amount of exercise equipment found in the home and reported level of physical activity among a sample of 96 women employed at one of two universities. There were no significant correlations found between reported physical activity and exercise equipment for the total sample or for men. Similarly, while proximity to exercise facilities from the home or work site has been found to be associated with greater reported physical activity levels, the strength of the association has been reasonably modest (61).

The few available experimental studies aimed at *increasing access* to exercise facilities have also demonstrated weak results. In addition to the Heirich et al work site study described earlier (31), a study by French et al (62) evaluated the effects of offering free access to university work site exercise facilities on subsequent physical activity participation levels in a sample of sedentary women employees randomly assigned to receive either free access or not. Facility access included receiving free lockers and passes (a $45 value) to all university sports facilities, including an indoor track, weight room, swimming pools, and tennis, squash, and racquetball courts, which were open from 7:00 AM to 9:00 PM. During the 8-week intervention and 6-month follow-up periods, physical activity levels among the group given free access to exercise facilities did not differ from groups not given free facility access. After the first month, the people with free facility access rarely used the facilities at all. The authors concluded that perceived lack of access to exercise facilities may actually reflect a lack of motivation to adopt a regular physical activity program as opposed to an important determinant of exercise participation (62).

As the above results demonstrate, the parameters and conditions underlying the importance of access to differing population segments remain unclear. While in more affluent communities neighborhood parks and other recreational facilities may be plentiful, in large urban centers and less affluent communities this is often not the case. In addition, such locations require a level of ongoing maintenance and safety features (open, well-lit, and utilized at a level that diminishes criminal elements) that may not exist in some communities. These issues may need to be addressed through local ordinances or grassroots organizations (e.g., neighborhood groups) before such facilities become readily usable by those who could particularly benefit from them (e.g., elderly adults and families). Safe, affordable, and dependable transportation to such facilities must be available throughout the community. The development of such transportation services may represent an opportunity for the formation of public-private sector partnerships. Additional exploration of how educational and behavioral approaches can be combined with increased environmental facilities access to promote optimal use of facilities is required.

In relation to this issue, resources must continue to be put into providing safe areas and open spaces in neighborhoods where children can play. Among the factors that parents rate as most important in selecting appropriate play spaces for their preschool children are safety, availability of toilets, drinking water, lighting, and shade (63). Such factors require ongoing community attention. Other potential venues for facilitating discretionary activity include the addition of outdoor paths or par courses on the grounds of government-subsidized housing facilities or other institutional settings such as hospitals or schools. In many communities, the grounds surrounding such facilities are often spacious and underutilized.

The second form of community facility is comprised of those structures or elements in a community that facilitate increases in outdoor, often routine or nondiscretionary, forms of physical activity. Examples include pedestrian malls, walking and bicycle lanes and paths, and the ready availability of stairs in addition to the escalators or elevators that are typically more physically attractive and accessible in public buildings. Examples also could potentially include parking facilities for public buildings that encourage walking or use of stairs. The presence, attractiveness, and safety of these types of facilities vary greatly by community and by state. For instance, in contrast to some European countries that locate bicycle and walking paths or lanes a safe and comfortable distance from streets and thoroughfares, in the U.S., bicycle lanes are often located on the street, with potential negative consequences with respect to safety, comfort, and health (e.g., on busy roads, bicyclists are exposed to what are typically uncomfortable levels of automobile emissions).

An example of a community-wide effort to increase both forms of physical activity facilities and structures as a means of promoting increases in physical activity has been reported by Linenger et al (64), who compared environmental and social changes enacted at a naval air base community (n = 1609) with a similar community not receiving the intervention over a 1-year period. Specific environmental and organizational interventions that occurred in the experimental community were the building of bicycle paths along roadways, the extension of hours at local recreation facilities, purchasing of new physical actvity equipment at gyms, scheduling of a variety of basewide athletic events, the opening of a women's fitness center, the designation of 1.5-mile run course at various sites throughout the community, and the organization of running and bicycle clubs. In addition, higher level commanding officers participated in encouraging release time for physical activity, setting explicit expectations for improved fitness, and initiating rewards for improved physical performance.

Significant improvements in fitness levels were reported in the intervention community, and the improvement was distributed throughout the community, including persons with substandard fitness levels at baseline (64). The results suggest that a combination of physical and social environmental changes that could be readily applied in a variety of settings may have a useful impact on physical activity fitness levels.

Media

Media, both electronic and print, have the potential for reaching large segments of the population with a rapidity unmatched by other intervention modalities. In addition, mass media also have the benefit of being viewed as a credible source for receiving health information, which often results in a low cost per person reached, and is in general an effective reinforcer of health messages (18). Among the disadvantages of media that have been noted are its potential for limited effectiveness when used alone; the fact that it can, in absolute terms, be expensive; the often limited control health professionals can exert with respect to the message and how or when it is relayed; and the difficulty in attempting to evaluate its effects in a systematic fashion (18). In addition, it is crucial that the media messages being delivered match the needs and educational level of the target audience. For instance, research is available indicating that many of the physical activity materials currently being offered in printed form require a reading level that is higher than the average reading level in this country (65).

Although a variety of mass media strategies have been incorporated into most of the public health campaigns that have included physical activity, including the community heart health projects described earlier, it has been difficult to disentangle the effects of media from other interventions focused on promoting physical activity in the target communities (27). Early studies evaluating the effectiveness of a U.S. Department of Health and Human Services–sponsored national health promotion media campaign, called Healthstyle (66), and an Australian national campaign for physical activity entitled Life—Be In It (55) suggested that mass media approaches might be most successful in increasing awareness and knowledge related to physical activity and less effective in promoting behavior change. Yet, more recent evidence from an Australian mass media campaign in which more moderate forms of physical activity, such as walking, were targeted have met with somewhat greater success in promoting reported physical activity behavior change, particularly among older segments of the population (19,67). Because of the small number of campaigns that have received even cursory evaluation, the potential promise of media for influencing both initial increases in and longer term maintenance of physical activity remains unclear. Systematic investigation of the communication parameters most likely to enhance physical activity levels among the population at large and specific audience segments is a necessary first step before the dissemination of further large-scale mass media initiatives in this area. Given the natural linkages between dietary and physical activity behaviors for weight control and blood lipid level management, it also makes sense to continue to systematically explore methods for utilizing national media campaigns surrounding other risk factors (e.g., cholesterol, dietary intake, and hypertension) to more prominently promote physical activity.

In addition to the continued exploration of mass media approaches for physical activity promotion, the field would benefit from a more systematic evaluation of the smaller forms of electronic media (e.g., exercise videotapes) that have proliferated over the past decade. While such forms of exercise programming appear to be preferred by women rather than by men (56), relatively little is known concerning which types of videotaped programs appeal to which segments of the population, as well as the frequency with which such videotapes are actually used. It would be worthwhile to explore whether such forms of media could be used to facilitate the increased use of home fitness equipment, which typically remains underused by a substantial proportion of owners. In addition, the few studies currently available that have used electronic mail, the Internet, or other forms of interactive electronic communication to increase physical activity levels have shown promising, although preliminary,

results (68,69). The potential future reach of such channels across the population as a whole is enormous.

LEGISLATION AND REGULATION

Although potentially the most far-reaching in terms of their effects on virtually all sectors of the American public, legislative and regulatory policies influencing the promotion of physical activity remain few.

Liability Legislation

Issues related to liability remain a troublesome area for most communities and municipalities. Liability difficulties have been noted with respect to the safety of sports equipment and products (e.g., helmets, weight-training equipment, treadmills); programs (e.g., how persons are screened before being allowed to participate in a program, whether the exercise leader is adequately trained and prepared to deal with emergencies if they arise); and facilities made available for public use. The enactment of local legislation to control liability costs in tandem with certification policies related to facilities and exercise personnel, as well as continued or increased federal consumer safety testing and evaluation of equipment and products, could reduce this potential barrier to physical activity promotion (24).

Zoning and Building Construction Legislation

In a growing number of communities in at least some regions of the country an increased environmental awareness has led to zoning restrictions that protect open spaces and other "green areas" that can subsequently be used for recreational pursuits. Such "greenways" are becoming particularly popular in urban areas as a means of connecting neighborhoods and promoting alternative modes of transportation (e.g., bicycling, walking) (24). The National Greenways Commission, organized under the auspices of the U.S. Department of the Interior, has been charged with the protection and connection of green strips for recreation as well as transportation use.

In addition to fostering such policies through the use of legislation, financial incentives, and similar strategies, it would be worthwhile to pursue how zoning and other policies governing building construction can be utilized to facilitate construction that encourages increases in energy expenditure throughout the day. Making stairs attractive and readily accessible, building parking lots that induce walking, and providing readily accessible and easy to use bicycle racks constitute three such methods.

In a similar vein, urban areas typically have large tracts of land, including disused factories and railway areas, gravel pits, urban redevelopment areas, and sanitary landfill sites, that could be used for the construction of small parks, swimming pools, skating arenas, and similar facilities (10). The currently high cost of urban land could potentially be reduced by legislation that curtailed speculation in land holdings in such areas coupled with policies targeting such sites for recreational activities. Other potential avenues for public sector financing include local bond issues, local or state lotteries, leaseback arrangements, revenues from concessions, bequests, and a specific recreational millage tax (10). Costs of building such facilities could also potentially be curtailed if the amount of land relegated to public parking for the facility was reduced in conjunction with the improvement of public transportation to the facility or by choosing sites within safe walking or cycling distance of the population segments being targeted (10).

State Educational Legislation

The types of state-mandated physical activity programs required in primary and secondary schools vary widely in terms of comprehensiveness (e.g., physical education require-ments only in elementary schools) and content (e.g., no specific amount of teaching time or program content) (29). Federal legislation outlining the minimum requirements for achieving appropriate physical education programming at both the elementary and secondary school levels could aid efforts to promote appropriate levels of physical activity among all of our nation's youth. In addition, the exploration of incentives or other policy-based programs that would encourage states to be innovative in developing physical education programming for the promotion of lifetime activities is indicated.

Similarly, continued evaluation of the types of physical education offerings and requirements currently available throughout state higher education systems (i.e., state colleges and universities) is suggested, particularly because young adulthood represents a period when decreases in physical activity and increases in body weight have been noted to occur (70).

Work Site Legislation

Work site legislation to promote physical activity could take a variety of forms, including policies mandating or encouraging, through economic incentives, the inclusion of appropriate facilities when new commercial buildings or government-supported housing structures are planned; break periods to allow for physical activity participation; economic incentives for commercial sponsorship of community facilities or programs; and the provision of adequate insurance or workers compensation coverage for injuries sustained during participation at on-site exercise facilities.

Insurance Policies, Regulation, and Legislation

As fiscal pressures increase to develop alternatives to the tradi-tional fee-for-service approach to health care disbursement and coverage, a movement is growing towards managed care systems and other alternatives enabling the provision of health care at more reasonable cost. Policy makers, corporate managers, health care proponents, and other interest groups must understand the important role of health promotion, including physical activity, in helping to curb or control health care utilization and costs (10). The development of explicit methods and structures for including the promotion of physi-cal activity and other health-enhancing behaviors in the cov-erage and disbursement of new health care delivery and insurance systems is essential. Such activities deserve a promi-nent place on the agendas developed by coalitions in the phys-ical activity area.

Transportation Policies and Legislation

With few exceptions (e.g., Rails to Trails legislation), trans-portation policies and legislation at all levels typically have ignored the nonmechanized forms of transportation (e.g., walking, biking) that are potentially available or relevant to the development of more cost-effective transportation systems. Linking the disbursement of highway funds to the develop-ment of such systems as part of the transportation network is likely to encourage the development of such alternatives. On the local level, it would be worthwhile to explore, as some communities have already begun, legislative or incentive-based strategies for facilitating walk- or bike-to-work programs. The existence of free loaner cars or bicycles for employees to use once at work may help to decrease employee resistance to such policies.

Policies for Training Health Care Providers to Deliver Physical Activity Advice

Although the U.S. Preventive Services Task Force has recom-mended that physicians provide regular advice supporting increases in regular physical activity among their patients (2), few U.S. physicians currently do so (71). Policies that would support the introduction of appropriate curricula in this area across the nation's medical and allied health schools as well as schools of public health would help to facilitate movement towards the Healthy People 2000 goals in this area, with benefits to patients' physical activity levels a probable outcome (71).

Federal Legislation

Among the types of federal legislation that have been enacted over the past 30 years are the National Trails System Act (PL 90-543, 1968), which has facilitated the development of aban-doned railroad tracks as part of the National Trails System, and several pieces of legislation that have explicitly or implic-itly supported the appropriation of resources for activities related to health promotion and disease prevention, including physical activity, e.g., the National Health Planning and Resources Development Act (PL 93-641, 1974) and the National Consumer Health Information and Health Promo-tion Act (PL-94-317, 1976). Unfortunately, many such pieces of legislation, e.g., the Health Services and Centers Amend-ments (PL 95-626, 1978), have not received appropriations or have been proposed but not passed.

A comparatively recent innovative piece of legisla-tion is the Intermodal Surface Transporation Efficiency Act (ISTEA). Passed in November 1991, federal transportation funds have been targeted for bicycle and pedestrian trans-portation projects. Authority is given to the states for local control, but each state is required to assign a bicycle or pedestrian coordinator (Moritz B, personal communication, 1992). However, ISTEA does not require that specific funding allocations be made for this purpose, making advocacy and other expressions of public support paramount to its success (24).

The Americans with Disabilities Act (ADA) of 1990 will continue to have an impact on the physical environment of most businesses, work sites, and commercial and public build-ings. Many of the necessary modifications for building and worksite access in response to this legislation can potentially enhance physical activity through the addition of sidewalks and ramps and enhance access to public transportation and appropriate places to park for persons with disabilities (24). In this manner, the ADA legislation could be used to the advantage of both persons with disabilities and the nondisabled.

A critical, currently missing aspect of legislative policy is a long-term plan or framework on which to build and direct national policy initiatives in the physical activity arena (24). Such a policy or plan should focus on developing the infrastructure that would support ongoing increases in the routine, transportation-based, or task-oriented forms of physical activity that are likely to result in the most significant increases in energy expenditure levels among the American people as a whole (72). Such a plan would be similar to legislative policy initiatives undertaken at the federal, state, and local levels to meet other public needs, such as the ongoing development of this nation's system of highways and other transportation services.

providers can do to fruitfully participate in this worthy endeavor. Worthwhile activities include increasing health provider knowledge and competence related to providing physical activity–related advice, support, and referrals to their clients; continued efforts to incorporate a standardized preventive medicine curriculum, including information pertaining to physical activity, as part of current medical and allied health professional training activities; and inclusion of health care professionals and organizations in the development of appropriate physical activity coalitions on the local, state, and national levels. Concerted efforts in many of these areas remain in their infancy. Yet, the critical importance of regular physical activity as a health promotion and maintenance tool, coupled with the aging of our society, brings a new sense of urgency to this endeavor, which hopefully will not be ignored.

SUMMARY

Although it may appear that instituting environmental and policy initiatives sufficient to move the U.S. population closer to the current national physical activity objectives is a daunting task, there is much that physicians and other health care

This chapter is adapted from a background paper presented at the Centers for Disease Control and Prevention Conference on Environmental and Policy Approaches to Prevention of Cardiovascular Disease, Sept. 1993, Atlanta. The author would like to acknowledge the input of Robert Jeffery, Ph.D., and Fred Fridinger, Ph.D., on the original background paper.

REFERENCES

1. U.S. Department of Health and Human Services. Physical activity and health: a report of the Surgeon General. Atlanta, GA: U.S. Department of Health and Human Services, Centers for Disease Control and Prevention, National Center for Chronic Disease Prevention and Health Promotion, 1996:1–277.

2. Harris SS, Caspersen CJ, DeFriese GH, et al. Physical activity counseling for healthy adults as a primary preventive intervention in the clinic setting. JAMA 1989; 261:3590–3598.

3. Bouchard C, Shephard RJ, Stephens T. Physical activity and health: international proceedings and consensus statement. Champaign, IL: Human Kinetics, 1994: 1–1055.

4. Kohl HW, LaPorte RE, Blair SN. Physical activity and cancer: an epidemiological perspective. Sports Med 1988;6:222–237.

5. Paffenbarger RSJ, Hyde RT, Wing AL, et al. Physical activity, all-cause mortality, and longevity of college alumni. New Engl J Med 1986;314:605–613.

6. U.S. Department of Health and Human Services. Healthy People

2000: national health promotion and disease prevention objectives. Washington, DC: U.S. Government Printing Office, 1990:1–112.

7. Klesges RC, Shelton ML, Klesges LM. Effects of television on metabolic rate: potential implications for childhood obesity. Pediatrics 1993;91:281–286.

8. McGinnis JM. The public health burden of a sedentary lifestyle. Med Sci Sport Exerc 1992;24 (suppl):S196–S200.

9. Blair SN, Kohl HWI, Paffenbarger RSJ, et al. Physical fitness and all-cause mortality: a prospective study of healthy men and women. JAMA 1989;262:2395–2401.

10. Shephard RJ. Economic benefits of enhanced fitness. Champaign, IL: Human Kinetics, 1986:1–209.

11. Berg RL, Casells JS, eds. The second fifty years: promoting health and preventing disability. Washington, DC: National Academy Press, 1990:1–332.

12. Trupin L, Rice DP, Max W. Medical expenditures for people with disabilities in the United States, 1987. Washington, DC: U.S. Department of Education, National

Institute on Disability and Rehabilitation Research, 1995:6–7.

13. Hoffman C, Rice D, Sung H. Persons with chronic conditions: their prevalence and costs. JAMA 1996;276:1478–1479.

14. World Health Organization. Prevention of cardiovascular diseases among the elderly: report of a WHO meeting. Geneva, Switzerland: World Health Organization, 1987:1–30.

15. Fries JW, Green LW, Levine S. Health promotion and the compression of morbidity. Lancet 1989;1:481–484.

16. Simonsick EM, Lafferty ME, Phillips CL, et al. Risk due to inactivity in physically capable older adults. Am J Public Health 1993;83:1443–1450.

17. Pate RR, Pratt M, Blair SN, et al. Physical activity and public health: a recommendation from the Centers for Disease Control and Prevention and the American College of Sports Medicine. JAMA 1995;273:402–407.

18. Flora JA, Cassidy D. Roles of media in community-based health promotion. In: Bracht NF, ed.

Health promotion at the community level. London: Sage, 1990: 143–157.

19. Owen N, Bauman A, Booth M, et al. Serial mass-media campaigns to promote physical activity: reinforcing or redundant? Am J Public Health 1995;85:244–248.

20. Marcus BH, Simkin LR. The transtheoretical model: applications to exercise behavior. Med Sci Sport Exerc 1994;26:1400–1404.

21. King AC, Blair SN, Bild DE, et al. Determinants of physical activity and interventions in adults. Med Sci Sport Exerc 1992;24(suppl): S221–S236.

22. Dishman RK, ed. Advances in exercise adherence. Champaign, IL: Human Kinetics, 1994:1–406.

23. Owen N, Lee C. Development of behaviorally based policy guidelines for the promotion of exercise. J Public Health Policy 1989;10: 43–61.

24. King AC, Jeffery RW, Fridinger F, et al. Environmental and policy approaches to cardiovascular disease prevention through physical activity: issues and opportunities. Health Educ Q 1995;22: 499–511.

25. Powell KE, Kreuter MW, Stephens T, et al. The dimensions of health promotion applied to physical activity. J Public Health Policy 1991;12:492–509.

26. Gritz ER, Berman BA, Read LL, et al. Weight change among registered nurses in a self-help smoking cessation program. Am J Health Promot 1990;5:115–121.

27. King AC. Community intervention for promotion of physical activity and fitness. Exerc Sport Sci Rev 1991;19:211–259.

28. Von Korff M, Wickizer T, Maeser J, et al. Community activation and health promotion: identification of key organizations. Am J Health Promot 1992;7:110–117.

29. Caspersen CJ, Heath GW. Priority strategies for the promotion of physical activity: a report to the Henry J. Kaiser Family Foundation. Menlo Park, CA: Henry J. Kaiser Family Foundation, 1986:1–46. Unpublished report.

30. King AC, Carl F, Birkel L, et al. Increasing exercise among blue-collar employees: the tailoring of work site programs to meet specific needs. Prev Med 1988; 17:357–365.

31. Heirich MA, Foote A, Konopka B. Work site physical fitness programs: comparing the impact of different program designs on cardiovascular risks. J Occup Med 1993;35:510–517.

32. Wilbur CS. The Johnson & Johnson program. Prev Med 1983;12:672–681.

33. Blair SN, Piserchia PV, Wilbur CS, et al. A public health intervention model for work site health promotion: impact on exercise and physical fitness in a health promotion plan after 24 months. JAMA 1986;255:921–926.

34. Felix MRJ, Stunkard AJ, Cohen RY, et al. Health promotion at the worksite: a process for establishing programs. Prev Med 1985;14:99–108.

35. Gray JAM, Young A, Ennis JR. Promotion of exercise at work. Brit Med J 1983;286:1958–1959.

36. Knadler GF, Rogers T. Mountain climb month program: a low-cost exercise intervention program at a high-rise work site. Fitness Business 1987;Oct:64–67.

37. Brownell KD, Stunkard AJ, Albaum JM. Evaluation and modification of exercise patterns in the natural environment. Am J Psychiatry 1980;137:1540–1545.

38. Blamey A, Mutrie N, Aitchison T. Health promotion by encouraged use of stairs. Brit Med J 1995; 311:289–290.

39. Mayer J, Geller ES. Motivating energy efficient travel: a community-based intervention for encouraging biking. J Environ Sys 1982; 12:99–112.

40. Oja P, Vuori I, Paronen O. Daily walking and cycling to work—their utility as health-enhancing physical activity. Patient Educ Counsel 1998;33:S87–S94.

41. Hammond SL, Long DM, Fowler K, et al. Centers for Disease Control and Prevention 1996 director's physical activity challenge evaluation report. Atlanta: Centers for Disease Control and Prevention, 1997:1–65.

42. Lasater TM, Wells BL, Carleton RA, et al. The role of churches in disease prevention research studies. Pub Health Rep 1986; 101:125–131.

43. Hatch JW, Cunningham WW, Woods WW, et al. The Fitness Through Churches project: description of a community-based cardiovascular health promotion intervention. Hygiene 1986;5:9–12.

44. Blair SN, Smith N, Collingwood TR, et al. Health promotion for educators: impact on absenteeism. Prev Med 1986;15:166–175.

45. Carnegie Council on Adolescent Development. A matter of time: risk and opportunity in the non-school hours. (Executive summary.) New York: Carnegie Corporation, 1990:1–7.

46. Nader PR, Sallis JF, Patterson TL, et al. A family approach to cardiovascular risk reduction: results from the San Diego family health project. Health Educ Q 1989;16: 229–244.

47. Jaycox S, Baranowski T, Nader PR, et al. Theory-based health education activities for third to sixth grade children. J School Health 1983;53:584–588.

48. Killen JD, Telch M, Robinson T, et al. Cardiovascular risk reduction for tenth graders: a multiple factor school-based approach. JAMA 1988;260:1728–1733.

49. Walter HJ. Primary prevention of chronic disease among children: the school-based 'Know Your Body' intervention trials. Health Educ Q 1989;16:201–214.

50. Steller JJ. Discover and understand Carolina, kids walking manual. Spartanburg, SC: South Carolina Public Schools, 1993: 1–12.

51. Simons-Morton BG, Parcel GS, O'Hara NM. Implementing organizational changes to promote

healthful diet and physical activity at school. Health Educ Q 1988;15:115–130.

52. Parcel GS, Simons-Morton BG, O'Hara NM, et al. School promotion of healthful diet and exercise behavior: an integration of organizational change and social learning theory. J School Health 1987;57:150–156.

53. Simons-Morton BG, Parcel GS, Baranowski T, et al. Promoting physical activity and a healthful diet among children: results of a school-based intervention study. Am J Pub Health 1991;81:986–991.

54. Luepker RV, Perry CL, McKinlay SM, et al. Outcomes of a field trial to improve children's dietary patterns and physical activity: the Child and Adolescent Trial for Cardiovascular Health (CATCH). JAMA 1996;275:768–776.

55. Iverson DC, Fielding ME, Crow RS, et al. The promotion of physical activity in the United States population: the status of programs in medical, work site, community, and school settings. Pub Health Rep 1985;100:212–224.

56. King AC, Taylor CB, Haskell WL, et al. Identifying strategies for increasing employee physical activity levels: findings from the Stanford/Lockheed exercise survey. Health Educ Q 1990;17:269–285.

57. Lewis CE, Raczynski JM, Heath GW, et al. Promoting physical activity in low-income African-American communities: the PARR project. Ethnic Dis 1993;3:106–118.

58. Godbey G, Graefe A, James SW. The benefits of local recreation and park services: a nationwide study of the perceptions of the American pubic. Washington, DC: National Recreation and Park Association, 1992:1–140.

59. Brown VA, Ritchie JE, Rotem A. Health promotion and environmental management: a partnership for the future. Health Promot Int 1992;7:219–230.

60. Jakicic JM, Wing RR, Butler BA, et al. The relationship between presence of exercise equipment in the home and physical activity level. Am J Health Promot 1997;11:363–365.

61. Sallis JF, Hovell MF, Hofstetter CR, et al. Distance between homes and exercise facilities related to frequency of exercise among San Diego residents. Pub Health Rep 1990;105:179–185.

62. French SA, Jeffery RW, Oliphant JA. Facility access and self-reward as methods to promote physical activity among healthy sedentary adults. Am J Health Promot 1994;8:257–262.

63. Sallis JF, McKenzie TL, Elder JP, et al. Factors parents use in selecting play spaces for young children. Arch Pediatr Adol Med 1997;151:414–417.

64. Linenger JM, Chesson CV, Nice DS. Physical fitness gains following simple environmental change. Am J Prev Med 1991;7:298–310.

65. Cardinal BJ, Sachs ML. An analysis of the readability of exercise promoting literature with implications and suggestions for practice. Res Q Exerc Sport 1992;63:186–190.

66. David MF, Iverson DC. An overview and analysis of the Health Style campaign. Health Educ Q 1984;11:253–272.

67. Booth M, Bauman A, Oldenburg B, et al. Effects of a national mass-media campaign on physical activity participation. Health Promot Int 1992;7:241–247.

68. Tate DF, Winett RA, Harris C. Promoting exercise adoption through computer networks. (International Congress Supplement.) Ann Behav Med 1996;(suppl). PA31A:S108.

69. Cullinane PM, Hyppolite K, Zastawney AL, et al. Telephone linked communication-activity counseling and tracking for older patients. J Gen Intern Med 1994;9:86A.

70. Williamson DF, Kahn HS, Remington PL, et al. The 10-year incidence of overweight and major weight gain in U.S. adults. Arch Intern Med 1990;150:665–672.

71. King AC, Sallis JF, Dunn AL, et al. Promoting physical activity in primary health care settings: rationale and methods of the Activity Counseling Trial (ACT) intervention. Med Sci Sport Exerc 1998;30:1086–1096.

72. Mittlemark MB, Hunt MK, Heath GW. Realistic outcomes: lessons from community-based research and demonstration programs for the prevention of cardiovascular diseases: public health approaches to community-based cardiovascular disease prevention programs. Paper prepared for the Conference entitled Public Health Approaches to Community-based Cardiovascular Disease Prevention Programs, Myrtle Beach, SC, 1992:1–35.

Chapter 115

Promoting Strategic Alliances to Increase Physical Activity

Elizabeth Harper Howze

Physical inactivity is a leading cause of preventable death, together with unhealthy eating and tobacco use, in the United States (1). *Physical Activity and Health: A Report of the Surgeon General*, which was released in the summer of 1996, documented numerous health risks associated with a sedentary lifestyle (2). Documentation of the health hazards associated with physical inactivity is an important public health function. However, it is not sufficient in itself to catapult the problem of physical inactivity to the top tier of public health priorities or to drive an investment in public health that will increase the level of physical activity in the United States. A strong knowledge base must be accompanied by the political will to address the problem and a social strategy to begin to resolve it (Figure 115-1) (3,4). The objective is to make the promotion of physical activity an enduring public health priority at the national, state, and local levels. This chapter discusses the role of strategic alliances in strengthening the knowledge base, developing the political will, and crafting a social strategy for the promotion of physical activity.

STRATEGIC ALLIANCES

A strategic alliance exists when two or more organizations or groups agree to work together, guided by an agreed-upon set of operating principles, to achieve an agreed-upon goal that neither could achieve alone (5,6). In their definition of an alliance, Mattessich et al refer not only to a shared interest in one or more outcomes, but to an expectation of mutual benefit and obligation: "Collaboration is a mutually beneficial and well-defined relationship entered into by two or more organizations to achieve common goals" (7).

The magnitude of the problem of physical inactivity and the limitations of the public health system in the United States make strategic alliances a matter of practical necessity. Formation of effective alliances becomes more urgent as governments decrease their role in financing new or existing programs for health promotion or risk reduction. Wandersman identified the advantages, in addition to practical necessity, for organizations that work together (6). Those advantages include the following abilities of coalitions of organizations:

- Work on an important issue without having to take sole responsibility for it.
- Create a critical mass of public opinion, money, and other resources to accomplish goals that any one organization could not achieve.
- Assemble a talent pool well beyond the resources of a single organization.
- Use scarce resources more appropriately by "minimiz(ing) duplication of effort" (6).

Alliances can provide stability and continuity when a member organization has budget, personnel, or other problems that might otherwise jeopardize its ability to advocate or to deliver programs and services. Simply stated, partnerships can provide added value. They can save time and money and bring energy and influence that no single organization can bring to a problem such as the promotion of physical activity. The resulting synergy is one of the central values of alliances—that 2 + 2 = 5 (5).

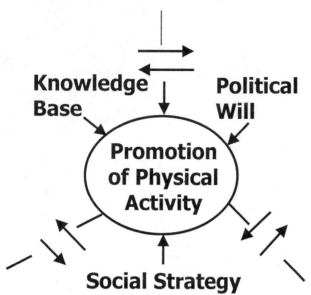

Figure 115-1 The health policy model applied to promotion of physical activity. (Reproduced by permission from Atwood K, Colditz GA, Kawachi I. From public health science to prevention policy: placing science in its social and political contexts. Am J Public Health 1997;87:1604. Copyright APHA.)

DEVELOPING THE KNOWLEDGE BASE

Atwood et al defined the knowledge base as "the scientific and administrative database upon which to make decisions" (4). The knowledge base linking physical activity and health has grown substantially in the last three decades. *Physical Activity and Health: A Report of the Surgeon General*, a review of that knowledge base, documented the numerous health benefits associated with regular, moderate physical activity (2). The report also identified many areas where research is needed to resolve important questions that remain (Table 115-1) (2). A quick review of the recommendations for research reveals a number of areas in which answers to the questions posed could generate additional support for the promotion of physical activity and suggest promising areas for intervention.

The determination of research priorities for physical activity should be guided by concern for translating science into public policy and improving public health. Public health research in recent years has been criticized for emphasizing "technical and methodological sophistication to the neglect of the broader mission of public health, much in the same way that economics, which began as an essentially moral endeavor . . . gradually evolved to become a highly technical discipline with diminishing relevance to the problems of society" (4). Alliances can articulate the need for investment across the spectrum of physical activity research while they advocate a course ensuring that the projects funded address the most salient research questions relevant to a larger public health agenda.

The Centers for Disease Control and Prevention (CDC) has established alliances with a number of schools of public health and their scientists to support the investigation of public health problems such as physical inactivity. A variety of mechanisms support these alliances—the CDC prevention centers program; grants and cooperative agreements; and programs for visiting scientists, expert consultants, and guest researchers (8). CDC collaborates with the University of South Carolina School of Public Health in Columbia to sponsor an annual research institute on physical activity for scientists who want to learn more about methodology, measurement, and other issues. In partnership with CDC, states track physical activity levels by using the Behavioral Risk Factor Surveillance System and the Youth Risk Behavior System. Data collected through these systems make it possible to estimate trends in the prevalence of physical activity across the United States, identify disparities in levels of physical activity by age, sex, race or ethnicity, and region of the country; generate research on the reliability and validity of physical activity measures; and provide data for development of interventions.

One notable example of an alliance to develop the knowledge base for physical activity is the physical activity research component of the Women's Health Initiative (WHI) (9), funded by the National Institutes of Health (NIH). NIH, in partnership with CDC and several of its university prevention centers, is tackling the problem of lower rates of physical activity in older women. Researchers participating in the WHI at the University of South Carolina School of Public Health, the University of New Mexico in Albuquerque, and the University of Texas School of Public Health in Houston are developing more valid and reliable measures to assess the physical activity behavior of African-American, Hispanic, and Native American women (9). WHI researchers at the St. Louis University School of Public Health Prevention Center in St. Louis, Missouri, are examining determinants of physical activity among low-income and minority women aged 40 to 75 years. The researchers are using their findings to develop programs tailored to meet the needs of these populations (10).

GENERATING POLITICAL WILL

Generating political will requires that those concerned with the issue of physical activity pay attention to the social and political contexts in which public health policy is set and take steps to ensure that the public understands the health issue (3). According to Atwood et al (4), political will can be defined as the expression "of society's desire and commitment to develop and fund new programs or to support or modify existing programs." Political will is required to accelerate the translation of the public health knowledge base into social action. Alliances have the potential to ratchet up the importance of physical activity in the public eye by increasing the visibility of this important public health issue in the media, through programs in communities and in myriad other ways. The American Heart Association, a strong advocate for promotion of physical activity, recognizes how important alliances are to generating political will. Its 1995 *Strategic Plan for Promoting Physical Activity* directs the American Heart Association to "promote partnerships (at the state level) between affiliates and state and local councils on health promotion and physical activity. (State health departments, state Governor's Councils on Physical Fitness and Sports, businesses

Table 115-1 Selected Recommendations for Strengthening the Science Base for Physical Activity

- Develop better methods for analysis and quantification of activity. These methods should be applicable to both work and leisure-time measurements and provide direct quantitative estimates of activity.
- Conduct research on the social and psychological factors that influence adoption of a more active lifestyle and the maintenance of that behavior change throughout life.
- Better characterize the mechanisms by which the musculoskeletal system responds differentially to endurance and resistance exercise.
- Better characterize the mechanisms by which physical activity reduces the risk of cardiovascular disease, hypertension, and non–insulin-dependent diabetes mellitus.
- Determine the minimal and optimal amount of exercise for disease prevention.
- Better characterize beneficial activity profiles for people with disabilities.
- Determine specific health benefits of physical activity for women, racial and ethnic minority groups, and people with disabilities.
- Examine the protective effects of physical activity in conjunction with other lifestyle characteristics and disease prevention behaviors.
- Examine the types of physical activity that preserve muscle strength and functional capacity in the elderly.
- Further study the relationship between physical activity in adolescence and early adulthood and the later development of breast cancer.
- Clarify the role of physical activity in preventing or reducing bone loss after menopause.
- Routinely monitor the prevalence of physical activity among children under age 12.
- Routinely monitor school policy requirements and students' participation in physical education classes in elementary, middle, and high schools.
- Assess the determinants of physical activity for various population subgroups (e.g., by age, sex, race, ethnicity, socioeconomic status, health and disability status, geographic location).
- Evaluate the interactive effects of psychosocial, cultural, environmental, and public policy influences on physical activity.
- Develop and evaluate the effectiveness of interventions that include policy and environmental supports.
- Develop and evaluate interventions designed to promote adoption and maintenance of moderate physical activity that addresses the specific needs and circumstances of population subgroups, such as racial or ethnic groups, men and women, girls and boys, elderly adults, disabled persons, overweight persons, low-income persons, and persons at life transitions, such as adolescence, early adulthood, family formation, and retirement.
- Develop and evaluate the effectiveness of interventions to promote physical activity in combination with healthy dietary practices that can be broadly disseminated to reach large segments of the population and can be sustained over time.

SOURCE: U.S. Department of Health and Human Services. Physical activity and health: a report of the Surgeon General. Atlanta: Centers for Disease Control and Prevention, 1996.

and corporations are essential members.)" (American Heart Association, 1995, unpublished document).

Collectively creating the political will to address the issue of physical inactivity ultimately can help to reduce health disparities by reaching populations that are underserved or at higher risk of disease associated with inactivity, or both. For example, in recent years, scientists from research institutions, professional associations, voluntary organizations, and the federal government have collaborated to develop physical activity guidelines, consensus statements, and a Surgeon General's report, all of which have provided a significant impetus for public health action (2,11–13).

How is political will generated? At times, political will is generated by what Bandura describes as fortuitous events or happenstance—chance events that can profoundly alter the course of events or arouse public interest or awareness about an issue in either a positive or negative direction. These events, in turn, may provide an opportunity for development of public policy (14,15). Former First Lady Nancy Reagan's diagnosis of breast cancer and the death of runner Jim Fixx had profound influence on public perceptions about the value of mammography and the health risk of exercise. Gray characterized the generation of political will as a function of three processes associated with the devel-

opment of an alliance: identifying stakeholders, creating a shared definition of the problem, and committing to collaborate (16).

Identifying Stakeholders

Collaboration to generate political will requires a strategic analysis of who the stakeholders are and what they can bring to the process of setting a research agenda, generating political will, or later, implementing a social strategy (16). Fortunately, the numerous determinants and consequences of physical inactivity provide a natural conjunction of shared interests for many organizations and, hence, many stakeholders who are potential partners.

Some considerations that help in identifying stakeholders are the following:

- Which populations are affected by determinants that diminish their opportunity to be physically active or are disproportionately affected by lack of rergular physical activity?

- Which organizations can provide access to specific target populations, such as adolescents, employees, older adults, racial or ethnic minorities, rural residents, or persons with chronic conditions or disabilities?

- Which organizations can provide the reach into diverse settings such as schools and workplaces that is ultimately required to create systems change?
- Which organizations that are not traditionally associated with promotion of physical activity have a stake in people becoming more active for reasons other than health (e.g., to reduce air pollution associated with vehicle emissions, reduce youth crime, or contain suburban sprawl)?
- Which organizations can provide access to gatekeepers and decision makers who can help shape public policy, budgets, and the ways in which issues are defined?
- Which organizations can furnish access to public and professional communications channels, such as television, radio, magazines, newspapers, newsletters, and conferences—media that provide continuous visibility for the issue of physical activity, make information available, and recommend actions?

Partnership opportunities with potential stakeholders should be evaluated on the basis of the following criteria (17,18):

- Will all parties benefit? In what ways?
- What is the fit with the alliance's mission and goals?
- What added value will accrue to the alliance?
- What are the risks, and are they sufficient to offset potential benefits?
- What will be the effect on the public's perception of the organization's image and mission?
- Will the public perceive the involvement of a for-profit organization in the alliance as a charitable activity or just a way to sell products or temper public criticism of its business practices?
- Will the public perceive the not-for-profit and government members of the alliance as having, in effect, given a product endorsement or "sold out" to corporate interests?

Creating a Shared Definition of the Problem

An alliance to promote physical activity may be seen by some partners as a way to reduce morbidity and mortality associated with inactivity-related conditions such as heart disease and diabetes. For other organizations, promoting physical activity may be seen as a means to other ends, such as increasing use of alternative transportation to improve air quality, reducing youth crime or substance abuse, creating more livable communities, or increasing employee productivity. Regardless of what brings them together, stakeholders must come to broad agreement on the problem and the goals of the alliance. It is perhaps just as important that partner organizations work together to define the problem and determine the desired outcomes of action to address it. Unilateral problem definition and goal setting by one organization short-circuits the dialogue and the engagement with the issue that must occur if participating organizations are to develop a sense of joint responsibility for the success of the alliance. "The recognition by stakeholders that their desired outcomes are inextricably linked to the

---

Table 115-2 Objectives of the *Jovenes Mejorando el Estado Fisico de la Comunidad* Program

- Establish partnerships between the chronic disease prevention and violence prevention communities.
- Improve youth access to physical activity programs and sites.
- Build youth leadership and advocacy skills, and provide youth mentorship and team leader opportunities.
- Increase multi-ethnic youth participation in organized sports programs that have little or no cultural diversity.
- Enhance intergenerational physical activity opportunities through adult mentoring programs.
- Create policies and organizational changes that increase access to physical activity programs for all youth.

SOURCE: C. Morrison, Director, ON THE MOVE, California Department of Health Services, personal communication, 1998.

actions of the other stakeholders is the fundamental basis for collaborating" (16).

The California Department of Health Services' ON THE MOVE! program and the department's Emergency Preparedness and Injury Control Branch joined forces with Hispanic communities in Fresno to creat the program *Jovenes Mejorando el Estado Fisico de la Comunidad* (Youth Improving the Physical State of the Community). This alliance consisted of the Fresno County Health Services Agency; La Vida Caminando Project; local schools; the Westside Youth Center; the Boys & Girls Club; the City of Fresno; California Project LEAN; United Health Clinic; California State University (Fresno); and the University of California Cooperative Extension Service (Morrison C, personal communication, February 1998). The objectives these organizations created for their programs are shown in Table 115-2. Physical activity was the common thread that linked sectors in this diverse community, providing a platform for youth mentoring and leadership development activities and expanding community programs to reach youth previously unserved by community programs.

This alliance of diverse stakeholders has yielded a number of benefits, including more resources and expertise to devote to the program, access to community youth, strengthened support and trust among community members, more rapid start-up, and greater overall effect. "Youth now play together on inter-racial sports teams, with conflict resolution activities, parent participation, and adult mentorship. The program increased access to physical activity programs by among other things providing reduced fees, improved transportation, and safe and convenient environments" (Morrison C, personal communication, February 1998).

Committing to Collaboration

The Committee on Medicine and Public Health, a collaboration of the American Medical Association and the American Public Health Association, cautions that "collaboration is damn tough" (19). Generating political will often is contingent on how well those with a common stake in the issue collaborate. Mutual respect, shared interest in the issue, and a clearly articulated mission or direction, such as establishing a policy, obtaining resources, or serving a particular population, are important elements of successful alliances (6,7,16). Makara and colleagues observed that commitment has several key dimensions: honesty about motivations for collaborating, shared goals and priorities, willingness to fulfill commitments in a timely manner, and an expectation of solid performance by all parties (20). Endorsement of these criteria can help avoid the pitfalls of poor strategy development. These pitfalls can occur when only a few members participate, information is inadequate or divergent views are not presented, or buy-in is insufficient to enable successful implementation of a strategy.

The potential benefits of collaboration must be weighed against potential disadvantages, including liabilities of and organizational impediments to joining an alliance (19). Potential disadvantages include the following:

- Opportunity costs (if an organization could be investing its resources elsewhere for other potential gains)
- Loss of autonomy that occurs when decision making is shared
- Loss of organizational identity or recognition
- The risk of organization members feeling unappreciated, uninvolved, or overworked
- A risk of being tarred with the same brush by unfavorable publicity that a partner organization receives
- Frustration with the process
- Impatience with the pace of the effort to meet the alliance's goals

In some circumstances, an organization's policy environment may impede development of an alliance by: 1) creating criteria that are too difficult, costly, or inflexible to accommodate alliance development within a reasonable time or 2) by implicitly or explicitly promoting an organizational ethic that discourages collaboration.

Collaboration within a sector, such as among public health agencies, may be easier than joint efforts across sectors, because collaborators within a sector share a common language and training. Cross-sector cooperation brings together people and organizations with diverse backgrounds, perspectives, idiosyncratic language of discipline or trade, and different approaches to management (19). A "boundary spanner" who has connections with each sector, knows the specific languages and cultures, and is seen as a leader in each sector can be enormously helpful as a leader and facilitator (20). Strong leadership can facilitate the work of a physical activity alliance. Leadership qualities include skills in administration, negotiation, conflict resolution, and problem solving; the ability to garner resources; access to media and decision makers; and proficiency in facilitating participation (inclusiveness) (21).

Objectives must be clearly stated and grounded in reasonable expectations for accomplishments over the short term and the long term. They must be perceived as achievable by the members of the alliance, considering

the skills and resources the members bring to bear on the problem. Operationally, responsibilities of each member for contribution of time, resources, and energy should be spelled out, and a process of ensuring accountability for those commitments should be implemented. Formal statement of responsibilities has been associated with greater satisfaction with an alliance; greater investment of time, money, and other resources; and other evidence of increased commitment. These factors, in turn, increase the likelihood that the alliance and its activities will be sustained (21). The planning process should be flexible and responsive, and having a skilled facilitator can be extremely helpful (21). As noted earlier, unilateral problem definition or decision-making should be avoided, because it may compromise the relationship and introduce difficult dynamics of power and communication. The glue that holds the alliance together and generates social capital has three components: trust, a spirit of cooperation, and agreement on one shared message rather than many messages (21,22). Establishing communications processes, such as regular conference calls and meetings, can serve as a valuable management tool for maintenance of the alliance (6). Finally, it is essential to find a way to share the credit for successes and to acknowledge each member's contributions.

The organization of the National Coalition to Promote Physical Activity (NCPPA) in 1994 in Dallas, Texas, was spearheaded by the American Heart Association, the American College of Sports Medicine, and the American Alliance of Health, Physical Education, Recreation, and Dance. The creation of NCPPA illustrates the leadership and commitment of diverse organizations to collaborate in promoting physical activity. NCPPA has established bylaws; strong organizational leadership in its steering committee; regular communications with its membership; and goals, objectives, and activities developed from the directives of its membership. The mission of NCPPA, as stated in one of its fact sheets, is "to unite the strengths of public, private, and industry efforts into a collaborative alliance to inspire Americans to lead physically active lifestyles to enhance their health and quality of life." One of its major initiatives is AIM 2010, which sets its sights on helping the nation achieve the Healthy People 2010 national objectives for physical activity through programs in worksites, schools, and communities (23).

IMPLEMENTING A SOCIAL STRATEGY

The third component of the health policy model is implementation of a social strategy. A social strategy is a blueprint for action, an application of the knowledge base and political will, to improve disease prevention and health promotion (4). "The social strategy requires the combined efforts of the many private and public agencies acting to bring better health information and programmes to all the people" (3). But a social strategy's aim is more than the provision of information and programs; it is behavior change, which ultimately results in altered behavioral and social norms across populations (4).

Models for Constructing a Social Strategy
A social strategy to promote physical activity should be devised to influence behavior change at several levels or in several domains. A single approach would be inadequate,

because the knowledge base describes a complex set of determinants for physical activity (2,24). The limited success observed in the field of health promotion when individuals have been the sole focus of change efforts with no attention given to the context in which their behavior occurs, has stimulated the development of more comprehensive approaches. The Ottawa Charter for Health Promotion, for example, defined five elements that should be included in any social strategy to achieve lasting behavior change (25):

- Build healthy public policy
- Create supportive environments
- Strengthen community action
- Develop personal skills
- Reorient health services toward prevention

To promote physical activity, strategic alliances could be formed around any one or more of these five elements.

McLeroy and associates proposed another ecologic framework for strategy development that has five levels of intervention: individual, interpersonal, community, institutional, and policy (26). These investigators advocate the importance of designing interventions that address policies, practices, and environments that support healthy behavior.

The current emphasis on multiple interventions at multiple levels of the "social ecology" is a response to the severity and complexity of chronic health problems that are rooted in a larger social, cultural, political, and economic fabric. The current wisdom in health promotion holds that targeting the behavior of individuals, without also intervening at these other social levels that shape behavior, will not have as great an impact on health status (21).

Makara and colleagues proposed a different approach. They defined seven domains that offer opportunities for fruitful collaboration: product dissemination, product development, service delivery, site development, issue exploration, message dissemination, and knowledge development (20). These domains, which are not mutually exclusive, are listed in Table 115-3 with examples of their relevance for promotion of physical activity.

CDC's National Physical Activity Initiative

CDC's comprehensive National Physical Activity Initiative, launched in October 1995 to address the public health problem of physical inactivity, exemplifies an ecologic approach to the creation of a social strategy (27). The initiative has seven components:

- Intervention research and program development
- Public information and education
- Professional education
- Policy and environmental guidelines development
- Promotion of partnerships
- Coordination and leadership
- Surveillance and evaluation

Since its inception, this initiative has served as an organizing framework for planning and capacity development within CDC. Table 115-4 provides examples of

collaboration of alliances with CDC in implementing component activities.

Cause Marketing

Alliances between not-for-profit organizations and government or the corporate sector for "cause marketing" offer each partner the opportunity to reach new customers, enhance their identities with established constituents, mobilize support for important issues, and access skills, media, and financial resources that otherwise would be out of reach. Three types of alliances are most common: transaction-based promotions, issue-based promotions, and product licensing (17). Typical transaction-based promotions involve a corporation contributing funds to a not-for-profit organization when consumers purchase that corporation's product or use its services. The American Express annual Charge Against Hunger, which occurs during the Christmas season, is a familiar example (17). Issue-based promotions include the CDC's alliance with the Young Women's Christian Association of the United States and Avon Corporation to increase mammography screening among low-income women aged 50 years or older and the CDC's Business Responds to AIDS campaign. To promote physical activity in the workplace, the National Association of Governor's Councils on Physical Fitness and Sports collaborates with The Sugar Association, Inc., on its annual National Employee Health and Fitness program (Porteus C, personal communication, January 1998).

Product licensing alliances may be more difficult to negotiate, but they can be powerful vehicles for conveying public health messages. Perhaps one of the better-known product licensing alliances in the public health arena is the alliance the National Cancer Institute has developed with the Produce for Better Health Foundation, Inc., for its "5 a Day—for Better Health" campaign to increase fruit and vegetable consumption by Americans (28). The foundation issues sublicenses for its logo and materials to industry partners, who clearly understand that established guidelines for their promotion must be strictly followed. Recently, CDC and NCPPA worked out an agreement in which NCPPA handles marketing and distribution of products such as T-shirts and water bottles that carry the public health message of CDC's national campaign: Ready. Set. Physical Activity: It's Everywhere You Go. This alliance provides a vehicle for the broad dissemination of a consistent public health message about physical activity and enables members of the alliance to have ready access to products to support their individual physical activity initiatives.

Another approach to cause marketing is to develop joint efforts with an entire industry. An industry-wide collaboration can be a powerful tool for raising public awareness, setting policy, and promoting change. For example, a not-for-profit organization might induce all manufacturers of baby strollers to agree to include printed materials with the stroller-assembly instructions on how new parents can get regular physical activity. Such a collaboration may have a greater effect on physical activity than the not-for-profit organization could have achieved through an alliance with a single business. At the same time, it reduces the organization's risk of appearing to have sold out to one company or of having its reputation tarnished if it is learned that the company engages in unacceptable business practices.

Table 115-3 Domains for Collaboration to Promote Physical Activity

DOMAIN	EXAMPLES OF OPPORTUNITIES FOR COLLABORATION
Product Dissemination	The state health department, the department of education, and a sporting goods manufacturer work together to distribute playground equipment to elementary schools at cost.
Product Development	A computer software company and a health care association team up to develop software that prompts employees to be active and helps to track their daily physical activity.
Service Delivery	Employers, insurers, and health care providers collaborate to develop and implement a protocol for physical activity counseling, reimbursement, and incentives.
Site Development	A school system and a parent-teacher organization implement a daily physical activity curriculum for kindergarten through grade 12.
Issue Exploration	The health department, the transportation department, community planners, and environmental and citizen groups organize a coalition to create a vision of a more livable community.
Messages	A state diabetes association and an Hispanic organization initiate a multimedia campaign on physical activity and diabetes management.
Knowledge Development	An organization for older adults, a consortium of universities, and a government agency collaborate on research to develop effective approaches to promote strength training among older adults.

Table 115-4 Examples of How Alliances Support the National Physical Activity Initiative of the Centers for Disease Control and Prevention (CDC)

COMPONENTS	EXAMPLES OF ALLIANCES
Intervention research and program development	CDC, the CDC Foundation, Emory University, and the International Life Sciences Institute are collaborating to improve physical activity and nutrition among children and adolescents.
Public information and education	CDC collaborated with the National Association of Governor's Councils on Physical Fitness and Sports, and Time-Warner of North Carolina to produce television public service announcements for "Ready. Set. Physical Activity, It's Everywhere You Go," a national campaign to promote physical activity.
Professional education	In partnership with the University of South Carolina School of Public Health and the South Carolina Department of Health and Environmental Control, CDC conducts annual training courses for researchers and practitioners to provide them with the skills to conduct physical activity research or promote physical activity in communities.
Development of policy and environmental guidelines	CDC collaborated with nearly 40 national organizations to develop *Guidelines for School and Community Programs to Promote Lifelong Physical Activity Among Young People* (13).
Promotion of partnerships	CDC encourages collaboration, such as with the National Association of State Legislators, to increase decision makers' awareness of the health and economic costs of physical inactivity, unhealthy diets, and obesity.
Coordination and leadership	CDC collaborates with federal, state, university, and private sector partners to evaluate the contributions of environmental and policy factors to levels of physical inactivity and explore prevention opportunities through environmental and policy modifications.
Surveillance and evaluation	CDC and state health departments monitor physical activity behavior in adults through the Behavioral Risk Factor Surveillance System. CDC and state departments of education monitor physical activity behavior of adolescents through the Youth Risk Behavior Survey.

EVALUATING THE EFFECTIVENESS OF STRATEGIC ALLIANCES

Tracking the effectiveness of a strategic alliance in developing a knowledge base, creating political will, or implementing a social strategy to increase levels of physical activity is important to each participating organization and to the alliance as a whole. Data on the activities of the alliance and its accomplishments enable member organizations to continuously assess the opportunity costs of participation, reaffirm their commitment to the alliance, and deal with performance pressures within their organizations (29). For the alliance as a whole, ongoing evaluation is important to

help partnerships review their progress and continually improve their efforts; gain community support, grant money, and donations; help overcome resistance to the initiative; determine whether the partnership has attained its goals; detect successful projects early in the life of the alliance; identify unforeseen challenges and side effects and redirect efforts of the alliance; acknowledge and celebrate small wins on the road to successful outcomes; [and] be more responsive and accountable to community members, grantmakers, and other constituents (30).

To use evaluation information as described here, an alliance should define short-term or intermediate objectives as well as long-term goals. Intermediate outcomes for a physical activity alliance might include a change in a school curriculum, an increase in public awareness of the benefits of being active, funds generated for construction of a walking path, the opening of a high school track after school hours for community use, an expanded range of options for after-school intramural physical activity for adolescents, or initiation of a community gardening project. If only long-term outcomes are defined, it becomes more difficult to evaluate the effectiveness of the alliance and to take any necessary corrective action. Most organizations have a short horizon for commitment of funds or other resources; they make commitments for 1 or 2 years, and if expected results have not been achieved they direct those resources elsewhere. Achieving rapid results is important, if not essential, to the health of the alliance. If short-term goals are not met, it becomes increasingly difficult for members to commit time and energy to the effort and to sustain the vision and momentum necessary for the alliance to achieve its long-term objectives.

Defining process objectives that are linked to achieving intermediate outcomes is another important component of an evaluation plan (29). For example, an alliance may determine that training its members in advocacy strategies, providing testimony to a legislative committee about the need for pedestrian-friendly transportation alternatives, and speaking to community groups about the need for walkways and bikeways will result in support for an urban trail and transit system. Process objectives define alliance activities and the responsibilities of individual members (e.g., which organization mails the newsletter or prepares materials for a legislative briefing). Such objectives help to ensure that the social strategy is being implemented as designed and that all partners are held accountable.

SUMMARY

A strong knowledge base, political will, and a social strategy are the three elements required to translate science into public health action to promote physical activity. Physical activity alliances can play an instrumental role in determining a research agenda with a public health focus, generating political will through advocacy and information dissemination, and devising a social strategy that addresses the problem of inactivity on multiple levels, in various setttings, and among different populations. Through collaboration to promote physical activity, progress will occur more rapidly and member organizations will experience the synergy and reap the benefits that working in partnership provides.

REFERENCES

1. McGinnis JM, Foege WH. Actual causes of death in the United States. JAMA 1993;270:2207–2212.

2. U.S. Department of Health and Human Services. Physical activity and health: a report of the Surgeon General. Atlanta: U.S. Department of Health and Human Services, Centers for Disease Control and Prevention, National Center for Chronic Disease Prevention and Health Promotion, 1996.

3. Richmond JB, Kotelchuck M. Coordination and development of strategies and policy for public health promotion in the United States. In: Holland WW, Detels R, Knox G, eds. Oxford textbook of public health. Oxford, England: Oxford Medical, 1991:441–454.

4. Atwood K, Colditz GA, Kawachi I. From public health science to prevention policy: placing science in its social and political contexts. A J Public Health 1997;87:1603–1606.

5. World Health Organization. Partnerships for health in the 21st century: 2 + 2 = 5. World Health Organization Fourth International Conference on Health Promotion, Jakarta, Indonesia, July 1997.

6. Wandersman A. Understanding coalitions and how they operate: an "open systems" perspective. WK Kellogg Foundation, 1993.

7. Mattessich PW, Monsey BR. Collaboration: what makes it work. St. Paul: Amherst H. Wilder Foundation, 1992.

8. Rugg DL, Levinson R, DiClemente R, et al. Centers for Disease Control and Prevention partnerships with external behavioral and social scientists: roles, extramural funding, and employment. Am Psychol 1997;52:147–153.

9. Masse LC, Ainsworth BE, Tortolero S, et al. Measuring physical activity in midlife, older, and minority women: issues from an expert panel. J Women Health 1998;7:57–67.

10. Howze E. No sweat: how research can increase women's physical activity. J Women Health 1997;6:623–625.

11. Pate RR, Pratt M, Blair SN, et al. Physical activity and public health: a recommendation from the Centers for Disease Control and Prevention and the American College of Sports Medicine. JAMA 1995;273:402–407.

12. National Institutes of Health. Physical activity and cardiovascular health. NIH Consens Statement 1995;13:1–33.

13. Centers for Disease Control and Prevention. Guidelines for school and community programs to promote lifelong physical activity among young people. MMWR 1997;46:RR-6.

14. Bandura A. Social foundations of thought and action. Englewood Cliffs, NJ: Prentice Hall, 1986:30–38.

15. Howze EH, Redman LJ. The uses of theory in health advocacy: policies and programs. Health Educ Q 1992;19:369–383.

16. Gray B. Collaborating: finding common ground for multiparty problems. San Francisco: Jossey-Bass, 1989:55–94.

17. Andreasen AR. Profits for non-profits: find a corporate partner. Harvard Bus Rev 1996;Nov–Dec: 47–59.

18. Centers for Disease Control and Prevention. Guidance for collaboration with the private sector. Atlanta: U.S. Department of Health and Human Services, Centers for Disease Control and Prevention, General Administration CDC-81, 1997.

19. Lasker RD, Committee on Medicine and Public Health. Medicine & public health: the power of collaboration. New York: The New York Academy of Medicine, 1997.

20. Makara P, Buchel B, Hagard S. Partnerships for health promotion. World Health Organization Fourth International Conference on Health Promotion, Jakarta, Indonesia, July 1997.

21. Butterfoss FD, Goodman RM, Wandersman A. Community coalitions for prevention and health promotion. Health Educ Res Theory Prac 1993;8:315–330.

22. Gillies P. The effectiveness of alliances or partnerships for health promotion. World Health Organization Fourth International Conference on Health Promotion, Jakarta, Indonesia, July 1997.

23. Pronk S, Couzelis P. AWHP partners with AIM 2010. Worksite Health 1998;1:2.

24. Schmid TL, Pratt M, Howze E. Policy as intervention: environmental and policy approaches to the prevention of cardiovascular disease. A J Public Health 1995;85: 1207–1211.

25. World Health Organization. Ottawa charter for health promotion. World Health Organization First International Conference on Health Promotion, Ottawa, Ontario, Canada, 1986.

26. McLeroy KR, Bibeau D, Steckler A, et al. An ecological perspective on health promotion programs. Health Educ Q 1988;15:351–377.

27. Marks JS. Letter announcing CDC national physical activity initiative. Centers for Disease Control and Prevention, Atlanta, Georgia, October 17, 1995.

28. Produce for Better Health Foundation, Inc. 5 a Day—for better health program guidebook. Newark, DE: Produce for Better Health Foundation 1991.

29. Francisco VT, Paine AL, Fawcett SB. A methodology for monitoring and evaluating community health coalitions. Health Educ Res Theory Prac 1993;8:403–416.

30. Fawcett SB, Sterling TD, Paine-Andrews A, et al. Evaluating community efforts to prevent cardiovascular diseases. Atlanta: Centers for Disease Control and Prevention, 1995.

Chapter 116

Obesity and Health: Public Policy Implications and Recommendations

James M. Rippe
Louis J. Aronne
Veronica F. Gilligan
Shiriki Kumanyika
Sanford Miller
Gary M. Owens
Charles P. Quesenberry, Jr.
Joseph E. Scherger
Madeleine Sigman-Grant

The United States and many other industrialized countries are in the midst of an alarming and rapidly growing epidemic of obesity. An estimated 35% of the adult population in the United States is obese (1). What is more, the prevalence of obesity *grew* a shocking 34% during the past decade (2).

Obesity ranks second to smoking as a preventable cause of death (3,4). Thus, an urgent need exists for all organizations and individuals concerned about the health and well-being of American citizens to sound the alarm and place obesity at the top of our health care agenda.

BACKGROUND

Obesity is a chronic disease caused by multiple factors. While recent scientific advances have elucidated a number of genetic components of obesity (5–11), environmental factors and lifestyle issues—primarily overconsumption of calories and a sedentary lifestyle—appear to dominate the recent explosive growth of obesity in the United States. In many people, these two factors are compounded by confusion (e.g., about the nature and content of fat in foods) and by discouragement with weight lost and regained. Unfortunately, the problem is not confined to adults. These same factors contribute to the dramatic increase in obesity recently seen in children and adolescents and promote the passage of an unhealthy legacy to the next generation.

Overconsumption of Calories

As mechanization has become the norm, it is no longer necessary to expend the same kind or amount of energy as once was required to keep food on our tables and roofs over our heads. Nowhere is this more evident than in the United States, where food is plentiful and obtainable with little or no physical effort. The food industry in the United States produces more than 3700 calories of food for every man, woman, and child in the country every day (12). This enormous quantity of food, which is typically high-fat, calorie-dense, good-tasting, and readily available, is then advertised with billions of dollars. Although Americans have access to a large variety of healthful foods year-round, we are credited with the invention of fast foods, take-out and delivery, snack foods, and numerous high-calorie, high-fat foods that are consumed each day in staggering quantities in every corner of the country.

Our Sedentary Lifestyle

Compounding the overconsumption of calorie- and fat-laden foods is the prevalence of a general lack of physical activity: we have become a nation of couch potatoes. Use of computers, automobiles, power-driven lawn mowers, and other time- and energy-saving devices and machines, along with sedentary leisure-time activities (e.g., television and video games), has become the norm, contributing to a further reduction in physical activity and calorie expenditure.

Physical Activity and Health: A Report of the Surgeon General estimates that only 24% of the US population engages in regular physical activity, 52% are intermittently active, and 25% are entirely sedentary (13). Inactivity contributes to a host of health problems, but most significantly, it plays a major role in the surge in obesity in the United States (4,13).

Confusion and Discouragement

A recent survey demonstrated that most people who are obese are concerned about the health implications of their weight and are trying to do something about it (14). However, incorrect information and discouragement abound.

A telephone survey conducted by Louis Harris and Associates of 2000 overweight or obese adults (body mass index, or BMI of more than 25) found that most appear to recognize the health risks of a high-fat diet and report that they try to limit their daily fat intake (14). For example, most say they rarely eat high-fat snacks or desserts. However, the majority of people surveyed are apparently unaware of the "hidden" sources of fat in the diet. In this population, daily fat intake more commonly comes from the consumption of what they consider to be "healthy" proteins, i.e., beef, cheese, and whole or 2% fat milk. Almost half the survey respondents report eating French fries often (daily or several times per week), and more than half eat vegetables with butter or sauce added.

The survey also highlights a disappointing lack of physician involvement in counseling concerning obesity and a troubling disparity between how physicians counsel men and women. Only 39% of women who are obese report that their physicians counsel them to lose weight for health reasons, while a mere 23% of men who are obese receive similar advice.

The findings also point to the inherent difficulties in weight loss through caloric restriction. Although many adults who are overweight have tried to lose weight, 75% are not currently trying to restrict caloric intake, according to this survey. Those who at some point successfully lost weight tended to regain the lost weight within a few years.

These findings present physicians and other health care professionals with an opportunity, and an obligation, to advise both male and female patients of the various risks associated with the consumption of a diet high in fat and calories and to attempt to alleviate patient confusion and discouragement in this area (14).

An Unhealthy Legacy

Unfortunately, the problem of obesity pervades all age groups in our society. The prevalence of obesity among children and adolescents more than doubled during the past decade (15,16). Unless this trend is reversed, our children are more at risk of becoming obese and experiencing negative health consequences than was any previous generation.

OBESITY: A PUBLIC HEALTH PROBLEM

The news about obesity in the United States is not good. Obesity ranks second only to smoking as a cause of preventable death (3). It has been described by the World Health Organization as "an escalating epidemic" as well as "one of the greatest neglected public health problems of our time with an impact on health which may well prove to be as great as that of smoking" (17). The United States government, in its 1995 *Dietary Guidelines for Americans*, lists obesity as one of the major nutrition-related health problems facing this nation (18).

This past decade has seen a substantial increase in the prevalence of obesity in the United States: today, one-third of adults (58 million) are obese (16). And of particular concern is that within the epidemic of obesity resides another: more than 50 million Americans are at greater than average risk for morbidity and mortality from obesity-related cardiovascular disease, type 2 diabetes, stroke, several types of cancer, gallbladder disease, and respiratory problems, such as sleep apnea (19–24). More than 70% of people who are obese have at least one of these co-morbid conditions (20).

In addition, there is a direct correlation between obesity and osteoarthritis, especially of the knees and hips (25). Osteoarthritis is a significant and costly problem for the elderly: among the "Medicare population," the third most common surgical procedure is total knee replacement and the fifth most common is total hip replacement (26). These procedures often might not have been required had early and aggressive weight-management measures been instituted.

The increase in prevalence of obesity has occurred across all age groups and in all ethnic, racial, and socioeconomic populations. However, minority populations, especially minority women, are at greatest risk for obesity, and hence, its co-morbidities. According to the National Health and Nutrition Examination Survey III (NHANES III), nearly 50% of African-American and Mexican-American women are obese. Between the ages of 45 and 55 years, the prevalence of obesity ranges from 60% to 70% in these groups (2).

Children and adolescents in the United States are also at risk of obesity, probably because their lifestyles are more sedentary than those of previous generations. NHANES III data show that more than 10% of 4- and 5-year-old children are obese, as are 21% of 12- to 19-year-old adolescents. These children and adolescents are also at increased risk of high cholesterol levels and generally poor physical condition, which may carry over into adulthood (27).

Adolescents who are obese experience discrimination on a variety of levels: they enter the job market at lower salaries than do peers who are not obese, and many never recover from this economic disadvantage (28). Furthermore, they are at increased risk for a variety of emotional problems, such as depression and low self-esteem, and are less likely to marry when they reach adulthood.

OBESITY: A CHRONIC DISEASE

By any criteria obesity must be considered a chronic disease. Obesity is multifactorial in origin, relapsing in nature, and associated with conditions that contribute overall to morbidity and mortality. Common co-morbid conditions include type 2 diabetes, dyslipidemias, hypertension, coronary artery disease, and osteoarthritis (19–24,29).

Like other chronic diseases, obesity also requires long-term therapy and a multidisciplinary approach to effective treatment. Prevention of obesity is of paramount importance but is frequently neglected. In addition to degree of obesity, weight gain during the adult years represents a strong and independent risk factor for the development of chronic disease in both men and women (19,20).

Maintenance of weight loss is also a critically important issue and has been historically hard to achieve. Long-term nonsurgical treatment of obesity in adults has largely been unsuccessful, regardless of whether the efforts have focused on diet, physical activity, behavior modification, or pharmacologic intervention (30). Unfortunately, at least 95% of people entering weight-loss programs regain the lost weight and within 5 years are back to their starting weight (21).

MEDICAL TREATMENT OF OBESITY

The medical community in the United States has not led the fight against obesity with the same vigor displayed for other chronic diseases, such as coronary artery disease, hypertension, and diabetes. Although this relative lack of enthusiasm for the treatment of obesity may be attributed to a variety of factors, several appear particularly noteworthy.

Historically, physicians have believed that obesity represents a relatively intractable condition for which effective therapies are lacking. Lifestyle interventions, such as increased physical activity and improved nutrition, have often appeared inadequate for the treatment of obesity and represent areas in which most physicians lack formal education and training.

Many physicians do not treat obesity because they mistakenly believe there are no effective treatments. Yet many devote considerable time and energy to treating the co-morbidities of coronary artery disease, type 2 diabetes, dyslipidemias, hypertension, or osteoarthritis in patients who are obese, without recognizing or treating the obesity as the underlying cause.

An additional and unfortunate reason why some physicians are reluctant to treat obesity or even to consider it a chronic disease is the possibility that they share (often without acknowledgment) the societal prejudices that obesity results from lack of discipline and self-control on the part of the person who is obese. This "blame the victim" attitude would not be tolerated in any other chronic disease and must be counteracted with effective medical education programs.

Currently compounding physician reluctance to treat obesity pharmacologically is a recent editorial in the *New England Journal of Medicine* that has been widely misinterpreted in the medical community and the popular press (31). The editorial emphasizes the legitimate use of pharmacotherapy as a component in the treatment of medically significant obesity rather than for the purpose of cosmetic weight loss.

Physician misperception about obesity and reluctance to treat it are further complicated by legitimate concerns about the serious side effects of, and conditions associated with, central nervous system–active agents (32–34). Recently, both dexfenfluramine (Redux) and fenfluramine (Pondimin) were voluntarily withdrawn from the market by their manufacturers, an action that may very well increase patient confusion and anxiety concerning the availability of effective treatments of obesity.

Physicians have a significant role to play in conjunction with other health care professionals in the treatment of obesity. Physician recommendation for lifestyle alteration has been shown in a number of studies to be a powerful motivator for behavioral change (35–37). Yet physicians currently counsel a distinct minority of patients, even those who are obese, on the health consequences of excess fat. As new understandings and treatment modalities emerge in the area of obesity, physician knowledge of this chronic disease and involvement in the treatment process will become even more critical.

DETERMINING WHO IS OBESE

Obesity is the excessive accumulation of body fat (38). Sedentary lifestyles and high-fat, energy-dense diets are the principal causes of the recent acceleration of the obesity problem. People who become obese do so partly because of a genetic predisposition to weight gain, but the combination of an unhealthful diet and lack of physical activity also plays a fundamental role.

In the past, standardized "desirable" weight and height tables were developed by the insurance industry to estimate obesity and to help determine eligibility and coverage risks. The industry's actuarial analyses of weights and death rates among policyholders formed the basis for these tables. The guidelines, notably those published by the Metropolitan Life Insurance Company in 1959, are still used by the American Heart Association (AHA), although the tables were revised upward by about 10% in 1983 to reflect the longer life span of policyholders who are overweight or obese (38–40). The AHA maintains that because the relation of weight to health and disease is complex, the revisions raised concerns that have yet to be addressed (38).

Move recently, BMI has been used to estimate degree of obesity and health risk and has become the recognized international standard among obesity researchers and health care providers (41,42). In addition to the overall estimate of level of obesity provided by BMI, distribution of body fat is also an important factor that independently contributes to health risk (43). Individuals with excessive accumulation of abdominal fat have been shown to have a significantly higher risk of coronary heart disease and type 2 diabetes compared with individuals with excessive fat accumulation in the hip area (29,43). Two widely used and validated measures of body fat distribution are waist-to-hip ratio and waist measurement (44).

Body Mass Index

BMI is defined as weight (in kilograms) divided by the square of the individual's height (in meters). In population studies, BMI has been shown to correlate with body fat in adults and also with health risk (29). Health risk based on BMI alone and BMI with the presence of at least one co-morbid condition is presented in the Table 116-1 (42). In addition to increased health risks, an elevated BMI is associated with higher health-care costs. A study by Kaiser Permanente in Oakland, California, demonstrated a clear association between BMI and outpatient visits, inpatient days, and total cost of care, including laboratory and pharmacy expenditures. Annual costs were 44% higher among those with a BMI greater than 35 and were 25% higher for those with a BMI of 30 to 35, compared with people with a BMI of 20 to 25 (45).

Table 116-1 Health Risk Associated with BMI

BMI Category	Health Risk Based on BMI	Risk Adjusted for Presence of Co-morbid Conditions and/or Other Risk Factors
<25	Minimal	Low
25–<27	Low	Moderate
27–<30	Moderate	High
30–<35	High	Very high
35–<40	Very high	Extremely high
≥40	Extremely high	Extremely high

Metric values must be used for proper calculation of BMI (kg/m²).
SOURCE: Guidance for treatment of adult obesity. Shape Up America!, 6707 Democracy Blvd., Ste. 306, Bethesda, MD 20817 (www.shapeup.org) and American Obesity Association, 1250 24th St. N.W., Ste. 300, Washington, DC 20037, 1996. Used by permission.

Waist-to-Hip Ratio

Waist-to-hip ratio is an accepted technique for assessing the pattern of body fat distribution. High waist-to-hip ratio suggests disproportionate accumulation of abdominal fat as opposed to a larger proportion of weight distributed on the thighs and hips. Waist-to-hip ratios greater than 1.0 in men and greater than 0.8 in women have been associated with increased risk of coronary artery disease (43).

Waist Circumference

Waist circumference provides an alternative method for assessing body fat distribution. Several recent studies have demonstrated that waist circumference alone correlates better with the amount of visceral abdominal fat than waist-to-hip ratio (44). A waist circumference of more than 39 inches (97.5 cm) has been shown to correlate with a significant increase in risk of both type 2 diabetes and coronary heart disease in both men and women (46–48).

HISTORICAL OVERVIEW OF THERAPY

Given the chronic, relapsing nature of obesity, effective long-term therapies are essential. A variety of lifestyle approaches have been tried, and some have achieved modest, short-term success. However, long-term success with lifestyle changes or commercial weight-loss programs has proved elusive (49,50).

Of individuals in weight-loss programs who lose weight through diet alone, 75% regain most of the weight within 1 year, and 85% to 90% regain most of the weight within 2 years (49). The situation is somewhat improved among individuals who have lost weight in programs that combined diet and behavior modification. Even with this combination, however, 71% regained most or all of the lost weight within 30 months, and virtually all regained some or all of the lost weight within 5 years (49).

The addition of exercise to diet and behavior modification yields further benefit, but results remain far from optimal. Of the people who used these three lifestyle mea-

sures in combination, 58% regained most or all of the weight lost within 2 years (49).

The absence of effective public health and societal strategies to deal with obesity and the emerging understanding of the limitations of lifestyle therapy have contributed to intense debate about the future of obesity treatment in the United States. As a clearer picture of the adverse health consequences of obesity has emerged and a more sophisticated understanding of the complex pathophysiology of obesity has been achieved, more attention has been focused on a possible role for pharmacotherapy as part of the treatment of chronic obesity.

It appears that pharmacologic therapy may be helpful in selected patients in combination with lifestyle modalities (3,51). A variety of novel pharmacologic approaches, including a partial blocker of fat absorption, obesity-related hormones such as leptin and its analogs and neuropeptide Y blockers, are at various stages of the development and approval processes (52,53).

Recent studies have demonstrated that weight loss may substantially decrease the risk factors associated with the co-morbidities of obesity (54,55). Promising information has been generated suggesting that loss of a relatively small amount of weight by obese individuals (5% to 10% of body weight) often yields substantial reductions in risk of obesity-associated co-morbidities (54). Although the reason why such small amounts of weight loss yield important health benefits is not fully understood, one explanation appears to be that modest weight loss results in a disproportionate loss of visceral abdominal fat (56–58). Visceral abdominal fat has been implicated in a cascade of metabolic abnormalities, including insulin resistance, glucose intolerance, and dyslipidemias (59).

The health benefits of small amounts of weight loss provide a potent impetus for physicians and other health care professionals to counsel people who are obese. Counseling should focus on the health benefits of realistic, modest weight loss rather than on the chimera of an "ideal" body weight or shape.

COST TO SOCIETY

The direct and indirect costs of obesity are staggering. In addition to the more than $30 billion spent each year in the United States on weight-loss treatment and diet products (most of which offer no demonstrable long-term success), an estimated $68 billion is spent on clinical complications directly related to obesity: diabetes, hypertension, and cardiovascular diseases (21,60). Approximately 52.6 million workdays are lost each year because of illness and disabilities directly related to obesity and inactivity (42). More than $68 billion in costs may be attributable to excess medical expenses and loss of income in the United States each year (3). More than $22 billion is spent each year on health care costs related to the cardiovascular complications of obesity (61).

FUTURE DIRECTIONS

The authors believe that because obesity is a chronic disease and this country is at a pivotal stage in combating this epidemic, it must be given a higher priority on the national health care agenda.

We believe that the responsibility to raise public consciousness of, and to take action against, obesity must now fall on the nation's well-respected health care providers. To be heard, these leaders in the medical and health care professions must be proactive as they provide substantive educational, preventive, and treatment programs for people of all ages and all socioeconomic groups.

Education

- Although some excellent health education materials on obesity have been developed, these materials must be made more easily accessible as well as appropriate to age and ethnicity, and they should be provided at all life stages, beginning with preschool. Particular attention must be focused on the link between obesity and the co-morbidities, i.e., hypertension, type 2 diabetes, dyslipidemias, and coronary heart disease.
- Parent programs should be provided that help children increase their physical activity and adopt healthy nutritional patterns (i.e., intake of dietary fat that does not exceed 30% of recommended daily calories).
- Most important of all, it is critical to educate or re-educate health care providers, teachers, and parents. Education must stress the importance of achievable and healthy rather than unattainable and unrealistic weight loss and must guard against attitudes that would inadvertently promote eating disorders or other unhealthy dietary restrictions.

Prevention

- Greater attention must be focused on the prevention of obesity in all age groups because it holds promise for lowering the incidence of obesity and for decreasing associated health risks.
- Among those who are already obese, attention must be paid to treatment, prevention of additional weight gain, maintenance of existing weight loss, and reaching attainable goals, such as "healthy weight," rather than seeking unrealistic goals for body types and body weight.
- Aspects of the culture, including general lifestyles and attitudes, that promote obesity should be challenged and reoriented or redirected toward more health-promoting patterns.
- National nutrition policies should be established that relate specifically to the prevention of obesity and support the *U.S. Dietary Guidelines*.

Treatment

- Treatment of obesity must begin with individualized programs developed by an interdisciplinary team following a chronic disease management model, similar to those used for hypertension and diabetes.
- The focus of treatment must be on obesity as a manageable disease, with realistic health-related goals established, beginning with loss of a modest amount of total body weight (5% to 10%), which can result in significant risk factor reduction and improvement in health.

- The important role of obesity in causing and perpetuating common conditions such as hypertension, type 2 diabetes, dyslipidemias, coronary disease, and osteoarthritis in people who are obese must be recognized. Moreover, the obesity must be treated as a significant underlying cause of these conditions.
- Treatment of obesity must promote proper nutrition, exercise, and a healthy lifestyle and must dispel misconceptions about obesity and available treatment options. When appropriate, pharmacotherapy may be used as adjunctive therapy in selected patients whose level of obesity or presence of co-morbid conditions creates significant health risks. The risk of pharmacotherapy must always be weighed against its potential health benefit. For extreme obesity, surgery may be considered in addition to lifestyle interventions.
- Healthy lifestyle modifications should include:
  - Dietary changes that result in the consumption of a diet that contains 30% or less of total calories from fat and 10% or less of total calories from saturated fats
  - Food plans that reduce the amount of energy-dense foods (i.e., fewer calories; more vegetables, fruits, grains, and cereals)
  - Increased physical activity, with an emphasis on moderate forms of exertion (e.g., walking rather than running or jogging) (62)
  - An emphasis on change in attitude that reflects a long-term weight-management focus rather than short-term extreme-weight reduction or practices that cannot be sustained
- Effective management of obesity must recognize the realities of the environment in which the patient lives. This includes an understanding on the part of the prescribing physician or other health care professional of the home, work, or education settings of the individual, as well has his or her cultural, societal, and family dynamics.
- Health-care delivery systems must recognize the health implications of obesity and its co-morbidities and work toward identification of clinically effective and cost-effective obesity-management strategies. Health-care delivery systems that currently do not cover treatment of obesity should carefully reassess this policy. Specifically they should evaluate the expenses they incur by treating the co-morbidities of hypertension, coronary heart disease, dyslipidemias, type 2 diabetes, and osteoarthritis in patients who are obese and reconsider the economic issues related to covering treatment of obesity.

RECOMMENDATIONS

To help combat the growing obesity epidemic in the United States, the authors submit the following recommendations to the groups involved in the public health problem of obesity:

Medical Professionals

- Encourage physician adoption of weight, BMI, and waist circumference in adults as the vital signs of obesity and as essential data to be recorded as a routine part of the office visits, in addition to measurement of blood pressure, blood glucose, and lipid levels.

- Motivate physicians to counsel all patients on the health risks of obesity and excessive weight gain throughout life, with a particular emphasis on the adult years.

- Encourage physicians to counsel all patients who are obese on the importance of prevention of further weight gain and the techniques for safe and effective weight loss.

- Educate physicians to discuss with their patients the health benefits of *modest* weight loss (i.e., 5% to 10% of body weight).

- Encourage physicians to discuss prevention of obesity with all adult patients, even those who are not currently obese.

- Provide physicians with supplemental or continuing medical education programs to better enable them to evaluate and treat obesity. These programs must provide physicians with cultural and social perspectives specific to their patient populations.

- Include registered dietitians, nutritionists, exercise physiologists, and psychologists as integral to the management team and as ongoing resources during the treatment process to facilitate and monitor progress as well as encourage positive behavior.

- Include obesity among the major chronic diseases worthy of discussion in various medical education settings, such as grand rounds, morbidity and mortality conferences, and other continuing medical education activities.

- Develop educational programs on the diagnosis and management of obesity to be delivered through the national medical associations, medical schools, and teaching hospitals.

- Take the opportunity to participate in randomized controlled clinical trials of the effectiveness of innovative prevention and treatment strategies for obesity.

Health Care Services

- Recognize that obesity is a disease and provide appropriate coverage and reimbursement for physician visits, dietitian or nutritionist and exercise physiologist referrals, and in appropriate patients, pharmacotherapy or surgery.

- Address the issue of obesity and provide incentives for the service provider physician networks to work toward the prevention of obesity in their patients and thereby reduce the risk of co-morbidities.

- Provide educational materials for their member-patients to inform them of the problem of obesity and to encourage them to seek appropriate individual evaluation by their primary care physician.

Employers

- Work with insurers, medical institutions, and others to develop healthy lifestyle programs that emphasize the reduction or prevention of obesity. Such programs can help increase productivity, reduce absenteeism, lower insurance premiums, and result in a healthier patient population and an overall increase in employee satisfaction.

- Make a commitment to combating obesity by offering and encouraging consumption of healthful cafeteria foods and by rewarding participation in readily available exercise programs associated with the workplace. Economic or other incentives for participation should be offered. Encourage distribution of materials on lifestyle options that can be incorporated easily into daily living.

- Ensure that employees have medical insurance coverage that reimburses for doctor visits, referrals to registered dietitians, and, when clinically indicated, appropriate pharmacotherapy or surgical intervention to treat obesity.

Government

- Establish a Surgeon General's Report on Obesity that publicly recognizes obesity as a chronic disease, encourages research into the metabolic basis of obesity, highlights effective preventive and treatment strategies, and establishes appropriate treatment guidelines.

- Amend Medicare regulations to ensure that examination, diagnosis, and treatment of obesity are available to all elderly or disabled people, regardless of income.

- Amend federal and state and Medicaid regulations to ensure the availability of obesity-related treatment to people of all ages with low incomes.

- Provide culturally sensitive client education materials for use by welfare and social service systems and other government agencies to advise clients of the problem of obesity and of the importance and efficacy of treatment of this disease.

- Encourage state medical associations to require completion of nutrition and exercise physiology courses by medical students and physicians as part of the process of obtaining a medical license and of securing license renewal, respectively.

- Establish meaningful outcome measures and performance criteria for safe and effective treatment of obesity and consider sanctions for unethical or unsafe treatment practices.

- Encourage food manufacturers to use their marketing acumen to develop and promote more nutritious and less calorically dense foods and food choices.

- Encourage school systems to serve healthful cafeteria foods; reward participation in physical activities; and educate children to make appropriate nutritional choices.

- Encourage state and local municipalities to expand the role of public health departments to collaborate with schools, service providers, and employers in the development and implementation of public education programs aimed at reducing obesity and increasing physical activity.

We fully endorse the objectives of Healthy People 2000. Although progress has been made in certain areas, ground has been lost in the area of obesity. In view of this, we ask that the government redouble its efforts in moving the nation toward a realization of the weight, nutrition, and physical activity objectives for Healthy People 2010. (For a list of nutrition- and physical activity–related Healthy People 2000 objectives, see Table 116-2.)

Table 116-2 Healthy People 2000: Objectives on Physical Activity and Nutrition

Physical Activity and Fitness
- Reduce overweight to a prevalence of 20% or less in people over age 20 and 15% or less in adolescents aged 12 to 19.
- Increase to at least 30% the proportion of people aged 6 and older who engage in regular light-to-moderate physical activity for at least 30 minutes a day.
- Increase to at least 20% the proportion of people 18 years and older and to at least 75% the proportion of children and adolescents aged 6 to 17 years who engage in vigorous physical activity that promotes cardiorespiratory fitness 3 or more days a week for at least 20 minutes per session.
- Reduce to 15% or less the proportion of people 6 years and older who engage in no leisure-time physical activity.
- Increase to at least 40% the proportion of people 6 years and older who regularly perform physical activities that enhance and maintain muscular strength, endurance, and flexibility.
- Increase to at least 50% the proportion of overweight people age 12 and older who have adopted sound dietary practices and regular physical activity to attain an appropriate weight.
- Increase to at least 50% the proportion of children and adolescents in first through twelfth grades who participate in daily physical activity at school.
- Increase to at least 50% the proportion of physical education class time that students spend in physical activity, preferably lifetime physical activities.
- Increase the proportion of work sites offering employer-sponsored physical activity and fitness programs.
- Increase availability and accessibility of community physical activity and fitness facilities, e.g., hiking, biking, and fitness trails; public swimming pools; and park and recreation spaces.
- Increase to at least 50% the proportion of primary care providers who routinely assess and counsel their patients regarding frequency, duration, type, and intensity of physical activities.

Nutrition
- Reduce dietary fat intake to an average of 30% or less of calories and saturated fat to 10% or less of calories for people over age 2 years.
- Increase ingestion of complex carbohydrate and fiber-containing foods for people age 2 or older to an average of 5 or more daily servings of vegetables and fruits and to an average of 6 or more daily servings of grain products.
- Increase to at least 85% the proportion of people over age 18 who use food labels to make nutritious selections.
- Achieve useful and informative nutrition labeling for virtually all processed foods and at least 40% of ready-to-eat carry-away foods. Achieve compliance by at least 90% of retailers with voluntary labeling of fresh meats, poultry, seafood, fruits, and vegetables.
- Increase the availability of processed food products that are reduced in fat and saturated fat to at least 5000 brand items.
- Increase to at least 90% the proportion of restaurants and institutional food service operations that offer identifiable low-fat, low-calorie food choices, consistent with the *Dietary Guidelines for Americans*.
- Increase to at least 90% the proportion of school lunch and breakfast services and child care food services with menus that are consistent with the nutrition principles in the *Dietary Guidelines for Americans*.
- Increase to at least 80% the receipt of home food services by people age 65 and older who have difficulty preparing their own meals or require home-delivered meals.
- Increase to at least 75% the proportion of the nation's schools that provide nutrition education from preschool through twelfth grade.
- Increase to at least 50% the proportion of work sites with 50 or more employees that offer nutrition education or weight-management programs for employees.
- Increase to at least 75% the proportion of primary care providers who provide nutrition assessment and counseling or referral to qualified nutritionists or dietitians.

CONCLUSION

Worldwide, obesity has been described by the World Health Organization as "an escalating epidemic" and "one of the greatest neglected public health problems of our time." That statement applies to the United States also, where approximately 58 million adults are obese, a number that is expected to increase across all age groups and all ethnic, racial, and socioeconomic populations unless we act to stem the tide. The direct and indirect costs of obesity are staggering: more than $30 billion is spent each year in the United States on weight-loss treatment and diet products, in addition to $68 billion spent on complications directly related to obesity and its co-morbidities. To make it clear that many individuals run significant health risks related to their obesity, we urge the adoption of the concept of "clinical," or "medical," obesity for these people.

People who are medically, or clinically, obese (i.e., have diabetes, hypertension, or abnormal lipid levels; are symptomatic or have risk factors for the development of diabetes, hypertension, or abnormal lipid levels; or have a chronic disease analogous to hypertension or diabetes) require long-term therapy using a multidisciplinary approach. The proper end points of this therapy are health, improvement in co-morbidities, and reduction in morbidity and mortality.

Physicians have a significant role to play in the management of patients with medical obesity. As new understandings and treatment modalities emerge, physician knowledge of obesity and involvement in the treatment process are critical.

Traditional approaches to weight loss—diet and exercise, behavior modification—are beneficial, but the results attained in the population who are clinically obese remain far from optimal. It appears that pharmacotherapy may be helpful in appropriately selected patients in combination with lifestyle changes.

The authors believe that responsibility to raise public awareness of and to take action against the ever-growing threat to our national health rests with the nation's well-respected health care leaders. These leaders must provide educational, preventive, and therapeutic programs that reach people of all ages and all socioeconomic groups in our schools, workplaces, and homes. The core messages of these programs should include the following:

- Recognition of clinical obesity as a disease that requires long-term therapy.

- Adoption of a nutritious diet that contains no more than 30% of daily calories from fat.

- Physical activities to increase energy expenditure.

- Adoption of weight, BMI, and waist circumference measurements as vital signs of obesity for all medical examinations.

- Physician education to enable counseling of patients concerning the health benefits of modest weight loss (i.e., 5% to 10% of baseline body weight).

- Consideration of pharmacotherapy for medically obese patients in whom diet, exercise, and lifestyle changes alone fail and of surgery for those with life-threatening obesity.

We urge leaders of the medical and health care communities, corporate America, and federal and state governments to sound the alarm and place obesity, particularly medical obesity, with its inherent dangers, at the top of our national health agenda. The time to act is now.

———————

This chapter was adapted with permission of the publisher and authors from Rippe J, Aronne L, Gilligan V, et al. Public policy statement on obesity and health. Nutr Clin Care 1998;1:34–47. Reprinted by permission of Blackwell Science, Inc.

REFERENCES

1. Update: prevalence of overweight among children, adolescents, and adults in the United States, 1988–1994. MMWR 1997;46:199–202.

2. Kuczmarski RJ, Flegal KM, Campbell SM, Johnson CL. Increasing prevalence of overweight among U.S. adults: the National Health and Nutrition Examination surveys, 1960–1991. JAMA 1994;272:205–211.

3. National Task Force on the Prevention and Treatment of Obesity. Long-term pharmacotherapy in the management of obesity. JAMA 1996;276:1907–1915.

4. McGinnis JM, Foege WH. Actual causes of death in the United States. JAMA 1993;270:2207–2212.

5. Bouchard C, ed. The genetics of obesity. Boca Raton, FL: CRC, 1994:2–3.

6. Leibel RL, Bahary N, Friedman JM. Genetic variation and nutrition in obesity. In: Simopoulous AP, Childs B, eds. Genetic variation and nutrition. World Rev Nutr Diet. Basel, Switzerland: S Karger, 1990.

7. Bouchard C. Genetics of obesity: an update on molecular market.

Int J Obes 1995;19(suppl):S10–S13.

8. Thompson DB, Janssen RC, Ossowski VM, et al. Evidence for linkage between a region on chromosome 1p and the acute insulin response in Pima Indians. Diabetes 1995;44:473–481.

9. Chung WK, Power-Kehoe L, Chua M, Leibel RL. Mapping of the OB receptor to 1p in a region of non-conserved gene order from mouse and rat to human. Genome Res 1996;6:431–438.

10. Montague CT, Farooqi IS, Whitehead JP, et al. Congenital leptin deficiency is associated with severe early-onset obesity in humans. Nature 1997;387:903–908. (Letter.)

11. Jackson RS, Creemers JWM, Ohagi S, et al. Obesity and impaired prohormone processing associated with mutations in the human prohormone convertase 1 gene. Nature Genet 1997;16:303–306. (Letter.)

12. Pi-Sunyer FX. Health implications of obesity. Am J Clin Nutr 1991;53:1595S–1603S.

13. U.S. Department of Health and Human Services. Physical activity and health: a report of the

Surgeon General. Atlanta: U.S. Department of Health and Human Services, Centers for Disease Control and Prevention, National Center for Chronic Disease Prevention and Health Promotion, 1996.

14. X-factor study. New York, NY: Louis Harris, 1997.

15. Troiano RP, Flegal KM, Kuczmarski RJ, et al. Overweight prevalence and trends for children and adolescents: the National Health and Nutrition Examination surveys, 1963 to 1991. Arch Pediatr Adolesc Med 1995;140:1085–1091.

16. National Institute of Diabetes and Digestive and Kidney Diseases. Statistics related to overweight and obesity. NIH Publication 96-4158. Rockville, MD: National Institutes of Health, July 1, 1996.

17. World Health Organization. Consultation on Obesity, Geneva, June 3–5, 1997.

18. Dietary guidelines for Americans. Washington, DC: U.S. Department of Health and Human Services, 1996.

19. Pi-Sunyer FX. Medical hazards of obesity. Ann Intern Med 1993;119:655–660.

20. 1997 heart and stroke statistical update. Dallas: American Heart Association, 1996.

21. National Task Force on Prevention and Treatment of Obesity. Towards prevention of obesity: research directions. Obes Res 1994;2:571–584.

22. VanItallie TB, Lew EA. Assessment of morbidity and mortality risk in the overweight patient. In: Wadden T, VanItallie T, eds. Treatment of the seriously obese patient. New York: Guilford, 1992:3–32.

23. Chan JM, Rimm EB, Colditz GA, et al. Obesity, fat distribution, and weight gain as risk factors for clinical diabetes in men. Diabetes Care 1994;17:961–969.

24. Colditz GA, Willett WC, Stampfer MJ, et al. Weight as a risk factor for clinical diabetes in women. Am J Epidemiol 1990;132:501–513.

25. Felson DT. Weight and osteoarthritis. Am J Clin Nutr 1996;63 (suppl):430S–432S.

26. Owens GM. Independence Blue Cross medical risk plan: internal keystone 65 data. Presented at the Interdisciplinary Council on Lifestyle and Obesity Management, New York, July 18, 1997.

27. Whitaker RC, Wright JA, Pepe MS, et al. Predicting obesity in young adulthood from childhood and parental obesity. N Engl J Med 1997;337:869–873.

28. Gortmaker SL, Must A, Perrin JM, et al. Social and economic consequences of overweight in adolescence and young adulthood. N Engl J Med 1993;329:1008–1012.

29. Thomas PR, ed. Weighing the options: criteria for evaluating weight-management programs. Washington, DC: National Academy, 1995:40–45.

30. NIH Technology Assessment Conference Panel. Methods for voluntary weight loss and control. Ann Intern Med 1993;119:764–770.

31. Curfman GD. Diet pills redux. N Engl J Med 1997;337:629–630. (Editorial.)

32. Abenhaim L, Moride Y, Brenot F, et al. Appetite-suppressant drugs and the risk of primary pulmonary hypertension. N Engl J Med 1996; 335:609–616.

33. Mark EJ, Patalas ED, Chang HT, et al. Fatal primary pulmonary hypertension associated with short-term use of fenfluramine and phentremine. N Engl J Med 1997;337:602–606.

34. Connolly HM, Crary JL, McGoon MD, et al. Valvular heart hisease associated with fenfluramine-phentermine. N Engl J Med 1997; 337:581–588.

35. Wilson DM, Taylor DW, Gibert JR, et al. A randomized trial of a family physician intervention for smoking cessation. JAMA 1988; 260:1570–1574.

36. Harris SS, Caspersen CJ, DeFriese GH, Estes GH Jr. Physical activity counseling for healthy adults as a primary preventive intervention in the clinical setting: report for the U.S. Preventive Services Task Force. JAMA 1989;261:3590–3598.

37. Campbell MK, DeVellis BM, Strecher VJ, et al. Improving dietary behavior: the effectiveness of tailored messages in primary care settings. Am J Public Health 1994;84:783–787.

38. American Heart Association. Heart and stroke A—Z guide. Available at: http://www.amhrt.org. Accessed June 1997.

39. New weight standards for men and women. Stat Bull 1959;40:1–5.

40. 1983 Metropolitan height and weight tables. Stat Bull 1983;64:2–9.

41. National Institute of Diabetes and Digestive and Kidney Diseases. Understanding adult obesity. NIH Publ. No. 94-3680. Rockville, MD: National Institutes of Health, 1993.

42. Guidance for treatment of adult obesity. Bethesda, MD: Shape Up America! and the American Obesity Association, 1996.

43. Björntorp P. Regional patterns of fat distribution. Ann Intern Med 1985;103:994–995.

44. Lemieux S, Prud'homme D, Bouchard C, Tremblay A, Després J-P. A single threshold value of waist girth identifies normal-weight and overweight subjects with excess visceral adipose tissue. Am J Clin Nutr 1996;64:685–693.

45. Quesenberry CP Jr, Caan B, Jacobson A. Obesity, health services utilization, and health care costs among members of a health maintenance organization. Arch Intern Med 1998;158:466–472.

46. Pouliot M-C, Després J-P, Lemieux S, et al. Waist circumference and abdominal sagittal diameter: best simple anthropometic indexes of abdominal visceral adipose tissue accumulation and related cardiovascular risk in men and women. Am J Cardiol 1994;73:460–468.

47. Després J-P. Abdominal obesity as important component of insulin-resistance syndrome. Nutrition 1993;9:452–459.

48. Pouliot M-C, Després J-P, Nadeau A, et al. Visceral obesity in men: associations with glucose tolerance, plasma insulin, and lipoprotein levels. Diabetes 1992;41:826–834.

49. Safer DJ. Diet, behavior modification, and exercise: a review of obesity treatments from a long-term perspective. South Med J 1991;84:1470–1474.

50. Goldstein F, Levine R, Troy L, et al. Three-year follow-up of participants in a commercial weight loss program: can you keep it off? Arch Intern Med 1996;156:1302–1306.

51. Silverstone T. Appetite suppressants: a review. Drugs 1992;43:820–836.

52. Guerciolini R. Mode of action of orlistat. Int J Obes 1997;21 (suppl):S12–S23.

53. James W, Avenell A, Broom J, Whitehead J. A one-year trial to assess the value of orlistat in the management of obesity. Int J Obes 1997;21(suppl):S24–S30.

54. Goldstein DJ, Potvin JH. Long-term weight loss: the effect of

pharmacologic agents. Am J Clin Nutr 1994;60:647–657.

55. Wing RR, Koeske R, Epstein LH, et al. Long-term effects of modest weight loss in type II diabetic patients. Arch Intern Med 1987; 147:1749–1753.

56. Després J-P. Dyslipidemia and obesity. Baillieres Clin Endocrinol Metab 1994;8:629–660.

57. Fujioka S, Matsuzawa Y, Tokunaga K, et al. Treatment of visceral fat obesity. Int J Obes 1991;15:59–65.

58. Ostman J, Arner P, Engfeldt P, Kager L. Regional differences in the control of lipolysis in human adipose tissue. Metabolism 1979; 28:1198–1205.

59. Després J-P, Marette A. Relation of components of insulin resistance syndrome to coronary disease risk. Curr Opin Lipidol 1994;5:274–289.

60. Wolf AM, Colditz GA. The cost of obesity: the U.S. perspective. Pharmaco Economics 1994; 5(suppl):34–37.

61. Carek PF, Sherer JT, Carson DS. Management of obesity: medical options. Am Fam Physician 1997; 55:551–558.

62. Pate RR, Pratt M, Blair SN, et al. Physical activity and public health: a recommendation from the Centers for Disease Control and Prevention and the American College of Sports Medicine. JAMA 1995;273:402–407.

Index

Index

M

Macrophages, aging and, 1160
Magnesium
  supplements, 783
  type 2 diabetes and, 878
Magnetic resonance imaging (MRI),
    meniscus tears, 256
Ma huang, 1054
Maintenance, theory of, 1106
Maintenance groups, for weight
    management, 533
Males. *See also* Gender differences
  bone mineral density, exercise and,
    238
  sterilization, 414
Malnutrition, forms of, 168, 169
Mammography, for breast cancer
    prevention, efficacy of, 292
Mammography Quality Standards Act,
    292
Managed care
  health promotion. *See* Health
    promotion, in managed care
  historical aspects, 912–913
Manipulation, chiropractic, 220
Manual therapy, for sports injuries, 220
Marasmus, 1245
Marfan's syndrome, 211
Marijuana use
  adolescent/child
    clustering, 567
    epidemiology, 566
    exercise and, 569
  conception attempts and, 377
Market
  forces, health promotion and, 941
  segmentation, health promotion and,
    941
Marketing, cause, 1314
MAS (maximal aerobic speed), 611
Massage, for sports injuries, 220
Mastitis, 398
Mature adults
  activities of daily living, nutrition and,
    161, 162
  nutrition
    activities of daily living and, 161,
    162
    physiologic factors and, 161
    psychosocial factors and, 161–162
    requirements, 162–163
  physiologic changes in, nutrition and,
    161
  physiologic disorders, common,
    163–165
  psychosocial factors, nutrition and,
    161–162
  RDAs for, 160–161
Maximal aerobic speed (MAS), 611
Maximal oxygen consumption (V_{O_2} max)
  adaptations to endurance training,
    1101–1102
  age and, 1108
  calculation, 1083
  cardiorespiratory endurance and,
    1083

cardiovascular fitness and, 226
exercise intensity and, 1107
gender differences in, 609–612
iron deficiency and, 643
Maximal oxygen consumption (V_{O_2MAX})
  abnormal, 455
The Mayo Clinic Family Pharmacist, 297
Mazindol, 1056
MCL (medial collateral ligament), 247
MCT (medium-chain triglycerides), 186
MDI (metered-dose inhaler), 486–487
Media
  campaign, to enhance exercise
    participation, 1022
  physical activity promotion,
    1303–1304
  programs, for smoking cessation, 526
  violence, 360
Medial collateral ligament (MCL), 247
Medical evaluation, for exercise
    prescription, 58
Medical history, preconceptional care
    and, 375–376
Medical models, shift to
    prevention/public health models,
    143
Medical problem history, in
    preparticipation examination, 680
Medical professionals. *See* Health care
    providers; Physician
Medical self-care
  physician-directed, 271–272
    delivery methods for, 272
    informed medical decision making
    and, 274
    interactive CD-ROM resources, 272
    potential for, 272–273
    telecommunication and, 273–274
    technology and, 271
Medications. *See* Drugs
Medium-chain triglycerides (MCT), 186
MEDLINE, 884
Medroxyprogesterone acetate (MPA)
  with conjugated equine estrogen, 307
    continuous, 307–308
    cyclic, 307
  effect on HDL, 305
Melanoma, malignant, 1261–1262
Memory disturbances, sleep loss and,
    1236
Menarche
  delayed
    bone mineral density and, 656–658
    breast cancer risk and, 658
  in female athletes, 654
  models for, 654–655
Meniscus injuries
  evaluation, 255
  history of, 255
  tears
    joint line tenderness and, 256
    provocative tests, 256–257
    range of motion and, 255–256
    surgical management, 256–257
Menke's hair syndrome, 1250
Menopause
  clinical findings, 304

epidemiology, 303
physiology, 303–304
Menstrual cycle
  bleeding
    intrauterine device and, 408
    reduction, DMPA and, 410
  disorders. *See also* Amenorrhea
    dysmenorrhea, oral contraceptives
    and, 405
    exercise and, 655
  irregularity
    DMPA and, 410
    levonorgestrel implants and, 409
    risk, physical activity and, 350–
    351
  oral contraceptive benefits for, 405
Mental health, conception attempts and,
    376
Mental illness, exercise prescription,
    702
Metabolic equivalents (METs)
  definition, 91, 343–344
  exercise intensity and, 761, 762
Metabolic rate, heat production and,
    1172–1173
Metabolic syndrome. *See* Syndrome X
Metered-dose inhaler (MDI), 486–487
Metronidazole, for bacterial vaginosis,
    428–429
METs. *See* Metabolic equivalents
Mφ adherence, exercise-induced
    changes, 1133
MHHP (Minnesota Heart Health
    Program), 122, 124, 125
MI. *See* Myocardial infarction
Micronutrients
  dietary intake, for adolescents,
    152–154
  type 2 diabetes and, 878
Migraine, oral contraceptive usage and,
    407
Migration studies, type 2
    diabetes/exercise association and,
    873
Miliaria, 1269–1270
Miliaria rubra (heat rash), 1179
Military groups, risk, dysthermia,
    1190–1191
Milk, composition, 589
Mind-body connection
  cognitive function and, 948–949
  emotions and, 949–951
  future research, 953
  historical aspects, 947–948
  patterns, 953
Minerals. *See also specific minerals*
  deficiencies, 169
  dietary intake, for adolescents,
    152–154
  excess of, 169
  requirements, for mature adult, 163
Minnesota Heart Health Program
    (MHHP), 122, 124, 125
Minnesota Longitudinal Study, 981
Miscarriage, second-trimester, 374
Mitogenesis, exercise-induced changes,
    1130–1131

Mo adherence, exercise-induced changes, 1133
Modeling, for enhancing exercise participation, 513–514
Moist heat, for sports injuries, 219
Moisturizers
  in skin cleansers, 1283–1284
  types, 1280–1282
Mold control, for asthma, 465
Molluscum contagiosum, 421, 1273–1274
Monocytes, exercise response, 1128
Monosodium glutamate (MSG), 472
Montreal Adoption Survey, family history of essential hypertension, 558
Mood
  changes, oral contraceptive usage and, 407
  exercise and, 959, 995
  overtraining and, 1000–1002
  sleep loss and, 1235, 1236
Morbidity, cardiac rehabilitation and, 743
"Morning after" pills. *See* Emergency contraception
Morning sickness, 385
Mortality rates
  all-cause, exercise and, 348
  cardiovascular disease, 90
  lipid lowering and, 98–99
  population-attributable, sedentary lifestyle and, 1296
  of spinal cord injured persons, 981–982
Mothers
  fatigue, breastfeeding and, 395
  working, breastfeeding and, 399
Motivational enhancement therapy, for adolescent/childhood substance use, 572–573
Motivational readiness, for physical activity, 691
Motor fitness skills, youth resistance training and, 628
Motor performance development
  gender differences, 616–618
  normal, 615–616
Mountain sickness, acute, 1201–1202, 1203
Mouth, age-related changes, 161
MPA. *See* Medroxyprogesterone acetate
MPQ (Multidimensional Personality Questionnaire), 981
MRFIT (Multiple Risk Factor Intervention Trial), 11, 44, 45, 91, 92, 1098–1099
MRI (magnetic resonance imaging), meniscus tears, 256
MSG (monosodium glutamate), 472
Multidimensional Personality Questionnaire (MPQ), 981
Multimedia, background information, 295–296
Multiple Risk Factor Intervention Trial (MRFIT), 11, 44, 45, 91, 92, 1098–1099

Muscle
  actions, types of, 222–223
  contraction
    concentric *vs.* eccentric, 223
    energy absorption and, 253
    isokinetic, 222, 223
    isometric, 222, 223
    isotonic, 222, 223
  endurance
    evaluation, 1086
    training, 225–226
  energy production, biochemistry of, 451, 452
  fatigue, 225–226
  flexibility. *See* Flexibility
  glycogen stores, 182–183
  mass, exercise and, 1090–1091
  passively stretched, energy absorption and, 253
  preparticipation evaluation, 212–213
  size, gender differences, 615
  sports injuries, rehabilitation, 216, 217
  strength, in injury prevention, 210
Muscle spasm, with dislocation, 251
Muscular strength. *See* Strength
Musculoskeletal system
  examination, for preparticipation examination, 682–683
  in exercise during pregnancy, 389–390
  fitness. *See also* Strength
    definition, 696
  history, for preparticipation examination, 678
  injury risk, exercise and, 349, 350
Musculotendinous injuries
  menicus tears, 255–257
  strains, 253–255
Myocardial contractility, cardiac rehabilitation and, 743
Myocardial infarction (MI)
  African-Americans and, 8
  aspirin prophylaxis, in women, 314
  C-reactive protein and, 12–13
  exercise and, 349
  exercise prescription, 701
  incidence, 14, 16
  in-hospital case fatality rates, temporal trends in, 16–17
  prediction, perioperative, 733
  risk, exercise and, 349
  smoking cessation and, 67–68
  treatment, in women, 316–317
  triggering agents, 6
  in women, 312, 346
Myocardial ischemia
  cardiac rehabilitation and, 743
  stress and, 792
Myocardial perfusion, cardiac rehabilitation and, 743
Myocardial revascularization procedures, for women, 317
Myocarditis, sudden cardiac death and, 780–781
Myocardium, exercise benefits, 854

N

Nadir, 1229, 1230
NAFTA (Northern American Free Trading Accord), 143, 146
National Cancer Institute (NCI), 291
National Children and Youth Fitness Study (NCYFS), 664
National Cholesterol Education Program (NCEP), 143
  cholesterol-lowering guidelines, 54–56, 99
  dietary fat intake recommendations, 856
  recommendations for childhood cholesterol levels, 594, 595
  Step I diet, 589
National Coalition to Promote Physical Activity (NCPPA), 1313
National Consumer Health Information and Health Promotion Act (PL 94-317), 1305
National Crime Victimization Survey (NCVS), 357
National Family Violence Survey, 359
National Health and Nutrition Examination Survey (NHANES), 15
  adolescent nutritional intake, 150
  calcium intake data, 153
  childhood obesity, 587, 1319
    energy intake in, 548
    prevalence, 546–547
  children's diets, 589
  dietary vitamin intake data, 153–154
  exercise benefits for depression, 351
  hypertension, lifestyle modification for, 109, 116
  iron intake data, 152
  leisure-time activities, 823, 824, 825
  obesity prevalence, 546–547, 1319
  Phase III data, 845
  physical activity measures, 847
National Health Interview Survey (NHIS)
  description, 823, 824, 844
  leisure-time activities
    exercise, 827–831, 834
    physical inactivity, 825
    stretching exercise, 833
  physical activity measures, 846
National Health Interview Survey-Youth Risk Behavior Survey (NHIS-YRBS), 823, 824, 835–842, 845, 847
National Health Planning and Resources Development Act (PL 93-641), 1305
National Heart, Lung and Blood Institute (NHLBI)
  Framingham Heart Study, 4
  obesity pharmacotherapy guidelines, 1055
National High Blood Pressure Education Program (NHBP), 143
National Institutes of Health (NIH), 879
National Runner's Health Study, 114

Stress (*cont.*)
  management, workplace health
      promotion program, effectiveness,
      921
  myocardial ischemia and, 792
  reduction
      coronary artery disease risk and, 61
      exercise and, 952, 958
      for hypertension treatment, 57
  reduction, for hypertension control,
      116
Stress fractures, 216, 349, 350
Stress relaxation, of viscoelastic
    materials, 221
Stretching exercises
  for elderly, 710
  forms of, 221–222
  as leisure-time activity, 833
  proprioceptive neuromuscular
      facilitation, 221–222
  static, 710
Stretch injury, 245
Stretch marks, 1267
Striae distensae, 1267
Stridor, 442
Stroke
  cardiorespiratory fitness, leisure-time
      activity and, 1100
  exercise prescription, 702, 704
  risk, exercise and, 346
Subcutaneous tissue, age-related
    changes, 1254
Substance abuse
  adolescent/child
      clustering, 566–568, 567
      epidemiology, 565–566, 566
      nutrition and, 568
      primary care
          screenings/interventions,
          571–573
  conception attempts and, 377
  sudden cardiac death and, 781
Subungual hemorrhage, 1267–1268
Sucrose, type 2 diabetes and, 877–878
Sudden cardiac death (SCD)
  in adolescent athletes, 681
  age ceiling, 783
  atherosclerosis and, 780
  average risk ratios, 782
  environmental factors, 782–783
  exercise and, 349
  incidence, 14
  pathologic mechanisms, 780–781
  type of exercise and, 783
  warning signs, 783
Sudden infant death syndrome (SIDS),
    520
Sulfur dioxide exposure, 1219, 1222
Sulfuric acid particles, in outdoor air,
    1218
Sunburn, 1258–1259, 1270
Sun exposure
  injuries induced by, 1270–1271
  physiologic reaction, 1258–1260
Sunscreens, 1260, 1262, 1287–1288
Suntanning, 1259, 1262–1263

Superficial heat, rationale for, 260
Supervision, for sports participation,
    212
Support
  problem-focused services, on Internet,
      287
  Web-based, for behavior change,
      288
Suprachiasmatic nucleus (SCN), 1229,
    1230
Surface area artifact, 1081
Surgery, for morbid obesity, 1066–1067
  body mass index criteria, 1061–1062
  duodenal switch, 1065–1066
  gastric bypass, 1062–1065
  intestinal bypass, 1062
  partial biliopancreatic bypass,
      1065–1066
  vertical banded gastroplasty,
      1062–1065
Sweat gland
  age-related changes, 1254
  fatigue, 1176
  heat-dissipating responses, 1175
Sweating
  defect, in cystic fibrosis, 478
  fluid/electrolyte loss, 1175–1176
Sweet eaters, gastric surgery for obesity
    and, 1062–1063
Swimmer's ear, 1272
Swimming, bone mineral density and,
    237
Switzerland National Research Program,
    122, 124, 125
Sympathetic-adrenal-medullary axis
    (SAM), 951
Symptom decrease, from cardiac
    rehabilitation, 742
Syndrome X
  characteristics, 47, 557
  childhood essential hypertension and,
      560
  childhood obesity and, 547
  coronary heart disease risk and, 10
  lifestyle measures for, 60–61
  vs. increased intra-abdominal
      pressure, 1061, 1063
Synthetic detergents, 1283
Syphilis, 424–425
Systolic blood pressure. *See* Blood
    pressure, systolic
Systolic Hypertension in the Elderly
    Program (SHEP), 313

T

Tachycardia, exercise testing, 734–735
Take Heart Program, 123, 124, 127
Talon noir (black heel), 1267
Tamoxifen, 307, 338
Tanner staging
  gender differences, 608
  for preparticipation examination,
      683–684
Tanning
  indoor

  acute effects, 1284–1285
  delayed effects, 1285–1286
  salons/parlors, 1262–1263, 1270
  self-tanning lotions, 1286–1287
  from sun exposure, 1259,
      1262–1263
Taping, of sports-related injuries,
    227–228
Target heart rate (THR), 761
Tartrazine, 473
TBI (Transition Dyspnea Index), 485
TBW (total body water), 608–609
TCA (trichloroacetic acid), 426
Telecommunication, physician-directed
    medical self-care and, 273–274
Telemedicine, technologic advances in,
    296
Telephone calls
  for enhancing exercise participation,
      513
  as exercise behavior prompts, 1033
  for smoking cessation counseling,
      525
Telepractice systems, 273–274
Temperature
  body. *See* Body temperature
  environmental. *See* Environment,
      temperature
Tendon injury rehabilitation, 216, 217
Tennis toe, 1267–1268
TENS (transcutaneous electrical nerve
    stimulation), 220
Teratogenicity
  anticonvulsants, 375
  of hyperthermia, 389
Tertiary prevention
  exercise risks/benefits, 783–785
  risks, 784
Testosterone
  libido and, 306–307
  production, after menopause, 304
  strength training and, 628
Thelarche, in female athletes, 654
Theophylline, for asthma, 466
Theory of Planned Behavior (TPB), 504
Theory of Reasoned Action (TRA), 504
Thermogenesis
  cold-enhanced, 1190
  cold exposure and, 1187–1188
Thermoreceptors, 1186–1187
Thermoregulation, control
  during exercise, 1178
  information integration, 1177–1178
Thiamin (vitamin B_1), 1247
Third International Study of Infarct
    Survival (ISIS-3), myocardial
    infarction outcome, gender
    differences in, 316–317
THR (target heart rate), 761
Throat examination, preparticipation,
    681
Thrombosis, coronary triggering, 5–7
Thromboxane A_2, platelet aggregation
    and, 33
Thymus gland
  exercise response, 1129

legislation, 1305
obesity problem recommendations,
    1323
organizational policy, for physical
    activity, 1299–1301
Wound healing. *See* Healing

X

Xenical (orlistat), 59–60, 1054, 1071

Y

Yeast vaginitis, 427–428
Yellow food dye No. 5, 473
Youth Risk Behavior Surveillance System
    (YRBSS), 664–666
Youth Risk Behavior Survey (YRBS),
    823, 824, 845, 1363847, 1017
Yuzpe method, 412, 413

Z

Zinc
    deficiency, 1250
        vegetarianism and, 188–189
        vitamin A deficiency and, 1246
    type 2 diabetes and, 878
Zoning legislation, 1304–1305
Zutphen Elderly Study, 873, 878
Zyban, 525